Pillitteri's Child and Family Health Nursing in Australia and New Zealand

Second Edition

Edited by

Christine Haley, RN, RM, BHSc (Nursing) GradCert (Women's Health), MPHC
Lecturer in Nursing, School of Nursing & Midwifery, Lithgow Campus
University of Western Sydney; Lecturer in Academic English
Health Science and Nursing, Lithgow Campus
UWS College

Original US edition
Maternal & Child Health Nursing: Care of the Childbearing and Childrearing Family

Adele Pillitteri, PhD, RN, PNP
Former Associate Professor
University of Southern California
Los Angeles, California

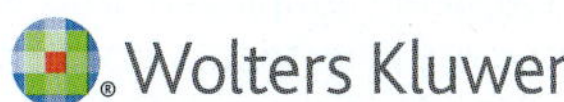

Philadelphia • Baltimore • New York • London
Buenos Aires • Hong Kong • Sydney • Tokyo

Wolters Kluwer Health
Two Commerce Square, 2001 Market Street, Philadelphia, PA 19103

Publisher: Julie Stegman
Product Manager: Caroline Hunter
Editor: Puddingburn Publishing Services
Proofreader: Puddingburn Publishing Services
Indexer: Puddingburn Publishing Services
Typesetter: Aptara, Inc.
Cover design: XouCreative
Printer: RR Donnelley, Shenzhen, China
Cover photograph © Lauren Kidziak

National Library of Australia cataloguing-in-publication entry

Creator: Haley, Christine, author.
Title: Child and family health nursing in Australia and New Zealand / by Christine Haley.
Edition: Second edition.
ISBN: 9781922228444 (paperback) 9781922228772 (ebook: epub)
Notes: Includes bibliographical references and index.
Subjects: Paediatric nursing–Australia–Textbooks.
Paediatric nursing–New Zealand–Textbooks.
Family nursing–Australia–Textbooks.
Family nursing–New Zealand–Textbooks.
Other creators/contributors: Pillitteri, Adele. Maternal & child health nursing.
Dewey number: 618.9200231

RRS1603

For my granddaughter Grace Elizabeth Kidziak.

This book would not have been possible without the love and support of my family.
To my husband Mark, children Lauren and Brent, their partners Nick and Claire, and my mother Norma.

Contributors

Laurin ALLEN **RN, GCert Mental Health (Child and Adolescent)**
Clinical Nurse Consultant, Child and Adolescent Mental Health Inpatient Unit, Orange Health Service, Orange
New South Wales
CHAPTER 54: Nursing care of a family when a young person has an intellectual or a mental health disorder

Carolyn BAILEY **RN, RM, MCMid, GDip (Midwifery) GCert (Health Professional Education), BN**
Lecturer, School of Nursing, Midwifery and Healthcare
Federation University Australia, Churchill, Victoria
CHAPTER 18: Nursing care of a family with a newborn

Sara BAYES **RN, RM, DipNurs (Adults) PGDip (Midwifery), MMidwifery, PhD**
Senior Lecturer (Midwifery)
School of Nursing and Midwifery, Edith Cowan University
Joondalup, Western Australia
CHAPTER 6: Assisting the family with contraception planning

Angela BULL **RN, RM, BN, Master ClinEd**
Lecturer in Midwifery, School of Health
Charles Darwin University, Darwin, Northern Territory
CHAPTER 17: Nursing care of a postnatal family
CHAPTER 26: Nursing care of a family with a high-risk newborn

Jane CONROY **RN, DipAppSci (Nursing) BHlthSci (Nursing), GCert (Emergency Nursing)**
Casual Lecturer/Marker, Bathurst Health Service
Bathurst Base Hospital, WNSWLHD
School of Nursing, Midwifery and Indigenous Health
Charles Sturt University, Bathurst, New South Wales
CHAPTER 40: Nursing care of a family when a child has a respiratory disorder
CHAPTER 45: Nursing care of a family when a child has a gastrointestinal disorder
CHAPTER 52: Nursing care of a family when a child has an unintentional injury

James DALEY **DipHlthSci (Nursing), GCert (Oncology) GCert (Palliative Care)**
Palliative Care WNSWLHD, Bathurst
Central West New South Wales
Clinical Nurse Consultant Palliative Care
WNSWLHD (Eastern and Southern Sectors)
Bathurst, New South Wales
CHAPTER 53: Nursing care of a family when a child has cancer
CHAPTER 56: Nursing care of a family when a child has a long-term or terminal illness

Miranda DALY **RN, DipAppSc (Nursing), GCert (HSM) GDip (AdvClinNur), MN**
Deputy Director of Clinical Education (Student Management); Teaching Focused Academic (Associate Lecturer), School of Nursing and Midwifery
University of Western Sydney, Hawkesbury Campus
Sydney, New South Wales
CHAPTER 50: Nursing care of a family when a child has a vision or hearing disorder

Carmel DAVIES **RN, RM, BA, Master of Tropical Health**
Lecturer, School of Nursing, Midwifery and Indigenous Health, Charles Sturt University
Wagga Wagga, New South Wales
CHAPTER 5: The nursing role in reproductive and sexual health
CHAPTER 15: Woman-centred care during labour and birth
CHAPTER 16: Providing comfort during labour and birth

Bill DEANS **MPH, RN (Child), RN (Adult), SCPHN (HV) DipClinHyp, DipHSM, TTCert**
Senior Lecturer, Faculty of Nursing and Health Studies
Manukau Institute of Technology
Manukau City, New Zealand
CHAPTER 4: Promoting family health in the community
CHAPTER 34: Child health assessment

Janet DeLANGE **MN (Ed), Post Grad Paeds, BN, RN**
Lecturer, School of Nursing and Midwifery, Monash University, Berwick, Victoria
CHAPTER 27: Care of the child born with a physical or developmental challenge

Sally-Ann DE-VITRY SMITH **RN, RM, PhD**
Midwifery Course Coordinator, School of Nursing Midwifery and Indigenous Health, Charles Sturt University, Wagga Wagga, New South Wales
CHAPTER 20: Care of a family experiencing a pregnancy complication from a pre-existing or newly acquired condition
CHAPTER 21: Sudden pregnancy complications
CHAPTER 22: Care of a pregnant family with special needs
CHAPTER 23: Care of a family experiencing a complication of labour or birth
CHAPTER 24: Care of a family during caesarean birth
CHAPTER 25: Care of a family experiencing a postpartum complication

Elaine DIETSCH **RN, RM, PhD, MN (Women's Health)**
Lecturer, School of Nursing and Midwifery
Griffith University, Logan, Queensland
CHAPTER 5: The nursing role in reproductive and sexual health
CHAPTER 15: Woman-centred care during labour and birth
CHAPTER 16: Providing comfort during labour and birth

Rakime ELMIR **RN, RM, BN (Hons), GCert Clinical Teaching, PhD**
Lecturer, School of Nursing and Midwifery, University of Western Sydney, Campbelltown, New South Wales
CHAPTER 12: Promoting fetal and maternal health
CHAPTER 14: Preparing a family for childbirth and parenting

Kirsteen FLEMING **Dip Nurs (Adult), Cert Sexual & Reproductive Health**
Clinical Nurse, Specialist Family Planning, New South Wales State Nurse Coordinator, Family Planning New South Wales, Sydney New South Wales
CHAPTER 37: Nursing care of a family when a child needs diagnostic or therapeutic modalities

Heather GALE **RN, MW, IBCLC, PGDip (Nurse Education), MN**
General Practice Nurse, Bowral Street Medical Practice
Bowral, New South Wales
CHAPTER *7: The nursing role in genetic assessment and counselling*

Christine HALEY **RN, RM, BHSC (Nursing) GCert (Women's Health), MPHC**
Lecturer in Nursing, School of Nursing and Midwifery
Lithgow Campus, University of Western Sydney
New South Wales; Lecturer in Academic English
Health Science and Nursing, Lithgow Campus
University of Western Sydney College, New South Wales
CHAPTER 38: Nursing care of a family when a child needs medication administration or intravenous therapy
CHAPTER 39: Pain management in children
CHAPTER 49: Nursing care of a family when a child has a neurological disorder

Janet JONES **RN, RM, BNurs, MClinMid GCert (Health Professional Education)**
Lecturer, Program Coordinator
Federation University, Churchill, Victoria
CHAPTER 19: Nutritional needs of a newborn

Sharon JONES **GDipSci (Mental Health)**
Formerly Infant Child Youth and Family MHDA Service Coordinator, CNC III, MHDA Services, WNSWLHD
Orange, New South Wales
CHAPTER 54: Nursing care of a family when a young person has an intellectual or a mental health disorder

Heather LATHAM **RN, Paed Nurs Cert, DNE (ACAE) BSocSci, MN**
Adjunct Senior Lecturer, School of Nursing Midwifery and Indigenous Health, Charles Sturt University
Bathurst, New South Wales
CHAPTER 2: Sociocultural aspects of child and family health nursing
CHAPTER 36: Nursing care of a family with an ill child

Tara LEWIS **RN, CNS (Surgical), BNurs GCert (Acute Care), Cert IV Training and Assessment**
Clinical Nurse Specialist (Surgical), Bathurst Health Service, Bathurst Base Hospital, Bathurst
New South Wales; Nursing Teacher, TAFE, Bathurst, New South Wales
CHAPTER 45: Nursing care of a family when a child has a gastrointestinal disorder

Rachel LOVETT **BN, GCert (Orthopaedic Nursing)**
Registered Nurse, Bathurst Base Hospital, Bathurst
New South Wales
CHAPTER 45: Nursing care of a family when a child has a gastrointestinal disorder

Cathy MAGINNIS **RN, RM, DipAppSci (Nurs) BAppSci (Nurs), GCert Child & Adol, MHlthSc (Nurs) PhD candidate**
Nursing Lecturer, School of Nursing, Midwifery and Indigenous Health, Charles Sturt University
Dubbo, New South Wales
CHAPTER 1: A framework for child and family health nursing
CHAPTER 3: The childbearing and childrearing family

Anne MARKS **RN, Nurse Practitioner, Credentialled Diabetes Educator, MN, BN (Hons), GCert (Diabetes, Child and Family Health, Cardiac), PhD candidate**
Lecturer, School of Nursing and Midwifery
University of Western Sydney, Penrith
New South Wales
CHAPTER 30: Nursing care of a family with a toddler

Renee McGILL **RN, MN (Education major) GCert (Critical Care), BSci (Nurs)**
Lecturer, Simulation Lead, School of Nursing Midwifery and Indigenous Health
Charles Sturt University, Bathurst, New South Wales
CHAPTER 40: Nursing care of a family when a child has a respiratory disorder
CHAPTER 52: Nursing care of a family when a child has an unintentional injury

Natalie MENZIES **RN, Cert Intensive Care MHlthSc (Nursing)**
CHAPTER 47: Nursing care of a family when a child has a reproductive disorder

Maureen MILES **RN, RM, MCN (MCHN), PhD**
Lecturer, School of Nursing and Midwifery
Deakin University, Burwood, Victoria
CHAPTER 10: Psychological and physiological changes of pregnancy

Anne MORRISON **BN (Hons), PIC Cert**
Nurse Unit Manager, ICU/HDU Bathurst Health Service
Bathurst, New South Wales
CHAPTER 48: Nursing care of a family when a child has an endocrine or a metabolic disorder
CHAPTER 55: Nursing care of a family in crisis: Abuse and violence in the family

Joanne PERKS **RN, RM, BHSc (Mid), GCert WHN MN (Nurse Practitioner), MMental Health Nursing (Distinction), Family Planning Cert, Cert 1V in TAE Cert 11 Continence Care, TAFE Attainment Aboriginal Cultural Awareness**
Advanced Childbirth Educator/Women's Health Nurse Practitioner, Liverpool and Penrith Women's Health Centres, Sydney, New South Wales
CHAPTER 8: Nursing care of the infertile couple

Suzanne QUERRUEL **BN, GDipNurs (Anaesthetics & Recovery), MN (Education), Cert IV Workplace Training & Assessment**
Sessional Tutor/ Registered Nurse, School of Nursing & Midwifery, University of Western Sydney, New South Wales; Academic Pathway Programs, University of Western Sydney College, Parramatta, Blacktown, New South Wales
CHAPTER 41: Nursing care of a family when a child has a cardiovascular disorder

Virginia SKINNER **MN (Hons), PhD**
Senior Lecturer, Midwifery Theme Leader
Charles Darwin University, Darwin, Northern Territory
CHAPTER 11: Assessing fetal and maternal health: Antenatal care
CHAPTER 13: Promoting nutritional health during pregnancy

Kylie SMITH
Clinical Nurse Specialist, Paediatric Unit
Dubbo Base Hospital, Dubbo, New South Wales
CHAPTER 46: Nursing care of a family when a child has a renal or urinary tract disorder

Lisa SPEEDIE **DipAppSci (Nursing), PGrad Paediatrics PGrad Women's Health**
Scholarly Teaching Fellow, School of Nursing Midwifery and Indigenous Health
Charles Sturt University, Albury, New South Wales
CHAPTER 28: Principles of growth and development
CHAPTER 29: Nursing care of a family with an infant
CHAPTER 31: Nursing care of a family with a preschool child
CHAPTER 32: Nursing care of a family with a school-aged child
CHAPTER 33: Nursing care of a family with an adolescent

Katie SULLIVAN **RN, RM, MM (Hons)**
Lecturer, School of Nursing and Midwifery
University of Western Sydney, New South Wales
CHAPTER 9: The growing fetus

Louise WELLS **BN, MN, GCerts Critical Care Nursing and Perioperative Nursing**
Lecturer in Nursing, School of Nursing, Midwifery and Indigenous Health, Charles Sturt University, Bathurst New South Wales
CHAPTER 35: Communication and teaching with children and families

Amanda WORTHINGTON **BA (Nursing), BA Clinical Practice (Paramedics), MA (International Public Health) MA (Environmental Health)**
CHAPTER 42: Nursing care of a family when a child has an immune disorder
CHAPTER 43: Nursing care of a family when a child has an infectious disorder
CHAPTER 44: Nursing care of a family when a child has a haematological disorder
CHAPTER 51: Nursing care of a family when a child has a musculoskeletal disorder

Reviewers

Regina BELSKI **BNutrDiet (Hons), GCertTertEd, PhD**
Senior Lecturer, School of Allied Health
La Trobe University, Melbourne, Victoria

Patricia BROMLEY **RN, Certs NICU, Midwifery Paediatric, MEd, EdD candidate**
Lecturer, Nursing & Midwifery, University of Tasmania, Hobart, Tasmania

Mandy EL ALI **BHS (Nursing), MN (Paediatric Specialisation), GDip (Paediatric Nursing) GCert (Paediatric Nursing), GCert (Higher Education)**
Lecturer, School of Nursing, Midwifery and Paramedicine
Australian Catholic University, St Patricks Campus, Melbourne, Victoria

Kristina GRIFFIN **RN, GCert (CCU), MN, PhD candidate**
Lecturer, School of Nursing, Midwifery and Indigenous Health, Charles Sturt University, Wagga Wagga
New South Wales

Kirsten GUNN **RN, RSCN, AdvDip Child Development MA (Education), PGCHE**
Senior Lecturer, Nursing, Christchurch Polytechnic Institute of Technology, Christchurch, New Zealand

Mary HUYNH **BN, GCert (Tertiary Education), GCertNurs (Research Methodologies), GDipAdvNurs (Paediatrics) MAdvNurs (Paediatrics)**
Lecturer, School of Nursing, Midwifery and Paramedicine
Australian Catholic University, Melbourne, Victoria

Jennifer JAMES **PhD, IBCLC, Midwife**
Senior Lecturer, Nursing & Midwifery
RMIT University, Bundoora, Victoria

Susie LE PAGE **RM, MN**
Nurse Educator, Primary Health
Health Care Development, Mid Central DHB
Palmerston North, New Zealand

Katie LUCAS **BN, GCert Health (Child, Adolescent and Family Health), GDip Clinical Education**
Lecturer, Nursing and Midwifery
University of South Australia, South Australia

Jane MATEER **RN, BA, GC Emerg, GD Nurse Practitioner GD Defence, MA International Security, MPH**
Lecturer, Nursing and Midwifery, RMIT University
Melbourne, Victoria

Kolleen MILLER-ROSSER **EN, RN, GDip (Pediatrics) MSN, PhD**
Lecturer, Health & Human Sciences (Nursing)
Southern Cross University, Coffs Harbour
New South Wales

Creina MITCHELL **RN, RM, MCH, DipAppSci (Nursing) BAppSci (Advanced Nursing), GDipComp, MPH, MACN**
Lecturer, School of Nursing and Midwifery
Griffith University, Gold Coast, Queensland

Ailsa MUNNS **RN, RM, CHN, BAppSci (Nursing) (Education major), MN**
Lecturer/Course Coordinator, Child and Adolescent Health Programs Coordinator Community Mothers Program (WA)
School of Nursing and Midwifery, Curtin University
Perth, Western Australia

Mimmie Claudine NGUM CHI WATTS **RN, MPH GCert (Tertiary Education), PhD**
Lecturer in Community Health, College of Health and Biomedicine, Victoria University, Melbourne
Victoria

Ibi PATANE **RN, BN, GCert (Infants, Children & Youth Health Nursing), GDip (EBP), MN**
Lecturer, School of Nursing, Queensland University of Technology, Kelvin Grove, Brisbane, Queensland

Geraldine REBEIRO **RN, Midwife, BAppSci (Adv Nursing), BEd Studs, MEd**
Lecturer, School of Nursing, Midwifery & Paramedicine,
Australian Catholic University, Melbourne, Victoria

Lael RIDGWAY **RN, MNSc, PgDipAdvNsg (ChildFamComm), Midwife, IBCLC**
Lecturer, Child Family and Community Nursing and Midwifery, Department of Nursing and Midwifery
La Trobe University, Melbourne, Victoria

Norma SCOBIE New Zealand Registered Obstetric and General Nurse, MNurs (Hons) (Child Health Endorsed)
Principal Lecturer, Bachelor of Nursing, NorthTec
Whangarei, New Zealand

Sue SHARRAD RN, BEd, GDip Intensive Care, MNurs
Lecturer, School of Nursing, The University of Adelaide
Adelaide, South Australia

Mercy THOMAS RN, BSc (Nursing), MSc (Paediatric Nursing), Cert Tertiary Teaching
Nurse Educator, Graduate Nurses
The Royal Children's Hospital Melbourne
Melbourne, Victoria

Preface

Maternal–newborn and child health nursing are expanding areas as a result of the broadening scope of practice within the nursing profession and the recognised need for better preventive and restorative care in these areas. At the same time that the information in these areas of nursing is increasing, less time is available in nursing programs for teaching it. It is difficult for students to read all of the material contained in overlapping textbooks.

Child and Family Health Nursing in Australia and New Zealand (second edition) is written with this challenge in mind. It views maternal–newborn and child healthcare not as two separate disciplines but as a continuum of knowledge. It is designed to present the content of the two disciplines comprehensively. It is based on a philosophy of nursing care that respects clients as individuals, yet views them as part of a family and society.

This book is designed for undergraduate student use, either in a combined course in maternal–newborn and child health or for a curriculum in which these courses are taught separately. It provides a comprehensive, in-depth discussion of the many facets of child and family health nursing, while promoting a sensitive, holistic outlook on nursing practice. As such, the book will also be useful for practising nurses or graduate students who are interested in reviewing or expanding their knowledge in these areas.

Basic themes that are integrated into this text include the experience of wellness and illness as family events, the perception of pregnancy and childbirth as periods of wellness, and the importance of knowing normal child development in the planning of nursing care. Also included are themes reflective of changes in healthcare delivery and the importance of meeting the needs of a culturally diverse population in Australia and New Zealand.

THE CHANGING HEALTHCARE SCENE

Managed care has drastically changed the healthcare delivery system, increasing the role of the nurse from a minor to a major player. It has made understanding multidisciplinary approaches to care more important than ever before. An increasingly multicultural population is reflected among both nurses and the clients they care for, necessitating fine-tuning of culturally sensitive care. In order for nurses to be prepared for this new level of responsibility, educational changes have to keep pace with healthcare reform by emphasising a primary healthcare (PHC) model of care and a greater focus on communication, nursing considerations and critical thinking.

Nursing issues that grow out of the current climate of change include:

- The importance of health promotion through education with families as a cornerstone of nursing responsibility. The teaching role of the nurse has greater significance in the new healthcare milieu as the emphasis on preventive care and short stays in the acute care setting creates the need for families to be better educated in their own care. The family teaching excerpts throughout the book present detailed health information for the family, emphasising the importance of a partnership between nurses and families in the management of health and illness. Understanding the challenges and changes experienced by parents and families during the childbearing years provides the nurse with skills to view more broadly the issues across the life span. Knowledge of the care of women (maternal care) and their partners through this period allows nurses to consider their ongoing health and wellbeing needs as they progress through the demanding years of parenting.
- The importance of individualising care according to sociocultural uniqueness. This is a reflection of both greater cultural sensitivity and an increasingly diverse population of carers and care recipients. Greater emphasis is being placed on the implications of multiple sociocultural factors in terms of how they affect responses to health and illness.
- The importance of basing nursing on evidence-based practice. The variety of new care settings, as well as the diversity of roles in which nurses practise, reflects the broadening scope of practice in contemporary nursing. This new edition places emphasis on the need for nurses to practise based on solid evidence in all settings. The focus on evidence-based practice excerpts in each chapter supply concrete examples of research and how it could be applicable to nursing practice.

Child and Family Health Nursing in Australia and New Zealand follows the family from the pregnancy period, through labour, delivery and the postpartum period; it then follows the child in the family from birth through to adolescence. It includes community and in-patient care and focuses on primary as well as secondary and tertiary care.

The book is organised in eight units:

- **Unit 1** provides an introduction to child and family health nursing. A framework for practice is presented, as well as current trends and the importance of considering childbearing and childrearing within a diverse socioeconomic and family/community context. A chapter on primary healthcare as a social model of care is included to develop students' understanding of working within a PHC framework to promote health and wellbeing of families in the community.
- **Unit 2** examines the nursing role in preparing families for childbearing and childrearing, and discusses reproductive and sexual health, the role of the nurse as a genetic counsellor, reproductive life planning and the concerns of the infertile family.
- **Unit 3** presents the nursing role in caring for a pregnant family during pregnancy, birth and the postnatal period and serving as a fetal advocate. A separate chapter details the role of the nurse in providing comfort during labour and birth.
- **Unit 4** addresses the nursing role when a woman develops a complication of pregnancy, labour or birth, or has a complication during the postnatal period. Separate chapters address the role of the nurse when a woman has a pre-existing illness, develops a complication during pregnancy or the postpartum period, has a special need or chooses or needs a caesarean birth. A final chapter details care of the high-risk newborn or a child born with a physical or developmental challenge.
- **Unit 5** discusses the nursing role in health promotion during childhood. The chapters in this unit cover principles of growth and development and care of the child from infancy through adolescence, including child health assessment and communication and health teaching with children and families.
- **Unit 6** presents the nursing role in supporting the health of children and their families. The effects of illness on children and their families, diagnostic and therapeutic procedures, medication administration and pain management are addressed with respect to care of the child and family in hospital, at home and in ambulatory settings.
- **Unit 7** examines the nursing role in restoring and maintaining the health of children and families when illness occurs. Disorders are presented according to body systems so that students have a ready orientation for locating content.
- **Unit 8** discusses the nursing role in restoring and maintaining the mental health of children and families. Separate chapters discuss the role of the nurse when domestic violence, child abuse or mental, long-term or fatal illness is present.

PEDAGOGICAL FEATURES

Each chapter in the text is organised to provide a complete learning experience for the student. Numerous pedagogical features are included to help students understand and increase retention. Important elements include:

- **Chapter objectives:** Learning objectives are included at the beginning of each chapter to identify outcomes expected after the material in the chapter has been mastered.
- **Key terms:** Terms that would be new to students are listed at the beginning of each chapter in a ready reference list. When the terms appear in the text, they are shown in boldface type and then defined. Definitions appear again in the Glossary.
- **Chapter opening case studies:** Short case studies appear at the beginning of each chapter. These are designed to help students appreciate that nursing care is always individualised and they provide a taste of what is to come in the chapter. At the end of the chapter, case study questions related to the scenario bring the chapter full circle.
- **Tables and boxes:** Numerous tables and boxes summarise important information or provide extra detail on topics so that students have ready references to this information.
- **Focus on assessment:** These visual guides provide head-to-toe assessment information for overall health status or specific disorders or conditions.
- **Focus on communication:** This feature presents case examples of less effective communication and more effective communication, illustrating for the student how an awareness of communication can improve the patient's understanding and positively impact outcomes.
- **Focus on evidence-based practice:** These boxes summarise research on topics related to child and family health nursing. They appear throughout the text to accentuate the use of evidence-based practice as the basis for nursing care.
- **Focus on family teaching:** These boxes present detailed health teaching information for the family, emphasising the importance of a partnership between nurses and clients in the management of health and illness.
- **Focus on pharmacology:** These boxes provide quick reference for medications that are commonly used for the health problems described in the text. They give the drug name (brand and generic, if applicable), dosage, pregnancy category, side effects and nursing considerations.
- **Checkpoint questions and case study questions:** Throughout the text, multiple-choice questions are inserted to help students check progress and comprehension. They ask students to use the knowledge just gained

in the last few pages, helping them retain this information. Answers are supplied on thePoint site for the text.

- **"What if" questions:** These questions ask students to apply the information just acquired to an "actual" situation. Students must process the information and apply it to the new situation, thus maximising learning and emphasising critical thinking. Suggested solutions are supplied on thePoint site for the text.
- **Key points for review:** A review of important points is highlighted at the end of each chapter to help students monitor their own comprehension.
- **Case study questions:** To involve students in the decision-making realities of the clinical setting, several thought-provoking questions are posed at the end of each chapter. These could also serve as a basis for conference or class discussion. Suggested considerations are supplied on thePoint site for the text.
- **References and suggested readings:** These provide students with the information needed to carry out more in-depth reading of the sources noted in the text, as well as other relevant articles on the topics included in the chapter.

Ancillary package

A learning and teaching package accompanies the text on thePoint. This resource contains useful lecture points in a PowerPoint presentation, a bank of questions and an image bank for each chapter, as well as Watch and Learn videos.

Christine Haley
RN, RM, BHSc (Nursing), GCert (Women's Health), MPHC
Lecturer in Nursing, School of Nursing & Midwifery, Lithgow Campus, University of Western Sydney, New South Wales; Lecturer in Academic English, Health Science and Nursing, Lithgow Campus, UWS College, New South Wales

Acknowledgements

In undertaking the second edition, I set out to broaden the nursing care perspective by encouraging contributors from across Australia and New Zealand. I would like to thank those new contributors who took on the challenge and therefore provided a more national and cross-cultural perspective to care of families in all communities.

A special acknowledgement must go to Caroline Hunter of Wolters Kluwer. It has been Caroline's considerable expertise, skill and knowledge that enabled the completion of this text. Finally, I would like to thank Michelle Forde and Sarah Plant at Puddingburn Publishing Services.

Christine Haley

Contents

UNIT 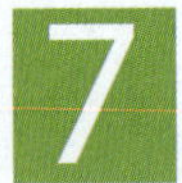

The nursing role in restoring and maintaining the health of children and families with physiological disorders 713

CHAPTER 40

Nursing care of a family when a child has a respiratory disorder 713

CHAPTER 41

Nursing care of a family when a child has a cardiovascular disorder 739

CHAPTER 42

Nursing care of a family when a child has an immune disorder 761

CHAPTER 43

Nursing care of a family when a child has an infectious disorder 777

CHAPTER 44

Nursing care of a family when a child has a haematological disorder 793

CHAPTER 45

Nursing care of a family when a child has a gastrointestinal disorder 811

CHAPTER **46**

Nursing care of a family when a child has a renal or urinary tract disorder 834

CHAPTER **47**

Nursing care of a family when a child has a reproductive disorder 853

CHAPTER **48**

Nursing care of a family when a child has an endocrine or a metabolic disorder 871

CHAPTER **49**

Nursing care of a family when a child has a neurological disorder 887

CHAPTER **50**

Nursing care of a family when a child has a vision or hearing disorder 916

CHAPTER **51**

Nursing care of a family when a child has a musculoskeletal disorder 932

Unit 1

Child and family health nursing practice

Chapter 1

A framework for child and family health nursing

This chapter discusses standards and philosophies of child and family healthcare and how these standards and philosophies affect care.

LEARNING OBJECTIVES

After studying this chapter, you should be able to:

1. Describe and understand the philosophy of child and family health nursing.
2. Describe strengths-based assessment and apply this model to practice.
3. Identify the goals and standards of child and family health nursing and apply these to practice.
4. Describe the evolution, scope, standards and professional roles for nurses in child and family health nursing.
5. Describe family-centred care and ways that child and family health nursing could be made more family-centred.
6. Define common statistical terms used in the field, such as infant and maternal mortality.
7. Identify legal and ethical issues important to child and family health nursing.
8. Use critical thinking to identify areas of care that could benefit from additional research or application of evidence-based practice.
9. Discuss the interplay of nursing process, evidence-based practice and nursing theory as they relate to the future of child and family health nursing practice.
10. Integrate knowledge of trends in child and family healthcare with the nursing process to achieve quality child and family health nursing care.

KEY TERMS

- child and family health nursing
- client advocacy
- evidence-based practice
- family-centred care
- infant mortality rate
- maternal, child and family health services
- maternal mortality
- nursing research
- scope of practice

CASE STUDY

Anna Chung is a premature neonate, born at 33 weeks' gestation, who will be transported to a hospital with a higher level neonatal intensive care unit in a large metropolitan city about 300 km from the hospital where she was born. Her parents, Melissa and Robert, are worried because their tiny daughter will be cared for a long way from home. Melissa, who is 41 years old, tells you that she feels too exhausted to leave the hospital only 2 days after having a caesarean birth. She wonders how her first child, Michael, now 6 years old, will react to having a hospitalised rather than a healthy baby sister. Michael has asthma and has been hospitalised previously for this condition and does not like hospitals.

CASE STUDY QUESTIONS

1. What are some healthcare issues evident for this family?
2. What is the nursing role here?

DEFINITIONS

Some definitions are required in this chapter due to a variety of specialist nurses being employed in child and family health nursing practice.

Registered midwives are people who have successfully completed a prescribed course of study to acquire the requisite qualification and registration to practise midwifery. Midwives provide a combination of primary and secondary care in both public and private areas of healthcare. These services are offered in community-based settings, including homes, as well as in hospital settings. Midwives in Australia and New Zealand have a strong focus on primary healthcare, encompassing social justice and empowering women and their families to make the best decisions for themselves and their families (Pairman et al., 2015).

Domiciliary midwives are part of home-based programs. These midwives provide support to parents of a newborn baby upon discharge from the hospital until care is transferred to the child and family health services in the family's local area. These services are managed by the facility where the woman has delivered her baby. The program aims to improve family and infant outcomes (Kralik & van Loon, 2011). The service differs in each state or territory of Australia as well as being different from what is offered in New Zealand.

Maternal, child and family health services offer a range of prevention and intervention programs for families. The target population is families with children up to 6 years of age (Schmied et al., 2011). This age limit differs, however, between Australia and New Zealand and within the states and territories of Australia and can encompass children up to 8 years of age (Kralik & van Loon, 2011). The staff who provide these services have different specialty qualifications and different titles. In NSW they are known as child and family health nurses while in Victoria they are known as maternal and child health nurses (Kruske & Grant, 2012; NSW Health, 2011). However, the roles they undertake are similar in their focus and are all based in community health. The New Zealand equivalent of child and family health nurses are known as Plunket nurses. This organisation aims to support the development of families to provide the best start possible for every child. The Plunket well child health service provides support for parents and children to ensure flexible models of care are available for supporting and developing healthy families, especially Māori and Pacific Islander families (Plunket, 2014).

Child and family health nurses are registered nurses with specialty qualifications in child and family health nursing (NSW Health, 2011). They work within a primary healthcare model with families that have infants and young children up to the age of 8 years. These nurses work in a range of settings including community health facilities, family homes and residential family care centres. The services they provide are ongoing and change based on the individual family's needs. These nurses use a strength-based and wellness approach in promoting the health and wellbeing of both families and children (NSW Health, 2011).

Family is defined in different ways by different organisations. Currently the ABS (2011) defines family as comprising two or more people related by blood, marriage, adoption, step or fostering, and who are usually resident in the same household. In New Zealand the term *family type* is adopted and is derived from the presence or absence of couples, parents and children but is explained as two or more people living in the same dwelling with or without children where a child can be any age, but a dependent child is under 18 years of age (Statistics NZ, 2012).

GOALS AND STANDARDS OF CHILD AND FAMILY HEALTH NURSING

The care of childbearing and childrearing families is a major focus of nursing practice, because to have healthy adults you must have healthy children. To have healthy children, it is important to promote the health of the childbearing woman and her family, from the time before children are born until they reach adulthood. The World Health Organization (WHO, 2014) advocates that early child development be adopted into all national and international policies to improve health and to enable children to achieve their optimal growth and development. Preconception and antenatal care are essential contributions to the health of a woman and fetus, and to a family's emotional preparation for childbearing and childrearing. As children grow, families need continued health supervision and support. As children reach maturity and plan for their own families, a new cycle begins and new support becomes necessary. A positive start in a child's life assists them to reach their full potential.

Families and communities have a crucial role in supporting children and determining their health and wellbeing (AIHW, 2013). Acknowledgement of the importance of families and communities in supporting and developing a child's health and wellbeing has been evidenced by a change in care delivery and a renewed focus on universal services, early contact and home visiting and acknowledgement of children's rights (AHMAC, 2011; NSW Health, 2011; Plunket, 2014). The nurse's role is central in all these phases focusing on promoting healthy growth and development of the child and family.

Although the field of nursing typically divides its concerns for families during childbearing and childrearing into two separate entities, maternity care and child healthcare, the full scope of nursing practice in this area is not actually two separate entities but rather a continuum: child and family health nursing (see Fig. 1.1).

The primary goal of **child and family health nursing** can be stated simply as the promotion and maintenance of optimal family health to ensure cycles of optimal childbearing and childrearing. Major philosophical assumptions about child and family health nursing are listed in Box 1.1. The goals of child and family health nursing care are necessarily broad because the **scope of practice** (the range of services and care that may be provided by a nurse based on state requirements) is so broad. The range of practice includes:

- Preconception healthcare
- Care of women, fetus and baby during three trimesters of pregnancy (antenatal) and the puerperium period (the 6 weeks after childbirth, sometimes termed the fourth trimester of pregnancy)
- Care of children from birth through to adolescence
- Care in settings as varied as the birthing room, the paediatric intensive care unit and the home.

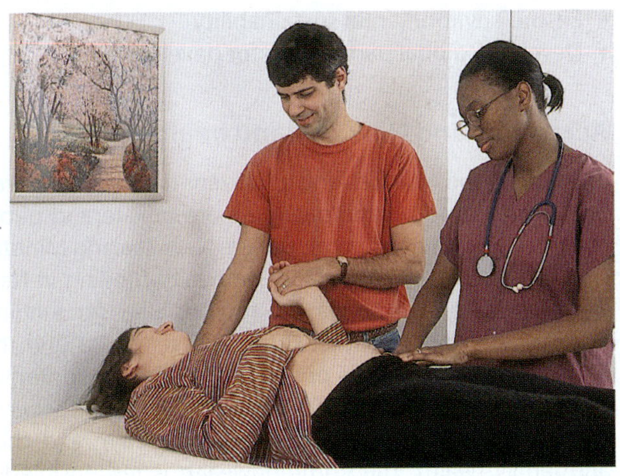

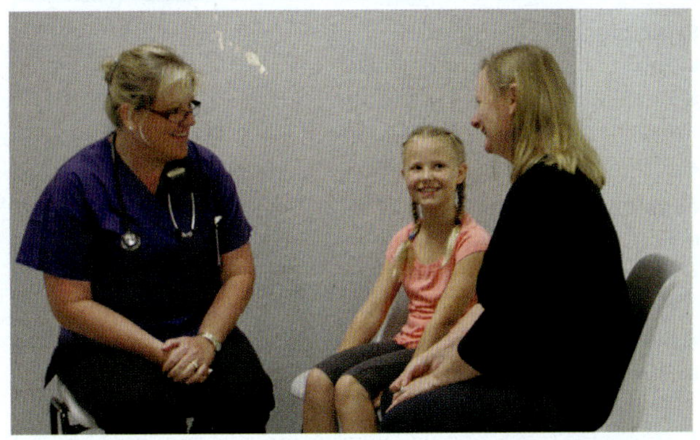

FIGURE 1.1 Child and family health nursing includes care of the pregnant woman, child and family. (**A**) During an antenatal visit, a nurse assesses that a pregnant woman's uterus is expanding normally. (**B**) During a health maintenance visit, a nurse assesses a child's growth and development. (**A** © Barbara Proud. **B** © Gavin Crawford.)

In all settings and types of care, keeping the family at the centre of care or considering the family as the primary unit of care is an essential goal. This is because the level of a family's functioning affects the health status of its members (Papp, 2012). If a family's level of functioning is low, the emotional, physical and social health of the family and potential of individuals in that family can be adversely affected. A healthy family, on the other hand, establishes an environment conducive to growth and health-promoting behaviours that sustain family members during crises. Similarly, the health and ability of an individual to function strongly influence the health of family members and overall family functioning.

Some men, for example, relate so closely during their wife's or partner's pregnancy, they experience morning sickness at the same level as she does (Paulson & Bazemore, 2010). For these reasons, a family-centred approach enables nurses to better understand individuals and their effect on others and, in turn, to provide holistic care (Hedges, Nichols & Filoteo, 2012). Box 1.2 provides a summary of key measures for the delivery of family-centred child and family healthcare.

BOX 1.1 ✻ Philosophy of child and family health nursing

- Child and family health nursing is family centred; assessment must include both family and individual assessment data.
- Child and family health nursing is community centred; the health of families depends on and influences the health of communities.
- Child and family health nursing is evidence-based, because this is the means whereby critical knowledge increases.
- A child and family health nurse serves as an advocate to protect the rights of all family members, including the fetus.
- Child and family health nursing includes a high degree of independent nursing functions, because teaching and counselling are major interventions.
- Promoting health and disease prevention are important nursing roles because these protect the health of the next generation.
- Child and family health nurses serve as important resources for families during childbearing and childrearing as these can be extremely stressful times in a life cycle.
- Personal, cultural and religious attitudes and beliefs influence the meaning and impact of childbearing and childrearing on families.
- Circumstances such as illness or pregnancy are meaningful only in the context of a total life.
- Child and family health nursing is a challenging role for nurses and a major factor in keeping families well and optimally functioning.

CHILD AND FAMILY HEALTH NURSING STANDARDS

Changes in social structure, family structure and function plus advanced healthcare technology have contributed to advancing child and family health nursing practice embedded within a primary healthcare philosophy to guide practice and optimise the health and wellbeing of children and families (MOHNZ, 2014b). Immunisation, childhood disease eradication, new fertility medications and technology are helping individuals and couples to conceive and have children, while the ability to delay preterm birth is improving the quality of life for babies born prematurely. In addition, advances have been made in the development of gene technology to identify and treat abnormalities and in the use of stem cell therapy to replace diseased cells with new growth cells and cure illnesses. These and other changes have expanded the role of the child and family health nurse while providing challenges in delivering quality care in a variety of settings to a diverse population. Australia and New Zealand have national health

BOX 1.2 * Common measures to ensure family-centred child and family healthcare

Principles

- The family is the basic unit of society.
- Families come in many different forms and sizes and represent racial, ethnic, cultural and socio-economic diversity.
- Children grow both individually and as part of a family.

Nursing interventions

- Consider the family as a whole as well as its individual members.
- Assess families for strengths as well as for specific needs or challenges.
- Respect diversity in families as a unique quality of that family.
- Share or initiate information on health planning with family members so that care is family oriented.
- Encourage family bonding through rooming-in in both child and family health hospital settings.
- Encourage families to give care to a newborn or ill child.
- Remember: family members affect other members; individual members affect the total family group.
- Encourage family and sibling visits in the hospital to promote family contacts.
- Participate in early hospital discharge programs to reunite families as soon as possible.
- Include developmental stimulation in nursing care.
- Encourage families to reach out to their community so that family members are not isolated from their community or from each other.

policies which determine the health priorities for each country. The Ministry of Health in New Zealand is responsible for health legislation and development of health strategies and policy (MOHNZ, 2014b). In Australia the federal government shares responsibility for health services with the states and territories as well as several national bodies. Some states and territories also involve local government funding and provision of services (Schmied et al., 2011). Both countries are closely associated with international organisations such as the WHO and the International Council of Nurses (ICN) to ensure their health policies are current and incorporate global policies and programs.

Global health goals

The United Nations (UN) and the WHO established millennium health goals in 2000 in an effort to improve health worldwide by decreasing poverty and the spread of diseases and providing universal primary education. All UN member states agreed to try to achieve these goals by 2015 (WHO, 2014). The global health goals are:

- End poverty and hunger
- Achieve universal primary education
- Promote gender equality and empower women
- Reduce child mortality
- Improve maternal health
- Combat HIV/AIDS, malaria and other diseases
- Ensure environmental sustainability
- Develop a global partnership for development.

Australian and New Zealand health goals

In Australia and New Zealand all citizens have access to free healthcare. In both countries there are private and publically funded healthcare options. The New Zealand Ministry of Health has the responsibility for health funding in New Zealand, while in Australia the responsibility for funding healthcare is split between states and territories and the Commonwealth divisions of health. The states and territories have responsibility for delivering public health services and community services such as dental health and child and family health. The Commonwealth is responsible for funding most hospital medical services via schemes such as Medicare and the Pharmaceutical Benefits Scheme (PBS). Each country has devised policies to address the cultural differences among the Indigenous populations, specifically the Māori and Aboriginal and Torres Strait Islander populations, to lessen the gap in healthcare provided and to ensure care is accessible, acceptable and affordable to all (Pairman et al., 2015).

Australia has developed a national framework for universal child and family health services with provision of universal no cost services provided for children and families from birth to 8 years of age (AHMAC, 2011). This document articulates objectives and principles for universal child and family health services. Another initiative in NSW is the development of the Child and Family Health Nursing Professional Practice Framework 2011–2016. This has been developed in the Australian context to provide support for child and family health nurses facilitating safe and effective primary healthcare for children and families in NSW (NSW Health, 2011, p. 7). In Victoria maternal and child health services provide universal primary care from birth to school age to promote healthy outcomes for children and their families (DEECD, 2014). The document titled 'Headline indicators for children's health, development and wellbeing' articulates priorities for health, development and wellbeing of children and their families from birth to 12 years of age (AIHW, 2011). The AIHW provides an overview of Australia's children in a comprehensive document on the health and wellbeing of children aged from birth to 14 years of age (AIHW, 2012). Other policies and regulations can be found at the Australian Government Department of Health and Ageing <www.health.gov.au/internet/main/publishing.nsf/Content/publications-Child+health> and the Australian Institute of Family Studies <www.aifs.gov.au>. All of these policies and frameworks deal with primary healthcare and the well child, with prevention of illness and promotion of health the focus as well as addressing inequalities in care and access to services. New Zealand is currently reviewing its child health strategy implemented in 1998 followed by a child health information strategy in 2003. The Well Child/Tamariki Ora quality improvement framework provides health education, promotion, protection, assessment and family support. These universal services are offered free of charge or with co-payments to all families from preconception until 6 years of age (MOHNZ, 2014b).

Both countries focus on the well child and maintaining and promoting the health of children through a variety of services and personnel to ensure health as children but also as adults (Schmied et al., 2014). Primary healthcare is the underlying philosophy behind many of the frameworks, policies, standards and strategies instigated to facilitate the well child and their family to maximise their health and wellbeing. The titles and roles of personnel providing care and support to children and families differ between states, territories and countries and this provides many challenges. Contemporary child and family health services have moved away from the biomedical model used in previous years to embrace models based on ecological and social models of health, incorporating a strengths-based framework (Briggs, 2013; Wells et al., 2014).

A FRAMEWORK FOR CHILD AND FAMILY HEALTH NURSING

Child and family health nursing can be visualised within a framework in which nurses, using nursing process, nursing theory and evidence-based practice, care for families during childbearing and childrearing years based on a strengths-based approach integrating family-centred care through four phases of healthcare:

- Health promotion
- Health maintenance
- Health restoration
- Health rehabilitation.

Examples of these phases of healthcare as they relate to child and family health are shown in Table 1.1.

Family-centred care

Family-centred care is a healthcare approach used throughout the world to provide a framework for planning, delivery and evaluation of healthcare for children and their families (Randall et al., 2013). It embodies a partnership approach between healthcare providers, individuals and their families. Key principles of family-centred care are dignity, respect, information sharing, participation and collaboration (Queensland Health, 2014). It is important to note that utilising this approach emphasises the need to negotiate care for each care episode. Expectations and roles should be discussed openly to empower families to plan and make decisions with the health professionals. In the hospital setting families can assist with nursing interventions and everyday care tasks, thus maintaining a sense of normality and continuity (Stuart & Melling, 2014). The underlying philosophy behind this approach is a belief that the child's emotional and developmental needs and the wellbeing of the child and the family will be best supported where the family is able to meet the needs of the child through involvement in the child's care (Watts et al., 2014).

Strengths-based approach

A strengths-based approach emphasises collaboration with families, children and healthcare professionals. This approach doesn't focus on weaknesses or deficits; rather, it aims to ascertain individual and family strengths and how individuals and families function (Gottlieb, 2014). All families have strengths and by working with this approach these strengths can be enhanced while at the same time increasing the parents' trust and confidence in their abilities (Wells et al., 2014). Using a strength-based approach promotes health and wellbeing of children and families while acknowledging differences in individual health and development and allowing for intervention when required (NSW Health, 2011). This approach can be used in acute and community settings and enhances the client–health

TABLE 1.1 Definitions and examples of phases of healthcare

Term	Definition	Examples
Health promotion	Educating individuals to be aware of good health through teaching and role modelling	Teaching women the importance of rubella immunisation before pregnancy; teaching children the importance of safer sex practices
Health maintenance	Intervening to maintain health when risk of illness is present	Encouraging women to come for antenatal care; teaching parents the importance of safeguarding their home by childproofing it against poisoning
Health restoration	Promptly diagnosing and treating illness using interventions that will return a person to wellness	Caring for a woman during a complication of pregnancy or a child during an acute illness
Health rehabilitation	Preventing further complications from an illness; bringing an ill person back to an optimal state of wellness or helping someone to accept inevitable death	Encouraging a woman with gestational trophoblastic disease to continue therapy or a child with a renal transplant to continue to take necessary medications

professional relationship while at the same time empowering families and individuals by focusing on positive, not negative, aspects.

An Australian research project identified eight strengths of Australian families (Geggie et al., 2000). The eight qualities identified assisted with families' abilities to cope with crisis and adversity and were used to develop the Australian Family Strengths (AFS) Nursing Assessment Guide. The eight qualities identified are:

- Communication
- Togetherness
- Sharing activities
- Affection
- Support
- Acceptance
- Commitment
- Resilience.

The AFS Nursing Assessment Guide can assist practitioners to engage in conversations with families regarding their strengths as a family and can be adapted to suit the family or the individual (Barnes & Rowe, 2013).

Evidence-based approach

Evidence-based practice is the conscientious, explicit and judicious use of current best evidence in making decisions about the care of individuals (Falk et al., 2012). Evidence can be a combination of research, clinical expertise and personal preferences when all three combine in decision making.

Use of evidence-based practice helps to move all healthcare actions to a more solid, and therefore safer, scientific base. The Cochrane Database of Systematic Reviews and the Joanna Briggs Institute are good sources for discovering evidence-based practice as they provide the best available evidence to inform clinical decision making.

Nursing research

Nursing research plays an important role in evidence-based practice as knowledge can grow only if the people within the profession are able to plan and engage in research (Christian, 2012). **Nursing research** is the controlled investigation of problems that have implications for nursing practice, providing evidence for practice and justification for implementing activities for outcome achievement, ultimately resulting in improved and cost-effective care.

A classic example of how the results of nursing research can influence nursing practice is the application of the research carried out by Rubin (1963) on a mother's approach to her newborn. Before the publication of this study, nurses assumed that a woman who did not immediately hold and cuddle her infant at birth was a "cold" or unfeeling mother. After observing a multitude of new mothers, Rubin concluded that attachment is not a spontaneous procedure; rather, it more commonly begins with only fingertip touching. Armed with Rubin's findings and integrating these findings into practice, nurses became better able to differentiate healthy from unhealthy bonding behaviour in postpartum women. Women who did not follow this step-by-step pattern of attachment were no longer categorised as unfeeling. By documenting these healthy and unhealthy parameters, nurses can identify women who do not follow a healthy pattern, and interventions can be planned and instituted to help these mothers gain a stronger attachment to their new infants. Additional nursing research in this area (discussed in Chapter 17) has provided further substantiation about the importance of this original investigation.

Evidence-based practice requires ongoing research to substantiate current actions as well as to provide guidelines for future actions. Some examples of current questions that warrant nursing investigation in the area of child and family health nursing include the following:

- What is the most effective stimulus to encourage women to come for antenatal care or parents to bring children for health maintenance care?
- What is the effect of market-driven healthcare on the quality of child and family nursing care?
- What active measures can nurses take to reduce the incidence of child or domestic partner abuse?
- What do child and family health nurses need to know about alternative therapies such as herbal remedies to keep their practices current?

The answers to these and other questions provided by research help to bolster a foundation for specific actions and activities that have the potential to improve child and family healthcare. Evidence-based practice boxes included in chapters throughout the text contain summaries of current child and family health research studies and are designed to assist you in developing a questioning attitude regarding current nursing practice and in thinking of ways to incorporate research findings into care (see Box 1.3).

Nursing theory

One of the requirements of a profession (together with other critical determinants, such as member-set standards, monitoring of practice quality and participation in research) is that the concentration of a profession's knowledge flows from a base of established theory. Nursing theorists offer helpful ways to view clients so that nursing activities can best meet client needs—for example, by seeing a pregnant woman not simply as a physical form but as a dynamic force with important psychosocial needs, or by viewing children as extensions or active members of a family as well as independent beings. Only with this broad theoretical focus can nurses appreciate the significant effect on a family of a child's illness or the

BOX 1.3 ❋ Focus on evidence-based practice

Breastfeeding

Research and expert opinion have established that breastfeeding is preferred over bottle feeding, with both short- and long-term benefits to mother and baby. Breast milk is viewed as the optimal feed for an infant. Exclusive breastfeeding can result in reduced infant gastrointestinal (GIT) problems, increased maternal weight loss and extended lactational amenorrhoea. In 1991 the WHO and the UN Children's Fund instigated a baby-friendly initiative with the aim to improve breastfeeding rates. These 10 steps to successful breastfeeding are the global standard.

A structured literature review using evidence-based healthcare databases has determined the following best practice recommendations:

- Babies should be breastfed exclusively for the first 6 months.
- Mothers and babies should have skin-to-skin contact and breastfeeding should be initiated within the first 30 minutes following birth.
- Healthcare workers need the skills to provide accurate and consistent information regarding breastfeeding.
- All maternity providers should be encouraged to be assessed as a baby-friendly centre.
- Breastfeeding information should be provided in the antenatal and postnatal periods.
- Midwives should provide information and support to couples and assist them to make informed choices regarding breastfeeding.

Providing evidence-based information can assist in dispelling myths and fallacies regarding many contentious topics in society. It is important as nurses that we provide accurate and factual information and support families to make decisions to assist their health and wellbeing.

Do the above recommendations provide you with information that you can share with your clients and the general public regarding breastfeeding?

Source: Jayasekara, R. (2014). Breastfeeding: Interventions to promote and best practice. The Joanna Briggs Institute.

introduction of a new member. Other issues most nursing theorists address are how nurses should be viewed and what the goals of nursing care should be. Extensive changes in the scope of child and family health nursing have occurred as health promotion, or keeping parents and children well, has become a greater priority (Salsman et al., 2012).

With health promotion as a major nursing goal, teaching, counselling, supporting and advocacy are also common roles (Woods, 2010). Nurses care for people who are more critically ill than ever before. Care of women during pregnancy and of children during their developing years helps protect not only current health but also the health of the next generation, and child and family health nurses fill these expanded roles to a unique and special degree.

CASE STUDY QUESTION

3. Suppose Melissa Chung asks you whether child health nursing is a profession. What qualifies as an activity of a profession?
   a. Members supervise other people
   b. Members use a distinct body of knowledge
   c. Members enjoy good working conditions
   d. Members receive relatively high pay

A CHANGING DISCIPLINE

Infant mortality rates have decreased with healthcare shifting from a treatment focus to a preventive one, dramatically changing the scope of child and family health nursing. Research on the benefits of early antenatal care has led to changes in providing antenatal care to all pregnant women through antenatal nursing services (home visits) and clinics and other community health measures (such as efforts to encourage breastfeeding, education on sudden infant death syndrome (SIDS) education, increased immunisation rates and injury prevention), as well as many technological advances (AIHW, 2012).

Medical technology has contributed to a number of important advances in child and family health: childhood diseases such as measles and poliomyelitis have been almost eradicated through immunisation; specific genes responsible for many inherited diseases have been identified; stem cell therapy may make it possible in the next few years to replace diseased cells with new growth cells; new fertility drugs and techniques allow more couples than ever before to conceive; and the ability to delay premature birth and improve life for premature infants has grown dramatically. In addition, a growing trend towards healthcare consumerism or self-care has made childbearing and childrearing families active participants in their own health monitoring and care. Healthcare consumerism has also moved care from hospitals to community and home care and from long-term hospital stays to overnight surgical and day-only procedures.

Even in the light of these changes, much more still needs to be done. Although healthcare may be more advanced, it is still not accessible to everyone. These and other social changes and trends have expanded the role of nurses in child and family health and, at the same time, have made the delivery of quality child and family health nursing care a continuing challenge. There are still discrepancies between health outcomes for Indigenous populations such as Māori and Indigenous Australians as opposed to their Caucasian counterparts (Pairman et al., 2015; Barnes & Rowe, 2013).

Further information on immunisation, SIDS and safety can be accessed from the New Zealand Ministry of Health (NZMOH) <www.moh.govt.nz> and in Australia from the Australian Government Department of Health (DoH)

TABLE 1.2 Trends in child and family healthcare and implications for nurses

Trend	Implications for nursing
Families are not as extended so are smaller than previously.	Fewer family members are present as support people in a time of crisis. Nurses are called on to fulfil this role more than ever before.
Single-parent families have increased.	A single parent may have fewer financial resources than two parents; this is more likely if the parent is a woman. Nurses can help by informing parents of care options and providing a backup opinion when needed.
Many women work outside the home at least part-time.	Healthcare must be scheduled at a time when a working parent can access care for herself or bring a child for care. Problems of latch-key (self-care) children and the selection of childcare centres need to be addressed.
Families are more mobile than previously; there is an increase in the number of homeless women and children.	Good interviewing and health monitoring are necessary with mobile families so a health database can be established and there can be continuity of care.
Both child and domestic partner abuse are increasing in incidence.	Screening for child or domestic partner abuse should be included in all family contacts. Nurses must be aware of the legal responsibilities for reporting abuse.
Families are more health conscious than ever before.	Families are ripe for health education; providing this can be a major nursing role.
Client advocacy is necessary as it is easy for families to feel lost in the healthcare system.	Advocacy is safeguarding and advancing the interests of clients and their families. Familiarity with the healthcare services available in a community, establishing and maintaining a relationship with families, as well as helping them make informed choices about what course of action to take or what services would be best to use are important nursing roles.

<www.immunise.health.gov.au>. SIDS information can be found at SIDS and KIDS <www.sidsandkids.org> and safety information at Safekids <www.kidsafensw.org>. The Children's Hospital at Westmead has a large amount of information available on its website <www.chw.edu.au>.

Trends in the child and family health nursing population

The population is constantly changing because of changes in social structure, variations in family lifestyle and changing patterns of illness. Table 1.2 summarises some of the social changes that are altering healthcare priorities for child and family health nurses. Client advocacy, participating in cost-containment measures, focusing on health education and creating new nursing roles are ways in which nurses have adapted to these changes. **Client advocacy** is safeguarding and advancing the interests of individuals and their families. The role includes knowing the healthcare services available in a community, establishing a relationship with families and helping them make informed choices about what course of action or service would be best for them.

Measuring child and family health

Measuring child and family health is not as simple as defining a person as ill or well because individuals and healthcare practitioners may have different perspectives on illness and wellness. For example, some children with chronic but controllable asthma think of themselves as well; others with the same degree of asthma consider themselves ill. Although pregnancy is generally considered a well state, some women think of themselves as ill during this period. A more objective view of health is provided by using national or regional health statistics.

A number of statistical terms are commonly used to express the outcomes of pregnancies and births and to describe child and family health; such statistics are useful for comparisons and for planning of future healthcare needs. Statistics require accurate recording, collection and analysis, and nurses play a major role in the accurate collection and recording of this data that allows the nation's present and future health to be described. Definitions and statistics can be accessed through the NZMOH website and the Statistics New Zealand website. In Australia these statistics can be accessed through the Australian Bureau of Statistics and the Australian Institute of Health and Welfare (AIHW). Another useful website for statistics is the WHO statistical information system. These websites also have specific statistics for Māori and Aboriginal Australians as well as main causes of death.

Birth and fetal death rates

Birth and fetal death rates correlate with the health of a nation as they reflect the overall quality of maternal health, preconception and antenatal care. The birth rate is defined as the number of live births per 1000 during the calendar year (ABS, 2013a). Fetal death is defined as the death of a baby of 20 or more completed weeks of gestation or at least 400 grams birth weight (ABS, 2013b; MOHNZ, 2014a).

Fertility rate

The fertility rate reflects what proportion of women who could have babies are having them. This is important as countries that experience famine, war or disease may have a low fertility rate. Australia's current fertility rate is 1.88, continuing a steady decline in the overall fertility rate (ABS, 2013a). In New Zealand the fertility rate was an average of 1.9 in 2012 (Statistics NZ, 2012).

Neonatal death rate

The neonatal death rate reflects not only the quality of care available to women during pregnancy and childbirth but also the quality of care available to infants during the first month of life. Some causes of infant mortality include prematurity (early gestational age or low birth weight of less than 2500 grams) and congenital malformations. The New Zealand neonatal death rate is down to 4.7/1000 live births (Statistics NZ, 2012).

Perinatal death rate

Perinatal deaths are defined as all fetal deaths (at least 20 weeks' gestation or at least 400 grams birth weight) plus all neonatal deaths per 1000 births. Australia's rate was 8.2 in 2012 (ABS, 2013b) and New Zealand's rate was 5.2 in 2009 (Statistics NZ, 2012).

Infant mortality rate

The **infant mortality rate** is defined as the number of deaths in a calendar year of children aged less than 1 year per 1000 live births in the same calendar year (ABS, 2013a). This is an important indicator of the general health and wellbeing of a population. A low infant mortality rate is associated with an increased life expectancy. This rate is the traditional standard used to compare the healthcare of a nation with that of previous years or of other countries. Australia's current infant mortality rate is 3.3/1000 (NHPA, 2014) and New Zealand is slightly higher at 4.7/1000 (Statistics NZ, 2012).

Some causes of infant mortality include prematurity, low birthweight, congenital malformations, infections, cardiovascular conditions and SIDS. SIDS remains the major cause of death in infants between 1 and 12 months of age (Pairman et al., 2015). SIDS deaths have decreased due to public health campaigns. Nurses have been instrumental in reducing deaths as they are the health professionals who most often discuss newborn care with new parents (AIHW, 2012; Pairman et al., 2015).

Maternal mortality rate

Maternal mortality can be described as the death of a woman who is pregnant or who dies within 42 days of giving birth or having a termination (Pairman et al., 2015). A decreased maternal mortality rate can be attributed to improved preconception, antenatal, labour, birth and postnatal care such as:

- Increased participation of women in antenatal care
- Greater detection of disorders such as ectopic pregnancy and prevention of related complications through the use of ultrasound
- Increased control of complications associated with hypertension of pregnancy
- Decreased use of anaesthesia with childbirth.

For most of the 20th century, uterine haemorrhage and infection were the leading causes of death during pregnancy and childbirth. This has changed because of the increased ability to prevent or control haemorrhage and infection. However, numbers of women suffering hypertensive disorders have increased with pregnancy-induced hypertension adding to pre-existing statistics relating to hypertensive disorders, especially in older women.

CASE STUDY QUESTION

4. Melissa Chung's doctor has told her that her baby's most dangerous time will be until the postnatal period ends. When does the postnatal period take place?
   a. From the day of birth until 1 month afterwards
   b. During the time the infant will be on ventilator support
   c. From birth until 6 weeks after birth
   d. Until the infant's body temperature stabilises following birth

Childhood mortality rate

The childhood mortality rate (under 5 years old) is declining worldwide (UNICEF, 2014). As shown in Figure 1.2, the most common causes in Australia include complications of pregnancy, labour and delivery, unknown causes such as SIDS, congenital malformations and disorders related to gestation and fetal growth (NHPA, 2014).

Childhood morbidity rate

Health problems commonly occurring in large proportions of children today include respiratory disorders, such as asthma; endocrine disorders, specifically diabetes; and cancers (AIHW, 2012). In New Zealand data highlights that 1:9 children aged 2–14 years were obese with a further 1:5 overweight, with an overall increase in childhood obesity of 11% (MOHNZ, 2014c). Obesity has become an increasing health problem and is a major contributor to the global burden of chronic disease. Levels of childhood obesity have been rising for several years correlating with an increased intake of foods that are high in sugar and fat and a reduction in the amount of time spent on physical activity (ABS, 2010). Obesity in school-aged children can lead to cardiovascular disorders, self-esteem issues and type 2 diabetes (Junnila et al., 2012). Nurses can be instrumental in teaching better nutrition and encouraging increased exercise to help decrease this incidence (AIHW, 2012).

As more immunisations become available, fewer children are affected by common childhood communicable diseases. The new vaccine against human papillomavirus (HPV) suggested for prepubertal girls should help prevent HPV infections (Nan, 2012). However, there is a potential for the

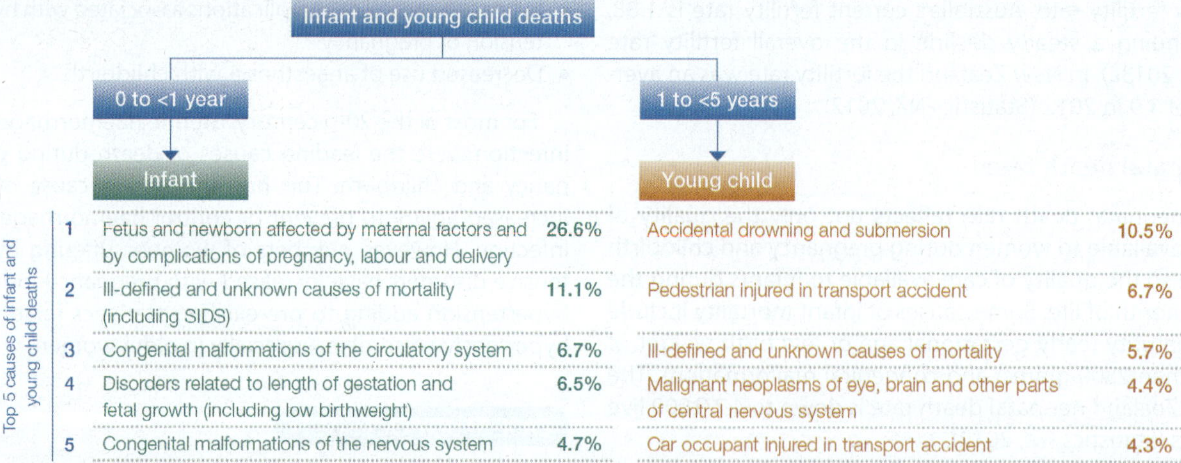

FIGURE 1.2 Most common causes and percentages of infant and young child deaths by category, Australia, 2010–2012. (This graphic is reproduced from the National Health Performance Authority's report *Healthy Communities: Child and Maternal Health in 2009–2012*, published July 2014 available at www.myhealthycommunities.gov.au.)

incidence of childhood infectious diseases to increase again if immunisation is not maintained as a high national priority.

Nurses play a vital role in helping prevent the spread of sexually transmitted infections (STIs) by educating adolescents and young adults about safer sexual practices (see Chapter 5). Nurses should follow standard infection precautions in child and family health nursing, as in other areas of nursing practice, to safeguard themselves, other healthcare providers and clients from the spread of infection.

The incidence of childhood injuries, child abuse, neglect and violence remains high despite a focus on early intervention for infants and an increased awareness in the community, changes in policy, practice and legislation (AIHW, 2012). A pregnancy can add stress to a family and these behaviours can often increase in this period (Brownridge et al., 2011).

Trends in healthcare environment

The settings and philosophy of child and family healthcare are both changing to better meet the needs of increasingly well-informed and vocal consumers. People have more understanding of the choices available as well as the need to ask questions when determining what is best for their individual family and situation (see Box 1.4).

Initiating cost containment

Cost containment refers to systems of healthcare delivery that focus on reducing the cost of healthcare by closely monitoring the cost of personnel, use and brands of supplies, length of hospital stays, number of procedures carried out and number of referrals requested while maintaining quality care (Saunier, 2011).

Increasing alternative settings and styles for healthcare

At the turn of the 19th century childbirth began to move into institutions throughout many countries including Australia and New Zealand. Prior to this most births took place in the home, with only the poor or very ill attending hospitals (Pairman et al., 2015). Today, a less dramatic but no less important trend that is occurring is an increase in the number of families once more choosing childbirth at home or in alternative birth settings rather than hospitals. Birth centres have developed in both Australia and New Zealand. These can be freestanding or located within hospitals. These centres assist women to achieve a "normal" birth but are intended only for pregnant women classified as "low risk" (Pairman et al., 2015). These alternative settings provide

BOX 1.4 ✻ Focus on family teaching

Tips for selecting a healthcare setting

Q. Melissa Chung asks you, "Where would we go for follow-up specialist paediatric care for our baby as she was born so early? Who can we go to closer to home if we have problems?"

A. When selecting a healthcare setting, asking the following questions can help you decide what is best for your family:

- Can it be reached easily? (Going for preventive care when well or for continuing care when ill should not be a chore.)
- Will the staff provide continuity of care so you will always see the same primary care provider if possible?
- Does the physical setup of the facility provide for a sense of privacy, yet a sense that healthcare providers share pertinent information so you do not have to repeat your history at each visit?
- Are preventive care and health education stressed (keeping well is as important as recovering from illness)?
- Is health education pitched at your learning level?
- Do healthcare providers respect your opinion and ask for your input on healthcare decisions?
- Do healthcare providers show a personal interest in you?
- Will the facility still be accessible if a family member becomes disabled?

families with increased control of the birth experience and options for birth surroundings that are unavailable in hospitals. A strength of this movement is its encouragement of family involvement in birth. It also increases nursing responsibility for assessment and professional judgement and provides expanded roles for advanced practice nurses such as the midwife practitioner (Comiskey et al., 2014).

Hospitals have responded to consumers' demands for a more natural childbirth environment by refitting labour and delivery suites as birthing rooms. Partners, family members and other support people are invited to stay with the woman in labour so they feel a part of the childbirth. The room is designed as a homelike environment. Couplet care—care for both the mother and newborn—is encouraged after the birth. Hospitals are continuing to search for the best labour, birth and postnatal options. Whether childbirth takes place at home, in a birthing centre or in a hospital, the goal is to keep it as natural as possible while ensuring the protection that experienced healthcare providers can provide.

Healthcare settings for children are also changing and include homes, community centres, pharmacies and school-based settings in which comprehensive healthcare may be administered. In these settings, a nurse may provide immunisations, screenings, health and safety education, counselling, crisis intervention, parenting classes and care of ill children and families. This form of community-based care can provide cost-effective health promotion, disease prevention and nursing care to a large number of children and families in an environment that is familiar to them.

Ambulatory or non-hospital-based care requires intensive health teaching by the nursing staff and follow-up by home care or community health nurses. Teaching parents of an ill child or a woman with a complication of pregnancy what danger signs to watch for that will warrant immediate attention includes not only imparting the facts of self-care but also providing support and reassurance that the child or parents are capable of this level of care.

> ***What if...***
>
> Melissa Chung has to remain in the hospital after the birth of her new baby while her baby is transported to a specialised hospital for neonatal care? How could you help her keep in touch with her new baby?

Including the family in healthcare

Health promotion and health education with families during pregnancy or childrearing are a family-centred event, because teaching health awareness and good health habits is accomplished chiefly by role modelling. When children must be admitted to hospital for extended stays, open visiting hours allow parents to visit as much as possible and perhaps even sleep overnight in a bed next to their child. Encourage parents in such a setting to do as much for their child as they wish, such as feeding and bathing their child or administering oral medicine. Most of a parent's time, however, should be spent simply being close by to provide a comfortable, secure influence on their child. For the same reasons, the most important role of parents in a maternity unit is to give total care to their newborn.

Family-centred nursing this way increases the number of people a nurse cares for—that is, not four children, for example, but four children plus four sets of parents; not just a single newborn, but his or her parents as well. Caring for families rather than individuals, however, has an immeasurable effect on the health of children and parents and client satisfaction (Stuart & Melling, 2014).

Illness in a child is automatically a family-centred event. Parents may need to adjust work schedules to allow one of them to stay with the ill child; siblings may have to sacrifice an activity such as a birthday party or having a parent watch their school play; and family finances may have to be readjusted. When a mother is pregnant, family roles or activities may have to change to safeguard her health. A family may feel drawn together by fear and concern related to an acute illness. On the other hand, if an illness becomes chronic, it may pull a family apart.

By adopting a view of pregnancy, childbirth or illness as a family event, nurses can be instrumental in including family members in events from which family members were once totally excluded, such as an unplanned caesarean birth. They can help child healthcare to be family-centred by consulting with family members about a plan of care and providing clear health teaching so that family members can monitor their own care (see Fig. 1.3).

Increasing the number of intensive care units

Over the past 20 years, care of infants and children has become extremely technical. It is generally assumed that newborns with a term birth weight (more than 2500 grams) will thrive at birth. However, many infants are born each year with birth weights lower than 2500 grams or

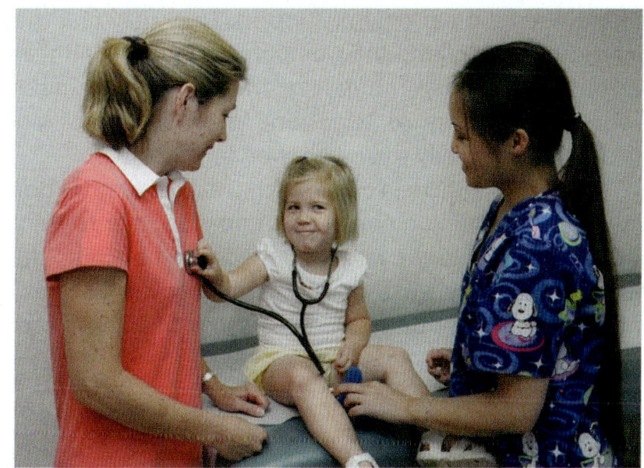

FIGURE 1.3 A nurse involves the mother in a physical examination to promote family-centred care. (Ricci, S. S. & Kyle, T. (2009). *Maternity and Pediatric Nursing*. Philadelphia: Lippincott Williams & Wilkins.)

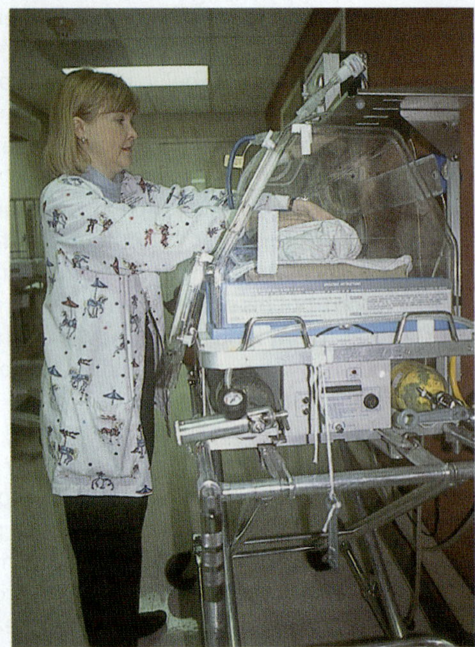

FIGURE 1.4 A nurse prepares an infant transport incubator to move a premature infant to a referral hospital. Helping with safe movement of pregnant women and ill newborns to referral centres is an important nursing responsibility. (© Caroline Brown, RNC, MS, DEd.)

who are ill at birth and do not thrive. Such infants are regularly transferred to a neonatal intensive care unit (NICU) or intensive care nursery (ICN). Children who are undergoing cardiac surgery or recovering from near-drowning or multi-injury accidents are cared for in a paediatric intensive care unit (PICU).

Regionalising intensive care

To avoid duplication of care sites, communities establish centralised maternal or paediatric health services. Such planning creates one site that is properly staffed and equipped for potential problems rather than a number of less well-equipped sites (see Fig. 1.4). When a newborn, older child or parent is hospitalised in a larger or specialised hospital, the family members who have been left behind need a great deal of support. They may feel they have lost their infant, child or parent unless healthcare personnel keep them abreast of the ill family member's progress by means of telephone calls or photos and encourage the family to visit as soon as possible.

Today, if it is known in advance that a child may be born with a life-threatening condition, it may be safer to transport the mother to the larger or specialised hospital during pregnancy, because the uterus has advantages as a transport incubator that far exceed those of any commercial incubator yet designed.

CASE STUDY QUESTION

5. Research by Blomqvist and colleagues (2012) shows that 'kangaroo care' (new fathers spending time skin-to-skin with their newborn) allows fathers to feel more in control and that they are doing something good for their infant. Based on this study, what action would you take with the Chungs?
   a. Assess whether Robert Chung is willing to try skin-to-skin care
   b. Suggest neither parent uses skin-to-skin care to prevent infection
   c. Encourage Robert Chung to praise his wife when she provides skin-to-skin care
   d. Apologise to Robert Chung's wife because men do skin-to-skin care more effectively than women

Increasing use of alternative treatment modalities

There is a growing tendency for families to use alternative forms of therapy, such as acupuncture or therapeutic touch, in addition to, or instead of, traditional healthcare. Nurses have an increasing obligation to be aware of complementary or alternative therapies as these have the potential to either enhance or detract from the effectiveness of traditional therapy (Adams et al., 2011). Healthcare providers who are unaware of the existence of some alternative forms of therapy may lose an important opportunity to capitalise on the positive features of that particular therapy. For instance, it would be important to know that an adolescent who is about to undergo a painful procedure is experienced at meditation, because asking the adolescent if she wants to meditate before the procedure could help her relax. Not only could this decrease her discomfort but it could also offer her a feeling of control over a difficult situation. People are using an increasing number of herbal remedies, so asking about these at a health assessment is important to prevent medication interactions. Ginger, for example, is frequently taken during pregnancy to relieve morning sickness (Dennehy, 2011).

Increasing reliance on home care

Shortened hospital stays have resulted in the return home of many women and children before they are optimally ready to care for themselves. Ill children and women with complications of pregnancy may choose to remain at home for care rather than be hospitalised. This has created a "second system" of care requiring many additional care providers (Turnbull & Osborn, 2012). Nurses are instrumental in assessing women and children on hospital discharge to help plan the best type of continuing care, devise and modify procedures for home care, and sustain morale. Because home care is a unique and expanding area in child and family health nursing, it is discussed in Chapter 4.

Increasing use of technology

The use of technology is increasing in all healthcare settings. The field of assisted reproduction technology such as in vitro fertilisation and the possibility of stem cell research are forging new pathways (Palermo, Nero, Monahan et al.,

2012). Charting by computer into electronic medical records by both consumers and health professional staff (Healthdirect Australia, 2012) and monitoring fetal heart rates by Doppler ultrasonography are other examples (Stewart et al., 2011). Technology can be used in any setting with a variety of practitioners able to access the information. One such system is the Australian Childhood Immunisation register, a national register to record vaccinations given to all Australian children under the age of 7 years (DoHS, 2014). Using electronic charting systems has the ability to allow different healthcare providers to share information. As long as privacy is maintained, the system allows for a coordination of care never before possible. In addition to learning these technologies, child and family health nurses must be able to explain their use and their advantages. Otherwise, individuals may find new technologies more frightening than helpful to them.

Antenatal healthcare concerns and attitudes

Healthcare has made great strides in the past century. As we progress through the 21st century, there are likely to be even more changes as Australia and New Zealand actively work towards effective health goals and improved healthcare for all citizens. These steps can create new concerns.

Increasing emphasis on preventive care

A generally accepted theory is that it is better to keep individuals well than to restore health after they have become ill. Counselling parents on ways to keep their homes safe for children is an important form of this type of prevention. Research supporting the facts that accidents are still a major cause of death in children and that many women still do not receive adequate preconception or antenatal care is testament to the need for much more anticipatory guidance in child and family health.

Increasing concern for the quality of life

In the past, healthcare of women and children was focused on maintaining physical health. Today, a growing awareness that quality of life is as important as physical health has expanded the scope of healthcare to include the assessment of psychosocial facets of life in such areas as self-esteem and independence. Good interviewing skills are necessary to elicit this information at healthcare visits. Nurses not only can help to obtain such information but also can plan ways to improve quality of life in the areas the client considers most important.

Increasing awareness of the individuality of clients

Children and families today do not fit easily into any set mould. Varying family structures, cultural backgrounds, socioeconomic levels and individual circumstances lead to unique and diverse clients. Women having children may range in age from 12 or 13 years up to and over the age of 40 (Johnson & Tough, 2012). Gay and lesbian couples raise families alongside traditional families, conceiving children through artificial insemination or adoption. As a result of advances in research and therapy, women who were once unable to have children, such as those with cystic fibrosis, are now able to achieve a full-term pregnancy. Individuals with cognitive and physical challenges who once would have been isolated from childbearing are now able to establish families and rear children.

Many families which have emigrated from other countries require sensitivity to sociocultural aspects of care as they may have different cultural beliefs about health and illness. As the level of violence in the world increases, more and more families are exposed to living in violent communities. All of these concerns require increased nursing attention.

Empowerment of healthcare consumers

In part because of the influence of market-driven care and a strengthened focus on health promotion and disease prevention, individuals and families have recently begun to take increased responsibility for their own health. This begins with learning preventive measures to stay well. For most families, this means following a more nutritious diet and planning regular exercise; and for some, this means adopting an entirely new lifestyle. When a family member is ill, empowerment means learning more about the illness, participating in the treatment plan and preventing the illness from returning. Parents want to stay with their ill child in the hospital. They are eager for information about their child's health and want to contribute to the decision-making process. They may question treatments or care plans that they believe are not in their child's best interest.

Nurses can promote empowerment of parents and children by respecting their views and concerns, regarding parents as important participants in their own or their child's health, and keeping them informed and helping them to make decisions about care.

ADVANCED-PRACTICE ROLES FOR NURSES IN CHILD AND FAMILY HEALTH

As trends in child and family healthcare change, so do the roles of child and family health nurses. In all settings, child and family health nurses function as carers, client advocates, researchers and educators. Many nurses with a specified number of years of direct client care, clinical expertise and validated completion of pertinent continuing education programs are registered in a specialty. Those with advanced education function in advanced-practice roles. Some definitions of these advanced nursing roles can be found in the Public Health System Nurses' and Midwives' (State) Award on the NSW Health website. The Australian Health Practitioner Regulation Agency (AHPRA) can provide information on legislation, regulation and registration. In New Zealand the National Framework for Nursing Professional Development and the New Zealand Nursing Council provide information on definitions, legislation, regulation and registration. Some of the advanced practice roles include clinical nurse specialist, clinical nurse consultant and nurse practitioners.

LEGAL CONSIDERATIONS OF MATERNAL-CHILD PRACTICE

Legal concerns arise in all areas of healthcare. Child and family health nursing carries legal concerns that extend above and beyond other areas of nursing, because care is often given to an "unseen client"—the fetus—or to individuals who are not of legal age for giving consent for medical procedures. Nurses and midwives are obliged to report all suspected or known cases of child abuse or neglect and failure to report is an offence under a specific act such as the Children and Young Persons (Care and Protection) Act 1998 (NSW) (McDonald & Then, 2014). Mandatory reporting is a legal requirement of registration as a nurse or midwife and is identified and discussed in competencies, codes of practice and guidelines in both Australia and New Zealand (AHPRA, 2014; NCNZ, 2014). Nurses are legally responsible for protecting the rights of their clients, including confidentiality, and they are accountable for the quality of their individual nursing care and that of other healthcare team members. New regulations on client confidentiality guarantee that individuals can see their medical records if they choose but health information must be kept confidential from others (Duffy, 2011).

Understanding the scope of practice and standards of care are crucial for nurses to practise within appropriate legal parameters. Competency standards in Australia and New Zealand are incorporated into registration requirements and provide a theoretical and practical base that guides nurses and midwives to practise within legal parameters (AHPRA, 2014; NCNZ, 2014). NSW has introduced a guide called "Keep them safe" that provides an overview to the mandatory reporting system and assists people who are considered to be mandatory reporters to notify authorities regarding suspected or actual children at risk. It advises them who they need to notify and how to report. Nurses and midwives can also call the child wellbeing units for assistance with their concerns (NSW Government, 2014).

Documentation is essential for protecting the nurse and justifying their actions. Nurses need to be conscientious about obtaining informed consent for invasive procedures and determining that pregnant women are aware of any risk to the fetus associated with a procedure or test. In divorced or blended families (those in which two adults with children from previous relationships now live together), it is important to establish who has the right to give consent for healthcare.

The National Ehealth Transition Authority Limited (NEHTA) was established in Australia in 2005 in an aim to collect and securely share electronic ehealth information (NEHTA, 2014). Individuals are encouraged to use Personally Controlled Electronic Health Records (PCEHR) as a means of collecting all their health information into one secure record that the individual controls and can share with different health professionals and systems. This new tool has been launched as "eHealth records" and is a key factor in national reform in the Australian health system (NEHTA, 2014).

The specific legal ramifications of procedures or care are discussed in later chapters that describe procedures or treatment modalities. Obstetric services are facing a crisis situation as more doctors and midwives find the cost of professional indemnity insurance to guard against malpractice or professional negligence suits prohibitive. However, professional indemnity is encouraged for nurse and midwife practitioners and midwives undertaking homebirths (Staunton & Chiarella, 2013).

ETHICAL CONSIDERATIONS OF PRACTICE

Some of the most difficult ethical quandaries in healthcare today are those that involve children and their families. Examples include:

- Conception issues, especially those related to in vitro fertilisation, embryo transfer, ownership of frozen oocytes or sperm, cloning, stem cell research and surrogate mothers
- Termination, particularly partial-birth terminations
- Fetal rights versus rights of the mother
- Use of fetal tissue for research
- Resuscitation (for how long should it be continued?)
- Number of procedures or degree of pain that a child should be asked to endure to achieve a degree of better health
- Balance between modern technology and quality of life.

Legal and ethical aspects of issues are often intertwined, which makes the decision-making process complex. As child and family health nursing is so strongly family-centred, it is common to encounter some situations in which the interests of one family member are in conflict with those of another. Maintaining privacy while aiding problem solving can be difficult (Clemens, 2012). It is not unusual for the values of an individual not to match those of a healthcare provider. For example, if a pregnancy causes a woman to develop a serious illness, the family must make a decision either to terminate the pregnancy and lose the child or to keep the pregnancy and work to support the mother through the crisis. If the fetus is also at risk from the illness, the decision may be easier to make; however, the circumstances are usually not clear cut and the decisions that need to be made are difficult. Nurses can help people who are facing such difficult decisions by providing factual information and supportive listening, helping the family clarify their values.

The Pregnant Woman's Bill of Rights and the United Nations Declaration of Rights of the Child provide guidelines for determining the rights of women in regard to healthcare.

✔ *Checkpoint question 1.1*

What is a legal implication pertinent to child and family health?

a. Informed consent is rarely needed as children are unable to understand this
b. All adolescents over age 14 are able to sign consent for their own healthcare
c. Children who feel they have been wronged can sue years into the future
d. Pregnant women are not legally mandated to protect the health of their fetus

Key points for review

- Nursing research and use of evidence-based practice are methods by which child and family health nursing expands and improves.
- The most meaningful and important measure of child and family health is the infant mortality rate. It is the number of deaths among infants from birth to 1 year of age per 1000 live births.
- Trends in child and family health nursing include changes in the settings of care, improved preventive care and family-centred care.
- Advanced-practice roles in child and family health nursing include women's health, family, neonatal and paediatrics. These expanded roles contribute to make child and family healthcare an important area of nursing and healthcare.
- Child and family healthcare has both legal and ethical considerations and responsibilities over and above those in other areas of practice because of the role of the fetus and child.

CASE STUDY QUESTIONS

6. How might family-centred care help the Chung family? How can you explain recent changes in healthcare so that Melissa might understand why her hospital stay is so short? How can you empower the family so that they feel more in control of what is happening to them?
7. The age at which women are having babies is increasing. For many women such as Melissa Chung, this age is now 35 years or older. How do you anticipate that this trend will change healthcare in the future? Are there special services that should be provided for such women? How will this trend influence childrearing in the future?
8. Examine your country's health goals related to maternal, newborn and child health. Most government-sponsored money for nursing research is allocated based on these goals. What would be a possible research topic to explore, pertinent to these goals, which would be applicable to the Chung family and could also advance evidence-based practice?
9. In your nursing practice with children and families such as the Chung family how would you implement a strengths-based approach and use a family-centred approach?

Resources

For an extensive range of additional resources to enhance teaching and learning and to facilitate understanding of this chapter, please see the text's accompanying website located on thePoint at http://thepoint.lww.com.

References

Adams, D., Cheng, F., Jou, H., et al. (2011). The safety of pediatric acupuncture: A systematic review. *Pediatrics, 128*(6), e1575–e1587.

Australian Bureau of Statistics (ABS). (2010). Measures of Australia's progress, 2013. Cat. no. 1370.0., accessed 17 December 2014, <www.abs.gov.au/ausstats/abs@.nsf/mf/1370.0>.

Australian Bureau of Statistics (ABS). (2011). Family, accessed 17 December 2014, <www.abs.gov.au/ausstats/abs@.nsf/0/014F8C1E2D27DFF8CA25720A0010F03D?opendocument>.

Australian Bureau of Statistics (ABS). (2013a). Births, Australia, 2013. Cat. no. 3301.0, accessed 17 December 2014, <www.abs.gov.au/AUSSTATS/abs@.nsf/Lookup/3301.0Main+Features12013?OpenDocument>.

Australian Bureau of Statistics (ABS). (2013b). Deaths, Australia, 2013. Cat. no. 3302.0, accessed 17 December 2014, <www.abs.gov.au/AUSSTATS/abs@.nsf/Lookup/3302.0Main+Features12013?OpenDocument>.

Australian Health Ministers' Advisory Council (AHMAC). (2011). *National Framework for Universal and Family Health Services*. Canberra: Department of Health and Ageing.

Australian Health Practitioner Regulation Agency (AHPRA). (2014). Guidelines for mandatory reporting, accessed 17 December 2014, <www.nursingmidwiferyboard.gov.au/Codes-Guidelines-Statements/Codes-Guidelines.aspx#practiceguide>.

Australian Institute of Family Studies (AIFS). (2012). Publications. Accessed 17 December 2014, <www.aifs.gov.au>.

Australian Institute of Health and Welfare (AIHW). (2011). Headline indicators for childrens's health, development and wellbeing. Cat. no. PHE 144. Canberra: AIHW.

Australian Institute of Health and Welfare (AIHW). (2012). A picture of Australia's children 2012. Cat. no. PHE 167. Canberra: AIHW.

Australian Institute of Health and Welfare (AIHW). (2013). Child health, development and wellbeing, accessed 17 December 2014, <www.aihw.gov.au/child-health-development-and-wellbeing/>.

Barnes, M. & Rowe, J. (Eds). (2013). *Child, Youth and Family Health: Strengthening Communities* (2nd ed.). Sydney: Churchill Livingstone Elsevier.

Blomqvist, Y. T., Rubertsson, C., Kylberg, E., et al. (2012). Kangaroo mother care helps fathers of preterm infants gain confidence in the paternal role. *Journal of Advanced Nursing, 68*(9), 1988–1996.

Briggs, C. (2013). Opportunities and challenges for maternal child and family health nursing. *Child and Family Nurses Association Journal, 24*(1), 9–14.

Brownridge, D. A., Taillieu, T. L., Tyler, K. A., et al. (2011). Pregnancy and intimate partner violence: Risk factors, severity and health effects. *Violence Against Women, 17*(7), 858–881.

Christian, B. J. (2012). Translating research into everyday practice: The essential role of pediatric nurses. *Journal of Pediatric Nursing, 27*(2), 184–185.

Clemens, N. A. (2012). Privacy, consent, and the electronic mental health record: The person vs. the system. *Journal of Psychiatric Practcie, 18*(1), 46–50.

Comiskey, C., Coyne, I., Lalor, J. & Begley, C. (2014). A national cross-sectional study measuring predictors for improved service user outcomes across clinical nurse or midwife specialist, advanced nurse practitioner and control sites. *Journal of Advanced Nursing, 70*(5), 1128–1137.

Dennehy, C. (2011). Omega-3 fatty acids and ginger in maternal health: Pharmacology, efficacy and safety. *Journal of Midwifery and Women's Health, 56*(6), 584–590.

Department of Education and Early Childhood Development (DEECD). (2014). Maternal and child health service, accessed 17 December 2014 <www.education.vic.gov.au/childhood/professionals/health/Pages/maternalchildhealth.aspx>.

Department of Health and Ageing. (2014). *Immunise Australia Program,* accessed 17 December 2014, <www.immunise.health.gov.au/>.

Department of Human Services (DoHS). (2014). Australian childhood immunisation register, accessed 17 December 2014, <www.humanservices.gov.au/customer/services/medicare/australian-childhood-immunisation-register>.

Duffy, M. (2011). iNurse: Patient privacy and company policy in online life. *American Journal of Nursing, 111*(9), 65–69.

Falk, J., Wongsa, S., Dang, J., et al. (2012). Using an evidence-based practice process to change visitation guidelines. *Clinical Journal of Oncology Nursing, 16*(1), 21–23.

Geggie, J., DeFrain, J., Hitchcock, S. & Silberberg, S. (2000). The family strengths research report. Newcastle: Family Action Centre, University of Newcastle.

Gottlieb, L. (2014). Strengths-based nursing. A holistic approach to care, grounded in eight core values. *AJN, 114*(8), 24–32.

Healthdirect Australia. (2012). eHealth, accessed 17 December 2014, <www.healthdirect.gov.au/ehealth?gclid=CIilwPfHhclCFcmTvQoda kcAdQ>.

Hedges, C. C., Nichols, A. & Filoteo, L. (2012). Relationship-based-nursing practice: Transitioning to a new care delivery model in maternity units. *Journal of Perinatal and Neonatal Nursing, 26*(1), 27–36.

Johnson, J. A. & Tough, S. (2012). Delayed child-bearing. *Journal of Obstetrics and Gynaecology Canada, 34*(1), 80–93.

Junnila, R., Aromaa, M., Heinonen, O. J., et al. (2012). The weighty matter intervention: A family-centred way to tackle an overweight childhood. *Journal of Community Health Nursing, 29*(1), 39–52.

Kidsafe The Child Accident Prevention Foundation of Australia. (2014). Accessed 17 December 2014, <www.kidsafe. com.au/>.

Kralik, D. & van Loon, A. (Eds). (2011). *Community Nursing in Australia* (2nd ed.). Milton, Qld Australia: John Wiley & Sons.

Kruske, S. & Grant, J. (2012). Educational preparation for maternal, child and family health nurses in Australia. *International Nursing Review, 59*(2), 200–207.

McDonald, F. & Then, S. (2014). *Ethics, Law and Health Care: A Guide for Nurses and Midwives.* South Yarra: Palgrave Macmillan.

Ministry of Health New Zealand (MOHNZ). (2011). Better, sooner, more convenient health care in the community, accessed 27 November 2014, <www.health.govt.nz/publication/better-sooner-more-convenient-health-care-community>.

Ministry of Health New Zealand (MOHNZ). (2014a). Fetal and infant deaths 2011. Wellington: Ministry of Health, <www.health.govt.nz/publication/fetal-and-infant-deaths-2011>.

Ministry of Health New Zealand (MOHNZ). (2014b). Well Child/Tamariki Ora services, accessed 17 December 2014, <www.health.govt.nz/our-work/life-stages/child-health/well-child-tamariki-ora-services>.

Ministry of Health New Zealand (MOHNZ). (2014c). Obesity data and stats, accessed 17 December 2014 <www.health.govt.nz/nz-health-statistics/health-statistics-and-data-sets/obesity-data-and-stats>.

Nan, X. (2012). Communicating to young adults about HPV vaccination. *Health Communications, 27*(1), 10–18.

National eHealth Transition Authority (NEHTA). (2014). The personally controlled eHealth record system, accessed 17 December 2014, <www.nehta.gov.au/>.

National Health Performance Authority (NHPA). (2014). *Healthy Communities: Child and Maternal Health in 2009–2012.* Sydney: National Health Performance Authority.

NSW Department of Health (NSW Health). (2011). Child and family health nursing professional practice framework 2011–2016. North Sydney: NSW Department of Health, <www.health.nsw.gov.au/nursing/projects/Publications/child-and-family-health-practice-framework.pdf>.

NSW Government. (2014). Keep them safe, accessed 17 December 2014, <www.keepthemsafe.nsw.gov.au/>.

Nursing Council of New Zealand (NCNZ). (2014). Continuing competence, accessed 17 December 2014, <www.nursingcouncil.org.nz/Nurses/Continuing-competence>.

Pairman, S., Tracy, S., Thorogood, C. and Pincombe, J. (2015). *Midwifery Preparation for Practice* (3rd ed.). Sydney: Churchill Livingstone Elsevier.

Palmero, G. D., Neri, Q. V., Monahan, D., et al. (2012). Development and current applications of assisted fertilization. *Fertility and Sterility, 97*(2), 248–259.

Papp, L. M. (2012). Longitudinal associations between parental and children's depressive symptoms in the context of intraparental relationship functioning. *Journal of Child and Family Studies, 21*(2), 199–207.

Paulson, J. F. & Bazemore, S. C. (2010). Prenatal and postpartum depression in fathers and its association with maternal depression. *Journal of the American Medical Association, 303*(19), 1961–1969.

Plunket. (2014). Our vision and mission, accessed 17 December 2014, <www.plunket.org.nz/what-we-do/who-we-are/our-vision-and-mission/>.

Queensland Health. (2014). Queensland clinical guidelines: Routine newborn assessment. Queensland Health: State of Queensland.

Randall, D., Munns, A. & Shields, L. (2013). Next steps: Towards child-focused nursing. *Neonatal, Paediatric and Child Health Nursing, 16*(2), 15–20.

Rubin, R. (1963). Maternal touch. *Nursing Outlook, 11*(2), 828–829.

Salsman, J. M., Grunberg, S. M., Beaumont, J. L. et al. (2012). Communicating about chemotherapy-induced nausea and vomiting: A comparison of patient and provider perspectives. *Journal of National Comprehensive Cancer Network, 10*(2), 149–157.

Saunier, B. (2011). The devil is in the details: Managed care and the unforeseen costs of utilization review as a cost containment mechanism. *Issues in Law and Medicine, 27*(1), 21–48.

Scmied, V., Donovan, J., Kruske, S., Kemp, L., Homer, C. & Fowler, C. (2011). Commonalities challenges: A review of Australian state and territory maternity and child health policies. *Contemporary Nurse, 40*(1), 106–117.

Scmied, V., Fowler, C., Rossiter, C., Homer, C., Kruske, S. & CHoRUS team. (2014). Nature and frequency of services provided by child and family health nurses in Australia: Results of a national survey. *Australian Health Review, 38*(2), 177–185.

Statistics New Zealand. (2012). Demographic trends: 2012, accessed 17 December 2014, <www.stats.govt.nz/browse_for_stats/population/estimates_and_projections/demographic-trends-2012/deaths%20and%20life%20expectancy.aspx>.

Statistics New Zealand. (2014). Family type, accessed 17 December 2014 <www.stats.govt.nz/methods/classifications-and-standards/classification-related-stats-standards/family-type/definition.aspx>.

Staunton, P. & Chiarella, M. (2013). *Nursing and the Law.* (7th ed.). Sydney: Churchill Livingstone Elsevier.

Stewart, M., Letourneau, N., Masuda, J. R., et al. (2011). Online solutions to support needs and preference of parents of children with asthma and allergies. *Journal of Family Nursing, 17*(8), 357–379.

Stuart, M. & Melling, S. (2014). Understanding nurses' and parents' perceptions of family-centred care, *Nursing, Children and Young People, 26*(7), 16–20.

Turnbull, C. & Osborn, D. A. (2012). Home visits during pregnancy and after birth for women with an alcohol or drug problem. *Cochrane Database of Systematic Reviews*, 2012(1), (CD004456).

UNICEF. (2014). Levels and trends in child mortality 2014, accessed 17 December 2104, <www.data.unicef.org/>.

Watts, R., Zhou, H., Shields, L., Taylor, M., Munns, A. & Ngune, I. (2014). Family-centred care for hospitalized children aged 0-12 years: A systematic review of qualitative studies. *JBI Database of Systematic Reviews and Implementation Reports, 12*(7), 204–283.

Wells, G., Hauck, Y., Bennett, E., Shields, L. & Johnson, K. (2014). Nurses' experience of using a strengths-based framework to facilitate change with families. *Australian Journal of Child and Family Health Nursing, 11*(1), 17–24.

Woods, M. A. (2010). Public health intervention model: Impact on Australian community and mental health nursing students' practice. *International Journal of Nursing Education Scholarship, 7*(1), 17–19.

World Health Organization (WHO). (2014). Maternal, newborn, child and adolescent health, accessed 17 December 2014, <www.who.int/maternal_child_adolescent/topics/maternal/en/>.

World Health Organization (WHO). (2014). Millenium development goals, accessed 17 December 2014, <www.who.int/topics/millennium_development_goals/en/>.

Suggested readings

Australian Research Alliance for Children and Youth <www.aracy.org.au>

Borrow, S., Munns, A. & Henderson, S. (2011). Community-based child health nurses: An exploration of current practice. *Contemporary Nurse, 40*(1), 71–86.

Child and Youth Health <www.cyh.com>.

Childrens Hospital at Westmead <www.chw.edu.au>.

Families NSW <www.families.nsw.gov.au>.

Jayasekara, R. (2014). Breastfeeding: Interventions to promote and best practice. The Joanna Briggs Institute.

Mikkelsen, G. & Frederiksen, K. (2010). Family-centred care of children in hospital: a concept analysis. *Journal of Advanced Nursing, 67*(5), 1152–1162.

Plunket New Zealand <www.plunket.org.nz>.

Rowe, J., Barnes, M. & Sutherns, S. (2013). Supporting maternal transition: Continuity, coaching and control. *The Journal of Perinatal Education, 22*(3), 145–155.

SIDS and Kids <www.sidsandkids.org/>.

Chapter 2

Sociocultural aspects of child and family health nursing

Chapter 1 described the standards and philosophy of maternal and child health nursing as well as family health. This chapter adds information on caring for families from diverse cultures. Such information can both enrich care and help improve the health of childbearing and childrearing families.

LEARNING OBJECTIVES

After studying this chapter, you should be able to:

1. Discuss cultural competence and explain its importance in the provision of child and family healthcare.
2. Critically analyse how the social determinants of health and cultural factors affect family functioning and health.
3. Plan and implement culturally competent and family-centred care to assist families to adapt to the changing sociocultural environment.
4. Analyse and discuss the social determinants of health and cultural factors that influence the way a family responds to childbearing and childrearing.
5. Develop outcomes to assist families with specific cultural needs to thrive in their community.
6. Evaluate expected outcomes for achievement and effectiveness of care.
7. Identify areas of care related to social determinants of health and cultural factors that could benefit from additional nursing research or application of evidence-based practice.
8. Integrate sociocultural aspects of care with the nursing process to achieve quality child and family health nursing care.

KEY TERMS

- assimilation
- cultural safety
- culture
- discrimination
- empowerment
- equity
- ethnicity
- ethnocentrism
- Indigenous
- minority
- multiculturalism
- prejudice
- racism
- respect
- social determinants of health
- social justice
- stereotyping
- xenophobic

CASE STUDY

Carleen is a young Māori woman who is the mother (*whaea*) of a 1-year-old boy Tama. She is also a sole parent. Carleen moved from her family (*whānau*) in the country to gain work in Auckland; however, prior to the birth of Tama she left work and now receives a benefit from the government. She is finding it a challenge to care for Tama without the support of her family. She is feeling socially isolated and is struggling to cope on a low income. Carleen remembers the special relationship she had with her grandparents (*tipuna*) who cared for her when she was young and taught her about her ancestors. Even though her grandparents live in Auckland they are both still working and she only sees them occasionally. Carleen recently visited a Well Child Centre but did not feel comfortable and probably won't return.

CASE STUDY QUESTION

1. What are the cultural factors to be considered when providing culturally competent healthcare to this family?

Culture is a view of the world and a set of traditions that a specific social group uses and transmits to the next generation. Cultural groups are characterised by inherent beliefs, values, traditions, customs, language, art and shared meaning about healing, health and illness. While there are strong influences that bind members of a cultural group, individuals within the group will express their attitudes, beliefs and behaviours according to their life experiences which include age, gender, situational, family group and community influences. Eckermann and colleagues (2010) remind us that cultures are adaptive and that, as people in the cultural group engage with their environments, there is a reciprocal effect on the environments and the people.

Culturally competent healthcare is a basic human right not a privilege, and should be the entitlement of every human. There is increasing evidence pointing to a strong link between culturally competent care and the achievement of improved health outcomes (Jeffreys, 2010).

Awareness, sensitivity and **respect** for the cultures of other people are essential in providing culturally competent child and family healthcare.

✔ *Checkpoint question 2.1*

Reflect on the beliefs, values, traditions and customs of your culture.

a. Are they strong influences that connect you to your cultural group?
b. Do they influence the way you respond in certain situations?

INDIGENOUS PEOPLES

The term **Indigenous** refers to the initial or earliest inhabitants of a place. They are also described as First Nations peoples (McMurray & Clendon, 2011, p. 335). Indigenous peoples have rich and diverse cultures and differing views of the world. The pattern of colonisation, segregation, oppression, **assimilation** and reconciliation of Indigenous peoples worldwide has been similar. However, Indigenous peoples in Australia and New Zealand have different histories and experiences.

The Treaty of Waitangi, which mandated recognition of all New Zealanders as equal before the law, was a significant development in demonstrating respect for New Zealand Indigenous people (New Zealand Ministry of Justice, 2014). New Zealand has advocated to be seen as a bicultural society reflecting an equal partnership between Māori and Pākeha (immigrant Europeans). Australia is yet to develop a treaty with its Indigenous peoples but recent initiatives by the government, such as Prime Minister Kevin Rudd's Apology to Australia's Indigenous People (Rudd, 2008) and the Closing the Gap: Prime Minister's Report 2011 (Attorney-General's Department, 2011), have emphasised the need for reconciliation between Indigenous Australian and non-Indigenous people. If Australia is to be reshaped as an inclusive society, much remains to be achieved for Aboriginal and Torres Strait Islander peoples, migrants and refugees. New Zealand is much clearer in the policy it has developed to provide a human rights approach to decision making.

As a nurse you must be fully informed of historical factors and current influences that impact on cultural groups, especially Indigenous peoples, which result in disproportionately high levels of disability and disease (McMurray & Clendon, 2011). This increased understanding will then provide you with an opportunity to use this knowledge to provide culturally competent care and increase awareness among the community by developing policy and practice based on primary healthcare and social justice (see Fig. 2.1).

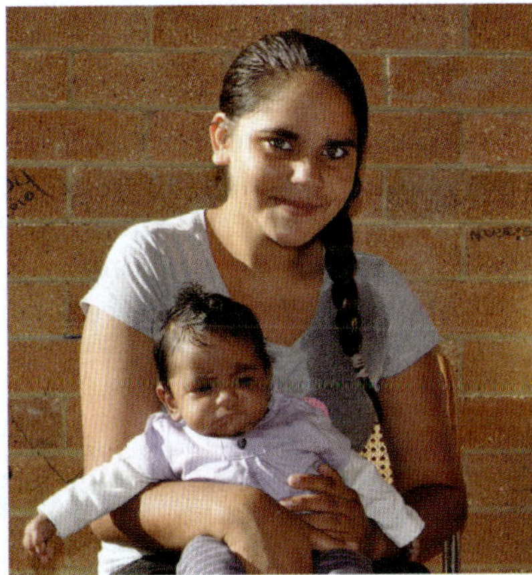

FIGURE 2.1 Nurses provide culturally competent child and family healthcare for Indigenous Australian families. (© Heather Latham.)

Indigenous Australian peoples

At 30 June 2011 Aboriginal and Torres Strait Islander peoples numbered 669,900 or 3% of the Australian population (ABS, 2013). Indigenous Australians die at a much younger age, have higher levels of disability and a significantly higher infant mortality rate than non-Indigenous Australians (AIHW, 2014). In 2010–2012 the life expectancy of an Indigenous female was 73.3 years; 9.5 years lower than for a non-Indigenous female. The life expectancy for an Indigenous male was 69.1 years; 10.6 years lower than for a non-Indigenous male living in Australia (AIHW, 2014). While these figures indicate a slight closing of the gap in life expectancy between Indigenous and non-Indigenous Australians there still remains much work to be done to reduce the inequality. During the period 2008–2012 the leading causes of death for Indigenous Australians included cardiovascular disease, cancers, external causes such as transport accidents, suicide and assault, diabetes and respiratory conditions (AIHW, 2014). Indigenous people are over-represented in the incidence of these diseases as a result of several factors, including difficulty or failure to access health services, biological and social disadvantage, geographical location and lack of health services, higher rates of unemployment, lower education levels and lower rates of home ownership than non-Indigenous Australians. Poor living conditions are not conducive to reducing the high rates of childhood infectious diseases and poor growth and development in Indigenous children (Taylor & Guerin, 2012).

New Zealand Māori

In 2013, people of Māori descent (a descendant of a person of the Māori race of New Zealand) made up 14.8% of the total New Zealand population (Statistics New Zealand, 2013a). Māori life expectancy is significantly lower than for non-Māori; however, the gap in life expectancy at birth has narrowed to 7.3 years compared to 8.2 years in 2005–2007. Māori women have a life expectancy of 76.5 years compared to 83.7 years for non-Māori, while Māori men have a life expectancy of 72.8 years compared with 80.2 years for non-Māori men (Statistics New Zealand, 2013b). Māori have the poorest health status of any ethnic group in New Zealand. Cardiovascular disease, cancer, respiratory disease, accidents, diabetes and suicide are the major causes of mortality for Māori (Tatau Kahukura, 2010). Other factors influencing Māori health include lower education levels, high unemployment and poor housing (Statistics New Zealand, 2013a). As mentioned previously, the Treaty of Waitangi provides the basis for Māori self-determination, the right to name themselves and be recognised as *tangata whenua* (people of the land) (New Zealand Ministry of Justice, 2014).

The development of Māori health services gained momentum in the 1980s where a Māori-centred approach to healthcare (*kaupapa* Māori services) has been successful in teaching Māori families or *whānau* (NZMOH, 2014). This is an excellent example of **empowerment** arising

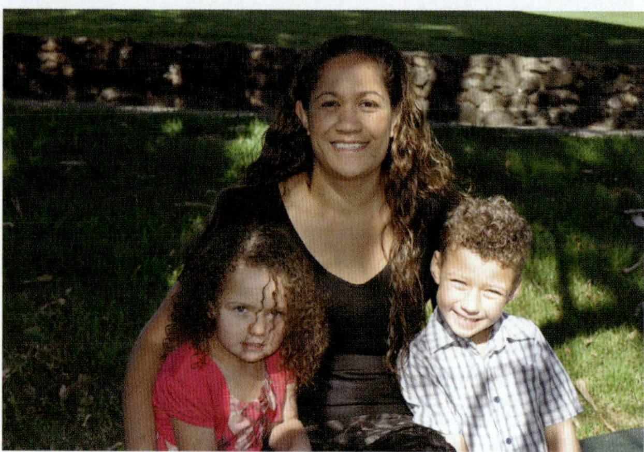

FIGURE 2.2 Nurses work in partnership with Māori families to provide culturally appropriate care. (© Heather Latham.)

from within the Māori to provide appropriate healthcare. Nurses, many of whom are Māori, have a leading role in providing services through kaupapa Māori health providers. Māori individuals and whānau receive culturally appropriate care when the Māori model of care is utilised. The central role in Māori wellbeing is the *whānau*. It is seen as the main source of strength, support, security and identity for Māori (NZMOH, 2014) (see Fig. 2.2).

CULTURAL SAFETY IN THE NEW ZEALAND CONTEXT

The concept of **cultural safety** originated in New Zealand and grew from dissatisfaction expressed by Māori consumers of nursing care. As they studied, Māori nursing students recognised the importance of safeguarding their culture. They wanted to be sure that Māori culture would be safe when nursing care was provided to Māori. Cultural safety was first described by Irithapeti Ramsden, a Māori nurse in the 1980s (Ramsden, 2001). It was held that cultural safety was already embedded in the Treaty of Waitangi where Māori are acknowledged as the first people of Aotearoa (New Zealand). The concept of cultural safety was meant to recognise power imbalances and inequity in social relationships. The Nursing Council of New Zealand recognises that cultural safety creates a safe environment for the interaction of all cultural groups where their understanding of cultural identity is acknowledged (Nursing Council of New Zealand, 2011).

The first step in achieving cultural safety is cultural awareness; recognition that authority exists in any relationship and can result in the nurse or health professional potentially holding power over the person receiving the care. Cultural sensitivity occurs when people explore their own life experiences and beliefs and think about how they might impact on other people. The nurse or health professional needs to make a conscious commitment to respect and preserve the cultures of other people. The Nursing Council of New Zealand maintains that "cultural safety education is focused on the understanding of self as a cultural bearer, the historical, social and political influences on health and the development of relationships that engender trust and respect" (Nursing Council of New Zealand, 2011, p. 5).

CULTURAL SAFETY IN THE AUSTRALIAN CONTEXT

The concept of cultural safety has been endorsed in a Cultural Safety Position Statement by The Congress of Aboriginal and Torres Strait Islander Nurses and Midwives (CATSINaM) in Australia. Cultural safety is viewed by CATSINaM as "the final step on a continuum of nursing and/or midwifery care that includes cultural awareness, cultural sensitivity, cultural knowledge, cultural respect and cultural competence" (CATSINaM, 2014). CATSINaM maintain that cultural safety is not something that can be defined by the carer; rather, it is the experience of the recipient of healthcare. CATSINaM promotes a framework of cultural safety to inform the attitudes and behaviours of health professionals in the provision of healthcare to Aboriginal and Torres Strait Islander individuals and communities so that they feel culturally secure, safe and respected. In order for nurses and midwives to achieve a state of cultural safety it must be embedded in every aspect of their practice (CATSINaM, 2014).

Taylor and Guerin (2012) maintain that the following principles of cultural safety identified by the Nursing Council of New Zealand (2011) have had a profound influence in focusing health professionals' understanding of cultural safety. The principles involve health professionals reflecting on their practice; seeking to minimise the power differentials between themselves and the client; engaging in discourse with the client to understand their unique needs, beliefs, understandings and preferred ways of doing things; undertaking a process of decolonisation where the role of colonising history on the health outcomes of Indigenous peoples is recognised; and ensuring that their actions do not diminish, demean or disempower others (Taylor & Guerin, 2012). Dunbar and Ford (2011, p. 35) believe that there is increasing recognition of the need for the health system to integrate cultural recognition and respect into the delivery of healthcare, organisational structure and the workforce to improve the health and wellbeing of Aboriginal and Torres Strait Islander peoples.

Understanding and respecting the cultures of others is particularly important in child and family health nursing care because childbearing and childrearing are times in life that are surrounded by many cultural traditions (Saggers, Walter & Gray, 2011, p. 2).

NURSING CONSIDERATIONS FOR RESPECTING SOCIOCULTURAL ASPECTS OF CARE

The importance of respecting sociocultural aspects of care is highlighted in research by Hoban and Liamputtong

(2013). This research demonstrates that the postpartum experiences of Cambodian migrant women in Victoria, Australia, who have no female kin support in the postpartum period, experience significant emotional stress, loneliness and social isolation and are at risk of developing postnatal depression. Hoban and Liamputtong (2013) point out that the postpartum period has been identified as the most important period of childbirth in cross-cultural studies and is a time where not only traditions are important but also appropriate social support to ensure the health and wellbeing of the mother and her newborn infant.

Assessment of the social determinants of health and cultural factors is important in planning care that is based not on predetermined assumptions but on the actual preferences and cultural needs of a family. To do this, you will need to assess each patient individually, not as one of a group. Note particularly any cultural characteristics that differ from the usual expectations of the setting in which care is being provided. In this way, potential conflicts can be acknowledged and culturally safe care can be offered.

Assessing the culture of a community is as important as assessing individual families because families are intrinsically joined to their community. An important area of assessment is determining whether the family matches the dominant culture in their community. This is important because the type of foods stocked in the local supermarkets, the type of entertainment events that are available, and the values and history that are stressed in local schools and work settings are all influenced by the dominant culture. The importance of community assessment is further discussed in Chapter 4.

Important nursing considerations resulting from culturally unsafe care include:

- Powerlessness related to expectations of care not being respected
- Powerlessness related to sociocultural isolation
- Impaired verbal communication related to limited English proficiency and educational level
- Poor nutrition related to unmet cultural food preferences
- Anxiety related to a cultural need that is not met
- Fear associated with possible discrimination related to **ethnicity**.

Planning needs to be specific to individual families because sociocultural preferences tend to be very personal. Care may begin with in-service education for healthcare providers who are unfamiliar with a particular cultural practice and its importance to the specific family involved. The plan of care may include arranging for variations in policy, such as the length of family visiting hours, types of food served or type of childcare provided. Such planning is beneficial not only because it can make healthcare more acceptable to a child or family but also because it can motivate providers to examine policies, question the rationale behind them and initiate more culturally safe care (see Fig. 2.3).

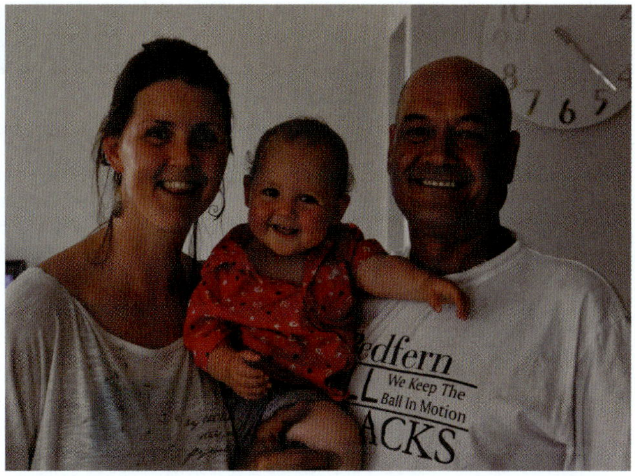

FIGURE 2.3 Multicultural families have traditions that strengthen and enrich family life and the community where they live. Nurses working with families should encourage them to share their cultural values so that these beliefs can be considered and respected and included in nursing care. (© Heather Latham.)

Safe Koori Kids is a project aimed to increase understanding of the factors involved in injury in Indigenous communities. It provides interactive web-based activities. This site can be accessed at <www.uow.edu.au/wic/safekoorikids>. Other reputable websites to use for additional information on the importance of culturally safe care include <www.temanutoroa.org.nz>, <www.naccho.org.au> and <www.health.qld.gov.au/multicultural/health_workers/ viet.pdf>.

Nurses must respect and understand the individual's cultural values. An example of implementing care might be to have the extended members of an Indigenous family present during the individual's hospitalisation. It might be to make arrangements for a female doctor to be available to conduct a Pap smear clinic for local Indigenous women or plan home care for a Chinese child whose family believes in herbal medicine. It might be to establish a network of health professionals or personnel from a nearby workplace to serve as interpreters. There may be situations, however, in which the hospital or community health centre is unable to adapt to the particular cultural situation. This may call for both sides to adjust (cultural negotiation).

Assessing whether expected outcomes have been met should reveal that a family's sociocultural preferences were considered and respected during care. If this was not achieved, procedures may need to be modified until this can be realised.

SOCIOCULTURAL DIFFERENCES AND IMPLICATIONS FOR DIVERSITY IN CHILD AND FAMILY HEALTH NURSING

Multiculturalism

Henry and Kurzak (2013, p. 1) believe that **multiculturalism** embodies "an ethic of acceptance of, and respect for cultural diversity, community harmony and inclusion". Koleth

CULTURAL DESTRUCTIVENESS	CULTURAL BLINDNESS	CULTURAL AWARENESS	CULTURAL SENSITIVITY	CULTURAL COMPETENCE
Making everyone fit the same cultural pattern, and excluding those who don't fit—forced assimilation. Emphasis on differences and using differences as barriers.	Do not see or believe there are cultural differences among people. Everyone is the same.	Being aware that we all live and function within a culture of our own and that our identity is shaped by it.	Understanding and accepting different cultural values, attitudes and behaviours.	The capacity to work effectively and with people, integrating elements of their culture—vocabulary, values, attitudes, rules and norms. Translation of knowledge into action.

FIGURE 2.4 Cultural competence continuum. (Courtesy of the National Council of La Raza.)

(2010, p. 3) has observed that multiculturalism includes "the pursuit of social justice, the recognition of identities and the appreciation of diversity, the integration of migrants, nation building, and attempts to achieve and maintain social cohesion". These values have been embraced with varying degrees of success by countries around the world.

Australia and New Zealand have been described in the past as cultural "melting pots" where all new arrivals gave up their native country's traditions and values to take on the traditions and values of their new home. However, this is not true for everyone. Some new arrivals have found themselves in communities that are inclusive of them and their culture. McMurray and Clendon (2011) nevertheless argue that the dominant culture will maintain its position of power and the less dominant or **minority** cultural groups will lose their languages and cultural attributes as they try to avoid feeling different and potentially excluded from mainstream society. McMurray and Clendon (2011, p. 333) suggest that "multiculturalism is a value-laden term that has sometimes been used as a panacea for intolerance". They believe that to advance multiculturalism, societies need to demonstrate understanding and tolerance of one another's cultural beliefs and practices in the hope that all cultures will prevail.

If this level of **equity** is not achieved individuals will tend to view and interpret the world through their own belief system and behaviours; they may believe that their own culture is superior to all others. This is known as **ethnocentrism** (Eckerman et al., 2010). If this view extends to an intolerance of other cultures the individual is described as **xenophobic**. This term is often used synonymously with **racism**, which usually involves the idea that one's birth-ascribed race or skin colour is superior to another (Eckermann et al., 2010). If an individual maintains feelings of superiority about another race or group it is called **stereotyping**, which can lead to **prejudice** that, when acted upon, results in **discrimination** (McMurray & Clendon, 2011). In addition to acknowledging and respecting cultural diversity it is essential that nurses and midwives incorporate cultural competence into their practice (see Fig. 2.4).

Cultural competence, or respecting cultural differences, allows you to plan culturally competent care and the integration of cultural elements into care is a goal worth achieving. A study of intercultural parenting by Crippen and Brew (2013, p. 263) explored the strategies used by intercultural parents to negotiate diversity based on cultural differences. The researchers suggest that health professionals can learn from these findings when working with intercultural couples and be aware of any cultural biases that they may have—in particular, recognising the importance of how individuals identify and situate their cultural context and that of their partner. Participants in this study demonstrated that there are multiple and interacting constructions of cultural difference (Crippen & Brew, 2013, p. 270). As a nurse, you will have the opportunity to meet many people who hold cultural values different from your own. When planning nursing care, try to not only respect people's cultural differences but also help people share their cultural values with healthcare providers so that their beliefs can be considered and respected (see Table 2.1).

Migrant families

The United Nations defines a migrant as "an individual who has resided in a foreign country for more than one year and irrespective of the causes, voluntary or involuntary and the means regular or irregular, used to migrate" (International Organization for Migration, 2011). Immigration has shaped and enriched Australian and New Zealand society for the past 200 years. Individuals and families have moved across the world to make their home in new countries. Developments such as gold rushes or to escape adverse conditions at home, world wars or more recently conflicts in Vietnam and Afghanistan have been the reasons for people seeking to make their home in countries such as Australia and New Zealand. Clearly these people contribute to the multicultural societies in these countries; however, this experience is often not without challenges and hardship.

Emigrating can be one of the most stressful events in a family's life, particularly if they then experience discrimination and feelings of isolation. A nationally representative cross-sectional survey of secondary school students in New Zealand found that there were significant ethnic

TABLE 2.1 Assessing for cultural values

Area of assessment	Questions to ask or observations to make
Ethnicity	What is the family's cultural preference?
Communication	What is the main language used in the home?
Touch	Do the family members typically touch each other? Do they use intimate or conversational space?
Time	How does the family value time in going about their everyday activities and planning for the future?
Occupation	What value does the family place on work? How do they utilise leisure time?
Pain	Does the family express pain or remain stoic when faced with it? What do they believe relieves pain best?
Family structure	Is the family nuclear? Extended? Single-parent? Are family roles clear? Can an individual name a family member he or she would call on for support in a crisis?
Male and female roles	Is the family male or female dominant?
Religion	What is the family's religion? Do they actively practise their religion?
Health beliefs	What does the family believe about health? What do they believe causes illness? Makes illness better? Do they use alternative therapies or traditional medical practices?
Nutrition	What types of food does the family eat on a weekly basis? Is this the cultural food that the family prefers or what is available?
Community	Is the predominant culture in the community the same as the family's? Can they name a neighbour they could call on in a crisis?

differences in the prevalence of ethnic discrimination. Ethnic discrimination was more commonly reported by Indigenous and minority group students. Ethnic group participants reporting ethnic discrimination were more likely to have adverse health outcomes than other students (Cringle et al., 2012). Terry, Le and Hoang (2012) report a study of the experiences of Asian migrants in a small rural, culturally and linguistically diverse community. An exploration of health risk behaviours found that physical engagement and food consumption were two predominant risk factors greatly influenced by migration to less dynamic culturally and linguistically diverse communities. Retaining ethnic traditions strengthens and enriches family life. It provides security to younger family members, realising that they are part of a continuing line of people who have both a past and a future.

Refugees

The United Nations Refugee Convention defines a refugee as "a person who is outside their own country and is unable or unwilling to return due to a well-founded fear of being persecuted because of their race, religion, nationality, membership of a particular social group or political opinion" (Australian Human Rights Commission, 2014). Many refugees experience torture, trauma and separation from or death of family members prior to or during their passage to a new country. Clearly these experiences will have a profound effect on the adjustment of family members to their new environment. A study by Niner, Kokanovic and Cuthbert (2013, p. 535) of the birth experiences of displaced Karen women from Burma both before and after resettlement in Australia were linked to those of persecution and displacement. The women were grateful for the security of resettlement in Australia; however, social inclusion was negligible. The women described how lack of interpreting services and an absence of the personal and communal care that they expected made childbirth more confusing and difficult. Lack of interpreting services impacted significantly on the healthcare these women received. The power relations inherent in the interactions between the women and the healthcare provider must be acknowledged and addressed. This study also points to the challenges beyond the health services to a view held by some Australians that "providing asylum is a charitable concession rather than an obligation to which forced migrants are entitled" (Niner, Kokanovic & Cuthbert, 2013, p. 549).

Australian law requires that all non-citizens who are in Australia without a valid visa must be held in detention centres. People arriving to seek asylum without a visa must stay in detention until their asylum claim has been finalised or a bridging visa is issued. Clearly this process may take a long time and the detrimental effect on these people, particularly children, is very significant (Australian Human Rights Commission, 2012). McMurray and Clendon (2011) point out that the New Zealand Government has one of the most open refugee policies in the western world, being one of only a few countries which accepts refugee quotas over and above those arriving spontaneously. This policy for "quota refugees" is characterised by a 6-week refugee resettlement program prior to transfer to their new home in locations throughout the country (Immigration New Zealand, 2013).

SOCIAL DETERMINANTS OF HEALTH

Social determinants of health (SDOH) include a vast number of interrelated factors that determine the health and wellbeing of individuals, families and communities. These factors range across biology, gender, culture, socio-economic resources, social support networks, services such as transport, access to food and water, and services for both healthcare and childcare.

As a nurse who adopts the "social determinants" approach to health, you should understand that the principle of **social justice**, which includes fair distribution of society's resources, underpins your practice. You have a responsibility to identify inequities and their underlying determinants, advocate for human rights and recognise the importance of economic, social and political factors impacting on health. In 2005, in recognition of the human rights implications of good health and the place of social determinants in supporting health and wellbeing, the World Health Organization assembled an international Commission on Social Determinants of Health (CSDH) (McMurray & Clendon, 2011). However, even though governments are now beginning to recognise the importance of SDOH in achieving good health for all people, progress is slow. It is essential for you as a nurse to understand the importance of primary healthcare as a framework for the care you provide. This approach will enable you to work in partnership with individuals, families and communities to achieve the best health outcomes in child and family healthcare.

CASE STUDY QUESTION

2. The nurse who Carleen and Tama met at the Well Child Centre made the following comments. Which is the most obvious example of stereotyping?
   a. Carleen is very serious, she never smiles.
   b. Māori women don't understand the importance of childcare.
   c. Carleen will accept my advice about how best to care for Tama.
   d. The nurse should be more assertive when communicating with Carleen.

SOCIOCULTURAL ASSESSMENT

When making assessments regarding whether there are socioeconomic or cultural influences that will make special considerations of care necessary, several categories of information related to the structure (composition) and function (roles and actions) of a family should be examined.

Communication patterns

Communication patterns (not only what people say but also how they say it) are culturally determined. People whose primary language is not English can have great difficulty detailing a health history in English to a healthcare provider. Language barriers can be particularly significant for people who must give health histories when they or their child is ill, because their ability to cope and express themselves when they are stressed may be at a low point (Taylor & Guerin, 2012, pp. 125–127). Even if people are able to converse well in English in social situations, they may still not be able to give a health history as well as they would like. They may have trouble recalling English words not commonly taught in English as a second language classes, such as words for nausea or dizziness. Children who are embarrassed or bashful about speaking another language may simply not talk, so their needs may go unmet. As a general rule, it is unfair to ask children to interpret for their parents.

Communication is also key in reducing the gap between Indigenous and non-Indigenous people. Feelings of powerlessness and the loss of control are clearly related to communication issues and are evident in the poor health status of Indigenous Australians (Taylor & Guerin, 2012, pp. 124–127).

There are many factors that affect the way Indigenous and non-Indigenous people communicate. They include:

- Dialect differences, although the majority of Indigenous people speak English
- Tonal differences, colloquialisms and other factors that can obscure "meaning"
- Gender and health beliefs
- Non-verbal communication, "unspoken messages"
- Using periods of silence
- Touching, eye contact and gestures which vary between and within cultures
- Exercising respect (Eckermann et al., 2010, pp. 128–136).

Cultural variations such as these should be respected in written as well as oral communications. In many instances, written communication is even more problematic: many people can speak a second language but cannot write or read it. Using short, easy sentences and taking care not to use words with double meanings are important techniques (see Box 2.1).

✔ *Checkpoint question 2.2*

a. How should you as the nurse communicate with Indigenous people who are accessing our dominant health system?
b. What non-verbal communication cues have you found to be important in your communication with Indigenous people and people from other cultures?
c. Think about your own communication style. How might this affect your communication with people from different cultures?

Use of conversational space

People of diverse cultures use the space around them differently. Being aware that use of space is culturally determined and can vary from person to person will help you to respect the use of space for individuals. Respect for modesty is one way to respect intimate space. Be aware that women from Middle Eastern cultures adhere to a level of modesty exceeding what you may be used to.

Time orientation

The cultural pattern for making and keeping appointments in Australia and New Zealand is geared towards punctuality. Other cultures, however, may not have this concern for time.

BOX 2.1 ✻ Improving healthcare when clients have limited English proficiency

1. Many people can speak a second language better than they can read it. Assess each person's reading level and rewrite information at an easier reading level if necessary.
2. Ask an interpreter to translate material into the family's primary language.
3. Be certain that rooms in your health facility, such as bathrooms, are labelled with international symbols.
4. Learn a few phrases, such as "Good morning" or "This won't hurt", from other languages, and use them in interactions with clients.
5. Use hand gestures or draw a figure, if need be, to communicate better. Imparting health information is what is important for safe care, not worrying how you look.
6. When using an interpreter, do not ignore the person seeking healthcare in preference to the interpreter. Observe their facial expressions for confirmation that they understand instructions. Use short sentences; avoid slang words that do not interpret cleanly.

You should expect to operate on their time not your time. Women from other cultures who do not have a strict time orientation may view the hospital's practice of feeding infants at designated times such as 10 a.m. or 2 p.m. as strange. People who are not accustomed to adhering to schedules in this way may have difficulty following a strict medical protocol. If they are told, for example, to give a child a medication at 8 a.m., noon and 6 p.m. daily and to return for another appointment at 2 p.m. in a week's time, you may have to stress that the medication should be taken three times a day, not necessarily at the specific times. Stating that returning for a checkup at a set time is important because the doctor is only in the hospital at that time is also helpful. Aboriginal Australians in particular have suffered from the pressure to use time according to western concepts. This has had a profound effect on the timing and duration of ceremonial life.

Work and school orientation

The predominant culture in Australia and New Zealand emphasises that everyone should be employed productively (called the protestant work ethic) and that work should be a pleasure and of intrinsic value (the occupation is as important as what it produces). In contrast, other cultures do not value work in itself but see it as only a means to an end (you work to get money or food, not satisfaction). Suppose that a pregnant woman you care for has been told that she must be at home on bed rest for the remainder of her pregnancy. It is easy to assume that she will be most concerned because she values the work she does as a primary school teacher. In another example, an Indigenous woman with a different work orientation might be more distressed to learn that she can't fulfil her ceremonial obligation by attending a funeral which is of great importance. This could be misconstrued as being unproductive when it is actually a cultural difference. Because people in Australia and New Zealand are expected to work, they also are expected to finish school so they can learn an occupation and support themselves in their adult life.

Family orientation

Family structure, the roles of family members and related lifestyle choices are often culturally determined. In some cultures, the nuclear family (mother, father and children) is most common. In other cultures, for example among Indigenous Australians, extended families (nuclear family plus grandparents, aunts, uncles and cousins) or single-parent families (one parent and child) may be more common. "The Māori regard the *whānau*/family as the principal source of strength, support, security and identity and they believe that it plays a central role in the well being of family members." (McMurray & Clendon, 2011, p. 342). Some cultures stress that information about a family should be carefully guarded (as a way of keeping the family intact and unique, and perhaps also as a reflection of mistrust of healthcare providers). Other cultures willingly share the same information. When caring for children, be certain to identify a child's primary carer before giving healthcare instructions because who cares for children in a family can vary by culture. Identifying the family decision-maker is also important, because this role can vary greatly among families.

Male and female roles

The roles of males and females within particular cultural groups vary considerably. For example, if approval for hospital admission or therapy is needed and the patient comes from a culture where males are the dominant figures, the man will be the one to give this approval. In a culture in which men are very dominant and women are extremely passive, a woman may be unable to offer an opinion of her own health or be embarrassed to submit to a physical examination, especially from a male doctor or nurse, unless a female nurse is also present. Indigenous Australian women hold an equal and interdependent role with men in maintaining tradition and family survival. Women hold dominant roles in childrearing and food gathering and they also share the roles of healers and custodians of traditions (Hampton & Toombs, 2013, p. 84).

It is important to evaluate male and female roles, because knowing the identity of the dominant person in the household also helps you to understand the impact of the illness on a family. If a woman is the family's dominant person and can no longer make her usual decisions, the entire family may be thrown into confusion. If the woman is a non-dominant member, you may have to act as an advocate for her rights with a more dominant person.

In most healthcare settings today, a father is expected to play an active role during labour, as well as during a child's hospital stay. However, a man who sees his role as a passive one may be uncomfortable participating in labour or visiting a hospital to play with an ill child. Awareness that male and female roles differ from country to country can help you find a middle ground for a parent's participation in pregnancy and childcare.

> ***What if...***
>
> Carleen is uncomfortable with the male doctor at the Well Child Centre? What could you do?

Religion

There are wide variations in religious practices, and many of these are culturally determined. Because religion guides a person's overall life philosophy, it influences how people feel about health and illness, what foods they eat, and their preferences about birth and death rituals. Indigenous Australian women have roles in religious activities, particularly in women's business (Dunbar & Ford, 2011, p. 31). Knowing the spiritual beliefs or the religion of a family helps you take the appropriate action. It also helps you in planning care. For example, many nutritional practices, such as whether the family eats meat, can be dictated by religious beliefs. Religion can also have important implications for decision making during a difficult pregnancy or for childhood terminal care.

Spirituality is a very significant part of Indigenous cultures. Indigenous Australians possess rich spiritual beliefs including remembrances of the past and the power of "clever" or "gundil" people. There are also special places and special signs that will bring them news (Eckermann et al., 2010). The Dreamtime, which refers to the creation period, is the basis of Aboriginal religion (Dunbar & Ford, 2011, p. 24). The spiritual connection with the land, described as "country" by Indigenous Australians, is the place that gives and receives life, and is part of the cycle of life–death–life. It provides the link to their ancestors (Dunbar & Ford, 2011, p. 27). The New Zealand Māori also describe a connection to the land, where they are recognised as *tangata whenua*. They regard the land as their spiritual, cultural and ancestral home. Information can be accessed at the following website <www.federation.Māori.nz/>.

Health beliefs

Health beliefs are not universal. It is generally assumed in developed countries that illness is caused by documented factors such as bacteria, viruses or trauma. In other cultures, however, illness may be viewed primarily as a punishment from God or an evil spirit, or as the work of a person who wishes harm to the sick person. Indigenous Australians' view of health is that it is multidimensional and embraces all aspects of living, recognising the importance of survival in harmony with the environment, in particular the land. There is a direct relationship for Aboriginal and Torres Strait Islander peoples between their connection with the land and their wellbeing (Dunbar & Ford, 2011, p. 27). Understanding different beliefs allows you to understand differing attitudes towards procedures and to work out mutual goals, even when the patient's views are not those you would choose for yourself or for a member of your family (see Box 2.2).

A study by Suwankhong, Liamputtong and Runbold, (2011) investigating cooperation between western and traditional medicine in Thailand identifies the differences between the systems that continue to keep them apart. One of the difficulties identified is that modern western health professionals try to motivate and require traditional healers to meet their standards. A big issue is that each group recognises health legalities differently. It is clear that in many societies traditional healers will continue to be a valuable resource for promoting healthcare and self-reliance (Suwankhong, Liamputtong & Runbold, 2011, p. 436).

> ***What if...***
>
> Carleen tells you that she thinks it will be too hard as a single parent to teach Tama about Māori culture so she won't bother about it? Reflect on how you would respond to Carleen and what strategies you might suggest to support her.

Nutrition practices

Foods and their methods of preparation are often strongly culturally related (see Fig. 2.5). In many instances, people cannot find any food on a hospital menu that appeals to them because of cultural preferences. When discussing nutrition with a woman during pregnancy, remember that respect for culturally preferred foods is important. People from some cultures, for example, tend to eat much less meat than do those from other cultures. Adequate protein can be ingested, however, by mixing sources of incomplete protein such as beans and rice. Be certain when discussing nutrition during pregnancy that you do not advise a woman who is lactose intolerant to drink milk. She can

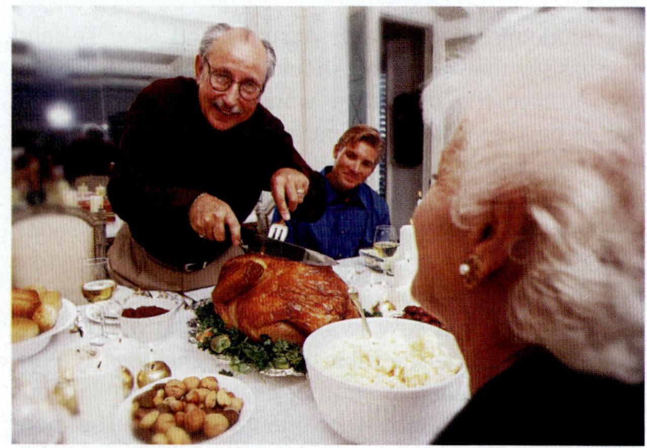

FIGURE 2.5 Families differ regarding what food selections they prefer because of sociocultural preferences. (Carter, P. J. & Goldschmidt, W. M. (2009). *Lippincott's Textbook for Long-Term Care Nursing Assistants*. Philadelphia: Lippincott Williams & Wilkins.)

BOX 2.2 ✻ Focus on nursing care planning

A multidisciplinary care map for a child needing sociocultural care

Maria Lee is a 12-year-old child who is hospitalised following surgical repair of a tibia that was broken when she rode her bicycle into a busy street. She has a cast on her right leg and will be on bed rest for 3 days and then allowed to learn crutch walking.

Family assessment ✻ Maria lives with her mother, Anna, her father, Sam, and a 4-year-old brother, James. She attends a local school and enjoys playing video games and reading Harry Potter books. Her mother is 4 months pregnant.

Patient assessment ✻ Temperature, 37.4°C; pulse, 86 beats/min; respirations, 24/min. Observed lying on side, gritting teeth as if in pain. Hands clenched and eyes tearing. When asked if she has pain, she quietly stated, "No. I'm okay." Father was overheard saying to her, "We're proud you're so brave." Cast on right leg dry and intact. Toes warm to touch. Intravenous fluid infusing without difficulty. Oral intake primarily tea and soup. Patient's mother states, "She needs 'hot' foods to get better. Don't you have anything hotter?"

Nursing diagnosis ✻ Pain related to tissue trauma of surgery, with cultural belief to not voice pain.

Outcome criteria ✻ Patient accepts pain medication when offered; non-verbal expressions of pain are minimal to absent. Patient begins to eat and manage self-care.

Team member responsible	Assessment	Intervention	Rationale	Expected outcome
		Self-care activities		
Nurse/physiotherapist	Assess what self-care activities child feels ready to begin.	Plan a program of self-care that is possible within constraints of limited ambulation.	Ability to complete self-care can add to self-esteem and supply physiological benefits.	Patient feeds self, is out of bed in 3 days, and completes hygiene measures at 12-year-old level.
		Consultations		
Nurse	Assess pain level on a 1-to-10 scale. Determine what child feels would relieve pain best.	Consult with pain management team to establish a total pain relief plan for patient.	Optimal healthcare is often a collaborative practice.	Child states that pain management plan is acceptable to her. Rates her pain level as below 2 on a 1-to-10 scale.
		Procedures/medications		
Nurse	Assess for both verbal and non-verbal indicators of pain.	Offer pain medication as prescribed before pain becomes acute.	Offering medications relieves the client of the need to ask for relief when her belief is that she should not express pain. It also allows the child to have some choice and control in her care.	Child's chart documents that pain medication was offered every 4 hours during waking hours throughout hospital stay.
		Nutrition		
Nurse/nutritionist	Assess whether the child has food preferences that are not being met by hospital service.	Encourage the family to bring in foods from home that meet their cultural preferences.	Allowing the family to bring in foods demonstrates respect for their culture and increases the child's sense of security and being cared for.	Patient increases nutrient intake by including foods brought from home.

(*continued*)

BOX 2.2 * Focus on nursing care planning (continued)

Team member responsible	Assessment	Intervention	Rationale	Expected outcome
		Patient/family education		
Nurse	Assess the child's knowledge of broken bones and of why trauma leads to pain.	Explain the physiology of pain to family members as a way of explaining why the client is experiencing it.	Explanations help a child of this age understand what is happening so minimise fear.	Patient describes what pain is and acknowledges that she will have some until healing is complete and that asking for something to relieve it is expected and acceptable.
		Spiritual/psychosocial/emotional needs		
Nurse	Assess whether child has unmet needs other than pain relief.	Explain to child that you want to help but that she needs to verbally express her needs to enable you to do so.	Children may imagine that healthcare providers are all-knowing.	Child agrees to participate in expressing the presence of other factors, such as loneliness or fear.
		Discharge planning		
Nurse	Assess with child what modifications she will need to make in her daily routine to adjust to cast.	Discuss with parents that their child may need modifications in daily routine to return to school.	Well-informed parents and children are able to make informed decisions.	Child attends school daily because of modifications in usual lifestyle.

obtain adequate calcium through supplements or other foods high in calcium such as dark-green vegetables. Adding a lactase additive to milk is another suggestion.

Pain responses

A person's response to pain is both individually and culturally determined. Narayan (2010) describes how and why culture affects both patients and nurses in the assessment and management of pain. She maintains that patients from minority groups are at high risk of their pain not being managed well (Narayan, 2010, p. 38). Her article suggests ways to provide culturally comfortable care, culturally sensitive pain assessment and culturally comfortable pain management. Although all people may have the same threshold sensation (the amount of stimulus that results in pain), their pain threshold (the point at which the individual reports that a stimulus is painful) and pain tolerance (the point at which an individual withdraws from a stimulus) may vary greatly.

Caring for a person experiencing pain can be problematic when the carer's concept of "proper" responses to pain differs from the patient's concept. One woman in labour might report labour contractions as "agonising" each time she feels one, whereas a woman in the room next to her, experiencing the same degree of pain, might report her pain as tolerable and barely change her facial expression with contractions. These differing responses may be the result of different cultural attitudes towards expressing pain. Because there are so many possible responses to pain, it is important to assess each person individually.

Strategies to help recognise cultural influences on pain perception are:

- Appreciate that the meaning of pain varies among cultures
- Appreciate that not all people communicate or express their level of pain in the same way
- Recognise that communication of pain may not be acceptable within a culture
- Develop an awareness of your personal values and beliefs and understand that they may affect how you respond to people in pain
- Use an assessment tool, such as a 1-to-10 scale, to assist in measuring pain so you are certain that you are being as objective as possible (Narayan, 2010, p. 45).

Further assessment of pain and its meaning to people is discussed in Chapters 16 and 39.

CASE STUDY QUESTION

3. Which statement by Carleen is the most obvious example of ethnocentrism?

a. "Māori people are more artistic than other people."
b. "Māori children like playing sport."
c. "Many non-Indigenous children live in my community."
d. "I am proud of my cultural heritage."

Key points for review

- Culture is an organised structure that guides behaviour into acceptable ways for that group.
- Stereotyping is expecting a person to act in a characteristic way without regard to his or her individual traits.
- Prejudice is thinking that people are different in some way.
- Discrimination is treating people differently based on their physical or cultural traits.
- Each culture differs to some degree from every other culture. Most people are proud of these differences or cultural traits.
- Cultural practices arise from environmental conditions and are transmitted in both formal and informal ways from generation to generation.
- Although cultural concepts adapt from time to time, they tend to remain constant.
- There is wide variation within a culture concerning values and actions, because individuals make up the group and individually express their cultural heritage.
- People bring cultural values and beliefs to nursing interactions, and these affect nursing and healthcare.
- Cultural aspects that are important to assess are communication patterns; use of conversational space; time, work, education, and family orientation; male and female roles; religion; response to pain; and social organisation including nutrition, family roles and health beliefs.

CASE STUDY QUESTIONS

4. What could the Well Child Centre do to make Carleen feel more comfortable when attending with her son Tama? If Carleen decides not to teach Tama about his Māori cultural heritage, how would you approach a discussion about this matter?
5. Carleen has regularly taken Tama for his growth and development checks and immunisations. During her visit to the Well Child Centre Carleen told the nurse that she is struggling to cope with the demands of a young child and feels depressed. What strategies could be implemented to assist Carleen and Tama?
6. Access the website for the Te Manu Toroa Trust—Kaupapa Māori Health Care Services <www.temanutoroa.org.nz> for examples of programs and support strategies for young Māori families. How might such programs assist Carleen and Tama?

Resources

For an extensive range of additional resources to enhance teaching and learning and to facilitate understanding of this chapter, please see the text's accompanying website located on thePoint at http://thepoint.lww.com.

References

Australian Bureau of Statistics. (2013). Estimates of Aboriginal and Torres Strait Islander Australians, June 2011, accessed 6 January 2015, <www.abs.gov.au/ausstats/abs@.nsf/mf/3238.0.55.001>.

Australian Government. (2013). Closing the Gap: Prime Minister's Report 2013, accessed 22 January 2015, <www.dss.gov.au/sites/default/files/documents/02_2013/00313-ctg-report_accessible11.pdf>.

Australian Human Rights Commission. (2012). A last resort? National inquiry into children in immigration detention, accessed 6 January 2015, <www.hreoc.gov.au/human_rights/children_detention_report/report/chap06.htm>.

Australian Human Rights Commission. (2014). Asylum seekers and refugees, accessed 6 January 2015, <www.humanrights.gov.au/our-work/asylum-seekers-and-refugees>.

Australian Institute of Health and Welfare (AIHW). (2014). Australia's Health 2014, accessed 6 January 2015, <www.aihw.gov.au/publication-detail/?id=60129547205>.

Centre for Interactive Development University of Wollongong. (2008). Safe Koori Kids, accessed 6 January 2015, <www.uow.edu.au/wic/safekoorikids>.

Congress of Aboriginal and Torres Strait Islander Nurses and Midwives (CATSINaM). (2014). Cultural safety position statement, accessed 6 January 2015, <http://catsinam.org.au/wp-content/uploads/2014/07/Cultural-Safety_Endorsed-March-2014.pdf>.

Cringle, S., Robinson, E., Ameratunga, S., Clark, T. & Raphael, D. (2012). Ethnic discrimination prevalence and associations with health outcomes: Data from a nationally representative cross-sectional survey of secondary school students in New Zealand. *BMC Public Health, 12*(45), 1–11.

Crippen, C. & Brew, L. (2013). Strategies of cultural adaption in intercultural parenting. *The Family Journal: Ccounselling & Therapy for Couples and Families, 21*(3), 263–271.

Dunbar, T. & Ford, L. (2011). New life: Conception, pregnancy and birthing. In R. Thackrah & K. Scott (Eds), *Indigenous Australian Health and Cultures* (pp. 22–42). Frenchs Forest: Pearson.

Eckermann, A., Dowd, T., Chong, E., Nixon, L., Gray, R. & Johnson, S. (2010). *Binan Goonj. Bridging Cultures in Aboriginal Health* (3rd ed.). Sydney: Elsevier.

Hampton, R. & Toombs, M. (2013). Indigenous Australian concepts of health and well-being. In R. Hampton and M. Toombs (Eds), *Indigenous Australians and Health: The Wombat in the Room* (pp. 73–90). South Melbourne, Victoria: Oxford University Press.

Henry, N. & Kurzak, K. (2013). The Australian collaboration. A collaboration of national community organisations. A multicultural Australia, accessed 6 January 2015, <www.australiancollaboration.com.au/pdf/FactSheets/Multicultural-Australia-FactSheet.pdf>.

Hoban, E. & Liamputtong, P. (2013). Cambodian migrant women's postpartum experiences in Victoria, Australia. *Midwifery, 29*, 772–778.

Immigration New Zealand. (2013). Refugee resettlement factsheet, accessed 6 January 2015, <www.immigration.govt.nz/migrant/general/generalinformation/media/refugeefactsheet.htm>.

International Organization for Migration. (2011). Key migration terms, accessed 6 January 2015, <www.iom.int/cms/en/sites/iom/home/about-migration/key-migration-terms-1.html>.

Jeffreys, M. (2010). *Teaching Cultural Competence in Nursing and Health Care.* (2nd ed.). New York: Springer Publishing Company.

Koleth, E. (2010). The Australian collaboration. A collaboration of national community organisations. A multicultural Australia, accessed 6 January 2015, <www.australiancollaboration.com.au/pdf/FactSheets/Multicultural-Australia-FactSheet.pdf>.

McMurray, A. & Clendon, J. (2011). *Community Health and Wellness. Primary Health Care in Practice.* Sydney: Elsevier.

Narayan, M. (2010). Culture's effects on pain assessment and management. *American Journal of Nursing, 110*(4), 38–47.

National Aboriginal Controlled Community Health Organisation, 2011, accessed 16 October 2011, <www.naacho.org.au>.

New Zealand Ministry of Health (NZMOH). (2014). He Korowai Oranga Māori Health Strategy, accessed 6 January 2015, <www.health.govt.nz/our-work/populations/Māori-health/he-korowai-oranga>.

New Zealand Ministry of Justice. (2014). The Treaty of Waitangi, accessed 6 January 2015, <www.justice.govt.nz/tribunals/waitangi-tribunal/treaty-of-waitangi>.

Niner, S., Kokanovic, R. & Cuthbert, D. (2013). Displaced mothers: Birth and resettlement, gratitude and complaint. *Medical Anthropology Cross-Cultural Studies in Health and Illness, 32*(6), 535–551.

Nursing Council of New Zealand (NCNZ). (2011). Guidelines for cultural safety, the Treaty of Waitangi and Māori health in nursing education and practice. Accessed 22 January 2015, <www.nursingcouncil.org.nz/Publications/Standards-and-guidelines-for-nurses>.

Ramsden, I. (2001). Improving practice through research. *Kai Tiaki Nursing New Zealand, 7*(1), 23–26.

Rudd, K. (2008). *Apology to Australia's Indigenous People.* Speech by Prime Minister Kevin Rudd to the Parliament. Department of Foreign Affairs and Trade, accessed 6 January 2015, <www.dfat.gov.au/indigenous/apology-to-stolen-generations/rudd_speech.html>.

Saggers, S., Walter, M. & Gray, D. (2011). Culture history and health. In R. Thackrah & K. Scott (Eds), *Indigenous Australian Health and Cultures* (pp. 1–21). Frenchs Forest: Pearson.

Statistics New Zealand. (2013a). 2013 Census QuickStats about Māori, accessed 6 January 2015, <www.stats.govt.nz/Census/2013-census/profile-and-summary-reports/quickstats-about-Māori-english.aspx>.

Statistics New Zealand. (2013b). New Zealand Period Life Tables: 2010–12, accessed 6 January 2015, <www.stats.govt.nz/browse_for_stats/health/life_expectancy/NZLifeTables_HOTP10-12.aspx>.

Suwankhong, D., Liamputtong, P. & Runbold, B. (2011). Traditional healers (*mor pheun baan*) in Southern Thailand: The barriers for cooperation with modern health care delivery. *Journal of Community Health, 36*, 431–437.

Tatau Kahukura. (2010). *Demographics and Socioeconomic Determinants of Health* (2nd ed.). Accessed 6 January 2015, <www.health.govt.nz/system/files/documents/publications/poster2-demographics-and-socioeconomic-determinants-of-health_0.pdf>.

Taylor, K. & Guerin, P. (2012). *Health Care and Indigenous Australians. Cultural Safety in Practice.* South Yarra: Palgrave Macmillan.

Te Manu Toroa—Kaupapa Māori Health Care Services, Bay of Plenty, New Zealand, accessed 16 October 2011, <www.temanutoroa.org.au>.

Terry, D., Le, Q. & Hoang, H. (2012). Migrants perceptions of health promotion messages in rural Tasmania. *Health Risk and Society, 14*, 1–11.

Vietnamese. (2011). A guide for health professionals, accessed 28 January 2015, <www.health.qld.gov.au/multicultural/health_workers/viet.pdf>.

Suggested readings

Australian Institute of Health and Welfare. (2012). A picture of Australia's children 2012, accessed 6 January 2015, <www.aihw.gov.au/WorkArea/DownloadAsset.aspx?id=10737423340>.

Federation of Māori Authorities <www.federation.Māori.nz>.

Hoban, E. & Liamputtong, P. (2013). Cambodian migrant women's postpartum experiences in Victoria, Australia. *Midwifery, 29*, 772–778.

National Aboriginal Community Controlled Health Organisation <www.naccho.org.au>.

New Zealand Ministry of Health. (2014). The health of New Zealand children 2011/12, accessed 6 January 2015, <www.health.govt.nz/publication/health-new-zealand-children-2011-12>.

Safe Koori Kids <www.uow.edu.au/wic/safekoorikids>.

Te Manu Toroa—Kaupapa Māori Health Care Services <www.temanutoroa.org.nz>.

Vietnamese. A Guide for Health Professionals <www.health.qld.gov.au/multicultural/health_workers/viet.pdf>.

Chapter 3

The childbearing and childrearing family

The previous chapters discussed the philosophy of child and family health nursing and how cultural mores affect care. This chapter adds information about families and how nurses can help ensure healthy outcomes for families. Inadequate family support, which can occur in a dysfunctional family, can contribute to poor pregnancy outcomes or poor childrearing practices.

LEARNING OBJECTIVES

After mastering the contents of this chapter, you should be able to:

1. Describe family structure, function, and roles and ways that these are changing.
2. Use critical thinking to analyse additional ways that nursing care can be more family-centred and strengths-based in approach to facilitate family members, integration into child and family healthcare.
3. Assess a family for structure and healthy function.
4. Formulate nursing considerations related to family health.
5. Develop expected outcomes to help a family achieve optimal health.
6. Plan health teaching strategies, such as helping a family to modify its lifestyle to adjust to a pregnancy, accommodate an ill child or face a major life event such as loss of a job.
7. Implement nursing care, such as teaching a family more effective wellness behaviours.
8. Evaluate outcome criteria for achievement and effectiveness of nursing care to be certain that expected outcomes have been achieved.
9. Identify areas of care related to family nursing that could benefit from additional nursing research or the application of evidence-based practice.
10. Integrate knowledge of family nursing with nursing process to promote quality child and family health nursing care.

KEY TERMS

- ecomap
- family
- family-centred care
- family nursing
- family of orientation
- family of procreation
- family theory
- family types
- genogram

CASE STUDY

Margo Hanovan is a 32-year-old woman who has a 13-year-old child, Carey, from a first marriage. Carey has been sick since birth with cystic fibrosis. He attends the local high school although he needs daily physiotherapy, sometimes twice daily when he has an infection. Steve, 33, Margo's present husband, has a 2-year-old son, Brian, from his first marriage who is also part of the family. Steve is currently unemployed because of an accident at work a year ago. He has some income from selling woodworking products at craft shows and markets. Margo, a freelance writer, is 6 months' pregnant with their first child. Finances are extremely tight as Carey requires regular trips to the children's hospital to access the cystic fibrosis specialist team: travelling for specialist care and to access the nearest hospital when he is sick are both costly activities. Margo and Steve do a home physiotherapy program as there is no physiotherapist close to their home. Carey has been hospitalised 10 times in the past 6 years. As the family live in a rural area they travel to the children's hospital which is several hours' drive away to attend the specialist cystic fibrosis clinic. Carey tires easily and is unable to participate in sporting activities. He has also missed large amounts of school due to hospitalisations and fatigue. He has a positive outlook and a friendly demeanour. He has a group of supportive friends at school who understand his condition. This family has not had a holiday for 5 years and Margo is finding herself tiring easily with her current pregnancy. They have no close family nearby, all relatives are interstate and they live an hour from the closest town which has a population of 3500.

CASE STUDY QUESTIONS

1. Is the Hanovan family a well family?
2. Is their structure typical of other Australian and New Zealand families?

Humans have always lived in families, but the types of families formed and family goals established have changed as the rest of the world has changed (see Fig. 3.1). The majority of people living in Australia and New Zealand live in a family structure, but the characteristics of this family have changed. For example, when the largest number of families lived on farms, families were extended or had a wealth of relatives close by for both physical and psychological support. As more people moved into higher populated urban areas, families became typically nuclear with only two parents and children present. Less support was available to families. Current trends indicate a reduction in the size of the family, an increase in the age when women have children and a rise in employment rates for mothers with dependent children (AIFS, 2014a). Numbers of single-parent families have increased, which has particular implications for nurses, as parents in this type of family may not have another adult to give them support (ABS, 2011). Thus families are looking

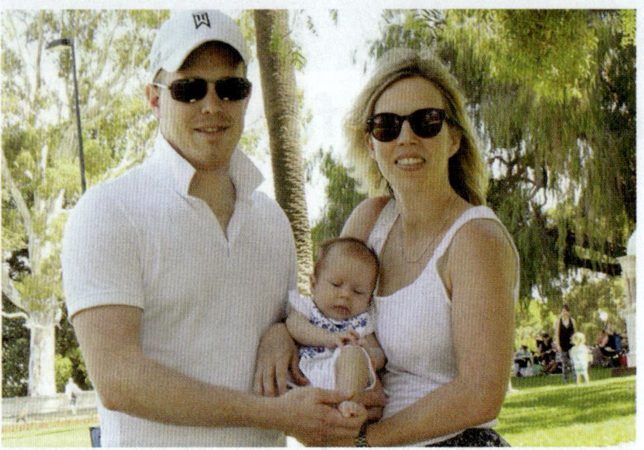

FIGURE 3.1 Families are a universal among almost all civilisations. (© Lauren Kidziak.)

more to healthcare providers for guidance when a problem with pregnancy or childrearing occurs.

Families are important to a country. No other social group has the potential to provide the same level of support and long-lasting emotional ties as a person's own family. What people learn in their family determines how they relate to people, what moral values they learn, and their perspective on both the present and the future (Parker et al., 2011). The family has such an influence on the individual, nursing care that considers the family, not the individual **(family nursing)** is a focus of modern nursing practice. **Family theory** details a set of perspectives from the family's point of view that can help nurses address the important health issues of childbearing and childrearing families.

For a family to adjust to a new member, particularly a baby, it must have a structure and roles that are flexible enough to adjust to the changes that pregnancy and a newborn will bring. An ill family member or one who is going through a difficult developmental period, such as adolescence, can put a tremendous strain on a family. The roles individuals assume in the family and their ability to adjust to new roles can influence a family's perception of the child's illness, as well as the family's ability to adjust to new situations and work through difficult times to reach a positive family outcome. As families do not live in isolation, their ability to thrive in a community and gain strength from the community is equally as important.

Family-centred child and family health nursing considers the strengths, vulnerabilities and patterns of families to support families during childbirth and childrearing and to encourage healthy coping mechanisms in families facing a crisis. Further research continues into the effectiveness of using a family-centred care approach for hospitalised children (Shields et al., 2012). Health assessment and intervention planning is best when it includes consideration of the family's social, emotional, spiritual and financial resources, as well as the physical and emotional condition of the home and the community.

PROMOTION OF FAMILY HEALTH

Assessment

Assessment of the structure, function, strengths and challenges of families provides information on the ability of a family to remain well during both calm and stressful times. It can reveal the meaning of a current health situation as well as the emotional support an individual family member can expect from other members or the community. This can be vital in understanding what a pregnancy or childhood illness will mean to different family members, especially if not all members appear to be in agreement.

Nursing considerations

Nursing considerations formulated for families generally relate to a family's ability to handle stress and to provide a positive environment for growth and development of members. Examples are:

- Parental role conflict related to prolonged separation from a child during a long hospital stay
- Interrupted family processes related to emergency hospital admission of oldest child
- Impaired parenting related to unplanned pregnancy
- Ineffective family coping related to inability to adjust to mother's illness during pregnancy
- Readiness for enhanced family coping related to improved perceptions of child's capabilities
- Health-seeking behaviours related to birth of first child.

"Impaired parenting" and "parental role conflict" are considerations that suggest parents need additional help with parenting. The first family coping consideration ("ineffective family coping") indicates that a family is not functioning at an optimal level; the second ("readiness for enhanced family coping") suggests a family that is ready for new growth because of a specific event, such as sudden illness in a child or discovery of an unplanned pregnancy. "Readiness for enhanced parenting" and "health-seeking behaviours" are considerations that apply to families who are investigating more effective ways to manage their present situation and improve family/community functioning.

Planning for nursing care is most effective if it includes a design that is family-centred and so is both appropriate and desired by the majority of family members. Be certain to also consider the community. For example, it is not helpful to suggest that a family take regular walks together to encourage shared decision making and improve family communication if walking in their neighbourhood park is unsafe.

Interventions to improve family health should flow smoothly if family members have agreed on a plan of action out of support for one another. It may be necessary in some instances, however, to encourage family members to agree on a plan or to abide by a chosen plan. Otherwise, they can expend needless energy carrying out an activity that is counterproductive or in direct opposition to their major goal.

Evaluation should reveal not only that a goal was achieved but also that the family feels more cohesive after working together towards the goal. If evaluation does not reveal these two factors, reassess the goal as necessary to determine whether further intervention is required.

THE FAMILY

How well a family works together and how well it can organise itself against potential threats depend on its structure (who its members are) and its function (the activities or roles family members carry out). Recognising different family structures can help you focus on **family-centred care** or provide a family-friendly environment for healthcare. It is important to remember that parents and family members are often the centre of a child's world and the care should be planned around the family, not just the child (Randall, Munns & Shields, 2013). It is important to discuss family-centred care and what this entails for the particular child and family as each child and family will opt to engage in different aspects of care. For example, most families of a hospitalised child are comfortable with engaging in basic care tasks for their child but not assisting or doing nursing interventions. These tasks would need to be negotiated on an individual basis (Stuart & Melling, 2014).

Defining the concept of family

A **family** is defined by the Australian Bureau of Statistics (ABS, 2011, p. 1) as "two or more people, one of whom is at least 15 years of age, who are related by blood, marriage (registered or de facto), adoption, step or fostering, and who are usually resident in the same household. The basis of a family is formed by identifying the presence of a couple relationship, lone parent–child relationship or other blood relationship. Some households will, therefore, contain more than one family". The New Zealand definition differs slightly with family defined as a couple with or without child(ren), or one parent and their child(ren) whose usual residence is in the same household. A child in a family can be of any age, but must not have a partner or child(ren) of their own living in the same household (Statistics New Zealand, 2013a, p. 1). This differs in that it excludes parents and children living in different households, thus the emphasis is on the household and not the child.

Family means different things to different people: marriage and children are not prerequisites for a family. There is an increasing trend for smaller families and an increase in couple and single-person households. Both the structure and the function of families have changed over the past few decades. Some changes are related to demographics with a declining fertility rate and ageing population, while other changes relate to choices of family members and emerging new family structures (ABS, 2011). Definitions may vary but it is important to consider the social, cultural and political factors that shape families. Diversity within families is a response to changing times (Barnes & Rowe, 2013).

Family types

Many types or structures of families exist and family structures change over time as they are affected by birth, work, death, divorce, illness and the growth of family members. For the purposes of assessing families in child and family health nursing, two basic **family types** can be described:

- **Family of orientation** (the family one is born into; or oneself, mother, father and siblings, if any)
- **Family of procreation** (a family one establishes; or oneself, spouse or significant other and children).

Almost all families, regardless of type, share common activities and they influence the health and activities of their members (Chapman et al., 2012). Specific descriptions of family types vary greatly depending on family roles, generational issues, means of family support and sociocultural influences.

Couple family

A couple family consists of two people living together. It can consist of a couple without children being present in the household. Newly married couples, as an example, are a couple family. Couple families are generally viewed as temporary arrangements, but if the couple chooses child-free living, this can also be a lifetime arrangement. This family type is increasing in popularity (AIFS, 2014a; Statistics New Zealand, 2013a).

The cohabitation family

Cohabitation families are composed of heterosexual couples, and perhaps children, who live together but remain unmarried. Although such a relationship may be temporary, it may also be as long-lasting and as meaningful as a more traditional alliance. Many couples choose cohabitation as a way of getting to know a potential life partner better before marriage. Statistically, however, couples who cohabit before marriage have a higher divorce rate than those who do not (Cherlin, 2012). When in place, an effective cohabitation arrangement offers psychological comfort, companionship and financial security similar to marriage.

The nuclear family

The traditional nuclear family structure is composed of husband, wife and children. In the past, it was the most common structure seen worldwide. However, the number of nuclear families has declined with an increase in divorce, acceptance of single parenthood and the greater acceptance of alternative lifestyles (AIFS, 2014a). One particular advantage of a nuclear family is its ability to provide support to family members; its small size means people know each other well and can feel genuine affection for each other. In a time of crisis, however, this same characteristic may become a challenge as there are few family members to share the burden and offer support.

The extended (multigenerational) family

An extended family includes not only the nuclear family but also other family members such as grandmothers, grandfathers, aunts, uncles, cousins and grandchildren. An advantage of such a family is that it contains more people to serve as resources during crises and provides more role models for behaviour or values (Keene, Prokos & Held, 2012). A possible disadvantage of an extended family is that family resources, both financial and psychological, must be stretched to accommodate all members. When assessing such families, remember that a parent's strongest support person may not be a spouse or intimate partner and a child's primary carer may not be his or her own mother or father. A grandparent or an aunt/uncle or another sibling, for example, may provide the largest amount of support or childcare.

The single-parent family

The incidence of single-parent families has increased. A health problem in a single-parent family is almost always compounded as there is no backup person for childcare and/or no close support person to give reassurance.

Single-parent families encounter higher levels of unemployment, partly due to the caring responsibilities inherent in this family type and are thus more likely to experience financial hardship (AIFS, 2014a). Single parents may have difficulty with role modelling or clearly identifying their role in the family (i.e. they must provide duplicate roles, or financial support as well as childcare). Trying to fulfil several central roles in this way is not only time-consuming but also mentally and physically exhausting. Such a parent may develop low self-esteem if things are not going well, especially if a spouse left them for another or if the other parent refuses to help with child support. Single-parent fathers may have difficulty with home management or childcare if they had little experience with these roles before the separation. Such feelings have the potential to interfere with decision making and impede daily functioning.

Single-parent families do, however, have a special strength in that such a family can offer the child a special parent–child relationship and increased opportunities for self-reliance and independence. If there has been a divorce, one parent may have been given legal custody of the children or both parents may have joint custody. Either way, both parents often participate in decision making. At a time of illness, both may stay with the ill child in the hospital and be eager to receive reports of the child's progress. Identifying who is the custodial parent is especially important when consent forms for care are signed.

The blended family

In a blended family, or a remarriage, a divorced or widowed person with children marries someone who also has children. Advantages of blended families include increased security and resources for the new family. Another benefit is that the children of blended families are exposed to different customs or culture and may become more adaptable to new situations.

Childrearing problems may arise in this type of family from rivalry among the children for the attention of a parent. In addition, each spouse may encounter difficulties in helping rear the other's children. Children may not welcome a step-parent because they have not yet resolved their feelings about the separation of their biological parents (through either divorce or death); the step-parent may differ from the biological parent, particularly in terms of discipline and caring; or they may believe that the step-parent threatens their relationship with their biological parent. They may also become distressed at seeing their other biological parent move into another home and become a step-parent to other children.

The gay or lesbian family

Gay is the socially acceptable term to describe men who have sex with other men; lesbian is the term used to describe women who have sex with women. Individuals of the same sex may live together as partners for companionship, financial security and sexual fulfilment. Laws are being revised to legally sanction gay marriage throughout the world and this type of family is increasing in number. Such a relationship offers support in times of crisis comparable to that offered by a nuclear or cohabitation family. Some lesbian and gay families include children from previous heterosexual marriages, adopted children or those born as the result of artificial insemination or surrogate motherhood. Laws governing homosexual partners can affect healthcare if they limit health insurance coverage. Lack of understanding by healthcare providers of the strength and richness of these unions can further impede healthcare (Chapman et al., 2012).

CASE STUDY QUESTION

3. The Hanovan family was a single-parent family before Margo remarried. What is a common concern of single-parent families?

a. Reading disorders are common
b. Finances may be inadequate
c. Children can't socialise with other children
d. Children do not know any other family like theirs

The foster family

Children whose parents can no longer care for them may be placed in a foster or substitute home by a child protection agency (Kubiak et al., 2012). Foster parents may or may not have children of their own. They receive remuneration for their care of the foster child. Foster home placement is theoretically temporary and only until children can be returned to their own parents. If return is impossible or is not imminent, children, unfortunately, may be raised to adulthood in foster care. Such children can experience almost constant insecurity, concerned that soon they will have to move again. In addition, they may have some emotional difficulties related to the reason they were removed from their original home (Taussig et al., 2012). When caring for children from foster homes, be certain to determine who has legal responsibility to sign for healthcare for the child as this may not be the foster parent.

The adoptive family

Many types of families (nuclear, extended, cohabitation, single-parent, gay and lesbian) adopt children today. No matter what the family structure, adopting brings several challenges to the adopting parents and the child, as well as to any other children in the family (Jones, 2012). Adoption information can be accessed at Adoption Australia <www.adoptionaustralia.com.au/> and the Australian Institute of Family Studies (AIFS) <www.aifs.gov.au>. In New Zealand, the Ministry of Social Development Area of Child, Youth and Family <www.cyf.govt.nz/adoption> and Adoption Option <http://adoptionoption.org.nz> offer information on adoption. There are different requirements for adopting in every country; this includes adoption within the same country and adopting from another country. Australia and New Zealand both have legislation in the form of Adoption Acts that must be adhered to.

Caring for adoptive families

- Regardless of the type of adoption, new parents should visit a healthcare facility shortly after a child is placed in their home so that a baseline of health information on the child can be obtained, potential problems can be discussed and solutions can be explored.
- Children from countries that are war-torn or poverty-stricken have a greater risk of having illnesses such as hepatitis B and intestinal parasites; they may also suffer from growth restriction and lack immunisations (Roeber et al., 2012).
- Determine the stage of parenting the parents have reached. There may be a need to explore their feelings about this change in their lives.
- With the increase in foreign adoptions, parents often express a conflict between trying to preserve the child's native culture and socialising the child into their community.
- Be sure to assess siblings' responses to the adopted child.
- It is generally accepted that adopted children should be told as early as they can understand that they are adopted. Knowing this from early childhood is not nearly as stressful as accidentally stumbling onto the information when they are school-aged or in adolescence. By 3 years of age, children are able to understand the story of their adoption.
- When children are first told they are adopted, they may exhibit "honeymoon behaviour" or try to behave perfectly for fear of being given away again. After this honeymoon period, children may then deliberately test their parents to see whether the parents will still keep them.
- Counselling an adopted child or forming a relationship with one as a healthcare provider carries the additional responsibility of making certain that the relationship does not end abruptly or without closure so the child does not feel abandoned.
- As adopted children enter puberty and begin to think about having children of their own, they may begin to worry whether they will make good parents. It is common for them to spend time tracing records and trying to locate their birth parents. Children seek their birth parents not because they do not love their adoptive parents but because they need that information to know where they fit into the scheme of life.

FAMILY FUNCTIONS AND ROLES

A family is a small community group and, as a group, it works best if it can designate certain people to complete certain tasks. The family roles that people view as appropriate are usually the ones they saw their own parents fulfilling. As each new generation takes on the values of the previous generation, family traditions and culture pass to the next generation. Family roles are flexible and often not as well defined as they might have been in the past. An important part of family assessment is to identify the roles of family members. Knowing who fulfils these roles in a family helps you to work most effectively with that family (see Fig. 3.2).

If a hospitalised child will need continued care after he or she returns home, for example, it is important to identify and contact the nurturing member of the family, because this person is probably the one who will supervise or give the needed care at home. Be careful not to make assumptions about role fulfilment based on gender or stereotyping.

Communication

Communication is the mutual exchange of information. It is a process of reciprocity and includes more than just language; it may incorporate signs, symbols, emotions and behaviours (O'Toole, 2012). Communicating with children of all ages and adolescents can be challenging.

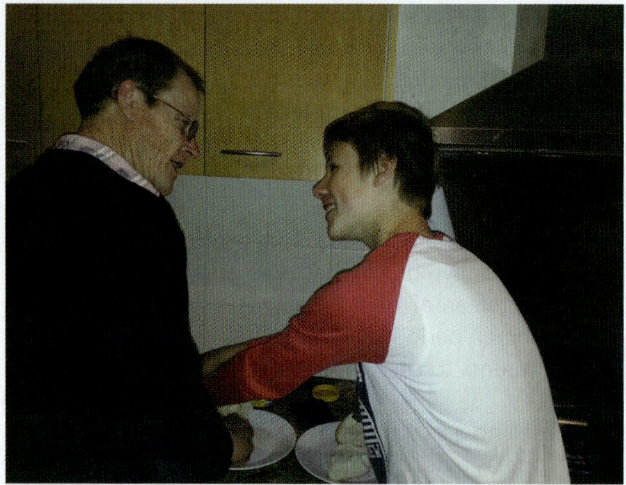

FIGURE 3.2 A healthy family supports each member and performs roles flexibly. Here, a father and son prepare lunch. (© Caroline Hunter.)

Differences in age, developmental stage, sociocultural experiences and personal perceptions can impact on the quality and quantity of information exchanged between health professionals and the child and family. Correcting fears, mistrust and wrong information is essential to facilitate effective communication. Using appropriate terminology and being on the same level as the child, being honest and listening are important techniques to enable effective communication and to form therapeutic relationships based on trust and respect (Stein-Parbury, 2013; see Box 3.1). Communicating with children and families is essential to empower them to make informed decisions to maintain their health and wellbeing. Incorporating a family-centred care approach where the child is acknowledged as a contributing member of the family and included in the communication process is important to achieve this aim (Lambert, Glacken & McCarron, 2010). Tips for communicating with children include:

- Gain the child's attention before talking
- Provide opportunities for children and young people to express themselves freely through play and art
- Speak kindly, be positive and be a good listener
- Respect children's privacy
- Be truthful
- Listen for, and to, children's communication
- Promote equity through communication with all children
- Display caring attributes
- Be aware that spaces and physical environments also communicate messages
- Be approachable (Barnes & Rowe, 2013, pp. 104–106).

Rights of the child

Children and young people have rights, just as adults do and as nurses we are bound to adhere to these rights and incorporate them in our practice. The UN Convention on the Rights of the Child sets out these basic rights including the right to develop to the fullest and to participate fully in family, cultural and social life (United Nations, 1989). Some of the specific articles within this Convention refer to respecting the view of children and the right to freedom of expression. Australia and New Zealand launched their own charters for the rights of children and young people in 2010 focusing on the right to both express their views and to be heard, their right to information and to participate in decision making appropriate to their capacity to do this (Children's Hospital Australasia, 2010a, 2010b).

Family tasks

Duvall and Miller (1990) identified eight tasks that are essential for a family to perform to survive as a healthy unit. These tasks differ in degree from family to family and depend on the growth stage of the family, but they are usually present to some extent in all families. Therefore, assessing families for these characteristics is helpful in establishing the extent of stress on a family and then empowering the family to move towards healthier behaviours.

- *Physical maintenance*: A healthy family provides food, shelter, clothing and healthcare for its members.

BOX 3.1 * Focus on family teaching

Tips to improve family communication

Q. Suppose Margo Hanovan tells you, "My family doesn't communicate well. How can I improve this?"

A. Traditionally, families gathered for an evening meal and this practice allowed a set period each day for interaction, problem solving and conflict resolution while problems were still small. If family meals are not possible because of busy work or school schedules, suggestions for better communication might include:

- Plan a time (even 15 minutes) daily when all family members "touch base" with each other.
- Use a telephone answering tape to leave daily messages.
- Set up a bulletin board or a chalk board that family members check each day for messages.
- Have all members check in daily by email or text message.
- Plan an earlier wake-up time two or three mornings a week so all family members can have breakfast together.
- Reserve one night a week as "family night", when the family plans a special activity to do together such as play a board game or watch a favourite movie.
- Agree that the night is off limits to mobiles, television, CDs, computers, iPods, etc., so family members are not distracted by outside sources.
- Plan special activities for holidays or weekends that involve the whole family.
- Participate in each other's activities (e.g. if one is playing in a ball game, all go and watch).

Being certain that a family has enough resources to provide for a new or ill member is an important assessment.

- *Socialisation of family members:* This task involves preparing children to live in the community and to interact with people outside the family. It means the family has an open communication system among family members and outwards to the community.
- *Allocation of resources:* Determining which family needs will be met and their order of priority is allocation of resources. In healthy families, there is justification, consistency and fairness in the distribution. Resources include not only material goods but also affection and space.
- *Maintenance of order:* This task includes establishing family values, instituting rules about expected family responsibilities and roles, and enforcing common regulations for family members such as using "time out" for toddlers.
- *Division of labour:* Healthy families evenly divide the workload among members and are flexible enough so that they can change workloads as needed. Pregnancy or the illness of a child may change this arrangement and cause the family to have to rethink family tasks.
- *Reproduction and recruitment of family members:* Often not a great deal of thought is given to this task; who lives in a family often happens more by changing circumstances than by true choice. Having to accept a new infant into an already crowded household may make a pregnancy a less-than-welcome event or cause reworking of this task.
- *Placement of members into the larger society:* Healthy families realise that they do not have to operate alone but can reach out to other families or their community for help when needed. Selecting a birth setting, or a special school setting or choosing a hospital or hospice setting is part of this task.
- *Maintenance of motivation and morale:* Healthy families are able to maintain a sense of unity and pride in the family. It means that parents are growing with and through the experience of their children, the same as children are growing through contact with the parents.

Family life cycles

Families, like individuals, pass through predictable developmental stages (Duvall & Miller, 1990). To assess whether a family is using stage-appropriate health promotion activities, it is helpful to first determine a family's developmental stage. The age of the oldest child marks the stage. As families are delaying the age at which they have a first child and parents are living longer, the lengths of stages 1, 7 and 8 are growing.

Stage 1: Marriage

Although Duvall referred to this stage as marriage, what occurs is also applicable to couples forming cohabitation, lesbian/gay or single families. During this first stage of family development, members work to:

- Establish a mutually satisfying relationship
- Learn to relate well to their families of orientation
- If applicable, engage in reproductive life planning.

Establishing a mutually satisfying relationship includes merging the values that the couple brings into the relationship from their families of orientation. This includes not only adjusting to each other in terms of routines (e.g. sleeping, eating, house cleaning) but also sexual and economic aspects.

Stage 2: The early childbearing family

The birth or adoption of a first baby is usually an exciting but at the same time a stressful event because it requires both economic and social role changes. An important nursing role during this period is health education about well-child care and how to integrate a new member into a family. It is a further developmental step for a family to change from being able to care for a well baby to being able to care for an ill one. Parents who have difficulty with this step need a great deal of support and counselling from healthcare providers to be able to care for an ill child at home or to manage a difficult pregnancy.

Stage 3: The family with a preschool child

A family with preschool children is a busy family because children at this age demand a great deal of time. Their imagination is at such a peak that safety considerations such as avoiding unintentional injuries (accidents) become a major health concern. If a child is hospitalised because of an accident, parents may have difficulty giving care because they feel they should have done more to prevent the child's injury. It may be difficult for parents to room-in at the hospital because they have other young children at home who need care. If the child returns home for further care, a family in this stage may need continued support and help from a community health nurse to provide necessary healthcare for the ill child.

Stage 4: The family with a school-aged child

Parents of school-aged children have the important responsibility of preparing their children to function in a complex world while at the same time maintaining their own satisfying marriage relationship. Illness imposed at this stage adds to the burdens already present and may be enough to dissolve a family. Important nursing concerns during this family stage are monitoring children's health in terms of immunisation, dental care and healthcare assessments; monitoring child safety related to home or vehicle accidents; and encouraging a meaningful school experience.

Stage 5: The family with an adolescent

The family must now loosen family ties to allow adolescents more freedom and prepare them for life on their own. As technology advances at a rapid rate, the gap between generations increases. Life when the parents were young was very different from what it is for their teenagers.

Violence, drug and alcohol abuse, accidents, homicide and suicide are major causes of death in this stage. As adolescents become sexually active they risk contracting sexually transmitted infections. A nurse working with families at this stage needs to spend time counselling members on safety (driving defensively and not under the influence of alcohol; safer sex practices) and the dangers of chemical abuse. If there is a "generation gap" between the parents and an adolescent, the adolescent may not be able to talk to the parents about these problems. A nurse can be a neutral person to assist families if communication is difficult, while also maintaining confidentiality.

Stage 6: The launching stage family: the family with a young adult

For many families, the stage at which children leave to establish their own households is the most difficult stage because it appears to represent the breaking up of the family. Parental roles change from those of mother or father to once-removed support people or guideposts. This stage may represent a loss of self-esteem for parents, who feel themselves being replaced by other people in their children's lives. They may feel old for the first time and less able to cope with responsibilities. Illness imposed on a family at this stage can be detrimental to the family structure, breaking up an already disorganised and non-cohesive group. It is important to reinforce to parents that a child leaving home is a positive, not a negative step.

Many young adults return home to live with their family after university until they can afford their own home or get married. These young adults are termed the "boomerang" generation. Another term applied when young adults return home is known as a "sandwich" family. This relates to a family that is taking care of both ageing parents and a returning young adult.

Stage 7: The family of middle years

When a family returns to a two-partner or single-person unit, as it was before childbearing, the partners may view this stage either as the prime time of their lives (an opportunity to travel, gain economic independence and spend time on hobbies) or as a period of gradual decline (lacking the constant activity and stimulation of children in the home, finding life boring without them or experiencing an "empty nest" syndrome). They may realise that they have both grown in such different ways that they have very little in common any more. Women tend to experience less "empty nest" feelings than previously because few women in developed countries now measure their worth only by their ability to care for children (Cherlin, 2012). At this stage some partners realise they have grown apart and have little in common, with the divorce rate the second highest at this stage. It is important to value the individual's personal worth when children leave home (Dare, 2011).

As the family has returned to a two-partner union or a one-person unit, support people may not be as plentiful as they were. Having children return home to live after living out of home can create the "sandwich" family, discussed above. When this happens parents may be squeezed into taking care of both their older and younger family members.

Stage 8: The family in retirement or older age

Although families at this stage are not having children, they remain important in child and family health because they can offer a great deal of support and advice to young adults who are just beginning their families. Many grandparents care for their grandchildren while parents are at work. This can be a strain on older adults as they struggle to meet young children's needs in relation to both energy level and finances.

CASE STUDY QUESTION

4. The Hanovan family consists of two parents plus Carey, age 13 and Brian, age 2. Margo is 6 months' pregnant. Which of Duvall's family life stages is the family currently experiencing?
   a. Pregnancy stage
   b. Preschool stage
   c. School-age stage
   d. Launching stage

Changing patterns of family life

Family life has changed significantly in the past 50 years because of many complex and interrelated factors, such as the increased mobility of families, an increase in the number of families in which both parents work outside the home (dual-earner families), an increase in the number of single-parent families and an increase in shared childrearing responsibilities. Many couples delay marriage and childrearing until they are completely finished with school and have established in their careers. This delay has implications for fertility and the need for assisted reproduction strategies. Understanding the impact these changes have on families can assist in creating care plans that are realistic and meet the needs of contemporary families. Some parents are surprised to find their grown children returning home after university to live with them again. Others find themselves playing duel rules by caring for both children and ageing parents.

Increasing mobility patterns

Population movement has an important influence on the quality of family life. During the 20th century, vast numbers of rural families moved to urban communities and many urban families moved to the suburbs. This has meant that some areas with many child and family healthcare facilities have found themselves with few women and children to use them while other areas with many women and children lack nearby facilities. This can cause problems as parents will travel a great distance to obtain healthcare for an ill child or during a pregnancy with complications, but they are less likely to do so for health maintenance or health promotion; therefore, antenatal care or routine immunisations may be neglected. When assessing families, always ask if a family has ready accessibility to healthcare.

Families of immigrants can have difficulty finding consistent healthcare because of their seasonal movement. Children from these families may also be at high risk of intestinal parasites, low socioeconomic status and lack of immunisations.

Changing cultural patterns

Although families are more mobile today than formerly, cultural values and characteristics remain constant. Knowing some of the basic norms and taboos of different cultural groups is important as it allows you to understand and accept different practices of families. It also helps you understand the family's value system and the degree of support family members are apt to have available.

Poverty tends to be a problem for non-dominant (minority) ethnic groups. Characteristic responses that are sometimes described as cultural limitations are actually the consequences of poverty—for example, a mother seeking medical care for her child late in the course of an illness or late in pregnancy for herself is just as apt to be a financial influence as a cultural one.

Fly-in fly-out (FIFO) families

Australia has a growing fly-in fly-out (FIFO) or drive-in drive-out (DIDO) workforce driven predominantly by the mining boom. This has associated impacts on lifestyles of the workers and their families and the communities where they live and work. These families have healthy functionality when there is a balanced work/family roster. Parenting can be challenging, especially for the parent at home as they function in a solo role then adjust to periods of co-parenting. The emphasis is on them to provide the physical, emotional and intellectual needs of the children without support of the partner. Potential impacts on the children include increased behaviour problems, more episodes of school bullying and increased pressure to succeed academically. It can also have positive effects on the children as they have more time at home with the FIFO parent. Communication is a crucial component of the effectiveness of the FIFO family. They need to be able to communicate regularly, privately, spontaneously and in an effective manner. The greatest challenge comes with childrearing and conflict over this issue, including daily routine and solo parenting that then changes to co-parenting when the FIFO parent returns. For these children there are negative emotions related to parent absence and restrictions to lifestyle and activities. Strategies have been developed to assist FIFO families to enhance family functioning and further research continues into this family type (Meredith, Rush & Robinson, 2014).

Aboriginal and Torres Strait Islander families

Aboriginal and Torres Strait Islander peoples have a multifaceted family structure as extended family relationships are core to their kinship systems and family relationships. The Australian Institute of Health and Welfare has published a report on the health and welfare of this population (AIHW, 2011). This has a lot of specific information that relates to families and childrearing practices. The report *Working and Walking Together* (SNAICC, 2010) provides a wealth of information relating to Aboriginal and Torres Strait Islander families. This report has been developed with the aim to assist non-Indigenous staff and organisations to provide culturally appropriate programs and services.

Social relationships are very important in Aboriginal culture. People belong to both "their family and clan as well as their traditional land" (SNAICC, 2010, p. 13). This includes the value of sharing, sharing a house, sharing wages and possessions; thus a group ownership ideal prevails as opposed to individual ownership. Aboriginal and Torres Strait Islander communities are built on "strong cross-generational relationships and on having access to well-developed kinship networks" (SNAICC, 2010, p. 20). This community approach means different people have different roles in the "upbringing and overall wellbeing of children and young people" (SNAICC, 2010, pp. 20–21).

Aboriginal and Torres Strait Islander families generally reside in one dwelling with extended family members. The parent/s rely on the extended family to assist in childrearing. These family members play a major role in parenting and decision making; there is an emphasis on culture and kin as passed on from the extended family and particularly the elders of the family. They face the challenge of bridging two cultures, trying to maintain links to their heritage and ancestry while living and adapting to non-Aboriginal and non-Torres Strait Islander ways. This population has significantly poorer health outcomes and lower socioeconomic outcomes. Infant mortality is high, as are levels of domestic violence, abuse and neglect (ABS, 2014). Along with lower levels of education and income, these factors all have an impact on the ability to parent. This can mean that younger parents do not access services as they rely on the support, advice and role modelling of the extended family members. Cultural sensitivity and cultural competence are required to assist Aboriginal and Torres Strait Islander families to make informed decisions regarding parenting and childrearing practices (Australian Government, 2012; Raising Children Network, 2006–2014).

Māori families

The report *Changes to the Well Child/Tamariki Ora Framework* (MOHNZ, 2010b) provides a comprehensive discussion on the framework being phased in from 2010 for New Zealand families with young children 0–5 years of age. The focus is on improving Māori health outcomes while reducing the inequalities in health in this population. The framework aims to improve program delivery by reducing fragmentation and inconsistencies in the delivery of services to Māori and Pacific Islander children, as these children continue to be identified as priority groups due to poor health outcomes when compared to other New Zealand children.

Refugees, families in detention and asylum seekers

Refugees, asylum seekers and families in detention require specialised services to support them in all areas of daily living. Common challenges associated with these populations are adapting to a new country and a new culture, changing family roles and dynamics, as well as family conflict and separation from other family members who remain in their homeland (Australian Refugee Rights Alliance, 2011; NSW Refugee Health Service, 2012). Some of the issues to be aware of when working with these families include: geographical isolation; loss of family networks and support, and difficulty in forming new social networks; communication and language barriers; lack of knowledge of the healthcare system and lack of confidence and/or fear of using health services; lack of education about individual rights and responsibilities; distrust and/or fear of healthcare professionals; traumatic experiences and post-traumatic stress disorder; differences in cultural practices and beliefs, especially relating to childbirth and childrearing practices; intergenerational conflict, domestic violence and financial pressure (NSW Refugee Health Service, 2012; NSW Health, 2011). Trust needs to be built when working with these families as they face many challenges. Often health professionals require specialised training to work with these families.

Migrant families

A migrant family is defined as one where one key member was born overseas (ABS, 2013b). Australian data shows a doubling of these families from the 1991–2000 census to the 2001–2010 census. Just under half of these families have children. This is important to note as families with children require provision of government and community services for housing, health, education and welfare. Language can be a barrier as often migrant families have one or more members for whom English is not their main language. The family unit provides the cultural context and teaches the traditions of the culture. These families may have migrated as individuals, marrying afterwards, or have arrived as a family unit. Many leave family members behind. Fewer migrant families with children have one or both parents employed, thus impacting on financial security and other social benefits. Migrants from different parts of the world contribute to the makeup of Australia's multicultural profile. The 2011 census identified the top five countries of birth for migrants as being the United Kingdom, New Zealand, China, India and Italy (ABS, 2013b). In New Zealand the term Asian refers to a group of people with origins in the Asian continent, including Afghanistan, Japan, China and Indonesia. Other migrants originate from Middle Eastern, Latin American and African populations (MOHNZ, 2012a).

Increasing poverty

Poverty exists in all countries including Australia and New Zealand. Living below the "poverty line" has ongoing health consequences due to a myriad of reasons. The Australian Council of Social Service (2014, p. 7) measures poverty by household income; the accepted standard for the poverty line is a disposable income less than $400 per week for a single adult and $841 for a couple with two children. People who live below the poverty line cannot afford the essentials that most people take for granted and they miss out on opportunities and resources such as adequate health and dental care, housing, education, food and recreation. They also struggle to find employment, especially sole parents and those born overseas. In 2012, 1 in 7 adults and 1 in 6 children lived below the poverty line in Australia. The Office of the Children's Commissioner New Zealand (2010) has produced a report on children and young people's views and experiences of poverty.

Increasing numbers of homeless families

Although there is diversity in homeless families, as in all families, many homeless families are headed by women, and an increasing number are headed by pregnant and parenting adolescents. In Australia, children under the age of 18 comprise 27% of homeless people and the majority are in a family group. For many, it is a single mother (Homelessness Australia, 2013). The frequency of drug and alcohol abuse and severe mental health problems is greater among homeless families. Many mothers of homeless families experience domestic and family violence. Such families may not use healthcare providers or community agencies as effectively as other families because of their inexperience in dealing with bureaucracies or their lack of transportation and money.

Homeless children younger than 5 years old have decreased environmental stimulation and lack of exposure to normal play activities as well as restricted opportunities to form friendships. They tend to have more physical illnesses, such as anaemia, pneumonia, dental problems and restricted growth.

When caring for homeless families, remember that every day represents a struggle. Specific information pertaining to homelessness in Australia and New Zealand can be found in the following reports: *Homelessness and*

Poverty available from Homelessness Australia <http://homelessnessaustralia.org.au> and *Definitions of Homelessness* available from Statistics New Zealand <www.stats.govt.nz>.

Increasing divorce rate

Divorce is rarely easy for anyone involved. As parents are so emotionally entangled and their perceptions of their roles are changing drastically, they may be unable to give their children the support they need (Velez et al., 2011). This can leave marked long-term, negative effects on children. Indeed, the loss of a parent through divorce can sometimes be little different from the loss of a parent through death. Severing ties with grandparents or other relatives can also be difficult.

Children react in different ways to divorce depending on their developmental age and the explanations that parents give them. Divorce, as a rule, has three separate phases, and children's responses follow a course similar to grief. The first phase for parents is an antagonistic phase when parents realise they are no longer compatible. This can be an upsetting period for children because they do not understand what is happening. They may react with denial or anger and may believe that the impending divorce is their fault. The second phase is the actual separation stage. Everyone in the family is asked to take on an unfamiliar role and perhaps a new home and/or marked difference in financial arrangements. It is a time for grieving for the missing parent. Although it is comforting to be free from a house filled with tension and arguing, children may also wish they had their old life back. The third phase involves reshaping: parents may remarry; financial arrangements may stabilise. Children realise that their lives are permanently changed and they cannot go back to the time before the divorce.

Often children may manifest their grief through physical symptoms such as nausea or fatigue. Their school performance may suffer. Most children report that when the non-custodial parent remarries, it is one of the hardest moments for them because at that point they have to accept the divorce is final (Angarne-Lindberg & Wadsby, 2012). Children need an explanation as to why the divorce has occurred and assurance that it was not their fault. Parents may also need help in avoiding making any derogatory comments about the former partner. Although a former spouse may not have been a good marriage partner, they may have been a good parent and may well be missed and loved by the children.

Decreasing family size

The birth rate in Australia is 12.19 births per 1000 population and in New Zealand it is 13.4 (Index Mundi, 2014a, 2014b). Although small families mean fewer childcare requirements for parents, this also limits the parents' experience in childrearing, so the amount of childrearing counselling time per parent may increase. There is a steady trend towards an increasing number of families with no children in both Australia and New Zealand.

Increasing dual-parent employment

Many women of childbearing age work at a paid job outside the home. The implication for healthcare providers is that healthcare facilities need to schedule appointments at times when parents are free to attend. In addition, parents may need help to tailor administration of medicine to the times that they will be with the child to supervise the administration (e.g. before breakfast, following after-school childcare, and at bedtime) rather than just being told to administer the medication "three times a day".

Dual-parent employment has increased the number of children attending daycare centres and after-school programs (Copeland et al., 2012). This may have an impact on healthcare, because children attending daycare centres have an increased incidence of illnesses (see Chapter 31). School-aged children often return home from school before their parents return from work. These are known as "latchkey" or "self-care" children (see Chapter 32).

> ***What if...***
>
> Margo, who works outside her home from 9 a.m. to 5 p.m., needs to supervise Carey taking medication four times a day? At what times would you suggest he take the medication?

Increasing family responsibility for health monitoring

In the past, parents relied on healthcare providers to monitor their children's health and they accepted advice about healthcare without asking many questions or expressing opinions. Today, most parents take an active role in monitoring their children's health and participating in planning and goal setting. Changes in healthcare such as short hospital stays and an increased focus on health promotion and maintenance add to the increased responsibility for families to be knowledgeable healthcare consumers. Child health services are dependent on policy and strategy at local, national and international levels with varying levels of involvement from child and family health nurses. Practice can be delivered through many portals including community and outreach centres and hospitals, telemedicine and schools. The challenge for nurses is how to maintain the balance between individual and family needs and provide targeted broad population practice (Borrow, Munns & Henderson, 2011).

Increasing technology

Children in the 21st century are considered to be the digital generation (ABS, 2014). Family life today is loaded with technological innovations such as television, computers, mobile phones and iPods. Children use this technology constantly, both at school and at home for entertainment, socialising and educational purposes. This includes playing games, listening to and downloading music, as well as social networking and school work requirements. Such technology has opened up a world to children that they were never exposed to in previous years—a world that brings encyclopaedias of knowledge to their fingertips but can also bring the danger of predators. In Australia a report discussing children and use of the internet and the statistics associated with using the different technology estimated that 79% of children aged 5–14 reported using the internet, increasing with age (ABS, 2011). In 2010 New Zealand published a report summarising children and young people's physical activity and dietary behaviours. Television watching for children aged 5–14 years highlighted that these children watched two or more hours of television daily. The Raising Children Network website recommends limiting children's screen time to 1 hour per day for 2–5-year-olds and 2 hours per day for children over 5. Screen time can be defined as including TV, DVD, gaming consoles and computer time <http://raisingchildren.net.au>.

It is important for children to learn to live in a fast-paced world; however, parents need to be certain they are monitoring how fast the world is being presented to their children. Discussing the importance of blocking inappropriate television programs and limiting and/or monitoring viewing time are important. An additional danger of too much technology is that it can interfere with communication in a family. Technology has the potential to enrich children's lives, but it also may limit their ability to interact with others.

Increasing obesity, reduced exercise and fast foods

The level of exercise of families today is greatly reduced when compared with what families enjoyed in the past. Children are often driven to school. They spend their time after school playing computer games instead of playing active games. After-school programs are structured around desk work rather than exercise. Families are busy and fast food is so available, families fix fast-food lunches and dinners. Although this type of food solves the problem of time management, it does cause families to ingest more fat daily than may be good for them. In Australia in 2011, 25.1% of children aged between 2 and 17 were classified as overweight or obese (ABS, 2013a). In a survey conducted in New Zealand in 2012–2013, 1 in 9 children aged 2–14 were classified as obese, with a further 1 in 5 overweight. The childhood obesity rate has increased from 8% in 2006–2007 to 11% in 2012–2013 (MOHNZ, 2014b). Childhood obesity can lead to long-term health problems such as diabetes, sleep apnoea and chronic tiredness as well as decreased self-esteem (Department of Health and Ageing, 2010). OECD obesity rates from 2011 show New Zealand as having the third highest rates of obesity of OECD countries, with Australia marginally behind on the fourth highest; statistics that need to be addressed in the light of the adverse health effects of obesity (Statistics New Zealand, 2013b).

It is important to remember that children are shaped not only by their family environment but also by their neighbourhood and wider environment. If children feel safe then this has a positive impact on their health and wellbeing. This can be evidenced by parents and carers encouraging children to engage in outdoor activities when they perceive the environment to be safe (AIHW, 2013).

Bullying

Bullying encompasses harassing, humiliating, embarrassing, tormenting, threatening and intimidating behaviour as well as picking on someone else and spreading rumours (Raising Children Network, 2010). Bullying is intentional and can involve physical, verbal or psychological harm. It can start as teasing that escalates, including extortion of money and possessions (Lyness, 2013). Bullying involves three core concepts: deliberate intent to harm; power imbalance between the perpetrator and the victim; and repeated behaviour. This behaviour can include misusing photographs and personal information, breaking up friendships, ostracising individuals and setting up fake accounts in the name of someone else.

Bullying has a detrimental effect on a child's safety and self-worth; in severe cases it has been linked to suicide and school shootings (Lyness, 2013). It is very hard to find statistics on the amount of bullying and how many suicides are related to bullying; however, research has shown anecdotal evidence of this. Cyberbullying has emerged as another option to engage in bullying behaviours. This can often be anonymous and is done through many social media forums (mobile phone, text messages, email and social networking sites such as facebook) to cause psychological harm (BoysTown, 2010).

Bullying for children and young people predominantly occurs in a school environment. An Australian mental health and wellbeing initiative known as Kids Matter has developed a series of programs to combat the rising incidence of bullying (Australian Government, 2012). It is set in primary schools and early childhood education and care services and helps these places and people to support children's mental health needs. It is important to assist children to deal with bullying, to discuss it and to discuss strategies to use to deal with it and who they can go to for assistance.

Increasing family violence

An alarming statistic in today's families is that the incidence and reports of family violence (both child and intimate partner) are common (AIFS, 2014b; MOHNZ, 2011). Detecting violence begins with the awareness that it does occur and that it has a cumulative effect. Both intimate partner and child abuse are discussed in Chapter 55. In Australia there is a national framework for protecting Australia's children (AIFS, 2014) that describes a shared approach to child protection as being everyone's business. The Australian and New Zealand governments have a statutory responsibility for protecting children from abuse and neglect and many programs have been developed to address this issue and family violence. Notifications of suspected or actual abuse and neglect have been increasing for several years; this may be due to more than one notification per child, an increase in awareness reflecting changes in legislation and public awareness (AIFS, 2014).

ASSESSMENT OF FAMILY STRUCTURE AND FUNCTION

Family characteristics can be assessed on a variety of levels and in varying degrees of detail. The type of family data collected and the method of collection should match the way in which the assessment data will be used. General characteristics of family type and functioning can be assessed using observation and general history questions. If more detailed information about family environment and roles is required, using an assessment tool specifically developed for that purpose is most effective.

Developmental surveillance, screening and monitoring

Child and family health services are delivered through a series of scheduled ongoing contacts with children aged from birth to school entry; this age differs between jurisdictions in Australia and New Zealand. The visits coincide with critical developmental periods to maximise parental guidance and to support developmental surveillance and health monitoring of the well child. Many different tools can be used to assess a child's health, development and wellbeing.

A key function of child and family nurses and midwives is the use of screening and assessment tools to assist in early identification of children who require monitoring or referral. Visits with midwives and child and family health nurses facilitate the opportunity to engage in and discuss developmental progression and concerns and promote wellbeing and health through observations and assessment in consultation and partnership with the parents and family members (AHMAC, 2011; MOHNZ, 2014a). Surveillance and health monitoring include a physical examination: head-to-toe physical assessment, growth assessment (height, weight and head circumference), vision, hearing and language assessment. Vision is targeted with school children aged 4 years and over for visual acuity and hearing screening is conducted on each newborn baby. Oral health is assessed through a visual examination such as the 'Lift the lip' campaign. Some populations have targeted surveillance and monitoring such as otitis media screening in the Aboriginal and Torres Strait Islander population to optimise speech and language development and decrease the amount of hearing loss in this population (AHMAC, 2011).

Australian tools that have been validated and that are used for general developmental monitoring are based on both parental reporting and direct contact and assessment by child and family health nurses. These include:

- Parents' Evaluation of Developmental Status (PEDS) for 0–8 years (see Appendix D)
- Ages and Stages Questionnaire (ASQ) for 3–60 months
- Brigance Screens for 21–90 months
- Child Development Inventory (CDI) for 3–72 months.

For monitoring child social and emotional wellbeing they include:

- Ages and Stages Social Emotional Questionnaire for 1 month–5 years
- Parents' Evaluation of Development Status (PEDS) for 0–8 years (see Appendix D)
- Neonatal Behavioural Assessment Scale for 0–2 months
- Strengths and Difficulties Questionnaire for 4–12 years
- Paediatric Symptom Checklist for 4–18 years
- NCAST Parent–Child Interaction Assessment Scales (Feeding and Teaching) for feeding 0–12 months and teaching 0–36 months
- Brigance Screens for 0–7 years
- Modified Checklist for Autism in Toddlers (M-CHAT) for 16–30 months (AHMAC, 2011, p. 22–23).

New Zealand has a Well Child/Tamariki Ora health book similar to the NSW blue book (see Fig. 3.3). This has a similar focus with 12 identified critical periods for a health

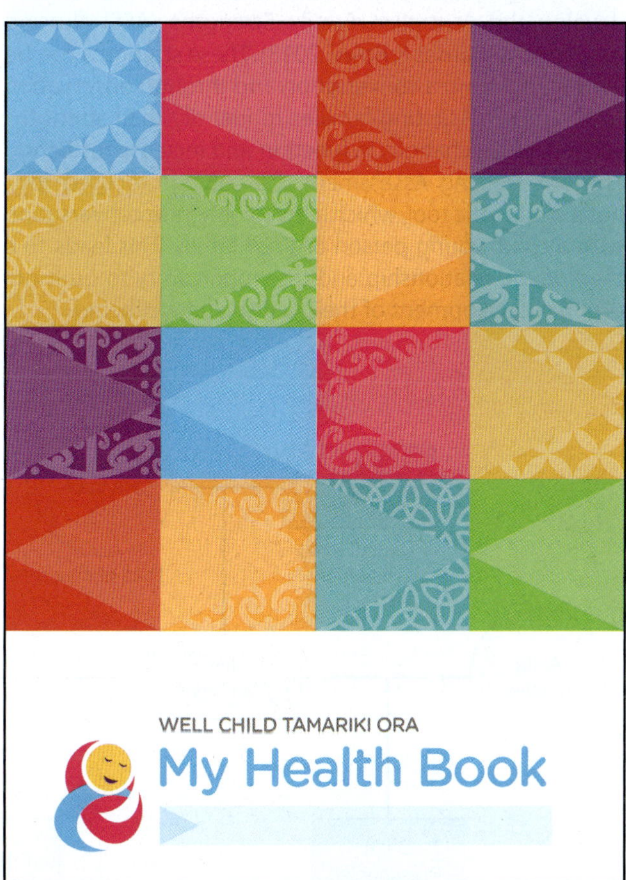

FIGURE 3.3 My Health Book. (© New Zealand Ministry of Health)

check between 0 and 5 years. The checks focus on assessment, health education, advice, family care and support and provide opportunities to discuss child health and development with families (MOHNZ, 2014a). New Zealand also offers universal services for child health surveillance and health monitoring. These include:

- Immunisations
- Vision and hearing
- Before school check
- Oral health
- Well Child Tamariki Ora.

These tools are used in conjunction with:

- Strengths and Difficulties Questionnaire (SDQ) (Youth*in*mind, 2014)
- Parents' Evaluation of Developmental Status (PEDS) (MOHNZ, 2012b; see Appendix D).

Family strengths assessment

Family strengths assessment, as discussed in Chapter 1, is an approach to guide nursing practice to facilitate empowerment, self-efficacy and hope with families (Gottlieb, 2014). It focuses on what the family can do and does best to assist them to deal with problems, rather than what they can't do. The eight core values of communication, togetherness, shared activities, affection, support, acceptance, commitment and resilience are the qualities used to develop the Australian Family Strengths (AFS) Nursing Assessment (Barnes & Rowe, 2013). These strengths can be identified during a conversation and through observation with families. Assisting families to identify their strengths can introduce changes in function and increase resilience. The AFS Nursing Assessment is a solution-focused tool, not a diagnostic tool, which aims to generate conversation with a child, young person or their family. This leads to a therapeutic relationship and the opportunity to promote optimal development of their health and wellbeing.

The well family

Assessment of psychosocial family wellness requires measurement of how the family relates and interacts as a unit, including communication patterns, bonding, roles and role relationships, division of tasks and activities, governance, decision making, problem solving and leadership within the family unit. Assessment also looks at how the family relates to the outside community.

The **genogram,** a diagram that details family structure, provides information about the family's history and the roles of various family members over time, usually through several generations. It can provide a basis for discussion and analysis of family interaction (see Fig. 3.4). Another aspect of family assessment is to document the "fit" of a family in its community. This is done by means of an **eco-map,** a diagram of family and community relationships (see Fig. 3.5). To construct such a map, first draw a circle in the centre to represent the family. Around the outside draw circles that represent the family's community contacts such as church, school, neighbours or other organisations. Families that "fit" well into their community usually have many outside circles or community contacts.

Although family assessment is best done when a family is managing well, assessment of a family often first occurs when a family is in crisis. The way families react to a crisis depends largely on the particular crisis, their past experiences with problem solving, their perception of the event and the resources available to them to help solve the problem. As a crisis can change a family's perceptions and the resources available to them, renewed assessment is necessary at the end of the crisis to see how the family has weathered the impact.

Listing a family's strengths and coping abilities as well as its possible challenges strengthens a family. It brings out insights and better prepares family members to cope with their current level of stress. Box 3.2 provides practical suggestions to help families endure periods of stress.

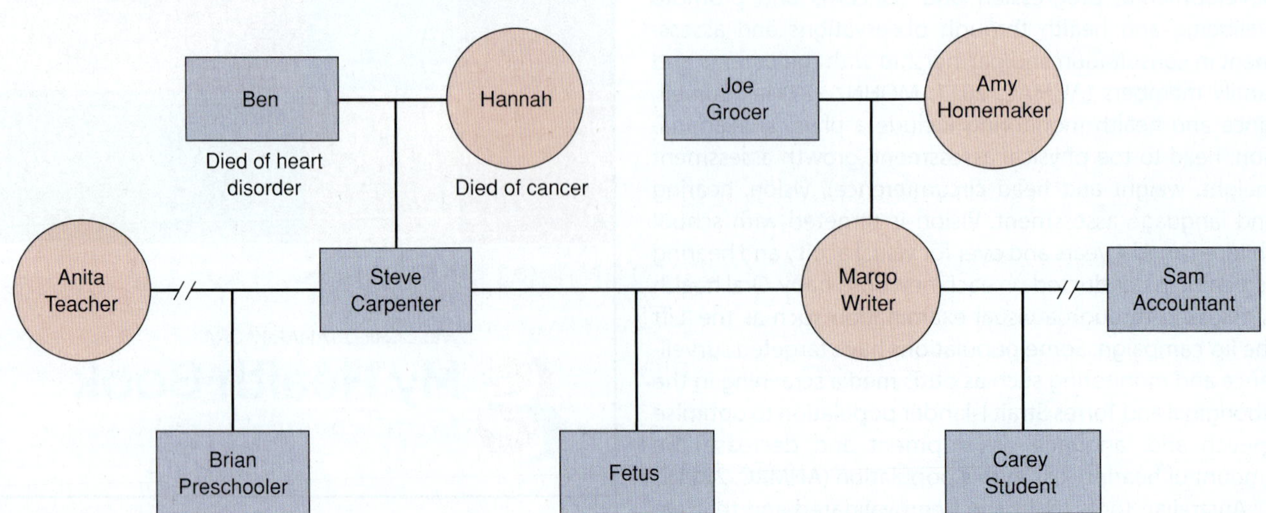

FIGURE 3.4 A Hanovan family genogram showing three generations. Males are shown by squares and females by circles.

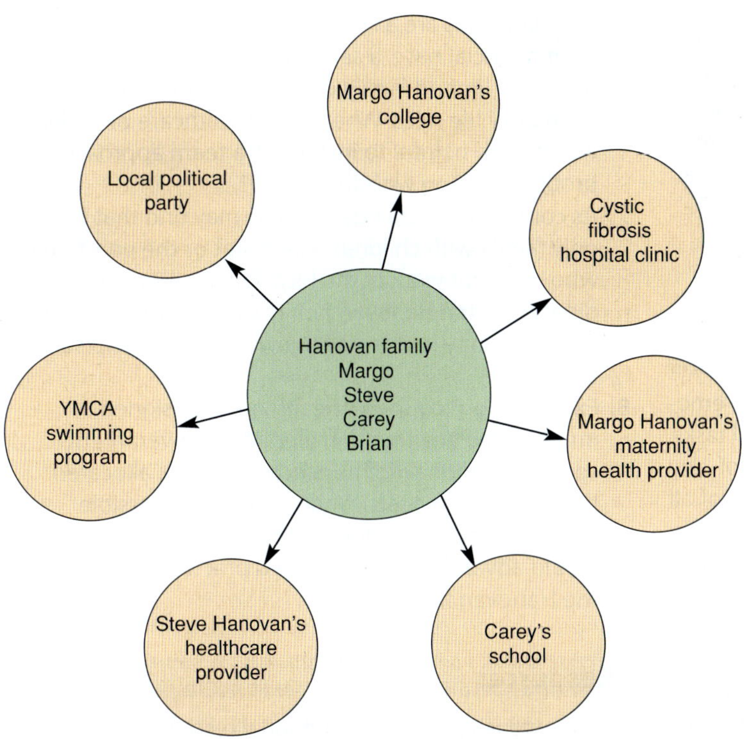

FIGURE 3.5 An ecomap of the Hanovan family's relationship to its community. The family members are shown in the centre circle; the outer circles show community contacts.

BOX 3.2 ✻ Focus on family teaching

Tips for reducing family stress

Q. Suppose Steve Hanovan tells you he is worried because the tension level in his family is growing. He asks you, "How can my family better manage stress?"

A. Managing stress calls for interventions specific to each family, but some general suggestions are:

1. Recognise that stress levels differ from person to person. Because one person is not upset by some condition does not mean that another person will not be. On the other hand, if a situation does not annoy a person, that person should not feel that he or she has to react to it just because someone else does.
2. Anticipate life events and plan for them to the extent possible. Anticipatory guidance will not totally prepare you for a coming event but will at least serve notice that distress over the situation is normal.
3. Face a situation as honestly as possible. As a rule, knowing the exact nature of a threat is less stressful than a "something-is-out-there" feeling. However, do not feel compelled to face intense threats, such as a serious complication of pregnancy or a fatal illness in a child, until you have had time to mobilise your defences, or you can feel overwhelmed.
4. Learn to change those things you cannot accept and accept those things you cannot change. Trial and error is often required to determine the difference.
5. Often a total change is unnecessary; a simple modification in one thing will be enough to make a difference.
6. Try to describe why you feel so stressed. Almost nothing limits the extent of a threat more than being able to describe it accurately. Detailing a problem is the beginning of problem solving.
7. Reach out for support. When you are under stress, it is easy to be so involved in the problem that you do not realise that people around you want to help. Sometimes people closest to you are under the same threat and so are no longer able to offer support. When this happens, you might have to call on second- or third-level support people (family or community) for help.
8. Reach out to give support when others are being threatened. Survival is a collaborative function of social groups; a favour offered now can be returned when you are in need at a later date.
9. Try to reduce the number of stressors that are coming at you by turning off television, dimming the lights and spending time with just your inner self.
10. Ask yourself if you really need to accomplish all the tasks that are piling up around you. Does the garage need to be cleaned this week?
11. Remember that unintentional injuries increase when people are under stress. A person worrying about a complication of pregnancy, for example, is more apt to have a car accident than a person who is stress-free. Children are more apt to poison themselves when the family is under stress because parents are more apt to leave medication on benches during this time.
12. Action feels good during stress because doing something brings a sense of control over feelings of helplessness and disorganisation. Action often is so satisfying that people do things such as write threatening letters or shout harmful remarks that they later regret. Channel your energy into therapeutic action (such as going for a long walk and quietly reflecting) instead.
13. Do not rush decisions or make final adaptive outcomes to a stressful situation. As a rule, major decisions should be delayed at least 6 weeks after an event; 6 months is even better.

What if...

Your assessment of one child who is ready for hospital discharge shows that his family has multiple connections with the community, but the assessment of Carey and the Hanovan family shows only the hospital as a connection? Which family might need more discharge planning?

Key points for review

- A family is a group of people who share a common emotional bond and perform certain interrelated social tasks.
- As families work as a unit, the unmet needs of any member can spread to become the unmet needs of all family members.
- Common types of families include nuclear, extended, single-parent, blended, cohabitation, gay and lesbian, foster and adopted families.
- Common family tasks are physical maintenance, socialisation of family members, allocation of resources, maintenance of order, division of labour, reproduction, placement of members into the larger society, and maintenance of motivation and morale.
- Common life stages of families are marriage; early childbearing; families with preschool, school-aged and adolescent children; launching stage; middle-year families; and the family in retirement.
- Changes in patterns of family life that are occurring are increased mobility; changing cultural patterns; social problems such as abuse, homelessness and poverty; increased divorce; reduced family size; dual-parent employment; increasing family responsibility for health monitoring; the addition of technology; and increasing obesity, reduced exercise and fast foods.
- Families with Aboriginal, Torres Strait Islander and Māori backgrounds, and refugees and asylum seekers have particular issues and needs that should be considered.
- Considering a family as a unit helps in planning nursing care that meets the family's total needs.
- Families exist within communities; assessment of the community and the family's place in the community yields further information on family functioning and abilities.
- Families do not always function at their highest level during periods of crisis; reassessing them during a period of stability may reveal a stronger family than appeared on first assessment.

CASE STUDY QUESTIONS

5. Why is this a challenging time for the Hanovans? Would their needs change if they were an extended family? A single-parent family? A cohabitation family?
6. The Hanovans are a family under stress because of a poor financial base, a serious and chronic family illness, and limited family communication stemming from busy life roles. What other healthcare providers would it be helpful to include in a team approach for problem solving with this family?
7. As communities change, a family may find that it is the only family with children on a street or the only family who does not work at the local factory. What if you discovered the Hanovan family was "out of sync" with its community in this way? How could you help such a family?
8. Examine your country's health goals designed to improve the health of families. Most government-sponsored money for nursing research is allocated based on these goals. What would be a possible research topic to explore pertinent to these goals that would advance evidence-based practice in relation to the Hanovan family?

Resources

For an extensive range of additional resources to enhance teaching and learning and to facilitate understanding of this chapter, please see the text's accompanying website located on thePoint at http://thepoint.lww.com.

References

Adoption Australia, accessed 8 December 2014, <http://adoptionaustralia.com.au>.

Adoption Option, accessed 8 December 2014, <http://adoptionoption.org.nz>.

Angarne-Lindberg, T. & Wadsby, M. (2012). Psychiatric and somatic health in relation to experience of parental divorce in childhood. *International Journal of Social Psychiatry*, *58*(1), 16–25.

Australian Bureau of Statistics (ABS). (2011). Family characteristics, Australia 2009–2010, Cat. no. 4442.0, accessed 7 January 2015, <www.abs.gov.au/ausstats/abs@.nsf/Latestproducts/4442.0Main%20Features22009-10?opendocument&tabname=Summary&prodno=4442.0&issue=2009-10&num=&view=>.

Australian Bureau of Statistics (ABS). (2013a). Australian health survey: updated results 2011–2012. Overweight and obesity, Cat. no. 4364.0.55.003, accessed 7 January 2015, <www.abs.gov.au/ausstats/abs@.nsf/Lookup/33C64022ABB5ECD5CA257B8200179437?opendocument>.

Australian Bureau of Statistics (ABS). (2013b). Perspectives on migrants, Cat. no. 3416.0, accessed 7 January 2015, <www.abs.gov.au/ausstats/abs@.nsf/mf/3416.0>.

Australian Bureau of Statistics (ABS). (2014). Australian Social Trends June 2011, Cat. no. 4102.0, accessed 7 January 2015, <www.abs.gov.au/AUSSTATS/abs@.nsf/mf/4102.0>.

Australian Council of Social Service (ACOSS). (2014). *Poverty in Australia 2014*, accessed 7 January 2015, <http://acoss.org.au/images/uploads/ACOSS_Poverty_in_Australia_2014.pdf>.

Australian Government. (2012). About kidsMatter, accessed 7 January 2015, <www.kidsmatter.edu.au/families/about-kidsmatter>.

Australian Government. (2013). Mychild website: programs for Indigenous families, accessed 7 January 2015, <www.mychild.gov.au>.

Australian Health Ministers' Advisory Council (AHMAC). (2011). *National Framework for Universal Child and Family Health Services.* Canberra: Department of Health and Aging.

Australian Institute of Family Studies (AIFS). (2012). *Past and Present Adoptions in Australia,* accessed 7 January 2015, <www.aifs.gov.au/institute/pubs/factssheets/2012/fs201202/fs201202.html>.

Australian Institute of Family Studies (AIFS). (2014a). Family facts and figures, accessed 7 January 2015, <www.aifs.gov.au/institute/info/charts/index.html>.

Australian Institute of Family Studies (AIFS). (2014b). Child abuse and neglect statistics fact sheet, accessed 7 January 2015, <www.aifs.gov.au/cfca/pubs/factsheets/a142086/>.

Australian Institute of Health and Welfare (AIHW). (2011). The health and welfare of Australia's Aboriginal and Torres Strait Islander people: An overview 2011, accessed 7 January 2015, <www.aihw.gov.au/publication-detail/?id=10737418989>.

Australian Institute of Health and Welfare (AIHW). (2013). Families and communities, accessed 7 January 2015, <www.aihw.gov.au/child-health/families-and-communities/>.

Australian Refugee Rights Alliance. (2011). Refugee families at risk in resettlement, accessed 7 January 2015, <www.arra.org.au/uploads/documents/2010_ARRA_Families_at_Risk.pdf>.

Barnes, M. & Rowe, J. (Eds). (2013). *Child, Youth and Family Health: Strengthening Communities* (2nd ed.). Sydney: Churchill Livingstone Elsevier.

Borrow, S., Munns, A. & Henderson, S. (2011). Community-based child health nurses: An exploration of current practice. *Contemporary Nurse, 40*(1), 71–86.

BoysTown (2010). Kids helpline information sheet: Bullying, harassment and physical violence, accessed 7 January 2015, <www.kidshelp.com.au>.

Chapman, R., Watkins, R., Zappia, T., et al. (2012). Second-level hospital health professionals' attitudes to lesbian, gay, bisexual and transgender parents seeking health for their children. *Journal of Clinical Nursing, 21*(5–6), 880–887.

Cherlin, A. J. (2012). *Public and Private Families* (2nd ed.). New York: McGraw-Hill.

Children's Hospital Australasia (2010a). *Charter on the Rights of Children and Young People in Healthcare Services in Australia.* Canberra: CHA/AWCH.

Children's Hospitals Australasia (2010b). *Charter on the Rights of Tamariki Children and Rangatahi Young People in Healthcare Services in New Zealand.* New Zealand: CHA/Paediatric Society.

Copeland, K. A., Sherman, S. N., Kendeigh, C. A., et al. (2012). Societal values and policies may curtail preschool children's physical activity in child care centers. *Pediatrics, 129*(2), 265–274.

Dare, J. S. (2011). Transitions in midlife women's lives: Contemporary experiences. *Health Care of Women International, 32*(2), 111–133.

Department of Health and Ageing. (2010). *Overweight and Obesity in Australia,* accessed 7 January 2015, <www.health.gov.au/internet/healthyactive/publishing.nsf/content/overweight-obesity>.

Duvall, E. M. & Miller, B. (1990). *Marriage and Family Development.* Philadelphia: Lippincott Williams & Wilkins.

Gottlieb, L. (2014). Strengths-based nursing. A holistic approach to care, grounded in eight core values. *Australian Journal of Nursing, 114*(8), 24–32.

Homelessness Australia. (2013). Homelessness and children fact sheet, accessed 2 December 2014, <http://homelessnessaustralia.org.au/index.php/about-homelessness/fact-sheets>.

Index Mundi. (2014a). Australia birth rate, accessed 7 January 2015, <www.indexmundi.com/australia/birth_rate.html>.

Index Mundi. (2014b). New Zealand birth rate, accessed 7 January 2015, <www.indexmundi.com/new_zealand/birth_rate.html>.

Jones, V. F. (2012). Comprehensive health evaluation of the newly adopted child. *Pediatrics, 129*(1), e214–e223.

Keene, J. R., Prokos, A. H. & Held, B. (2012). Grandfather caregivers: Race and ethnic differences in poverty. *Sociological Inquiry, 82*(1), 49–77.

Kubiak, S. P., Kasiborski, N., Karim, N., et al. (2012). Does subsequent criminal justice involvement predict foster care and termination of parental rights for children born to Incarcerated women? *Social Work in Public Health, 27*(1–2), 129–147.

Lambert, V., Glacken, M. & McCarron, M. (2010). Communication between children and health professionals in a child hospital setting: A child transitional communication model. *Journal of Advanced Nursing, 67*(3), 569–582.

Lyness, D. (2013). Helping kids deal with bullies. Kidshealth, accessed 7 January 2015, <http://kidshealth.org/parent/emotions/behavior/bullies.html>.

Meredith, V., Rush, P. & Robinson, E. (2014). Fly-in fly-out workforce practices in Australia: The effects on children and family relationships. CFCA paper no. 19. Canberra: Australian Institute of Family Studies.

Ministry of Social Development, Area of Child, youth and family. (n.d). Adoption, accessed 7 January 2015, <www.cyf.govt.nz/adoption/index.html>.

Ministry of Health New Zealand (MOHNZ). (2010a). A national survey of children and young people's physical activity and dietary behaviours in New Zealand: 2008/09 key findings, accessed 7 January 2015, <www.health.govt.nz/publication/national-survey-children-and-young-peoples-physical-activity-and-dietary-behaviours-new-zealand-2008>.

Ministry of Health New Zealand (MOHNZ). (2010b). Changes to the well child/tamariki ora framework, accessed 7 January 2015, <www.health.govt.nz/publication/changes-well-child-tamariki-ora-framework>.

Ministry of Health New Zealand (MOHNZ). (2011). Family violence. Part one: Why should health services respond to victims of family violence. accessed 7 January 2015, <www.health.govt.nz/our-work/preventative-health-wellness/family-violence/establishing-vip-programme/part-one-why-should-health-services-respond-victims-family-violence>.

Ministry of Health New Zealand (MOHNZ). (2012a). Asian and migrant health, accessed 7 January 2015, <www.health.govt.nz/our-work/populations/asian-and-migrant-health>.

Ministry of Health New Zealand (MOHNZ). (2012b). New Zealand's maternity and child health services: Preconception to 6 years, accessed 7 January 2015, <www.health.govt.nz/our-work/life-stages/child-health/new-zealands-maternity-and-child-health-services-preconception-6-years>.

Ministry of Health New Zealand (MOHNZ). (2014a). About the well child/tamariki ora health checks, accessed 7 January 2015, <www.health.govt.nz/your-health/services-and-support/health-care-services/well-child-tamariki-ora/about-well-child-tamariki-ora-health-checks>.

Ministry of Health New Zealand (MOHNZ). (2014b). Obesity data and stats, accessed 7 January 2015, <www.health.govt.nz/nz-health-statistics/health-statistics-and-data-sets/obesity-data-and-stats>.

New South Wales (NSW) Health. (2011). Refugee health plan 2011–2016, accessed 7 January 2015, <www.health.nsw.gov.au/policies/pd/2011/PD2011_014.html>.

NSW Refugee Health Service. (2010). Working with refugee families and children, accessed 6 February 2012, <www.mncdgp.org.au/system/ files/Working%20with%20Refugees%20Resource.pdf>.

NSW Refugee Health Service. (2012). Aiming to improve and protect the health of refugees in NSW. NSW Ministry of Health, accessed 7 January 2015, <www.swslhd.nsw.gov.au/refugee/>.

Office of the Children's Commissioner New Zealand. (2010). "This is how I see it." Children, young people and young adults' views and experiences of poverty, accessed 7 January 2015, <www.occ.org.nz/assets/Uploads/Reports/Poverty/This-is-how-I-see-it.pdf>.

O'Toole, G. (2012). *Communication. Core Interpersonal Skills for Health Professionals* (2nd ed.). Sydney: Elsevier.

Parker, J. A., Mandleco, B., Olsen Roper, S., et al. (2011). Religiosity, spirituality, and marital relationships of parents raising a typically developing child or a child with a disability. *Journal of Family Nursing, 2*(17), 82–104.

Raising Children Network. (2006–2014). The Australian parenting website: Indigenous parents, accessed 7 January 2015, <www.raisingchildren.net.au/articles/indigenous_parents.html>.

Randall, D., Munns, A. & Shields, L. (2013). Next steps: Towards child-focused nursing. *Neonatal, Paediatric and Child Health Nursing, 16*(2), 15–20.

Roeber, B. J., Tober, C. L., Bolt, D. M et al. (2012). Gross motor development in children adopted from orphanage settings. *Developmental Medicine and Child Neurology, 54*(6), 527–531.

Secretariat of National Aboriginal and Islander Child Care Inc. (SNAICC). (2010). Working and Walking Together, accessed 7 January 2015, <www.snaicc.asn.au/tools-resources/dsp-default-e.cfm?loadref=150&txnid=983&txnctype=resource&txncstype=document>.

Shields, L., Zhou, H., Pratt, J., Taylor, M., Hunter, J. & Pascoe, E. (2012). Family-centred care for hospitalised children aged 0–12 years. *Cochrane Database of Systematic Reviews,* Issue 10. Art. No.: CD004811.

Statistics New Zealand (nd). Family type, accessed 7 January 2015, <www.stats.govt.nz/methods/classifications-and-standards/classification-related-stats-standards/family-type/glossary-and-references.aspx>.

Statistics New Zealand. (2013a). Census quickstats about families and households, accessed 7 January 2015, <www.stats.govt.nz/Census/2013-census/profile-and-summary-reports/qstats-families-households/definitions-data.aspx>.

Statistics New Zealand, (2013b). NZ social indicators - obesity, accessed 7 January 2015, <www.stats.govt.nz/browse_for_stats/snapshots-of-nz>.

Stein-Parbury, J. (2013). *Patient and Person: Interpersonal Skills in Nursing* (5th ed.). Sydney: Churchill Livingstone Elsevier.

Stuart, M. & Melling, S. (2014). Understanding nurses' and parents' perceptions of family-centred care. *Nursing Children and Young People, 26*(7), 16–20.

Taussig, H. N., Culhane, S. E., Garrido, E., et al. (2012). RCT of a mentoring and skills group program: Placement and permanency outcomes for foster youth. *Pediatrics, 130*(1), e33–e39.

United Nations (UN). (1989). *Convention on the Rights of the Child.* New York: United Nations General Assembly.

Velez, C. E., Wolchik, S. A., Tein., J. Y., et al. (2011). Protecting children from the consequences of divorce: A longitudinal study of the effects of parenting on children's coping processes. *Child Development, 82*(1), 244–257.

Youth*inmind*. (2014). SDQ Information for researchers and professionals about the Strengths & Difficulties Questionnaires, accessed 12 January 2015, <www.sdqinfo.org>.

Suggested readings

Association for The Wellbeing of Children In Healthcare <www.awch.org.au>.

Australian Institute of Health and Welfare (AIHW). (2013). Overweight and obese, accessed 26 November 2014 <www.aihw.gov.au/overweight-and-obesity/>.

Carter, B., Coad, J., Bray, L. et al. (2012). Homebased care for special healthcare needs: Community children's nursing services. *Nursing Research, 61*(4), 260–268.

Munns, A., Hegney, D. & Walker, R. (2014). Effectiveness and experiences of families participating in peer led parenting support programs delivered as home visiting programs and the meaning they attribute to these support programs: A systematic review protocol. *JBI Database of Systematic Reviews & Implementation Reports, 12*(3), 1–13.

Social and Emotional Wellbeing: Bullying at School <www.abs.gov.au/AUSSTATS/abs@.nsf/lookup/4704.0Chapter460Oct+2010>.

Watts, R., Zhou, H., Shields, L., Taylor, M., Munns, A. & Ngune, I. (2014). Family-centred care for hospitalized children aged 0–12 years: A systematic review of qualitative studies. *JBI Database of Systematic Reviews & Implementation Reports, 12*(7), 204–283.

Chapter 4

Promoting family health in the community

This chapter discusses the primary healthcare (PHC) model of health service delivery and the role of community-based nursing in the prevention of disease and the promotion of health and wellbeing.

LEARNING OBJECTIVES

After mastering the contents of this chapter, you should be able to:

1. Discuss primary healthcare (PHC) as a social model of care for contemporary families and communities.
2. Develop an understanding of family functioning abilities.
3. Discuss the varied role of the nurse providing holistic healthcare for families in the community.
4. Critically analyse the importance of undertaking family and community needs assessment.
5. Develop an understanding of the role of health education in promoting health.
6. Develop an understanding of the provision of health services based on a PHC model.
7. Identify areas of community nursing that could benefit from additional nursing research or application of evidence-based practice.

KEY TERMS

- community
- community assessment
- community engagement
- cultural competence
- determinants of health
- family assessment
- family-centred policies
- health literacy
- health promotion
- primary healthcare (PHC)
- vulnerable individuals or families

CASE STUDY

Aata is 23 years of age and of Māori descent. Her partner works in the mining industry, which requires him to work away from home for 3-week periods, with a 7-day break in between. The family live in a remote rural community and have no family nearby. Aata has recently had a baby (now 6 weeks old) and also has an older child aged 4 years. The older child has asthma and has had several acute episodes recently. Aata has been feeling lonely and isolated since the birth of her baby and is finding it difficult to manage both children, especially when her partner is away.

CASE STUDY QUESTIONS

1. How will a health assessment assist to improve the wellbeing of this family?
2. What are the immediate risk factors for this family?
3. What is the main focus of a primary healthcare (PHC) approach to families such as Aata's?

Contemporary societal and economic changes have presented new challenges for nurses working in communities. The pressure of living in a community isolated from support systems, with the stress of meeting financial requirements, impacts on the health and wellbeing of each family member. The role of the community nurse now requires a thorough understanding of individual and family health assessment and the importance of community development strategies designed to support and improve the health of individuals and families.

PRIMARY HEALTHCARE, A SOCIAL MODEL OF HEALTH FOR FAMILIES AND COMMUNITIES

"The world is ageing. With people living longer and fewer children being born, the absolute number of older people is increasing. Today, worldwide, there are some 600 million persons aged 60 and over; this total will double by 2025 and will reach virtually two billion by 2050 when there will be more people aged 60 and over than children under the age of 15. The vast majority of older persons will be living in developing countries, which are often least prepared to meet the challenges of the rapidly ageing population" (World Health Organization [WHO], 2004). Australia and New Zealand are part of a global move away from a "medical" model of healthcare delivery to a **primary healthcare (PHC)** model, with an emphasis on health equality and the delivery of healthcare closer to where people live (Australian Government Department of Health, 2013; New Zealand Ministry of Health, 2001). This realignment of health service provision has been promoted by the WHO since the 1970s in response to:

- Rapid social and economic growth resulting in an increase in the number of elderly people who are prone to degenerative and chronic conditions such as dementia and depression (WHO, 2004)
- New patterns of illnesses brought on by social and economic factors, many resulting in an increase in chronic illness such as childhood obesity, type 2 diabetes and mental health problems
- Large numbers of people with minimal or no healthcare because they cannot afford it or are unable to access it
- An increase in public concern about access to and the quality, cost and fragmentation of healthcare (WHO, 2008; New Zealand Ministry of Health, 2014a).

The WHO Declaration of the Alma-ata in 1978 was the first step in the creation of a PHC movement, which energised health professionals, service providers, community and government organisations. There is a sense that the Alma-ata values have changed the way healthcare systems operate, and real progress is being made to harness the potential of other sectors (WHO, 2008 cited in Keleher & MacDougall, 2011). The WHO goal for PHC is to provide better health for everyone. It is envisaged that countries can achieve this by addressing the following five key areas:

- Reducing exclusion and social disparities in health (universal coverage reforms)
- Organising health services around people's needs and expectations (service delivery reforms)
- Integrating health into all sectors (public policy reforms)
- Pursuing collaborative models of policy dialogue (leadership reforms)
- Increasing stakeholder participation (WHO, 2015).

The PHC model utilises an interdisciplinary approach to individual and family care. However, it has been acknowledged that community nurses have a pivotal role in the re-shaped healthcare service, with particular focus on social justice, equity and health promotion. The escalating need for reform in healthcare and the economic pressures for cost-effective, multidisciplinary, high-quality care place nurses in a unique position to make changes in the community healthcare system (Pender, Murdaugh & Parsons, 2014). The reorientation of such services includes a health promotion and education approach, emphasising individual and community wellness rather than a disease-management focus. Berman and colleagues (2012) describe **health promotion** as being behaviour directed towards developing wellbeing and actualising human health potential.

CASE STUDY QUESTION

4. What key factors in Aata's circumstances would be addressed by a PHC approach to the family's situation?
   a. Aata's and her son's asthmatic condition
   b. Assessing her mental health status after the birth of her baby
   c. Her loneliness and her living environment
   d. All of the above

Aata would require a holistic approach to her health needs. The nurse can provide asthma education and medication compliance checks. As well, the nurse would have a local knowledge of specific allergens commonly identified in the area. Having just given birth to a second child, Aata could be experiencing symptoms of postnatal depression. This can be addressed by a mental health status assessment and investigation. Her current social factors can impact on the family's health and wellbeing. Aata could be given information about the local area that would provide the names for contact groups such as mother clubs, playgroups, cultural gatherings and preschools.

THE FAMILY AS PART OF A COMMUNITY

Families rarely live in isolation and need to get food, use transportation and receive wages for work (Monsen & Finley, 2007). A **community** can be defined in many ways, but it is generally accepted as being a defined geographical area where residents relate to and interact with each other (Allender & Spradley, 2008). When asked to describe their community, people may mention their local suburb, or an entire city, region, territory or state. Communities are also defined by what they have in common, including shared goals, relationships and physical, social and political environments, which may cross boundaries and borders depending on their individual circumstances (Allender & Spradley, 2008).

Australia and New Zealand are multicultural societies that include Indigenous peoples with rich cultures, languages, histories and their own concepts of health and healing. However, Indigenous people continue to be among the most marginalised populations in the world (WHO, 2007). While there are significant social and political differences between both countries, they also share much in common in terms of current community structures. For communities to be successful in promoting health and wellbeing it is essential that community members and groups are actively involved from the very beginning. This is particularly important when working with Indigenous peoples who have the greatest health disparity as a consequence of colonisation. In New Zealand, the Treaty of Waitangi (*te Tiriti o Waitangi*) identifies partnership, participation and protection as the primary principles for ensuring that the Māori world view has been acknowledged (Barnes, 2012). Similarly, in Australia the importance of engaging and working in partnership with Aboriginal and Torres Strait Islander peoples is an explicit element of the National Aboriginal and Torres Strait Islander Health Plan 2013–2023 (Australian Government, 2013; Women's and Children's Health Network, 2015). Having control over the decisions that affect you is a pivotal health promotion concept. Individuals, families and communities that have the relevant knowledge and skills are better equipped to make the behaviour changes necessary to improve their health and wellbeing.

Conway, McClune and Nosel (2007) suggest that a community assessment helps examine the various systems that are present in almost all communities, and assesses whether they are functioning adequately. All nurses, hospital and community-based, should have knowledge of the type and range of resources that are available in the communities they serve. This is especially important when working with Indigenous peoples to ensure that culturally appropriate care and services are provided (Nursing and Midwifery Board of Australia, 2008; Nursing Council of New Zealand, 2011). Examples of such care are the Orongomai Marae Health Services for Māori clients in Upper Hutt, New Zealand and the Aboriginal community-controlled organisations such as the Derbarl Yerrigan Health Service in Perth, Western Australia.

Drawing an ecomap or a diagram of a family's relationship with its community (see Chapter 3) can help identify what community contacts are available for a family. Different communities may or may not have resources for families with special needs such as home physiotherapists or occupational therapists to assist children whose growth or development is delayed.

Assessing family health needs requires close collaboration between the community nurse, the family and other relevant people/agencies (e.g. social worker, teacher, GP). Determining family roles (see Chapter 3), such as who is the wage earner, the decision maker and the nurturer, is important for nursing or healthcare planning. Community family care is most successful when family roles are not disrupted but strengthened to support whatever new activities or concerns need to be addressed. Typically, the initial referral from a clinician or an agency provides the foundation from which the community health nurse will decide on the appropriate nursing intervention or plan of care. As indicated previously, any planning will involve the family in what their needs are, what will be expected of them and what they can expect of the nurse. The agreed plan will outline the key objectives, the implementation and evaluation process and include a timescale. Finally, the nurse and family should reflect on health outcomes to meet ongoing needs. The nurse's knowledge of the community is fundamental in identifying resources, such as support groups for parents or people with chronic conditions.

COMMUNITY ASSESSMENT

One method of **community assessment** is undertaking a windshield and/or walking survey. As the names indicate, one is a systematic observation of a community through the windscreen of a moving vehicle and the other is undertaken on foot. Each has a slightly different value. A windshield survey is clearly more useful when observing a large area and a walking survey is of more value when observing what is not visible from the road, for example public spaces and gardens. Both surveys can be used to assess general community needs. Indeed, an examination of the physical, social and economic characteristics of a community could provide an insight into, for example, the quality and availability of housing (Community Tool Box, 2014). Both surveys can also be used to examine different aspects of a community, including:

- Age, type, design and condition of available housing (e.g. terraced, apartments, rented, owner occupied, etc.)
- Infrastructure (e.g. roads, streetlights, medical centres, etc.)
- Type and range of local businesses (e.g. cafes, large employers, charity shops, etc.)
- Quality and availability of public spaces (e.g. parks, pedestrian only areas, etc.)
- Amount of activity on the streets (e.g. age groups, ethnicity, traffic volume, etc.)
- Environmental issues (e.g. noisy industrial areas, pollution, heavy traffic, etc.)
- Location and condition of public buildings (e.g. libraries, council buildings, etc.).

A systematic assessment of a community in this way can provide a means of comparing different parts of a community to determine the disparity of services and resources, and also provide an indication regarding the state of the community's health.

McDonald, Bailie and Michel (2013) developed and trialled a tool to measure, monitor and evaluate key social determinants of health at a community level in remote Indigenous communities in the Northern Territory of Australia. The infrastructure and programs considered important to promote good health and prevent chronic disease include food supply, water supply, electricity supply, a sewage system, pest control, air quality, drainage, healthy housing and the promotion of physical activity. Although a trial, the authors concluded that this tool provided "benefits for community leaders, government officers and others seeking to measure environmental health conditions and address inequities in the social determinants of health in remote communities" (McDonald, Bailie & Michel, 2013). In New Zealand similar work has been undertaken, resulting in the development of the Health Equity Assessment Tool (HEAT) to assist and guide District Health Boards in addressing health inequalities (Signal et al., 2008).

CASE STUDY QUESTION

5. After identifying Aata's needs the community nurse will develop strategies with the family and then identify resources that would be used appropriately for improving the wellbeing of the family. Which of the following might support the family in their current situation?

a. Providing health information and general information of what is available in the local region for the family
b. Enrolling the toddler in preschool, to provide Aata with some personal time
c. Arranging a family meeting, including Aata's husband, to discuss Aata's situation

FAMILY HEALTH ASSESSMENT

A family health assessment is essential prior to any nursing interaction with a family, especially where a long-term relationship or treatment plan is required; for example, provision of child developmental services or long-term care provision for a chronic condition. The **family assessment** helps the nurse, in partnership with the family, to identify family strengths (knowledge, skills and resilience) and barriers that could impact on the family's ability to function effectively or prevent them accessing healthcare,

BOX 4.1 * Areas of family assessment

What is the family structure?
- Who are the family members?
- What are the roles within the family?
- What are the ages and sex of the family members?
- What are their occupations?
- What is the health status of family members?
- Does any member of the family have an impairment or a disability?

What resources does the family have?
- What is the financial situation?
- Is the family home safe and does it have appropriate facilities (e.g. heating)?
- Can the family afford healthcare?
- What community resources are available?
- What support systems does the family have (e.g. friends, church or community groups)?

What is the family's educational and cultural background?
- What is the family's attitude towards learning?
- Do family members have basic literacy and numeracy skills?
- Are there any language barriers?
- What is the family's cultural background and health beliefs?
- Does the family have any traditional healing or medicine beliefs?
- What is the family's lifestyle (e.g. dietary patterns)?
- Is the family open to new information?
- What is the family's level of health literacy?

How does the family function?
- Are family members sensitive to the needs of each other?
- Do family members appear to communicate with each other?
- Does the family accept help from others when needed?
- Do family members support each other in times of need?
- What experience does the family have in handling crisis situations?
- Does the family demonstrate resilience in times of crisis?

What are the family's health information needs?
- What does the family already know about their health and health needs?
- What does the family think are the most important things they still need to know?
- Does the family have experience of caring for someone with a health problem?
- Are there any barriers to learning (e.g. physical or cognitive limitations, cultural conflicts)?
- Is the family willing to participate in self-care strategies in collaboration with the healthcare team?
- Do family members share the same understanding about what needs to be done?

Adapted from Rankin, S. H. & Stallings, K. D. (1996). *Patient Education: Issues, Principles, Practices* (3rd ed.). Philadelphia: Lippincott-Raven, pp. 128–129.

or other services, when required. It is important to remember that in many cultures the indiviudal is a member of an extended family and community, who are often involved with decisions on healthcare and healthcare management. It is common in Pacific cultures, for example, for the extended family to be involved in the provision of care while a family member is in hospital. Consequently, the nurse needs to understand the family and extended family relationships in order to provide culturally appropriate care (New Zealand Ministry of Health, 2008). A family health assessment, therefore, is an opportunity for the nurse to get to know the family, their beliefs and values, and begin to develop a therapeutic relationship, aimed at enabling the family to make better health decisions (Lewis & Foley, 2014).

An effective nursing care/intervention plan requires a thorough and accurate assessment. The nurse needs to have good observation and listening skills when gathering information about the structure, function and health needs of the family. The assessment does not need to be restricted to structured interviews and information can be obtained as part of other interactions with the family; for example, when undertaking clinical procedures such as dressings, tube feeds or child developmental screening. Box 4.1 identifies what might be included in a baseline family health assessment.

In the immediate period, after the first consultation, the community nurse should provide health information and educational resources for the family. For example, Aata should participate in all strategy development and decision-making processes. Healthcare resources are utilised to promote independence and autonomy as the community nurse and family work towards improving the overall wellbeing of the family situation.

Current healthcare provision places greater emphasis on support for families in communities. Being able to access community health resources becomes more and more important because of shorter hospital stays and increased community-based services, resulting in individuals spending more time at home recuperating from illness than ever before. The term "resources" refers not only to material objects (e.g. hospital beds, oxygen, home monitors) but also to whether a family can deal with the chronic stress of home care. Women often have to leave work to become carers for children and older parents. This can reduce a family's income dramatically and cause financial problems.

Availablity of, or access to, important resources can be problematic, especially in rural communities. Does Aata's home have adequate facilities (e.g. water, electricity, refrigeration)? Are there resources in the community that will provide additional support (e.g. an asthma support group)? Is the house safe or are there potential health risks for the family?

THE ROLE OF NURSES IN COMMUNITY AND FAMILY HEALTH

Community and family nursing roles are varied and, as mentioned previously, are in a stage of transition to a PHC model of healthcare delivery where accessibility, equity, culturally appropriate care, intersectoral collaboration, community participation, and patient and family empowerment are cornerstone principles (Earl, Terblanche & Patten, 2012). McMurray and Clendon (2014) cite the following community-developed models as examples of PHC practice: the original baby health centres in Australia and the Well Child (Plunket and Tamariki Ora) clinics in New Zealand, women's health and reproductive services, gay and lesbian health services, community crisis and mental health services, and services for refugees, immigrants and asylum seekers. It can be identified from these programs that nurses have been pivotal in developing or participating in the provision of these fundamental community-based health services.

Implementation of community-based nursing care, especially in someone's home, is different from that performed in an acute care facility. The nurse's role can range from teaching and counselling, lobbying and advocating to hands-on care, depending on the geographical location and role and availability of healthcare and other relevant services. To do this, community nurses need to have the same level of specialised knowledge and expertise as acute care nurses. In addition, they may need to be more flexible and adaptable because each home visit may be very different. All nurses should be involved in health promotion and patient education. Community nurses will also be involved in screening, early detection and prevention-focused nursing activities, as well as undertaking rehabilitative and curative activities with individuals and groups (Kralik & van Loon, 2011).

Figure 4.1 provides a representation of the different levels of prevention. This model is often used for specific health concerns (e.g. asthma and diabetes), but can be applied to health issues generally.

✔ Checkpoint question 4.1

a. With reference to the levels of prevention (see Fig. 4.1), how do different community nurses (e.g. public health, home care, school and practice nurses) contribute to the prevention of illness and disease?
b. What health promotion interventions and strategies are in place for asthma in each of the levels of prevention?

When undertaking a home visit, it is important to remember that you are a guest in someone's home and that you must respect their privacy, beliefs, lifestyles, routines and culture. Keep in mind the ethical and legal aspects of nursing care, such as confidentiality, informed consent, decision making and client rights. This must also be remembered when taking notes or when discussing the visit with others. Because home care visits are often made alone, measures must be taken to ensure personal safety on the way to a client's home, during a visit and afterwards.

Knowing the individual aspects of families or a community can help the nurse to understand why some people reach the illness level they do before they come for healthcare; for example, a woman has no transport available to her until her husband comes home from work so this prevents her from attending daytime prenatal care; a 5-year-old child develops measles because there are no free immunisation services in the community. Children with chronic illnesses who need monitoring but not

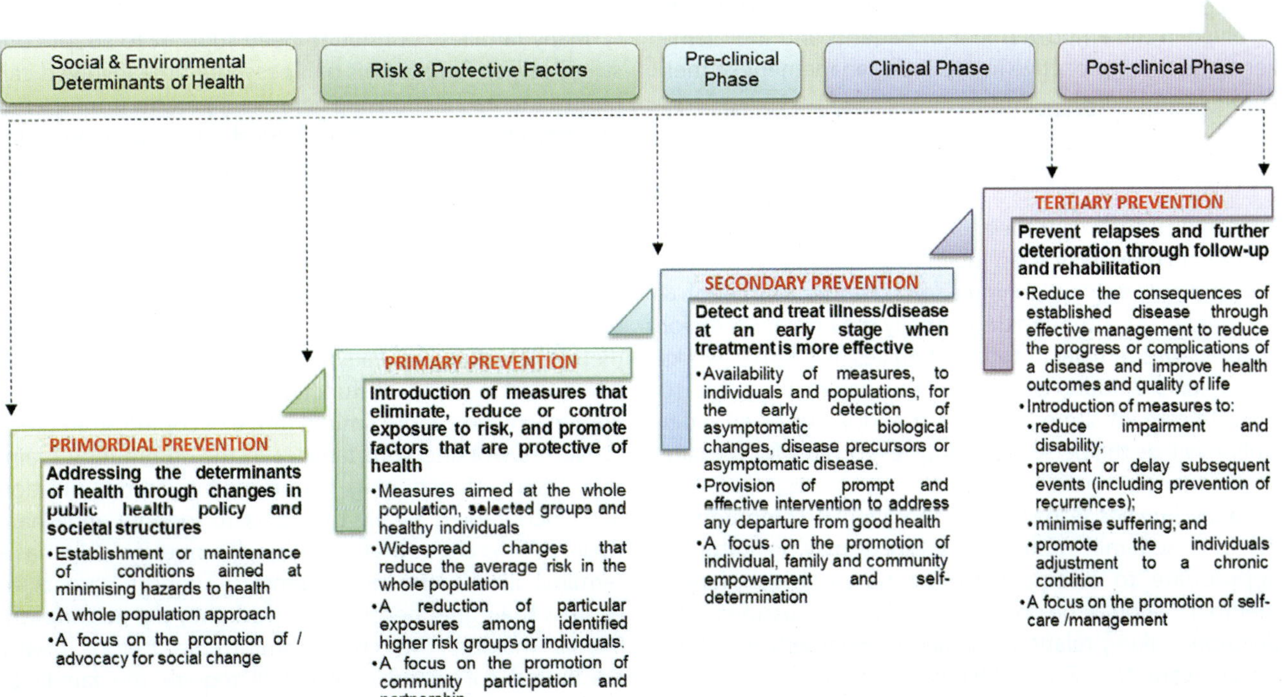

FIGURE 4.1 Levels of prevention. (© Bill Deans.)

critical care are equally good candidates. It is possible that having a caring person such as a community health nurse visit frequently and take an interest in a family could have long-term effects, such as lowering the incidence of child abuse and child injury.

Having regular contact with a family, at home and/or at the clinic, allows the nurse to observe any possible signs of stressors in individual family members or changes in health status that may place an individual or a family at risk. This is especially important for community nurses working with **vulnerable individuals or families**; for example, a family with a member who has a chronic illness, a disability or drug/alcohol issues can place individuals at higher risk of neglect and/or abuse (Barlow et al., 2007).

A first home visit usually includes documenting a family's current status and an environmental, community and social assessment. The community nurse is able to observe the family in their personal environment and assess the factors that impact on their ability to manage their health or condition (Kralik & van Loon, 2011). The assessment may look at specific areas such as: adherence to medical, preventive or medication regimens; whether the family will be able to continue to address health issues at home; and what other services or resources the family needs, such as the services of home help or further nursing visits to ensure that healthcare is optimal.

For individuals with a chronic condition or illness to function effectively at home, it is essential that the individual and/or their family have the relevant knowledge and skills. For example: Do they know the signs of an acute asthma attack? Do they know how to care for a spacer device? Can they explain the possible side effects of their medication?

All nurses, inpatient and community, need to be involved in the empowerment of patients and their families to be more proactive in the self-management of their chronic conditions.

PROMOTING HEALTHY FAMILIES

The family is the major social unit responsible for socialisation of children, so it is an ideal target for health promotion and prevention planning efforts (Pender, Murdaugh & Parsons, 2014). Although traditionally the primary carer for children was female, in today's families, if a father works more flexible hours, he may be the parent best able to provide care. In some homes, a grandparent or an older sibling will be the person primarily responsible for the care of younger siblings.

Many families, especially in Indigenous communities, live in close family groups. Therefore, it may be culturally appropriate to discuss with the family which family members should be included in any discussions and decision making relating to a family member's health or nursing care (New Zealand Ministry of Health, 2008). Both Australia and New Zealand have a diverse range of ethnic and cultural communities. Both countries have large communities that originated in the Pacific Islands. The New Zealand Ministry of Health's literature review (2008) highlights **cultural competence** as "a key tool for making health services more responsive to Pacific peoples, Māori and other groups". Although commissioned by the Ministry of Health in New Zealand this publication has implications for Australian service providers working with families with their own traditional health belief system.

A functional family supports family members and provides a supportive environment within which family members can grow and develop. Families that have been exposed to normal everyday challenges and have developed healthy coping responses will be able to overcome most obstacles. However, families can be faced with very difficult situations, for example the death of a child, that may test the family's resilience and ability to cope. Dysfunctional families and those with complex health problems are at greater risk.

CASE STUDY QUESTION

6. What family goals could you assist Aata to establish to promote wellness in the family?

a. Increase communication with her husband about her current circumstances
b. Increase physical exercise by daily walks with the children to assist with depression
c. Develop an asthma management plan for both Aata and her son
d. Identify a social activity that Aata can undertake to meet other community members
e. All of the above goals would enhance Aata's and her family's physical, mental and social wellbeing

Many families continue to need support to adapt constructively to family crisis or illness. The time involved can harm a marital relationship or prevent parents from spending time with their children. Physical care requirements for an ill family member can disrupt the normal family routines and shift the focus of attention away from other children in the family. The challenge for the nurse is to assist the family unit in identifying relevant health goals, planning for positive lifestyle changes and capitalising on their strengths to achieve desired health outcomes (Pender, Murdaugh & Parsons, 2014). This is especially true when working with dysfunctional or vulnerable families, who may have a more limited range of coping strategies.

Nurses working with families in the community maintain healthy functioning by promoting communication and encouraging family members to identify and share their feelings about their situation at home. If a child has a terminal illness, the nurse aims to support parents to express their grief because the work they are accomplishing is making the child comfortable before death. Continued successful coping will require the family to acknowledge and take seriously the impact on each family member and work together to solve identified problems. They may need to renegotiate roles and responsibilities within the family or seek outside help. When a family is not functioning well, supportive measures for family functioning become even more important. A family whose coping strategies are maladaptive and ineffective may not be able to consider the implications on the health and wellbeing of each family member.

Research now shows that many challenges in adult society—mental health problems, obesity, stunted growth, heart disease, criminality, competence in literacy and numeracy—have their roots in early childhood. The early years of life are crucial in influencing a range of health and social outcomes across the life-course (Middlebrooks & Audage, 2008; Center on the Developing Child Harvard University, 2015). Consequently, the Australian and New Zealand governments have introduced a range of inter-agency, cross-departmental and health promotion strategies, aimed primarily at supporting parents to develop skills in effective childrearing. Examples of this include: the New Zealand Government website, SKIP Strategies for Kids/Information for Parents at <www.skip.org.nz>; and the Australian Government website, Raising Children Network at <http://raisingchildren.net.au>.

This focus on early-years development has re-emphasised the important role of the well child nurse in both countries. In Australia, Child Health Centres, staffed by registered nurses with qualifications in child and family health, provide a range of services in partnership with parents and carers of babies and young children up to the age of 4 years. In New Zealand, Well Child (Tamariki Ora) services offer a similar range of services for children up to 5 years (New Zealand Ministry of Health, 2013). Historically, the New Zealand Well Child service was provided by Plunket Nurses—registered nurses with qualifications in child and family health. However, in recent years a range of Māori and Pacific Well Child service providers have been established to represent these communities. "A healthy start in life gives each child an equal chance to thrive and grow into an adult who makes a positive contribution to the community—economically and socially" (Irwin, Siddiqi & Hertzman, 2007).

Child and family healthcare is more successful if there is effective support from the family or community. Otherwise, both women and children can experience loneliness and low self-esteem which interferes with their ability to manage any health issues they may have. Community nurses, with their local knowledge of the community, can often identify and access resources. School nurses work in partnership with school principals and staff, parents, students and other health professionals to help promote the healthy development of school children (Francis et al., 2013). Voluntary agencies often provide services such as transportation to and from healthcare agency assessments or respite care so parents can have time, free from continual care (Yantzi, Rosenberg & McKeever, 2007). Advantages of community care for a family include the following:

- It prevents extensive disruption to the family unit. For those who are chronically ill or dying, being close to their family and friends may be the most important aspect of their care; for these children, home care is ideal (Tuffrey, Finlay & Lewis, 2007)
- It increases the self-confidence of family members, because it allows for more self-care and often more control of their circumstances.
- Families are better assessed in their own environment than in a health facility, because family interactions, values and priorities are more obvious than in a healthcare setting.
- Home visits provide a private, one-on-one opportunity for health education.
- In most instances, it is less costly to the healthcare delivery system to provide community care for families at home rather than in a hospital setting, especially when the care is underpinned by a health education and promotion philosophy (New Zealand Ministry of Health, 2014a).

COMMUNITY DEVELOPMENT AND MOBILISATION

Changing the health behaviour of communities, rather than individuals, is based on the premise that community development and mobilisation are central to community health education and promotion (Pender, Murdaugh & Parsons, 2014). The health information requirements to meet the education needs of families and communities will be varied and depend largely on community **health literacy** levels. Health education is any combination of learning experiences designed to help individuals and communities improve their health by increasing their knowledge or influencing their attitudes (Keleher & MacDougall, 2011). Assessing the level of health literacy about a specific illness or health issue prevalent in the community will assist in the maintenance and improvement of overall health. In providing health information, the community nurse develops an understanding of local and regional statistical data, to assist in providing education about health-impacting conditions. An essential role of the nurse is as a broker of knowledge. The community nurse builds relationships and networks to share and disseminate research (Kralik & van Loon, 2011).

It is also important for health professionals to be aware of the barriers to providing effective health information and education. Poverty, low literacy levels, lower socioeconomic status, geographical remoteness and unemployment are just some examples of the social **determinants of health** (see also Chapter 2) which can have a significant impact on individual and community health literacy (WHO, 2013). An understanding of the social determinants is important for the nurse and other healthcare professionals to effectively intervene in neighbourhoods, communities and organisations to improve individual health (Pender, Murdaugh & Parsons, 2014). Marginalised groups within a community may provide a greater challenge to effective health education. Keleher and MacDougall (2011) argue that empowering community groups through education requires an all-inclusive approach. An example is a community of Indigenous people with diabetes where the approach will require both individual and group education, organisational change, **community engagement** and policy change in partnership with community members, community elders and other relevant parties (Australian Government Department of Health, 2013; New Zealand Ministry of Health, 2014b).

One major advancement in overcoming some of these barriers to health literacy and access to health information is the use of the internet. Utilising new technology appropriately and efficiently is a key strategy in the provision of PHC. Good internet referral sites regarding care for families are now an essential resource for promoting health through education. The information can be accessed in almost any geographical location. This has important implications for people living in rural or inaccessible areas, who are at home or who work (Pender, Murdaugh & Parsons, 2014). Examples of internet-based resources developed to help improve health literacy can be found at South Australia Health <www.sahealth.sa.gov.au> and Health Navigator New Zealand <www.healthnavigator.org.nz>. In some settings, telephone, email and social media are used to link healthcare providers with families receiving home care. In many instances, nurses need to advocate on behalf of families to secure adequate funding and resources to provide these services.

Although providing access to health information is a key focus of PHC, often families require a more direct approach to self-manage personal health situations. Typically, family members with medical conditions may need to self-assess various health parameters such as blood pressure, temperature, pulse and perhaps urine for protein or glucose. Parents or the carer of an ill child may need to assess vital signs, comfort level and side effects of medications. Before initiating a health education program, it is critical to assess the client's current level of knowledge and skill, their learning style and their motivation to learn. Acknowledging that people already have knowledge and skills is a core concept of person-/family-centred care (Pender, Murdaugh & Parsons, 2014).

CASE STUDY QUESTION

7. For which aspects of Aata's current circumstances could a community nurse provide health information?

a. Postnatal mental and physical health
b. Asthma and allergens
c. Promotion of wellness through social interactions
d. Available resources in the community
e. All of the above

Community nurses are well placed as healthcare professionals to undertake a holistic assessment of individuals, families and communities. They are also able to use their knowledge and skills to improve health literacy, including the provision of health information, teaching self-care skills and advocating for better access to healthcare services for vulnerable populations. Health promotion and education is now an essential role for nurses and a key strategy in implementing a PHC model of healthcare.

SERVICE PROVISION TO PROMOTE HEALTHY FAMILIES AND COMMUNITIES

Nurses are active in providing health promotion services across the age span of the community and the opportunity to promote health to families in communities has never been more achievable. Policy development that now employs a PHC model of care for the provision of universal assessment, coordinated care and home visiting for all new parents is now firmly on government agendas. A range of **family-centred policies** and programs are being implemented across Australia and New Zealand aimed at improving child and family health, promoting positive parenting and addressing family relationship issues, such as domestic violence (Francis et al., 2013).

Research confirms that all families require support to raise their children at some point, with some families requiring additional support. This includes working with the family and facilitating the development of parent-healthy relationships. Both Australia and New Zealand have well-developed child and family health services that provide equitable access to health education and promotion as well as well-child screening programs. Services such as "Closing the Gap" specifically developed by, and for, Indigenous people, are predominately underpinned by a PHC model of care. Indigenous Australians view their health quite differently from mainstream western society, and they have developed a model of primary healthcare that reflects their holistic view of health and a process whereby they have control over it. This is also the case for a wide range of other ethnic groups living in both countries who have their own world views of health and healthcare (Talemaitoga, 2010).

Central to health service provision for individuals, families and communities is the concept of self-determination, self-management and community activation through the development of health-promoting partnerships. Using a PHC model of healthcare enables the identification of health needs, the allocation of appropriate funding and resources, plus the development of specialised services aimed at preventing disease and disability, improving health and wellbeing, and empowering individuals and communities to manage their own healthcare needs.

Key points for review

- Primary healthcare (PHC) is a social model of health that best provides a holistic approach to healthcare in Australia and New Zealand.
- Health needs assessment of individuals and families provides invaluable information about health status, health literacy, risks to health and protective factors, such as coping strategies.
- Community assessment helps identify resources that may help, or barriers that may hinder, the individual or family to achieve optimum health and wellbeing.
- Using a person-/family-/community-centred approach will aid engagement and empowerment, promote self-determination and ensure culturally congruent care is delivered.
- A new way of thinking is required for nurses working within a PHC framework of healthcare to meet health needs, with a greater emphasis on problem solving, health promotion, interdisciplinary/agency collaboration and the use of technology (e.g. telehealth and telephone triage).
- Community-based healthcare has the advantage of being a more cost-effective and flexible form of care that focuses on empowering families and communities.
- Meeting the health needs of a family requires close collaboration between the family, the healthcare provider and other relevant agencies.
- PHC requires careful planning and an interdisciplinary approach to healthcare provision to ensure collaboration and continuity of care.
- Policy development now employs a PHC model of care for the provision of services that promotes universal assessment, equity of services and coordinated care.

CASE STUDY QUESTIONS

8. When assessing families in their homes, why is it important for nurses to be considerate of working in this environment?
9. Identify services in your local community that you feel would provide support for a family in Aata's situation.
10. What health promotion strategies would you consider to address this family's health needs?
11. To promote wellness through health promotion activities for Aata and her family, what consideration would you give to her cultural needs?

Resources

For an extensive range of additional resources to enhance teaching and learning and to facilitate understanding of this chapter, please see the text's accompanying website located on thePoint at http://thepoint.lww.com.

References

Allender, J. A. & Spradley, B. W. (2008). *Community Health Nursing: Concepts and Practice* (6th ed.). Philadelphia: Lippincott Williams & Wilkins.

Australian Government. (2013). *National Aboriginal and Torres Strait Islander Health Plan 2013–2023.* Accessed 9 February 2015, <www.health.gov.au/internet/main/publishing.nsf/content/B92E980680486C3BCA257BF0001BAF01/$File/health-plan.pdf>.

Australian Government Department of Health. (2013). *National Primary Health Care Strategic Framework.* Canberra: Australian Government Department of Health.

Barlow, J., Davis, H., McIntosh, E., Jarrett, P., Mockford, C. & Stewart-Brown, S. (2007). Role of home visiting in improving parenting and health in families at risk of abuse and neglect: Results of a multicentre randomised controlled trial and economic evaluation. *Archives of Disease in Childhood, 92*(3), 229–233.

Barnes, H. M. (2012). Better Indigenous policies: The role of evaluation. Accessed 9 February 2015, <www.pc.gov.au/research/completed/better-indigenous-policies>.

Berman, A., Snyder, S., Kozier, B., Erb, G. L., Levett-Jones, T., Dwyer, T., Hales, M., Harvey, N., Luxford, Y., Moxham, L., Park, T., Parker, B., Reid-Searl, K. & Stanley, D. (2012). *Kozier and Erb's Fundamentals of Nursing* (2nd Australian ed.). Sydney: Pearson.

Center on the Developing Child Harvard University. (2015). Key concepts: Toxic stress. Accessed 9 February 2015, <http://developingchild.harvard.edu/key_concepts/toxic_stress_response/>.

Community Tool Box. (2014). Windshield and walking surveys. Accessed 9 February 2015, <http://ctb.ku.edu/en/table-of-contents/assessment/assessing-community-needs-and-resources/windshield-walking-surveys/main>.

Conway, A. E., McClune, A. J. & Nosel, P. (2007). Down on the farm: Preventing farm accidents in children. *Pediatric Nursing, 33*(1), 45–48.

Earl, C., Terblanche, J. & Patten, E. (2012) Health and the living environment. In Liamputtong, P., Fanany, R. & Verrinda, G. (Eds). *Health, Illness and Wellbeing: Perspectives and Social Determinants.* Melbourne: Oxford University Press.

Francis, K., Chapman, Y., Hoare, K. & Mills, J. (2013). *Australian and New Zealand Community as Partner: Theory and Practice in Nursing* (2nd ed.). Sydney: Lippincott Williams & Wilkins.

Irwin, L. G., Siddiqi, A. & Hertzman, C. (2007). *Early Child Development: A Powerful Equalizer. Final Report for the World Health Organization's Commission on Social Determinants of Health.* Accessed 9 February 2015, <http://whqlibdoc.who.int/hq/2007/a91213.pdf>.

Keleher, H. & MacDougall, C. (2011). *Understanding Health* (3rd ed.). South Melbourne: Oxford University Press.

Kralik, D. & van Loon, A. (Eds). (2011). *Community Nursing in Australia* (2nd ed.). Brisbane: John Wiley & Sons.

Lewis, P. & Foley, D. (2014). *Health Assessment in Nursing* (2nd ed.). Sydney: Lippincott Williams & Wilkins.

McDonald, E. L., Bailie, R. & Michel, T. (2013). Development and trialling of a tool to support a systems approach to improve social determinants of health in rural and remote Australian communities: The healthy community assessment tool. *International Journal for Equity in Health, 12*(15), 3–10.

McMurray, A. & Clendon, J. (2014). *Community Health & Wellness: Primary Health Care in Practice.* NSW: Churchill Livingstone.

Middlebrooks, J. S. & Audage, N. C. (2008). *The Effects of Childhood Stress on Health Across the Lifespan.* Atlanta: Centers for Disease Control and Prevention, National Center for Injury Prevention and Control.

Monsen, R. B. & Finley, S. (2007). The child in the community: Nursing makes a difference. Shortages of nurses and child health. *Journal of Pediatric Nursing: Nursing Care of Children and Families, 22*(3), 231–232.

New Zealand Ministry of Health. (2001). *The Primary Health Care Strategy.* Wellington: New Zealand Ministry of Health.

New Zealand Ministry of Health. (2008). *Pacific Cultural Competencies: A Literature Review.* Wellington: Ministry of Health.

New Zealand Ministry of Health. (2013). *Well Child/Tamariki Ora programme Practitioner Handbook: Supporting Families and Whānau to Promote their Child's Health and Development.* Wellington: Ministry of Health.

New Zealand Ministry of Health. (2014a). *Care Closer to Home.* Wellington: Ministry of Health.

New Zealand Ministry of Health. (2014b). *He Korowai Oranga: Maori Health Strategy 2014.* Wellington: Ministry of Health.

Nursing and Midwifery Board of Australia. (2008). *Code of Professional Conduct for Nurses in Australia.* Melbourne: Nursing and Midwifery Board of Australia.

Nursing Council of New Zealand. (2011). *Cultural Safety, the Treaty of Waitangi and Māori Health.* Wellington: Nursing Council of New Zealand.

Pender, N. J., Murdaugh, C. L. & Parsons, M. (2014). *Health Promotion in Nursing Practice* (7th ed.). Upper Saddle River, N.J.: Pearson.

Rankin, S. H. & Stallings, K. D. (1996). *Patient Education: Issues, Principles, Practices* (3rd ed.). Philadelphia: Lippincott-Raven, pp. 128–129.

Signal, L., Martin, J., Cram, F. & Robson, B. (2008). *The Health Equity Assessment tool: A User's Guide.* Wellington: New Zealand Ministry of Health.

Talemaitoga, A. (2010). The health of Pacific peoples in Aotearoa is "everybody's business". *Best Practice Journal, 32*, 5–9.

Tuffrey, C., Finlay, F. & Lewis, M. (2007). The needs of children and their families at end of life: An analysis of community nursing practice. *International Journal of Palliative Nursing, 13*(2), 64–71.

Women's and Children's Health Network. (2015). *Consumer and Community Participation.* Accessed 9 February 2015, <www.wchn.sa.gov.au/Content.aspx?p=492>.

World Health Organzation (WHO). (2004). *Towards Age-Friendly Primary Health Care.* Geneva: World Health Organization, p. IV.

World Health Organization (WHO). (2007). *Health of Indigenous Peoples. Fact sheet no. 326.* Accessed 9 February 2015, <www.who.int/mediacentre/factsheets/fs326/en/>.

World Health Organization (WHO). (2008). *The World Health Report 2008. Primary health care (now more than ever).* Geneva: World Health Organization.

World Health Organization (WHO). (2013). *Health Literacy. The Solid Facts.* Copenhagen: World Health Organization.

World Health Organization. (2015). *Health Topics: Primary Health Care.* Accessed 5 March 2015, <www.who.int/topics/primary_health_care/en>.

Yantzi, N. M., Rosenberg, M. W. & McKeever, P. (2007). Getting out of the house: The challenges mothers face when their children have long-term care needs. *Health and Social Care in the Community, 15*(1), 45–55.

Suggested readings

Australian Government Department of Health and Aging. (2011). *National Framework for Universal Child and Family Health Services.* Accessed 9 February 2015 <www.health.gov.au/internet/main/publishing.nsf/Content/AFF3C1C460BA5300CA257BF0001A8D86/$File/NFUCFHS.PDF>.

McBain-Rigg, K. E. & Veitch, C. (2011). Cultural barriers to health care for Aboriginal and Torres Strait Islanders in Mount Isa. *Australian Journal of Rural Health, 19*, 70–74.

National Aboriginal Community Controlled Health Organisation (NACCHO) and the Royal Australian College of General Practitioners (RACGP). (n.d.). *National Guide Lifecycle Chart: Child.* Accessed 9 February 2015, <www.naccho.org.au/download/aboriginal-health/3.Child%20preventive%20health%20life%20cycle%20summary%20chart.pdf>.

National Aboriginal Community Controlled Health Organisation (NACCHO) and the Royal Australian College of General Practitioners (RACGP). (2011). *National Guide to a Preventive Health Assessment for Aboriginal and Torres Strait Islander People* (2nd ed.). Accessed 9 February 2015, <www.racgp.org.au/your-practice/guidelines/national-guide/>.

New Zealand Ministry of Health. (2012). *Māori Health Models: Te Whare Tapa Whā.* Accessed 9 February 2015, <www.health.govt.nz/our-work/populations/maori-health/maori-health-models/maori-health-models-te-whare-tapa-wha>.

Women's and Children's Health Network. (n.d.). *Parenting and Child Health.* Accessed 9 February 2015, <www.cyh.com/SubDefault.aspx?p=98>.

Unit 2

The nursing role in preparing families for childbearing and childrearing

Chapter 5

The nursing role in reproductive and sexual health

Previous chapters presented the scope of child and family health and how the structure, function and culture of families can have an impact on health. This chapter discusses the nurse's role in promoting sexual and reproductive health, providing the nurse with essential background information and strategies that can be used in health education to communicate with individuals about their sexuality and reproductive health. While sexual and reproductive health is the focus of women's and sexual health nursing, as well as midwifery practice, it is an integral part of all nursing. Promoting sexual health is a core component of holistic nursing care but most nurses do not feel confident discussing sexuality with clients (Saunamaki, Andersson & Engstrom, 2010). The purpose of this chapter is to enable nurses to feel more confident in this important aspect of their role.

LEARNING OBJECTIVES

After studying this chapter, you should be able to:

1. Consider how nurses can use a specific sexual counselling model (PLISSIT) to optimise sexual and reproductive health education, promotion and communication.
2. Use reflective and critical thinking to analyse the nurse's role in providing reproductive and sexual healthcare.
3. Formulate nursing diagnoses related to reproductive and sexual health.
4. Identify appropriate outcomes for reproductive and sexual health education.
5. Implement nursing care related to reproductive and sexual health, such as educating adolescents about menstruation.
6. Evaluate expected outcomes for achievement and effectiveness of care.
7. Identify areas of care in relation to reproductive and sexual health that could benefit from additional nursing research or application of evidence-based practice.
8. Integrate knowledge of reproductive health and sexuality with nursing process to achieve quality child and family health nursing care.

KEY TERMS

- biological gender
- dysmenorrhoea
- dyspareunia
- erectile dysfunction (ED)
- gender identity
- gender role
- menarche
- menopause
- menorrhagia
- metrorrhagia
- premature ejaculation (PE)
- vaginismus

CASE STUDY

You have just facilitated a clinic to provide immunisation against human papillomavirus (HPV) to 13-year-old students at a girls' boarding school. You are enjoying morning tea and conversation with the students when Violet confides that she is very worried because most of her friends have breasts, pubic hair, regular periods and boyfriends and she feels like a freak because she does not. You make an appointment for Violet to see you after school.

CASE STUDY QUESTION

1. How do you plan to respond to Violet?

Although the general public is becoming increasingly sophisticated about their bodies, misunderstandings about sexuality, conception, contraception and childbearing still abound. Sexuality may be a major area of concern for school-aged children and adolescents. When caring for children of these ages, you may be asked a variety of detailed questions about sexuality or reproductive health. For instance, many young adults want to know what is considered a "normal" sexual response or the "normal" expected frequency for sexual relations. A general rule in answering this question is that normal sexual behaviour includes any consensual act mutually satisfying to both sexual partners. Actual frequency and type of sexual activity vary widely (Aruda, 2011).

One of the greatest contributions nurses can make is to encourage people to ask questions about sexual and reproductive functioning. With this attitude, problems of sexuality and reproduction are brought out into the open and made as resolvable as other health concerns or problems. If this is an area that you were raised to not discuss freely, learning to be comfortable with the topic and your own sexuality can be the first step needed.

REPRODUCTIVE AND SEXUAL HEALTH PROMOTION

Assessment

Problems of sexuality or reproductive health may not be evident on a first meeting, because it may be difficult for a person to bring up the topic until they feel more secure. This makes good follow-through and planning important, because a person may find the courage to discuss a problem once but then be unable to do so again. If the problem is ignored or forgotten through a change in carers, it may never be addressed again.

Any change in physical appearance can intensify or create a sexual or reproductive concern. The person who has a sexually transmitted infection (STI); excessive weight loss or gain; a disfiguring scar from surgery or an accident; hair loss such as occurs with chemotherapy, surgery or inflammation or infection of reproductive organs; chronic fatigue or pain; spinal cord injury; or a retention catheter needs to be assessed for sexual and reproductive health problems. While reproductive health issues cease to be applicable for women following menopause, sexual health is of lifelong significance.

Assessing sexuality may not be appropriate as a routine part of every health assessment; however, it should be included when appropriate, such as when discussing adolescent development or providing preconception counselling. At all times, it is wise to listen for verbal or non-verbal clues that suggest a person wants to discuss a sexual or reproductive concern. These clues are often subtle: "I guess marriage isn't for everyone"; "I'm not the woman I used to be"; "Are there ever funny effects from this medicine I'm taking?" Telling a seemingly inappropriate sexual joke may be yet another clue. Non-verbal clues may include extreme modesty or obvious embarrassment in response to questions, for example, about voiding. All sexual and reproductive health information sharing must be culturally sensitive so that any misunderstanding can be explored and clarified (Ngum Chi Watts, Liamputtong & Carolan, 2013).

Sexual and reproductive health assessment begins with interviewing to determine what a person knows. Any concerns they might have about their own sexual health and/or reproductive functioning such as safer sex practices should be explored. This area of health interviewing takes practice and the conviction that exploring sexual health is as important as exploring less emotionally involved areas of health, such as dietary intake or activity level. The 14-year-old girl who is not yet menstruating, for instance, may be anxious about that fact but may be reluctant to say so unless asked directly. A statement such as the following invites discussion: "Although many of your friends at school may be menstruating, it's not at all uncommon for some girls not to begin their periods until age 15 or 16. How do you feel about not yet having your period?" This combination of providing information and questioning may encourage an adolescent to discuss not only her possible concern about delayed **menarche** (the beginning of menstruation) but also other areas that will show her knowledge or lack of knowledge about reproductive health.

It is important to include in a physical examination observation for normal distribution of body hair (remembering that hair distribution varies between people of different race and age in both sexes), normal genital and breast development, and signs and symptoms of STIs. Many STIs are asymptomatic, so it is important to assess whether the person is at risk of contracting an STI rather than relying on visual signs (see Chapters 33 and 47 for documentation of stages of sexual development and signs of STIs).

Nursing considerations

Common nursing considerations used in regard to reproductive health include:

- Health-seeking behaviour related to reproductive functioning
- Anxiety related to inability to conceive after 6 months without contraception
- Pain related to uterine cramping prior to and/or during menstruation
- Disturbance in body image related to early development of secondary sex characteristics.

Considerations relevant to sexuality could include:

- Sexual dysfunction related to as-yet-unknown cause
- Altered sexuality patterns related to chronic illness
- Self-esteem disturbance related to recent surgery
- Altered sexuality patterns related to fear of harming the fetus during pregnancy
- Anxiety related to fear of unplanned pregnancy or contracting an STI
- Health-seeking behaviour related to learning responsible sexual practices.

A major part of nursing care in this area is to empower individuals to feel control over their bodies. Plan health teaching to provide people with knowledge about their reproductive system and specific information about ways to alleviate discomfort or prevent ill health. It may also be important to plan interventions to strengthen the person's gender identity or role behaviour. It is essential to design care that demonstrates acceptance of all gender-related lifestyles.

A primary nursing role concerning sexual and reproductive health is education as both females and males may feel comfortable asking questions of nurses and expect them to have sexual and reproductive health information. To help people understand sexual and reproductive health throughout their lives, specific teaching might include:

- Teaching an early adolescent what is normal and abnormal in relation to menstrual function
- Explaining to adolescents that sexual daydreaming, sexual desire, nocturnal ejaculations and the like are normal
- Providing adolescents with information about safer sex practices
- Encouraging women to have regular cervical and breast screening
- Explaining reproductive physiology to a couple who wish to become pregnant.

Health education, either to individuals or in groups, is often enhanced by the use of illustrations from books or journals, clips from the Internet or DVDs, or anatomical models of internal and external reproductive organs. Nursing interventions in this area, however, include much more than just distributing educational materials. For example, empathy for a woman's concern about increased irritability before menstruation may help validate her concern that she has premenstrual syndrome (PMS). Discussing the subject of sexual and reproductive health in a matter-of-fact way, and treating menstruation as a positive sign of maturation in a woman rather than as a burden, is helpful. An individual's sense of masculinity or femininity is important and the nurse may need to ensure that a person's gender identity or gender role is maintained in the hospital or community care setting. For example, a woman who values being assertive and sees it as being part of her female role needs opportunities in her care plan for making decisions and self-care and having her assertions respected; a hospitalised adolescent male who views watching Monday night football as part of his masculinity needs time structured for this activity at the same priority level as other activities. Unless such activities are structured, they can be easily omitted by busy nurses.

Men who have sex with men (MWM), women who have sex with women (WWW) and bisexual individuals may reveal their sexual orientation to nurses because they want help dealing with friends or family who are having difficulty accepting their gender identity. Nurses need to be aware of relevant support groups in their local area or helpful websites to which they may refer people. Helpful websites may include but are not limited to <www.gaynz.com/>, which is the leading lesbian, gay, bisexual and transgender community news website for New Zealand, and <www.livingproud.org.au>, which is the Australian gay and lesbian community services website, Living Proud. For same-sex parents, the Rainbow Families Council provides services and resources <www.rainbowfamilies.org.au> and the Australian Raising Children Network is useful for same-sex parents or their children <www.raisingchildren.net.au>. In addition to support, health education must address potential concerns whatever a person's sexual orientation; for example, including a discussion about anal or oral-genital sex practices whenever presenting information on safer sex practices.

Evaluation in the area of sexual and reproductive health must be ongoing, because health education needs change with circumstances and increasing maturity. For example, the sexual and reproductive health concerns of a woman at the beginning of a pregnancy may be totally different from her needs at the end.

How people feel about themselves sexually may impact on their motivation to maintain sexual health, for example practising safer sex in contrast to unsafe sex, or how quickly they recover from an illness. The nurse can play an invaluable role in promoting sexual and reproductive health.

EDUCATION ABOUT MENSTRUATION

Menstruation is the periodic (approximately monthly) shedding of blood and tissue from the lining of the uterus which has been prepared to accept a fertilised ovum. Education about menstruation is an important component of comprehensive sexuality education as many myths about menstruation still exist. Early preparation for menstruation to dispel myths is important to a girl's concept of herself as a woman, because it teaches her to trust her body and to think of menstruation as a mark of pride and growing up rather than a burden. Education regarding menstruation is also important for boys so they can appreciate the cyclic process that a woman's reproductive system activates and can be active participants in helping plan or prevent the conception of children.

Girls who are well prepared for menstruation and view it as a positive happening are more likely to cope with any menstrual discomfort effectively, which results in fewer missed school days than those who view menstruation as an ill time. Menstrual disorders, including **dysmenorrhoea** (painful menstruation), **menorrhagia** (abnormally heavy menstrual flows), **metrorrhagia** (bleeding between menstrual periods), menstrual migraines and premenstrual syndrome, are discussed in Chapter 47 with other reproductive system disorders.

CASE STUDY QUESTION

2. During your discussion with Violet, she discloses that she is quite scared of experiencing her first period. What would be an appropriate reply?
   a. 'Don't worry: it all comes naturally to girls.'
   b. 'What concerns you the most about commencing to menstruate?'
   c. 'Ask someone to assist you when it happens.'
   d. 'I have some pamphlets for you to read.'

MENOPAUSE

Menopause is the cessation of the menstrual cycle. Perimenopause is a term used to denote the period during which menopausal changes occur. Postmenopause describes the time of life following the final menses. The age range at which menopause occurs is wide, between approximately 40 and 55 years of age with a mean age of 51.3.

The age at which menopause symptoms begin appears to be genetically influenced and is not associated with the age of menarche. Women who smoke tend to have earlier menopause (Hayatbakhsh et al., 2012). For some women, menopause can be emotionally and/or physiologically distressing; for many others, it is a welcomed life phase. While many signs and symptoms are attributed to menopause, not all are menopause related and it is very important that nurses and/or women do not negate the significance of bodily changes simply because of a woman's age or menopausal status. For example, while heart palpitations can accompany hot flushes and be physiological for some women, they can also be a sign of underlying cardiac/haematological pathology and always warrant medical referral and investigation.

SEXUALITY AND SEXUAL IDENTITY

Sexuality is a multidimensional phenomenon that includes feelings, attitudes and actions. It has both biological and cultural components. It encompasses and gives direction to a person's physical, emotional, social and intellectual responses throughout life.

For most individuals, the family is the dominating factor in their development, including their sexual development. Simons, Burt and Tambling (2013) argue that two aspects of family life will influence sexual development and behaviour—that is, family structure and parenting style. Individuals from continuously married families are more likely to have more commitment to lifelong sexual relationships. However, parenting style, no matter what the family type, plays a more significant role in sexual behaviours and risk-taking. Sexual risk-taking includes early sexual debut, low rates of condom use and multiple casual partners. Parental warmth and support are a protective factor against risky sexual behaviour. Supportive parenting leads to individuals believing that sensitivity and sharing of values are more important in partner selection than physical attractiveness. Conversely, harsh or rejecting parenting is more likely to lead to individuals developing a cynical, distrustful view of others and engaging in sexual relationships that tend to be superficial and volatile (Simons et al., 2013).

Biological gender is the term used to denote a person's chromosomal sex: male (XY) or female (XX). **Gender identity** or sexual identity is the inner sense a person has of being male or female, which may be the same as or different from biological gender. **Gender role** is the male or female behaviour a person exhibits, which again, may or may not be the same as biological gender or gender identity and can be culturally specific. Gender role is culturally and time influenced. While pregnancy, childbirth and breastfeeding are exclusive to women, historically, in western society, women were viewed as having intrinsic nurturing qualities with primary responsibility for childrearing and homemaking. Men were viewed as financial providers and protectors of their families. Gender roles today are more interchangeable: women pursue all types of jobs and careers without loss of femininity, and men participate in childrearing and household duties without loss of masculinity.

Infancy

From the day of birth, female and male babies are often treated differently by their parents. Girls and boys are often provided with stereotypically gender-particular clothes and toys. By the end of the first year, differences in play are usually strongly evident. Boys can demonstrate more innate aggression, even at this early stage, than do girls. For more about the infant period, see Chapter 29.

Preschool period

Children can distinguish between males and females as early as 2 years of age. By age 3 or 4 years, they can say what sex they are, and they have absorbed many of the cultural expectations of that sex role. Often, boys will play rough-and-tumble games with other boys, and girls will play more quietly, although the two frequently mix at this age.

Sex role modelling is reinforced through behaviour towards and expectations of the child, as well as from such things as the colour and décor of the child's room and the child's clothing. Social contacts between the child and significant adults contribute to sexual identification and should be encouraged in this developmental period. A positive self-concept grows from parental love, effective relationships with others, success in play activities and gaining skills and self-control. Preschooler development is further discussed in Chapter 31.

School-aged child

Early school-aged children typically spend playtime imitating adult roles as a way of learning gender roles (see Fig. 5.1). They form strong impressions of what a female or male role should be. Where once schools promoted differences between males and females by separating activities into those for girls and those for boys and promoting beliefs such as expecting boys to be poorer readers, to write less neatly and to act rougher in the school hallways, primary schools have become more attuned to unisex activities. For more information about school-age development, see Chapter 32.

Adolescent

At puberty, the adolescent begins the process of establishing a sense of identity. It is during this time that family

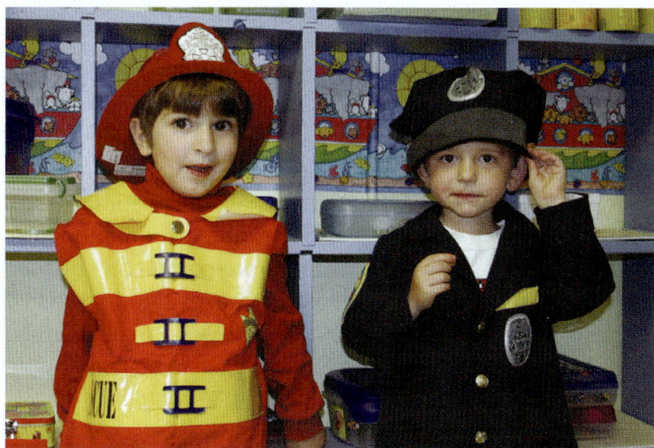

FIGURE 5.1 Early school-aged children imitate adult roles to learn more about them and whether they will "fit" the role. Here, children pretend to be a fireman and a policeman.

influences on sexual behaviour are reduced and community influences, especially those of their peer community, come to the fore.

Most early adolescents maintain strong ties to their gender group, boys with boys and girls with girls. The advent of menstruation may provide a common bond for girls at this stage. Some adolescents choose a person of their own gender a few years older than themselves to use as their model of gender role behaviour. This is a way that adolescents can be certain that they understand and feel comfortable with their own sex before they reach out and interact with members of the opposite sex.

When interviewing adolescents for a sexual history, appreciate that this is a new and sensitive area for them, so they may feel embarrassed at being questioned about this area of their life. Median age of first penis-vagina sexual Intercourse in Australia is 13–17 years, with no significant difference between males and females (Department of Education and Early Childhood Development, 2013). This means that adolescents as young as the early teen years need information on safer sex practices. One of the reasons that preventive measures for human immunodeficiency virus (HIV) and other STIs have not been as successful as first predicted may be that adolescents' total lifestyle and interpretation of sexuality have not been adequately considered.

CASE STUDY QUESTION

3. Violet informs you that many of her girlfriends are sexually active. As a nurse, your role in providing advice on sexual activity is to:

a. Inform Violet that sexual health is her own responsibility
b. Ask Violet to talk to her parents
c. Inform Violet's teachers about her comments
d. Provide health promotion education and information about the topic and discuss any further concerns that Violet may have

Adolescence can be a very stressful time for the boy who first realises that he is gay or the girl who first realises that she is a lesbian. Part of the reason for the high suicide rate in adolescence may be because homosexual teenagers feel so lost in a heterosexual-dominant culture (Hetzenbuehler & Keyes, 2013). For more information about adolescence, see Chapter 33.

Young adult

It is during young adulthood that most people choose the way they will express their sexuality along with other life patterns. Many young adults make a commitment to one sexual partner through marriage or in a de facto, cohabiting relationship. Others establish relationships that are less binding by legal definitions but perhaps equally binding in concern and support. Young adults may view cohabitation as a means of learning more about a possible marriage partner on a day-to-day basis, in the hope that a future marriage will then be stronger and more lasting. Homosexuality or bisexuality may be expressed openly for the first time during this period.

Conflicts in parenting can occur if an individual's gender role does not meet the expectations of a family, or if an individual's partner has different expectations regarding gender role. It is time well spent for parents-to-be to take time to discuss with each other the views they have on parenting to see whether they agree on male and female roles and their relationship with their children. A single parent may be concerned about how both roles can be fulfilled and can appreciate talking with a nurse about this area of concern. Conflicts in the roles parents have chosen often come to light for the first time during pregnancy, as they worry about what type of parents they are going to be or whether they are adequately prepared to be parents.

Young adulthood is the time when many couples begin childbearing. Early in pregnancy, a woman may experience a decreased desire for coitus because of tiredness, mastalgia, nausea and vomiting, and other accompanying signs of pregnancy. As pregnancy advances and her abdomen increases in size, she and her sexual partner may need to use new positions for penis-vagina intercourse such as a side-by-side position or the woman in a superior position. Oral sex continues to be safe during pregnancy as long as a partner does not have oral herpes or a sore throat or forcefully blows air into the vagina (risk of infection and air embolism, respectively). Women with more than one sexual partner or a non-monogamous sexual partner need to practise safer sex, including using condoms for penis-vagina intercourse to prevent transmission of an STI during pregnancy.

Middle-aged adult

For many women and men in midlife, sexuality has achieved a degree of stability. A sense of masculinity or femininity and comfortable patterns of behaviour have been established.

This increased security in identity can promote greater intimacy in sexual and social relationships. This may also be a time when adults allow themselves more freedom in exploring and satisfying sexual needs.

Although menopause alters reproductive functioning, it does not physically inhibit sexual functioning. Generally, a woman with a strong self-image, positive sexual and social relationships, and knowledge regarding her body and menopause is likely to progress through this natural biological stage without problems and remain sexually active and satisfied. Nurses can be instrumental in teaching women what to expect at menopause so that it is not a surprise and in helping them maintain self-esteem through this natural process.

During midlife, men may begin to experience changes in sperm production, erectile power, achievement of orgasm and sex drive, although these changes usually do not significantly alter reproductive or sexual functioning. Some men feel that these changes threaten their sexuality and "maleness" and may respond negatively. Other men feel that these changes make sex more pleasurable and intimate and often respond positively. Actual sexual dysfunctions, as a result of physical or psychosocial changes, may arise at this time. For example, a man's erectile dysfunction may have an underlying pathology such as circulatory changes secondary to undiagnosed diabetes and should be investigated. Teaching men about normal biophysical changes, providing them with methods to improve sexual functioning and offering them support are important health education roles.

Midlife is often a time when both men and women reexamine life goals, careers, accomplishments, value systems, and familial and social relationships. As a result, some people adapt and enjoy, whereas others experience stress or a crisis. This reflection can positively or negatively affect an individual's gender identity and sexuality. The increased incidence of sexual encounters with younger partners at this time may be a person's way of reassuring themselves of their attractiveness and denial of ageing.

Certain medications, such as anti-hypertensives, antianxiety agents and narcotics, may diminish sexual desire and response in both men and women. Being aware of this fact is important not only for individuals, so that they can understand that it is an expected response, but also for their partners.

The individual who comments about the need to maintain a reduced activity level at work or a reduced social schedule may also be seeking information and direction in other important areas of life, such as in their sexual relationship(s).

Some women have surgery at midlife such as a hysterectomy (removal of the uterus). If both ovaries are also removed (bilateral oophorectomy), an immediate surgical menopause occurs. For some women, the loss of their uterus and ovaries can be synonymous with the loss of their femininity. Women who have such surgery need sensitive nurses to listen to their concerns about the meaning of the experience for them.

Older adult

Both male and female older adults continue to enjoy active sexual relationships. Some men experience less erectile firmness or ejaculatory force than when they were younger, but others discover that they are able to maintain an erection for longer. Older women may have less vaginal secretions because they have less oestrogen after menopause. Use of a water-soluble lubricant before coitus can enhance their comfort and enjoyment. Both sexes need to follow safer sex practices throughout life. Because males remain fertile throughout life, they must continue to be responsible sex partners in terms of reproductive planning.

The individual who has a physical or cognitive disability

Individuals who are physically or cognitively challenged have sexual desires and needs the same as all others (Franco, Cardoso & Neto, 2012). However, they may have difficulty with sexual identity or sexual fulfilment because of their disability. Males with upper spinal cord injury may have difficulty with erection and ejaculation, because these actions are governed at the spinal level. Physical stimulation of the penis or psychological stimulation achieves erection in most men with spinal cord lesions and satisfying sexual relationships are very possible. Most women with spinal cord injuries cannot experience orgasm but are able to conceive and have children.

Anyone who interprets a procedure such as a colostomy as disfiguring may be reluctant to participate in sexual activities, fearing that the sight of an apparatus will diminish their partner's satisfaction or enjoyment. People with chronic pain (e.g. arthritis) may be too uncomfortable to enjoy sexual relations. Individuals with urinary catheters may be concerned about their ability to enjoy coitus with the catheter in place. For women, a retention catheter should not interfere with sexual intercourse. Men can be taught how to replace their own catheter, so that they can remove it when desired. In all instances in which one sexual partner is disabled in some way, the response of a loving partner does much to enhance body image and feelings of adequacy of a mate. Encouraging these individuals to ask questions and work on specific difficulties is a nursing role.

Sexuality is a facet of rehabilitation that has not always received attention. If a person can accomplish activities of daily living such as eating, elimination and mobility, then they are considered to be leading a normal or near-normal life. Establishment of a satisfying sexual relationship is an important part of living, however, so should be included in assessments of people in rehabilitation programs.

HUMAN SEXUAL RESPONSE

Sexuality has always been a part of human life, but it is only in the past few decades that it has been studied scientifically. One common finding of researchers has been that feelings and attitudes about sex vary widely: the sexual experience is unique to each individual, but sexual physiology (i.e. how the body responds to sexual arousal) has common features (Georgiadis & Kringelbach, 2012).

Sexual response cycle

Two of the earliest researchers of sexual response were Masters and Johnson. In 1966, they published the results of a major study of sexual physiology based on more than 10,000 episodes of sexual activity among more than 600 men and women (Masters & Johnson, 1966). In this study, they described the human sexual response as a cycle with four discrete stages: excitement, plateau, orgasm and resolution. The Masters and Johnson Sexual Response Cycle has been critiqued and stages may actually be more individualised than Masters and Johnson proposed; they may blend together much more into one smooth process of desire, arousal and orgasm (Paterson et al., 2014).

Excitement

Excitement occurs with physical and psychological stimulation (i.e. sight, sound, emotion or thought) that causes parasympathetic nerve stimulation. This leads to arterial dilation and venous constriction in the genital area. The resulting increased blood supply leads to vasocongestion and increasing muscular tension. In women, this vasocongestion causes the clitoris to increase in size and mucoid fluid to appear on vaginal walls as lubrication. The vagina widens in diameter above the introitus and increases in length. The nipples become erect. In men, penile erection occurs, as well as scrotal thickening and elevation of the testes. In both sexes, there is an increase in heart and respiratory rates and blood pressure.

Plateau

The plateau stage is reached just before orgasm. In women, the clitoris is drawn forwards and retracts under the clitoral prepuce; the lower part of the vagina becomes extremely congested (formation of the orgasmic platform) and there is increased nipple elevation. In men, the vasocongestion leads to distension of the penis. Heart rate increases to 100 to 175 beats per minute and respiratory rate to approximately 40 respirations per minute.

Orgasm

Orgasm occurs when stimulation proceeds through the plateau stage to a point at which the body suddenly discharges accumulated sexual tension. A vigorous contraction of muscles in the pelvic area expels or dissipates blood and fluid from the area of congestion. The average number of contractions for a woman is 8 to 15 contractions at intervals of 1 every 0.8 seconds. In men, muscle contractions surrounding the seminal vessels and prostate project semen into the proximal urethra. These contractions are followed immediately by 3 to 7 propulsive ejaculatory contractions, occurring at the same time interval as in the woman, which force semen from the penis.

As the shortest stage in the sexual response cycle, orgasm is usually experienced as intense pleasure affecting the whole body, not just the pelvic area. It is also a highly personal experience: descriptions of orgasms vary greatly from person to person.

Resolution

Resolution is a period of approximately 30 minutes during which the external and internal genital organs return to an unaroused state. For the male, a refractory period occurs during which further orgasm is impossible. Women do not go through this refractory period, so it is possible for women who are interested and properly stimulated to have additional orgasms immediately after the first (Paterson et al., 2014).

Controversies about female orgasm

The female orgasm has been a topic of much controversy over the years, beginning with Freud, who deducted that there were two types of female orgasms: clitoral and vaginal. He believed that clitoral orgasms (originating from masturbation or other non-coital acts) represented sexual immaturity and that only vaginal orgasms were the authentic, mature form of sexual behaviour in women. Accordingly, he considered women to be neurotic if they could not achieve orgasm through intercourse (Colson, 2010).

Colson (2010) showed that there is no physiological difference between an orgasm achieved through intercourse and one achieved by direct stimulation of the clitoris. Women have reported a difference in intensity and character between orgasms achieved through coitus and through other means, and some prefer one to the other, but there is no physiological difference between them. For most women, adequate time for foreplay is essential for them to be orgasmic.

In recent years, a subject of controversy regarding female sexuality has arisen: the existence or not of the G-spot. First described in 1950 by the German physician, Gräfenberg, not as a spot but as an area of urethral tissue presumably locatable on the inner anterior portion of the vaginal wall, halfway between the pubic bone and the cervix, the G-spot has been promoted as an area of heightened erotic sensitivity (Gräfenberg, 1950). Several studies carried out in the past 10 years have not been able to verify the existence of this particular anatomical site, although some women do claim to possess such an erotic trigger (Burri, Cherkas & Spector, 2010) with or without an emission of fluid accompanying orgasm.

Influence of the menstrual cycle on sexual response

During the second half of the menstrual cycle—the luteal phase—there is increased fluid retention and vasocongestion in a woman's lower pelvis. Because some vasocongestion is already present at the beginning of the excitement stage of the sexual response, some women appear to reach the plateau stage more quickly and achieve orgasm more readily during this time. Women may also be more interested in initiating sexual relations at this time.

Influence of pregnancy on sexual response

Pregnancy is another time in life when there is vasocongestion of the lower pelvis because of the blood supply needed by a rapidly growing fetus. This causes some women to experience orgasm for the first time during a pregnancy. Following pregnancy, some women experience increased sexual interest because of the effect of oxytocin during breastfeeding and because the new growth of blood vessels during pregnancy lasts for some time and continues to facilitate pelvic vasocongestion. For others, especially those who are experiencing nausea or extreme tiredness, sexual interest can decrease dramatically. This is why discussing sexual relationships and the huge continuum of "normal" is an important part of health teaching during and after pregnancy, as it is at any other time. At a time when a woman may want sexual contact, she needs to be free of myths and misconceptions, such as the notion that orgasm might cause a miscarriage. Although the level of oxytocin does peak in women and men during orgasm, this rise is not sufficient to lead to worry that orgasm or sexual activity will lead to preterm labour in the healthy woman.

For some women, the increased breast engorgement that accompanies pregnancy results in extreme breast sensitivity. Foreplay that includes sucking or massaging the breasts may cause the release of oxytocin, but it is not contraindicated unless the woman has a history of preterm labour or is experiencing threatened preterm labour (Chapman et al., 2013).

Types of sexual orientation

Sexual gratification is experienced in several ways. What is considered normal varies greatly among cultures, although general components of accepted sexual activity are that it is an activity of adults and privacy, consent and lack of force are included. Most individual value systems are closely aligned to these cultural norms.

Heterosexuality

A heterosexual is a person who finds sexual fulfilment with a member of the opposite gender. Because interest in sexual activity and relationships may begin as early as the beginning of puberty, it is important that information on safer sex practices, including issues of choice and consent, is provided early. Otherwise, this knowledge comes too late to be most helpful.

Homosexuality

A homosexual is a person who finds sexual fulfilment with a member of their own sex. Many homosexual men prefer to use the term "gay". "Lesbian" refers to a homosexual woman. More recent terms are MWM and WWW.

Why homosexual gender identity develops is unknown, although evidence that this orientation is genetically determined or develops because of the effect of an unusual level of oestrogen or testosterone in utero is increasing. Even before puberty, most individuals who are homosexual know they are "different" in that they are not sexually interested in opposite sex classmates. It is usually during adolescence, in seeking a sense of identity, that they realise the reason they feel "different" is because they are homosexual. This can be a stressful time, because a homosexual identity may not be easy to reveal to family or friends. Although attitudes are changing, some people stigmatise or fear homosexuality to the extent that homophobia still exists (Lee, 2013).

Although MWM and WWW have often demonstrated behaviour that is inconsistent with expected gender roles from early childhood, young adulthood is the time most people begin to identify as homosexual or bisexual (Rosario, Schrimshaw & Hunter, 2011). Some young adults are worried about the stigma of being labelled homosexual and therefore keep their identity secret from heterosexual friends, family, acquaintances and nurses. Others "commit" or "come out" and are more comfortable revealing their sexual identity.

Because a period of identity confusion during adolescence can be traumatic, it is important for nurses to be extremely sensitive to needs in this area. MWM may need additional counselling to help them avoid acquiring HIV and other STIs, because issues such as safer anal intercourse may not be routinely covered in sex education classes. If WWW have sexual contact with bisexual women, they have the same risk of STIs as the heterosexual/bisexual population. Although not immune to STIs, lesbian women tend to be at less risk of STIs because of the lower incidence of these infections in the lesbian population.

Bisexuality

People are said to be bisexual if they achieve sexual satisfaction from both homosexual and heterosexual relationships. Like MWM, bisexual men may be at greater risk of HIV and other STIs than are others. Female partners of bisexual men need to be aware that they are also at increased risk of HIV and other STIs.

Transsexuality

A transsexual or transgender person is an individual who, although of one biological gender, feels as if they are of the opposite gender (McQueen, 2014). Such people may have sex-change operations so that they appear cosmetically as the gender they feel they are. Such operations do not change the person's chromosomal structure, however, so although capable of sexual relations in this new role (a vagina or penis is surgically created), the person is incapable of reproduction. The incidence of sex change operations has decreased in recent years because of potential disappointment after the surgery: despite a new outward appearance, people realise that they are still not totally the person they wished to become. Children of a transsexual parent may have a great deal of difficulty understanding why their parent changed from male to female or female to male (Veldorale-Griffin, 2014).

CASE STUDY QUESTION

4. Violet asks you during one of your interviews to explain what transgender means. Your best response would be that a transgender person would:
   a. Be more likely homosexual
   b. Be more likely bisexual
   c. Be of one biological gender but identify with another
   d. Be asexual

DISORDERS OF SEXUAL FUNCTIONING

Disorders involving sexual functioning can be lifelong (primary) or acquired (secondary). They can have a psychogenic origin (produced by psychic rather than organic factors), a biogenic origin (produced by biological processes), or both. They can be universal or specific. They occur in both men and women.

Strategies are available for nurses to use to assist them whenever they are communicating with individuals about disorders of sexual functioning or any sexual or reproductive health issue. These strategies are useful during health education, health promotion and sexual counselling. One strategy is the PLISSIT model of sexual counselling, first presented by Annon (1981) and of proven effectiveness for nurses (Huang et al., 2013). The PLISSIT model involves nurse counselling at an increasing level of complexity and can be outlined as follows:

P **P**ermission
LI **L**imited **i**nformation
SS **S**pecific **s**uggestions
IT **I**ntensive **t**herapy

- *Permission.* The nurse ensures the person knows they have permission to discuss any aspect of their sexuality that might be a concern to them. Equally important, the person knows they have the right not to discuss any issue with the nurse that they do not feel secure in doing so. This is especially important in the early part of a nurse–client relationship, where the person may not feel safe enough to share their thoughts and concerns about sensitive issues. By providing permission to discuss sexual issues, the nurse should never take on an interrogatory, interview style. It is the nurse's role to create a safe environment and relationship, so the person feels safe to discuss their sexual and reproductive health if, when and with whom they choose.
- *Limited information.* The nurse provides the level of information they are competent and confident to share with the person. Importantly, the information should not be limited by the nurse's knowledge base as the nurse has a responsibility to find out required information and/or refer the person to another health professional who can assist. The information should be limited to that which is appropriate, relevant and applicable to the person's needs, questions and concerns.
- *Specific suggestions.* It is the nurse's responsibility to ensure that any specific suggestions they may make are based on best evidence, and are relevant and appropriate for that individual.
- *Intensive therapy.* Most nurses do not have the experience, qualifications, confidence or competence to provide intensive therapy for individuals who have concerns of a sexual nature and it is important they do not attempt to provide nursing care beyond their scope of practice. Where intensive therapy is required, the nurse should refer the person to a suitably qualified and experienced nurse specialist (e.g. in women's or sexual health) or to a counsellor/clinical psychologist. The PLISSIT model is a very suitable tool to use when working with people who express concerns in regard to sexual difficulties, some of which are outlined below.

Inhibited sexual desire

Inhibited sexual desire can be a very normal phenomenon related to attributes in a sexual partner that are perceived as unattractive; for example, poor personal hygiene or halitosis. It may also reflect other difficulties within a relationship; for example, when a person feels neglected or abused by their partner. Or the cause may simply be tiredness; for example, one partner has the primary responsibility for the childrearing and household chores. Lessened interest in sexual relations is normal in some circumstances, such as after the death of a family member, a divorce or a stressful job change. The support of a caring sexual partner or relief of the tension causing the stress allows a return to sexual interest.

Decreased sexual desire can also be a side effect of many medicines. Chronic diseases such as peptic ulcers or chronic pulmonary disorders that cause frequent pain or discomfort may interfere with a person's overall wellbeing and interest in sexual activity. An individual with an STI such as genital herpes may choose to forgo sexual relations rather than inform a partner of the disease.

What if...

Marella Jube, who has brought her 2-month-old baby for her initial immunisation to the child and family health clinic where you are nursing, bursts into tears during her baby's pre-immunisation assessment and tells you that she and her partner are experiencing sexual difficulties as she is just not interested in having sex with him? Marella tells you she is feeling depressed and has recently been prescribed anti-depressants by her general practitioner. Marella is breastfeeding her baby daughter and is using the progestogen-only pill for contraception. All of the above factors may inhibit sexual desire. Using the PLISSIT model described above, how would you respond to Marella?

Anorgasmia

A woman's inability to reach orgasm can be a result of relationship problems, poor sexual technique, concentrating too hard on achievement or negative attitudes towards sexual expression. Treatment is aimed at relieving the underlying cause. It may include providing limited information, specific suggestions and counselling for the couple about sexual functioning and needs.

Erectile dysfunction

Erectile dysfunction (ED), formerly referred to as impotence, is the inability of a man to produce or maintain an erection long enough for vaginal penetration or partner satisfaction (Lewis et al., 2010). Most causes of ED are physical, such as ageing, atherosclerosis or diabetes, which limit blood supply. It may also occur as a side effect of certain medications. The problem is compounded by doubt about the ability to perform and reluctance to discuss the problem with healthcare providers. Examples of medications prescribed for ED are sildenafil citrate (Viagra), tadalafil (Cialis) and vardenafil (Levitra), which are taken up to once a day to stimulate penile erection (McKenna & Mirkov, 2014). However, these should not be prescribed without thorough investigations to ensure there is no co-morbidity as they are contraindicated in men with a risk of cardiovascular illness and also in those who are taking medications that contain nitrates. A surgical implant to aid erection, penile injections or the use of vacuum pressure are possible alternative medical/surgical options. Testosterone injections may be helpful in some men. In all instances, frank discussion about the cause of the problem and currently available therapies is helpful.

Premature ejaculation

Premature ejaculation (PE) is ejaculation before penile-vaginal contact (Lewis et al., 2010). The term is also often used to mean ejaculation before the sexual partner's satisfaction has been achieved. Premature ejaculation can be unsatisfactory and frustrating for both partners. The cause, like that of ED, can be psychological. Masturbating to orgasm (in which orgasm is achieved quickly because of lack of time) may exacerbate PE. Other reasons suggested are doubt about masculinity and fear of impregnating or infecting a partner which may increase anxiety and, therefore, PE. Specific suggestions may be for the man/couple to practise a squeeze technique of his penis to delay ejaculation, and sexual counselling for both partners to reduce stress. Medical options include the prescription of serotonergic anti-depressants such as mirtazapine. However, side effects are common and may be serious; for example, exacerbation of existing depression or suicidal ideation.

Persistent sexual arousal syndrome

Persistent sexual arousal syndrome (PSAS) is excessive and unrelenting sexual arousal in the absence of desire (Lewis et al., 2010). It may be triggered by medications or psychological factors. When assessing someone with the disorder, be certain to ask if they are taking any herbal remedies such as Ginkgo biloba as some of these can have arousal effects.

Pain disorders

Because the reproductive system has a sensitive nerve supply, when pain occurs in response to sexual activities, it can be acute and severe and impair a person's ability to enjoy sexual activity.

Vaginismus

Vaginismus is involuntary contraction of the muscles at the outlet of the vagina that prohibits penetration. It may be primary, when a woman has never been able to tolerate vaginal penetration, or secondary, as occurs when she has once enjoyed vaginal penetration which is now impossible due to pain. The vaginismus may be universal, when the woman is not able to tolerate vaginal penetration with any object, for example a tampon, or it may be specific and relate to penile penetration only. On rarer occasions, a woman is able to tolerate penile penetration by one man but not another. Vaginismus may be iatrogenic and occur in women following medical/surgical/obstetric procedures or may occur following trauma such as sexual assault; or the cause may be unknown. Whatever the type or the cause of the woman's vaginismus, intensive and long-term therapy is often required to alleviate the problem and, for most nurses, their role will be to refer the woman/couple for sexual counselling.

Dyspareunia

Dyspareunia is pain during coitus. It may be shallow and occur simultaneously with vaginal penetration or it may be deep and associated with penile thrusting. There are many causes and one of the most common is attempted vaginal penetration before the woman is fully aroused. For this reason, it is important that the female partner with dyspareunia takes charge of when the penis penetrates and the position that the couple assumes so that the depth of penetration can be controlled. Other causes may be endometriosis (abnormal placement of endometrial tissue), vestibulitis (inflammation of the vestibule), vaginal infection or hormonal changes such as those that occur with menopause and cause vaginal drying. A psychological component may be present. Limited information provided by the nurse may relate to sexual techniques to ensure adequate arousal; specific suggestions might be for the couple to ensure that depth of penetration can be controlled by female superior coital positions. Medical/surgical options include treating any underlying cause for example, the prescription of azithromycin to treat chlamydial infection or laser to remove endometriosis surgically.

CASE STUDY QUESTION

5. Violet asks you about sexual harassment. You tell her that sexual harassment:
   a. Is a form of sexual assault
   b. Occurs between both genders
   c. Is illegal
   d. Is all of the above

Critical thinking exercises

1. Providing individuals with limited information is an integral part of sexual and reproductive health education and promotion. What resources do you have to ensure all individuals are able to receive holistic nursing care that addresses their sexual and reproductive health needs?
2. Intensive therapy/counselling may sometimes be needed, for example when a woman is experiencing vaginismus. Many women's and sexual health nurses have postgraduate qualifications and experience in sexual counselling. Identify health professionals in your local area to whom you might be able to refer individuals if they require intensive sexual therapy.

Resources

For an extensive range of additional resources to enhance teaching and learning and to facilitate understanding of this chapter, please see the text's accompanying website located on thePoint at http://thepoint.lww.com.

References

Annon, J. (1981). PLISSIT therapy. In R. Corsini (Ed.). *Handbook of Innovative Psychotherapies* (pp. 626–639). New York: Wiley & Sons.

Aruda, M. (2011). Predictors of unprotected intercourse for female adolescents measured at their request for a pregnancy test. *Journal of Pediatric Nursing, 26*(3), 216–223.

Burri, A., Cherkas, L. & Spector, T. (2010). Genetic and environmental influences on self-reported G-spots in women: A twin study. *Journal of Sexual Medicine, 7*, 1842–1852.

Chapman, T., Pincombe, J., Harris, M. & Fereday, J. (2013). Antenatal breast expression: Exploration and extent of teaching practices amongst International Board Certified Lactation Consultant midwives across Australia. *Women & Birth, 26*(1), 41–48.

Colson, M. (2010). Female orgasm: Myths, facts and controversies. *Sexologies, 19*(1), 8–14.

Department of Education and Early Childhood Development. (2013). Age of initiation of sexual intercourse in young people (mean). Melbourne, Vic, accessed 19 February 2015, www.education.vic.gov.au/about/research/pages/146intercourse.aspx.

Franco, D., Cardoso, J. & Neto, I. (2012). Attitudes toward affectivity and sexuality of people with intellectual disability. *Sexuality and Disability, 30*(3), 261–267.

Georgiadis, J. & Kringelbach, M. (2012). The human response cycle: Brain imaging evidence linking sex to other pleasures. *Progress in Neurobiology, 98*(1), 49–81.

Gräfenberg, E. (1950). The role of the urethra in female orgasm. *International Journal of Sexology, 3*(3), 145–148.

Hayatbakhsh, M., Clavarino, A., Williams, G., Sina, M. & Najam, J. (2012). Cigarette smoking and age at menopause: A large prospective study. *Maturitas, 72*(4), 346–352.

Hetzenbuehler, M. & Keyes, K. (2013). Inclusive anti-bullying policies and reduced risk of suicide attempts in lesbian and gay youth. *Journal of Adolescent Health, 53*(1), S21–S26.

Huang, C., Tsai, L., Tseng, T., Li, C. & Lee, S. (2013). Nursing students' attitudes towards provision of sexual health care in clinical practice. *Journal of Clinical Nursing, 22*(23/24), 3577–3586.

Lee, J. (2013). *Torn: Rescuing the Gospel from the Gays-vs-Christian Debate*. New York: Hachette Book Group.

Lewis, R., Fugi-Meyer, K., Corona, G., Hayes, R., Lauman, E., Moreira Jr, L., Rellini, A. & Segraves, T. (2010). Definitions/epidemiology/risk factors for sexual dysfunction. *Journal of Sexual Medicine, 7*(4pt2), 1598–1607.

McKenna, L. & Mirkov, S. (2014). *McKenna's Drug Handbook for Nursing and Midwifery* (7th ed.). Sydney: Lippincott Williams & Wilkins.

McQueen, P. (2014). Enslaved by one's body? Gender, citizenship and the 'wrong body' narrative. *Citizenship Studies, 18*(5), 533–548.

Masters, W. & Johnson, V. (1966). *Human Sexual Response*. Boston, MA: Little, Brown.

Ngum Chi Watts, M., Liamputtong, P. & Carolan, M. (2013). Contraception knowledge and attitudes: Truths and myths among African Australian teenage mothers in Greater Melbourne, Australia. *Journal of Clinical Nursing, 23*, 2131–2141.

Paterson, L., Jin, E., Amsel, R. & Binik, Y. (2014). Gender similarities and differences in sexual arousal, desire and orgasmic pleasure in the laboratory. *Journal of Sex Research, 51*(7), 801–813.

Rizvi, S. & Kennedy, S. (2013). Psychopharmacology for the clinician. *Journal of Psychiatry and Neuroscience, 38*(5), E27–E28.

Rosario, M., Schrimshaw, E. & Hunter, J. (2011). Different patterns of sexual identity development over time: Implications for the psychological adjustment of lesbian, gay and bisexual youths. *Journal of Sex Research, 48*(1), 3–5.

Saunamaki, N., Andersson, M. & Engstrom, M. (2010). Discussing sexuality with patients: nurses' attitudes and beliefs. *Journal of Advanced Nursing, 66*(6), 1308–1316.

Simons, L., Burt, C. & Tambling, R. (2013). Identifying mediators of the influence of family factors on risky sexual behavior. *Journal of Child and Family Studies, 22*, 460–470.

Veldorale-Griffin, A. (2014). Transgender parents and their adult children's experiences of disclosure and transition. *Journal of GLBT Family Studies, 10*(5), 475–501.

Suggested readings

Olsson, A., Robertson, E., Falk, K. & Nissen, E. (2011). Assessing women's sexual life after childbirth: The role of the postnatal check. *Midwifery*, 27(2), 195–202.

O'Maley, D. & Smith, V. (2013). Altered sexual health after childbirth: Part 2. *Practising Midwife*, 16(2), 27–29.

Chapter 6

Assisting the family with contraception planning

This chapter adds information about supporting individuals and couples to prevent pregnancy in a planned way and in an emergency situation. Unwanted unplanned pregnancy is also discussed.

LEARNING OBJECTIVES

After mastering the contents of this chapter, you should be able to:

1. Describe common methods of contraception used in Australia and New Zealand and understand the advantages, disadvantages, side effects and failure rates associated with each method.
2. Use critical thinking to analyse ways that contraception planning can be accomplished.
3. Assess clients for contraception needs.
4. Identify expected outcomes for couples desiring contraception planning.
5. Plan nursing care related to contraception planning.
6. Evaluate expected outcomes for achievement and effectiveness of care.
7. Integrate knowledge of contraception planning with nursing considerations to achieve quality child and family health nursing care.

KEY TERMS

- abstinence
- barrier methods
- coitus
- coitus interruptus
- condom
- contraceptive
- diaphragm
- elective termination of pregnancy
- emergency contraception
- fertile days
- implantation contraception
- intrauterine device
- laparoscopy
- male condom
- natural family planning
- tubal ligation
- vaginal ring
- vasectomy

CASE STUDY

Seventeen-year-old Lena Crews presents at your Community Health Centre for contraception advice. Lena has been sexually active for two months and has had one sexual partner; her current boyfriend who is 18 years old. They occasionally use condoms but they also practise sex without condoms. When they don't use a condom, Lena says her boyfriend "pulls out", but she knows this puts her at risk of pregnancy, which she doesn't want at this stage of her life. Lena is worried that she may fall pregnant and wants to discuss her options.

CASE STUDY QUESTION

1. What education and support about choosing a contraceptive method would you give Lena?

Contraceptive planning includes all the decisions an individual or couple make about whether and when to have children, how many children to have and how they are spaced. Some people you meet, like Lena in the case study, will want to know how to avoid conceiving; others will need advice and support because their contraceptive efforts have failed (Bond, 2013).

It is important for the health of children that as many pregnancies as possible be intended, because when a pregnancy is unintended or mistimed, both short-term and long-term consequences may occur. These include women being less likely to seek antenatal care, being less likely to breastfeed and being less careful to protect their fetus from harmful substances. A disproportionate number of women who bear children whose conception was unintended are adolescent; women in this group are less likely to complete high school or university and more likely to require government assistance and to live in poverty than are their peers who are not mothers. Children born to adolescent mothers are at greater risk of low birth weight, dying in the first year, being abused and not receiving sufficient resources for healthy development (Centers for Disease Control and Prevention, 2012).

CONTRACEPTIVE PLANNING

Reproductive and sexual health assessment

Humans are sexual beings and there will come a time in life when the people you care for will need accurate information on their reproductive cycles, contraception choices and sexual health needs. Prior to providing contraceptive information, it is important to conduct a reproductive and sexual health assessment. Because of changing societal values, it is far more acceptable for people to discuss issues of a sexual nature than ever before and this means that many people who require help with contraception will ask for it. There will, however, also be people who are not comfortable to start a conversation with a health professional about their contraceptive concerns and needs. To give those people an opportunity to voice their needs in this regard, the topic should also be incorporated whenever a health history is taken in a primary care setting. This assessment should include the following:

- General health (age, current medications, past surgeries, allergies, mental health history)
- Social history (tobacco, alcohol and/or recreational drug use, distance from health facilities, social support, living conditions, ethnic background, history of tattoos and piercings)
- Family history (cancer, heart disease, clotting disorders, venous thromboembolic diseases)
- Breast history (previous breast problems, breast screening, cosmetic surgery/implants, breastfeeding)
- Contraception history (current method if any, past use of contraceptives, history of any problems associated with contraception)
- Sexual history (previous sexually transmitted infections [STIs], last STI screen, sexual practices, frequency, number of partners)

For women, the assessment should also include:

- Menstrual history (age at menarche, last menstrual period, length and flow of cycle, premenstrual symptoms)
- Obstetric history (number of pregnancies, number of live births, miscarriages, terminations)
- Gynaecological history (vaginal discharge, genital lesions or lumps, pelvic inflammatory disease, endometriosis, pelvic or lower back pain, date of last Pap smear, history of abnormal pap smears, pain or bleeding with intercourse) (Collier, 2011).

Nursing considerations

Contraception planning touches so many facets of life, the nurse's approach to these consultations can differ greatly depending on the circumstances. Examples of factors that will influence the consultation might include:

- Readiness for/capacity to understand information about contraception options
- Spiritual, cultural and/or emotional dissonance or distress related to own or partner's preferences for contraception
- Decisional conflict regarding choice of birth control because of health concerns
- Powerlessness related to failure of chosen contraceptive
- Compromised sexual activity pattern related to fear of pregnancy
- Physical or dexterity limitations due to illness or disability
- Decisional conflict in the case of unintended pregnancy.

When establishing expected outcomes for care in this area, be certain that they take account of and are realistic for the factors and considerations relevant to the individual. As outlined above, contraception decisions are influenced by many factors; the nurse's role is to educate and to support the choice an individual or couple comes to decide is right for her/him/them. For example, if a woman identifies difficulties in taking regular medications it might not be realistic for her to plan to take an oral contraceptive at the same time every day. Be certain to be sensitive to a person or couple's religious, cultural, social and moral beliefs before suggesting possible methods. It is equally important to explore your own beliefs and values. This not only helps develop self-awareness of how these beliefs affect nursing care, but it allows you to become more sensitive to the beliefs of others.

Some couples cannot make realistic plans about contraception because they do not have all the information about the available options. It is vital, when counselling on this topic to be certain to emphasise safer sex considerations (see Chapter 5) as well as contraceptive ones. For example, although many contraceptive options offer reliable pregnancy prevention, only condoms provide protection against STIs, which is an important concern if the person is not practising monogamy. Two very helpful resources people can refer to for more information are the "advice" section of the New Zealand Family Planning website (www.familyplanning.org.nz), and the "publications" section of the Sexual Health and Family Planning Australia (SHFPA) website (www.shfpa.org.au). Additionally, further information about emergency contraception is available at the Family Planning NSW website (www.fpnsw.org.au/422437_8.html).

Evaluation is important in contraceptive planning, because anything that causes a person or couple to discontinue or misuse a particular method will leave them at risk of pregnancy. Reassess early (within 1 to 3 weeks) after a new method of contraception is started, to ensure its use is working for the person or couple, and that it is being used effectively.

METHODS OF CONTRACEPTION

There are several methods of contraception available in Australia and New Zealand and the widespread use of contraceptives today points to both an increased awareness of responsibility for contraception and the wider range of options available (see Table 6.1). The nurse's role in relation to this topic is to educate individuals and couples on what methods are available, how various methods of contraception work, how they compare in terms of benefits and disadvantages, and how to use them effectively.

Natural family planning

Natural family planning can be used to prevent pregnancy or to assist a couple to conceive. Natural family planning involves no introduction of chemicals or foreign material into the body. Many people hold religious beliefs that rule out the use of birth control pills or devices; others simply prefer natural methods because no expense or foreign substance is involved; still others believe that a

TABLE 6.1 Overview of contraceptive choices

Contraception - Your Choice

Contact Family Planning for detailed information on any of these methods

POSITIVE SEXUAL HEALTH
Family Planning
familyplanning.org.nz

Method	What is it? How does it work?	Chance of getting pregnant	Health concerns	Advantages	Disadvantages
LONG ACTING REVERSIBLE CONTRACEPTION					
IMPLANT	• progestogen is released from 1 or 2 rods implanted under the skin of the arm • by thickening mucus in cervix and may stop ovaries from releasing an egg each month	• less than 1%	• no serious risk	• lasts 3 - 5 years - fit and forget • useful for women who can't take combined pill • useful for women who forget pills or injection appointments	• irregular bleeding often gets better with time and can be controlled with medication
INTRA UTERINE DEVICE - IUD	• Put inside the womb • Copper IUD or progestogen-releasing Mirena (IUS) • stops sperm reaching an egg	• IUD and Mirena – less than 1%	• very small chance of pelvic infection when IUD put in	• can stay in place for 5 years or more - fit and forget • doesn't interfere with sexual intercourse • IUS – lighter periods or no period at all, suitable for women with heavy periods	• needs to be inserted by an experienced doctor or nurse • IUD may cause heavier periods or cramping • IUS may cause irregular bleeding in the first few months
DEPO PROVERA	• an injection of progestogen • stops ovaries from releasing an egg each month	• typically 3% but less than 1% if next injection given on time	• no serious concerns	• one injection lasts 12 weeks • doesn't interfere with sexual intercourse • usually no periods • useful for women who can't take combined pill	• irregular bleeding, no periods or occasional heavy bleeding • periods and fertility take an average of 6 months to return after stopping the injection • may have change in weight
CONTRACEPTIVE PILLS AND RING					
COMBINED PILL	• pill made of two hormones, oestrogen and progestogen • stops ovaries from releasing an egg each month	• typically 8% but less than 1% if used perfectly	• very small chance of blood clots, heart attacks and strokes. More likely in women over 35 who smoke, are obese or have a family history of the above conditions • very slight increased risk of cervical cancer	• simple and easy to take • doesn't interfere with sexual intercourse • periods usually regular, shorter, lighter and less painful • less chance of cancer of lining of the womb or ovaries • can be taken up to menopause if a healthy non smoker	• should not be used by women over 35 who smoke • must remember to take it daily • may have irregular bleeding
PROGESTOGEN ONLY PILL	• pill made of one hormone – progestogen • by thickening mucus in cervix and may stop ovaries from releasing an egg each month	• typically 8% but less than 1% if used perfectly	• no serious risk	• doesn't interfere with sexual intercourse • can be used at any age • can be used by breast-feeding women • useful for women who can't take combined pill	• may have irregular bleeding
VAGINAL RING	• NuvaRing contains two hormones, oestrogen and progestogen • Sits inside vagina • Stops ovaries from releasing an egg each month	• typically 8% but less than 1% if used perfectly	• very small chance of blood clots, heart attacks and strokes. More likely in women over 35 who smoke, are obese or have a family history of the above conditions	• Lasts for 3-4 weeks • Useful for those who forget pills	• Should not be used by women over 35 who smoke
BARRIERS					
MALE CONDOM	• a thin rubber barrier • fits over erect penis and catches sperm when the man ejaculates • best used with lubricant (water based)	• typically 15% but 2% if used perfectly every time • DO NOT USE oil-based lubricant or some anti thrush creams	• none known	• easy to use, easy to carry • used only when needed • helps protect against STIs • available from Family Planning clinics and other health care providers • can buy from pubs, clubs, pharmacies and many shops • cheaper on prescription	• some people are allergic to rubber • must be put on when penis is erect and before sexual intercourse • some people say it reduces sexual feeling • can slip off or break
FEMALE CONDOM	• a thin polyurethane barrier • goes into the vagina and prevents sperm entering the woman's body	• typically 21% but 5% if used perfectly	• none known	• helps protect against STIs • women can use it • easy to use	• relatively expensive • can be noisy • can get them from the internet • need to insert every time
DIAPHRAGM	• dome shaped silicone barrier fits inside vagina over the cervix • used with spermicide jelly that kills sperm	• typically 16% but can be 6% if using spermicide and following instructions perfectly	• more bladder infections for some women	• can be put in several hours before sexual intercourse • used only when needed • helps protect against STIs	• first fitting should be by an experienced nurse or doctor • some women find it hard to put in and take out • can be messy • spermicide may irritate vagina or penis • must be left in place at least 6 hours after sexual intercourse
FERTILITY AWARENESS					
	• woman checks body temperature, cervical mucus and periods. These body signs show when you are more likely to get pregnant	• typically 25% but can be 3% if used perfectly	• none	• after learning method, no further costs or visits to health professionals required • helps you understand how your body works	• expert instruction needed to learn method • no sexual intercourse during fertile time • must chart temperature and cervical mucus daily • body signs can be difficult to recognise and may vary
EMERGENCY CONTRACEPTION					
	• Emergency Contraceptive Pills (ECP) or copper IUD used after unprotected sexual intercourse • delays ovulation or stops sperm reaching an egg	• ECP – 2% for women of average weight, 6% if overweight • IUD – less than 1%	• ECP – none known • IUD – risk of pelvic infection if STI present	• reduces chance of pregnancy after unprotected sexual intercourse • ECP – can be used up to 72 hours after unprotected sexual intercourse • can have ECP at home for future use • can be used if other method fails, eg. broken condom or missed pill • can buy from pharmacies	• ECP should be started within 72 hours of unprotected sexual intercourse • ECP may not be effective for heavier women • IUD needs to be fitted by an experienced doctor or nurse and can be uncomfortable
PERMANENT CONTRACEPTION					
VASECTOMY & TUBAL LIGATION	• permanent contraception • an operation • vasectomy – male tubes cut to stop the sperm getting to the penis • tubal ligation – clips put on female tubes to stop the egg getting to the uterus	• less than 1%	• vasectomy – rare possibility of long term scrotal pain • tubal ligation – very slight risk from reaction to anaesthetic or damage to internal organs	• once only • permanent	• not easily reversible • requires an operation • may have short term side effects, eg. pain, bruising

CYC Chart JUNE2014

Source: Thanks to Family Planning for permission to reproduce this material, which is taken from the Contraception Your Choice pamphlet (February 2015).

"natural" way of planning pregnancies is simply best for them. The effectiveness of these methods varies greatly from 25% to 85%, depending mainly on the couple's ability to refrain from having sexual intercourse on **fertile days** or days on which the woman has the most likely chance to become pregnant (Schorge et al., 2008). Natural family planning is undertaken by committed couples and involves recognising the signs of ovulation. To avoid pregnancy, sexual intercourse is avoided during the fertile part of the female cycle or another form of contraception, such as condoms or diaphragms, is used.

There are a variety of ways, or methods, to determine a woman's fertile period such as calculating the period based on a set formula, measuring the woman's body temperature, observing the consistency of cervical mucus, using an over-the-counter ovulation test kit, or using a combination of these methods. It is important to note that natural family planning should be taught only by those with extensive knowledge and training in this area. Always refer people who are interested in this method to either their local GP, Family Planning Association or a natural family planning educator for more information.

The following methods of contraception can encompass natural family planning but deserve more detail as some couples use them as a stand-alone method.

Lactation amenorrhoea method (LAM)

As long as a woman is breastfeeding an infant, there is some natural suppression of ovulation. Because women may ovulate, however, but not menstruate, a woman may still be fertile even if she has not had a period since childbirth. When correctly used LAM is 98% effective. For this, three criteria must be met:

- Menstrual periods have not commenced since delivery
- The baby is not being fed supplements (still solely breastfeeding) and there are no long intervals between feeds day or night (for instance more than 4 hours during the daytime and more than 6 hours at night)
- It has been less than 6 months since the birth (Family Planning NSW, 2011).

Coitus interruptus

Coitus interruptus is one of the oldest known methods of contraception. The couple proceeds with **coitus** until the moment of ejaculation. Then the man withdraws and spermatozoa are emitted outside the vagina. Unfortunately, ejaculation may occur before withdrawal is complete and, despite the care used, some spermatozoa may be deposited in the vagina. Furthermore, because there may be a few spermatozoa present in pre-ejaculation fluid, fertilisation may occur even if withdrawal seems controlled. For these reasons, coitus interruptus is only about 75% effective (Stubblefield, Carr-Ellis & Kapp, 2007).

Postcoital douching

Douching following intercourse, no matter what solution is used, is ineffective as a contraceptive measure as sperm may be present in cervical mucus as quickly as 90 seconds after ejaculation.

Abstinence

Abstinence, or refraining from sexual intercourse, has a theoretical 0% failure rate and is also the most effective way to prevent STIs. However, clients, particularly adolescents, may find it difficult to adhere to abstinence, or they may completely overlook it as an option. Use of no contraceptive has a failure rate of 85% (Cunningham et al., 2008). In a moment of passion, many otherwise responsible people are unable to remain abstinent. Only 67% of women still use the method after a year. Many sex education classes advocate abstinence as the only contraceptive measure, so adolescents who take these courses may know little about other options. When discussing abstinence as a contraceptive method, be sure to provide information not only on the method but suggestions of ways to comply with this method. A worry is that adolescents who make "abstinence pledges" to not have sexual intercourse until they are married may "tune out" not only on additional information on contraception but on safer sex practices as well. Then, if they break their pledge (about 50% do), that could leave them more vulnerable to STIs and pregnancy than others (Cherlin, 2008).

Barrier methods

Barrier methods are forms of contraception that work by the placement of a barrier between the cervix and advancing sperm so that sperm cannot enter the uterus or fallopian tubes and fertilise the ovum. A major advantage of barrier methods is that they lack the hormonal side effects associated with hormonal methods of contraception. However, compared with hormonal methods, their failure rates are higher and sexual enjoyment may be lessened. Barrier methods include male and female **condoms** and **diaphragms**.

Male condoms

A **male condom** is a synthetic sheath that is placed over the erect penis before coitus to trap sperm (see Fig. 6.1). Condoms have an ideal failure rate of 2% and a typical failure rate of about 15%, because breakage or spillage occurs in up to 15% of uses (Shoupe & Kjos, 2010). A major advantage of condoms is that they are one of the few "male-responsibility" birth control measures available, and no healthcare visit or prescription is needed. Condoms have the additional potential of preventing the spread of STIs, and their use has become a major part of the fight to prevent infection with human immunodeficiency virus

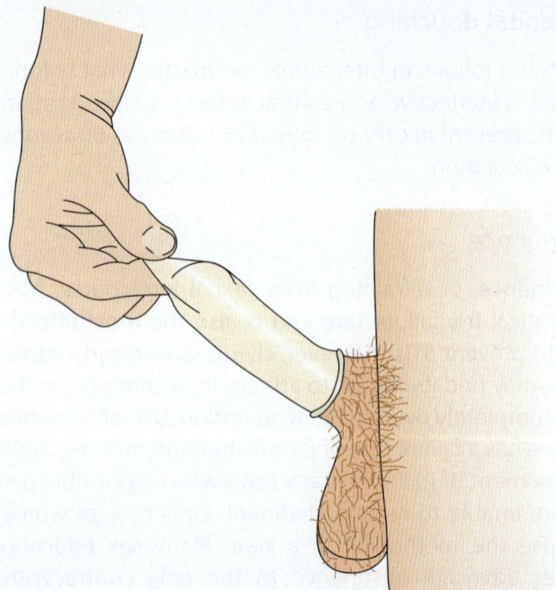

FIGURE 6.1 Male condom. Being certain that space is left at the tip helps to ensure the condom will not break with ejaculation.

(HIV). Recommend them for any partners who do not maintain a monogamous relationship.

Side effects and contraindications

There are no contraindications to the use of condoms except for an allergy to latex. If either the male or his partner has a latex allergy they can use latex free condoms.

Female condoms

Female condoms are made from polyurethane. The inner ring (closed end) covers the cervix and the outer ring (open end) rests against the vaginal opening (see Fig. 6.2). The sheath may be inserted any time before sexual activity begins and then removed after ejaculation occurs. Like male condoms, they are intended for one-time use and offer protection against both conception and STIs. Female condoms can be purchased without a prescription but are more expensive than male condoms. Male and female condoms should not be used together. Advantages of the female condom are similar to that of the male condom; they can be used by breastfeeding women, they require no prescription and there is no delay in a return to a woman's fertility. Although female condoms may reduce the risk of acquiring an HIV infection by as much as 90%, they have not gained great popularity, because of their bulk and difficulty in use (Burkman, 2007).

Side effects and contraindications

There are no known side effects or contraindications of the female condom.

CASE STUDY QUESTION

2. Lena wants to try female condoms as her reproductive planning method. Which instruction would you give her?
   a. The hormone the condom releases may cause mild weight gain
   b. She should insert the condom before any penile penetration
   c. Female condoms, unlike male condoms, can be reused
   d. Female condoms require a prescription

Diaphragms

Diaphragms, also a barrier method of contraception, are a circular bowl-shaped silicone disc that is placed over the

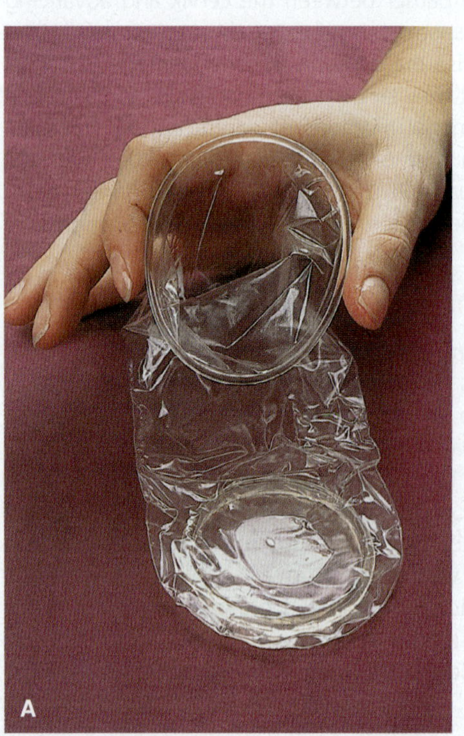

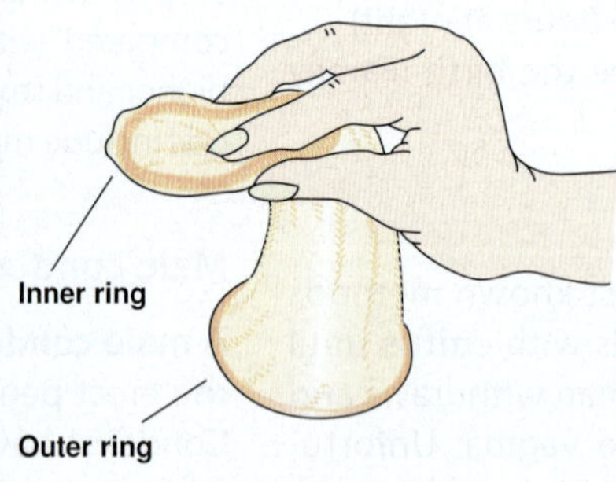

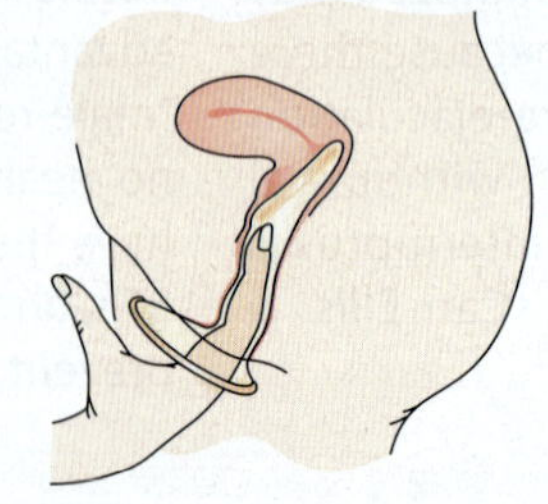

FIGURE 6.2 A female condom. Such a device is effective protection against both STIs and pregnancy. (**A**) The REALITY (WP-333) female condom (© Barbara Proud.) (**B**) Insertion technique (Courtesy of Wisconsin Pharmaceutical Company, Inc.)

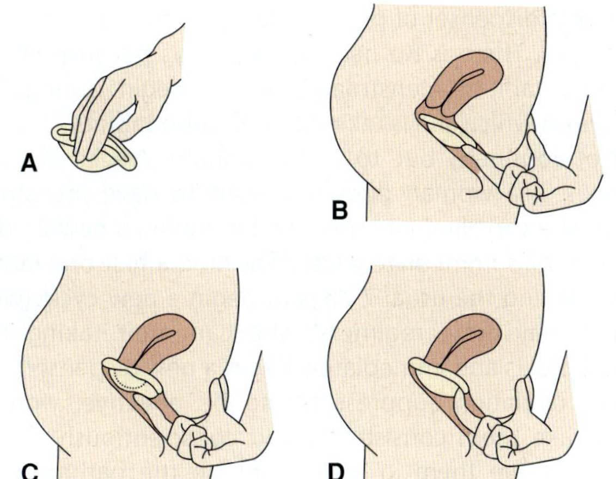

FIGURE 6.3 Proper insertion of a diaphragm. (**A**) The diaphragm is pinched between the fingers and thumb. (**B**) The folded diaphragm is then inserted into the vagina and pushed backwards as far as it will go. (**C**) To check for proper positioning, the woman should feel the cervix to be certain it is completely covered by the soft rubber dome of the diaphragm. (**D**) To remove the diaphragm, a finger is hooked under the forward rim and the diaphragm is pulled down and out.

cervix before intercourse. A diaphragm is prescribed and fitted (diaphragms come in four sizes and it is important for the correct size to be used) initially by a doctor, midwife or women's health nurse to ensure a correct fit. Because the shape of a woman's cervix changes with pregnancy, miscarriage, cervical surgery (dilation and curettage [D&C]), or elective termination of pregnancy, teach women to return for a second fitting if any of these circumstances occur. A woman should also have the fit of the diaphragm checked if she gains or loses more than 3 kg, because this could also change her pelvic and vaginal contours.

A diaphragm is inserted into the vagina, by sliding it along the posterior wall and pressing it up against the cervix so that it is held in place by the vaginal fornices (see Fig. 6.3). A woman should check her diaphragm with a finger after insertion to be certain that it is fitted well up over the cervix; she can palpate the cervical os through the diaphragm. Research indicates the use of spermicide with diaphragms does not increase efficacy and spermicide is no longer available in Australia (Family Planning NSW, 2011). However, Family Planning New Zealand (2012) still recommends the use of spermicides with diaphragms.

A diaphragm should remain in place for at least 6 hours after coitus, because spermatozoa remain viable in the vagina for that length of time. It may be left in place for as long as 24 hours. If it is left in the vagina longer than this, the stasis of fluid may cause cervical inflammation (erosion) or urethral irritation. A diaphragm is removed by inserting a finger into the vagina and loosening the diaphragm by pressing against the anterior rim and then withdrawing it vaginally. After use, a diaphragm should be washed in mild soap and water, dried gently and stored in its protective case. With this care, a diaphragm will last for 2 to 3 years.

Side effects and contraindications

Diaphragms may not be effective if the uterus is prolapsed, retroflexed or anteflexed to such a degree that the cervix is also displaced in relation to the vagina. Intrusion on the vagina by a cystocele or rectocele, in which the walls of the vagina are displaced by bladder or bowel, may make insertion of a diaphragm difficult. Users of diaphragms may experience a higher number of urinary tract infections (UTIs) than non-users; probably because of pressure on the urethra. Diaphragms should not be used in the presence of acute cervicitis or a papillomavirus infection, because the close contact of the rubber and the use of a spermicide can cause additional irritation. Other contraindications include:

- History of toxic shock syndrome (TSS; staphylococcal infection introduced through the vagina)
- Allergy to rubber or spermicides
- History of recurrent UTIs.

To prevent TSS while using a diaphragm, advise women to:

1. Wash their hands thoroughly with soap and water before insertion or removal
2. Not use a diaphragm during a menstrual period
3. Not leave a diaphragm in place longer than 24 hours
4. Be aware of the symptoms of TSS, such as elevated temperature, diarrhoea, vomiting, muscle aches and a sunburn-like rash
5. Immediately remove the diaphragm and call a healthcare provider if symptoms of TSS should occur.

> ***What if...***
>
> Lena tells you that she and a friend intend to share a diaphragm because they do not have enough money to each buy one. Is this good planning?

Hormonal contraception

Hormonal contraceptives are, as the name implies, hormones that cause such fluctuations in a normal menstrual cycle that ovulation does not occur. Hormonal contraceptives may be administered orally, vaginally, by implantation or through injection.

Oral route

Oral contraceptives (OCs), commonly known as the pill, or combination oral contraceptives (COCs), are composed of varying amounts of synthetic oestrogen combined with a small amount of synthetic progesterone (progestin). The oestrogen acts to suppress follicle-stimulating hormone (FSH) and LH, thereby suppressing ovulation. The progesterone action complements that of oestrogen by causing a decrease in the permeability of cervical mucus, thereby limiting sperm motility and access to ova. Progesterone also interferes with tubal transport and endometrial proliferation to such degrees that the possibility of implantation is significantly decreased.

Popular COCs prescribed in Australia are monophasic or provide fixed doses of both oestrogen and progestin throughout a 21-day cycle. Biphasic preparations deliver a constant amount of oestrogen throughout the cycle but an increased amount of progestin during the last 11 days. Triphasic preparations vary in both oestrogen and progestin content throughout the cycle. Triphasic types more closely mimic a natural cycle, thereby reducing breakthrough bleeding (bleeding outside the normal menstrual flow). Caution women to always take pills in the order designated by the dispenser or the progesterone level could be inaccurate and ineffective for that day.

COCs are prescribed by a doctor or nurse practitioner and when used correctly, they are 99.7% effective in preventing conception. Evidence suggests that despite their effectiveness, women harbour significant concerns about their safety (Nelson, 2011). Further, women who forget to take them as scheduled experience a failure rate of 95% (Schorge et al., 2008).

Oral contraceptives have non-contraceptive benefits such as decreased incidences of:

- Dysmenorrhoea, because of lack of ovulation
- Premenstrual dysphoric syndrome and acne, because of the increased progesterone levels
- Iron deficiency anaemia, because of the reduced amount of menstrual flow
- Acute pelvic inflammatory disease (PID) and the resulting tubal scarring
- Endometrial and ovarian cancer, ovarian cysts and ectopic pregnancies
- Fibrocystic breast disease
- Possibly osteoporosis, endometriosis, uterine myomata (fibroid uterine tumours) and progression of rheumatoid arthritis
- Colon cancer (Schindler, 2010).

Because oestrogen interferes with lipid metabolism, it may lower the concentration of low-density lipoproteins (LDL) and increase the high-density lipoprotein (HDL) level.

As COCs are not effective for the first 7 days, advise women to use a second form of contraception during the initial 7 days on which they take the hormone pills. COCs are packaged with 21 or 28 pills in a convenient dispenser. Twenty-one-day cycle pills contain 21 hormone pills whereas the 28-day cycle of pills contain 21 hormone pills and 7 placebo or sugar pills. A woman prescribed a 21-day cycle brand takes a pill at the same time every day for 21 days, then does not take any pills for seven days. A woman taking a 28-day package of pills takes 21 hormone pills and seven sugar pills. This allows her to continuously take pills so she cannot forget when to resume pill taking. Once a woman stops taking the hormone pills her menstrual flow will then begin about 4 days after she finishes a cycle of pills.

To eliminate having to count days between pill cycles, most brands of OCs are packaged with 28 pills—21 active pills and 7 placebo pills. With these brands, a woman starts a second dispenser of pills the day after finishing the first dispenser. There is no need to skip days because of the placebo tablets. Menstrual flow will begin during the 7 days on which she is taking the placebo tablets.

Not routinely, but to accommodate special circumstances, if a woman does not want to have menstrual flows, she can eliminate them by beginning a new 21-day cycle of pills immediately after finishing a first one rather than waiting the usual 7 days to begin a new cycle (with the 28-day cycle regimens, she can omit taking the placebo pills and immediately begin a new dispenser).

For ovulation suppressants to be effective, women must take them consistently and conscientiously. Some women leave them in plain sight on the bathroom or kitchen counter so that they are easily reminded to take them. Caution women with young children in the house that this is a potentially dangerous practice. Poisoning with increased blood clotting from the high oestrogen content could result if a small child ingested the pills accidentally. Women who have difficulty remembering to take a contraceptive in the morning may find it easier to take a daily pill at bedtime or with a meal (the time of day makes no difference; it is the consistency that is important). Also, some women find that taking pills at bedtime rather than in the morning eliminates any nausea they otherwise experience.

Side effects and contraindications

The main side effects that women may experience from taking OCs and COCs are:

- Nausea
- Weight gain
- Headache
- Breast tenderness
- Breakthrough bleeding (spotting outside the menstrual period)
- Yeast vaginal infections (thrush)
- Mild hypertension
- Depression.

Side effects such as nausea and breakthrough bleeding usually subside after a few months of use. They may be lessened by using a different routine or brand of contraceptive.

It is no longer believed that the use of COCs leads to an increased risk of myocardial infarction, and the risk of increased clotting or blood pressure elevation is low. Nevertheless, COCs are not routinely prescribed for women with a history of thromboembolic disease, or a family history of cerebral or cardiovascular accident, who are over 40 years of age, or who smoke because of the increased tendency towards clotting as an effect of increased oestrogen (McKenna & Mirkov, 2014).

There are several contraindications for COCs. Advise all women taking COCs to notify their healthcare provider if symptoms of myocardial or thromboembolic complications occur. These are:

- Chest pain (pulmonary embolus or myocardial infarction)
- Shortness of breath (pulmonary embolus)
- Severe headache (cerebrovascular accident)
- Severe leg pain (thrombophlebitis)
- Eye problems such as blurred vision (hypertension, cerebrovascular accident).

Early studies of birth control pills found that breastfed infants had lower weight gains when the mother was taking an OC because the oestrogen content decreased the woman's milk supply. Although there is less oestrogen in today's preparations, it is still not recommended that breastfeeding women take oestrogen-based COCs until their milk supply is well established. Women may take progesterone-only pills (mini-pills) during breastfeeding (see later discussion).

COCs can interfere with glucose metabolism. For this reason, women with diabetes mellitus or a history of liver disease, including hepatitis, are evaluated individually before COCs are prescribed. COCs apparently do not increase the risk of breast cancer as was once feared (Stubblefield, Carr-Ellis & Kapp, 2007).

When discussing COCs, be certain to assess both a woman's ability to pay for them and her ability to follow instructions faithfully. Women using COCs should return for a follow-up visit yearly (for a pelvic examination, pap smear and breast examination), as long as they continue to use this form of birth control. Women without risk factors may continue to take low-dose OCs until they reach menopause.

Mini-pills

Oral contraceptives containing only progestins are popularly called mini-pills. The progesterone content thickens cervical mucus and helps prevent sperm entry into the uterine cervix. Ovulation may occur but, because the endometrium does not develop fully, implantation will not take place. Such a pill has advantages for the woman who cannot take an oestrogen-based pill because of the danger of thrombophlebitis but who wants high-level contraception assurance (they are as effective as oestrogen/progestin pills). They have the disadvantage of causing more breakthrough bleeding than combination pills. They are taken every day, even through the menstrual flow. Because it does not interfere with milk production, they may be taken during breastfeeding.

Vaginal insertion

A **vaginal ring** (NuvaRing) is a soft plastic ring that is inserted into the vagina (see Fig. 6.4). The vaginal ring contains the hormones oestrogen and progestogen and these two hormones are continually released. Once inserted into the vagina it is left in place for 3 weeks, then removed for 1 week (Roumen, 2007). Menstrual bleeding occurs during the ring-free week. The hormones released are absorbed directly by the mucous membrane of the vagina, thereby avoiding a "first pass" through the liver, as happens with COCs; this is an advantage for women with liver disease. The effectiveness is equal to that of COCs. Fertility returns immediately after discontinuing using the ring. Women may need to make out a calendar that they post conspicuously to remind themselves to remove and replace the ring. Alternatively, the company that makes the NuvaRing offers a reminder system either as an email alert or as a text message. Some women experience vaginal discomfort, which makes a ring not a desirable contraceptive for them. While rings do not need to be removed for intercourse, if a woman senses that a vaginal ring is in place, this could interfere with sexual enjoyment.

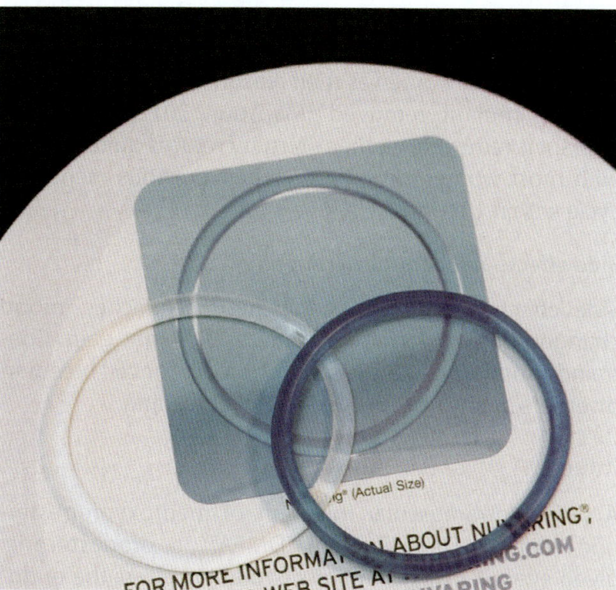

FIGURE 6.4 A vaginal ring. Both oestrogen and progesterone are gradually released to be absorbed by the vaginal walls.

Side effects and contraindications

Contraindications include a history of previous leg clots, stroke, heart attack, liver disease, migraines or breast cancer. Some side effects include increased vaginal secretion, vaginal irritation, headache, nausea and weight gain.

Implantation

Implanon NXT® is the brand name for the progestogen **implantation contraception** available in Australia and New Zealand. The implant is a small, flexible rod which is inserted under the skin of the upper arm by a doctor under local anaesthetic. It slowly releases the hormone progestogen to prevent pregnancy for up to 3 years. Implanon is a very effective form of contraception and is over 99% effective as women cannot forget to take it. A common disadvantage is that many women will experience vaginal bleeding after the insertion of the implant and this tends to occur in the first 4 months of the implant being inserted. Side effects include headaches, breast tenderness, acne, mood changes and weight gain (Sexual

Health and Family Planning Australia, 2008). Bleeding problems can also occur, and in one study this was cited by one-third of women as their reason for having a contraceptive implant removed (Mansour, 2012). Once the implant is removed, women's fertility returns quite quickly, with most women returning to their previous menstrual cycle within 1 month.

Side effects and contraindications

Side effects of the implant include headaches, mood changes, breast tenderness, acne and weight gain. Contraindications include a history of breast cancer, bleeding disorders or any unexplained vaginal bleeding.

Injection

A single intramuscular injection of medroxyprogesterone acetate (Depo-Provera [DMPA]), a progesterone, given every 12 weeks inhibits ovulation, alters the endometrium and changes the cervical mucus (Perry, 2014). The effectiveness rate of this method is almost 100%, making it an increasingly popular contraceptive method (Chrousos, 2008). Because Depo-Provera contains only progesterone, it can be used during breastfeeding. Advantageous effects are reduction in ectopic pregnancy, endometrial cancer, endometriosis, and, for unknown reasons, reduction in the frequency of sickle cell crises (Burkman, 2007). Potential side effects are similar to those of subdermal implants: irregular menstrual cycle, headache, weight gain and depression. Depo-Provera may impair glucose tolerance in women at risk of diabetes. Because there may also be an increase in the risk of osteoporosis from loss of bone mineral density, advise women to include an adequate amount of calcium in their diet (up to 1200 milligrams per day) and to engage in weight-bearing exercise daily to minimise this risk; rules that are good for all women. Depo-Provera is not routinely prescribed to adolescents, to protect their bone mineral density (Glasier, Yan & Wellings, 2007).

Intramuscular injections have the advantage of longer-term reliability without many of the side effects and contraindications associated with COCs. An advantage of intramuscular injections over implants is that there is no visible sign that a birth control measure is being used; this makes them attractive to adolescents (Rickert et al., 2007). Two disadvantages are that a woman must return to a healthcare provider for a new injection every 4 to 12 weeks for the method to remain reliable, and the return to fertility is often delayed by 6 to 12 months. A reminder system, such as a postcard mailed by the prescribing agency, may be necessary to be certain that women return on time for their next injection (see Box 6.1).

BOX 6.1 ❊ Focus on pharmacology

Medroxyprogesterone acetate (Depo-Provera)
Classification: Contraceptive
Action: Medroxyprogesterone acetate (Depo-Provera or DMPA) is a progesterone derivative that inhibits the secretion of pituitary gonadotropins, thereby altering the endometrium and preventing follicular maturation and ovulation (McKenna & Mirkov, 2014)
Pregnancy category: X
Dosage: 150 mg intramuscular injection every 3 months
Possible adverse effects: Spotting, breakthrough bleeding, amenorrhoea, irregular menstrual flow, headaches, weight fluctuations, fluid retention, oedema, rash or acne, abdominal discomfort, glucose intolerance, pain at injection site or osteoporosis (loss of bone density)

Nursing implications

- Advise the woman to have an annual physical examination that includes breast examination, pelvic examination and Pap smear.
- Caution that potential side effects may occur
- Advise the woman to maintain a high calcium intake to reduce development of osteoporosis
- Advise the woman to report pain or swelling of the legs, acute chest pain or shortness of breath, tingling or numbness in the extremities, loss of vision, sudden severe headaches, dizziness or fainting; these are signs of potentially serious cardiovascular complications

Intrauterine devices

An **intrauterine device** (IUD) is a small plastic object that is inserted into the uterus through the vagina (see Fig. 6.5). IUDs became popular as a method of birth control in the 1980s, and although still a popular choice worldwide, IUDs are used by only a small number of women. Few manufacturers continue to provide them since several lawsuits were filed in association with the increased incidence of pelvic inflammatory disease (PID) in women using one particular brand, now no longer available.

Although the insertion of foreign objects into the uterus for contraceptive purposes dates back thousands of years (ancient camel drivers used the technique on their animals), the mechanism of action for the method is still not fully understood. Originally, it was thought that the presence of a foreign substance in the uterus interfered with the ability of an ovum to develop as it traversed the fallopian tube. Today, the IUD is thought to prevent fertilisation as well as creating a local sterile inflammatory condition that prevents implantation. When copper is added to the device, sperm mobility appears to be affected as well. This decreases the possibility that sperm will successfully cross the uterine space and reach the ovum.

An IUD must be fitted by a doctor who first performs a Pap test and pelvic examination. The device is inserted before a woman has had coitus after a menstrual flow, so the healthcare provider can be assured that the woman is not pregnant at the time of insertion.

The insertion procedure is performed in an ambulatory setting such as a doctor's office or family planning clinic. The device is inserted in a collapsed position, then enlarged to its final shape in the uterus when the inserter

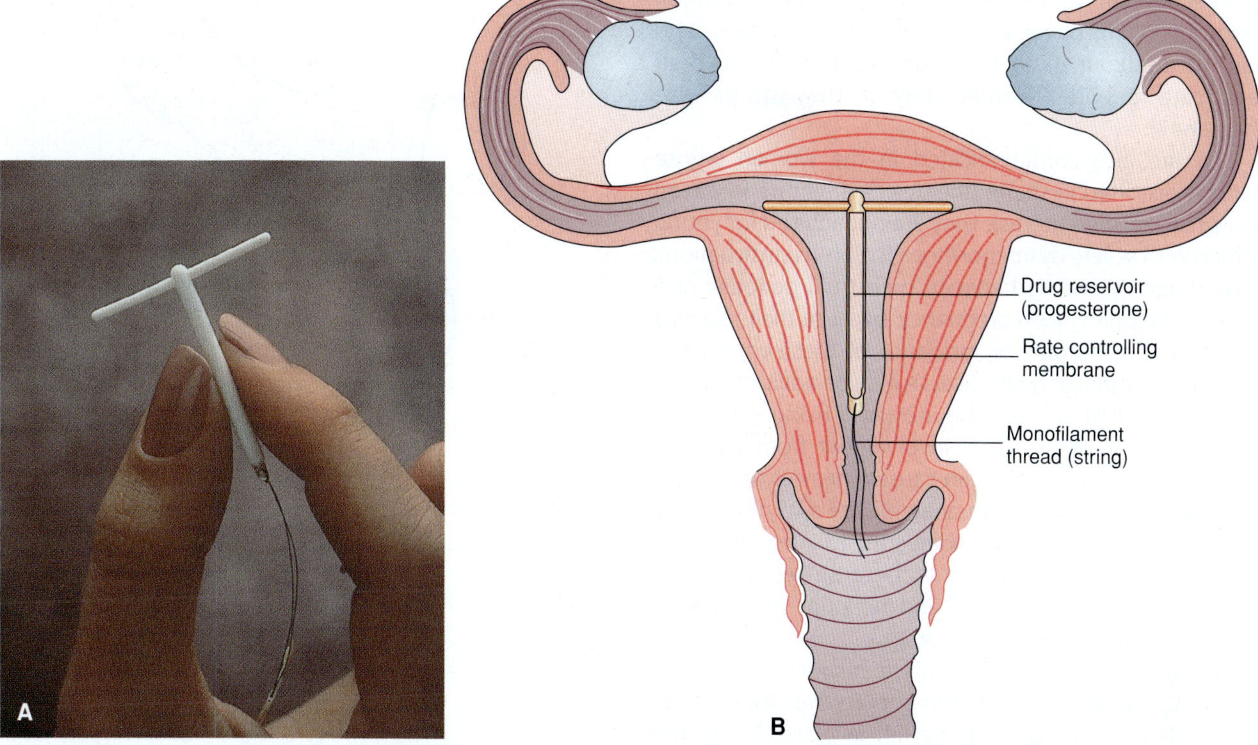

FIGURE 6.5 (**A**) Intrauterine device. (**B**) An IUD in place in the uterus. (Courtesy of ALZA Pharmaceuticals, Palo Alto, CA.)

is withdrawn. The woman may feel a sharp cramp as the device is passed through the internal cervical os, but she will not feel the IUD after it is in place. Properly fitted, such devices are contained wholly within the uterus, although the attached string protrudes through the cervix into the vagina (Burkman, 2007).

Two common types of IUDs used in Australia and New Zealand are the copper IUD and the hormone releasing IUD (Mirena), which holds a medication reservoir of progesterone in the stem. The progesterone in the medication reservoir gradually diffuses into the uterus through the plastic; it both prevents endometrium proliferation and thickens cervical mucus. The Mirena type is effective for 5 years (possibly as long as 7 years). It has a failure rate as low as 0.1% to 1.5%. The copper IUD because of the added copper, has a comparable failure rate (Cunningham et al., 2008). It is effective for 5–10 years (depending on the type), after which it should be removed and replaced with a new one.

IUDs have several advantages over other contraceptives. Only one insertion is necessary, so there is no continuing expense. The device does not require daily attention or interfere with sexual enjoyment. It is appropriate for women who are at risk of complications associated with COCs or who wish to avoid some of the systemic hormonal side effects. They may create lighter or fewer periods.

Teach women to regularly check after each menstrual flow to make sure the IUD string is in place, and to obtain a yearly pelvic examination.

Side effects and contraindications

A woman may notice some spotting or uterine cramping the first 2 or 3 weeks after IUD insertion; as long as this is present, she should use an additional form of contraception, such as vaginal foam. Theoretically, a woman with an IUD in place has a higher-than-usual risk for pelvic inflammatory disease (PID), although this does not bear out in practice (Campbell, Cropsey & Matthews, 2007). This may be because copper wound around the device may help resist infection. Some women have a heavier than usual menstrual flow for 2 or 3 months and experience more dysmenorrhoea than other women. Ibuprofen, a prostaglandin inhibitor, is helpful in relieving the pain. Occasionally, a woman continues to have cramping and spotting after insertion; in such instances, she is likely to expel the device spontaneously. Women with IUDs in place should take active steps to avoid toxic shock syndrome (TSS; a staphylococcal infection introduced through the vagina), because infection might travel by the IUD string into the uterus to cause uterine infection. TSS is discussed in Chapter 47.

IUDs are not recommended for women with an increased risk of contracting STIs, such as those who have multiple sexual partners, because this combination could lead to pelvic infection (Stubblefield, Carr-Ellis & Kapp, 2007). They are also not recommended for women who have never been pregnant (their small uterus could be punctured with insertion) or who have a history of having had PID. If PID is suspected, the device should be removed and the woman should receive antibiotic therapy to treat the infection. All women need to know the most common symptoms of PID (fever, lower abdominal tenderness and pain on intercourse) so they can report these to their healthcare provider immediately if they occur (see Chapter 47).

IUDs are also contraindicated in the woman whose uterus is distorted in shape (the device might perforate an abnormally shaped uterus). They are not advised for young women with severe dysmenorrhoea (painful menstruation), menorrhagia (bleeding between menstrual periods), or a history of ectopic (tubal) pregnancy, because their use may increase the symptoms or incidence of these conditions. Women with valvular heart disease may be advised against the use of an IUD because the increased risk of PID could lead to accompanying valve involvement from bacterial endocarditis. Because IUDs can cause a heavier than usual menstrual flow, women with anaemia are also not usually considered to be good candidates for IUD use. IUDs are rarely prescribed for adolescents, because teens tend to have variable sexual partners and no prior pregnancies, both contraindications to IUD use.

If a woman with an IUD in place suspects that she is pregnant, she should alert her primary healthcare provider. Although the IUD may be left in place during the pregnancy, it is usually removed vaginally to prevent the possibility of infection or spontaneous miscarriage during the pregnancy. The woman should receive an early ultrasound to document placement of the IUD. This can also rule out ectopic pregnancy, which has an increased incidence among IUD users who become pregnant with the IUD in place.

Surgical methods

Surgical methods of contraception, often called "sterilisation", include tubal ligation for women and vasectomy for men. Many people choose these surgical methods because they are the most effective methods of contraception besides abstinence, because there are no further costs and because they have no effect on sexual enjoyment.

Although reversal procedures are possible, such techniques are much more complicated and expensive than the sterilisation itself and success rates are only 70% to 80%. For this reason, surgical methods should be chosen with great thought and care and should be considered permanent. Counselling should be especially intensive for men and women younger than 25 years of age, because the possibility of divorce, death of a sexual partner, loss of a child or remarriage could change a person's philosophy towards childbearing in the future. In addition, sterilisation is not recommended for individuals whose fertility is important to their self-esteem.

Vasectomy

In a **vasectomy**, a small incision or puncture wound is made on each side of the scrotum. The vas deferens on each side are then pulled forwards, cut and tied, cauterised or plugged, blocking the passage of spermatozoa (Cameron & Glasier, 2012) (see Fig. 6.6). Vasectomy can be carried out under local anaesthesia in an ambulatory setting, such as a doctor's office or a family planning clinic. The man experiences a small amount of local pain afterward, which can be managed by taking a mild analgesic and applying ice to the site. The procedure is 99.5% effective (MacKay, 2009). Spermatozoa that were present in the vas deferens at the time of surgery can remain viable for as long as 6 months. Therefore, although the man can resume sexual intercourse within 1 week, an additional birth control method should be used until two negative sperm reports have been obtained (proof that all sperm in the vas deferens have been eliminated, usually requiring 10 to 20 ejaculations).

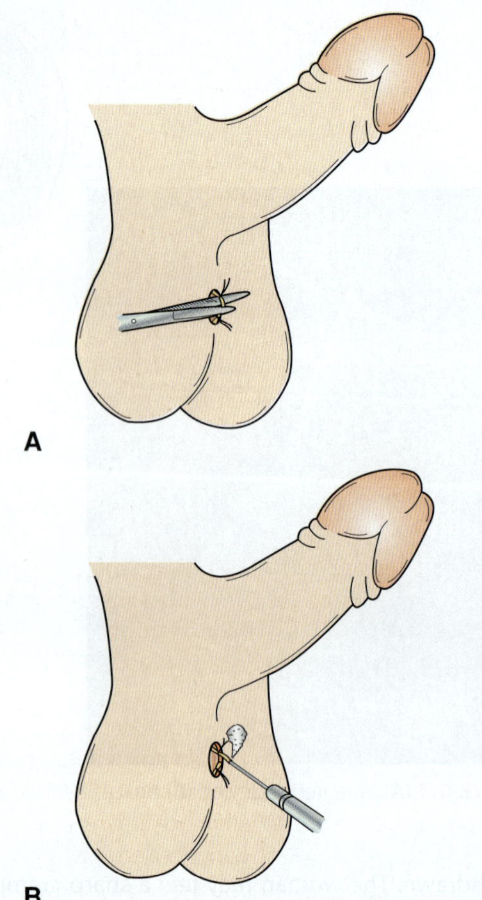

FIGURE 6.6 Vasectomy. (**A**) The left vas deferens being cut with surgical scissors. (**B**) The cut ends of the vas deferens are cauterised or clamped to completely ensure blockage of the passage of sperm.

Some men resist the concept of vasectomy because they are not sufficiently aware of their anatomy to know exactly what the procedure involves. They can be assured that vasectomy does not interfere with the production of sperm; the testes continue to produce sperm as always, but the sperm simply do not pass beyond the severed vas deferens and are absorbed at that point. The man will still have full erection capacity. Because he also continues to form seminal fluid, he will ejaculate seminal fluid—it will just not contain sperm.

There are very few complications associated with vasectomy. A haematoma at the surgical site may occur, although this is seen less frequently with "no scalpel" or puncture incisions (Cook et al., 2009). The procedure may be associated with the development of urolithiasis (kidney stones). A few men develop chronic pain after vasectomy (post vasectomy pain syndrome); having the procedure reversed relieves this pain. Some men develop autoimmunity or form antibodies against sperm, so that even if reconstruction of the vas deferens is successful, the sperm they produce do not have good mobility and are incapable of fertilisation. It should be explained to men that although techniques are advancing for reversal of vasectomy, the procedure is only effective in 90% of cases and in those, fertility can take up to two years to be restored (Schwarzer & Steinfatt, 2013). Men who feel a need to have their sperm available for the future can have it stored in a sperm bank before vasectomy.

Tubal ligation

Sterilisation of women could include removal of the uterus or ovaries (hysterectomy), but it usually refers to a minor surgical procedure, such as **tubal ligation**, where the fallopian tubes are occluded by cautery, crushing, clamping or blocking, thereby preventing passage of both sperm and ova. A fimbriectomy, or removal of the fimbria at the distal end of the tubes, is another possible, but little used technique. Tubal ligation has a 99.5% effectiveness rate (Shoupe & Kjos, 2010). Although the reason is not clear, tubal ligation is associated with a decreased incidence of ovarian cancer.

The most common operation to achieve tubal ligation is **laparoscopy** (see Fig. 6.7). After a menstrual flow and before ovulation an incision as small as 1 centimetre is made just under the woman's umbilicus, with the woman under general or local anaesthesia. A lighted laparoscope is inserted through the incision. Carbon dioxide is then pumped into the incision to lift the abdominal wall upwards and out of the line of vision. The surgeon locates the fallopian tubes by viewing the field through a laparoscope. An electrical current to coagulate tissue is then passed through the instrument for 3 to 5 seconds, or the tubes are clamped by plastic, metal or rubber rings, then cut or filled with a silicone gel to seal them. The procedure provides immediate contraception.

The procedure can also be done by culdoscopy (a tube inserted through the posterior fornix of the vagina) or colpotomy (incision through the vagina), but the incidence of pelvic infection is higher with these procedures and visualisation is less.

The woman is discharged from the hospital a few hours after the procedure. She may notice abdominal bloating for the first 24 hours, until the carbon dioxide infused at the beginning of the procedure is absorbed. This can also cause sharp diaphragmatic or shoulder pain if some of the carbon dioxide escapes under the diaphragm and presses on ascending nerves. Complications include bowel perforation, haemorrhage and the risks of general anaesthesia with the procedure (Warehime, Bass & Pedulla, 2007). A woman may notice a day or two of abdominal discomfort caused by local necrosis if clips were used.

A system called Essure, which consists of a spring-loaded mechanism that, when inserted through the vagina and uterus into the outer end of a fallopian tube (a hysteroscopy procedure), releases a soft micro-insert into the tube that effectively seals the tube (Pavone & Burke, 2007). This can be carried out as an office procedure. Women must use a second form of contraception afterwards, until, at 3 months, a hysterosalpingogram is carried out to confirm that the fallopian tubes are blocked.

A woman may return to having coitus as soon as 2 to 3 days after the procedure. Be certain that they understand that tubal ligation, unlike a hysterectomy, does not affect the menstrual cycle, so they will still have a monthly

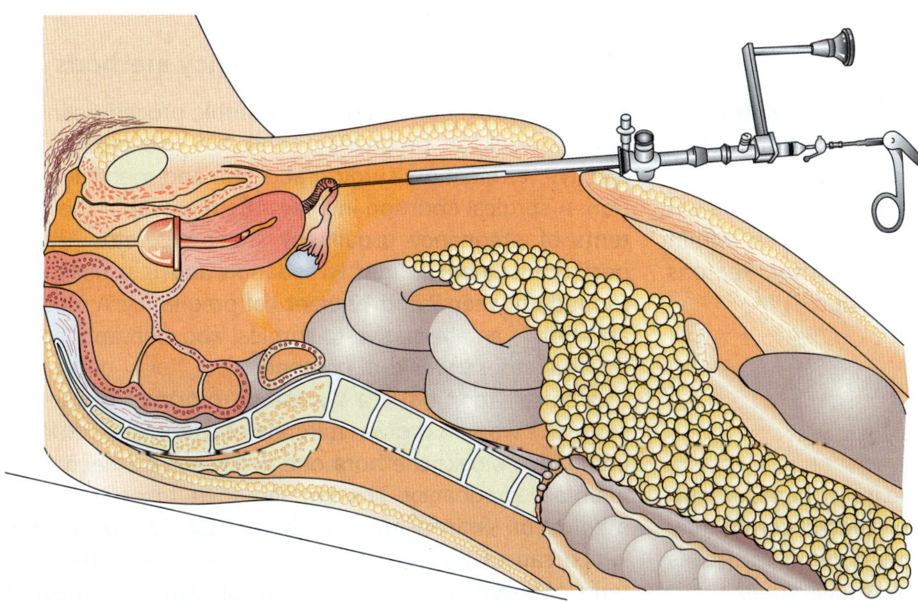

FIGURE 6.7 Laparoscopy for tubal sterilisation. (From Richard Wolf Medical Instruments Corporation, with permission).

menstrual flow. Be certain that women know to have no unprotected coitus before a tubal ligation (sperm trapped in the tube could fertilise an ovum there and cause an ectopic pregnancy). Tubal ligation has been found to have no detrimental effect on, and possibly is beneficial to, women's libido (Smith et al., 2010).

Contraindications to tubal ligation surgery, if performed by laparoscopy, are an umbilical hernia, because bowel perforation might result, and extensive obesity, which would probably require a full laparotomy to allow adequate visualisation. Some women develop vaginal spotting, intermittent vaginal bleeding and even severe lower abdominal cramping after tubal ligation; these symptoms are labelled post-tubal ligation syndrome. Removal of the fallopian tubes appears to relieve the symptoms.

Not only is it difficult to reconstruct fallopian tubes after they have been cauterised, but there is also a possibility that afterward, the anastomosis site, because of its irregular surface, could cause an ectopic (tubal) pregnancy. If a silicone gel has been instilled into the tubes as a blocking agent, it can be removed at a later date to reverse the procedure. As with vasectomy, however, women should view tubal ligation as a permanent, irreversible procedure. Otherwise, they can regret having the procedure. This happens most in women under 30 years (Pavone & Burke, 2007).

CASE STUDY QUESTION

3. Lena asks you how a tubal ligation prevents pregnancy. Which would be the best answer?

a. Sperm can no longer reach the ova, because fallopian tubes are blocked
b. Sperm cannot enter the uterus, because the cervical entrance is blocked
c. Prostaglandins released from the cut fallopian tubes effectively kill sperm
d. The ovary no longer releases ova, as there is nowhere for them to go

Emergency contraception pill

The most common form of **emergency contraception** is a single pill containing a 1.5 mg dose of a hormone called levonorgestrel (LNG). Emergency contraception reduces the chance of an unintended pregnancy after unprotected sex. Emergency contraception should be taken within 72 hours of intercourse, the sooner the better. Reasons for taking emergency contraception include:

- Missed contraceptive pills
- Condom breakage or slippage
- Unplanned intercourse
- Sexual assault.

Emergency contraception is available from chemists, family planning clinics, women's health centres, community health centres, emergency departments and local GPs (Sexual Health and Family Planning Australia, 2008).

It is important for nurses working in emergency departments and rural and remote hospitals to understand that women who have been admitted for a sexual assault need to be referred to relevant sexual assault services as soon as possible, keeping in mind that emergency contraception is more effective the sooner it is taken after unprotected intercourse. It may be timely for the nurse on duty to also offer emergency contraception if there is a delay in the woman being referred to the sexual assault service.

ELECTIVE TERMINATION OF PREGNANCY (INDUCED ABORTION)

For some women, an unplanned pregnancy may occur. This may be because the woman or couple has failed to use contraception, their contraception method may have failed (such as a broken condom) or the women may have had non-consensual intercourse (i.e. sexual assault). In this case the woman has a few choices. She may proceed with the pregnancy and either raise the child alone or with a partner; she may proceed with the pregnancy and then choose to have the baby adopted; she may choose to proceed with the pregnancy and have the baby fostered out until she can care for the baby; or she may seek an elective termination of the pregnancy (Collier, 2011). An **elective termination of pregnancy** is a procedure performed to end a pregnancy before fetal viability. Elective termination of pregnancy is also referred to as therapeutic, medical or induced abortion. Having such a procedure is a woman's choice; nurses employed in healthcare agencies where induced elective terminations are performed are asked to assist with and offer support as a part of their role. Elective terminations in Australia and New Zealand are legal to protect the life and health of a woman. This encompasses a woman's physical and mental health including social and economic health. In New Zealand elective termination is the subject of national law, whereas in Australia abortion is the subject of state law.

Elective termination of pregnancy methods

Elective termination is a safe and simple procedure in the first 12 weeks of pregnancy. There are two methods of elective termination; surgical abortion and medical abortion. A surgical abortion involves the removal of the contents of pregnancy usually by suction curette. This is performed under a light IV sedation and is usually performed between 7 and 12 weeks of pregnancy. A medical abortion is an alternative to surgical abortion and is performed under 9 weeks of pregnancy.

Medical abortion is a two stage process. In the first stage the women is given mifepristone (known as RU486) orally; this blocks the hormone progesterone needed to maintain pregnancy. The woman then takes a second medication (misoprostol) at home, 24–72 hours later, which causes the uterus to contract and expel the contents of pregnancy. In Australia, the availability of medical abortions is limited as RU486 is not commercially available and requires an application to the Therapeutic Goods Administration (Collier, 2011). In New Zealand, medical abortions are available in selected clinics.

Psychological aspects of elective termination of pregnancy

Women of all ages, married or unmarried, with or without children, request elective terminations. The usual profile of a woman who is having such a procedure is a woman who:

- Is young and unmarried
- Has no previous live births
- Undergoes the procedure to end an unwanted pregnancy
- Has not taken any or adequate protection against becoming pregnant.

Adolescents, often blamed for not using contraception responsibly, do not appear to have been any more careless than adult women at the time they ask for an elective termination of pregnancy (Harvey & Gaudoin, 2007). Be certain to give women of all ages having elective termination the same kind of explanations and support that women in labour receive (women do not share termination experiences with each other the same way as they share labour experiences, so women usually have received little advanced preparation).

Most women feel anxious when they appear at the hospital or clinic for an elective termination procedure. Some of the anxiety comes from having made a difficult decision to reach this step; some comes from having to face the unknown; some may come from feelings of loss or shame and sadness that they have had to make a decision with which they are not totally comfortable. Remembering that this is not a decision taken lightly helps in planning nursing care aimed at making an elective termination as non-traumatic as possible.

Women may express sadness and guilt after abortion; however, this may not be apparent at the time or may develop later. All women undergoing termination of pregnancy should be provided with the details of accessible counselling services so that they may be assisted to integrate this often enormously disruptive and potentially distressing event in their lives.

Key points for review

- Contraceptive choices involve personal decisions based on each individual's background, experiences and sociocultural beliefs. It involves thorough planning to be certain that the method chosen is acceptable and can be used effectively.
- Natural family planning methods are varied but involve determining the fertile period each month and then avoiding sexual intercourse during that time.
- Oral contraceptives provide one of the most reliable forms of contraception outside of abstinence. Women older than 40 years of age who smoke are not candidates for oral contraceptive use because of the danger of cardiovascular complications. They should be counselled to find a form of contraception that is reliable and allows them to remain sexually active.
- Contraceptive implants (renewed every 3 months), intramuscular injections (renewed every 1 or 3 months) and vaginal rings are as equally effective as oral contraceptives, if not more effective, as women cannot forget to take them daily.
- Intrauterine devices are placed in the uterus to prevent fertilisation and implantation. Women with intrauterine devices should limit their number of sexual partners to help prevent sexually transmitted infections, and be aware of the signs and symptoms of pelvic inflammatory disease.
- Barrier methods of contraception include diaphragms and condoms (male and female). Such methods are low in cost but are not as effective as ovulation suppressant methods. Use of diaphragms may be associated with urinary tract infections.
- Emergency contraception involves administration of a high dose of oestrogen or progesterone that prevents follicle-stimulating hormone release, preventing ovulation in case unprotected intercourse occurred. It must be given up to 72 hours after unprotected intercourse, the sooner the better.
- Surgical methods of contraception are tubal ligation in women and vasectomy in men.
- Elective termination of pregnancy can be accomplished surgically or medically by administration of mifepristone and misoprostol.

CASE STUDY QUESTIONS

4. What patient education information would you provide for Lena? What method of contraception would you recommend for her? Would your recommendation be different if she had a guaranteed monogamous relationship?
5. Suppose Lena was 39 years old, had high blood pressure and smoked. Would your teaching and recommendations differ?
6. If a woman presents to the emergency department or small rural hospital where you work, who has been sexually assaulted, what actions would you take in regards to emergency contraception and counselling?

Resources

For an extensive range of additional resources to enhance teaching and learning and to facilitate understanding of this chapter, please see the text's accompanying website located on thePoint at http://thepoint.lww.com.

References

Bond, S. (2013). No-cost contraceptive reduces unintended pregnancies and abortion rates at a population level. *Journal of Midwifery and Women's Health, 58*(2), 226–227.

Burkman, R. T. (2007). Contraception & family planning. In DeCherney, A. H. & Nathan, L. (Eds). *Current Diagnosis & Treatment in Obstetrics & Gynecology* (10th ed.). Columbus, OH: McGraw-Hill.

Cameron, S. T. & Glasier, A. (2012). Contraception and sterilization. In D. K. Edmonds (Ed.), *Dewhurst's Textbook of Obstetrics & Gynaecology* (8th ed.), pp. 495–512. Oxford, UK: John Wiley & Son.

Campbell, S. J., Cropsey, K. L. & Matthews, C. A. (2007). Intrauterine device use in a high-risk population: Experience from an urban university clinic. *American Journal of Obstetrics & Gynecology, 197*(2), 193–197.

Centers for Disease Control and Prevention. (2012). *Unintended Pregnancy Prevention.* Washington, DC: Centers for Disease Control and Prevention.

Cherlin, A. J. (2008). *Public and Private Families.* New York: McGraw-Hill Publishing Company.

Chrousos, G. P. (2008). The gonadal hormones and inhibitors. In Katzung, P. B. G. (Ed). *Basic and Clinical Pharmacology* (10th ed.). Columbus, OH: McGraw-Hill.

Collier, M. (Ed). (2011). *Reproductive & Sexual Health. An Australian Clinical Practice Handbook* (2nd ed.). Ashfield: Family Planning NSW.

Cook, L., et al. (2009). Vasectomy occlusion techniques for male sterilization. *Cochrane Database of Systematic Reviews, 2009*(1), (CD003991).

Cunningham, F. G., et al. (2008). Contraception. In Cunningham, F. G., et al. (Eds). *Williams Obstetrics* (22nd ed.). Columbus, OH: McGraw-Hill.

Family Planning NSW. (2011). *SAHRNI Update Spring Edition.* Ashfield: Family Planning NSW.

Family Planning New Zealand. (2012). Positive Sexual Health—Diaphragms, accessed 18 February 2015, <www.familyplanning.org.nz/advice/contraception/diaphragms>.

Glasier, A., Yan, Y. & Wellings, K. (2007). How do healthcare professionals respond to advice on adverse side effects of contraceptive methods? The case of Depo Provera. *Contraception, 76*(1), 18–22.

Harvey, N. & Gaudoin, M. (2007). Teenagers requesting pregnancy termination are no less responsible about contraceptive use at the time of conception than older women. *BJOG: An International Journal of Obstetrics and Gynaecology, 114*(2), 226–229.

MacKay, H. T. (2009). Gynecologic disorders. In McPhee, S. J., et al. (Eds). *Current Medical Diagnosis & Treatment.* Columbus, OH: McGraw-Hill.

McKenna, L. & Mirkov, S. (2014). *McKenna's Drug Handbook for Nursing & Midwifery* (7th ed.). Sydney: Lippincott Williams & Wilkins.

Mansour, D. (2012). European experience of Implanon. *European Journal of Contraception and Reproductive Health Care. 17*(20).

Nelson, A. L. (2011). What women want from their oral contraceptives. *Expert Review of Obstetrics and Gynecology, 6*(5), 509–523.

Pavone, M. E. & Burke, A. (2007). Fertility control: Contraception, sterilization, and abortion. In Fortner, K. B., et al. (Eds). *The Johns Hopkins Manual of Gynecology and Obstetrics* (3rd ed.). Philadelphia: Lippincott Williams & Wilkins.

Perry, M. (2014). Depo-Provera: A review of contraceptive efficacy. *Practice Nursing, 25*(2), 77–80.

Rickert, V. I., et al. (2007). Depo Now: Preventing unintended pregnancies among adolescents and young adults. *Journal of Adolescent Health, 40*(1), 22–28.

Roumen, F. J. (2007). The contraceptive vaginal ring compared with the combined oral contraceptive pill: A comprehensive review of randomized controlled trials. *Contraception, 75*(6), 420–429.

Schindler, A. E. (2010). Non-contraceptive benefits of hormonal contraceptives. *Minerva Ginecologica, 62*(4), 319–329.

Schorge, J. O., et al. (2008). Contraception and sterilization. In Schorge, J. O., et al. (Eds). *Williams Gynecology.* Columbus, OH: McGraw-Hill.

Schwarzer, J. U. & Steinfatt, H. (2013). Current status of vasectomy reversal. *Nature Reviews Urology, 10*(4), 195–205.

Sexual Health and Family Planning Australia, (2008). *Contraception: An Australian Clinical Practice Handbook.* Sexual Health and Family Planning Australia.

Shoupe, D. & Kjos, S. L. (Eds). (2010). *The Handbook of Contraception.* Totowa, NJ: Humana Press.

Smith, A., Lyons, A., Ferris, J., Richters, J., Pitts, M. and Shelley, J. (2010). Are sexual problems more common in women who have had a tubal ligation? A population-based study of Australian women. *BJOG: An International Journal of Obstetrics and Gynaecology, 117*(4), 463–468.

Stubblefield, P. G., Carr-Ellis, S. & Kapp, N. (2007). Family planning. In Berek, J. S. (Ed). *Berek & Novak's Gynecology.* Philadelphia: Lippincott Williams & Wilkins.

Warehime, M. N., Bass, L. & Pedulla, D. (2007). Effects of tubal ligation among American women. *Journal of Reproductive Medicine, 52*(4), 263–272.

Suggested readings

Cheng, L., et al. (2009). Interventions for emergency contraception. *Cochrane Database of Systematic Reviews, 2009*(1), (CD001324).

Children By Choice <www.childrenbychoice.org.au>.

Family Planning NSW <www.fpnsw.org.au/index.html>.

Halpern, V., et al. (2009). Strategies to improve adherence and acceptability of hormonal methods of contraception. *Cochrane Database of Systematic Reviews, 2009*(1), (CD004317).

New Zealand Family Planning <www.familyplanning.org.nz>.

Sexual Health and Family Planning Australia <www.shfpa.org.au>.

Chapter 7

The nursing role in genetic assessment and counselling

Previous chapters described common family types and how they are affected by sociocultural and community influences. This chapter discusses the basic principles by which disorders can be inherited and the necessary assessments, care and guidelines for counselling of families with the potential for a genetic disorder. Such information can influence the health of a family for generations to come.

LEARNING OBJECTIVES

After mastering the contents of this chapter, you should be able to:

1. Use critical thinking to analyse ways that nurses can make genetic assessment or education more family-centred.
2. Assess a family for its adjustment to the probability of inheriting a genetic disorder.
3. Discuss expected outcomes that meet the needs of the family undergoing genetic assessment and counselling.
4. Discuss nursing care planning related to a potential alteration in genetic health, such as assisting with an amniocentesis.
5. Implement nursing care such as counselling a family with a genetic disorder.
6. Discuss expected outcomes for achievement and effectiveness of care.
7. Identify areas related to genetic assessment that could benefit from additional nursing research or application of evidence-based practice.

KEY TERMS

- chromosomes
- cytogenetics
- dermatoglyphics
- genes
- genetic counselling
- genetics
- genome
- genotype
- karyotype

CASE STUDY

Amy de Sousa, 26 years old, is a woman you meet at a genetic counselling centre. She was adopted as a newborn and never felt a need to locate her birth parents because her adoptive parents provided a "close to perfect" childhood for her. After university, she married Dan from her local community. She is now pregnant with her first child. At 15 weeks into her pregnancy, after serum and ultrasound testing, she has been advised that her child may have Down syndrome. She asks you, "How could this happen? There's no condition like that in either of our families."

CASE STUDY QUESTION

1. How would you answer Amy?

As many as one in 20 newborns inherit a genetic disorder, while as many as 70% of paediatric hospital admissions may be for genetic-influenced disorders (Simpson, Holzgreve & Driscoll, 2012). The possibility that a child could have a genetic disorder crosses the minds of most pregnant women and their partners at some point in a pregnancy, whether or not there is any family history of such disorders. This causes pregnant couples to ask healthcare providers about their chances of having a child with a genetic disorder and about genetic testing.

GENETIC ASSESSMENT AND COUNSELLING

Assessment

Assessment measures for genetic disorders include:

- A detailed family history, preferably covering three generations
- Physical examination of both the parents and any affected children
- An ever-growing series of laboratory tests of blood, amniotic fluid, and maternal and fetal cells.

For example, women are offered routine screening of maternal serum levels of alpha-fetoprotein (MSAFP) early in pregnancy to evaluate for neural tube or chromosomal disorders in the fetus. Chorionic villi sampling (CVS) and amniocentesis are follow-up techniques that may be offered to women who are older than 35 years of age, or to those whose MSAFP level is abnormal, to further screen for genetic disorders. Couples who already know of the existence of a genetic disorder in their family or those who have had a previous child born with a congenital anomaly can have additional, more extensive testing. Nurses serve as members of genetic assessment and counselling teams to help obtain the initial family history, assist with physical examination, obtain blood serum for analysis and assist with procedures such as amniocentesis in this process.

Certain genetic disorders are more commonly found in some ethnic groups than in others, because people often marry within their own racial or ethnic group.

β-thalassaemia, for example, a blood dyscrasia, occurs most frequently in families of Greek or Italian heritage, whereas α-thalassaemia occurs most often in persons from the Philippines or Southeast Asia. Sickle cell anaemia occurs most often in African-Americans. Tay-Sachs disease occurs most often in people of Jewish ancestry.

Identifying which families might be at risk of particular genetic disorders because of their ethnic heritage and being certain they are informed of the incidence of these disorders and that genetic screening is available is a nursing responsibility.

Nursing considerations

The following are typical nursing considerations related to the area of genetic disorders:

- Decisional conflict related to testing for an untreatable genetic disorder
- Fear related to outcome of genetic screening tests
- Situational low self-esteem related to identified chromosomal abnormality
- Deficient knowledge related to inheritance pattern of the family's inherited disorder
- Health-seeking behaviours related to potential for genetic transmission of disease
- Altered sexuality pattern related to fear of conceiving a child with a genetic disorder. Families undergoing genetic assessment differ according to the types of assessments performed and the results obtained.

Nursing care may include determining what information the couple needs to know before testing can proceed or helping couples arrange for further assessment measures. The nurse must ensure that goals are realistic and consistent with the individual's or couple's lifestyle (not all people want to be totally informed about family illnesses). Helpful websites to use for referral are:

- Raising Children Network <http://raisingchildren.net.au/articles/disabilities_genetic_counselling.html>
- The Fragile X Association of Australia <http://fragilex.org.au/>
- The Paediatric Society of New Zealand Kids Health <http://kidshealth.org.nz/>
- New Zealand Down Syndrome Association <http://nzdsa.org.nz/>.

Parental reactions to the knowledge that their child has a possible genetic disorder or to the birth of a child with a genetically-inherited disorder usually involves grief, similar to that experienced by parents whose child has died at birth (their "perfect" child is gone). Both parents may pass through stages of shock and denial ("this cannot be true"), anger ("it's not fair that this happened to us") and bargaining ("if only this would go away") before they reach reorganisation and acceptance ("it has happened to us and it is all right"). For some couples, a genetic disorder is diagnosed during the pregnancy; for others, it may not be discovered until birth, or possibly not even until the child is of school age. For these parents, the reaction will occur at that later point of diagnosis.

As a rule, when parents are under stress, it is most helpful to guide them to concentrate on short-term goals and actions. Help them look first at the immediate needs of their family, the fetus, or the newborn, and later on at what type of continued follow-up will be necessary. For instance, after the birth, will the baby need to be hospitalised for immediate surgical correction of accompanying congenital anomalies, or will the parents be able to take the baby home? These decisions must be made immediately. What kind of special schooling the child will need is a decision that can wait until later.

It is important to identify support people who can be helpful to the parents during their time of uncertainty. These people may be usual family resources, such as grandparents or other family members. In some families however, these people are as disturbed by the diagnosis as the parents and therefore cannot offer their usual support. There are a number of organisations that can be of assistance to families. Yet, not all parents are ready to talk to members of such organisations at the time of diagnosis. Contacting an appropriate organisation should be done on a case-by-case basis. Some families will need more time to come to terms with the diagnosis than others. Identify healthcare personnel with whom the parents will need to maintain contact during the next few months such as a surgeon or other healthcare services. Ensuring that the parents have healthcare providers they know they can turn to, especially when they are moving out of denial, helps them move forward to the next step in accepting their child's diagnosis.

A couple's decisions about genetic testing and childbearing can change over time. For example, a decision made at age 25 not to have children because of a potential genetic disorder may be difficult to maintain at age 30, as the couple sees many of their friends with growing families. A nurse should ensure that such couples have the telephone number of a genetic counsellor.

GENETIC DISORDERS

Inherited or genetic disorders are disorders that can be passed from one generation to the next. They result from some disorder in **gene** or chromosome structure and occur in 5% to 6% of newborns. **Genetics** is the study of the way such disorders occur. **Cytogenetics** is the study of chromosomes by light microscopy and the method by which chromosomal aberrations are identified.

A phenotype is a person's outward appearance. **Genotype** refers to the actual gene composition. A person's **genome** is the complete set of genes present. A **karyotype** is a graphic representation of the chromosomes that are present.

Genetic disorders may occur at the moment an ovum and sperm fuse or even earlier, in the meiotic division phase of the gametes (ovum and sperm). Some genetic abnormalities are so severe that normal fetal growth cannot continue past that point. This early cell division is so precarious a process, in fact, that up to 50% of first-trimester spontaneous miscarriages may be the result of chromosomal abnormalities (McNair & Altman, 2011). Other genetic disorders do not affect life in utero, so the result of the disorder becomes apparent only at the time of fetal testing or after birth. Women having in vitro fertilisation (IVF) can have both the egg and sperm examined for genetic disorders of single gene or chromosome concerns before implantation. In the near future, it may be possible not only to identify aberrant genes for disorders this way but also to insert healthy genes in their place using stem cell implantation (Harper et al., 2012). Gene replacement therapy is encouraging in the treatment of blood, spinal cord and immunodeficiency syndromes (Domen, Gandy & Dalal, 2012; Mele, 2012). Women are able to arrange to have a newborn's cord blood frozen and reserved for bone marrow or other cell transplantation procedures in the future. Stem cells from menstrual blood and human breast milk are showing promise for replacement therapy and may be a future contribution source (Allickson et al., 2011; Twigger et al., 2013).

GENETIC COUNSELLING

Any individual concerned about the possibility of transmitting a disease to his or her children should have access to **genetic counselling** for advice on the inheritance of disease. Such counselling can serve to:

- Provide concrete, accurate information about the process of inheritance and inherited disorders
- Reassure people who are concerned that their child may inherit a particular disorder that the disorder will not occur
- Allow people who are affected by inherited disorders to make informed choices about future reproduction
- Offer support to people who are affected by genetic disorders.

Genetic counselling can make individuals feel "well" or free of guilt for the first time in their lives, particularly if they discover that the disorder they were worried about was not an inherited one but rather a chance occurrence.

In other circumstances, counselling results in informing individuals that they are carriers of a trait that is responsible for a child's condition. Even when people understand that they have no control over this, knowledge about passing a genetic disorder to a child can cause guilt and self-blame. This has the potential to destroy marriages and relationships unless both partners receive adequate support.

It is essential that information revealed in genetic screening be kept confidential, because such information could be used to damage a person's reputation or harm a future career or relationship. This necessity to maintain confidentiality prevents healthcare providers from alerting other family members about the inherited characteristic unless the member requesting genetic assessment has given consent for the information to be revealed. In some instances, a genetic history reveals information that a family doesn't want revealed, such as that a child has been adopted or is the result of artificial insemination, or that a current husband is not the child's father. The person seeking counselling has the right to decide whether this information may be shared with other family members.

The ideal time for counselling is before a first pregnancy. Some couples take this step even before committing themselves to marriage so both parties can make informed choices if counselling reveals that children of the marriage would be subject to a serious inherited disorder. Other couples first become aware of the need for genetic counselling after the birth of a first child with a disorder. It is best if these couples receive counselling before a second pregnancy. A couple may not be ready for this, however, until the initial shock of their first child's condition and the grief reaction that may accompany it have run their course. Only then may they be ready for information and decision making.

Even if a couple decides not to have any more children, it is important that they know that genetic counselling is available should their decision change. The nurse's role is also to be certain that they are aware that as their children reach reproductive age, they, too, may benefit from genetic counselling.

Nursing considerations

Nurses play important roles in assessing for symptoms and signs of genetic disorders, in offering support to individuals who seek genetic counselling and in helping with reproductive genetic testing procedures by such actions as:

- Explaining to a couple what procedures they can expect to undergo
- Explaining how different genetic screening tests are done and when they are usually offered
- Supporting a couple during the wait for test results
- Assisting couples in values clarification, planning and decision making based on test results.

A great deal of time may need to be spent offering support to a grieving couple confronted with the reality of how tragically the laws of inheritance have affected their lives. Genetic counselling is a role for nurses, however, only if they are adequately prepared in the study of genetics; without this background, genetic counselling can be dangerous and destructive.

Whether one is acting as a nursing member of a genetic counselling team or as a genetic counsellor, some common principles apply. First, the individual or couple being counselled needs a clear understanding of the information provided. People may listen to the statistics of their situation ("Your child has a 25% chance of having this disease") and construe a "25% chance" to mean that if they have one child with the disease, they can then have three other children without any worry. A 25% chance, however, means that with each pregnancy there is a 25% chance that the child will have the disease (chance has no "memory" of what has already happened). It is as if the couple had four cards, all aces, with the ace of spades representing the disease. When a card is drawn from the set of four, the chance of it being the ace of spades is 1 in 4 (25%). When the couple is ready to have a second child, it is as if the card drawn during the first round is returned to the set, so the chance of drawing the ace of spades in the second draw is exactly the same as in the first draw. Similarly, the couple's chances of having a child with the disease remain 1 in 4 in each successive pregnancy.

Second, it is never appropriate for any healthcare provider to impose his or her own values or opinions on others. Individuals with known inherited diseases in their family must face difficult decisions, such as how much genetic testing to undergo or whether to terminate a pregnancy that will result in a child with a specific genetic disease. Be certain that couples have been made aware of all the options available to them; then leave them to think about the options and make their own decisions by themselves. See also Boxes 7.1 and 7.2.

BOX 7.1 * Focus on family teaching

Genetic screening

Q. Amy is anxious to have her fetus' health confirmed. She asks you, "Why do I have to wait so late in pregnancy for genetic studies by amniocentesis?"

A. Genetic analysis is done on skin cells obtained from amniotic fluid. The test cannot be scheduled until enough amniotic fluid is present for analysis. Fortunately, this analysis can now be done as early as the 12th week of pregnancy.

Q. Why do laboratories take so long to return karyotyping results?

A. Karyotyping has traditionally (and by necessity) been done on cells at the metaphase (centre phase) of division, so the laboratory had to delay testing until the cells had grown to reach this phase. New techniques now allow analysis to be done immediately so that results are available much sooner.

Q. If there are no inherited diseases in a couple's family, should the couple have a karyotype done "just to be sure" before they have their first baby?

A. A genetic analysis is not routinely recommended unless there is evidence or suspicion of genetic disease in the family. Remember that karyotyping reveals only diseases that are present on chromosomes. A "perfect" karyotype does not guarantee that a newborn will not be ill in a non-inherited way.

Q. If chorionic villi are part of the placenta, how does testing them reveal the chromosome picture of the fetus?

A. Because the fetus and all accessory structures arise from the same single ovum and sperm, the placenta contains the same cells as the fetus.

BOX 7.2 * Focus on communication

Amy tells you that her mother has advised her not to have more children, rather than risk having a child with Down syndrome.

Less effective communication

Nurse: Hello, Amy. What's the reason you've come to the clinic today?

Amy: I need to know what chance there is that all my children will have Down syndrome.

Nurse: You're only 26, far too young to be worrying about that. Down syndrome only occurs in older women.

Amy: Thanks. It's good to get good information.

More effective communication

Nurse: Hello, Amy. What's the reason you've come to the clinic today?

Amy: I need to know what chance there is that all my children will have Down syndrome.

Nurse: That isn't the kind of question I can answer off the top of my head. Let me ask you some questions about your family to get started towards an answer.

Because we live in an age in which information can be obtained quickly, people may believe that predictions about the inheritance of disorders can also be supplied quickly. More important than getting information to people quickly is being certain they are getting it accurately. Because Amy is a balanced translocation carrier, more aspects than her age must be considered.

CASE STUDY QUESTION

2. Amy was told at a genetic counselling session that she is a chromosomal disorder carrier for Down syndrome. What would be your best action regarding this information?
   a. Be certain all of her family members understand what this means
   b. Discuss the cost of various abortion techniques with Amy
   c. Be sure Amy knows that she should not have any more children
   d. Ask Amy if she has any questions that you could answer for her

Assessment for genetic disorders

Genetic assessment begins with careful study of the pattern of inheritance in a family. A health history, physical examination of family members and laboratory analysis, such as karyotyping or DNA analysis, are performed to define the extent of the problem and the chance of inheritance.

History

Taking a health history for a genetic diagnosis is often difficult because the facts detailed may evoke uncomfortable emotions such as sorrow, guilt or inadequacy in parents. The genetic nurse should obtain information and document diseases in family members for a minimum of three generations, remembering to include half brothers and sisters or anyone related in any way as family. The nurse should also document the mother's age because some disorders increase in incidence with age. Important information includes whether the parents are consanguineous or related to each other.

Documenting the family's ethnic background can reveal risks for certain disorders that occur more commonly in some ethnic groups than others. If the couple seeking counselling is unfamiliar with their family history, ask them to talk to senior family members about other relatives (grandparents, aunts, uncles) before they come for an interview. Have them ask specifically for instances of spontaneous miscarriage or children in the family who died at birth. In many instances, these children died of unknown chromosomal disorders or were miscarried because of one of the 70 or more known chromosomal disorders that are inconsistent with life. Many people have only sketchy information about their families, such as, "The baby had some kind of nervous disease" or "Her heart didn't work right." Attempt to obtain more information by asking the couple to describe the appearance or activities of the affected individual or by requesting permission to obtain health records.

An extensive prenatal history of any affected person should be obtained to determine whether environmental conditions could account for the condition. Based on the above information, draw a family genogram. Such a diagram helps to not only identify the possibility of a chromosomal disorder occurring in a particular couple's children but also helps to identify other family members who might benefit from genetic counselling.

When a child is born dead, parents are advised to have a chromosomal analysis and autopsy performed. If at some future date they elect to have genetic counselling, this would allow their genetic counsellor to access additional medical information.

Physical assessment

Because genetic disorders often occur in varying degrees of expression, a careful physical assessment of any family member with a disorder, that child's siblings and the couple seeking counselling is needed. It is possible for an individual to have a minimal expression of a disorder that has gone previously undiagnosed. During inspection, pay particular attention to certain body areas, such as the space between the eyes; the height, contour and shape of ears; the number of fingers and toes and the presence of webbing. Dermatoglyphics (the study of surface markings of the skin) can also be helpful. Note any abnormal fingerprints or palmar creases as these are present with some disorders. Abnormal hair whorls (a patch of hair growing in the opposite direction to the rest of the hair), or colouring of hair can also be present.

TABLE 7.1 Common physical characteristics of children with chromosomal syndromes

Characteristic	Probable syndrome
Late closure of fontanelles	Down syndrome
Bossing (prominent forehead)	Fragile X syndrome
Microcephaly	Trisomy 18, trisomy 13
Low-set ears	Trisomy 18, trisomy 13
Slant of eyes	Down syndrome
Epicanthal fold	Down syndrome
Abnormal iris colour	Down syndrome
Large tongue	Down syndrome
Prominent jaw	Fragile X syndrome
Low-set hairline	Turner's syndrome
Multiple hair whorls	Trisomy 18, trisomy 13
Webbed neck	Turner's syndrome
Wide-set nipples	Trisomy 13
Heart abnormalities	Many syndromes
Large hands	Fragile X syndrome
Clinodactyly	Down syndrome
Overriding of fingers	Trisomy 18
Rocker-bottom feet	Trisomy 13
Abnormal dermatoglyphics	Down syndrome
Simian crease on palm	Down syndrome
Absence of secondary sex characteristics	Klinefelter and Turner's syndromes

Careful inspection of newborns is often sufficient to identify a child with a potential chromosomal disorder. Infants with multiple congenital anomalies, those born at less than 35 weeks' gestation, and those whose parents have had other children with chromosomal disorders need extremely close assessment. Table 7.1 lists the physical characteristics suggestive of some common inherited syndromes in children.

Diagnostic testing

Many diagnostic tests are available to provide important clues about possible disorders.

Karyotyping

For karyotyping, a sample of peripheral venous blood or a scraping of cells from the buccal membrane is taken. Cells are allowed to grow until they reach metaphase, the most easily observed phase. Cells are then stained, placed under a microscope and photographed. **Chromosomes** are identified according to size, shape and stain; they are cut from the photograph and arranged. Any additional, lacking or abnormal chromosomes can be visualised by this method.

Maternal serum screening

Alpha-fetoprotein (AFP) is a glycoprotein produced by the fetal liver that reaches a peak in maternal serum between the 13th and 32nd week of pregnancy. The level is elevated where there is fetal spinal cord disease (more than twice the value of the mean for that gestational age) and decreased in a fetal chromosomal disorder such as trisomy 21 (Down syndrome). Most pregnant women have an MSAFP test done routinely at the 15th week of pregnancy. If the result is abnormal, amniotic fluid is then assessed. Unfortunately, the MSAFP test has a false-positive rate of about 30% if the date of conception is not well-documented. Use of a "triple study" (AFP, estriol and hCG) reduces this false-positive rate, although false-positive reports still occur.

Analysis of a pregnancy-associated plasma protein A, which is also increased with a Down syndrome pregnancy, and measurement of the fetal neck thickness by ultrasound are other measures used for analysis if an MSAFP test is positive. Women with an elevated serum result need support while they wait for ultrasound or amniocentesis confirmation as they are facing what may be very grave information. Receiving a false-positive report is unfortunate as it can potentially interfere with the mother's bonding with her infant.

Chorionic villi sampling

Chorionic villi sampling (CVS) is a diagnostic technique that involves the retrieval and analysis of chorionic villi from the growing placenta for chromosome or DNA analysis (Katorza & Achiron, 2012). The test is highly accurate and yields no more false-positive results than does amniocentesis. Although this procedure may be done as early as week 5 of pregnancy, it is more commonly done at 8 to 10 weeks. With this technique, the chorion cells are located by ultrasound. A thin catheter is then inserted vaginally, or a biopsy needle is inserted abdominally or intravaginally, and a number of chorionic cells are removed for analysis (see Fig. 7.1). CVS carries a small risk (less than 1%) of causing excessive bleeding, leading to pregnancy loss. There have been some instances of children being born with missing limbs after the procedure (limb reduction syndrome). This has occurred with a high enough frequency that women need to be well-informed of these risks beforehand.

After CVS, instruct the woman to report chills or fever suggestive of infection or symptoms of threatened miscarriage (uterine contractions or vaginal bleeding). Women with an Rh-negative blood type need Rh immune globulin administration after the procedure to guard against isoimmunisation in the fetus.

The cells removed in CVS are karyotyped or submitted for DNA analysis to reveal whether the fetus has a genetic disorder. Because chorionic villi cells are rapidly dividing, results are available quickly, perhaps as soon as the next day. If a twin or multiple pregnancy is present, with two or more separate placentas, cells should be removed separately from each placenta. Because fraternal twins are derived from separate ova, one twin could have a chromosomal abnormality while the other does not.

Not all inherited diseases can be detected by CVS. Be certain that parents understand that only those disorders involving abnormal chromosomes or non-disjunction, and

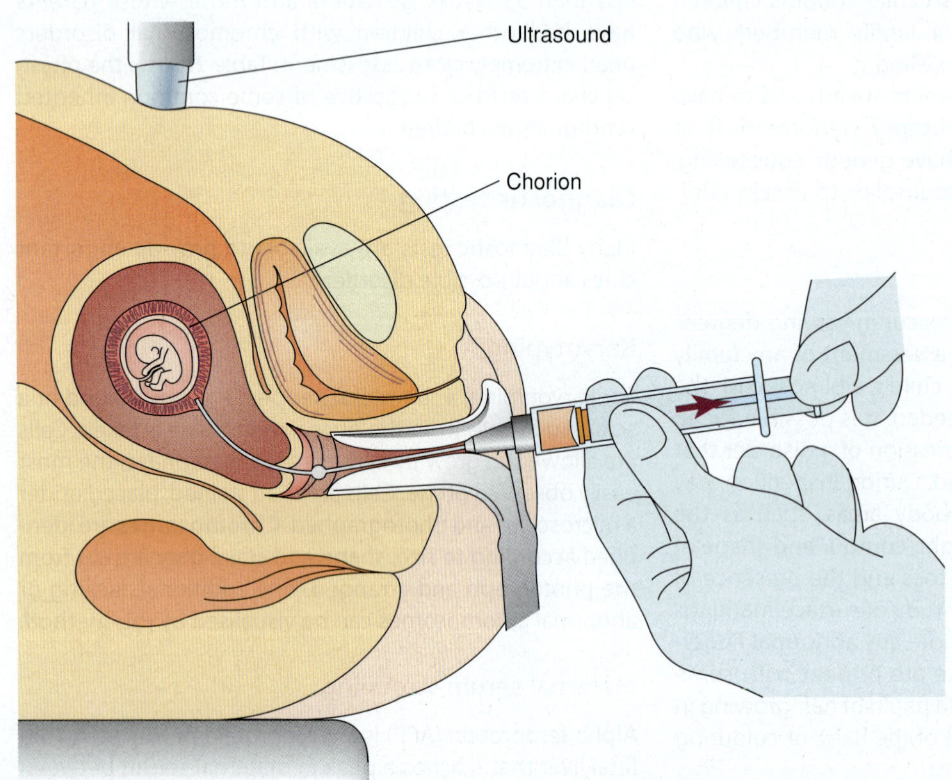

FIGURE 7.1 Chorionic villi sampling. Since the villi arise from trophoblast cells, their chromosome structure is the same as the fetus.

those whose specific gene location is known, can be identified by CVS. The test is not apt to reveal the extent of spinal cord abnormalities, for example.

Common chromosomal disorders that can be diagnosed prenatally through karyotyping are discussed below. Additional disorders that can be identified by DNA analysis are retinoblastoma, myotonic dystrophy, Huntington disease, sickle cell anaemia, thalassaemia and Duchenne's muscular dystrophy.

The decision to undergo CVS is a major one for a couple. As a rule, they are not making a decision simply for CVS. If the CVS reveals that their child is abnormal, they then have to make a second decision about the future of the pregnancy. Deciding to terminate a pregnancy based on a laboratory finding is rarely easy. The couple may need a great deal of support with their decision, both to carry it through and to live with it afterwards. If they decide not to terminate, they will need support during the remainder of the pregnancy and in the days following birth. It may be difficult for a couple to believe that what the test showed is true. Only when they inspect the baby and see that the test was accurate—the child does have a genetic disorder—will they see the reality. This can result in long-lasting depression.

Amniocentesis

Amniocentesis is the withdrawal of amniotic fluid through the abdominal wall for analysis between the 14th and 16th week of pregnancy (Simpson et al., 2012). Because amniotic fluid has reached about 200 mL at this point, enough fluid can be withdrawn for karyotyping of skin cells found in the fluid as well as an analysis of AFP or acetylcholinesterase. If no acetylcholinesterase, a breakdown product of blood, is found in the specimen, it confirms that an elevated AFP level is not a false-positive reading caused by blood in the fluid.

For the procedure, a pocket of amniotic fluid is located by ultrasound. A needle is then inserted transabdominally and about 20 mL of fluid is aspirated. Skin cells in the fluid are karyotyped for chromosomal number and structure. The level of AFP is analysed. Some disorders, such as Tay-Sachs disease, can be identified by the lack of a specific enzyme, such as hexosaminidase A, in amniotic fluid.

Amniocentesis has the advantage over CVS of carrying only a 0.5% risk of spontaneous miscarriage. Unfortunately, it usually is not done until the 14th to 16th week of pregnancy. This may prove to be a difficult time because, by this date, a woman is beginning to accept her pregnancy and bond with the fetus. In addition, termination of pregnancy during the second trimester is more difficult than during the first trimester. Parents will need support while they wait for test results and also when making decisions about the pregnancy. Women with a Rh-negative blood type need Rh immune globulin administration after the procedure to protect against isoimmunisation in the fetus. All women need to be observed for about 30 minutes after the procedure to be certain that labour contractions are not beginning and that the fetal heart rate remains within normal limits. Because amniocentesis is also a common assessment for fetal maturity, it is discussed further in Chapter 9.

Percutaneous umbilical blood sampling

Percutaneous umbilical blood sampling (PUBS), or cordocentesis, is the removal of blood from the fetal umbilical cord at about 17 weeks using an amniocentesis technique (see Fig. 7.2). This allows analysis of blood components as well as more rapid karyotyping than is possible when only skin cells are removed. PUBS is discussed further in Chapter 9.

Fetal imaging

Magnetic resonance imaging (MRI) and ultrasound are diagnostic tools used to assess a fetus for general size and structural disorders of the internal organs, spine and limbs. Because some genetic disorders are associated with physical appearance, both of these methods may be helpful (Collins & Limpey, 2012). Ultrasound is used concurrently with amniocentesis.

Fetoscopy

Fetoscopy is the insertion of a fibreoptic fetoscope through a small incision in the mother's abdomen into the uterus

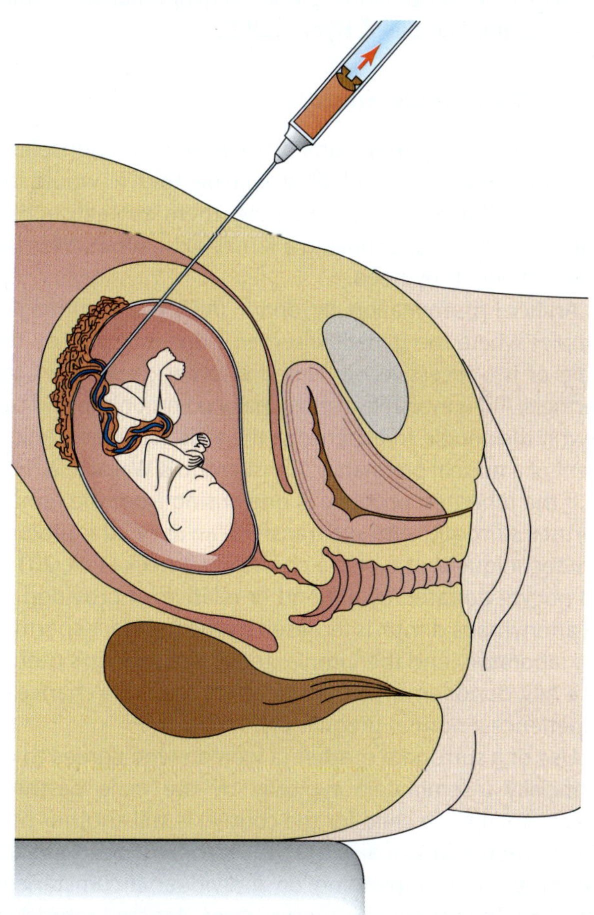

FIGURE 7.2 Percutaneous umbilical blood sampling. Blood is withdrawn from the umbilical cord using an amniocentesis technique.

and membranes to visually inspect the fetus for gross abnormalities. It can be used to confirm an ultrasound finding, to remove skin cells for DNA analysis, or to perform surgery for a congenital disorder such as a stenosed urethra.

Preimplantation diagnosis

Preimplantation diagnosis is possible for in vitro fertilisation procedures. It may be possible in the future for a naturally fertilised ovum to be removed from the uterus by lavage before implantation and studied for DNA analysis in the same way. The ovum would then be reinserted or not, depending on the findings and the parents' wishes. This would provide genetic information extremely early in a pregnancy.

Nuchal translucency screening

A number of genetic disorders such as Down syndrome and Turner's syndrome can be detected on a sonogram taken during the first trimester of pregnancy (11 to 13 weeks) because of unusual fat or fluid deposits at the back of the fetal neck, which show on a sonogram as excessive thickening. Such findings are then followed by a chromosome or gene analysis to confirm the finding. Nuchal translucency may also suggest congenital heart defects because it can be caused from interference of lymphatic or vascular flow (Mogra, Alabbad & Hyett, 2012).

Reproductive alternatives

Some couples are reluctant to seek genetic counselling because they are afraid they will be told it would be unwise to have children. Helping them to realise that viable alternatives for having a family exist allows them to seek the help they need.

Artificial insemination by donor (AID) is an option for couples where the genetic disorder is one inherited by the male or is a recessively inherited disorder carried by both partners. AID is available in most major communities and can permit the couple to experience the satisfaction and enjoyment of a normal pregnancy (Christianson & Wallach, 2011).

If the inherited problem is one arising from the female partner, surrogate embryo transfer is an assisted reproductive technique that is also a possibility (Check et al., 2012). An oocyte donated by a friend or relative, or provided by an anonymous donor, is fertilised by the partner's sperm in the laboratory and then implanted into a woman's uterus. Like AID, donor embryo transfer offers couples a chance to experience a normal pregnancy.

Use of a surrogate mother (a woman who agrees to be artificially inseminated, typically by the male partner's sperm and bear a child for the couple) is still another possibility (Golombok et al., 2011). All of these procedures are expensive and, depending on individual circumstances, may have disappointing success rates. Assisted reproductive techniques are discussed in more detail in Chapter 8.

Adoption is an alternative many couples can find rewarding (see Chapter 3). Choosing to remain child free should also not be discounted as a viable option. Many couples who have every reason to think they would have children without a genetic disorder choose this alternative because they believe their existence is full and rewarding without the presence of children.

Diagnosis of a disorder during pregnancy with prompt treatment at birth to minimise the prognosis and outcome of the disorder is another route to explore. Termination of a pregnancy that reveals a chromosomal or metabolic abnormality should be a final option.

Future possibilities

Stem cell research is looking at the possibility that immature cells (stem cells) could be implanted into an embryo with a known abnormal genetic makeup, replacing the abnormal cells or righting the affected child's genetic composition (Rodts, 2012). Although presently possible, stem cell research is costly and produces some ethical questions (e.g. although stem cells can be harvested from cord blood, adult skin cells, menstrual blood and human breast milk, will these be able to serve as main sources of donor DNA for the new technology?).

Legal and ethical aspects of genetic screening and counselling

Nurses can be instrumental in seeing that couples who seek genetic counselling receive results in a timely manner and with compassion and understand what those results may mean to future childbearing. You should always keep in mind the legal responsibilities of genetic testing, counselling and therapy, including:

- Participation by couples or individuals in genetic screening must be elective
- People desiring genetic screening must sign an informed consent for the procedure
- Results must be interpreted correctly yet provided to the individuals as quickly as possible
- The results must not be withheld from the individuals and must be given only to those persons directly involved
- After genetic counselling, persons must not be coerced to undergo procedures such as abortion or sterilisation. Any procedure must be the result of a free and individual decision.

Failure to heed these guidelines could result in charges of invasion of privacy, breach of confidentiality, or psychological injury caused by "labelling" someone or imparting unwarranted fear and worry about the significance of a disease or carrier state. If couples are identified as being at risk of having a child with a genetic disorder and are not informed of the risk and offered appropriate diagnostic procedures (e.g. amniocentesis) they can bring a "wrongful birth" lawsuit if their child is born with the detected genetic disorder.

COMMON CHROMOSOMAL DISORDERS RESULTING IN PHYSICAL OR COGNITIVE DEVELOPMENTAL DISORDERS

Several chromosomal disorders are easily detected at birth upon physical examination. Many of these disorders leave children cognitively challenged. Care of the child who is cognitively challenged is discussed in Chapter 54.

Trisomy 13 syndrome (47XY131 or 47XX131)

In trisomy 13 syndrome (Patau syndrome), the child has an extra chromosome 13 and is severely cognitively challenged. The incidence of the syndrome is low, approximately 0.45 per 1000 live births. Midline body disorders such as cleft lip and palate (see Fig. 7.3), heart defects, particularly ventricular septal defects and abnormal genitalia are present. Other common findings include microcephaly with abnormalities of the forebrain and forehead; eyes that are smaller than normal (microphthalmos) or absent; and low-set ears. Most of these children do not survive beyond early childhood.

Trisomy 18 syndrome (47XY181 or 47XX181)

Children with trisomy 18 syndrome have three copies of chromosome 18. The incidence is approximately 0.23 per 1000 live births. These children are severely cognitively challenged and tend to be small for gestational age at birth, have markedly low-set ears, a small jaw, congenital heart defects, and usually misshapen fingers and toes (the index finger deviates or crosses over other fingers). Also, the soles of their feet are often rounded instead of flat (rocker-bottom feet). As in trisomy 13 syndrome, most of these children do not survive beyond early infancy.

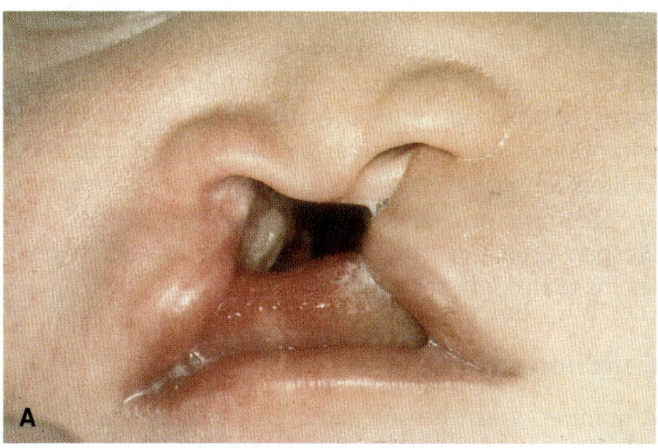

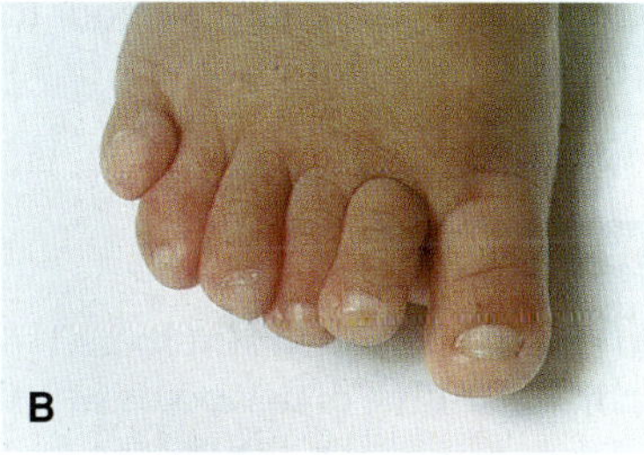

FIGURE 7.3 An infant with trisomy 13 has (**A**) a cleft lip and palate and (**B**) supernumerary digits (polydactyly). (© NMSB/Custom Medical Stock Photograph.)

Cri-du-chat syndrome (46XX5p2 or 46XY5P2)

Cri-du-chat syndrome is the result of a missing portion of chromosome 5. In addition to an abnormal cry, which sounds much more like the sound of a cat than a human infant's cry, children with cri-du-chat syndrome tend to have a small head, wide-set eyes and a downward slant to the palpebral fissure of the eye. They are severely cognitively challenged.

Turner's syndrome (45X0)

The child with Turner's syndrome (gonadal dysgenesis) has only one functional X chromosome. The child is short in stature and has only streak (small and non-functional) ovaries. She is sterile and with the exception of pubic hair, secondary sex characteristics do not develop at puberty. The hairline at the nape of the neck is low set, and the neck may appear to be webbed and short. A newborn may have appreciable oedema of the hands and feet and a number of congenital anomalies, most frequently coarctation (stricture) of the aorta and kidney disorders. The incidence of the syndrome is approximately 1 per 10,000 live births. The disorder can be identified with an ultrasound during pregnancy because of the presence of increased neck folds.

Although children with Turner's syndrome may be severely cognitively challenged, difficulty in this area is more commonly limited to learning disabilities. Socio-emotional adjustment problems may accompany the syndrome because of the lack of fertility and if the nuchal folds are prominent.

Klinefelter syndrome (47XXY)

Infants with Klinefelter syndrome are males with an extra X chromosome. Characteristics of the syndrome may not be noticeable at birth. At puberty, secondary sex characteristics do not develop; the child has small testes that produce ineffective sperm (Jospe, 2011). Affected individuals tend to develop gynecomastia (increased breast size) and have an increased risk of male breast cancer (Brinton, 2011). The incidence is about 1 per 1000 live births. Karyotyping can be used to reveal the additional X chromosome.

Fragile X syndrome (46XY23q2)

Fragile X syndrome is the most common cause of cognitive challenge in males. It is an X-linked disorder in which one long arm of an X chromosome is defective and results in inadequate protein synaptic responses (Wang, Bray & Warren, 2012). The incidence is about 1 in 1000 live births.

Before puberty, boys with fragile X syndrome typically may demonstrate maladaptive behaviours such as hyperactivity and autism. They may have reduced intellectual functioning, with marked deficits in speech and arithmetic (Lubs, Stevenson & Shwartz, 2012). They may be identified by the presence of a large head, a long face with a high forehead, a prominent lower jaw and large protruding ears. Hyperextensive joints and cardiac disorders may also be present. After puberty, enlarged testicles may become evident. Affected individuals are fertile and can reproduce.

Carrier females may show some evidence of the physical and cognitive characteristics. Although intellectual function from the syndrome cannot be improved, both folic acid and an antipsychotic drug such as phenothiazines may improve symptoms of poor concentration and impulsivity (McLennan et al., 2011).

Down syndrome (Trisomy 21) (47XY211 or 47XX211)

Trisomy 21, the most frequently occurring chromosomal abnormality, occurs in about 1 in 800 pregnancies. The number of children born with the disorder is now considerably less as many women choose to end pregnancies when the diagnosis is made (Natoli et al., 2012; see Box 7.3).

BOX 7.3 ✻ Focus on evidence-based practice

Having a child with Down syndrome

If it is predicted during a pregnancy that a couple will have a child with Down syndrome, the couple is asked to make a choice as to whether they want to continue the pregnancy or terminate it at that point. To discover how couples feel about having a child with Down syndrome, researchers surveyed 2044 parents on the mailing lists of six, non-profit Down syndrome organisations. The majority of parents reported that they are happy with their decision to have their child and find their son or daughter a great source of love and pride. Ninety-nine percent reported they love their affected son or daughter, 97% reported being proud of them, 79% felt their outlook on life was more positive because of them, only 5% felt embarrassed by them and only 4% regretted having them. In a following study, siblings also reported their relationship with their affected sibling as a positive one. Less than 10% felt embarrassed and less than 5% expressed a desire to trade their sibling in for another brother or sister.

Would the above findings be helpful to you when talking to Amy about her concerns of having a child with Down syndrome?

Source: Skotko, B. G., Levine, S. P. & Goldstein, R. (2011a). Having a brother or sister with Down syndrome: Perspectives from siblings. *American Journal of Medical Genetics, 155*(10), 2335–2347; and Skotko, B. G., Levine, S. P. & Goldstein, R. (2011b). Having a son or daughter with Down syndrome: Perspectives from mothers and fathers. *American Journal of Medical Genetics, 155*(10), 2348–2359.

The physical features of children with Down syndrome are so marked that fetal diagnosis is possible by ultrasound in utero. The nose is broad and flat. The eyelids have an extra fold of tissue at the inner canthus (an epicanthal fold) and the palpebral fissure (opening between the eyelids) tends to slant laterally upward. The iris of the eye may have white specks, called Brushfield spots. The tongue may protrude from the mouth because the oral cavity is smaller than usual. The back of the head is flat, the neck is short and an extra pad of fat at the base of the head causes the skin to be so loose it can be lifted easily. The ears may be low-set. Muscle tone is poor, giving the baby a rag-doll appearance. This can be so lax that the child's toe can be touched against the nose (not possible in the average mature newborn). The fingers of many children with Down syndrome are short and thick, and the little finger is often curved inward. There may be a wide space between the first and second toes, and between the first and second fingers. The palm of the hand shows a peculiar crease (a simian line), which is a single horizontal palm crease rather than the usual three creases in the palm (see Fig. 7.4).

Children with Down syndrome are usually cognitively challenged to some degree. The challenge can range from an intelligence quotient (IQ) of 50 to 70 to a child who is profoundly affected (IQ less than 20). The extent of the cognitive challenge is not evident at birth. The fact that the brain is not developing well is evidenced by a head size that is usually smaller than the 10th or 20th percentile when measured at healthcare visits.

These children also appear to have altered immune function as they are prone to upper respiratory tract infections. Congenital heart disease, especially atrioventricular defects, is common. Stenosis or atresia of the duodenum, strabismus and cataract disorders are also common. For as yet undetected reasons, acute lymphocytic leukaemia occurs approximately 20 times more frequently in children with Down syndrome than in the general population (Buitenkamp et al., 2012). Even if children are born without an accompanying disorder such as heart disease, their lifespan usually is only 50 to 60 years, because ageing seems to occur faster than normal.

Childhood tumours

A number of cancers in children are also associated with chromosomal aberrations. Chief among these are retinoblastoma (chromosome 13), Wilms' tumour (chromosome 11) and neuroblastoma (chromosome 1 or 11) (Nicholson & Cimini, 2011).

CASE STUDY QUESTION

3. Amy's child is born with Down syndrome. What is a common physical feature of newborns with this disorder?

a. Spastic and stiff muscles
b. Loose skin at back of neck
c. A white lock of forehead hair
d. Wrinkles on the soles of the feet

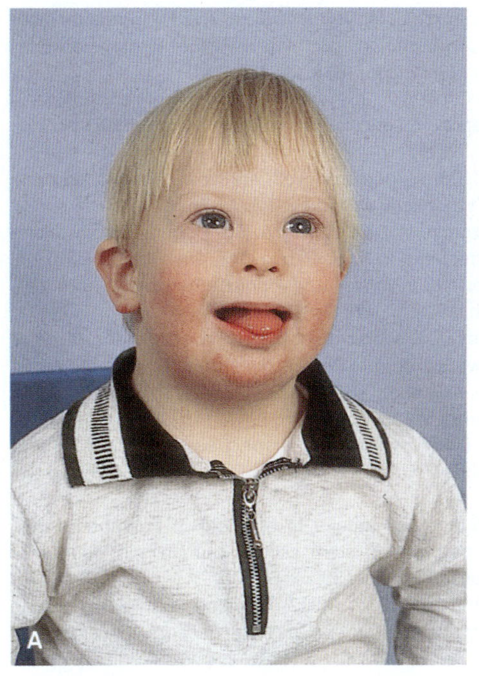

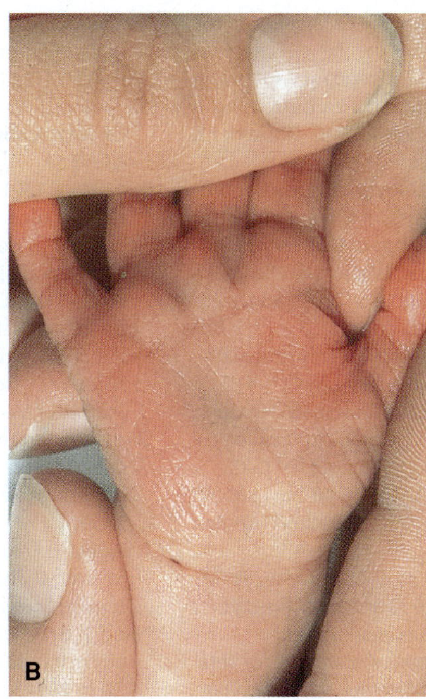

FIGURE 7.4 (**A**) Typical facial features of a child with Down syndrome. (**B**) A simian line, a horizontal crease seen in children with Down syndrome. (SPL/Custom Medical Stock Photograph.)

Key points for review

- Genetic disorders are disorders resulting from a defect in the structure or number of genes or chromosomes. Genetics is the study of how and why such disorders occur.
- A phenotype is a person's outward appearance. **Genotype** refers to the actual gene composition. A person's **genome** is the complete set of genes present. A **karyotype** is a graphic representation of the chromosomes that are present.
- Genetic counselling can be a role for nurses with advanced preparation and education. Assessment of genetic disorders consists of a health history, physical examination, and diagnostic studies such as chorionic villi sampling, amniocentesis and maternal serum levels of alpha-fetoprotein analysis.
- Some karyotyping tests, such as chorionic villi sampling and amniocentesis, introduce a risk of spontaneous or threatened miscarriage. Be certain that women undergoing these tests remain in the healthcare facility for at least 30 minutes after the procedure to be sure that any complications such as vaginal bleeding, uterine cramping or abnormal fetal heart rate are not present. Women with an Rh-negative blood type need Rh immune globulin administration after these procedures.
- An important aspect of genetic counselling is respecting a couple's right to privacy. Be certain that information gained from testing remains confidential and is not given indiscriminately to others, including other family members.
- People who are told that a genetic abnormality does exist in their family may suffer a loss of self-esteem. Offering support to help them deal with the feelings they experience is an important nursing intervention.

CASE STUDY QUESTIONS

4. Amy doesn't know her family history so is unable to answer questions about family members. What questions would you want to ask about her husband's family? Suppose Mr de Sousa tells you he had two brothers who died at birth. Would that finding be important?
5. Suppose Amy's husband's sister and her husband both carry a gene for a recessively inherited disorder, yet they have had five children and none of the children shows symptoms of the disorder. Is it possible for them to have had five children without any symptoms of the disease? What are the chances that their sixth child will also be disease free?
6. Amy tells you, "My family will be so ashamed if a genetic defect happens in our family." What does her statement tell you about her family's knowledge of genetic disorders?

Resources

For an extensive range of additional resources to enhance teaching and learning and to facilitate understanding of this chapter, please see the text's accompanying website located on thePoint at http://thepoint.lww.com.

References

Allickson, J. G., Sanchez, A., Yefimenko, N., et al. (2011). Recent studies assessing the proliferative capability of a novel adult stem cell identified in menstrual blood. *Open Stem Cell Journal, 3*(2011), 4–10.

Brinton, L. A. (2011). Breast cancer risk among Klinefelter syndrome patients. *Acta Paediatrica, 100*(6), 814–818.

Buitenkamp, T. D., Pieters, R., Gallimore, N. E., et al. (2012). Outcome in children with Down syndrome and acute lymphoblastic leukaemia:

Role of IKZF1 deletions and CRLF2 aberrations. *Leukaemia, 26*(10), 2204–2211.

Check, J. H., Katsoff, B., Wilson, C., et al. (2012). Pregnancy following fresh vs frozen embryo transfer into gestational carriers using a simplified slow freeze protocol. *Clinical & Experimental Obstetrics & Gynaecology, 39*(1), 23–24.

Christianson, M. S. & Wallach, E. E. (2011). Infertility and assisted reproductive technologies. In K. J. Hurt, M. W. Guile, J. L. Bienstock et al. (Eds), *The Johns Hopkins Manual of Gynaecology and Obstetrics* (4th ed.), pp. 421–437. Philadelphia, PA: Lippincott Williams & Wilkins.

Collins, S. L. & Limpey, L. (2012). Prenatal diagnosis: Types and techniques. *Early Human Development, 88*(1), 3–8.

Domen, J., Gandy, K. & Dalal, J. (2012). Emerging uses for paediatric haematopoietic stem cells. *Paediatric Research, 71*(4–2), 411–417.

Golombok, S., Readings, J., Blake, L., et al. (2011). Families created through surrogacy: Mother-child relationships and children's psychological adjustment at age 7. *Developmental Psychology, 47*(6), 1579–1588.

Harper, J., Magli, M. C., Lundin, K., et al. (2012). When and how should new technology be introduced into the IVF laboratory? *Human Reproduction, 27*(2), 303–313.

Jospe, N. (2011). Disorders of puberty. In K. J. Marcdante, R. M., Kliegman, H. B., Jenson, et al. (Eds), *Nelson Essentials of Paediatrics* (6th ed.), pp. 645–653. Philadelphia, PA: Saunders/Elsevier.

Katorza, E. & Achiron, R. (2012). Early pregnancy scanning for fetal anomalies – The new standard? *Clinical Obstetrics & Gynaecology, 55*(1), 199–216.

Lubs, H. A., Stevenson, R. E. & Schwartz, C. E. (2012). Fragile X and X-linked intellectual disability: Four decades of discovery. *American Journal of Human Genetics, 90*(4), 579–590.

McLennan, Y., Polussa, J., Tassone, F., et al. (2011). Fragile X syndrome. *Current Genomics, 12*(3), 216–224.

McNair, T. & Altman, K. (2011). Miscarriage & recurrent pregnancy loss. In K. J. Hurt, M. W. Guile, J. L. Bienstock, et al. (Eds), *The Johns Hopkins Manual of Gynaecology and Obstetrics* (4th ed.), pp. 438–447. Philadelphia, PA: Lippincott Williams & Wilkins.

Mele, C., (2012). Gene therapy; A genetic era of technological development to treat pediatric genetic disorders. *Journal of Pediatric Nursing, 27*(2), 180–183.

Mogra, R., Alabbad, N. & Hyett, J. (2012). Increased nuchal translucency and congenital heart disease. *Early Human Development, 88*(5), 261–267.

Natoli, J. L., Ackerman, D. L., McDermott, S., et al. (2012). Prenatal diagnosis of Down syndrome: A systematic review of termination rates (1995-2011). *Prenatal Diagnosis, 32*(2), 142–153.

Nicholson, J. A. & Cimini, D. (2011). How mitotic errors contribute to karyotypic diversity in cancer. *Advances in Cancer Research, 112*(4), 43–75.

Rodts, M. F. (2012). Cord blood stem cells and cord tissue to aid bone regeneration. *Orthopaedic Nursing, 31*(1), 35–36.

Simpson, J. L., Holzgreve, W. & Driscoll, D. A. (2012). Genetic counselling and genetic screening. In S. G. Gabbe, J. R. Niebyl, J. L. Simpson, et al. (Eds), *Obstetrics: Normal and Problem Pregnancies* (6th ed.), pp. 193–209. Philadelphia, PA: Elsevier/Saunders.

Skotko, B. G., Levine, S. P. & Goldstein, R. (2011a). Having a brother or sister with Down syndrome: Perspectives from siblings. *American Journal of Medical Genetics*, 155(10), 2335–2347.

Skotko, B. G., Levine, S. P. & Goldstein, R. (2011b). Having a son or daughter with Down syndrome: Perspectives from mothers and fathers. *American Journal of Medical Genetics, 155*(10), 2348–2359.

Twigger, A. J., Hodgetts, S., Filgueira, L., et al. (2013). From breast milk to brains: The potential of stem cells in human milk. *Journal of Human Lactation, 29*(2), 136–139.

Wang, T., Bray, S. M. & Warren, S. T. (2012). New perspectives on the biology of fragile X syndrome. *Current Opinion in Genetics & Development, 22*(3), 256–263.

Suggested readings

Chismark, E. & Evans, D. D. (2012). Adverse drug events in the emergency department: Why genetics matters in practice. *Advances in Emergency Nursing Journal, 34*(1), 3–9.

Daack-Hirsch, S., Driessnack, M., Perkhounkova, Y., et al. (2012). A practical first step to integrating genetics into the curriculum. *Journal of Nursing Education, 9*(3), 1–5.

Natoli, J. L., Ackerman, D. L., McDermott, S., et al. (2012). Prenatal diagnosis of Down syndrome: A systematic review of termination rates (1995-2011). *Prenatal Diagnosis, 32*(2), 142–153.

Tonkin, E., Calzone, K., Jenkins, J., et al. (2011). Genomic education resources for nursing faculty. *Journal of Nursing Scholarship, 43*(4), 330–340.

Chapter 8

Nursing care of the infertile couple

Previous chapters described normal anatomy and physiology and ways to prevent pregnancy. This chapter adds information to expand your knowledge base about care of the couple who is unable to conceive.

LEARNING OBJECTIVES

After studying this chapter, you should be able to:

1. Describe common causes of infertility in both men and women.
2. Use critical thinking to analyse ways that a fertility assessment can be more family-centred.
3. Describe common assessments necessary to detect infertility.
4. Formulate nursing considerations related to infertility.
5. Identify appropriate outcomes for the infertile couple.
6. Plan nursing interventions to meet the needs of a couple with a diagnosis of infertility.
7. Implement nursing care associated with the diagnosis of infertility or measures to promote fertility, such as health teaching.
8. Evaluate outcomes for achievement and effectiveness of care.
9. Identify areas of nursing care related to fertility that could benefit from additional nursing research or application of evidence-based practice.
10. Integrate knowledge about infertility with the nursing process to achieve quality child and family health nursing care.

KEY TERMS

- anovulation
- artificial insemination
- cryptorchidism
- endometriosis
- erectile dysfunction
- in vitro fertilisation
- infertility
- pelvic inflammatory disease
- sperm count
- sperm motility
- spermatogenesis

CASE STUDY

Cheryl and Bob Carl married when they were both 25 and planned to wait 5 years before beginning their family so they could save money for a house. At the end of 5 years they bought the house. On the day they moved in, Mrs Carl stopped taking her contraception. At the end of a year, however, she still was not pregnant. Three years later, the Carls began fertility testing. They are now undergoing their second cycle of in vitro fertilisation and embryo transfer. The Carls have applied for a second mortgage on their house to finance the fertility testing and fertilisation procedures. At her last visit, Mrs Carl stated, "This is my fault because I'm so rigid. I can't relax enough to get pregnant. Look how I had to buy the house before I could even consider getting pregnant and now we'll probably lose it. Besides that, it feels like our whole life revolves around trying to get pregnant."

CASE STUDY QUESTION

1. How could you best help the Carls?

Infertility is a term used to describe the inability to conceive a child, sustain a pregnancy to birth or the potential to conceive with additional help. Infertility affects as many as 11–14% of couples who desire children (Sheaves, 2013). Couples exploring fertility testing come in all different types: many are married couples who are having trouble conceiving; some desire to remain single or partner with someone of their own sex and bear a child through an assisted fertility method.

When a couple first pursues fertility counselling, they usually have fears and anxieties not only about their inability to conceive but also about what this condition will mean to their future lifestyle and family. Without information about the cause of their infertility, partners can blame themselves or carry unexpressed anger towards a partner. Some couples may strongly desire a child but also feel anxious about impending parenthood, which would bring with it loss of independence and their established lifestyle. For all these reasons, infertility screening and counselling can be an emotionally difficult and physically demanding process, often creating a high level of strain on a couple's relationship, especially if they don't maintain open communication (Chachamovich et al., 2010).

Because most fertility tests are conducted in primary healthcare settings, nurses play a key role in educating couples about the variety of tests and procedures that may be performed. Nurses are important members of fertility healthcare teams, often assuming responsibility for health assessment, client education and counselling and helping clients identify and express their feelings about their desire to have a child, express how far they are willing to go in terms of testing and procedures to achieve this desire, and how they might feel if they are not able to have a child.

FOR THE COUPLE WITH INFERTILITY

Assessment

Infertility assessment and infertility investigation is usually limited to three assessments: semen analysis, ovulation monitoring and tubal patency.

Nursing considerations

Nursing considerations related to infertility are likely to focus on psychosocial issues associated with the inability to conceive and the process of fertility testing and management. Examples of possible considerations include:

- Fear related to possible outcome of infertility studies
- Situational low self-esteem related to the apparent inability to conceive
- Anxiety related to what the process of fertility testing will entail
- Deficient knowledge related to measures to promote fertility
- Anticipatory grieving related to failure to conceive or sustain a pregnancy
- Powerlessness related to repeated unsuccessful attempts at achieving conception
- Hopelessness related to perception of no viable alternatives to usual conception.

In establishing expected outcomes with a couple undergoing fertility testing and counselling, be certain that the couple realises that results may not be instantaneous. A couple may need to change or modify their goals if tests begin to show that what they first wanted—to have a child without medical intervention—is impossible. Participation in a support group may allow a couple to work through the stress that fertility testing places on their lives. Access Australia <www.access.org.au> an Australian support group or Fertility NZ <http://fertilitynz.org.nz> a New Zealand support group can be helpful in offering referral sources and support that a couple can use in planning.

Fertility testing can be costly. Couples need to be informed beforehand of specific estimates of the cost of testing or therapy. Throughout testing, couples need thorough education about the various procedures. Make sure to review any specific instructions about preprocedural and postprocedural care. Depending on their motivations, a couple's reaction to study results may vary from relief, to stoic acceptance, to grief for children never to be born. Each partner may wonder whether the other will be able to continue the relationship if he or she turns out to be the "infertile" one. Couples need the active support of healthcare personnel from the first day they brace themselves to ask, "Exactly why are we childless?" until the end, regardless of the results.

Examples of expected outcomes in this area include:

- Client rearranges work shifts to manage fertility testing routine by 1 month's time.
- Couple verbalises that they understand their individual infertility problem after preliminary testing.

For the couple with the problem of infertility, evaluation is best if it is ongoing because, as circumstances around them change, so may their goals and desires. Until they can accept an alternative method of having children—adoption or an assisted reproductive technique such as **artificial insemination** (deposition of sperm into a woman's cervix or uterus) or **in vitro fertilisation** (IVF; the union of sperm and ovum under laboratory conditions)—former plans have been crushed. It is not unusual to see a couple move through steps of denial, anger, bargaining and depression before they reach a level of acceptance that they are different in this one area of life from others. Only after acceptance are they able to make adjustments in their wants or plans to feel fulfilled again.

Future evaluation is also important, because a couple who decide at age 20 to choose child-free living may change their minds at a later date. A couple who chooses an assisted reproductive technique may decide after several unsuccessful attempts that they are no longer interested in this method of conception. Keeping evaluation an ongoing process allows such plans to be modified as necessary.

INFERTILITY

Infertility is said to exist when a pregnancy has not occurred after at least 1 year of engaging in unprotected coitus. In primary infertility, there have been no previous conceptions; in *secondary* infertility, there has been a previous viable pregnancy but the couple is unable to conceive at present. Sterility is the inability to conceive because of a known condition, such as the absence of a uterus.

In about 40% of couples with an infertility problem, the cause of infertility is multifactorial; in about 30% of couples, it is the man who is infertile. In women seen for a fertility concern, 20% to 25% experience ovulatory failure and another 20% experience tubal, vaginal, cervical or uterine problems. In about 10% of couples, no known cause for the infertility can be discovered despite all the diagnostic tests currently available. Such couples are categorised as having unexplained infertility (Rybak & Wallach, 2007).

Some couples, because they are unaware of the average length of time it takes to achieve a pregnancy, may worry that they are infertile when they are not. When engaging in coitus an average of four times per week, 50% of couples will conceive within 6 months and 85% within 12 months. These periods will be longer if sexual relations are less frequent (Burney, Schust & Yao, 2007).

Couples who engage in coitus daily, hoping to cause early impregnation, may actually have more difficulty conceiving than those who space coitus to every other day. This is because too-frequent coitus can lower a man's **sperm count** (number of sperm in a single ejaculation) to a level below optimal fertility. Also, couples who focus their sexual relations on trying to increase sperm/ovum exposure may find their lives governed by temperature charts and "good days" and "bad days" to such an extent that their relationship suffers. Precise timing of intercourse is not important provided it is regular and occurs around ovulation time (Jenkins & Jenkins, 2006).

The chance of infertility increases with age. Because of this gradual decline in fertility, women who defer pregnancy to their late 30s are apt to have more difficulty conceiving than their younger counterparts. Women who are using oral and injectable hormones for contraception may have difficulty becoming pregnant for several months after discontinuing these medications, because it takes that long for the body to restore normal functioning.

Male infertility factors

Several factors typically lead to male infertility:

- Disturbance in **spermatogenesis** (production of sperm cells)
- Obstruction in the seminiferous tubules, ducts or vessels preventing movement of spermatozoa
- Qualitative or quantitative changes in the seminal fluid preventing **sperm motility** (movement of sperm)
- Development of autoimmunity that immobilises sperm
- Problems with ejaculation or deposition preventing spermatozoa from being placed close enough to a woman's cervix to allow ready penetration and fertilisation.

Inadequate sperm count

The sperm count is the number of sperm in a single ejaculation or in a millilitre of semen. The minimum sperm count considered normal is 20 million per millilitre of seminal fluid, or 50 million per ejaculation. At least 50% of sperm should be motile and 30% should be normal in shape and form. Spermatozoa must be produced and maintained at a temperature slightly lower than body temperature to be fully motile. This is why the testes, in which sperm are produced and stored, are suspended in the scrotal sac away from body heat. Any condition that significantly increases body temperature, such as a chronic infection from tuberculosis or recurrent sinusitis, can lower a sperm count. Actions that increase scrotal heat, such as working at desk jobs or driving a great deal every day (e.g. salesmen, motorcyclists) may produce lower sperm counts compared with men whose occupations allow them to be ambulatory at least part of each day.

Congenital abnormalities such as **cryptorchidism** (undescended testes) may lead to lowered sperm production if surgical repair of this problem was not completed until after puberty or if the spermatic cord became twisted after the surgery.

A worry is that a varicocoele (varicosity of the spermatic vein) could increase temperature within the testes and slow and disrupt spermatogenesis although whether this actually causes much difference is in doubt (Evers & Collins, 2009). If this is happening, surgery to repair the varicocoele has the potential to increase the chance for conception (Miyaoka & Esteves, 2012).

Other conditions that may inhibit sperm production are trauma to the testes; surgery on or near the testicles that results in impaired testicular circulation; and endocrine imbalances, particularly of the thyroid, pancreas or pituitary glands. Drug use or excessive alcohol use and environmental factors such as exposure to x-rays or radioactive substances have also been found to negatively affect spermatogenesis. Men who are exposed to radioactive substances in their work environment should be provided adequate protection of the testes.

Obstruction or impaired sperm motility

Obstruction may occur at any point along the pathway that spermatozoa must travel to reach the outside: the seminiferous tubules, the epididymis, the vas deferens, the ejaculatory duct or the urethra. Diseases such as mumps orchitis (testicular inflammation and scarring because of the mumps virus), epididymitis (inflammation of the epididymis) and tubal infections such as gonorrhoea or ascending urethral infection can result in this type of obstruction because adhesions form and occlude sperm transport (Hedger, 2011). Congenital stricture of a spermatic duct may occasionally be seen. Benign hypertrophy of the prostate gland occurs in most men beginning at about 50 years of age. Pressure from the enlarged gland on the vas deferens can interfere with sperm transport. Infection of the prostate, through which the seminal fluid must pass, or infection of the seminal vesicles (spread from urinary tract infections) can change the composition of the seminal fluid enough to reduce sperm motility (Parsons, 2007).

A few men who have vasectomies develop an autoimmune reaction or form antibodies that immobilise their own sperm; they also may experience long-term pain unless the procedure is reversed (Horovitz et al., 2012). It is also conceivable that men with obstruction in the vas deferens from other causes, such as scarring after an infection, could also develop an autoimmune reaction that immobilises sperm in the same way.

Anomalies of the penis, such as hypospadias (urethral opening on the ventral surface of the penis) or epispadias (urethral opening on the dorsal surface), can cause sperm to be deposited too far from the sexual partner's cervix to allow optimal cervical penetration. Extreme obesity in a male may also interfere with effective penetration and deposition (Hammoud et al., 2012).

Ejaculation problems

Psychological problems, diseases such as a cerebrovascular accident, diabetes or Parkinson's disease, and some medications (e.g. certain antihypertensive agents) may result in **erectile dysfunction** (formerly called impotence or the inability to achieve an erection). This condition is *primary* if the man has never been able to achieve erection and ejaculation and *secondary* if the man has been able to achieve ejaculation in the past but now has difficulty. Erectile dysfunction can be a difficult problem to solve if it is associated with stress, because this is not easily relieved.

Solutions to the problem can include psychological or sexual counselling as well as use of a drug such as sildenafil (Viagra).

Premature ejaculation (ejaculation before penetration) is another factor that may interfere with the proper deposition of sperm. It is another problem often attributed to psychological causes.

CASE STUDY QUESTION

2. The Carls are undergoing testing for infertility. Infertility is said to exist when:

   a. A couple has been trying to conceive for 1 year
   b. A woman has no children from a marriage
   c. A woman has no uterus or fallopian tubes
   d. A couple has wanted a child for over 6 months

Female infertility factors

The factors that cause infertility in women are similar to those causing infertility in men: anovulation (faulty or inadequate production of ova), problems of ova transport through the fallopian tubes to the uterus, uterine factors such as tumours or poor endometrial development, and cervical and vaginal factors that immobilise spermatozoa. In addition, nutrition, body weight and exercise may be responsible.

Anovulation

Anovulation (absence of ovulation), the most common cause of infertility in women, may occur from a genetic abnormality such as Turner's syndrome (hypogonadism) in which there are no ovaries to produce ova. More often it results from a hormonal imbalance caused by a condition such as hypothyroidism that interferes with hypothalamus-pituitary-ovarian interaction. Ovarian tumours may also produce anovulation because of feedback stimulation on the pituitary. Chronic or excessive exposure to x-rays or radioactive substances, general ill health, poor diet and stress may all contribute to poor ovarian function.

Nutrition, body weight and exercise all influence the blood glucose/insulin balance. When either glucose or insulin levels are too high, they can disrupt the production of follicle-stimulating hormone (FSH) and luteinising hormone (LH) leading to infertility from ovulation failure.

Women should try to maintain an ideal body weight and height, as represented by a body mass index (BMI) of 20 to 24.9 (Chavarro et al., 2007). This ideal BMI may also apply to men, as excessive weight may alter testosterone production and sperm production.

The most frequent cause, however, is naturally occurring variations in ovulatory patterns or polycystic ovary syndrome, a condition in which the ovaries produce excess testosterone, lowering FSH and LH levels. Polycystic ovary syndrome is associated with the metabolic syndrome (a waist circumference of 90 cm or above in women; a fasting blood glucose over 100 mg/dL; serum triglycerides over 150 mg/dL; blood pressure over 135/85 mmHg; and high-density lipoprotein cholesterol over 50 mg/dL), plus the development of hirsutism (unwanted body hair) (Smith & Schust, 2011). Metabolic syndrome is associated with increased cardiac disease, so efforts to reduce weight and lower triglycerides and cholesterol can improve heart health as well as promote fertility.

Some women ovulate only a few times a year because of polycystic ovary syndrome. The condition can usually be detected by examining the menstrual history, but even if a woman experiences regular monthly menstruation, it does not necessarily indicate that she is ovulating on a regular basis (DuRant & Leslie, 2007).

Tubal transport problems

Difficulty with tubal transport usually occurs because scarring has developed in the fallopian tubes. Typically this is caused by chronic salpingitis (chronic pelvic inflammatory disease). It can result from a ruptured appendix or from abdominal surgery involving infection that spread to the fallopian tubes and left adhesion formation in the tubes. Tubal transport is the chief problem if a woman had a tubal ligation in years past but now wants to become pregnant.

Pelvic inflammatory disease (PID) is infection of the pelvic organs: the uterus, fallopian tubes, ovaries and their supporting structures. The initial source of the infection is usually a sexually transmitted infection. In some women, infection can spread even further than reproductive organs or involve the pelvis, causing pelvic peritonitis. Many organisms can cause PID, but chlamydia and gonorrhoea are among those most frequently seen. PID occurs at a rate of 25 per 100 women; in other words, one fourth of all women will experience this type of infection in a lifetime. About 12% of those who acquire PID are left infertile because of tubal scarring (Guile & Keller, 2011).

Uterine problems

Tumours such as fibromas (leiomyomas) may be a rare cause of infertility if they block the entrance to the fallopian tubes into the uterus or limit the space available on the uterine wall for effective implantation. A congenitally deformed uterine cavity may also limit implantation sites, but this is rare.

Poor secretion of oestrogen or progesterone from the ovary can result in inadequate endometrium formation (over production or underproduction), interfering with implantation and embryo growth. Endometriosis also can interfere with uterine fertility. **Endometriosis** refers to the implantation of uterine endometrium, or nodules, that have spread from the interior of the uterus to locations outside the uterus (Gunderson & Yates, 2011). The most common sites of endometrium spread include Douglas' cul-de-sac, the ovaries, the uterine ligaments and the outer surface of the uterus and bowel. Some evidence of endometriosis occurs in as many as 50% of women, most probably from regurgitation through the fallopian tubes at the time of menstruation. Symptoms of endometriosis can begin in adolescence. The condition can be treated both medically and surgically (see Chapter 47).

Cervical problems

At the time of ovulation, the cervical mucus is thin and watery and can be easily penetrated by spermatozoa for a period of 12 to 72 hours. If coitus is not synchronised with this time period, the cervical mucus may be too thick to allow spermatozoa to penetrate the cervix. Infection or inflammation of the cervix (erosion) is another reason that cervical mucus can thicken so much that spermatozoa cannot penetrate it easily or survive in it. A stenotic cervical os or obstruction of the os by a polyp may further compromise sperm penetration. However, this is rarely enough of a problem to be the sole cause of infertility. A woman who has undergone dilatation and curettage (D&C) procedures several times or cervical conisation (cervical surgery) should be evaluated in light of the possibility that scar tissue and tightening of the cervical os has occurred.

Vaginal problems

Infection of the vagina can cause the pH of the vaginal secretions to become acidotic, limiting or destroying the motility of spermatozoa. Some women appear to have sperm-immobilising or sperm-agglutinating antibodies in their blood plasma that act to destroy sperm cells in the vagina or cervix. Either of these problems can limit the ability of sperm to survive in the vagina and enter the uterus.

Unexplained infertility

In a small proportion of couples, no known cause for infertility can be discovered. Possibly the problems of either partner alone are not significant, but when these are combined they become sufficient to create infertility. It is obviously discouraging for couples to complete a fertility evaluation and be told that their inability to conceive cannot be explained. Offer active support to help the couple find alternative solutions, such as continuing to try to conceive, using an assisted reproductive technique or considering adopting or fostering.

CASE STUDY QUESTION

3. Cheryl Carl is diagnosed as having endometriosis. This condition interferes with fertility because:

a. The ovaries stop producing adequate oestrogen
b. The uterine cervix becomes inflamed and swollen
c. Pressure on the pituitary leads to decreased FSH levels
d. Endometrial implants can block the fallopian tubes

FERTILITY ASSESSMENT

Not all couples who desire fertility testing want to have children immediately. Some just want to know for their own peace of mind that they are fertile. The age of the couple and the degree of apprehension they feel about possible infertility make a difference in determining when they should be referred for fertility evaluation. Some fertility clinics set limits on the age range in which fertility testing can be scheduled (e.g. not before age 18 years and not after age 45 years). As a rule, if a woman is younger than 35 years of age, it is usually suggested that she have an evaluation after 1 year of infertility; if older than 35 years, after 6 months of infertility. Referral is recommended sooner for older women because of possible age limitations associated with adoption, assisted reproductive strategies such as in vitro fertilisation (IVF) and embryo transfer, common alternatives to natural childbearing. Basic fertility assessment begins with a health history and physical examination of both sexual partners.

Health history

Nurses often assume the responsibility for initial history taking with an infertile couple. Because of the wide variety of factors that may be responsible for infertility, a minimum history for the man should include:

- General health
- Nutrition
- Alcohol, drug or tobacco use
- Congenital health problems such as hypospadias or cryptorchidism
- Illnesses such as mumps orchitis, urinary tract infection or sexually transmitted infections
- Radiation to his testes because of childhood cancer or another cause
- Operations such as surgical repair of a hernia, which could have resulted in a blood compromise to the testes
- Current illnesses, particularly endocrine illnesses or low-grade infections
- Past and current occupation and work habits (e.g. does his job involve sitting at a desk all day or exposure to x-rays or other forms of radiation?)
- Sexual practices such as the frequency of coitus and masturbation, failure to achieve ejaculation, premature ejaculation, coital positions used and use of lubricants
- Past contraceptive measures and existence of any children produced from a previous relationship
- Any complementary alternative therapies such as herbal additives the man is using.

For a thorough women's health history, ask about:

- Current or past reproductive tract problems, such as infections
- Overall health, emphasising endocrine problems such as galactorrhoea (breast nipple secretions) or symptoms of thyroid dysfunction

- Abdominal or pelvic operations that could have compromised blood flow to pelvic organs
- Past history of a childhood cancer treated with radiation that might have reduced ovarian function
- The use of douches or intravaginal medications or sprays that could interfere with vaginal pH
- Exposure to occupational hazards such as x-rays or toxic substances
- Nutrition, including an adequate source of folic acid and avoidance of trans-fats
- If she can detect ovulation through such symptoms as breast tenderness, midcycle "wetness" or lower abdominal pain (mittelschmerz).

Also obtain a menstrual history including:

- Age of menarche
- Length, regularity and frequency of menstrual periods
- Amount of flow
- Any difficulties experienced, such as dysmenorrhoea or premenstrual dysphoric disorder (PDD) (see Chapter 47)
- History of contraceptive use
- History of any previous pregnancies or abortions.

While obtaining the history, take time with each partner individually and as a couple to encourage questions about pregnancy and parenting. A frank discussion centred on resolving the couple's fears and clearing up any long-standing confusion or misinformation will help set a positive tone for future interactions, establish a feeling of trust with healthcare personnel and increase self-esteem. Talking with both partners can also help them clarify their feelings about infertility and why they are seeking help in this area.

Obtaining a sexual history is often difficult because cultural taboos can make couples feel uncomfortable discussing this part of their life. Simple factors, such as how often couples engage in sexual intercourse, for example, are influenced by culture and religion. Some cultures forbid artificial insemination because preserving male lineage is so important. Being aware of cultural differences this way can influence how a couple reacts to a diagnosis of infertility and help you appreciate the meaning of this diagnosis to an individual couple.

Physical assessment

After a thorough history, both men and women need a complete physical examination. For the man, important aspects of this are detection of the presence of secondary sexual characteristics and genital abnormalities, such as the absence of a vas deferens or the presence of undescended testes or a varicocoele (enlargement of a testicular vein). The presence of a hydrocoele (collection of fluid in the tunica vaginalis of the scrotum) is rarely associated with infertility but should be documented if present.

For a woman, a thorough physical assessment including breast and thyroid examination is necessary to rule out current illness. Of particular importance are secondary sex characteristics, which indicate maturity and good pituitary function. A complete pelvic examination including a pap smear (see Chapter 11) is needed to rule out anatomical disorders and infection.

Fertility testing

Basic fertility testing involves only three tests: semen analysis in the male and ovulation monitoring and tubal patency assessment in the female. Nurses play a key role in preparing couples for these tests, helping them schedule the studies appropriately and supporting them while they wait for results.

Additional testing for men, if warranted, can include urinalysis; a complete blood count; blood typing, including Rh factor; a serological test for syphilis; a test for the presence of human immunodeficiency virus (HIV); erythrocyte sedimentation rate (an increased rate indicates inflammation); protein-bound iodine (a test for thyroid function); cholesterol level (arterial plaques could interfere with pelvic blood flow) and gonadotropin and testosterone levels.

Advanced testing for a woman may include a rubella titre, a serological test for syphilis and an HIV evaluation. If a woman has symptoms of thyroid dysfunction, a thyroid uptake determination and thyroid-stimulating hormone level may be ordered. If a woman has a history of menstrual irregularities, blood may be assayed for FSH, oestrogen, LH and progesterone levels. If a woman has a history of galactorrhoea, a serum prolactin level will be obtained. A pelvic ultrasound may be performed to rule out ovarian, tubal or uterine structural disorders.

Semen analysis

For a semen analysis, after 2 to 4 days of sexual abstinence, the man ejaculates by masturbation into a clean, dry specimen jar. The number of sperm in the specimen are counted and then examined under a microscope within 1 hour (see Box 8.1). An average ejaculation should produce a minimum of 1.4 to 1.7 mL of semen and should contain a minimum of 33 to 46 million spermatozoa per mL of fluid (World Health Organization, 2010) (the average normal sperm count is 50 to 200 million per millilitre). The analysis may need to be repeated after 2 or 3 months, because spermatogenesis is an ongoing process and 30 to 90 days is needed for new sperm to reach maturity.

Ovulation monitoring

Ovulation monitoring is most commonly undertaken with regular blood tests to determine the phase of the cycle and increase in frequency as ovulation gets closer. Blood results then determine what other action is needed and when. Usually blood tests are used in conjunction with ultrasound to determine ovum maturation.

BOX 8.1 ✻ Focus on family teaching

Tips for ensuring an accurate semen analysis

Q. Bob Carl asks you, "What can I do to make sure that the analysis of my semen sample is as accurate as possible?"

A. When obtaining a semen sample for analysis:

- Use a clean, dry plastic or glass container with a secure lid to collect the sample.
- Collect the specimen as close as possible to your usual schedule of sexual activity.
- Avoid using any lubricants when you collect the specimen.
- After you have collected the specimen in the container, close it securely and write down the time you collected it.
- Keep the specimen at body temperature while transporting it. Carrying it next to your chest is one way to do this.
- Take the specimen to the fertility clinic immediately so that it can be analysed within 1 hour of collection. For accurate results a referral to a fertility clinic for semen analysis is advised.

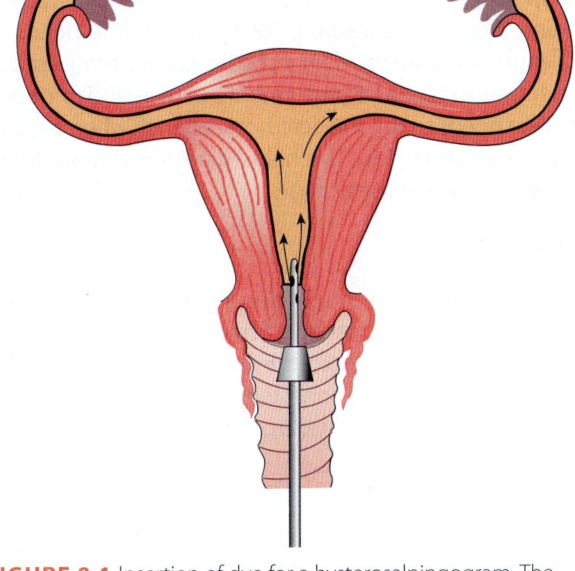

FIGURE 8.1 Insertion of dye for a hysterosalpingogram. The contrast dye outlines the uterus and fallopian tubes on radiographs to demonstrate patency.

What if...

Cheryl Carl tells you that she works nights as a cocktail waitress, goes to bed at 4 a.m., then wakes at 6 a.m. to drive her husband to work? Starting at noon, she sleeps for 4 or 5 hours before getting up to go to work. When, during the day, should she record her basal body temperature?

Tubal patency

Both ultrasound and x-ray imaging can be used to determine the patency of fallopian tubes and assess the depth and consistency of the endometrial lining.

Sonohysterography

Sonohysterography is an ultrasound technique designed for inspecting the uterus. The uterus is filled with sterile saline, introduced through a narrow catheter inserted into the uterine cervix. A transvaginal ultrasound transducer is then inserted into the vagina to inspect the uterus for abnormalities such as septal deviation or the presence of a myoma. Because this is a minimally invasive technique, it can be done at any time during the menstrual cycle.

Hysterosalpingography

Hysterosalpingography (uterosal pingography), a radiological examination of the fallopian tubes using a radiopaque medium, is a second frequently used technique. The procedure is scheduled immediately after a menstrual flow to avoid reflux of menstrual debris up the tubes and unintentional irradiation of a growing zygote. It is contraindicated if infection of the vagina, cervix or uterus is present (infectious organisms might be forced into the pelvic cavity). For the procedure, iodine-based radiopaque material is introduced into the cervix under pressure. The radiopaque material outlines the uterus and both tubes, provided that the tubes are patent. Because the medium is thick, it distends the uterus and tubes slightly, causing momentary painful uterine cramping. After the study, the contrast medium drains out through the vagina (see Fig. 8.1).

Advanced surgical procedures

If common assessments do not reveal the cause of infertility, several surgical procedures may be scheduled.

Uterine endometrial biopsy

Uterine endometrial biopsy may be used to reveal an endometrial problem such as a luteal phase defect. If the endometrium removed by biopsy resembles a corkscrew (a typical progesterone-dominated endometrium) in the second half of a menstrual cycle, this suggests that ovulation has occurred. Endometrial biopsies are being performed less commonly than previously, having been replaced with serum progesterone level evaluations that also suggest that ovulation occurred.

Endometrial biopsies are carried out 2 or 3 days before an expected menstrual flow (day 25 or 26 of a typical 28-day menstrual cycle). After a paracervical block, a thin probe and biopsy forceps are introduced through the cervix. A woman may experience mild to moderate discomfort from the manoeuvring of the instruments. There may be a moment of sharp pain as the biopsy specimen is taken from the anterior or posterior uterine wall. Possible complications include pain, excessive bleeding, infection and uterine perforation. This procedure is contraindicated if pregnancy is suspected (although the chance that it would interfere with a pregnancy is probably less than 10%) or if an infection such as acute PID or cervicitis is present. Caution a woman that she might notice a small amount of vaginal spotting after the procedure. For follow-up, she needs to call her primary care provider if she develops a temperature greater than 38°C, has a large amount of bleeding or passes clots. She needs to call the healthcare agency when she has her next menstrual flow. This helps "date" the endometrium and the accuracy of the analysis.

Hysteroscopy

Hysteroscopy is visual inspection of the uterus through the insertion of a hysteroscope, a thin hollow tube, through the vagina, cervix and into the uterus. This is helpful to further evaluate uterine adhesions or other abnormalities that were discovered on hysterosalpingogram.

Laparoscopy

Laparoscopy is the introduction of a thin, hollow, lighted tube (a fibreoptic telescope or laparoscope) through a small incision in the abdomen, just under the umbilicus, to examine the position and state of the fallopian tubes and ovaries. It allows the examiner to view the proximity of the ovaries to the fallopian tubes. If this distance is too great, the discharged ovum cannot enter the tube. It is rarely done unless the results of uterosalpingography are abnormal. It is scheduled during the follicular phase of a menstrual period and is done under general anaesthesia because of the pain caused by extensive manoeuvring. This also allows for good relaxation and a steep Trendelenburg position (which brings the reproductive organs down out of the pelvis). Carbon dioxide is introduced into the abdomen to move the abdominal wall outward and offer better visualisation. Women may feel bloating of the abdomen from the infusion of the carbon dioxide after such a procedure. If some carbon dioxide escapes under the diaphragm, there may be extremely sharp shoulder pain from pressure.

During the procedure, dye can be injected into the uterus through a polyethylene cannula placed in the cervix to assess tubal patency. Tubes are patent if the dye appears in the abdominal cavity. A scope may be passed directly into a fallopian tube to reveal information about the presence and condition of the fimbria and endometrium lining the tube. If the fimbria have been destroyed by PID, the chance for a normal conception is in doubt, because ova seem to be unable to enter a tube if fimbrial currents are absent.

CASE STUDY QUESTION

4. Cheryl is scheduled to have a hysterosalpingogram. Which of the following instructions would you give her regarding this procedure?
   a. She may feel some mild cramping when the dye is inserted
   b. The ultrasound of the uterus will reveal any tumours present
   c. She will not be able to conceive for 3 months after the procedure
   d. Many women experience mild bleeding as an after effect

INFERTILITY MANAGEMENT

Management of infertility focuses on correction of any underlying problem that was discovered during assessment. All couples can benefit from some practical information on how to increase the chances of achieving conception on their own (see Box 8.2).

Correction of the underlying problem

Underlying causes, such as chronic disease, inadequate hormone production, endometriosis or infection need to be treated. If correction of these problems does not yield success, infertility management focuses on achieving conception through an assisted reproductive technology such as IVF or sperm donation.

BOX 8.2 * Focus on family teaching

Suggestions to aid conception

Q. Cheryl Carl asks, "Is there anything we can do to help increase our chances for conception?"

A. The following are time-honoured suggestions to help aid conception:

- Although frequent intercourse may stimulate sperm production, men need sperm recovery time after ejaculation to maintain an adequate sperm count. Regular intercourse particularly around the time of ovulation will enhance the chances of achieving pregnancy.
- The male-superior position is the best position for intercourse to achieve conception because it places sperm closest to the cervical opening.
- The male should try for deep penetration so ejaculation places sperm as close as possible to the cervix. Elevating a woman's hips on a small pillow can facilitate sperm collection near the opening to the cervix.
- A woman should remain on her back with knees drawn up for at least 20 minutes after ejaculation to help sperm remain near the cervix.
- Do not use douching or lubricants before or after intercourse so vaginal pH is unaltered, which could interfere with sperm motility.
- Eat a diet high in slowly digested carbohydrates, low in saturated or trans-fatty acids and moderate in protein.
- Maintain a body weight that results in a body mass index between 20 and 24.
- Exercise about 30 minutes a day to help keep blood glucose and insulin levels stabilised.
- Choose a new activity the two of you can do together, such as learning how to bowl or ballroom dance, so you create an activity separate from planning a baby. This can help to pass the time in a positive way and also offer a positive outlook for a month when you do not conceive.

Increasing sperm count and motility

If sperm are not motile because the vas deferens is obstructed, the obstruction is most likely to be extensive and difficult to relieve by surgery. If sperm are present but the total count is low, a man may be advised to abstain from coitus for 7 to 10 days at a time to increase the count.

Sperm can be extracted by syringe from a point proximal to the vas deferens blockage and used for intrauterine insemination (Verhulst et al., 2009). If the problem appears to be that sperm are immobilised by vaginal secretions because of an immunological factor, the response can be reduced by abstinence or condom use for about 6 months. However, to avoid this prolonged time interval, washing of the sperm and intrauterine insemination may be preferred. The administration of corticosteroids to a woman may have some effect in decreasing sperm immobilisation because it reduces her immune response and antibody production.

Reducing the presence of infection

If a vaginal infection is present, the infection will be treated according to the causative organism based on culture reports (see Chapter 47). Vaginal infections such as bacterial vaginosis and moniliasis tend to recur, requiring close supervision and follow-up. Caution women who are prescribed metronidazole (Flagyl) for a bacterial vaginosis infection that it can be teratogenic early in pregnancy and therefore should not be continued if a pregnancy is suspected (McKenna & Mirkov, 2014).

Hormone therapy

If the problem appears to be a disturbance of ovulation, administration of GnRH is a possibility. Therapy with drugs used to stimulate ovulation may be used. In other women, ovarian follicular growth can be stimulated by the administration of human menopausal gonadotropins, combinations of FSH and LH derived from postmenopausal urine in conjunction with administration of human chorionic gonadotropin (hCG) to produce ovulation. If increased prolactin levels are identified, bromocriptine is added to the medication regimen to reduce prolactin levels and allow for the rise of gonadotropins (McKenna & Mirkov, 2014).

Administration of either clomiphene citrate or human menopausal gonadotropins may overstimulate an ovary, causing multiple ova to come to maturity and possibly resulting in multiple births. Counsel women who receive these agents that this is a possibility.

If the problem appears to be a luteal phase defect, this can be corrected by progesterone vaginal suppositories begun on the third day of the temperature rise and continued for the next 6 weeks (if pregnancy occurs) or until a menstrual flow begins.

Surgery

Fallopian tubes that have been ligated can be reopened surgically but the success of the operation is not greater than 70% to 80%. Also, the irregular line left by the surgery may result in an ectopic pregnancy (a tubal pregnancy) if a fertilised ovum is stopped at the irregular point (Ahmad et al., 2009). Intrauterine insemination is more commonly used today and more likely to result in a viable pregnancy.

If a myoma (fibroid tumour) is interfering with fertility, a myomectomy, or surgical removal of the tumour, can be scheduled (Gambadauro, Gudmundsson & Torrejón, 2012). Myomectomy can be done via a hysteroscopic ambulatory procedure if the growth is small. Uterine adhesions may also be lysed by hysteroscopy. After this procedure, a woman is prescribed oestrogen for 3 months to prevent adhesions from reforming and an IUD may be inserted to help prevent the uterine sides from touching. This treatment can be difficult for a woman to accept, because preventing pregnancy (using an IUD) is exactly what she does not want to do.

For problems of abnormal uterine formation, such as a septate uterus, surgery is also available. However, these defects are usually related to early pregnancy loss not infertility.

If the problem is tubal insufficiency from inflammation, diathermy or steroid administration may be helpful in reducing adhesions. Hysterosalpingography can be repeated to determine whether these produce a therapeutic effect. Canalisation of the fallopian tubes and plastic surgical repair (microsurgery) are possible treatments. If peritoneal adhesions or nodules of endometriosis are holding the tubes fixed and away from the ovaries, these can be removed by laparoscopy or laser surgery (Jacobson et al., 2009). Additional hormonal therapy for endometriosis is discussed in Chapter 47.

Assisted reproductive techniques

If ovulation, sperm production or sperm motility problems cannot be corrected, assisted reproductive strategies are the next step.

Artificial insemination

Artificial insemination is the instillation of sperm into the female reproductive tract to aid conception. The sperm is instilled into the cervix (intracervical insemination) or directly into the uterus (intrauterine insemination). Either the partner's sperm or donor sperm can be used. Artifical insemination is used if the man has an inadequate sperm count or a woman has a vaginal or cervical factor that interferes with sperm motility. Donor insemination can be used if the man has a known genetic disorder that he does not want transmitted to children, if a woman has no male partner or for same-sex couples who wish to have a child. It is a useful procedure for men who, feeling their family was complete, underwent a vasectomy but now wish to have children. In the past, men who underwent chemotherapy or radiation for testicular cancer had to accept being child-free afterwards as they were no longer able to produce sperm.

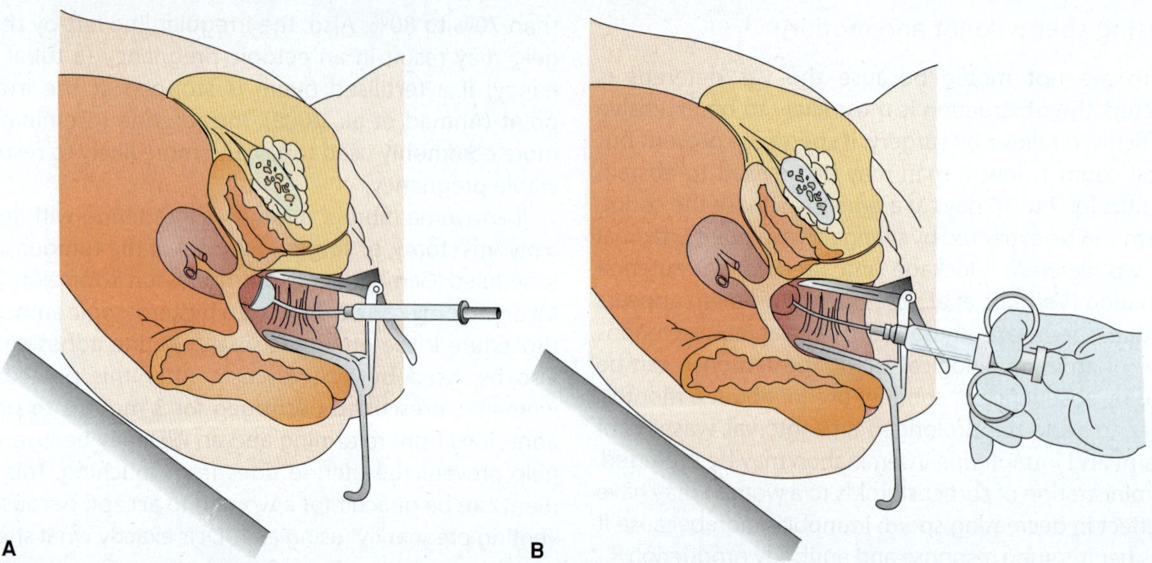

FIGURE 8.2 Therapeutic insemination. Sperm are deposited next to the cervix (**A**) or injected directly into the uterine cavity (**B**).

Today, sperm can be cryopreserved (frozen) in a sperm bank before radiation or chemotherapy and then used for insemination afterwards (Dillon & Gracia, 2012).

One disadvantage of using frozen sperm is that it tends to have slower motility than unfrozen specimens. However, although the rate of conception may be lower from this source, there appears to be no increase in the incidence of congenital anomalies in children conceived by this method. An advantage of cryopreserved sperm is that it can be used even after years of storage.

To prepare for artificial insemination, a woman must undertake blood tests to determine her BBT, assess her cervical mucus, or use an ovulation predictor kit to predict her likely day of ovulation. On the day after ovulation, the selected sperm are instilled into her cervix using a device similar to a cervical cap or diaphragm, or they are injected directly into the uterus using a flexible catheter (see Fig. 8.2).

If artificial donor insemination is selected, the donors are volunteers who have no history of disease and no family history of possible inheritable disorders. The blood type, or at least the Rh factor, can be matched with the woman's to prevent incompatibility. Sperm from sperm banks can be selected according to desired physical or mental characteristics.

CASE STUDY QUESTION

5. Bob Carl asks you what therapeutic insemination by donor entails. Which would be your best answer?
   a. Therapeutic sperm are injected vaginally to test tubal patency
   b. Donor sperm are introduced vaginally into the uterus or cervix
   c. The husband's sperm is administered intravenously weekly
   d. Donor sperm are injected intra-abdominally into each ovary

What if...

Bob Carl has some sperm cryopreserved so that Cheryl could become pregnant, but he and Cheryl divorce before it is used? To whom would the cryopreserved sperm belong at that point?

In vitro fertilisation

In in vitro fertilisation (IVF), one or more mature oocytes are removed from a woman's ovary by laparoscopy and fertilised by exposure to sperm under laboratory conditions outside a woman's body. After fertilisation, the laboratory-grown fertilised ova are inserted into a woman's uterus, where ideally one or more of them will implant and grow. Usually embryos are implanted on day 2, 3 or 5, depending on the clinical process.

IVF is most often used for couples who have not been able to conceive because a woman has blocked or damaged fallopian tubes. IVF may be helpful to couples when an absence of cervical mucus prevents sperm from travelling to or entering the cervix, or antisperm antibodies cause immobilistion of sperm. In addition, couples with unexplained infertility of long duration may be helped by IVF.

Before the procedure, a woman is given an ovulation-stimulating agent. Beginning about the tenth day of the menstrual cycle, the ovaries are examined daily by ultrasound to assess the number and size of developing ovarian follicles. When at least one follicle appears to be mature, a woman is given an injection of hCG, which causes ovulation in 38 to 42 hours.

A needle is then introduced intravaginally, guided by ultrasound, and the oocyte is aspirated from its follicle. Because of the drugs given to induce ova maturation, many oocytes may ripen at once, and perhaps as many as

3 to 12 can be removed. The oocytes are incubated for at least 8 hours to ensure viability. In the meantime, the woman's partner supplies a fresh semen specimen or donor sperm is thawed. The sperm cells and oocytes are mixed and allowed to incubate in a growth medium. Genetic analysis to reveal chromosomal abnormalities can be completed at this point.

In the past, many sperm were necessary even under laboratory conditions to allow sufficient sperm to make their way through the resistant zona pellucida surrounding the ovum. Several techniques, such as creating passages through the resistant cells (zona drilling), have been discovered to help sperm cross the zona. In some instances, it has been possible to inject sperm directly under the zona pellucida (intracytoplasmic sperm injection or ICSI). This is the technique that makes it possible for fertilisation to take place with only one sperm.

After fertilisation of the chosen oocytes occurs, the zygotes formed almost immediately begin to divide and grow. By 40 hours after fertilisation, they will have undergone their first cell division. In the past, multiple eggs were chosen and implanted to ensure a pregnancy resulted but this technique also resulted in many multiple births. Newborns from multiple births have a much lower chance of surviving the neonatal period than others. For that reason, today, only one or two fertilised eggs are chosen and transferred back to the uterine cavity through the cervix by means of a thin catheter.

If the couple desires, any embryos not used can be frozen for use at a later time. As with sperm cryopreservation, embryo cryopreservation presents a range of ethical and religious dilemmas regarding who would "own" them if the couple should divorce; as well as whether the embryo should be saved, donated or discarded.

A lack of progesterone can occur if the corpus luteum was injured by the aspiration of the follicle. Therefore, progesterone may be given to a woman if it is believed that she will not produce enough on her own to support implantation. Proof that the zygote has implanted can be demonstrated by a routine serum pregnancy test as early as 11 days after transfer (see Fig. 8.3).

In all centres, nurses need to support and counsel the couple through the process. The recovery rate for harvesting ripened eggs is high (about 90%), as is the ability to fertilise eggs by sperm in vitro. The overall pregnancy rate by IVF is as low as 38% to 42% per treatment cycle (Van Voorhis, 2007). Although IVF programs do not result in an increase in birth defects, about 25% of pregnancies end in spontaneous abortion (the same rate as for natural pregnancies). Once a pregnancy has been successfully established, a woman's prenatal care is the same as that for any pregnancy. Research has shown that, because the couple was so committed to the procedure, they adjust to pregnancy and parenthood well. Following an uncomplicated birth, postnatal care should be the same as for any pregnancy and breastfeeding should be encouraged (see Box 8.3).

If an ultrasound reveals that a multiple pregnancy of more than two zygotes has been achieved, selective termination of gestational sacs until only two are remaining may be recommended. IVF is expensive and is available only at specialised centres. There is a risk of maternal infection if bacteria are introduced at any point in the transfer. Waiting for the steps of obtaining the oocyte, laboratory growth and pregnancy success is a major psychological strain. Couples report a feeling of social isolation during this time and weariness answering friends' and family's questions about the procedure.

Gamete intrafallopian transfer

In gamete intrafallopian transfer (GIFT) procedures, ova are obtained from ovaries exactly as in IVF. Instead of waiting for fertilisation to occur in the laboratory, however, both ova and sperm are instilled within a matter of hours, using a laparoscopic technique, into the open end of a patent fallopian tube. Fertilisation then occurs in the tube and the zygote moves to the uterus for implantation. This procedure has a pregnancy rate equal to that of IVF. The procedure is contraindicated if a woman's fallopian tubes are blocked, because this could lead to ectopic (tubal) pregnancy.

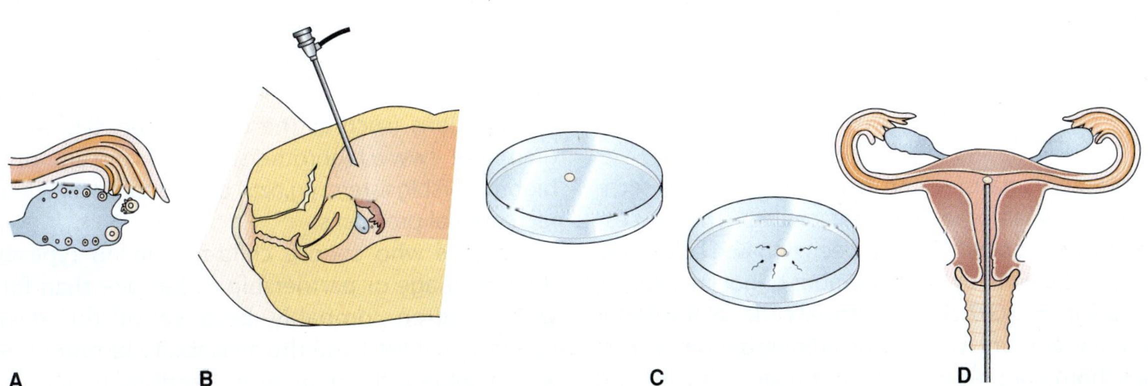

FIGURE 8.3 Steps involved with in vitro fertilisation. (**A**) Ovulation. (**B**) Capture of ova (done here intra-abdominally). (**C**) Fertilisation of ova and growth in culture medium. (**D**) Insertion of fertilised ova into uterus.

BOX 8.3 ✻ Focus on evidence-based practice

Breastfeeding after successful IVF

It is generally agreed that breast milk is the natural and best food for babies for the entire first year or at least for 6 months. To see if women who had babies through assisted reproductive techniques such as IVF choose to breastfeed as much as women having babies without an assisted technique, researchers interviewed 183 women who conceived using an assisted technique as to whether they breastfed their baby or not. Results showed that more women who conceived with the help of an assisted technique began breastfeeding than others (89.3% versus 83.3%). By 3 months, however, a smaller number of women who had used an assisted technique were exclusively breastfeeding (46% versus 57%) and at 8 months, only 23% were still breastfeeding versus 57% of non-assisted women. Researchers attributed the decline in breastfeeding among women who used an assisted technique to more anxiety late in pregnancy and possibly to receiving suboptimal advice about assisted reproduction and breastfeeding from healthcare providers.

How could you use the results of this study to educate a couple whose IVF has been successful?

Source: Hammarberg, K., Fisher, J. R., Wynter, K. H., et al. (2011). Breastfeeding after assisted conception: A prospective cohort study. *Acta Paediatrica, 100*(4), 529–533.

Zygote intrafallopian transfer

Zygote intrafallopian transfer (ZIFT) involves oocyte retrieval by transvaginal, ultrasound-guided aspiration, followed by culture and insemination of the oocytes in the laboratory. Within 24 hours, the fertilised eggs are transferred by laparoscopic technique into the end of a waiting fallopian tube. ZIFT differs from GIFT in that fertilisation takes place outside the body, allowing healthcare providers to be certain that fertilisation has occurred before the growing structure is reintroduced. As in GIFT, a woman must have one functioning fallopian tube for the technique to be successful, because the zygotes are implanted into the fimbriated end of a tube rather than into the uterus. This technique allows for genetic analysis the same as IVF.

Surrogate embryo transfer

Surrogate embryo transfer is an assisted reproductive technique for a woman who does not ovulate. The process involves use of an oocyte that has been donated by a friend or relative or provided by an anonymous donor (van Berkel, Candido & Pijffers, 2007). The menstrual cycles of the donor and recipient are synchronised by administration of gonadotropic hormones. At the time of ovulation, the donor's ovum is removed by a transvaginal, ultrasound-guided procedure. The oocyte is then fertilised in the laboratory by the recipient woman's male partner's sperm (or donor sperm) and placed in the recipient woman's uterus by embryonic transfer. Once pregnancy occurs, it progresses the same as an unassisted pregnancy. This is still relatively rare in Australia and New Zealand.

ALTERNATIVES TO CHILDBIRTH

For some couples, even treatments for infertility with procedures such as IVF are not successful. These couples need to consider other options. Adoption is an alternative for infertile couples, although today there are fewer children available for adoption from official agencies than formerly. The process of adoption is discussed in Chapter 3. Both long- and short-term fostering of children are also an alternative for infertile couples. Long-term fostering tends to focus on permanent placements, in many cases until the child is an adult and able to care for themselves. In some cases, long-term fostering can progress to adoption.

Child-free living is an alternative lifestyle available for both fertile and infertile couples. For many infertile couples who have been through the rigours and frustrations of infertility testing and unsuccessful treatment regimens, child-free living may emerge as the option they finally wish to pursue. A couple in the midst of fertility testing may begin to reexamine their motives for pursuing pregnancy and may decide pregnancy and parenting are not worth the emotional or financial cost of future treatments. They may decide the additional stress of going through an adoption is not for them either, or they may simply decide children are not necessary for them to complete their family unit.

Child-free living can be as fulfilling as having children because it allows a couple more time to help other people and contribute to society through personal accomplishments. It has advantages for a couple in that it also allows time for both members to pursue careers. They can travel more or have more time and money to pursue hobbies or continue their education. If a couple still wishes to include children in their lives in some way, many opportunities are available for them to do this through family connections (most parents welcome offers from siblings or other family members to share in childrearing), through volunteer organisations (such as the Big Brothers Big Sisters program; see <www.bigbrothersbigsisters.org.au> or <www.bigbrothersbigsisters.org.nz>) or through local schools and recreational programs.

Couples who choose child-free living typically rate their marriage or partnership as happier than for those with children, probably because of the decreased expense involved and the availability of more free time, which allows them greater freedom in life (Cherlin, 2012).

CASE STUDY QUESTION

6. Cheryl is having a GIFT procedure. What makes her a good candidate for this procedure?
   a. She has patent fallopian tubes, so fertilised ova can be implanted into them
   b. She is Rh negative, a necessary requirement to rule out Rh incompatibility
   c. She has a normal uterus, so sperm can be injected through the cervix into the uterus
   d. Her husband is taking sildenafil (Viagra), so all sperm will be motile

Key points for review

- Infertility is said to exist when a pregnancy has not occurred after 1 year of unprotected coitus. Sterility refers to the inability to conceive because of a known condition.
- Approximately 14% of couples today experience infertility. The incidence increases with the age of the couple.
- Infertility testing can be an intense psychological stressor for couples. Help couples not only to persist through the experience but also help them maintain their relationship as a couple.
- Couples who are told that an infertility problem has been discovered are apt to suffer a loss of self-esteem. Offer support to help them look at other aspects of their lives in which they do achieve and to recognise that they are productive, healthy people in other ways.
- Male factors that contribute to Infertility are inadequate sperm count, obstruction or impaired sperm motility and problems with ejaculation. Female factors that cause infertility are problems with ovulation, tubal transport or impaired implantation.
- Basic infertility assessment procedures consist of a health history, physical examination, laboratory tests to document general health and specific tests for semen, ovulation and tubal patency.
- Measures to induce fertility are aimed at improving sperm number and transport, decreasing infections, stimulating ovulation, improving nutrition and regulating hormones.
- Artificial insemination, donor egg transfer, in vitro fertilisation, adoption, surrogate motherhood and child-free living are all possible solutions for infertility.

CASE STUDY QUESTIONS

7. Cheryl stated that she believed her infertility problem was her fault because she was too rigid. She said, "It feels like our whole life revolves around trying to get pregnant." Does a rigid personality affect infertility? Does relaxation aid conception?
8. The Carls want to have a child as soon as possible. In addition to their infertility assessment, what advice would you give them to help increase their chances of conceiving quickly?
9. Cheryl tells you that she eats a lot of "fast foods". Could this be creating a risk factor for infertility?

Resources

For an extensive range of additional resources to enhance teaching and learning and to facilitate understanding of this chapter, please see the text's accompanying website located on thePoint at http://thepoint.lww.com.

References

Ahmad, G., et al. (2009). Techniques for pelvic surgery in subfertility. *Cochrane Database of Systematic Reviews, 2009*(1), (CD000221).

Burney, R. O., Schust, D. J. & Yao, M.W.M. (2007). Infertility. In Berek, J. S. (Ed). *Berek & Novak's Gynecology.* Philadelphia: Lippincott Williams & Wilkins.

Chachamovich, J. R., Chachamovich, E., Ezer, H., et al. (2010). Agreement on perceptions of quality of life in couples dealing with infertility. *Journal of Obstetric, Gynecologic, & Neonatal Nursing, 39*(5), 557–565.

Chavarro, J. E., et al. (2007). Dietary fatty acid intakes and the risk of ovulatory infertility. *American Journal of Clinical Nutrition, 85*(1), 231–237.

Cherlin, A. J. (2012). *Public and Private Families*. New York: McGraw-Hill.

Dillon, K. E. & Gracia, C. R. (2012). Pediatric and young adult patients and oncofertility. *Current Treatment Options in Oncology, 13*(2), 161–173.

DuRant, E. & Leslie, N. S. (2007). Polycystic ovary syndrome: A review of current knowledge. *Journal for Nurse Practitioners, 3*(3), 180–185.

Evers, J. L. & Collins, J. A. (2009). Surgery or embolisation for varicocele in subfertile men. *Cochrane Database of Systematic Reviews, 2009*(1), (CD000479).

Gambadauro, P., Gudmundsson, J. & Torrejón, R. (2012). Intrauterine adhesions following conservative treatment of uterine fibroids. *Obstetrics & Gynecology International, 2012*, 853269.

Guile, M. W. & Keller, J. (2011). Infections of the genital tract. In K. J. Hurt, M. W. Guile, J. L. Bienstock, et al. (Eds), *The Johns Hopkins Manual of Gynecology and Obstetrics* (4th ed., pp. 322–339). Philadelphia, PA: Lippincott Williams & Wilkins.

Gunderson, C. & Yates, M. (2011). Menstrual disorders: Endometriosis, dysmenorrhea & premenstrual dysphoric syndrome. In K. J. Hurt, M. W. Guile, J. L. Bienstock, et al. (Eds.), *The Johns Hopkins Manual of Gynecology and Obstetrics* (4th ed., pp. 454–463). Philadelphia, PA: Lippincott Williams & Wilkins.

Hammarberg, K., Fisher, J. R., Wynter, K. H., et al. (2011). Breastfeeding after assisted conception: A prospective cohort study. *Acta Paediatrica, 100*(4), 529–533.

Hammoud, A. O., Meikle, A. W., Reis, L. O., et al. (2012). Obesity and male infertility: A practical approach. *Seminars in Reproductive Medicine, 30*(6), 486–495.

Hedger, M. P. (2011). Immunophysiology and pathology of inflammation in the testis and epididymis. *Journal of Andrology, 32*(6), 625–640.

Horovitz, D., Tjong, V., Domes, T., et al. (2012). Vasectomy reversal provides long-term pain relief for men with the post-vasectomy pain syndrome. *Journal of Urology, 187*(2), 613–617.

Jacobson, T. Z., et al. (2009). Laparoscopic surgery for subfertility associated with endometriosis. *Cochrane Database of Systematic Reviews, 2009*(1), (CD001398).

Jenkins, G. & Jenkins, J. (2006). *Issues Relating to Infertility*. Philadelphia: USA.

McKenna, L. & Mirkov, S. (2014). *McKenna's Drug Handbook for Nursing and Midwifery* (7th ed.). Sydney: Lippincott Williams & Wilkins.

Miyaoka, R. & Esteves, S. C. (2012). A critical appraisal on the role of varicocele in male infertility. *Advances in Urology, 5*(1), 1–9.

Parsons, J. K. (2007). Modifiable risk factors for benign prostatic hyperplasia and lower urinary tract symptoms: New approaches to old problems. *Journal of Urology, 178*(2), 395–401.

Rybak, E. A. & Wallach, E. E. (2007). Infertility and assisted reproductive technologies. In Fortner, K., et al. (Eds). *The Johns Hopkins Manual of Gynecology and Obstetrics* (3rd ed.). Philadelphia: Lippincott Williams & Wilkins.

Sheaves, C. (2013). Advances in endometriosis treatment. *Nurse Practitioner, 38*(5), 42–47.

Smith, M. L. & Schust, D. J. (2011). Endocrinology and recurrent early pregnancy loss. *Seminars in Reproductive Medicine, 29*(6), 482–490.

van Berkel, D., Candido, A. & Pijffers, W. H. (2007). Becoming a mother by non-anonymous egg donation: Secrecy and the relationship between egg recipient, egg donor and egg donation child. *Journal of Psychosomatic Obstetrics & Gynecology, 28*(2), 97–104.

Van Voorhis, B. J. (2007). In vitro fertilization. *New England Journal of Medicine, 356*(4), 379–386.

Verhulst, S. M., et al. (2009). Intra-uterine insemination for unexplained subfertility. *Cochrane Database of Systematic Reviews, 2009*(1), (CD001838).

World Health Organization. (2010). *WHO Laboratory Manual for the Examination & Processing of Human Semen* (5th ed.). Geneva, Switzerland.

Suggested readings

Andrology Australia <www.andrologyaustralia.org>.

Bunker, K. (2010). PCOS and infertility. *Diabetes Forecast, 63*(8), 46.

Child, T. (2013). Optimising the management of patients with infertility, *Practitioner, 257*(1759), 19–22.

Ficorelli, C. T. & Weeks, B. (2007). Health matters. Untangling the complexities of male infertility. *Nursing, 37*(1), 24–26.

Jean Hailes for Women's Health <www.jeanhailes.org.au>.

McCarthy, M. P. (2008). Women's lived experience of infertility after unsuccessful medical intervention. *Journal of Midwifery & Women's Health, 53*(4), 319–324.

Naab, F., Brown, R. & Heidrich, S. (2013). Psychosocial health of infertile Ghanaian women and their infertility beliefs. *Journal of Nursing Scholarship, 45*(2), 132–140.

Norcross, S. (2007). Premature menopause: Recognition and effects. *Practice Nursing, 18*(6), 281–285.

Your Fertility <www.yourfertility.org.au>.

Unit 3

Caring for families during normal pregnancy, birth, the postpartum and newborn period

Chapter 9

The growing fetus

A previous chapter described reproductive anatomy. This chapter adds information about fetal growth and development and assessment of fetal health.

LEARNING OBJECTIVES

After mastering the contents of this chapter, you should be able to:

1. Describe the growth and development of a fetus by gestation week.
2. Use critical thinking to analyse ways to make care family-centred, even at this early point in life.
3. Assess fetal growth and development through maternal and pregnancy landmarks.
4. Provide nursing care that promotes healthy fetal growth and development such as nutrition counselling.
5. Provide nursing care to help ensure both a safe fetal environment and a safe pregnancy outcome.
6. Identify areas of fetal health that could benefit from additional nursing research or application of evidence-based practice.
7. Integrate knowledge of fetal growth and development with nursing process to achieve quality child and family health nursing care.

KEY TERMS

- amniocentesis
- amniotic membrane
- chorionic membrane
- chorionic villi
- decidua
- embryo
- estimated date of birth
- fertilisation
- fetus
- foramen ovale
- hydramnios
- implantation
- McDonald's rule
- meconium
- oligohydramnios
- surfactant
- trophoblast
- umbilical cord
- zygote

CASE STUDY

Liz Calhorn, an 18-year-old, is 20 weeks' pregnant. Although she says she knows she should have stopped smoking during pregnancy, she has not been able to do this. Twice during the pregnancy (at the fourth and tenth week), she drank beer at summer picnics. Today, at a hospital visit, she tells you she has felt her baby move. She states, "Feeling the baby move made me realise there's someone inside me, you know what I mean? It made me know it's time I started being more careful with what I do." Her boyfriend (the father of the baby) is supportive, but the couple has no plans to marry. Liz states, "I'm not ready for that big a commitment."

Feeling a baby move is often the trigger that makes having a baby "real" for many women. The more women know about fetal development before and after this event, the easier it is for them to begin to think of the pregnancy not as something interesting happening to them but as an act that is producing a separate life.

CASE STUDY QUESTION

1. In the light of Liz's realisation, how would you modify your health teaching with her?

Although the care of women during pregnancy requires specialist care by a registered midwife, registered nurses are often involved in providing nursing care in a variety of circumstances. For example, Australia has many rural and remote communities and in these communities registered nurses may need to assist women and their families with health education and promotion, as well as emergency care. Registered nurses therefore need to have a sound knowledge and an ability to provide nursing assistance to women and their families across the life span, including the childbearing years. When care is required in the absence of a registered midwife, it is important to have formal communication pathways with specialists in maternal care to provide appropriate and safe practices.

In the opening scenario, the registered nurse must remain within the boundaries of the scope of practice as set by the Australian Nursing and Midwifery Accreditation Council (ANMAC). In addition, it would be important to refer Liz to a registered midwife or local general practitioner. Nurses have the skill to identify immediate general health needs. The cues given by Liz suggest that she is identifying the importance of providing a safe and healthy environment for her baby while in utero. Although Liz has stated that she has a partner, there is an opportunity for the nurse to discuss this further to ensure that Liz will have the ongoing support required during the later months of her pregnancy. As nurses are knowledgeable and skilled on the need for health promotion and education, it is then timely during this discussion for the nurse to provide Liz with reading material that will assist her to understand the growth and development of her baby, as well as indentifying substances and environments that should be avoided. Nursing expertise at this time of Liz's pregnancy can provide strong foundational knowledge and support to ensure a healthy outcome at birth.

TO HELP ENSURE FETAL HEALTH

Assessment

Assessing fetal growth throughout pregnancy, by such means as fundal height and fetal heart rate, is important because these predictable signs of fetal development provide guides for determining the wellbeing of fetuses. For the expectant family, knowledge about fetal growth and development can provide an important frame of reference, helping a mother to understand some of the changes going on in her body and allowing all family members to begin thinking about and accepting the newest member of the family before the baby is actually born. For this reason, convey the findings gained from fetal assessment at antenatal visits in as much detail as the parents' request.

Nursing considerations

Common considerations related to growth and development of the fetus focus on the mother and family as well as on the fetus. Examples might include:

- Health-seeking behaviours related to knowledge of normal fetal development
- Anxiety related to lack of fetal movement
- Deficient knowledge related to need for good antenatal care for healthy fetal wellbeing

BOX 9.1 * Focus on family teaching

Teratogens at work

Q. Liz Calhom tells you, "I have to work. How can I guard against fetal teratogens at work?"

A. Here are some helpful tips:

- Ask your employer for a statement on hazardous substances at your work site; discuss your need to avoid these substances during pregnancy.
- Ask your employer to maintain a smoke-free site if that is not already a rule.
- Avoid any room, such as a coffee room, where smokers gather.
- Refrain from drinking alcohol, a frequent accompaniment to work lunches or social functions; ask for non-alcoholic drinks to be available at such events.

Be certain that plans for care include ways to educate potential parents about teratogens (any substance that could be harmful to a fetus) that might interfere with fetal health (see Box 9.1). Be certain that outcome criteria established for teaching about fetal growth are realistic and based on the parents' previous knowledge and desire for information.

Most expectant parents are interested in learning about how mature their baby is at various points in pregnancy because this helps them visualise their coming newborn. This, in turn, helps them to understand the importance of implementing healthy behaviours, such as eating well and avoiding substances that may be dangerous to a fetus such as recreational drugs. Viewing an ultrasound and learning the fetal sex can be steps to help initiate bonding between the parents and the infant.

STAGES OF FETAL DEVELOPMENT

In just 38 weeks, a fertilised egg (ovum) matures from a single cell to a fully developed fetus ready to be born. Table 9.1 lists common terms used to describe the fetus at various stages in this growth.

TABLE 9.1 Terms used to denote fetal growth

Name	Time period
Ovum	From ovulation to fertilisation
Zygote	From fertilisation to implantation
Embryo	From implantation to 5–8 weeks
Fetus	From 5–8 weeks until term
Conceptus	Developing embryo or fetus and placental structures throughout pregnancy
Age of viability	The earliest age at which fetuses could survive if they were born at that time, generally accepted as 24 weeks, or fetuses weighing more than 400 grams

Fertilisation: The beginning of pregnancy

Fertilisation (also referred to as conception and impregnation) is the union of an ovum and a spermatozoon. This usually occurs in the outer third of a fallopian tube, the ampullar portion (Taylor & Badell, 2011). Usually only one of a woman's ova will reach maturity each month. Once the mature ovum is released, fertilisation must occur fairly quickly because an ovum is capable of fertilisation for only 24 hours (48 hours at the most). After that time, it atrophies and becomes non-functional. Because the functional life of a spermatozoon is also about 48 hours, possibly as long as 72 hours, the total critical time span during which sexual relations must occur for fertilisation to be successful is about 72 hours (48 hours before ovulation plus 24 hours afterwards).

As the ovum is extruded from the graafian follicle of an ovary with ovulation, it is surrounded by a ring of mucopolysaccharide fluid (the zona pellucida) and a circle of cells (the corona radiata). The ovum and these surrounding cells (which increase the bulk of the ovum and serve as protective buffers against injury) are propelled into a nearby fallopian tube by currents initiated by the fimbriae—the fine, hair-like structures that line the openings of the fallopian tubes. A combination of peristaltic action of the tube and movements of the tube cilia help propel the ovum along the length of the tube.

Normally, an ejaculation of semen averages 2.5 mL of fluid containing 50 to 200 million spermatozoa per millilitre, or an average of 400 million sperm per ejaculation. At the time of ovulation, there is a reduction in the viscosity (thickness) of the cervical mucous, which makes it easy for spermatozoa to penetrate it. Sperm transport is so efficient close to ovulation that spermatozoa deposited in the vagina generally reach the cervix within 90 seconds and the outer end of a fallopian tube within 5 minutes after deposit. This is one reason why douching is not an effective contraceptive measure (Burkman, 2007).

The mechanism whereby spermatozoa are drawn towards an ovum is probably a species-specific reaction, similar to an antibody-antigen reaction. Spermatozoa move through the cervix and the body of the uterus and into the fallopian tubes, towards the waiting ovum by the combination of movement by their flagella (tails) and uterine contractions. Capacitation is a final process that sperm must undergo to be ready for fertilisation. This process, which happens as the sperm move towards the ovum, consists of changes in the plasma membrane of the sperm head, which reveal the sperm-binding receptor sites.

All of the spermatozoa that achieve capacitation reach the ovum and cluster around the protective layer of corona cells. Hyaluronidase (a proteolytic enzyme) is released by the spermatozoa and dissolves the layer of cells protecting the ovum. One reason that an ejaculation contains such a large number of sperm is probably to provide sufficient enzymes to dissolve the corona cells. Under ordinary circumstances, only one spermatozoon is able to penetrate the cell membrane of the ovum. Once it penetrates the cell, the cell membrane changes composition to become impervious to other spermatozoa.

Immediately after penetration of the ovum, the chromosomal material of the ovum and spermatozoon fuse to form a zygote. Because the spermatozoon and ovum each carried 23 chromosomes (22 autosomes and 1 sex chromosome), the fertilised ovum has 46 chromosomes. If an X-carrying spermatozoon entered the ovum, the resulting child will have two X chromosomes and will be female (XX). If a Y-carrying spermatozoon fertilised the ovum, the resulting child will have an X and a Y chromosome and will be male (XY).

Fertilisation is never a certain occurrence because it depends on at least three separate factors: equal maturation of both sperm and ovum, the ability of the sperm to reach the ovum and the ability of the sperm to penetrate the zona pellucida and cell membrane and achieve fertilisation.

From the fertilised ovum **(zygote)**, both the future child and the accessory structures needed for support during intrauterine life (e.g. placenta, fetal membranes, amniotic fluid and umbilical cord) are formed.

Implantation

Once fertilisation is complete, a zygote migrates over the next 3 to 4 days towards the body of the uterus, aided by the currents initiated by the muscular contractions of the fallopian tubes. During this time, mitotic cell division, or cleavage, begins. The first cleavage occurs at about 24 hours; cleavage divisions continue to occur at a rate of about one every 22 hours. By the time the zygote reaches the body of the uterus, it consists of 16 to 50 cells. At this stage, because of its bumpy outward appearance, it is termed a morula (from the Latin word *morus,* meaning "mulberry").

The morula continues to multiply as it floats free in the uterine cavity for 3 or 4 additional days. Large cells tend to collect at the periphery of the ball, leaving a fluid space surrounding an inner cell mass. At this stage, the structure becomes a blastocyst. It is this structure that attaches to the uterine endometrium. The cells in the outer ring are **trophoblast** cells. They are the part of the structure that will later form the placenta and membranes. The inner cell mass (embryoblast cells) is the portion of the structure that will form the **embryo**.

Implantation, or contact between the growing structure and the uterine endometrium, occurs approximately 8 to 10 days after fertilisation. After the third or fourth day of free floating (about 8 days since ovulation), the blastocyst sheds the last residues of the corona and zona pellucida. The structure brushes against the rich uterine endometrium (in the second [secretory] phase of the menstrual cycle), a process termed *apposition*. It attaches to the surface of the endometrium (adhesion) and settles down into its soft folds (invasion).

The touching or implantation point is usually high in the uterus, on the posterior surface. If the point of implantation is low in the uterus, the growing placenta may occlude the cervix and make birth of the child impossible (placenta previa). The blastocyst is able to invade the endometrium because, as the trophoblast cells on the outside of the structure touch the endometrium, they produce proteolytic enzymes that dissolve any tissue they touch. This action allows the blastocyst to burrow deeply into the endometrium and receive some basic nourishment of glycogen and mucoprotein from the endometrial glands. As invasion continues, the structure establishes an effective communication network with the blood system of the endometrium.

Implantation is an important step in pregnancy, because as many as 50% of zygotes never achieve it (Knuppel, 2007). In these instances, the pregnancy ends as early as 8 to 10 days after conception, often before a woman is even aware she was pregnant. Occasionally, a small amount of vaginal spotting appears on the day of implantation because capillaries are ruptured by the implanting trophoblast cells. A woman who normally has a particularly scant menstrual flow may mistake implantation bleeding for her menstrual period. If this happens, the predicted date of birth of her baby (based on the time of her last menstrual period) will be calculated 4 weeks late. Once implanted, the zygote becomes an embryo.

CASE STUDY QUESTION

2. Liz asks how much longer her midwife will refer to the baby inside her as an embryo. The conceptus is an embryo:
   a. Until the time of fertilisation
   b. Until the placenta forms
   c. From implantation until 20 weeks
   d. From implantation until 5 to 8 weeks

EMBRYONIC AND FETAL STRUCTURES

The placenta, which will serve as the fetal lungs, kidneys and digestive tract in utero, begins growing in early pregnancy in coordination with embryo growth.

The decidua

After fertilisation, the corpus luteum in the ovary continues to function rather than atrophying, because of the influence of human chorionic gonadotropin (hCG), a hormone secreted by the trophoblast cells. This causes the uterine endometrium to continue to grow in thickness and vascularity, instead of sloughing off as in a usual menstrual cycle. The endometrium is now termed the **decidua** (the Latin word for "falling off"), because it will be discarded

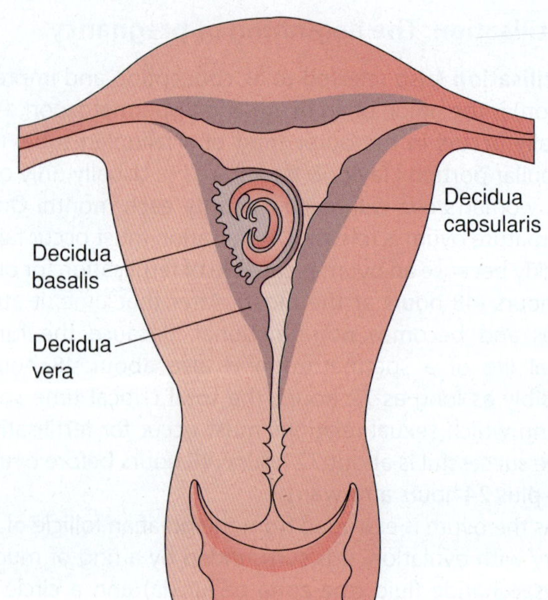

FIGURE 9.1 The three areas of uterine decidua.

after the birth of the child. The decidua has three separate areas (see Fig. 9.1):

1. Decidua basalis
2. Decidua capsularis
3. Decidua vera.

As the embryo continues to grow, it pushes the decidua capsularis before it like a blanket. Eventually, the embryo enlarges so much that this action brings the decidua capsularis into contact with the opposite uterine wall (the decidua vera). Here, the two decidua areas fuse, which is why, at birth, the entire inner surface of the uterus is stripped away, leaving the organ highly susceptible to haemorrhage and infection.

Chorionic villi

Once implantation is complete, the trophoblastic layer of cells of the blastocyst begins to mature rapidly. As early as the 11th or 12th day, miniature villi that resemble probing fingers, termed **chorionic villi**, reach out from the single layer of cells into the uterine endometrium to begin formation of the placenta. At term, almost 200 such villi will have formed (Knuppel, 2007). All chorionic villi have a central core of connective tissue and fetal capillaries. A double layer of trophoblast cells surrounds these. The outer of the two covering layers is the *syncytiotrophoblast*, or the syncytial layer. This layer of cells produces various placental hormones, such as hCG, somatomammotrophin (human placental lactogen [hPL]), oestrogen and progesterone. (Ainbinder, Ramin & DeCherney, 2007)

The placenta

The placenta (Latin for "pancake," which is descriptive of its size and appearance at term) arises out of the continuing growth of trophoblast tissue. Its growth parallels that of the fetus, growing from a few identifiable cells at the beginning of pregnancy to an organ 15 to 20 cm in diameter and 2 to 3 cm in depth, covering about half the surface area of the internal uterus at term (Huppertz & Kingdom, 2012).

Circulation

Placental circulation is shown in Figure 9.2. As early as the 12th day of pregnancy, maternal blood begins to collect in the intervillous spaces of the uterine endometrium surrounding the chorionic villi. By the third week, oxygen and other nutrients, such as glucose, amino acids, fatty acids, minerals, vitamins and water, osmose from the maternal blood through the cell layers of the chorionic villi into the villi capillaries. From there, nutrients are transported to the developing embryo.

Placental osmosis is so effective that all except a few substances are able to cross from the mother into the fetus. Because almost all medications are able to cross into the fetal circulation, it is important that a woman take no non-essential medications (including alcohol and nicotine) during pregnancy (Rogers-Adkinson & Stuart, 2007). Alcohol, as an example of a drug which can cause fetal growth disorders, perfuses across the placenta so well that pregnant women are advised to drink no alcohol at all during pregnancy (Crombleholme, 2009).

As the number of chorionic villi increases with pregnancy, the villi form an increasingly complex communication network with the maternal blood. Intervillous spaces grow larger and larger, becoming separated by a series of partitions or septa. In a mature placenta, there are as many as 30 separate segments, or *cotyledons*. These compartments are what make the maternal side of the placenta look rough and uneven.

As the blood circulates around the villi and nutrients osmose from maternal blood into the villi, the maternal blood gradually loses its momentum and settles to the floor of the cotyledons. From there, it enters the orifices of maternal veins located in the cotyledons and is returned to the maternal circulation. Braxton Hicks contractions, the barely noticeable uterine contractions that are present from about the 12th week of pregnancy, aid in maintaining

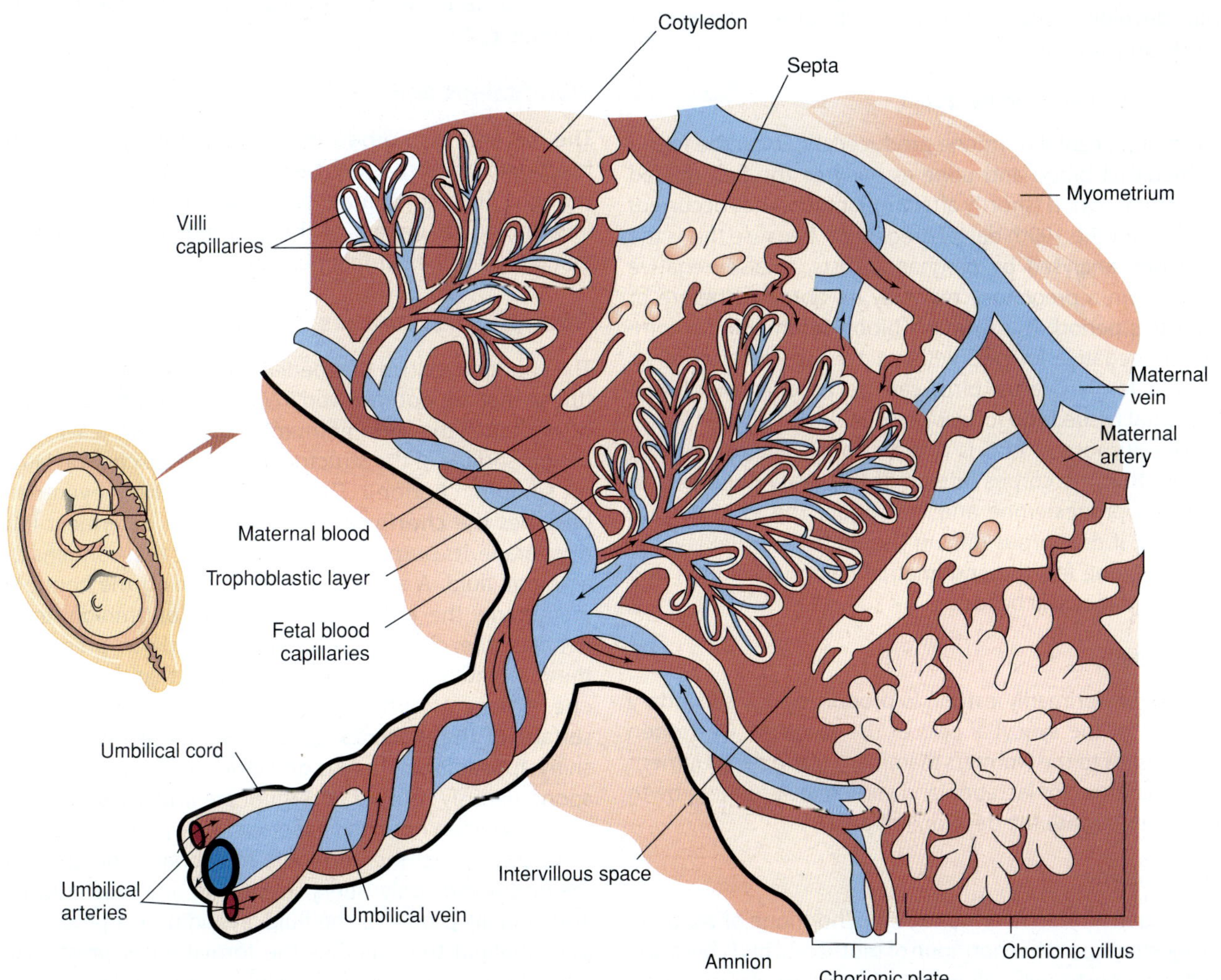

FIGURE 9.2 Placental circulation

pressure in the intervillous spaces by closing off the uterine veins momentarily with each contraction.

Uterine perfusion, and thus placental circulation, is most efficient when the woman lies on her left side. This position lifts the uterus away from the inferior vena cava, preventing blood from being trapped in the woman's lower extremities. If the woman lies on her back and the weight of the uterus compresses the vena cava, placental circulation can be so sharply reduced that supine hypotension (very low maternal blood pressure and poor uterine circulation) occurs (Coad & Dunstall, 2011).

At term, the placental circulatory network has grown so extensively that a placenta weighs 400 to 600 grams, one-sixth the weight of the baby. If a placenta is smaller than this, it suggests that circulation to the fetus may have been inadequate. A placenta larger than this may also indicate that circulation to the fetus was threatened, because it suggests that the placenta was forced to spread out in an unusual manner to maintain a sufficient blood supply.

Endocrine function

Aside from serving as the conduit for oxygen and nutrients for the fetus, the syncytial (outer) layer of the chorionic villi develops into a separate, important hormone-producing system.

Human chorionic gonadotropin

The first placental hormone produced, hCG, can be found in maternal blood and urine as early as the first missed menstrual period (shortly after implantation has occurred) until about the 100th day of pregnancy. Because this is the hormone analysed by pregnancy tests, a false-negative result from a pregnancy test may be obtained before or after this period. The woman's blood serum will be completely negative for hCG within 1 to 2 weeks after birth. Testing for hCG after birth can be used as proof that placental tissue is no longer present.

The purpose of hCG is to act as a fail-safe measure to ensure that the corpus luteum of the ovary continues to produce progesterone and oestrogen. This is important because, if the corpus luteum should fail and the level of progesterone fall, the endometrial lining will slough and the pregnancy will be lost.

Oestrogen

Oestrogen (primarily estriol) is produced as a secondary product of the syncytial cells of the placenta. Oestrogen contributes to the woman's mammary gland development in preparation for lactation and stimulates uterine growth to accommodate the developing fetus.

Progesterone

Oestrogen is often referred to as the "hormone of women"; progesterone as the "hormone of mothers". This is because, although oestrogen influences a female appearance, progesterone is necessary to maintain the endometrial lining of the uterus during pregnancy. It is present in serum as early as the fourth week of pregnancy, as a result of the continuation of the corpus luteum. After placental synthesis begins (at about the 12th week), the level of progesterone rises progressively during the remainder of the pregnancy. This hormone also appears to reduce the contractility of the uterus during pregnancy, preventing premature labour. Such reduced contractility is probably produced by a change in electrolytes (notably potassium and calcium), which decreases the contraction potential of the uterus.

Human placental lactogen (human chorionic somatomam-motrophin)

Human placental lactogen (hPL) is a hormone with both growth-promoting and lactogenic (milk-producing) properties. It is produced by the placenta beginning as early as the sixth week of pregnancy, increasing to a peak level at term. It can be assayed in both maternal serum and urine. It promotes mammary gland (breast) growth in preparation for lactation in the mother. It also serves the important role of regulating maternal glucose, protein and fat levels so that adequate amounts of these nutrients are always available to the fetus (Taylor & Lebovic, 2007).

Placental proteins

The placenta also produces several plasma proteins. The function of these has not been well documented, but it is thought that they may contribute to decreasing the immunological impact of the growing placenta through being part of the complement cascade (Knuppel, 2007).

Amniotic membranes

The chorionic villi on the medial surface of the trophoblast (those that are not involved in implantation because they do not touch the endometrium) gradually thin, leaving the medial surface of the structure smooth (the chorion laeve, or smooth chorion). The smooth chorion eventually becomes the **chorionic membrane**, the outermost fetal membrane. Its purpose is to form the sac that contains the amniotic fluid. A second membrane lining the chorionic membrane, the **amniotic membrane** or amnion, forms beneath the chorion (see Fig. 9.3). Early in pregnancy, these membranes become so adherent that they seem as one at term. At birth they can be seen covering the fetal surface of the placenta, giving that surface its typically shiny appearance. There is no nerve supply, so when they spontaneously rupture at term or are artificially ruptured, neither woman nor child experiences any pain.

In contrast to the chorionic membrane, the amniotic membrane not only offers support to amniotic fluid but also actually produces the fluid. In addition, it produces a phospholipid that initiates the formation of prostaglandins, which can cause uterine contractions and may be the trigger that initiates labour. Occasionally, fibrous amniotic

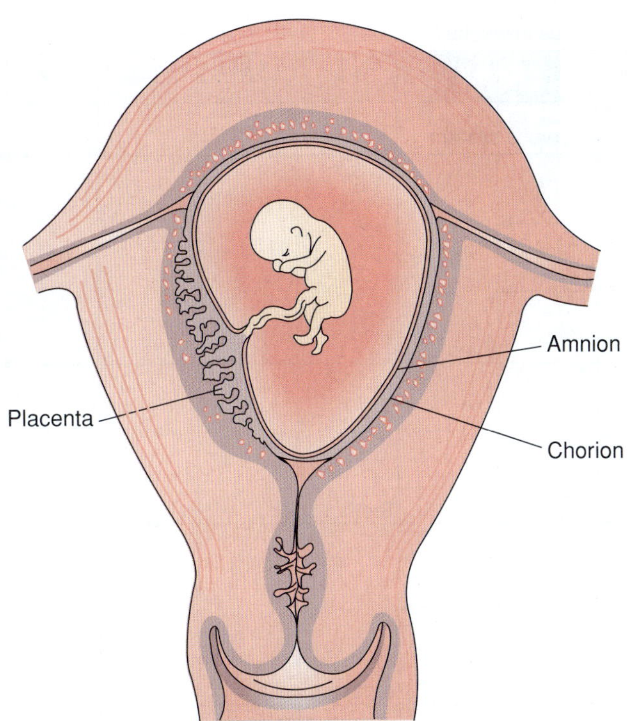

FIGURE 9.3 Membranes, with embryo lying within amniotic sac.

bands can form in utero. These amniotic bands range in severity but can close off the blood supply to the distal extremity causing growth of the extremity to halt at that point (Kumar, Das & Kumar, 2007).

Amniotic fluid

Amniotic fluid is constantly being newly formed and reabsorbed by the amniotic membrane, so it never becomes stagnant. Some of it is absorbed by direct contact with the fetal surface of the placenta. The major method of absorption, however, occurs because the fetus continually swallows the fluid. In the fetal intestine, it is absorbed into the fetal bloodstream. From there, it goes to the umbilical arteries and to the placenta, and it is exchanged across the placenta. At term, the amount of amniotic fluid has increased so much it ranges from 800 to 1200 mL. If for any reason the fetus is unable to swallow (oesophageal atresia or anencephaly are the two most common reasons) excessive amniotic fluid, or polyhydramnios (more than 2000 mL in total, or pockets of fluid larger than 8 cm on ultrasound), will result. Hydramnios also tends to occur in women with diabetes, because hyperglycaemia causes excessive fluid shifts into the amniotic space (Perovià et al., 2011). Early in fetal life, as soon as the fetal kidneys become active, fetal urine adds to the quantity of the amniotic fluid. A disturbance of kidney function may cause **oligohydramnios**, or a reduction in the amount of amniotic fluid (Petrozella et al., 2011).

The most important purpose of amniotic fluid is to shield the fetus against pressure or a blow to the mother's abdomen. Because liquid changes temperature more slowly than air, it also protects the fetus from changes in temperature. As yet another function, it aids in muscular development, because it allows the fetus freedom to move. Finally, it protects the umbilical cord from pressure, protecting the fetal oxygen supply. Even if the amniotic membranes rupture before birth and the bulk of amniotic fluid is lost, some will always surround the fetus in utero, because new fluid is constantly formed.

The umbilical cord

The **umbilical cord** is formed from the fetal membranes (amnion and chorion) and provides a circulatory pathway that connects the embryo to the chorionic villi of the placenta. Its function is to transport oxygen and nutrients to the fetus from the placenta and to return waste products from the fetus to the placenta. It is about 53 cm in length at term and about 2 cm thick. The bulk of the cord is a gelatinous mucopolysaccharide called Wharton's jelly, which gives the cord body and prevents pressure on the vein and arteries that pass through it. The outer surface is covered with amniotic membrane.

An umbilical cord contains only one vein (carrying blood from the placental villi to the fetus) but two arteries (carrying blood from the fetus back to the placental villi). The number of veins and arteries in the cord is always assessed and recorded at birth. Because the rate of blood flow through the cord is so rapid, it is unlikely that a cord will twist or knot enough to interfere with the fetal oxygen supply. In about 20% of all births, a loose loop of cord is found around the fetal neck (nuchal cord) at birth. It is recommended to leave the nuchal cord regardless of whether it is loose or tight (Reed, Barnes & Allan, 2009). If this loop of cord is removed before the newborn's shoulders are born, so that there is no traction on it, the oxygen supply to the fetus remains unimpaired (Jackson, Melvin & Downe, 2007).

The walls of the umbilical cord arteries are lined with smooth muscle. Constriction of these muscles after birth contributes to haemostasis and helps prevent haemorrhage of the newborn through the cord. Because the umbilical cord contains no nerve supply, it can be cut at birth without discomfort to either the child or mother.

ORIGIN AND DEVELOPMENT OF ORGAN SYSTEMS

Following the moment of fertilisation, the zygote, which later becomes an embryo and then a fetus, begins to grow at an active pace (see Fig. 9.4).

Cardiovascular system

Fetal circulation

As early as the third week of intrauterine life, fetal blood begins to exchange nutrients with the maternal circulation

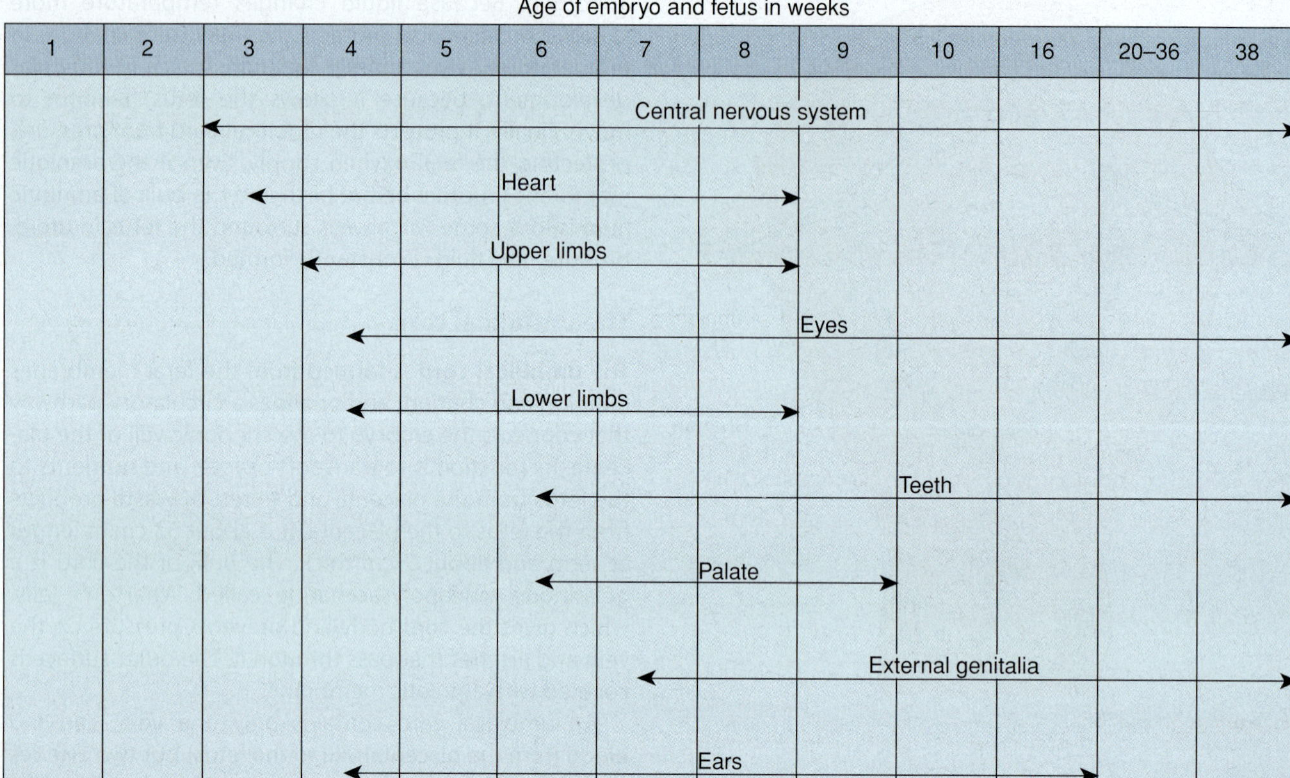

FIGURE 9.4 Critical periods of fetal growth.

across the chorionic villi. Fetal circulation differs from extrauterine circulation because the fetus derives oxygen and excretes carbon dioxide not from gas exchange in the lung but from gas exchange in the placenta.

Blood arriving at the fetus from the placenta is highly oxygenated. This blood enters the fetus through the umbilical vein (called a vein even though it carries oxygenated blood, because the direction of the blood is towards the fetal heart). Specialised structures present in the fetus then shunt blood flow to first supply the most important organs of the body: the brain, liver, heart and kidneys. Blood flows from the umbilical vein to the *ductus venosus*, an accessory vessel that directs oxygenated blood directly to the fetal liver. Blood then empties into the fetal inferior vena cava so oxygenated blood is directed to the right side of the heart. Because there is no need for the bulk of blood to pass through the lungs, it is shunted, as it enters the right atrium, into the left atrium through an opening in the atrial septum, called the **foramen ovale.** From the left atrium, it follows the course of adult circulation into the left ventricle and into the aorta.

A small amount of blood that returns to the heart via the vena cava does leave the right atrium via the adult circulatory route—that is, through the tricuspid valve into the right ventricle, and then into the pulmonary artery and lungs to service the lung tissue. However, the larger portion of even this blood is shunted away from the lungs through an additional structure, the *ductus arteriosus*, directly into the descending aorta.

Most of the blood flow from the descending aorta is transported by the umbilical arteries (called arteries, even though they are now transporting deoxygenated blood, because they are carrying blood away from the fetal heart) back through the umbilical cord to the placental villi, where new oxygen exchange takes place.

The blood oxygen saturation level of the fetus is about 80% of a newborn's saturation level. The rapid fetal heart rate during pregnancy (110–160 beats per minute) is necessary to supply oxygen to cells, because the red blood cells are never fully saturated. Despite this low blood oxygen saturation level, carbon dioxide does not accumulate in the fetal system because it rapidly diffuses into maternal blood across a favourable placental pressure gradient.

Fetal haemoglobin

Fetal haemoglobin differs from adult haemoglobin in several ways. It has a different composition (two alpha and two gamma chains, compared with two alpha and two beta chains of adult haemoglobin). It is also more concentrated and has greater oxygen affinity, two features that increase its efficiency. So much haemoglobin is present at birth that a newborn's haemoglobin level is about 170–180 g/mL, compared with an adult normal level of 110 g/mL; a newborn's haematocrit is about 53%, compared with an adult normal level of 45%. The change from fetal to adult haemoglobin levels begins before birth and accelerates after birth (Rees, 2007).

Respiratory system

At the third week of intrauterine life, the respiratory and digestive tracts exist as a single tube. Like all body tubes, initially this forms as a solid structure, which then canalises (hollows out). By the end of the fourth week, a septum begins to divide the oesophagus from the trachea. At the same time, lung buds appear on the trachea. Until the seventh week of life, the diaphragm does not completely divide the thoracic cavity from the abdomen. This causes lung buds to extend down into the abdomen, re-entering the chest only as the chest's longitudinal dimension increases and the diaphragm becomes complete (at the end of the seventh week) (Moyer et al., 2009). Other important respiratory developmental milestones include:

- Alveoli and capillaries begin to form between the 24th and 28th weeks. Both capillary and alveoli development must be complete before gas exchange can occur in the fetal lungs.
- Spontaneous respiratory practice movements begin as early as 3 months' gestation and continue throughout pregnancy.
- Specific lung fluid with a low surface tension and low viscosity forms in alveoli to aid in expansion of the alveoli at birth; it is rapidly absorbed after birth.
- **Surfactant**, a phospholipid substance, is formed and excreted by the alveolar cells at about the 24th week of pregnancy. This decreases alveolar surface tension on expiration, preventing alveolar collapse and improving the infant's ability to maintain respirations in the outside environment (Soll, 2009).

Surfactant has two components: lecithin and sphingomyelin. Early in the formation of surfactant, sphingomyelin is the chief component. At about 35 weeks, there is a surge in the production of lecithin, which then becomes the chief component by a ratio of 2:1. As a fetus practises breathing movements, surfactant mixes with amniotic fluid. Respiratory distress syndrome, a severe breathing disorder, can develop if there is lack of surfactant or it has not changed to its mature form at birth (see Chapter 26). Any interference with the blood supply to the fetus, such as occurs with placental insufficiency from hypertension, appears to enhance surfactant development (Roberts & Dalziel, 2009).

CASE STUDY QUESTION

3. Liz asks you why her doctor is so concerned about whether her fetus is producing surfactant. Your best answer would be:

   a. Surfactant keeps lungs from collapsing on expiration and so aids newborn breathing
   b. Surfactant is produced by the fetal liver, so its presence reveals liver maturity
   c. Surfactant is the precursor to IgM antibody production, so it prevents infection
   d. Surfactant reveals mature kidney function, as it is produced by kidney glomeruli

Nervous system

Like the circulatory system, the nervous system begins to develop extremely early in pregnancy. During the third and fourth weeks of intrauterine life, possibly before the woman even realises she is pregnant, active formation of the nervous system and sense organs has already begun.

- A neural plate (a thickened portion of the ectoderm) is apparent by the third week of gestation. The top portion differentiates into the neural tube, which will form the central nervous system (brain and spinal cord) and the neural crest, which will develop into the peripheral nervous system.
- All parts of the brain (cerebrum, cerebellum, pons and medulla oblongata) form in utero, although none are completely mature at birth. Growth proceeds rapidly during the first year and continues at high levels until 5 or 6 years of age.
- The eye and inner ear develop as projections of the original neural tube.
- By 24 weeks, the ear is capable of responding to sound; the eyes exhibit a pupillary reaction, indicating that sight is present.
- Brain waves can be detected on an electroencephalogram (EEG) by the eighth week.

The neurological system seems particularly prone to insult during the early weeks of the embryonic period. Spinal cord disorders such as meningocele (herniation of the meninges) may occur because of lack of folic acid (contained in green leafy vegetables and pregnancy vitamins) (Lumley et al., 2009). During pregnancy and at birth, the nervous system is vulnerable to damage from anoxia.

Endocrine system

As soon as endocrine organs mature in intrauterine life, function begins.

- The fetal adrenal glands supply a precursor necessary for oestrogen synthesis by the placenta.
- The fetal pancreas produces insulin needed by the fetus (insulin is one of the few substances that does not cross the placenta from the mother to the fetus).
- The thyroid and parathyroid glands play vital roles in fetal metabolic function and calcium balance.

Digestive system

The digestive tract separates from the respiratory tract at about the fourth week of intrauterine life and, after that, begins to grow extremely rapidly. Initially solid, the tract canalises (hollows out) to become patent. Later, the endothelial cells of the gastrointestinal tract proliferate extensively, occluding the lumen once more and the tract must canalise again. Atresia (blockage) or stenosis (narrowing) can develop if either the first or second canalisation does not occur. The proliferation of cells shed in the second recanalisation forms the basis for meconium (see below).

Because of this rapid intestinal growth, by the sixth week of intrauterine life, the intestine becomes too large to be contained by the abdomen. A portion of the intestine, guided by the vitelline membrane (a part of the yolk sac), is pushed into the base of the umbilical cord, where it remains until about the tenth week, when the abdominal cavity has grown large enough to accommodate the intestinal mass again. A defect, *gastroschisis*, occurs when the original midline fusion that occurred at the early cell stage is incomplete (Thilo & Rosenberg, 2011).

Meconium, a collection of cellular wastes, bile, fats, mucoproteins, mucopolysaccharides and portions of the vernix caseosa, the lubricating substance that forms on the fetal skin, accumulates in the intestines as early as the 16th week. Meconium is sticky in consistency and appears black or dark green (obtaining its colour from bile pigment).

The gastrointestinal tract is sterile before birth. Because vitamin K is synthesised by the action of bacteria in the intestines, vitamin K levels are low in the newborn. Sucking and swallowing reflexes are not mature until the fetus is at about 32 weeks' gestation or weighs 1500 grams. The ability of the gastrointestinal tract to secrete enzymes essential to carbohydrate and protein digestion is mature at 36 weeks. However, amylase, an enzyme found in saliva that is necessary for digestion of complex starches, is not mature until 3 months after birth. Many newborns have not yet developed lipase, an enzyme needed for fat digestion.

The liver is active throughout gestation, functioning as a filter between the incoming blood and the fetal circulation and as a deposit site for fetal stores such as iron and glycogen, but is still immature at birth. This can possibly lead to hypoglycaemia and hyperbilirubinaemia, two serious problems, in the first 24 hours after birth. The liver does not prevent recreational drugs or alcohol ingested by the mother from entering the fetal circulation.

Musculoskeletal system

During the first 2 weeks of fetal life, cartilage prototypes provide position and support. Ossification of this cartilage into bone begins at about the 12th week. Ossification continues all through fetal life and actually until adulthood. Carpals, tarsals and sternal bones generally do not ossify until birth is imminent. A fetus can be seen to move on an ultrasound as early as the 11th week, although the woman usually does not feel this movement until almost 20 weeks of gestation.

Reproductive system

A child's sex is determined at the moment of conception by a spermatozoon carrying an X or a Y chromosome and can be ascertained as early as 8 weeks by chromosomal analysis. At about the sixth week of life, the gonads (ovaries or testes) form. If testes form, testosterone is secreted, apparently influencing the sexually neutral genital duct to form other male organs (maturity of the wolffian or mesonephric duct). In the absence of testosterone secretion, female organs will form (maturation of the müllerian or paramesonephric duct).

The testes first form in the abdominal cavity and do not descend into the scrotal sac until the 34th to 38th week. Because of this, many male preterm infants are born with undescended testes. These children need follow-up care to be certain that their testes do descend when they reach what would have been the 34th to 38th week of gestational age, because testicular descent does not occur as readily in extrauterine life as it would in utero. Surgery is necessary as undescended testes are associated with poor sperm production and testicular cancer (Zeitler et al., 2011).

Urinary system

Although rudimentary kidneys are present as early as the end of the fourth week of intrauterine life, the presence of kidneys does not appear to be essential for life before birth because the placenta clears the fetus of waste products. Urine is formed by the 12th week and is excreted into the amniotic fluid by the 16th week of gestation. At term, fetal urine is being excreted at the rate of 500 mL/day. An amount of amniotic fluid that is less than normal (oligohydramnios) suggests that fetal kidneys are not secreting adequate urine and that there is a kidney, ureter or bladder disorder (Kumar, 2012). The complex structure of the kidneys is gradually developed during intrauterine life and continues for months afterwards. The loop of Henle, for example, is not fully differentiated until the child is born. Glomerular filtration and concentration of urine in the newborn are not efficient, because the kidney function is still not mature at birth.

Integumentary system

The skin of a fetus appears thin and almost translucent until subcutaneous fat begins to be deposited at about 36 weeks. Skin is covered by soft downy hairs (lanugo) that serve as insulation to preserve warmth in utero and a cream cheese-like substance, vernix caseosa, which is important for lubrication and for keeping the skin from macerating in utero.

Immune system

Immunoglobulin G (IgG) maternal antibodies cross the placenta into the fetus as early as the 20th week and certainly by the 24th week of intrauterine life, to give a fetus temporary passive immunity against diseases for which the mother has antibodies. These often include poliomyelitis, rubella (German measles), rubeola (regular measles), diphtheria, tetanus, infectious parotitis (mumps), hepatitis B and pertussis (whooping cough). Little or no immunity to the herpes virus (the virus of chickenpox, cold sores and genital herpes) is transferred to the fetus, so the average newborn is potentially susceptible to these diseases. The recommended immunisation for teenagers against the virus should reduce the incidence of this in newborns.

The passive immunity received by the newborn has already declined substantially by about 2 months. Immunisation against diphtheria, tetanus, pertussis, poliomyelitis, rotovirus, *Haemophilus influenzae* and pneumococcus is typically started at this time. Passive antibodies to measles have been demonstrated to last for longer than 1 year. Consequently, the immunisation for measles is not given until an extrauterine age of 12 months.

MILESTONES OF FETAL GROWTH AND DEVELOPMENT

When fetal milestones occur can be confusing, because the life of the fetus is typically measured from the time of ovulation or fertilisation (ovulation age), but the length of a pregnancy is more commonly measured from the first day of the last menstrual period (gestational age). Because ovulation and fertilisation take place about 2 weeks after the last menstrual period, the ovulation age of the fetus is always 2 weeks less than the length of the pregnancy or the gestational age.

The following discussion of fetal developmental milestones is based on gestational weeks, because it is helpful when talking to expectant parents to be able to correlate fetal development with the way they measure pregnancy—from the first day of the last menstrual period. Figure 9.5 illustrates the comparative size and appearance of human embryos and fetuses at different stages.

End of 4th gestational week

At the end of the fourth week of gestation, the human embryo is a group of rapidly growing cells but does not yet resemble a human being.

- Length: 0.75–1 cm
- Weight: 400 mg
- The spinal cord is formed and fused at the midpoint
- Lateral wings that will form the body are folded forwards to fuse at the midline
- The head folds forwards and becomes prominent, representing about one-third of the entire structure
- The back is bent so that the head almost touches the tip of the tail
- The rudimentary heart appears as a prominent bulge on the anterior surface
- Arms and legs are budlike structures
- Rudimentary eyes, ears and nose are discernible

End of 8th gestational week

- Length: 2.5 cm
- Weight: 20 grams
- Organogenesis is complete

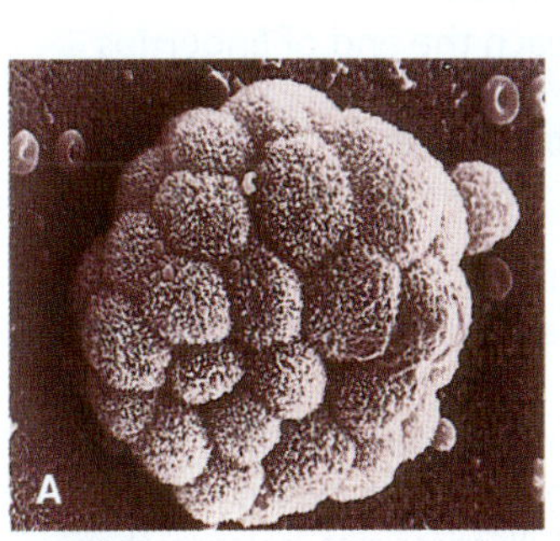

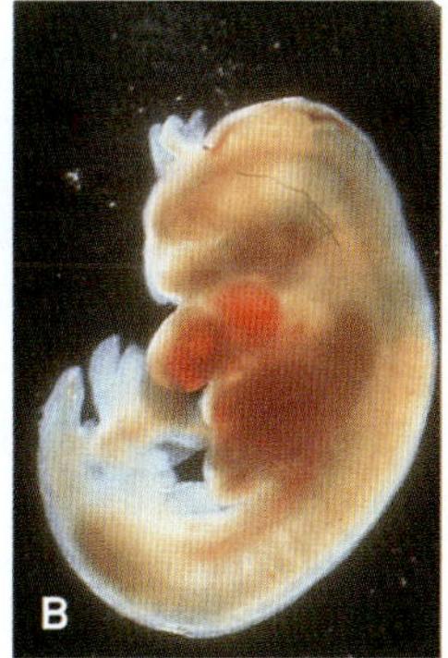

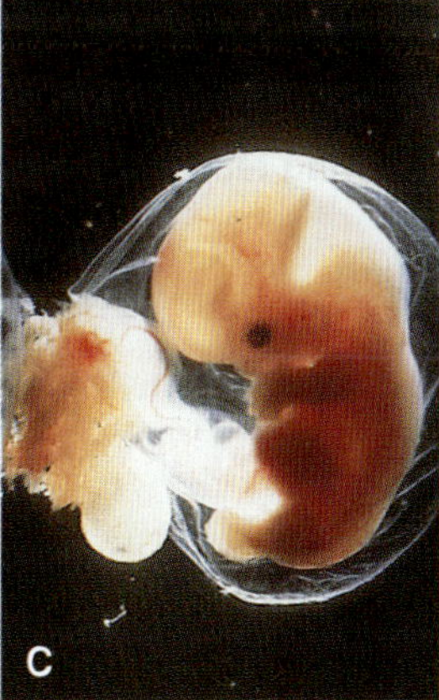

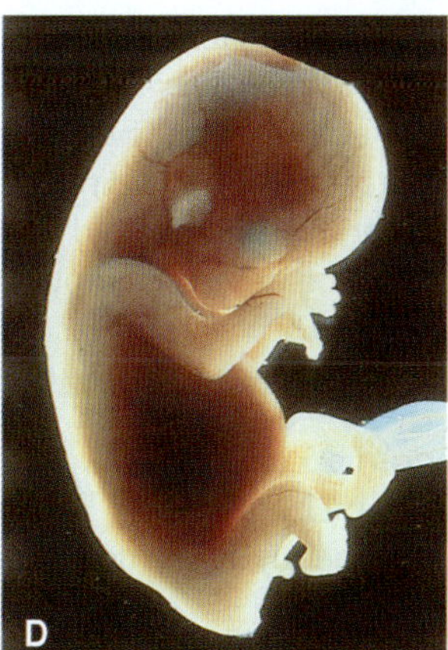

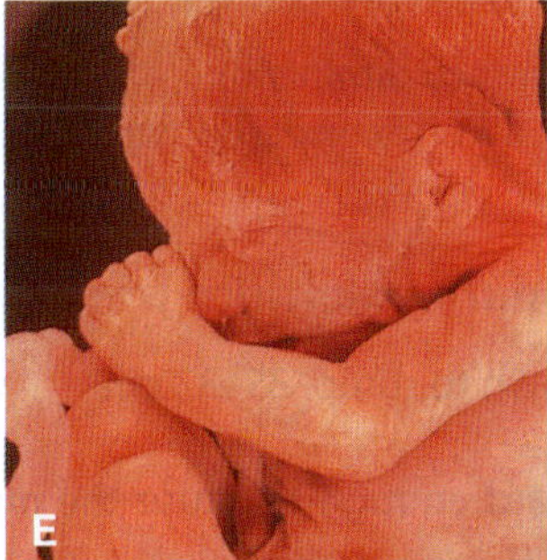

FIGURE 9.5 Human embryos at different stages of life: (**A**) implantation in uterus 7–8 days after conception. (**B**) Embryo at 32 days. (**C**) At 37 days. (**D**) At 41 days. (**E**) Between 12 and 15 weeks. (From Petit Format/Nestle/Science Source/Photo Researchers.)

- The heart, with a septum and valves, is beating rhythmically
- Facial features are definitely discernible
- Arms and legs have developed
- External genitalia are forming, but sex is not yet distinguishable by simple observation
- The primitive tail is regressing
- The abdomen bulges forwards because the fetal intestine is growing so rapidly
- An ultrasound shows a gestational sac, diagnostic of pregnancy

End of 12th gestational week (first trimester)

- Length: 7–8 cm
- Weight: 45 grams
- Nail beds are forming on fingers and toes
- Spontaneous movements are possible, although they are usually too faint to be felt by the mother
- Some reflexes, such as the Babinski reflex, are present
- Bone ossification centres begin to form
- Tooth buds are present
- Sex is distinguishable by outward appearance
- Urine secretion begins but may not yet be evident in amniotic fluid
- The heartbeat is audible through Doppler technology

End of 16th gestational week

- Length: 10–17 cm
- Weight: 55–120 grams
- Fetal heart sounds are audible by an ordinary stethoscope
- Lanugo is well formed
- Liver and pancreas are functioning
- Fetus actively swallows amniotic fluid, demonstrating an intact but uncoordinated swallowing reflex; urine is present in amniotic fluid
- Sex can be determined by ultrasound

End of 20th gestational week

- Length: 25 cm
- Weight: 223 grams
- Spontaneous fetal movements can be sensed by the mother
- Antibody production is possible
- The hair forms on the head, extending to include eyebrows
- Meconium is present in the upper intestine
- Brown fat, a special fat that will aid in temperature regulation at birth, begins to be formed behind the kidneys, sternum and posterior neck
- Vernix caseosa begins to form and cover the skin
- Passive antibody transfer from mother to fetus begins
- Definite sleeping and activity patterns are distinguishable (the fetus has developed biorhythms that will guide sleep/wake patterns throughout life)

End of 24th gestational week (second trimester)

- Length: 28–36 cm
- Weight: 550 grams
- Meconium is present as far as the rectum
- Active production of lung surfactant begins
- Eyebrows and eyelashes become well defined
- Eyelids, previously fused since the 12th week, now open
- Pupils are capable of reacting to light
- Hearing can be demonstrated by response to sudden sound

End of 28th gestational week

- Length: 35–38 cm
- Weight: 1200 grams
- Lung alveoli begin to mature and surfactant can be demonstrated in amniotic fluid
- Testes begin to descend into the scrotal sac from the lower abdominal cavity
- The blood vessels of the retina are formed but are thin and extremely susceptible to damage from high oxygen concentrations (an important consideration when caring for preterm infants who need oxygen)

End of 32nd gestational week

- Length: 38–43 cm
- Weight: 1600 grams
- Subcutaneous fat begins to be deposited (the former stringy, "little old man" appearance is lost)
- Fetus responds by movement to sounds outside the mother's body
- Active Moro reflex is present
- Iron stores, which provide iron for the time during which the neonate will ingest only milk after birth, are beginning to be developed
- Fingernails grow to reach the end of fingertips

End of 36th gestational week

- Length: 42–48 cm
- Weight: 1800–2700 grams
- Body stores of glycogen, iron, carbohydrate and calcium are deposited
- Additional amounts of subcutaneous fat are deposited
- Sole of the foot has only one or two crisscross creases, compared with the full crisscross pattern that will be evident at term
- Amount of lanugo begins to diminish
- Most babies turn into a vertex (head down) presentation during this month

End of 40th gestational week (third trimester)

- Length: 48–52 cm (crown to rump, 35–37 cm)
- Weight: 3000 grams
- Fetus kicks actively, hard enough to cause the mother considerable discomfort

- Fetal haemoglobin begins its conversion to adult haemoglobin. The conversion is so rapid that, at birth, about 20% of haemoglobin will be adult in character
- Vernix caseosa is fully formed
- Fingernails extend over the fingertips
- Creases on the soles of the feet cover at least two thirds of the surface

In primiparas (women having their first baby), the fetus often sinks into the birth canal during the last 2 weeks, giving the mother a feeling that the load she is carrying is less. This event, termed *lightening*, is a fetal announcement that the third trimester of pregnancy has ended and birth is at hand.

DETERMINATION OF ESTIMATED BIRTH DATE

It is impossible to predict the day an infant will be born with a high degree of accuracy. Traditionally, this date was referred to as the estimated date of confinement (EDC). Because women are no longer "confined" after childbirth, the abbreviation EDB **(estimated date of birth)** or EDD (estimated date of delivery) is more commonly used today. Fewer than 5% of pregnancies end exactly 280 days from the last menstrual period or exactly on this date; fewer than half end within 1 week of the 280th day. If fertilisation occurred early in a menstrual cycle, the pregnancy will probably end "early"; if ovulation and fertilisation occurred later in the cycle, the pregnancy will end "late." Because of these normal variations, a pregnancy ending 2 weeks before or 2 weeks after the calculated EDB is considered well within the normal limit (37–42 weeks). Gestational age wheels or birth date calculators that can be used to predict a birth date are available, but calculation by Nagele's rule is the standard method used to predict the length of a pregnancy (see Box 9.2).

ASSESSMENT OF FETAL GROWTH AND DEVELOPMENT

Fetal growth and development can be compromised if a fetus has a metabolic or chromosomal disorder that interferes with normal growth, if the supporting structures such as the placenta or cord do not form normally or if environmental influences such as cigarette smoking (the nicotine in cigarettes causes fetal growth restriction) or alcohol consumption (alcohol causes severe cognitive challenge) interfere with fetal growth. Much information regarding whether a baby is growing and is healthy can be gathered through a variety of assessment techniques.

Consent to perform a procedure is necessary if the procedure poses any risk to the mother or fetus that would not otherwise be present.

BOX 9.2 ✻ Nagele's rule

To calculate the date of birth by this rule, count backwards 3 calendar months from the first day of a woman's last menstrual period and add 7 days. For example, if the last menstrual period began 15 May, you would count back 3 months (15 April, 15 March, 15 February) and add 7 days, to arrive at a date of birth of 22 February.

Health history

Like all assessments, fetal assessment begins with a health history. Ask specifically about nutritional intake, because, if a woman is not eating a well-balanced diet, she may not be taking in sufficient nutrients for fetal growth. Be certain to ask also about personal habits such as cigarette smoking, recreational drug use and exercise, because all of these influence glucose/insulin balance and fetal growth. Most women actively protect a fetus growing inside them. Asking if the woman has had any accidents or experienced domestic violence helps reveal whether the fetus could have suffered any trauma (domestic violence tends to increase during pregnancy because of the stress a pregnancy can create) (Dalton, 2012).

CASE STUDY QUESTION

4. Which statement by Liz would make you most worried she might have difficulty quitting smoking during the remainder of her pregnancy?
   a. "I don't have a lot of spare cash, just like everyone else in my family."
   b. "When I feel tense, I like to shop. It really takes away that bad feeling."
   c. "I'm trying to stop smoking so I won't have to smoke around my baby."
   d. "My mother had five children with no trouble; why am I so different?"

Estimating fetal growth

McDonald's rule, a symphysis-fundal height measurement, although not documented to be thoroughly reliable, is an easy method of determining during mid-pregnancy that a fetus is growing in utero. Typically, the distance from the uterine fundus to the symphysis pubis in centimetres is equal to the week of gestation between the 20th and 31st weeks of pregnancy. Make the measurement from the notch of the symphysis pubis to over the top of the uterine fundus as a woman lies supine. A fundal height much greater than this standard suggests multiple pregnancy, a miscalculated due date, a large-for-gestational-age infant, **hydramnios** (increased amniotic fluid volume), or possibly even hydatidiform mole (see Chapter 21). A fundal measurement much less than this suggests that the fetus is failing to thrive (intrauterine growth restriction), the pregnancy length was miscalculated or an anomaly, such as anencephaly, has developed.

Assessing fetal wellbeing

Several actions or procedures are helpful in detecting and documenting that the fetus is not only growing but apparently healthy.

Fetal movement

Fetal movement that can be felt by the mother occurs at approximately 18 to 20 weeks of pregnancy and peaks in intensity at 28 to 38 weeks. A healthy baby moves with a degree of consistency, or at least 10 times a day. In contrast, a fetus not receiving enough nutrients because of placental insufficiency has greatly decreased movements (Chang & Blakemore, 2007). Make sure to assure a woman that fetal movements do vary, especially in relation to sleep cycles of the baby, her activity and the time since she last ate. Otherwise, she can become unduly worried that her baby may be in jeopardy when the baby is just having an inactive time.

Fetal heart rate

Fetal hearts beat at 110 to 160 beats per minute throughout pregnancy. Fetal heart sounds can be heard and counted as early as the tenth to eleventh week of pregnancy by the use of an ultrasonic Doppler technique.

Electronic fetal monitoring or cardiotocography

A cardiotocography (CTG) measures the response of the fetal heart rate to fetal movement. Position a woman and attach both a fetal heart rate and a uterine contraction monitor. Instruct a woman to push a button attached to the monitor (similar to a call bell) whenever she feels the fetus move. This will create a dark mark on the paper tracing at these times. When the fetus moves, the fetal heart rate should increase about 15 beats per minute and remain elevated for 15 seconds. It should decrease to its average rate again as the fetus quietens. If no increase in beats per minute is noticeable on fetal movement, poor oxygen perfusion of the fetus is suggested.

A CTG is usually carried out for 10 to 20 minutes. The test is said to be reactive if two accelerations of fetal heart rate (by 15 beats or more) lasting for 15 seconds occur after movement within the chosen time period. The test is non-reactive if no accelerations occur with the fetal movements. The results can also be interpreted as non-reactive if no fetal movement occurs or if there is low short-term fetal heart rate variability (less than 6 beats per minute) throughout the testing period (Chang & Blakemore, 2007). If a 20-minute period passes without any fetal movement, it may mean only that the fetus is sleeping. Other reasons for lessened variability are maternal smoking, drug use or hypoglycaemia. Because a CTG is a non-invasive procedure and causes no risk to either the mother or fetus, it can be used as a screening procedure.

If a CTG is non-reactive, additional fetal assessment will be scheduled. CTG monitoring should always be discussed with a trained maternity care provider such as a midwife or trained medical officer.

Ultrasonography

Ultrasonography, which measures the response of sound waves against solid objects, is a much-used tool in modern obstetrics, although the recommendations for its use are being questioned because of unproven benefits in the face of added expense (Neilson, 2009). It can be used to:

- Diagnose pregnancy as early as 6 weeks' gestation
- Confirm the presence, size and location of the placenta and amniotic fluid
- Establish that a fetus is growing and has no gross anomalies, such as hydrocephalus, anencephaly, or spinal cord, heart, kidney and bladder defects
- Establish sex if a penis is revealed
- Establish the presentation and position of the fetus
- Predict maturity by measurement of the biparietal diameter of the head.

Ultrasonography can also be used to discover complications of pregnancy, such as the presence of an intrauterine device, hydramnios or oligohydramnios, ectopic pregnancy, missed miscarriage, abdominal pregnancy, placenta praevia, premature separation of the placenta, coexisting uterine tumours, multiple pregnancy or genetic disorders such as Down syndrome. Fetal anomalies such as neural tube disorders, diaphragmatic hernia or urethral stenosis also can be diagnosed. Fetal death can be revealed by a lack of heartbeat and respiratory movement. A parent who is in doubt that her fetus is well or whole can be greatly reassured by viewing a real-time ultrasound image (see Fig. 9.6).

Before an ultrasound examination, be sure that a woman has received a good explanation of what will happen and reassurance that the process does not involve x-rays. This means it is also safe for the father of the child to remain in the room during the test. For the sound waves to reflect best and the uterus to be held stable, it is helpful if the woman has a full bladder at the time of the procedure.

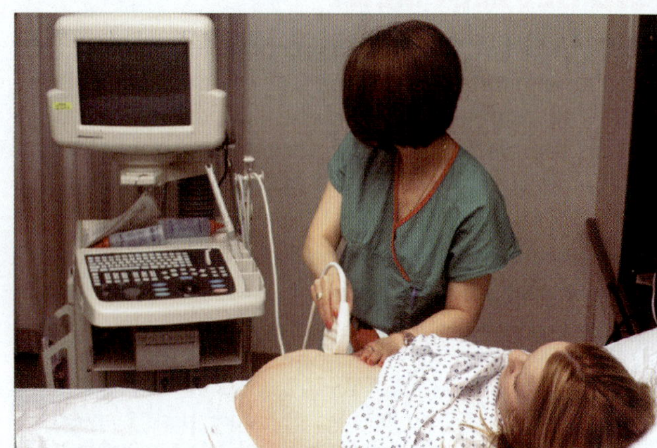

FIGURE 9.6 An ultrasound being recorded. Notice the mother's interest in being able to see her baby's first photograph.

Although the long-term effects of ultrasound are not yet known, the technique appears to be safe for both mother and fetus and involves no discomfort for the fetus. Usually, the only discomfort for the woman is that the contact lubricant may be messy and she may experience a strong desire to void before the scan is completed. Taking home a photograph of the ultrasound image can enhance bonding because it is proof that the pregnancy exists and the fetus appears well.

CASE STUDY QUESTION

5. Liz is scheduled to have an ultrasound examination. What instruction would you give her before her examination?
   a. "Void immediately before the procedure to reduce your bladder size."
   b. "The intravenous fluid infused to dilate your uterus does not hurt the fetus."
   c. "You will need to drink at least 3 glasses of fluid before the procedure."
   d. "You can have medicine for pain for any contractions caused by the test."

Biparietal diameter

Ultrasonography may be used to predict fetal maturity by measuring the biparietal diameter (side-to-side measurement) of the fetal head. In 80% of pregnancies in which the biparietal diameter of the fetal head is 8.5 cm or greater, it can be predicted that the infant will weigh more than 2500 grams or is at a fetal age of 40 weeks. Two other measurements commonly made by ultrasound to predict maturity are head circumference (34.5 cm indicates a 40-week fetus) and femoral length.

Amniotic fluid volume assessment

The amount of amniotic fluid present is yet another way to estimate fetal health because a portion of the fluid is formed by fetal kidney output. If a fetus is becoming stressed in utero so that circulatory and kidney functions are failing, urine output and, consequently, the volume of amniotic fluid will also decrease. A decrease in amniotic fluid volume puts the fetus at risk for compression of the umbilical cord and interference with nutrition. The average index is approximately 12–15 cm between 28 and 40 weeks. An index greater than 20–24 cm indicates polyhydramnios (excessive fluid, perhaps caused by inability of the fetus to swallow); an index less than 5–6 cm indicates oligohydramnios (decreased amniotic fluid, perhaps caused by poor perfusion and kidney failure).

Invasive fetal testing

If a genetic or growth concern is identified by non-invasive measures, a number of invasive measures allow for more refined investigation.

Amniocentesis

Amniocentesis (from the Greek *amnion* for "sac" and *kentesis* for "puncture") is the aspiration of amniotic fluid from the pregnant uterus for examination. The procedure can be carried out in a doctor's surgery. It is typically scheduled between the 14th and 16th weeks of pregnancy to allow for a generous amount of amniotic fluid to be present. The technique can be used again near term to test for fetal maturity.

Amniocentesis is a technically easy procedure, but it can be frightening to a woman. Because it involves penetration of the integrity of the amniotic sac, there also are risks to the fetus, although the incidence of these is low (less than 0.5%). Fetal complications range from haemorrhage from penetration of the placenta, infection of the amniotic fluid and puncture of the fetus. If it leads to irritation of the uterus, it can initiate premature labour (Alfirevic, 2009).

An ultrasound is carried out to determine the position of the fetus and the location of a pocket of amniotic fluid and the placenta. The abdomen is then washed with an antiseptic solution and a local anaesthetic is injected. The woman may feel a sensation of pressure as the needle used for aspiration, an 8 or 10 cm, 20- to 22-gauge spinal needle, is introduced.

The needle is inserted until it reaches the amniotic cavity and a pool of amniotic fluid, carefully avoiding the fetus and placenta. A syringe is attached and about 15 mL of amniotic fluid is withdrawn. The needle is then removed and the woman rests quietly for about 30 minutes. During the procedure and for the 30 minutes afterwards, observe the fetal heart rate monitor to be certain the rate remains within normal values and observe the uterine contraction monitor to be sure that no contractions are occurring.

Amniotic fluid is analysed for:

- Alpha-fetoprotein (AFP)
- Bilirubin determination
- Chromosome analysis
- Colour fetal fibronectin
- Inborn errors of metabolism
- Lecithin/sphingomyelin ratio
- Phosphatidyl glycerol and desaturated phosphatidyl choline.

Percutaneous umbilical blood sampling

Percutaneous umbilical blood sampling (PUBS) (also called cordocentesis or funicentesis) is the aspiration of blood from the umbilical vein for analysis. After the umbilical cord is located by ultrasound, a thin needle is inserted by amniocentesis technique into the uterus and is guided by ultrasound until it pierces the umbilical vein. A sample of blood is then removed for blood studies, such as a complete blood count, direct Coombs' test, blood gases and karyotyping. To ensure that the blood obtained is fetal blood, it is submitted to a Kleihauer-Betke test which measures the difference between adult and fetal blood.

Key points for review

- The union of a single sperm and egg (fertilisation) signals the beginning of pregnancy.
- The fertilised ovum (zygote) travels by way of a fallopian tube to the uterus, where implantation takes place in about 8 days.
- From implantation to 5 to 8 weeks, the growing structure is called an embryo. The period after 8 weeks until birth is the fetal period.
- Growth of the umbilical cord, amniotic fluid and amniotic membranes proceeds in concert with fetal growth. The placenta produces several important hormones: oestrogen, progesterone, human placental lactogen and human chorionic gonadotropin.
- Various methods to assess fetal growth and development include fundal height, fetal movement, fetal heart tones, ultrasonography, amniocentesis and percutaneous umbilical blood sampling.

CASE STUDY QUESTIONS

6. Liz has stated that her feelings have changed since she felt her baby move. Would you modify your health teaching with her because of this statement?
7. When Liz is scheduled for an ultrasound examination at 20 weeks' gestation, she tells you she does not want to know the sex of her fetus. Why do some women want to know this, whereas some do not? Is there an advantage to knowing or not knowing?
8. Late in pregnancy, Liz is scheduled for weekly CTG's. She invariably comes late for these tests because they are "time-consuming and boring." How could you make such tests more appealing to help increase her cooperation?

Resources

For an extensive range of additional resources to enhance teaching and learning and to facilitate understanding of this chapter, please see the text's accompanying website located on thePoint at http://thepoint.lww.com.

References

Ainbinder, S. W., Ramin, S. M. & DeCherney, A. H. (2007). Sexually transmitted diseases and pelvic infections. In A. H. DeCherney & L. Nathan (Eds). *Current Considerations and Treatment in Obstetrics and Gynecology* (10th ed.). Columbus, OH: McGraw-Hill.

Alfirevic, Z. (2009). Early amniocentesis versus transabdominal chorion villus sampling for antenatal considerations. *Cochrane Database of Systematic Reviews, 2009*(1), (CD000077).

Burkman, R. T. (2007). Contraception and family planning. In A. H. DeCherney & L. Nathan (Eds). *Current Considerations and Treatment in Obstetrics and Gynecology* (10th ed.). Columbus, OH: McGraw-Hill.

Chang, D. & Blakemore, K. (2007). Fetal assessment. In K. B. Fortner et al. (Eds). *The Johns Hopkins Manual of Gynecology and Obstetrics*. Philadelphia: Lippincott Williams & Wilkins.

Coad, J. & Dunstall, M. (2011). Physiological adaptation to pregnancy. In J. Coad & M. Dunstall (Eds), *Anatomy & Physiology for Midwives*, pp. 257–288. London, England: Elsevier/Churchill Livingstone.

Crombleholme, W. R. (2009). Obstetrics. In S. J. McPhee & M. A. Papadakis (Eds). *Current Medical Diagnosis and Treatment*. Columbus, OH: McGraw-Hill.

Dalton, M. (2012). Domestic violence and sexual assault. In D. K. Edmonds (Ed), *Dewhurst's Textbook of Obstetrics & Gynaecology* (6th ed.), pp. 798–804. Oxford: John Wiley & Son.

Huppertz, B. & Kingdom, J. C. P. (2012). The placenta and fetal membranes. In D. K. Edmonds (Ed), *Dewhurst's Textbook of Obstetrics & Gynaecology* (6th ed.), pp. 16–25. Oxford: John Wiley & Son.

Jackson, H., Melvin, C. & Downe, S. (2007). Midwives and the foetal nuchal cord: A survey of practices and perceptions. *Journal of Midwifery & Women's Health, 52*(1), 49–55.

Knuppel, R. A. (2007). Maternal-placental-foetal unit: Foetal and early neonatal physiology. In A. H. DeCherney & L. Nathan (Eds). *Current Considerations and Treatment in Obstetrics and Gynecology* (10th ed.). Columbus, OH: McGraw-Hill.

Kumar, S. (2012). Fetal anomalies. In D. K. Edmonds (Ed.), *Dewhurst's Textbook of Obstetrics & Gynaecology* (6th ed.). Oxford: John Wiley & Son.

Kumar, M., Das, S. & Kumar, B. (2007). Amniotic band syndrome. *Ultrasound, 15*(2), 96–98.

Lumley, J., et al. (2009). Periconceptional supplementation with folate and/or multivitamins for preventing neural tube defects. *Cochrane Database of Systematic Reviews, 2009*(1), (CD001056).

Moyer, V., et al. (2009). Late versus early surgical correction for congenital diaphragmatic hernia in newborn infants. *Cochrane Database of Systematic Reviews, 2009*(1), (CD001695).

Neilson, J. P. (2009). Ultrasound for foetal assessment in early pregnancy. *Cochrane Database of Systematic Reviews, 2009*(1), (CD000182).

Peroviá, M., Garalejiá, E., Gojniá, M., et al. (2011). Sensitivity and specificity of ultrasonography as a screening tool for gestational diabetes mellitus. *Journal of Maternal–Fetal & Neonatal Medicine, 25*(8), 1348–1353.

Petrozella, L. N., Dashe, J. S., McIntire, D. D., et al. (2011). Clinical significance of borderline amniotic fluid index and oligohydramnios in preterm pregnancy. *Obstetrics & Gynecology, 117*(2, Pt. 1), 338–342.

Reed, R., Barnes, M. & Allan, J. (2009). Nuchal cords: Sharing the evidence with parents. *British Journal of Midwifery, 17*(2), 106–110, accessed 9 February 2015, <https://dl.dropboxusercontent.com/u/19684636/Publications/2009_ncord_bjm.pdf>.

Rees, D. C. (2007). Neonatal sickle cell disease and thalassaemia. *Infant, 3*(1), 31–35.

Roberts, D. & Dalziel, S. (2009). Antenatal corticosteroids for accelerating foetal lung maturation for women at risk of preterm birth. *Cochrane Database of Systematic Reviews, 2009*(1), (CD004454).

Rogers-Adkinson, D. L. & Stuart, S. K. (2007). Collaborative services: Children experiencing neglect and the side effects of antenatal alcohol exposure. *Language, Speech, and Hearing Services in Schools, 38*(2), 149–156.

Soll, R. F. (2009). Prophylactic synthetic surfactant for preventing morbidity and mortality in preterm infants. *Cochrane Database of Systematic Reviews, 2009*(1), (CD001079).

Taylor, R. N. & Badell, M. L. (2011). The endocrinology of pregnancy. In D. G. Gardner & D. Shoback (Eds), *Greenspan's Basic & Clinical Endocrinology* (9th ed.), pp. 553–572. New York: McGraw-Hill.

Taylor, R. N. & Lebovic, D. I. (2007). The endocrinology of pregnancy. In Gardner, D. G. & Shoback, D. (Eds). *Greenspan's Basic and Clinical Endocrinology* (8th ed.). New York: McGraw-Hill.

Thilo, E. H. & Rosenberg, A. A. (2011). The newborn infant. In W. Hay, M. J. Levin, J. M. Sondheimer, et al. (Eds), *Current Diagnosis & Treatment Pediatrics* (20th ed.), pp. 1–63. New York: McGraw-Hill Publishing.

Zeitler, P. S., Travers, S. H., Nadaou, K., et al. (2011). Endocrine disorders. In W. Hay, M. J. Levin, J. M. Sondheimer, et al. (Eds), *Current Diagnosis & Treatment Pediatrics* (20th ed.), pp. 943–983. New York: McGraw-Hill Publishing.

Suggested reading

East, C., et al. (2009). Vibroacoustic stimulation for foetal assessment in labour in the presence of a nonreassuring foetal heart rate trace. *Cochrane Database of Systematic Reviews*, (1), (CD004664).

Chapter 10

Psychological and physiological changes of pregnancy

Previous chapters discussed the anatomy and physiology of women. This chapter adds information about the physical and psychological changes that occur in both a woman and her partner during pregnancy. Knowing such information can help you protect the health of both women and their growing baby for the next 9 months.

LEARNING OBJECTIVES

After mastering the contents of this chapter, you should be able to:

1. Describe common psychological and physiological changes that occur with pregnancy and the relationship of the changes to pregnancy diagnosis.
2. Use critical thinking to analyse how the physiological and psychological changes of pregnancy affect family functioning, and develop ways to make nursing care more family-centred.
3. Assess a woman's psychological and physiological changes that have occurred with pregnancy.
4. Identify potential problems related to the psychological and physiological changes of pregnancy.
5. Identify expected outcomes for a family's psychological and physical adaptation to pregnancy.
6. Plan nursing care for the woman and her family related to the changes and diagnosis of pregnancy.
7. Implement health promotion related to the expected changes of pregnancy.
8. Evaluate outcomes of care.
9. Identify areas of nursing care related to the psychological and physiological changes of pregnancy that could benefit from additional research or application of evidence-based practice.
10. Integrate knowledge of the psychological and physiological changes of pregnancy to achieve quality child and family health nursing care.

KEY TERMS

- ballottement
- Braxton Hicks contractions
- Chadwick's sign
- couvade syndrome
- diastasis
- Goodell's sign
- Hegar's sign
- lightening
- linea nigra
- melasma
- Montgomery's tubercles
- multipara
- operculum
- primigravida
- quickening
- striae gravidarum

CASE STUDY

Lauren Maxwell has come to your clinic for her first antenatal visit. She tells you she missed her period 4 weeks ago and immediately took a home pregnancy test. She's both excited and anxious that it was positive, because she and her partner, John, have been trying for several months to get pregnant. Lauren and John are particularly worried about doing the right things during pregnancy and becoming good parents. They are keen to learn as much as they can during the pregnancy.

In addition to the positive home pregnancy test, Lauren presents with amenorrhoea, breast tenderness, fatigue and morning sickness. She is interested in knowing when she will begin to look pregnant and what she can do for the morning sickness.

CASE STUDY QUESTIONS

1. What psychological and physical development challenges of pregnancy will Lauren need to complete?
2. How can health professionals support Lauren in addressing her concerns about being a good parent?

Women and their partners are often interested in learning more about the physical or psychological changes that pregnancy brings, because these changes verify the reality of pregnancy and its subsequent progress.

Physiological changes of pregnancy occur gradually but eventually affect all the organ systems of a woman's body. The changes are necessary to allow a woman to be able to provide oxygen and nutrients for her growing baby as well as extra nutrients for her own increased metabolism during the pregnancy. They also prepare her body for labour and birth and for lactation (breastfeeding) once the baby is born. Because the physiological changes that occur with pregnancy are extensive, women are usually happy to learn that they are also temporary. When pregnancy ends, a woman's body will return virtually to its prepregnant state.

Psychological changes of pregnancy occur in response not only to the physiological alterations that are happening but also to the increased responsibility associated with welcoming a new and completely dependent person into a family.

Despite the magnitude of some of these changes, they are all extensions of normal physiology and psychology; pregnancy represent a time of wellness, not of illness. A major responsibility of healthcare personnel caring for pregnant women and their families is to help the family maintain a state of wellness throughout the pregnancy and into early parenthood (Crombleholme, 2013) or identify early any deviations that may occur.

HEALTHY ADAPTATION TO PREGNANCY

Assessment

Ideally, assessment for pregnancy begins before the pregnancy with preconception counselling. The preconception assessment is an evaluation of a woman's overall health status which includes nutritional intake (e.g. sufficient intake of folic acid and protein) and lifestyle (e.g. drinking, recreational drugs and smoking habits); identification of any potential problems (e.g. pre-existing medical conditions); and identifying a woman's understanding and expectations of conception, pregnancy and parenthood.

In early pregnancy, the health professional's role is to establish a partnership with the woman, a relationship that ensures she is central to her care. Woman-centred care is "focused on the woman's individual, unique needs, expectations and aspirations, rather than the needs of institutions or maternity services professionals. This type of care recognises the woman's right to self-determination in terms of choice, control and continuity of care" (NHMRC, 2010, p 14).

Within this trusting relationship, information sharing takes place to enable informed decision-making to occur. It is expected that during the woman's pregnancy the health professional will:

- Assess the woman's health and nutritional status
- Assess the wellbeing of the developing baby
- Document the physiological adaptations and the family's psychological adaptations to pregnancy and
- Identify and refer any abnormal findings throughout her pregnancy.

Physical findings are gained through the health history, physical assessment and laboratory tests. Assessment of a woman's psychological health is usually performed through interviewing and will enable the health professional to gain some insight into the woman's social, cultural, family and personal influences that could affect her adaptation to pregnancy.

Nursing considerations

Examples of nursing considerations involving the changes that occur with pregnancy include:

- Anxiety related to unexpected pregnancy
- Altered breathing pattern related to respiratory system changes of pregnancy
- Disturbed body image related to weight gain with pregnancy
- Knowledge deficit related to normal changes of pregnancy
- Imbalanced nutrition, less than body requirements, related to early morning nausea.

Planning nursing care in connection with the physiological and psychological changes of pregnancy should involve a plan to review these types of concerns with the woman. Reliable resources on antenatal care should be provided. For example:

- Home Birth Aotearoa <www.homebirth.org.nz>
- Lead Maternity Carers Freephone New Zealand: 0800 MUM 2 BE (0800 686 223)
- Mothers Online <www.mothersonline.co.nz>
- National Institute for Health and Clinical Excellence <www.nice.org.uk>
- National Support Team Parents Centre <www.parentscentre.org.nz>
- NHMRC National Guidance on Collaborative Maternity Care <www.nhmrc.gov.au>
- Plunket <www.plunket.org.nz>
- Plunket Freephone New Zealand: 0800 933 922
- The 3centres guidelines <www.3centres.com.au>
- The Women's Pregnancy and Birth Information Sheets <www.thewomens.org.au>.

The changes in pregnancy are many and often appear insignificant, but when they occur in combination they could be a substantial concern.

Body image changes caused by changing body shape and weight gain can also impact on how a woman feels about herself and her self-image. At the beginning of pregnancy, she may feel constantly nauseated. Towards the end, the extra weight and the strain of waiting may make her feel tired and short of breath. Endocrine changes can make her feel emotional and out of control. She may never have been concerned with her health before; now, every month (and towards the end of pregnancy, every week), she reports to a healthcare provider for antenatal assessments. She may worry that she will never lose all the weight she has gained, that the stretch marks on her abdomen will remain forever and that she will always be as tired or as nauseated as she feels during various stages of her pregnancy.

Women need assistance to voice their concerns about their physical and psychological changes. They may need suggestions on exercise and nutrition and where to find support and information. Educating women on the assessments to be undertaken during antenatal visits can be instrumental to guiding a woman safely through a pregnancy, and enabling her to take control of future healthcare concerns.

PSYCHOLOGICAL CHANGES OF PREGNANCY

Pregnancy is such a huge change in a woman's life that it brings about more psychological changes than any other life event besides puberty (Rojas, Wood & Blakemore, 2007). A woman's attitude towards a pregnancy depends a great deal on psychological aspects such as the environment in which she was raised, the messages about pregnancy her family communicated to her as a child, the society and culture in which she lives as an adult and whether the pregnancy has come at a good time or less than a good time in her life (Darby, 2007).

Social influences

Today, healthcare settings view pregnancy as a healthy event in a family's life. Health professionals have played an important role in helping bring about this change by convincing agencies that long-standing protocols of the 20th century that separated women from their families are not appropriate. As a result, from the early 1960s, instead of coming alone for antenatal care, women now bring their families. Instead of being given general anaesthetics so they can "sleep through" labour and birth, they participate actively in the experience. Women can make choices about pain relief, positions to birth, method of birth, place of birth and how she wants to feed her baby.

How well a pregnant woman and her partner feel during pregnancy and childbirth is related to their cultural background, their personal experiences and the experiences of friends and relatives. Women are also influenced by the current public philosophy of childbirth and childbirth education and information that highlights social issues that are seen by the public as priority. People's opinions about adolescent pregnancies, "late in life" pregnancies or whether women who have sex with women should have children, have been highlighted and have changed markedly over time. Informing women about their healthcare options and continuing to work with other healthcare providers contribute in the "demedicalisation" of childbirth. Midwives and nurses can assist in making pregnancy and childbirth a natural, normal and empowering event for women and their families.

Cultural influences

A woman's cultural background may strongly influence how active a role she wants to take in her pregnancy, because certain beliefs and taboos may place restrictions on her behaviour and activities (Andrews & Boyle, 2011). To learn about the beliefs of a particular woman and her partner, it is important to ask at antenatal visits if there is anything they believe should or should not be done to make the pregnancy successful and keep the baby healthy. Supporting these beliefs and helping to dispel myths shows respect for the individuality of a woman and her knowledge of good health.

The role of the midwife and nurse is to maintain cultural safety for all individuals, to listen and to hear what the family want and need for their pregnancy. The midwife is required to provide contemporary and accessible information that enables the woman and her family to make informed decisions about her care (Pairman et al., 2014).

Family influences

The family of origin has a huge influence on the pregnant woman's perception of pregnancy, birth and the rearing of children. Family stability or instability affects the woman and her future choices and beliefs about her ability to adapt to motherhood, her self-confidence and successfully raising a family. Women with disabilities may have specific concerns. They will need careful assessment regarding their feelings about having a baby along with assessment of special adjustments to make during their pregnancy (Smeltzer, 2007). However, these can all be overcome with good support, including family, friends and social services.

Individual influences

Maternal role attainment and transition occurs during pregnancy and postpartum, the transition to motherhood is significant and researchers have discussed this time as one of crisis for woman (Mercer, 1986; Rubin, 1984; Tulman & Fawcett, 2002). According to contemporary midwifery, however, this is a time that is commonly accepted as normal, a healthy event that requires an accepted transition (Parratt & Fahy, 2011). Most women welcome the experience to become mothers but it is also a time of high anxiety and depression (Tulman & Fawcett, 2003; Mortazavi et al., 2013). A woman's ability to cope with or adapt to stress plays a major role in how she will resolve this time of transition and adapt to the new life contingencies that are coming (see Box 10.1).

The woman's awareness of her own needs and ability to provide support for them and the competing needs of her new baby and family are vital in achieving this important transition. Discussing these are important in her pregnancy

BOX 10.1 ✻ Focus on evidence-based practice

Reducing maternal stress

Pregnancy can be a stress-filled time because of the added responsibility that a coming child will bring. At the same time, finding time to relax can be difficult for busy women. Researchers, who were interested in whether teaching a pregnant woman to truly relax by using guided imagery could have an effect on her fetus as well as provide additional relaxation for her, recorded fetal responses to induced maternal relaxation during the 32nd week of pregnancy for 100 women. Changes documented in the fetus over an 18-minute relaxation time period were decreased fetal heart rate, increased fetal heart rate variability, and lower umbilical and uterine artery resistance. The researchers concluded that induced relaxation effects can be noted in the fetus. Such effects as creating reduced artery resistance could help improve fetal circulation for a compromised fetus.

Could you use the above results to help a pregnant woman plan to take deliberate time every day to rest and relax?

Source: DiPietro, J. A., et al. (2008). Fetal responses to induced maternal relaxation during pregnancy. *Biological Psychology, 77*(1), 11–19.

journey and preparation for motherhood. Being able to articulate her own losses and gains from being single, a couple and now becoming a mother enables her to plan and balance her future needs and requirements. These may include time out, support, playtime, work, childcare and so on. The free Mindfulness Meditation App from beyondblue and Smiling Mind (2014) (www.mindthebump.org.au) helps individuals and couples and supports their mental and emotional wellbeing in preparation for having a baby and becoming new parents.

PSYCHOLOGICAL TASKS OF PREGNANCY

During the 9 months of pregnancy, a woman and her partner run a gamut of emotions ranging from the surprise at finding out she is pregnant (or wishing she were not), the pleasure and acceptance of the fact as they begin to identify with the coming child, the worry for themselves and the child, as well as the acute impatience near the end of pregnancy (see Table 10.1). Once the child is born, surprise and excitement may be experienced again as the reality sinks in.

From a physiological standpoint, it takes 9 months for the fetus to mature and be prepared for life outside the protective uterine environment. From a psychological standpoint, this period provides the woman and her family with time to prepare emotionally. How well a woman adjusts to the potential stress of pregnancy can affect her relationship with the child and may even influence whether she is able to carry the pregnancy to term. These psychological changes are frequently termed "guaranteeing safe passage" for the fetus.

TABLE 10.1 Common psychosocial changes that occur with pregnancy

Psychosocial change	Description
First trimester Task: Accepting the pregnancy	The woman and her partner both spend time recovering from shock of learning they are pregnant and concentrate on what it feels like to be pregnant. A common reaction is ambivalence, or feeling both pleased and not pleased about the pregnancy.
Second trimester Task: Accepting the baby	The woman and her partner move through emotions such as narcissism and introversion as they concentrate on what it will feel like to be a parent. Role-playing and increased dreaming are common.
Third trimester Task: Preparing for the baby and end of pregnancy	The woman and her partner prepare clothing and sleeping arrangements for the baby but also grow impatient with pregnancy as they ready themselves for birth.

First trimester: Accepting the pregnancy

The first task of a woman and her partner during the first trimester is to accept the reality of the pregnancy.

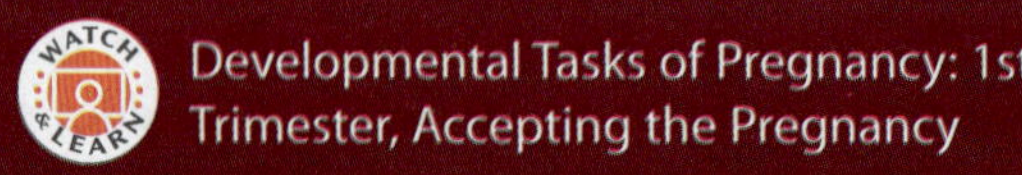

The woman

Most cultures structure their celebrations around important life events—coming of age, marriages, birthdays and deaths. These all have rituals to help individuals take a step forwards or accept the coming change in their lives. A diagnosis of pregnancy is a similar rite of passage. This aura of initiation into one of the large mysteries of life gives special meaning to the healthcare visit in which the diagnosis of pregnancy is confirmed, making it more than an ordinary visit to a healthcare facility. Receiving confirmation of pregnancy, at her healthcare provider's office, makes the mother feel "more pregnant".

The availability of reproductive planning measures today, in theory, would seem to prevent the diagnosis of pregnancy from being a surprise. Every pregnancy is a surprise to some extent, however, either because a woman had not planned on becoming pregnant or because she had been looking forward to being pregnant but the reality of it happening came too quickly. If pregnancy announces itself with more reliable signs than a missed period, slight breast tenderness, or vague nausea and tiredness, women could become more certain how they feel about being pregnant sooner. Home pregnancy test kits have helped women in this regard by confirming pregnancy as early as the first missed menstrual period. Until it is verified by a home test or a healthcare visit, however, the uncertainty of the symptoms makes pregnancy only a vague theoretical possibility that leaves room for denial. As almost all medications cross the placenta and many can cause fetal harm, the earlier that a woman realises that she is pregnant, the sooner she can safeguard fetal health by discontinuing all medications not specifically prescribed or approved by her doctor or midwife (Cunningham et al., 2014).

Often women immediately experience something less than pleasure and closer to disappointment, or anxiety or a feeling of ambivalence at the news that they are pregnant. Ambivalence towards pregnancy does not mean that positive feelings counteract negative feelings so the woman is left feeling nothing towards her pregnancy.

Instead, it refers to the interwoven feelings of wanting and not wanting that can exist at high levels. When talking to pregnant women, emphasise that this ambivalence is normal. Otherwise, if a poor outcome should result, a woman may recall her ambivalence and feel guilty.

By the fourth month and feeling the baby's movements, women exchange ambivalence and guilt with anticipation and feelings of protection towards the baby. Some healthcare plans provide for a routine ultrasound at 4 months of pregnancy. Seeing a beating heart or a fetal outline on the monitor screen during an ultrasound can be a major step in promoting acceptance (Matsui & Gardiner, 2007).

The partner

Once partners, whether male or female, were forgotten persons in the childbearing process. Today, it is recognised that all partners are important and should be encouraged to play an emotional role in the pregnancy. This means that, as a woman adapts to pregnancy, her partner may go through some of the same psychological changes (Finnbogadottir, Svalenius & Persson, 2003).

For partners, accepting the pregnancy means not only accepting the certainty of the pregnancy and the reality of the child to come but also accepting the woman in her changed state. Partners' feelings regarding the pregnancy often vary. Some partners are proud and happy about the pregnancy. However, partners may experience overwhelming feelings, with concerns about financial loss. Some may experience a feeling close to jealousy of the growing baby, who, although not yet physically apparent, seems to be taking up a great deal of the woman's time and thought.

Partners also experience ambivalence, sometimes more so than pregnant women. The feeling of ambivalence can be compounded if partners are afraid to voice their concerns. This happens if they do not want to intensify the pregnant woman's anxieties by appearing anxious themselves. Partners may also feel ambivalent if they are not well prepared for parenthood or have had little experience with children. Finnbogadottir, Svalenius and Persson (2003) in their study on first time father's experiences reported that fathers experienced a variety of feelings including exclusion, unreality, inadequacy and responsibility. Some of the partners were disregarded by health professionals which exacerbated their feelings of ambivalence. It is the role of health professionals to assist partners to resolve some of these issues and provide an outlet for them to discuss their concerns and offer information.

CASE STUDY QUESTION

3. Due to her morning sickness, Lauren sometimes feels ambivalent about being pregnant. What psychological tasks would you like to see her complete during the first trimester of pregnancy?

a. Asks why morning sickness occurs and if treatments are available
b. Accepts the fact that she's pregnant
c. Discusses names for her baby with her partner
d. Asks about body changes in the first trimester

Second trimester: Accepting the baby

As soon as fetal movements can be felt, psychological responses of both partners are apt to change.

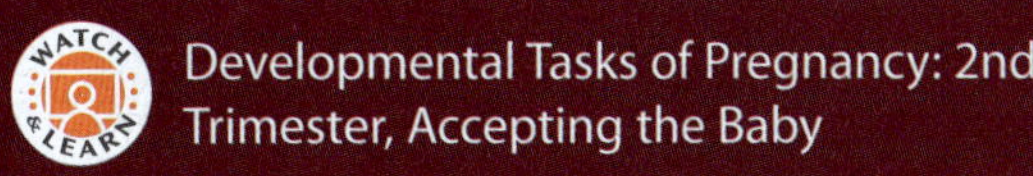

Developmental Tasks of Pregnancy: 2nd Trimester, Accepting the Baby

The woman

During the second trimester, the psychological task of a woman is to accept that she is having a baby, a second step to accepting the pregnancy. This change usually happens at **quickening,** or the first moment a woman feels fetal movement. Until a woman experiences for herself this proof of the child's existence, she may think of the life inside her as an integral part of herself rather than as a separate entity. She knows it is there; she eats to meet its needs and takes special vitamins to help it grow, but it seems more like just another part of her body. With quickening, however, the fetus assumes a separate identity. She begins to imagine how she will feel at the birth. She begins to imagine herself as a mother, perhaps teaching her child the alphabet or how to ride a bicycle. This anticipatory role-playing is an important activity for mid-pregnancy. It leads her to a larger concept of her condition and helps her realise that not only is she pregnant but also there is a child inside her.

Women often use the term "it" to refer to the child inside them. This does not mean that they have not yet accepted the pregnancy or still consider the baby an inanimate object. Some parents want the gender of the child to be a surprise at birth, while it is more common today for couples to find out at their 20-week ultrasound scan. Seeing their child on the ultrasound scan enables them to realise the reality of the big event that will inevitably occur for most women.

Most women can pinpoint a moment during the pregnancy when they knew definitely that they wanted their child. For a woman who carefully planned the pregnancy, this moment of awareness may occur as soon as she recovers from the surprise of learning she has actually conceived. For others, it may come when she announces the news to her parents and hears them express their joy or when she sees a look of pride on her partner's face. It might be the moment of quickening, when she realises that the fetus inside her is not passive but is an active being. Shopping for baby clothes for the first time, setting up the bassinet, seeing a blurry outline on an ultrasound screen; any of these small actions may suddenly make the coming baby seem real and desired (see Fig. 10.1).

On the other hand, accepting the baby as a welcome family addition might not come until labour has begun or after several hours of labour. It might even be the moment a woman first hears her baby's cry or first touches or feeds

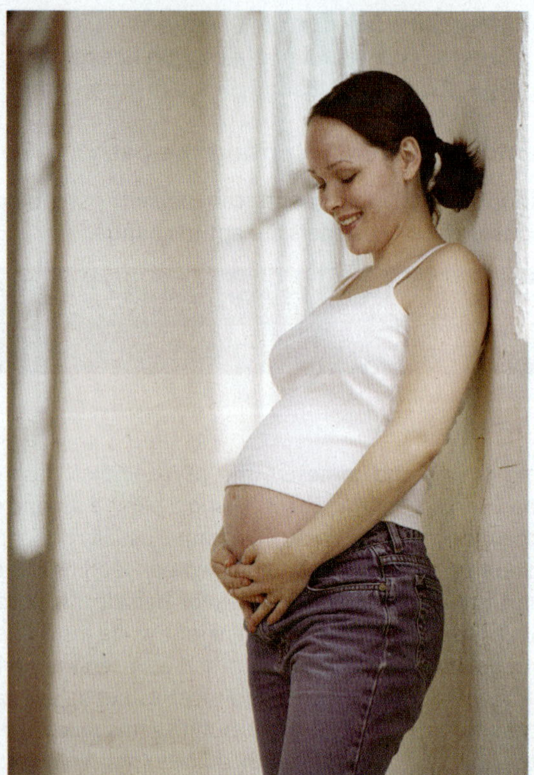

FIGURE 10.1 A growing abdomen and fluttering fetal movements help to make a pregnancy a reality.

her newborn. If a woman has a complication of pregnancy, is having financial difficulties or lacks emotional support, it could take several weeks after the baby is born for her to accept her new reality and come to terms with motherhood (see Box 10.2). The pregnancy hormonal changes are powerful and affect women's health both physically and emotionally. There is no clear understanding why some women become depressed or anxious when others do not. Some theories suggest it is brain chemistry, or a reaction to the hormonal changes occurring in the pregnant body. Everyday activities may suddenly get on top of some women and then there are specific circumstances that make it more difficult to cope for example:

- Previous depression or mental health problems, or depression during pregnancy
- Not having a supportive partner, or not having family or friends living close by
- Troubles with money, housing, work or their relationship
- A difficult birth or health problems afterwards
- Having a baby who was born prematurely or is not well
- Finding it hard to breastfeed
- Sad memories being stirred up, such as the death of one of your parents when you were a child (McCauley-Elsom & Hopkins, 2011; Paradice, 2002).

For some women these changes are so tremendous that they can lead not only to poor acceptance of the child but also to postpartum depression (Westdahl et al., 2007).

Asking the woman questions about her pregnancy and listening to the answers will provide cues to how she may be adapting and accepting of the pregnancy and if she requires further supports.

BOX 10.2 ✻ Events that could contribute to difficulty accepting a pregnancy

- Learning that the pregnancy is a multiple one
- Learning that the fetus has a developmental abnormality
- Pregnancy less than 1 year after a previous one
- Relocation during pregnancy (involves a need to find new support people)
- Moving away from the family or back to the family for economic reasons
- Role reversal (a previously supporting person who becomes dependent or vice versa)
- Job loss
- Marital infidelity
- Illness in self, partner or a relative
- Loss of a significant other
- Complications of pregnancy such as severe hypertension
- Having friends or relatives who have had children born with health disorders
- Series of devaluing experiences (e.g. failure in school or work)
- History of previous miscarriages, fertility problems, traumatic births
- Previous fetal or neonatal loss
- History of rape, incest or domestic violence

The partner

As the woman starts to prepare for the coming baby, the partner also experiences a time of transition as they also seem to experience psychological, social and for some physical changes during pregnancy. Finnbogadottir, Svalenius & Persson (2003, p. 98) express this as a "transition from being a man to being a father", a "life world" change that occurs during their partner's pregnancy. It is therefore imperative to have partners and fathers involved in antenatal care. They can participate in supporting the woman to make important decisions and become informed about the care that will be provided as well as important environmental issues that may impact on the health and wellbeing of both the woman and the baby during pregnancy (AHMAC, 2012). These could include lifestyle factors as diet, exercise, smoking and drug usage. Antenatal and childbirth health education and information needs to be available to women and their partners. Other vital information such as mental health and immunisation and the available interventions should also be available (AHMAC, 2012). Fathers and partners need to be actively involved in the care of the woman and their unborn children so that their full participation in parenting will be able to continue throughout infancy, childhood and adolescence (McLeod et al., 2014).

Third trimester: Preparing for parenthood

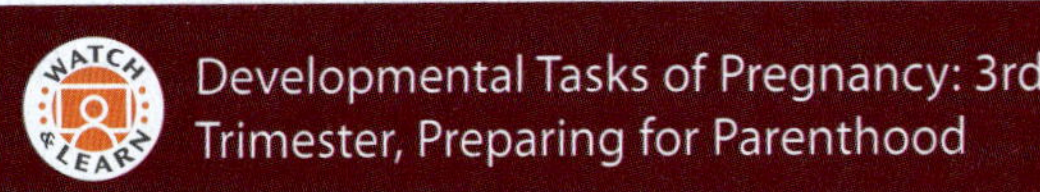

During the third trimester, couples usually begin "nest-building" activities, such as planning the infant's sleeping arrangements, buying clothes, choosing a name for the baby and "ensuring safe passage" by learning about birth. These preparations are evidence that women are completing the third trimester task of pregnancy or preparing for parenthood.

Couples at this point are interested in attending antenatal classes or preparation for childbirth classes. Certain external life contingencies may slow the mental work of pregnancy on the part of a woman or her partner. It is helpful to ask a couple what specifically they are doing to get ready for birth to see if they are interested in taking such a class and to document how well prepared they will be for the baby's arrival.

During antenatal visits, ask such questions as, "How does your partner feel about you being pregnant?" or "Has anything changed in your home life since you last came to the clinic?" to reveal if any situation that could interfere with bonding is present. It is unrealistic to believe that one healthcare professional has all the solutions to the problems that couples reveal when asked these questions. A multidisciplinary approach (e.g. referral to the nutritionist, nurse practitioner or social services) is often necessary to help solve some of these multifaceted problems.

It is helpful for most couples to attend childbirth education classes or classes on preparing for parenthood, as attending these classes can help a couple accept the pregnancy, expose them to other parents as role models and provide practical information about pregnancy and childcare. It is best if these classes are conducted in small groups so they can meet the individual needs of couples. (See Chapter 14 for more information on childbirth education classes and planning for parenthood.)

Additional preparation work to complete in pregnancy

In addition to the three main tasks of pregnancy, more subtle emotions also surface or need to be worked through.

Reworking developmental tasks

An important task to complete during pregnancy is working through previous life experiences. Needs and wishes that have been repressed for years may surface to be studied and reworked, for some to an extreme extent. Primary among these life experiences is a woman's relationship with her parents, particularly her mother. For the first time in her life, she finds she can empathise with her mother and the way her mother used to worry when she came home later than expected. The pregnant woman has already begun to worry about her child, feeling protective towards her baby. Her mother may become more significant to her and changes in their relationship can often develop.

For a woman to work through past fears and conflicts of this kind, she may need a variety of opportunities to discuss or think about them, from spending time alone thinking about them, to discussing them with others, partner, friends, or healthcare professionals and qualified counsellors. If the feelings are negative and/or traumatic, they may impact on the woman's ability to transition to motherhood.

Fear of being separated from family or dying are common childhood fears that can be revived during pregnancy. A clue that might signal a woman's distress over this could be, "Am I ever going to make it through this?" This expression might mean simply that she is tired of her backache, but it also might be a plea for reassurance that she will survive this event in her life.

A woman needs to have confidence in those who provide healthcare for her during pregnancy, so that she can express some of these disturbing thoughts and work through them. As a rule, a woman who is comfortable seeking information experiences less anxiety than one who feels unable to do this.

A pregnant woman's partner needs to do the same reworking of old values and forgotten developmental tasks. A man may rethink his relationship with his father to understand better what kind of father he will be. Some men may have had emotionally distant fathers and wish to be more emotionally available to their own children. These men have to reconcile feelings towards their fathers and learn a new pattern of behaviour.

Role-playing and fantasising

Another step in preparing for parenthood is role-playing or fantasising about what it will be like to be a parent. Just as a child learns what to do by following her mother, a pregnant woman begins to spend time with other pregnant women or mothers of young children to learn how to be a mother. She is drawn into a world of talk about babies and pregnancy with these women. A pregnant woman may offer to babysit for a neighbour or relative so she can "practise" caring for a new baby. As a part of the role-playing process, women's dreams tend to focus on the pregnancy and concerns about keeping herself and her coming child safe.

Although role-playing may be difficult for a pregnant teen who has not yet made the transition to adulthood, it is important in helping her become a mother. If the only role models she has are other girls her age, who typically are not interested in the commitment to mothering—or if her role model is her own mother, who might be unable to cope with problems such as poverty, too many children or an ineffectual partner—a worry is that the young girl will assume the same role. Try to locate good role models (in classes for mothers, at the healthcare agency or from a social agency) for adolescents so they can find a good maternal role to copy and integrate into their own behaviour.

The father-to-be also has role-playing to do during pregnancy. He has to imagine himself as the father of a boy or as the father of a girl. A first-time father may have to change his view of himself from being a carefree individual to being a significant member of a family unit. Opportunities to join in conversations with other fathers or join the 'daddy's club' will offer occasions for the first time father to hear other fathers' experiences (Finnbogadottir, Svalenius & Persson, 2003). If he already is a father, he has to cast aside a father-of-one identity to accept a father-of-two image and so forth. Many fathers want or need to take on the role of nurturer but have had little or no experience caring for newborns or infants. Newborn care classes provided before or after the birth can help fathers grow comfortable with this role.

Other support persons who will have an active role in raising the child (e.g. grandparents, close friends) also have to work out their roles in regard to the pregnancy and impending parenthood. This may be particularly difficult, because the roles for these support persons may not be clearly defined and no role model may be apparent.

Emotional responses to pregnancy

Because of all the tasks that need to be worked through during a pregnancy, emotional responses can vary greatly. Common reactions include grief, narcissism, introversion or extroversion, body image and boundary concerns, couvade syndrome (somatic experiences of father during pregnancy simulating those of the pregnant mother), stress, mood swings and changes in sexual desire. It is helpful to caution a pregnant woman and her partner about common changes they may expect. Otherwise they can misinterpret the woman's mood swings, decreased sexual interest, introversion or narcissism not as changes of pregnancy but as a loss of interest in their relationship.

Grief

The thought that grief could be associated with such a positive process as childbirth seems at first incongruent. But before a woman can take on a mothering role, she has to give up or alter her present roles. She will never be a daughter in exactly the same way again. She will never be as irresponsible and carefree as she is now again. She may not even sleep soundly for the next few years. She must incorporate her new role as a mother into her other roles as a daughter, wife or friend. Her partner must incorporate a new role as a father into his other roles of son, husband or friend.

Narcissism

Self-centredness (narcissism) is generally an early reaction to pregnancy. A woman who previously was barely conscious of her body suddenly begins to concentrate on how her body feels or reacts to changes that are occurring. She dresses so her pregnancy will or will not show, making dressing a time-consuming, mirror-studying procedure. Nutrition and diet changes for some become central as there can be anxiety about what to eat and drink. Daily events may lose their importance as she focuses on her new role of growing a baby.

Narcissism may be manifested by a change in activity. A woman may stop playing tennis, for example, even though her doctor tells her it will do no harm in moderation. She may criticise her partner's driving, although it never bothered her before. She does these things to unconsciously protect her body and her baby. Men may demonstrate the same behaviour by reducing risky activities such as mountain biking, trying to ensure that they will be present to raise their child.

This need of a woman to protect her body has implications for nursing care. It means she may regard unnecessary nudity as a threat to her body (be sure to drape properly for pelvic and abdominal examinations). She may resent casual remarks such as, "Oh my, you've gained weight" (a threat to her appearance) or "You don't like milk?" (a threat to her judgement).

There is a tendency to organise health instructions during pregnancy around the baby: "Be sure and keep this appointment. You want to have a healthy baby." "You really ought to eat more protein for the baby's sake." This approach may be particularly inappropriate early in pregnancy, before the fetus stirs and before a woman is convinced not only that she is pregnant but also that there is a baby inside her. At early stages, a woman may be much more interested in doing things for herself because it is her body, her tiredness and her wellbeing that will be directly affected ("Eat protein because it keeps your fingernails from breaking" or "Protein will give you more energy").

Introversion versus extroversion

Introversion, or turning inwards to concentrate on oneself and one's body, is a common finding during pregnancy. Some women, however, react in an entirely opposite fashion and become more extroverted. They become more active, appear healthier than ever before and are more outgoing. This tends to occur in women who are finding unexpected fulfilment in pregnancy, perhaps who had seriously doubted that they would be lucky enough or fertile enough to conceive. Although such a woman may become more varied in her interests during pregnancy, she may be puzzling to those around her who previously regarded her as quiet and self-contained.

Body image and boundary

Body image (the way your body appears to yourself) and body boundary (a zone of separation you perceive between yourself and objects or other people) change during pregnancy as a woman begins to envision herself as a mother. In addition to being a daughter or wife, she begins to see herself becoming "bigger" in many different ways. This change in body image is part of the basis for narcissism and introversion. Changes in concept of body boundaries leads to a firmer distinction between objects, yet at the same time her body boundary is perceived as extremely vulnerable, as if her body were delicate and easily harmed. This change in boundary perception is so startling that pregnant women may walk far away from an object such as a table to avoid bumping against it.

CASE STUDY QUESTION

4. Lauren is aware that she's been showing some narcissistic tendencies since becoming pregnant. Which of her actions best describes narcissism?
   a. She feels pulled in multiple directions
   b. Her thoughts tend to be mainly about herself
   c. She feels a need to sleep a lot more than usual
   d. She often feels "numb" or as if she's taken a narcotic

Stress

Because pregnancy brings with it such a major role change, it can cause extreme stress in a woman. This stress of pregnancy, like any stress, can make it difficult for a woman to make decisions, be as aware of her surroundings as usual or maintain time management with her usual degree of skill. Determining whether the twinges she feels in her back are beginning labour contractions or just backache and whether she should call her primary care provider are difficult decisions to make for someone who is stressed. This may cause people who were dependent on a woman before pregnancy to feel neglected, because now that she is pregnant she seems to have strength only for herself. If a woman was in an abusive relationship before the pregnancy, the increased stress of pregnancy is apt to cause even more abuse. Asking whether intimate partner abuse has ever occurred in the past to help predict if it could occur during pregnancy is an important part of antenatal interviewing (Casanueva & Martin, 2007).

To help families keep their perspective for the full length of a pregnancy, remind them that any decrease in the ability to function that happens to a pregnant woman is a reaction to the stress of pregnancy, not the pregnancy itself. Many non-pregnant women and men function at work under just as much stress because of marital discord or a loved one's illness or death and have just as much difficulty with making decisions. Pregnancy may actually be less stressful than those situations because of its predictable 9 month outcome.

A woman with fewer support people around her almost automatically has more difficulty adjusting to and accepting a pregnancy and a new child than do women who have more support. A woman who begins a pregnancy with a strong support person and then loses that person through trauma, illness, separation or divorce needs special attention in regard to loneliness and depression. Evaluate her carefully regarding how she is managing and give her extra support because her feeling of loss is likely to be extremely acute. A loss of this kind has the potential to interfere not only with her own health but also with parent–child bonding. Knowing that she has supportive healthcare providers she can call on when needed is the one thing that may make this pregnancy tolerable.

Couvade syndrome

Many men experience physical symptoms such as nausea, vomiting and backache to the same degree or even more intensely than their partners during a pregnancy. These symptoms apparently result from stress, anxiety and empathy for the pregnant woman. This is common enough that it has been given a name: **couvade syndrome**. The more the partner is involved in or attuned to the changes of the pregnancy, the more symptoms they may experience. As a woman's abdomen begins to grow, the partner may perceive himself as growing larger too, as if he is experiencing changing boundaries the same as his partner. For the most part, these are healthy happenings and require psychological attention only if the man becomes emotionally stressed or delusional (Brennan et al., 2007).

Emotional lability

Mood changes occur frequently in a pregnant woman, partly as a manifestation of narcissism (her feelings are easily hurt by remarks that would have been laughed off before) and partly because of hormonal changes, particularly the sustained increase in oestrogen and progesterone (see Box 10.3). Mood swings may be so common that they make a woman's reaction to her family and to healthcare routines unpredictable. What she finds acceptable one week she may find intolerable the next. She may cry over her children's bad table manners at one meal and find the situation amusing and even charming at the next.

BOX 10.3 ✻ Focus on family teaching

Mood swings during pregnancy

Q. Lauren Maxwell tells you she has noticed extreme mood swings since she has been pregnant. She asks you how she can reduce them.

A. Try these measures:

- Avoid fatigue, because when you are tired, your normal defences are most likely to be down.
- Reduce your level of stress by setting priorities. Ask yourself if everything you are doing really needs to be done.
- Do not let little problems grow into big ones; attack them when they first occur.
- Try to view situations from other people's perspective. They are not as involved in your pregnancy as you are. Things that do not seem important to you may be important to them.
- Let others know you are aware that you are having trouble with emotions since you became pregnant. Your family and friends will be more than willing to help you through this time if they realise that your shifting emotions are of concern to you.

Women and their partners and families need to be cautioned that such mood swings occur, beginning with early pregnancy, so that they can accept them as part of pregnancy.

Changes in sexual desire

Most women report that their sexual desire changes, at least to some degree, during pregnancy. Women who formerly were worried about becoming pregnant may truly enjoy sexual relations for the first time during pregnancy. Others might feel a loss of desire because of their oestrogen increase, or they might unconsciously view sexual relations as a threat to the fetus they must protect. Some may worry that having sexual relations could bring on early labour.

During the first trimester, most women report a decrease in libido because of the nausea, fatigue and breast tenderness that accompany early pregnancy. During the second trimester, as blood flow to the pelvic area increases to supply the placenta, libido and sexual enjoyment rise markedly. During the third trimester, sexual desire may remain high or it may decrease because of difficulty finding a comfortable position and increasing abdominal size. When a couple knows early in pregnancy that such changes may occur, they can be interpreted in the correct light (i.e. as a difference, not as loss of interest in the sexual partner). Suggestions for helping women and their partners adjust to these circumstances are discussed in Chapter 12.

Changes in the expectant family

Most parents are aware that their older children need preparation when a new baby is on the way; however, knowing that preparation is needed and being prepared to do this are two different things. For this reason, some couples appreciate suggestions from healthcare personnel regarding how this task can be accomplished. Both preschool and school-age children may need to be reassured periodically during pregnancy that a new baby will be an addition to the family and will not replace them in their parents' affection. Preparing a child for the birth of a sibling is discussed in Chapters 14 and 31.

The psychological transition to motherhood consists of acceptance, control, support and forming a family. For most women there is some loss of control over their lives, especially in early pregnancy and after the birth. There is a refocusing during the pregnancy from themselves, their self-image, to the needs of the fetus. Being pregnant for the first time situates the woman and her partner into unfamiliar territory: to assist in normalising their feelings and experiences there is a need for a mentor or mentors to help guide them through the transition (Darvill, Skirton & Farrand, 2010). The implications for practice include providing information about early pregnancy to enable couples to form more realistic expectations of the stages in pregnancy and facilitating contact between pregnant mothers to establish support networks prior to the birth.

Useful websites:

- beyondblue clinical practice guidelines (www.beyondblue.org.au)
- Perinatal mental health introductory session for nurses and midwives (http://perinatal.med.monash.edu.au).

DIAGNOSIS OF PREGNANCY

The diagnosis of pregnancy serves to estimate the date when the birth will occur and also helps predict the existence of a high-risk status. A planned pregnancy diagnosis brings a sense of fulfilment and achievement. If this is an unexpected pregnancy, however, it can result in an equally extreme crisis state.

Once the pregnancy is confirmed, most women try to eat a more nutritious diet, give up cigarette smoking and alcohol ingestion, and stop taking non-essential medications. Because a woman may not take these measures before confirmation of her pregnancy, early confirmation of pregnancy is important. If a woman does not wish to continue the pregnancy, early diagnosis is also imperative: therapeutic termination of pregnancy should always be carried out at the earliest stage possible for the safest outcome.

If a sexually active woman is scheduled for diagnostic testing that includes a pelvic x-ray you should investigate the possibility if she could be pregnant and suggest a rapid serum pregnancy test to rule this out, thereby avoiding the exposure of a fetus to radiation.

Most women who come to a healthcare facility for a diagnosis of pregnancy have already guessed that they are pregnant based on a multitude of subjective signs. Most have already used a home pregnancy test to confirm the pregnancy for themselves.

Pregnancy is officially diagnosed on the basis of the symptoms reported by the woman and the signs elicited by a healthcare provider. These signs and symptoms are traditionally divided into three classifications: presumptive or subjective, probable or objective, and positive or documented (see Table 10.2).

Presumptive (subjective) signs of pregnancy

Presumptive signs of pregnancy are those that are least indicative of pregnancy; taken as single entities, they could easily indicate other conditions (Rojas, Wood & Blakemore, 2007). These findings, discussed in connection with the body system in which they occur, are experienced by the woman but cannot be documented by an examiner (see Box 10.4).

Probable signs of pregnancy

In contrast to presumptive signs, probable signs of pregnancy are objective so can be documented by an examiner.

TABLE 10.2 Presumptive, probable and positive signs of pregnancy

Time from implantation (weeks)	Presumptive finding	Probable finding	Positive finding	Description
1		Serum laboratory tests		Tests of blood serum reveal the presence of human chorionic gonadotropin hormone
2	Breast changes			Feeling of tenderness, fullness or tingling; enlargement and darkening of areola
2	Nausea, vomiting			Nausea or vomiting on arising
2	Amenorrhoea			Absence of menstruation
3	Frequent urination			Sense of having to void more often than usual
6		Chadwick's sign		Colour change of the vagina from pink to violet
6		Goodell's sign		Softening of the cervix
6		Hegar's sign		Softening of the lower uterine segment
6		Evidence on ultrasound of		Characteristic ring is evident
8			Evidence on ultrasound of fetal outline	Fetal outline can be seen and measured by ultrasound
10–12			Fetal heart audible	Doppler ultrasound reveals heartbeat
12	Fatigue			General feeling of tiredness
12	Uterine enlargement			Uterus can be palpated over symphysis pubis
16		Ballottement		When lower uterine segment is tapped on a bimanual examination, the fetus can be felt to rise against abdominal wall
18	Quickening			Fetal movement felt by woman
20			Fetal movement felt by examiner	Fetal movement can be palpated through abdomen
20		Braxton Hicks contractions		Periodic uterine tightening occurs
20		Fetal outline felt by examiner		Fetal outline can be palpated through abdomen
24	Linea nigra			Line of dark pigment on the abdomen
24	Melasma			Dark pigment on face
24	Striae gravidarum			Red streaks on abdomen

Although they are more reliable than presumptive signs, they are still not positive or true diagnostic findings. They are also discussed in connection with the body system in which they occur.

Laboratory tests

The commonly used laboratory tests for pregnancy are based on detecting the presence of human chorionic gonadotropin (hCG), a hormone created by the chorionic villi of the placenta, in the urine or blood serum of the pregnant woman. Because all laboratory tests for pregnancy are accurate in diagnosing pregnancy only 95% to 98% of the time, positive results from these tests are considered probable rather than positive signs.

These tests are performed by radioimmunoassay (RIA), enzyme-linked immunosorbent assay (ELISA), or radioreceptor assay (RRA) techniques. For these tests, hCG is measured in international units. In the non-pregnant woman, no units are detectable because there are no trophoblast cells producing hCG. In the pregnant woman, trace amounts of hCG appear in the serum as early as 24 to 48 hours after implantation. They reach a measurable level (about 50 mIU/mL) 7 to 9 days after conception. Levels peak at about 100 mIU/mL between the 60th and 80th day of gestation. After that point, the concentration of hCG declines again, so that at term it is barely detectable in serum or urine.

Home pregnancy tests

Several kits for pregnancy testing based on immunological reactions are available over-the-counter. These tests have a high degree of accuracy (about 97%) if the instructions are followed exactly. They are convenient to

BOX 10.4 Assessment ✻ **Assessing the pregnant woman for presumptive signs of pregnancy**

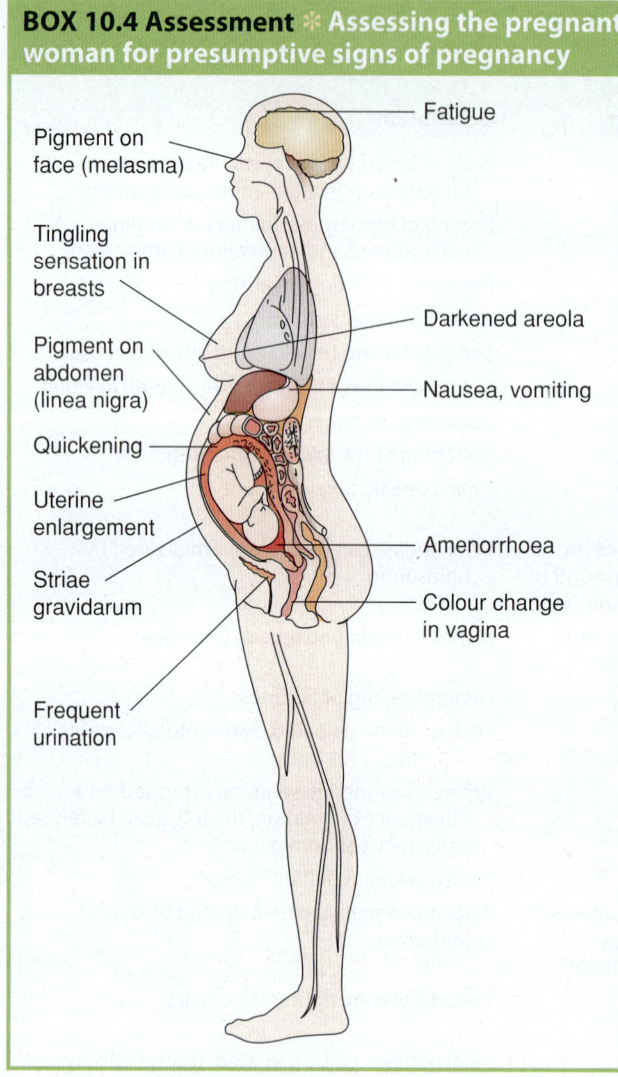

use. For this type of test, a woman dips a reagent strip into her stream of urine. A colour change on the strip denotes pregnancy. Home tests can detect as little as 35 mIU/mL of hCG. They take 3 to 5 minutes to perform. Most manufacturers suggest that women wait until the day of the missed menstrual period to test. Advise any woman who thinks she might be pregnant but gets a negative result from a home pregnancy test to repeat the test one week later if she is still experiencing amenorrhoea. If symptoms persist after two tests, she needs to see a healthcare provider.

Women taking psychotropic medication (e.g. anti-anxiety agents) may have false positive results on pregnancy tests. Women taking oral contraceptives may also have false positive results; for such a test to be accurate, oral contraceptives should have been discontinued 5 days before the test. Women who have proteinuria, are postmenopausal or have hyperthyroid disease may also show false positive results.

Once pregnancy has been diagnosed, early and regular antenatal care needs to be commenced. After a positive pregnancy test, the first step should be to arrange for antenatal care (Bernstein & Weinstein, 2007).

Positive signs of pregnancy

There are only three documented or positive signs of pregnancy:

- Demonstration of a fetal heart separate from the mother's
- Fetal movements felt by an examiner
- Visualisation of the fetus by ultrasound.

Demonstration of a fetal heart separate from the mother's

The fetal heart can be shown to be beating on ultrasound as early as the sixth to seventh week of pregnancy. Ultrasonic monitoring systems that convert ultrasonic frequencies to audible frequencies (Doppler technique) can detect fetal heart sounds as early as the tenth to twelfth week of gestation. Echocardiography can demonstrate a heartbeat as early as 5 weeks.

Although the fetal heart has been beating since the 24th day after conception, it is audible by auscultation of the abdomen with an ordinary stethoscope only at about 18 to 20 weeks of pregnancy. Fetal heart sounds are difficult to hear if a woman's abdomen has a great deal of subcutaneous fat or if a larger than normal amount of amniotic fluid is present (hydramnios). They are heard best when the position of the fetus is determined by palpation and the stethoscope is placed over the area of the fetal back. The fetal heart rate usually ranges between 110 and 160 beats per minute as per Royal Australian and New Zealand College of Obstetricians and Gynaecologists (RANZCOG, 2006).

Fetal movements felt by an examiner

Fetal movements may be felt by a woman as early as 16 to 20 weeks of pregnancy. Those felt by an objective examiner are considered much more reliable because a woman could mistake the movement of gas through her intestines for fetal movement. Fetal movements can be felt by an examiner at the 20th to 24th week of pregnancy unless a woman is extremely obese.

Visualisation of fetus by ultrasound

High-frequency sound waves projected towards a woman's abdomen are useful in diagnosing pregnancy. If a woman is pregnant, a characteristic ring, indicating the gestational sac, will be revealed on an oscilloscope screen as early as the fourth to sixth week of pregnancy. This method also gives information about the site of implantation and whether a multiple pregnancy exists. By the eighth week, a fetal outline can be seen so clearly within the sac that the crown-to-rump length can be measured to establish the gestational age of the pregnancy. Seeing the fetal outline on an ultrasound is clear proof for a couple that a woman is pregnant if they had any doubt up to that point.

CASE STUDY QUESTION

5. Lauren Maxwell used a urine pregnancy test but was surprised to learn that a positive result is not a sure sign of pregnancy. She asks you what would be a positive sign. Your best answer would be:
   a. She is having consistent uterine growth
   b. She feels the fetus move especially after meals
   c. hCG can be found in her bloodstream
   d. The fetal heart can be seen on ultrasound

PHYSIOLOGICAL CHANGES OF PREGNANCY

Physiological changes that occur during pregnancy can be categorised as local (confined to the reproductive organs) or systemic (affecting the entire body). Both symptoms (subjective findings) and signs (objective findings) of the physiological changes of pregnancy are used to diagnose and mark the progress of pregnancy. Table 10.3 summarises the physiological changes that occur in body organs or systems during a typical 40-week pregnancy.

Reproductive system changes

Reproductive tract changes are those involving the uterus, ovaries, vagina and breasts.

Uterine changes

The most obvious alteration in a woman's body during pregnancy is the increase in the size of the uterus to accommodate the growing fetus. Over the term (40–42 weeks) of pregnancy, the uterus increases in length, depth, width, weight, wall thickness and volume:

- Length increases from approximately 6.5 to 32 cm.
- Depth increases from 2.5 to 22 cm.
- Width expands from 4 to 24 cm.
- Weight increases from 50 to 1000 g.
- Early in pregnancy, the uterine wall thickens from about 1 cm to about 2 cm; towards the end of pregnancy, the wall thins to become supple and only about 0.5 cm thick.
- The volume of the uterus increases from about 2 mL to more than 1000 mL. The uterus can hold a 3175-g fetus plus 1000 mL of amniotic fluid for a total of about 4000 g at term.

This great uterine growth is due partly to formation of a few new muscle fibres in the uterine myometrium but principally to the stretching of existing muscle fibres; by the end of pregnancy, muscle fibres in the uterus have become two to seven times longer than they were before pregnancy. The uterus is able to withstand this stretching of its muscle fibres because of the formation of extra fibroelastic tissue between fibres, which binds them closely together. Because uterine fibres simply stretch during pregnancy and are not newly built, the uterus is able to return to its prepregnant state at the end of the pregnancy with little difficulty and almost no destruction of tissue (Kahn & Koos, 2007).

A woman becomes aware of her growing uterus early in pregnancy; by the end of the 12th week, the uterus is large enough to be palpated as a firm globe under the abdominal wall, just above the symphysis pubis. An important factor to assess regarding uterine growth is its constant, steady, predictable increase in size. By the 20th or 22nd week of pregnancy, for example, it should reach the level of the umbilicus. By the 36th week, it should touch the xiphoid process and can make breathing difficult. About

TABLE 10.3 Timetable for physiological changes of pregnancy

Location of change	1st trimester	2nd trimester	3rd trimester
Circulatory system	Blood volume increasing Pseudoanaemia Clotting factors increasing	Blood pressure slightly decreased	Blood pressure returns to prepregnancy levels
Ovary	Corpus luteum active	Corpus luteum fading	
Uterus	Increased growth	Placenta forming oestrogen and progesterone	
Cervix	Softening progressive		"Ripe"
Vagina	White discharge present		Increasing in amount
Musculoskeletal system		Progressive cartilage softening Lordosis increasing	
Pigmentation		Progressively increasing	
Kidney	Maternal glomerular filtration rate increasing Aldosterone increased, retaining sodium and fluid	Glycosuria	
Gastrointestinal system		Slowed peristalsis	
Thyroid	Increased metabolic rate		

two weeks before term (the 38th week) for a **primigravida**, a woman in her first pregnancy, the fetal head settles into the pelvis to prepare for birth and the uterus returns to the height it was at 36 weeks. This event is termed **lightening**, because a woman's breathing is so much easier it seems to lighten a woman's load. When lightening will occur is not predictable in a **multipara** (a woman who has had one or more children). In these women, it may not occur until labour begins.

Changes in fundal height during pregnancy are shown in Fig. 10.2. Uterine height is measured from the top of the symphysis pubis to over the top of the uterine fundus (Neilson, 2009). The exact shape of the expanding uterus is influenced by the position of the fetus inside. The fundus of the uterus usually remains in the midline during pregnancy, although it may be pushed slightly to the right side because of the larger bulk of the sigmoid colon on the left. As the uterus increases in size, it pushes the intestines to the sides of the abdomen, elevates the diaphragm and liver, compresses the stomach and puts pressure on the bladder. A woman may worry that there will not be enough room inside her abdomen for this increase in size. You can assure her that the abdominal contents will shift readily to accommodate uterine enlargement (Fig. 10.3).

Uterine blood flow increases during pregnancy as the placenta grows and requires more blood for perfusion. Doppler ultrasonography has shown that, before pregnancy, uterine blood flow is 15 to 20 mL/min. By the end of pregnancy, it expands to as much as 500 to 750 mL/min, with 75% of that volume going to the placenta. Measuring

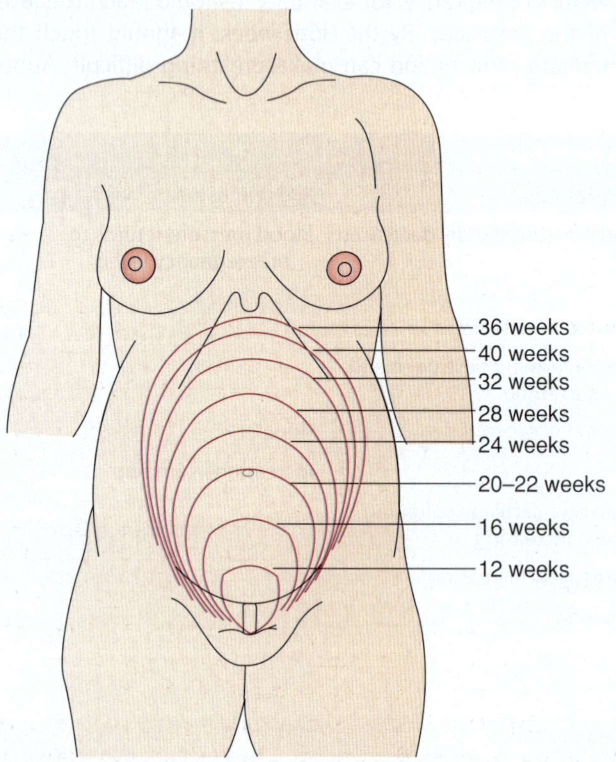

FIGURE 10.2 Fundus height at various weeks of pregnancy.

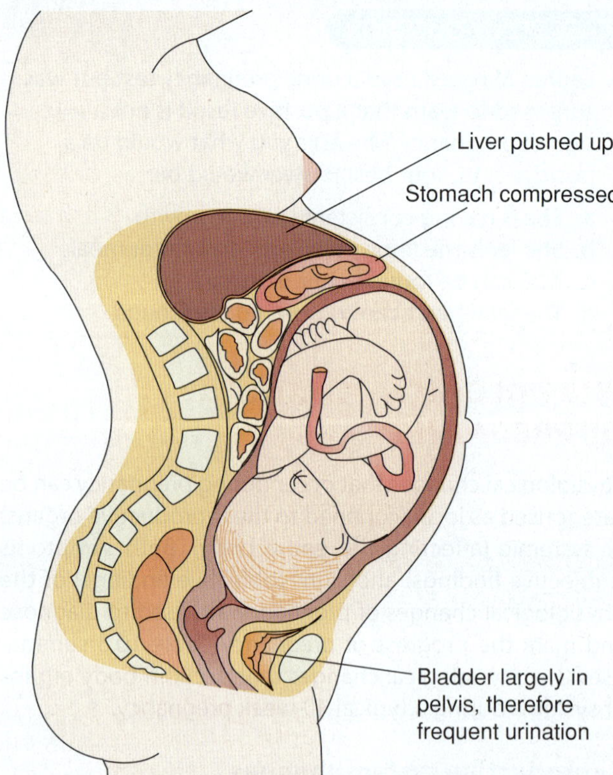

FIGURE 10.3 Crowding of abdominal contents late in pregnancy.

that placenta blood volume and velocity is increasing this way is one of the most important gauges of fetal health (Gonzalez et al., 2007).

Towards the end of pregnancy, one-sixth of a woman's blood supply is circulating through the uterus at any given time; therefore, uterine bleeding in pregnancy is always potentially serious because it could result in a major blood loss. Vaginal blood loss, which suggests uterine bleeding, could pose a major health risk. Women should always contact their healthcare practitioner if such bleeding occurs.

A bimanual examination (one finger of an examiner is placed in the vagina, the other hand on the abdomen) can demonstrate that, with pregnancy, the uterus feels more anteflexed, larger and softer to the touch than usual. At about the sixth week of pregnancy (at the time of the second missed menstrual period), the lower uterine segment just above the cervix becomes so soft that when it is compressed between examining fingers on bimanual examination, the wall cannot be felt or feels as thin as tissue paper. This extreme softening of the lower uterine segment is known as **Hegar's sign**. It is a probable sign of pregnancy (Rojas, Wood & Blakemore, 2007).

During the 16th to 20th week of pregnancy, when the fetus is still small in relation to the amount of amniotic fluid present, **ballottement** (from the French word balloter, meaning "to toss about") may be demonstrated. On bimanual examination, if the lower uterine segment is tapped sharply by the lower hand, the fetus can be felt to bounce or rise in the amniotic fluid up against the top examining hand. Between the 20th and 24th week of pregnancy, the uterine wall has become thinned to such a degree that a fetal outline within the uterus may be palpated by a skilled examiner. Uterine contractions begin early in pregnancy, at least by the 12th week and are present throughout the rest of pregnancy, becoming stronger and harder as the pregnancy advances. They may be felt by a woman as waves of hardness or tightening across her abdomen. An examining hand may be able to feel a contraction as well, and an electronic monitor will be able to measure the frequency and length of such contractions. These "practice" contractions, termed **Braxton Hicks contractions**, serve as warm-up exercises for labour and also increase placental perfusion. They may become so strong and noticeable in the last month of pregnancy that they are mistaken for labour contractions (false labour). They can be differentiated from true labour contractions on internal examination because they do not cause cervical dilation (Bernstein & Weinstein, 2007).

Amenorrhoea

Amenorrhoea (absence of menstruation) occurs with pregnancy because of the suppression of follicle-stimulating hormones (FSH) by rising oestrogen levels. In a healthy woman who has menstruated previously, the absence of menstruation strongly suggests that impregnation has occurred. Amenorrhoea, however, also heralds the onset of menopause or could result from delayed menstruation because of unrelated reasons, such as uterine infection, worry (perhaps over becoming pregnant), a chronic illness such as severe anaemia, or stress. It occurs in athletes who train strenuously, especially in long-distance runners whose percentage of body fat drops below a critical point. Amenorrhoea is, therefore, only a presumptive sign of pregnancy.

Cervical changes

In response to the increased level of circulating oestrogen from the placenta during pregnancy, the cervix of the uterus becomes more vascular and oedematous. Increased fluid between cells causes it to soften in consistency and increased vascularity causes it to darken from a pale pink to a violet hue. The glands of the endocervix undergo both hypertrophy and hyperplasia as they increase in number and distend with mucus. A tenacious coating of mucus fills the cervical canal. This mucus plug, called the **operculum**, acts to seal out bacteria during pregnancy and therefore helps prevent infection in the fetus and membranes.

Softening of the cervix in pregnancy **(Goodell's sign)** is marked at 4 to 6 weeks. The consistency of a non-pregnant cervix may be compared with that of the nose, whereas the consistency of a pregnant cervix more closely resembles that of an earlobe. This softening is so marked it is rated as a probable diagnostic sign of pregnancy. Just before labour, the cervix becomes so soft that it takes on the consistency of butter or is said to be "ripe" for birth (Kahn & Koos, 2007).

Vaginal changes

Under the influence of oestrogen, the vaginal epithelium and underlying tissue become hypertrophic and enriched with glycogen; structures loosen from their connective tissue attachments in preparation for great distension at birth. This increase in the activity of the epithelial cells results in a white vaginal discharge throughout pregnancy.

An increase in the vascularity of the vagina, beginning early in pregnancy, parallels the vascular changes in the uterus. The resulting increase in circulation changes the colour of the vaginal walls from the normal light pink to a deep violet **(Chadwick's sign)** at 8–12 weeks.

Vaginal secretions during pregnancy fall from a pH of greater than 7 (an alkaline pH) to 4 or 5 (an acid pH). This occurs because of the action of Lactobacillus acidophilus, bacteria that grow freely in the increased glycogen environment and by so doing increase the lactic acid content of secretions. This changing acid content helps to make the vagina resistant to bacterial invasion for the length of the pregnancy. This change in pH also, unfortunately, favours the growth of Candida albicans, a species of yeast-like fungi. A Candida infection is manifested by an itching, burning sensation in addition to a cream cheese–like discharge. A non-pregnant woman needs medication for such an infection to relieve discomfort. A pregnant woman needs medication not only to relieve discomfort but also to prevent transmission of the infection to the newborn as it passes through the birth canal at term. Candida infection in the newborn is termed thrush or oral monilia. Therapy for this infection is discussed in Chapter 43.

CASE STUDY QUESTION

6. Lauren's doctor told her she had a positive Chadwick's sign. She asks you what this means and you tell her that:
   a. Her abdomen is soft and tender
   b. Her uterus has tipped forwards
   c. Her cervical mucus is clear but sticky
   d. Her vagina has darkened in colour

Ovarian changes

Ovulation stops with pregnancy because of the active feedback mechanism of oestrogen and progesterone produced by the corpus luteum early in pregnancy and by the placenta later in pregnancy. This feedback causes the pituitary gland to halt production of FSH and luteinising hormone (LH). Without stimulation from FSH and LH, ovulation does not occur.

The corpus luteum that was created after the ovulation that led to the pregnancy continues to increase in size on the surface of the ovary until about the 16th week of pregnancy, by which time the placenta takes over as the chief provider of progesterone and oestrogen. The corpus luteum, no longer essential for the continuation of the pregnancy, regresses in size and appears white and fibrous on the surface of the ovary (a corpus albicans).

Changes in the breasts

Subtle changes in the breasts may be one of the first physiological changes of pregnancy a woman notices (at about 6 weeks). She may experience a feeling of fullness, tingling or tenderness in her breasts because of the increased stimulation of breast tissue by the high oestrogen level in her body. As the pregnancy progresses, breast size increases because of hyperplasia of the mammary alveoli and fat deposits. The areola of the nipple darkens and its diameter increases from about 3.5 cm to 5 or 7.5 cm. There is additional darkening of the skin surrounding the areola in some women, forming a secondary areola. As vascularity of the breasts increases, blue veins may become prominent over the surface of the breasts. The sebaceous glands of the areola **(Montgomery's tubercles)** enlarge and become protuberant. The secretions from these glands are what keeps the nipple supple and helps to prevent nipples from cracking and drying during lactation.

Early in pregnancy, the breasts begin readying themselves for the secretion of milk. By the 16th week, colostrum, the thin, watery, high-protein fluid that is the precursor of breast milk, can be expelled from the nipples. Talking to women during pregnancy about breast changes and breastfeeding for their infant's health can be the trigger that alerts them to the importance of breastfeeding (Mattar et al., 2007).

Systemic changes

Although the physiological changes first noticed by a woman are apt to be those of the reproductive system and breasts, changes are occurring in almost all body systems.

Integumentary system

As the uterus increases in size, the abdominal wall must stretch to accommodate it. This stretching (plus possibly increased adrenal cortex activity) can cause rupture and atrophy of small segments of the connective layer of the skin. This leads to pink or reddish streaks **(striae gravidarum)** appearing on the sides of the abdominal wall and sometimes on the thighs. During the weeks after birth, striae gravidarum lighten to a silvery-white colour (striae albicantes or atrophicae) and, although permanent, they become barely noticeable. Occasionally, the abdominal wall has difficulty stretching enough to accommodate the growing fetus, causing the rectus muscles to actually separate, a condition known as **diastasis**. If this happens, it will appear after pregnancy as a bluish groove at the site of separation.

The umbilicus is stretched by pregnancy to such an extent that by the 28th week, its depression becomes obliterated and smooth because it has been pushed so far outward. In most women, it may appear as if it has turned inside out, protruding as a round bump at the centre of the abdominal wall.

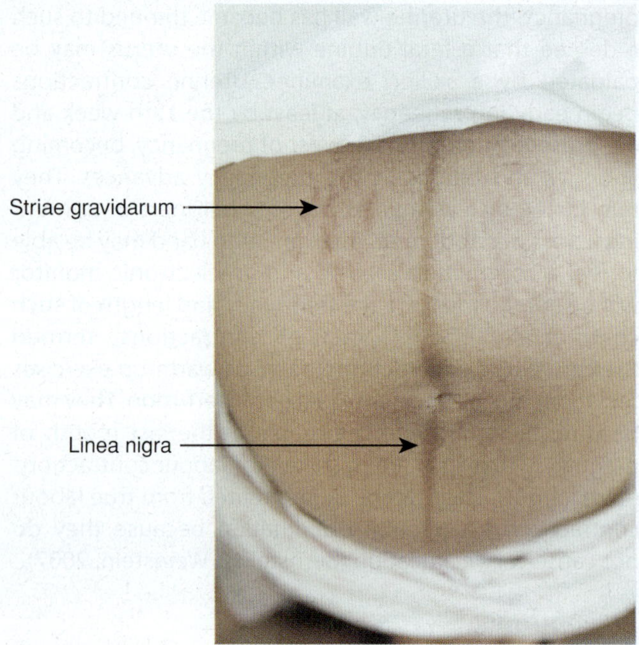

FIGURE 10.4 Skin changes in pregnancy: striae gravidarum and linea nigra. (From Klossner, N. J. & Hatfield, N. T. [2010]. *Introductory Maternity & Pediatric Nursing.* Lippincott Williams & Wilkins.)

Extra pigmentation generally appears on the abdominal wall. A narrow, brown line **(linea nigra)** may form, running from the umbilicus to the symphysis pubis and separating the abdomen into right and left hemispheres (see Fig 10.4). Darkened areas may appear on the face as well, particularly on the cheeks and across the nose. This is known as **melasma** (chloasma), or the "mask of pregnancy". These increases in pigmentation are caused by melanocyte-stimulating hormone, which is secreted by the pituitary. With the decrease in the level of the hormone after pregnancy, these areas lighten and again disappear.

Vascular spiders or telangiectases (small, fiery-red branching spots) are sometimes seen on the skin of pregnant women, particularly on the thighs. These probably result from the increased level of oestrogen in the body. They may fade but not completely disappear after pregnancy. The activity of sweat glands increases throughout the body during pregnancy. Women notice this as an increase in perspiration. Palmar erythema (redness and itching) may occur on the hands from the increased oestrogen level. Fewer hairs on the head enter a resting phase because of overall increased metabolism, so scalp hair growth is increased.

Respiratory system

A local change that often occurs in the respiratory system is marked congestion, or "stuffiness", of the nasopharynx, a response to increased oestrogen levels. Some women may use over-the-counter medications to relieve the congestion.

Ask all women at antenatal visits if they are taking any kind of medicine or if they have noticed nasal stuffiness to detect this possibility.

As the uterus enlarges during pregnancy, a great deal of pressure is put on the diaphragm and, ultimately, on the lungs. This can displace the diaphragm by as much as 4 cm upwards. This crowding of the chest cavity causes an acute sensation of shortness of breath late in pregnancy, until lightening relieves the pressure. Even with all this crowding, a woman's vital capacity (the maximum volume exhaled after a maximum inspiration) does not decrease during pregnancy because, although the lungs are crowded in the vertical dimension, they can still expand horizontally. Residual volume (the amount of air remaining in the lungs after expiration) is decreased up to 20% by the pressure of the diaphragm. Tidal volume (the volume of air inspired) is increased up to 40% as a woman draws in extra volume to increase the effectiveness of air exchange. Total oxygen consumption increases by as much as 20%.

The cumulative effect of respiratory changes is often experienced by a woman as chronic shortness of breath. Although her breathing rate is more rapid than usual (18–20 breaths per minute), this is normal for pregnancy. The total respiratory changes and the compensating mechanisms that occur in the respiratory system can be described as a chronic respiratory alkalosis fully compensated by a chronic metabolic acidosis. Changes in respiratory function during pregnancy are summarised in Table 10.4.

Temperature

Early in pregnancy, body temperature increases slightly because of the secretion of progesterone from the corpus luteum (the temperature, which increased at ovulation, remains elevated). As the placenta takes over the function of the corpus luteum at about 16 weeks, the temperature usually decreases to normal. Explaining the reason for these changes allows a woman to accept them without thinking she is unwell.

TABLE 10.4 Respiratory changes during pregnancy

Variable	Change
Vital capacity	No change
Tidal volume	Increased by 30% to 40%
Respiratory rate	Increased by 1–2/min
Residual volume	Decreased by 20%
Plasma Pco_2	Decreased to about 27–32 mmHg
Plasma pH	Increased to 7.40–7.45
Plasma Po_2	Increased to 104–108 mmHg
Respiratory minute	Increased by 40% volume
Expiratory reserve	Decreased by 20%

TABLE 10.5 Changes in the cardiovascular system during pregnancy

Assessment factor	Pre-pregnancy	Pregnancy
Cardiac output		25% to 50% increase
Heart rate (bpm)	70–80	80–90
Plasma volume (mL)	2600	3600
Blood volume (mL)	4000	5250
Red blood cell mass (mm^3)	4.2 million	4.65 million
Leucocytes (mm^3)	7000	20,500
Total protein (g/dL)	7.0	5.5–6.0
Fibrinogen (mg/dL)	300	450
Blood pressure		Decreases in second trimester, at pre-pregnancy level in third trimester

Cardiovascular system

Changes in the circulatory system are extremely significant to the health of the fetus because they are necessary for adequate placental and fetal circulation (see Table 10.5).

Blood volume

To provide for an adequate exchange of nutrients in the placenta and to provide adequate blood to compensate for blood loss at birth, the total circulatory blood volume of a woman's body increases by at least 30% (and possibly as much as 50%) during pregnancy. Blood loss at a normal vaginal birth is about 300 to 400 mL; blood loss from a caesarean birth can be as high as 800 to 1000 mL. The increase in blood volume occurs gradually, beginning at the end of the first trimester. It peaks at about the 28th to the 32nd week and then continues at this high level throughout the third trimester. Because the plasma volume increases faster than red blood cell production, the concentration of haemoglobin and erythrocytes may decline, giving a woman pseudoanaemia early in pregnancy. A woman's body compensates for this change by producing more red blood cells, creating near-normal levels of red blood cells again by the second trimester.

Iron, folic acid and vitamin needs

Almost all women need some iron supplementation during pregnancy because of a variety of factors. The fetus requires a total of about 350 to 400 mg of iron to grow. The increases in the mother's circulatory red blood cell mass require an additional 400 mg of iron. This is a total increased need of about 800 mg. Because the average woman's store of iron is less than this amount (about 500 mg) and because iron absorption may be impaired during pregnancy as a result of decreased gastric acidity (iron is absorbed best from an acid medium), additional iron is often prescribed during pregnancy to prevent a true anaemia.

Either a haemoglobin concentration of less than 11 g/100 mL or a haematocrit value below 33% in the first or third trimester of pregnancy or a haemoglobin concentration of less than 10.5 g/dL (haematocrit, 32%) in the second trimester is considered true anaemia, for which iron therapy above normal supplementation is advocated (Arnett & Greenspoon, 2007).

Recommendations from the Royal Women's Hospital, Victoria suggest an iron-rich diet that include at least two serves of the following foods: meat, chicken, fish, legumes or nuts. Some women, however, find it difficult to meet their iron requirements through diet alone and an iron supplement will be recommended. Women who are vegetarian, have pregnancies close together, have a poor diet, a history of anaemia or severe morning sickness may have an increased risk of iron deficiency. Side effects from iron supplements include constipation and stomach irritation. These can be overcome by increasing fluid and fibre intake and participating in gentle exercise (Pena-Rosas & Viteri, 2009). (See Chapter 20 for additional information on anaemia in pregnancy.) The need for folic acid increases even more during pregnancy. If the intake of folic acid is not great enough, megalohemoglobinaemia (large, non-functioning red blood cells) will result. Inadequate folic acid levels have also been linked to an increased risk for neural tube disorders in fetuses (Lumley et al., 2009). Encourage women to eat foods that are high in folic acid (e.g. spinach, asparagus, legumes) both during the prepregnancy period and during pregnancy. Antenatal vitamins that contain folic acid are routinely prescribed. However, an association between multivitamin supplementation during pregnancy and reduced rates of cancers in children, such as neuroblastoma, leukaemia and brain tumours, can be documented (Goh et al., 2007).

Heart

To handle the increase in blood volume in the circulatory system, a woman's cardiac output increases significantly, by 25% to 50%, and the heart rate increases by 10 beats per minute. Like the circulating volume increase, the bulk of the cardiac work increase occurs during the second trimester, with a small increase in the third trimester. An average woman is unaware of the significant circulatory system changes that are occurring inside her to supply adequate blood to the placenta.

Palpitations of the heart are not uncommon during pregnancy, particularly on quick motion. You can caution women not to feel frightened if palpitations do occur. Palpitations in the early months of pregnancy are probably caused by sympathetic nervous system stimulation; in later months, they may result from increased thoracic pressure caused by the pressure of the uterus against the diaphragm.

Blood pressure

Despite the hypervolaemia of pregnancy, the blood pressure does not normally rise because the increased heart action takes care of the greater amount of circulating blood. In most women, blood pressure actually decreases slightly during the second trimester because the peripheral resistance to circulation is lowered as the placenta expands rapidly. During the third trimester, the blood pressure rises again to first trimester levels.

Peripheral blood flow

During the third trimester of pregnancy, blood flow to the lower extremities is impaired by the pressure of the expanding uterus on veins and arteries. This resistance to blood flow in the venous system can lead to oedema and varicosities of the vulva, rectum and legs.

Supine hypotension syndrome

When a pregnant woman lies supine, the weight of the growing uterus presses the vena cava against the vertebrae, obstructing blood flow from the lower extremities. This causes a decrease in blood return to the heart and, consequently, decreased cardiac output and hypotension (see Fig. 10.5). A woman experiences this hypotension as

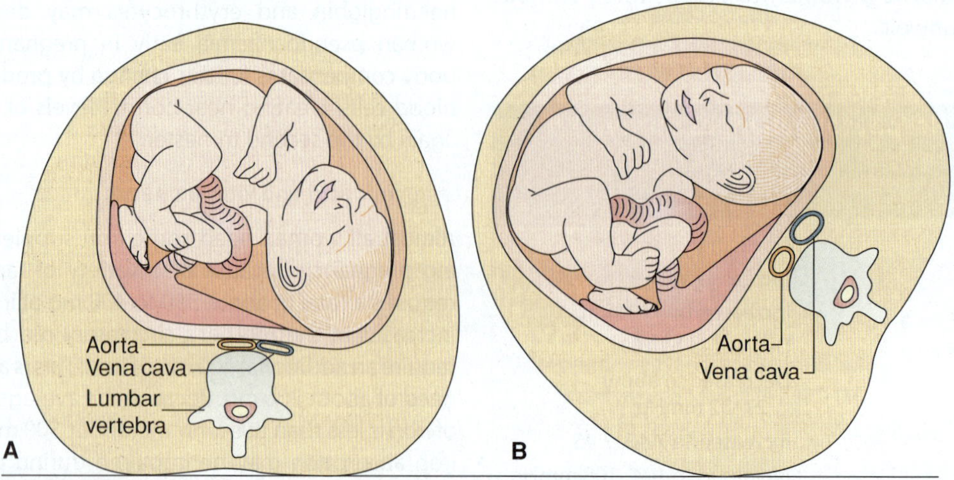

FIGURE 10.5 Supine hypotension can occur if a pregnant woman lies on her back. (**A**) The weight of the uterus compresses the vena cava, trapping blood in the lower extremities. (**B**) If a woman turns on her side, pressure is lifted off of the vena cava.

light-headedness, faintness and palpitations (Bernstein & Weinstein, 2007). The condition is potentially dangerous because it can cause fetal hypoxia.

Supine hypotension syndrome can easily be corrected by having a woman turn onto her side (preferably the left side), so that blood flow through the vena cava increases again. To lessen the possibility of occurrence of this phenomenon, women develop an increase in collateral blood circulation during pregnancy. Teach women always to rest on the left side rather than the back, because even with additional collateral circulation, a supine position tends to lead to hypotension.

Blood constitution

The level of circulating fibrinogen, a constituent of the blood that is necessary for clotting, increases as much as 50% during pregnancy, probably because of the increased level of oestrogen. Other clotting factors, such as factors VII, VIII, IX and X, and the platelet count also increase. These increases are a safeguard against major bleeding should the placenta be dislodged and the uterine arteries or veins be opened. Total white blood cell count rises slightly, both as a protective mechanism and as a reflection of a woman's increased total blood volume (up to about 20,000 cells/mm^3). The total protein level of blood decreases, perhaps indicating the amount of protein being used by the fetus. Because the circulating system has a lower total protein load and hypervolaemia, fluid readily leaves the blood for institial tissue vessels to equalise osmotic and hydrostatic pressure. This causes the common ankle and foot oedema of pregnancy (not to be confused with non-dependent or generalised oedema, which is a symptom of pregnancy-induced hypertension).

Blood lipids increase by one-third and the cholesterol serum level increases by 90% to 100%. These increases provide a ready supply of available energy for the fetus.

Gastrointestinal system

At least 50% of women experience some nausea and vomiting early in pregnancy. This is one of the first sensations a woman may experience with pregnancy (sometimes it is noticed even before the first missed menstrual period). It is most apparent early in the morning, on rising, or if a woman becomes fatigued during the day. It is more frequent in women who smoke cigarettes. Known as morning sickness, nausea and vomiting begin to be noticed at the same time levels of hCG and progesterone begin to rise so these may contribute to its cause. It may occur as a systemic reaction to increased oestrogen levels or decreased glucose levels, because glucose is being used in such great quantities by the growing fetus. Many alternative or complementary methods to help reduce nausea with pregnancy are available such as acupuncture or wrist bands, or drinking ginger or peppermint tea.

This common feeling of nausea usually subsides after the first 3 months, after which time a woman may have a voracious appetite. Although the acidity of stomach secretions decreases during pregnancy, heartburn may result from reflux of stomach contents into the oesophagus, caused by upward displacement of the stomach by the uterus and a relaxed cardioesophageal sphincter, caused by the action of relaxin, an enzyme produced by the ovary. Interventions for heartburn are also discussed in Chapter 13.

As the uterus increases in size, it pushes the stomach and intestines towards the back and sides of the abdomen. At about the midpoint of pregnancy, this pressure may be sufficient to slow intestinal peristalsis and the emptying time of the stomach, leading to increased heartburn, constipation and flatulence. Relaxin may contribute to decreased gastric motility; this natural slowing can be helpful, because the blood supply may be reduced to the gastrointestinal tract (i.e. blood is drawn to the uterus). Progesterone also has an effect on smooth muscle, such as that in the intestine, making the gastrointestinal tract less active.

Women with chronic gastric reflux usually find their condition improves during pregnancy because the acidity of the stomach is decreased. Because of the gradual slowing of the gastrointestinal tract, decreased emptying of bile from the gallbladder may result. This can lead to reabsorption of bilirubin into the maternal bloodstream, giving rise to a symptom of generalised itching (subclinical jaundice). A woman who has had gallstones may have an increased tendency to stone formation during pregnancy as a result of the increased plasma cholesterol level and additional cholesterol incorporated in bile. Pressure from the uterus on veins returning from the lower extremities can lead to haemorrhoids.

Some pregnant women notice hypertrophy at their gumlines and bleeding of gingival tissue when they brush their teeth. There may be increased saliva formation (hyperptyalism), probably as a local response to increased levels of oestrogen. This is an annoying but not serious problem. A lower than normal pH of saliva may lead to increased tooth decay if tooth brushing is not done conscientiously. This can be a problem for women who do not have frequent access to a place to brush their teeth (Agueda et al., 2008).

What if...

Lauren asks you what to do for morning sickness and fatigue? What if you discovered she was homeless? Would your advice for her be any different?

Urinary system

Like other systems, the urinary system undergoes many physiological changes during pregnancy. These include alterations in fluid retention and renal, ureter and bladder function. Changes in the urinary system are summarised in Table 10.6.

TABLE 10.6 Urinary tract changes during pregnancy

Variable	Change
Glomerular filtration rate	Increased by 50%
Renal plasma flow	Increased by 25% to 80%
Blood urea nitrogen	Decreased by 25%
Plasma creatinine level	Decreased by 25%
Renal threshold for sugar	Decreased to allow slight spillage
Bladder capacity	Increased by 1000 mL
Diameter of ureters	Increased by 25%
Frequency of urination	Increased first trimester, last 2 weeks of pregnancy to 10–12 times/day

These changes result from:

- Effects of high oestrogen and progesterone levels
- Compression of the bladder and ureters by the growing uterus
- Increased blood volume
- Postural influences

Fluid retention

To provide sufficient fluid volume for effective placental exchange, total body water increases to 7.5 L; this requires the body to increase its sodium reabsorption in the tubules to maintain osmolarity. Under the influence of progesterone, there is an increased response of the angiotensin-renin system in the kidney, which leads to an increase in aldosterone production. Aldosterone aids sodium reabsorption. Progesterone appears to be potassium-sparing, so that even with an increased urine output, potassium levels remain adequate.

Water is retained during pregnancy to aid the increase in blood volume and to serve as a ready source of fluid for the fetus. Because nutrients can pass to the fetus only when dissolved in or carried by fluid, this ready fluid supply is a fetal safeguard. In addition, the excess fluid can serve to replenish the mother's own blood volume, should haemorrhage occur.

Renal function

During pregnancy, a woman's kidneys must excrete not only the waste products from her body but also those of the growing fetus. Also, her kidneys must be able to excrete additional fluid and manage the demands of increased renal blood flow. The kidneys may increase in size, changing their structure and ultimately affecting their function.

Ureter and bladder function

During pregnancy, urinary output gradually increases (by about 60% to 80%). A pregnant woman may notice an increase in urinary frequency during the first 3 months of pregnancy, until the uterus rises out of the pelvis and relieves pressure on the bladder. Frequency of urination may return at the end of pregnancy, as lightening occurs and the fetal head exerts renewed pressure on the bladder.

Because of the increased level of progesterone during pregnancy, the ureters increase in diameter and the bladder capacity increases to about 1500 mL. The uterus tends to rise on the right side of the abdomen because it is pushed slightly in that direction by the greater bulk of the sigmoid colon. As a result, pressure on the right ureter may lead to urinary stasis and pyelonephritis if not relieved. Pressure on the urethra may lead to poor bladder emptying and bladder infection. Such infections are potentially dangerous to the pregnant woman, because they can progress to become kidney infections. They are potentially dangerous to the fetus too, because urinary tract infections are associated with preterm labour (Cootauco & Althaus, 2007).

Skeletal system

Calcium and phosphorus needs are increased during pregnancy, because the fetal skeleton must be built. As pregnancy advances, there is a gradual softening of a woman's pelvic ligaments and joints to create pliability and to facilitate passage of the baby through the pelvis at birth. This softening is probably caused by the influence of both the ovarian hormone relaxin and placental progesterone. Excessive mobility of the joints can cause discomfort. A wide separation of the symphysis pubis, as much as 3 to 4 mm by 32 weeks of pregnancy, may occur. Referral to a physiotherapist may assist with the discomfort.

Endocrine system

Almost all aspects of the endocrine system change during pregnancy (see Table 10.7).

Placenta

The most striking change in the endocrine system during pregnancy is the addition of the placenta as an endocrine organ that produces large amounts of oestrogen, progesterone, hCG, human placental lactogen (hPL), relaxin and prostaglandins. Oestrogen causes breast and uterine enlargement. Palmar erythema during early pregnancy may also be a response to the high circulating oestrogen levels. Progesterone has a major role in maintaining the endometrium, inhibiting uterine contractility and aiding in the development of the breasts for lactation. Relaxin, secreted primarily by the corpus luteum, is responsible for helping to inhibit uterine activity and to soften the cervix and the collagen in joints. Softening of the cervix allows for dilatation at birth; softening of collagen allows for laxness in the lower spine and helps enlarge the birth canal. hCG is secreted by the trophoblast cells of the placenta in early pregnancy. It stimulates progesterone and oestrogen synthesis in the ovaries until the placenta can assume

TABLE 10.7 Endocrine gland changes and effects during pregnancy

Gland	Change	Effect
Thyroid gland	Slight enlargement Increased basal metabolism rate	Increased thyroid hormone production Increased oxygen consumption
Parathyroid gland	Slight enlargement Increased parathyroid hormone production	Better utilisation of calcium and vitamin D
Pancreas	Early in pregnancy, decreased insulin production because of heavy fetal demand After first trimester, increased insulin production because of insulin antagonist properties of oestrogen, progesterone and human placental lactogen	Additional glucose is available for fetal growth for glucose
Pituitary gland	FSH and LH decrease Prolactin increases Melanocyte-stimulating hormone increases Human growth hormone increases	Anovulation Breasts prepared for lactation Increased skin pigment Aids fetal growth
Placenta	Oestrogen and progesterone produced Relaxin increased Human placental lactogen	Uterine and breast enlargement, fat deposits Increased blood coagulation, sodium and water retention Softening of cervix and collagen of joints Increases glucose available for fetus Decreases utilisation of protein for energy, increasing availability for fetal growth

this role. hPL, also known as human chorionic somatomammotropin, is also produced by the placenta. It serves as an antagonist to insulin, making insulin less effective, which allows more glucose to become available for fetal growth.

In addition to these changes, prostaglandins are found in high concentrations in the female reproductive tract and the decidua during pregnancy. Prostaglandins affect smooth muscle contractility to such an extent they may be the trigger that initiates labour at term.

Pituitary gland

The pituitary gland is affected by pregnancy because there is a halt in the production of FSH and LH brought on by the high oestrogen and progesterone levels of the placenta. There is increased production of growth hormone and melanocyte-stimulating hormone (which causes skin pigment changes). Late in pregnancy, the posterior pituitary begins to produce oxytocin, which will be needed to aid labour. Prolactin production is also begun late in pregnancy, as the breasts prepare for lactation.

Thyroid and parathyroid glands

The thyroid gland enlarges in early pregnancy to such an extent that the basal metabolic rate increases by about 20%. Levels of protein-bound iodine, butanol-extractable iodine and thyroxine are all elevated in blood serum. If a sufficient supply of iodine is not present during pregnancy, goitre (thyroid hypertrophy) can occur as the gland intensifies its productive effort. These thyroid changes, along with emotional lability, tachycardia, palpitations and increased perspiration, may lead to a mistaken diagnosis of hyperthyroidism if pregnancy has not been determined.

The parathyroid glands, which are necessary for the metabolism of calcium, also increase in size during pregnancy. Because calcium is important for fetal growth, the hypertrophy is probably necessary to satisfy the increased requirement for this.

Adrenal glands

Adrenal gland activity increases in pregnancy as increased levels of corticosteroids and aldosterone are produced. It is assumed that these increased levels aid in suppressing an inflammatory reaction or help reduce the possibility of a woman's body rejecting the foreign protein of the fetus, the same as it would a foreign-tissue transplant. They also help to regulate glucose metabolism in a woman. The increased level of aldosterone aids in promoting sodium reabsorption and maintaining osmolarity in the amount of fluid retained. This indirectly helps to safeguard the blood volume and to provide adequate perfusion pressure across the placenta.

Pancreas

The pancreas increases production of insulin in response to the higher levels of glucocorticoid produced by the adrenal glands. Insulin is less effective than normal, however, because oestrogen, progesterone and hPL are all antagonists to insulin. Therefore, a woman who is diabetic and taking insulin before pregnancy will need more insulin during pregnancy. A woman who is prediabetic may develop overt diabetes for the first time during pregnancy.

Overall, the effect of diminishing the action of insulin is beneficial because it ensures a ready supply of glucose for fetal growth.

The glucose level of a fetus is about 30 mg/100 mL lower than the maternal glucose level. To prevent fetal hypoglycaemia, with resultant cell destruction or lack of fetal growth, the maternal glucose level is usually at a higher than normal level during pregnancy. Several fail-safe physiological measures are initiated to achieve this.

As mentioned, although the pancreas secretes an increased level of insulin throughout pregnancy, it appears to be not as effective. With insulin that is less effective, fat stores of a woman are utilised, as well as available glucose. This maintains maternal glucose levels at a fairly steady level despite long intervals between meals or days of increased activity. To ensure against hypoglycaemia, a pregnant woman should keep her diet high in calories and should never go longer than 12 hours between meals. Because the rapidly developing fetus uses so much glucose in early pregnancy, a fasting blood glucose level at this time is usually low (80–85 mg/100 mL).

Immune system

Immunological competency during pregnancy apparently decreases, probably to prevent a woman's body from rejecting the fetus as if it were a transplanted organ. Immunoglobulin G (IgG) production is particularly decreased, which can make a woman more prone to infection during pregnancy. A simultaneous increase in the white blood cell count may help to counteract the decrease in IgG response.

CASE STUDY QUESTION

7. Lauren Maxwell overheard her doctor say that insulin is not as effective during pregnancy as usual. How would you explain how decreased insulin effectiveness safeguards the fetus?
   a. Decreased effectiveness prevents the fetus from being hypoglycaemic
   b. If insulin is ineffective, it cannot cross the placenta and harm the fetus
   c. The lessened action prevents the fetus from gaining too much weight
   d. The mother, not the fetus, is guarded by this decreased insulin action

Key points for review

- The ability of a woman to accept her pregnancy depends on social, cultural, family and individual influences.
- The psychological tasks of pregnancy are centred on ensuring safe passage for the fetus. These consist of, in the first trimester, accepting the pregnancy; in the second trimester, accepting the baby; and in the third trimester, preparing for parenthood.
- Common emotional responses that occur with pregnancy include grief, narcissism, introversion or extroversion, stress, couvade syndrome, body image and boundary confusion, emotional lability and changes in sexual desire.
- Physiological changes that occur with pregnancy are both local (uterine, ovarian and vaginal changes) and systemic (respiratory, cardiovascular, urinary and skin changes).
- Women may have read about the expected psychological and physiological changes of pregnancy, but once these changes are actually being experienced, they may find them more intense than anticipated.
- The positive signs of pregnancy are demonstration of a fetal heartbeat separate from the mother's, fetal movement felt by an examiner and visualisation of the fetus by ultrasound.
- Although a woman may be in a doctor's office or antenatal clinic for only an hour, if her pregnancy was confirmed at that visit, she invariably feels "more pregnant" when she leaves. Early diagnosis is important so that a woman can begin to change unhealthy habits or, if she desires, have adequate time to carry out a therapeutic termination of pregnancy.

CASE STUDY QUESTIONS

8. Lauren said she is worried about being pregnant because she "would die" if she thought she might be the same type of parent as her parents. Is this type of worry a common reaction to learning about a pregnancy? She says her partner is not worried. Would it be better or worse if he felt the same way? Has she completed the psychological development tasks of pregnancy? What suggestions could you make to help her be a better parent?
9. Lauren used a home test kit to determine that she was pregnant. She did not schedule an antenatal visit, because the most important reason for going would have been to learn whether she was pregnant and she already knew that. What argument could you use to convince her that antenatal care is important for more than pregnancy diagnosis?
10. You notice that Lauren's husband (35 years old) does not come with her on antenatal visits. He says this is because doing that is only for "young guys". How would you advise him?

Resources

For an extensive range of additional resources to enhance teaching and learning and to facilitate understanding of this chapter, please see the text's accompanying website located on thePoint at http://thepoint.lww.com.

References

Agueda, A., et al. (2008). Periodontal disease as a risk factor for adverse pregnancy outcomes: a prospective cohort study. *Journal of Clinical Periodontology, 35*(1), 16–22.

Andrews, M. & Boyle, J. (2011). *Transcultural Concepts in Nursing Care* (6th ed.). Philadelphia: Lippincott Williams & Wilkins.

Arnett, C. & Greenspoon, J. S. (2012). Hematologic disorders in pregnancy. In A. H. DeCheney, L. Nathan & T. Murphy Goodwin (Eds). *Current Diagnosis and Treatment in Obstetrics and Gynecology* (11th ed.). Columbus, OH: McGraw-Hill.

Australian Health Ministers' Advisory Council (AHMAC). (2012). Clinical practice guidelines: Antenatal care – Module 1. Australian Government Department of Health and Ageing, Canberra, accessed 17 February 2015, <www.health.gov.au/antenatal>.

Bernstein, H. B. & Weinstein, M. (2012). Normal pregnancy and antenatal care. In A. H. DeCheney, L. Nathan & T. Murphy Goodwin (Eds). *Current Diagnosis and Treatment in Obstetrics and Gynecology* (11th ed.). Columbus, OH: McGraw-Hill.

Brennan, A., et al. (2007). A qualitative exploration of the Couvade syndrome in expectant fathers. *Journal of Reproductive and Infant Psychology, 25*(1), 18–39.

Casanueva, C. E. & Martin, S. L. (2007). Intimate partner violence during pregnancy and mothers' child abuse potential. *Journal of Interpersonal Violence, 22*(5), 603–622.

Cootauco, A. C. & Althaus, J. E. (2010). Preterm labour and premature rupture of membranes. In F. B. Fortner, et al. (Eds). *The Johns Hopkins Manual of Gynecology and Obstetrics* (4th ed.). Philadelphia: Lippincott Williams & Wilkins.

Crombleholme, W. R. (2013). Obstetrics. In S. J. McPhee & M. A. Papadakis (Eds). *Current Medical Diagnosis and Treatment* (53rd ed.). Columbus, OH: McGraw-Hill.

Cunningham, F. G., et al. (2014). Antenatal care. In F. G. Cunningham, et al. (Eds). *Williams Obstetrics* (24th ed.). Columbus, OH: McGraw-Hill.

Darby, S. B. (2007). Pre- and perinatal care of Hispanic families: Implications for nurses. *Nursing for Women's Health, 11*(2), 160–169.

Darvill, R., Skirton, H. & Farrand, P. (2010). Psychological factors that impact on women's experiences of first-time motherhood: A qualitative study of the transition. *Midwifery* (2010) *26*, 357–366.

DiPietro, J. A., et al. (2008). Fetal responses to induced maternal relaxation during pregnancy. *Biological Psychology, 77*(1), 11–19.

Finnbogadottir, H., Svalenius, E. & Persson, E. (2003) Expectant first time fathers' experiences of pregnancy. *Midwifery. 19*, 96–105.

Goh, Y. I., et al. (2007). Antenatal multivitamin supplementation and rates of pediatric cancers: A meta-analysis. *Clinical Pharmacology and Therapeutics, 81*(5), 685–691.

Gonzalez, J. M., et al. (2007). Relationship between abnormal fetal testing and adverse perinatal outcomes in intrauterine growth restriction. *American Journal of Obstetrics and Gynecology, 196*(5), e48–e51.

Kahn, D. A. & Koos, B. J. (2012). Maternal physiology during pregnancy. In A. H. DeCheney, L. Nathan & T. Murphy Goodwin (Eds). *Current Diagnosis and Treatment in Obstetrics and Gynecology* (11th ed.). Columbus, OH: McGraw-Hill.

Lumley, J., et al. (2009). Periconceptional supplementation with folate and/or multivitamins for preventing neural tube defects. *Cochrane Database of Systematic Reviews, 2009*(1), (CD001056).

Matsui, H. & Gardiner, H. M. (2007). Examination of the fetal heart: making a diagnosis and avoiding pitfalls. *Ultrasound, 15*(2), 62–67.

Mattar, C. N., et al. (2007). Simple antenatal preparation to improve breastfeeding practice: A randomised controlled trial. *Obstetrics and Gynecology, 109*(1), 73–80.

McCauley-Elsom, K. & Hopkins, F. (Chapter 23, p. 463). In K. L. Edward, I. Munro, A. Robins & A. Welch (2011). *Mental Health Nursing – Dimensions of Praxis*. New York: Oxford University Press.

McLeod, M., Miles, M., Rosenberg, J. & Gale, P. (2014). Pregnancy, paternity and parenting in rural communities (Chapter 5). In K. Francis, Y. Chapman & C. Davies. *Rural Nursing: The Australian Context*. Melbourne: Cambridge University Press.

Mercer, R. T. (1986). Predictors of maternal role attainment at one year postbirth. *Western Journal of Nursing Research, 8*, 9–32.

Mortazavi, F., Charman, R., Mousavi, S. A., Khosravi, A. & Ajami, M. E. (2013). Maternal psychological state during the transition to motherhood: A longitudinal study. *Asia Pacific Psychiatry*. June; *5*(2): E49–57

Neilson, J. P. (2009). Symphysis-fundal height measurement in pregnancy. *Cochrane Database of Systematic Reviews, 2009*(1), (CD000944).

NHMRC (National Health and Medical Research Council) (2010). *National Guidance on Collaborative Maternity Care*. NHMRC: Canberra.

Pairman, S., Tracy, S., Thorogood, C. & Pincombe, J. (2014) (Eds). *Midwifery: Preparation for practice,* (3rd ed.*)*. Australia: Churchill Livingstone.

Paradice, R. (2002). *Psychology for Midwives*. Mark Allen Publishing, Wiltshire.

Parratt, J. & Fahy, K. (2011). A feminist critique of foundational nursing research and theory on transition to motherhood. *Midwifery, 27*(4), pp. 445–451.

Pena-Rosas, J. P. & Viteri, F. E. (2009). Effects of routine oral iron supplementation with or without folic acid for women during pregnancy. *Cochrane Database of Systematic Reviews, 2009*(1), (CD004736).

Price, S. (2006). *Mental Health in Pregnancy and Childbirth*. Edinburgh: Churchill Livingstone, Elsevier.

RANZCOG. (2006). *Intrapartum fetal surveillance clinical guidelines*. Royal Australian and New Zealand College of Obstetricians and Gynaecologists (2nd ed.), accessed 18 February 2015, <www.ranzcog.edu.au>.

Rojas, F., Wood, E. & Blakemore, K. (2007). Preconception counseling and prenatal care. In F. B. Fortner, et al. (Eds). *The Johns Hopkins Manual of Gynecology and Obstetrics* (4th ed.). Philadelphia: Lippincott Williams & Wilkins.

Rubin, R. (1984). *Maternal Identity and Maternal Experience*. New York: Springer Publishing Co.

Smeltzer, S. C. (2007). Pregnancy in women with physical disabilities. *JOGNN: Journal of Obstetric, Gynecologic, and Neonatal Nursing, 36*(1), 88–96.

Tulman, L. & Fawcett, J. (2003). *Women's Health During and After Pregnancy: A Theory-based Study of Adaptation to Change*. New York: Springer Publishing Co.

Westdahl, C., et al. (2007). Social support and social conflict as predictors of antenatal depression. *Obstetrics and Gynecology, 110*(1), 134–140.

Suggested readings

Dowswell, T., Carroli, G., Duley, L., Gates, S., Gülmezoglu, A. M., Khan-Neelofur, D. & Piaggio, G. G. P. (2010). Alternative versus standard packages of antenatal care for low-risk pregnancy. *Cochrane Database of Systematic Reviews*, 10, (CD000934).

Jaafar, S. H., Lee, K. S. & Ho, J. J. (2012). Separate care for new mother and infant versus rooming-in for increasing the duration of breastfeeding. *Cochrane Database of Systematic Reviews*, 9, (CD006641).

National Support Team Parents Centre <www.parentscentre.org.nz>

NHMRC National Guidance on Collaborative Maternity Care <www.nhmrc.gov.au>.

Sandall, J., Soltani, H., Gates, S., Shennan, A. & Devane, D. (2013). Midwife-led continuity models versus other models of care for childbearing women. *Cochrane Database of Systematic Reviews*, 8, (CD004667).

The 3centres guidelines <www.3centres.com.au>

The Women's Pregnancy and Birth Information Sheets <www.thewomens.org.au>.

Chapter 11

Assessing fetal and maternal health: Antenatal care

Previous chapters described normal anatomy and physiology of the reproductive tract and the psychological and physiological changes that occur during pregnancy. This chapter adds information about care needed during pregnancy to help ensure a healthy outcome for both a woman and her child.

LEARNING OBJECTIVES

After mastering the contents of this chapter, you should be able to:

1. Describe the areas of health assessment commonly included in antenatal visits.
2. Use critical thinking to analyse ways to ensure that antenatal care is family centred.
3. Discuss the assessment of a pregnant woman's health status and readiness for pregnancy.
4. Nursing considerations related to women's health status during pregnancy.
5. Nursing care such as preparing a woman for a fundal measurement.
6. Nursing care such as establishing a risk score for pregnancy.
7. Identify areas of antenatal care that could benefit from additional nursing research or application of evidence-based practice.
8. Integrate knowledge of pregnancy health assessment with nursing process to achieve quality child and family healthcare.

KEY TERMS

- chloasma
- gravida
- para

CASE STUDY

Sandra Czerinski is a 29-year-old woman, 12 weeks' pregnant, who comes for a first antenatal visit. She is concerned because she did not realise she was pregnant until a week ago. Because of this, she has been actively dieting (two diet drinks plus one meal of mainly vegetables daily) plus lifting weights at a health club. She is worried she has a urinary tract infection now because she has to "go all the time". She does not want any blood tests done because she is scared of needles.

CASE STUDY QUESTIONS

1. What type of care does Sandra need?
2. Is Sandra high risk or low risk?

Antenatal care, essential for ensuring the overall health of newborns and their mothers, is a major strategy for helping to reduce complications of pregnancy by establishing a relationship and planned journey between the woman and her care provider (Grigg, 2010). Ideally, antenatal care begins during a woman's childhood. It includes balanced nutrition with adequate intake of calcium and vitamin D during childhood to prevent rickets (which can distort pelvic size); adequate immunisation against contagious diseases so a woman has protection against viral diseases such as rubella during pregnancy; and maintenance of an overall healthy lifestyle to ensure the best state of health possible for a woman and her partner when entering pregnancy.

An overall healthy lifestyle includes a positive attitude about sexuality, womanhood and childbearing. Once a woman becomes sexually active, preparation for a successful pregnancy includes practising safer sex, regular Pap smears and prompt treatment of any sexually transmitted infection to prevent complications that could lead to subfertility (Katsufrakis & Workowski, 2008). It includes not smoking or using recreational drugs. Acquisition and use of reproductive life planning information can help to ensure that each pregnancy is planned.

Women who maintain a healthy lifestyle this way come to a first antenatal visit prepared to follow health-promotion strategies. For many women this visit is the first time they have been to a healthcare facility since their routine health maintenance visits of childhood. It also may be the first time they have had an appointment that focuses more on health promotion than on the diagnosis of a disease. A woman may have a specific reason (her agenda) for coming to a first antenatal visit (e.g. to confirm the diagnosis of pregnancy). An antenatal visit encompasses more than this, though. It is also a time for additional health promotion, pregnancy education and development of a positive pattern of healthy behaviours for the family to use in the future (your agenda). What and how much is needed vary depending on the lifestyle, age and parity of a woman and her degree of family support (Kingston et al., 2012).

Lack of antenatal care is associated with the birth of preterm infants and various complications for a woman such as complications associated with a preterm birth (Attilakos & Overton, 2012).

ANTENATAL CARE

Assessment

The first antenatal visit is a time to establish baseline data relevant to health assessment and health-promotion strategies that will be important at every antenatal visit. This begins with obtaining a health history, including screening for the presence of teratogens (any factor that may adversely affect the fetus) and any concerns a woman may be experiencing. Explaining why specific assessment data is relevant to the pregnancy is important. Relating assessment information and health-promotion activities this way throughout the pregnancy helps keep a woman and her family well informed and eager to comply with further healthcare recommendations.

Nursing considerations

Be certain to reserve sufficient time at antenatal visits so care can be thorough and there is enough time to set realistic goals and expected outcomes with both a woman and her partner, if desired. Make sure that a woman leaving an initial antenatal visit schedules an appointment for a following visit, as this may not occur to a woman who may be extremely excited or overwhelmed by all the new things that are happening to her and her family; establishing a pattern of regular appointments is crucial to providing effective antenatal care. Antenatal visits are recommended as first contact with a health professional, then a booking in and screening appointment. The subsequent visit should be 16 weeks; then an 18 to 20 week visit for a morphology scan; next visit at 25 weeks for a nulliparous woman, otherwise 28 weeks; 31 weeks for a nulliparous woman, otherwise 34 weeks. Final visits should then be every two weeks until birth (40th week only for nulliparous) and 41 and 42 weeks (NICE Guidelines, 2014). Women categorised as high risk are followed more closely.

An important nursing intervention at antenatal visits is teaching women and their families about a safe pregnancy lifestyle. It may be helpful to give a woman and her partner pamphlets or books that cover the same topics. Be certain that you have read all the printed material you give families. This helps to ensure that a pamphlet's advice is consistent with what you have said and with the views of a woman's primary care doctor or nurse-midwife.

BOX 11.1 ✻ Focus on evidence-based practice

Continuity of in the antenatal setting

In many antenatal settings, women see either one caregiver (usually a midwife) for the majority of their antenatal visits or see a multitude of care providers (midwives, doctors). To investigate whether continuity of care with one provider made a difference, researchers randomised two groups of women, one to standard low-risk antenatal care and one to a caseload model of care. This trial found that women who were provided continuity of care in the caseload model of care for their pregnancy visits were less likely to have a caesarean section (19.4%) compared with those who had standard care (24.9%). No differences were detected in Apgar scores, low birth weight, stillbirths or neonatal deaths. They were more likely to be pleased with their antenatal, intrapartum and postnatal care.

Would the above study influence the decisions you would make if you had the chance to reorganise an antenatal clinic?

Source: Davey, M-A., McLachlan, H. L., Forster, D. & Flood, M. (2013). Influence of timing of admission in labour and management of labour on method of birth: results from a randomised controlled trial of caseload midwifery (COSMOS trial). *Midwifery, 29*(12), 1297.

HEALTH PROMOTION DURING PREGNANCY

The purposes of antenatal care are to:

- Establish a baseline of present health
- Determine the gestational age of the fetus
- Monitor fetal development and maternal wellbeing
- Identify women at risk of complications
- Minimise the risk of possible complications by anticipating and preventing problems before they occur
- Provide time for education about pregnancy, lactation and newborn care.

If a woman has good health coming into a pregnancy, it helps to ensure a good pregnancy outcome.

Choosing a healthcare provider for pregnancy and childbirth

Once a woman is or suspects that she may be pregnant, her next step is to choose a primary healthcare provider to care for her throughout the pregnancy and birth. Various options are available, including an antenatal clinic, a registered midwife, an obstetrician or a family practitioner. Regardless of the type of healthcare provider chosen, antenatal care needs to be initiated early and continued throughout pregnancy (see Box 11.1). Nurses contribute to the success of antenatal care by listening, counselling and teaching, three areas of nursing expertise.

HEALTH ASSESSMENT DURING THE FIRST ANTENATAL VISIT

The major causes of death during pregnancy today are ectopic pregnancy, hypertension, haemorrhage, embolism, infection and anaesthesia related complications such as intrapartum cardiac arrest. An important focus of all antenatal visits, therefore, in addition to education about pregnancy, is to screen for danger signs that might reveal any of these conditions. Screening includes an extensive health history, a complete physical examination and blood and urine specimens for laboratory tests.

CASE STUDY QUESTION

3. Sandra feels well so she asks you why she needs to come for antenatal care. The best reason for her to receive regular care is:
   a. Discovering allergies can help eliminate early birth
   b. It helps document how many pregnancies occur each year
   c. It provides time for education about pregnancy and birth
   d. It will give her something to look forward to every month

The initial interview

Because initial health history taking is often time-consuming, a woman may be asked to complete some of the forms. Good interviewing technique, however, is important to obtain thorough and meaningful health histories. The rapport established by face-to-face interviewing gives a woman a feeling that she is more than just a client number or chart. It may be as much a reason she returns for follow-up care as her desire to be assured that her pregnancy is progressing normally (see Box 11.2).

Interviewing expectant women often elicits contradictory information. Women are likely to want to talk about their past health and current pregnancy, so interviewing them should go smoothly and be productive. On the other hand, pregnancy symptoms are subtle, so a woman may not regard certain information as important, providing vague answers instead of specific information to questions about these areas. She may be unaware that she is the only person who knows the answers to several vital questions ("How do you feel about being pregnant?" or "Have you been taking anything for your morning nausea?"). Outside pressures, such as having to report for work or older children coming home from school, can limit the length of an interview. Late in pregnancy, a woman may feel uncomfortable sitting for a long interview.

Interviewing is best accomplished in a private, quiet setting. It is helpful if the person scheduling appointments cautions a woman that a first visit may be lengthy. This prevents a woman from trying to fit the visit in between other errands or from having to terminate the interview because of another appointment. Be certain to ask what name a woman wants you to use when addressing her in an antenatal setting (Mrs, Miss, Ms or her first name) and make certain that she knows your name and understands your role correctly.

BOX 11.2 ✻ Focus on communication

Sandra has come to her obstetrician's office for a first antenatal visit.

Less effective communication

Nurse: Tell me what a typical day is like for you.
Sandra: I don't usually have typical ones. Or very interesting ones.
Nurse: What about yesterday? Could you describe that to me?
Sandra: Okay. I was up at 7 a.m. and at work by 9 a.m. A friend picked me up after work and we celebrated his birthday. I was back home and in bed by 10 p.m. That's pretty much the day.
Nurse: You're right. It doesn't sound too interesting. Next, let me ask you about your family medical history.

More effective communication

Nurse: Tell me what a typical day is like for you.
Sandra: I don't usually have typical ones. Or very interesting ones.
Nurse: What about yesterday? Could you describe that to me?
Sandra: Okay. I was up at 7 a.m., was at work by 9 a.m. A friend picked me up after work and we celebrated his birthday. I was back home and in bed by 10 p.m. That's pretty much the day.
Nurse: What did you have for breakfast?
Sandra: Nothing. I was too rushed to eat.
Nurse: Dinner?
Sandra: We went to a bar to celebrate. Cheese pancakes, I think. And beer. A lot of beer.

Most people are not aware how much information can be revealed by a day history, so they give only a scant description of their day. Asking additional questions to make them elaborate on various parts often reveals poor nutrition, poor exercise or risky pregnancy patterns.

Components of the health history

An initial interview serves several purposes:

- Establishing rapport
- Gaining information about a woman's physical and psychosocial health
- Obtaining a basis for anticipatory guidance for the pregnancy.

Included in the following section are the elements pertinent to a pregnancy history.

Demographic data

Demographic data obtained usually includes name, age, address, telephone number, email address, religion and health insurance information.

Chief concern

The chief concern is the reason a woman has come to the healthcare setting—in this instance, the fact that she is or thinks she is pregnant. To help confirm pregnancy, inquire about the date of her last menstrual period and whether she has had a pregnancy test or used a home test kit. Elicit information about the signs of early pregnancy, such as nausea, vomiting, breast changes or fatigue. Ask if she has any discomforts of pregnancy, such as constipation, backache or frequent urination. Also, ask about any danger signs of pregnancy, such as bleeding, continuous headache, visual disturbances or swelling of the hands and face.

Family profile

In the past, the social history or family setting history (family profile) was left until the end of a health interview. However, obtaining this information early in an interview can help you get to know a woman earlier, identify important support persons, shape the nature and kind of questions to be asked and evaluate the possible impact of a woman's culture on care. It also lays a foundation for health teaching, as before you can begin to offer a woman any more than stereotyped healthcare instructions, you need to know her age and that of her sexual partner, their educational levels (offers an estimation of the level of teaching you will plan) and occupation (does a woman's work involve heavy lifting, long hours of standing in one position, handling of a toxic substance, actions that may need to be modified during pregnancy?).

Be certain to ask about marital status and support people available as part of the information obtained. As a rule, both married and unmarried women want you to know their marital status as they want to alert you if they do not have support people readily available.

Adaptation to pregnancy is highly individualised. A change in status from independence to dependence because of stopping work, chronic illness at home, the death or loss of a significant person during pregnancy, geographical moves, financial hardship and lack of support people are examples of situations that can hinder a woman's ability to accept her pregnancy and child. No-one in the healthcare setting will be aware of these potentially harmful situations unless questions of this kind about family profile are asked.

History of past illnesses

Questions about a woman's past medical history are an important part of an interview because a past condition can become active during or immediately following pregnancy. Representative diseases that pose potential difficulty during pregnancy include kidney disease, heart disease (coarctation of the aorta and heart valve problems from rheumatic fever cause problems most often), hypertension, sexually transmitted infections (including hepatitis B and human immunodeficiency virus [HIV]), diabetes, thyroid disease, recurrent seizures, gallbladder disease, urinary tract infections, varicosities, phenylketonuria, tuberculosis and asthma. It is important to find out whether a woman had childhood diseases such as chickenpox (varicella), mumps (epidemic parotitis), measles (rubella), German measles (rubella) or poliomyelitis and whether she has had immunisations against these. Ask also about HPV (human papillomavirus) vaccine as many women are not yet aware there is a vaccine for this. The vaccine has the potential to prevent not only HPV infections but the development of cervical cancer (Centers for Disease Control and Prevention, 2012).

Ask also about any allergies, including any medication sensitivities. Although not well-proven, encouraging women with allergies of any magnitude to breastfeed rather than bottle-feed may help avoid milk or protein allergy in their infants (Kramer, 2011). Any past surgical procedures are also important to know about, because adhesions resulting from past abdominal surgery such as appendicitis could interfere with uterine growth.

What if...

Sandra tells you she has no idea what childhood diseases or immunisations she has had? How would you suggest that she obtain this information?

History of family illnesses

A family history documents illnesses that occur frequently in the family and so can help identify potential problems in a woman during pregnancy or in her infant at birth. Ask specifically about cardiovascular and renal disease, cognitive impairment, blood disorders, or any known genetically inherited diseases or congenital anomalies (Grigg, 2010).

Day history/social profile

Information about a woman's current nutrition, elimination, sleep, recreation and interpersonal interactions can be elicited best by asking her to describe a typical day of her life. If any of this information is not reported spontaneously as she describes her day, ask for additional details (see Box 11.2). Nutrition is an important part of a day history, particularly in the light of the number of young adults with eating disorders today. Ask about the type, amount and frequency of exercise to determine a woman's routine pattern and whether it will be consistent with a recommended level for pregnancy as this varies greatly among women (Grigg, 2010).

Because smoke, whether first-hand or second-hand, has been shown to be harmful to fetal growth, obtain information about a woman and her family's smoking habits. Excessive alcohol intake can not only lead to poor nutrition but can be directly responsible for fetal alcohol spectrum disorders and preterm birth so also record the amount of alcohol a woman consumes (Grigg, 2010). Pregnant women, especially adolescents, are at an increased risk of domestic violence (Grigg, 2010). Ask enough questions to be certain a woman is not involved in an abusive partnership with questions such as, "Have

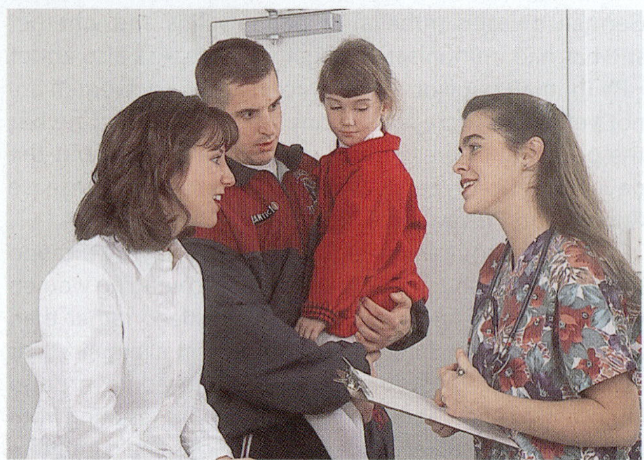

FIGURE 11.1 A woman should be given the choice of who she wants to bring with her for each antenatal visit, keeping in mind the screening for domestic violence and drugs and alcohol in the first few visits.

you ever been hurt by someone?" or "Are you afraid of anyone?" (see Fig. 11.1).

It is also important to obtain a medication history. Ask whether a woman takes any medications, prescribed or over-the-counter, because their effect on a growing fetus will have to be evaluated (McKenna & Mirkov, 2014). Many women use herbal supplements to relieve the nausea of early pregnancy, for example ginger, that may be detrimental to pregnancy as it causes anticoagulation (Tiran, 2012).

Cocaine use during pregnancy puts the fetus at risk of low birthweight. There is good evidence to show that cocaine can cause neurological and behavioural defects in the developing fetal brain. Opioid use during pregnancy is associated with an increased risk of prematurity, fetal growth restriction, sudden infant death syndrome and neonatal abstinence syndrome. The effects of heroin are very difficult to determine as most heroin users also use tobacco, having a profound effect on low birthweight. Women who are on a methadone program have fewer complications than those women who continue to use heroin. Pregnant women who are drug-dependent during pregnancy should be informed of the associated risks. In Australia, methadone is the only approved treatment for pregnant women and it is not without its risks. Methadone use is still associated with low birthweight and neonatal withdrawal from the drug (Thorogood, 2010).

Gynaecological history

A woman's past experience with her reproductive system may have some influence on how well she accepts a pregnancy so obtain information about her age of menarche (first menstrual period) and how well she was prepared for it as a normal part of life. Ask about her usual cycle, including the interval, duration, amount of menstrual flow and any discomfort she feels. Ascertain if she has discomfort with periods, including when the discomfort occurs, how long it lasts and what she does to relieve it. If she describes menstrual cramps as "horrible" and wonders "how I live through them some months", anticipate the need for additional counselling to help her prepare for labour. Some women with severe dysmenorrhoea are looking forward to pregnancy as it will mean 9 months without discomfort.

Ask about past surgery on the reproductive tract. For example, if a woman has had tubal surgery following an ectopic pregnancy, her statistical risk of another tubal pregnancy is increased because of the tubal scarring present. If she has had uterine surgery, a caesarean birth may be necessary because her uterus may not be able to expand and contract as efficiently as usual because of the surgical scar.

Ask also about what reproductive planning methods, if any, have been used. Occasionally, a woman may become pregnant with an intrauterine device (IUD) in place. If this occurs, it will be removed to prevent infection during pregnancy. Another woman, not realising she is pregnant, may continue to take an oral contraceptive for some time into her pregnancy. Document whether such use occurred, because some evidence suggests that oestrogen can harm fetal growth.

As part of any woman's gynaecological history, assess for the possibility of stress incontinence (incontinence of urine on laughing, coughing, deep inspiration, jogging or running). Stress incontinence occurs from lack of strength in the perineal muscles and bladder supports. Commonly, this weakness has occurred from difficult births, the birth of large infants, grand multiparity and instrumental births. During pregnancy, stress incontinence can become intensified from the increasing abdominal pressure. Women can relieve stress incontinence to some degree by strengthening the perineal muscles with the use of Kegel exercises (periodic tightening of the perineal muscles; see Chapter 12).

Obstetric history

Do not assume that the current pregnancy is a woman's first pregnancy simply because she is very young or says she has only recently been married. She may have had an adolescent pregnancy or this could be a second marriage. For each previous pregnancy, document the child's sex and the place and date of birth. Review the pregnancy briefly for:

- Was it planned?
- Did she have any complications, such as vaginal spotting, swelling of her hands or feet, falls or surgery?
- Did she take any medication? If so, what and why?
- Did she receive antenatal care? If so, when did she start?
- What was the duration of the pregnancy?
- What was the duration of labour?
- Was labour what she expected? Worse? Better?
- What was the type of birth? Vaginal or caesarean? Vertex or breech? In a hospital or at home?
- What type of anaesthesia, if any, was used?

- Did she have perineal stitches following birth?
- Did she have any complications, such as excessive bleeding or infection following the birth?
- What was the infant's birth weight and sex?
- What was the condition of the infant at birth? Did the infant cry right away?
- What was the infant's Apgar score? (Most mothers know this.)
- Was any special care needed for the baby, such as suctioning, oxygen or an incubator?
- Was the baby discharged from the healthcare setting with her?
- What is the child's present state of health?
- How was the pregnancy overall for her?

Ask about any previous miscarriages or terminations of pregnancies and whether she had any complications during or following these. If a woman's blood type is Rh negative, ask if she received Rh immune globulin (RhIG [RhoGAM]) (Anti-D) after miscarriages or terminations or previous births so you will know whether Rh sensitisation could have occurred. Ask if she has ever had a blood transfusion to establish possible risk of hepatitis B or HIV exposure or Rh sensitisation from a blood transfusion.

After a history of previous pregnancies is obtained, determine a woman's status with respect to the number of times she has been pregnant, including the present pregnancy **(gravida)** and the number of children above the age of viability she has previously borne **(para)** with each pregnancy being counted as para 1 even if she has a multiple pregnancy. For example, a woman who has had two previous pregnancies, has given birth to two term children and is again pregnant, is gravida 3, para 2. A woman who has had two miscarriages at 12 weeks (under the age of viability) and is again pregnant is a gravida 3, para 0. If a woman has been pregnant twice and has birthed her first pregnancy with two live viable twin infants and she is pregnant again now, she would be classed as G 2, P 1.

A review of systems helps women recall concerns they forgot to mention earlier, such as a urinary tract infection, a disease that can influence the outcome of pregnancy and so would be important to your history taking. The following body systems and questions about conditions constitute the minimum information to be addressed in a review of systems for a first antenatal visit:

- *Head:* Headache? Head injury? Seizures? Dizziness? Fainting?
- *Eyes:* Vision? Glasses needed? Diplopia or double vision? Infection? Glaucoma? Cataract? Pain? Recent changes?
- *Ears:* Infection? Discharge? Earache? Hearing loss? Tinnitus? Vertigo?
- *Nose:* Epistaxis (nose bleeds)? Discharge? How many colds a year? Allergies? Post nasal drainage? Sinus pain?
- *Mouth and pharynx:* Dentures? Condition of teeth? Toothaches? Any bleeding of gums? Hoarseness? Difficulty in swallowing? Tonsillectomy? Last dental examination?
- *Neck:* Stiffness? Masses?
- *Breasts:* Lumps? Secretion? Pain? Tenderness?
- *Respiratory system:* Cough? Wheezing? Asthma? Shortness of breath? Pain? Serious chest illness, such as tuberculosis or pneumonia?
- *Cardiovascular system:* History of heart murmur? History of heart disease such as rheumatic fever or Kawasaki disease? Hypertension? Any pain? Palpitations? Anaemia? Does she know her blood pressure? Has she ever had a blood transfusion?
- *Gastrointestinal system:* What was her pre-pregnancy weight? Vomiting? Diarrhoea? Constipation? Change in bowel habits? Rectal pruritus? Haemorrhoids? Pain? Ulcer? Gallbladder disease? Hepatitis? Appendicitis?
- *Genitourinary system:* Urinary tract infection? Haematuria? Frequent urination? Sexually transmitted infection? Pelvic inflammatory disease? Hepatitis B? HIV? Was subfertility a concern? Did she have a problem getting pregnant?
- *Extremities:* Varicose veins? Pain or stiffness of joints? Any fractures or dislocations?
- *Skin:* Any rashes? Acne? Psoriasis?

Conclusion

End an interview by asking if there is something you have not covered that a woman wants to discuss. This gives her one more chance to ask any questions she has about this new life experience.

Support person's role

Both partners and young children may accompany women for antenatal care. Some women bring a female friend or their mother as their best support person. If family members are present, should they be included in an initial interview? As a whole, interviewing is most effective if it is a one-to-one interaction. A woman may be unwilling to mention certain concerns when her family is present for fear of worrying them. A husband may not be the father of her child, for example, and she would be unable to voice her concern over this or alert you to the possibility she is worried about blood incompatibility because another man is the father.

If childbearing is to be a family affair, however, it is important to determine a partner's degree of acceptance of the pregnancy and of assuming a new parenting role. Including siblings in an antenatal visit provides you with an opportunity to involve them with the pregnancy planning and coming baby from the very beginning. See Box 11.3.

CASE STUDY QUESTION

4. Why is it important to ask Sandra about past surgery in a pregnancy health history?

a. To test both her recent and long-term memory
b. Adhesions from surgery could limit uterine growth
c. To assess whether she could be allergic to any medication
d. To determine if she has effective health insurance

BOX 11.3 * Focus on family teaching

Suggestions for encouraging partner participation in antenatal visits

Q. Sandra asks you, "What can I do to make sure that my boyfriend feels involved with antenatal care?"

A. Here are some suggestions for encouraging your partner's participation:

- Ask for appointments to be scheduled at a time that is convenient for both of you.
- Be certain that your partner reserves enough time so the visit does not become more of an inconvenience than an enjoyable event. An antenatal visit can be lengthy.
- Ask your partner to accompany you into the examining room at visits so you can share progress or decisions.
- Be certain that your partner listens to the fetal heart at visits as soon as it can be heard.
- If an ultrasound is scheduled, ask your partner to view it with you (it is an exciting moment for both of you to see your fetus moving).

Physical examination

The next step in health assessment is a physical examination. Ask a woman to void for a clean-catch urine specimen. A urinalysis is performed for evaluation of leucocytes, protein, glucose and ketones. A physical examination at a first antenatal visit typically includes inspection of major body systems, with emphasis on the changes that occur with pregnancy or that could signal a developing problem. General techniques of physical examination are discussed in Chapter 34.

Baseline height/weight and vital sign measurement

Measure a woman's weight and height at a first antenatal visit to establish a baseline for future comparison. Record this assessment with her pre-pregnancy BMI, if available, to calculate an acceptable weight gain during pregnancy. When weighing, be certain to convey an air of "weight gain is healthy" so the woman feels comfortable gaining 8 to 12 kg during pregnancy.

Measure vital signs, including blood pressure, respiratory rate and pulse rate, for a baseline level as well. A sudden increase in blood pressure, the same as a sudden weight gain, is a danger sign of hypertension of pregnancy. NICE Guidelines (2011) define hypertension as ≥140 mmHg systolic and ≥90 mmHg diastolic. If you are able to ascertain information about the woman's blood pressure prior to pregnancy, the woman's systolic blood pressure increase of 30 mmHg and the woman's diastolic blood pressure increase of 15 mmHg or above would also be classified as hypertension. So, for example, if the woman's blood pressure was 90/60 mmHg pre-pregnancy, and it is currently 120/75 mmHg, this would be classified as hypertension. A sudden increase in pulse or respirations can suggest bleeding and anxiety.

Assessment of systems

General appearance and mental status

Physical examination always begins with an inspection of general appearance to form an overall impression of a woman's health and wellbeing. General appearance is important because the manner in which people dress, the way they speak and the body posture they assume all suggest how they feel about themselves. Not all women are happy about being pregnant. Closely inspect for signs such as careless hygiene, unwashed hair, inappropriate or soiled clothing and sad facial expression that may suggest fatigue or depression about their pregnancy.

Head and scalp

Examine a woman's head for symmetry, normal contour and tenderness and the hair for presence, distribution, thickness, excessive dryness or oiliness, cleanliness, or the use of hair dye (hair dye may be carcinogenic over an extended period of time). Look for **chloasma** (extra pigment on the face that occurs from melanocyte-stimulating hormone), which may accompany pregnancy. Hair growth speeds up during pregnancy as a result of the overall increased metabolic rate and women may comment they have noticed this. Dryness or sparseness of hair suggests poor nutrition whilst lack of cleanliness may suggest fatigue, reflecting that a woman has not felt well enough to wash it recently.

Eyes

Oedema of the eyelids combined with a swollen optic disk (identified on ophthalmoscopic examination) suggests oedema from pregnancy-induced hypertension, a potentially dangerous condition in pregnancy. On interview, women with pregnancy-induced hypertension also usually report spots before their eyes or diplopia (double vision) and blurred vision. Teach pregnant women to recognise symptoms of changing vision as a potential danger sign of pregnancy that should be reported as soon as possible.

Nose

The increased level of oestrogen associated with pregnancy may cause nasal congestion or the appearance of swollen nasal membranes. Even topical medicines such as nose drops or nasal sprays used to reduce this are absorbed to some degree. Advise a woman to avoid these during pregnancy without her doctor's or midwife's knowledge and consent.

Ears

The nasal stuffiness that accompanies pregnancy may lead to blocked eustachian tubes and therefore a feeling of "fullness" in the ears or dampening of sound during early pregnancy. Usually this disappears as the body adjusts to the new oestrogen level.

Sinuses

Sinuses should feel non-tender. Establishing that tenderness over sinuses does not exist helps to evaluate that a woman's report of headache during pregnancy (a danger sign until ruled otherwise) is probably not sinus related.

Mouth, teeth and throat

Gingival (gum) hypertrophy may result from oestrogen stimulation during pregnancy. The gums become slightly swollen and tender to the touch, but not reddened. Pregnant women are prone to vitamin deficiency because of the rapid growth of the fetus. Assess carefully for cracked corners of the mouth, which would reveal vitamin A deficiency. Assess carefully for pinpoint lesions with an erythematous base on the lips; these suggest a herpes infection (a herpes lesion on the gumline is more often a shallow ulcer). As newborns are susceptible to any infection in the first 6 weeks due to low immunity levels, lesions present at birth may necessitate a woman needing to wear a mask to breastfeed her newborn.

Teach all women not to neglect good dental hygiene or yearly dental visits while pregnant. They should maintain thorough toothbrushing (some stop thorough brushing because they notice slightly blood-tinged saliva because of gingival hypertrophy).

Breasts

Breast changes may be one of the first things women notice in pregnancy:

- Areolae darken
- Secondary areolae develop
- Montgomery tubercles (sebaceous glands in the areolae) become prominent
- Overall breast size increases
- Breast consistency firms
- Blue streaking of veins becomes prominent
- Colostrum may be expelled as early as the 16th week of pregnancy
- Any supernumerary nipple also may become darker and enlarge in size.

Heart

Heart rate typically ranges from 60 to 90 beats per minute in pregnant women and no accessory sounds or murmurs should be present. Many women notice occasional palpitations (heart skipping a beat) during pregnancy, especially when lying supine. Teach pregnant women always to rest or sleep on their side (left side is best) to help avoid this problem.

Lungs

Assess respiratory rate and rhythm. Although lung tissue assumes a more horizontal position during pregnancy, vital capacity is not reduced. Late in pregnancy, diaphragmatic excursion (diaphragm movement) is lessened because the diaphragm cannot descend as fully as usual because of the distended uterus. This causes women to feel short of breath.

Back

The lumbar curve in many pregnant women is accentuated on standing so that they can maintain body posture in the face of increasing abdominal size. This response can cause considerable back pain during pregnancy. This is known as lumbar lordosis as body weight is redistributed to accommodate the large growing uterus. Progesterone and relaxin also increase during pregnancy, which causes relaxation of muscles and laxation of discs. Lumbar disc prolapse may cause sciatica and referred pain travelling down the leg, accompanied by pins and needles in the foot. Assess a woman's spine for any abnormal curve that would suggest scoliosis.

Extremities and skin

Assess the lower extremities carefully for varicosities, filling time of the toenails (which should be under 5 seconds) and the presence of oedema caused by impaired venous return from the lower extremities. Any oedema more than ankle swelling may be a danger sign of pregnancy.

Measurement of fundal height and fetal heart sounds

At about 12 to 14 weeks of pregnancy, the uterus becomes palpable as a firm globular sphere over the symphysis pubis. It reaches the umbilicus at 24 weeks and the xyphoid process at 36 weeks, and then often returns to about 4 cm below the xyphoid because of "lightening" at 40 weeks. If a woman is past 12 weeks of a pregnancy, palpate the fundus location, measure the fundal height (from the notch above the symphysis pubis to the superior aspect of the uterine fundus) and plot the height on a graph such as the one shown in Fig. 11.2. Plotting uterine growth at each visit this way can help detect any unusual variation in fetal growth. If an abnormality is detected, further investigation with ultrasound can be carried out to determine the cause of the unusual increase or decrease in growth.

Auscultate for fetal heart sounds (110 to 160 beats per minute). These can be heard at 10 to 12 weeks if a Doppler technique is used. Palpate for fetal outline and position after the 30th week as a further estimation of fetal size and growth.

Pelvic size

The pelvis is a bony ring formed by four united bones: the two innominate (flaring hip) bones, which form the anterior and lateral portion of the ring, and the coccyx and sacrum, which form the posterior aspect. It serves both to support and protect the pelvic organs. Important terms in relation

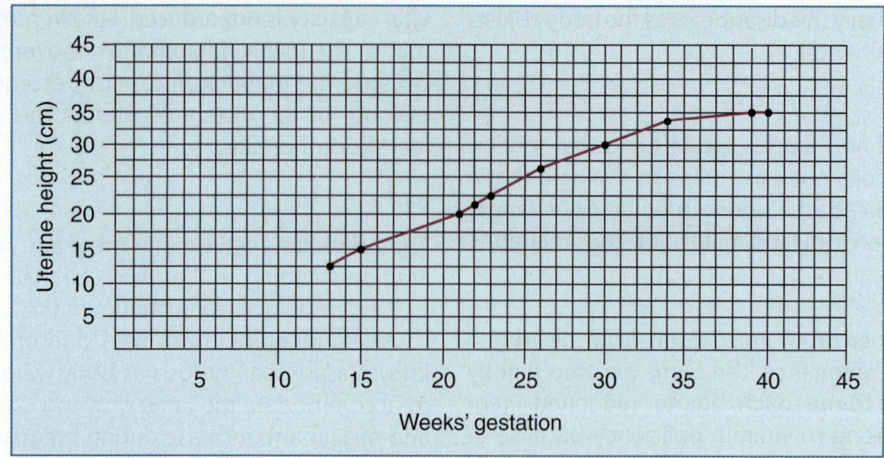

FIGURE 11.2 Plotting uterine height on a uterine height graph at antenatal visits (typically after 12 weeks' gestation) helps to monitor whether fundal height is increasing.

to the pelvis are the inlet, the pelvic cavity and the outlet. The inlet is the entrance to the true pelvis, or the upper ring of bone through which the fetus must pass to be born vaginally. The pelvic cavity is the space between the inlet and the outlet.

Establishing adequacy for childbirth

The pelvis is a bony ring formed by four united bones: the two innominate (flaring hip) bones, which form the anterior and lateral portion of the ring, and the coccyx and sacrum, which form the posterior aspect (see Fig. 11.3). The pelvis serves both to support and protect pelvic organs.

- Each innominate bone is divided into three parts: ilium, ischium and pubis.
- The ilium forms the upper and lateral portion. The flaring superior border forms the prominence of the hip (the crest of the ilium).
- The ischium is the inferior portion.
- At the lowest portion of the ischium are two projections: the ischial tuberosities, or the part of the bone on which a person sits. These projections are important markers used to determine lower pelvic width.
- The ischial spines are small projections that extend from the lateral aspects of the pelvis into the pelvic cavity. They mark the midpoint of the pelvis. Their location is

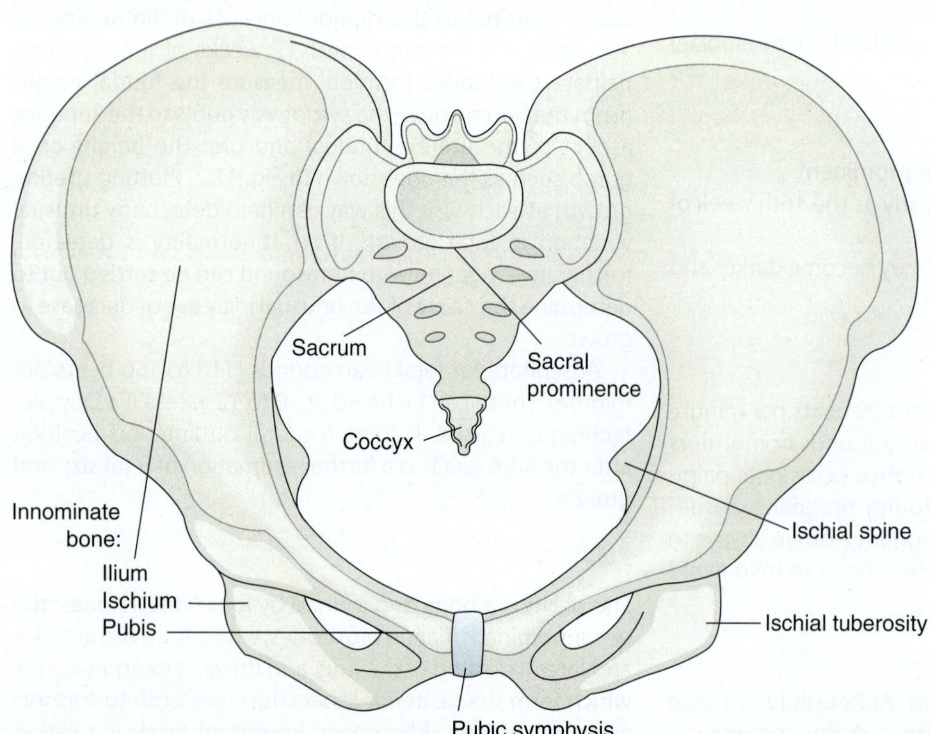

FIGURE 11.3 Structure of the pelvis.

used to assess the level to which a fetus has descended into the birth canal just before or during labour.

- Where the two anterior portions of the innominate bone meet is the symphysis pubis.
- The sacrum is the upper posterior portion of the pelvic ring. There is a marked anterior projection of this bone at the point where it touches the lower lumbar vertebrae (the sacral prominence), which is used as a landmark when securing pelvic measurements.
- The coccyx, just below the sacrum, is composed of five very small bones fused together. Although the bone itself is stiff, there is a degree of movement possible in the joint between the sacrum and the coccyx (the sacrococcygeal joint). This movement is important during labour because it permits the coccyx to be pressed backwards, allowing more room for the fetal head to pass through the bony pelvic ring at birth. For obstetric purposes, the pelvis is further divided into the false pelvis (the superior half) and the true pelvis (the inferior half) (see Fig. 11.4). The false pelvis supports the uterus during the late months of pregnancy and aids in directing the fetus into the true pelvis for birth. The false pelvis is divided from the true pelvis only by an imaginary line, the linea terminalis. This imaginary line is drawn from the sacral prominence at the back of the pelvis to the superior aspect of the symphysis pubis at the front.

Other important terms in relation to the pelvis are the *inlet*, the *outlet* and the *pelvic cavity*:

- The *inlet* is the entrance to the true pelvis, or the upper ring of bone through which the fetus must pass to be born vaginally. It is at the level of the linea terminalis or is marked by the sacral prominence in the back, the ilium on the sides and the superior aspect of the symphysis pubis in the front. If you looked down at the pelvic inlet, the passageway would appear heart-shaped because of the jutting sacral prominence. It is wider transversely (sideways) than in the anteroposterior dimension.
- The *outlet* is the inferior portion of the pelvis, or that portion bounded in the back by the coccyx, on the sides by the ischial tuberosities and in the front by the inferior aspect of the symphysis pubis. In contrast to the inlet of the pelvis, the greatest diameter of the outlet is its anteroposterior diameter.
- The *pelvic cavity* is the space between the inlet and the outlet. This space is not a straight but a curved passage; the purpose of its curve is to slow and control the speed of birth. This helps reduce sudden pressure changes in the fetal head, lowering the danger of ruptured cerebral arteries. The snugness of the cavity also serves to compress the chest of the fetus as he or she passes through. This helps to expel lung fluid and mucus and thereby better prepare lungs for good aeration at birth. For a baby to be born vaginally, he or she must be able to pass through the inlet, the cavity and the outlet of the pelvic bone. This is not a problem for the average fetus; it may, however, be a problem if the mother is a young adolescent who has not yet achieved full pelvic growth (girls younger than age 14 years are most prone to this difficulty) or a woman who has had a pelvic injury from something such as an automobile accident. A macrosomic or baby weighing >4000 g has a much higher percentage of experiencing shoulder dystocia or difficulty birthing the shoulders than a normal sized baby, 2500 g to 4000 g.

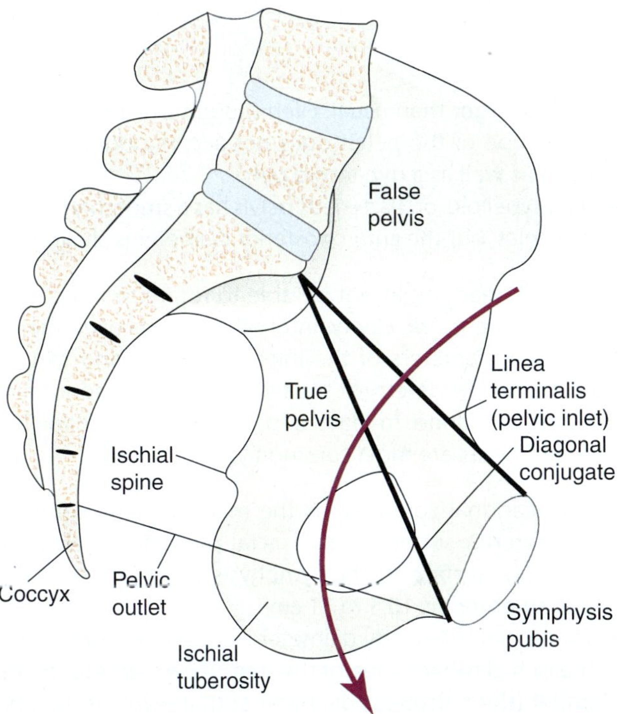

FIGURE 11.4 True and false pelvis. Portion above linea terminalis is false pelvis; portion below is true pelvis. Arrow shows "stovepipe" curve the fetus must follow to be born.

Estimating pelvic size

It is impossible to predict from the outward appearance of a woman whether her pelvic ring will be adequate for a fetus to pass through its centre without difficulty. This is because some women appear to have a wide pelvis but, in reality, have only wide iliac crests and a normal or even smaller-than-usual internal ring. Other women look as if their pelvis will be small because the iliac crests are non-flaring, but the internal pelvis, the part that must be sufficiently large for childbirth, is of average size, allowing them to give birth vaginally without difficulty. Differences in pelvic contour occur mainly because of hereditary factors, but diseases such as rickets, now rarely seen in Australia and New Zealand but still a concern in undeveloped countries, may cause contraction of the pelvis and severely narrow the pelvic outlet (Mughal, 2011).

If on an initial prenatal visit, the primary care provider establishes that a woman is pregnant, and if she has never given birth vaginally before, pelvic measurements may be taken. Some care providers prefer, however, to take these measurements later in pregnancy, when a woman's pelvic

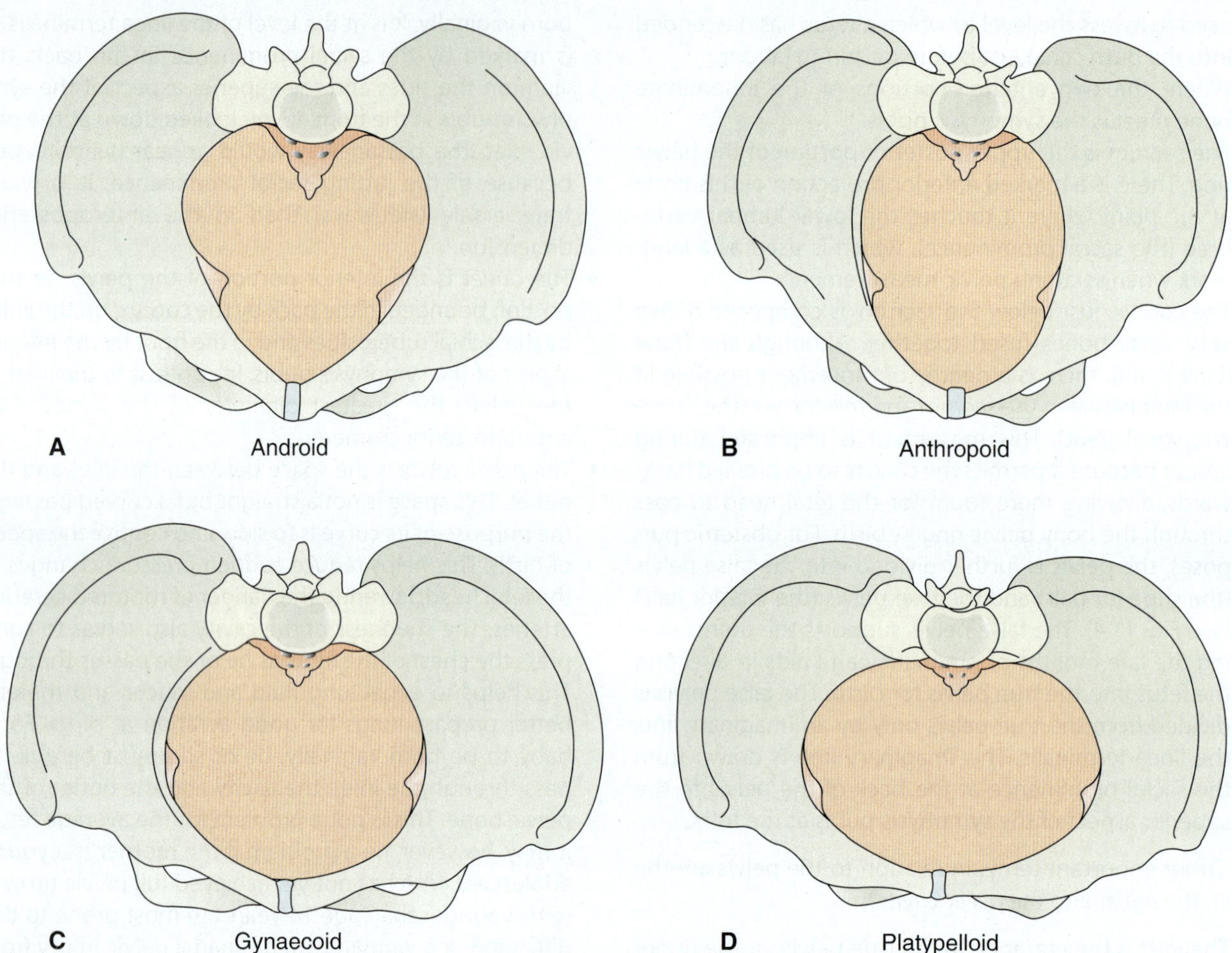

FIGURE 11.5 Types of pelves. (**A**) *Android*, or "male", pelvis. (**B**) *Anthropoid*, or "ape-like", pelvis. (**C**) *Gynaecoid*, or "female", pelvis. (**D**) *Platypelloid*, or "flattened", pelvis.

muscles are more relaxed, making measurement easier. Estimation of pelvic adequacy must be done at least by the 24th week of pregnancy, because by this time there is danger that the fetal head has reached a size that would interfere with safe passage and birth if the pelvic measurements are small. Once a woman has given birth vaginally, her pelvis has been proven adequate for vaginal birth, so it is unnecessary for pelvic measurements to be repeated unless she had an intervening history or trauma to the pelvis between pregnancies.

Types of pelves found in women can be categorised into four groups: gynaecoid, android, anthropoid and platypelloid (see Fig. 11.5):

- A gynaecoid, or "female", pelvis has an inlet that is well rounded forwards and backwards and has a wide pubic arch. This pelvic type is ideal for childbirth.
- In an android, or "male", pelvis, the pubic arch forms an acute angle, making the lower dimensions of the pelvis extremely narrow. A fetus may have difficulty exiting from this type of pelvis.
- In an anthropoid, or "ape-like", pelvis, the transverse diameter is narrow; the anteroposterior diameter of the inlet is larger than usual. Even though the inlet is large, the shape of the pelvis does not accommodate a fetal head as well as a gynaecoid pelvis.
- A platypelloid, or "flattened", pelvis has a smoothly curved oval inlet, but the anteroposterior diameter is shallow.

A fetal head might not be able to rotate to match the curves of the pelvic cavity. Internal pelvic measurements reveal the diameters of the inlet and outlet and can be obtained by pelvimetry at the time of a routine sonogram examination done to date a pregnancy. The following measurements are most commonly determined:

- The diagonal conjugate is the measurement between the anterior surface of the sacral prominence and the posterior surface of the symphysis pubis. The average measurement is 10.5 to 11 cm.
- The ischial tuberosity diameter is the distance between the ischial tuberosities, or the transverse diameter of the outlet (the narrowest diameter at that level, or the one most apt to cause a misfit). It is made at the medial and lowermost aspect of the ischial tuberosities at the level of the anus. A diameter of 11 cm is considered adequate

because it will allow the widest diameter of the fetal head, or 9 cm, to pass freely through the outlet.

Pap smear

A Pap smear is taken for early detection and diagnosis of precancerous and cancerous conditions of the uterine cervix, vulva or vagina; the test also reveals inflammatory and infectious diseases (MacKay, 2009).

Laboratory assessment

Several laboratory studies are included in assessment measures at a first antenatal visit to confirm general health and screen for HIV, hepatitis B, sexually transmitted infections, rubella, antibodies, and genetic disorders such as Down syndrome (Trisomy 21) and spina bifida.

Blood studies

The following blood studies are usually obtained at a first antenatal visit:

1. A complete blood count, including haemoglobin or haematocrit, a red cell index to determine the presence of anaemia, a white blood cell count to determine infection and a platelet count to estimate clotting ability.
2. A serological test for syphilis (VDRL or rapid plasma reagin test). If syphilis is present, it must be treated early in pregnancy before fetal damage occurs. A blood sample for a serological test for gonorrhoea may be drawn as well.
3. Blood typing (including Rh factor). Blood type is documented because blood may have to be made available if a woman experiences bleeding during pregnancy and to detect the possibility of Rh isoimmunisation.
4. Antibody titres for rubella and hepatitis B (HBsAg). These tests determine whether a woman is protected against rubella if exposure should occur during pregnancy and whether a newborn will have a chance of developing Hepatitis B. HBsAg testing may be repeated at about 36 weeks. Antibodies for varicella (chickenpox) may also be assessed. Vaccines against these diseases can then be offered in the postpartum period.
5. HIV screening. Screening is carried out by an enzyme-linked immunosorbent assay (ELISA) on a blood sample. If this is positive, the finding is confirmed by a second test (a Western blot). Testing for HIV early in pregnancy allows a woman who is found to be HIV antibody positive the opportunity to begin therapy with zidovudine (AZT), which can decrease the risk of her infant acquiring the virus. It also allows a woman the option of choosing to terminate a pregnancy to avoid giving birth to an infant who has a high risk of HIV infection. Because HIV testing is controversial, be certain that the information given about test results is accurate (a high blood antibody titre means the person has been exposed to the virus, not that he or she necessarily is infected) and findings are presented with tact and compassion, with respect to the meaning of the results to a woman. Results of HIV testing are kept confidential; be certain not to report this information to anyone other than the woman.
6. A low level of maternal alpha fetoprotein in pregnancy may indicate Down syndrome or Trisomy 21. The Bart's test may also be used to determine other disorders which includes levels of oestriol, hCG and Pregnancy Associated Plasma Protein A (PAPP-A).
7. Women are scheduled for a 75-gram oral glucose challenge test towards the end of the first trimester to rule out gestational diabetes. This will be carried out routinely at the 24th to 28th week to evaluate insulin-antagonistic effects of placental hormones, which can register a noticeable effect at this time.

Urinalysis

A urinalysis is performed to test for proteinuria, glycosuria and leucocytes. All three of these can be carried out by means of test strips or microscopic examination of the urine.

Ultrasonography

If the date of the last menstrual period is unknown, the earliest ultrasound date will be the most accurate. The woman can be provided with information about the nuchal translucency test at 11 to 13 weeks' gestation and a morphology ultrasound at 18 to 20 weeks' gestation. The morphology scan is the best time to visualise the spine in order to screen for spina bifida. Be certain that women know that an ultrasound performed this early in pregnancy will show only the presence of a gestation sac, not a moving, kicking fetus, so that their expectations of what they will see are realistic (Grigg, 2010).

Risk assessment

After the first antenatal visit assessment, findings are analysed and discussed with the woman so that she can make an informed decision about screening and possible termination. A woman identified as being at high risk will need close observation during pregnancy to see that the pregnancy is progressing well; the infant born of a woman identified this way needs close observation in the neonatal period until it is confirmed that no anomalies exist. Risk assessment should be updated at each pregnancy visit, as the failure to identify risk potential in pregnancy leads to increased perinatal mortality. See Chapters 20–22 for discussion of high-risk pregnancy and its management. A woman can be provided with options for antenatal care throughout her pregnancy that includes continuity of care models (see Box 11.4).

SIGNS INDICATING COMPLICATIONS OF PREGNANCY

Although most signs indicating complications of pregnancy occur towards the end of pregnancy, women can be

BOX 11.4 ✻ Assessments and care for continuing antenatal visits

Mother's health

Health interview

Interim history or new personal or family developments since last visit
Review danger signs of pregnancy
Review symptoms of beginning labour

Physical examination

Blood pressure (every visit)
Clean-catch urine for glucose, protein and leucocytes (every visit)
Blood serum level for alpha-fetoprotein (MSAFP) (16 weeks)
VDRL test for syphilis if possibility of new exposure
Glucose screen (28 weeks)
Glucose challenge (24–28 weeks) if warranted
Anti-Rh titre (28 weeks)
Anti-Rh titre (34 weeks)
Group B streptococci (GBS) (35–37 weeks)

Fetal health

Fetal heart rate
Fundal height
Quickening or fetal movement
Ultrasound dating of pregnancy

provided with education from the outset. The woman can be educated about pregnancy as a normal event and if any deviations occur, she can notify her carer.

Vaginal bleeding

A woman should report vaginal bleeding, no matter how slight, because some of the serious bleeding complications of pregnancy begin with only slight spotting. When talking with a woman, ask her how she discovered the spotting. If she discovered it on toilet paper following a bowel movement, she is probably reporting spotting from haemorrhoids. Until the bleeding is found to be innocent, however, all women with spotting need further evaluation.

Persistent vomiting

Once- or twice-daily vomiting is not uncommon during the first trimester of pregnancy. However, persistent, frequent vomiting is not normal. Vomiting that continues past the 12th week of pregnancy is also extended vomiting. Persistent or extended vomiting depletes the nutritional supply available to a fetus so is a danger to the pregnancy. (See Chapter 13 for an in-depth discussion of persistent vomiting [hyperemesis gravidarum].)

Chills and fever

Chills and fever may be symptoms of a relatively benign gastroenteritis, but they may also indicate an intrauterine infection, a potentially serious complication for both a woman and a fetus. Because a woman cannot make a definite determination about the cause of a fever, further evaluation by a healthcare provider is necessary.

Sudden escape of clear fluid from the vagina

When a gush of clear fluid is discharged suddenly from the vagina, it means the membranes have ruptured and provides an avenue of infection. The woman should go to hospital to have the fetal heart rate checked, but she may be discharged 18 hours post-rupture if no labour ensues. She is less likely to harbour infection at home compared to the hospital environment. One of the risks of a high fetal head that does not fit snugly into the lower pole of the uterus or apply well to the cervix is that the umbilical cord may prolapse following membrane rupture. If the cord is then compressed by the fetal head, oxygenation is compromised and will be viewed as variable decelerations on a cardiotocograph (CTG). Occasionally, a woman confuses stress incontinence (involuntary loss of urine on coughing or sneezing or lifting a heavy object) with this. In this situation, speculum examination typically reveals that the membranes are still intact.

Abdominal or chest pain

Abdominal pain at any time is a signal that something is abnormal, so a woman should report it immediately. Some women may think that this is normal because the growing uterus is deflecting their other organs from their usual alignment, but a pregnant uterus normally expands painlessly. Abdominal pain is therefore a sign of some other problem, such as a tubal (ectopic) pregnancy, separation of the placenta, preterm labour or something unrelated to the pregnancy but perhaps equally as serious, such as appendicitis, an ulcer or pancreatitis. Chest pain may indicate a pulmonary embolus, a complication that can follow thrombophlebitis.

Pregnancy-induced hypertension

Pregnancy-induced hypertension (PIH) refers to a potentially severe and even fatal elevation of blood pressure that occurs during pregnancy. Several symptoms signal that PIH is developing:

- Rapid weight gain (over 4 kg/week in the second trimester, over 2 kg/week in the third trimester)
- Swelling of the face or fingers
- Flashes of light or dots before the eyes
- Dimness or blurring of vision
- Severe, continuous headache
- Decreased urine output
- Blood pressure increased ≥140/≥90 mmHg
- Indigestion that could mean epigastric pain from enlargement of the liver.

Individually, these symptoms can sometimes be vague so a woman may need some help appreciating that they are important to report during pregnancy. Some oedema of the ankles during pregnancy is normal, for example, particularly if it occurs after a woman has been on her feet for a long period. Swelling of the hands (ask if she has noticed if her rings are tight) or face (difficulty opening eyes in the morning because of oedema of the eyelids), however, indicates oedema that is more extensive than usual. Visual disturbances or a continuous headache may signal cerebral oedema or acute hypertension. Be certain a woman is not reporting symptoms she had before she became pregnant. If she had the same visual difficulties and headaches before pregnancy as she is reporting now, she may need to see an ophthalmologist rather than her obstetrician for help with the problem. (See Chapter 21 for more on PIH.)

Increase or decrease in fetal movement

A fetus normally moves more or less the same amount every day, an unusual increase or decrease in movement suggests that a fetus is responding to a need for oxygen. Be sure to ask a woman about typical fetal movements and whether she has noticed any increase or decrease in this rate. If there has been a change, she is a candidate for further testing and follow-up.

CASE STUDY QUESTION

5. You tell Sandra about the danger signs of pregnancy. Which of the following would you tell her to report if it should occur?
   a. Her uterus becomes palpable over the symphysis pubis at 12 weeks
   b. Blue veins can be readily observed on both of her breasts
   c. She gains more weight than 1 kilogram a week beginning at 20 weeks
   d. Her uterus is growing so slowly the growth is not causing any pain

Key points for review

- Antenatal care has the potential to reduce the incidence of preterm birth and congenital anomalies and the infant mortality rate.
- The purpose of antenatal care is to establish a baseline of present health, determine the gestational age of the fetus, monitor fetal development, identify women at risk of complications, minimise the risk of possible complications by anticipating and preventing problems before they occur and provide time for education about pregnancy and possible dangers.
- A first antenatal visit confirms a pregnancy, but it is also a time for important assessments such as a health history, physical examination and laboratory tests. The physical examination includes measurement of fundal height and assessment of fetal heart sounds if the pregnancy is beyond 12 weeks.
- A first antenatal visit sets the tone for visits to follow. Maintaining a supportive manner is helpful to establish rapport and allow a woman to feel comfortable to return for future care.
- Danger signs for women to report during pregnancy are vaginal bleeding, persistent vomiting, chills and fever, escape of fluid from the vagina, abdominal or chest pain, swelling of the face and fingers, vision changes or continuous headache, burning with urination or a pronounced decrease in fetal movement.
- Remember that a family, not a woman alone, is having a baby, and include family members in procedures and health teaching as desired.

CASE STUDY QUESTIONS

6. Sandra was worried about having a pelvic examination. How could you help relieve her concern?
7. Sandra works at a commercial laundry ironing sheets. Is this a job that probably keeps her on her feet for long periods? Is she apt to be exposed to toxic substances at work? Is there a greater opportunity than usual for her to develop upper respiratory infections?
8. Sandra's boyfriend rarely comes with her to antenatal visits. Another woman has a supportive husband who always comes. Would your role be different in these two situations?

Resources

For an extensive range of additional resources to enhance teaching and learning and to facilitate understanding of this chapter, please see the text's accompanying website located on thePoint at http://thepoint.lww.com.

References

Attilakos, G. & Overton, T. G. (2012). Antenatal care. In D. K. Edmonds (Ed). *Dewhurst's Textbook of Obstetrics & Gynaecology* (8th ed., pp. 42–52). Oxford, UK: John Wiley & Sons.

Centers for Disease Control and Prevention. (2012). Human papillomavirus—associated cancers: United States, 2004–2008. *MMWR: Morbidity & Mortality Weekly Report, 20*(61), 258–261.

Cootauco, A. C. & Althaus, J. E. (2007). Preterm labour and premature rupture of membranes. In K. B. Fortner et al. (Eds). *The Johns Hopkins Manual of Gynecology and Obstetrics.* Philadelphia: Lippincott Williams & Wilkins.

Davey, M-A., McLachlan, H. L., Forster, D. & Flood, M. Influence of timing of admission in labour and management of labour on method of birth: Results from a randomised controlled trial of caseload midwifery (COSMOS trial). *Midwifery*, ISSN 0266-6138, 12/2013, Volume 29, Issue 12, p. 1297.

Grigg, C. (2010). Working with women in pregnancy. In S. Pairman, S. Tracy, C. Thorogood & C. Pinombe. 2010, *Midwifery Preparation for Practice*, (2nd ed.). Sydney: Churchill Livingstone Elsevier.

Katsufrakis, P. J. & Workowski, K. A. (2008). Sexually transmitted diseases. In J. E. South Paul, S. Matheny & E. L. Lewis (Eds). *Current Diagnosis and Treatment in Family Medicine* (2nd ed.). Columbus, OH: McGraw-Hill.

Kingston, D., Heaman, M., Fell, D., et al. (2012). Comparison of adolescent, young adult, and adult women's maternity experiences and practices. *Pediatrics, 129*(5), e1228–e1237.

Kramer, M. S. (2011). Breastfeeding and allergy: The evidence. *Annals of Nutrition & Metabolism, 59*(Suppl. 1), 20–26.

MacKay, H. T. (2009). Gynecology. In S. J. McPhee & M. A. Papadakis (Eds). *Current Medical Diagnosis and Treatment*. Columbus, OH: McGraw-Hill.

McKenna, L. & Mirkov, S. (2014). *McKenna's Drug Handbook for Nursing and Midwifery* (7th ed.). Sydney: Lippincott Williams & Wilkins.

Mughal, M. Z. (2011). Rickets. *Current Osteoporosis Reports, 9*(4), 291–299.

NICE (National Institute for Health and Clinical Excellence) Guideline 107, (2011). Hypertension in pregnancy. The management of hypertensive disorders during pregnancy, accessed 17 January, <www.nice.org.uk/cg107>.

NICE Guidelines. (2014). Schedule of appointments in routine antenatal care, accessed 13 January 2015, <http://pathways.nice.org.uk/pathways/antenatal-care>.

Thorogood, C. (2010). Challenges to womens' health. In S. Pairman, S. Tracy, C. Thorogood & C. Pinombe (2010). *Midwifery Preparation for Practice*, (2nd ed.). Churchill Livingstone Elsevier: Sydney.

Tiran, D. (2012). Ginger to reduce nausea and vomiting during pregnancy: Evidence of effectiveness is not the same as proof of safety. *Complementary Therapies in Clinical Practice, 18*(1), 22–25.

Suggested readings

Bar-Zeev, S., Barclay, L., Kruske, S. & Kildea, S. (2014). Factors affecting the quality of antenatal care provided to remote dwelling Aboriginal women in northern Australia, *Midwifery, 30*(3), 289–296.

Brown, M. J., Sinclair, M., Liddle, D., Hill, A. J., Stockdale, D. J. & Madden, N. E. (2013). Motivating pregnant women to eat healthily and engage in physical activity for weight management: An exploration of routine midwife instruction. *Evidence Based Midwifery, 11*(4), 120–127.

Foster, C. E. & Hirst, J. (2014). Midwives' attitudes towards giving weight-related advice to obese pregnant women. *British Journal of Midwifery, 22*(4), 254–262.

Powers, J., McDermott, L., Loxton, D. & Chojenta, C. (2013). A prospective study of prevalence and predictors of concurrent alcohol and tobacco use during pregnancy. *Maternal & Child Health Journal, 17*(1), 76–84.

Wilkes, L., Mannix, J. & Jackson, D. (2012). 'I am going to be a dad': Experiences and expectations of adolescent and young adult expectant fathers. *Journal of Clinical Nursing, 21*(1/2), 180–188.

Chapter 12

Promoting fetal and maternal health

Previous chapters discussed normal anatomy and physiology and the changes that occur with pregnancy. This chapter adds information about the health teaching that women need during pregnancy to ensure a healthy outcome for themselves and their child.

LEARNING OBJECTIVES

After mastering the contents of this chapter, you should be able to:

1. Describe health behaviours important for a healthy pregnancy outcome.
2. Use critical thinking to analyse ways to promote both individualised and family-centred antenatal care.
3. Assess a woman for healthy practices and concerns during pregnancy.
4. Develop nursing considerations related to a healthy pregnancy.
5. Encourage health-promotion strategies to limit exposure to teratogens or reduce the minor discomforts of pregnancy.
6. Apply nursing care to promote positive health practices during pregnancy.
7. Identify areas of antenatal care that could benefit from additional nursing research or the application of evidence-based practice.

KEY TERMS

- cytomegalovirus
- fetal alcohol syndrome
- leucorrhoea
- Sims' position
- teratogen
- toxoplasmosis

CASE STUDY

Melissa Adams, a single woman, is 4 months' pregnant when you see her in an antenatal clinic. She works as a curator for an art gallery but has missed work this past week because of nausea. She is worried she will not be able to work past 6 months of her pregnancy because her job involves a great deal of walking. She wonders how she will be able to afford her apartment if she has to quit work. She has already stopped volunteer work teaching children's swimming. She wants to travel to see her sister in Sydney because her sister is very ill but has heard that pregnant women should not drive more than 100 km. She asks you if marijuana would help reduce her early pregnancy nausea.

CASE STUDY QUESTION

1. What additional health teaching does Melissa need?

The health of a fetus and the health of the mother are inextricably linked. Generally, a woman who eats well and takes care of her own health during pregnancy provides a healthy environment for fetal growth and development. However, she may need instructions on exactly what constitutes a healthy lifestyle for herself and her baby. Most women have questions regarding how much extra rest they need, what type of exercise they can continue, and whether all the changes going on in their bodies, some of which bring them daily discomfort, are normal. Therefore, a major role in promoting maternal and fetal health is education. Providing empathetic advice about ways to alleviate the minor discomforts of pregnancy, alerting a woman to the danger signs in pregnancy, and keeping abreast of the latest evidence-based practice studies done on maternal exposure to **teratogens** (factors detrimental to fetal health) are all part of this role (Knopik, 2009), because effective antenatal care is vital to healthy fetal growth.

HEALTH PROMOTION OF A FETUS AND MOTHER

Assessment

A thorough health history, physical evaluation and initial laboratory data are obtained at the first antenatal visit. Continuing assessment concentrates on screening for any abnormalities in physical or emotional health that might be occurring and for the possibility of teratogens in the pregnant woman's environment. Encourage a pregnant woman to discuss whatever concerns she is having during all visits. Although some of these concerns may represent minor common discomforts associated with normal pregnancy, others may be early indicators of potential problems (see Box 12.1). Early problem identification allows you to provide information and guidance on ways to alleviate the discomforts of pregnancy. Early detection and continued monitoring of conditions such as pregnancy-induced hypertension (PIH) and gestational diabetes reduce their risks.

Unless women bring problems to the attention of their healthcare provider early in pregnancy, they do not have the opportunity to take the necessary measures to prevent further discomfort during or after the pregnancy. Many women do not mention any concerns or discomforts unless specifically asked because they may not be aware of their significance or are reluctant to take up a busy healthcare provider's time for these things. For example, women experiencing constipation may not take care of

BOX 12.1 Assessment * Assessing a woman for discomforts of pregnancy

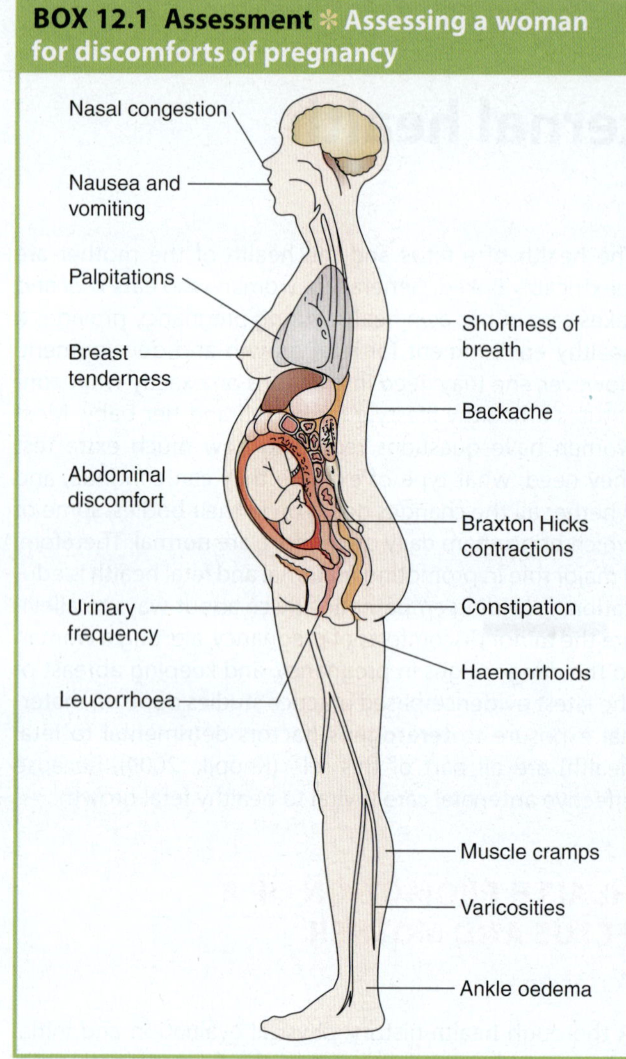

the problem early or well enough to prevent the occurrence of haemorrhoids, which can then become a long-term problem not only throughout the pregnancy but afterwards as well.

Nursing considerations

Examples of nursing considerations related to health promotion of the pregnant woman and fetus are:

- Health-seeking behaviours related to interest in maintaining optimal health during pregnancy
- Anxiety related to minor discomforts of pregnancy
- Risk of deficient fluid volume related to nausea and vomiting of pregnancy
- Disturbed body image related to change of appearance with pregnancy
- Risk of altered sexual patterns related to fear of harming fetus during pregnancy
- Disturbed sleep pattern related to frequent need to empty bladder during night
- Risk of fetal injury related to maternal cigarette smoking
- Risk to fetus from alcohol use.

When establishing goals and outcomes, be certain that plans are realistic for a woman's situation and family lifestyle. Try to turn long-term goals into realistic and more manageable short-term ones if possible; for instance, you cannot set a goal for a woman to be free of the nausea of early pregnancy. The best you can expect to accomplish is to be certain that she maintains good nutrition and adequate weight gain in the face of it. Nor can you do much about the frequency of urination, backache or fatigue that occur with pregnancy except to help a woman adapt her lifestyle to these symptoms (e.g. encourage her to drink more liquids during the day and less in the early evening; schedule regular rest periods when possible).

Often, helping a woman plan to avoid teratogens is difficult because a total change in lifestyle, such as not smoking, not drinking alcohol or changing a work environment, may be involved. Fortunately, most women are highly motivated to have a healthy baby. With this level of motivation, planning the best route to achieve a goal becomes the focus rather than educating about the need for goal achievement.

The major intervention associated with health promotion during pregnancy is education. Although the average woman is aware that some discomforts may occur, these discomforts may seem extreme when they are happening to her. It is crucial to all teaching to be certain all women understand that they should double-check with their midwife, obstetrician or general practitioner before taking any non-essential medication during pregnancy. Other important interventions include good role modelling, such as not smoking in antenatal settings, and exhibiting a healthy lifestyle through adequate nutrition and exercise.

Cultural beliefs play a large role in how teaching is structured. Teaching can be challenging if a woman has limited English proficiency. Women from cultures that view pregnancy as a wellness state may not seek care because they do not view pregnancy as a time when medical intervention is necessary. Some women may rely on herbs and home remedies to manage the common discomforts of pregnancy, so they do not feel a need for medical management. This variety of cultural backgrounds makes individualised assessment and education mandatory.

Implementing antenatal care to meet the needs of all of the different cultures represented in Australia and New Zealand may include furnishing interpreters to aid in communication, providing classes in antenatal health, explaining how health-promotion regimens fit with women's cultural belief systems, and maintaining an attitude of advocacy to help women adjust to a formal healthcare system.

When planning teaching strategies, a woman's receptiveness to instruction is key. Regardless of how excited and pleased a woman is about being pregnant, she can assimilate only so much information at one particular time. Therefore, be selective about the health information you provide and include those points most relevant to the individual woman.

More information on current practices and choices that a woman and her family have for antenatal care can be found at the following useful sites: <www.midwife.org.nz>, <www.maternity.org.nz>, <www.midwivesaustralia.com.au>.

HEALTH PROMOTION DURING PREGNANCY

Health promotion during pregnancy begins with reviewing aspects of self-care.

Self-care needs

Because pregnancy is not an illness, few special care measures other than common sense about self-care are required. Many women, however, have heard different warnings about what they should or should not do during pregnancy, so they may need some help separating fact from fiction so that they can enjoy their pregnancy unhampered by unnecessary restrictions. In no other area of nursing, except possibly infant feeding, does there seem to be as many misconceptions or inappropriate information available to women.

Bathing

During pregnancy, sweating tends to increase because a woman excretes waste products for herself and her fetus. She also has an increase in vaginal discharge. For these reasons, daily baths or showers are recommended. Women should not soak for long periods in extremely hot water or hot baths as heat exposure for a lengthy time could lead to hyperthermia in the fetus and birth defects, specifically oesophageal atresia, omphalocele and gastroschisis (Duong et al., 2011). As pregnancy advances, a woman may have difficulty maintaining her balance when getting in and out of the bath. If so, she should change to showering or sponge bathing for her own safety.

Breast care

A few precautions during pregnancy are helpful to prevent breast discomfort. A general rule is for a woman to wear a firm, supportive bra with wide straps to spread breast weight across the shoulders. A woman may need to buy a larger bra halfway through pregnancy to accommodate her increasing breast size. If she plans on breastfeeding her newborn, she might choose bras suitable for breastfeeding so she can continue to use them after the baby's birth.

Dental care

Gingival tissue tends to hypertrophy during pregnancy. Unless a pregnant woman brushes her teeth well, pockets of plaque form readily between the enlarged gumline and teeth. In addition to promoting brushing, encourage pregnant women to see their dentist regularly for routine examination and cleaning because 9 months is a long time to be without preventive dental care. Remind women that x-ray examinations are often included as a part of routine dental health. A pregnant woman may want to consider delaying these until after her baby is born. In the few instances when x-ray examinations are necessary for dental health, they can be done safely as long as a woman's abdomen is shielded with a lead apron.

Perineal hygiene

Most women have an increased vaginal discharge during pregnancy and may desire to cleanse with a douche. Douching is contraindicated during pregnancy. The force of the irrigating fluid could cause it to enter the cervix and lead to infection. In addition, douching alters the pH of the vagina, leading to an increased risk of bacterial growth (Guile & Keller, 2011).

Clothing

Women have a multitude of clothing options to wear during pregnancy. Recommend loose-fitting, comfortable garments. Caution women to avoid tight-fitting items such as garters, girdles with panty legs and knee-high stockings during pregnancy. These items impede lower-extremity circulation. Suggest wearing shoes with a moderate to low heel to minimise pelvic tilt and possible backache. Otherwise, the rules are common sense and comfort.

Sexual activity

Some women are embarrassed to ask questions about sexual relations during pregnancy. However, most women are concerned about whether sexual intercourse should be restricted. Many need information to refute some of the myths about sexual relations in pregnancy that still exist, such as:

- Coitus on the expected date of her period will initiate labour
- Orgasm will initiate preterm labour, but participating in sexual relations without orgasm will not
- Coitus during the fertile days of a cycle will cause a second pregnancy or twins
- Coitus might cause rupture of the membranes.

None of the above are true. Asking a woman at an antenatal visit if she has any questions about sexual activity allows her to voice such concerns (see Box 12.2). By dispelling these myths, you allow her to feel more comfortable and secure that coitus is not harming her child.

There are a few situations when sexual relations during a pregnancy are contraindicated. Women with a history of spontaneous miscarriage may be advised to avoid coitus during the time of the pregnancy when a previous miscarriage occurred. Women whose membranes have ruptured or who have vaginal spotting should be advised against coitus until examined, to prevent possible

BOX 12.2 * Focus on communication

Melissa Adams is 4 months' pregnant and no longer lives with the father of her baby.

Less effective communication

Nurse: Do you have any questions, Mrs Adams?
Melissa: I'm not Mrs Adams.
Nurse: I'm sorry, Ms Adams. Do you have any questions?
Melissa: How long into pregnancy can I have sex?
Nurse: Well, since you're single, you don't really need that kind of advice. Let's talk about exercise and nutrition instead.

More effective communication

Nurse: Do you have any questions, Mrs Adams?
Melissa: I'm not Mrs Adams.
Nurse: I'm sorry, Ms Adams. Do you have any questions?
Melissa: How long into pregnancy can I have sex?
Nurse: Basically, as long as you're comfortable and you don't have any complications.
Melissa: Good. My new boyfriend made me promise to ask today.

Health teaching is an art separate from teaching morality. In the first scenario, the nurse cuts off communication by making a judgement to supply only information that the nurse thinks that her client needs. In the second scenario, the nurse actively listens to the client, focuses on her needs and concerns, and supplies the information the client has requested.

infection. Otherwise, there are no sexual restrictions during pregnancy.

CASE STUDY QUESTION

2. Which statement by Melissa would alert you that she needs more teaching about self-care practices during pregnancy?
   a. "I take either a shower or bath, because I know both are safe."
   b. "I wash my breasts with clear water, not with soap, every day."
   c. "I'm glad I don't have to ask my boyfriend to use condoms anymore."
   d. "I'm wearing low-heeled shoes to try to avoid backache."

Exercise

Extreme exercise has been associated with lower birth weight but moderate exercise is healthy during pregnancy. It can help prevent circulatory stasis in the lower extremities. It also can offer a general feeling of wellbeing. For some women, teaching about exercise focuses on helping them realise the need for exercise and urging them to get enough. Others may need to be cautioned to restrict exercise or participation in contact sports.

The average, well-nourished woman should aim to meet the prescribed physical activity levels of the Australian Physical Activity and Sedentary Behaviour Guidelines–that is, 150 minutes of moderate-intensity exercise or 75 minutes of vigorous-intensity exercise, or a combination of both, each week (Better Health Channel, 2015).

In addition to being healthy during pregnancy, a planned exercise program may have long-term benefits such as:

- Lowering cholesterol level
- Reducing risk of osteoporosis
- Increasing energy level
- Maintaining a healthy body weight
- Decreasing risk of heart disease
- Increasing self-esteem and wellbeing.

As a rule, a woman can continue any sport she participated in before pregnancy unless it was one that involved body contact, such as soccer. If a woman is a competent horsewoman, for example, there is little reason for her to discontinue riding until it becomes uncomfortable. Pregnancy is not the time to learn to ride, however, because a beginning rider is at greater risk for being thrown than is an experienced rider.

Walking is the best exercise during pregnancy, and women should be encouraged to take a walk daily unless inclement weather, many levels of stairs or an unsafe neighbourhood are contraindications (Kramer & McDonald, 2009).

Swimming is a good activity for pregnant women and, like bathing, is not contraindicated as long as the membranes are intact. It may help relieve backache during pregnancy (Young & Jewell, 2009). General guidelines for exercise during pregnancy are highlighted in Box 12.3.

Sleep

The optimal condition for body growth occurs when growth hormone secretion is at its highest level—that is, during sleep. This, plus the overall increased metabolic demand of pregnancy, appears to be the physiological reason that pregnant women need an increased amount of sleep or at least need rest to build new body cells during pregnancy.

Late in pregnancy, a woman often finds herself awakened from sleep at short, frequent intervals by the activity of her fetus. Frequent waking this way leads to loss of rapid eye movement (REM) sleep. This can cause a woman to feel anxious or not well-rested, although she has slept her usual number of hours. Pyrosis (heartburn) or dyspnoea (shortness of breath) also can cause her to wake, especially if she has been lying flat. In this instance, sleeping with two pillows or on a couch with an armrest may be helpful.

To obtain enough sleep and rest during pregnancy, most pregnant women need a rest period during the afternoon as well as a full night of sleep. Be certain a woman knows to avoid resting on her back, as supine hypotension syndrome (faintness, diaphoresis and hypotension from the pressure of the expanding uterus on the inferior vena cava) can develop in this position.

BOX 12.3 ✻ Focus on family teaching

Guidelines for exercise in pregnancy

Q. Melissa Adams asks you, "Now that I'm pregnant, can I still do aerobic exercises?"

A. New and intense exercise should never be started for the first time during pregnancy. Use the following recommendations as guidelines for safe exercise:

1. Perform regular exercise (about three times per week) rather than engaging in intermittent activity.
2. Do not perform vigorous exercise in hot, humid weather or if you have a fever to avoid overexerting yourself or developing hyperthermia.
3. Avoid activities that require jumping, jarring motions or rapid changes in direction such as jogging, because your joints may be unstable.
4. Exercise on a wooden floor or a tightly carpeted surface to reduce shock to the abdomen or knees and provide a sure footing.
5. To avoid muscle cramping, avoid exercises and motions that involve deep flexion or joint extension, such as stretching with the toes extended.
6. Always start your exercise program by warming up for approximately 5 minutes with activities such as slow walking or stationary cycling with low resistance.
7. End your exercise program with a period of gradually declining activity that includes gentle, stationary stretching. Because of the increased risk of joint injury, do not stretch to the point of maximum resistance.
8. Measure your heart rate at times of peak activity. Talk with your primary care provider about target heart rate and limits, and do not exceed them.
9. When getting up from lying on the floor, do so gradually to prevent dramatic blood pressure changes or stretching of the round ligament that can lead to sharp abdominal pain.
10. Drink liquids liberally before and after exercise to prevent dehydration. If necessary, interrupt your activity to replenish fluids.
11. If you were sedentary before pregnancy, begin your exercise program with physical activity of very low intensity and advance your activity level gradually.
12. Stop any activity and contact your primary care provider if any unusual symptoms appear.
13. Perform strenuous activities for no longer than 20 minutes.
14. To prevent supine hypotension do not exercise in the supine position (lying down flat) after the fourth month of pregnancy.
15. Avoid exercises that employ a Valsalva manoeuvre (holding your breath, bearing down) because these actions decrease blood supply to the fetus.
16. Make sure your kilojoule intake is adequate to meet not only the extra energy needs of pregnancy but also those of the exercise performed.

CASE STUDY QUESTION

3. Melissa describes her typical day to you. What would alert you that she may need further pregnancy advice?
   a. "I jog rather than walk to get an increased amount of exercise."
   b. "I always go to sleep on my side, not on my back."
   c. "I pack a lunch every day so I know I won't eat junk food."
   d. "I walk around my desk every hour to help leg circulation."

Travel

Because we live in a mobile society, many women have questions about travel during pregnancy. Early in a normal pregnancy, there are no restrictions. If a woman is susceptible to motion sickness, advise her not to take any medication for this unless it is specifically prescribed or approved by her doctor or nurse-midwife. Suggest that she use a "sea-sick" wrist or acupuncture band instead. Late in pregnancy, travel plans should take into consideration the possibility of early labour, requiring birth at a strange setting where a woman's obstetric history will be unknown. Regardless of the month of her pregnancy, if a woman plans to spend time at a remote location, such as a campsite, be certain she knows the location of a nearby healthcare facility should an unexpected complication occur.

Advise a woman who is taking a long trip by car to plan for frequent rest or stretch periods. Preferably every hour, but at least every 2 hours, she should get out of the car and walk a short distance. This break relieves stiffness and muscle aches and improves lower extremity circulation, helping prevent varicosities, haemorrhoids and thrombophlebitis. Pregnant women may drive as long as they fit comfortably behind the steering wheel. They are required to use seatbelts like everyone else. Occasionally, uterine rupture has been reported from seatbelt use, but overall evidence suggests that seatbelts reduce mortality among pregnant women in car accidents, as they do for everyone (Russell, Denne & Schwartz, 2011). Both shoulder harnesses and lap belts should be used. The lap belt should be worn as snugly as comfortable so that it fits under the abdominal bulge and across the pelvic bones. The shoulder harness should be snug but comfortable, worn across the shoulder, chest and upper abdomen. A pad may be placed under the shoulder harness at the neck to avoid chafing (see Fig. 12.1).

Pregnancy is also a time for a family to think about transportation safety for the newborn. Purchasing a car child restraint is an investment that not only is legally required for transporting infants but also helps guarantee their safety. Families who cannot afford to purchase an infant car restraint may want to consider hiring one, or asking friends or relatives about the possibility of borrowing one no longer needed.

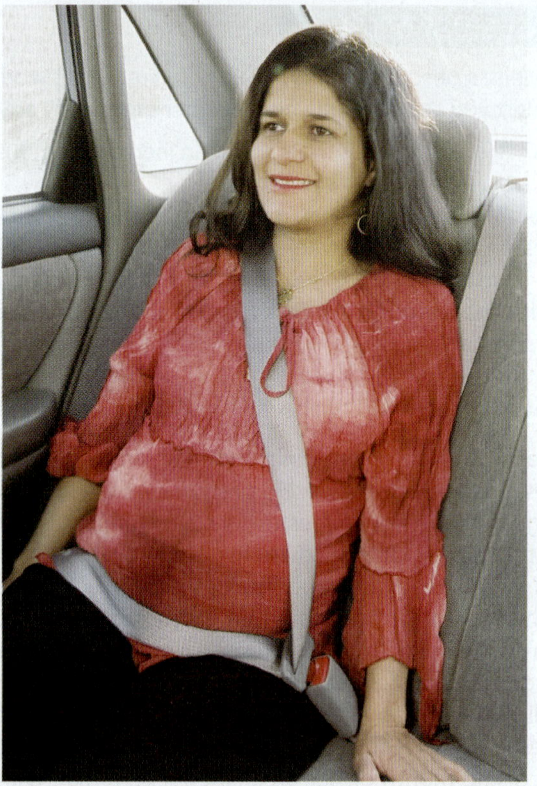

FIGURE 12.1 The law requires women to wear a seatbelt while pregnant.

Travelling by plane for women is not contraindicated during pregnancy as long as the plane has a well-pressurised cabin (true of commercial airlines but not of all small private planes) and a woman walks the length of the plane every hour to help prevent thrombophlebitis. Some airlines do not permit women who are more than 7 months pregnant to board; others require written permission from a woman's primary care provider. Advise a woman to investigate these restrictions by calling the airline or a travel agency before making such travel plans.

Discomforts of early pregnancy

Early pregnancy symptoms can often cause discomfort in an expectant woman. Providing empathic and sound advice about measures to relieve these discomforts helps promote overall health and wellbeing (see Box 12.4). Although these symptoms are classified as minor, they may not seem minor to a woman who wakes up each morning feeling nauseated, wondering if she will ever feel like herself again. Also, each of these symptoms has the potential to lead to problems that are more serious.

Midwifery considerations and related interventions

Most women will experience at least one minor discomfort of pregnancy. Because each woman's experience is unique, nursing considerations and care must be developed according to each woman's individual needs. Examples of nursing considerations that might be developed for women experiencing the discomforts of early pregnancy are:

- Constipation related to reduced peristalsis in pregnancy
- Fatigue related to increased physiological need for sleep and rest during pregnancy
- Acute pain related to frequent muscle cramps secondary to physiological changes of pregnancy
- Disturbed sleep pattern related to frequent need to empty bladder during night.

> **BOX 12.4 * Focus on evidence-based practice**
>
> **The minor discomforts of pregnancy**
>
> Almost all women experience a number of minor discomforts during pregnancy. To investigate whether these symptoms are serious enough to lead to depression, researchers scored 1507 Australian women during their first pregnancy on a depression inventory questionnaire. The women were also asked what minor body changes they were experiencing. The most frequent body changes reported were exhaustion (86.9%), morning nausea (64.3%), back pain (45.6%), constipation (43.5%) and severe headache or migraine (29.5%). Women who reported five or more physical health problems were three times more likely to also report depressive symptoms.
>
> *Would the results of this study be useful when assessing a pregnant woman at her next prenatal visit?*
>
> *Source:* Perlen, S., Woolhouse, H., Gartland, D., et al. (2013). Maternal depression and physical health problems in early pregnancy: Findings of an Australian nulliparous pregnancy cohort study. *Midwifery, 29*(3) 233–239.

Breast tenderness

Breast tenderness is often one of the first symptoms noticed in early pregnancy; it may be most noticeable on exposure to cold air. For most women, the tenderness is minimal and transient, something they are aware of but not something that overly concerns them.

Palmar erythema

Palmar erythema, or palmar pruritus, occurs in early pregnancy and is probably caused by increased oestrogen levels. Constant redness or itching of the palms can make a woman believe she has developed an allergy. Explain that this type of itching in early pregnancy is normal. As soon as a woman's body adjusts to the increased level of oestrogen, the erythema and pruritus disappear.

Constipation

As peristalsis slows and the weight of a growing uterus presses against the bowel, constipation can occur (Bernstein & Weinstein, 2007). Discuss preventive measures with a woman early in pregnancy to help her avoid this problem. Increase the amount of fibre in her diet by eating raw fruits, bran and vegetables and encourage her to drink water daily.

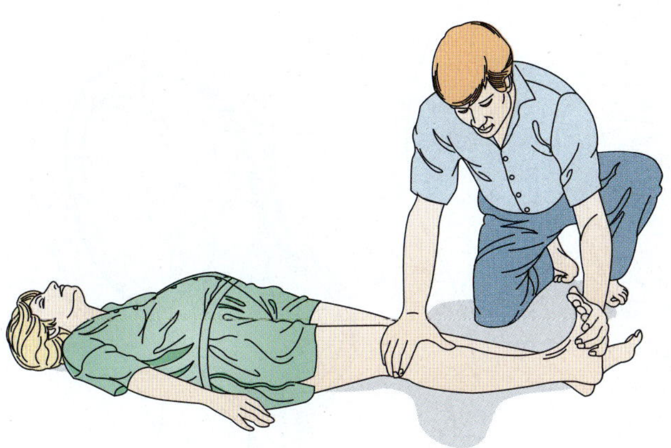

FIGURE 12.2 Relieving a leg cramp in pregnancy. Pressing down on the knee and pressing the toes backwards (dorsiflexion) relieves most cramps. Here, a woman's partner helps.

Nausea, vomiting and pyrosis

At least half of pregnant women experience other gastrointestinal symptoms such as nausea, vomiting and pyrosis (heartburn). Because these symptoms also interfere with nutrition, they are discussed in Chapter 13.

Fatigue

Fatigue is extremely common in early pregnancy, probably because of increased metabolic requirements. Much of it can be relieved by increasing the amount of rest and sleep. Some women, however, are reluctant to take time out of their day for rest. They know that pregnancy is not an illness, and so they proceed as if nothing is happening to them. Rarely is there justification during a normal pregnancy for women to take extra days off from work because of their condition, but it is also unrealistic to proceed as if nothing is different. Fatigue can increase the amount of morning sickness a woman experiences. If she becomes too tired, she may not eat properly and nutrition can suffer. If she remains on her feet without at least one break during a day, the risk for varicosities and the danger of thromboembolic complications increase.

Muscle cramps

Decreased serum calcium levels, increased serum phosphorus levels and, possibly, interference with circulation commonly cause muscle cramps of the lower extremities during pregnancy. This problem is best relieved if a woman lies on her back momentarily and extends her involved leg while keeping her knee straight and dorsiflexing the foot until the pain disappears (see Fig. 12.2).

If a woman is experiencing frequent leg cramps, she may be advised to take magnesium citrate. Elevating lower extremities frequently during the day to improve circulation and avoiding full leg extension, such as stretching with the toes pointed, may also be helpful. Typically, muscle cramps are a minor symptom of pregnancy, but the pain is extreme and the intensity of the contraction can be frightening.

Hypotension

Supine hypotension is a symptom that occurs when a woman lies on her back and the uterus presses on the vena cava, impairing blood return to her heart. A woman experiences an irregular heart rate and a feeling of apprehension. The method of relieving the problem is simple: if a woman turns or is turned onto her side, pressure is removed from the vena cava, blood flow is restored, and the symptoms quickly fade. To prevent the syndrome, advise pregnant women to always rest or sleep on their side, not their back. If they can only fall asleep on their back, they should insert a small firm pillow under their right hip to cause the weight of their uterus to shift off their vena cava.

If a woman rises suddenly from a lying or sitting position or stands for an extended time in a warm or crowded area, she may faint from the same phenomenon (blood pooling in the pelvic area or lower extremities). Rising slowly and avoiding extended periods of standing prevent this problem. If a woman should feel faint, sitting with her head lowered—the same action as for any person who feels faint—alleviates the problem.

Varicosities

Varicosities, or the development of tortuous leg veins, are common in pregnancy because the weight of the distended uterus puts pressure on the veins returning blood from the lower extremities. This causes pooling of blood and distension of the vessels. The veins become engorged, inflamed and painful. Although usually confined to the lower extremities, varicosities can extend up to and include the vulva. They occur most frequently in women with a family history of varicose veins and those who have a large fetus or a multiple pregnancy.

Resting in a **Sims' position** or on the back with the legs raised against the wall (with a small firm pillow under their right hip) or elevated on a footstool for 15 to 20 minutes twice a day is a good precaution (see Fig. 12.3). Some women, especially those who developed varicosities during

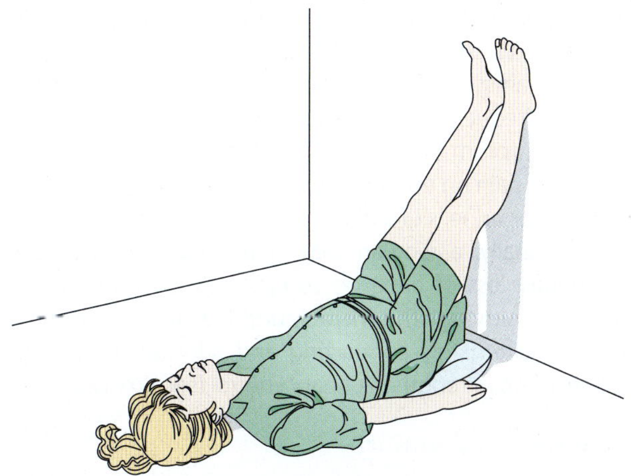

FIGURE 12.3 Position to relieve varicosities. The mother keeps a pad under her right hip to prevent supine hypotensive syndrome.

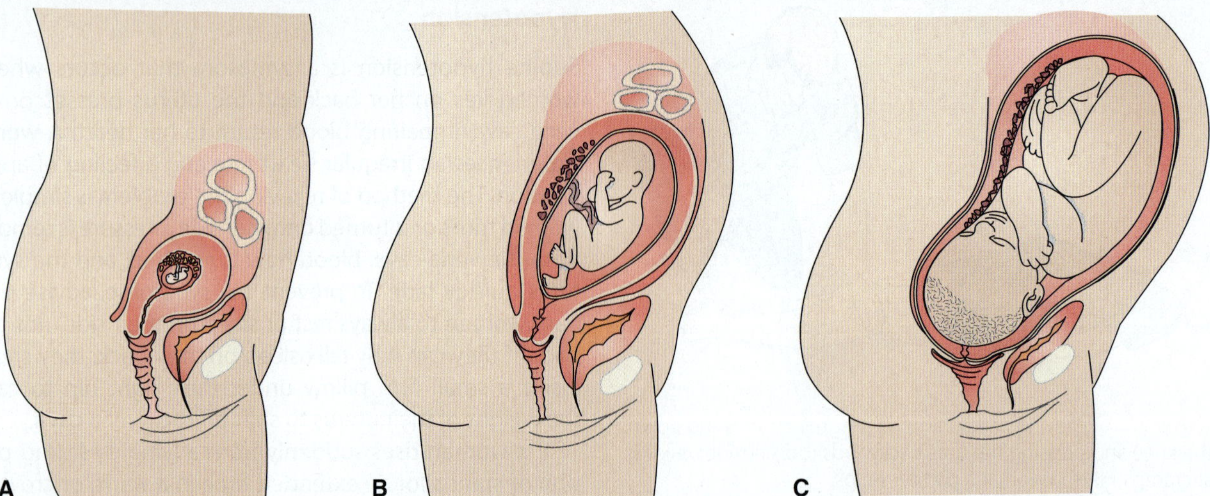

FIGURE 12.4 Bladder changes during pregnancy. (**A**) Early pregnancy: the uterus presses against the bladder, causing frequent urination. (**B**) Middle pregnancy: urinary frequency is relieved. (**C**) Late pregnancy: the uterus is again pressing on the bladder, leading to the recurrence of urinary frequency.

a previous pregnancy, may need elastic support stockings such as T.E.D. stockings for relief of varicosities in a second pregnancy. Urge a woman to put on support stockings before she gets up in the morning as once she is on her feet, the pooling of blood begins, and the stockings will be less effective. Because it stimulates venous return, exercise is as effective as rest periods for alleviating varicosities.

Haemorrhoids

Haemorrhoids (varicosities of the rectal veins) occur commonly in pregnancy because of pressure on these veins from the bulk of the growing uterus (Quijano & Abalos, 2009). Daily bowel evacuation to relieve constipation and resting daily, in a modified Sims' position, are both helpful.

Frequent urination

Frequent urination occurs in early pregnancy because of the pressure of the growing uterus on the anterior bladder. The sensation may last for about 3 months, sometimes beginning as early as the first or second missed menstrual period, disappear in mid pregnancy when the uterus rises above the bladder, and return again in late pregnancy as the fetal head presses against the bladder (see Fig. 12.4). When a woman describes frequency of urination, be certain this is the only urinary symptom she is experiencing. Ask her about any burning or pain on urination or whether she has noticed any blood in her urine, signs of urinary tract infection.

Occasionally, a woman may notice stress incontinence (involuntary loss of urine on coughing or sneezing) during pregnancy. Although this is largely unpreventable, doing Kegel exercises (alternately contracting and relaxing the perineal muscles) helps strengthen urinary control (see Box 12.5).

Abdominal discomfort

Some women experience uncomfortable feelings of abdominal pressure early in pregnancy. Women with a multiple pregnancy may notice this throughout pregnancy. Typically, pregnant women stand with their arms crossed in front of them because the weight of their arms resting on their abdomen relieves this discomfort.

Leucorrhoea

Leucorrhoea, a whitish, viscous vaginal discharge or an increase in the amount of normal vaginal secretions, occurs in response to the high oestrogen levels and the increased blood supply to the vaginal epithelium and cervix in pregnancy. A daily bath or shower to wash away accumulated secretions and prevent vulvar excoriation usually controls this problem. Wearing cotton underpants

BOX 12.5 ✻ Kegel exercises

Kegel exercises are exercises designed to strengthen the pubococcygeal muscles. Each is a separate exercise and should be done about three times a day.

1. Squeeze the muscles surrounding the vagina as if stopping the flow of urine. Hold for 3 seconds. Relax. Repeat this sequence 10 times.
2. Contract and relax the muscles surrounding the vagina as rapidly as possible 10 to 25 times.
3. Imagine that you are sitting in a bathtub of water and squeeze muscles as if sucking water into the vagina. Hold for 3 seconds. Relax. Repeat this action 10 times.
4. Caution: Do not regularly start and stop the flow of urine during urination to try and strengthen muscles as this can lead to incomplete emptying of the bladder.

It may take as long as 6 weeks of exercise before pubococcygeal muscles are strengthened. In addition to strengthening urinary control and preventing stress incontinence, Kegel exercises can lead to increased sexual enjoyment because of the tightened vaginal muscles.

and sleeping at night without underwear can be helpful to reduce moisture and possible vulvar excoriation. Some women may need to wear a perineal pad to control the discharge. Caution women not to use tampons because this could lead to stasis of secretions and subsequent infection. Advise women to contact their doctor or midwife if there is a change in the colour, odour or character of this discharge, as these suggest infection.

What if...

Melissa tells you she has urinary frequency and also reports a white vaginal discharge? How would you go about evaluating whether she is experiencing a normal discomfort of pregnancy or a urinary tract infection?

Discomforts of mid to late pregnancy

At about 20 to 24 weeks, the midpoint of pregnancy, a woman is usually ready for further health teaching that relates to the new developments that will occur in the latter half of pregnancy. As she starts to view the child within her as a separate person, she becomes interested in discussing and making plans for the signs and symptoms of beginning labour, birth and the infant's care. The midpoint of a pregnancy is also a good time to describe the new minor symptoms that may occur and to review the precautionary measures to prevent constipation, varicosities and haemorrhoids, as these increase in intensity late in pregnancy.

Backache

As pregnancy advances, a lumbar lordosis develops and postural changes necessary to maintain balance lead to backache. Wearing shoes with low to moderate heels reduces the amount of spinal curvature necessary to maintain an upright posture. Encouraging a woman to walk with her pelvis tilted forwards (putting pelvic support under the weight of the fetus) is also helpful. In addition, applying local heat may aid in relieving backache.

Headache

Many women experience headache during pregnancy, apparently from their expanding blood volume, which puts pressure on cerebral arteries. Trying to reduce any possible causative situations, such as eye strain or tension, may lessen the number of headaches they experience. Resting with cold towels on their forehead and taking usual adult doses of paracetamol usually furnishes adequate relief. Although a few women who have migraine headaches find these worsen during pregnancy, most women notice considerable improvement with this type of headache during pregnancy. Caution women that if a headache is unusually intense or continuous, they should report it. A continuous sharp headache may be a danger sign of high blood pressure during pregnancy.

Dyspnoea

As the expanding uterus places pressure on the diaphragm, lung compression and shortness of breath result. A woman will notice this primarily at night if she lies flat. She also will definitely notice it on exertion. To relieve night time dyspnoea, advise her to sleep with her head and chest elevated so the weight of the uterus falls away from her diaphragm. As pregnancy progresses, she may require two or more pillows to sleep at night to avoid the problem.

Ankle oedema

Most women experience some swelling of the ankles and feet during late pregnancy, most noticeably at the end of the day. Women are often first conscious of this when they kick off their shoes to rest and then cannot put them on again comfortably. As long as proteinuria and hypertension are absent, ankle oedema of this nature is a normal occurrence of pregnancy. This simple oedema can be relieved best by resting. Sitting for half an hour in the afternoon and again in the evening with the legs elevated is helpful.

Some women need reassurance that ankle oedema is normal during pregnancy. Otherwise, they worry that it is a beginning sign of PIH (Menzies et al., 2007). On the other hand, do not dismiss a report of lower extremity oedema lightly until you are certain a woman does not exhibit any signs of proteinuria or oedema of other, non-dependent parts, or has had a sudden increase in weight indicative of PIH.

Braxton Hicks contractions

Beginning as early as 8 to 12 weeks of pregnancy, the uterus periodically contracts and then relaxes again (Coad & Dunstall, 2011). Early in pregnancy, these sensations, termed Braxton Hicks contractions, are not noticeable. By mid or late pregnancy, the contractions become stronger, and a woman who tenses at the sensation may even experience some minimal pain, similar to a hard menstrual cramp. Although these contractions are not a sign of beginning labour, women should inform their primary care provider about them so that they can be evaluated. A rhythmic pattern of even very light but persistent contractions could be a beginning sign of labour.

CASE STUDY QUESTION

4. Melissa has ankle oedema by the end of each day. Which statement by her would reveal that she understands what causes this?

a. "I know this is a beginning complication; I'll call my doctor tonight."
b. "I understand this is from eating too much salt; I'll restrict that more."
c. "I'll rest in a Sims' position to take pressure off lower extremity veins."
d. "I know this is from gaining too much weight. I'll start to diet tomorrow."

PREVENTING FETAL EXPOSURE TO TERATOGENS

A *teratogen* is any factor, chemical or physical, that adversely affects the fertilised ovum, embryo or fetus.

Effects of teratogens on a fetus

Several factors influence the amount of damage a teratogen can cause. The strength of the teratogen is one of these. For example, radiation is a known teratogen. In small amounts (everyone is exposed to some radiation every day, such as from sun rays), it causes no damage. However, in large doses (e.g. the amount of radiation necessary to treat cancer of the cervix), serious fetal defects or death can occur.

The timing of the teratogenic insult makes a significant impact on damage done to the fetus. If a teratogen is introduced before implantation, either the zygote is destroyed or it appears unaffected. If the insult occurs when the main body systems are being formed (in the second to eighth weeks of embryonic life), a fetus is very vulnerable to injury. During the last trimester, the potential for harm again decreases because all the organs of a fetus are formed and are merely maturing. The times when different anatomical areas of a fetus are most likely to be affected by teratogens are shown in Chapter 9. Two exceptions to the rule that deformities usually occur in early embryonic life are the effects caused by the organisms of syphilis and toxoplasmosis. These two infections can cause abnormalities in organs that were originally formed normally.

A third factor determining the effects of a teratogen is the teratogen's affinity for specific tissue. Lead and mercury, for example, attack and disable nervous tissue. Thalidomide, a medication once used to relieve nausea in pregnancy, causes limb defects. Tetracycline, a common antibiotic, causes tooth enamel deficiencies and, possibly, long-bone deformities. The rubella virus can affect many organs: the eyes, ears, heart and brain are the four most commonly attacked.

Teratogenic maternal infections

Teratogenic maternal infections can involve either sexually transmitted or systemic infections. These organisms that cross the placenta can be viral, bacterial or protozoan. Most infections important to a healthy pregnancy outcome cause relatively mild, flu-like symptoms in a woman but can have much more serious effects on a fetus or newborn. Preventing and predicting fetal injury from infection is complicated because a disease may be subclinical (without any symptoms in the mother) and yet may injure a fetus.

Several diseases that are commonly known to cross the placenta and cause fetal harm are tested for and are described collectively under the umbrella term TORCH, an abbreviation for *t*oxoplasmosis, *r*ubella, *c*ytomegalovirus, *h*erpes simplex virus and syphilis.

Toxoplasmosis

Toxoplasmosis, a protozoan infection, is spread most commonly through contact with uncooked meat, although it may also be contracted through handling cat stool in soil or cat litter (Friars, 2007). A woman experiences almost no symptoms of the disease except for a few days of malaise and posterior cervical lymphadenopathy. Even in the light of these mild symptoms, if the infection crosses the placenta, the infant may be born with central nervous system damage, hydrocephalus, microcephaly, intracerebral calcification and retinal deformities.

Rubella

The rubella virus usually causes only a mild rash and mild systemic illness in a woman, but the teratogenic effects on a fetus can be devastating, such as hearing impairment, cognitive and motor challenges, cataracts, cardiac defects (most commonly patent ductus arteriosus and pulmonary stenosis), restricted intrauterine growth (i.e., small for gestational age), thrombocytopenic purpura, and dental and facial clefts, such as cleft lip and palate (White et al., 2012). Fetal damage from maternal infection with rubella (German measles) includes hearing impairment, cognitive and motor challenges, cataracts, cardiac defects (most commonly patent ductus arteriosus and pulmonary stenosis), intrauterine growth restriction (IUGR), thrombocytopenic purpura, and dental and facial clefts such as cleft lip and palate.

Typically, a rubella titre from a pregnant woman is obtained on the first antenatal visit. After a rubella immunisation, a woman is advised not to become pregnant for 3 months, until the rubella virus is no longer active. Immediately after a pregnancy, assess whether a woman with low rubella titres would like to be immunised to provide protection against rubella in future pregnancies (Johnson & Ross, 2007).

Cytomegalovirus

Cytomegalovirus (CMV), a member of the herpes virus family, is another teratogen that can cause extensive damage to a fetus while causing few symptoms in a woman (Stohl & Satin, 2011). It is transmitted from person to person by droplet infection such as occurs with sneezing. If a woman acquires a primary CMV infection during pregnancy and the virus crosses the placenta, the infant may be born severely neurologically challenged (hydrocephalus, microcephaly, spasticity) or with eye damage (optic atrophy, chorioretinitis), hearing impairment or chronic liver disease. The child's skin may be covered with large petechiae ("blueberry-muffin" lesions). Because a woman has almost no symptoms, she may not be aware that she has contracted an infection. However, diagnosis in the mother or infant can be established by the isolation of CMV antibodies in blood serum. Unfortunately, there is no treatment for the infection even if it presents in the mother with enough symptoms to allow detection. Because there is no treatment or vaccine for the disease, routine screening for CMV during pregnancy is not recommended. Women can help prevent exposure by thorough handwashing before eating and avoiding crowds of young children at daycare or nursery settings.

Herpes simplex virus (genital herpes infection)

The first time a woman contracts a genital herpes infection, systemic involvement occurs. The virus spreads into the bloodstream (viraemia) and crosses the placenta to a fetus, posing substantial fetal risk (ACOG, 2007; Jaiyeoba et al., 2012). If the infection takes place in the first trimester, severe congenital anomalies or spontaneous miscarriage may occur. If the infection occurs during the second or third trimester, there is a high incidence of premature birth, intrauterine growth restriction, and continuing infection of the newborn at birth. Unless recognised and treated, the fetal mortality and morbidity rates are as high as 80% (ACOG, 2007).

If a woman has had herpes simplex virus type 1 infections before the genital herpes invasion or if the genital herpes (type 2) infection is a recurrence, antibodies to the virus in her system prevent spread of the virus to a fetus across the placenta. If genital lesions are present at the time of birth, however, a fetus may contract the virus from direct exposure during birth. For women with a history of genital herpes and existing genital lesions, caesarean birth is often advised to reduce the risk of this route of infection. Intravenous or oral acyclovir (Zovirax) can be administered to women during pregnancy (McKenna & Mirkov, 2014). The primary mechanism for protecting a fetus, however, focuses on disease prevention. Urging women to practise safe sex is important to lessen their exposure to this and other sexually-transmitted infections. Advising adolescents to obtain a vaccine against HPV (Gardasil) should lessen the incidence of genital herpes infection in the future.

Syphilis

Syphilis, a sexually transmitted infection, is of great concern for the maternal–fetal population despite the availability of accurate screening tests and proven medical treatment, as it is growing in incidence and places a fetus at risk for intrauterine or congenital syphilis (Walker, 2009). If syphilis is detected and treated with an antibiotic such as benzylpenicillin in the first trimester, a fetus is rarely affected. If left untreated beyond the 18th week of gestation, hearing impairment, cognitive challenge, osteochondritis and fetal death are possible. For this reason, serological screening (by either a VDRL or a rapid plasma reagin test) should be done at a first antenatal visit.

The newborn with congenital syphilis may have congenital anomalies, extreme rhinitis (sniffles) and a characteristic syphilitic rash, all of which identify the baby as high risk at birth (Follett & Clarke, 2011). When the baby's primary teeth come in, they are oddly shaped (Hutchinson teeth). As the infant requires long-term follow-up, medical and nursing care of the newborn with congenital syphilis is discussed in Chapter 47.

Infections that cause illness at birth

Several infections are not teratogenic to a fetus during pregnancy but are harmful if they are present at the time of birth. Gonorrhoea, candidiasis, *Chlamydia, Streptococcus* B and hepatitis B infections are examples of these. Chapters 26 and 43 discuss the effects of these infections on maternal, fetal and neonatal health.

Teratogenic medications

Many women, assuming that the rule of being cautious with medications during pregnancy applies only to prescription medications, take over-the-counter medications or herbal supplements freely. Although not all medications cross the placenta (heparin, for example, does not because of its large molecular size), most do. Also, even though most herbs are safe, ginseng, for example, used to improve general wellbeing, or senna, used to relieve constipation, may not be safe (Der Marderosian & Beutler, 2007).

The use of recreational drugs during pregnancy puts a fetus at risk in two ways: the drug may have a direct teratogenic effect, and intravenous drug use risks exposure to diseases such as HIV and hepatitis B (Donnelly et al., 2008). Narcotics, such as heroin, have long been implicated as causing intrauterine growth restriction (IUGR). The use of marijuana alone apparently does not, although the long-term effects of marijuana during pregnancy are still unstudied. Cocaine, particularly its crack form, is potentially harmful to a fetus because it causes severe vasoconstriction in the mother, compromising placental blood flow and perhaps dislodging the placenta. Its use is associated with spontaneous miscarriage, preterm labour, meconium staining and IUGR (Rojas, Wood & Blakemore, 2007; Bernstein & Weinstein, 2007). See Chapter 22 for more information on the potential hazards of cocaine or heroin use during pregnancy.

Teratogenicity of alcohol

Evidence over the years has shown that when women consume a large quantity of alcohol during pregnancy, their babies show a high incidence of congenital deformities and cognitive impairment. It was assumed in the past that these defects were the result of the mother's poor nutritional status (drinking alcohol rather than eating food), not necessarily the direct result of the alcohol. However, alcohol has now been firmly isolated as a direct teratogen. Fetuses cannot remove the breakdown products of alcohol from their body. The large buildup of this leads to vitamin B deficiency and accompanying neurological damage.

Women during pregnancy should be screened for alcohol use because an infant born with **fetal alcohol syndrome** (FAS) not only is small for gestational age but can be cognitively challenged (Shankar, Ronis & Badger, 2007). The infant typically has a characteristic craniofacial deformity including short palpebral fissures, a thin upper lip and an upturned nose. Because of individual variations in metabolism it is impossible to define a safe level of alcohol consumption. Women are best advised, therefore, to abstain from alcohol completely. Be certain to ask about binge drinking (consuming more than five alcoholic drinks in an evening) as women may refer to this as only "occasional drinking". Refer women with alcohol addiction to an alcohol treatment program as early in pregnancy as possible to help them reduce their alcohol intake.

Teratogenicity of cigarettes

Cigarette smoking is associated with infertility in women. Cigarette smoking by a pregnant woman has been shown to cause fetal growth restriction (Lawrence & Haslam, 2007). In addition, a fetus may be at greater risk for being stillborn and, after birth, may be at greater risk than others for sudden infant death syndrome (Treyster & Gitterman, 2011). Low birth weight in infants of smoking mothers results from vasoconstriction of the uterine vessels, an effect of nicotine. This limits the blood supply to a fetus. Another contributory effect may be related to inhaled carbon monoxide. Secondary smoke, or inhaling the smoke of another person's cigarettes, may be as harmful as actually smoking the cigarettes. All antenatal healthcare settings should be smoke-free environments for this reason.

If a woman cannot stop smoking during pregnancy (and, realistically, many women cannot), reducing the number of cigarettes smoked per day should help diminish adverse effects on a fetus as well as also protect a woman's health from long-term illnesses such as chronic respiratory diseases. There are several smoking cessation aids women can use during pregnancy to reduce cigarette consumption. Nicotine replacement therapy (NRT) is most commonly used and works by replacing nicotine from cigarettes in the form of gum, patches, nasal spray, an inhaler, tablet or a lozenge (Pairman et al., 2010).

Environmental teratogens

Teratogens from environmental sources can be as damaging to a fetus as those that are directly or deliberately ingested. Women can be exposed through contact at home or at work sites.

Metal and chemical hazards

Pesticides and carbon monoxide, such as from car exhaust, should be avoided as these are examples of chemical teratogens. Teratogens that can be contacted at work sites include arsenic, a by-product of copper and lead smelting, used in pesticides, paints and leather processing; formaldehyde, used in paper manufacturing; and mercury, used in the manufacture of electrical apparatuses and found in swordfish and tuna fish. Lead poisoning is generally considered a problem of young children eating lead-based paint chips, but it also can be a fetal hazard (Maloney, 2007).

Radiation

Rapidly growing cells are extremely vulnerable to destruction by radiation. That makes radiation a potent teratogen to unborn children because of their high proportion of rapidly growing cells. Radiation produces a range of malformations depending on the stage of development of the embryo or fetus and the strength and length of exposure. If the exposure occurs before implantation, the growing zygote apparently is killed. If the zygote is not killed, it survives apparently unharmed. The most damaging time for exposure and subsequent damage is from implantation to 6 weeks after conception (when many women are not yet aware that they are pregnant). The nervous system, brain and retinal innervation are most affected. Radiation of the pelvis should be avoided during pregnancy if possible. It should be undertaken only at term if the data obtained are important for birth and cannot be obtained by any other means.

In addition to immediate fetal damage, evidence exists that radiation can have long-lasting effects on the health of a child. There appears to be an increased risk of cancer in children who are exposed to radiation in utero. Exposure of the fetal gonads could lead to a genetic mutation that will not be evident until the next generation (Pavone & Hueppchen, 2007).

Hyperthermia and hypothermia

Hyperthermia to a fetus can be detrimental to growth because it interferes with cell metabolism. This can occur from the use of saunas, hot tubs or tanning beds; from a work environment next to a furnace, such as in welding or steel making; or from a high maternal fever early in pregnancy (4–6 weeks). For this reason, after exercise programs, advise pregnant women not to use hot tubs or saunas. The effect of hypothermia on pregnancy is not well known. Because the uterus is an internal organ, a woman's body temperature would have to be lowered significantly before a great deal of fetal temperature change would result.

CASE STUDY QUESTION

5. Melissa Adams makes the following statements. Which one is the safest practice?

a. "My brother takes medicine for heartburn; if I get that, I'll just borrow his."
b. "I'm going to get a measles shot; I don't want measles while I'm pregnant."
c. "There are so many medicines for headache, I have to ask my doctor what to take."
d. "I know all over-the-counter medicine is safe; it's why it's over the counter."

PREPARATION FOR LABOUR

At about the midpoint of pregnancy, along with cautioning women about discomforts of pregnancy and possible teratogenic situations, it is time to review the events that signal the beginning of labour so that women will not be surprised by these happenings or dismiss them as something other than what they are.

Lightening

Lightening is the settling of the fetal head into the inlet of the true pelvis. It occurs approximately 2 weeks before labour in primiparas but at unpredictable times in multiparas, either before or during labour. A woman notices she is not as short of breath as she was before. Her abdominal contour is definitely changed, and on standing she may experience frequency of urination or sciatic pain (pain across a buttock radiating down her leg) from the lowered fetal position.

Show

Show is the common term used to describe the release of the cervical plug (operculum) that formed during pregnancy. It consists of mucus, often blood-streaked vaginal discharge, and indicates the beginning of cervical dilation.

Rupture of the membranes

A sudden gush of clear fluid (amniotic fluid) from the vagina indicates rupture of the membranes. A woman should telephone her primary care provider immediately when this occurs as after rupture of the membranes, there is a danger of uterine infection and cord prolapse if the fetal head is not well engaged or there is a malpresentation such as breech presentation.

Excess energy

Feeling extremely energetic is a sign of labour important for women to recognise. It occurs as part of the body's physiological preparation for labour. If a woman does not recognise the sensation for what it is, she may use this burst of energy to clean her house or finish paperwork at the office and exhaust herself before labour begins. If she can recognise this symptom as an initial sign of labour, she can conserve her energy in preparation for labour.

Uterine contractions

For most women, labour begins with contractions. True labour contractions usually start in the back and sweep forwards across the abdomen like the tightening of a band or similar to mild menstrual cramps. They gradually increase in frequency and intensity. Advise a woman to call her primary care provider when contractions begin, to alert healthcare personnel that she is in labour.

Key points for review

- Antenatal education is an important part of antenatal care. The more women know about measures they should take during pregnancy to safeguard their health, the more likely it is that they will avoid substances or activities harmful to fetal growth.
- Urge women to find the best way for them to modify their lifestyle for pregnancy. The average length of pregnancy is 40 weeks, so modifications must be agreeable to a woman or she will not maintain them over such a long time span.
- Women need to make provisions for rest periods during their day and to be aware of any potential teratogens at a work site, such as exposure to radiation or heavy metals.
- Women who travel should plan for break periods to avoid congestion in their lower extremities. Seatbelts must be used when travelling by car.
- Common discomforts of early pregnancy include breast tenderness, constipation, palmar erythema, nausea and vomiting, fatigue, muscle cramps, pain from varicosities or haemorrhoids, heart palpitations, frequency of urination and leucorrhoea. If women know that these symptoms may occur, they will not interpret them as complications.
- Minor discomforts of mid or late pregnancy include backache, dyspnoea, ankle oedema and Braxton Hicks contractions. Caution women that contractions could be a sign of labour.
- Women should take active measures to avoid exposure to infectious diseases such as rubella, HIV, cytomegalovirus, herpes simplex virus, syphilis and toxoplasmosis during pregnancy.
- Counsel women about the necessity to avoid the use of any medications or herbal supplements not specifically approved by their doctor or midwife during pregnancy, as well as alcohol and cigarettes.
- Beginning signs of labour for which the pregnant woman should be alert include lightening, show, excess energy, rupture of membranes and uterine contractions.

CASE STUDY QUESTIONS

6. Melissa voiced several concerns, including whether she should stop work and whether it would be safe to take a long trip. What advice would you give her regarding these questions?
7. Although Melissa describes a day she says involves a lot of walking, she also has long periods of sitting with almost no exercise. What would be some recommendations you could make to help her prevent blood clots from the sharp bend in her knee while sitting?

Resources

For an extensive range of additional resources to enhance teaching and learning and to facilitate understanding of this chapter, please see the text's accompanying website located on thePoint at http://thepoint.lww.com.

References

American College of Obstetricians and Gynecologists (ACOG). (2007). Management of herpes in pregnancy. *Obstetrics and Gynecology, 109*(6), 1489–1498.

Bernstein, H. B. & Weinstein, M. (2007). Normal pregnancy and antenatal care. In A. H. DeCheney & L. Nathan (Eds). *Current Diagnosis and Treatment in Obstetrics and Gynecology* (10th ed.). Columbus, OH: McGraw-Hill.

Better Health Channel (2015). Pregnancy and exercise, accessed 23 February 2015, <www.betterhealth.vic.gov.au/bhcv2/bhcarticles.nsf/pages/pregnancy_and_exercise>.

Coad, J. & Dunstall, M. (2011). Physiological adaptation to pregnancy. In J. Coad & M. Dunstall (Eds), *Anatomy & Physiology for Midwives* (pp. 257–288). London, England: Elsevier/Churchill Livingstone.

Der Marderosian, A. & Beutler, J. A. (2007). *Review of Natural Products.* New York: Facts & Comparisons.

Donnelly, J. C., et al. (2008). Illegal drug use, smoking and alcohol consumption in a low-risk Irish primigravid population. *Journal of Perinatal Medicine, 36*(1), 70–72.

Duong, H. T., Shahrukh-Hashmi, S., Ramadhani, T., et al. (2011). Maternal use of hot tub and major structural birth defects. *Birth Defects Research, 91*(9), 836–841.

Follett, T. & Clarke, D. F. (2011). Resurgence of congenital syphilis: Diagnosis and treatment. *Neonatal Network, 30*(5), 320–328.

Friars, C. (2007). Toxoplasmosis and pregnancy. *Practising Midwife, 10*(4), 20–21.

Guile, M. W. & Keller, J. (2011). Infections of the genital tract. In K. J. Hurt, M. W. Guile, J. L. Bienstock, et al. (Eds). *The Johns Hopkins Manual of Gynecology and Obstetrics* (4th ed.), pp. 322–348. Philadelphia, PA: Lippincott Williams & Wilkins.

Jaiyeoba, O., Amaya, M. I., Soper, D. E., et al. (2012). Preventing neonatal transmission of herpes simplex virus. *Clinical Obstetrics & Gynecology,* 55(2), 510–520.

Johnson, A. & Ross, B. (2007). Perinatal infections. In K. B. Fortner et al. (Eds). *The Johns Hopkins Manual of Gynecology and Obstetrics.* Philadelphia: Lippincott Williams & Wilkins.

Knopik, V. S. (2009). Maternal smoking during pregnancy and child outcomes: Real or spurious effect? *Developmental Neuropsychology, 34*(1), 1–36.

Kramer, M. S. & McDonald, S. W. (2009). Aerobic exercise for women during pregnancy. *Cochrane Database of Systematic Reviews, 2009*(1), (CD000180).

Lawrence, W. T. & Haslam, C. (2007). Smoking during pregnancy: Where next for stage-based interventions? *Journal of Health Psychology, 12*(1), 159–169.

McKenna, L. & Mirkov, S. (2014). *McKenna's Drug Handbook for Nursing & Midwifery* (7th ed.). Sydney: Lippincott Williams & Wilkins.

Maloney, G. (2007). Lead poisoning. In J. Schaider et al. (Eds). *Rosen & Barkin's 5-minute Emergency Medicine Consult.* Philadelphia: Lippincott Williams & Wilkins.

Menzies, J., et al. (2007). Instituting surveillance guidelines and adverse outcomes in preeclampsia. *Obstetrics and Gynecology, 110*(1), 121–127.

Pairman, S., Tracy, S., Thorogood, C. & Pincombe, J. (2010). *Midwifery Preparation for Practice* (2nd ed.). Churchill Livingstone: Elsevier Australia.

Pavone, M. E. & Hueppchen, N. A. (2007). Surgical disease and trauma in pregnancy. In K. B. Fortner et al. (Eds). *The Johns Hopkins Manual of Gynecology and Obstetrics.* Philadelphia: Lippincott Williams & Wilkins.

Perlen, S., Woolhouse, H., Gartland, D., et al. (2013). Maternal depression and physical health problems in early pregnancy: Findings of an Australian nulliparous pregnancy cohort study. *Midwifery, 29*(3), 233–239.

Quijano, C. E. & Abalos, E. (2009). Conservative management of symptomatic and/or complicated haemorrhoids in pregnancy and the puerperium. *Cochrane Database of Systematic Reviews, 2009*(1), (CD004077).

Rojas, F., Wood, E. & Blakemore, K. (2007). Preconception counseling and prenatal care. In K. B. Fortner et al. (Eds). *The Johns Hopkins Manual of Gynecology and Obstetrics.* Philadelphia: Lippincott Williams & Wilkins.

Russell, J. B., Denne, E. W. & Schwartz, D. (2011). Preconception counseling and prenatal care. In K. J. Hurt, M. W. Guile, J. L. Bienstock, et al. (Eds.), *The Johns Hopkins Manual of Gynecology and Obstetrics* (4th ed., pp. 56–72). Philadelphia, PA: Lippincott Williams & Wilkins.

Shankar, K., Ronis, M.J.J. & Badger, T. M. (2007). Effects of pregnancy and nutritional status on alcohol metabolism. *Alcohol Research & Health, 30*(1), 55–59.

Stohl, H. & Satin, A. J. (2011). Perinatal infections. In K. J. Hurt, M. W. Guile, J. L. Bienstock, et al. (Eds), *The Johns Hopkins Manual of Gynecology and Obstetrics* (4th ed.), pp. 137–153. Philadelphia, PA: Lippincott Williams & Wilkins.

Treyster, Z., & Gitterman, B. (2011). Second hand smoke exposure in children: Environmental factors, physiological effects, and interventions within pediatrics. *Reviews on Environmental Health, 26*(3), 187–195.

Walker, G.J.A. (2009). Antibiotics for syphilis diagnosed during pregnancy. *Cochrane Database of Systematic Reviews, 2009*(1), (CD001143).

White, S. J., Boldt, K. L., Holditch, S. J., et al. (2012). Measles, mumps, and rubella. *Clinical Obstetrics & Gynecology, 55*(2), 550–559.

Young, G. L. & Jewell, D. (2009). Interventions for leg cramps in pregnancy. *Cochrane Database of Systematic Reviews, 2009*(1), (CD000121).

Suggested readings

Alcohol and pregnancy: A practical guide for health professionals <www.moh.govt.nz>.

Australian Government Quit Line <www.quitnow.gov.au/internet/quitnow/publishing.nsf/content/warnings-b-babies>.

Australian Indigenous Health Bulletin <http://healthbulletin.org.au>.

Guidelines on weight management, Society of Obstetric Medicine of Australia and New Zealand <https://somanz.org/guidelines.asp>.

Health Direct Australia <www.pregnancybirthbaby.org.au>.

Willix, C., Rasmussen, S., Evans, S., & Walshe, V. (2015). A comparison of vitamin D levels in two antenatal populations in regional Western Australia: 'Tjindoo Ba Thonee Thurra': sunshine for the pregnant belly <http://healthbulletin.org.au/articles/a-comparison-of-vitamin-d-levels-in-two-antenatal-populations-in-regional-western-australia-tjindoo-ba-thonee-thurra-sunshine-for-the-pregnant-belly>.

Chapter 13

Promoting nutritional health during pregnancy

Previous chapters described the changes associated with pregnancy, common discomforts and danger signs of pregnancy. This chapter adds information about antenatal nutrition, an important aspect to help ensure a healthy outcome for both a woman and her child. Inadequate nutrition during pregnancy can affect not only fetal health but also the child's health for years to come.

LEARNING OBJECTIVES

After mastering the contents of this chapter, you should be able to:

1. Discuss the recommendations for healthy nutrition during pregnancy.
2. Use critical thinking to analyse the effects of different life situations on nutrition patterns to create ways nutritional health can be both improved and family-centred.
3. Assess a woman for nutritional adequacy during pregnancy.
4. Develop expected outcomes to assist a pregnant woman achieve optimal nutrition during pregnancy.
5. Discuss teaching strategies, such as ways to increase folic acid and calcium intake to promote optimal nutritional intake during pregnancy.
6. Discuss nursing care that encourages healthy nutritional practices during pregnancy.
7. Identify areas related to nutrition and pregnancy that could benefit from additional nursing research or application of evidence-based practice.

KEY TERMS

- body mass index
- food standards
- heartburn (dyspepsia)
- hyperemesis gravidarum
- obese
- pica

CASE STUDY

Renee Davidson is 4 months pregnant. She works at a fast-food restaurant and eats her breakfast and lunch at the restaurant where she works. Her husband works 4 evenings per week, so she cooks for herself on those evenings. She dislikes milk, so she takes milkshakes as a source of calcium. She is concerned because she has already gained 10 kg. She asks, "What's wrong with me?"

CASE STUDY QUESTION

1. What nutritional counselling does Renee need?

Although adequate nutrition during pregnancy cannot guarantee a good pregnancy outcome, it does make an important contribution. Both the nutritional state that a woman brings into pregnancy and her nutrition during pregnancy have a direct bearing on her health and on fetal growth and development. A poor diet, such as one deficient in folic acid, for example, is associated with birth anomalies such as neural tube defects. To ensure that early pregnancy deficiencies do not occur, encourage women of childbearing age to follow a healthy nutrition plan before pregnancy (preconception care) that specifically supplies adequate folic acid (400 mcg/0.4 mg per day). Otherwise, in the time before a woman recognises that she is pregnant (about 6 weeks), her poor diet and lack of important nutrient stores could seriously impair fetal growth (Fowles & Murphey, 2009).

PROMOTING NUTRITIONAL HEALTH IN A PREGNANT WOMAN

Assessment

Assessment begins with a woman's preconception nutrition patterns. From this assessment, determine whether she is eating healthy food sources as represented by the food pyramid and evaluate any cultural, environmental, or social lifestyles that could affect eating habits. A 24-hour recall history is the quickest way to secure necessary information, confirm well-balanced nutrition, and identify areas for teaching and learning. Once the woman has built rapport with the midwife during the antenatal period, the woman may want to write a journal of her daily intake over the course of a week so that the midwife can advise her of any nutritional requirements.

Nursing considerations

In relation to nutritional status of the pregnant woman, consider the desired health and growth of both the fetus and the woman. Both a woman who is eating large amounts of nutritionally inferior food and a woman who has a problem eating because of fatigue or nausea and vomiting may be at risk of the same problem: fetal growth restriction. Nursing considerations would be:

- Nutritional requirements due to an increase in physiological needs

- Nutritional imbalance due to nausea and vomiting every morning
- Promoting best food choices in pregnancy
- Nutritional education regarding appropriate intake of nutrients and kilojoules during pregnancy.

In large health centres, nutritionists are available to meet with women prenatally and help them plan nutrition during pregnancy. In other settings, a nutritionist may be available only for women with special needs, so the responsibility for nutrition advice falls directly on the midwife or medical practitioner. Many families in Australia and some areas of New Zealand live in rural or remote regions. Geographical isolation often requires long-distance travel to seek advice from the nearest health practitioners.

Social and cultural considerations

There are a number of considerations when assisting women to set expected outcomes for improving nutritional patterns. You must be certain to consider all the cultural and lifestyle factors that give different meanings to food. Food Standards Australia New Zealand (FSANZ) is a bi-nation government agency. The Food Standards Code was developed to ensure that food is suitable to eat in these countries. The code includes **food standards** for food additives, food safety, labelling and foods that need pre-approval such as genetic modification (FSANZ, 2014). Because food is an expensive commodity, consider financial resources as well. The purchase of food in rural and remote communities is often made more difficult as it is substantially more expensive due to transport costs. Indigenous communities also require special dietary considerations; health promotion and education are essential to ensure that healthy eating choices are made. Teaching about long-term outcomes such as building iron stores or bone mass is as important as short-term goals such as eating better for the upcoming week. Continuing a healthy eating pattern throughout the pregnancy (and maintaining it throughout life) will bring about important changes and help prepare the woman for feeding her family nutritionally for the future. Further Australian and New Zealand websites for nutritional information include:

- Food Standards Australia New Zealand <www.foodstandards.gov.au/Pages/default.aspx>
- Dietitians Association of Australia <http://daa.asn.au/for-the-public/smart-eating-for-you/nutrition-a-z/pregnancy/>
- National Health and Medical Research Council, Nutrient Reference Values for Australia and New Zealand Including Recommended Dietary Intakes <www.nhmrc.gov.au/guidelines-publications/n35-n36-n37>
- New Zealand Food Safety Authority <www.foodsafety.govt.nz>.

As everyone who has tried to change a nutritional pattern knows, this can be a lonely and seemingly unrewarding endeavour as results occur slowly. Begin by emphasising the physiological basis for nutritional needs in pregnancy (a woman is building a whole new person). Based on this the midwife would explain what nutritional deficits have been identified and work in partnership with the woman to assist her to alter her nutritional intake accordingly. In addition, when the midwife or doctor is determining the nutritional needs of pregnant women, they rely on the most important assessments: weight, energy level, general appearance, bowel function, and, when available, haemoglobin and urinalysis findings.

RELATIONSHIP OF MATERNAL NUTRITION TO INFANT HEALTH

During pregnancy, a woman must eat adequately to supply enough nutrients to the fetus so it can grow, as well as to support her own nutrition (Crombleholme, 2009). Adequate protein intake is vital because so much is needed by the fetus to build a body framework. Adequate protein may also help prevent complications of pregnancy such as pregnancy-induced hypertension or preterm birth. Either deficiencies or overuse of vitamins may contribute to birth anomalies (Subramanian et al., 2008). Remember that people have some degree of "backsliding", especially on holidays and at special events. Positive reinforcement, a basic rule of teaching, enhances learning, self-esteem and compliance more than criticism.

Recommended weight gain during pregnancy

A gain of 11.3 to 15.9 kg is recommended as an average weight gain in pregnancy. If a woman is at high risk of nutritional deficits, a more precise estimation of adequate weight gain can be calculated (Rode et al., 2007). This is done by calculating the **body mass index** (BMI), the ratio of weight to height (see Box 13.1). Women who are high or low in weight for their height (BMI below 18.5 or above 25 kg/m^2) need to have their expected outcomes for weight gain adjusted. The woman's BMI should be calculated at the initial antenatal visit so that a plan can be devised for normal weight gain during pregnancy. Repeated weighing in pregnancy should be undertaken only if this impinges on clinical practice (Australian Health Ministers' Advisory Council, 2012).

Weight gain in pregnancy occurs from both fetal growth and accumulation of maternal stores (see Box 13.2). It occurs at approximately 0.4 kg per month during the first trimester and then 0.4 kg per week during the last two trimesters. As a general rule, in the average woman, weight gain is considered excessive if it is more than 3 kg a month during the second and third trimesters; it is less than usual if it is less than 1 kg per month during the second and third trimesters. Women can be reassured that most of the weight gained with pregnancy will be lost afterwards (Bernstein & Weinstein, 2007). Women's appetites may increase due to increased circulation of human

BOX 13.1 Calculating body mass index

A body mass index calculator is available online at the Heart Foundation website <www.heartfoundation.org.au/healthy-eating/Pages/bmi-calculator.aspx>.

BMI also can be calculated using the formula: bodyweight in kilograms divided by height in metres squared.

For example: Renee Davidson is 165 cm tall and weighs 68 kg. To determine her BMI:

1. Weight in kilograms: 68 kg.
2. Height in centimetres: 165 cm.
3. Convert centimetres into metres: 165 ÷ 100 = 1.65 m.
4. Square height in metres (1.65 x 1.65 = 2.72).
5. Divide weight (kg) by m^2 (68 ÷ 2.72 = 25 BMI).

Normal pre-pregnancy BMI

Underweight	Under 18.5
Severe thinness	Less than 16.00
Moderate thinness	6.00–16.99
Mild thinness	17.00–1849
Normal weight	18.5–24.9
Overweight	≥25.0
Pre-obese	25.00–29.99
Obese	Above 30.0
Class I	30.00–34.99
Class II	35.00–39.99
Class III	≥40

With a BMI of 25, Renee enters pregnancy slightly overweight.

Source: Adapted from WHO 1995, WHO 2000 and WHO Expert Consultation 2004.

BOX 13.2 Assessment Sources of maternal weight gain

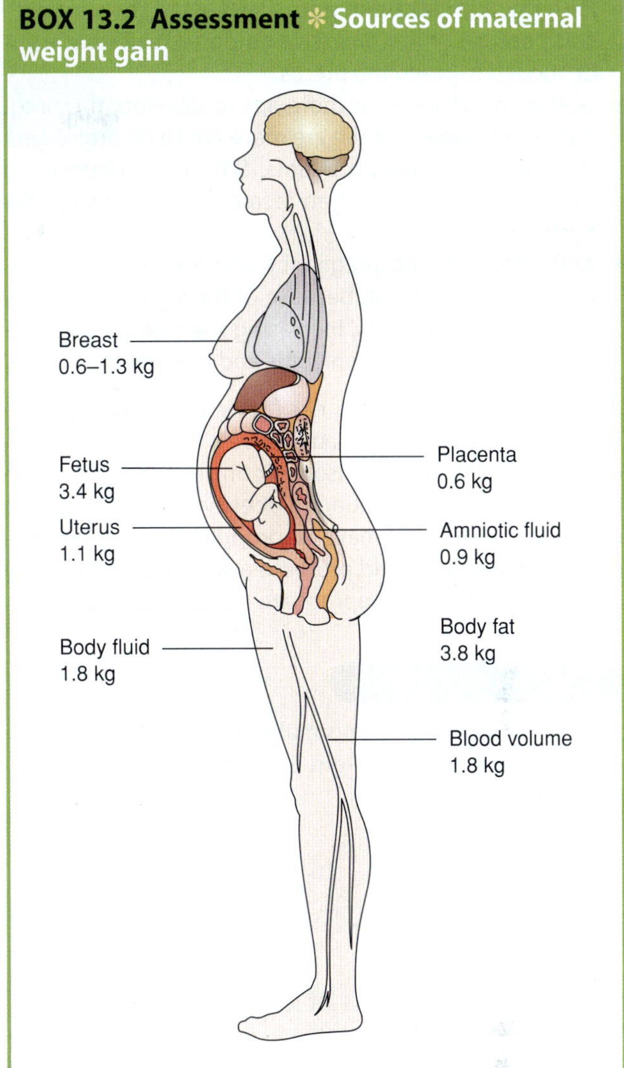

chorionic gonadatrophin (HCG) and thyroxine (T4). The US Institute of Medicine (IOM) provides guidance on weight gain in pregnancy as indicated in Table 13.1.

Women who are underweight coming into pregnancy should gain slightly more weight than the average woman (0.5 kg per month or week rather than 0.4). An obese woman might be advised to gain less than the average (0.3 kg). Weight gain will be higher for a multiple pregnancy than for a single pregnancy.

Obesity in pregnancy

A woman is considered **obese** if her BMI is above 30 kg/m^2. Rates of obesity are rising worldwide, including in pregnancy (Gratton, 2008 as cited in Pairman et al., 2010, p. 423). Less-educated women and those living in poverty tend to be more overweight than others. Obesity in pregnancy is serious because it is associated with an increased incidence of gestational diabetes and pregnancy-induced hypertension (Rode et al., 2007). Obesity also becomes a problem during pregnancy for a variety of reasons:

- Pregnancy causes circulatory volume to increase 20% to 50% and metabolism to increase to meet the demands of the pregnancy, placing additional stress on a possibly already overworked body. Hypertension and thrombophlebitis are more likely to occur.
- It is often difficult to hear fetal heart tones in an obese woman; palpating for position and size of a fetus at birth is also difficult.
- Obese women are at an increased risk for giving birth to infants with *macrosomia* (excessive fetal growth); this increases the incidence of caesarean births.

TABLE 13.1 Recommended weight gain during pregnancy based on BMI pre-pregnancy

Underweight	Normal	Pre-obese	Obese class I	Obese class II	Obese class III
<18.5 BMI	18.5 to 24.9 BMI	25.0 to 29.9 BMI	30.0 to 34.9 BMI	35.0 to 39.9 BMI	≥40 BMI
12.7–18.1 kg	11.3–15.9 kg	6.8–11.3 kg	5–9 kg	5–9 kg	5–9 kg

Source: Australian Health Ministers Advisory Council, 2012, *Clinical Practice Guidelines: Antenatal Care—Module 1.*

- Performing a caesarean birth, if necessary, may be difficult because of the excessive adipose tissue that must be incised to reach the uterus.
- Gestational diabetes is more apt to develop; the pregnancies of obese women are more apt to be prolonged, leading to postmature infants. Soft-tissue deposits in the vagina may present an increased risk for shoulder dystocia.
- Ambulating during pregnancy and immediately afterwards is more difficult because of the increased energy expenditure necessary, increasing the risk of complications such as thrombophlebitis and pneumonia.

As well as obesity being a risk factor in pregnancy, conversely, extreme thinness can also be a risk factor (Australian Health Ministers' Advisory Council 2012). The main focus of the nurse in relation to obesity in pregnancy is to empower women to make appropriate health choices. Health education should promote a sound mix of healthy eating, exercising and appropriate rest and relaxation.

CASE STUDY QUESTION

2. Suppose Renee has a normal BMI. What would be the recommended weight gain for her during pregnancy?
   a. 4 kg
   b. 9 kg
   c. 13 kg
   d. 27 kg

Essential components of healthy nutrition for the pregnant woman

Energy (kilojoule) needs

Pregnant women's requirements per day during pregnancy include:

- Five serves of 75 g of vegetables, beans and legumes for all ages
- Two serves of 150 g of fruit for all ages
- Eight 500-kJ servings of wholegrain cereals for women aged under 18 years and 8.5 servings for women 19 years or older
- 3.5 500-kJ serves of fish, eggs, tofu, nuts, lean meat, poultry, legumes, seeds, beans for all ages
- 3.5 500-kJ servings of milk, cheese or yoghurt for women aged under 18 years and 2.5 servings for women 19 years or older.

Taller or more active women may need extra kilojoule requirements, but generally the woman should follow the above requirements (Australian Government Department of Health & Ageing & National Health & Medical Research Council, 2013). Figure 13.1 illustrates the Australian Guide to Healthy Eating, a food selection guide that visually represents the proportion of the five food groups recommended for daily consumption.

Protein needs

The daily recommended intake (DRI) for protein in women is 46 g/d. During pregnancy, the need for protein increases to 58–60 g daily (Australian Government Department of Health & Ageing & National Health & Medical Research Council, 2013). If protein needs are met, overall nutritional needs are likely to be met as well (with the possible exceptions of vitamins C, A and D) because of the high incorporation of other nutrients with protein foods. If protein intake is inadequate, iron, B vitamins, calcium and phosphorus will also probably be inadequate. Vitamin B_{12} is found almost exclusively in animal protein, so if animal protein is excluded from the diet, vitamin B_{12} deficiency can occur unless supplemented.

Fat needs

Only linoleic acid, an essential fatty acid necessary for new cell growth, cannot be manufactured in the body from other sources. Because linoleic acid must be obtained from food, women must be sure to consume a source of this nutrient during pregnancy. Vegetable oils are a good source. In addition, using vegetable oils (e.g. olive, sunflower and canola oil) that have a low cholesterol content rather than animal oils (butter) is recommended for all adults as a means of preventing hypercholesterolaemia and coronary heart disease. Women should also try and ingest omega-3 oils, found primarily in fish, omega-3–fortified eggs and the newer omega-3–fortified spreads (Bourre, 2007).

Vitamin needs

The intake of vitamins as a daily dietary supplement has become so common that their importance may be underestimated by some women. Requirements for both fat-soluble and water-soluble vitamins increase during pregnancy to support the growth of new fetal cells. However, it is important that vitamin supplementation only be taken under medical supervision. This is to ensure that the recommended dosage of vitamin A is provided. Some supplement products contain high levels of vitamin A, which is contraindicated in pregnancy.

Vitamin deficiency can result in several common problems. For example, vitamin D, essential for calcium absorption, when lacking, can begin to diminish both fetal and maternal mineral bone density. Pregnant women should thus be encouraged to have time in the sun. This could be combined with periods of exercise.

Although folic acid (folacin) belongs to the B-vitamin group, its importance during pregnancy warrants a separate discussion. Found predominantly in fresh fruits and vegetables, folic acid is necessary for red blood cell formation. As a woman's blood volume doubles during pregnancy, this substantially increases her folic acid needs. Without adequate folic acid, a megaloblastic anaemia (large but ineffective red blood cells) may develop. If a woman has this blood pattern at the time of birth, the infant may be affected as well.

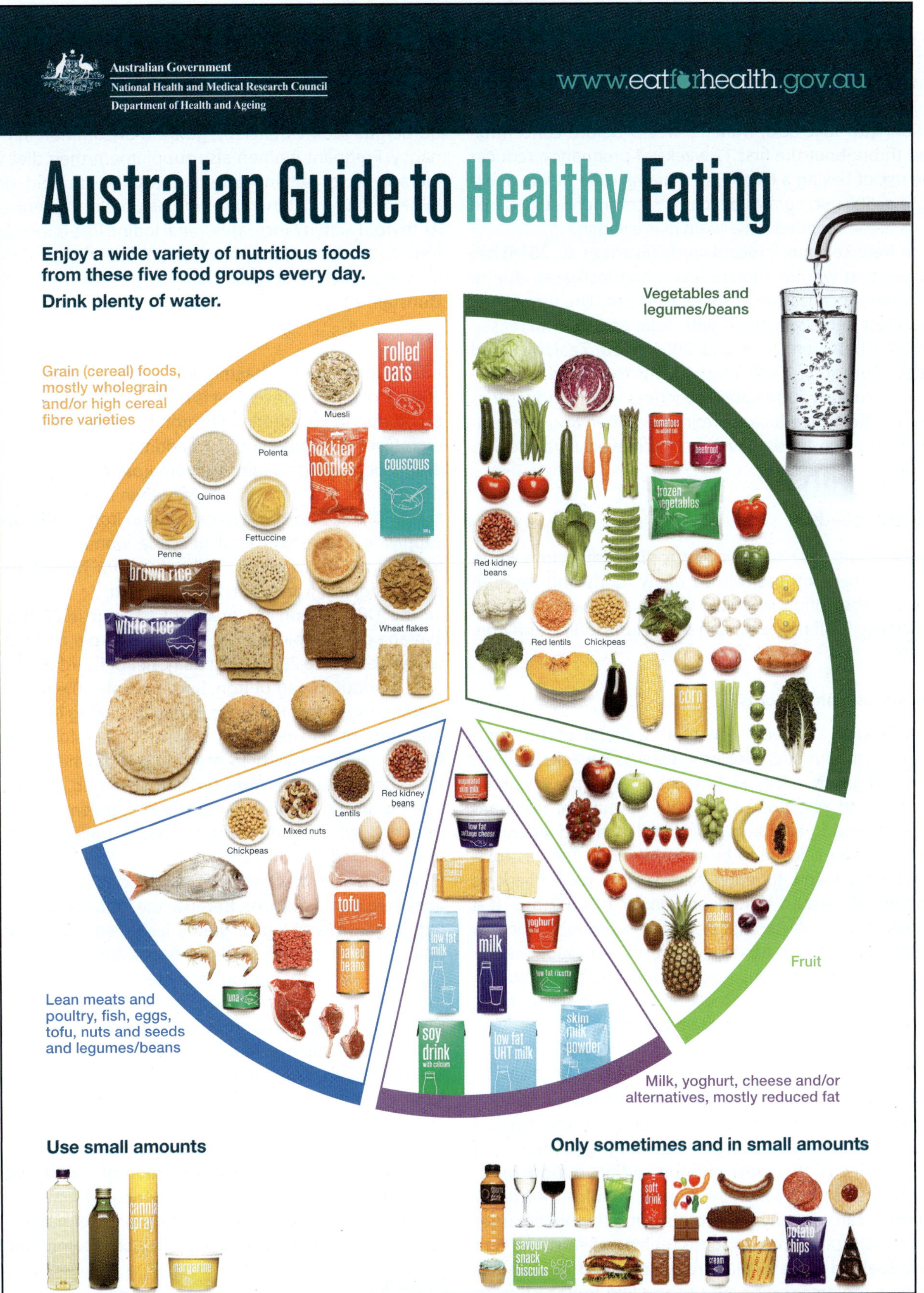

FIGURE 13.1 Australian Guide to Healthy Eating (National Health and Medical Research Council and DHA) (2013). *Eat for Health Australian Dietary Guidelines: Summary*. Canberra: NHMRC and DHA.)

For this reason, as well as its importance in preventing neural tube defects, women should eat foods high in folic acid such as vegetables and fruit, and should take an antenatal vitamin that contains a folic acid supplement of 0.4 to 1.0 mg (Subramanian et al., 2008). Dietary supplementation with folic acid, from 12 weeks before conception and throughout the first 12 weeks of pregnancy, reduces the risk of having a baby with a neural tube defect and a dose of 500 micrograms per day is recommended. Vitamin B_{12} is recommended if the woman is a vegan.

In New Zealand, a recent study (Evans et al., 2014) has shown that women's folate levels had increased due to voluntary fortification of folate in bread. The number of breakfast cereals fortified with folic acid has increased by 30% between 2003 and 2006 (New Zealand Food Safety Authority, 2009). Mechanisms to extend and promote voluntary fortification practices within industry as well as efforts to educate pregnant women about choosing folate rich foods have been achieved (Evans et al., 2014).

Mineral needs

Minerals are necessary for new cell building in a fetus. Because they are found in so many foods and because mineral absorption improves during pregnancy, mineral deficiency, with the exception of calcium, iodine and iron, is rare.

Calcium and phosphorus

The skeleton and teeth constitute a major portion of a fetus. Tooth formation begins as early as 8 weeks in utero. Bones begin to calcify at 12 weeks. To supply adequate calcium and phosphorus for bone formation, pregnant women need to eat foods high in calcium and vitamin D (necessary for calcium to be absorbed from the gastrointestinal tract and to enter bones). The recommended amount of calcium during pregnancy is 1300 mg. If a woman cannot drink milk or eat milk products such as cheese, she can be prescribed a daily calcium supplement. Most foods high in protein are also high in phosphorus, so by eating high-protein foods, women receive enough phosphorus, also important for bone growth.

Iodine

Iodine is essential for the formation of thyroxine and, therefore, for the proper functioning of the thyroid gland. As thyroid function increases during pregnancy, a woman needs to ingest enough iodine during pregnancy to supply this increased need. If iodine deficiency occurs, it can cause hypothyroidism and thyroid enlargement (goitre). Women in some regions of Australia and New Zealand in particular are encouraged to consider iodine supplementation due to the low iodine content in the soil.

The hypothalamic-pituitary-thyroid axis undergoes marked changes in pregnancy. Both oestrogen and hCG cause changed levels of tri-iodothyronine (T3) and thyroxine (T4) which supports the altered metabolism of pregnancy. Pregnancy runs parallel with hyperthyroidism in relation to increasing body temperature and appetite and feelings of fatigue. Unless pregnant women are borderline iodine deficient, goitre is uncommon in pregnancy. Pregnant women also supplement their diet with iodized table salt in current times. The thyroid gland hypertrophies at it increases iodine uptake in pregnancy. As thyroid activity increases, renal iodine loss is increased. Nausea and vomiting have been linked not only to increased hCG but also the rise in free T4 (Coad & Dunstall, 2011).

Iron

A fetus at term has a haemoglobin level of 17 to 21 g per 100 mL of blood, a level that is necessary to oxygenate the blood during intrauterine life. Iron is needed to build this high level of haemoglobin. In addition, after week 20 of pregnancy, a fetus begins to store iron in the liver to last through the first 3 months of life, when intake will consist mainly of milk, which is typically low in iron. In addition to supplying these high fetal needs, a woman needs iron to build an increased red cell volume for herself and to protect against iron lost in blood at birth.

The DRI for iron for pregnant women is 27 mg. An average diet supplies about 6 mg of iron per 4100 kJ. If a woman eats a 10,250-kJ diet daily, her daily intake, therefore, is about 15 mg of iron. Because only 10% to 20% of dietary iron is absorbed, she is actually taking in less than this amount (closer to 1.5 to 3 mg). Therefore, dietary supplementation with 15 mg iron per day helps ensure that adequate iron is ingested and absorbed. It is important to stress to women that iron supplementation is intended as a supplement to, not a replacement for, iron-rich foods.

Women with low incomes may find it difficult to eat adequate iron-rich foods, because the foods richest in iron (e.g. organ meats; eggs; green, leafy vegetables; whole grains; enriched breads; dried fruits) are also the most expensive. Iron absorption increases in an acid environment, so eating iron-rich foods or swallowing iron tablets with ascorbic acid (found in orange juice) may increase absorption. Oral iron compounds turn stools black or blackish green. The compounds can be irritating to the stomach or cause constipation in some women.

Fluoride

Because fluoride aids in the formation of sound teeth, a pregnant woman should drink fluoridated water. In an area where the water is not fluoridated either naturally or artificially, supplemental fluoride may be recommended.

Sodium

Sodium is the major electrolyte that acts to maintain fluid in the body: when sodium is retained rather than excreted by the kidneys, an equal or balancing amount of fluid is also retained. Retaining enough fluid in the maternal circulation is important to ensure a pressure gradient and allow optimal exchange of nutrients across the placenta. Sodium is controlled by aldosterone that is produced in the adrenal cortex gland. Aldostrone works in conjunction with the renin-angiotensin regulation cycle that regulates blood pressure and reabsorbs more sodium to enhance vasoconstriction.

Zinc

Zinc is necessary for the synthesis of DNA and RNA. Although not proved, zinc deficiency may be associated with preterm birth. The DRI for zinc during pregnancy is 12 mg, or an increase of 3 mg over pre-pregnancy needs. Most people who take in adequate protein also take in adequate zinc because zinc is contained in foods such as meat, liver, eggs and seafood. It is also a component of antenatal vitamins to help ensure an adequate intake (Rolfes, Pinna & Whitney, 2009).

Fluid needs

Extra amounts of water are needed during pregnancy to promote kidney function because a pregnant woman must excrete waste products for two. Two or three glasses of water daily over and above the DRI is recommended. The intake of additional fluid also helps to avoid constipation due to decreased gastric motility. Water balance is controlled by the posterior pituitary gland that produces anti-diuretic hormone (ADH) and has the same function as oxytocin which retains fluid. Oxytocin is also produced by the posterior pituitary gland.

Fibre needs

Constipation can occur during pregnancy from slowed peristalsis because of progesterone that enhances relaxation and decreases GIT activity, thereby reducing peristaltic activity. Eating fibre-rich foods, regular exercise and increasing water intake all aid in reducing constipation in pregnancy. Fibre also has the advantage of lowering cholesterol levels and may remove carcinogenic contaminants from the intestine. Therefore, encourage women to eat plenty of fresh fruits and vegetables, especially green, leafy vegetables, to provide fibre. Eating fibre-rich foods is a better choice for preventing constipation than taking a fibre laxative. Doing so allows a woman to receive nutrients from the food as well as preventing constipation (Derbyshire, 2007).

Foods to avoid or limit in pregnancy

Soft cheese, pâté and unpasteurised dairy products can cause listeriosis which may cause septicaemia in the baby. Shark, marlin and swordfish should be avoided due to the increased mercury content (Baston & Hall, 2009). Not drinking alcohol during pregnancy is the safest option (Australian Government Department of Health & Ageing & National Health & Medical Research Council, 2013).

Foods with caffeine

Caffeine is thought by many to be just an incidental ingredient in beverages. Actually, it is a central nervous system stimulant capable of increasing heart rate, urine production in the kidney and secretion of acid in the stomach (Rolfes, Pinna & Whitney, 2009). A daily intake of caffeine such as two or three cups of coffee has not been associated with low birth weight; however, drinking more than three cups per day is associated with an increased rate of early miscarriage (Applebee, 2008). To limit their caffeine intake, women may need to limit not only the amount of coffee they drink but also other sources of caffeine such as chocolate, soft drinks and tea. If a woman has difficulty omitting these common foods from her diet, she can still reduce the amount of caffeine she ingests. Decaffeinated coffee, as the name implies, contains almost no caffeine. Due to the popularity of coffee within our contemporary culture, Food Standards Australia New Zealand provides the following advice. It is best to limit the daily amount of caffeine to:

- 1 regular espresso style coffee or
- 3 cups of instant style coffee
- 4 cups of tea or
- 4 cans of diet/regular cola drink (FSANZ, 2014).

Artificial sweeteners

Artificial sweeteners are used to improve the taste and to limit the kilojoule content of foods. It is probably safest for pregnant women to reduce their intake of these. The use of saccharine is not recommended during pregnancy because it is eliminated slowly from the fetal bloodstream. In any event, pregnant women need carbohydrates furnished by sugar rather than artificial substances (Rolfes, Pinna & Whitney, 2009) and simple and complex carbohydrates.

What if...

Renee states, "I love coffee. There's always a pot brewing where I work. And I love a cup of cappuccino for lunch." What suggestions could you make to help her reduce her caffeine intake?

CASE STUDY QUESTION

3. Which statement by Renee lets you know she understands how iron is best absorbed?

a. "I always take my iron pills with milk."
b. "I crush my iron pills to disguise the taste."
c. "I take the pills with a carbonated beverage."
d. "I swallow my iron pills with orange juice."

ASSESSMENT OF NUTRITIONAL HEALTH

Women who follow good nutrition practices before pregnancy come into pregnancy in better health and better prepared to avoid pregnancy complications. The best method for assessing a woman's nutritional intake is to ask for a "typical day" history or a 24-hour nutrition recall to isolate usual patterns and possible nutritional risk factors. First, ask if yesterday was a typical day. If it was, then ask the woman to list all the food she ate within the past 24 hours, from when she awakened until she went to sleep. Be certain she includes all the snack foods she ate, as well as sit-down meals. This method of history taking yields much more accurate information than if a woman is asked how often during the week she eats citrus fruit or how much milk she drinks every day; most people eat automatically with little thought to their food intake (Cohen & Farley, 2008).

Haemoglobin or haematocrit determinations are also important assessments of good nutrition. These may reveal smoking habits, as cigarette smokers have lower haemoglobin levels than non-smokers. These values are measured early in pregnancy and then usually repeated close to term and again at birth. A urinalysis can also be important. A finding such as elevated urine specific gravity could suggest a less-than-adequate fluid intake and elevated urine glucose levels could suggest gestational diabetes (see Chapter 20).

PROMOTING NUTRITIONAL HEALTH DURING PREGNANCY

Be certain that plans for improving nutritional patterns take into account a woman's lifestyle, family preferences, financial resources, customs and cultural desires, because she and her family must follow them for 9 months.

Family considerations

Meal planning is best if it involves the entire family. Even if a woman is receptive to changing her eating habits, she may have difficulty carrying out recommendations if her family resists the change. In families where a member has a special nutritional need, change may be even more difficult.

Financial considerations

Food is costly; however, in promoting healthy food choices women require an understanding that with the need of only an additional 1230 kJ per day in pregnancy, the additional cost is minimal. There are three different requirements: first trimester, no extra kJ; second trimester, 1400 extra kJ; and third trimester, 1900 extra kJ. However, a woman of lower socioeconomic status may have difficulty actually planning with a nutritional variety of foods. If this occurs, review what foods the woman is eating to be certain she is not buying only energy-dense and nutritionally poor food. Provide advice and healthy food choices that are achievable with limited financial circumstances. Many communities provide social and financial assistance programs to support lower income members in their local environment. Networking with these support groups is an essential component of the role of a contemporary nurse.

BOX 13.3 ✻ Focus on evidence-based practice

Gestational diabetes

What women eat during pregnancy certainly influences their serum glucose levels. Interested in learning if a diet high in total fatty acids, saturated fatty acids and red meat increases women's risk of developing diabetes during pregnancy, researchers asked 1733 women to record everything they ate during the first trimester of their pregnancies. At 26 to 28 weeks, a glucose tolerance test was done to assess if gestational diabetes had occurred. Of the 1733 women studied, 91 (5%) developed gestational diabetes (a fasting serum glucose over 126 mmol/L) and 206 (11%) developed impaired glucose tolerance or a blood glucose 100 to 125 mmol/L. The types of food women ate, however, did not influence these results, and the type of nutrient or food intake in early pregnancy was not linked to a risk of gestational diabetes. Nutritional status entering pregnancy, as reflected by the women's pre-pregnancy BMI, appeared to be more predictive than was food eaten during pregnancy.

Would the results of this study be helpful in pre-pregnancy or adolescent counselling?

Source: Radesky, J. S., et al. (2008). Diet during early pregnancy and development of gestational diabetes. *Paediatric and Perinatal Epidemiology, 22*(1), 47–59.

CASE STUDY QUESTION

4. You need to obtain a nutrition history from Renee. What is the best way to do this?
   a. Ask her to tell you how much protein she eats daily
   b. Assess if Renee feels satisfied with her nutrition
   c. Ask Renee to describe what she ate in the last 24 hours
   d. Tell Renee to describe her concept of ideal nutrition

Managing common problems affecting nutritional health

Specific nutritional problems may result during pregnancy because of several factors or circumstances. Discomfort resulting from food choices, such as constipation, has been discussed (see Chapter 12).

Nausea and vomiting

As many as 50% of pregnant women report nausea and vomiting (Rojas, Wood & Blakemore, 2007). No definite cause has been established for this symptom of early pregnancy, but it may be related to:

- Sensitivity to the high level of chorionic gonadotropin hormone produced by the trophoblast cells
- High oestrogen or progesterone levels
- Lowered maternal blood sugar caused by the needs of the developing embryo
- Lack of pyridoxine (vitamin B_6)
- Increased circulating thyroxine (T4) levels
- Diminished gastric motility.

Nausea is aggravated by fatigue and may also be aggravated by emotional disturbance. Most women notice the sensation as early as the first missed menstrual period and experience it throughout pregnancy. The sensation is usually most intense on arising but may occur while a woman is preparing meals or smelling food. Vomiting at least once a day is common. Women who work nights and sleep days often experience "evening sickness", because that is when they arise.

Methods such as acupressure, anti–motion sickness wrist bands, or avoiding fluid with meals are effective for some women. Mild-flavoured ginger tea may also be helpful (White, 2007). Increasing carbohydrate intake seems to relieve nausea better than any other nutritional remedy. The traditional solution is for women to keep dry crackers by their bedside and to eat a few before rising. A woman can then eat a light breakfast or delay breakfast until 10 or 11 a.m., past the time her nausea seems to persist. To be certain she maintains a good food intake during pregnancy even in the presence of nausea, she should compensate for any missed meals later in the day. It is a good rule for women not to go longer than 12 hours between meals during pregnancy to prevent hypoglycaemia. A woman may need to eat a late-evening snack to compensate for a late breakfast. She may be able to tolerate fruit and raw vegetables during the morning before other food. Urge her to experiment with soups or vegetable drinks that she may not usually think of as breakfast foods but that will give her early-morning kilojoules.

Caution

Women should be cautioned against self-medicating for nausea by taking antacids. Excessive use of antacids containing sodium bicarbonate may cause fluid retention because of the sodium content. Fortunately, nausea usually disappears spontaneously as a woman enters her fourth month of pregnancy. If it persists beyond this month or is so extreme in early pregnancy that it interferes with nutrition, it may indicate the development of hyperemesis gravidarum, a serious complication of pregnancy.

Cravings

Cravings for food or aversions to certain foods during pregnancy are so common that they are considered a normal part of adaptation to pregnancy. It was formerly considered that these strange desires for food reflected a woman's need to call attention to her pregnancy or were a reaction to her imposed dependent state. However, cravings are actually more likely the result of a physiological need for more carbohydrates or particular vitamins and minerals such as iron.

During pregnancy, some women report an abnormal craving for non-food substances (termed **pica** from the Latin word for "magpie", a bird that is an indiscriminate eater). Because pica is a symptom that often accompanies iron deficiency anaemia, correcting this underlying problem with an iron supplement may correct the pica. At subsequent visits, be certain to assess if a woman's haemoglobin is increasing and ask if she notices any difference in her cravings.

Heartburn (dyspepsia)

Heartburn (dyspepsia) is a burning sensation along the oesophagus caused by regurgitation of gastric contents into the lower oesophagus. In pregnancy, it may accompany early nausea, but it may persist beyond the resolution of nausea and even increase in severity as pregnancy advances.

Dyspepsia is probably caused by decreased gastric motility, which slows gastric emptying, and pressure of the expanding uterus pushing up against the stomach and increased production of progesterone. It is noticed by at least 50% of pregnant women (Orr, 2007). Common suggestions to help prevent reflux into the oesophagus are:

- Eat small meals frequently rather than large meals.
- Sleep on the left side with two pillows to elevate the upper torso.
- Do not lie down immediately after eating; try and wait at least 2 hours.
- Avoid fatty and fried foods, coffee, carbonated beverages, tomato products and citrus juices.

CASE STUDY QUESTION

5. Which statement by Renee would best suggest she has pica?

a. "I cannot stand smell of cooked vegetables in the evening."
b. "I feel like eating chalk."
c. "I notice I've been eating more sweet stuff than usual."
d. "I crave oranges; can't get enough of them every day."

Hyperemesis gravidarum

Hyperemesis gravidarum (sometimes called *pernicious* or *persistent vomiting*) is nausea and vomiting of pregnancy that is prolonged past week 12 or is so severe that dehydration, ketonuria and significant weight loss occur within the first 12 weeks (Alalade, Khan, & Dawlatly, 2007). It occurs at an incidence of 1 in 200 to 300 women. The cause is unknown, but women with the disorder may have increased thyroid function because of the thyroid-stimulating properties of

BOX 13.4 ✻ Focus on communication

Renee comes to your antenatal clinic for her first visit. You want to obtain a nutrition history from her.

Less effective communication

Nurse: Hi, Renee. Are you eating a nutritious diet?

Renee: I'm always hungry since I've been pregnant. No problem.

Nurse: Have you ever compared what you eat to a food pyramid to see if you're eating all the different types of food it shows?

Renee: Sure. Grain is on one side; meat is on the other. I eat both of those.

Nurse: It's important to drink at least a litre of milk a day during pregnancy. Are you doing that?

Renee: I'm drinking milkshakes so I not only get calcium but extra kilojoules.

Nurse: That's great. Good nutrition is so important during pregnancy. I'm glad you're so aware of it.

More effective communication

Nurse: Hi, Renee. Tell me about your diet.

Renee: I'm always hungry since I've been pregnant. No problem.

Nurse: Tell me what you ate yesterday.

Renee: A muffin and coffee for breakfast, a milkshake for lunch, a hamburger and fries for supper. A soft drink before bed. And ice cubes. I suck on them all day like lollies.

Nurse: Let's talk about ways you might get some fruit and vegetables into your day.

Most people believe they eat well, so if just asked general questions about nutrition, they respond that their nutrition is adequate. Only when they are asked to actually describe what they ate during one day is the truth revealed.

human chorionic gonadotropin. Some studies reveal that it is associated with *Helicobacter pylori*, the same bacteria that causes peptic ulcers (Golberg, Szilagyi & Graves, 2007).

With hyperemesis gravidarum, a woman's nausea and vomiting are so severe that she cannot maintain her usual nutrition. Always try to determine exactly how much nausea and vomiting women are experiencing during pregnancy. Ask a woman to describe the events of the day before if she says it was a typical day. How late into the day did the nausea last? How many times did she vomit and how much? What was the total amount of food she was able to eat? Women with hyperemesis gravidarum may need to be hospitalised for about 24 hours to monitor intake, output and blood chemistry, and to restore hydration with intravenous fluids.

CASE STUDY QUESTION

6. Suppose Renee is a vegetarian. What is her greatest nutritional risk?
   a. Lack of iron
   b. Lack of vitamin C
   c. Lack of folic acid
   d. Lack of vitamin B_{12}

Key points for review

- Assessment of nutritional health should include a diet history (24-hour recall and week-long diary) and physical examination.
- Nutrition during pregnancy should include about 1230 additional kJ daily to provide energy, spare protein and provide for fetal growth requirements.
- Important minerals necessary for pregnancy include iron, iodine, calcium, fluoride, sodium and zinc.
- Most women need to take an iron supplement to prevent iron deficiency anaemia.
- Women should monitor their intake of caffeine, fish and artificial sweeteners during pregnancy.
- Antenatal vitamins contain additional folic acid supplements and iron, so these should be used instead of over-the-counter vitamins during pregnancy.
- Advise pregnant women not to go longer than 12 hours between meals, to avoid hypoglycaemia.
- Common nutrition concerns associated with pregnancy include nausea and vomiting, constipation, cravings (including pica) and pyrosis.
- Hyperemesis gravidarum is nausea and vomiting of pregnancy that extends past 12 weeks or is too extreme to allow for adequate nutrition.

CASE STUDY QUESTIONS

7. Renee drinks milkshakes as a source of calcium. Is this a wise choice? Why do you think she craves oranges?
8. Renee works at a fast-food restaurant. She states she is too nauseated in the morning to eat before she leaves for work and is too tired of seeing food all day to prepare a good meal after work. What suggestions could you make to help her increase her food intake?
9. Renee rarely eats vegetables; when she does, she fries them in butter. How would you use a food pyramid to explain better pregnancy nutrition to her?
10. What would be a possible research topic to explore pertinent to the Food Standards Australia New Zealand Guidelines that would be applicable to the Davidson family and also advance evidence-based practice?

Resources

For an extensive range of additional resources to enhance teaching and learning and to facilitate understanding of this chapter, please see the text's accompanying website located on thePoint at http://thepoint.lww.com.

References

Alalade, A. O., Khan, R. & Dawlatly, B. (2007). Day-case management of hyperemesis gravidarum: Feasibility and clinical efficacy. *Journal of Obstetrics & Gynaecology, 27*(4), 363–364.

Applebee, B. K. (2008). The deleterious effects of caffeine on pregnancy. *Nutritional Perspectives, 3*(3), 23–25.

Australian Government Department of Health & Ageing & National Health & Medical Research Council, (2013), *Healthy eating during your pregnancy*, accessed 5 June 2015 at <www.eatforhealth.gov.au>.

Australian Health Ministers' Advisory Council (2012). *Clinical practice guidelines: Antenatal care – module 1*. Australian Government Department of Health and Ageing, Canberra, accessed 5 June 2015 at <www.health.gov.au/antenatal>.

Baston, H. & Hall, J. (2009). *Midwifery Essentials Antenatal* (Vol. 3). London: Churchill Livingstone.

Bernstein, H. B. & Weinstein, M. (2007). Normal pregnancy and prenatal care. In A. H. DeCheney & L. Nathan (Eds). *Current Diagnosis and Treatment in Obstetrics and Gynecology* (10th ed.). Columbus, OH: McGraw-Hill.

Bourre, J. M. (2007). Dietary omega-3 fatty acids for women. *Biomedicine & Pharmacotherapy, 61*(2–3), 105–112.

Coad, J. & Dunstall, M. (2011), *Anatomy and Physiology for Midwives*. (3rd ed.). Edinburgh: Elsevier Churchill Livingstone.

Cohen, D. & Farley, T. A. (2008). Eating as an automatic behavior. *Preventing Chronic Disease, 5*(1), A23.

Crombleholme, W. R. (2009). Obstetrics. In S. J. McPhee & M. A. Papdakis (Eds). *Current Medical Diagnosis and Treatment*. Columbus: McGraw-Hill.

Derbyshire, E. (2007). The importance of adequate fluid and fibre intake during pregnancy. *Nursing Standard, 21*(24), 40–43.

Evans, S. E., Mygind, V. L., Peddie, M. C., Miller, J. C. & Houghton, L. A. (2014). Effect of increasing voluntary folic acid food fortification on dietary folate intakes and adequacy of reproductive-age women in New Zealand. *Public Health Nutrition*, 17, 1447–1453.

Food Standards Australia New Zealand (FSANZ) (2014). *Caffeine*, accessed 5 June 2015 at <www.foodstandards.gov.au/consumer/generalissues/Pages/Caffeine.aspx>.

Fowles, E. R. & Murphey, C. (2009). Nutrition and mental health in early pregnancy: A pilot study. *Journal of Midwifery & Women's Health, 54*(1), 73–77.

Golberg, D., Szilagyi, A. & Graves, L. (2007). Hyperemesis gravidarum and *Helicobacter pylori* infection: A systematic review. *Obstetrics & Gynecology, 110*(3), 695–703.

New Zealand Food Safety Authority (2009) *Fortification overages of the food supply, Folate,* accessed 5 June 2015 at <www.foodsafety.govt.nz/elibrary/search.htm?audience=industry&keywords=folate&publication_type=>.

Orr, W. C. (2007). Consequences of nighttime heartburn: Quality of life and sleep disturbances *Sleep Medicine, 11*(2), 1–5.

Pairman, S., Tracey, S., Thorogood, C. & Pincombe, J. (2010). *Midwifery Preparation for Practice* (2nd ed.). Sydney: Churchill Livingstone Elsevier.

Radesky, J. S., et al. (2008). Diet during early pregnancy and development of gestational diabetes. *Paediatric and Perinatal Epidemiology, 22*(1), 47–59.

Rode, L., et al. (2007). Association between maternal weight gain and birth weight. *Obstetrics and Gynecology, 109*(6), 1309–1315.

Rojas, F., Wood, E. & Blakemore, K. (2007). Preconception counseling and prenatal care. In K. B. Fortner et al. (Eds). *The Johns Hopkins Manual of Gynecology and Obstetrics*. Philadelphia: Lippincott Williams & Wilkins.

Rolfes, S. R., Pinna, K. & Whitney, E. (2009). *Understanding Normal and Clinical Nutrition* (8th ed.). New York: Wadsworth/Cengage Learning.

Subramanian, A., et al. (2008). *Drug Facts and Comparisons*. St Louis: Wolters Kluwer Health.

White, B. (2007). Ginger: An overview. *American Family Physician, 75*(11), 1689–1691.

Suggested readings

Boland, R. & Gibbons, M. (2009). The cost of healthy eating for pregnant and breastfeeding women in Otago. *New Zealand College of Midwives Journal, 41*, 26–28.

Charlton, K. E., Gemming, L., Yeatman, H. & Ma, G. (2010). Suboptimal iodine status of Australian pregnant women reflects poor knowledge and practices related to iodine nutrition. *Nutrition, 26*(10), 963–968.

Cox, S. R. (2008). Staying healthy on a vegetarian diet during pregnancy. *Journal of Midwifery & Women's Health, 53*(1), 91–92.

Chapter 14

Preparing a family for childbirth and parenting

Previous chapters discussed normal anatomy, physiology and nursing care necessary during pregnancy. This chapter adds information about ways that couples can make labour and birth a more satisfying experience. Such information helps protect the mental as well as physical health of both women and children throughout the continuum of pregnancy, birth and childrearing.

LEARNING OBJECTIVES

After mastering the contents of this chapter, you should be able to:

1. Describe common preparations for childbirth and parenting including common settings for birth.
2. Use critical thinking to analyse ways that birth can be made more family-centred through the use of prepared childbirth classes and alternative birth settings.
3. Assess a couple for readiness for childbirth in regard to choice of birth attendant, preparation for labour and setting.
4. Plan nursing care such as teaching exercises for strengthening abdominal and perineal muscles for childbirth.
5. Identify areas related to preparation for childbirth that could benefit from additional nursing research or application of evidence-based practice.
6. Integrate the principles of prepared childbirth with nursing process to achieve quality child and family health nursing care.

KEY TERMS

- birth centres
- birthing bed
- birthing room
- distraction
- doula
- multipara
- primipara
- vaginal birth after caesarean (VBAC)

CASE STUDY

Julia Marco is pregnant with her second child. During her first pregnancy, she did not attend any childbirth classes and received an epidural for the birth. During an antenatal visit for this pregnancy, Julia tells you that she would now like to have a natural birth in a birth centre. She asks you for information on childbirth education classes. Her husband, Joe, wants Julia to go to the hospital and have an epidural like the last time. He insists, "The doctors know what they're doing. We should just let them do their job." After speaking further with Joe, you discover he does not want Julia to go through the pain of natural childbirth because he fears he will not be able to help her during labour.

CASE STUDY QUESTION

1. How can you help alleviate some of Joe's concerns and best advise the Marcos on preparations for childbirth?

As active consumers of healthcare, expectant families can find themselves faced with a wide array of choices about the childbirth experience and preparation for parenting. Three of the most important decisions they need to make involve the choice of birth attendant and setting and how much or what type of analgesic they want to use in labour. For example, a woman may elect to have her family doctor, obstetrician or midwife attend the birth and to be supported by her husband, partner, family member, friend or **doula** (a woman who is experienced in childbirth and provides continuous emotional and physical support). Most women choose to give birth in a birth centre or a hospital. Birth centres and birthing rooms within hospitals both provide environments for families who desire a childbirth experience that is relaxed, "homey" and "family-centred" yet close to medical assistance should any complication arise during the birth or early postpartum period. Families who are rated as low risk may plan a home birth (Olsen & Jewell, 2009).

No matter what setting a woman or couple chooses, expectant parents are well advised to be as prepared as possible for the physical and emotional aspects of childbirth and non-pharmacological methods of pain relief during labour such as aromatherapy. Preparation for childbirth courses that teach this material can be individualised to meet parents' needs by being structured for women with special needs such as adolescents, career women, women who are physically challenged, or those experiencing a high-risk pregnancy. Women having a **vaginal birth after caesarean (VBAC)** or women who know they will have a caesarean birth also can attend specially designed classes for this.

CHILDBIRTH AND PARENTING EDUCATION

Assessment

Some couples have a clear idea of where and how they wish their child's birth to occur from the moment they realise they are pregnant. Others cannot even consider the actual birth until they have adjusted to the idea of pregnancy. Assessing each woman's or couple's readiness for decision making, as well as providing information early in the process, can help a woman or couple make this kind of decision. Whether women want or are able to take a childbirth and parenting preparation course depends a great deal on cultural and socioeconomic factors and individual choices. In some cultures, for example, the advice of a friend or family member carries more weight than the advice of a professional healthcare practitioner. Asking each woman separately whether she is interested in a course and being certain that women are fully informed about the options available to them are two ways to ensure all women receive as much advice and knowledge as they wish about childbirth.

Childbirth education is not just for **primiparas** (a woman who experiences pregnancy for the first time) because if a woman expecting her second or third child has waited several years between children, she usually appreciates refresher information as much as a primipara hungers for new information. Always, therefore, whether a woman is a primipara or **multipara** (experiencing a subsequent pregnancy), ask whether either she or her support person wants to attend childbirth or parenting courses. Provide appropriate information on what classes are available and how and when they could enrol. Childbirth and parenting education classes are normally run by the institution a woman is booked into to have her baby.

Nursing considerations

Nursing considerations tend to cluster around whether a couple is sure of their decision about a birth setting or preparation.

Planning and interventions

Be certain when planning with couples for labour and birth that the goals they set not only seem realistic but also flexible. Not all women want to go through labour without any analgesia, so setting a goal to do so would not be realistic for such a woman. Most women want to participate as fully as possible, however, so setting a goal for them to do that would be very realistic. Some women may be reluctant to attend a childbirth preparation course because they fear that would mean they are committing themselves to a medication-free birth. You can assure them that learning about methods of making childbirth easier does not preclude them learning about what medications are available for pain relief and using those medications if desired. At the same time a couple is planning goals for childbirth, encourage them to be flexible in their expectations. A woman who has decided ahead of time that she absolutely does not want any medication during labour and birth may find the intensity or duration of labour to be so severe that she will need an analgesic or epidural block to make the experience tolerable. If she and her support person have made the goal of medication-free labour too strict, they may believe they have failed when medication becomes necessary. A birth plan (discussed later) that includes information regarding the woman's or couple's preferences for labour, birth, immediate care of the newborn and actions to be taken if complications should arise can help the woman and her support person set realistic expected outcomes. Finally, talk to the woman or couple about the ultimate goal of childbirth: a healthy baby and healthy parents.

Culture is a major determinant of the plans that women make for childbirth. A woman from a culture in which modesty is stressed, for example, may not want to have a mirror positioned over a birthing bed. Demonstrating cultural sensitivity or an understanding of one's culture can prevent any miscommunication issues.

It is important to provide a woman and her partner with information on the benefits and drawbacks of birthing options, without influencing them in a particular direction. To remain objective, examine your own attitudes, cultural influences and values related to childbirth and explore how these beliefs might differ from those of the woman and her partner. Referring couples to a childbirth preparation course can answer many of their questions in a sympathetic group setting, where feelings and anxieties can be shared as well. Be familiar with the content of courses in your community so you can be certain that the courses you suggest present adequate and accurate information and are appropriate for individual couples. Be certain that a woman has thought through arrangements for transportation to the hospital or birth centre and has arranged for childcare if she has other children at home. Be certain that a woman who anticipates a home birth has organised her home and purchased supplies for birth well in advance of her expected due date.

Evaluate whether expected outcomes for childbirth education have been achieved during the last few antenatal visits. By this time, a woman or couple should know where the baby will be born and should have worked out transportation and childcare details. Final evaluation regarding whether the couple was satisfied with their birth setting or preparation choices takes place after the birth.

CHILDBIRTH EDUCATION

Although parenting is unarguably an important occupation, it is one of the few that requires no formal education, no examination to test a person's ability to take on such a role and no refresher course to ensure that a parent is following healthy standards of childrearing. Assessing whether couples need a preparation for childbirth or parenting class or encouraging them to take one, therefore, can be extremely important to make childbirth a satisfying experience, help a family bond with its new member and become effective parents.

BOX 14.1 Assessment ✻ Assessing a woman's preparation for labour

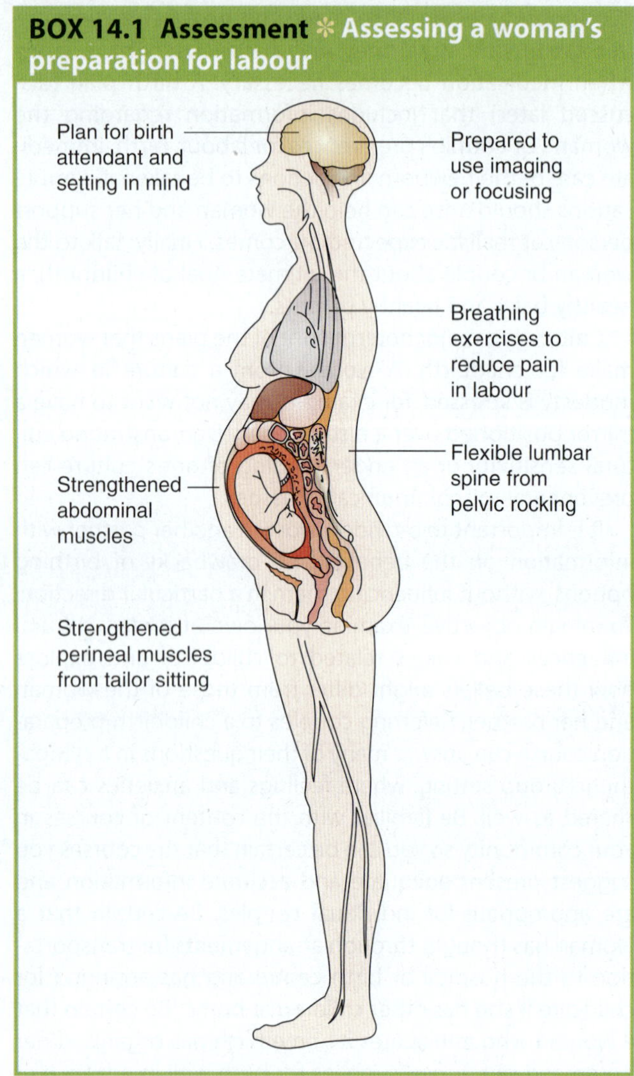

BOX 14.2 ✻ Focus on communication

You care for Julia Marco at an antenatal clinic visit. She is in the 24th week of an uncomplicated pregnancy.

Less effective communication

Nurse: Have you signed up for a childbirth preparation class yet, Julia?
Julia: No.
Nurse: Don't wait too much longer. You're already in your sixth month.
Julia: I don't really need to go to one.
Nurse: Okay. You know best.

More effective communication

Nurse: Have you signed up for a childbirth preparation class yet, Julia?
Julia: No.
Nurse: Don't wait too much longer. You're already in your sixth month.
Julia: I don't really need to go to one.
Nurse: Why is that?
Julia: Classes are all at the wrong time. And cost too much.
Nurse: Let's work together to find a course that's right for you. We can use the internet to find out what options are available.

It is important for couples to attend preparation for labour classes but, also, it is easy to ignore the reasons couples present for not wanting to go. Careful listening often reveals that time or money concerns are often the basis. Helping to investigate the many options is the beginning of problem solving.

Box 14.1 provides an overview of assessing a woman's preparation for labour. As many as 7–11% of women voice that they are afraid of the unknown and what will happen in labour. Those who are young, have a low education level, low self-rated health and lack a social network express this concern often (Laursen, 2008). Fear of labour and birth may occur in women experiencing birth for the first time and for women having their subsequent child. Fear may be associated with unrealistic expectations, particularly for the first time mother as they have no prior experience. Fear of labour and birth may also result from lack of childbirth education, preparation, information, communication and support (Dahlen et al., 2010). A woman's previous birth experience has the potential to influence feelings and emotions about her current pregnancy, labour and birth. Fear of childbirth is more prevalent among women with psychological symptoms such as depression and anxiety. The overall goals of childbirth education are to prepare expectant parents emotionally and physically for childbirth while promoting wellness behaviours that can be used by parents and families for life. Women often enjoy such classes because they offer a sense of empowerment and confirm that they can have direct input into their labour experience (see Box 14.2).

Childbirth educators and methods of teaching

Childbirth education is historically associated with midwifery and midwives play a major role in designing and teaching such courses. Most classes are taught in a group format; most incorporate a variety of teaching techniques such as videos and slides, lecture and demonstration (especially for content on relaxation and breathing techniques). One of the most important aspects of these courses, however, is group interaction. Women and their partners enjoy the opportunity to share their fears and hopes about their pregnancy and upcoming birth with others as they learn together.

Efficacy of childbirth education courses

Many studies have been done to determine just how effective childbirth courses are in reducing the pain of childbirth, shortening the length of labour, decreasing the amount of medication used and increasing overall enjoyment of the experience. Because of the variability in courses offered, however, it is often difficult to compare results of attending childbirth classes versus not attending classes. This is partly because people who volunteer to attend classes already have a high degree of positive motivation, which may skew the results. Despite these difficulties with measurement, it is generally accepted that preparation courses can increase satisfaction, reduce the amount of reported pain and increase feelings of control during childbirth (Al-Sahab et al., 2010; Records & Wilson, 2011). It is documented that by discussion of breastfeeding, classes can increase the proportion of new mothers who breastfeed (Johnson & Strube, 2011).

THE CHILDBIRTH PLAN

Most antenatal classes for expectant parents urge couples to make a written childbirth plan or spell out their choice of setting, birth attendant, special needs such as the extent of family participation they wish during labour, birthing positions, medication options, plans for the immediate postpartum period and baby care, and family visitation. Urge couples to make informed decisions about these issues before the day of birth to avoid feeling stressed by last minute decisions. Box 14.3 lists questions a couple might want to discuss about birth.

BOX 14.3 ❋ Focus on family teaching

Choosing a birth setting

Q. Julia and her husband Joe ask you, "There are so many options available for a birth setting. How do we decide which one to choose?"

A. Choosing a birth setting is a personal decision. Some questions to ask yourself to help with the decision are:

- What type of carer do I want to supervise my antenatal care and labour and birth? Midwife? Family doctor? Obstetrician?
- What settings does a particular childbirth provider let me choose from? A birthing room? A birth centre? My home?
- Will the same person be present at antenatal visits as for birth? Does the setting offer preparation for childbirth or childrearing classes?
- Will I be allowed to choose a birth position? Will I have input into the amount of anaesthesia used? Will I have an opportunity for immediate and uninterrupted skin-to-skin contact after birth? Can I begin breastfeeding immediately? Will nurses who are supportive and informed be available? Can I use a doula?
- Will the setting allow my partner to participate? Will they be allowed to be with me throughout labour and birth? Could they cut the cord or help with the birth? Can older children participate? Can I record the birth on video or by photograph?
- Is early discharge available? Will a follow-up home visit be included in care?
- If I should have a complication during labour or birth, is there adequate equipment and personnel available for emergency care? If our baby should have a complication, is there provision for immediate emergency care or transport to a high-risk facility?

Be certain all couples understand, however, that the birth plan should be flexible in case a complication or change of plans arises. For example, in the event of a complication of labour or birth that requires an emergency caesarean birth, a preference to have the baby without anaesthesia will need to be modified.

ANTENATAL CLASSES

Expectant parenting classes are designed for couples who are already pregnant. They focus on family health during a pregnancy, covering such topics as the psychological and physical changes of pregnancy, pregnancy nutrition, routine healthcare such as dental checkups and newborn care. A typical course plan for 8 weeks is shown in Box 14.4.

Included in these classes is information about breastfeeding which helps women learn more about it so they can appreciate the advantages of breastfeeding over formula feeding. Such classes cover the physiology of breastfeeding as well as psychological aspects. They stress that women should try to breastfeed exclusively for the first 6 months and find ways to fit breastfeeding into busy schedules so they can continue it for the full 2 years (World Health Organization (WHO), 2011).

Common goals of antenatal classes are to:

- Prepare an expectant woman and her support person for the childbirth experience
- Create clients who are knowledgeable consumers of obstetric care
- Help women reduce and manage pain with both medication and medication-free methods
- Help increase a couple's overall enjoyment of and satisfaction with the childbirth experience.

BOX 14.4 ❋ Sample content for expectant parents' class

- **Class 1** Review of physiological changes of pregnancy and fetal growth
- **Class 2** Personal care during pregnancy
  Nutrition
  Hygiene such as bathing, dental care
  Exercise
  Rest
- **Class 3** Emotional changes during pregnancy
- **Class 4** Labour and birth
  The process of birth
  Exercises and breathing techniques
  Medication in labour
- **Class 5** Plans for birth
  Birth settings available
  Supplies to take to birth settings
  Tour or film of a typical setting
- **Class 6** The postpartum period
- **Class 7** Infant care
  Nutrition
  Hygiene
- **Class 8** Reproductive life planning

In addition to teaching about normal labour, they include several exercises to ready the body for labour, as well as methods of pain prevention or pain relief in labour.

> ***What if...***
>
> Julia tells you her husband won't be coming to class with her because he won't be able to be with her during labour? She asks you if it is really important to have someone with her. How would you advise her?

EXERCISE DURING PREGNANCY

Antenatal yoga

Antenatal yoga classes are aimed at helping a woman relax and manage stress better for all times in her life, not just pregnancy. Yoga exercises help a woman stay fit by focusing on gentle stretching and deep breathing. Yoga can also help a woman feel a high level of self-esteem as she masters difficult levels or positions. Yoga breathing techniques can be used in labour to help with relaxation and pain management.

Perineal and abdominal exercises

In addition to encouraging an overall exercise program, antenatal classes teach women specific exercises to strengthen pelvic and abdominal muscles and make these muscles stronger and more supple. Supple perineal muscles allow for stretching during birth, reduce discomfort and help muscles revert more quickly to pre-birth state and function more efficiently after childbirth, which helps reduce the possibility of urinary incontinence (Hay-Smith et al., 2011).

A woman may begin exercises as early in pregnancy as she likes. Many exercises to strengthen abdominal or perineal muscles can be incorporated into daily activities so they take little time from a woman's day. It is best, however, for a woman to set aside a specific time each day to practise; otherwise, her participation is apt to be sporadic. Initially, women should do each exercise only a few times, gradually increasing the number per session.

Squatting

Squatting (see Fig. 14.1) also stretches perineal muscles and can be a useful position for second-stage labour, so a woman should also practise this position for about 15 minutes a day. Most women need a demonstration of effective squatting; otherwise, they tend to squat on their tiptoes. For pelvic muscles to stretch, a woman should keep her feet flat on the floor. Incorporating squatting into daily activities such as picking up toys from the floor or weeding in the garden reduces the amount of time a woman must devote to daily exercises.

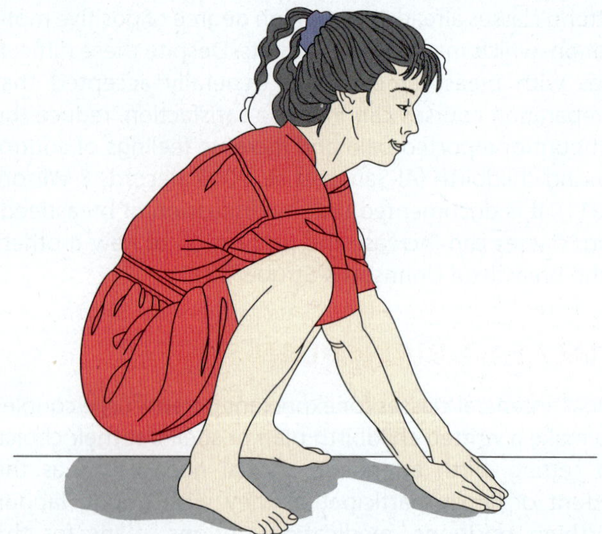

FIGURE 14.1 Squatting helps to stretch the muscles of the pelvic floor. Notice that the feet are flat on the floor for optimal perineal stretching.

Pelvic floor contractions (Kegel exercises)

Pelvic floor contractions can be done easily during daily activities. While sitting at her desk or working around the house, a woman can tighten the muscles of her perineum by doing Kegel exercises (see Chapter 12). Such perineal muscle-strengthening exercises are helpful in the postpartum period to reduce pain and promote perineal healing. They have long-term effects of increasing sexual responsiveness and helping prevent stress incontinence (Allahdin & Kambhampati, 2012).

Abdominal muscle contractions

Abdominal muscle contractions help strengthen abdominal muscles during pregnancy and therefore may help prevent constipation as well as help restore abdominal tone after pregnancy. Strong abdominal muscles can also contribute to effective second-stage pushing during labour. Abdominal contractions can be done in a standing or lying position along with pelvic floor contractions. A woman merely tightens her abdominal muscles, then relaxes them. She can repeat the exercise as often as she wishes during the day.

Another way to do the same thing is to practise "blowing out a candle". A woman takes a fairly deep inspiration, then exhales normally. Holding her finger about 15 centimetres in front of herself, as if it were a candle, she then exhales forcibly, pushing out residual air from her lungs as if her finger were a lit candle. She can feel her abdominal muscles contract as she reaches the end of a forcible exhalation.

Pelvic rocking

Pelvic rocking (see Fig. 14.2) helps relieve backache during pregnancy and early labour by making the lumbar spine more flexible. It can be done in a variety of positions: on hands and knees, lying down, sitting or standing. A woman

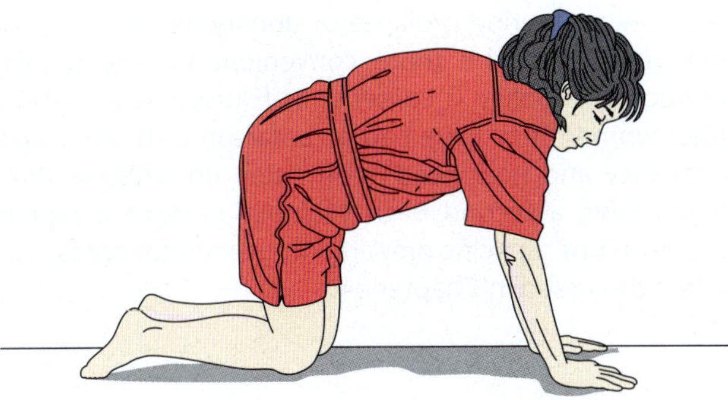

FIGURE 14.2 Pelvic rocking is helpful in relieving backache during pregnancy and labour. To do this, a woman first hollows her back and then arches it.

arches her back, trying to lengthen or stretch her spine. She holds the position for 1 minute, then hollows her back. If a woman does this at the end of the day about five times, it not only increases flexibility but also helps relieve back pain and make her more comfortable for the night.

CASE STUDY QUESTION

2. Julia asks you which type of exercise is best to strengthen perineal muscles. Your best answer would be:
   a. Walk 20 minutes daily at a fairly rapid pace
   b. Tighten and relax perineal muscles as if stopping voiding
   c. Periodically push as if you're moving your bowels
   d. Lift both legs into the air while you lie supine

Methods for managing pain in childbirth

Beginning in the late 1950s, many specific methods for non-pharmacological pain reduction during labour were developed. More recently, childbirth education has moved away from a strict method approach like these to more eclectic ones. Many educators teach a variety of approaches, including the use of complementary or herbal therapies. Most approaches are based on three premises:

1. Discomfort during labour can be minimised if a woman comes into labour informed about what is happening and prepared with breathing exercises to use during contractions. In classes, therefore, a woman learns about her body's response in labour, the mechanisms involved in childbirth and breathing exercises she can use to aid relaxation.
2. Discomfort during labour can be minimised if a woman's abdomen is relaxed and the uterus is allowed to rise freely against the abdominal wall with contractions. Childbirth methods differ only in the manner by which they achieve this relaxation.
3. Pain perception can be altered by **distraction** techniques that effectively move a woman's concentration to other things than pain (see Box 14.5).

The position in which the women gives birth can impact the birthing process (see Box 14.6).

BOX 14.5 ❊ Gate control mechanisms to reduce pain

Pain flows through pathways because:

1. The endings of small peripheral nerve fibres detect a stimulus.
2. They transmit it to cells in the dorsal horn of the spinal cord.
3. Impulses pass through a dense, interfacing network of cells in the spinal cord (the substantia gelatinosa).
4. Immediately, a synapse occurs that returns the transmission to the peripheral site through a motor nerve. For example, a person touches a candle flame; the impulse travels to the spinal cord and back, and the person jerks his or her hand away from the flame.
5. After this short-circuit synapse, the impulse then continues in the spinal cord to reach the hypothalamus and cortex of the brain.
6. The impulse is interpreted (the candle is hot) and perceived as pain.

Gating theory of pain control

The gating theory of pain refers to gate control mechanisms in the substantia gelatinosa that are capable of halting an impulse at the level of the spinal cord so the impulse is never perceived at brain level as pain: a process similar to closing a gate.

Techniques to assist gating mechanisms

- **Cutaneous stimulation.** If large peripheral nerves next to an injury site are stimulated, the ability of the small nerve fibres at the injury site to transmit pain impulses appears to decrease. Therefore, rubbing an injured part or applying transcutaneous electrical nerve stimulation (TENS) or heat or cold to the site (cutaneous stimulation) are effective manoeuvres to suppress pain. Effleurage, or light massage used in the Lamaze method, also accomplishes this.
- **Distraction.** If the cells of the brain stem that will register an impulse as pain are preoccupied with other stimuli, a pain impulse cannot register. Different childbirth classes use different breathing, vocalisation or focusing techniques such as imaging to accomplish this. Breathing techniques not only provide distraction but can increase oxygenation to the mother and fetus.
- **Reduction of anxiety.** Pain impulses are perceived more quickly if a woman is anxious. The third technique of gating, therefore, is to reduce her anxiety as much as possible. Teaching a woman what to expect during labour is a means of achieving this.

Focusing or imagery

Focusing intently on an object (sometimes called "sensate focus") is a method of keeping sensory input from reaching the cortex of the brain. A woman brings into labour a photograph of her partner or children, a graphic design or just something that appeals to her. She concentrates on it during contractions. Be careful not to step into a woman's line of vision during a contraction and break this focused concentration. Other women use imagery by imagining they are in a calm place such as on a beach watching waves rolling in or relaxing on a swing. Try not to ask

BOX 14.6 * Focus on evidence-based practice

The birth position

One of the most controversial aspects of childbirth addresses the question of the best birth position for women to use. To evaluate the impact of birth position on maternal and newborn wellbeing, researchers reviewed 40 studies on birth position published over a period of 15 years. The results showed both physical and psychological benefits for women when they are able to adopt positions other than on their back for labour. Women allowed to birth in an upright position had a shorter duration of the first and second stages of labour, experienced less medical intervention and reported less severe pain; they also had an increased rate of satisfaction with their childbirth experience than women who gave birth in a semi-recumbent or supine/lithotomy position. The only disadvantage identified of an upright position was increased blood loss during the third stage of labour, which may be due to increased perineal oedema caused by the upright position.

When writing out a curriculum for a preparation for childbirth class, would this information be important to include?

Source: Priddis, H., Dahlen, H. & Schmied, V. (2011). What are the facilitators, inhibitors, and implications of birth positioning? *Women & Birth, 25*(3), 100–106.

questions or talk to women using this technique because you may break their concentration.

Second-stage breathing

During the second stage of labour, when the baby will be actually pushed down the birth canal, the type of breathing that is best to use is controversial. In the past, women were told to hold their breath while they pushed. Now it is believed that holding the breath for a prolonged time impairs blood return from the vena cava (a Valsalva manoeuvre), so this is now discouraged. Most classes suggest that women breathe any way that is natural for them, except holding their breath, during this stage of labour. Women should not practise pushing. The possibility that they could rupture membranes by doing this is too great. They can practise assuming a good position for pushing (squatting, sitting upright, leaning on partner) but should always be cautioned not to actually push during pregnancy.

Preparation for caesarean birth

The fact that caesarean birth may become necessary during labour to ensure a safe birth and what a couple can expect if this happens is covered in most childbirth classes, although as vaginal birth is encouraged, this may be done to varying degrees. Some women need this information because they know from the beginning of pregnancy that they will have a caesarean birth as these are offered in some communities as an alternative to vaginal birth to help prevent uterine prolapse or urinary incontinence in later years or to be more convenient for the family, although this policy is contentious (Dursun et al., 2011). Other women may have had a caesarean birth for a first pregnancy and now need information on whether they should have a second birth vaginally or have a repeat caesarean one. Specific preparation needed for caesarean birth is discussed in Chapter 24.

THE BIRTH SETTING

Another important decision that a couple needs to make during pregnancy is choosing a birth setting. The decision they make depends on a woman's health and that of her fetus, as well as the couple's preferences for how much and what kind of supervision they desire for the birth. Although hospitals are the usual site for birth today in Australia, that has not always been true. Up until the late 1800s, childbirth was conducted in the home. Analgesia or anaesthesia for childbirth was unpopular until Queen Victoria delivered Prince Leopold under chloroform in 1853. Birth at that point became more complicated and less natural because extensive levels of anaesthesia led to additional interventions. Women were not only asleep for one of the most memorable moments of their life, but under anaesthesia they were no longer able to push effectively during the second stage of labour. That made it necessary to use a lithotomy position and an episiotomy and forceps for birth.

Part of the reason for the use of so much anaesthesia during birth can be attributed to doctors misinterpreting the type of pain of childbirth. It was assumed that the moment of birth was the major time of discomfort. As a result, women were allowed to labour without any pain medication and then were given anaesthesia or analgesia right before the baby was born. Although the pain felt at birth is intense, it is also over quickly, unlike the hours of labour that precede it, so in reality women may not be as uncomfortable during the actual birth as they are during labour. Birth is also such an exhilarating time that the excitement of the moment can mask pain.

Fortunately, birthing practices have changed to better meet women's needs based on their descriptions of the pain of childbirth. If women choose doctors or hospitals who subscribe to more progressive birth practices over the services of more traditional facilities, the overall standard of care in communities leans towards the more progressive settings. The addition of birthing rooms to hospitals in the past 20 years is an example of this. Midwives are in a strong position to advocate for making childbirth a "natural" process in the least restrictive setting possible. At the same time, midwives have a strong responsibility to encourage parents to maintain enough restrictions that birth remains safe.

In Australia less than 1% of births are planned home births, while in New Zealand approximately 4–6% of women have a home birth, attended by a midwife. Women need to be aware of their choices when making this decision. The following websites provide further information and assistance: <www.midwife.org.nz>, <www.maternity.org.nz>, <www.midwives.org.au>.

Choosing the appropriate setting

Women with uncomplicated pregnancies may choose hospitals, birth centres or their homes as settings for birth. Women with high-risk pregnancies have less choice; women with potential complications are advised to give birth at hospitals where immediate emergency care will be available.

Choosing a birth attendant and support person

In Australia and New Zealand most births are supervised by an obstetrician or a registered midwife. It is also becoming more common for registered midwives to be involved both within the hospital environment as well as at birth centres or homes. In addition to selecting who will medically supervise her baby's birth, a woman needs to choose who will support her in labour. In years past, this support was offered by experienced women in the community. In the 1960s, the role was given to the father of the baby. Today, many different family members offer this type of support.

Hospital birth

Maternity services of hospitals have changed a great deal in recent years and a woman has the opportunity to:

- Experience a healthy and joyous birth experience, regardless of her age or circumstances
- Give birth as she wishes in an environment in which she feels nurtured and secure
- Have access to the full range of options for pregnancy, birth and nurturing her baby
- Receive accurate and up-to-date information about the benefits and risks of all procedures, medications and tests suggested for use during pregnancy, birth and the postpartum period, with the rights to informed consent and informed refusal
- Receive support for making informed choices about what is best for her and her baby based on her individual values and beliefs (CIMS, 2012).

Based on the above criteria,10 characteristics of a mother- and baby-friendly hospital climate have been identified (see Box 14.7). Urge women to ask hospitals in their community if they are rated as mother-friendly as this may influence their choice of hospital or birth attendant.

Advantages and disadvantages of hospital birth are summarised in Box 14.8. The major advantage of a hospital is that equipment and expert personnel are readily available if the mother, fetus or newborn should have a complication.

BOX 14.7 ✻ Characteristics of a mother- and baby-friendly hospital

Mother-friendly hospitals:

1. Have a written breastfeeding policy that is routinely communicated to all healthcare staff.
2. Train all healthcare staff in skills necessary to implement this policy.
3. Inform all pregnant women about the benefits and management of breastfeeding.
4. Help mothers to initiate breastfeeding within a half-hour of birth.
5. Show mothers how to breastfeed and how to maintain lactation, even if they should be separated from their infants.
6. Give newborn infants no food or drink other than breast milk unless medically indicated.
7. Practice rooming-in allow mothers and infants to remain together 24 hours a day.
8. Encourage breastfeeding on demand.
9. Give no artificial teats or dummies to breastfeeding infants.
10. Foster the establishment of breastfeeding support and refer mothers to them on discharge from the hospital or clinic. (Baby Friendly Health Initiative (BFHI) Australia, 2014)

In evaluating studies that compare the complications of birth centres or home births with those of hospitals, women who gave birth in hospitals invariably have more complications than those who give birth in other settings,

BOX 14.8 ✻ Advantages and disadvantages of hospital birth

Advantages

- A woman is encouraged to be prepared to control the discomfort of labour through non-medication measures such as controlled breathing, although anaesthesia such as an epidural is readily available.
- A woman is encouraged to be knowledgeable about the labour process and make decisions about procedures performed.
- A woman is encouraged to consider breastfeeding to aid uterine contraction and infant bonding after birth.
- Labour, birth and immediate postnatal care can all be scheduled in a single room.
- A woman is attended by skilled professionals during labour, birth and the postnatal period.
- Emergency care and extended high-risk care are immediately available.

Disadvantages

- Separation of the family for at least one night.
- Mother may not feel as much in control of the childbirth experience as she may wish.
- Care may be fragmented, particularly if a woman's doctor is not present during the entire labour and birth, or if the midwife changes shifts in the middle of labour. (Many midwives make it a point, however, to remain with the mother throughout the entire childbirth.)

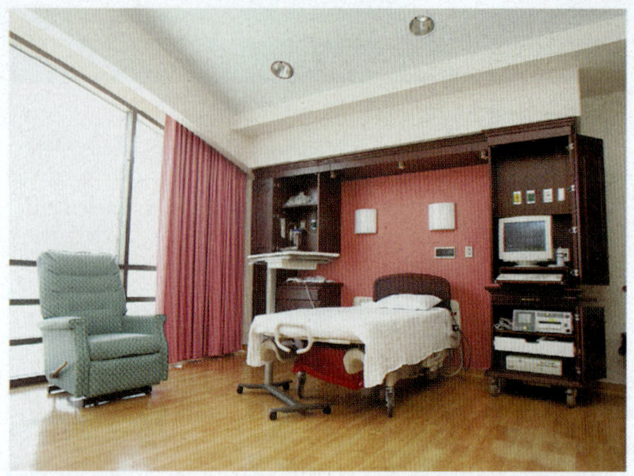

FIGURE 14.3 A birthing room designed to maintain a home-like atmosphere in a hospital setting.

but that happens because high-risk mothers give birth at hospitals so the number of complications in hospital settings is bound to be higher than in other settings.

A woman usually comes to the hospital when her contractions are approximately 5 minutes apart and regular. If she has preregistered at the hospital, she is admitted to a **birthing room** without any separation time from her support person. Such rooms are decorated in a home-like way; couples can bring favourite music or reading materials with them to use during labour; and the bed can be used as a labour bed until birth, when it converts into a **birthing bed** or a lithotomy position bed (see Fig. 14.3). Women are expected to use a prepared method of childbirth with a minimum of analgesia and anaesthesia (although an advantage of a hospital birth is that anaesthesia such as an epidural is readily available if needed). An important aspect of birthing rooms is that the support person and often other family members can stay with a woman throughout labour and birth, allowing a couple and their families to feel that they have control over their birth experience. Women report greater satisfaction with birth when they use a more home-like setting than a bare, functional labour room for birth (Hodnett et al., 2010).

At the time of birth, additional cabinets in the room are opened and converted into a space for baby care. Women can choose a birthing position: lithotomy, squatting, supine recumbent or side-lying. A support person remains with a woman during birth and in some settings can cut the umbilical cord if desired.

Most hospitals screen women in early labour with an external monitor for both fetal heart rate and uterine contractions. If the fetal heart rate is good, such a monitor can usually be removed and used again only for intermittent auscultation as labour progresses. Alternatively, a Doppler can also be used. Women are encouraged to remain upright and ambulate during labour. There are various positions women can assume to ease labour such as pelvic rocking, squatting, using a ball or deep bath for pain management.

Postpartum care

After giving birth women will be transferred to a postpartum unit and will remain there for the remainder of their hospital stay. After birth, encourage mothers to breastfeed immediately. Urge a couple to keep their newborn with them in their hospital room so they have ample time to become acquainted. Breastfeeding on demand for infants should be the rule. There should be no restrictions on visiting for the primary support person; in many institutions, a rollaway bed is provided so he or she can remain constantly. Siblings should be allowed to visit at least once and touch and become acquainted with the newborn.

Birth centres

Birth centres are wellness-oriented childbirth facilities designed to remove childbirth from the acute care hospital setting while still providing enough medical resources for emergency care should a complication of labour or birth arise. Such a setting is established within, or at least within an easy distance of a hospital. Because it is located outside an acute care setting, where infections abound, the risk of hospital-acquired infection to a woman is thought to be reduced. The birth attendants are midwives. Women who give birth in birth centres are screened for complications before being admitted. Because women are carefully screened, the mortality rate of mothers and infants is no higher and may be lower in these out-of-hospital settings than in hospital settings. Advantages and disadvantages of birth centres are summarised in Box 14.9.

BOX 14.9 ✻ Advantages and disadvantages of birth centres

Advantages

- A woman is encouraged to be prepared to control the discomfort of labour through non-medication measures such as controlled breathing.
- A woman is encouraged to be knowledgeable about the labour process and to help care providers with decision making.
- A woman is encouraged to breastfeed to aid uterine contraction and infant bonding after birth.
- Family integrity can be maintained because family members may accompany a woman to the birth centre.
- A woman is attended by skilled professionals during labour and birth.
- Emergency care is immediately available. Extended high-risk care is easily arranged.

Disadvantages

- Extended high-risk care is not immediately available.
- A woman may be fatigued after birth because of brief healthcare setting stay.
- She must independently monitor her postnatal status because of her brief healthcare setting stay.

Home birth

Home birth is the usual mode of birth in developing countries. It is also a popular choice for birth in Europe. Home birth may be supervised by a doctor, but midwives are the more likely choice as birth attendants in this setting. The main advantage of a home birth is that it encourages family integrity: a woman and her family are not separated so the baby can be immediately integrated into the family. On the other hand, it puts responsibility on a woman to prepare her home for the birth (which is difficult if she is exhausted towards the end of pregnancy) and to take care of the infant after birth. Some people, however willing, may be unable to take on these roles in a crisis situation such as childbirth. Many women passing through their first postpartum or "taking-in" phase may be happier maintaining a dependent passive role than immediately taking responsibility for the infant's care.

To be a candidate for a home birth, a woman must be in good health, must be able to adjust to changing circumstances, and must have adequate support people who will sustain her during labour and assist her for the first few days after birth. Women who have pregnancy complications may still choose a home birth. It is important for the attending midwife to explain clearly the risks associated with birth in a home environment. Unfortunately, some women may choose to birth at home without a qualified birth attendant if a home birth midwife is unable to care for her.

Advantages and disadvantages of home birth are summarised in Box 14.10.

BOX 14.10 Advantages and disadvantages of home birth

Advantages

- A woman is more relaxed and confident in her own surroundings; she also has control over who is with her when she gives birth.
- A woman is encouraged to become knowledgeable about the birth process and be an active participant in independently reducing the discomfort of labour.
- A woman has the greatest freedom for expressing her individuality.
- There is no separation of the family at birth.
- A skilled professional can attend the birth.

Disadvantages

- Adequate equipment other than first-line emergency equipment is unavailable.
- An abrupt change of goals is necessary if hospitalisation is required.
- A woman and support person may become exhausted because of the responsibility placed on them.
- Interference with the "taking-in phase" may occur postpartally because a woman must "take hold."
- A woman must independently monitor her postpartal status.

What if...

Julia and her husband have a serious disagreement about whether to plan for a home birth or hospital birth? What issues would you suggest they explore? If they cannot agree, how could they compromise?

Children attending the birth

Most birth centres and some hospitals allow children to view the birth of a sibling. Attendance at sibling classes designed to prepare children to witness the birth is often required. If children will be present, a person separate from the main support person needs to be designated to provide entertainment, explanations, food and a place for them to sleep. A child who is without supervision during this time could remember the experience as a time of rejection rather than an exciting, happy experience. The mother should not be expected to provide such supervision during labour.

ALTERNATIVE METHODS OF BIRTH

In addition to varied settings, several different methods of childbirth have become popular in the past 15 to 20 years. These include alternative birth methods such as the Leboyer method and water birth.

Leboyer method

Frederick Leboyer was a French obstetrician who postulated that moving from a warm, fluid-filled intrauterine environment to a noisy, air-filled, brightly lit birth room creates a major shock for a newborn (Leboyer, 1975). With the Leboyer method, the birthing room is darkened so there is no sudden contrast in light; it is kept pleasantly warm, not chilled. Soft music is played, or at least harsh noises are kept to a minimum. The infant is handled gently; the cord is cut late; and the infant is placed immediately after birth into a warm-water bath. Some neonatologists question the wisdom of a warm bath because it could reduce spontaneous respirations and allow a high level of acidosis to occur. Late cutting of a cord can lead to excess blood viscosity in a newborn. Certainly, soft music, gentle handling and a welcoming atmosphere are important ingredients for all birth attendants to try to incorporate into birth. Providing dim lights (or at least not bright, glaring ones) and providing a warm temperature could be given more consideration in most institutions.

Hydrotherapy and water birth

Reclining or sitting in warm water during labour can be soothing; the feeling of weightlessness that occurs under water as well as the relaxation from the warm water can contribute to reducing discomfort in labour. Using this principle, many birth centres allow women to labour in warm showers or give birth in spa tubs of warm water

(Cluett & Burns, 2012). The baby is born underwater and then immediately brought to the surface for a first breath. Most women who choose underwater birth are very pleased that they chose this method. A potential difficulty is contamination of the bath water with faeces expelled with pushing efforts during the second stage of labour. This could lead to uterine infection in the mother or aspiration of contaminated bath water by a newborn, which could lead to pneumonia. Maternal chilling when a woman leaves the water is another factor to consider and prevent.

CASE STUDY QUESTION

3. Suppose Julia decides on a hospital birth. What is an advantage of hospital birth over other settings?
   a. Women can use breathing exercises
   b. Labour and childbirth can be pain free
   c. Extended high-risk care is available
   d. The cost of a hospital stay is low

Key points for review

- Couples should be encouraged to make a childbirth plan early in pregnancy that includes birth attendant, setting, desired method of pain management and any special wishes.
- Common exercises taught in pregnancy to strengthen perineal muscles include squatting and Kegel exercises. Abdominal muscle-contraction and pelvic-rocking strengthen the abdominal muscles and help relieve backache.
- Some commonly used non-pharmacological techniques for pain relief in labour are focusing, imagery, breathing and hydrotherapy.
- Classes for expectant parents provide information on pregnancy, birth and childcare.
- Common sites for childbirth include hospitals, birth centres and at home.
- Couples should consider if birth settings are rated as mother-friendly before choosing them as a birth site.

CASE STUDY QUESTIONS

4. Joe wants his wife to have their baby at a hospital and have epidural anaesthesia for pain relief. He insists, "The doctors know what they're doing. We should just let them do their job." After further speaking with Joe, you discover he does not want Julia to go through the pain of natural childbirth because he fears he will not be able to help her during labour. How would you convey to Joe that natural childbirth can be a positive experience for him and his wife? How would you assure him that he and Julia can play a safe and active part in the birth of their child?
5. Suppose Julia told you she does not intend to do antenatal classes because she wants to have epidural anaesthesia as soon as she is admitted to the hospital in labour. Would you advise her to attend a class?

Resources

For an extensive range of additional resources to enhance teaching and learning and to facilitate understanding of this chapter, please see the text's accompanying website located on thePoint at http://thepoint.lww.com.

References

Allahdin, S. & Kambhampati, L. (2012). Stress urinary incontinence in continent primigravidas. *Journal of Obstetrics & Gynaecology, 32*(1), 2–5.

Al-Sahab, B., Saqib, M., Hauser, G., et al. (2010). Prevalence of smoking during pregnancy and associated risk factors among Canadian women: A national survey. *BMC Pregnancy & Childbirth*, *10*(5), 24–25.

Baby Friendly Health Initiative (BFHI) Australia (2014), accessed 21 February 2015, <www.babyfriendly.org.au>.

Coalition for Improving Maternity Services (CIMS). (2012). The mother friendly childbirth initiative, accessed February 2015, <www.motherfriendly.org/MFCI>.

Cluett, E. R. & Burns, E. (2012). Immersion in water in pregnancy, labour and birth. *Cochrane Database of Systematic Reviews, 2012*(7), (CD000111).

Dahlen, H. G., Barclay, L. M. & Homer, C.S.E. (2010). The novice birthing: Theorising first-time mothers' experiences of birth at home and in hospital in Australia. *Midwifery, 26*(1), 53–63.

Dursun, P., Yanik, F. B., Zeyneloglu, H. B., Baser, E., Kuscu, E. & Ayhan, A. (2011). Why women request cesarean section without medical indication? *Journal of Maternal-Fetal & Neonatal Medicine, 24*(9), 1133–1137.

Hay-Smith, E. J., Herderschee, R., Dumoulin, C. & Herbison, G. P. (2011). Comparisons of approaches to pelvic floor muscle training for urinary incontinence in women. *Cochrane Database of Systematic Reviews, 2011*(12), (CD009508).

Hodnett, E. D., Downe, S., Walsh, D. & Weston, J. (2010). Alternative versus conventional institutional settings for birth. *Cochrane Database of Systematic Reviews, 2010*(9), (CD000012).

Johnson, T. S. & Strube, K. (2011). Breast care during pregnancy. *Journal of Obstetric, Gynecologic, & Neonatal Nursing, 40*(2), 144–148.

Laursen, M., Hedegaard, M. & Johansen, C. (2008). Fear of childbirth: Predictors and temporal changes among nulliparous women in the Danish National Birth Cohort. *BJOG: An International Journal of Obstetrics & Gynaecology, 115*(3), 354–360.

Leboyer, F. (1975). *Birth Without Violence*. New York: Alfred A. Knopf.

Olsen, O. & Jewell, M. D. (2000). Home versus hospital birth. *Cochrane Database of Systematic Reviews, 2000*(1), (CD000352).

Pitiphat, W., Joshipura, K. J., Gillman, M. W., Williams, P. L., Douglass, C. W. & Rich-Edwards, J. W. (2008). Maternal periodontitis and adverse pregnancy outcomes. *Community Dentistry & Oral Epidemiology, 36*(1), 3–11.

Records, K. & Wilson, B. L. (2011). Reflections on meeting women's childbirth expectations. *Journal of Obstetric, Gynecologic & Neonatal Nursing, 40*(4), 394–398.

World Health Organization (WHO). (2011). Exclusive breastfeeding for six months best for babies everywhere, accessed 5 June 2015 at <www.who.int/mediacentre/news/statements/2011/breastfeeding_20110115/en/>.

Suggested readings

Dumoulin, C. & Hay-Smith, J. (2009). Pelvic floor muscle training versus no treatment, or inactive control treatments, for urinary incontinence in women. *Cochrane Database of Systematic Reviews, 2009*(1), (CD005654).

Pairman, S., Pincombe, J., Thorogood, C. & Tracy, S. (2014). *Midwifery: Preparation for Practice* (3rd ed.). Churchill Livingstone: Elsevier Australia.

Chapter 15

Woman-centred care during labour and birth

Previous chapters described the anatomical and physiological changes that occur in pregnancy as well as effective steps women can take to prepare for labour. This chapter adds information about the actual labour process and will be useful for the nurse considering a career change to midwifery.

LEARNING OBJECTIVES

After mastering the contents of this chapter, you should be able to:

1. Describe the philosophy of woman-centred care during labour.
2. Identify strategies to increase the number of women who give birth vaginally.
3. Use critical thinking to analyse ways that labour and birth can become more woman-centred.
4. Outline the steps the midwife takes to identify the woman's readiness, stage and progression in labour.
5. Promote optimal outcomes for a woman and her newborn.
6. Identify areas related to labour and birth that could benefit from additional research.

KEY TERMS

- abdominal palpation
- attitude
- breech presentation
- cephalic presentation
- crowning
- dilation
- effacement
- engagement
- fetal descent
- lie
- mechanisms of labour
- moulding
- position
- ripening of the cervix
- shoulder presentation
- station
- transition

CASE STUDY

Cath Bailey is a 26-year-old woman you welcome into the birthing room. She has been having labour contractions 45 seconds long and 3 minutes apart for the last 6 hours. She tells you she wants to have her baby "naturally" without any analgesia or anaesthesia. Her husband is in the Army and assigned overseas, so he is not with her. Although her sister lives only two blocks from the hospital, Cath does not want her called. She asks if she can talk to her mother on the telephone instead. As you finish assessing contractions, she screams with pain and shouts, "I'm doing everything I'm supposed to do! How much longer does this go on?"

CASE STUDY QUESTION

1. How can you best support Cath during her labour and birth?

Prior to 1 August 2004, midwifery in Australia was considered a nursing specialty but, since the passing of the *Nurses and Midwives Act* in 2004, they are two discrete professions. A registered midwife no longer has to be a registered nurse. In Australia, only registered midwives and medical practitioners (and midwifery and medical students under the direct supervision of a registered midwife or medical practitioner) are legally entitled to be responsible for professional care for labouring and birthing women. As well as the possibility of a career change to midwifery, there may be occasions when a nursing student or registered nurse acts as a support person or has the privilege of being with a labouring woman. This chapter provides valuable information on what they are likely to observe as well as strategies a person can use to provide optimal support. For these reasons, this chapter and the next do not adhere to the formatting of other chapters and will not include sections on nursing diagnoses and the like.

Throughout this chapter and the next, the concept of woman-centred care during labour and birth will be discussed. By definition, woman-centred care includes any person (usually her partner, family or close friend) who the woman identifies as being significant to her (Australian College of Midwives, 2011).

More New Zealand women are able to access home birth with a midwife than Australian women. The majority of Australian women birth in a hospital maternity unit and around 5% birth in a birth centre—with many more women stating that a birth centre would be their first option if it were available. Compared with New Zealand, only a very small proportion of women will birth at home with a midwife in Australia but, again, this is because there are very few midwives who have home-birthing practices. On very rare occasions a woman will choose to give birth unassisted by a midwife or medical practitioner. This is called "freebirth" and is almost always due to women not having the option of a midwife who will assist them to have a home birth. Some women, most often those living in rural and remote areas, will give birth en route to the maternity unit because many maternity units in rural and remote areas of Australia have closed (Dietsch et al., 2011). As the majority of women in Australia give birth in a maternity unit, this is the assumed place of birth in this chapter.

Woman-centred care is a concept that is based on feminist ethics and implies that care:

- Is focused on the woman's individual, unique needs, expectations and aspirations, rather than the needs of the institutions or professions
- Is holistic in approach and recognises each woman's emotional, physical, spiritual, social and cultural needs as she defines them
- Recognises the woman's right to self-determination in terms of choice, control and continuity of care
- Recognises the woman's right to make informed choices (and refusals) with assistance, when requested by health professionals
- Is informed by scientific evidence, by collective and individual expertise and by intuition
- Encompasses the needs of the baby (born and unborn), the woman's family, significant others and community, as identified and negotiated by the woman herself
- Includes collaboration and consultation between health professionals as required and while focusing on the woman herself, rather than institutions or the professionals involved (Australian College of Midwives, 2011).

Like pregnancy and breastfeeding, labour and childbirth are essentially normal and significant life experiences for the woman. Labour is much more than the series of events by which uterine contractions and abdominal pressure expel a fetus and placenta from a woman's body. Labour is more than regular contractions that cause progressive dilation (enlargement of the cervical canal) and create sufficient muscular force to enable a baby to be pushed from the vagina. It is a time of exquisite change, both an ending and a beginning for a woman, a baby and those who are important to her.

Labour and birth require a woman to utilise all her emotional and physical strength. For many women, the experience of labour and birth has significant spiritual meaning and the birth of their baby is perceived as a sacred time. Labour is not a pathology requiring nursing diagnoses but rather the most intense, demanding and usually painful experience a woman will ever journey through. In an institutional setting, it is very possible that the environment and those in it (professional and support people) may inhibit the progress of labour, making it more difficult for the labouring woman. Prior to being with the woman, it is important for a nurse (or any person supporting the woman) to ask themselves a number of questions, including:

1. Do you have trust in the woman and her ability to birth well? Lack of trust and fear of giving birth by you or any person with her, will be unintentionally conveyed to the woman and may lead her to doubt herself.
2. Is it appropriate for you to be with the labouring woman? Will your nurturing, respect and gentleness enhance the woman's birthing experience or will you be an unnecessary distraction? The presence of unnecessary people with the labouring woman is an intervention. Any additional people that the woman does not specifically wish to be present should not be permitted without a great deal of thought on behalf of those accompanying the labouring woman and, of course, the express consent of the woman herself.
3. Is the labouring environment being made as safe, comfortable, private and familiar as possible? Simple strategies such as a sign on the door that says, "Please knock and wait before entering" can do much to help the woman's labour progress well.

The best outcomes for a woman and her newborn arise when she has had continuity of care from a known midwife during her pregnancy and that same midwife supports her during her labour and birth. Continuity of midwifery care includes assessments of the woman's physical, emotional, spiritual and social wellbeing. The woman should be provided with individualised education, counselling and antenatal care as well as continuous presence and support during labour, birth and the immediate postpartum period. Unnecessary technological, midwifery and obstetric interventions should be avoided and the woman referred for obstetric or other specialist attention if her situation becomes complex (Sandall et al., 2013).

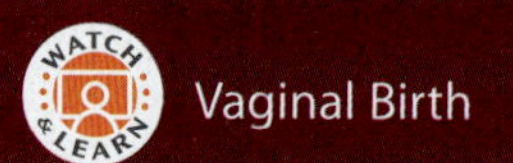

Vaginal Birth

ONSET OF LABOUR

Labour normally begins when a fetus is sufficiently mature to cope with extrauterine life yet not too large to cause mechanical difficulty with birth. Although the exact cause of the onset of labour is not fully understood, it is thought that the fetus triggers the onset of labour through a complex interplay of hormones (McNabb, 2011). In a healthy pregnancy, this means that labour starts at the optimal time for the fetus and is a factor to consider when discussing the benefits and risks of induction of labour with women.

SIGNS OF LABOUR

A common concern of women as they near the end of pregnancy is how they will know if they are beginning labour.

Preliminary signs of labour

Before labour, a woman often experiences subtle signs that signal labour is imminent. It is important to review these with women during the last trimester of pregnancy so they can more easily recognise beginning signs.

Lightening

In women expecting their first baby (primiparas), *lightening*, or descent of the fetal presenting part into the pelvis, usually occurs approximately 10 to 14 days before labour begins. This **fetal descent** changes a woman's abdominal contour, because it positions the uterus lower and more anterior in the abdomen. Lightening gives a woman relief from the diaphragmatic pressure and shortness of breath that she has been experiencing and in this way "lightens" her load. Lightening probably occurs early in primiparas because of tight abdominal muscles. In multiparas (women having their second or subsequent baby), it is not as dramatic and usually occurs on the day of labour or even after labour has begun.

Increase in level of activity

Immediately before labour starts, a woman may be full of energy, in contrast to the feeling of fatigue she felt during the previous month. This increase in activity is related to an increase in adrenaline release initiated by a decrease in progesterone levels. This additional adrenaline prepares a woman's body for the work of labour ahead.

Braxton Hicks contractions

Up to the 30th week of pregnancy, uterine activity consists of slight, short, localised contractions. As pregnancy progresses, palpable contractions which are usually but not always painless occur with increasing frequency and intensity and are known as Braxton Hicks contractions. Braxton Hicks contractions are thought to help facilitate the circulation of blood in the placental site and also play some part in the development of the lower uterine segment. These contractions result in a lowering of oxygen content in the fetal blood. When the myometrium contracts, it squeezes the uterine arteries and reduces the amount of blood flowing through them to the placenta. The fetus responds by reducing/eliminating its fetal breathing movements (Mander, 2011). In addition to fetal hypoxaemia, the fetus is squeezed by the contraction. In late pregnancy, when not completely surrounded by amniotic fluid, the fetus is in contact with the uterine wall over large portions of the body surface. The degree of squeezing (hugging) exerted on the fetus not only varies with the strength of the contraction, and with the amount of amniotic fluid in the uterus, but also with the position that the fetus has most recently assumed in the uterus. A contraction may decrease the front-to-back measurement of the fetal chest by up to 30%. This squeezing sends a large number of nerve impulses to the fetal brain. Many parts of the brain only develop correctly if they have constant stimulation and are constantly active. McNamara (2012) has hypothesised that the stimulation provided by Braxton Hicks contractions is part of this activity-dependent brain maturation process.

Although some women may mistake these Braxton Hicks contractions for established labour, it is important not to discourage the woman by referring to them as false labour. Rather, she can be encouraged to see them as important preparation for labour and as fetal growth enhancers (Mander, 2011). Women can be reassured that the Braxton Hicks contractions will become longer, stronger and closer together as early labour becomes established.

Ripening of the cervix

Ripening of the cervix is an internal sign seen only on pelvic examination. Throughout pregnancy, the cervix feels softer than pre-pregnancy, and when palpated, it feels similar to the consistency of an earlobe. At term, the cervix becomes still softer (feeling more like pursed lips) and tips forwards.

Signs of established labour

Signs of established labour involve uterine and cervical changes. The more a woman knows about these labour signs, the better she will be able to recognise and accommodate them.

Uterine contractions

Most women will refer to contractions but some will refer to them as waves or pains or another term. It is important to reflect back the words the woman herself is using as a form of validation. In established labour, contractions will gradually increase in length and intensity, as well as in strength and frequency. Women can be assured that the increasing intensity of contractions is accompanied by an increasing secretion of endorphins. Endorphins mediate the stress and pain of contractions with their analgesic properties; they alter perception of time and help increase the woman's self-confidence (Mander, 2011).

Show

As the cervix softens and ripens, the mucus plug that filled the cervical canal during pregnancy (operculum) is expelled. The exposed cervical capillaries seep blood as a result of pressure exerted by the fetus. This blood, mixed with mucus, takes on a pink tinge and is referred to as a "show" or a "bloody show". Women need to be aware of this event so that they do not think they are bleeding abnormally.

Rupture of the membranes

Labour may begin with rupture of the membranes, experienced either as a sudden gush or as a scanty, slow seeping of clear fluid from the vagina. Some women may worry if their labour begins with rupture of the membranes, because they have heard that labour will then be "dry" causing it to be difficult and long. Actually, amniotic fluid continues to be produced until delivery of the membranes after the birth of a fetus, so no labour is ever "dry". Physiologically, the membranes usually spontaneously rupture at full dilation of the cervix. These intact membranes can protect the fetal head (or presenting part) as it descends and dilates the cervix. Routine amniotomy (artificial rupture of the membranes) is not recommended.

It is important that the woman's membranes rupture spontaneously, rather than being artificially ruptured which can lead to a cascade of other interventions. Risks associated with artificially rupturing the membranes include increased pain for the woman, intrauterine infection and prolapse of the umbilical cord, which could cut off the oxygen supply to the fetus. In most instances, if labour has not spontaneously occurred by 24 hours after membrane rupture and the pregnancy is at term, induction of labour will be considered to reduce the risk of infection for the woman and her newborn.

CASE STUDY QUESTION

2. Cath had limited support from a familiar person during her labour. This is often associated with:

a. a shorter labour as there will be less people to interfere with her midwifery care
b. a more painful labour if she feels lonely or neglected
c. a longer labour that should be augmented so she doesn't become exhausted
d. less suffering because there will no one to talk her out of having an epidural

For a woman in labour

Assessment

Assessment of a woman in labour must be done quickly yet thoroughly and gently. A woman is keenly aware of words spoken around her and the manner with which procedures are carried out. Because of this, she may have difficulty relaxing for any physical examination, especially a vaginal examination if she fears pain from the procedure or a lack of sensitivity from the health professional. For this reason, vaginal examinations are no longer considered routine to be conducted at regular time intervals during the woman's labour. Rather, they are carried out as an assessment only when essential information cannot be ascertained in any other way. It is likely that nurses will observe that the more experienced and woman-centred the midwife, the fewer vaginal examinations will be conducted.

Pain is a very subjective symptom and will be discussed in more depth in the next chapter. It is important, however, to mention that assessment of the woman may induce discomfort or pain and the significance of gentleness, kindness and respect for the labouring woman can never be overestimated. Only the woman can evaluate how much pain she is experiencing or how much she wants to endure. Mander (2011, p. 7) offers this health warning to midwives that everyone supporting the labouring woman can learn from: "Do not allow yourself to be lulled into assuming that you know what another person's pain is—that way lies danger!"

A woman's pain or discomfort can be assessed not only by what she tells you or scores on a pain scale but also by subtle signs of pain such as facial tenseness, flushing or paleness of the face, hands clenched in a fist, rapid breathing or rapid pulse rate. Considering the extent of a woman's discomfort helps you to provide optimal support. Although the discomfort of labour is commonly referred to as "contractions" rather than "pain," unless requested by the woman, do not omit the word "pain" from your communication with her, because the term strengthens an understanding of the problem.

It is important not to project time limits for labour to be completed, because the length of labour can vary from woman to woman and still be within normal limits. It is necessary to appreciate the magnitude and significance of labour. While it is unlikely that all the fear or anxiety experienced during a woman's labour can be alleviated, those supporting her can do much to encourage her to feel confident and to sustain the energy she needs. Because it is such a significant experience, many couples appreciate the support of other caring people who will assist them to experience the labour and birth in the way that they had hoped and planned.

Both the woman and her support person are ideally involved in her birth planning, so that the experience is a shared one. Planning may include review and education about what might be expected during labour. Although a couple may have learned this information during pregnancy, the reality of labour may seem very much different from what they had imagined. So planning also must be flexible, changing with the progress of labour, and individualised, enabling a woman to experience the significance of the event as she chooses. There are many excellent websites available to assist women in writing a birthing and/or breastfeeding plan; some are associated with lobby groups and others are government sponsored. Comfort promotion is a vital part of care. A plan that addresses the discomforts of labour includes planning for education, validation and response to a woman's pain to help her maintain realistic perceptions about it. Whether in a written plan or not it is important to provide simple, non-pharmacological comfort measures such as offering a moisturising cream for dry lips or encouraging the woman to labour in the bath or shower with plenty of fluids to maintain hydration.

Interventions in labour must always be carefully considered before being implemented. The question needs to be asked: Do the benefits of this intervention outweigh the disadvantages or risks? In keeping with best available evidence, the Australian Government and states are issuing policy directives aimed at reducing unnecessary interventions in labour and birth. For example, NSW Health (2010) published *Maternity—Towards Normal Birth in NSW*. This is a very useful document that aims to:

- Increase the vaginal birth rate and decrease the caesarean section rate
- Develop, implement and evaluate strategies to support women to have a positive experience of pregnancy and birth

- Ensure midwives and doctors have the knowledge and skills to support women who choose to give birth without technological interventions unless necessary, use non-pharmacological interventions, use birthing pools and different positions for labour and birth.

The purpose of the action plan, *Towards Normal Birth in NSW* (NSW Health, 2010), is to:

- Increase the number of women starting labour spontaneously
- Increase the number of women receiving support at home in early labour
- Reduce the use of interventions that women experience in labour, particularly augmentation of labour, analgesia and electronic fetal monitoring
- Enhance experiences and satisfaction with care during pregnancy and childbirth, including social and emotional aspects of care
- Enable women to be better prepared for birth and early parenting with increased participation in decision making
- Increase women's sense of self-confidence and self-esteem in the early postnatal period which may have an important role in the prevention of postnatal distress or depression.

When interventions are deemed necessary, they are best carried out between contractions, if possible, so as not to add to the pain of contractions. This calls for good coordination of care among healthcare providers and planning with the woman and her support person. The person a woman chooses to stay with her during childbirth can be a partner, the father of the child, a sister or parent, or a close friend. How many support people a woman has and who is there is often a cultural preference and must be respected.

It is important for women to be able to understand what is happening to them during labour. If the woman is not proficient in English, arrangements must be made to engage an interpreter. If she is hearing challenged, it is the hospital's responsibility to provide an interpreter for her so that she can receive adequate explanations of her progress and support. Whether a woman enjoys being touched or not during labour is in part culturally determined and in part very individualistic. It should be assessed early in a woman's labour whether she might benefit from such caring measures as having her hand held or her back rubbed and by whom.

Outcome evaluation

During labour, evaluation must be ongoing to preserve the safety of a woman and her baby. After birth, evaluation helps to determine a woman's opinion of her experience with labour and birth. Ideally, the experience should be not only one that she was able to endure but one that enabled her self-esteem to grow and relationships with those who were with her to deepen through a shared experience. It is advantageous to talk to women in the early postpartum period about their labour. However, where a woman has experienced a traumatic birth, her immediate perception of her experience may be very different after an extended period of time. Providing formal debriefing in the immediate postpartum enables the woman the chance to "work through" her experience and incorporate it into her self-image, which may require referral to a professional counsellor. However, most women find it more helpful to debrief with someone, weeks—even months rather than days—after birth. Longer term counselling may be beneficial for the woman who has experienced a traumatic labour and birth.

COMPONENTS OF LABOUR

It has often been taught that a successful labour depends on four integrated concepts:

1. A woman's pelvis (the *passage*) is of adequate size and contour.
2. The *passenger* (the fetus) is of appropriate size and in an advantageous position and presentation.
3. The *powers* of labour (uterine factors) are adequate; this is also interpreted as the woman's ability to push. (The powers of labour are strongly influenced by the woman's position during labour.)
4. A woman's *psychological outlook* is preserved, so that afterwards labour can be viewed as a positive experience.

However, these concepts have been critiqued for a number of reasons, including that they are over-simplistic, paternalistic and reductionist and focus on the biomechanics of birth. Downe and Dykes (2010) argue that referring to the powers of the uterus infers that the woman's uterus functions separately from her mind and emotions. The baby, considered an inert passenger, passes passively through the maternal passage to be born, and the environment in which the woman labours and births can be ignored (Downe & Dykes, 2010). With this caveat in mind, it is useful to consider the following factors which have an impact on the progression of labour.

Attitude describes the degree of flexion a fetus assumes during labour or the relation of the fetal parts to each other. A fetus in *good* attitude is in complete flexion: the spinal column is bowed forwards, the head is flexed forwards so much that the chin touches the sternum, the arms are flexed and folded on the chest, the thighs are flexed onto the abdomen, and the calves are pressed against the posterior aspect of the thighs. This "fetal position" is advantageous for birth because it helps a fetus present the smallest diameter of the skull to the pelvis and also because it puts the whole body into an ovoid shape, occupying the smallest space possible (see Fig. 15.1).

Engagement refers to the settling of the presenting part of a fetus far enough into the pelvis to be at the level

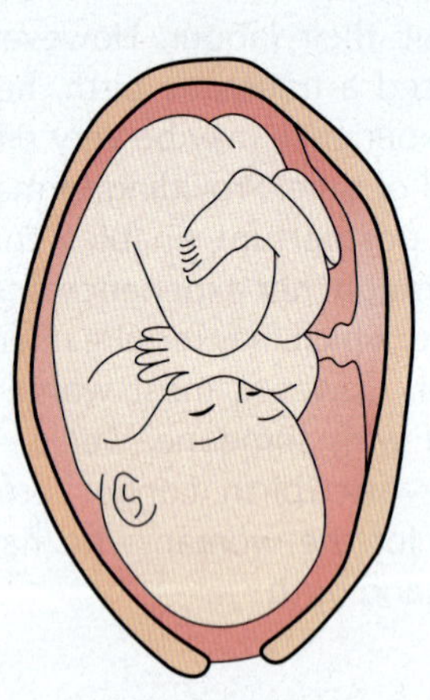

A Vertex (full flexion)

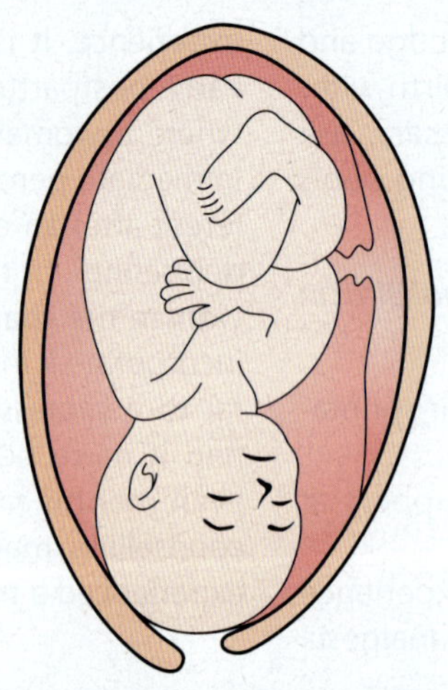

B Sinciput (moderate flexion [military attitude])

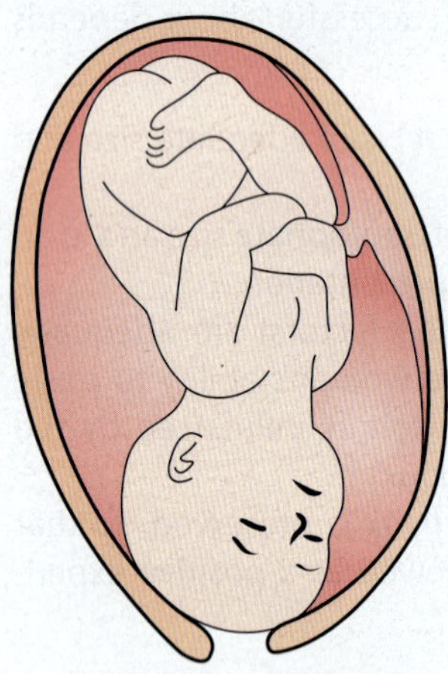

C Brow (partial extension)

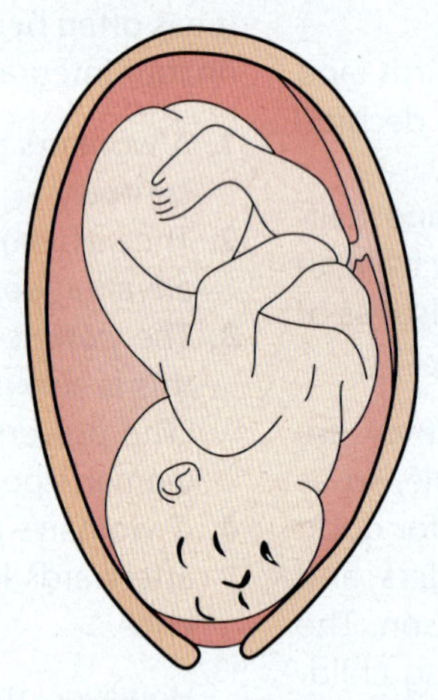

D Face (poor flexion, complete extension)

FIGURE 15.1 Fetal attitude. (**A**) Fetus in full flexion presents smallest (suboccipitobregmatic) anteroposterior diameter of skull to inlet in this good attitude (vertex presentation). (**B**) The fetus is not as well flexed (military attitude) and presents the occipitofrontal diameter to the inlet (sinciput presentation). (**C**) The fetus in partial extension (brow presentation). (**D**) The fetus in complete extension presents a wide (occipitomental) diameter (face presentation).

of the ischial spines, a midpoint of the pelvis. Descent to this point means that the widest part of the fetus (the biparietal diameter in a cephalic presentation) has passed through the pelvis inlet and the pelvic inlet has been proved adequate for birth. In a primiparous woman, engagement of the head normally occurs before labour starts. In multiparous women, engagement may or may not be present at the beginning of labour. The degree of engagement is assessed by **abdominal palpation** and vaginal examination.

Station refers to the relationship of the presenting part of a fetus to the level of the ischial spines. When the presenting fetal part is at the level of the ischial spines, it is at a 0 station (synonymous with engagement). If the presenting part is above the spines, the distance is measured and described as minus stations. If the presenting part is below the ischial spines, the distance is stated as plus stations (see Fig. 15.2).

Lie is the relationship between the long axis of the fetal body and the long axis of a woman's body; in other words, whether the fetus is lying in an oblique, horizontal (transverse) or a vertical (longitudinal) position. Approximately 99% of fetuses assume a longitudinal lie (with their long axis parallel to the long axis of the woman). Longitudinal lies are further classified as cephalic, which means the head will be the first part to contact the cervix, or breech, with the buttocks as the first portion to contact the cervix.

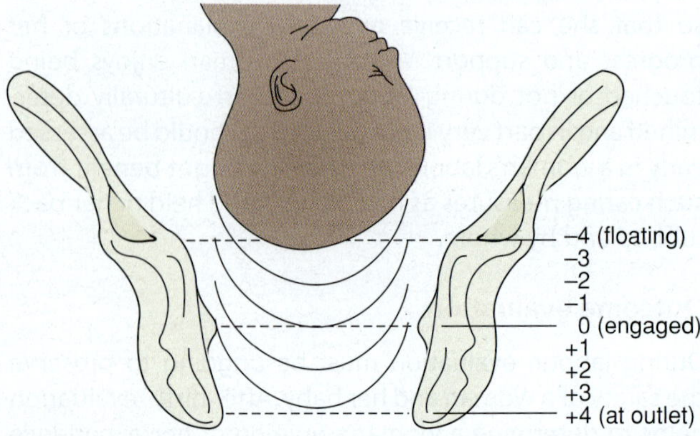

FIGURE 15.2 Station (anteroposterior view). Station, or degree of engagement, of the fetal head is designated by centimetres above or below the ischial spines. At –4 station, the head is "floating"; at 0 station, the head is "engaged"; and at +4 station, the head is "at outlet".

TABLE 15.1 Types of cephalic presentation

Type	Lie	Attitude	Description
Vertex	Longitudinal	Good (full flexion)	The head is sharply flexed, making the parietal bones or the space between the fontanelles (the vertex) the presenting part. This is the most common presentation and allows the suboccipitobregmatic diameter to present to the cervix.
Brow	Longitudinal	Moderate (military)	Because the head is only moderately flexed, the brow or sinciput becomes the presenting part.
Face	Longitudinal	Poor	The fetus has extended the head to make the face the presenting part. From this position, extreme oedema and distortion of the face may occur. The presenting diameter is so wide that birth may be impossible.
Mentum	Longitudinal	Very poor	The fetus has completely hyperextended the head to present the chin. The widest diameter (occipitomental) is presenting. As a rule, a fetus cannot enter the pelvis in this presentation.

Types of fetal presentation

Fetal presentation denotes the body part that will first contact the cervix or be born first. This is determined by a combination of fetal lie and the degree of fetal flexion (attitude).

A **cephalic presentation** is the most frequent type of presentation, occurring as often as 95% of the time. With this type of presentation, the fetal head is the body part that will first contact the cervix. The vertex is the ideal presenting part, because the skull bones are capable of effectively **moulding** to accommodate the cervix. This aids in cervical dilation and prevents complications such as a prolapsed cord (i.e. a portion of the cord passing between the presenting part and the cervix and entering the vagina before the fetus). During labour, the area of the fetal skull that contacts the cervix often becomes oedematous from the continued pressure against it. This oedema is called a *caput* succedaneum and parents can be reassured that it will disappear within 24 hours (see Table 15.1).

A **breech presentation** means that either the buttocks or the feet are the first body parts that will contact the cervix. Breech presentations occur in approximately 3% of births. Three types of breech presentation (complete, frank and footling) are possible (see Table 15.2).

A **shoulder presentation** occurs in a transverse lie, when a fetus lies horizontally in the pelvis so that the longest fetal axis is perpendicular to that of the mother. The presenting part is usually one of the shoulders (acromion process), an iliac crest, a hand or an elbow (see Fig. 15.3). Less than 1% of fetuses lie transversely.

Types of fetal position

Position is the relationship of the presenting part to a specific quadrant of a woman's pelvis. For convenience, the maternal pelvis is divided into four quadrants according to the mother's right and left: (a) right anterior, (b) left anterior, (c) right posterior and (d) left posterior. Four parts of a fetus have been chosen as landmarks to describe the relationship of the presenting part to one of the pelvic quadrants. In a vertex presentation, the occiput is the chosen point; in a face presentation, it is the chin (mentum); in a breech presentation, it is the sacrum; and in a shoulder presentation, it is the acromion process.

Position is indicated by an abbreviation of three letters. The middle letter denotes the fetal landmark (O for occiput, M for mentum or chin, Sa for sacrum and A for acromion process). The first letter defines whether the landmark is pointing to the mother's right (R) or left (L). The last letter defines whether the landmark points anteriorly (A), posteriorly (P) or laterally (L). If the occiput of a fetus points to the left anterior quadrant in a vertex position, for example, this is a left occipitoanterior (LOA) position. If the occiput points to the right posterior quadrant, the position is right occipitoposterior (ROP). LOA is the most common fetal position, and right occipitoanterior (ROA) the second most frequent.

Position is important, because it can influence the process and efficiency of labour. Typically, a fetus is born fastest from an ROA or LOA position. Labour is usually considerably extended if the position is posterior (ROP or LOP). Posterior positions may also be more painful for a woman, because the rotation of the fetal head puts pressure on sacral nerves, causing sharp back pain. Encouraging a woman to be upright and mobile may encourage rotation from an occipitoposterior to an occipitoanterior position before and during labour (DiFranco & Curl, 2014) and being on hands and knees in labour can reduce backache that accompanies a posterior labour.

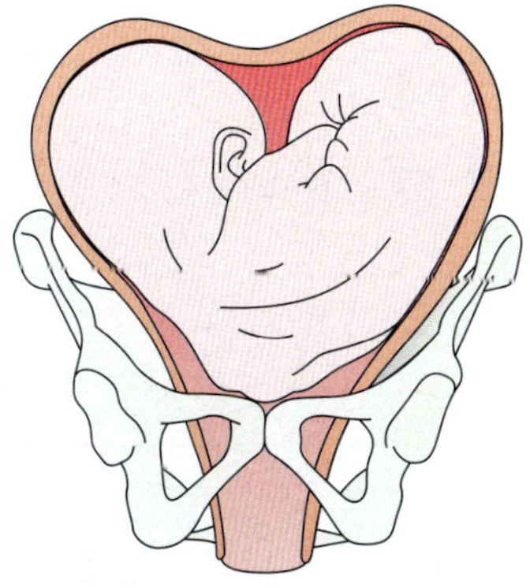

FIGURE 15.3 Transverse or shoulder presentation.

TABLE 15.2 Types of breech presentation

Type	Lie	Attitude	Description
Complete	Longitudinal	Good (full flexion)	The fetus has thighs tightly flexed on the abdomen; both the buttocks and the tightly flexed feet present to the cervix.
Frank	Longitudinal	Moderate	Attitude is moderate because the hips are flexed but the knees are extended to rest on the chest. The buttocks alone present to the cervix.
Footling	Longitudinal	Poor	Neither the thighs nor lower legs are flexed. If one foot presents, it is a single-footling breech; if both present, it is a double-footling breech.

CASE STUDY QUESTION

3. A midwife attends a vaginal examination at Cath's request and tells Cath that her baby is in an ideal position to birth. This means that her baby is:
   a. Right occipitoanterior and fully flexed
   b. Left mento lateral with moderate flexion
   c. Right occipitoposterior and partly deflexed
   d. Left sacroanterior and fully flexed

Importance of determining fetal presentation and position

It is important to document fetal presentation and position, because these help determine if the progress of labour is optimal for the woman and her baby. Knowing fetal presentation and position also helps the midwife to assist the woman into positions of comfort, usually upright positions which enable the woman to be more easily mobile. Three methods are used to determine fetal position, presentation and lie in labour: (a) combined abdominal inspection and palpation, (b) auscultation of fetal heart tones, and (c) vaginal examination when being attended for another purpose.

Mechanisms of labour

To better understand birth, it is important to know the mechanisms of labour and birth. In a normal labour and birth, the fetal head descends through the pelvis and, as it does so, it rotates to ensure optimum positioning for birth. These are called the **mechanisms of labour**.

- **Descent** of the fetus takes place throughout.
- **Flexion** (increases with descent). The fetal head flexes to allow its descent through the pelvic inlet and engagement to occur.
- **Internal rotation** of the head follows engagement and allows the fetal head to align with the diameter of the pelvic outlet.
- **Crowning** occurs when the occiput is seen bulging at the vaginal introitus.
- **Extension** of the head allows the head to be born as the face sweeps over the perineum.
- **Restitution** occurs after the birth of the head as the head returns to the side (left or right) where it was in the pelvis.
- **Internal rotation** of the shoulders, with simultaneous **external rotation** of the head, occurs when the shoulders turn to fit the diameter of the pelvis.
- **Lateral flexion** of the body occurs with the shoulders usually born sequentially.

Cervical changes

Cervical changes include effacement (thinning out) and dilation (opening up) of the cervix. **Effacement** is shortening and thinning of the cervical canal. Normally, the canal is approximately 1 to 2 cm long, at the start of labour. With effacement, the canal virtually disappears (see Fig. 15.4).

In women who are primiparas, effacement is accomplished before dilation begins. It is important that women are informed of this, otherwise, they can become discouraged if, for example, at noon after a vaginal examination a woman is told she is 2 cm dilated and then at 4 p.m. is told she is still 2 cm dilated. This type of report makes it seem as if nothing has happened in 4 hours. However, effacement will have been occurring and, when it is complete, dilation will then progress rapidly. In women who are multiparas, dilation may proceed before effacement is complete.

Dilation refers to the enlargement or widening of the cervical canal from an opening a few millimetres wide to one large enough (approximately 10 centimetres) to permit passage of the fetus (see Fig. 15.4). As dilation begins, there is an increase in the amount of vaginal secretions (show), because the last of the operculum or mucus plug in the cervix is dislodged and minute capillaries in the cervix rupture. Contrary to the popularly held belief, cervical dilation is not necessarily linear, but on occasions a woman's cervical dilation may actually regress, especially if the woman is feeling frightened or anxious (Wickham, 2011).

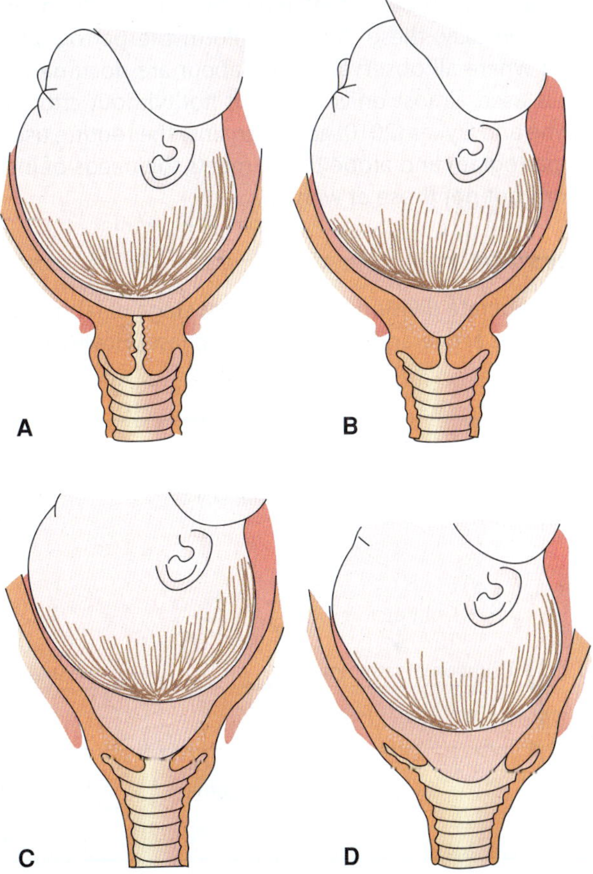

FIGURE 15.4 Effacement and dilation of cervix. (**A**) Beginning labour. (**B**) Effacement is beginning; dilation is not apparent yet. (**C**) Effacement is almost complete. (**D**) After complete effacement, dilation proceeds rapidly.

STAGES OF LABOUR

Labour is traditionally divided into three stages but this concept has been criticised as labour is actually much more of a continuum than a staged process. Defining the stages of labour in relation to cervical dilation encourages unnecessary and potentially harmful vaginal examinations. Vaginal examinations are not only uncomfortable for some women, especially those who have survived sexual assault, but also can be deeply traumatising and increase the risk of infection. Furthermore, assessment of cervical dilation is a very subjective skill and its accuracy has often been questioned (Davies, 2011).

Nevertheless, labour continues to be defined in terms of stages in most textbooks. The first stage of labour begins with the initiation of labour contractions and ends when the cervix is fully dilated; the second stage extends from the time of full dilation until the infant is born; and the third stage lasts from the time the infant is born until the delivery of the placenta. The first 1 to 4 hours after birth of the placenta is sometimes termed the "fourth stage" to emphasise the importance of not inhibiting attachment and bonding between the parents and newborn and the close maternal observation needed at this time.

Friedman (1978), a doctor who studied the process of labour extensively, used data to divide the first two stages of labour into phases: latent and active labour. When plotted graphically, these divisions inform the partogram, a graph where all observations of labour are documented, that is used almost universally but not without criticism. Downe and Dykes (2010) advise against the routine use of the partogram and argue that it meets the needs of institutions but not those of women.

First stage

Three separate divisions mark the first stage of labour: the latent, the active and the transition phase. However, it is very important not to consider the woman is in labour until it is established during the active phase so as to reduce the likelihood of unnecessary intervention.

Latent phase

The latent phase begins at the onset of regularly perceived uterine contractions and ends when rapid cervical dilation begins. The mark of effective uterine contractions is their rhythmicity and progressive lengthening and intensity. Contractions during the latent phase tend to be mild and short. Cervical effacement occurs and the cervix dilates from 0 to 3 cm. The phase lasts approximately 6 hours in a primipara and 4.5 hours in a multipara, but there are wide variations. A woman who enters labour with a "non-ripe" cervix will have a longer than usual latent phase. A woman can be encouraged to continue to walk about and make preparations for birth, such as doing last-minute packing for her stay at the maternity unit.

Active phase

During the active phase of labour, cervical dilation occurs more rapidly, increasing from 4 to 7 cm. Contractions grow stronger, longer and closer together (see Fig. 15.5). This phase lasts approximately 3 hours in a primipara and 2 hours in a multipara but can vary greatly and still be normal. Women can be safely encouraged to remain active participants in labour by assuming the most comfortable position for them during this time (Priddis, Dahlen & Schmied, 2012).

Transition phase

During the **transition** phase, contractions reach their peak of intensity, often occurring every 2 to 3 minutes with a duration of 60 to 90 seconds (these times are approximate) and causing maximum cervical dilation of 8 to 10 cm. Many women find water immersion during this phase especially

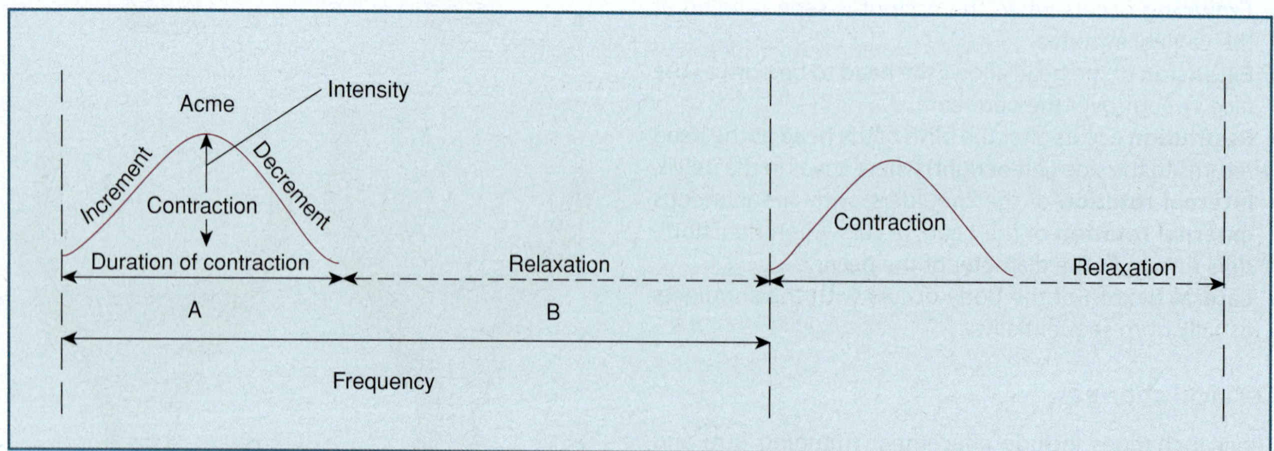

FIGURE 15.5 The interval and duration of uterine contractions. The frequency of contractions is the time from the beginning of one contraction to the beginning of the next contraction. It consists of two parts: (A) the duration of the contraction and (B) the period of relaxation. The broken line indicates an indeterminate period because the relaxation time (B) is usually of longer duration than the actual contraction (A).

helpful (NSW Health, 2010). If the membranes have not previously ruptured, they will usually rupture at full dilation (10 cm). By the end of this phase, both full dilation and complete cervical effacement have occurred.

During this phase, a woman may experience intense discomfort, so strong that it is accompanied by nausea and vomiting which is a vagal nerve response. Because of the intensity and duration of the contractions, a woman may also experience a feeling of loss of control, anxiety, panic or irritability. A few minutes before, she enjoyed having her forehead wiped with a cool cloth. Now she may knock a partner's hand away. A moment before, she enjoyed having her partner rub her back. Now she may resist being touched and push that person away. Her focus is entirely inwards on the task of giving birth to her baby.

The peak of the transition phase can be identified by a slight slowing in the rate of cervical dilation when 9 cm is reached. As a woman reaches the end of this stage at 10 cm of dilation, a new sensation (i.e. an irresistible urge to push) may occur.

Second stage

The second stage of labour is the period from full cervical dilation to birth of the infant; with an uncomplicated birth, this stage usually takes about 1 hour but there is no evidence to support placing time limitations on the second stage of labour (Cooke, 2010). Some women feel an overwhelming urge to push before full dilation and in most instances this need not be discouraged (Downe & Dykes, 2010). Other women do not feel an urge to push until long after the cervix is fully dilated. It is not uncommon for contractions to slow down at the beginning of the second stage and women should be encouraged to conserve their energy ("rest and be grateful") and push only when they have an overwhelming desire to do so. A woman's contractions may slow or she may feel contractions change from the characteristic crescendo–decrescendo pattern to an overwhelming, uncontrollable urge to push or bear down with each contraction as if to move her bowels. There is no evidence to support instructing women when and how to push (but there is evidence against it!), and directing women to push during second stage is a common practice that should be abandoned (Cooke, 2010).

As the fetal head touches the internal side of the perineum, the perineum begins to bulge and appears tense. The anus may become everted and faeces may be expelled. As the fetal head pushes against the perineum, the vaginal introitus opens and the fetal scalp appears at the opening to the vagina. The circle enlarges and **crowning** occurs.

It may take a few contractions of this new type for a woman to realise everything is still all right, just different, and to appreciate that it feels good, not frightening, to push with contractions. In fact, the need to push becomes so intense that she cannot stop herself. She barely hears the conversation in the room around her. All of her energy, her thoughts, her being are directed towards giving birth. As she pushes, using her abdominal muscles to aid the involuntary uterine contractions, the fetus is pushed out of the vagina.

Third stage

The third stage of labour begins with the birth of the baby and ends with the expulsion of the placenta, membranes and the achievement of haemostasis. This stage can be physiological; cord clamping is delayed and the woman expels the placenta aided by her baby nuzzling on her breast (to increase oxytocin levels) and possibly gravity. Or the expulsion of the placenta can be actively managed when a uterotonic drug, usually syntocinon is given. The timing of the administration of the drug may vary but is usually given when the first shoulder of the baby is born. The woman then has a contraction and the placenta begins to separate. At this stage the midwife or doctor guards the uterus (places a hand on the abdomen above the symphysis pubis) and gently applies traction to the cord. In Australia, almost all third stages of labour are actively managed in the belief it will reduce the risk of serious haemorrhage.

For some women, the placenta has emotional, cultural or spiritual significance. For this reason, women may ask if they can take it home with them. It is important that parents are asked whether saving the placenta is important to them before it is destroyed. Infection control processes must be adhered to whether the placenta is destroyed or given to the parents.

MATERNAL AND FETAL RESPONSES TO LABOUR

Because labour is such an intense process, it has systemic physiological effects on both a woman and her fetus.

Physiological effects of labour on a woman

Labour is a local process that involves the abdomen and reproductive organs, but its intensity is so great that almost all body systems are affected by it.

Cardiovascular system

Labour involves strenuous work and effort and requires a response from the cardiovascular system. The healthy labouring woman is well able to tolerate cardiovascular changes. If a woman is frightened, anxious, embarrassed or even cold, she will produce excessive levels of adrenaline that will not only put additional strain on her cardiovascular system, but also inhibit oxytocin release and the progress of labour.

With the increased cardiac output caused by contractions during labour, systolic blood pressure rises an average of 15 mmHg with each contraction. Higher increases could be a sign that the woman's pregnancy is complicated by hypertension or possibly, pre-eclampsia. When a woman lies in a supine position and pushes during the second stage of labour, the pressure of the uterus on the vena cava causes her blood pressure to drop precipitously, leading to hypotension. An upright or side-lying position during the second stage of labour not only makes pushing more effective but also can help avoid such a problem (Priddis et al., 2012).

Respiratory system

Whenever there is an increase in cardiovascular parameters, the body responds by increasing the respiratory rate to supply additional oxygen.

Temperature regulation

The increased muscular activity associated with labour can result in a slight elevation (1°C) in temperature. Diaphoresis occurs with accompanying evaporation to cool and limit excessive warming.

Fluid balance

Because of the increase in rate and depth of respirations (which causes moisture to be lost with each breath) and diaphoresis, insensible water loss, increases during labour. Fluid balance is further affected if a woman takes nothing but sips of fluid or ice cubes or lollies. Women should be encouraged to drink and eat light nourishing foods as desired during labour (Singata, Tranmer & Gyte, 2013).

Urinary system

Women should be encouraged to void regularly during labour. Pressure of the fetal head as it descends in the birth canal against the anterior bladder reduces bladder tone or the ability of the bladder to sense filling. Therefore, unless the woman is asked to void approximately every 2 hours during labour, overfilling may occur, possibly decreasing bladder tone in the postpartum period.

Musculoskeletal system

During pregnancy, relaxin, an ovarian-released hormone, has acted to soften the cartilage between bones. In the week before labour, considerable additional softening causes the symphysis pubis and the sacral/coccyx joints to become even more relaxed and movable, allowing them to stretch apart to increase the size of the pelvic ring by as much as 2 cm. A woman may report this increased pubic flexibility as increased back pain or irritating, nagging pain at the pubis as she walks or turns in labour.

Gastrointestinal system

The gastrointestinal system slows during labour, probably because of the shunting of blood to more life-sustaining organs and also because of pressure on the stomach and intestines from the contracting uterus. Digestive and emptying time of the stomach become prolonged. At the beginning of labour, under the influence of prostaglandin, many women experience loose bowel movements which serve the function of emptying the bowel and allowing more room for the baby to pass through the pelvis. Once advised not to eat or even drink in labour, that advice is no longer considered evidence-based, and women should be encouraged to eat and drink if they choose to do so (Singata et al., 2013). Very light nourishment is preferable because of the delayed gastric emptying time and because of the energy required to labour and birth.

Neurological and sensory responses

The neurological responses that occur during labour are responses related to pain. Early in labour, the contraction of the uterus and dilation of the cervix cause discomfort. This pain is registered at uterine and cervical nerve plexuses (at the level of the 11th and 12th thoracic nerves). At the moment of birth, the pain is centred on the perineum as it stretches to allow the fetus to move past it. Perineal pain is registered at S2 to S4 nerves. It too is functional as the perineal pain causes the woman to instinctively stop pushing and she will intuitively "breath her baby out" which helps protect her perineum. This is another reason why it is important not to instruct women how and when to push or not push as it can be confusing for the woman and counterproductive.

Emotional responses of a woman to labour

Labour is an emotional challenge (and opportunity for tremendous emotional growth) for all women. Even for the most patient woman, pain reduces the ability to cope and may make her short-tempered or quick to criticise things around her.

Fatigue

As term approaches, a woman is generally tired from the burden of carrying so much extra weight. In addition, most women do not sleep well during the last month of pregnancy. They have a backache in a side-lying position; they turn on their back and the fetus kicks and wakens them to ensure adequate placental perfusion; they turn to their side and their back aches again; and so on. Sleep hunger from this discomfort can make it difficult for them to perceive situations clearly or to adjust rapidly to new situations. It can make a little deficiency such as a wrinkled sheet appear as a threatening discrepancy in their care. It can make the process of labour loom as an overwhelming, unendurable experience unless they have competent support people with them.

Fear

Most women appreciate a quick review of the labour process early in labour and a brief discussion of how their birth plan is respected and can best be implemented. Being taken by surprise—labour moving faster or slower than the woman thought it would or contractions harder and longer than she remembers from last time—can lead a woman to feel out of control and increase the pain she experiences (see Box 15.1). It may exacerbate worry that her infant may die or be born with an abnormality; it may make her afraid that she will not meet her own behavioural expectations. Women can be assured that their bodies will provide them with an optimum cocktail of naturally-produced hormones to help them to cope and respond well; they can also be assured that, in a normal labour, they will have a pain-free period between contractions.

Cultural influences

Cultural factors can strongly influence a woman's experience of and response to labour. In the past, Australian and New Zealand women were accustomed to following hospital procedures and the medical model of care; therefore, they followed instructions during labour with few questions. Today, women are educated to help plan their care. In addition, every woman responds to cultural cues in some way. This makes her response to pain, her choice of nourishment, her preferred birthing position, the proximity and involvement of a support person, and customs related to the immediate postpartum period individualised (Phiri, Dietsch & Bonner, 2010).

To make labour a positive experience, be prepared to adapt your care to the woman's specific circumstances. A woman may have traditions that run counter to maternity unit protocols. Address these differences, and make arrangements to accommodate her beliefs or customs if possible (e.g. providing warm food or fluids during labour, saving the placenta for her to take home). If the woman is not proficient in English, arranging for an interpreter or working closely with a family member who can interpret is important.

Physiological effects of labour on a fetus

The fetus is not a passive participant in labour (Bergman & Bergman, 2013) and the pressure and circulatory changes that occur with contractions cause detectable physiological changes all of which are preparing the fetus for transition to newborn, extrauterine life. The way a baby is born has immediate and long term effects on their health and wellbeing even into adulthood (Harman & Wakeford, 2014). To give babies the very best start in life, they require:

- To be born vaginally, rather than by caesarean section
- Labour to start and continue without the use of syntocinon being used to induce or augment labour
- Antibiotics and other drugs to be avoided during labour
- Uninhibited skin-to-skin contact with their mothers (while both are kept warm)
- Unrestricted access to their mother's breast so they receive colostrum and then breast milk.

BOX 15.1 ✻ Focus on evidence-based practice

Fear of labour and birth

The increasing emphasis on risk assessment in maternity care has not seen improved outcomes for women and newborns. The unacceptable rise in the number of caesarean sections has not resulted in improved outcomes and in fact pregnancy and childbirth have become inherently riskier due to unanticipated secondary health problems.

Ironically, as childbirth becomes safer for women and their infants in Western countries, the fear of childbirth is increasing. Increasing medicalisation of birth with its accompanying focus on biomedical risk assessment and management is leading to women and their midwifery/obstetric carers becoming more fearful.

Women and their carers, particularly in Australia, have come to fear that their baby may die in utero if they go past their due date (usually determined by ultrasound, which is accurate to only plus or minus 5 to 10 days, depending on how early the ultrasound was taken) but they do not fear the risks of inducing labour. Women and their carers fear the pain of labour but not the side effects of an epidural. Women and their carers feel reassured by continuous fetal monitoring and do not fear the unnecessary caesarean section the monitoring often leads to. Women and their carers fear that birth in a small rural town is unsafe and so without hesitation risk travelling on long, dangerous roads (often in labour) to birth in a larger hospital where there is 24-hour obstetric and anaesthetic cover.

You are encouraged to do your own literature search or to retrieve, read and review:

Dahlen, H. (2014). Managing risk or facilitating safety? *International Journal of Childbirth, 4*(2), 66–68.

Dietsch, E., Shackleton, P., Davies, C., Alston, M. & McLeod, M. (2010). 'Mind you, there's no anaesthetist on the road': women's experiences of labouring en route. *Rural and Remote Health, 10*, 1371 (online).

Hildingsson, I., Nilsson, C., Karlström, A. & Lundgren, I. (2011). A longitudinal survey of childbirth-related fear and associated factors. *Journal of Obstetric, Gynecologic and Neonatal Nursing, 40*(5), 532–543. DOI: 10.1111/j.1552-6909.2011.01274.x.

Jordan, R. & Aikins Murphy, P. (2009). Risk assessment and risk distortion: finding the balance. *Journal of Midwifery and Women's Health, 54*(3), 191–200.

Lothian, J. (2012). Risk, safety, and choice in childbirth. *Journal of Perinatal Education, 21*(1), 45–47.

Scammell, M. & Alaszewski, A. (2012). Fateful moments and the categorisation of risk: midwifery practice and the ever-narrowing window of normality during childbirth. *Risk and Society, 14*(2), 207–221.

How could you use these studies to guide your actions when caring for women during pregnancy or supporting them during labour and birth?

Neurological system

Uterine contractions exert pressure on the fetal head, so the same response that is involved with any instance of increased intracranial pressure occurs. The fetal heart rate (FHR) decreases slightly and as long as it remains within normal limits with good variability it is considered a physiological response and is to be expected, especially during second stage labour. The function of these anticipated decelerations is for the fetus to conserve oxygen.

Cardiovascular system

The ability to respond to cardiovascular changes is usually developed enough so that the fetus is unaffected by the continual variations of heart rate that occur with labour—a slight slowing and then a return to normal (baseline) levels. During a contraction, the arteries of the uterus are sharply constricted and the filling of cotyledons almost completely halts. The amount of nutrients, including oxygen, exchanged during this time is reduced, causing a slight but inconsequential fetal hypoxia. Increased intracranial pressure caused by uterine pressure on the fetal head serves to keep circulation from falling below normal during the duration of a contraction.

Integumentary system

The pressure involved in the birth process is often reflected in minimal petechiae or ecchymotic areas on a fetus (particularly the presenting part). There may also be oedema of the presenting part (caput succedaneum).

Musculoskeletal system

The force of uterine contractions tends to push a fetus into a position of full flexion, the most advantageous position for birth.

Respiratory system

The process of labour appears to aid in the maturation of surfactant production by alveoli in the fetal lung. The pressure applied to the chest from contractions and passage through the birth canal helps to clear it of lung fluid. For this reason, an infant born vaginally is usually able to establish respiration more easily than a fetus born by caesarean birth.

BOX 15.2 Assessment * Assessing for danger signs in labour

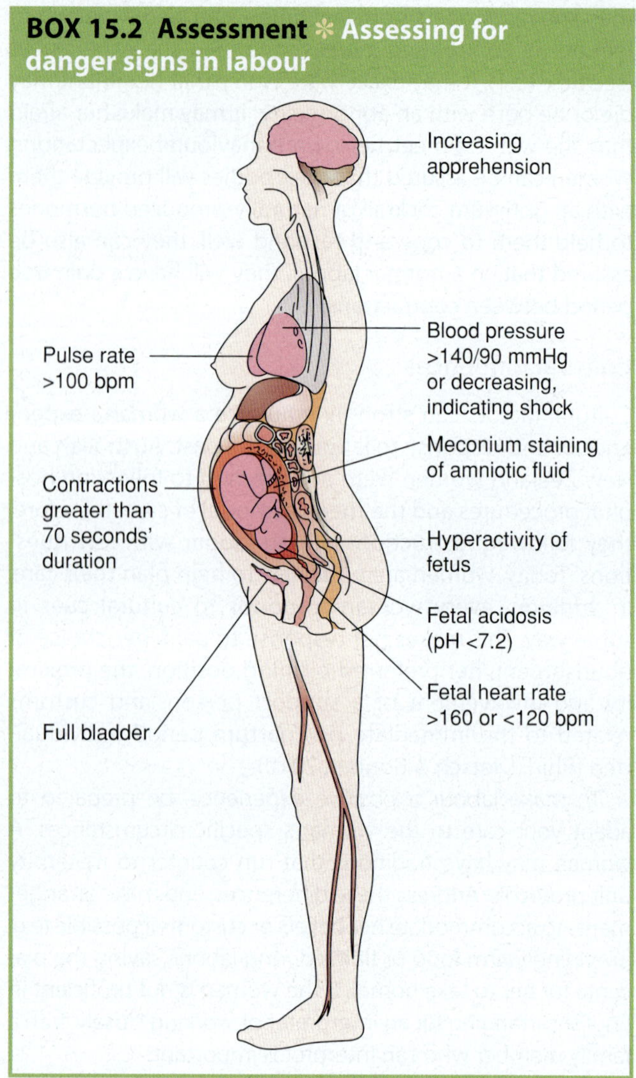

DANGER SIGNS IN LABOUR

Wide variation exists among individuals in their patterns of labour contractions and in maternal responses to labour and birth. Certain signs, however, indicate that the course of events is deviating from normal. These signs, both fetal and maternal, are described in Box 15.2. It is essential that the midwife knows the parameters of normal labour very well so they can respond appropriately to ensure that unnecessary interventions are not considered while, at the same time, they can refer when appropriate to ensure the best possible outcomes for the woman and her newborn (NSW Health, 2010).

Maternal danger signs

High or low blood pressure

Normally, a woman's blood pressure rises slightly in the second stage of labour because of her spontaneous pushing effort. A systolic pressure greater than 140 mmHg and a diastolic pressure greater than 90 mmHg, or an increase in the pressure of more than 15 mmHg should be reported. Just as important to report is a falling blood pressure, because it may be the first sign of shock from epidural anaesthesia or intrauterine haemorrhage. A falling blood pressure is often associated with other clinical signs of shock, such as apprehension, increased pulse rate and pallor.

Abnormal pulse

Most pregnant women have a pulse rate of 70 to 80 bpm. This rate normally increases slightly during the second stage of labour because of the exertion involved. A maternal pulse rate greater than 100 bpm during the normal course of labour is unusual and should be reported. It may be another indication of haemorrhage.

Inadequate or prolonged contractions

Uterine contractions normally become more frequent, intense and longer as labour progresses. If they become less frequent, less intense or shorter in duration, this may indicate uterine exhaustion (inertia). Once labelled, "failure to progress", this term is no longer acceptable as it is derogatory to the labouring woman. The phenomenon is now termed, labour dystocia and the most common cause is that the woman is releasing adrenaline because she is frightened or does not feel safe in the birthing environment or secure with the health professionals supporting her. Adrenaline, in turn, has a negative impact on the release of oxytocin. Labour dystocia, often iatrogenic, is one of the main causes of the increasing caesarean section rate in Australia (Sandstrom et al., 2012).

A period of relaxation must be present between contractions so that the intervillous spaces of the uterus can fill and maintain an adequate supply of oxygen and nutrients for the fetus. Uterine contractions that are excessively long and/or strong (hypertonic) are usually associated with syntocinon infusion (induction or augmentation of labour). The syntocinon infusion must be reviewed as a matter of urgency as hypertonic contractions may compromise fetal wellbeing by interfering with adequate uterine artery filling or increase the risk of a uterine rupture.

Abnormal lower abdominal contour

If a woman has a full bladder during labour, a round bulge on her lower anterior abdomen may appear. This is a danger signal for two reasons: first, the bladder may be injured by the pressure of the fetal head; second, the pressure of the full bladder may not allow the fetal head to descend. To avoid a full bladder, women need to try to void about every 2 hours during labour.

Increasing apprehension

Warnings of psychological danger during labour are as important to consider in assessing maternal wellbeing as physical signs. A woman who is becoming increasingly apprehensive despite clear explanations of unfolding events may only be approaching the second stage of labour. She may, however, not be "hearing" because she has a concern that has not been met. Using an approach such as, "You seem more and more concerned. Could you tell me what is worrying you?" may be helpful or it may be counterproductive and distracting to the woman experiencing normal labour. Caution must be exercised before engaging the woman in cognitive thought once she is in established labour and especially around transition. Increasing apprehension also needs to be investigated for physical reasons as it can be a sign of oxygen deprivation or internal haemorrhage.

Fetal danger signs

High or low fetal heart rate

As a rule, a fetal heart rate (FHR) of more than 160 bpm (fetal tachycardia) or less than 110 bpm (fetal bradycardia) is a sign of possible fetal compromise.

Meconium staining

Meconium staining, a green colour in the amniotic fluid, is not always a sign of fetal compromise but is a warning sign, especially if the meconium is thick and fresh. It reveals that the fetus has had loss of rectal sphincter control, allowing meconium to pass into the amniotic fluid. It may indicate that a fetus has or is experiencing hypoxia, which stimulates the vagal reflex and leads to increased bowel motility. Although meconium staining may be normal in a breech presentation, because pressure on the buttocks causes meconium loss, it should always be reported immediately so that its cause can be investigated.

Hyperactivity

Ordinarily, a fetus is relatively quiet during labour. Fetal hyperactivity may be a sign that hypoxia is occurring, because frantic motion is a common reaction to the need for oxygen.

CASE STUDY QUESTION

4. Suppose Cath is having long and hard uterine contractions. What length of contraction would you report as abnormal?
   a. Any length over 30 seconds
   b. A contraction over 70 seconds in length
   c. A contraction that peaks at 20 seconds
   d. A contraction shorter than 60 seconds

MATERNAL AND FETAL ASSESSMENT DURING LABOUR

Immediate assessment of a woman in first stage

Several immediate assessment measures are necessary to safeguard maternal and fetal health when a woman first arrives at a birthing facility. All women should be encouraged to bring a support person with them into labour (Madden et al., 2013). After the woman and her support person are orientated to the area, vital assessment data can be obtained.

Initial interview and physical examination

Important data that need to be obtained include a description of the woman's labour thus far, her general physical condition, and her preparedness for labour and birth, including her birth plan.

The woman is asked about:

- Expected date of birth
- Frequency, duration and intensity of contractions and time they commenced
- Amount and character of show

- Whether rupture of membranes has occurred and the colour of any liquor
- Any known drug allergies
- Previous pregnancy history
- Her birth plan or what individualised measures she has planned, such as no analgesia or who will cut the umbilical cord.

The woman is assessed:

- Vital signs—temperature, pulse, respiration and blood pressure (assessed between contractions)
- Contractions (frequency, duration and intensity)
- Her preparedness and readiness for labour.

This amount of information is scant but helps to establish whether the woman is in active labour and needs immediate preparation for birth or whether she has arrived at the birthing setting at an early stage of labour and therefore can benefit most from paced support. Many women have hand-held records of their antenatal care which can be reviewed to give an idea of the course of antenatal care.

Detailed assessment during the first stage of labour

If the woman is in active labour, the history taken on arrival may be the only history obtained until after her baby is born. If birth is not imminent, her extensive history documented during pregnancy can be reviewed and a physical examination conducted.

History

The full history should include a review of the woman's pregnancy, including both physical and psychosocial events, and a review of past pregnancies, her general health and family medical information. However, it is important that this history be taken and documented during the woman's pregnancy. It is not conducive for labour for a woman to be engaged cognitively and to have to share this information during her labour. The history taken and revisited during the woman's pregnancy should include the following:

Current pregnancy history

Important information needed for a complete history includes documentation of gravida (the number of pregnancies she has had) and para (the number of births after 20 weeks' gestation) status; a description of this pregnancy (planned or not, pattern and place of antenatal care, adequacy of nutrition, whether any complication such as spotting, falls, hypertension of pregnancy, infection, or alcohol or drug ingestion has occurred); plans for labour (does she want medication for pain, will she use breathing exercises, will she have a support person with her, does she want a water birth etc?); and her breastfeeding (or formula-feeding) plans.

Past pregnancy history

Document prior pregnancies, including number, dates, types of birth, any complications and outcomes, including sex and birth weights of children. What is the current health status of the children?

Past health history

Document any previous surgeries; heart disease or diabetes; anaemia; tuberculosis; kidney disease or hypertension; or if she has ever had a sexually transmissible infection such as herpes. All of these may have a detrimental effect on the woman's pregnancy and childbirth or, conversely, pregnancy and childbirth may have an adverse effect on these morbidities. Determine also whether a woman's lifestyle places her at high risk for prescription or non-prescription drug use or blood borne diseases such as human immunodeficiency virus (HIV).

Family medical history that may have a hereditary component

During pregnancy, the woman should have been asked if any family member is cognitively challenged or has a condition such as heart disease, a blood dyscrasia, diabetes, kidney disease, cancer, allergies, seizures or a congenital disorder.

Physical examination

After reviewing the woman's history, if she is not in active labour, the woman receives a thorough physical examination. Physical assessment during labour begins, as does all physical assessment, with the woman's overall appearance: Does she appear tired? Pale? Ill? Frightened? Is there obvious oedema or dehydration? Does she have open lesions anywhere? The examination will need to be adapted to meet a woman's stage of labour, frequency of contractions and labour progression.

After the woman has emptied her bladder, her abdomen is inspected, palpated and fetal heart auscultation is attended. The examination also usually includes a vaginal examination, to confirm the presentation and position of the fetus and the stage of cervical dilation.

Assessing rupture of membranes

When the membranes spontaneously rupture, a woman feels a sudden gush or a gradual leakage of amniotic fluid from her vagina. This is a startling sensation because it feels as if she has lost bladder control. She may feel embarrassed before she realises that the warm fluid on her perineum and legs is not urine but a sudden announcement that labour is imminent. When there is a slow loss of fluid (which happens if the leak is from the hindwaters), there may be a question of whether the membranes have ruptured.

If there is doubt, after vaginal secretions are obtained (usually with the use of a sterile, cotton-tipped applicator), they can be tested with a strip of Nitrazine paper (brand names include *amnisure, amnitest* and *amnicheck*). Vaginal secretions are usually acidic; amniotic fluid, in contrast, is alkaline. If amniotic fluid has passed through the vagina recently, the pH of the vaginal fluid will probably be alkaline (6.5) when tested by Nitrazine paper (appears blue-green or grey to deep blue). A false reading may occur in a woman with intact membranes who has a heavy, bloody show, because blood is also alkaline.

If the woman's membranes ruptured at home, ask her to describe the colour of the amniotic fluid. It should be as clear as water. Yellow-stained fluid may indicate a blood incompatibility between mother and fetus (the amniotic fluid is bilirubin stained from the breakdown of red blood cells). Green fluid suggests meconium (first bowel action) staining. Although meconium staining is normal in breech births because of buttocks compression, in a vertex presentation it may indicate fetal compromise.

Vaginal examination

A vaginal examination is often but not always necessary to determine the extent of cervical effacement and dilation and to confirm the fetal presentation, position and degree of descent. The woman's express consent is of course required before a vaginal examination and it must always be attended with respect and as much gentleness as possible. The woman should receive an explanation about her progress immediately after an examination. Most women are aware of dilation but not the word "effacement". It is important that women are told in a positive way; there is never an excuse for the woman to be told, "You're only x centimetres dilated." In many but not all units, after the vaginal examination results have been explained to the woman, they will be documented on a partogram.

Vital signs

Vital signs are taken at the beginning and then periodically during labour.

Temperature

Temperature is usually obtained every 4 hours during labour. A woman with a temperature greater than 37.2°C may need to be referred to a medical practitioner because it may indicate the development of infection. Unless there are accompanying symptoms, however, temperature elevation in a woman who is taking no fluids by mouth usually reflects dehydration and she should be encouraged to take fluids. Hyperthermia may also be an artefact from epidural anaesthesia (Segal, 2010). After rupture of the membranes, temperature should be taken every 2 hours, because the possibility of infection increases markedly after this time.

Pulse and respiration

Pulse and respiration rate should be measured and recorded every 4 hours during labour. A woman's pulse may be rapid on admission because she is nervous and anxious. After she has become better acquainted with her surroundings and has been assured that everything is going well, her pulse usually ranges between 70 and 80 bpm. A persistent pulse rate of more than 100 bpm suggests tachycardia from dehydration or haemorrhage. Respiratory rate during labour is usually 18 to 20 breaths per minute. Do not count respirations during contractions, because women tend to breathe rapidly from pain. Conversely, if a woman is using controlled breathing to decrease pain in labour, her respirations could be abnormally slow.

Observe for hyperventilation (rapid, deep respirations). Prolonged hyperventilation leads to the "blowing off" of carbon dioxide and accompanying symptoms of dizziness and tingling of hands and feet and tetany. Breathing into a paper bag and being reassured help to reverse this process. An even easier way is to encourage the woman to inhale through her nose.

Blood pressure

Blood pressure is usually measured and recorded every 2 to 4 hours during labour (much more frequently following an epidural because of the risk of hypotension caused by peripheral vasodilation). Always measure blood pressure between contractions, both for a woman's comfort and for accuracy, because blood pressure tends to rise 5 to 15 mmHg during a contraction. An increase in blood pressure may indicate the development of pregnancy-induced hypertension. A decrease in blood pressure or a decrease in the pulse pressure (the difference between the systolic and diastolic pressures) may indicate haemorrhage. If a woman receives an analgesic agent (such as pethidine) that tends to be hypotensive, her blood pressure should be checked approximately 15 minutes after administration to be certain that extreme hypotension is not occurring.

Urinalysis

Urine is tested for protein, ketones and glucose. If a woman reports any symptoms that suggest a urinary tract infection (e.g. burning on urination, blood in urine, extreme frequency, flank pain), a clean-catch specimen of urine is taken for culture and sensitivity.

Assessment of uterine contractions

Uterine contractions may be monitored intermittently by hand (preferred method) or continuously by an internal or external system (not recommended during normal labour). There is no evidence to support a routine electronic monitoring of the fetus or uterine contraction either on admission or during normal labour and this practice should be avoided. Continuing to monitor the duration, strength and interval between contractions by electronic monitoring during normal birth leads to an increase in caesarean birth without improving outcomes for the woman or her newborn (NSW Health, 2010).

Length of contractions

To determine the beginning of a contraction without a monitor, rest a hand on a woman's abdomen at the fundus of the uterus very gently to sense the gradual tensing and upward rising of the fundus that accompanies a contraction. It is possible to palpate this tensing approximately 5 seconds before the woman is able to feel the contraction. (Contractions are palpable when the intrauterine pressure reaches approximately 20 mmHg. The pain of a contraction is not usually felt until pressure reaches approximately 25 mmHg.) The duration of a contraction can be timed from the moment the uterus first tenses until it has relaxed again but this can be extremely annoying to the labouring woman. If the woman and fetus are coping well with the contractions, there is no syntocinon infusion or the woman is not using inhalational anaesthesia (nitrous oxide and oxygen) it is usually an unnecessary intrusion.

Intensity of contractions

In addition to observing the duration of contractions, estimate the intensity or strength. If contractions are being assessed manually, they are described as mild if the uterus does not feel more than minimally tense, as moderate if the uterus feels firm, and as strong if the uterus feels as hard as a wooden board at the peak of the contraction.

The fundus can be checked at the conclusion of the contraction, to be certain that it is relaxing and becoming soft to the touch again. This demonstrates that the uterus is not in continuous contraction but is providing a relaxation time during which blood vessels can fill to supply the fetus with adequate oxygen. This is particularly important if the woman's labour is being induced or augmented with syntocinon that can lead to uterine hyperstimulation and hypertonia.

Frequency of contractions

The frequency is timed from the beginning of one contraction to the beginning of the next. Use as light a touch as possible on a woman's abdomen while timing contractions or estimating their strength manually. The fundus of the uterus becomes tender if it has to push against the extra weight of a hand with each contraction. This is an unnecessary discomfort for a woman and will be exacerbated if the woman is labouring lying on her back or semi-sitting (not recommended).

Initial fetal assessment

The fetus is subjected to extreme pressure by uterine contractions and passage through the birth canal, so it is important to ascertain that the FHR remains within normal limits despite these pressures.

Auscultation of fetal heart sounds

In an ROA position, the fetal heart sounds are heard best in the right lower quadrant; in an LOA position, in the left lower quadrant. In posterior positions (LOP or ROP), heart sounds are loudest at a woman's side. Figure 15.6 shows how to locate heart sounds for various fetal positions. Hearing fetal heart sounds in these positions provides confirmatory information about fetal position. Conversely, recognising fetal position aids in locating fetal heart sounds.

Determine the FHR every 30 minutes during beginning labour, every 15 minutes during active labour and every 5 minutes during the second stage of labour. Intermittent auscultation of the fetal heart is the preferred method of fetal heart assessment in normal labour. Continuous electronic fetal heart rate monitoring is not recommended during normal labour and there is no evidence to support its use during normal labour (NSW Health, 2010).

To auscultate fetal heart sounds, a Pinnard's stethoscope can be used (but this means that the woman and other people in the room cannot hear it), or the fetal heart can be heard with a hand-held Doppler unit, which uses ultrasound waves that bounce off the fetal heart to produce echoes or clicking noises.

CASE STUDY QUESTION

5. You assess Cath's contractions and fetal heart rate. As Cath is experiencing a normal labour, evidence-based practice for assessing the fetal heart rate is to:
   a. Do a twenty minute CTG trace when Cath first comes into the birth suite
   b. Use CTG continuously throughout Cath's labour
   c. Don't listen to the fetal heart rate at all
   d. Listen intermittently to the fetal heart rate with a Doppler or Pinard's fetal stethoscope

SUPPORT OF A WOMAN DURING THE FIRST STAGE OF LABOUR

Labour is a natural process and should be kept free of unnecessary interventions (NSW Health, 2010). Six major principles to make labour and birth as natural as possible are:

1. Labour should begin on its own, not be artificially induced.
2. Women should be able to move about freely throughout labour or rest immersed in water but not be confined to bed (see Fig. 15.7).
3. Women should receive continuous support during labour.
4. No interventions such as intravenous fluid should be used routinely.
5. Women should be enabled to assume a non-supine (e.g. upright, side-lying, all-fours) position for birth.
6. Mother and baby should be together after the birth, with unlimited opportunity for breastfeeding (Bergman & Bergman, 2013).

Most women have had labour contractions for hours before they arrive at a maternity unit, because they

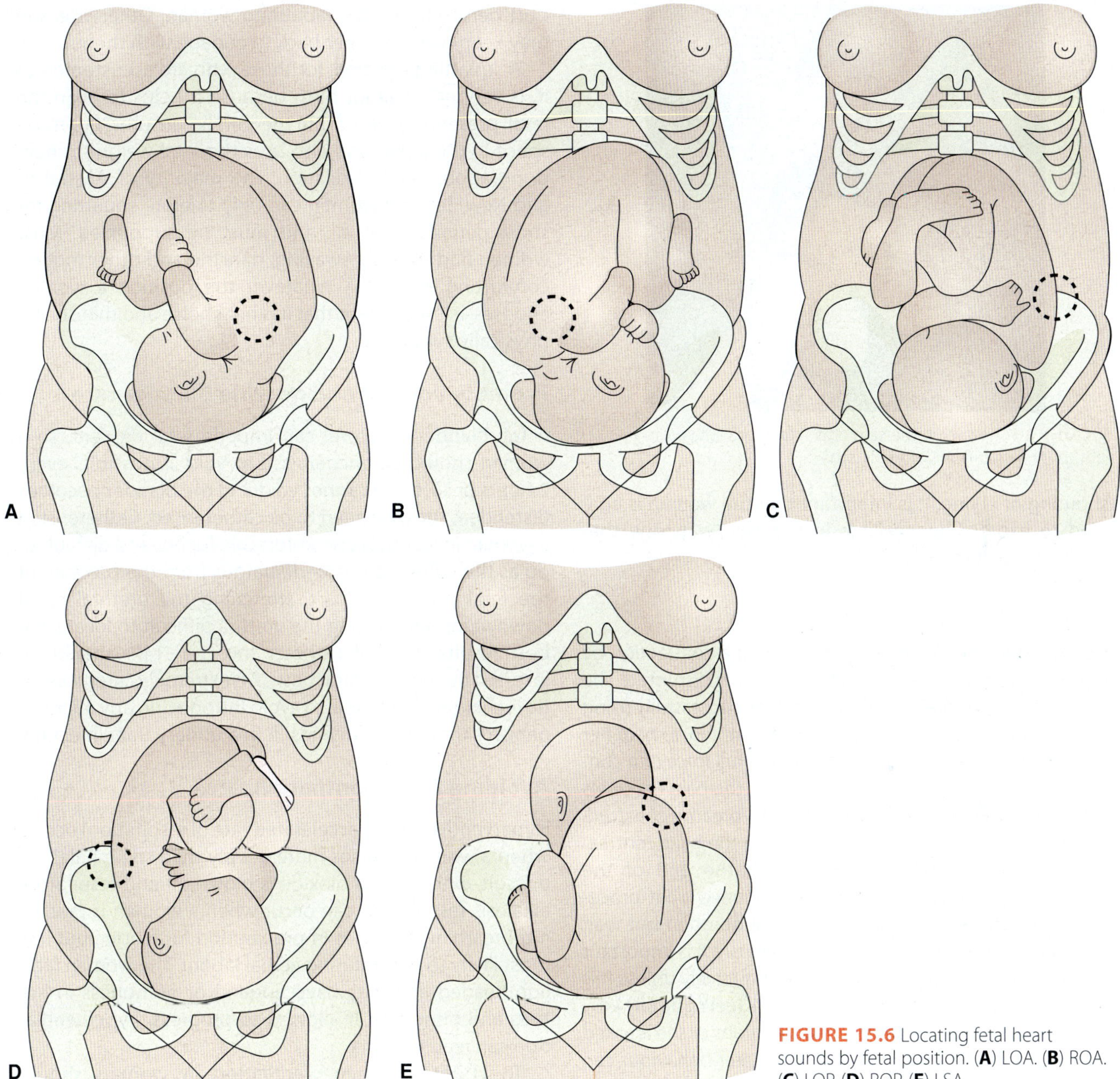

FIGURE 15.6 Locating fetal heart sounds by fetal position. (**A**) LOA. (**B**) ROA. (**C**) LOP. (**D**) ROP. (**E**) LSA.

deliberately stay at home until they are well into the first stage. This means that, most likely, they have been experiencing pain and relying on their own judgement that everything is going well for a long time. One of their chief needs when they arrive at the maternity unit, therefore, is to be reassured that everything is going well. For a woman who has been unable to manage the pain of contractions at home, pain relief may be her priority need.

Care during the first stage of labour centres on helping a woman feel confident in her ability to work with the pain and progress of labour, and maintain physiological stability. At first, it is exciting for a woman to feel labour contractions. They are little more than menstrual cramps and project a "this-is-really-happening" sensation. Soon, however, despite the fact that she is becoming more and more uncomfortable, it may seem that nothing is happening. A woman can begin to worry that something is going wrong. Giving women frequent progress reports during labour so they do not become discouraged or fearful at this seeming lack of progress can be very reassuring.

While labour is essentially an uncontrollable experience, a woman needs to feel and be in control of those aspects that she can control. Most women accomplish this by stating their preferences, for example, experiencing birth *without* pharmacological pain relief, having a water birth, using inhalational analgesia but not narcotics, or having an epidural as soon as possible in labour. Some women handle the stress of labour by becoming extremely quiet and passive. Others feel most comfortable when they can show their emotions and work with their pain by

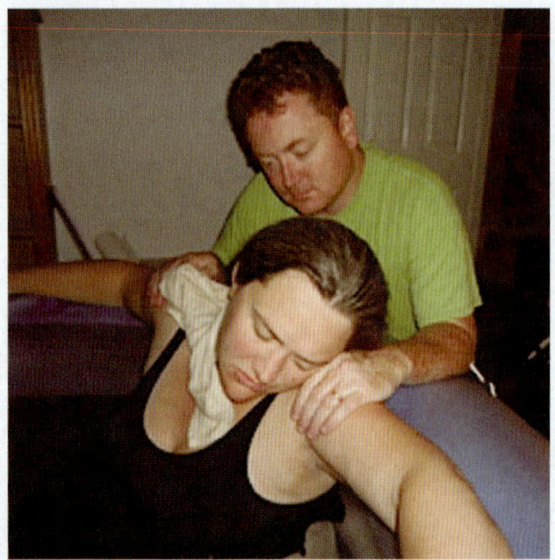

FIGURE 15.7 Water immersion offers many advantages in labour. (© Nathan and Cathy Dietsch.)

shouting or crying. It is important that the woman is enabled to express her feelings in her own way, one that works the best for her.

Respect contraction time

Do not interrupt a woman who is having a contraction by talking to her, as once her concentration is disrupted, she will experience more pain. If she has been successfully using her own strategies, for example deep breathing, to help her work with the pain, suddenly feeling the full force of a contraction can be frightening. If she tenses, the pain becomes worse, and she may doubt her ability to breathe constructively in the face of such sharp pain with the next contraction. Instead of interrupting, wait till the end of the contraction, then ask questions or announce what procedure needs to be done next, or ask the question but wait patiently for the answer. As stated previously, it is important not to expect the woman to engage cognitively unless it is essential during labour. Most women will feel rightfully very annoyed if there is idle chatter or distractions or she is asked unnecessary questions in labour. Such carer behaviour can inhibit the process of labour.

Promote change of positions

Because the bed is the main piece of furniture in a birthing room, many women assume that they are expected to lie quietly in bed during labour. However, a woman is best out of bed or sitting in a chair, kneeling, squatting or in whatever position she prefers. Encourage the woman to move around as much as she desires.

If medication such as a narcotic is given, the woman may feel dizzy and less able to move around. If a woman is in bed, encourage her to lie on her side, preferably the left side. This position causes the heavy uterus to tip forwards, away from the vena cava, allowing free blood to return from the lower extremities and adequate placental filling and circulation. Most women are comfortable in this position and adjust to it readily. Position the chair for the support person facing the labouring woman. Otherwise, she may keep turning to her back to engage with them.

A squatting position, for those who are accustomed to it, is very effective for birth because it helps to align the fetal presenting part with the cervix, ensures optimum space in the pelvis and also uses the fetal weight to help bring about cervical dilation. The majority of Australian and New Zealand women can only tolerate squatting for short periods, if at all, and must be supported. Most women find rocking, swaying, dancing and other motion comforting in labour. Whatever the position a woman chooses, it is important that it is her choice and that she be physically supported.

Promote voiding and provide bladder care

A full bladder or bowel can impede fetal descent, so a woman should be encouraged to void, if possible, every 2 hours or so. If she cannot void and the bladder becomes distended, she may need to be catheterised. Catheterising a woman in labour is uncomfortable for her and difficult to do as the vulva may be oedematous from the pressure of the fetal presenting part, stretching the urethral canal downwards and making the urethra difficult to locate. For best results, a small catheter (no. 12F–14F) should be inserted between contractions. An extremely careful aseptic technique is essential to avoid introducing any microorganisms that might then result in a urinary tract infection.

Avoiding hyperventilation

Hyperventilation (an accelerated rate of respiration) occurs when a woman exhales more deeply than she inhales. As a result, extra carbon dioxide is blown off and respiratory alkalosis results. This can occur when a woman is practising breathing exercises in preparation for labour, but it is most likely to occur during actual labour. The woman feels lightheaded and may have tingling or numbness in her toes and fingertips. If allowed to progress, hyperventilation can lead to coma.

To counteract hyperventilation, a woman should breathe in and out into a paper bag which will cause her to rebreathe the carbon dioxide she has exhaled, replacing the carbon dioxide lost. If a paper bag is unavailable, she can use her cupped hands instead.

The best way to handle hyperventilation is to prevent it by encouraging the woman to breathe slowly through her nose. Be certain when a woman is breathing rapidly that she is not hyperventilating and that she ends all breathing sessions with a long cleansing breath to help restore carbon dioxide balance. Pregnant women were once taught to use psychoprophylaxis in labour that utilised a series of prescribed breathing techniques to help her cope with the pain of contractions. Hyperventilation was not uncommon when women used psychoprophylaxis. Most childbirth educators in Australia and New Zealand now inform women about active birth strategies and the importance of following their own intuitive cues in labour.

Ensure support

Most but not all women appreciate personal touch and contact during labour. A gentle back, sacrum or foot massage can be useful. Patting a woman's arm while whispering to her that she is progressing well in labour, brushing a wisp of hair off her forehead, wiping her forehead with a cool cloth—these are indispensable methods of conveying concern. This caring attitude has several benefits including that it may make the difference in helping a woman to feel safe and able to continue in control. On the other hand, not all women care for physical contact during labour, or they want contact only from some people but not others, as enjoyment of touch is culturally and individually determined. Anyone supporting the woman must be careful to observe subtle body language as well as verbal cues to learn if, when, by whom and how the woman wants to be touched in labour.

Respect and promote the support person(s)

It is essential to respect and promote the woman's support persons. Having someone with the woman during labour is important. Everyone needs to be acquainted with the physical facilities, for example, where supplies such as towels, washcloths and ice chips are stored, so the support person can get them when required. Support people may need to be reassured that they are not only welcome, but also play an invaluable role in labour.

Encouragement, affirmation and support, not only for the woman but also for the support person, is essential because being with a labouring woman is a physically and emotionally demanding (as well as rewarding) experience. If older children are present, it is important they have a carer with them so they can be reassured about what they are experiencing and the woman and her partner are not distracted. In addition to having the father of their baby and/or a close friend or family member present, some women choose a doula or another woman to be with them in labour. This is because fathers may find it hard to provide doula-type support during labour because of their own emotional involvement in the birth. Research demonstrates that rates of syntocinon augmentation, epidural anaesthesia and caesarean birth can be reduced by doula support (Kozhimannil et al., 2014).

Support a woman's birth plan

Many women plan on using non-pharmacological pain relief measures during labour. Birth plans have many advantages and are a very useful point of discussion with the woman during pregnancy (Whitford et al., 2014) to ensure she can make truly informed choices to accept or decline what is offered. If a woman says she does not want to use pharmacological analgesia/anaesthesia in labour, she should be encouraged to write it in her birth plan and state that she does not want anyone to offer her pharmacological analgesia/anaesthesia in labour and she will ask for it if she needs it. It is imperative that health professionals and support people respect a woman's birth plan.

Avoiding dehydration

Unless "high risk", there is no justification for withholding food or fluids from a labouring woman (Singata et al., 2013). The amount and type of oral fluids a woman has in labour, should be in response to her own desires and not prescribed. As labour progresses, many women feel like eating or drinking less. Ice chips or sips of fluid through a straw may be useful. A woman's mouth and lips may become uncomfortably dry from mouth breathing. Applying a cream to her lips or suggesting that she suck on ice chips to relieve this discomfort can be helpful.

CARE OF A WOMAN DURING THE SECOND STAGE OF LABOUR

The second stage of labour is the time from full cervical dilation to birth of the newborn. Even women who have taken childbirth education classes may be surprised at the intensity of the contractions in this phase of labour. As stated above, at the start of the second stage, some women's contractions will slow down and they may or may not have an overwhelming urge to push with these contractions. In the past, women were instructed when and how to push and even to hold their breath while they pushed. This is no longer recommended. It is best practice that women are no longer instructed when and how to push; rather, they are encouraged to assume any position which is comfortable for them and push in response to their own intuition (Holvey, 2014).

A support person plays a vital role during this time. Their gentle affirmation and physical and emotional support can be energising. As well, their participation creates an important sharing time, after the birth, that gives them a sense of family for the first time (Kozhimannil et al., 2014).

Positioning for birth

Women can choose a variety of positions for birth. At one time, the lithotomy or semi-recumbent/semi-sitting positions were the preferred positions for birth, but this is no longer so. Given the choice and left to their own intuition, women will usually select a more upright, forward leaning position such as on all-fours to give birth. Women experience side-lying, kneeling, sitting on a birth stool or upright positions as more comfortable. There is less risk of perineal trauma and the baby has better APGAR scores (is in good condition at birth) when the woman has not been made to be on her back for birth (DiFranco & Curl, 2014).

Promoting effective second-stage pushing

For the most effective pushing during the second stage of labour, a woman should wait to feel the urge to push even

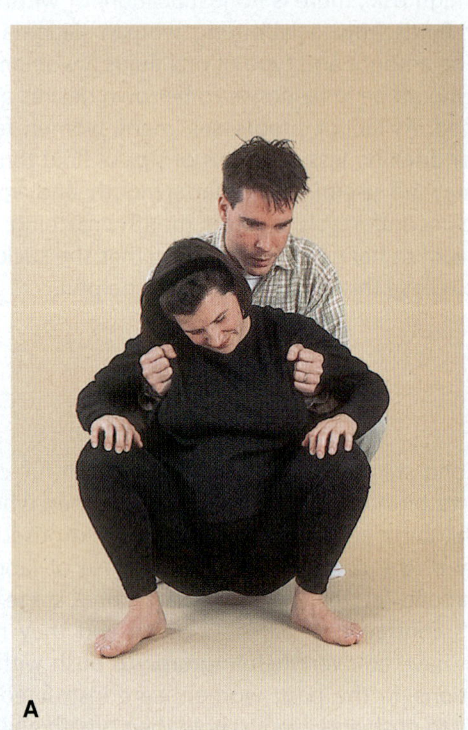

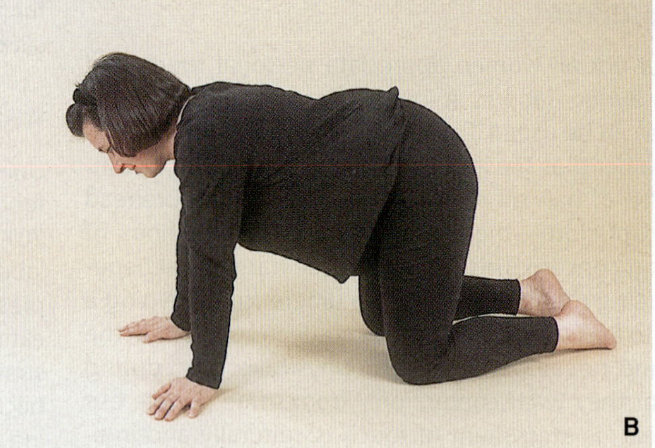

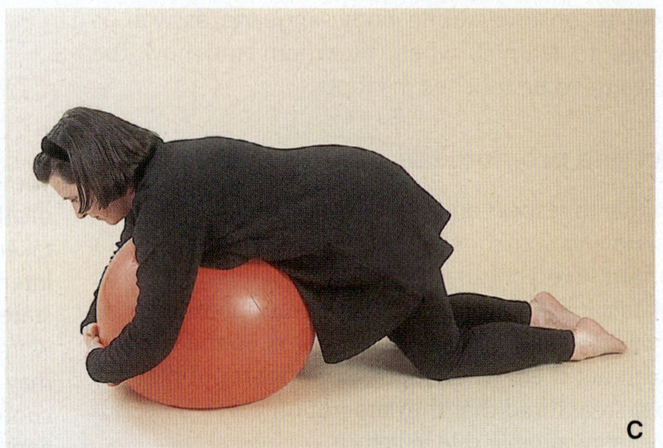

FIGURE 15.8 Positions for pushing during second stage labour. (**A**) Squatting with support person. (**B**) All-fours. (**C**) All-fours with chest support. (© Barbara Proud.)

if a vaginal examination has revealed that she is fully dilated. She will intuitively push with contractions and rest between them. Pushing is usually best done in an upright, squatting or all-fours position rather than lying flat, to allow gravity to aid her effort (DiFranco & Curl, 2014; Holvey, 2014) (see Fig. 15.8).

Perineal cleaning

As the woman pushes, the pressure of the fetal head on the bowel may cause faecal material to be expelled from the rectum. This can easily be sponged away if it is a problem but do not use antiseptics (Harman & Wakeford, 2014).

Birth

As stated at the beginning of the chapter, only a registered midwife or medical practitioner (or a supervised midwifery or medical student) is legally permitted to act as the professional assisting the woman to give birth.

A woman who has not had anaesthesia experiences the birth of the head as a flash of pain or a burning sensation, as if someone had momentarily poured hot water on her perineum. It is a short-lived but intense sensation and prompts the woman to stop pushing.

A baby is considered born when the whole body is born. This is the time that should be noted and recorded as the time of birth. It is essential that the moment of birth be respected. No-one but the woman or her partner should announce the sex of the baby as most parents enjoy discovering the gender of the baby for themselves, so this should be respected. Many parents are so enamoured with their new baby that it takes them a little while to even think about checking the sex. With the birth of the infant, the second stage of labour is complete.

THE THIRD AND FOURTH STAGES OF LABOUR

The third stage of labour is the time from the birth of the baby until the placenta and membranes are delivered. For most women, this is a time of excitement, because the infant has safely been born. The fourth stage includes the first few hours after birth. It signals the beginning of dramatic changes because it marks the beginning of a new family.

Clamping and cutting the cord

The cord continues to pulsate for a few minutes after birth, and then the pulsation ceases. Delaying the cutting until pulsation ceases allows as much as 100 mL of blood to pass from the placenta into the newborn; this helps ensure an adequate red blood cell count in the newborn. There is no evidence to support cutting the cord before it stops pulsating (but there is much evidence against it); both term and preterm infants benefit from delayed cord clamping (Hanson & Simkin, 2011; McAdams, 2014).

Skin-to-skin contact

Even before the cord is cut, the new parents can start to enjoy time and skin-to-skin contact with their newborn (Harman & Wakeford, 2014). Both the mother and her partner usually want to see and touch their newborn immediately; this assures them the baby is well and is an important step in establishing a parent–child relationship. When a woman does not have an epidural in place, the physiological surge of adrenaline that occurs late in second stage ensures that both the mother and newborn are energised, with dilated pupils eager to make eye contact with one another. The adrenaline surge helps the newborn adapt to extrauterine life and prepares them to breastfeed. If left undisturbed and skin-to-skin with their mother, the newborn can "crawl" from their mother's abdomen to the breast and attach and suckle without assistance (Henderson, 2011). Skin-to-skin contact promotes breastfeeding and is associated with longer duration of breastfeeding.

Immediate postpartum assessment

Following expulsion of the placenta, the woman's vital signs are checked regularly. The woman's fundus is palpated for size, consistency and position. The midwife will observe the amount and characteristics of lochia (vaginal loss), her perineum is checked and repaired if needed and she is given a perineal pad to apply.

The woman is encouraged to shower *only* after she has spent time with her baby skin-to-skin *and* the baby has breastfed (Harman & Wakeford, 2014). While a support person has the baby, the woman can shower and change into warm, clean clothes. A woman often experiences a chill and shaking sensation minutes after birth. This may be because of the low temperature of the birthing room but may also be a result of the sudden release of pressure on pelvic nerves, from having an epidural or as the adrenaline levels slowly decrease. In any event, it is a normal phenomenon but it can be frightening to the woman. She may associate the shaking chill with fever or infection and worry she will be ill at a time when she most wants to be well to care for her new child. She can be reassured that this is a normal, transitory sensation.

Aftercare

It is the beginning of the postpartum period or the fourth stage of labour when the woman is at particular risk of postpartum haemorrhage, whether her third stage was physiological or managed actively. Women who have syntocinon during their labour (induction or augmentation) are at particular risk of haemorrhage (as are women who have undergone a caesarean section). In addition, a woman may be so exhausted, or under the influence of narcotics, that she may be unable to assess her own condition or report any changes. Specific assessments done during this time are continued throughout the postpartum period.

UNIQUE CONCERNS OF A WOMAN IN LABOUR

A woman without a partner

Some women have chosen to labour without their partner. Such women may appreciate having a family member or close friend act as their support person. A woman who has no support person especially needs a supportive professional to be with her (Kozhimannil et al., 2014).

A woman who will be placing her baby for adoption

If a woman has decided to place her baby for adoption, she needs to be an active participant in her labour and birth experience and be enabled to hold and care for her child as desired. Although this decision may have been made during pregnancy, once the woman holds the baby in her arms, the prospect of giving up the child may be more painful than she realised. The woman needs unbiased and non-directional support no matter what decision she eventually makes.

A woman whose baby will be an "assumption of care" (taken from her)

If a woman's baby is to be taken from her soon after birth to protect the baby, this is called being an "assumption of care" and is an extremely traumatic experience for everyone. Women have every right and their baby will benefit from skin-to-skin contact with their mother and receiving colostrum from her breast. It needs to be the woman's choice as to whether she does this or not and it is the midwife's role never to coerce the woman but to support her in the decision she makes (Everitt, Homer & Fenwick, 2013).

Vaginal birth after caesarean birth

Women who have had a previous caesarean birth that involved a low transverse uterine incision can plan for vaginal birth with their next pregnancy (Qazi, Akhtar & Khan, 2013). The length of labour for vaginal birth after caesarean birth is usually comparable to that of primiparas (women having their first baby) if they have not laboured with their first birth, not multiparas (subsequent babies), because it is the first vaginal birth. Most women are anxious for vaginal birth to be successful so that they do not have to undergo surgery again.

CASE STUDY QUESTION

6. Cath has birthed her baby and both are healthy. The most important care is now to:
   a. Attach the baby to her breast to prevent bleeding and ensure the baby receives colostrum
   b. Weigh the baby and provide the necessary immunisations
   c. Ensure skin-to-skin contact can occur for Cath and her newborn in a warm environment (e.g. a warm blanket placed over both)
   d. Inform Cath of the sex of her baby

Key points for review

Woman-centred care is at the core of labour and birth. Woman-centred care is a concept that is based on feminist ethics and implies that care:

- Is focused on the woman's individual, unique needs, expectations and aspirations, rather than the needs of the institutions or professionals
- Is holistic in approach and recognises each woman's emotional, physical, spiritual, social and cultural needs as she defines them
- Recognises the woman's right to self-determination in terms of choice, control and continuity of care
- Recognises the woman's right to make informed choices (and refusals) with assistance, when requested by health professionals
- Is informed by scientific evidence, by collective and individual expertise and by intuition
- Encompasses the needs of the baby (born and unborn), the woman's family, significant others and community, as identified and negotiated by the woman herself
- Includes collaboration and consultation with health professionals as required and while focusing on the woman herself, rather than institutions or the professionals involved (Leap, 2009).

Critical thinking exercises

1. Describe the philosophy of woman-centred care during labour.
2. From your reading and observation to date, why do you think continuity of care with a known midwife is likely to bring about best outcomes for the woman and her newborn?
3. List strategies that a support person, midwives and students can use to help facilitate normal birth.

Resources

For an extensive range of additional resources to enhance teaching and learning and to facilitate understanding of this chapter, please see the text's accompanying website located on thePoint at http://thepoint.lww.com.

References

Australian College of Midwives. (2011). *Philosophy of the midwife.* Canberra: Australian College of Midwives.

Bergman, J. & Bergman, N. (2013). Whose choice? Advocating birthing practices according to baby's biological needs. *Journal of Perinatal Education, 22*(1), 8–13.

Cooke, A. (2010). When will we change practice and stop directing pushing in labour? *British Journal of Midwifery, 18*(2), 76–81.

Davies, L. (2011). Vaginal examinations in normal labour. *Essentially MIDIRS, 2*(4), 38–41.

Dietsch, E., Martin, T., Shackleton, P., Davies, C., McLeod, M. & Alston, M. (2011). Australian Aboriginal kinship: A means to enhance maternal well-being. *Women and Birth, 24*(2), 58–64.

DiFranco, J. & Curl, M. (2014). Healthy birth practice # 5: Avoid giving birth on your back and follow your body's urge to push. *Journal of Perinatal Education, 23*(4), 207–210.

Downe, S. & Dykes, F. (2010). Counting time in pregnancy and labour. In C. McCourt (Ed.). *Childbirth, Midwifery and Concepts of Time.* New York: Berghahn Books, pp. 61–83.

Everitt, L., Homer, C. & Fenwick, J. (2013). Assumption of care of a newborn: How can you be prepared? *Women and Birth, 26*(1), S6.

Friedman, E. (1978). *Labor, Clinical Evaluation and Management* (2nd ed.). New York: Appleton-Century-Crofts.

Hanson, L. & Simkin, P. (2011). Optimal newborn transition and third and fourth stage labor management. In P. Simpkin & R. Anchets (Eds.). *The Labor Progress Handbook: Early Interventions to Prevent and Treat Dystocia* (3rd ed.). Chichester, UK: Wiley-Blackwell, pp. 224–241.

Harman, T. & Wakeford, A. (Producers). (2014). *Microbirth* [DVD]. Available from <www.oneworldbirth.net>.

Henderson, A. (2011). Understanding the breast crawl. *Nursing for Women's Health, 15*(4), 296–307.

Holvey, N. (2014). Supporting women in the second stage of labour. *British Journal of Midwifery, 22*(3), 182–186.

Kozhimannil, K., Attansio, L., Jou, J., Joarnt, L., Johnson, P. & Gjerdingen, D. (2014). Abstracts for web exclusive content. Potential benefits of increased access to doula support in childbirth. *American Journal of Managed Care, 20*(8), 610.

Leap, N. (2009). Woman-centred or women-centred care: Does it matter? *British Journal of Midwifery, 17*(1), 12–16.

McAdams, R. (2014). Time to implement delayed cord clamping. *Obstetrics & Gynecology, 123*(3), 549–552.

McNabb, M. (2011). Fertilization embryonic, fetal and placental development. In S. Macdonald & J. Magill Cuerden (Eds.). *Mayes' Midwifery* (14th ed.). London: Bailliere Tindall, pp. 353–378.

McNamara, P. (2012). Fetal sleep. *International Journal of Childbirth Education, 27*(1), 58–63.

Madden, K., Turnbull, D., Cyna, A., Adelson, P. & Wilkinson, C. (2013). Pain relief for childbirth: The preferences of pregnant women, midwives and obstetricians. *Women and Birth, 26*(1), 33–40.

Mander, R. (2011). *Pain in Childbearing and Its Control: Key Issues for Midwives and Women.* Chichester, UK: Wiley-Blackwell.

NSW Health. (2010). Maternity–towards normal birth in NSW. Policy Directive PD2010_45. North Sydney: Department of Health, accessed 5 June 2015 at <www.health.nsw.gov.au/policies/pd/2010/pdf/ PD2010_045.pdf>.

Phiri, J., Dietsch, E. & Bonner, A. (2010). Cultural safety and its importance for Australian midwifery practice. *Collegian, 17*(3), 105–111.

Priddis, H., Dahlen, H. & Schmied, V. (2012). What are the facilitators, inhibitors and implications of birth positioning? A review of the literature. *Women and Birth, 25*(3), 100–106.

Qazi, Q., Akhtar, Z. & Khan, A. (2013). Maternal and foetal outcome in successful vaginal birth after caesarean section versus repeat caesarean section. *Journal of Postgraduate Medical Institute, 27*(4), 414–418.

Sandall, J., Soltani, H., Gates, S., Shennan, A. & Devane, D. (2013). Midwife-led continuity models versus other models of care for childbearing women. *Cochrane Database of Systematic Reviews 2013,* Issue 8. Art. No.: CD004667.

Sandstrom, A., Cnattingius, S., Wikstrom, A. & Stephansson, O. (2012). Labour dystocia – risk of recurrence and instrumental delivery in following labour – a population-based cohort study. *BJOG: An International Journal of Obstetrics and Gynaecology, 119*(13), 1648–1656.

Segal, S. (2010). Labor epidural analgesia and maternal fever. *Anesthesia and Analgesia. 111*(6), 1467–1475.

Singata, M., Tranmer, J. & Gyte, G. (2013). Restricting oral fluid and food during labour. *Cochrane Database of Systematic Reviews 2013,* Issue 8. Art. No.: CD003930.

Whitford, H., Entwistle, V., van Teijlingen, E., Aitchison, P., Davidson, T., Humphrey, T. & Tucker, J. (2014). Use of a birth plan within woman-held maternity records: A qualitative study with women and staff in Northeast Scotland. *Birth, 41*(3), 283–289.

Wickham, S. (2011). Plenary session. *Passage to Motherhood Conference,* Brisbane, 4–7 May.

Suggested readings

Dahlen, H. (2014). Managing risk or facilitating safety? *International Journal of Childbirth, 4*(2), 66–68.

Dietsch, E., Shackleton, P., Davies, C., Alston, M. & McLeod, M. (2010). 'Mind you, there's no anaesthetist on the road': Women's experiences of labouring en route. *Rural and Remote Health, 10,* 1371 (online).

Lothian, J. (2012). Risk, safety, and choice in childbirth. *Journal of Perinatal Education, 21*(1), 45–47.

O'Hare, J. & Fallon, A. (2011). Women's experience of control in labour and childbirth. *British Journal of Midwifery, 19*(3), 164–169.

Stevens, J., Dahlen, H., Peters, K. & Jackson, D. (2011). Midwives' and doulas' perspectives on the role of the doula in Australia: A qualitative study. *Midwifery, 27,* 509–516.

Chapter 16

Providing comfort during labour and birth

Chapter 15 discussed the process of labour and care for a woman in labour. This chapter adds information to your knowledge base about how to work with and support women experiencing pain in labour.

LEARNING OBJECTIVES

After mastering the contents of this chapter, you should be able to:

1. Describe the physiological basis of contractions during labour and how analgesia, anaesthesia and alternative therapies can be used to promote a woman's comfort during labour and birth.
2. Compare and contrast the concepts of pain and suffering in labour.
3. Use critical thinking to analyse ways in which to maintain woman-centred care when analgesia and anaesthesia are used in childbirth.
4. Consider interventions to promote comfort during labour and birth.
5. Evaluate common complementary and pharmacological measures used by women during labour and birth.
6. Identify areas related to promoting comfort during labour that could benefit from additional research or application of evidence-based practice.

KEY TERMS

- anaesthesia
- analgesia
- doula
- endorphins
- epidural anaesthesia
- pain
- transcutaneous electrical nerve stimulation (TENS)
- water immersion

CASE STUDY

Susan Baranca is a primipara (experiencing her first labour and birth) and she has been admitted to the birthing suite in early labour. Susan is experiencing slight, irregular contractions and her cervix is dilated to 3 cm. She tells you her sister had an epidural when in labour for the birth of her baby 3 months ago but following the epidural which was only partially effective, her sister's baby was born via forceps and her sister developed a serious post-epidural headache. Based on her sister's experience and what she learnt in childbirth classes, Susan is reluctant to have an epidural but otherwise says she will "just go with the flow" as far as strategies to work with the pain of labour are concerned.

CASE STUDY QUESTION

1. What are some immediate strategies you could use to support Susan and her partner as she works with the pain in labour?

From Chapter 15 you will recall that, in Australia, only registered midwives and medical practitioners (and midwifery and medical students under the direct supervision of a registered midwife or medical practitioner) are legally entitled to be responsible for professional care for labouring and women giving birth. There may be occasions when a nursing student or registered nurse acts as a support person or they have the privilege of being with a labouring woman, and this chapter provides valuable information on what they are likely to observe as well as strategies that can be used to provide optimal support. Throughout this chapter the concept of woman-centred care during labour and birth will be discussed. By definition, woman-centred care includes any person (usually her partner, family or close friend) the woman identifies as being significant to her (Australian College of Midwives, 2011).

Many women (and midwives) prefer the concept of "working with pain/working through pain" rather than pain management (Leap, Dodwell & Newburn, 2010). The Leap model of working with women experiencing pain in labour has thus been more influential on contemporary Australian midwifery practice than a pain management model per se (Mander, 2011).

Before discussing the strategies that women can use to help them work with pain in labour, it is important to compare and contrast two important concepts—pain and suffering in labour. Pain in labour is physiological, not pathological and helps to create strong, confident, competent mothers. Labour is not just about making babies, it is about making mothers (Leap, Dodwell & Newburn, 2010). Pain causes labouring women to seek a place of safety and the support of those she knows will support and protect her and her newborn (Leap et al., 2010). Pain in labour not only provides feedback to the woman and her midwife about her progress in labour, it also marks the occasion of labour as one of life's most challenging but also empowering experiences. Pain causes women to pause and gives them time to prepare emotionally as well as physically for the birth of their baby: a newborn who will not survive without protection and nurturing (Candib & Shields, 2010). Pain leads to avoidance behaviour; for example, guiding the woman to mobilise and adopt physiological positioning. Burning perineal pain will stop the woman from forcefully pushing her baby out of her vagina, which helps to maintain her perineal integrity and ensures a more gentle birth. Pain in labour triggers the neurohormonal cascade of oxytocin and endorphin, and the release of adrenalin in second stage labour (Buckley, 2011).

Pain and suffering are not synonymous (Mander, 2011). Although pain and suffering often occur together, a woman in labour can suffer without experiencing pain or can experience pain with co-existing satisfaction and empowerment but no suffering. A woman who is feeling powerless or helpless when others are not respecting her wishes, or who fears that she has insufficient resources to cope with labour, or that she or her baby are at risk of harm or death will experience suffering. Suffering in labour will increase if the woman is feeling lonely, isolated or alone; this commonly occurs when women living in rural and remote areas of Australia are forced to leave their local communities to give birth. Suffering is increased when the woman is treated unkindly or with disrespect or she feels ignored, bullied or misunderstood (Dietsch et al., 2010). The physical sensation of pain is magnified when it is accompanied by suffering. Ironically, the intention to eliminate pain in labour may exacerbate suffering if the woman experiences a sense of helplessness or believes that others have made the decision for her to have pain relief. A woman's satisfaction with her labour and birth is correlated with the quality of support she receives, involvement in decision making and her personal expectations of childbirth (Jones et al., 2011).

The focus of medicalised labour and birth is to eliminate or at least significantly reduce pain in labour through pharmacological means. The focus of the midwifery model of care is to prevent suffering in labour (Nolan, 2010). Woman-centred midwifery support of women experiencing pain in labour does not argue against pharmacological analgesia and anaesthesia. It argues for a woman's right to receive accurate, unbiased information about all strategies a woman experiencing pain in labour might utilise, and then for her to be fully supported to experience labour and birth as she chooses.

Concerns about the pain that accompanies labour and birth can dominate a pregnant woman's thoughts about childbirth during pregnancy and particularly as the baby's due date approaches. Providing information during antenatal visits about how labour works naturally to provide women with endorphins that help to increase their coping skills can help allay some of these fears. As well, information about the numerous non-pharmacological and pharmacological strategies available to assist women to cope with pain can also be helpful. However, for some women, the labour experience is so overwhelming, or so much greater than expected, that they elect to use an analgesic or a regional anaesthetic, even if they had not originally planned to use pharmacological strategies. For other women, their ability to work with the pain in labour and the support they receive means that their plan to use analgesia or anaesthesia becomes redundant and the experience itself becomes incredibly empowering. Only the woman herself knows the pain she is experiencing and her ability to work with that pain.

WOMEN WORKING WITH PAIN IN LABOUR

Pain is a subjective, personal symptom; it is what the person says it is and is present when the person says it is (Kaviani et al., 2014). It is unique to each individual, so a woman is the only person who can describe or know the extent of her own pain. To assess the amount of pain a woman is experiencing in labour, those who are supporting her need to listen carefully to what she is saying as well as looking for subtle signs such as facial tension, flushing or pallor, hands clenched in fists, rapid breathing or rapid pulse rate (see Box 16.1).

BOX 16.1 Assessment ✻ Assessing pain level for a woman in labour

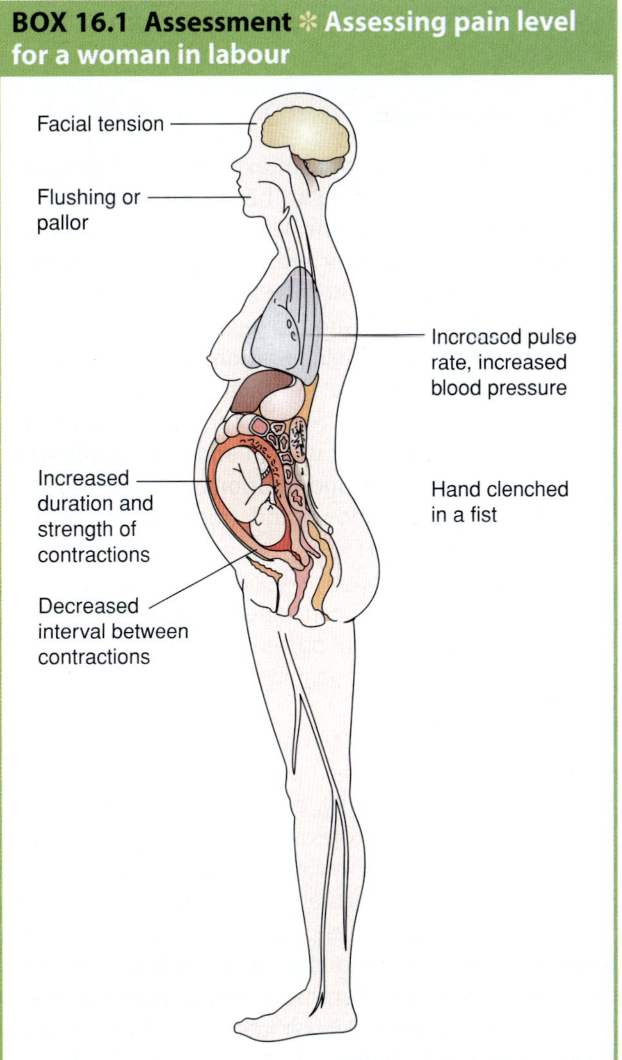

Experience of pain during childbirth

Pain accompanies labour contractions for several different reasons and is manifested in different ways in individual women. The perception of pain is, in part, culturally determined. Some women believe that being stoic and nonverbal is what is expected of them. Others believe that expressing their pain by screaming or verbalising their feelings is the best way to work with their pain. If a woman is not proficient in English, it may be particularly difficult for her to describe her level of pain.

Many women elect to work with the pain of labour by adopting physiological positioning, breathing calmly and deeply, using water immersion and the like. Other women elect to use pharmacological strategies to either assist them to work with pain or in an attempt to reduce or eliminate labour pain. Whether or not a woman elects to use pharmacological and/or non-pharmacological strategies is both situationally and culturally determined. In a culture in which birth is seen as a "natural" process, less analgesia is generally desired. Women who have an effective support person and a known midwife with them generally request less pharmacological pain relief than those who do not (Hodnett et al., 2011; Sandall et al., 2013).

Perception of pain

The amount of pain a woman experiences during contractions differs according to her expectations of and preparation for labour; the length of her labour; the position of her fetus; the presence of fear, anxiety or worry; her body image; her self-efficacy; and the availability of support people around her. Women who believe that they can control their situation (have self-efficacy) are more apt to report a satisfactory birth experience than those who do not feel in control. However, the most important mediator of pain and suffering is when the woman feels safe and supported in her birthing environment with a known and trusted carer (Homer, 2013; Sandall et al., 2013).

Fetal position is a physical variable that can influence the degree of pain a woman experiences. For example, if the fetus is in an occipital posterior position, the woman often reports intense or nagging back pain, even between contractions.

Pain is perceived differently by different individuals because of psychosocial, physiological and cultural responses and importantly, because of the environment that maternity care professionals provide. The body's ability to produce and maintain **endorphins** (naturally occurring opiate-like substances) influences a labouring woman's overall pain threshold, tolerance and perception. Some women who come into labour believing the pain will be horrible may be surprised afterwards to realise that the agony they expected never materialised. On the other hand, women who thought that pain would be minimal can be overwhelmed by its intensity.

INTERVENTIONS FOR WOMEN IN LABOUR

The pattern of interventions to assist women to work with pain in labour has undergone a process of change in industrialised societies. Historically, there was a philosophy of no intervention (none given because it was unavailable or it was believed that pain in labour was a "woman's lot"). In the middle of last century, the philosophy changed so that pharmacological intervention was thought to be in a woman's best interest and always required. The current philosophy is that a woman should be provided with unbiased, accurate and evidence-based information on her own physiological power, and pharmacological and non-pharmacological interventions. It is the woman herself who should be enabled to choose how she would best like to work with her pain during labour, within the limits of safety.

The overriding principle is that pain in normal labour and birth is physiological and it is the woman herself who knows how she would like to work with that pain. For those women who would prefer to use interventions to assist them, the following information provides a brief outline of non-pharmacological and pharmacological interventions.

Support from a doula

A woman's partner or the father of her child has traditionally served as the chief support person in labour. However, some husbands or fathers find it difficult to provide effective support in labour because of their emotional involvement in the birth. Women who are aware that they may not have effective one-to-one support in labour should be encouraged to identify an additional person who could come with them and provide support. A **doula** is a woman who is experienced in childbirth, but without professional credentials; she guides and assists women in labour. Having a doula can increase a woman's self-esteem as well as decrease rates of syntocinon augmentation, epidural anaesthesia and caesarean birth (Green & Hotelling, 2014).

CASE STUDY QUESTION

2. Susan asks you to explain the purpose of a doula in labour. Your best answer would be:
   a. "She can time contractions to keep them from becoming too long."
   b. "She can cook you something to keep you from becoming dehydrated."
   c. "She can serve as a support person during your labour."
   d. "She replaces your husband as your support person during labour."

Non-pharmacological interventions

Non-pharmacological measures may be used on their own or to complement a woman's own physiological coping strategies or pharmacological interventions. Although not exhaustive or complete, a list of non-pharmacological strategies is presented below.

Acupressure and acupuncture

These interventions involve the activation of acupressure and acupuncture points. This results in the release of endorphins which can be helpful, especially in the first stage of labour (Smith et al., 2011).

Aromatherapy

This is the use of aromatic oils to complement emotional and physical wellbeing. Their use is based on the principle that the sense of smell plays a significant role in overall health. When an essential oil is inhaled, its molecules are transported via the olfactory system to the limbic system in the brain. The brain responds to particular aromas with emotional responses. When applied externally in a diluted form (non-diluted essential oils should never be applied directly to the skin), the oils are absorbed by the skin and carried throughout the body. Oils used may be able to penetrate cell walls and transport nutrients or oxygen to the inside of cells. Jasmine and lavender are oils thought to be especially useful in labour to reduce anxiety (Jones et al., 2011; Smith, Collins & Crowther, 2011).

Biofeedback

Biofeedback is based on the belief that people have control and can regulate internal events such as heart rate and pain responses. Women who are interested in using biofeedback for pain relief in labour must attend several sessions during pregnancy to condition themselves to regulate their pain response. During these sessions, a biofeedback apparatus is used to measure muscle tone or the woman's ability to relax (Barragán Loayza, Solà & Juandó Prats, 2011).

Doula support

Doula support involves using a female support person, usually employed (although may be voluntary) by the woman to provide her with support or to provide additional support for both her and her partner during labour. Having a doula can increase a woman's self-esteem as well as decrease the rates of syntocinon augmentation, epidural anaesthesia and caesarean birth (Hodnett et al., 2011; Green & Hotelling, 2014).

Heat or cold application

Both of these can be of particular assistance in relieving back pain. Women who experience back pain in labour may find the application of heat to the lower back, by a heating pad or moist compress, comforting. Women who become warm from the exertion of labour can find application of a cool washcloth to the forehead comforting. When a woman would prefer not to drink fluids in labour, ice chips to suck on to relieve mouth dryness are also refreshing. Some women find the administration of hot, wet compresses to their perineum very helpful in the second stage of labour (Chaillet et al., 2014).

Herbal preparations

Herbs have traditionally been used to reduce pain with dysmenorrhoea or labour, although there is little factual support for their effectiveness. Examples include raspberry leaves, fennel and life root. Some herbs (and essential oils) are contraindicated in labour, for example, clary sage that can cause hypertonic uterine contractions and fetal compromise (Tiran, 2011).

Massage, therapeutic touch and reflexology

These are all used to help relax tense muscles and convey caring, kindness, support and compassion to the labouring woman. Although the action is not well-documented, touch and massage probably work to relieve pain by increasing the release of endorphins. Massage, especially, can be helpful in the first stage of labour (Tiran, 2011) (see Fig. 16.1).

Relaxation strategies

Relaxation strategies may include yoga, meditation, music therapy, prayer, deep breathing, hypnosis and/or visualisation or any combination. Some women use relaxation strategies as a distraction technique. Concentrating intently on an object is another method of distraction. A woman may choose to use a photograph of someone important to her or some other image she finds appealing. She concentrates on it during contractions (focusing). Other women concentrate on a mental image, such as waves rolling onto a beach (imagery). Whether a woman is using relaxation strategies or not, it is important not to ask unnecessary questions or engage a woman in cognitive

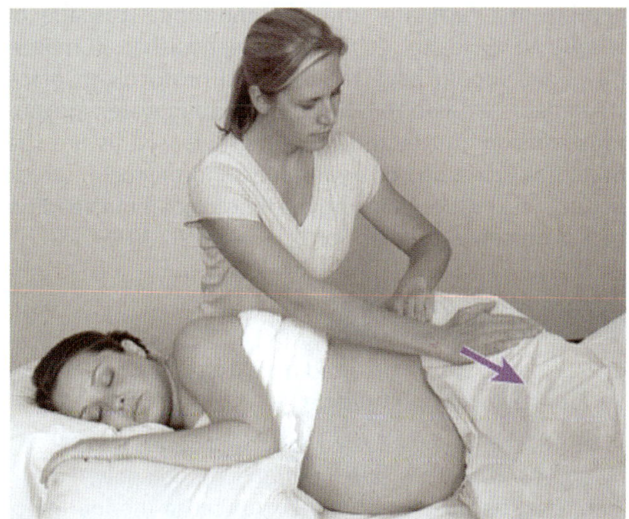

FIGURE 16.1 Massage may be helpful in the first stage of labour. (Stager, L. (2009). *Nurturing Massage for Pregnancy*. Philadelphia: Lippincott Williams & Wilkins.)

activity while she has a contraction or when her labour is established and claiming her concentration. Calmbirthing© is a particular relaxation strategy often used by Australian women and their midwives. In addition to conscious relaxation, having a woman mobilise and find the position in labour that is most comfortable for her can also be helpful. Many women find their own choice of music in labour to be very helpful (Beckett, 2011).

Sterile water injections

Sterile water injections is a technique some women find helpful while others prefer not to submit to injections. Intracutaneous nerve stimulation (INS) is a technique of counter-irritation involving the intradermal injection of sterile water or saline along the borders of the sacrum to relieve low back pain during labour. The sterile water injections, which cause a short-lived but intense stinging sensation, are thought to be effective by "closing the gate" to the perception of pain in labour (gate control theory of pain) and enhancing endorphin secretion (Jones et al., 2011).

Transcutaneous electrical nerve stimulation (TENS)

Transcutaneous electrical nerve stimulation (TENS) utilises a device that emits low voltage electrical impulses which serve to "close the gate" to the perception of labour pain and also to increase endorphin secretion. It is most useful when the woman starts the TENS intervention early in labour. Many women like a strategy that they can control while others do not like the sense that they are attached to a machine, especially one that cannot be used in the shower or bath. TENS may reduce anxiety and increase a sense of wellbeing which in turn can help labour to progress (Jones et al., 2011).

Water immersion

Water immersion aids relaxation, mobility and pain perception and facilitates the neurohormonal cascade of labour. NSW Health (2010) recommends that all maternity units should have facilities and protocols in place that enable women to labour and birth in water. Placental perfusion and fetal flexion are increased as are the maternal secretions of endorphins and oxytocin, which in turn help reduce pain and the length of labour, leading to less obstetric interventions (Jones et al., 2011).

CASE STUDY QUESTION

3. Susan asks you if she could have a bath during labour. Your best answer would be:
   a. "No. No-one is allowed to bathe during labour."
   b. "Yes, absolutely, and I will run it for you now."
   c. "No, because warm water can cause uterine infections."
   d. "Yes, as long as you know that warm water has no effect."

Pharmacological interventions

Pharmacological interventions include **analgesia**, which reduces or decreases awareness of pain, and **anaesthesia**, which causes partial or complete loss of sensation. Virtually all medication given during labour crosses the placenta and has some effect on the fetus, which makes it important for a woman to receive as little medication as possible. On the other hand, labour should not test a woman beyond what she envisages as her own limits of endurance. There is no perfect analgesic agent for labour or birth that does not have an effect on labour, the mother and the fetus. A brief list of common pharmacological interventions used by Australian and New Zealand women in labour is presented below.

Inhalational analgesia

This can be used by women to help them work with the pain of labour. In Australia, nitrous oxide (in 50% oxygen) is commonly used. Having been instructed on how to use it, the woman can easily administer it herself while experiencing contractions. Maternal side effects may include drowsiness, hallucinations, nausea and vomiting, hyperventilation and tetany. Maternal and fetal hypoxia are rare, but possible effects, especially if someone other than the mother is administering the inhalational analgesia (Jones et al., 2011). There is concern for the wellbeing of health professionals including midwives who are exposed to nitrous oxide and oxygen for prolonged periods of time, especially in a poorly ventilated room as it is associated with lowered fertility, spontaneous abortion, preterm birth and lowered concentrations of vitamin B12 (Jordan, 2010).

Narcotics (opioids)

These medications may be given during labour because of their potent analgesic and sedative effects. However, all drugs in this category cause fetal central nervous system depression to some extent so need to be used cautiously (McKenna & Mirkov, 2014). Narcotics can be given via intravenous, epidural, intrathecal, buccal, oral, transdermal or intramuscular routes. Morphine and pethidine are the most common opioids used in labour and are advantageous because they have additional sedative and antispasmodic actions. Most commonly given by intramuscular (IM) injection, these narcotics begin to act about 20–30 minutes after IM injection and the duration of action is 2 to 3 hours (McKenna & Mirkov, 2014). Their sedative effect is thought to be stronger than their analgesic effect and many women report inadequate pain relief following their administration (Jordan, 2010).

Maternal and fetal/newborn side effects are common. Maternal side effects include sedation, drowsiness, impaired cognition, hypoventilation, hypotension, prolonged labour, urinary retention, delayed gastric emptying, and nausea and vomiting. All of which make it less likely that the woman will mobilise and use upright positioning which may result, paradoxically, in an increase in the length of labour and the pain she experiences (Jones et al., 2011). Narcotics readily cross the placenta affecting fetal heart rate variability and consequent obstetric interventions. Newborn side effects include respiratory depression, inhibited sucking at the breast, decreased alertness and subtle behavioural changes (Jordan, 2010). The fetus and newborn will excrete opioids more slowly than adults and neonatal behaviour is adversely affected for approximately 3 days following their administration during labour (Jordan, 2010).

Narcotics, though usually administered intramuscularly, can also be given intrathecally or as an epidural. Fentanyl is a common narcotic given in this way. However, once a woman has an effective epidural block, she will no longer secrete endorphins. Endorphins not only alter pain perception but also play an integral role in early maternal/infant attachment (see Fig. 16.2). Fentanyl also has the potential to cause respiratory depression in both the woman and the newborn (Jordan, 2010).

Regional anaesthesia

This includes epidural anaesthesia, spinal anaesthesia and, rarely, paracervical and pudendal nerve blocks. Regional anaesthesia involves the injection of a local anaesthetic to block specific nerve pathways. Because regional anaesthetics are not introduced into the maternal circulation, it was once believed that they had no effect on a fetus. However, research has demonstrated that there is some uptake of these drugs by the fetus, possibly resulting in fetal heart rate decelerations and symptoms of flaccidity, bradycardia and hypotension in the newborn (Jordan, 2010). Adverse effects are less than those of systemic anaesthetic and analgesic agents. Most importantly, regional anaesthesia allows a woman to be completely awake and aware of what is happening during birth. It does not depress uterine tone, so the uterus remains capable of optimal contraction after birth, thereby helping to prevent postpartum haemorrhage.

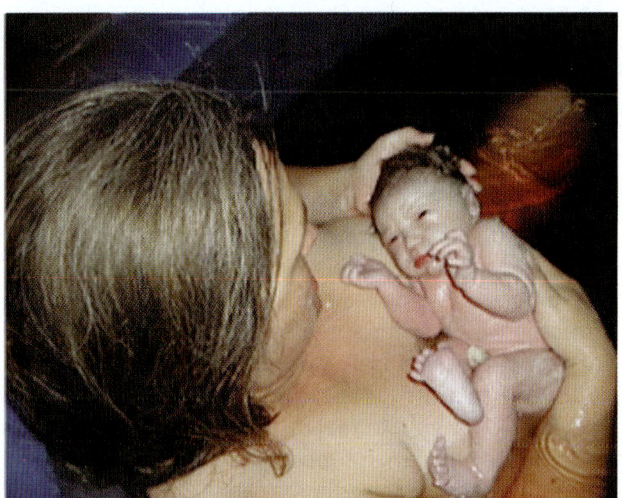

FIGURE 16.2 Endorphin and oxytocin secretion continue following an unmedicated birth and enhance maternal/infant connection. (© Nathan and Cathy Dietsch.)

Epidural anaesthesia

An **epidural anaesthesia** provides pain relief for both labour and birth (Jordan, 2010) but, as a form of regional anaesthetic, also stops the secretion of endorphins. An anaesthetic and/or narcotic agent is placed in the epidural space at the L4–5, L3–4, or L2–3 interspace. Epidural solutions are administered either by bolus, top-ups, continuous infusion or "patient-controlled" pumps (see Fig. 16.3).

Epidural blocks, administered by an anaesthetist, are suitable for almost all women who desire to use them. They are advantageous for women with heart disease, pulmonary disease, diabetes and sometimes severe pregnancy-induced hypertension, because they make labour virtually pain free and thereby reduce stress caused by the pain of labour. Because the woman does not feel contractions, her physical energy is preserved. Epidural blocks are acceptable for use in preterm labour because the drug has scant effect on a fetus and allows for a controlled and gentle birth with less trauma to an immature fetal skull. Because the woman receives no systemic medication, the infant responds more quickly after birth than if systemic narcotic analgesics are used.

The chief concern with epidural anaesthesia is its tendency to cause hypotension because of its blocking effect on the sympathetic nerve fibres in the epidural space. The combined use of fentanyl and a local anaesthetic can lower but not eliminate the risk of hypotension. In addition, the risk also can be reduced by being sure a woman is well-hydrated with 500 to 1000 mL of IV fluids, before the anaesthetic is given. It is important that a woman does not lie supine but moves from side to side after an epidural block, to help prevent supine hypotension syndrome. If hypotension should occur, raising the woman's legs and administering oxygen and additional IV fluid, along with an agent such as ephedrine to elevate blood pressure, may be necessary to stabilise cardiovascular status.

The use of an epidural block may prolong the second stage of labour, making an instrumental delivery more likely (Jones et al., 2011). However, the question of whether epidurals lead to an increase in caesarean births is controversial. Relaxation of the levator ani muscle may impede internal rotation of the fetal head, further slowing labour or making the use of forceps necessary to effect rotation. This occurs primarily when the fetus is in an occipito-posterior position. Syntocinon may be given to shorten labour but how one intervention necessitates the need for additional intervention (referred to as the cascade of interventions) is obvious. Allowing an epidural to wear off by the second stage of labour, so that a woman can push with contractions, is another option. However, experiencing contractions at this point can be overwhelming for a woman whose endorphin secretion has ceased and can

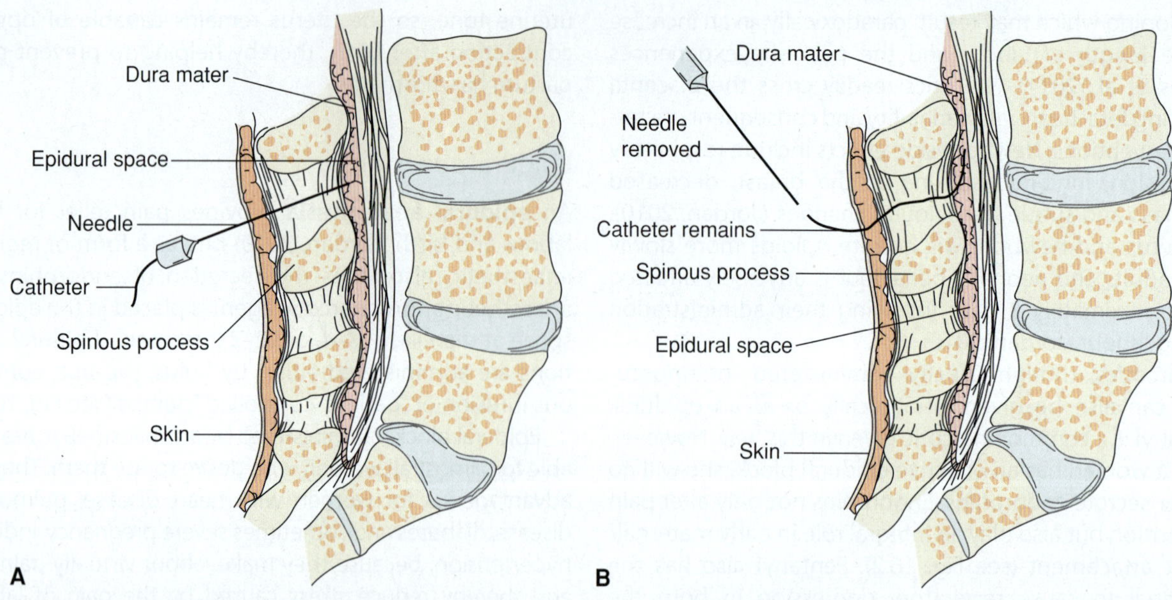

FIGURE 16.3 Epidural anaesthesia. (**A**) A needle is inserted into the epidural space. (**B**) A catheter is threaded into the epidural space; the needle is then removed. The catheter allows medication to be administered intermittently or continuously to relieve pain during labour and childbirth.

counteract the original reason for giving the anaesthetic: to reduce pain in labour.

Maternal side effects from epidural anaesthesia include loss of sensation of bladder filling: the woman needs to be reminded to void every 2 hours to avoid urinary retention. Vasodilation and hypotension mentioned above are common. Other reported side effects include shivering, fever, tinnitus, tremor and respiratory and cardiovascular depression. Neuroaxial administration is a very rare but serious adverse effect with the possible introduction of infection and nerve root damage (Jones et al., 2011). In rare instances, the anaesthetic enters the blood circulation. This occurrence is manifested as drowsiness, a metallic taste on the tongue, slurred speech, blurred vision, unconsciousness and seizure leading to cardiac arrest. If such symptoms occur, it is an emergency situation requiring immediate resuscitation of the woman and prompt birth of the fetus.

Epidural anaesthesia increases the risk of neonatal hypoglycaemia, tachypnoea and a disturbance of lipid metabolism. With an epidural block, there are subtle neurobehavioural effects on the neonate which are undetectable at 18 months (Jordan, 2010).

Spinal (subarachnoid) anaesthesia

Spinal anaesthesia is used less frequently than epidural blocks. It may be used by some GP anaesthetists or in an emergency, however, because the administration technique is simpler than an epidural and can be accomplished more rapidly.

For spinal anaesthesia, a local anaesthetic agent is injected using lumbar puncture technique into the subarachnoid space (into the CSF) at the third or fourth lumbar interspace. A narcotic agonist such as morphine or fentanyl may be added for additional pain relief. Intrathecal fentanyl will take effect in approximately 15 minutes or less and pain relief lasts 4 to 7 hours. A woman is able to feel the urge to push at the second stage of labour, allowing her to actively participate in the birth.

CASE STUDY QUESTION

4. Susan's sister chose to have epidural anaesthesia. What are two risks associated with this?
   a. Hypotension and prolonged second stage of labour.
   b. Severe headache and coldness of all extremities.
   c. Continued back pain and short first stage of labour.
   d. Hypertension and a reduced red blood cell count.

Key points for review

- Pain and suffering are not synonymous although one may exacerbate the other in labour.
- Each person perceives pain differently. Only a woman herself can describe the extent of her pain and know best how she would like to work with it.
- It is the midwife's role to provide unbiased, accurate, evidence-based information to women (ideally during pregnancy) and then support them in how they would like to work with the pain they are experiencing.
- There is no perfect analgesic/anaesthetic agent and all have possible adverse effects on the woman, her labour and her fetus/newborn.

CASE STUDY QUESTION

5. Susan did not want an epidural block during labour. If you had met her during pregnancy, instead of when she was beginning labour, what information would you have provided to her about working with pain in labour, complementary and alternative therapies as well as epidural anaesthesia to enable her to make an informed choice and birth plan?

Resources

For an extensive range of additional resources to enhance teaching and learning and to facilitate understanding of this chapter, please see the text's accompanying website located on thePoint at http://thepoint.lww.com.

References

Australian College of Midwives. (2011). *Philosophy of the midwife.* Canberra: Australian College of Midwives.

Barragán Loayza, I., Solà, I. & Juandó Prats, C. (2011). Biofeedback for pain management during labour. *Cochrane Database of Systematic Reviews 2011*, Issue 6. Art. No.: CD006168.

Beckett, R. (2011). The use of music during labour and birth. *MIDIRS Midwifery Digest, 21*(4), 471–474.

Buckley, S. (2011). Undisturbed birth. *AIMS Journal, 23*(4), 4–7.

Candib, L. & Shields, S. (2010). Being realistic–an uphill battle. In S. Shields & L. Candib (Eds). *Woman-centered Care in Pregnancy and Childbirth* (pp. 431–439). Oxford, UK: Radcliffe.

Chaillet, N., Belaid, L., Crochetière, C., Roy, L., Gagné, G., Moutquin, J., Rossignol, M., Dugas, M., Wassef, M. & Bonapace, J. (2014). Nonpharmacologic approaches for pain management during labor compared with usual care: A meta-analysis. *Birth: Issues in Perinatal Care, 41*(2), 122–137.

Dietsch, E., Shackleton, P., Davies, C., McLeod, M. & Alston, M. (2010). 'You can drop dead': Midwives bullying women. *Women and Birth, 23*(2), 53–59.

Green, J. & Hotelling, B. (2014). Healthy birth practice #3: Bring a loved one, friend or doula for continuous support. *Journal of Perinatal Education, 23*(4), 194–197.

Hodnett, E., Gates, S., Hofmeyr, G., Sakala, C. & Weston, J. (2011). Continuous support for women during childbirth. *Cochrane Database of Systematic Reviews 2011*, Issue 2. Art. No.: CD003766.

Homer, C. (2013). Home-like environments for labour and birth: Benefits for women and babies. *Evidence-Based Medicine, 18*(4), e32.

Jones, L., Othman, M., Dowsell, T., Alfirevic, Z., Gates, S., Newburn, M., Jordan, S., Lavender, T. & Neilson, J. (2011). Pain management for women in labour: An overview of systematic reviews. *Cochrane Database of Systematic Reviews 2011*, Issue 7. Art No.: CD009234.

Jordan, S. (2010). *Pharmacology for Midwives: The Evidence for Safe Practice* (2nd ed.). London: Palgrave Macmillan.

Kaviani, M., Azima, S., Alavi, M. & Tabaei, M. (2014). The effect of lavender aromatherapy on pain perception and intrapartum outcome in primiparous women. *British Journal of Midwifery, 22*(2), 124–129.

Leap, N., Dodwell, M. & Newburn, M. (2010). Working with pain in labour: An overview of the evidence. *Perspective, 6*, 9–12.

Leap, N., Sandall, J., Buckland, S. & Huber, U. (2010). Journey to confidence: Women's experiences of pain in labour and relational continuity of care. *Journal of Midwifery and Women's Health, 55*(3), 234–242.

Mander, R. (2011). *Pain in childbearing and its control: Key issues for midwives and women.* Chichester, UK: Wiley-Blackwell.

McKenna, L. & Mirkov, S. (2014). *McKenna's Drug Handbook for Nursing & Midwifery* (7th ed.). Sydney: Lippincott Williams & Wilkins.

NSW Health. (2010). *Maternity–towards normal birth in NSW.* North Sydney: Department of Health, accessed 14 January 2015, <www.health.nsw.gov.au/policies/pd/2010/pdf/PD2010_045.pdf>.

Nolan, M. (2010). Childbirth education: Politics, equality and relevance. In D. Walsh & S. Downe (Eds). *Essential Midwifery Practice: Intrapartum Care* (pp. 31–44). Oxford, UK: Wiley-Blackwell.

Sandall, J., Soltani. H., Gates, S., Shennan, A. & Devane, D. (2013). Midwife-led continuity models versus other models of care for childbearing women. *Cochrane Database of Systematic Reviews 2013*, Issue 8. Art. No.: CD004667.

Smith, C., Collins, C. & Crowther, C. (2011). Aromatherapy for pain management in labour. *Cochrane Database of Systematic Reviews 2011*, Issue 7. Art. No.: CD009215.

Smith, C., Collins, C., Crowther, C. & Levett, K. (2011). Acupuncture or acupressure for pain management in labour. *Cochrane Database of Systematic Reviews 2011*, Issue 7. Art. No.: CD009232.

Tiran, D. (2011). Smell's good! Aromatherapy in midwifery. *Practising Midwife, 14*(10), 11–15.

Suggested readings

Burns, E., Boulton, M., Cluett, E., Cornelius, V. & Smith, L. (2012). Characteristics, interventions, and outcomes of women who used a birthing pool: A prospective observational study. *Birth, 39*(3), 192–202.

Garland, D. (2011). Exploring carers views and attitudes towards the use of water during labour and birth. *MIDIRS, 21*(2), 193–196.

Madden, K., Turnbull, D., Cyna, A., Adelson, P. & Wilkinson, C. (2013). Pain relief for childbirth: The preferences of pregnant women, midwives and obstetricians. *Women and Birth, 26*(1), 33–40.

Rooks, J. (2012). Labor pain management other than neuraxial: What do we know and where do we go next? *Birth, 39*(4), 318–322.

Chapter 17

Nursing care of a postnatal family

Previous chapters discussed caring for the pregnant woman and her family during the antenatal and intrapartum periods. This chapter adds information about caring for a postnatal woman and family. Midwives and child and family health nurses are able to play major roles in assessment, promoting comfort and education during this period. They can help a new family adjust to the many physiological and psychological changes that occur.

LEARNING OBJECTIVES

After mastering the contents of this chapter, you should be able to:

1. Describe the psychological and physiological changes that occur in a postnatal woman.
2. Use critical thinking to analyse ways that postpartum nursing care can be more family-centred.
3. Assess a woman and her family for physiological and psychological changes after childbirth and make referrals as necessary.
4. Identify nursing considerations for a postnatal woman and family related to the changes during this period.
5. Discuss nursing care measures to encourage bonding.
6. Implement nursing care to aid the progression of physiological and psychological transitions occurring in a postnatal woman and family.
7. Identify areas related to care of the postnatal family that could benefit from additional nursing research or application of evidence-based practice.

KEY TERMS

- afterpains
- engorgement
- involution
- letting-go phase
- lochia
- postnatal depression
- puerperium
- rooming-in
- taking-hold phase
- taking-in phase
- uterine atony

CASE STUDY

As the nurse working in a postnatal unit, you care for Mike and Jae Cooper, who have just become parents of a 3.5-kg baby girl. Jae is on maternity leave from her job as a sales assistant. Mike plans to take a week off work to spend time with Jae and the new baby. As you prepare them for discharge, you notice they seem overwhelmed with the amount of information they have been given. Jae says, trying to get the baby to breastfeed, "She always seems to be hungry, will she get enough milk? I was hoping by breastfeeding I wouldn't have to worry about contraception for a while, but I'm having so much trouble maybe that won't work out." Mike pulls you aside and says, "Sometimes I see my wife crying for no reason. Why isn't she as happy as I am?"

CASE STUDY QUESTION

1. What additional postnatal teaching does the Cooper family need?

The postnatal period, or **puerperium** (from the Latin *puer,* for "child", and *parere,* for "to bring forth"), refers to the 6-week period after childbirth. It is a time of maternal changes that are both retrogressive (involution of the uterus and vagina) and progressive (production of milk for breastfeeding, beginning of a parenting role and where the woman is not fully breastfeeding, restoration of the normal menstrual cycle). Protecting a woman's health as these changes occur is important for preserving her future childbearing function and for ensuring that she is physically well enough to incorporate her new child into her family. The physical care a woman receives during the postnatal period can influence her health for the rest of her life. The emotional support she receives can influence her own mental health and the emotional health of her child and family so much that it can be felt into the next generation (McGarry et al., 2009).

CARING FOR A POSTNATAL WOMAN AND FAMILY

Assessment

In the immediate hours after birth, postnatal assessment of a woman is implemented by a midwife or medical practitioner. Later in the puerperium the midwife or nurse assesses the woman through a health interview, physical examination and, if necessary, analysis of laboratory data. It is important to ensure that physical changes, such as uterine involution, are occurring by evaluating uterine size and consistency and lochia flow amount.

Assessment of a woman's psychological adjustment begins with her reaction at birth. Each woman is different and her reaction may be influenced by her beliefs, values and culture, and that of her family (Holden, 2010). Assessment of the woman's psychological adjustment can be made by observing the extent and quality of the woman's interaction with her child, including whether she holds and talks to the infant, whether her overall mood seems appropriate and whether she feels comfortable to begin infant care. Observing the woman for self-care is important when assessing her psychological adjustment. For example, a woman who feels good about herself will be more confident in caring for herself and her baby, whereas a woman who is feeling overwhelmed may have difficulty achieving this.

Nursing considerations

Nursing considerations during the postnatal period are usually concerned with supporting the woman and her family to make the normal physiological and psychological adjustments to parenting or with managing actual or potential problems, such as a family's inability to accept and bond with a new child and physiological complications of the puerperium. Most postnatal families remain in the hospital for a relatively short time, only 48 to 72 hours. The postpartum stay can be as short as 4 hours. That means outcomes must be devised that can be accomplished and evaluated during this short period of contact. If an outcome cannot be evaluated within this short timeframe, follow-up visits by the community midwife will be provided to ensure women and their partners receive the education required in regard to postnatal health, wellbeing and parenting.

When planning care in the postnatal period, the midwife or nurse should try to arrange procedures to allow optimal time for family–infant interaction and yet also provide adequate time for a woman to rest, to prevent exhaustion. Prevention of exhaustion can improve coping ability and plans for self-care. After adequate instruction, a woman should be prepared to monitor her own health after she returns home.

Planning should also include ample time for health teaching. To be effective, teaching should be individualised and take into account the beliefs, values and culture of the woman and family. In a study by Crippen and Brew (2013), intercultural couples were found to be at risk of marital disharmony where their cultural influences around parenting were misaligned. To interact effectively midwives and nurses need to be aware how the family situates their parenting practices within their culture (Crippen & Brew, 2013). For Aboriginal and Torres Strait Islander parents, the involvement of family in parenting is vital, with shared responsibilities including roles for aunties, uncles and grandparents that in other cultures would normally fall to the parents (Heath et al., 2011). For example, in many Aboriginal cultures, the grandmother or another family member names the child. It is also important to remember that cultural differences exist within Aboriginal and Torres Strait Islander groups, so a blanket approach to care may not be appropriate. Respecting the woman and her family by individualising care and asking what is important for them will enable effective communication and better reception of parenting education.

Midwives and nurses play a pivotal role in educating families about caring for their baby. An important part of teaching related to care of the newborn is preparation for the unexpected and the need for flexibility. New parents do not yet know what their life will be like and that there will be changes to their relationship and the relationships within their family (Parker & Hunter, 2011). Empowering strategies should be geared towards increasing a woman's self-esteem and allowing her to view herself as a new mother and her new infant as part of her family. Parenting education involving family members is also important. Exploring what the woman and family already know about childcare can be empowering for the family and beneficial in enabling individualised parenting education. This can be achieved by giving them scenarios and asking them what they think would be the best choice for themselves and their baby.

Failure to make an adequate adjustment to new life changes may lead to difficulty integrating an infant into the family. This could affect the child's mental health, self-esteem and later ability to trust. Evaluation in the postnatal period involves being certain not only that a woman and her baby are safe but also that the woman knows how to maintain her own health. Such follow-up evaluation can be done during home visits, or during postnatal and well-child assessments.

PSYCHOLOGICAL CHANGES OF THE POSTNATAL PERIOD

A transition is a movement or passage from one position or concept to another, or a pause between what was and what is to be. It represents the internal process experienced by people when change occurs. In a classic presentation of what transition entails, Bridges (1994) stated that change is something that happens to people and transition is how they respond to that change.

People move through several predictable stages during transition: first, is the act of ending old ways of thinking or believing; next, there is a neutral zone, during which the old way is gone but the new way is not yet comfortable; and finally, there is a new beginning, during which new ideas and concepts are put into action (Bridges, 1994). The postnatal period is a time of transition, during which a couple gives up concepts such as "childless" or "parents of one" and moves to the beginning of new parenthood. The immediate postnatal period is a neutral time during which a couple tries out their new roles and attempts to "fit" their expectations. Opening channels for communication, anticipating new needs and highlighting potential gains that will occur because of the change are important actions.

Phases of the puerperium

In her classic work on maternal behaviour, Reva Rubin, a nurse, divided the puerperium into three separate phases (Rubin, 1977). She viewed the first of these as a

taking-in phase, or a time when the new parents review their pregnancy and the labour and birth. The subsequent phases, called the **taking-hold phase** and the **letting-go phase**, are times of renewed action and forward movement. At the time these phases of the puerperium were identified, women were hospitalised for 5 to 7 days after childbirth and moved in a paced manner from one step to the next. Today, with hospitalisation potentially as short as a few hours, women appear to move through these phases much more quickly and may even experience two different phases at once.

Taking-in phase

The taking-in phase is a time of reflection. During this period some women can be largely passive. Nurses, midwives and family members need to understand that new mothers require additional attention to enable them to physically and psychologically care for a new baby. A woman may allow others to care for her basic needs and make decisions for her, rather than do these things herself. This dependence results partly from her physical discomfort because of muscle fatigue and pain (such as afterpains, haemorrhoids or perineal pain), partly from her uncertainty in caring for her newborn and partly from the tiredness that follows childbirth.

As a part of thinking about her new role, the woman will usually want to talk about her pregnancy, especially about her labour and birth. During the taking-in phase, she rests to regain her physical strength and considers the events of the pregnancy and birth. Encouraging her to talk about the birth helps her integrate it into her life experiences.

Taking-hold phase

After a time of passive dependence, the woman begins to initiate action. She may prefer to make her own decisions. Women who give birth without any medical intervention may reach this second phase in a matter of hours after birth. During the taking-in phase, a woman may have felt unable to take a lead role in caring for her child. In the taking-hold phase, she will begin to take a stronger interest. Care is provided depending on individual needs. Some women may require brief demonstrations of baby care to build confidence; however, many are already active at this stage. Although a woman's actions suggest strong independence during this time, she may still feel insecure about her ability to care for her new child. Facilitating the woman's ability to care for her baby by working with her to assist her when she feels necessary will build her confidence. Encouragement and positive reinforcement begin in the healthcare facility and continue after discharge, at home and during well-child visits.

Letting-go phase

In the third phase, called the letting-go phase, a woman finally redefines her new role. She is able to integrate her new baby into her family and her broader life with confidence and purpose. This process requires readjustment of relationships, similar to what occurred during pregnancy. This phase is extended and continues during the child's growing years.

CASE STUDY QUESTION

2. Which of the following actions would alert you that Jae, 2 days' postpartum, is entering a postnatal taking-hold phase?

a. She tells you she has painful contractions for 8 hours
b. She sleeps as if exhausted from the effort of her labour
c. She appears to need little support with breastfeeding her baby
d. She displays an unwillingness to assume baby care needs

Development of parental love and positive family relationships

Bonding

During pregnancy, almost every woman worries about her ability to be a "good" mother: This concern does not evaporate as soon as the baby is born. Some women seem able to recognise a newborn's needs immediately and to give care with confident understanding right from the start, whereas other women enter into a relationship with their newborn tentatively and with qualms and conflicts that must be addressed before the relationship can be meaningful. This is because parental love is only partly instinctive. Parental love develops gradually and in stages such as: planning the pregnancy, or adjusting to an unplanned pregnancy, hearing the pregnancy confirmed, feeling the child move in utero, giving birth, seeing the baby, touching the baby and, finally, giving total care to the child. Factors such as a difficult labour or separation from the newborn may lead to symptoms of a traumatic stress disorder that slows the bonding process or interferes with the ability to bond warmly (Johnson, 2013).

Many women may not experience maternal feelings for their infants until days or even weeks after giving birth. Some fathers admit they have difficulty "claiming" or bonding with an infant (feeling fatherly towards the new child) until as late as 3 months after the birth, when the child begins to smile or coo and interact more directly with them. It is important that these parents are informed that their feelings are normal. The ability of both parents to reach out to their child can be strengthened by allowing them to touch and spend as much time as possible with their new child during the first few hours of life (see Fig. 17.1).

Forming a strong bond with a child is not a problem found only in first-time parents. Experienced parents can have just as much difficulty. Because of these mixed feelings, parents may not show genuine warmth the first

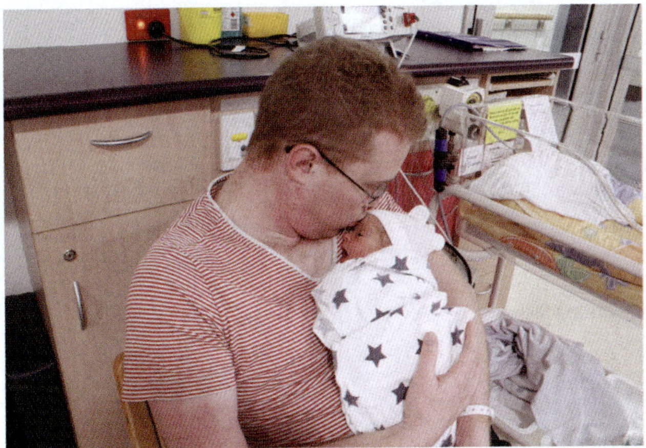

FIGURE 17.1 A father interacts and bonds with his newborn. (© Lauren Kidziak.)

time they hold their infant. They may only touch the blanket and not make close physical contact. This identification process is termed *claiming* or *bonding*. Looking directly at her newborn's face, with direct eye contact (termed an en face position), is a sign a woman is beginning effective interaction. Many fathers can be observed staring at a newborn for long intervals in this same way. Often termed *engrossment*, this action alerts carers to how actively the father, as well as the mother, is beginning to bond. The length of time parents take to bond with a child depends on the circumstances of the pregnancy and birth, the wellness and ability of the child to meet the parent's expectations, reciprocal actions by the newborn and the opportunities the parents have to interact with the child. Freedom from stringent health agency rules helps good parent–child relationships to develop.

CASE STUDY QUESTION

3. You observe Jae holding her newborn. Which reaction to her baby would best reassure you that she is relating well to her newborn?
   a. She looks directly at her infant's face and talks to him
   b. She is reluctant to have additional time nursing her infant other than when feeding
   c. She leaves the infant in the care of family and friends as often as possible
   d. She appears despondent when the nurses are providing assistance with baby care

Rooming-in

The more time a woman has to spend with her baby the sooner she may feel competent in child care and the more likely she may be to form a sound mother–child relationship (Jaafar, Lee & Ho, 2012). **Rooming-in** is the term given to the practice of babies staying in the room with the mother. This enables the mother to become better acquainted with her child and begin to feel more confident in her ability to care for him or her after discharge (Jafaar et al., 2012). Rooming-in has also been shown to improve breastfeeding rates as the woman can learn and respond early to her baby's hunger cues (Walker, 2013). In many settings, the father can stay overnight in the room, or room-in, as well.

Sibling visitation

Separation from children is often as painful for a mother as it is for her children. Waiting at home, separated from their mother and listening only to telephone reports of what a new brother or sister looks like, can be very difficult for older children. A chance to visit the hospital and see the new baby and their mother can reduce feelings of displacement or resentment. It can help to relieve some of the impact of separation (see Fig. 17.2).

Maternal concerns and feelings in the postnatal period

Traditionally, it is assumed that the bulk of a woman's concerns in the postnatal period centre on the care of her new infant. Based on this, classes in the postnatal period have traditionally focused on teaching how to breastfeed and bathe infants. Although these acts are concerns for many mothers, they are not necessarily every new mother's chief concern. A woman has come through a tremendous psychological experience during pregnancy and the birth of a child. She is in the middle of a complete role change. It can be expected, therefore, that some of her attention and interest during this time will be directed inwards as she tries to view herself in this new role. Typical issues identified by postnatal

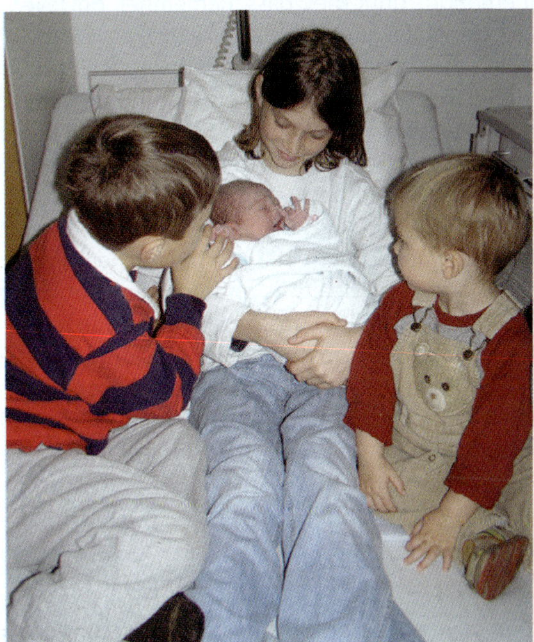

FIGURE 17.2 Sibling visiting is important to bring a family together. (Ricci, S. S. & Kyle, T. (2009). *Maternity and Pediatric Nursing*. Philadelphia: Lippincott Williams & Wilkins.)

women include breast soreness; regaining their figure; regulating the demands of housework, their partner and their children; coping with emotional tension and sibling jealousy; and fatigue.

Postnatal blues

During the postnatal period, as many as 84% of women experience some feelings of crying and mood lability (O'Hara & Wisner, 2014). They may burst into tears easily or feel let down or irritable. This temporary feeling after birth has long been known as the "baby blues". This phenomenon may be caused by hormonal changes, particularly the decrease in oestrogen and progesterone that occurs with delivery of the placenta. For some women, it may be a response to dependence and low self-esteem caused by exhaustion, being away from home, physical discomfort and the tension engendered by assuming a new role, especially if a woman is not receiving support from her partner. Typically the baby blues manifests through tearfulness, feelings of inadequacy, mood changes, anorexia and sleep disturbance.

Anticipatory guidance, education and individualised support from healthcare personnel are all important to help the parents understand that this response is normal. Women should be reassured that sudden crying episodes may occur as they may have difficulty understanding why this is happening. Their support person also needs reassurance. It is important to give the woman a chance to verbalise her feelings. Statements such as "I know there's absolutely no reason for me to be crying, but I cannot stop" are common. Reassurance and assisting her to make as many decisions as possible can help give her a sense of control over her life and help her cope with these postnatal emotions until they pass. Remember, however, that not all postnatal women cry because they have baby blues. A woman sometimes has other reasons to feel sad during this time. For example, problems at home may have become overwhelming. Keeping lines of communication open is important to help differentiate between problems that can be handled best with discussion and concerned understanding, and those that should be referred to a social service department or a community health agency.

Perinatal mental health is an important public health issue. The beyondblue postnatal depression screening program found that **postnatal depression** affects up to 16% of women (Buist, 2014). Because these are deeper level concerns, postpartum depression and psychosis are discussed in Chapter 25.

PHYSIOLOGICAL CHANGES OF THE POSTNATAL PERIOD

Retrogressive physiological changes that occur during the postnatal period include those related specifically to the reproductive system as well as other systemic changes (see Box 17.1).

BOX 17.1 Assessment ✻ Assessing the postnatal woman

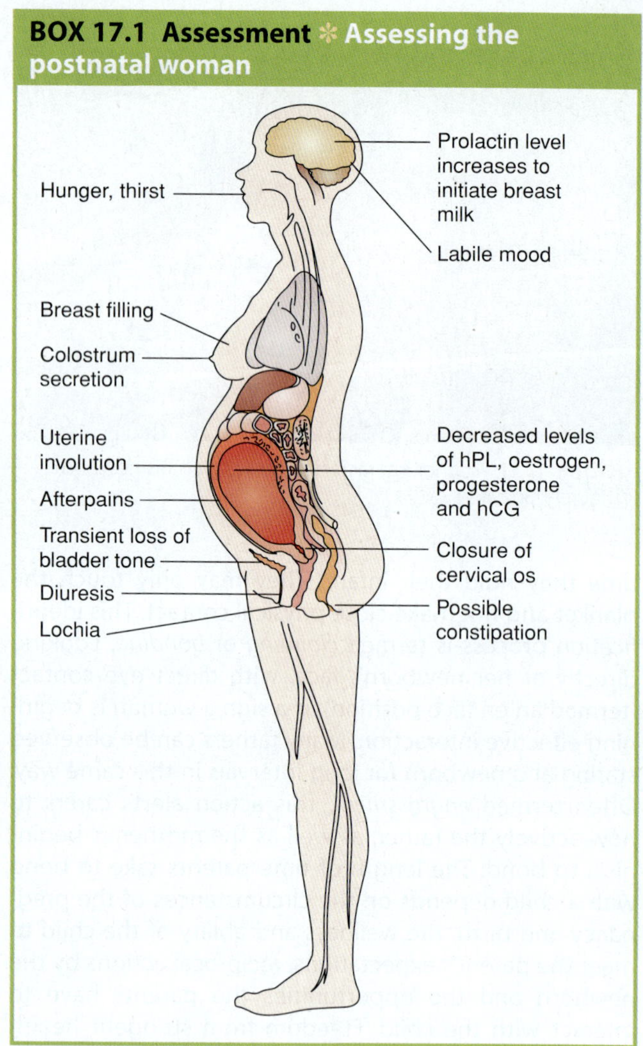

Reproductive system changes

The uterus

Involution is the process whereby the reproductive organs return to their non-pregnant state. A woman is in danger of haemorrhage from the placental site until involution is complete, which takes a matter of weeks. Involution of the uterus involves two main processes. First, the area where the placenta was implanted is sealed off to prevent bleeding. Second, the organ is reduced to its approximate pre-gestational size.

The sealing of the placenta site is accomplished by rapid contraction of the uterus immediately after delivery of the placenta. This contraction occludes the blood vessels supplying the placental site to stop bleeding. Additionally, the opposing walls of the contracted uterus apply pressure to the placental site and clotting mechanisms are activated (Stables & Rankin, 2010). With time, thrombi form within the uterine sinuses and permanently seal the area. Eventually, endometrial tissue undermines the site and obliterates the organised thrombi, covering and healing the area so completely that the process leaves no scar

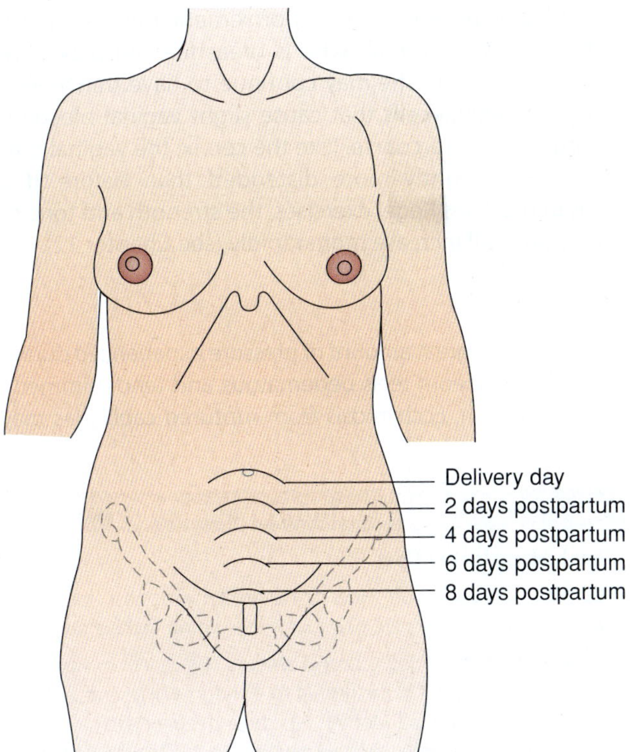

FIGURE 17.3 Uterine involution. The uterus decreases in size at a predictable rate during the postnatal period. After 10 days, it recedes under the pubic bone and is no longer palpable.

tissue within the uterus and does not compromise future implantation sites.

The same contraction process reduces the bulk of the uterus. Devoid of the placenta and the membranes, the walls of the uterus thicken and contract, gradually reducing the uterus from a container large enough to hold a full-term fetus to one the size of a grapefruit (see Fig. 17.3). Over a period of weeks the uterus undergoes a process of involution which includes ischaemia, autolysis and phagocytosis. Thus the uterine muscle cells reduce to their pre-pregnant size, and excess fibrous and elastic tissue is removed (Stables & Rankin, 2010). The main mechanism that reduces the bulk of the uterus, however, is contraction, a phenomenon that can be compared with a rubber band which has been stretched for many months and now is regaining its normal contour. Although the uterus will never completely return to its pre-pregnancy state, its reduction in size is dramatic. Immediately after birth, the uterus weighs about 1000 grams. At the end of the first week, it weighs 500 grams. By the time involution is complete (6 weeks), it weighs approximately 50 grams, similar to its pre-pregnancy weight.

Because uterine contraction begins immediately after placental delivery, the fundus of the uterus may be palpated by a midwife or medical practitioner through the abdominal wall, halfway between the umbilicus and the symphysis pubis, within a few minutes after birth. One hour later, it will have risen to the level of the umbilicus, where it remains for approximately the next 24 hours. From then on, it decreases one fingerbreadth per day—on the first postnatal day, it will be palpable one fingerbreadth below the umbilicus; on the second day, two fingerbreadths below the umbilicus; and so on. Because a fingerbreadth is about 1 centimetre (cm), this can be recorded as 1 cm below the umbilicus, 2 cm below it and so forth. In the average woman, by the ninth or tenth day, the uterus will have contracted so much that it is withdrawn into the pelvis and can no longer be detected by abdominal palpation. The uterus of a breastfeeding mother may contract even more quickly, because oxytocin, which is released with breastfeeding, stimulates uterine contractions. However, breastfeeding alone is not sufficient to protect against postpartum haemorrhage.

A midwife or medical practitioner should assess fundal height shortly after a woman has emptied her bladder for the most accurate results. A full bladder can keep the uterus from contracting, pushing it upwards and possibly deviating it from the midline, because of the laxness of the uterine ligaments. Contraction may be difficult if there is retained placenta or membranes. Involution will occur most dependably in a woman who is well-nourished and who ambulates early after birth (gravity may also play a role).

An estimation of the consistency of the postnatal uterus made by the midwife or medical practitioner is as important as measurement of its height. A well-contracted fundus feels firm. It can be compared with a grapefruit in both size and tenseness. Whenever the fundus feels boggy (soft or flabby), it is not as contracted as it should be, despite its position in the abdomen. The first hour after birth is potentially the most dangerous time for a woman. If her uterus should become relaxed during this time **(uterine atony)**, she will lose blood very rapidly, because no permanent thrombi have yet formed at the placental site.

In some women, contraction of the uterus after birth causes intermittent cramping termed **afterpains**, similar to that accompanying a menstrual period. Afterpains tend to be noticed most by multiparas rather than primiparas and by women who have given birth to large babies or multiple births. In these situations, the uterus must contract more forcefully to regain its pre-pregnancy size and has difficulty maintaining a steady contracted state. These sensations are noticed most intensely with breastfeeding, when the infant's sucking causes a release of oxytocin from the posterior pituitary, increasing the strength of the contractions.

Lochia

The separation of the placenta and membranes occurs in the spongy layer or outer portion of the decidua basalis of the uterus. By the second day after birth, the layer of decidua remaining under the placental site and throughout the uterus differentiates into two distinct layers. The inner layer attached to the muscular wall of the uterus remains, serving as the foundation from which a new layer of endometrium will be formed. The layer adjacent to the uterine cavity becomes necrotic and is cast off as a uterine

TABLE 17.1 Characteristics of lochia

Type of lochia	Colour	Postpartal day	Composition
Lochia rubra	Red	1–3	Blood, fragments of decidua and mucus
Lochia serosa	Pink	3–10	Blood, mucus and invading leucocytes
Lochia alba	White	10–14 (may last 6 weeks)	Largely mucus; leucocyte count high

discharge similar to a menstrual flow. This uterine flow, consisting of blood, fragments of decidua, white blood cells, mucus and some bacteria, is known as **lochia** (see Table 17.1 and Box 17.2).

The portion of the uterus where the placenta was not attached is so fully cleansed by this sloughing process that it will be in a reproductive state in about 3 weeks' time. It takes approximately 6 weeks (the entire postnatal period) for the placental implantation site to be healed. For the first 3 days after birth, a lochia discharge consists almost entirely of blood, with only small particles of decidua and mucus. Because of its mainly red colour, it is termed *lochia rubra*. As the amount of blood involved in the cast-off tissue decreases (about the fourth day) and leucocytes begin to invade the area, as they do with any healing surface, the flow becomes pink or brownish (*lochia serosa*). On about the tenth day, the amount of the flow decreases and becomes colourless or white (*lochia alba*). Lochia alba is present in most women until the third week after birth, although it is not unusual for a white discharge to continue for up to 6 weeks.

The cervix

Immediately after birth, a uterine cervix is soft and malleable. Both the internal and external os are open. Like contraction of the uterus, contraction of the cervix towards its pre-pregnant state begins at once. By the end of 7 days, the external os has narrowed to the size of a pencil opening; the cervix feels firm and non-gravid again. Like the fundus, the cervix does not return exactly to its pre-pregnancy state. The internal os closes as before, but after a vaginal birth the external os usually remains slightly open and appears slit like or stellate (star-shaped), whereas previously it was round. Finding this pattern on pelvic examination suggests that childbearing has taken place.

The vagina

After a vaginal birth, the vagina is soft, with few rugae, and its diameter is considerably greater than normal. The hymen is permanently torn and heals with small, separate tags of tissue. It takes the entire postnatal period for the vagina to involute (by contraction, as with the uterus) until it gradually returns to its approximate pre-pregnancy state. Because a woman who is breastfeeding may have delayed ovulation, she may continue to have thin-walled or fragile vaginal cells that cause slight vaginal bleeding during sexual intercourse. Like the cervix, the vaginal outlet remains slightly more distended than before. If a woman practises Kegel exercises, the strength and tone of the vagina will increase more rapidly (see Chapter 12).

The perineum

Because of the great amount of pressure experienced during birth, the perineum feels oedematous and tender immediately after birth. Ecchymosis from ruptured capillaries may

BOX 17.2 ✻ Focus on family teaching

Evaluating lochia flow

Q. Jae Cooper asks you, "How do I know if my lochia is normal?"

A. Several guidelines are helpful for evaluating lochia flow:

- *Evaluate the amount:* Lochia amount will vary from woman to woman but in the first 24 to 48 hours will resemble that of a heavy period. Mothers who breastfeed tend to have less lochial discharge than those who do not, because the natural release of the hormone oxytocin during breastfeeding strengthens uterine contractions. Conservation of fluid for lactation may also be a factor. Lochial flow increases on exertion, especially the first few times a woman is out of bed, but decreases again with rest. The increase in amount that occurs with ambulation is the result of vaginal discharge of pooled lochia, not a true increase in amount. However, lochia amount does increase with strenuous exercise, such as lifting a heavy weight or walking up stairs. Saturating a perineal pad in less than 1 hour is considered an abnormally heavy flow and should be reported.
- *Check the consistency:* Lochia should contain no large clots. Clots may indicate that a portion of the placenta has been retained and is preventing closure of the maternal uterine blood sinuses. In any event, large clots denote poor uterine contraction, which needs to be corrected.
- *Observe the pattern:* Lochia is red for the first 1 to 3 days (lochia rubra), pinkish-brown from days 4 to 10 (lochia serosa) and then white (lochia alba) for as long as 6 weeks after birth. The pattern of lochia (rubra to serosa to alba) should not reverse. A red flow after a pink or white flow may indicate that placental fragments have been retained, infection is present or uterine contraction is decreasing and new bleeding is beginning.
- *Assess the odour:* Lochia should not have an offensive odour. Lochia has the same odour as menstrual blood. An offensive odour usually indicates that the uterus has become infected. Immediate intervention is needed to treat postnatal infection.
- *Watch for absence:* Lochia should never be absent during the first 1 to 3 weeks. Absence of lochia, like the presence of an offensive odour, may indicate postnatal infection. Lochia may be scant in amount after caesarean birth, but it is never altogether absent.

show on the surface. The labia majora and labia minora typically remain atrophic and softened after birth, never returning to their pre-pregnancy state.

Systemic changes

The same body systems that were involved in pregnancy are also involved in changes as the body returns to its pre-pregnancy state.

The hormonal system

Pregnancy hormones begin to decrease as soon as the placenta is no longer present. Levels of human chorionic gonadotrophin (hCG) and human placental lactogen (hPL) are almost negligible by 24 hours. By the end of the first week, progesterone, oestrogen and oestradiol are all at pre-pregnancy levels. Prolactin is the hormone responsible for lactogenesis, which is the onset of milk secretion. Its level rises during pregnancy; however, in the presence of progesterone, lactogenesis is prevented. Lactogenesis occurs postpartum, correlating with the fall in progesterone. In addition, the release of oxytocin occurs as a result of sucking, which enables milk to be ejected from the breast.

The urinary system

During pregnancy, as much as 2000 to 3000 mL excess fluid accumulates in the body. An extensive diuresis begins to take place almost immediately after birth to rid the body of this fluid. This easily increases the daily output of a postnatal woman from a normal level of 1500 mL to as much as 3000 mL/day during the second to fifth day after birth. This marked increase in urine production causes the bladder to fill rapidly.

During a vaginal birth, the baby's head exerts a great deal of pressure on the maternal bladder and urethra as it passes on the bladder's underside. This pressure may leave the bladder with a transient loss of tone that, together with the oedematous tissue surrounding the urethra, decreases a woman's ability to sense when she has to void. A woman who has undergone epidural or spinal anaesthesia will feel no sensation in the bladder area until the anaesthetic has worn off.

The circulatory system

The diuresis that is evident between the second and fifth days after birth, as well as the blood loss at birth, acts to reduce the added blood volume a woman accumulated during pregnancy. This reduction occurs so rapidly, in fact, that the blood volume returns to its normal pre-pregnancy level by the first or second week after birth. The usual blood loss with a normal vaginal birth is minimal (Pairman et al., 2015). Women usually continue to have the same high level of plasma fibrinogen during the first period. Any varicosities that are present will recede, but they rarely return to a completely pre-pregnant appearance. Although vascular blemishes, such as spider angiomas, fade slightly, they may not disappear completely.

The gastrointestinal system

Digestion and absorption begin to be active again soon after birth unless a woman has had a caesarean birth. Almost immediately, the woman feels hungry and thirsty and she can usually eat without difficulty from nausea or vomiting during this time.

The integumentary system

After birth, the stretch marks on a woman's abdomen (striae gravidarum) still appear reddened and may be even more prominent than during pregnancy, when they were tightly stretched. Typically, in a Caucasian woman, these will fade to a pale white over the next 3 to 6 months; in Aboriginal women or women with a darker complexion, they may remain as areas of slightly darker pigment. Excessive pigment on the face and neck (chloasma) and on the abdomen (linea nigra) will become barely detectable in 6 weeks' time. Both the abdominal wall and the ligaments that support the uterus, which were obviously stretched during pregnancy, usually require the full 6 weeks of the puerperium to return to their former state.

Effects of post-birth changes

Fatigue

As soon as birth is completed, some women experience total exhaustion. For the last several months of pregnancy, a woman may have experienced some difficulty sleeping. Near the end of pregnancy, she probably was unable to find a comfortable position to sleep because of the fetus' activity or the presence of back or leg pain. During labour, she worked hard with little or no sleep. The resulting sleep deprivation may make it difficult for her to cope with new experiences and stressful situations until she has enjoyed a sustained period of sleep (see also Box 17.3).

Weight loss

The rapid diuresis and diaphoresis during the second to fifth days after birth usually result in a weight loss of 2 to 4 kg, in addition to the approximately 5 kg lost at birth. Lochia flow causes an additional 1 kg loss, for a total weight loss of about 8 to 9 kg. Additional weight loss is most dependent on the amount of pregnancy weight gain and on whether a woman takes active measures to lose weight. It is also influenced by nutrition, exercise and breastfeeding. The weight a woman reaches at 6 weeks after birth becomes her baseline postnatal weight unless she takes active measures to lose the weight.

BOX 17.3 ✻ Focus on evidence-based practice

The effect of newborn crying on maternal and infant wellbeing

Many new mothers are not prepared for how much time newborns spend crying (as many as 16 out of 24 hours). Trying to quiet a newborn can lead to extreme fatigue in a postpartal parent. To investigate the effect of newborn crying on new mothers' ability to rest, researchers conducted a systematic review of studies concerned with newborn crying. Results of the literature review revealed that infant crying during the first 3 months postpartum is responsible for disrupting new mothers' circadian rhythms, reducing opportunities to rest and exacerbating tiredness. Incremental exhaustion from infant crying diminishes a parent's ability to concentrate, raises the fear of harming the child, triggers depressive symptoms and burdens parent–child interaction.

How could you use the results of this study to help new mothers after they return home from hospital?

Source: Kurth, E., Kennedy, H. P., Spichiger, E., et al. (2011). Crying babies, tired mothers: What do we know? A systematic review. *Midwifery, 27*(2), 187–194.

Vital signs changes

Vital signs changes in the postpartum period reflect the internal adjustments that occur as a woman's body returns to its pre-pregnant state.

Temperature

A woman may show a slight increase in temperature during the first 24 hours after birth because of dehydration that occurred during labour. If she receives adequate fluid during the first 24 hours, this temperature elevation will return to normal. Most women are thirsty immediately after birth and are able to drink adequate quantities of fluid unless they are nauseated from a birth anaesthetic. Any woman whose axillary temperature rises above 38°C is considered to be febrile. In such women, a postnatal infection may be present. Occasionally, when a woman's breasts fill with milk on the third or fourth postpartum day, her temperature rises for a period of hours because of the increased vascular activity involved.

Pulse

A woman's pulse rate during the postnatal period is usually slightly slower than during pregnancy. During pregnancy, the distended uterus obstructed the amount of venous blood returning to the heart; after birth, to accommodate the increased blood volume returning to the heart, stroke volume increases. This increased stroke volume reduces the pulse rate to between 60 and 70 beats per minute. As diuresis diminishes the blood volume and causes blood pressure to fall, the pulse rate increases accordingly. By the end of the first week, the pulse rate will have returned to the normal pre-pregnancy rate. Evaluate the pulse rate conscientiously in the postnatal period, because a rapid and thready pulse during this time could be a sign of haemorrhage. It is important to compare a woman's pulse rate with the slower range expected in the postnatal period, not with the normal pulse rate in the general population.

Blood pressure

Blood pressure should also be monitored carefully during the postnatal period, because a decrease can indicate bleeding. In contrast, an elevation above 140 mmHg systolic or 90 mmHg diastolic may indicate the development of pre-eclampsia, a serious complication of the puerperium which requires immediate referral to medical staff (see Chapter 21). To evaluate blood pressure, compare a woman's blood pressure with her pregnancy level, rather than with standard blood pressure ranges; otherwise, a significant increase or decrease in blood pressure could be missed and may be life-threatening.

A major complication in women who have lost an appreciable amount of blood with birth is orthostatic hypotension, or dizziness that occurs on standing because of the lack of adequate blood volume to maintain nourishment of brain cells. To test whether a woman will be susceptible to orthostatic hypotension, assess her blood pressure and pulse while she is lying supine. Advise her to always sit up slowly and "dangle" on the side of her bed before attempting to walk. Caution her not to attempt to walk carrying her newborn until her cardiovascular status adjusts to her blood loss.

Progressive changes

Two physiological changes that occur during the puerperium involve progressive changes or the building of new tissue. Because building new tissue requires good nutrition, caution women against strict dieting that would limit cell-building ability during the first 6 weeks after childbirth (Rolfes, Pinna & Whitney, 2009).

Breastfeeding

The formation of breast milk (lactation) begins in a postnatal woman whether or not she plans to breastfeed (Walker, 2013). Early in pregnancy, the increased oestrogen level produced by the placenta stimulates the growth of milk glands; breasts increase in size because of the larger glands, accumulated fluid and some extra adipose tissue. For the first 2 days after birth, women will notice little change in their breasts from the way they were during pregnancy. From midway through pregnancy, women may experience secretion of colostrum—a thick, yellowish fluid. Colostrum will continue to be secreted during the first 2 to 3 days postpartum and is the baby's first milk. Frequent feeding encourages the production of mature breast milk that is produced from about 3 days postpartum. The production of mature breast milk will result in the woman's breasts feeling full and tense or tender.

Breast milk forms in response to the decrease in oestrogen and progesterone levels that follows delivery of the placenta (which stimulates prolactin production and, consequently, milk production). When breast milk first begins to form, the milk ducts become distended. The nipple secretion changes from the creamy colostrum to bluish white, the typical colour of breast milk. A woman's breasts become fuller, larger and firmer. In many women, breast distension becomes marked and this often is accompanied by a feeling of heat or throbbing pain. Breast tissue may appear reddened, simulating an acute inflammatory or infectious process. The distension is not limited to the milk ducts but occurs in the surrounding tissue as well, because blood and lymph enter the area to contribute fluid to the formation of milk. This feeling of tension in the breasts on the third or fourth day after birth is termed primary **engorgement** and can be minimised by early and frequent breastfeeding. It fades as the infant begins effective sucking and empties the breasts of milk. Whether milk production continues depends on the sucking of the infant at the breasts as this releases oxytocin and causes new milk to form.

Whether women continue to breastfeed after hospital discharge is influenced by such factors as breastfeeding support both in hospital and in the community, employment, personal habits and how important they view breastfeeding to be (Abdulwadud & Snow, 2009). Adequate support systems to ensure that individual needs are being met also influence the duration of breastfeeding. Women must be certain to drink adequate fluid daily, eat a nutritious diet and check with their healthcare provider before ingesting medications or alternative therapies such as herbs as most of these can be found in breast milk and could be toxic to a newborn (Riordan & Wambach, 2010). Techniques for breastfeeding are discussed in Chapter 19.

Return of menstrual flow

With the delivery of the placenta, the production of placental oestrogen and progesterone ends. The resulting decrease in hormone concentrations causes a rise in production of follicle-stimulating hormone (FSH) by the pituitary, which leads, with only a slight delay, to the return of ovulation. This initiates the return of the normal menstrual cycle. A woman who is not breastfeeding can expect her menstrual flow to return in 7 to 9 weeks after birth. If she is breastfeeding, her menstrual flow may not return for 3 or 4 months (lactational amenorrhoea) or, in some women, for the entire lactation period. However, the absence of a menstrual flow does not guarantee that a woman will not conceive during this time, because she may ovulate before menstruation returns (Pairman et al., 2015).

NURSING CARE OF A WOMAN AND FAMILY DURING THE FIRST 24 HOURS AFTER BIRTH

Ideally, a woman remains in a birthing room for at least the first hour after birth so she can be monitored for uterine involution and normal blood loss, and undergo perineal repair where necessary. In addition, the initiation of breastfeeding within the first hour after birth is encouraged and the woman has time to become acquainted with her newborn. After this initial hour, it is helpful for the woman to be educated about perineal care and the risk of haemorrhage post-birth. She then remains in the room as a postnatal patient or is transferred to a separate postnatal room. Primary postpartum haemorrhage is possible for the first 24 hours after birth, until the myometrial vessels have sclerosed. Secondary postpartum haemorrhage (up to 6 weeks) is still a potential risk and one that nurses may encounter while the woman is either in hospital or in the community.

Laboratory data

Women who experienced excessive blood loss or underwent caesarean section routinely have their haemoglobin and haematocrit levels measured 12 to 24 hours after birth, to determine whether blood loss at birth has left them anaemic. If the haemoglobin finding is lower than 10 g/100 mL, supplementary iron is usually prescribed. Take note of the laboratory reports on a postnatal woman and make certain that any abnormal finding, such as low haemoglobin, is brought to the attention of the woman's doctor or midwife. The responsibilities of being a new mother, coupled with the additional burden of an undetected low haemoglobin level, can severely tax a woman's energy levels (Dodd, Dare & Middleton, 2009).

Postnatal physical assessment

During the postnatal period, repetition of a complete examination is not necessary. Crucial assessments examining particular aspects of health, such as an estimation of nutrition and fluid state, energy level, presence or absence of pain, breast health, fundal height and consistency, lochia amount and character, perineal integrity and circulatory adequacy are required. With early discharge, women require postnatal education on self-assessment to ensure they will seek medical assistance should abnormalities occur.

General appearance

A woman's general appearance in the postnatal period reveals a great deal about her energy level, her self-esteem and whether she is moving into the taking-hold phase of recovery. The postnatal period is generally regarded as a time of wellness; early ambulation and eating a varied diet are encouraged. In some cultures, the period after childbirth may be regarded primarily as a time of rest. Cultural differences include restricting certain foods, reducing activity levels, or both; taboos and rituals are not uncommon. Assessing women in the postnatal period for cultural variations of these types is important, because such variations can explain why a woman might be reluctant to ambulate or why she leaves food she views as unacceptable uneaten although she says she is hungry.

Breasts

Breast tissue increases in size as breast milk forms, so a bra that was adequate during pregnancy may no longer be adequate by the second or third postnatal day. Use of a bra supports breast tissue that feels heavy because of increased fluid accumulation and aids comfort. Advise women to buy a maternity bra for the postnatal period that is one to two sizes larger than their pregnancy size to allow for this increase. Properly fitted, a bra should sit firmly and snugly. The straps should not leave erythematic marks on a woman's shoulders and there should be no underwires.

Breast tissue should feel soft on palpation on the first and second postnatal day. Towards the third day, it should begin to feel firm and warm (described as *filling*). With each day, breasts will appear larger and firmer. On palpation, they will feel hard and irregular and may be painful. If engorgement occurs the entire breast may feel warm or appear reddened. Many women experience little discomfort during this period. If only one segment of a breast is warm or reddened, inflammation or, possibly, infection of glands or milk ducts (mastitis) is suggested (Walker, 2013). The midwife will assess for inverted nipples, cracks, fissures or the presence of caked milk. Avoid squeezing the nipples because this can be painful.

Uterus

Before performing a uterine assessment it is helpful to ask the woman to void to minimise discomfort and ensure the fundus can be correctly palpated. To correctly palpate the fundal height the midwife or medical practitioner will ask the woman to lie supine so that the height of the uterus is not influenced by an elevated position. Observation of her abdomen for contour, to detect distension and for the appearance of striae or a diastasis, is useful.

The midwife will palpate the fundus of the uterus by placing the dominant hand at or below the umbilicus (see Fig. 17.4). The midwife will press in and downwards with the hand at the umbilicus until a "bump" against a firm globular mass in the abdomen is felt. Consistency (firm, soft or boggy), location (midline) and height are assessed. For the first hour after birth, the height of the fundus is at the umbilicus or even slightly above it, decreasing about one fingerbreadth in size daily. The height is measured in fingerbreadths or centimetres (e.g. 2 fingerbreadths equals 2 cm) beneath the umbilicus.

Palpation of a fundus should not cause pain as long as the action is done gently (unless the woman is recovering from caesarean section where adequate pain relief is required). If the uterus is not firm on palpation, the midwife will massage it gently with the examining hand. This usually causes the uterus to contract and become firm immediately. A gentle rotating motion is used to minimise pain. If the uterine fundus does not grow firm with massage, extreme atony, possibly retained placental fragments or an excess amount of blood loss may be occurring. Placing the woman's infant at the breast will cause endogenous release of oxytocin which will assist in uterine involution; however, breastfeeding is not adequate to manage a postpartum haemorrhage.

If massage appears ineffective, a clot may be present in the cavity of the uterus. The clot may be expressed from the uterus by gentle pressure on the fundus, but only after the uterus has been massaged. This can be painful for the woman. Another reason the uterus may not be well contracted is that a rapidly filling bladder is preventing contraction.

A woman who received no oxytocin after birth to help her uterus contract is at greater risk of poor uterine contraction than a woman who did. If no oxytocin was given, the midwife should assess the woman's uterine fundus every 10 to 15 minutes immediately after birth, to evaluate and assist the fundus to contract, should it become soft or relaxed. Once the first hour after birth has passed, a woman's uterus may be evaluated for height and consistency less frequently, depending on institutional policy. By the ninth or tenth day after delivery, the uterus will have

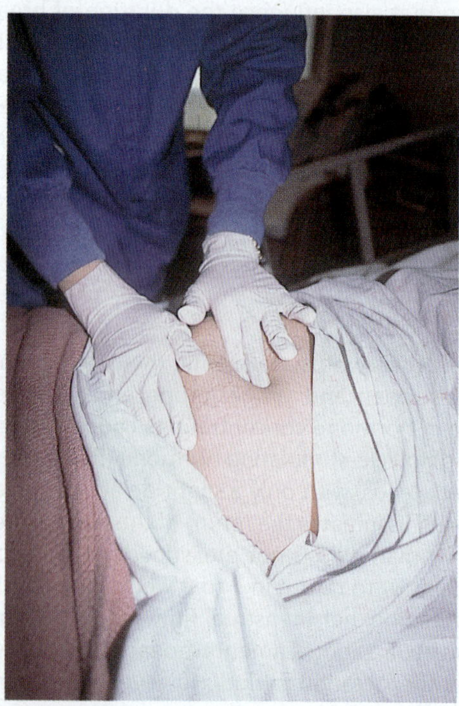

FIGURE 17.4 To palpate a uterus, be certain to place one hand at the base of the uterus. This fundus measures about two fingerbreadths below the umbilicus.

become so small it is no longer palpable above the symphysis pubis.

Lochia

During the first hour the midwife will inspect the mother's perineal pad and evaluate lochia character, amount, colour (rubra, serosa or alba), odour and presence of any clots. When the midwife asks a woman to turn so she can inspect her perineum, she will check under her buttocks to observe any blood that may be pooling beneath her. If there is a constant trickle of vaginal flow or the soaking through of a thick maternity pad every 60 minutes, the woman needs to be checked for the cause of excessive bleeding and a referral to the medical officer is required urgently.

Perineum

While evaluating lochia, also inspect the perineum. If perineal trauma has occurred or an episiotomy was performed, position the woman on her side. Gently lift the upper buttock and inspect the perineum. Observe for ecchymosis, haematoma, erythema, oedema, intactness and the presence of drainage or bleeding from any sutures.

An episiotomy is usually 2–4 cm long. A haematoma (blood-filled, protruding sphere) could be present if surface capillaries were broken during the pressure of birth; this should be noted as a potential complication. If there is clotted lochia along the incision line, re-educate the woman about the importance of hygiene and perineal care so that this does not continue to occur. Before discharge, teach a woman who has perineal sutures how to lie on her back and view her perineum with a handheld mirror so that, once a day while at home, she can inspect her perineum for redness, sloughing of sutures, pus formation or drainage at the suture line. After perineal assessment, assess the rectal area for the presence of haemorrhoids. If any are present, document their number, appearance and size in centimetres.

> ***What if...***
>
> Jae, at 18 hours postpartum, states that she has had to change her maternity pads twice in the last 30 minutes because they were saturated? She noticed two large clots on the last pad. What assessment should you first perform on her and why?

Nursing considerations

Pain relief for afterpains

Pain from uterine contractions can be intense, but you can assure a woman that this type of discomfort is normal and rarely lasts longer than a week. If necessary, an anti-inflammatory or a common analgesic is effective for pain relief. In addition, applying heat to the abdomen can be comforting (Thorpe & Anderson, 2010).

Muscular aches

Many women feel sore and aching after labour and birth because of the excessive energy they used for pushing during birth. Often rest or a mild analgesia is sufficient.

Cold and hot therapy

Applying an ice or cold pack to the perineum for the first 2 to 3 days reduces perineal oedema and the possibility of haematoma formation, thereby reducing pain and promoting healing and comfort. Be certain not to place ice or plastic directly on the woman's perineum. Commercial cold packs combined with perineal pads are available. For a low-cost alternative, a rubber glove may be partially filled with ice chips, provided latex allergy is not a concern. After this time healing is enhanced if circulation to the area is encouraged by the use of heat. Dry heat in the form of a perineal hot pack or moist heat with a bath is an effective way to increase circulation to the perineum, provide comfort, reduce oedema and promote healing.

Pelvic floor exercises

Some women find that carrying out pelvic floor (Kegel) exercises three or four times a day can greatly relieve perineal oedema. This aids comfort by improving circulation to the area and decreasing oedema. When repeated frequently, Kegel exercises also help a woman regain her pre-pregnant muscle tone and help prevent urinary incontinence (Hay-Smith & Dumoulin, 2009).

Education for care of perineal trauma

Although relatively small in size, perineal sutures can cause considerable discomfort, because the perineum is an extremely tender area and the muscles of the perineum are involved in many activities such as sitting, walking, stooping, squatting, bending, urinating and defecating. Because the perineal area heals rapidly, women can be assured that this discomfort is normal and does not usually last longer than 5 or 6 days. A woman may worry that she will experience additional discomfort when the sutures are removed. Explain that the sutures are made of an absorbable material so will not need to be removed. Sutures usually dissolve within 10 days.

Rest

Few women are prepared for the degree of fatigue they experience after childbirth. Try to do all procedures swiftly yet gently, to allow as much time for sleep as possible. Some women experience shaking chills immediately or within a half-hour after birth. This is caused in part by the pressure changes in the abdomen that occur with reduction in the bulk of the uterus and temperature readjustment in response to the diaphoresis of labour. It also may result from the exhilaration the woman is feeling, combined with exhaustion. In any event, shaking chills at this point are common. Reassure the woman that chills are common, so that she will not attribute them to a developing cold or infection.

Many women do not realise how long it will take to fully return to their previous level of functioning. When families were closely knit and neighbourhoods were smaller, new mothers often had support to look after the baby while they rested. Today, many couples do not have family or close friends nearby. If the parents have not thought through this problem before birth, you can help them look at their situation and see what is available to them. A woman without support has many demands arising from her new role. If she is overcome by fatigue, her judgement and sense of balance can be blurred.

Adequate fluid intake

Women often feel thirsty during this period of rapid fluid loss and want additional fluid. It seems a paradox that while the body is ridding itself of unwanted fluid, it should also demand fluid. Part of this paradox stems from a woman having had little to drink during labour. Part of the need for fluid stems from the increased amount of nitrogen being released from catabolised uterine cells. A woman needs to increase her fluid intake to rid her body of these wastes.

Urinary elimination

Because the diuresis of the postnatal period begins almost immediately after birth, a woman's bladder begins filling almost immediately. A full bladder puts pressure on the uterus and causes difficulty with uterine contraction. An over-distended bladder may also damage bladder function. Women who have had epidural anaesthesia are particularly prone to developing urinary retention (Simmons et al., 2012).

Encourage a woman to walk to the bathroom and void at the end of the first hour after birth, to help prevent bladder distension. Some women have too much perineal oedema to be able to void this early. A woman with perineal trauma may be reluctant to void because she knows that acid urine against her sutures will sting. If the woman still has not been able to void by 4 to 8 hours after birth and bladder distension is present, she will need to be catheterised. Fortunately for most women who must be catheterised, the procedure needs to be done only once after birth. Usually, after another 6 to 8 hours have passed and the bladder has filled again, some of the perineal oedema has subsided, the bladder has achieved better tone and the woman is able to void by herself. Some women report urinary incontinence during the postnatal period, resulting from poor perineal tone and sensation. Kegel exercises are helpful to strengthen perineal muscles and eliminate incontinence in the future.

BOX 17.4 ✻ Focus on pharmacology

Docusate sodium (Coloxyl)

Classification: Docusate sodium is a stool softener

Action: Used in the postpartum period to prevent constipation. It works by lowering the surface tension of faeces, allowing water and lipids to penetrate the stool and soften it (McKenna & Mirkov, 2014)

Pregnancy risk category: C

Dosage: 50–100 mg PO daily

Possible adverse effects: Occasional abdominal pain and diarrhoea

Nursing implications

- Encourage a woman to swallow the medication with a full glass of water or juice
- Instruct a woman to consume high-fibre foods to encourage elimination
- Encourage activity to promote intestinal motility

Constipation

Many women have difficulty moving their bowels during the first week of the puerperium, a condition that can be concerning and uncomfortable. Constipation occurs because of relaxation of the abdominal wall and the intestine, now that they are no longer compressed by the bulky uterus, and the use of pain relief containing codeine. For a bowel movement, the abdominal wall must exert pressure. In its relaxed state, the pressure is not strong enough to be effective. Also, if haemorrhoids or perineal sutures are present, a woman may decline to try to move her bowels for fear of pain.

To prevent constipation, many women are prescribed a stool softener, beginning with the first day after birth (see Box 17.4). If a woman has not moved her bowels by the third postpartum day, a mild laxative may be prescribed. Early ambulation, a good diet with adequate roughage and an adequate fluid intake all aid in preventing the problem of constipation. Bowel evacuation may also be difficult because of the pain of perineal sutures and/or other perineal trauma or haemorrhoids.

Haemorrhoids

The pressure of the fetal head on the rectal veins during birth tends to aggravate or produce haemorrhoids (swollen rectal veins) to such an extent that some women find haemorrhoidal discomfort to be their chief discomfort in the first few days after birth (Quijano & Abalos, 2009). This discomfort can be relieved by baths, anaesthetic sprays, witch hazel or astringent preparations.

Peripheral circulation

The midwife will assess for oedema at the ankle and over the tibia on the lower leg. In addition, the midwife can also assess for thrombophlebitis by palpating the calf area for heat and examining the lower legs for signs of inflammation or distension. Be certain to allow a woman to dangle her legs on the edge of the bed for a few minutes to prevent dizziness before she gets up for the first time. Then assist her as needed to take the few steps to a nearby bathroom. Remain with her to be certain that dizziness does not occur. After this, she may be up on her own as she wishes.

Breast hygiene

If a woman is breastfeeding, encouraging her newborn to suck at the breast will reduce the risk of engorgement. Similarly, breastfeeding is the main treatment for relief of the tenderness and soreness of primary breast engorgement (techniques of breastfeeding are discussed in Chapter 19). Many women find the application of warm compresses or standing under a warm shower beneficial to relieve engorgement discomfort. Good support from a maternity bra also offers relief because it prevents unnecessary strain on the supporting muscles of the breasts, positions the breasts in good alignment and diminishes the amount of engorgement caused by blocked milk ducts. A woman who is not breastfeeding may experience even stronger discomfort. However, when little or no milk is removed from the breasts, the accumulation of milk inhibits further milk formation and engorgement subsides in about 2 days. Cold compresses, applied to the breasts three or four times a day during the period of engorgement, or an oral analgesic, or both, provide relief. Wearing a snug-fitting bra and avoiding nipple stimulation may help. Restricting fluid and expressing milk from the breasts are not effective measures to manage engorgement and are to some degree harmful, so these actions should be avoided.

It is not necessary for women to wash their breasts more often than daily. They should avoid using soap, because it tends to dry the nipples, possibly leading to nipple trauma. A woman who secretes a considerable amount of colostrum or milk from her breasts (whether breastfeeding or not) should insert clean gauze squares or commercial breastfeeding pads into her bra to absorb the moisture, changing them as often as necessary to keep the nipples dry. If the nipples remain wet for any length of time, nipple trauma may form and lead to infection.

Postnatal exercise

A woman can best help her abdominal wall to return to good tone by using proper body mechanics and posture, getting adequate rest and performing prescribed exercises. Exercises to strengthen the abdominal and pelvic muscles may be started, on advice from the woman's doctor, physiotherapist or midwife, as early as the first day after birth. She should continue these exercises until the end of the puerperium to derive the maximum benefit from them. Many women find commercial abdominal exercisers helpful to fully strengthen their abdominal wall.

Sexual relationships in the postnatal period

At one time, women were cautioned not to resume sexual relations after the birth of a baby until after their medical check-up at 6 weeks. However, there is no apparent physiological reason to delay sexual relations this long. For most couples, coitus may be resumed as soon as lochia serosa has stopped. Caution women, however, that intercourse may be somewhat uncomfortable if it is begun too early. Tissue at a perineal wound site may be sensitive. Perineal trauma should be healed before resumption of intercourse. Because the vaginal epithelium is still thin, vaginal tenderness may be noticed. Use of a lubricant will help any mucosal dryness. A woman who is breastfeeding may notice that milk is released from her nipples with sexual arousal. Women may already be aware that their degree of exhaustion can make them less receptive to sexual arousal than before. Be sure that women receive adequate reproductive planning information, if desired, before they resume sexual relations (see Chapter 6).

BOX 17.5 * Signs of good parent–child adaptation

Good parent–child adaptation is demonstrated when a parent:

- Speaks of the baby as desirable and attractive
- Is not upset by vomiting, drooling and the like
- Holds the baby warmly
- Makes eye contact with the baby
- Plays with and soothes the baby
- Talks or sings to the baby
- Expresses confidence that the baby is well
- Finds physical or psychological attributes to admire about the baby
- Is able to discriminate between the baby's signs of hunger, sleep and so on.

Bonding

To assess that bonding is occurring, observe parenting behaviours and listen to what parents say about their newborn in the immediate postnatal period (see Box 17.5). First impressions may not be lasting ones; however, negative comments need to be identified, so that extra discussion can take place. Although brief hospital stays are advantageous in many ways, if such discussion does not occur, a family may be discharged from the healthcare agency with their needs unmet (Brown et al., 2009). At home, away from healthcare personnel who are attuned to how disappointment can interfere with parent–child interaction, parents may have great difficulty adjusting to and relating to this new child.

NURSING CARE OF A WOMAN AND FAMILY IN PREPARATION FOR DISCHARGE

The greatest need of a postnatal woman before discharge from a healthcare agency is education to prepare her to care for herself and her newborn at home. She must be aware of signs and symptoms of complications for herself and her baby and know whom to call if she notices any of them. She must understand safe baby care. Because of shortened lengths of stay, every contact with women during their hospital stay should include some education. At the same time, be aware that learning does not take place if the learner is overwhelmed and hurried. Use common sense to determine when it is time to teach and when it is time to observe or listen.

Many women attend classes in newborn care during their pregnancies. They remember many points from these classes, but when they actually have a newborn they can become worried that they do not remember enough. Many mothers say that childcare did not seem real during pregnancy. The postnatal period is a time for teaching, re-teaching and offering anticipatory guidance to help in the new situations a family can expect when they go home.

Some nurses assume that multiparas will react negatively to childcare suggestions. However, most women appreciate up-to-date information about baby care and parenting. For example, a mother of girls may feel insecure about the care of her new baby boy, or a woman whose next youngest child is 5 years old may admit that in 5 years she has forgotten much about care of the newborn. The nurse who is comfortable with newborn care is able to reassure the woman that she is competently caring for her own baby. All mothers, whether primiparas or multiparas, need to be evaluated individually and helped whenever they ask or you find that they need guidance.

Group classes

Providing group classes on topics such as bathing infants, breastfeeding techniques, minimising jealousy in older children and maintaining health in the newborn can be helpful to parents. In many settings, referral of families to community health services who provide postnatal parenting classes may be useful, as in the immediate postnatal period, there is often too much to take in. In these settings they can learn not only from the instructor but also from other parents, and develop long-term friendships with other young families. During their hospital stay or postnatal home visiting by midwives, time for questions should be planned so parents can apply what is being taught to their individual circumstances. Urging fathers/partners to attend classes is helpful, because many fathers/partners give direct childcare for at least part of every day. Including the father/partner in teaching is also important, because the problems that arise with newborn care are, by their nature, family problems, and every effort should be made by nursing personnel to help both parents prepare to deal with them.

Discharge planning

Before a postnatal family is discharged from hospital, a woman will be given instructions by her doctor or midwife concerning her care at home. These instructions differ among healthcare providers.

Before discharge, make sure a woman is aware that she must see her medical practitioner for an examination 6 weeks after birth. Women whose blood group is Rh-negative and who have had an Rh-positive infant will receive Rh(D) Immunoglobulin (anti-D) to prevent problems in a future pregnancy (Crowther & Middleton, 2009). In addition, they may be advised to update their immunisations for illnesses such as pertussis that can be fatal for babies.

Discharge instructions for the family are given both verbally and in writing. Getting ready to go home, dressing the baby, seeing him or her in new clothes for the first time and experiencing the thrill of realising the baby is really theirs to take home is so exciting that oral instructions may go unheard. On the other hand, parents should not simply be handed a list of printed material. Review the instructions with the parents to be sure they understand them.

The Australian Institute of Family Studies is Australia's key research body on families and conducts social research about Australian families to make recommendations to government for policy and strategy direction. Each state and territory has overarching policy frameworks to support families. These can be accessed through various government websites:

- New South Wales: www.families.nsw.gov.au
- Queensland: www.qld.gov.au/families/babies/advice
- Victoria: www.dhs.vic.gov.au/for-individuals/children,-families-and-young-people/family-and-parenting support
- Northern Territory: http://childrenandfamilies.nt.gov.au/Families
- South Australia: www.parenting.sa.gov.au
- Tasmania: www.dhhs.tas.gov.au/children/child_health
- Australian Capital Territory: www.parentlink.act.gov.au
- Western Australia: www.communities.wa.gov.au/communities-in-focus/parenting_and_children/Pages/default.aspx

Linking women and families to resources in the community is vital in enabling them to make a smooth transition to parenthood. Community Health Centres are often the first service that can give advice on parenting or link women to other services on a needs basis. Each jurisdiction has various programs to help new parents and some programs are nationally accessible. For example, the Raising Children website (<http://raisingchildren.net.au>) is an Australian parenting website which provides information for day-to-day parenting decisions. In some jurisdictions face-to-face or over-the-phone parenting programs exist to support parenting, such as the Bupa parent and baby wellbeing program (over the phone and email); Relaxing into parenting (face-to-face in the ACT); and Baby makes 3 (face-to-face in Victoria).

NURSING CARE OF A WOMAN AND FAMILY AFTER DISCHARGE

Postnatal home visits

In today's healthcare climate of cost containment, most women are discharged from a healthcare facility 2 to 3 days after childbirth. Such a practice has the advantage of allowing the family unit to be interrupted as little as possible. A new mother may rest better at home than in a strange setting and she may eat better if she has cultural preferences for specific foods. The infant can be more quickly exposed to family routines rather than a superficial facility schedule. However, early discharge has the disadvantage of not allowing a new family to have the ready support of healthcare personnel if they have questions about their newborn or about the woman's condition.

In New Zealand, all pregnant women choose a lead maternity care (LMC) person. Part of the LMC role is to assess postnatal requirements and implement care. The Maternity Facility Service Specifications are national documents that describe the service that maternity facilities are required to provide to women and their families. However, this differs in Australia where postnatal visits in women's homes after discharge from hospital are limited according to models of care and funding (Dixon, 2010, pp. 577, 578).

The purposes of a home visit for the well postpartum woman and her newborn are to help integrate the infant into the family and to provide the family with additional information on newborn care that they may not have been able to learn during a brief hospital stay. Such a visit also allows for physical examination of the woman and newborn, and for newborn screening procedures or bilirubin testing if these were not done before hospital discharge.

Families NSW has proposed a new component to healthcare policy to ensure a consistent state-wide approach to the provision of primary healthcare (PHC) to parents expecting or caring for a new baby. This policy utilises a PHC model of care for the provision of universal assessment, coordinated care and home visiting, by NSW Health's maternity and community health services, for all parents expecting or caring for a new baby. This policy recognises that all families require support to raise their children with health services working with the family and facilitating the development of healthy relationships. You can obtain a copy of this policy at the NSW Health website <www.health.nsw.gov.au>.

NURSING CARE OF A POSTNATAL WOMAN AND FAMILY WITH UNIQUE NEEDS

A woman who chooses not to keep her child

Although the availability of contraception information and the ability of women to secure abortions have reduced the number of unwanted or unplanned children, some women still may complete a pregnancy and then give up their child for adoption. There are numerous reasons for this decision and the decision should be respected.

The decision to place a child for adoption may be a mutual decision made by both parents. In New Zealand, the mother is always the guardian and the father is a guardian if he has lived with the mother at any time during the pregnancy and/or his name is on the birth registration (New Zealand Government Ministry for Social Development, 2011). The NSW Government provides guidelines for adoption: Adoption of a Child—Guidelines for Hospitals & Maternity Staff in Response To Parents Considering. Details are available from the NSW Health website.

For a woman who chooses not to keep her child, the wait in the birthing room for preparations to transfer the baby to a nursery may seem unusually long. She may also be alone and have no partner or support person with her during this time. Every woman has a right to see, hold and feed her child if she wishes. A woman who is not going to keep her child may still feel proud that she has produced a healthy baby. Nurses must not attempt to change a woman's mind about keeping her child or placing the child for adoption during the postnatal period. Women are extremely vulnerable to suggestion at this time and such decisions are too long range and too important to be made at such an emotional time. A woman's earlier conclusions may be the most sound ones. Instead, you should offer non-judgemental support. Be especially aware of your own feelings about this issue, to avoid influencing a woman's decision making unnecessarily.

A woman who is discharged but whose child remains hospitalised

Newborns that are premature or ill at birth are often transported to a regional centre or to a neonatal intensive care nursery for care, a move that automatically separates them from their parents, particularly if they live in a remote or regional part of the country. In 2011 in Australia, 8.3% of births were premature, with the highest incidence in the Northern Territory (11.1%) and the lowest in New South Wales (7.5%). Babies can spend days, weeks and even months separated from their parents in the neonatal nursery.

To help the mother with the issue of separation many transport teams and neonatal nursery nurses take a photograph of the baby and leave it with her. They also leave the nursery telephone number and the name of a nurse or doctor to contact for questions or information. Most transport teams call the mother after they arrive at the distant hospital to assure her that her infant has managed the stress of transport well.

Maintaining communication with the nursery is important so that parents can begin to bond with their child. Parents are encouraged to call the nursery frequently to ask about their infant. If the infant is hospitalised in the same hospital, mothers are encouraged to spend as much time in the nursery as possible, and in some cases, the baby may be able to room in with the mother for periods of time. Assuring the mother that her telephone calls and visits are encouraged will enable her to feel more confident in caring for her baby in the nursery. It is easy for a woman who is separated from her newborn to feel highly stressed (Lee & O'Brien, 2014). Some mothers whose infants are ill at birth may feel uncomfortable sharing a hospital room with a postnatal roommate who is caring for a well baby. When this happens it is often a good time to arrange for a visit to the nursery or to suggest that you and the woman take a walk in the hallway to increase her amount of ambulation.

A family who is adopting a child

A family who is adopting an infant may come into the hospital or birthing centre to meet their new infant for the first time. Such a couple needs the same introduction to newborn care as biological parents. Additional needs of adopting parents are discussed in Chapter 3.

CASE STUDY QUESTION

4. You care for Jae at a 6-week postpartum visit. What should an estimation of her fundal height be at this time?
   a. Six fingerbreadths below the umbilicus
   b. No longer palpable on her abdomen
   c. 1 cm above the symphysis pubis
   d. Inverted and palpable at the cervix

Key points for review

- The postnatal period (puerperium) is the 6-week period after childbirth. This is an important period, because it marks the child's introduction to the family. Women move through an initial "taking-in" phase, in which they are dependent; a "taking-hold" phase, in which they manifest independence; and a "letting-go" phase, in which the mother role is finally defined.
- Rooming-in is the preferred arrangement for postnatal families, because it allows a new family the best chance for quality interaction. The more time new parents spend with a newborn, the more likely it is that effective bonding will occur. Help parents to feel comfortable with their newborn by offering anticipatory guidance and role modelling infant care.
- "Postnatal blues" are a normal accompaniment to childbirth. You can assure a woman that her feelings are normal and offer supportive care until the emotion passes.
- Uterine involution is the process whereby the uterus returns to its pre-pregnant state. A uterus decreases in size one fingerbreadth a day until it disappears under the pubic bone at about day 10.
- Lochia is the name of the vaginal flow after childbirth: the flow is lochia rubra (red) for the first 1 to 3 days, lochia serosa (pink to brown) on days 4 to 10 and lochia alba (white) until 2 to 6 weeks after the birth.
- A woman is at risk of haemorrhage in the postnatal period, so assessments done during this time are some of the most critical assessments made in nursing. Do not discount the importance of these assessments because the overall content of the postnatal period is so focused on wellness.
- Lactation is the production of breast milk. Colostrum is present immediately after birth; milk forms on the third to fourth postnatal day. A feeling of fullness and firmness on this day is termed filling; if warmth and discomfort occur, it is termed engorgement.
- Women may need various comfort measures to alleviate pain from sutures, uterine pain (afterpains) and breast tenderness. Application of cold or heat and administration of analgesics are important nursing interventions.
- Nurses need to work in partnership with women to ensure they have the necessary self-care knowledge before discharge. All women should seek a postnatal medical assessment visit at 6 weeks after childbirth, to be certain their reproductive organs have returned to their pre-pregnant state. A menstrual flow should return within 6 to 10 weeks in the non-breastfeeding mother, or 3 to 4 months in the breastfeeding mother.

CASE STUDY QUESTIONS

5. Jae is unsure of how she will cope once discharged from hospital. Identify strategies that Jae and her husband can utilise to ensure there is a smooth transition period to returning home and beginning family life.
6. Suppose because Jae does not have an episiotomy incision, you expect her to have little perineal discomfort but instead, she states that her perineal pain is excruciating. You notice she has haemorrhoids. You overhear her tell her husband that he is acting selfishly by paying more attention to their new daughter than to her. You also observe her handing her baby roughly to her husband. What could you suggest to make her more comfortable?

Resources

For an extensive range of additional resources to enhance teaching and learning and to facilitate understanding of this chapter, please see the text's accompanying website located on thePoint at http://thepoint.lww.com.

References

Abdulwadud, O. A. & Snow, M. E. (2009). Interventions in the workplace to support breastfeeding for women in employment. *Cochrane Database of Systematic Reviews,* (1), (CD006177).

Bridges, W. (1994). *Job Shift: How to Prosper in a Workplace Without Jobs.* Menlo Park, CA: Addison-Wesley.

Brown, S., et al. (2009). Early postnatal discharge from hospital for healthy mothers and term infants. *Cochrane Database of Systematic Reviews,* (1), (CD002958).

Buist, A. (2014). Perinatal mental health: Identifying problems and managing medications. *Australian Family Physician, 43*(4), 182–185.

Buultjens, M. & Liamputtong, P. (2007). When giving life starts to take the life out of you: Women's experiences of depression after childbirth. *Midwifery, 23*(1), 77–91.

Corwin, E. J. & Arbour, M. (2007). Postpartum fatigue and evidence-based interventions. *MCN: The American Journal of Maternal/Child Nursing, 32*(4), 215–222.

Crippen, C. & Brew, L. (2013). Strategies of cultural adaptation in intercultural parenting. *The Family Journal: Counseling and Therapy for Couples and Families, 21*(3), 263–271.

Crowther, C. & Middleton, P. (2009). Anti-D administration after childbirth for preventing Rhesus alloimmunisation. *Cochrane Database of Systematic Reviews,* (1), (CD000021).

Dixon, L. (2015). Supporting women becoming mothers. In S. Pairman, S. Tracy, C. Thurgood & J. Pincombe (Eds). *Midwifery Preparation for Practice* (3rd ed.). Sydney: Churchill Livingstone Elsevier.

Dodd, J., Dare, M. R. & Middleton, P. (2009). Treatment for women with postpartum iron deficiency anaemia. *Cochrane Database of Systematic Reviews,* (1), (CD004222).

Engqvist, I., et al. (2007). Strategies in caring for women with postpartum psychosis—an interview study with psychiatric nurses. *Journal of Clinical Nursing, 16*(7), 1333–1342.

Fontenot, H. B. (2007). Transition and adaptation to adoptive motherhood. *Journal of Obstetric, Gynecologic and Neonatal Nursing, 36*(2), 175–182.

Hay-Smith, E.J.C. & Dumoulin, C. (2009). Pelvic floor muscle training versus no treatment, or inactive control treatments, for urinary incontinence in women. *Cochrane Database of Systematic Reviews,* (1), (CD005654).

Holden, G. W. (2010). *Parenting: A Dynamic Perspective.* Los Angeles: Sage Publications.

Jaafar, S. H., Lee, K. S. & Ho, J. J. (2012). Separate care for new mother and infant versus rooming-in for increasing the duration of breastfeeding. *Cochrane Database of Systematic Reviews,* (9), (CD006641).

Johnson, K. (2013). Maternal – infant bonding: A review of the literature. *International Journal of Childbirth Education, 28*(3), 17–22.

Lee, S. & O'Brien, K. (2014). Parents and primary caregivers in the neonatal intensive care unit. *Canadian Medical Association Journal, 186*(11), 845.

Lipscomb, K. & Novy, M. J. (2007). The normal puerperium. In A. H. DeCherney & L. Nathan (Eds). *Current Diagnosis and Treatment in Obstetrics and Gynecology* (10th ed.). Columbus, OH: McGraw-Hill.

McGarry, J., et al. (2009). Postpartum depression and help-seeking behavior. *Journal of Widwifery & Women's Health, 54*(1), 50–56.

McKenna, L. & Mirkov, S. (2014). *McKenna's Drug Handbook for Nursing & Midwifery* (7th ed.). Sydney: Lippincott Williams & Wilkins.

Moore, E. R., Anderson, G. C. & Bergman, N. (2009). Early skin-to-skin contact for mothers and their healthy newborn infants. *Cochrane Database of Systematic Reviews,* (1), (CD003519).

New Zealand Government Ministry of Social Development. (2014). Child youth and family. Accessed 17 December 2014, <www.cyf.govt.nz/adoption/placing-your-child-for-adoption/index.html>.

NSW Pregnancy and Newborn Services Network. (2014). Accessed 17 December 2014, <www.psn.org.au/index.php?option=com_contact&task=view&contact_id=1&Itemid=30>.

O'Hara, M. & Wisner, K. (2014). Perinatal mental illness: Definition, description and aetiology. *Best Practice & Research Clinical Obstetrics and Gynaecology, 28*(1), 3–12.

Pairman, S., Pincombe, J., Thorogood, C. & Tracey, S. (2015). *Midwifery Preparation for Practice* (3rd ed.). Australia: Elsevier.

Parker, R. & Hunter, C. (2011). *Supporting Couples across the Transition to Parenthood.* Australian Family Relationships Clearing House. No. 20.

Pavone, M. E., Purinton, S. C. & Petersen, S. M. (2007). Postpartum care and breast-feeding. In Fortner, K. B., et al. (Eds). *The Johns Hopkins Manual of Gynecology and Obstetrics.* Philadelphia: Lippincott Williams & Wilkins.

Poggi, S.B.H. (2007). Postpartum hemorrhage and the abnormal puerperium. In DeCherney, A. H. & Nathan, L. (Eds). *Current Diagnosis and Treatment in Obstetrics and Gynecology* (10th ed.). Columbus, OH: McGraw-Hill.

Quijano, C. E. & Abalos, E. (2009). Conservative management of symptomatic and/or complicated haemorrhoids in pregnancy and the puerperium. *Cochrane Database of Systematic Reviews,* (1), (CD004077).

Riordan, S. & Wambach, K. (2010). *Breastfeeding and Human Lactation.* Sudbury: Jones and Bartlett Publishers.

Rolfes, S. R., Pinna, K. & Whitney, E. (2009). Life cycle nutrition: Pregnancy and lactation. In S. R. Rolfes, K. Pinna & E. Whitney (Eds). *Understanding Normal and Clinical Nutrition* (8th ed.). Columbus, OH: McGraw-Hill.

Rubin, R. (1977). Binding-in in the postpartum period. *Maternal Child Nursing Journal, 6*(2), 67–69.

Simmons, S. W., Taghizadeh, N., Dennis, A. T., Hughes, D. & Cyna, A. M. (2012). Combined spinal-epidural versus epidural analgesia in labour. *Cochrane Database of Systematic Reviews,* (10), (CD003401).

Stables, D. & Rankin, J. (2010). *Physiology in Childbearing.* Edinburgh: Bailliere Tindall Elsevier.

Subramanian, A., et al. (Eds). (2008). *Drug Facts and Comparisons.* St Louis, MO: Wolters Kluwer Health.

Thorpe, J. & Anderson, J. (2010). Supporting women in labour and birth. In S. Pairman, S. Tracy, C. Thurgood & J. Pincombe (Eds). *Midwifery: Preparation for Practice* (2nd ed.), 486–511. Sydney: Churchill Livingstone Elsevier.

Van der Wijden, C., Kleijnen, J. & Van den Berk, T. (2009). Lactational amenorrhea for family planning. *Cochrane Database of Systematic Reviews,* (1), (CD001329).

Walker, M. (2013). *Breastfeeding Management for the Clinician: Using the Evidence* (3rd ed.). London: Jones and Bartlett Publishers.

Suggested readings

AIFS. (2014). Supporting couples across the transition to parenthood. AFRC Briefing No. 20. Accessed 28 January 2015, <www3.aifs.gov.au/cfca/publications/supporting-couples-across-transition-parenthood/key-factors-affecting-relationship>.

Kurth, E., Kennedy, H. P., Spichiger, E., et al. (2011). Crying babies, tired mothers: What do we know? A systematic review. *Midwifery, 27*(2), 187–194.

Lawrence, R. (2012). Breastfeeding triumphs. *Birth, 39*(4), 311–314.

Poh, H. & Koh, S. (2014). An integrative review of fathers' experiences during pregnancy and childbirth. *International Nursing Review, 61*(4), 543–554.

Vennemann, M., Hense, H., Bajanowski, T., Blair, P., Complojer, C., Moon, R. & Kiechl-Kohlendorfer, U. (2012). Bed sharing and the risk of sudden infant death syndrome: Can we resolve the debate? *The Journal of Pediatrics, 160*(1), 44–48.

Chapter 18

Nursing care of a family with a newborn

Previous chapters described the care of a pregnant woman and family during the antenatal, intrapartum and postnatal periods. This chapter adds information about caring for a newborn and family. The newborn period is important to a family's wellbeing because it lays the foundation for the rest of the family's childrearing years.

LEARNING OBJECTIVES

After mastering the contents of this chapter, you should be able to:

1. Describe the normal characteristics of a term newborn.
2. Use critical thinking to analyse ways that the care of a term newborn can be more family-centred.
3. Assess a newborn for normal growth and development.
4. Identify expected outcomes for a newborn and family during the first 4 weeks of life.
5. Discuss nursing care planning to augment normal development of a newborn, such as ways to aid parent–child bonding.
6. Implement nursing care of a normal newborn, such as instructing parents on the daily requirements of their newborn.
7. Identify areas related to newborn assessment and care that could benefit from additional nursing research or application of evidence-based practice.

KEY TERMS

- acrocyanosis
- caput succedaneum
- central cyanosis
- cephalhaematoma
- conduction
- convection
- erythema toxicum
- evaporation
- jaundice
- kernicterus
- lanugo
- macrosomia
- meconium
- neonate
- radiation
- vernix caseosa

CASE STUDY

Cassandra Phillips has just given birth to her second child, a 2.7-kg baby girl she named Beth. Apgar scores at 1 and 5 minutes were 6 and 8. Vital signs are temperature (axillary), 36.8°C; heart rate, 136 beats per minute; and respirations, 74 breaths per minute. She is 47 cm long, with a head circumference of 34 cm. She has a small port-wine birthmark on her right thigh. While Ryan, Cassandra's husband, is in the room, Cassandra tells you she is a "veteran" at baby care. Ryan adds, "Little Jordan [their 3-year-old] will be so excited to see his new sister. That's all he's been talking about lately." However, when Cassandra is alone, you notice she seems a little apprehensive about caring for her new daughter. She tells you, "She's so much smaller than Jordan was. And why does it sound like she has a cold? And what is this rash all over her? Isn't it bad enough she has a birthmark?"

CASE STUDY QUESTIONS

1. Does Cassandra know as much about newborns as she thought?
2. What additional teaching does this family need?

Newborns undergo profound physiological changes at the moment of birth (and, probably, psychological changes as well), as they are released from a warm, snug, dark, liquid-filled environment that has met all of their basic needs into a chilly, unbounded, brightly lit, gravity-based outside world. Within minutes of being plunged into this strange environment, a newborn has to initiate respirations and adapt a circulatory system to extrauterine oxygenation. Within 24 hours, neurological, renal, endocrine, gastrointestinal and metabolic functions must be operating competently for life to be sustained.

How well a newborn makes these major adjustments depends on his or her genetic composition, the competency of the recent intrauterine environment, the care received during the labour and birth period, and the care received during the newborn or *neonatal period* (from birth through the first 28 days of life) (Walsh & Goser, 2013). Two-thirds of all deaths that occur during the first year of life occur in the neonatal period. More than half occur in the first 24 hours after birth—an indication of how hazardous a time this is for an infant.

HEALTH PROMOTION OF THE TERM NEWBORN

Assessment

Assessment of a newborn or **neonate** (a baby in the neonatal period) includes a review of the mother's pregnancy history; physical examination of the infant; analysis of laboratory reports such as haematocrit and blood type, if indicated; and assessment of parent–child interaction for the beginning of bonding. Assessment begins immediately after birth and is continued at every contact during a newborn's hospital or birthing centre stay, early home visits and early childhood health centre visits. Teaching parents to make assessments concerning their infant's temperature, respiratory rate and overall health is crucial so that they can continue to monitor their infant's health at home.

Nursing considerations

Nursing considerations associated with a newborn often centre on the problems of establishing respirations, beginning nutrition and assisting with parent–newborn bonding. Examples are:

- Ineffective airway clearance related to mucus in airway
- Ineffective thermoregulation related to heat loss from exposure in birthing room
- Imbalanced nutrition, less than body requirements, related to poor sucking reflex
- Readiness for enhanced family coping related to birth of planned infant
- Health-seeking behaviours related to newborn needs.

Planning nursing care should take into account both the newborn's needs during this transition period and the mother's need for adequate rest during the postnatal period. Try to adapt teaching time to the schedules of the mother and her newborn. Although the woman must learn as much as possible about newborn care, she must also go home from the healthcare setting with enough energy to practise what she has learned. Important planning measures for newborns include helping them regulate their temperature and helping them grow accustomed to breastfeeding or bottle feeding. A helpful Internet site to recommend to parents is the Raising Children Network <http://raising children.net.au>.

A major portion of implementation in the newborn period is role modelling to help new parents grow confident with their newborn. Be aware how closely parents observe you for guidance in newborn care. Conserving newborn warmth and energy, to help prevent hypoglycaemia and respiratory distress, should be an important consideration to accompany all interventions.

Evaluation of expected outcomes should reveal that parents are able to give newborn care with confidence. The nurse will ensure that parents are provided with a referral to a community-based child and family health nurse for continued health supervision for their newborn, so that evaluation can be continued and the family's long-term health needs can be met.

PROFILE OF A NEWBORN

Every child is born with individual physical and personality characteristics that make him or her unique right from the start (see Fig. 18.1).

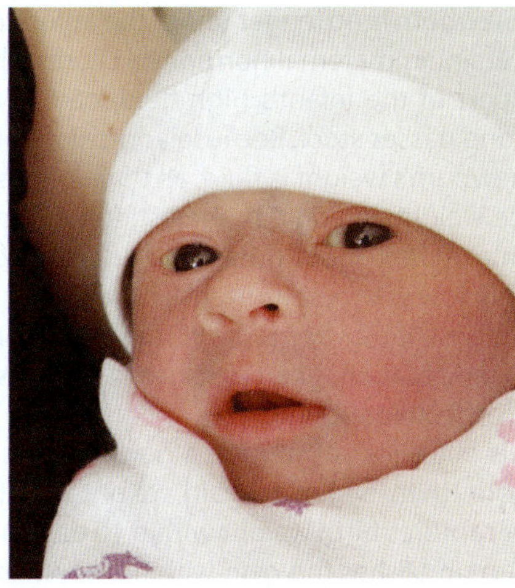

FIGURE 18.1 Personality is apparent in a newborn from the start. Note the alert, searching interest. (© Lauren Kidziak.)

General measurements

Baseline measurements in a newborn are weight, length and head circumference. The technique for obtaining these is shown in Chapter 34, along with other aspects of health assessment. Be sure all healthcare providers involved with newborns are aware of safety issues specific to newborn care when taking these measurements, such as not leaving a newborn unattended on a bed or scale.

Weight

The birth weight of newborns varies depending on the racial, nutritional, intrauterine and genetic factors that were present during conception and pregnancy. The weight in relation to the gestational age should be plotted on a standard neonatal graph, such as the one shown in Appendix B. Plotting weight helps identify newborns who are at risk because of their small size. This information also separates those who are small for their gestational age (newborns who have suffered intrauterine growth restriction) from preterm infants (infants who are healthy but small only because they were born early). These first measurements also establish a baseline for future evaluation.

Plotting weight in conjunction with height and head circumference is helpful because it highlights disproportionate measurements. All three of these measurements should fall near the same percentile in an individual child. For example, a newborn who falls within the 50th percentile for height and weight but whose head circumference is in the 90th percentile may have abnormal head growth. A newborn who is in the 50th percentile for weight and head circumference but in the 3rd percentile for height may have a growth problem.

The average birth weight (50th percentile) for a term newborn is 3.5 kg. The arbitrary lower limit of normal for all term babies is 2.5 kg. Birth weight exceeding 4.7 kg is unusual. If a newborn weighs more than 4.7 kg, the baby is said to be macrosomic. **Macrosomia** is a condition that usually occurs in conjunction with a maternal illness, such as gestational diabetes (Song, Zhang & Song, 2013).

During the first few days after birth, a newborn loses up to 10% of his or her birth weight. This weight loss occurs because a newborn is no longer under the influence of salt- and fluid-retaining maternal hormones. Diuresis begins to remove a part of the infant's high fluid load. A newborn also voids and passes stool. Because approximately 75% to 90% of a newborn's weight is fluid, all three of these measures reduce weight. In addition, breastfed newborns have a limited intake until about the third day of life because of the relatively low kilojoule content and amount of colostrum they ingest. If newborns are formula-fed, their intake during this time is also limited because of the time needed to establish effective sucking.

After this initial loss of weight, a newborn has 1 day of stable weight, then begins to gain weight. The breastfed newborn recaptures birth weight within 10 days; a formula-fed infant accomplishes this gain within 7 days. After this, a newborn begins to gain about 0.5–1.0 kg per month for the first 6 months of life.

Length

The average birth length (50th percentile) of a term neonate is 50 cm; however, this can range from 46 to 56 cm.

Head circumference

In a mature newborn, the head circumference is usually 34 to 36 cm. A term newborn with a head circumference greater than 37 cm or less than 33 cm should be carefully assessed for neurological involvement, although occasionally a well newborn falls within these limits. Head circumference is measured with a tape measure drawn across the centre of the forehead and around the most prominent portion of the posterior head (the occiput).

Vital signs

Vital sign measurements begin to change from those present in intrauterine life at the moment of birth.

Temperature

The temperature of newborns is about 37.2°C at birth because they have been confined in an internal body organ. The temperature falls almost immediately to below normal because of heat loss and immature temperature-regulating mechanisms. The temperature of birthing rooms, approximately 21°C to 22°C, can add to this loss of heat. Newborns lose heat by four separate mechanisms: convection, conduction, radiation and evaporation (see Fig. 18.2).

- **Convection** is the flow of heat from the newborn's body surface to cooler surrounding air. The effectiveness of convection depends on the velocity of the flow (a current of air cools faster than non-moving air). Eliminating drafts from windows or air conditioners reduces convection heat loss.
- **Conduction** is the transfer of body heat to a cooler solid object in contact with a baby. For example, a baby

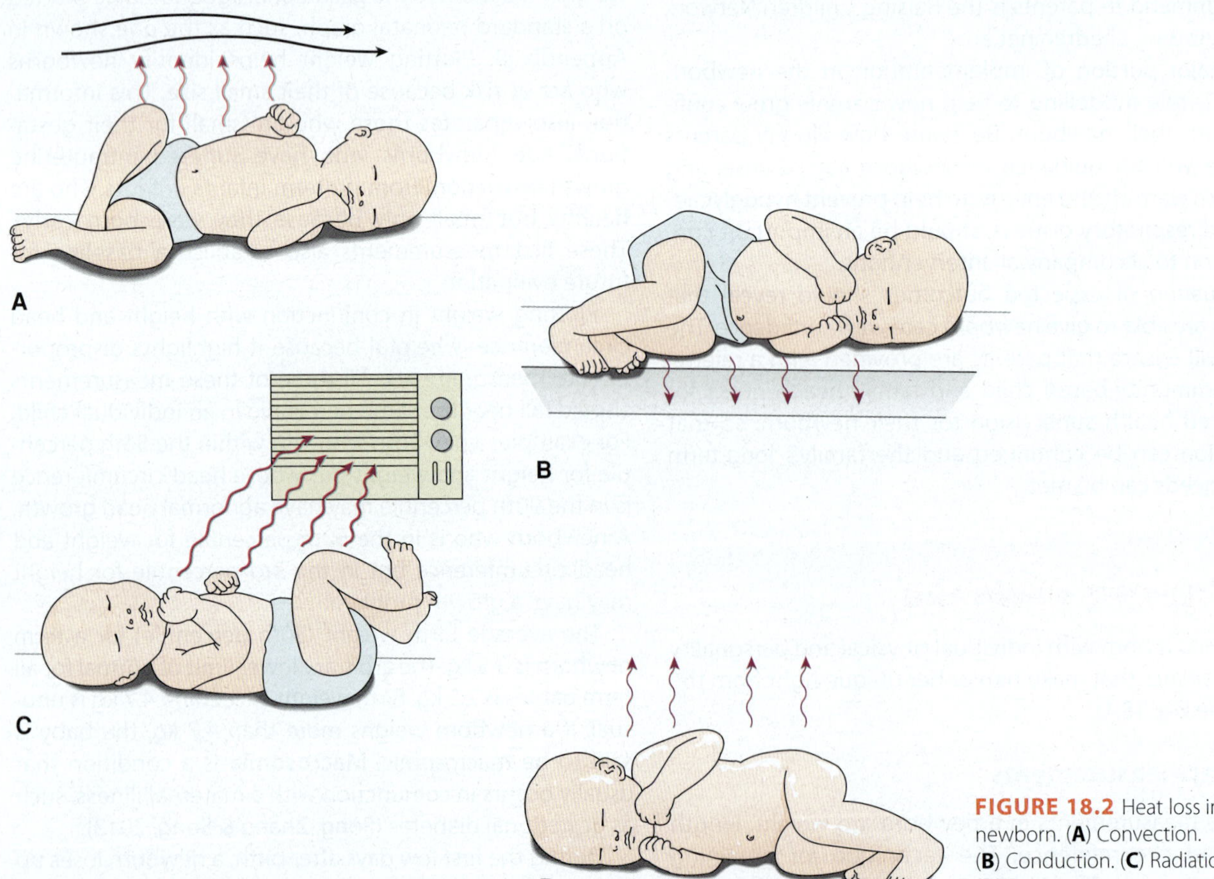

FIGURE 18.2 Heat loss in the newborn. (**A**) Convection. (**B**) Conduction. (**C**) Radiation. (**D**) Evaporation.

placed on a cold counter or on the cold base of a warming unit quickly loses heat to the colder metal surface. Covering surfaces with a warmed blanket or towel helps to minimise conduction heat loss.

- **Radiation** is the transfer of body heat to a cooler solid object not in contact with the baby, such as a cold window or air conditioner. Moving an infant as far away from the cold surface as possible helps reduce this type of heat loss.
- **Evaporation** is loss of heat through conversion of a liquid to a vapour. Newborns are wet, so they lose a great deal of heat as the amniotic fluid on their skin evaporates. To prevent this heat loss, dry newborns as soon as possible, especially their face and hair because the head, a large surface area in a newborn, can be responsible for a great amount of heat loss. Covering the hair with a hat after drying it further reduces the possibility of evaporation cooling. Be certain to remove any wet blankets used to dry the infant immediately and place the infant on a warm, dry blanket.

A newborn not only loses heat easily but also has difficulty conserving heat under any circumstance.

Pulse

The heart rate of a fetus in utero averages 110 to 160 beats per minute (bpm). Immediately after birth, as the newborn begins to initiate respirations, the heart rate may be as rapid as 180 bpm. Within 1 hour after birth, the heart rate stabilises to an average of 120 to 140 bpm.

The heart rate of a newborn often remains slightly irregular because of immaturity of the cardiac regulatory centre in the medulla. Transient murmurs may result from the incomplete closure of fetal circulation shunts. During crying, the rate may rise again to 180 bpm. In addition, heart rate can decrease during sleep, ranging from 90 to 110 bpm.

You should be able to palpate brachial and femoral pulses in a newborn, but the radial and temporal pulses are more difficult to palpate with any degree of accuracy. Therefore, a newborn's heart rate is always determined by listening for an apical heartbeat for a full minute, rather than assessing a pulse in an extremity. Always palpate for femoral pulses, however, because their absence suggests possible coarctation (narrowing) of the aorta, which is a possible cardiovascular abnormality (Schneider, 2011).

Respiration

The respiratory rate of a newborn in the first few minutes of life may be as high as 80 breaths per minute. As respiratory activity is established and maintained, this rate settles to an average of 30 to 60 breaths per minute when the newborn is at rest. Respiratory depth, rate and rhythm are likely to be irregular and short periods of apnoea (without cyanosis) which last less than 15 seconds, sometimes called *periodic respirations,* are normal. Respiratory rate can be observed most easily by watching the movement of a newborn's abdomen, because breathing primarily involves the use of the diaphragm and abdominal muscles.

Coughing and sneezing reflexes are present at birth to clear the airway. Newborns are obligatory nose-breathers, however, and show signs of acute distress if their nostrils become obstructed. Short periods of crying, which increase the depth of respirations and aid in aerating deep portions of the lungs, may be beneficial to a newborn. Long periods of crying, however, can exhaust the cardiovascular system.

Blood pressure

The blood pressure of a newborn is approximately 80/46 mmHg at birth. By the tenth day, it rises to about 100/50 mmHg. Because measurement of blood pressure in a newborn is somewhat inaccurate, it is not routinely measured unless a cardiac anomaly is suspected. For an accurate reading, the cuff width used must be no more than two-thirds the length of the upper arm or thigh. Blood pressure tends to increase with crying (and a newborn cries when disturbed and manipulated by such procedures as taking blood pressure). A Doppler method may be used to take blood pressure. Haemodynamic monitoring is helpful when continuous assessment is necessary.

CASE STUDY QUESTION

3. Beth Phillips, like all newborns, can lose body heat by conduction. Under which condition is conduction most apt to occur?

a. The nursery is cooled by air conditioning
b. The infant is wet from amniotic fluid
c. There is a breeze from an open window
d. Beth is placed in a cold bassinet

Physiological functions

Just as changes occur in vital signs after birth, so do changes occur in all the major body systems.

Cardiovascular system

Changes in the cardiovascular system are necessary after birth because the lungs must oxygenate the blood that was formerly oxygenated by the placenta. When the cord is clamped, a neonate is forced to take in oxygen through the lungs. As the lungs inflate for the first time, pressure decreases in the pulmonary artery (the artery leading from the heart to the lungs). This decrease in pressure plays a role in promoting closure of the ductus arteriosus, a fetal shunt. As pressure increases in the left side of the heart from increased blood volume, the foramen ovale between the two atria closes because of the pressure against the lip of the structure (permanent closure does not occur for weeks). With the remaining fetal circulatory structures (umbilical vein, two umbilical arteries and ductus venosus) no longer receiving blood, the blood within them clots and the vessels atrophy over the next few weeks.

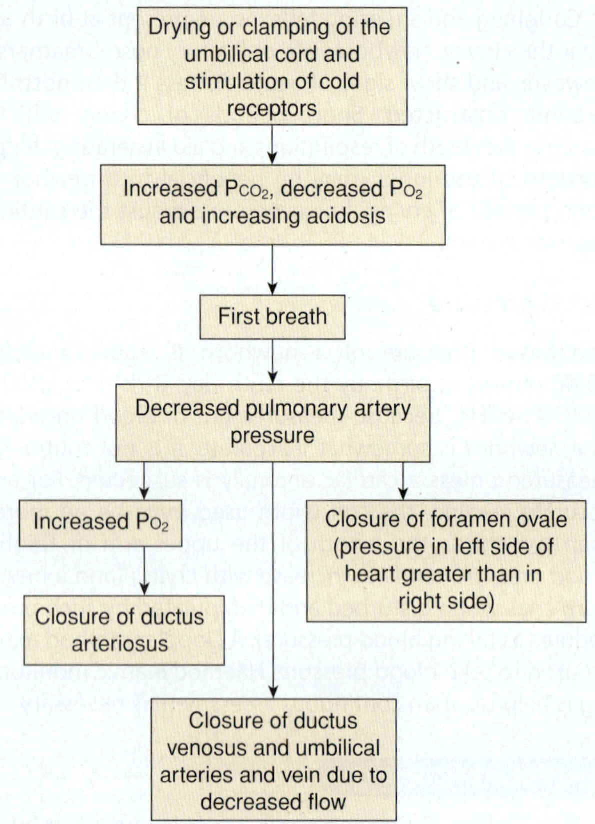

FIGURE 18.3 Circulatory events at birth.

Figure 18.3 shows the respiratory and cardiovascular changes that occur at birth, beginning with the first breath. The peripheral circulation of a newborn remains sluggish for at least the first 24 hours. It is common to observe cyanosis in the infant's feet and hands **(acrocyanosis)** and for the feet to feel cold to the touch at this time.

Blood values

A newborn's blood volume is 80 to 110 mL/kg of body weight, or about 300 mL in total. The oxygen dissociation curve is shifted to the left; that is, the quantity of oxygen bound to haemoglobin and the partial pressure of oxygen are greater in newborn blood than in an adult's blood, or a newborn's haemoglobin carries a greater proportion of oxygen than adult haemoglobin. Haemoglobin level averages 17 to 18 g/100 mL of blood. The haematocrit is between 45% and 50%. A newborn also has an elevated red blood cell count, about 6 million cells per cubic millimetre. Capillary heel-sticks may reveal a falsely high haematocrit or haemoglobin value because of sluggish peripheral circulation. Before obtaining a blood specimen from a heel, warm the foot by wrapping it in a warm cloth. This increases circulation and improves the accuracy of this value.

Once proper lung oxygenation has been established, the need for the high red cell count diminishes. Therefore, within a matter of days, a newborn's red cells begin to deteriorate. Bilirubin is a by-product of the breakdown of red blood cells. An indirect bilirubin level at birth is 17.1 to 68.4 mmol/L. Any increase over this amount reflects the release of bilirubin as excessive red blood cells begin their breakdown (Chetham, 2007).

A newborn has an equally high white blood cell count at birth, about 15,000 to 30,000 cells/mm^3. Values as high as 40,000 cells/mm^3 may be seen if the birth was stressful. Polymorphonuclear cells (neutrophils) account for a large part of this leucocytosis, but by the end of the first month, lymphocytes become the predominant cell type. This leucocytosis is a response to the trauma of birth and is non-pathogenic; an increased white blood cell count should not be taken as evidence of infection. On the other hand, although the high white blood cell count makes infection difficult to prove in a newborn, infection must not be dismissed as a possibility if other signs of infection such as pallor, respiratory difficulty or cyanosis are present.

Blood coagulation

Because most newborns are born with a lower than normal level of vitamin K, they have a prolonged coagulation or prothrombin time. Vitamin K, synthesised through the action of intestinal flora, is necessary for the formation of factor II (prothrombin), factor VII (proconvertin), factor IX (plasma thromboplastin component) and factor X (Stuart-Prower factor). A newborn's intestine is sterile at birth, unless membranes were ruptured more than 24 hours before birth, and it takes about 24 hours for flora to accumulate and for vitamin K to be synthesised. Because almost all newborns can be predicted to have this diminished blood coagulation ability, vitamin K (phytomenadione) is usually administered intramuscularly into the lateral anterior thigh, the preferred site for all injections in a newborn, immediately after birth.

Respiratory system

A first breath is a major undertaking because it requires a tremendous amount of pressure (about 40 to 70 cm H_2O). It is initiated by a combination of cold receptors; a lowered partial pressure of oxygen (P_{O_2}), which falls from 80 to as low as 15 mmHg before a first breath; and an increased partial carbon dioxide pressure (P_{CO_2}), which rises as high as 70 mmHg before a first breath. All newborns have some fluid in their lungs from intrauterine life that will ease the surface tension on alveolar walls and allows alveoli to inflate more easily than if the lung walls were dry. About a third of this fluid is forced out of the lungs by the pressure of vaginal birth. Additional fluid is quickly absorbed by lung blood vessels and lymphatics after the first breath.

Once the alveoli have been inflated with a first breath, breathing becomes much easier for a baby, requiring only about 6 to 8 cm H_2O pressure. Within 10 minutes after birth, most newborns have established a good residual volume. By 10 to 12 hours of age, vital capacity is established at newborn proportions. The heart in a newborn takes up proportionately more space than in an adult, so the amount of lung expansion space available is proportionately limited.

A baby born by caesarean does not have as much lung fluid expelled at birth as one born vaginally and so may have more difficulty establishing effective respirations, because excessive fluid blocks air exchange space. Newborns who are immature and whose alveoli collapse each time they exhale (because of the lack of pulmonary surfactant) have difficulty establishing effective residual capacity and respirations. If the alveoli do not open well, a newborn's cardiac system becomes compromised, because closure of the foramen ovale and ductus arteriosus depends on free blood flow through the pulmonary artery and good oxygenation of blood. Therefore, a newborn who has difficulty establishing respirations at birth should be examined closely in the postnatal period for a cardiac murmur or other indication that he or she still has patent fetal cardiac structures, especially a patent ductus arteriosus.

Gastrointestinal system

Although the gastrointestinal tract is usually sterile at birth, bacteria may be cultured from the intestinal tract in most babies within 5 hours after birth and from all babies at 24 hours of life. Most of these bacteria enter the tract through the newborn's mouth from airborne sources. Others may come from vaginal secretions at birth, from hospital bedding and from contact at the breast. Accumulation of bacteria in the gastrointestinal tract is necessary for digestion and for the synthesis of vitamin K.

Although a newborn's stomach holds about 60 to 90 mL, a newborn has limited ability to digest fat and starch because the pancreatic enzymes, lipase and amylase, remain deficient for the first few months of life. A newborn regurgitates easily because of an immature cardiac sphincter between the stomach and the oesophagus. Immature liver functions may lead to lowered glucose and protein serum levels.

Stools

The first stool of a newborn is usually passed within 24 hours after birth. It consists of **meconium**, a sticky, tarlike, blackish-green, odourless material formed from mucus, vernix, lanugo, hormones and carbohydrates that accumulated during intrauterine life. If a newborn does not pass a meconium stool by 24 to 48 hours after birth, the possibility of some factor such as meconium ileus, imperforate anus or volvulus should be suspected.

About the second or third day of life, newborn stool changes in colour and consistency, becoming green and loose. This is termed *transitional stool* and it may resemble diarrhoea to the untrained eye. By the fourth day of life, breastfed babies pass three or four light-yellow stools per day. They are sweet-smelling, because breast milk is high in lactic acid, which reduces the amount of putrefactive organisms in the stool. A newborn who receives formula usually passes two or three bright-yellow stools a day. These have a slightly more noticeable odour, compared with the stools of breastfed babies.

A newborn placed under phototherapy lights as a treatment for jaundice has bright-green stools because of increased bilirubin excretion. Newborns with bile duct obstruction have clay-coloured (grey) stools, because bile pigments are not entering the intestinal tract. Blood-flecked stools usually indicate an anal fissure. Occasionally, a newborn has swallowed some maternal blood during birth and either vomits fresh blood immediately after birth or passes a black tarry stool after 2 or more days. Maternal blood may be differentiated from fetal blood by a dipstick Apt test. If the stools remain black or tarry, intestinal bleeding should be suspected. If mucus is mixed with stool or the stool is watery and loose, a milk allergy, lactose intolerance or some other condition interfering with digestion or absorption should be suspected.

Urinary system

The average newborn voids within 24 hours after birth. A newborn who does not take in much fluid for the first 24 hours may void later than this, but the 24-hour point is a good general rule. Newborns who do not void within this time should be examined for the possibility of urethral stenosis or absent kidneys or ureters. The possibility of obstruction of the urinary tract can be assessed by observing the force of the urinary stream in both male and female infants. Males should void with enough force to produce a small projected arc; females should produce a steady stream, not just continuous dribbling. Projecting urine further than normal may signal urethral obstruction, because it indicates that urine is being forced through a narrow channel.

The kidneys of newborns do not concentrate urine well, making newborn urine usually light-coloured and odourless. The infant is about 6 weeks of age before much control over reabsorption of fluid in tubules and concentration of urine becomes evident.

A single voiding in a newborn is only about 15 mL and may be easily missed in a thick nappy. Specific gravity ranges from 1.008 to 1.010. The daily urinary output for the first 1 or 2 days is about 30 to 60 mL in total. By week 1, total daily volume rises to about 300 mL. The first voiding may be pink or dusky because of uric acid crystals that were formed in the bladder in utero; this is an innocent finding. A small amount of protein may be normally present in voidings for the first few days of life, until the kidney glomeruli are more fully mature. Nappies can be weighed to determine the amount of urine output.

Immune system

Because they have difficulty forming antibodies against invading antigens until about 2 months of age, newborns are prone to infection. This inability to form antibodies is the reason that most immunisations against childhood diseases are not given to infants younger than 2 months of age.

Newborns do have some immunological protection, because they are born with passive antibodies (immunoglobulin G) from their mother that crossed the placenta. In most instances, these include antibodies against poliomyelitis, measles, diphtheria, pertussis, chickenpox, rubella and tetanus. Newborns are routinely administered hepatitis B vaccine soon after birth to protect against this disease (Australian Government Department of Health and Ageing 2014; NZMOH, 2014). Little natural immunity is transmitted against herpes simplex. Any healthcare personnel with herpes simplex eruptions (cold sores) should not care for newborns until the lesions have crusted. Without antibody protection, herpes simplex infections can become systemic or create a rapidly fatal form of the disease in a newborn.

Neuromuscular system

Mature newborns demonstrate neuromuscular function by moving their extremities, attempting to control head movement, exhibiting a strong cry and demonstrating newborn reflexes. Limpness or total absence of a muscular response to manipulation is never normal and suggests narcosis, shock or cerebral injury. A newborn occasionally makes twitching or flailing movements of the extremities in the absence of a stimulus because of the immaturity of the nervous system. Newborn reflexes can be tested for consistency by using simple manoeuvres.

Blink reflex

A blink reflex in a newborn serves the same purpose as it does in an adult—to protect the eye from any object coming near it by rapid eyelid closure. It may be elicited by shining a strong light such as a flashlight or an otoscope light on an eye. A sudden movement towards the eye can sometimes elicit the blink reflex.

Rooting reflex

If the cheek is brushed or stroked near the corner of the mouth, a newborn infant will turn the head in that direction. This reflex serves to help a newborn find food: when a mother holds the child and allows her breast to brush the newborn's cheek, the reflex makes the baby turn towards the breast. The reflex disappears at about the sixth week of life. At about this time, newborn eyes focus steadily, so a food source can be seen and the reflex is no longer needed.

Sucking reflex

When a newborn's lips are touched, the baby makes a sucking motion. The reflex helps a newborn find food: when the newborn's lips touch the mother's breast or a bottle, the baby sucks and so takes in food. The sucking reflex begins to diminish at about 6 months of age. It disappears immediately if it is never stimulated, such as in a newborn with a tracheo-oesophageal fistula who cannot take in oral fluids. It can be maintained in such an infant by offering the child a non-nutritive sucking object such as a dummy (after the fistula has been corrected by surgery and until oral feedings can be given).

Swallowing reflex

The swallowing reflex in a newborn is the same as in the adult. Food that reaches the posterior portion of the tongue is automatically swallowed. Gag, cough and sneeze reflexes are also present in newborns to maintain a clear airway in the event that normal swallowing does not keep the pharynx free of obstructing mucus.

Extrusion reflex

A newborn extrudes any substance that is placed on the anterior portion of the tongue. This protective reflex prevents the swallowing of inedible substances. It disappears at about 4 months of age. Until then, the infant may seem to be spitting out or refusing solid food placed in the mouth.

Palmar grasp reflex

Newborns grasp an object placed in their palm by closing their fingers on it (see Fig. 18. 4). Mature newborns grasp so strongly that they can be raised from a supine position and suspended momentarily from an examiner's fingers. This reflex disappears at about 6 weeks to 3 months of age. A baby begins to grasp meaningfully at about 3 months of age.

Step-(walk)-in-place reflex

Newborns who are held in a vertical position with their feet touching a hard surface will take a few quick, alternating steps (see Fig. 18.5). This reflex disappears by 3 months of age. By 4 months, babies can bear a good portion of their weight unhindered by this reflex.

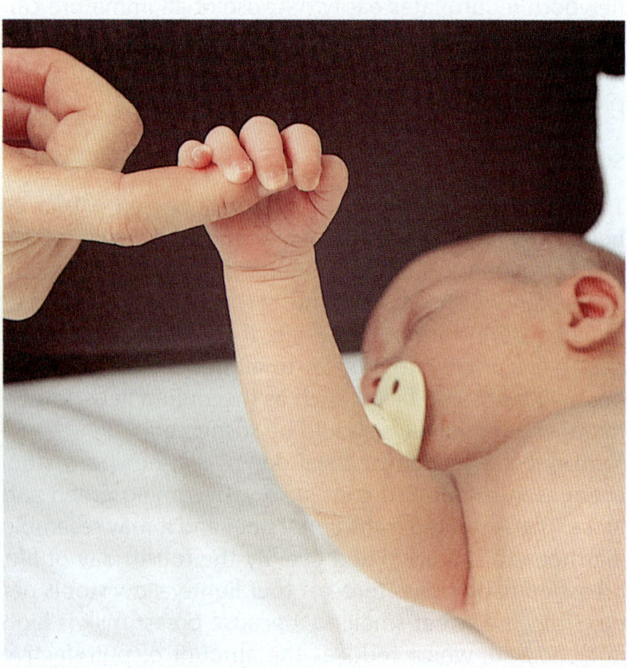

FIGURE 18.4 Palmar grasp reflex.

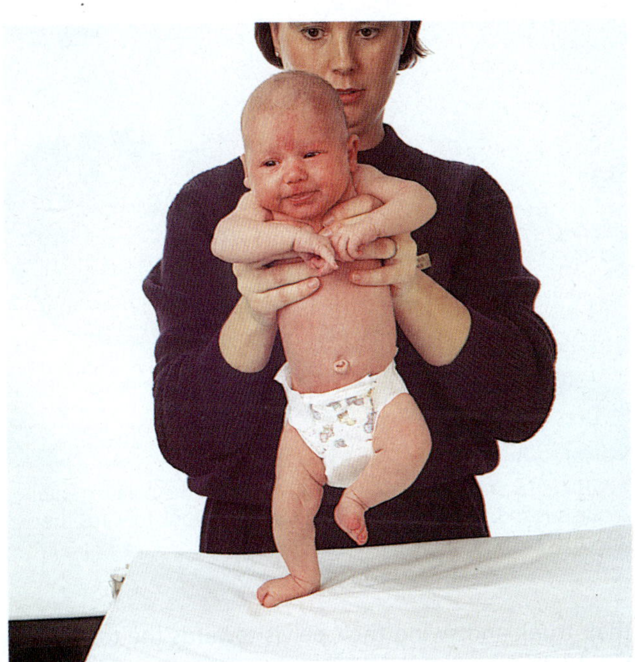

FIGURE 18.5 Step-in-place reflex.

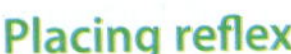

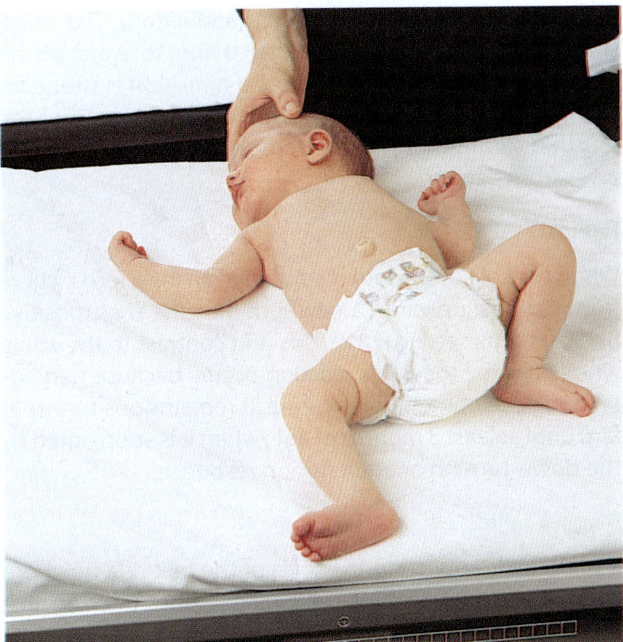

FIGURE 18.6 Tonic neck reflex.

Placing reflex

The placing reflex is similar to the step-in-place reflex, except that it is elicited by touching the anterior surface of the lower part of a newborn's leg against a hard surface such as the edge of a bassinet or table. The newborn makes a few quick lifting motions, as if to step onto the table, because of the reflex.

Plantar grasp reflex

When an object touches the sole of a newborn's foot at the base of the toes, the toes grasp in the same manner as do the fingers. This reflex disappears at about 8 to 9 months of age in preparation for walking. However, it may be present during sleep for a longer period.

Tonic neck reflex

When newborns lie on their backs, their heads usually turn to one side or the other. The arm and the leg on the side towards which the head turns extend and the opposite arm and leg contract (see Fig. 18.6). The movement is most evident in the arms but may also be observed in the legs. If you turn a newborn's head to the opposite side, he or she will often change the extension and contraction of legs and arms accordingly. This is also called a boxer or fencing reflex, because the position simulates that of someone preparing to box or fence. Unlike many other reflexes, the tonic neck reflex does not appear to have a function. It does stimulate eye coordination, because the extended arm moves in front of the face. It may signify handedness. The reflex disappears between the second and third months of life.

Moro reflex

A Moro (startle) reflex (see Fig. 18.7) can be initiated by startling a newborn with a loud noise or by jarring the bassinet. The most accurate method of eliciting the reflex is to hold newborns in a supine position and allow their heads to drop backwards about 2.5 cm. In response to this sudden head movement, they abduct and extend their arms and legs. Their fingers assume a typical "C" position. Finally, they swing their arms into an embrace position and pull up

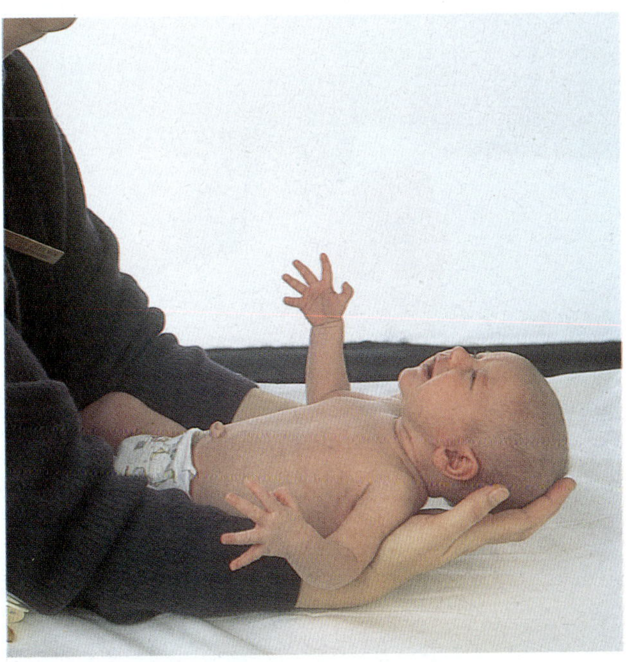

FIGURE 18.7 Moro reflex.

their legs against their abdomen (adduction). The reflex simulates the action of someone trying to ward off an attacker, then covering up to protect himself. It is strong for the first 8 weeks of life and then fades by the end of the fourth or fifth month, at the same time an infant can roll away from danger.

Babinski reflex

When the sole of the foot is stroked in an inverted "J" curve from the heel upwards, a newborn fans the toes (positive Babinski sign; see Fig. 18.8). This is in contrast to the adult, who flexes the toes. This reaction occurs because nervous system development is immature. It remains positive (toes fan) until at least 3 months of age, when it is supplanted by the down-turning or adult flexion response.

Magnet reflex

If pressure is applied to the soles of the feet of a newborn lying in a supine position, he or she pushes back against the pressure. This and the two following reflexes are tests of spinal cord integrity.

Crossed extension reflex

If one leg of a newborn lying supine is extended and the sole of that foot is irritated by being rubbed with a sharp object, such as a thumbnail, the infant raises the other leg and extends it, as if trying to push away the hand irritating the first leg.

Trunk incurvation reflex

When newborns lie in a prone position and are touched along the paravertebral area by a probing finger, they flex their trunk and swing their pelvis towards the touch (see Fig. 18.9).

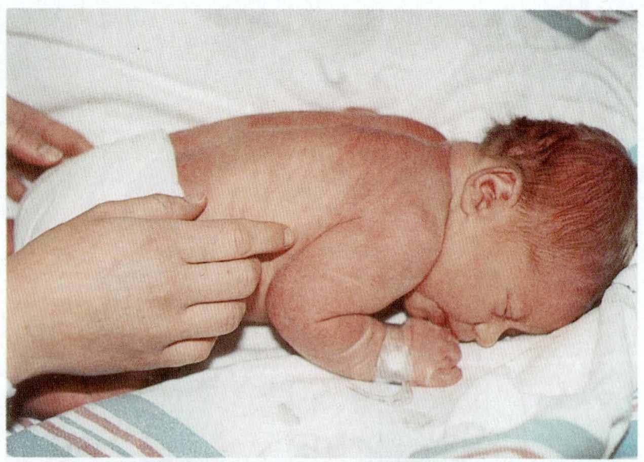

FIGURE 18.9 Trunk incurvation reflex. When the paravertebral area is stroked, the newborn flexes his or her trunk towards the direction of the stimulation.

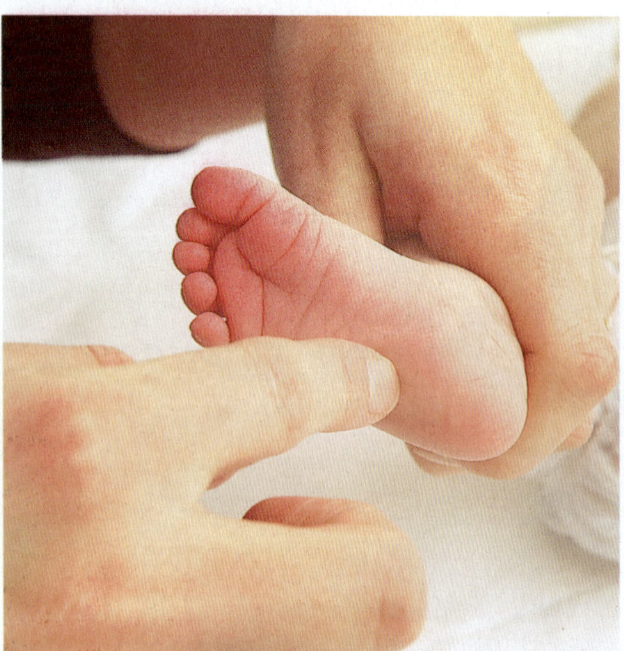

FIGURE 18.8 Babinski reflex. When the examiner moves her finger upwards, the newborn's toes will fan outwards.

Deep tendon reflexes

A patellar reflex can be elicited in a newborn by tapping the patellar tendon with the tip of the finger. The lower leg moves perceptibly if the infant has an intact reflex. To elicit a biceps reflex, place the thumb of your left hand on the tendon of the biceps muscle on the inner surface of the elbow. Tap the thumb as it rests on the tendon. You are more likely to feel the tendon contract than to observe movement. A biceps reflex is a test for spinal nerves C5 and C6; a patellar reflex is a test for spinal nerves L2–L4.

CASE STUDY QUESTION

4. A Moro reflex is the single best assessment of neurological ability in a newborn. What is the best way to test this reflex?
   a. Observe Beth while she is on her abdomen to see whether she can turn her head
   b. Lift Beth's head while she is supine and allow it to fall back 2.5 cm
   c. Shake Beth's cot until she responds by flailing her arms
   d. Make a sharp noise, such as clapping your hands, to wake Beth

The senses

The senses in newborns are already developed at birth.

Hearing

A fetus is able to hear in utero even before birth. As soon as amniotic fluid drains or is absorbed from the middle ear by way of the eustachian tube—within hours after birth—hearing becomes acute. Newborns appear to have difficulty locating sound, however, and so do not turn towards it consistently. Perhaps they must learn to interpret small differences among sounds arriving at their ears at different times. They respond with generalised activity to a sound such as a bell ringing a short distance from their ear. A newborn who is actively crying when a bell is rung stops crying and seems to attend. Similarly, newborns calm in response to a soothing voice and startle at loud noises. They recognise their mother's voice almost immediately, as if they have heard it in utero.

Vision

Newborns see as soon as they are born and possibly have been "seeing" light and dark in utero for the last few months of pregnancy, as the uterus and the abdominal wall were stretched thin. Newborns demonstrate sight at birth by blinking at a strong light (blink reflex) or by following a bright light or toy a short distance with their eyes. Because they cannot follow past the midline of vision, they lose track of objects easily. This is why parents sometimes think and report that their newborn does not see. Newborns focus best on black and white objects at a distance of 20–30 cm. A pupillary reflex or ability to contract the pupil is present from birth.

Touch

The sense of touch is also well developed at birth. Newborns demonstrate this by quieting at a soothing touch and by sucking and rooting reflexes, which are elicited by touch. They also react to painful stimuli.

Taste

A newborn has the ability to discriminate taste because taste buds are developed and functioning even before birth. A fetus in utero, for example, will swallow amniotic fluid more rapidly than usual if glucose is added to sweeten its taste. The swallowing decreases if a bitter flavour is added. A newborn turns away from a bitter taste such as salt but readily accepts the sweet taste of milk or sucrose.

Smell

The sense of smell is present in newborns as soon as the nose is clear of lung and amniotic fluid. Newborns turn towards their mother's breast partly out of recognition of the smell of breast milk and partly as a manifestation of the rooting reflex. Their ability to respond to odours can be used to document alertness.

Physiological adjustment to extrauterine life

All newborns seem to move through periods of irregular adjustment in the first 6 hours of life, before their body systems stabilise. These periods were first described by Desmond and colleagues in 1963 and are termed periods of reactivity (Desmond et al., 1963). The first phase lasts about half an hour. During this time, the baby is alert and exhibits exploring, searching activity, often making sucking sounds. Heart beat and respiratory rate are rapid. This is called the *first period of reactivity.* Next comes a quiet *resting period.* Heartbeat and respiratory rates slow and the newborn typically sleeps for about 90 minutes. The *second period of reactivity,* between 2 and 6 hours of life, occurs when the baby wakes again, often gagging and choking on mucus that has accumulated in the mouth. He or she is again alert and responsive and interested in surroundings.

Newborns who are ill or who had difficulty at birth may not pass through these typical stages; they may never have periods of alertness or periods of quiet. Their vital signs may not fall and rise again but remain rapid; their temperature may remain subnormal. Demonstration of this typical reactivity pattern, therefore, is an indication that a newborn is healthy and adjusting well to extrauterine life. The ability to transition from one period to another is an important indicator of neurological status.

APPEARANCE OF A NEWBORN

Although all newborns have similar physical findings, there are individual differences.

Skin

General inspection of a newborn's skin reveals many characteristic findings.

Colour

Most term newborns have a ruddy complexion because of the increased concentration of red blood cells in blood vessels and a decrease in the amount of subcutaneous fat, which makes the blood vessels more visible. This ruddiness fades slightly over the first month. Infants with poor central nervous system control may appear pale and cyanotic. A grey colour in newborns generally indicates infection. Twins may be born with a twin transfusion phenomenon, in which one twin is larger and has good colour and the smaller twin has pallor (Roberts et al., 2014).

Cyanosis

Generalised mottling of the skin is common. A newborn's lips, hands and feet are likely to appear blue from immature peripheral circulation initially. Acrocyanosis (blueness of hands and feet) is so prominent in some newborns that it appears as if some stricture were cutting off circulation, with usual skin colour on one side and blue on the other. Acrocyanosis is a normal phenomenon in the first 24 to 48 hours after birth; however, **central cyanosis**, or cyanosis of the trunk, is always a cause for concern. Central cyanosis indicates decreased oxygenation. It may be the result of a temporary respiratory obstruction or an underlying disease state and requires immediate medical referral.

What if...

Cassandra inspects her new baby and says to you, "Her hands are cold and blue. Is something wrong with her hands?" How should you answer?

Hyperbilirubinaemia

Hyperbilirubinaemia leads to **jaundice**, or yellowing of the skin. This occurs on the second or third day of life in about 50% of all newborns, as a result of a breakdown of fetal red blood cells (physiological jaundice). The infant's skin and the sclera of the eyes appear noticeably yellow. This happens because the high red blood cell count built up in utero is destroyed, and haem and globin are released. Globin is a protein component that is reused by the body and is not a factor in the developing jaundice. Haem is further broken down into iron (which is also reused and not involved in the jaundice) and protoporphyrin. Protoporphyrin is further broken down into indirect bilirubin. Indirect bilirubin is fat soluble and cannot be excreted by the kidneys in this state. For removal from the body, it is converted by the liver enzyme glucuronyl transferase into direct bilirubin, which is water soluble. This is incorporated into stool and then excreted in faeces. Many newborns have such immature liver function that indirect bilirubin cannot be converted to the direct form; it therefore remains indirect. As long as the buildup of indirect bilirubin remains in the circulatory system, the red colouring of the blood cells covers the yellow tint of the bilirubin. After the level of this indirect bilirubin has risen to more than 7 mg/100 mL, however, bilirubin permeates the tissue outside the circulatory system and causes the infant to appear jaundiced.

Observe infants who are prone to extensive bruising (large, breech or immature babies) carefully for jaundice, because bruising leads to haemorrhage of blood into the subcutaneous tissue or skin. A **cephalhaematoma** is a collection of blood under the periosteum of the skull bone. As the bruising in these locations heals and the red blood cells are haemolysed, additional indirect bilirubin is released and can be another cause of jaundice (Nelson et al., 2012). If intestinal obstruction is present and stool cannot be evacuated, intestinal flora may break down bile into its basic components, leading to the release of indirect bilirubin into the bloodstream again. Early feeding of newborns promotes intestinal movement and excretion of meconium and helps prevent indirect bilirubin buildup from this source.

The level of jaundice in newborns may be judged grossly by estimating the extent to which it has progressed on the surface of the infant's body, as it is noticed first in the head and then spreads to the rest of the body. Various commercial devices (transcutaneous bilirubinometry devices) are available to measure skin tone for jaundice and help in estimating jaundice levels. Although use of these devices rarely replaces serum measurements, they can be used to identify infants who need serum bilirubin determinations. Treatment for physiological jaundice or the routine rise in bilirubin in newborns is rarely necessary, except for measures such as early feeding to speed passage of faeces through the intestine and prevent reabsorption of bilirubin from the bowel.

Above-normal indirect bilirubin levels are potentially dangerous because, if enough indirect bilirubin (about 342.0 mmol/L) leaves the bloodstream, it can interfere with the chemical synthesis of brain cells, resulting in permanent cell damage, a condition termed **kernicterus**. If this occurs, permanent neurological damage, including cognitive challenge, may result. There is no set level at which indirect serum bilirubin requires treatment, because other factors, such as age, maturity and breastfeeding status, affect this determination. If the level rises to more than 171.0–205.2 mmol/L, treatment is usually considered. Phototherapy (exposure of the infant to light to initiate maturation of liver enzymes) is a common therapy (see Chapter 26). If this is necessary, the incubator and light source can be moved to the mother's room so that the mother is not separated from her baby.

Compared with formula-fed babies, a small proportion of breastfed babies may have more difficulty converting indirect bilirubin to direct bilirubin because breast milk contains pregnanediol (a metabolite of progesterone), which depresses the action of glucuronyl transferase. However, breastfeeding alone rarely causes enough jaundice to warrant therapy (Thilo & Rosenberg, 2011).

Pallor

Pallor in newborns is usually the result of anaemia. This may be caused by (a) excessive blood loss when the cord was cut, (b) inadequate flow of blood from the cord into the infant at birth, (c) fetal–maternal transfusion, (d) low iron stores caused by poor maternal nutrition during pregnancy or (e) blood incompatibility in which a large number of red blood cells were haemolysed in utero. It also may be the result of internal bleeding. A baby who appears pale should be watched closely for signs of blood in stool or vomitus.

Birthmarks

Several common types of birthmarks occur in newborns. Most are of cosmetic significance only and will improve over time. There are a small amount of lesions that require further identification and management, and may be associated with systemic conditions or complications (Ryan & Warren, 2012).

Mongolian spots

Mongolian spots are collections of pigment cells (melanocytes) that appear as slate-grey patches across the sacrum or buttocks and possibly on the arms and legs (see Fig. 18.10). They tend to occur in children of Asian, southern European or African ethnicity (Thilo & Rosenberg, 2011). This may

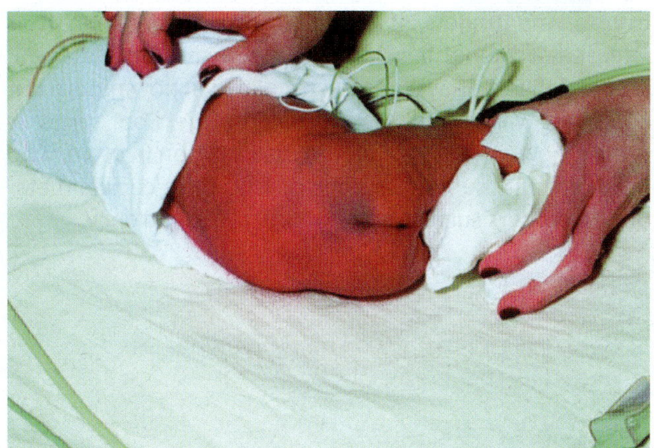

FIGURE 18.10 Mongolian spot. (Klossner, N. J. & Hatfield, N. [2009]. *Introductory Maternity and Pediatric Nursing* (2nd ed.). Philadelphia: Lippincott Williams & Wilkins.)

include infants with Māori, Pacific Islander and Indigenous Australian parents. They disappear by school age without treatment. Be sure to inform parents that these are not bruises; otherwise, they may worry their baby sustained a birth injury.

Vernix caseosa

Vernix caseosa is a white, cream cheese–like substance that serves as a skin lubricant in utero. Usually, it is noticeable on a term newborn's skin, at least in the skin folds, at birth. Until the first bath, when vernix is washed away, handle newborns with gloves to protect yourself from exposure to this body fluid. Never use harsh rubbing to wash away vernix. A newborn's skin is tender and breaks in the skin caused by too vigorous attempts at removal may open portals of entry for bacteria.

Lanugo

Lanugo is the fine, downy hair that covers a newborn's shoulders, back and upper arms. It may also be found on the forehead and ears. A baby born between 37 and 39 weeks of gestation has more lanugo than a newborn of 40 weeks gestational age. Postmature infants (more than 42 weeks of gestation) rarely have lanugo. Lanugo is rubbed away by the friction of bedding and clothes against the newborn's skin. By 2 weeks of age it has disappeared.

Desquamation

Within 24 hours after birth, the skin of most newborns has become extremely dry. The dryness is particularly evident on the palms of the hands and soles of the feet. This results in areas of peeling similar to those caused by sunburn. This is normal, however, and needs no treatment. Parents may apply hand lotion to prevent excessive dryness if they wish. Newborns who are post-mature and have suffered intrauterine malnutrition may have extremely dry skin, with a leathery appearance and cracks in the skin folds. This should be differentiated from normal desquamation.

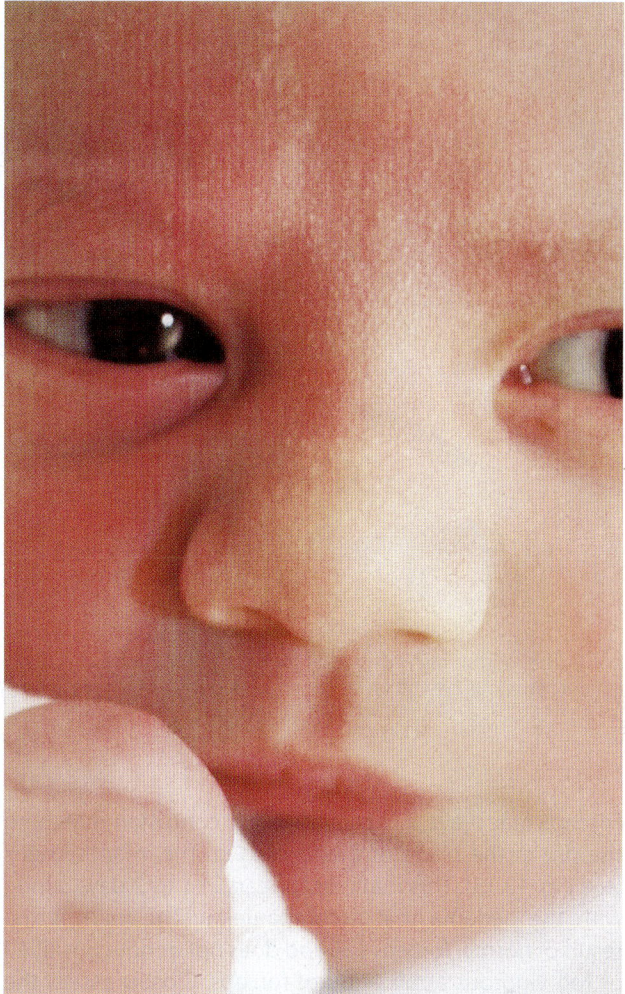

FIGURE 18.11 Milia are unopened sebaceous glands frequently found on the nose, chin or cheeks of a newborn.

Milia

All newborn sebaceous glands are immature. At least one pinpoint white papule (a plugged or unopened sebaceous gland) can be found on the cheek or across the bridge of the nose of almost every newborn. Such lesions, termed milia, disappear by 2 to 4 weeks of age, as the sebaceous glands mature and drain (see Fig. 18.11). Teach parents to avoid scratching or squeezing the papules, to prevent secondary infections.

Erythema toxicum

In most normal mature infants, a newborn rash called **erythema toxicum** can be observed (see Fig. 18.12). This usually appears in the first to fourth day of life but may appear up to 2 weeks of age. It begins with a papule, increases in severity to become erythema by the second day, and then disappears by the third day. One of the chief characteristics of the rash is its lack of pattern. It occurs sporadically and unpredictably and may last hours rather than days. It is caused by a newborn's eosinophils reacting to the environment as the immune system matures. It requires no treatment.

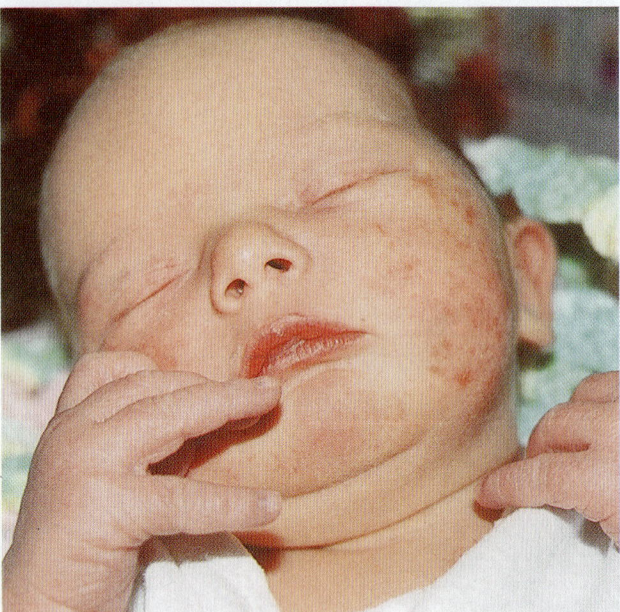

FIGURE 18.12 Erythema toxicum is found on almost all newborns. The reddish rash consists of sporadic pinpoint papules on an erythematous base. It fades spontaneously in a few days.

Forceps marks

Forceps may leave a circular or linear contusion matching the rim of the blade of the forceps on the infant's cheek (see Fig. 18.13). This mark disappears in 1 to 2 days, along with the oedema that accompanies it. The mark is the result of normal forceps use and does not denote unskilled or too vigorous application of forceps. Closely assess the facial nerve while a newborn is at rest and during crying episodes to detect any potential facial nerve compression requiring further evaluation.

Skin turgor

Newborn skin should feel resilient if the underlying tissue is well hydrated. If a fold of the skin is grasped between the thumb and fingers, it should feel elastic. When it is released, it should fall back to form a smooth surface. If severe dehydration is present, the skin will not smooth out again but will remain in an elevated ridge. Poor turgor is seen in newborns who suffered malnutrition in utero, who have difficulty sucking at birth or who have certain metabolic disorders such as adrenocortical insufficiency.

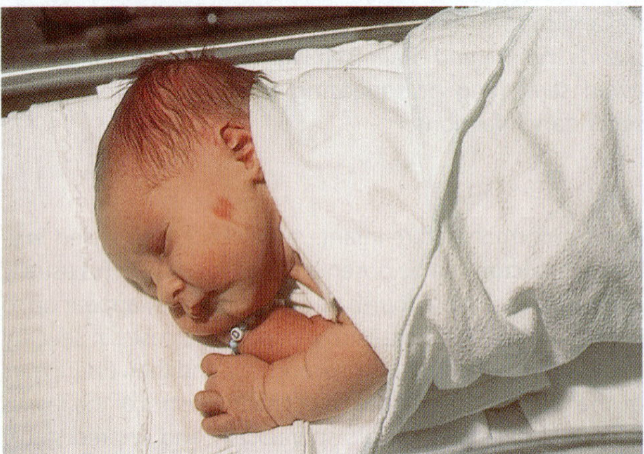

FIGURE 18.13 Forceps marks are commonly found in newborns born by forceps. Such marks are transient and disappear in a day or two.

CASE STUDY QUESTION

5. Beth Phillips has milia on her nose. What is the necessary therapy for this?
   a. Ice packs to reduce inflammation
   b. Warm heat to increase circulation
   c. No therapy is necessary for milia
   d. Lancing the lesions so they drain

Head

A newborn's head appears disproportionately large because it is about one-quarter of the total body length; in an adult, the head is one-eighth of total height. The forehead of a newborn is large and prominent. The chin appears to be receding and it quivers easily if an infant is startled or cries.

Fontanelles

The fontanelles are the spaces or openings where the skull bones join. The anterior fontanelle is located at the junction of the two parietal bones and the two fused frontal bones. It is diamond shaped and measures 2 to 3 cm in width and 3 to 4 cm in length. The posterior fontanelle is located at the junction of the parietal bones and the occipital bone. It is triangular and measures about 1 cm in length. The anterior fontanelle can be felt as a soft spot. It should not appear indented (a sign of dehydration) or bulging (a sign of increased intracranial pressure) when the infant is held upright. The fontanelle may bulge if the newborn strains to pass a stool, cries vigorously or is lying supine. With vigorous crying, a pulse may additionally be seen in the fontanelle. The anterior fontanelle normally closes at 12 to 18 months of age. In some newborns, the posterior fontanelle is so small that it cannot be palpated readily. The posterior fontanelle closes by the end of the second month.

Sutures

The skull sutures, the separating lines of the skull, may override at birth because of the extreme pressure exerted on the head during passage through the birth canal. If the sagittal suture between the parietal bones overrides, the fontanelles are less perceptible than usual. The overriding subsides within 24 to 48 hours. Suture lines should never appear widely separated in newborns. Wide separation suggests increased intracranial pressure because of abnormal brain formation, abnormal accumulation of

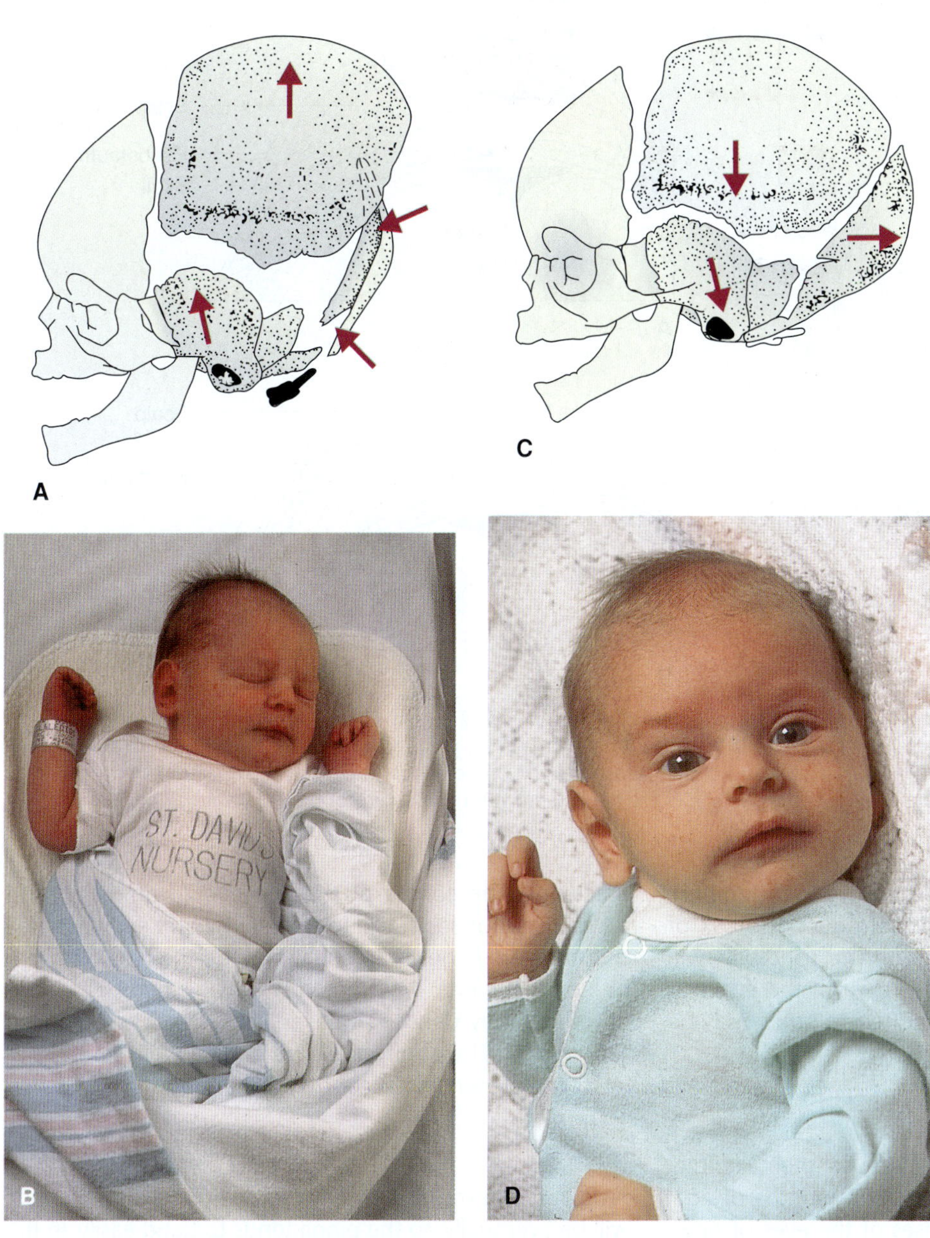

FIGURE 18.14 Moulding. (**A, B**) The infant head moulds to fit the birth canal more easily. On palpation, the skull sutures will be felt to be overriding. (**C, D**) The head shape returns to normal within 1 week.

cerebrospinal fluid in the cranium (hydrocephalus) or an accumulation of blood from a birth injury such as subdural haemorrhage. Fused suture lines are also abnormal; they require radiographic confirmation and further evaluation because they will prevent the head from expanding with brain growth.

Moulding

The part of the infant's head that engaged the cervix (usually the vertex) moulds to fit the cervix contours during labour. After birth, this area appears prominent and asymmetrical. The head will revert to its normal shape within a few days after birth (see Fig. 18.14).

Caput succedaneum

Caput succedaneum is oedema of the scalp at the presenting part of the head. It may involve wide areas of the head or it may resemble a large egg (see Fig. 18.15a). The oedema, which crosses the suture lines, is gradually absorbed and disappears at about the third day of life. It needs no treatment (Wisser et al., 2012).

Cephalohaematoma

A cephalohaematoma, a collection of blood between the periosteum of the skull bone and the bone itself, is caused by rupture of a periosteal capillary because of the pressure of birth (see Fig. 18.15b). Swelling usually appears 24 hours after birth. Although the blood loss is negligible, the swelling is usually severe and is well outlined as an egg shape. It may be discoloured (black and blue) because of the presence of coagulated blood. A cephalohaematoma is confined to an individual bone, so the associated swelling stops at the bone's suture line. It often takes weeks for a cephalohaematoma to be absorbed. It might be supposed

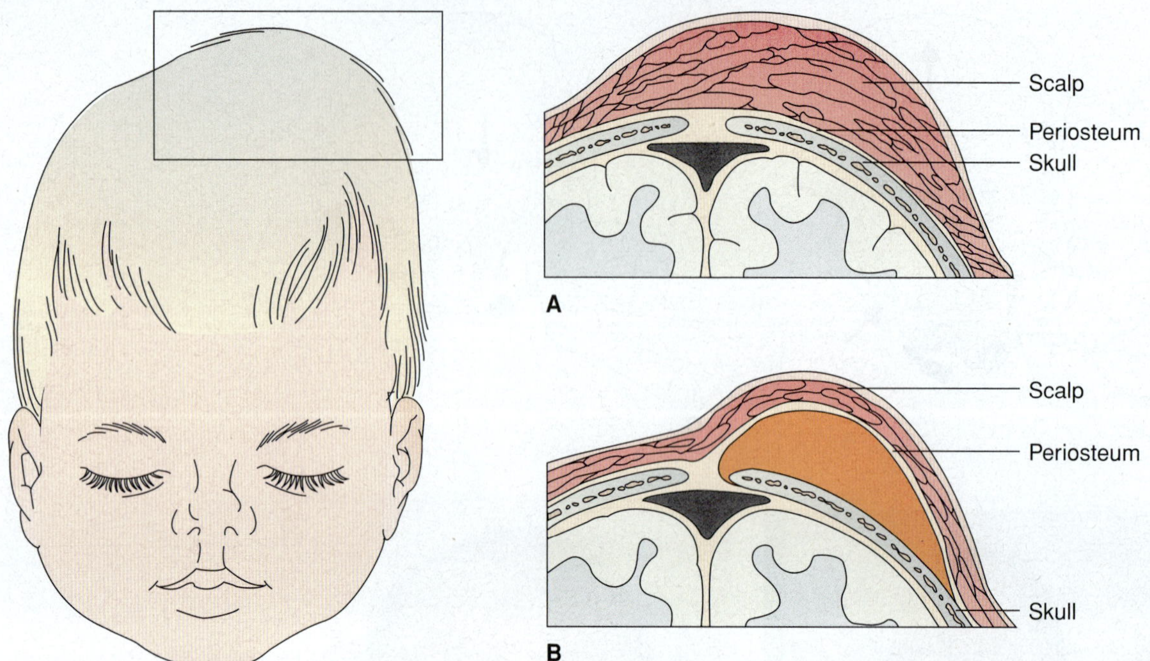

FIGURE 18.15 (**A**) Caput succedaneum. From pressure of the birth canal, an oedematous area is present beneath the scalp. Note how it crosses the midline of the skull. (**B**) Cephalohaematoma. A small capillary beneath the periosteum of the skull bone has ruptured and blood has collected under the periosteum of the bone. Note how the swelling now stops at the midline. Because the blood is contained under the periosteum, it is necessarily stopped by a suture line.

that the blood could be aspirated to relieve the condition. However, such a procedure would introduce the risk of infection and is unnecessary because the condition will subside by itself. As the blood captured in the space is broken down, a great amount of indirect bilirubin may be released, leading to jaundice.

Eyes

Newborns usually cry tearlessly because their lacrimal ducts do not fully mature until about 3 months of age. Almost without exception, the irises of the eyes of newborns are grey or blue; the sclera may be blue because of its thinness. Infant eyes assume their permanent colour between 3 and 12 months of age.

To inspect the eyes, lay the newborn in a supine position and lift the head. This manoeuvre causes the baby to open the eyes. A newborn's eyes should appear clear, without redness or purulent discharge. Pressure during birth sometimes ruptures a conjunctival capillary of the eye, resulting in a small subconjunctival haemorrhage. This appears as a red spot on the sclera, usually on the inner aspect of the eye, or as a red ring around the cornea. The bleeding is slight, requires no treatment and is completely absorbed within 2 or 3 weeks. You can assure parents that these haemorrhages are normal variations. Otherwise, they may assume that their baby is bleeding from within the eye and that vision will be impaired. Oedema is often present around the orbit or on the eyelids. This remains for the first 2 or 3 days, until the newborn's kidneys are capable of evacuating fluid more efficiently. The cornea of the eye should appear round and proportionate in size to that of an adult eye. A cornea that appears larger than usual may be the result of congenital glaucoma. An irregularly shaped pupil or discoloured iris may denote disease such as a coloboma (see Chapter 50). The pupil should be dark. A white pupil suggests the presence of a congenital cataract.

Ears

A newborn's external ear is not as completely formed as it will be eventually, so the pinna tends to bend easily. In the term newborn, however, the pinna should be strong enough to recoil after bending. The level of the top part of the external ear should be on a line drawn from the inner canthus to the outer canthus of the eye and back across the side of the head. Ears that are set lower than this are found in infants with certain chromosomal abnormalities, particularly trisomy 18 and 13, syndromes in which low-set ears and other physical defects are coupled with varying degrees of cognitive challenge (see Chapter 7).

A small tag of skin is sometimes found just in front of the newborn's ear. Although these tags may be associated with chromosomal abnormalities or kidney disease, they usually are isolated findings that are of no consequence. They can be removed by ligation immediately or when the child is 1 week old. A preauricular dermal sinus may be present directly in front of the ear as well. Always inspect in front of newborns' ears for pinpoint-size openings that reveal these sinuses. Visualisation of the tympanic membrane of the ear in a newborn is difficult and usually is not attempted because amniotic fluid and flecks of vernix still fill the canal, obliterating the drum and its accompanying landmarks. In many healthcare facilities, newborns are tested by a commercial standardised response to sound before discharge.

Nose

A newborn's nose tends to appear large for the face. As the infant grows, the rest of the face grows more than the nose does, and this discrepancy disappears. Choanal atresia is the most common congenital anomaly of the nose, either unilateral or bilateral, which may be associated with increased work of breathing or poor feeding.

Mouth

A newborn's mouth should open evenly when he or she cries. If one side of the mouth moves more than the other, cranial nerve injury is suggested. A newborn's tongue appears large and prominent in the mouth. Inspect the palate of a newborn to be sure it is intact. Occasionally, one or two small, round, glistening, well-circumscribed cysts (Epstein's pearls) are present on the palate, a result of extra calcium that was deposited in utero. Be sure to inform parents that these pearl-like cysts are insignificant, require no treatment and will disappear spontaneously within 1 week. Otherwise, a parent may mistake them for thrush, a *Candida* infection, which usually appears on the tongue and sides of the cheeks as white or grey patches and needs therapy with an antifungal drug (Subramanian et al., 2014).

All newborns have some mucus in their mouths. Newborns delivered by caesarean usually have an increased amount. If a newborn is placed on the side, the mucus drains from the mouth and results in no distress. If the mouth is filled with so much mucus that a neonate seems to be blowing bubbles, a tracheo-oesophageal fistula is suspected. This must be confirmed or ruled out before the newborn is fed; otherwise, formula can be aspirated into the lungs from the inadequately formed oesophagus.

Small, white epithelial pearls (benign inclusion cysts) may be present on the gum margins. No therapy is necessary for these. It is unusual for a newborn to have teeth, but sometimes one or two (called natal teeth) will have erupted. Any teeth that are present must be evaluated for stability. If loose, they should be extracted to prevent possible aspiration during feeding.

Neck

The neck of a newborn is short and often chubby, with creased skin folds. The head should rotate freely on it. If there is rigidity of the neck, congenital torticollis, caused by injury to the sternocleidomastoid muscle during birth, might be present (see Chapter 27). In newborns whose membranes were ruptured more than 24 hours before birth, nuchal rigidity suggests meningitis.

The neck of a newborn is not strong enough to support the total weight of the head but in a sitting position, a newborn should make a momentary effort at head control. When lying prone, newborns can raise the head slightly, usually enough to lift the nose out of mucus or spit-up formula or milk. If they are pulled into a sitting position from a supine position, the head will lag behind considerably. Again, however, they should make some effort to control and steady the head as they reach a sitting position.

The trachea may be prominent on the front of the neck and the thymus gland may be enlarged because of the rapid growth of glandular tissue (in comparison with other body tissues) early in life. The thymus gland will triple in size by 3 years of age; it remains at that size until the child is about 10 years old and then shrinks. Although the thymus may appear to be bulging in a newborn, it is rarely a cause of respiratory difficulty, as was once believed.

Chest

The chest in some newborns looks small because the head is large in proportion. It is actually smaller in circumference and as wide in the anteroposterior diameter as it is across. Not until a child is 2 years of age does the chest measurement exceed that of the head. The clavicles should be straight. Overall, a newborn's chest should appear symmetrical side to side. Respirations are normally rapid (30 to 60 breaths per minute) but not distressed. A supernumerary nipple (usually found below and in line with the normal nipples) may be present. If so, it may be removed later for cosmetic purposes although this is not necessary.

In both female and male infants, the breasts may be engorged. Occasionally, the breasts of newborn babies secrete a thin, watery fluid popularly termed *witch's milk*. Engorgement develops in utero as a result of the influence of the mother's hormones. As soon as the hormones are cleared from the infant's system (about 1 week), the engorgement and any fluid that is present subside. Fluid should never be expressed from infants' breasts because the manipulation could introduce bacteria and lead to mastitis. *Retraction* (drawing in of the chest wall with inspiration) should not be present. An infant with retractions is using such strong force to pull air into the respiratory tract that he or she is pulling in the anterior chest muscle. Because a newborn's lung alveoli open slowly over the first 24 to 48 hours and the baby invariably has mucus in the back of the throat, listening to lung sounds often reveals the sounds of rhonchi—the harsh, innocent sound of air passing over mucus. An abnormal sound, such as grunting, suggests respiratory distress syndrome; a high, crowing sound on inspiration suggests stridor or immature tracheal development.

Abdomen

The contour of a newborn abdomen looks slightly protuberant. A scaphoid or sunken appearance may indicate missing abdominal contents or a diaphragmatic hernia (bowel positioned in the chest instead of the abdomen). Bowel sounds should be present within 1 hour after birth. The edge of the liver is usually palpable 1 to 2 cm below the right costal margin. The edge of the spleen may be palpable 1 to 2 cm below the left costal margin. Tenderness is difficult to determine in a newborn. If it is extreme, however, palpation will cause the infant to cry, thrash about or tense the abdominal muscles to protect the abdomen.

For the first hour after birth, the stump of the umbilical cord appears as a white, gelatinous structure marked with the blue and red streaks of the umbilical vein and arteries. When the cord is first cut, the vessels are counted to be certain that one vein and two arteries are present. In 0.5% of births (3.5% of twin births), there is only a single umbilical artery, and in one-third of such infants, this single artery is associated with a congenital heart or renal abnormality. Because these heart and kidney anomalies may not be readily apparent, any child with a single umbilical artery needs close observation and assessment until anomalies are ruled out.

Inspect the cord clamp to be certain it is secure. After the first hour of life, the cord begins to dry and shrink. By the second or third day, it has turned black. It breaks free by day 6 to 10, leaving a granulating area a few centimetres wide that heals during the following week. There should be no bleeding at the cord site. Bleeding suggests that the cord clamp has become loosened or the cord has been tugged loose by the friction of clothing. The base of the cord should appear dry. A moist or odorous cord suggests infection. If present, infection should receive immediate treatment or it may enter a newborn's bloodstream and cause septicaemia. Moistness at the base of the cord may also indicate a patent urachus (a canal that connects the bladder and the umbilicus), which will drain urine at the cord site until it is surgically repaired.

Inspect the base of the cord to be certain no abdominal wall defect such as an umbilical hernia is present. Because a newborn's voiding only demonstrates there is at least one kidney functioning, but not two, attempt to verify the presence of kidneys by deep palpation of the right and left abdomen within the first few hours after birth. After this time, the intestines fill with air, making palpation more difficult. The right kidney (at least its lower pole) can usually be palpated readily, because it is located lower than the left; the left kidney is more difficult to locate, because the intestine is bulkier on the left side and the kidney is higher in the retroperitoneal space. Nonetheless, try to locate both of them. Placing one hand behind the infant while you palpate offers a firmer base and helps when evaluating kidney size (newborn kidneys are about the size of a walnut). An enlarged kidney suggests a polycystic kidney or pooling of urine from a urethral obstruction.

Anogenital area

Inspect the anus of a newborn to be certain it is present, patent and not covered by a membrane (imperforate anus).

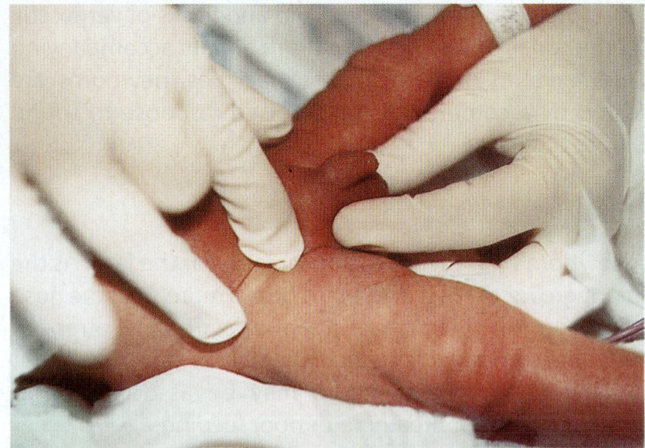

FIGURE 18.16 Press the non-dominant hand against the inguinal ring when palpating testes.

Also note the time after birth at which the infant first passes meconium. If a newborn does not do so in the first 24 hours, suspect imperforate anus or meconium ileus.

Male genitalia

The scrotum in most male newborns is oedematous and has rugae (folds in the skin). It may be deeply pigmented in dark-skinned newborns. Make a practice of pressing your non-dominant hand against the inguinal ring before palpating for testes, so they do not slip upwards and out of the scrotal sac as you palpate (see Fig. 18.16).

Both testes should be present in the scrotum. If one or both testicles are not present (cryptorchidism), referral is needed to establish the extent of the problem. This condition could be caused by agenesis (absence of an organ), ectopic testes (the testes cannot enter the scrotum because the opening to the scrotal sac is closed) or undescended testes (the vas deferens or artery is too short to allow the testes to descend). Newborns with agenesis of the testes are usually referred for investigation of kidney anomalies, because the testes arise from the same germ tissue as the kidneys. The penis of newborns appears small, approximately 2 cm long. If it is less than this, the newborn should be referred for evaluation by an endocrinologist to be certain there aren't other occurring anomalies. Inspect the tip of the penis to see that the urethral opening is at the tip of the glans, not on the dorsal surface (epispadias) or on the ventral surface (hypospadias). In most newborns, the prepuce (foreskin) is adherent and slides back poorly from the meatal opening, so no attempt to retract the foreskin should be made.

Female genitalia

The vulva in female newborns may be swollen because of the effect of maternal hormones. Some female newborns have a mucus vaginal secretion, which is sometimes blood-tinged (pseudomenstruation). Again, this is caused by the action of maternal hormones. The discharge disappears as soon as the infant's system has cleared the hormones. The discharge should not be mistaken for an infection or taken as an indication that trauma has occurred.

Back

The spine of a newborn typically appears flat in the lumbar and sacral areas. The curves seen in an adult appear only after a child is able to sit and walk. Inspect the base of a newborn's spine carefully to be sure there is no pinpoint opening, dimpling or sinus tract in the skin, which would suggest a dermal sinus or spinal bifida occulta. True neural tube defects in newborns have been greatly decreased in incidence because of the recognition that folic acid supplementation during pregnancy can prevent these (Wallingford et al., 2013).

A newborn normally assumes the position maintained in utero, with the back rounded and the arms and legs flexed on the abdomen and chest. A child who was born in a frank breech position tends to straighten the legs at the knee and bring their feet up next to the face. The position of a baby with a face presentation sometimes simulates opisthotonos or extreme hyperextension for the first week because the curve of the back is deeply concave.

Extremities

The arms and legs of a newborn appear short. The hands are plump and clenched into fists. Newborn fingernails are soft and smooth, and usually long enough to extend over the fingertips, with post-term infants often having longer nails. Test the upper extremities for muscle tone by unflexing the arms for approximately 5 seconds. If tone is good, the arm should return immediately to its flexed position after being released. Hold the arms down by the sides and note their length. The fingertips should reach the proximal thigh. Unusually short arms may signify achondroplastic dwarfism. Observe for unusual curvature of the little finger and inspect the palm for a simian crease (a single palmar crease, in contrast to the three creases normally seen in a palm). Although curved fingers and simian creases can occur normally, they are commonly associated with Down syndrome (Haldeman-Englert, Saitta & Zackai, 2012).

A newborn's arms and legs should move symmetrically (unless the infant is demonstrating a tonic neck reflex). An arm that hangs limply and unmoving suggests possible birth injury, such as injury to a clavicle or to the brachial or cervical plexus or fracture of a long bone. Assess for webbing (syndactyly), extra toes or fingers (polydactyly), or unusual spacing of toes, particularly between the big toes and the others (this finding is present in certain chromosomal disorders, although it is also a normal finding in some families). Test to see whether the toenails fill immediately after blanching from pressure.

Normally, newborn legs are bowed as well as short. The sole of the foot appears flat because of an extra pad of fat in the longitudinal arch. The foot of a term newborn has many crisscrossed lines on the sole, covering approximately two-thirds of the foot. If these creases cover less than two-thirds of the foot or are absent, suspect immaturity.

The feet of many newborns turn in (varus deviation) because of their former intrauterine position. This simple deviation needs no correction if the feet can be brought into the midline position by easy manipulation. When the infant begins to bear weight, the feet will align themselves. If a foot does not align readily (will not turn to a definite midline position), a talipes deformity (clubfoot) may be present. This condition needs further investigation because congenital problems of this kind are best treated in the immediate newborn period.

With a newborn in a supine position, both hips can be flexed and abducted to such an extent (180°) that the knees touch or nearly touch the surface of the bed (see Fig. 18.17). If the hip joint seems to lock short of this distance (160 to 170°), hip subluxation (a shallow and poorly formed acetabulum) is suggested (Gulati et al., 2013). Examination of the hips can begin with observation for signs of dislocation, for example unequal leg length and asymmetry of the thigh creases. Further testing for subluxation can be elicited by holding the infant's leg with the fingers on the greater and lesser trochanter and then abducting the hip; if subluxation is present, a "clunk" of the femur head striking the shallow acetabulum can be heard (Ortolani's sign). If the hip can be felt to actually slip in the socket, this is Barlow's sign. Subluxated hip may be bilateral but is usually unilateral. It is important that hip subluxation be discovered as early as possible because correction is most successful if it is initiated early.

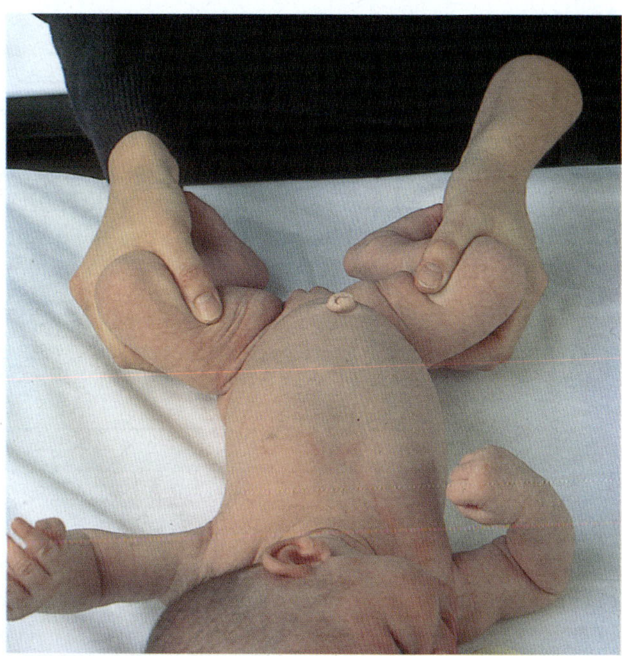

FIGURE 18.17 Hip abduction in a newborn—both hips should abduct so completely they lie almost flat against the mattress (180°).

When lying on the abdomen, newborns are capable of bringing their arms and legs underneath them and raising their stomach off the bed high enough for a hand to be slipped underneath. The preterm newborn does not have this ability, so it is an indication of maturity.

ASSESSMENT FOR WELLBEING

There are several traditional standardised assessments to evaluate a newborn quickly at birth.

Apgar scoring

At 1 minute and 5 minutes after birth, newborns are observed and rated according to an Apgar score, an assessment scale used as a standard since 1958 (Apgar et al., 1958). As shown in Table 18.1, the newborn's heart rate, respiratory effort, muscle tone, reflex irritability and colour are rated 0, 1 or 2; the five scores are then totalled. A newborn whose total score is less than 4 is in serious danger of respiratory or cardiovascular failure and needs resuscitation. A score of 4 to 6 means that the infant's condition is guarded and the baby may need clearing of the airway and supplementary oxygen. A score of 7 to 10 indicates that the infant scored as high as 70% to 90% of all infants at 1 to 5 minutes after birth or is adjusting well to extrauterine life (10 is the highest score possible). The Apgar score is repeated every additional 5 minutes, until a minimum score of 7 is reached. The Apgar score standardises infant assessment at birth and serves as a baseline for future evaluations. There is a high correlation between low 5-minute Apgar scores and neurological illness (Wiberg et al., 2010). The following points should be considered in obtaining an Apgar rating.

Heart rate

Auscultating a newborn heart with a stethoscope is the best way to determine heart rate; however, heart rate also may be obtained by observing and counting the pulsations of the cord at the abdomen if the cord is still uncut. Once the cord has been cut and clamped, a pulse may often be palpated by placing an index finger and thumb at the base of the cord.

Respiratory effort

Respirations are counted by watching respiratory movements. A mature newborn usually cries and aerates the lungs spontaneously at about 30 seconds after birth. By 1 minute, he or she is maintaining regular, although rapid, respirations. A depressed respiratory effort might be anticipated in a newborn whose mother received large amounts of analgesia or a general anaesthetic during labour or birth.

Muscle tone

Mature newborns hold their extremities tightly flexed, simulating their intrauterine position. Muscle tone is tested by observing their resistance to any effort to extend their extremities. Poor muscle tone is observed when the infant shows no flexion of the arms and legs, and extremities "flop" back to the mattress when manipulated or flexed.

Reflex irritability

Reflex irritability in a newborn is the response to stimulation. A good response to these actions would be vigorous crying or a strong facial grimace. A baby whose mother was heavily sedated will probably demonstrate a low score in this category.

Colour

All infants appear cyanotic at the moment of birth. They grow pink with or shortly after the first breath, which makes the colour of newborns correspond to how well they are breathing. Acrocyanosis (cyanosis of the hands and feet) is so common in newborns that a score of 1 in this category can be thought of as normal.

Respiratory evaluation

Good respiratory function obviously has the highest priority in newborn care, so assessment for it is ongoing at

TABLE 18.1 Apgar scoring system

Sign	Score 0	Score 1	Score 2
Heart rate	Absent	<100 bpm	>100 bpm
Respiratory effort	Absent	Slow (irregular)	Good crying
Muscle tone	Limp	Some flexion of extremities	Active motion
Reflex irritability	No response	Grimace	Cough or sneeze
Colour	Blue, pale	Pink body, blue extremities	All pink

Source: From Cloherty, J.P., Eichenwald, E.C., Hansen, A.R., Stark, A.R. (2011). *Manual of Neonatal Care* (7th ed.). Philadelphia: Lippincott Williams & Wilkins. Adapted from Apgar V. (1953). A proposal for a new method of evaluation of the newborn infant. *Current Researches in Anesthesia & Analgesia, 32,* 260–267.

every newborn contact. At birth most newborn infants will commence movement of all extremities, start breathing and have a heart rate over 100 bpm. If these signs aren't evident tactile stimulation by drying with a towel should be initiated. If the infant does not breathe then assisted ventilation should be commenced.

CASE STUDY QUESTION

6. Beth Phillips had Apgar scores of 6 at 1 minute of age and 8 at 5 minutes of age. What are the five components of the Apgar score?
   a. Heart rate, respiratory effort, muscle tone, reflex irritability and colour
   b. Respiratory rate, abdominal tone, reflex irritability, colour and head circumference
   c. Colour, breathing rate, cry, amount of brown fat and response to an adult voice
   d. Abdominal tone, persistence, gastric acidity, arterial pressure and response to pain

Physical examination

A newborn is given a preliminary physical examination immediately after birth to establish gestational age and to detect any observable condition such as difficulty breathing, a congenital heart anomaly, meningocele, cleft lip or palate, hydrocephalus, a birthmark, imperforate anus, tracheo-oesophageal atresia or bowel obstruction. This assessment may be the responsibility of the delivering doctor, midwife, paediatrician or nurse. This health assessment is done quickly, to prevent overexposing a newborn, yet not so swiftly that important findings are overlooked.

Height and weight

Assuming newborns are breathing well, they are weighed nude and without a blanket soon after birth in the birthing room (see Fig. 18.18). Measurements such as body length and head circumference can be obtained later. A newborn's weight is important because it helps to determine maturity as well as establish a baseline against which all other weights can be compared. Following this initial weight, an infant is weighed nude again on day 3 of life to ensure the infant is not losing more than the normal physiological amount (10% of birth weight). Abnormal loss of weight may be the first indication that a newborn has an inborn error of metabolism, such as adrenocortical insufficiency (salt-dumping type) or is becoming dehydrated.

Assessment of gestational age

Specific findings on physical assessment provide clues to a newborn's gestational age. Ballard modified the Dubowitz scale (Ballard et al., 1991) to an assessment scale that can be completed in 3 to 4 minutes (see

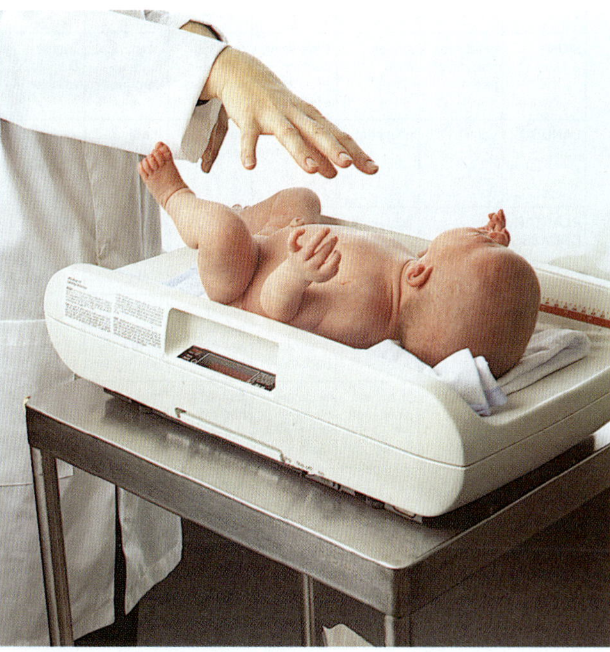

FIGURE 18.18 Weighing a newborn. Notice the protective hand held over the infant.

Fig. 18.19). The assessment consists of two portions: physical maturity and neuromuscular maturity. The first is a series of observations about skin texture, colour, lanugo, foot creases, genitalia, ear and breast maturity. Each designated body part is inspected and given a score of 0 to 5. This observational scoring should be done as soon as possible after birth because skin assessment becomes much less reliable after 24 hours.

Using such a standard method to rate maturity is helpful in detecting infants who are small for gestational age (they are light in weight, but the neuromuscular and physical observation scales are adequate for their weeks in utero) and differentiating them from newborns who are immature because of a miscalculated due date. An infant who is found to be less than 35 weeks' gestation requires close observation, usually in a special care nursery.

Assessment of behavioural capacity

Term newborns are physically active and emotionally prepared to interact with the people around them (see Fig. 18.20). They are people oriented from the beginning—how much so can be demonstrated by the way they immediately attune to human voices or concentrate on their mother's face.

CARE OF A NEWBORN AT BIRTH

Newborn identification and registration

Infant identification is important, because there always exists the possibility that a newborn may be handed to the wrong parents or be switched or kidnapped from a healthcare facility, although these events are rare.

A

	0	1	2	3	4	5
SKIN	gelatinous red, trans-parent	smooth pink, visible veins	superficial peeling &/or rash, few veins	cracking pale area, rare veins	parchment, deep cracking, no vessels	leathery, cracked, wrinkled
LANUGO	none	abundant	thinning	bald areas	mostly bald	
PLANTAR CREASES	no crease	faint red marks	anterior transverse crease only	creases ant. 2/3	creases cover entire sole	
BREAST	barely percept.	flat areola, no bud	stippled areola, 1–2 mm bud	raised areola, 3–4 mm bud	full areola, 5–10 mm bud	
EAR	pinna flat, stays folded	sl. curved pinna, soft with slow recoil	well-curv. pinna, soft but ready recoil	formed & firm with instant recoil	thick cartilage, ear stiff	
GENITALS Male	scrotum empty, no rugae		testes descend-ing, few rugae	testes down, good rugae	testes pendulous, deep rugae	
GENITALS Female	prominent clitoris & labia minora		majora & minora equally prominent	majora large, minora small	clitoris & minora completely covered	

B

	0	1	2	3	4	5
Posture						
Square Window (Wrist)	90°	60°	45°	30°	0°	
Arm Recoil	180°		100°-180°	90°-100°	<90°	
Popliteal Angle	180°	160°	130°	110°	90°	<90°
Scarf Sign						
Heel to Ear						

C

Score	Wks
5	26
10	28
15	30
20	32
25	34
30	36
35	38
40	40
45	42
50	44

FIGURE 18.19 Ballard's assessment of gestational age criteria. (**A**) Physical maturity assessment criteria. (**B**) Neuromuscular maturity assessment criteria. *Posture:* With infant supine and quiet, score as follows: arms and legs extended = 0; slight or moderate flexion of hips and knees = 2; legs flexed and abducted, arms slightly flexed = 3; full flexion of arms and legs = 4. *Square window:* Flex hand at the wrist. Exert pressure sufficient to get as much flexion as possible. The angle between hypothenar eminence and anterior aspect of forearm is measured and scored. Do not rotate wrist. *Arm recoil:* With infant supine, fully flex forearm for 5 sec, then fully extend by pulling the hands and release. Score as follows: remain extended or random movements = 0; incomplete or partial flexion = 2; brisk return to full flexion = 4. *Popliteal angle:* With infant supine and pelvis flat on examining surface, flex leg on thigh and fully flex thigh with one hand. With the other hand, extend leg and score the angle attained according to the chart. *Scarf sign:* With infant supine, draw infant's hand across the neck and as far across the opposite shoulder as possible. Assistance to elbow is permissible by lifting it across the body. Score according to location of the elbow: elbow reaches opposite anterior axillary line = 0; elbow between opposite anterior axillary line and midline of the thorax = 1; elbow at midline of thorax = 2; elbow does not reach midline of thorax = 3; elbow at proximal axillary line = 4. *Heel to ear:* With infant supine, hold infant's foot with one hand and move it as near to the head as possible without forcing it. Keep pelvis flat on examining surface. (**C**) Scoring for a Ballard assessment scale. The point total from assessment is compared to the left column. The matching number in the right column reveals the infant's age in gestation weeks. (From Ballard, J. L., Khoury, J. C., Wedig, K., et al. [1991]. New Ballard score expanded to include extremely premature infants. *Journal of Pediatrics*, *119*(3), 417–424.)

Identification band

One traditional form of identification used with newborns is a plastic bracelet with permanent locks that require cutting to be removed. A number that corresponds to the mother's hospital number, the mother's full name, and the sex, date and time of the infant's birth are printed on the band. If an identification band is attached to a newborn's arm or leg, two bands should be used. This is because a newborn's wrist and hand, as well as the ankle and foot, are not very different in width and bands can slide off easily.

Birth registration

The doctor or midwife who supervised the birth of an infant has the responsibility to see that the parents receive birth registration forms that are filed with the Registry of Births, Deaths and Marriages in the state/region in which the infant was born. A report is sent from the place of birth each month to the Registry to ensure parents have lodged the forms. The infant's name, the mother's name and the birth date and place are recorded. Official birth information is important in proving eligibility for school and, later, for voting, passports and social security benefits.

Birth record documentation

The infant's chart is also a vital piece of documentation. It serves as a baseline indicating whether the infant was well at birth. Be certain a newborn chart contains the following information:

- Time of birth
- Time the infant breathed
- Whether respirations were spontaneous or aided
- Apgar score at 1 minute and at 5 minutes of life

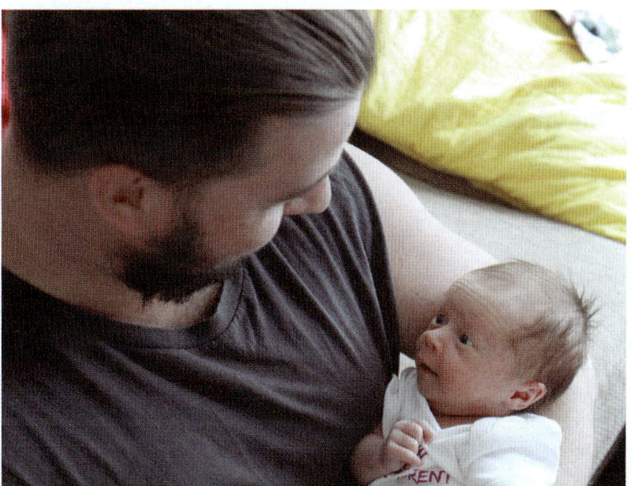

FIGURE 18.20 A newborn recognises her parent's face. (© Lauren Kidziak.)

- Whether vitamin K was administered
- General condition of the infant
- Number of vessels in the umbilical cord
- Whether cultures were taken (they are taken if the mother has a history of vaginal or uterine infection)
- Whether the infant voided and whether he or she passed a stool (this information is helpful if, later on, the diagnosis of bowel obstruction or absence of a kidney is considered).

Potential problems

Temperature regulation

There is a risk of ineffective thermoregulation related to a newborn's transition to the extrauterine environment and care should be aimed at maintaining the newborns' axillary temperature at 37°C by 1 hour after birth. Several procedures help a baby to conserve body heat at birth.

Keep newborn warm

Gently rub a newborn dry, remove the wet linen, then swaddle the infant loosely with a clean, warm and dry blanket. Be certain to place a hat on the infant's head. Alternatively the infant may be dried off on the mother's chest then remain skin-to-skin with her; both are covered with a blanket. This has the additional benefit of allowing the infant to initiate breastfeeding and encourages bonding. These actions all help to prevent heat loss (see Fig. 18.21).

During the first day of life, a newborn's temperature is usually taken hourly for the first 4 hours. Thereafter, unless the temperature is elevated or subnormal, or the infant appears to be in distress, measurement once a day while in the healthcare facility is enough.

Effective respiration

There is a risk of ineffective airway clearance related to the presence of mucus in the mouth and nose at birth. Care should be aimed at the neonate's ability to maintain a respiratory rate of 30 to 60 breaths per minute without evidence of retraction or grunting by 5 minutes after birth.

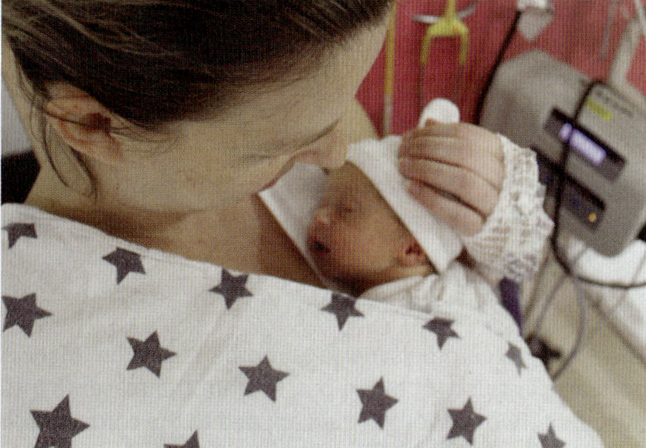

FIGURE 18.21 A newborn is wrapped and capped to conserve body heat. (© Lauren Kidziak.)

Record the first cry

A crying infant is a breathing infant, because the sound of crying is made by a current of air passing over the larynx. The more lusty the cry, the greater the assurance the newborn is breathing deeply and forcefully. Vigorous crying also helps blow off the extra carbon dioxide that makes all newborns slightly acidotic and so helps to correct this condition. Although gentleness is necessary to make an infant's transition from intrauterine life to extrauterine life as untraumatic as possible, there is no need to completely halt the initial crying of a newborn.

A newborn who does not breathe spontaneously or who takes a few quick, gasping breaths but is unable to maintain respirations needs resuscitation as an emergency measure. An infant with grunting respirations needs careful observation for respiratory distress syndrome (see Chapter 26).

Promote adequate breathing pattern and prevent aspiration

Normal newborn infants do not require suctioning of the nose, mouth or pharynx after birth as they can effectively clear their airways. Suction should be used only if the infant shows obvious signs of obstruction either to spontaneous breathing or positive pressure ventilation. If suctioning is required a large-bore suction catheter (size 10–12 Fg) should be passed not more than 5 cm from the term infant's lips, with suction time limited to a few seconds and negative pressure not exceeding 100 mmHg (Australian Resuscitation Council, 2010).

Brisk suctioning has also been associated with bradycardia in newborns because of vagal nerve stimulation. Although the effectiveness of the procedure is not well documented, when an infant is born with meconium-stained amniotic fluid and is non-vigorous, intubation may be performed so that deep tracheal suction can be accomplished before respirations are established, to help prevent meconium aspiration (ARC, 2010).

Umbilical cord care

There is a risk of infection related to a newly clamped umbilical cord. The area around the cord should be dry and free of erythema.

Inspection and care of an umbilical cord

The umbilical cord pulsates for a moment after an infant is born as a last flow of blood passes from the placenta into the infant. Two clamps are then applied to the cord and the cord is cut between the clamps. Some fathers choose to do this as their responsibility. The infant cord is then clamped again by a permanent cord clamp.

Every time you handle a newborn, inspect the cord to be certain it is clamped securely. If a clamp loosens before thrombosis obliterates the umbilical vessels, haemorrhage could result. As previously mentioned, the number of cord vessels should be counted and noted immediately after the cord is cut. Cords begin to dry almost immediately and the vessels may be obscured by the time of the infant's first thorough physical examination. The cord falls off at about day 6 to 10 of life.

Remind parents to continue to keep the cord dry until it falls off after they return home. The use of creams, lotions and oils near the cord should be discouraged because they tend to slow drying of the cord and invite infection. Some healthcare agencies recommend rubbing alcohol on the cord site once or twice a day to hasten drying. Others prefer the cord be left strictly alone because manipulation could invite infection. After the cord falls off, a small, pink, granulating area may remain. This should also be left clean and dry until it has healed (about 24 to 48 additional hours).

NURSING CARE OF A NEWBORN AND FAMILY IN THE POSTPARTUM PERIOD

Initial feeding

A term newborn who is to be breastfed may be fed within the first hour after birth. A baby who is to be formula-fed may receive a first feeding at about 2 to 4 hours of age. Both formula-fed and breastfed infants do best on a demand schedule; many need to be fed as often as every 2 hours in the first few days of life. Chapter 19 covers the elements of breastfeeding and formula feeding in detail. Encouraging women to not only begin breastfeeding but also to continue for a minimum of 6 months is important (see Box 18.1).

BOX 18.1 ✻ Focus on evidence-based practice

The influence of self-efficacy on breastfeeding

The World Health Organization recommends that infants should be breastfed exclusively until 6 months of age, and breast milk should remain in the infant's diet until 2 years of age. Many women try breastfeeding in the hospital, then stop breastfeeding shortly after they return home; while others continue for the recommended time. To discover if a feeling of self-efficacy (the belief that one can bring about positive results) is important in determining whether women will continue breastfeeding, many researchers have assessed general self-efficacy in pregnant women. A longitudinal study looking at the effect of psychosocial variables including self-efficacy, body image, psychological adjustment, and intention, motivation and confidence to exclusively breastfeed were assessed at 32 weeks' gestation, 2 months' postpartum and 6 months' postpartum. Analysis of the results of the study showed that confidence to achieve exclusive breastfeeding, self-efficacy and psychological adjustment were predictors for exclusive breastfeeding duration. The researchers recommend individual antenatal breastfeeding education and support, implementing psychosocial supports and methods of providing positive feedback which increases a woman's self-efficacy to breastfeed to 6 months.

Based on this study, would you include efforts to increase a mother's self-efficacy when helping her begin breastfeeding?

Source: de Jager, E., Broadbent, J., Fuller-Tyszkiewicz, M., Nagle, C., McPhie, S. & Skouteris, H. (2015). A longitudinal study of the effect of psychosocial factors on exclusive breastfeeding duration. *Midwifery 31*(2015), 103–111.

Bathing

Bathing of an infant is best done by the parents under a midwife's or nurse's supervision. Be sure the room is warm (about 24°C) to prevent chilling. Bath water should be approximately 37°C to 38°C, a temperature that feels pleasantly warm to the elbow or wrist. Equipment necessary for an infant's bath consists of a basin of water, soap, washcloth, towel, comb, and clean nappy and clothing. Assemble these items beforehand, so the baby is not left exposed or unattended while you go for more equipment.

Bathing should proceed from the cleanest to the most soiled areas of the body—that is, from the eyes and face to the trunk and extremities and, last, to the nappy area. Wipe a newborn's eyes with clear water from the inner canthus outwards, using a clean portion of the washcloth for each eye to prevent spread of infection to the other eye. Wash the face with clear water only (no soap) to avoid skin irritation; soap may be used on the rest of the body. Wash each area of the baby's body, rinse so no soap is left on the skin (soap is drying and newborns are susceptible to desquamation) and then dry the body part. Give particular care to the creases of skin, where milk tends to collect if the child regurgitates after feedings. In male infants, the foreskin of the penis should not be forced back, or constriction of the penis may result. Wash the vulva of a female infant, wiping from front to back to prevent contamination of the vagina or urethra by rectal bacteria.

Do not apply powder or lotion to newborns because some infants are allergic to these products. In addition, many adult talcum powders contain zinc stearate, which is irritating to the respiratory tract; such preparations should always be avoided. If a newborn's skin seems extremely dry and portals for infection are becoming apparent, a natural lubricant may be added to the bath water or applied directly to the baby's skin, which should relieve the condition.

Sleeping position

Stress to parents the need for safe sleeping strategies. Sudden infant death syndrome (SIDS) is the sudden, unexplained death of an infant younger than 1 year of age during sleep that remains unexplained after a thorough investigation (AIHW, 2012). With the introduction of safe sleeping campaigns the rate of SIDS has decreased across both Australia and New Zealand (AIHW, 2012; Mitchell & Blair, 2012). Further information for both health professionals and parents can be found at: <www.sidsandkids.org; www.sids.org.nz/site>. The SIDS and Kids safe sleeping message is to:

1. Sleep baby on the back from birth, not on the tummy or side.
2. Sleep baby with face uncovered (no doonas, pillows, lambs' wool, cot bumpers or soft toys).
3. Avoid exposing baby to tobacco smoke before birth and after.
4. Provide a safe sleeping environment (safe cot, safe mattress, safe bedding).
5. Sleep baby in their own safe sleeping environment next to the parent's bed for the first 6 to 12 months of life.

Nappy area care

Preventing nappy dermatitis is a practice that parents need to start from the very beginning with their newborn. Regular nappy changes, washing the area with clear water and drying the area well, can aid to prevent the ammonia in urine from irritating the infant's skin, causing a nappy rash. Wear gloves for nappy care as part of standard precautions. For breastfed babies, parents should be educated to expect 5 to 6 wet disposable nappies, or 6 to 8 wet cloth nappies each day and loose, grainy, mustard-coloured stools. Once breastfeeding is established breastfed babies can have no bowel actions for 5 to 6 days, as long as the infant is otherwise well, settled between feeds, breastfeeding regularly and having plenty of wet nappies. Infants being formula fed will have the same number of wet nappies; however, the stool will be more formed and vary in colour from yellow to brown.

Newborn screening tests

Infants are screened for phenylketonuria (PKU; a disease of defective protein metabolism), hypothyroidism, cystic fibrosis and many rarer metabolic disorders. Screening is done by means of a simple blood test in which drops of blood from the heel are dropped onto a special filter paper. Ideally, the baby should have received formula or breast milk for 24 hours (providing an intake of phenylalanine, an essential amino acid found in milk) before the test for PKU to be accurate. If the infant has not received adequate milk before the blood sample is taken, the results may be falsely negative (a child with PKU will test as if normal). However, it is recommended that this test is taken between 48 to 72 hours of age for all newborn infants regardless of gestational age, weight, feeding or health status.

If blood testing is not done before discharge, the tests may be done at a home health visit by the domiciliary midwife, child and family health nurse, or in a health clinic with a GP. Always assess at the first newborn health visit whether these procedures were done. As with any heel-prick for blood, sampling of this nature is best done by a spring-activated lancet rather than a regular lancet, so that the skin incision is made as quickly and painlessly as possible. Allowing a newborn to breastfeed during painful procedures may be helpful. (Further information for health professionals including testing procedures, pain relief and eLearning tools can be found in Australia at <www.vcgs.org.au/pathology/sections/NewbornScreening/?docid=aa3a4d81-d44b-42ff-8340-99360112c7a7> or in New Zealand at <www.nsu.govt.nz/health-professionals/newborn-metabolic-screening-programme/procedures-guidelines-and-reports>.)

Hepatitis B vaccination

All newborns receive a first vaccination against hepatitis B at birth; a second dose is administered at 2 months and a third at 6 months. Infants whose mothers are positive for the hepatitis B surface antigen (HBsAg) also receive hepatitis B immune globulin (HBIG) at birth (Australian Government Department of Health and Ageing, 2014). Immunisation schedules for Australia and New Zealand are covered in Chapter 34.

Vitamin K administration

Newborns are at risk of bleeding disorders during the first week of life because their gastrointestinal tract is sterile at birth and unable to produce vitamin K and vitamin K crosses the placenta poorly. Vitamin K is necessary for blood coagulation. A single dose of 0.5 to 1.0 mg of vitamin K is administered intramuscularly within the first hour of life to prevent such problems (see Box 18.2). Parents can also choose to give vitamin K orally with three doses of 2 mg, one at birth, one at 3 to 5 days of age and a final dose at 4 weeks of age (NHMRC, 2010).

Nursing considerations

Before discharge, the parents should think through how they are going to care for their child at home (see also

BOX 18.2 ✻ Focus on pharmacology

Vitamin K (phytonadione)

Action: Vitamin K is used to prevent and treat vitamin K deficiency bleeding (VKDB). It is a necessary component for the production of certain coagulation factors (II, VII, IX, and X) and is produced by microorganisms in the intestinal tract (McKenna & Mirkov, 2014).

Pregnancy risk category: C

Dosage: Prophylaxis—0.5 to 1.0 mg IM one time immediately after birth; or orally 2 mg × 3 doses.

Possible adverse reactions: Local irritation, such as pain and swelling at the site of injection.

Nursing implications

- Anticipate the need for injection immediately after birth.
- Administer IM injection into large muscle; the lateral anterior thigh is the preferred site for all injections in a newborn.
- If giving for treatment, obtain prothrombin time before administration (the single best indicator of vitamin K–dependent clotting factors).
- Assess for signs of bleeding, such as black, tarry stools (different from meconium stools, which have a greenish shade), haematuria, decreased haemoglobin and haematocrit levels, and bleeding from any open wounds or base of the cord. (These signs would indicate that more vitamin K is necessary, because bleeding control has not been achieved.)

Box 18.3). Many parents have been mulling over these concerns throughout the pregnancy, whereas others may not yet have addressed some or any of these important issues. Young mothers without family support and mothers who did not seek regular antenatal care in particular may be unprepared for newborn care. With all parents, try to anticipate problems that may be relevant to them. If there are other children at home, discuss whether the parents are aware that sibling jealousy may occur. Pets can also become jealous. Discuss with a mother who is formula feeding, how to prepare the equipment and strategies for feeding. Be sure the parents have been advised on the domiciliary midwife's or nurse's role and the referral to the child and family health nurse. Check the child's identification band against the mother's one final time before discharge to help prevent the possibility of wrong identification of the infant.

Daily home care

Newborns thrive on a gentle rhythm of care, a sense of being able to anticipate what is to come next. Based on this, parents can decide what is the best daily at-home routine for them and their new child. There are no fixed rules. There is no set time at which an infant must be bathed, nor even a rule that requires a bath every day. All infants do not have to be in bed for the night by 8.00 p.m. Your aim in helping parents plan their schedule of care is to arrive at one that:

- Offers a degree of consistency
- Appears to satisfy the infant

BOX 18.3 ✻ Focus on family teaching

Determining if a newborn is well

Q. Cassandra Phillips asks you, "Could you review with me how to know if a newborn is well?"

A. The following items are helpful to determine your newborn is well:

- Sucks as if she is hungry
- Possibly regurgitates a slight amount after feeding, but has no vomiting
- Moves bowels approximately three to four times per day (may be more often if breastfed), with stools that are loose or semi-formed but not runny and watery
- Appears happy overall (despite a fussy period during the day) and sleeps for 2 to 3 hours at a time
- Has a normal temperature
- Breathes more rapidly than an adult, but breathing is easy and not stressed
- Skin is neither yellow nor blue in tone.

- Gives the parents a sense of wellbeing and contentment with their child.

Sleep patterns

A newborn sleeps for an average of 16 out of every 24 hours during the first week home, for an average of 4 hours at a time. By 4 months of age, an infant sleeps for an average of 15 hours out of every 24 and through the night. A baby probably wakes every 4, 5, 6 or 8 hours because of a physiological need for fluid. Advise parents that, because of this fluid need, they should not try to eliminate night feedings. Knowing their baby is not sick, that you are concerned and willing to listen to their questions, and that every other parent of a newborn is also up at night does not solve the difficulty of interrupted sleep, but it may help parents adjust to parenthood.

Crying

Many new parents are not prepared for the amount of time a newborn spends crying. Infants, however, typically cry an average of 2 out of every 24 hours during the first 7 weeks of life. The frequency seems to peak at age 6 or 7 weeks and then tapers off. Almost all infants have a period during the day when they are wide awake and invariably fussy. New parents need to recognise this as normal and not worry that it means their child is ill. Parents might use this fussy time for bathing or playing with the infant, arranging their schedules accordingly. It is important to learn the infant's cues and to help the infant learn to self-quiet. The most typical time for wakefulness is between 6.00 p.m. and 11.00 p.m., which, unfortunately, is when parents may be tired and least able to tolerate crying.

Parental concerns related to breathing

Some parents report that their newborns have stuffy noses or make snoring noises in their sleep and that they sneeze frequently. This occurs because most newborns continue to have some mucus in the upper respiratory tract and posterior pharynx for up to 2 weeks after birth. The snoring noise is a result of this mucus, not a cold. In addition, infants continue to breathe irregularly for about the first month. A new parent may wake at night, notice this breathing pattern, and grow alarmed that the baby is in respiratory distress. If these are the only symptoms, this is a normal newborn respiratory pattern. If the child has rhinitis (nasal discharge) or a fever, he or she needs to be seen by a healthcare professional because these symptoms suggest an upper respiratory tract infection.

Continued health maintenance for a newborn

Parents do not need to continue to weigh a newborn or take the newborn's temperature at home. These practices only cause worry, because weight fluctuates day by day, and infant activity and clothing can influence temperature. Teach parents to judge their infant's state of health by overall appearance, eagerness to feed, general activity and disposition. Make certain that parents make and keep a healthcare appointment for a first newborn assessment according to their primary care provider's schedule (2 to 6 weeks). The national healthcare program of key ages and stages that the primary health nurse assesses are to keep the child well and refer early if deviations occur.

Car safety

Motor vehicle accidents are a safety problem throughout childhood. For protection while in vehicles, newborns should always be transported in car seats. Without this protection, if a car stops suddenly, an infant can be thrown onto the floor or, in a collision, thrown out of the car or through the windscreen. When purchasing a car seat, parents should look at the label to be sure the seat meets the requirements of the Australian/New Zealand Standard (AS/NZS) 1754. Infants should sit in a backward-facing seat until they are 6 months of age (see Fig. 18.22).

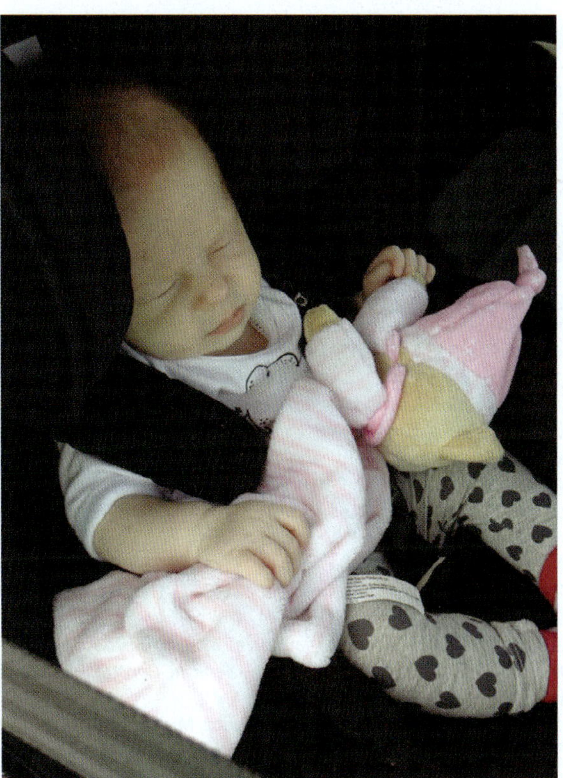

FIGURE 18.22 A newborn should always be transported in a backward-facing car seat. (© Lauren Kidziak.)

CASE STUDY QUESTION

7. Cassandra is preparing to take her new daughter home. On about what day of life can she expect her baby's umbilical cord to fall off?

   a. Day 1
   b. Days 2 to 3
   c. Days 6 to 10
   d. Day 30

Key points for review

- Converting from fetal to adult respiratory function is a major step in adaptation to extrauterine life. Newborns need particularly close observation during the first few hours of life to determine that this adaptation has been made.
- Maintaining body heat is a second major problem of newborns. The temperature of the term baby's environment should be about 24°C. When procedures that require undressing an infant for an extended period are being carried out a radiant heat source should be used.
- Identification bands should be attached securely to newborns; assess these bands carefully before hospital discharge. To help prevent the possibility of kidnapping, be certain of the identification of anyone to whom you give a newborn.
- To feel confident with newborn care, parents need to hold and give care in the hospital. Encouraging them to spend as much time as possible with a newborn is a major nursing role. Be certain parents have a car seat to use at discharge.

CASE STUDY QUESTIONS

8. Cassandra is concerned because Beth seems small, is covered by erythema toxicum and has noisy respirations. You discover that the family has no car seat to transport the baby home. What would you teach the mother to make her feel more comfortable with her newborn? What would you do about the car seat—ask that they stay until they can arrange to rent or borrow one, or discharge them?
9. When you are assessing Beth in her mother's room, what newborn reflexes would you assess? Suppose it is so cold in the room that you test only one reflex. Which one would you test and why?

Resources

For an extensive range of additional resources to enhance teaching and learning and to facilitate understanding of this chapter, please see the text's accompanying website located on thePoint at http://thepoint.lww.com.

References

Apgar, V., Holaday, D. A., Stanley James, L., et al. (1958). Evaluation of a newborn infant: Second report. *Journal of the American Medical Association, 168*(15), 1985–1988.

Australian Government Department of Health and Ageing. (2014). *The Australian Immunisation Handbook* (10th ed.). Canberra: Department of Health and Ageing.

Australian Institute of Health and Welfare (AIHW) (2012). *A Picture of Australia's Children 2012*. Cat. no. PHE 167. Canberra: AIHW.

Australian Resuscitation Council (ARC) (2010). *Guideline 13.4 - Airway Management and Mask Ventilation of the Newborn Infant.* East Melbourne: ARC.

Ballard, J. L., Khoury, J. C., Wedig, K., et al. (1991). The new Ballard Scale. *Journal of Paediatrics, 119*(3), 417–424.

Chetham, M. (2007). Neonatal jaundice. In S. R. Hayden et al. (Eds). *Rosen & Barkin's 5-Minute Emergency Medicine Consult*. Philadelphia: Lippincott Williams & Wilkins.

de Jager, E., Broadbent, J., Fuller-Tyszkiewicz, M., Nagle, C., McPhie, S. & Skouteris, H. (2015). A longitudinal study of the effect of psychosocial factors on exclusive breastfeeding duration. *Midwifery, 31*(2015), 103–111.

Desmond, M. N., Franklin, R. D., Valbona, C., et al. (1963). The hospital behavior of the newly born: The term infant. *Journal of Paediatrics, 62*(3), 307–309.

Gulati, V., Eseonu, K., Sayani, J., Ismail, N., Uzoigwe, C., Choudhury, M.Z., Gulati, P., Aqil, A., and Tibrewal, S. (2013). Developmental dysplasia of the hip in the newborn: A systematic review. *World Journal of Orthopedics*, *4*(2), 32–41.

Haldeman-Englert, C. R., Saitta, S. C. & Zackai, E. H. (2012). Specific chromosome disorders in newborns. In C. A. Gleason & S. U. Devaskar (Eds), *Avery's Diseases of the Newborn* (9th ed, pp. 196–208). Philadelphia: Elsevier/Saunders.

McKenna, L. & Mirkov, S. (Eds). (2014). *McKenna's Drug Handbook for Nursing and Midwifery* (7th ed.). Sydney: Lippincott, Williams & Wilkins.

Mitchell, E. A. & Blair, P. S. (2012). SIDS prevention: 3000 lives saved but can we do better. *The New Zealand Medical Journal, 125*(1359).

National Health and Medical Research Council (NHMRC) (2010). *Joint Statement and Recommendations on Vitamin K Administration to Newborn Infants to Prevent Vitamin K Deficiency Bleeding in Infancy*. Canberra: NHMRC.

Nelson, L., Doering, J. J., Anderson, M., et al. (2012). Outcome of clinical nurse specialist-led hyperbilirubinemia screening of late preterm newborns. *Clinical Nurse Specialist, 26*(3), 164–168.

New Zealand Ministry of Health (NZMOH). (2014). *Immunisation Handbook 2011*. Wellington: Ministry of Health.

Roberts, D., Gates, S., Kilby, M. & Neilson, J. P. (2014). Interventions for twin-twin transfusion syndrome: A Cochrane review. *Ultrasound Obstetrics Gynecology, 31*(6), 701–711.

Ryan, E. & Warren, L. (2012). Birthmarks: Identification and management [online]. *Australian Family Physician, 41*(5), 274–277.

Schneider, D. S. (2011). The cardiovascular system. In K. J. Marcdante & R. M. Kliegman (Eds), *Nelson Essentials of Pediatrics* (7th ed.) (pp. 525–554). Philadelphia: Saunders/Elsevier.

Song, Y., Zhang, S. & Song, W. (2013). Significance of neonatal body indices in identifying fetal macrosomia. *Journal of Perinatology, 33*(2), 103–106.

Subramanian, A., et al. (Eds). (2014). *Drug Facts and Comparisons.* (68th ed.). St Louis: Wolters Kluwer Health.

Thilo, E. H. & Rosenberg, A. A. (2011). The newborn infant. In W. W. Hay, M. J. Levin, J. M. Sondheimer et al. (Eds) *Current Diagnosis & Treatment: Pediatrics* (21st ed.), pp. 1–63. Columbus, OH: McGraw-Hill.

Wallingford, J. B., Niswander, L. A., Shaw, G. M. & Finnell, R. H. (2013). The continuing challenge of understanding, preventing, and treating neural tube defects. *Science*, *339*.

Walsh, J. & Goser, L. (2013). Development of an innovative NICU teen parent support program: One unit's experience. *Journal of Perinatal & Neonatal Nursing, 27*(2), 176–183.

Wiberg, N., Kallen, K., Herbst, A. and Olofsson, P. (2010). Relation between umbilical cord blood pH, base deficit, lactate, 5-minute Apgar score and development of hypoxic ischemic encephalopathy. *Acta Obstetricia et Gynecologica*, *89*, 1263–1269.

Wisser, M., Rothschild, M. A., Schmolling, J. C., et al. (2012). Caput succedaneum and facial petechiae—birth-associated injuries in healthy newborns under forensic aspects. *International Journal of Legal Medicine*, *126*(3), 385–390.

Suggested readings

Raising Children Network <http://raising children.net.au>.

Ruiz, M. J., Thatch, K. A., Fisher, J. C., Simpson, L. L., et al. (2009). Neonatal outcomes associated with intestinal abnormalities diagnosed by fetal ultrasound. *Journal of Paediatric Surgery*, *44*(1), 71–74.

Chapter 19

Nutritional needs of a newborn

Previous chapters described the care of a woman and family during the antenatal, intrapartum, postnatal and newborn periods. This chapter adds information about the nutritional needs of a newborn. A newborn's nutritional needs are high during this time because of a rapid rate of growth and development. Knowing these needs fortifies you to play a key role in educating parents about how to provide optimal nutrition to meet physiological, developmental and psychological needs of their infants.

LEARNING OBJECTIVES

After mastering the contents of this chapter, you should be able to:

1. Describe nutritional requirements for a term newborn.
2. Use critical thinking to assist parents with nutritional problem solving and be sure newborn nutrition is family-centred.
3. Assess nutritional intake and feeding method of a newborn to determine adequate nutritional status.
4. Identify outcomes for a newborn and parents related to nutrition.
5. Support a woman's choice in infant feeding.
6. Implement midwifery/nursing care such as supporting a new mother while breastfeeding.
7. Evaluate effectiveness of care.
8. Identify areas related to nutrition and newborns that could benefit from additional research or application of evidence-based practice.
9. Integrate knowledge of normal newborn nutrition with practice to achieve quality child and family healthcare.

KEY TERMS

- areola
- bifidus factor
- colostrum
- engorgement
- interferon
- lactoferrin
- let-down reflex
- lysozyme

CASE STUDY

Linda Smith is a new mother of a term baby girl. During the pregnancy, she and her husband, Paul, both agreed Linda would breastfeed. Linda will be returning to work as an executive assistant after her maternity leave. She attempted to breastfeed her newborn in the birthing room with minimal success. As you offer to help her feed her baby for the second time, she says, "Do you think I made the right choice? Maybe I should formula feed her. Paul could help that way and I won't have to worry about what to do when I go back to work."

CASE STUDY QUESTION

1. How would you answer Linda?

Proper nutrition is essential for optimal growth and development, especially in the first few months of life, because brain growth proceeds at such a rapid rate during this time. The *Global Strategy for Infant and Young Child Feeding* (2003) produced by the World Health Organization recommends that infants should be exclusively breastfed for the first six months of life, followed by the gradual introduction of nutritionally adequate and safe complementary foods to meet nutritional needs. Breastfeeding should still continue until two or more years of age. This will facilitate optimal growth, development and health for the infant.

Providing adequate nutrition for an infant extends beyond physiological needs, however; it also fulfils important psychological needs. During feeding, a parent is close to the infant and a baby is apt to be particularly sensitive to the parent's demonstration of affection or lack of warmth. An infant who does not experience a warm relationship with a mother or primary carer may fail to thrive as surely as one who is denied sufficient protein or kilojoules (Britton et al., 2009).

PROMOTING NUTRITIONAL HEALTH IN A NEWBORN

Assessment

Assessment of infant nutrition begins during pregnancy with assessment of the mother's and father's attitudes and choices about infant feeding. Breastfeeding is widely accepted as the best method of human newborn nutrition, and it is the role of the health professional to ensure parents make fully informed decisions based on current evidence. However, if a mother chooses not to breastfeed because of her individual circumstances, it is important that she not be made to feel guilty for her choice, because formula feeding can be substituted. Most important, parents need to feel comfortable with, and confident about, the feeding method they choose.

Teach parents how to recognise signs of hunger in a newborn such as restlessness, tense body posture, smacking lips and tongue thrusting. Otherwise, they may wait for their infant to cry, which is a late sign of hunger. Once infant feeding begins, teach parents to assess whether the amount the infant is receiving is adequate—not by how long the newborn breastfeeds at a time or by how much

BOX 19.1 Assessment ✻ Assessing the newborn for adequate nutrition

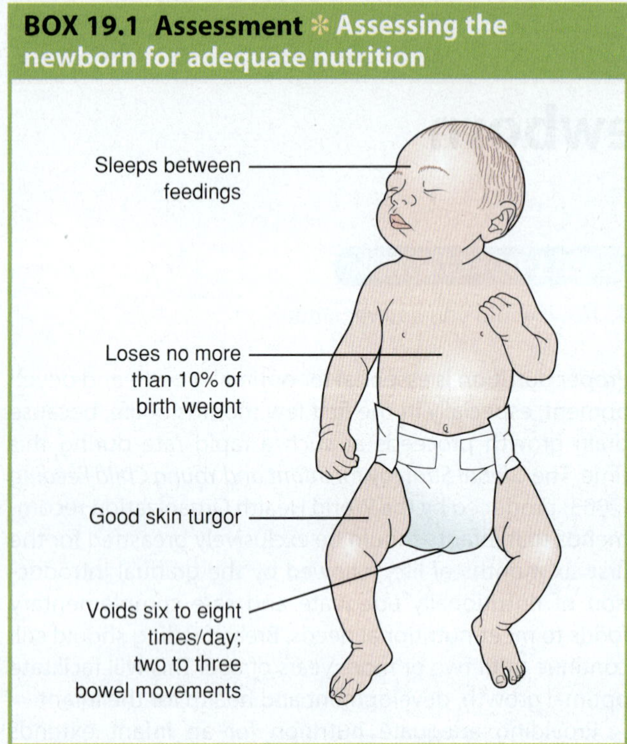

formula is taken at a feeding, but by a larger measure, such as whether the baby is voiding, growing and alert (see Box 19.1). After the mother's milk comes in, usually days 3–5, the breastfed baby will get a full feed more quickly and will generally settle and sleep for longer periods. Before this time it is normal for newborns to feed 8–12 times in a 24-hour period. A formula-fed infant regains birth weight at about 10 days, a breastfed infant at about 14 days.

Nursing diagnoses

Nursing care in relation to nutrition usually centres on a woman's choice regarding method of feeding or a newborn's nutritional intake and feeding patterns. As breastfeeding is best for newborns, planning begins while a woman is still pregnant, focusing on providing her with the information necessary to allow her to become familiar and comfortable with breastfeeding. After birth, a teaching plan addressing the nutritional needs of both the woman and her newborn can be developed. Helpful Internet sites for referral are the Australian Breastfeeding Association (ABA) <www.breastfeeding.asn.au> and the International Lactation Consultant Association <www.ilca.org>. Despite the advantages of breastfeeding, some parents still choose artificial feeding because of their individual preferences. When parents choose to formula feed they need to plan ways to make feeding time special for both themselves and the baby. The Raising Children Network is a useful and reliable Internet site offering information on many aspects of infant care, including formula feeding, and can be found at <http://raisingchildren.net.au/nutrition/newborns_nutrition.html>.

Evaluation is important to ensure that a newborn receives adequate nutrition, because unforeseen circumstances, such as an unsuspected milk allergy or mastitis (breast infection) may interfere and drastic changes may then be required to reach desired outcomes. Help parents appreciate that newborns are very adaptive and can adjust to another feeding method if necessary. Examples suggesting successful expected outcomes related to newborn feeding are:

- A breastfed infant breastfeeds every 2 to 3 hours; is content and sleeps between feedings
- A formula-fed infant ingests a total of 150 mL per kilogram of body weight of formula every 24 hours
- The mother states she feels satisfied with her chosen method of infant feeding
- The infant voids six times daily, as a measure of adequate hydration, by 1 week
- The infant's bowel actions change in colour and consistency from sticky green-black meconium on day one, to lighter greenish-brown that may be seedy or watery on day four, through to a mustard-yellow soft or liquid stool after day five.

NUTRITIONAL ALLOWANCES FOR A NEWBORN

Nutritional allowances for a newborn need to take into account total kilojoules, protein, vitamins, minerals and fluid. Breast milk supplies all nutritional requirements for the first six months of life and the breastfed infant requires no additional dietary supplements at all.

Kilojoules

Growth in the neonatal period and early infancy is more rapid than at any other period of life (Krebs & Primak, 2011). The kilojoule requirements exceed those at any other age. An infant up to 2 months of age requires 460 to 500 kJ per kilogram of body weight every 24 hours to provide an adequate amount for maintenance and growth. After 2 months of age, this amount gradually declines until the requirement at 1 year is 420 kJ/kg per day. In contrast, the adult requirement is 175 kJ/kg per day. The actual energy requirement, of course, depends on an infant's individual activity level and growth rate. For example, an active infant, one who cries frequently and squirms constantly, needs more kilojoules than one who is more passive, content to spend long hours playing quietly or just studying the environment. During growth spurts, more kilojoules are needed to supply additional energy.

Commercial infant formulas provide basic nutritional elements for infants up to the age of 1 year. They contain about 9% to 12% of their kilojoules as protein and 45% to 55% of their kilojoules as lactose carbohydrate. The balance is fat, of which about 10% (4% of the kilojoules) is linoleic acid.

Protein

Protein, necessary for the formation of new cells, has a high requirement during the newborn and infancy periods to provide for rapid growth of new cells as well as maintenance of existing cells. Both breast milk and commercial formulas provide all the essential amino acids necessary to form protein. Unaltered cow's milk is not recommended for newborns because it contains about 16% of its kilojoules as protein, whereas breast milk contains about 8%. This means that cow's milk can create such a rich solute load (the amount of urea and electrolytes that must be excreted in the urine) that a newborn's kidneys could be overwhelmed. In addition, the protein in cow's milk (casein), differs from that in breast milk (lactalbumin), both in composition and amount. The amount of casein present in milk determines its curd tension. The curd in cow's milk is large, tough and difficult to digest, whereas in breast milk the curd is softer and easier to digest. This is the rationale for formula-fed infants to be given a commercial formula containing albumin rather than cow's milk. Cow's milk products, such as yoghurt and cottage cheese, should not be introduced until 9 to 12 months of age for the same reason.

Fat

Linoleic acid, an essential fatty acid necessary for growth and skin integrity in infants, is found in both breast milk and commercial formulas. Use of fat-free milk for long periods (when other sources of food are not being offered) can result in linoleic acid deficiency. Therefore, parents should not feed fat-free milk as a means of preventing obesity in a young infant. In addition, fat-free milk does not contain sufficient kilojoules for a newborn; it has only about half as many kilojoules as commercial formulas or breast milk.

Carbohydrate

Lactose, the disaccharide found in breast milk and added to commercial formulas, appears to be the most easily digested of the carbohydrates. Lactose also improves calcium absorption and aids in nitrogen retention. It produces stools consisting predominantly of gram-positive rather than gram-negative bacteria and therefore decreases the possibility of gastrointestinal illness (which usually results from gram-negative organisms). Adequate lactose also allows protein to be used for building new cells rather than for kilojoules, encouraging normal water balance and preventing abnormal metabolism of fat. Lactose intolerance, which can occur in older children, is rarely present in newborns; they typically use the kilojoules provided by lactose well.

Fluid

It is important to maintain a sufficient fluid intake in newborns because their metabolic rate is so high (and metabolism requires water). In addition, a newborn's body surface area is large in relation to body mass. This means that a baby loses water by evaporation much more readily than an adult. Because the kidneys of a newborn are not yet capable of fully concentrating urine, a newborn cannot conserve body water by this mechanism to prevent dehydration. Another difference between newborns and adults is that body water is distributed differently. In a newborn, 30% to 35% of body weight is extracellular fluid; in an adult, this proportion is only 20%. Consequently, if a newborn's extracellular fluid store is depleted through loss of fluid or inadequate fluid intake, as much as 35% of a newborn's fluid component may be lost.

Because of all these factors, a newborn needs 150 to 200 mL/kg of water intake every 24 hours (adults require 2400 mL/day). This requirement can be supplied completely by breastfeeding or formula feeding. For the first few days, however, the capacity of the newborn's stomach is only 3–5 mL, which is approximately the volume of **colostrum** a breastfed baby will receive at each feed. Initially a formula-fed infant should be expected to take similar amounts at each feed, however, as formula is not as easily digested as breast milk the infant may not demand to feed as frequently. As they feed more the capacity of their stomach will increase.

Minerals

A number of minerals are particularly important to early growth.

Calcium

Calcium is an important mineral in the newborn period because a newborn's skeleton is growing so rapidly. Because milk is high in calcium, tetany resulting from a low calcium level seldom occurs in infants who suck well, regardless of whether they are fed breast milk or commercial formula.

Iron

A full term newborn of a mother who had an adequate iron intake during pregnancy will be born with iron stores that, theoretically, last for the first 6 months of life, until the newborn begins to produce adult haemoglobin. In Australia, every formula available to buy meets strict standards and supplementation is not usually needed. Similarly, supplements are unnecessary for breastfed infants because breast milk usually provides an adequate amount of iron.

Fluoride

Fluoride is essential for building sound teeth and for preventing tooth decay. Because teeth grow into their primary form during pregnancy, it is important for women to drink fluoridated water during pregnancy. A lactating mother should continue drinking fluoridated water (although only a small amount of fluoride passes into breast milk) and formulas should be prepared with fluoridated water. This is an essential point to remember, because a mother may think she is helping her child by using bottled water in formula, rather than chlorinated (and fluoridated) water from a tap.

If a mother is breastfeeding and a source of fluoridated water is not available (the family drinks well, spring or bottled water, or the tap water is not fluoridated), a fluoride supplement (0.25 mg daily) may be given to the infant beginning at 6 months of age. Remind parents that too much fluoride can be detrimental or cause staining of the teeth, to prevent them from giving infants unnecessary fluoride supplements.

Vitamins

Because vitamins are naturally included in breast milk, supplementation is not necessary for breastfed infants. Likewise, vitamin additives are unnecessary for a formula-fed infant because vitamins A, C and D are incorporated into commercial formula. If a newborn will not be exposed to sunlight for some reason, 400 IU of vitamin D daily may be either prescribed for the breastfeeding mother, to increase the level of the vitamin in breast milk, or given to the formula-fed infant. Additional vitamins are not usually begun until the infant approaches 6 months of age.

CASE STUDY QUESTION

2. Newborns need more fluid than adults, because their extracellular fluid component differs from that of adults. How much of a newborn's body weight is extracellular fluid?
   a. 20%, compared with 35% in an adult
   b. 35%, compared with 20% in an adult
   c. 50%, compared with 70% in an adult
   d. 70%, compared with 40% in an adult

BREASTFEEDING

It is universally agreed that breast milk is the optimal nutrition for an infant because it provides numerous health benefits to both a mother and her baby; it remains the ideal nutritional source for infants through the first year of life (American College of Obstetricians & Gynecologists, 2007) and to 2 years and beyond (WHO, 2015).

Women are recognised as the "keepers of the culture" or the main people who transmit customs to the next generation. Chief among these customs is the method for feeding newborns. The rate of breastfeeding varies in communities and over time. Data from the Australian Bureau of Statistics from the 2011–2012 health survey indicates that although breastfeeding was initiated in over 92% of babies, only 50.2% were still receiving breast milk at 6 months of age and less than 28% at 12 months of age (Australian Bureau of Statistics, 2013). Data from the Royal New Zealand Plunket Society indicate that although over 80% of babies begin breastfeeding at birth, by 6 months of age only around 20% are still exclusively breastfed (New Zealand Breast Feeding Association, 2014). If a woman comes from a family where no-one has ever breastfed, she may be very interested in being a "pioneer" in her family or, on the other hand, she may be more interested in following her family's tradition of formula feeding.

How soon women want to begin breastfeeding after birth is also culturally determined. Although it is the usual practice in hospitals to begin immediately after birth, some cultures believe that colostrum is not appropriate for newborns and they have a cultural preference not to begin breastfeeding until milk is present, at about 3 days of age. It is necessary therefore to assess each family individually to recognise cultural preferences such as these. Ask all women during pregnancy about their plans for feeding their newborn, as thinking about feeding in advance allows couples to make informed choices. As stated above, over 90% of women in Australia start to breastfeed. Offering them the opportunity to explore this issue further, prior to the birth, may increase the number of women who continue to breastfeed beyond the newborn period.

Some fathers experience jealousy at the thought of breastfeeding. Early discussion can help them work through this natural sensation, with the eventual realisation that parenting will involve many other opportunities for interaction with their child.

What if...

Linda told you that she doesn't want to breastfeed but her husband is insisting that she do so? What would you do?

Advantages of breastfeeding

Little controversy exists about breastfeeding as the best nutrition for human infants, but the ultimate decision to breastfeed should depend on what would please the mother and her infant most. If the mother is pleased with what she is doing, her infant will be comfortable and content, will enjoy being fed and will thrive. Nurses and midwives are in a prime position to teach women about the benefits of breastfeeding and provide anticipatory guidance for problems that may occur (Li, Rock & Grummer-Strawn, 2007). Implementing the World Health Organization's "Ten steps for successful breastfeeding" can also help create an atmosphere conducive to breastfeeding success in healthcare facilities (see Box 19.2). The Baby Friendly Health Initiative (BFHI) offers a lot of advice in implementing these steps.

According to the National Health and Medical Research Council (NHMRC) Infant Feeding Guidelines for Health Workers, breastfeeding is contraindicated in only a few circumstances. Absolute contraindications include:

BOX 19.2 ✻ Ten steps to successful breastfeeding

Every facility providing maternity services and care for newborn infants should:

1. Have a written breastfeeding policy that is routinely communicated to all healthcare staff.
2. Train all healthcare staff in skills necessary to implement this policy.
3. Inform all pregnant women about the benefits and management of breastfeeding.
4. Help mothers initiate breastfeeding within half an hour of birth.
5. Show mothers how to breastfeed, and how to maintain lactation even if they should be separated from their infants.
6. Give newborn infants no food or drink other than breast milk, unless medically indicated.
7. Practise rooming-in - that is, allow mothers and infants to remain together - 24 hours a day.
8. Encourage breastfeeding on demand.
9. Give no artificial teats or pacifiers (also called dummies or soothers) to breastfeeding infants.
10. Foster the establishment of breastfeeding support groups and refer mothers to them on discharge from the hospital or clinic.

Source: World Health Organization. (1989). *Protecting, Promoting and Supporting Breast-feeding: The Special Role of Maternity Services.* A Joint WHO/UNICEF statement. Geneva: World Health Organization.

- Active pulmonary tuberculosis
- Brucellosis
- Syphilis
- Breast cancer
- HIV infection
- Infant conditions such as galactosaemia and maple urine disease.

Relative contraindications include:

- Phenylketonuria
- HBV and HBC
- Some maternal medications (further information can be found at <http://toxnet.nlm.nih.gov/newtoxnet/lactmed.htm>.

A number of situations call for individual planning, such as a mother or an infant too ill for breastfeeding, or a mother who has undergone breast-reduction surgery where the nipples were detached during surgery.

Advantages for a mother

A woman gains several physiological benefits from breastfeeding:

- Breastfeeding may provide a protective function in preventing breast cancer
- The release of oxytocin from the posterior pituitary gland aids in uterine involution and may reduce the risk or severity of postpartum haemorrhage (PPH)
- Successful breastfeeding can have an empowering effect, because it is a skill only a woman can master
- Breastfeeding reduces the cost of feeding and preparation time
- Breastfeeding provides an excellent opportunity to enhance a true symbiotic bond between mother and child. (Although this does occur readily with breastfeeding, a woman who holds her baby to formula feed can form this bond as well.)

Advantages for an infant

Breastfeeding has major physiological advantages for an infant as well. Breast milk contains secretory immunoglobulin A (IgA), which binds large molecules of foreign proteins, including viruses and bacteria, keeping them from being absorbed from the gastrointestinal tract into the infant.

Lactoferrin is an iron-binding protein in breast milk that interferes with the growth of pathogenic bacteria. The enzyme lysozyme in breast milk actively destroys bacteria by lysing (dissolving) their cell membranes, possibly increasing the effectiveness of antibodies. Leucocytes in breast milk provide protection against common respiratory infectious invaders. Macrophages, responsible for producing interferon (a protein that protects against viruses), help interfere with virus growth. The **bifidus factor** is a specific growth-promoting factor for the beneficial bacteria *Lactobacillus bifidus*. The presence of *L. bifidus* in breast milk interferes with the colonisation of pathogenic bacteria in the gastrointestinal tract, reducing the incidence of diarrhoea.

In addition to these anti-infective properties, breast milk contains the ideal electrolyte and mineral composition for human infant growth. It is high in lactose, an easily digested sugar that provides ready glucose for rapid brain growth. The protein in breast milk is easily digested and the ratio of cysteine to methionine (two amino acids) favours rapid brain growth in the early months. It contains nitrogen in compounds other than protein, so that an infant can receive cell-building materials from sources other than just protein.

Breast milk contains more linoleic acid, an essential fatty acid for skin integrity, and less sodium, potassium, calcium and phosphorus than do many formulas. Breast milk also has a better balance of trace elements, such as zinc. These levels of nutrients are enough to supply the infant's needs, yet they spare the infant's kidneys from having to process a high renal solute load of unused nutrients. Women who have a familial history of allergy are usually encouraged to breastfeed to try and eliminate the possibility of exposing their infant to cow's milk protein, which could be allergenic this early in life (Hampton, 2008).

Yet another advantage is that breastfed newborns appear to be able to regulate their calcium/phosphorus levels better than infants who are formula fed. Decreased

BOX 19.3 ✻ Focus on evidence-based practice

Breastfeeding and the obesity epidemic in children

A number of studies have looked at whether breastfeeding can help reduce the epidemic of obesity in children and have come to similar conclusions: that breastfeeding reduces the risk of obesity in children and in later life. Breastfeeding has also been identified as a protective factor in reducing the risk or severity of a number of other diseases (NHMRC, 2012).

Would this information be helpful when discussing the advantages of breastfeeding and the risks associated with not breastfeeding?

Source: National Health and Medical Research Council. (2012). Infant feeding guidelines. Information for health workers, <www.nhmrc.gov.au/guidelines-publications/n56>.

calcium levels in a newborn can lead to tetany (muscle spasm). The increased concentration of fatty acid in commercial formulas may bind calcium in the gastrointestinal tract, increasing the danger of tetany. Breastfeeding may also help prevent excessive weight gain in infants (see Box 19.3).

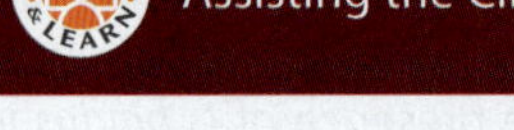

Assisting the Client with Breastfeeding

Learning to breastfeed

In cultures where breastfeeding is practised by almost all mothers, the technique is learned early in life by observation. Some women, however, may have had few, if any, opportunities to observe breastfeeding. Midwives are in a unique position to help new mothers. All should be able to assist a woman to begin breastfeeding and manage some of the difficulties commonly encountered. Lactation consultants are healthcare professionals especially educated to assist women with breastfeeding. Making a referral to such a person can be extremely helpful, particularly if the woman is experiencing problems or difficulties that are not easily overcome.

If the woman is tense and anxious, she may have difficulty achieving a **let-down reflex** and her infant may have difficulty obtaining adequate milk. This can lead to increasing tension and anxiety because the infant does not seem content. As a result, the infant becomes hungrier and is left even more unsatisfied, creating a vicious circle of events. Support, adequate instruction and reassurance from healthcare personnel are important in helping a woman feel secure enough to be able to relax (Furber & Thomson, 2007). Rooming-in is ideal for breastfeeding because it allows a woman to sense when her infant is hungry, resulting in her feeding before the infant grows fatigued from crying or her breasts grow uncomfortable from filling.

Many women who are breastfeeding sleep with their infant at night so they can easily breastfeed (bed sharing). However, as studies as to whether bed sharing increases the incidence of sudden infant death are contradictory, bed sharing should not be recommended (Ateah & Hamelin, 2008). Keeping the baby in the same room, but in its own separate bed at night, will maximise the woman's sleep opportunities.

Provide information regarding lactation and proper positioning techniques. Mature breast milk looks like non-fat milk. It is thin and almost blue-tinged in appearance. Some women may need assurance that this colour and consistency are normal; otherwise, they may think their milk is not nutritious enough. Before breastfeeding, recommend that a woman wash her hands to be sure they are free of pathogens picked up from handling perineal pads or other sources. Washing her breasts is not necessary unless she notices caked colostrum on the nipples. When she is first attempting to breastfeed, lying on her side with a pillow under her head is a good position to use. This relieves fatigue because it allows her baby to rest on the bed.

There are various holds or positions that can be used when breastfeeding:

- Side-lying position: The mother lies on her side with her baby on his side facing her. The mother supports her baby's back with either of her arms (see Fig. 19.1).
- Cradle hold: The baby's head rests in the bend of the mother's arm, near her elbow. The mother's other arm and hand can be used to support her breast or the baby's body. The mother brings the baby up to the level of her breast so that the baby lies on his side with his body facing her (see Fig. 19.2).

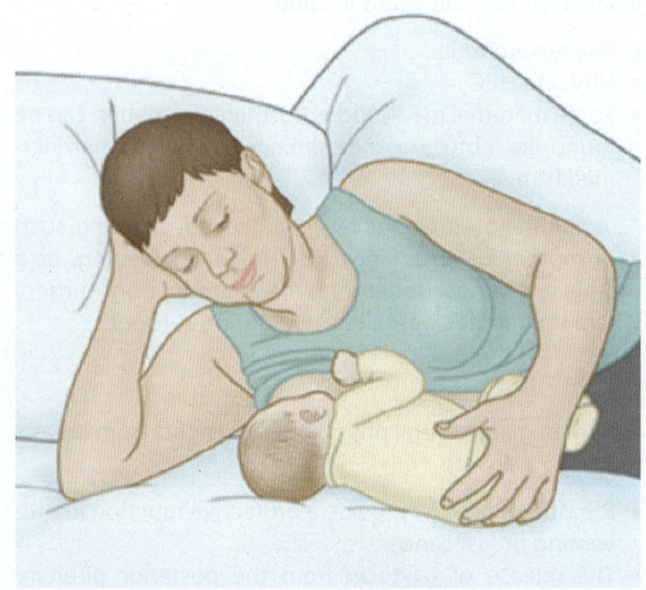

FIGURE 19.1 Side-lying position. (www.drugs.com/cg/how-to-hold-and-breastfeed-your-baby.html)

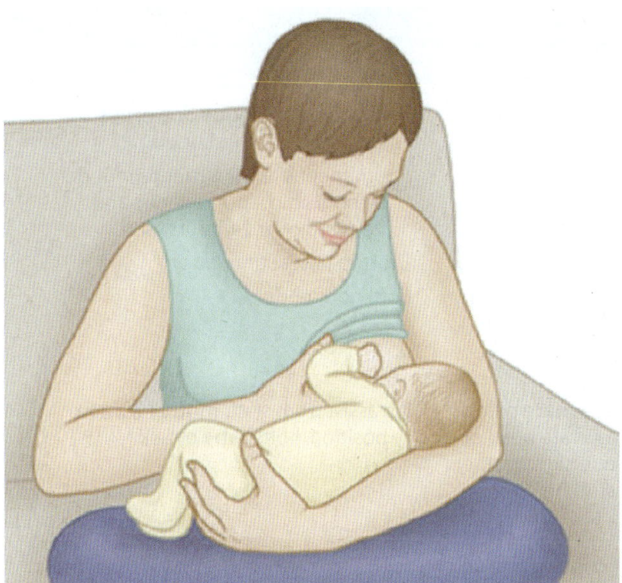

FIGURE 19.2 Cradle hold. (www.drugs.com/cg/how-to-hold-and-breastfeed-your-baby.html.)

- Cross-cradle hold: The mother supports or cradles her baby with the arm that is on the opposite side of the breast she uses to feed. For example, if the mother is going to breastfeed her baby with her right breast, she supports his body with her left arm. The mother uses her left hand to support his head, while her right arm and hand can be used to support her breast (see Fig. 19.3). The cross-cradle hold is often used when a baby is born early, is very small or has a weak neck or upper body. It may also be helpful to use this position for newborns.
- Football or underarm hold: This position works best when the mother is in a sitting position. The baby lies on his back and the mother tucks his body under her arm on the same side as the breast she uses to feed. The mother supports the baby's body with her arm and his head with her hand. She can support her breast with her other hand (see Fig. 19.4).

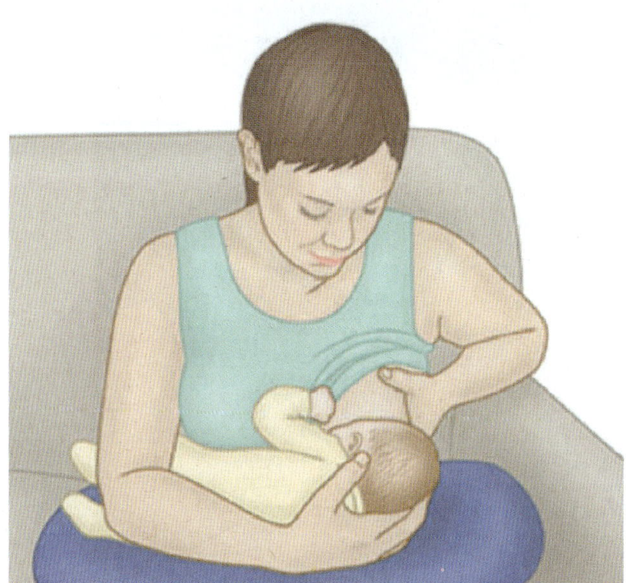

FIGURE 19.3 Cross-cradle hold. (www.drugs.com/cg/how-to-hold-and-breastfeed-your-baby.html.)

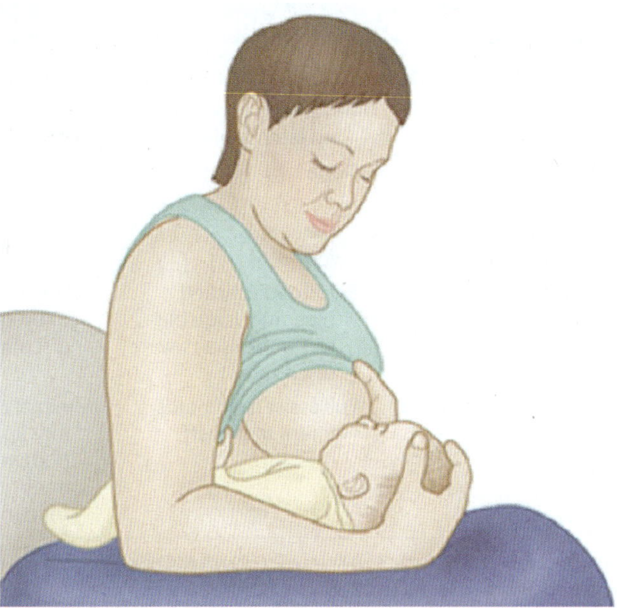

FIGURE 19.4 Football hold. (www.drugs.com/cg/how-to-hold-and-breastfeed-your-baby.html.)

Although not well documented as to efficiency or reliable results, an assessment tool such as the LATCH assessment (see Table 19.1) can provide measures to help evaluate a newborn's breastfeeding effectiveness (Howe et al., 2008).

During the first few days of life, because they are receiving colostrum and need the nutrients and fluid obtained by frequent sucking, babies should be fed as often as they seem hungry (every 2 to 3 hours). Frequent feeding also is advantageous to establish a milk supply, because the more often breasts are emptied, the more efficiently they fill and continue to maintain a good supply of milk.

Techniques of breastfeeding

Promote adequate sucking

Often, a newborn being breastfed drops off to sleep while feeding during the early days after birth. To both stimulate milk production effectively and ensure adequate fluid intake, a woman may need to keep the infant awake and urge him or her to suck. Advise mothers to be sure to awaken newborns fully before feeding by handling them, stroking their backs, changing their position, rubbing their arms and chest or changing their nappy. Gently tickling the bottom of a baby's feet will also wake a baby effectively. If an infant is not sucking well, a woman can use breast massage after feeding to empty her breasts manually. This helps ensure good milk production for the time when the infant is ready to suck.

TABLE 19.1 Latch breastfeeding charting system

	0	1	2
Latch	Too sleepy or reluctant; no latch achieved	Repeated attempts; hold nipple in mouth; stimulate to suck	Grasps breast; tongue down; lips flanged; rhythmic sucking
Audible swallowing	None	A few with stimulation	Spontaneous and intermittent under 24 hours old; spontaneous and frequent over 24 hours old
Type of nipple	Inverted	Flat	Everted (after stimulation)
Comfort (breast/nipple)	Engorged; cracked, bleeding, large blisters or bruises; severe discomfort	Filling; reddened/small blisters or bruises; mild/moderate discomfort	Soft, non tender
Hold (positioning)	Full assist (staff holds infant at breast)	Minimal assist (i.e. place pillows for support, elevate head of bed); teach one side, mother does other; staff holds and then mother takes over	No assist from staff; mother able to position/hold baby by self

Source: Jensen, D., Wallace, S., & Kelsey, P. (1994). LATCH: a breastfeeding charting system and documentation tool. *Journal of Obstetric, Gynecologic, and Neonatal Nursing*, *23*(1) , 27-32

Provide immediate support if problems arise

When managed well by healthcare personnel, the common problems that arise with breastfeeding can usually be resolved. Handled otherwise, they can complicate breastfeeding and discourage a woman from continuing.

Provide information regarding techniques for burping the breastfed baby

Some infants seem to swallow little air when they breastfeed, whereas others swallow a great deal. As a rule, it is helpful to burp newborns after they have emptied the first breast and again after the total feeding. Holding the baby in a sitting position on the lap, then leaning the child forwards against one hand, with the index finger and thumb supporting the head, is often the best position to use. This position provides head support but leaves the other hand free to pat the baby's back (see Fig. 19.5). Laying the baby prone across the lap is another alternative position.

Provide support for a mother who is breastfeeding multiple infants

Because of in vitro fertilisation, many more women today, than previously, give birth to twins or multiple infants. You can assure women that the average woman can easily produce enough milk to feed multiple infants. Because of the time involved, however, fewer women with multiple infants choose to breastfeed than do mothers of single infants (Moore, 2007). Support those who want to breastfeed multiple infants: eating and drinking adequately is important for all breastfeeding mothers but when there is more than one infant this is even more important. Also, refer women to the Multiple Birth Association in their region, their local council for any support services that may be available, the local branch of the Australian Breastfeeding Association or La Leche League.

Beginning breastfeeding

Breastfeeding should begin as soon after birth as possible, ideally within the first hour while the woman is still in the birthing room and while the infant is in the first reactivity period (Forster & McLachlan, 2007). The release of oxytocin by breastfeeding at this time begins the let-down of milk and also stimulates uterine contraction.

Most women enjoy having an experienced midwife or nurse with them for a first feeding to offer suggestions. Placing the baby skin-to-skin with its mother immediately

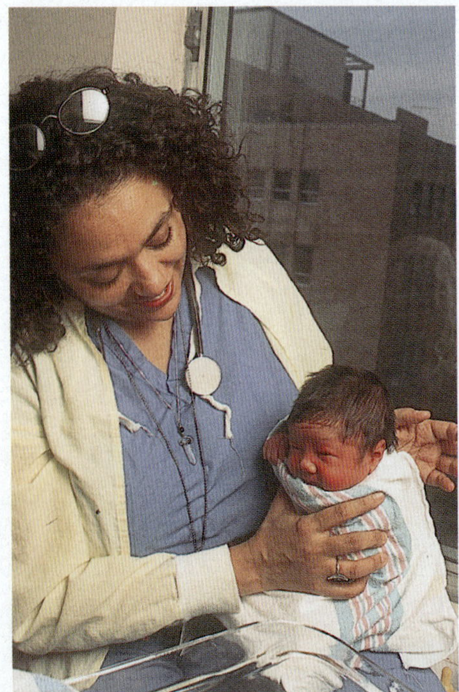

FIGURE 19.5 A midwife burps a newborn using a sitting position. The infant's head is supported by the nurse's hand.

after birth is important for a number of reasons: it allows unrestricted access to the breast and facilitates baby-led attachment, and is beneficial for the physiological stability of the newborn. Babies placed skin-to-skin with their mothers are better able to regulate their temperature, blood sugar levels, heart rate and breathing. Baby-led attachment generally results in better attachment, fewer problems and increases maternal confidence. Not every woman will desire to be skin-to-skin with her baby however, so it is important to determine the mother's preference.

Physical preparation such as nipple rolling, advised in the past as a way of making a woman's nipples more protuberant, is not necessary because most nipple issues will resolve during the pregnancy and/or during breastfeeding, when the baby is well attached to the breast. It is important that infants open their mouths wide enough to grasp both the nipple and the **areola** (the pigmented circle surrounding the nipple) when sucking. This facilitates effective sucking action and helps to empty the breast completely. As important as making certain that infants grasp the breast areola, is helping them to break away from the breast when they have finished feeding or if they need to reattach to improve latch. If a woman needs to remove her baby from the breast, teach her to insert a finger in the corner of the infant's mouth or pull down the infant's chin to release suction. Otherwise, the baby may pull too hard on the nipple, causing cracking or soreness. Most babies, however, will relax their jaw and come off the breast spontaneously when they have finished feeding.

A woman should always place her infant first at the breast at which the infant fed last in the previous feeding, to help ensure that each breast is completely emptied at every other feeding. Milk forms in response to being used. If breasts are completely emptied, they completely fill again. If half emptied, they only half fill, and, after a time, milk production will be insufficient for proper nourishment (see Box 19.4).

Assessing adequate infant intake

Some breastfeeding mothers wonder whether their infant is getting enough to eat. They watch a woman formula feed and listen to her report, "He took 60 millilitres this feed", and wish they could tell as surely whether their infant's intake is adequate. Assure them that the ultimate test with either breastfeeding or formula feeding is not how much an infant swallows at one time but whether the infant seems content between feedings. Acceptable criteria by the end of the first week of life are wetting 6–8 nappies within 24 hours; bowel actions changing from meconium, in the first 2–3 days, to mustard-yellow in the second week; and losing no more than 10% of birth weight. After the first week, growth, voiding 6–8 times and at least one good-sized bowel motion each 24 hours are good criteria. Once breastfeeding is properly established breastfed babies can go 5–6 days without a bowel action, which is acceptable so long as the baby is otherwise settled and well.

Although the formula-feeding mother measures the amount of formula as a way of determining adequate feeding in the early weeks, soon she too, begins to use the alternative criteria: her baby is happy, voids an adequate number of times and is gaining weight. Helping a woman use these criteria allows her to develop confidence in her judgement to evaluate her child's health, a role that will be hers for the next 18 or more years.

Medications, alcohol and breastfeeding

For years it was believed that a placental barrier protected a fetus from exposure to medication taken by a woman during pregnancy; a similar protection was postulated for breast milk. However, it is clear a fetus is extremely susceptible to medication ingested by a woman and the same is true of breastfed infants. Almost any medicine may cross into the acinar cells and be secreted in breast milk. The rule during pregnancy, that a woman should take no medication unless prescribed or approved by her primary care provider continues to apply during breastfeeding. There are few medications that are contraindicated during breastfeeding however professional advice should always be sought.

Alcohol also will pass into a mother's breast milk and will pass out again as it does in her bloodstream when metabolised in her liver. Women may be advised that drinking small amounts of alcohol while breastfeeding poses little or no risk of harm to their infants. The amount and type of alcohol must be considered in relation to when the baby breastfeeds, however. One serving of alcohol may pass into breast milk within 30 to 60 minutes, and may be eliminated from the mother's body within 3 hours of consumption, therefore feeding outside this time frame will pose little risk of transfer of alcohol to her infant. If the baby requires a feed within this time period previously expressed breast milk may be given. The safest option is to advise against drinking alcohol when breastfeeding even though this may be imposing further restrictions on breastfeeding women (ABA, 2014; La Leche League International, 2014).

Potential breastfeeding concerns and strategies to address them

Common concerns that can arise with breastfeeding once a mother returns home are summarised in Table 19.2. Women who do not remember to begin feeding the baby at the breast the infant finished on the last time, may find their milk supply decreasing in one breast. Although changing breasts may be easy to remember in the hospital, distractions at home can make the sequence difficult to remember. Pinning a safety pin to the bra strap on the side to start with at the next feeding is a useful way to help remember this.

BOX 19.4 Nursing procedure ✻ Manual breast milk expression

Purpose: To assist the woman to manually express milk so she can increase her milk supply and supply milk for her newborn should they be separated.

Procedure	Principle
1. Explain the procedure to the woman.	**1.** Explanations help decrease anxiety and enhance learning; they also provide information for the client to carry out the procedure on her own.
2. Assemble equipment, including a clean towel and collection container.	**2.** Assembling equipment aids in organisation and efficiency.
3. Wash your hands and put on clean gloves; have the woman wash her hands.	**3.** Handwashing prevents the transmission of infection; use of gloves protects self and mother from possible infection.
4. Provide privacy and place the woman in a comfortable sitting position.	**4.** The let-down reflex may not occur readily if the woman is tense or nervous.
5. Instruct the woman to place her right hand on her right breast, with her right thumb on the top of the breast at the outer limit of the areola and her right fingers underneath the breast. Tell the woman to press inwards towards the chest wall.	**5.** Milk is expressed by pressure on the breast, not the nipple.
6. Help the woman hold the collecting jar just under her nipple.	**6.** Collecting bottles should be made of plastic to preserve antibodies found in milk; having the container close by prevents waste of any breast milk that is expressed.
7. Have the woman move her thumb and fingers around her breast, repeating the technique.	**7.** Repeating the technique ensures that all breast lobes are emptied.
8. Caution the woman not to use excess force.	**8.** Excess force will damage sensitive breast tissue.
9. After collection, refrigerate milk if it will be used within 24 hours; freeze if this time is longer.	**9.** Breast milk should be stored appropriately
10. Reinforce the woman's success with this manoeuvre, regardless of the amount of breast milk expressed.	**10.** Manual breast milk expression is an easy technique to carry out once it is learned, but it can be difficult to grasp at first. Positive reinforcement enhances progress and self-esteem.

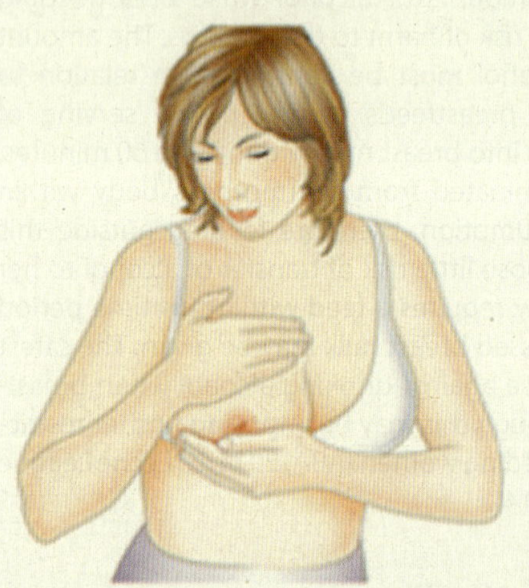

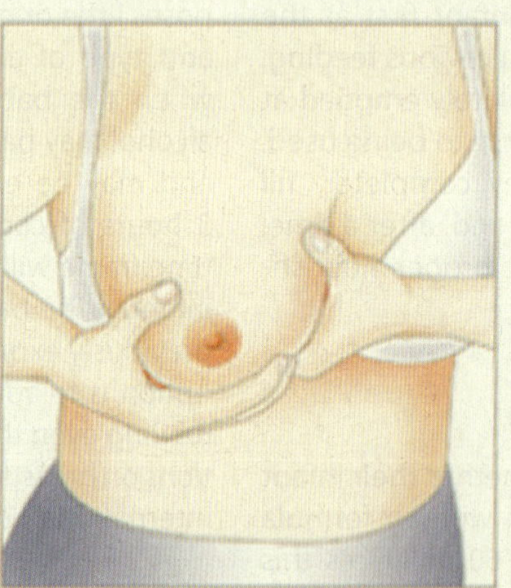

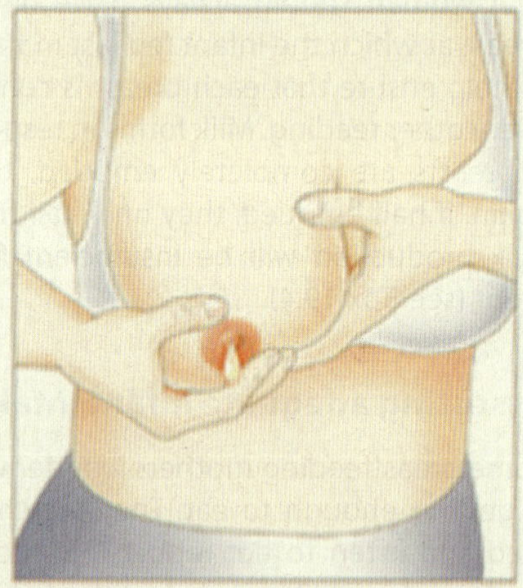

Source: www.nhs.uk/Conditions/pregnancy-and-baby/pages/expressing-storing-breast-milk.aspx#close.

Fatigue can be another issue on returning home if a woman does not take adequate measures to conserve her energy. Sitting relaxed in a comfortable chair with her feet elevated, feeding her baby or side-lying on her bed and enjoying this time is an excellent way to rest.

Remind women that adequate maternal fluid intake is necessary to maintain an adequate milk supply. Women who are breastfeeding should drink at least four 250-mL glasses of fluid a day and many need to drink six glasses. They need to increase their kilojoule intake by about 2000 kJ a day. For a daily diet plan for woman who is breastfeeding see Table 19.3.

At one time, women were given a list of foods not to eat while they were breastfeeding because it was thought they caused diarrhoea, constipation or colic in infants. Today, there are no rules other than to use common sense.

TABLE 19.2 Common concerns of breastfeeding mothers

Concern	Cause	Nursing interventions
Mother worries about amount of milk being taken	Mother cannot see the amount taken	Assure mother that the best way to judge amount taken is to note whether infant appears content between feedings and is wetting nappies.
Infant does not suck well	Possible effect of analgesia from labour Infant brought to mother when not hungry Infant exhausted by crying from hunger	Adjust feeding pattern to infant's needs; assure mother that effect of analgesia is temporary. Encourage rooming-in. Encourage feeding on demand.
Mother reports infant's stools are loose and thin	Stools normally looser and lighter in colour than in formula-fed babies	Examine stools; explain normal stool pattern and transitions.
Father feels shut out of parent–child relationship	Father does not participate in infant feeding	Show other ways of interacting with infant than through feeding.
Sore nipples	Infant not gripping entire areola Nipple kept wet	Help infant to grasp nipple correctly; expose nipple to air between feedings; hospital grade lanolin applied to nipples helps heal tissue. Avoid using anything on nipples that needs to be removed prior to the next breastfeed.
Engorgement	Lymphatic filling as milk production begins	Encourage infant to suck (engorgement subsides best if infant can be encouraged to suck); apply warm packs to breasts or have mother take a warm shower before feeding to help soften breast tissue. Apply cold packs to the breast after feeds.
Breastfeeding in public	Some people make a woman feel uncomfortable breastfeeding at work or other public places	Encourage a woman to use discretion to avoid confrontation (unless she wants to make a point that breastfeeding is a natural action) and to speak to work site administrator about comfortable arrangements.

A woman can eat anything that agrees with her, that is taken in moderation and to which she is not allergic.

Some women stop breastfeeding because they have no-one to talk to about a problem or to give them support. A midwife or nurse working as a hospital community liaison person, child and family health nurse or lactation consultant can be a valuable resource to provide answers and support while a woman is at home.

Provide information on expressed breast milk feedings

A breastfeeding woman may leave her child during the day or evening in the care of a babysitter or another care provider, just as a formula-feeding woman may. She can express breast milk manually and leave it in a bottle in the refrigerator. Bottles used for storage should be washed using normal dishwashing practice. Breast milk that has been freshly expressed may be stored in the following manner:

- 6–8 hours at room temperature
- Up to 72 hours in the body of the refrigerator (not the door) at 4°C or below
- Up to 3 months in the freezer section of a refrigerator
- Up to 12 months in a deep freeze at -18°C or lower.

The bottle used should be glass or opaque, non-shiny plastic, as shiny types may contain polycarbonate, a compound that can leech into stored milk and is associated with chromosomal aberrations (Raloff, 2007).

TABLE 19.3 Daily quantities of food necessary for a woman during breastfeeding

Food group	Quantities for active non-pregnant woman	Quantities for breastfeeding woman
Meat, poultry or fish	2 servings daily	2–3 servings daily
Vegetables	3–5 servings daily	4 servings daily
Fruits	2–4 servings daily	4 servings daily
Breads, cereals, rice, pasta	6–11 servings daily	6–12 servings daily
Milk	2 glasses (250 mL) daily	4–6 glasses (250 mL) daily
Fats, oils, sweets	Use sparingly	1 serving daily
Additional fluid	As desired	4–6 glasses daily

Once breastfeeding has been established (after about 6 weeks), missing one feed will not affect milk production enough to make a difference at the next feeding. There is no need for a mother to express milk manually to safeguard a supply, although she may prefer to do so to reduce tension and discomfort.

Provide information for a mother who works outside the home

Many women return to work while continuing to breastfeed by bringing their infant with them to their workplace. Others express breast milk for a carer to give by bottle while they work. As there are many considerations to think about, women should review with an employer the best way for them to continue breastfeeding at their worksite (Abdulwadud & Snow, 2009) (see Box 19.5).

Provide information on weaning

It is best for infants if they are exclusively breastfed for at least 6 months (Kramer & Kakuma, 2009). Women breastfeed for varying lengths of time, however; some do it for 1, 2 or 3 months and then wean their children from breast to formula. Others continue until their children are 6 to 12 months of age and then wean directly to a small cup or glass. Some continue to breastfeed until the child is of toddler age. The World Health Organization (2002) recommends exclusive breastfeeding for 6 months and continuation for 2 years or more. Discontinuing breastfeeding may make infants more susceptible to infection as infants are no longer receiving immune protection (Akus & Bartick, 2007) which continues for as long as the child is being breastfed.

At any age, breastfeeding should be discontinued gradually to prevent engorgement and pain in a mother's breasts while still providing satisfaction for the infant. To do this, a woman could first omit one breastfeed a day, substituting a formula feeding or milk from a glass or cup. Then she could omit two breastfeeds, then three and so on, until her infant is feeding entirely from a bottle, glass or cup. If breasts are not emptied by regular feedings, the resulting pressure leads to milk suppression and natural, gradual discontinuance of milk secretion. If weaned before 12 months, infants should be weaned to formula, not cow's milk, so that they continue to receive the added vitamins and the low solute load of commercial formulas.

Potential problems

Breast engorgement and sore nipples

On the third or fourth day after birth, when breast milk forms, some women may notice breast distension, accompanied by hardness, tenderness and perhaps heat in their breasts. The skin appears red, tense and shiny. This is primary **engorgement**, caused by vascular and lymphatic congestion arising from an increase in the blood and lymph supply to the breasts. Infants have difficulty attaching to engorged breasts, because the areola is too hard to grasp (see Fig. 19.6). A woman also may have difficulty breastfeeding her infant, because her breasts feel so tender.

BOX 19.5 * Focus on family teaching

Suggestions for returning to work while breastfeeding

Q. Linda Smith tells you, "I'm going to be returning to work in 6 weeks. How can I continue to breastfeed my baby?"

A. Here are some suggestions for returning to work while breastfeeding:

- Some women are able to arrange for childcare near or at their worksite so they can breastfeed at lunch or during a morning or afternoon break. Discuss with your employer or your immediate work supervisor whether this would be a possibility for you.
- Breastfeeding can be done in a public place, such as a lounge area, without undue exposure if you wear a smock-type or buttoned blouse that you lift or unfasten only as far as necessary; covering any bared breast with a shawl or towel ensures modesty.
- If you are not able to breastfeed during work hours, you will need to express milk manually at least once during the day to maintain a milk supply. You might want to rent an electric pump to keep at work. Expressed breast milk can be safely stored in the refrigerator or in an iced container for 24 to 48 hours and used by your carer to feed the infant the next day.
- Any reminder of a baby may cause leaking of milk from breasts. Wear breast pads inside your bra to prevent stains on your clothing, and keep an extra change of clothing at work. Pressing against your breasts with the heel of your hands may be helpful in halting leakage.
- Drink four to six 250-mL glasses of fluid during the day to ensure a high fluid intake.
- Try to arrive early at your day-care centre or carer so you can breastfeed just before leaving the baby.
- Fatigue can interfere with breastfeeding. Relax and enjoy your baby during the time you are home.

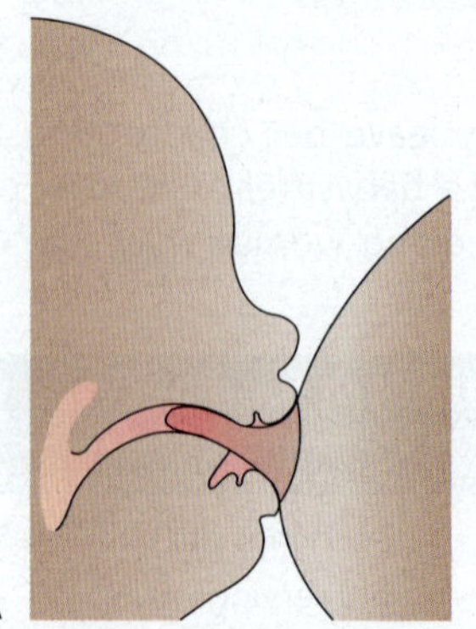

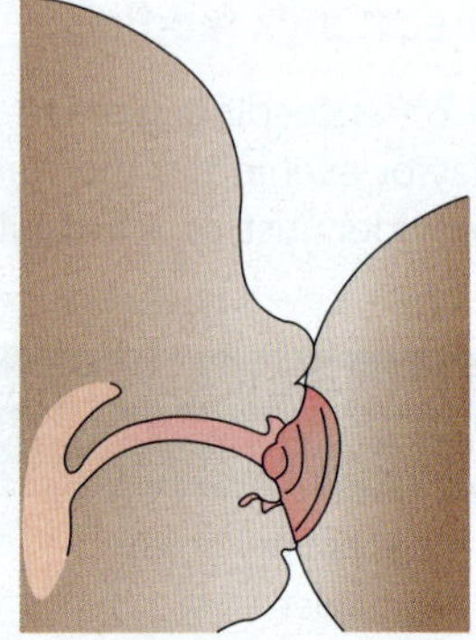

FIGURE 19.6 The problem that breast engorgement causes to breastfeeding. (**A**) When sucking at a normal breast, the infant's lips compress the areola and fit neatly against the sides of the nipple. The infant also has adequate room to breathe. (**B**) When a breast is engorged, the infant has difficulty grasping the nipple. Breathing ability is compromised.

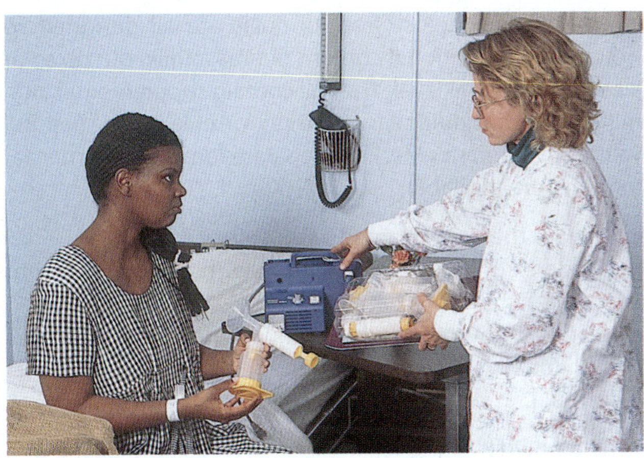

FIGURE 19.7 A midwife and mother discuss the advantages and disadvantages of an electric breast pump (shown on the table) and a manual pump (shown in the mother's hands).

The primary method for relieving engorgement is emptying the breasts of milk by having the infant suck more often, or at least continue to suck as much as before. Unfortunately, a woman's breasts are sometimes so painful that it is difficult for her to continue to breastfeed unless she is given something for pain relief. Good breast support from a firm-fitting bra helps prevent a pulling, heavy feeling. Early, effective, frequent breastfeeding will reduce the severity of primary engorgement for most women.

If an infant cannot grasp a nipple to suck strongly because of engorgement, warm packs applied to both breasts or standing under a warm shower for a few minutes before feeding, combined with massage to begin milk flow, often promotes breast softness so an infant can attach. Manual expression or the use of a breast pump to empty the breasts as much as possible after the baby has fed can help maintain or promote a good milk supply during a period of engorgement (see Fig. 19.7). Full breasts will inhibit further milk production.

Some level of nipple tenderness or sensitivity in the first few weeks is normal; however, painful nipples result from poor attachment of a newborn at the breasts. This may be worsened by:

- Improper positioning of an infant (failure to grasp the areola as well as the nipple)
- Forcefully pulling an infant from a breast
- Permitting a nipple to remain wet from leaking milk.

Normally, nipples are kept supple from the secretions of the Montgomery tubercles in the areola. They can become sore when they are excessively dry or wet, which makes them crack or fissure. To help prevent soreness, encourage a mother to position her baby slightly differently for each feeding. This helps prevent the same area of the nipple from receiving the majority of pressure. Discourage the use of plastic liners that come with nursing bras; change breast pads if wet; and encourage the mother to air dry her nipples before replacing her bra. Applying a few drops of breast milk to the nipples after feeding and gently massaging it into the areola is also recommended.

Women should be taught to hand express until their milk comes in. Advise women with sore nipples not to use a hand pump, because the pressure may cause fissures to worsen. An electric or battery-operated pump (standard equipment in most maternity or paediatric hospitals) usually can be used once the milk comes in; these devices exert less pressure on the nipples.

Sore nipples, like engorgement, are not a contraindication to breastfeeding. If steps to prevent sore nipples are followed, the problem is unlikely to become acute again.

Prolonged jaundice in breastfed infants

Jaundice occurs in as many as 15% of breastfed infants. This is because pregnanediol (a breakdown product of progesterone) in breast milk depresses the action of glucuronyl transferase, the enzyme that converts indirect bilirubin to the direct form, which is then readily excreted in bile (Huether & McCance, 2013). To prevent hyperbilirubinaemia in their infant, women should feed frequently in the immediate birth period, because colostrum is a natural laxative and helps promote the passage of meconium and bile. Newborns who are discharged early need to be observed for jaundice while at home. However, breastfeeding rarely results in a serum bilirubin level high enough to warrant therapy or to require discontinuation of breastfeeding, because pregnanediol remains in breast milk for only 24 to 48 hours (Thilo & Rosenberg, 2008).

CASE STUDY QUESTION

3. How does breast milk help prevent infection in a newborn?
   a. It is rich in fatty acid, so bacteria are destroyed by it
   b. It is always flowing forwards in the breast, so it is not static
   c. It contains maternal antibodies and viral binding factors
   d. It is low in lactose, so it becomes a poor culture medium

ARTIFICIAL FEEDING

There is little opposition to the concept that breastfeeding is the best method for feeding human infants unless it is contraindicated. Formulas that provide the basic nutritional elements are available for infants who will be formula-fed and formula feeding still allows women to establish a close bond with their infant. Support a woman's informed choice by helping her adjust to formula feeding (Gomella & Haist, 2007; see Box 19.6).

BOX 19.6 ✻ Focus on communication

Carolyn Morgan, Linda's roommate in the hospital, is a new mother who has chosen to formula feed her newborn. You notice on the second day after birth that she is studying her baby closely.

Less effective communication

Midwife: Is everything all right? You look worried.
Carolyn: I feel guilty I'm not breastfeeding.
Midwife: Breastfeeding would be better for your baby.
Carolyn: I can't. I'm going back to work next week.
Midwife: You really should breastfeed. It's so much better for the baby.
Carolyn: I guess I'm not going to be a very good mother.

More effective communication

Midwife: Is everything all right? You look worried.
Carolyn: I feel guilty I'm not breastfeeding.
Midwife: What made you decide not to do that?
Carolyn: I work as an electrician at a construction site. I can't breastfeed on a scaffold a hundred metres in the air in freezing weather.
Midwife: Your work situation definitely sounds like an exception to the rule. Infant formula may be the best option for you.
Carolyn: I'm trying to be a good mother. Thanks for the support.

Imposing your opinions on someone is not therapeutic. Allowing a woman to explain her individual situation permits a midwife to understand the woman's decision and support her in it.

Preparing for formula feeding

Carers should use only commercial infant formulas for formula feeding. Occasionally, an infant is allergic to the protein in infant formulas. This can lead to such severe intestinal inflammation, diarrhoea and vomiting that the infant becomes anaemic and dehydrated from loss of blood and inability to absorb nutrients. In these instances, the infant needs to be reviewed by a medical practitioner.

Commercial formulas

The contents of commercial formulas are regulated by the Australian New Zealand Food Standards Code. Formulas are available in three types: milk based, soy based and elemental (fat, protein and carbohydrate content is modified, such as in lactose-free formula). Milk-based formulas are used for the average newborn; lactose-free formulas are used for infants with lactose intolerance or galactosaemia (inability to use sugar). Soy formulas were devised for infants who are allergic to cow's milk protein. Today, such infants may be given casein hydrolysate formulas, which have protein particles too small to be recognised by the immune system, rather than soy formulas. Elemental formulas are used for infants with protein allergies or fat malnutrition. Milk-based, soy-based and lactose-free formulas are all designed to simulate the nutritional content of breast milk, but do so at a basic nutritional level. They all contain supplemental vitamins. Parents should plan on using formula for the first full year of their infant's life. Four separate forms of commercial formulas are available:

- Powder that is combined with water
- Condensed liquid that is diluted with an equal amount of water
- Ready-to-pour type, which requires no dilution
- Individually pre-packaged and prepared bottles of formula.

The powder is the least expensive. A single bottle at a time is easy to prepare by vigorous shaking. The pre-packaged type does not need refrigeration or preparation but is the most expensive. Cost should not be the only basis for a parent's choice, however; tolerance of the formula by the infant and convenience for the parents are also important.

Calculating a formula's adequacy

To calculate the adequacy of a formula, remember these two rules of thumb:

1. The total fluid ingested in a 24-hour period must be sufficient to meet the infant's fluid needs: 150 to 200 mL/kg per day.
2. The number of kilojoules required per day is 460 to 500 kJ/kg.

If an infant is taking a commercial formula, only total fluid needs to be calculated. For example, a baby weighing 3 kg requires 450–600 mL of fluid per day (3×150–200 mL). The total volume can be divided into six feeds of 75–100 mL each. A 3.5 kg infant would need 525–700 mL of fluid per day, divided into six feeds of approximately 90–120 mL each.

As infants change from six to five feeds a day (at about 4 months of age, when they may begin to sleep through the night), they begin to take more at each feeding, keeping their total intake the same. Knowing the minimum requirements for fluid and kilojoules per day, being able to calculate whether formula is adequate and remembering to assess an infant's intake over 24 hours, allow evaluation of the adequacy of an infant's intake.

Preparing formula

Most parents today do not prepare a full day's supply of formula at once but prepare it bottle by bottle, as needed. Caution parents to keep opened cans of liquid formula covered and refrigerated, discarding any unused formula within 24 hours. They should use glass or non-shiny plastic bottles as these do not contain polycarbonate, a chemical that is capable of leeching into stored milk and possibly causing chromosomal aberrations (Raloff, 2007).

Teats for bottles should be firm enough so an infant sucks vigorously. A soft, flabby teat allows a baby to suck in milk so rapidly that the need for sucking may not be satisfied. A way to judge a teat's adequacy is to hold a bottle of milk with teat attached upside down. The milk should drip from it at a rate of about one drop a second. Bottle caps to cover teats are helpful to keep teats clean when outdoors or during transport.

Infant formula of any type must be prepared with careful attention to cleanliness to prevent pathogenic microorganisms from growing in it. Accuracy when measuring powder or water is also important to prevent under or over concentration: parents must be advised to adhere to the instructions on the formula container, including using the correct measuring scoop provided in each tin of powder. Health professionals must demonstrate and monitor the correct method of formula preparation by parents.

Principles of preparing formula

- All equipment and preparation surfaces must be thoroughly clean: wash bottles and teats in hot soapy water, rinse well.
- Sterilise by boiling for 5 minutes in water or using a steam or microwave steriliser (follow the manufacturer's instructions).
- Boil fresh water and allow to cool to just warm.
- Wash hands with soap and running water; clean preparation surface.
- Following instructions on the formula tin add the required amount of cooled boiled water to a bottle followed by the appropriate number of scoops of formula powder. The full scoop should be tapped on the side to expel pockets of air and levelled across the top using a clean flat blade.
- Put the teat and lid on the bottle, tap gently to loosen powder then shake to thoroughly mix the formula and water.
- Refrigerate until required if not for immediate use. Discard all prepared formula 24 hours after being made up.
- To heat a bottle of prepared formula stand in a jug of warm water until heated through to the required temperature. Do not use a microwave as heating occurs unevenly and increases the risk of burns to the infant.

Feeding techniques

Whether to warm formula or not is a parental decision: infants who are fed cooled formula directly from the refrigerator thrive as well as those who are fed warmed formula. The best method to warm formula is to stand the bottle in a bowl of warm water or hold it under a tap of running hot water for a few minutes. Caution parents not to use a pan on the stove to warm formula because if the pan boils dry, the bottle of milk will burst. Disposable bottles with plastic liners should definitely not be heated on the stove; the liner tends to melt and then leak during feeding.

It also is not recommended to warm bottles in a microwave oven, because the milk in the centre of the bottle can become hotter than that near the sides. If parents do not follow this recommendation, caution them to heat no longer than 30 seconds for a 160-mL bottle and 45 seconds for a 260-mL bottle (Goldenring, 2007). After warming, they should add the teat and shake the bottle well to mix the cool and warm portions. Finally, with all warming methods parents should test the temperature of the formula by allowing a drop or two to fall onto the inside of a wrist, to make sure it is not hot enough to burn the baby's mouth.

With any type of bottle, any contents remaining after a feed should be thrown away, not stored and reused. When sucking, an infant exchanges a small amount of saliva for milk. Because formula is a good growth medium for bacteria and the baby's mouth harbours many bacteria, the bacterial content in reused formula is likely to be high. Feeding the baby such contaminated milk may cause a catastrophic infection.

Like breastfeeding, formula feeding an infant is a skill that must be learned. A parent needs a comfortable chair (as does a nurse or midwife who feeds babies) and adequate time (at least half an hour) to enjoy the process and not rush the baby (see Fig. 19.8). The baby should be held close in to the parent's body with his or her head slightly elevated, which reduces the danger of aspiration and retention of air bubbles. A parent should be sure the teat is kept filled so that the baby is sucking milk, not air. He or she can be assured a baby is sucking effectively if small bubbles rise in the bottle. Babies in the early weeks should be burped after every 30 mL of milk taken. The technique for burping is the same as that used for breastfed infants.

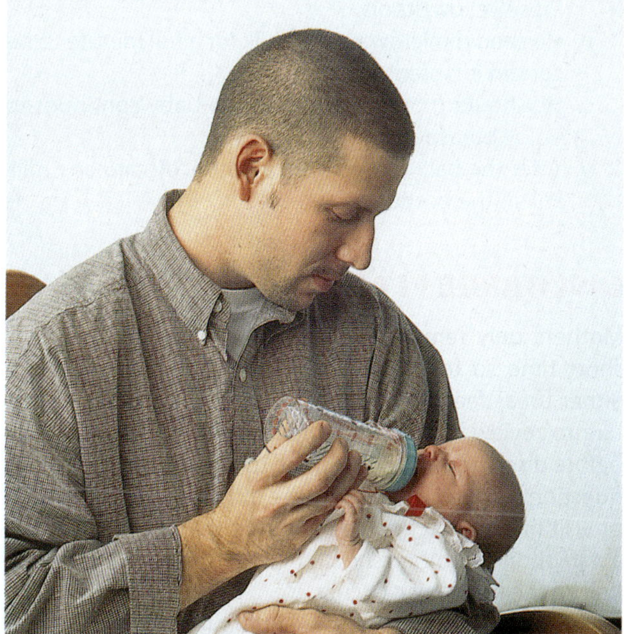

FIGURE 19.8 A newborn receives a bottle feeding from her father. Notice the *en face* position: the father and baby are both looking directly at each other.

TABLE 19.4 Common concerns of formula-feeding parents

Concern	Possible causes	Nursing interventions
Infant sucks for a few minutes, then stops and cries	Either teat is blocked and infant is unable to get milk or flow is too fast and baby has choking sensation.	Show parent how to test flow of milk from the teat (hold bottle upside down); milk should flow from teat at rate of about 1 drop/sec.
Infant does not burp well after feeding	Some infants swallow little air with feeding. Parent may be handling infant too tentatively or not burping effectively.	Observe baby feeding and parent's technique of handling; rubbing newborn's back may be more effective than patting it.
Parent reports constipation	Bowel movements from formula-fed infants are not as loose as those from breastfed infants, so parents may be concerned.	Examine stools; assure parent and explain normal stool pattern and that straining to pass stool is normal.

Remind parents not to prop up bottles, because babies are in danger of aspiration if a bottle is propped. In addition, an increased incidence of otitis media has been associated with bottle-propping, because the infant's head is not upright and formula may enter the eustachian tube. Propping can also limit the amount of parent–child interaction. Also remind parents not to put a baby to bed with a bottle of formula, because this can lead to "baby-bottle syndrome" or cavities of the lower teeth (see Chapter 29). Some common problems that can arise with formula feeding are summarised in Table 19.4.

CASE STUDY QUESTION

4. Linda's husband will offer their baby bottled breast milk once a day when Linda returns to work. Which of the following would you teach him?
   a. He should stop feeding bottled milk if the baby has loose yellow stools
   b. He should microwave the milk for a full minute to be certain it is sterile
   c. He should prop the bottle so the baby continues to enjoy breastfeeding
   d. After the baby drinks from a bottle, discard any milk still in the bottle

DISCHARGE PLANNING

Mothers only remain in a hospital or birthing centre a short time so teaching a mother and her family about either breastfeeding or formula feeding is crucial. Be certain to review a mother's plans for feeding her baby just before discharge, so there is time to answer any remaining questions. If needed, check to see that a home care referral or visit has been scheduled and that the new mother has a telephone number she can call if she has a question before the home visit occurs.

Review with a mother the criteria for adequate nutrition (6–8 heavy wet nappies a day, sleeping between feedings, no excessive crying). Supply the telephone number of the local breastfeeding association, lactation consultants and other local support groups in her area.

Ensure a woman has an appointment with a primary care provider for her infant or the telephone number of this person to call for an appointment. Remind her that infant nutrition is an important topic and one she should always feel free to discuss at healthcare visits. Babies experience growth spurts during the first year at about 3 months, 6 months and 9 months; during these times, they need to be fed more frequently to meet their nutritional needs.

No-one can anticipate all of the questions or problems regarding feeding that will arise in the next few months. Empowering women to learn to make decisions regarding feeding and not be reluctant to ask for help when they need it will go a long way towards solving these problems.

Key points for review

- Breastfeeding is the preferred feeding method for newborns, because it supplies antibodies as well as nutrients. Urge all women at least to try breastfeeding unless they are taking a medication that would be a contraindication, or there is a potential for spreading a microorganism through the breast milk.
- Linoleic acid is an essential fatty acid that is necessary for growth and skin integrity and cannot be manufactured by the body. It is supplied by both breast milk and infant formula but not by non-fat milk.
- Both breast milk and commercial formulas contain similar energy. A term newborn requires 500 kJ/kg per day and 150 to 200 mL of fluid per kilogram of body weight.
- Encourage mothers who are breastfeeding to drink fluoridated water and formula-feeding mothers to prepare formula using fluoridated water to help build strong teeth in the infant. If a newborn will not have exposure to sunlight, the breastfeeding mother may need to take a supplement of vitamin D; formula-fed infants may need supplemental oral vitamin D.

- Almost all medication passes into breast milk. A breast-feeding mother must be certain not to take any medication without contacting her primary care provider to be certain it is compatible with breastfeeding.
- If a baby will be formula-fed, be certain the parents understand the potential danger of warming bottles in a microwave oven (the inner core of milk may grow very hot).
- Caution parents not to prop bottles, because it increases the risk for aspiration and otitis media. It also deprives infants of the pleasure of being held for feedings.
- To avoid baby-bottle syndrome (cavities of the lower teeth), infants should not be put to bed with a bottle.

CASE STUDY QUESTIONS

5. Linda is unsure whether she wants to breastfeed, especially because she does not know how she will manage breastfeeding when she returns to work. How would you advise her?
6. Linda worries that her 1-day-old newborn is not receiving enough milk. How could you assure her that her baby is receiving enough?
7. Linda's grandmother tells you that she always changed her babies to fat-free milk at 3 months to keep them from gaining too much weight. Would you support this practice?

Resources

For an extensive range of additional resources to enhance teaching and learning and to facilitate understanding of this chapter, please see the text's accompanying website located on thePoint at http://thepoint.lww.com.

References

Abdulwadud, O. A. & Snow, M. E. (2009). Interventions in the workplace to support breastfeeding for women in employment. *Cochrane Database of Systematic Reviews, 2009*(1), (CD006177).

Akus, M. & Bartick, M. (2007). Lactation safety recommendations and reliability compared in 10 medication resources. *Annals of Pharmacotherapy, 41*(9), 1352–1360.

American College of Obstetricians & Gynecologists (ACOG). (2007). Special report from ACOG. Breastfeeding: Maternal and infant aspects. *ACOG Clinical Review, 12*(1), 1S–16S.

Ateah, C. A. & Hamelin, K. J. (2008). Maternal bedsharing practices, experiences, and awareness of risks. *JOGNN: Journal of Obstetric, Gynecologic, and Neonatal Nursing, 37*(3), 274–281.

Australian Breastfeeding Association (2014). Alcohol and breastfeeding. Accessed 10 February 2015, <www.breastfeeding.asn.au/bf-info/safe-when-breastfeeding/alcohol-and-breastfeeding>.

Australian Bureau of Statistics (ABS). (2013). Australian health survey: Health service usage and health related actions, 2011-12. Accessed 10 February 2015, <www.abs.gov.au/ausstats/abs@.nsf/Lookup/6664B939E49FD9C1CA257B39000F2E4B?opendocument>.

Britton, C., et al. (2009). Support for breastfeeding mothers. *Cochrane Database of Systematic Reviews, 2009*(1), (CD001141).

Forster, D. A. & McLachlan, H. L. (2007). Breastfeeding initiation and birth setting practices: A review of the literature. *Journal of Midwifery and Women's Health, 52*(3), 273–280.

Furber, C. M. & Thomson, A. M. (2007). Midwives in the UK: An exploratory study of providing newborn feeding support for postpartum mothers in the hospital. *Journal of Midwifery & Women's Health, 52*(2), 142–147.

Goldenring, J. M. (2007). What to tell parents before they leave the hospital. *Contemporary Pediatrics, 24*(4), 74–79.

Gomella, L. G. & Haist, S. A. (2007). *Clinician's Pocket Reference* (11th ed.). Columbus, OH: McGraw-Hill.

Hampton, T. (2008). Report assesses effects of early nutrition options on atopic diseases. *Journal of the American Medical Association, 299*(6), 621.

Howe, T., et al. (2008). A review of psychometric properties of feeding assessment tools used in neonates. *JOGNN: Journal of Obstetric, Gynecologic, and Neonatal Nursing, 37*(3), 338–349.

Huether, S. E. & McCance, K. L. (2013). *Understanding Pathophysiology.* (6th ed.). New York: Elsevier.

Jensen, D., Wallace, S. & Kelsey, P. (1994). LATCH: A breastfeeding charting system and documentation tool. *Journal of Obstetric, Gynecologic, and Neonatal Nursing, 23*(1), 27–32.

Kramer, M. S. & Kakuma, R. (2009). Optimal duration of exclusive breast-feeding. *Cochrane Database of Systematic Reviews, 2009*(1), (CD003517).

Krebs, N. F. & Primak, L. E. (2011). Diet of the normal infant. In K. J. Marcdante, R. M. Kliegman, H. B. Jenson, et al. (Eds), *Nelson Essentials of Pediatrics* (6th ed.), pp. 103–107. Philadelphia: Saunders/Elsevier.

La Leche League International (2014). What about drinking alcohol and breastfeeding? Accessed 10 February 2015, <www.llli.org/faq/alcohol.html>.

Li, R., Rock, V. J. & Grummer-Strawn, L. (2007). Changes in public attitudes toward breastfeeding in the United States, 1999–2003. *Journal of the American Dietetic Association, 107*(1), 122–127.

Moore, J. E. (2007). Multiple births: The art and science of caring for twins, triplets, and more. *Pediatrics in Review, 28*(3), e9–e15.

National Health and Medical Research Council. (2012). Infant feeding guidelines. Information for health workers. Accessed 10 February 2015, <www.nhmrc.gov.au/guidelines-publications/n56>.

New Zealand Breast Feeding Association. (2014). Baby Friendly Initiative for Aotearoa New Zealand. Breastfeeding data. Accessed 10 February 2015, <www.babyfriendly.org.nz/going-baby-friendly/breastfeeding-data/>.

New Zealand Ministry of Health. (2008). Food and nutrition guidelines for healthy infants and toddlers (aged 0–2): A background paper - partially revised August 2012, accessed 10 February 2015, <www.health.govt.nz/publication/food-and-nutrition-guidelines-healthy-infants-and-toddlers-aged-0-2-background-paper-partially>.

Raising Children Network. (2006–2012). Newborns nutrition, accessed 10 February 2015, <http://raisingchildren.net.au/nutrition/newborns_nutrition.html>.

Raloff, J. (2007). Bad for baby: New risks found for plastic constituent. *Science News, 7*(11).

Thilo, E. H. & Rosenberg, A. A. (2008). The newborn infant. In W. W. Hay, et al. (Eds). *Current Pediatric Diagnosis and Treatment* (18th ed.). Columbus, OH: McGraw-Hill.

World Health Organization. (2015). Breast feeding. Accessed 10 February 2015, <www.who.int/>.

Suggested readings

Australian Breastfeeding Association <www.breastfeeding.asn.au>.

Australian National Breastfeeding Strategy <www.health.gov.au/internet/main/publishing.nsf/Content/aust-breastfeeding-strategy-2010-2015>.

Baby Friendly Health Initiative Australia <www.babyfriendly.org.au>.

Baby Friendly: New Zealand <www.babyfriendly.org.nz>.

Ingram, J., Johnson, D., Copeland, M., Churchill, C. & Taylor, H. (2015). The development of a new breast feeding assessment tool and the relationship with breast feeding self-efficacy. *Midwifery*, *31*(1), 132–137.

Moore, E. (2010). Mothers bottle feeding their babies feel negative emotions such as guilt and worry, and receive little information about bottle feeding. *Evidence Based Nursing*, *13*(1), 27–28.

National Health Service, United Kingdom: Expressing and storing breastmilk <www.nhs.uk/Conditions/pregnancy-and-baby/pages/expressing-storing-breast-milk.aspx#close>.

New Zealand National Strategic Plan of Action for Breastfeeding 2008–2012 <www.health.govt.nz/publication/national-strategic-plan-action-breastfeeding-2008-2012>.

Unit 4

Caring for a family when pregnancy, birth or the postnatal period becomes complex

Chapter 20

Care of a family experiencing a pregnancy complication from a pre-existing or newly acquired condition

Previous chapters discussed normal pregnancy and the minor discomforts that may occur. This chapter adds information about illnesses and other events that can complicate pregnancy when they occur prior to or during pregnancy.

LEARNING OBJECTIVES

After mastering the contents of this chapter, you should be able to:

1. Define high-risk pregnancy and pre-existing risk factors.
2. Describe the pathophysiology, diagnosis and treatment of pregnancy complications from pre-existing or newly acquired conditions.
3. Use critical thinking to analyse strategies for family-centred care of women with pre-existing or newly acquired conditions during pregnancy.
4. Plan and implement safe evidence-based, collaborative care for a woman with complications.
5. Identify areas related to pre-existing or newly acquired conditions during pregnancy that could benefit from additional research or application of evidence-based practice.

KEY TERMS

- deep vein thrombosis
- glycosuria
- glycosylated haemoglobin
- high-risk pregnancy
- hyperglycaemia
- hypoglycaemia
- megaloblastic anaemia
- orthopnoea
- paroxysmal nocturnal dyspnoea
- peripartum cardiomyopathy
- proteinuria

CASE STUDY

Angelina Little, 22, is pregnant with her first child. She had rheumatic fever with mitral stenosis as a child. She developed gestational diabetes early in her pregnancy. By the 34th week, she has been hospitalised twice for hyperglycaemia. She fainted this afternoon while participating in her weekly hour-long aerobics class. When seen in the emergency department, her serum glucose is 11 mmol/L. Her blood pressure is 90/40 mmHg; her pulse is 130/min; the fetal heart rate is 180/min. An abdominal monitor shows moderate-strength uterine contractions 7 minutes apart. The attending doctor asks for an echocardiogram to see if her mitral stenosis is contributing to her low blood pressure. Angelina says to you, "If exercise is supposed to be good for you, why did this happen?"

CASE STUDY QUESTIONS

1. How would you answer Angelina?
2. Do you think she realises that pregnancy often becomes high-risk not because of any one factor, but an accumulation of them?

When a woman enters pregnancy with a chronic condition such as cardiovascular or kidney disease, both she and the fetus can be at risk of complications because either the pregnancy can complicate the disease or the disease can complicate the pregnancy. Care for a woman with a pre-existing condition focuses on close observation of maternal health and fetal wellbeing, education of the woman and her family about special danger signs to watch for during pregnancy and actions to minimise complications whenever possible.

In addition to pre-existing conditions, a pregnant woman, like any person, may develop a new disorder during pregnancy. This can adversely affect not only the woman but also her unborn child. Caring for the well, pregnant woman focuses on preventing illness by promoting a healthy lifestyle. When accidents and complications occur, despite these safeguards, care focuses on:

- Preventing such disorders from affecting the health of the fetus
- Helping a woman regain her health as quickly as possible so she can continue a healthy pregnancy and prepare herself psychologically and physically for labour and birth
- Facilitating a woman to learn more about her chronic condition so she can continue to safeguard her health.

Conditions that cause severe symptoms such as a marked change in fluid and electrolyte balance, altered cardiovascular or respiratory function, or severe blood loss are especially dangerous to a fetus. Therefore careful assessment and monitoring are essential.

CARE OF A WOMAN WITH A PRE-EXISTING OR NEWLY ACQUIRED ILLNESS

Assessment

Accurate antenatal assessment of a woman with a pre-existing or newly acquired illness requires a thorough understanding of the signs and symptoms of her pre-existing or acquired conditions as well as understanding normal pregnancy. Assessment includes objective measures such as establishing baseline vital signs plus subjective factors, for example, the level of fatigue a woman describes (see Fig. 20.1). Continuity of care during pregnancy enables detection of subtle changes in condition and provides opportunities for health education. This assists women to be aware of any changes they notice and to report them. For example, in relation to daily activity a woman may notice that, "Two weeks ago I could walk a block without being short of breath. Today I could walk only half a block"; "I wasn't noticing my oedema until bedtime. Now I notice it every afternoon, by the time my son comes home from school."

Nursing considerations

It is important to be aware of specific, disease-related conditions as well as any therapeutic restrictions. For example:

- Ineffective tissue perfusion (cardiopulmonary) related to poor heart function secondary to mitral valve prolapse during pregnancy
- Pain related to pyelonephritis secondary to pressure on ureters

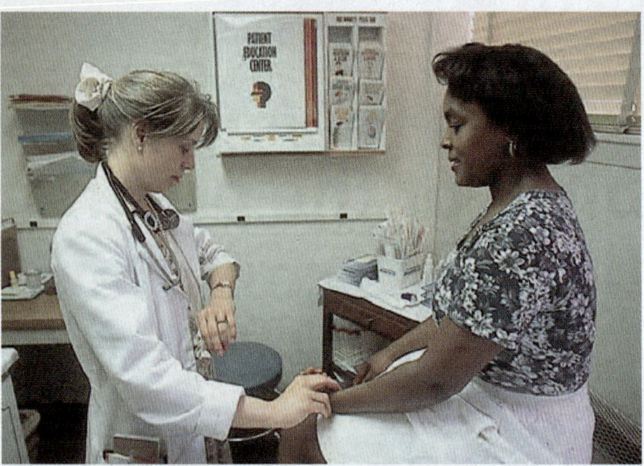

FIGURE 20.1 It is important to establish baseline vital signs to later identify a complication related to a pre-existing condition.

- Social isolation related to prescribed bed rest during pregnancy secondary to concurrent illness
- Ineffective role performance related to increasing level of daily restrictions secondary to chronic illness and pregnancy
- Knowledge deficit related to normal changes of pregnancy versus illness complications
- Fear regarding pregnancy outcome related to chronic conditions
- Health-seeking behaviours related to the effects of illness on pregnancy
- Situational low self-esteem related to illness during pregnancy.

IDENTIFYING A HIGH-RISK PREGNANCY

It is important to understand and protect normal pregnancy and birth, however sometimes pregnancies become high risk (see Table 20.1). This may result from pre-existing conditions superimposed on the pregnancy; complications resulting from pregnancy; new conditions acquired during pregnancy; and external factors. These complications can jeopardise the health of the woman, the fetus, or both. Multiple factors may contribute to making pregnancy high risk including psychological, social and physical factors. These include poverty, lack of social support, poor coping mechanisms, genetic inheritance, adolescence, illicit drugs, pre-existing conditions or past history of pregnancy complications. A great deal of emotional support is required for women who have been identified as having a **high-risk pregnancy**.

CARDIOVASCULAR DISORDERS AND PREGNANCY

Cardiovascular disease complicates 0.5–4% of all pregnancies. Women with heart disease require careful monitoring by a multidisciplinary team during pregnancy and

TABLE 20.1 Factors that categorise a pregnancy as high risk

Psychological	Social	Physical
Prepregnancy		
History of drug dependence (including alcohol) History of intimate partner abuse History of mental illness History of poor coping mechanisms Cognitively challenged Survivor of childhood sexual abuse	Occupation involving handling of toxic substances (including radiation and anaesthesia gases) Environmental contaminants at home Isolated Lower economic level Poor access to transportation for care High altitude Highly mobile lifestyle Poor housing Lack of support people	Visual or hearing challenges Pelvic inadequacy or misshape Uterine incompetency, position or structure Secondary major illness (heart disease, diabetes mellitus, kidney disease, hypertension, chronic infection such as tuberculosis, haemopoietic or blood disorder, malignancy) Poor gynaecological or obstetric history History of previous poor pregnancy outcome (miscarriage, stillbirth, intrauterine fetal death) History of child with congenital anomalies Obesity (BMI >30) Underweight (BMI <18.5) Pelvic inflammatory disease History of inherited disorder Small stature Potential of blood incompatibility Younger than age 18 years or older than 35 years Cigarette smoker Substance abuser
Pregnancy		
Loss of support person Illness of a family member Decrease in self-esteem Drug abuse (including alcohol and cigarette smoking) Poor acceptance of pregnancy	Refusal of or neglected prenatal care Exposure to environmental teratogens Disruptive family incident Decreased economic support Conception less than 1 year after last pregnancy	Subject to trauma Fluid or electrolyte imbalance Intake of teratogen such as a drug Multiple gestation A bleeding disruption Poor placental formation or position Gestational diabetes Nutritional deficiency of iron, folic acid or protein Poor weight gain Pregnancy-induced hypertension Infection Amniotic fluid abnormality Postmaturity
Labour and birth		
Severely frightened by labour and birth experience Inability to participate because of anaesthesia Separation of infant at birth Lack of preparation for labour Birth of infant who is disappointing in some way (such as sex, appearance or congenital anomalies) Illness in newborn	Lack of support person Inadequate home for infant care Unplanned caesarean birth Lack of access to continued healthcare Lack of access to emergency personnel or equipment	Haemorrhage Infection Fluid and electrolyte imbalance Dystocia Precipitous birth Lacerations of cervix or vagina Cephalopelvic disproportion Internal fetal monitoring Retained placenta

the postpartum period. The improved management of women with cardiac disorders has resulted in women who previously may have avoided pregnancy being able to complete pregnancies successfully (Swan, 2014). The number of women with congenital heart defects who become pregnant is increasing due to improvements in medical care. Congenital heart disease is now responsible for 80% of cardiac disease in pregnancy (Lam, 2012). Effective treatment of rheumatic fever has resulted in a dramatic decline in the numbers of women entering pregnancy with rheumatic heart disease in Australia, with the notable exception of Indigenous and Torres Strait Islanders. Mitral valve stenosis is the most common heart disorder complicating pregnancy worldwide and is usually a result of rheumatic fever (Mohan & Nelson-Piercy, 2014). The increasing age of mothers at their first pregnancy has resulted in higher numbers of women with acquired heart disease due to diabetes, hypertension and obesity (Mohan & Nelson-Piercy, 2014). In the report on maternal deaths in Australia in 2006–2010, cardiac conditions were the major cause of indirect maternal death (Johnson et al., 2014).

Septal defects are one of the most common congenital heart diseases. Other disorders include tetralogy of

Fallot, pulmonary stenosis, left ventricular outflow obstruction, aortic valve disease, (most of which is congenital), coarctation of the aorta, transposition of the great arteries, cyanotic cardiac defects, Eisenmenger's physiology and Ebstein's anomaly (Swan, 2014). Marfan's syndrome is hereditary connective tissue disorder which includes cardiac involvement in around 80% of those affected, the most common being valve prolapse. Marfan's syndrome increases the risk of aortic dissection (Curry et al., 2014). As the number of women delaying their first pregnancy until later in life is increasing, there is a corresponding increase in the incidence of coronary artery disease and varicosities during pregnancy. In contrast, heart disease that occurs specifically with pregnancy (peripartum heart disease) occurs rarely and is unrelated to age.

A woman with cardiovascular disease needs an interprofessional team approach to care during pregnancy. Ideally, a woman should visit her pregnancy care provider for preconception care so her state of health and baseline data prior to pregnancy can be evaluated. A woman should begin antenatal care as soon as she suspects she is pregnant (1 week after the first missed menstrual period) so that her general condition and circulatory system can be monitored from the beginning of pregnancy.

During pregnancy both the blood volume and cardiac output increase by 30–50%. Half of this increase occurs by 8 weeks; it is maximised by mid pregnancy (Gilbert, 2011). Because of the increased blood flow past valves, functional (innocent) or transient murmurs can be heard in many women during pregnancy. Heart palpitations on sudden exertion are also common in pregnancy. Neither of these symptoms is a sign of cardiovascular disease, but merely an indication of the normal physiological adjustment to pregnancy. These symptoms disappear after pregnancy.

The danger of pregnancy in a woman with cardiac disease occurs primarily because of the increase in circulatory volume. The most dangerous time for a woman is between weeks 28 to 32, just after the blood volume peaks. However, if heart disease is severe, symptoms can occur as early as the beginning of pregnancy. A woman's heart may become so overwhelmed by the increase in blood volume towards the end of pregnancy that her cardiac output falls to the point that vital organs (including the placenta) are no longer perfused adequately. When this happens, neither the oxygen nor nutritional requirements of her cells nor those of the fetus are met.

The estimation of whether a woman with cardiovascular disease can complete a pregnancy successfully depends on the type and extent of her disease. Women with a mechanical prosthetic heart valve have an increased risk of mortality which is also related to adherence to anticoagulation therapy and the underlying cardiac pathology (Vause & Clarke, 2014). The majority of women with an artificial but well-functioning heart valve, a pacemaker and even a heart transplant can be expected to successfully complete pregnancy if consistent antenatal and postpartum care is provided (Humphreys et al., 2012).

TABLE 20.2 Classification of heart disease

Class	Description
I	Person has cardiac disease but general physical activity does not cause fatigue, palpitations, dyspnoea or angina pain.
II	Person has cardiac disease and is comfortable at rest but general physical activity results in fatigue, palpitations, dyspnoea or angina pain.
III	Person has cardiac disease and is comfortable at rest but less than ordinary physical activity causes fatigue, palpitations, dyspnoea or angina pain.
IV	Person has cardiac disease with symptoms of cardiac insufficiency or angina even at rest. Discomfort increases with physical activity.

Source: Heart Foundation. (2013). *A Systematic Approach to Chronic Heart Failure Care: A Consensus Statement*. Available at <www.heartfoundation.org.au/SiteCollectionDocuments/HF_CHF_consensus_web_FINAL_SP.pdf>.

To predict pregnancy outcome, heart disease is divided into four categories based on criteria established by the New York State Heart Association (see Table 20.2). A woman with class I or II heart disease can expect to experience a normal pregnancy and birth. Women with class III can complete a pregnancy by maintaining almost complete bed rest. Women with class IV heart disease are poor candidates for pregnancy because they are in cardiac failure even at rest and when they are not pregnant. They are usually advised to avoid pregnancy.

A woman with cardiac disease

Cardiac disease affects either the left or right side of the heart. In women with cardiac disease the most common complication is heart failure which occurs in 13% of women and incurs maternal and fetal mortality and morbidity (Ruys et al., 2014). Heart failure occurs more commonly in women with cardiomyopathy or pulmonary hypertension and women with cardiac conditions, who develop preeclampsia, have a 30% risk of heart failure (Ruys et al., 2014). Peak onsets are the end of the second and beginning of the third trimester and at birth.

Left-sided heart failure

Left-sided heart failure occurs in conditions such as mitral stenosis, mitral insufficiency and aortic coarctation. In these instances, the left ventricle cannot move the volume of blood forwards that it has received by the left atrium from the pulmonary circulation. The resulting back pressure distends the left side of the heart, decreases cardiac output and systemic blood pressure resulting in pulmonary hypertension. The normal physiological tachycardia of pregnancy shortens diastole (atrial contraction) and decreases the time available for blood to flow across this valve. The inability of the mitral valve to push blood forwards causes back-pressure on the pulmonary circulation, causing it to become distended; systemic blood pressure decreases in the face of lowered cardiac output and pulmonary hypertension occurs. When pressure in the pulmonary vein reaches a point of about 25 mmHg, fluid begins to pass from the pulmonary capillary membranes into the interstitial spaces surrounding the alveoli and then into the alveoli themselves (pulmonary oedema). Pulmonary oedema produces profound dyspnoea as it interferes with oxygen–carbon dioxide exchange (Brushers, 2012). If pulmonary capillaries rupture under the pressure, small amounts of blood leak into the alveoli and a productive cough of blood-speckled sputum develops. Because of the limited oxygen exchange, women with left-sided heart failure are at extremely high risk of spontaneous miscarriage, preterm labour or maternal death.

As the oxygen saturation of the blood decreases from dysfunction of the alveoli, chemoreceptors stimulate the respiratory centre to increase respiratory rate. At first this is noticeable only on exertion, then finally with rest also. As the systemic fall in blood pressure is registered with the renin-angiotensin system, retention of sodium and water occurs. A woman experiences increased fatigue, weakness and dizziness (specifically from lack of oxygen in brain cells). The placenta may not receive adequate blood because of the decreased peripheral circulation.

As pulmonary oedema becomes severe, a woman cannot sleep in any position except with her chest and head elevated **(orthopnoea)**. Elevating her chest allows fluid to settle to the bottom of her lungs and frees space for gas exchange. She may also notice **paroxysmal nocturnal dyspnoea**—suddenly waking at night short of breath. This occurs because heart action is more effective when she is at rest. With the more effective heart action, interstitial fluid returns to the circulation. This overburdens the circulation, causing increased left-side failure and increased pulmonary oedema.

If mitral stenosis is present, it is difficult for blood to leave the left atrium and thrombus formation can occur from non-circulating blood. If coarctation of the aorta is causing the difficulty, dissection of the aorta from high blood pressure from trying to push blood past the constriction can occur. To prevent thrombus formation anticoagulants may be prescribed. To decrease the strain on the aorta, antihypertensives may be prescribed to control blood pressure, diuretics to reduce blood volume and beta-blockers to improve ventricular filling. A woman will be scheduled for serial ultrasound and non-stress tests after weeks 30 to 32 of pregnancy to monitor fetal health and rule out poor placental perfusion. A balloon valve angioplasty to loosen mitral valve adhesions can be performed safely during pregnancy (Traill, 2012).

If an anticoagulant is required, low-molecular-weight heparin (LMWH) is the drug of choice for early pregnancy because it does not cross the placenta and so does not have teratogenic effects.

Right-sided heart failure

Right-sided heart failure occurs when the output of the right ventricle is overwhelmed by the amount of blood received by the right atrium from the vena cava. It can be caused by an unrepaired congenital heart defect such as pulmonary valve stenosis, but the anomaly most apt to cause right-sided heart failure in women of reproductive age is Eisenmenger's syndrome, a right-to-left arterial or ventricular septal defect with an accompanying pulmonary valve stenosis (Wolff & Weitzel, 2011).

With this, congestion of the systemic venous circulation and decreased cardiac output to the lungs occurs. Blood pressure decreases in the aorta because less blood is able to reach it; in contrast, pressure is high in the vena cava from back pressure of blood. Both jugular venous distention and increased portal circulation are evident. The liver and spleen both become distended. Extreme liver enlargement can cause dyspnoea and pain in a pregnant woman because the enlarged liver, as it is pressed upwards by the enlarged uterus, puts extreme pressure on the diaphragm. Distention of abdominal and lower extremity vessels can lead to excudation of fluid from the vessels into the peritoneal cavity (i.e. ascites) or peripheral oedema.

Women who have an uncorrected anomaly of this type may be advised not to become pregnant. If they do plan a pregnancy, they can expect to be hospitalised for some time, during the latter part of pregnancy, for oxygen administration and arterial blood gas assessments, to ensure adequate fetal growth. During labour, they may need a pulmonary artery catheter inserted to monitor pulmonary pressure. They need extremely close monitoring after epidural anaesthesia to minimise the risk of hypotension.

Cardiomyopathy

Cardiomyopathy during pregnancy is an extremely rare but serious condition accounting for up to 11% of maternal deaths (Lewey & Haythe, 2014). **Peripartum cardiomyopathy** occurs in women with no history of heart disease one month before birth and up to five months after birth (Lewey & Haythe, 2014). The cause is unknown, however, it is linked to pregnancy-related circulatory changes. Identified risk factors include hypertension preeclampsia and maternal age. In some women hypertrophic cardiomyopathy is first diagnosed during pregnancy (Mohan & Nelson-Piercy, 2014). Symptoms of cardiomyopathy include shortness of breath, chest pain, dizziness and oedema. Cardiomegaly, pulmonary oedema and arrhythmias can also occur. Management may include diuretics, vasodilators and low-molecular-weight heparin. Seriously affected women may need ICU care and a heart transplant. A normal vaginal birth is preferable because a caesarean section carries more risk due to haemodynamic changes, anaesthesia, increased blood loss and increased risk of infection (Lewey & Haythe, 2014).

Women with a history of cardiomyopathy require pre-conception assessment to determine their level of risk in another pregnancy. Approximately 50% of women fully recover; those who have abnormal ventricular function 6 months postpartum have a 50% risk of more severe heart failure and a 25% risk of death in future pregnancy (Mohan & Nelson-Piercy, 2014). Up to 10% of women with cardiomyopathy during pregnancy develop heart failure and eventually require a heart transplant (Lewey & Haythe, 2014). Contraception discussion is important, as combined oral contraceptives which contain oestrogen are contraindicated because of the increased risk of thromboembolism.

Cardiac disease

Cardiovascular disease requires continuous assessment of a woman's health status, health education and health-promoting activities. Assessment of a woman with cardiac disease begins with a thorough health history to document her pre-pregnancy cardiac status (see Box 20.1). This includes exercise tolerance, which is the level achieved before growing short of breath and the occurrence of physical symptoms, such as cyanosis of the lips or nail beds. Also note if she normally has a cough or oedema because pulmonary oedema from heart failure may first manifest itself as a simple cough.

Assessment of oedema in women with heart disease is important because systemic oedema is a sign of heart failure. Oedema can begin at any time and other symptoms will probably also be present: irregular pulse, rapid or difficult respirations and perhaps chest pain on exertion. At the first antenatal visit record a baseline blood pressure, pulse rate and respiratory rate in either a sitting or lying position; then, at future visits, always take these in the same position for the most accurate comparison. For additional cardiac status assessment, a woman may need an electrocardiogram (ECG), chest radiograph or echocardiogram performed at periodic points in the pregnancy. Assure her that an ECG merely measures cardiac electrical discharge and so cannot harm her fetus in any way. Echocardiography uses ultrasound and so will also not harm her fetus. Chest radiography is considered safe as long as a woman's abdomen is covered by a lead apron during the exposure. An ECG may become less accurate late in pregnancy (demonstrates left axis deviation) because the enlarged uterus presses upwards on the diaphragm and displaces the heart laterally.

Fetal assessment

Cardiac failure can affect fetal growth when maternal blood pressure becomes insufficient to provide an adequate supply of blood and nutrients to the placenta. For this reason, the infants of women with severe heart disease tend to have low birth weights. A poor perfusion level may also lead to an acidotic fetal environment if the blood flow becomes inadequate for carbon dioxide exchange. This can result in preterm labour, exposing an infant to the hazards of immaturity as well as low birth weight. An infant may not respond well to labour (evidenced by late deceleration patterns on a fetal heart monitor) and a caesarean birth may need to be performed which increases the risk for mother and fetus. Fetal assessment includes CTG, Doppler assessment and biophysical profiles.

BOX 20.1 Assessment ✻ Assessing a pregnant woman with cardiac disease

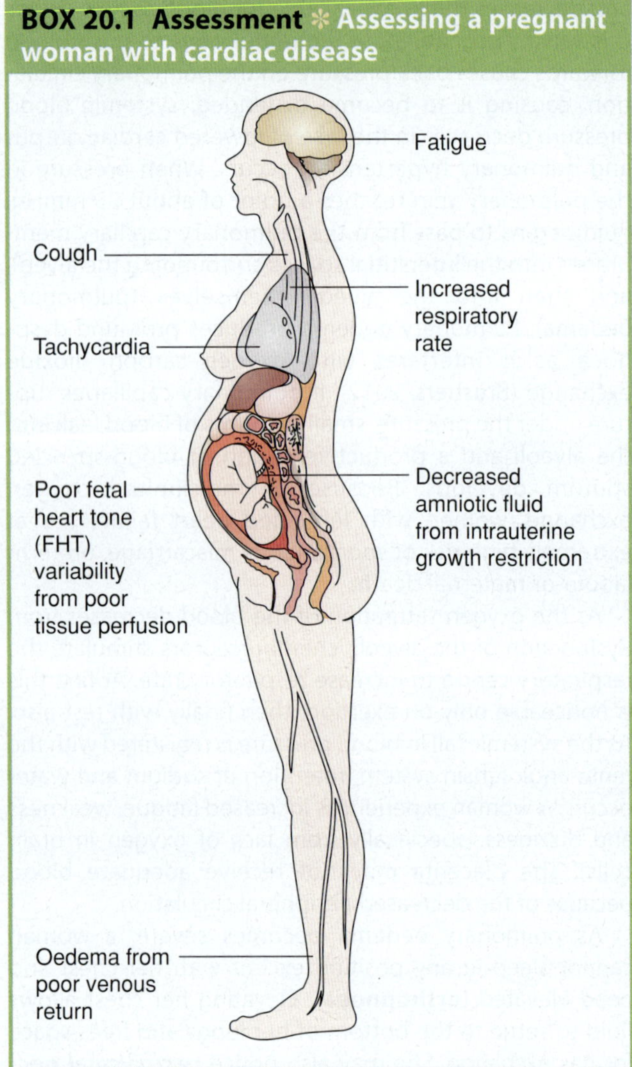

Management

Maternal blood pressure should be maintained above 100/60 mmHg and fetal heart rate should remain in the normal range of 110 to 160 beats per minute. Women need to be aware of danger signs and the steps to take if they occur. The goals and outcomes established in collaboration with a woman with heart disease should be realistic. Not all women with heart disease will be able to complete a pregnancy successfully; some infants of women with severe involvement will be born with the effects of placental insufficiency, such as neurological involvement or cognitive challenge.

When cardiac output is not enough to meet systemic body demands, peripheral vasoconstriction occurs. Because the uterus is a peripheral organ, this causes uterine/placental constriction. Therefore, a rest program must be carefully designed so a woman stops exercising before this point is reached. The most appropriate amount of rest and activity needs to be individualised and detailed. Women may interpret recommendations for rest and reduced activities very differently.

A woman with cardiac disease may need closer supervision of nutrition during pregnancy because she must gain enough weight to ensure a healthy pregnancy and a healthy baby, but not so much weight that she has to supply additional cells with nutrients. This could overburden her heart and circulatory system. If anaemia is present it should be treated, as anaemia places an extra burden on the heart because it requires the body to circulate blood more vigorously to distribute oxygen to all body cells. If a woman was following a sodium-restricted diet before pregnancy, this may be continued during pregnancy, although typically a woman's sodium intake is only limited, not severely restricted, during pregnancy. Sodium is necessary for maintaining fluid volume and balance and thus is necessary to allow a woman's body to retain enough blood volume to supply blood to the fetus.

Women with heart disease may need supplemental oxygen if they over exert, as could happen during an antenatal visit. Cardiac resuscitation in women who are pregnant is the same as adult resuscitation with the addition of a 15–30% uterine tilt to prevent caval compression (Australian Resuscitation Guidelines, 2015); see Box 20.2.

Labour and birth

Careful planning and monitoring during labour is important as cardiac output is increased. A rapidly increasing pulse rate is an indication that the heart is pumping ineffectively and has increased its rate in an effort to compensate. If pulmonary oedema is present, breathing may be easier if the chest and head are elevated (semi-Fowler's position). A side-lying position or tilt of the uterus with a towel promotes optimum perfusion and avoids supine hypotension syndrome. Women with severe heart disease need oxygen administered during labour, to compensate for the added oxygen required for the exertion of labour, as well as continuous haemodynamic monitoring such as by a Swan-Ganz catheter. Epidural anaesthesia using fentanyl is appropriate as it does not decrease peripheral vascular resistance. A vaginal birth is generally preferred, however, second stage pushing may be very taxing and an instrumental birth may be required.

BOX 20.2 Nursing procedure ✻ CPR during pregnancy

Purpose: To restore respiratory and cardiac function.

Plan	Principle
1. Shake the woman's shoulders and shout.	1. Shaking the shoulders and shouting are an attempt to determine unconsciousness and to rouse a woman who may have fainted or be asleep.
2. Phone or call for help.	2. The woman may need more than simple resuscitation.
3. Place a rolled or folded towel under the woman's right hip.	3. A towel placed under one hip helps to prevent uterine compression on the vena cava or helps prevent supine hypotension syndrome.
4. Lift the chin to position the airway.	4. Lifting the chin aids in straightening the airway to ensure that it is patent.
5. Establish lack of respirations by listening and feeling for air movement.	5. Listening and feeling for air movement provides evidence of breathing.
6. Begin rescue breathing with administration of two quick breathing-bag breaths.	6. Rescue breathing introduces oxygen for gas exchange.
7. Assess carotid pulse.	7. Presence of carotid pulse indicates cardiac function.
8. Begin chest compressions if there is no carotid pulse. Place both hands on the lower sternum just above xiphoid process and deliver 30 chest compressions followed by 2 rescue breaths (1 second each) until cardiopulmonary function returns.	8. External chest compressions stimulate the action of the heart to maintain tissue perfusion. They should be at a rate of 100 bpm and allow the chest to rise between compressions.
9. If an automated external defibrillator (AED) is necessary, remove any fetal or uterine monitors if these are in place. Follow standard application and procedure according to agency protocol.	9. AED is effective in stimulating heart action and is not detrimental to pregnancy or a fetus.

Source: www.resus.org.au.

Postpartum

Third stage may be actively managed with controlled cord traction and an oxytocic to reduce the risk of postpartum haemorrhage. With birth of the placenta, the blood that supplied the placenta is now released into general circulation, subsequently increasing blood volume 20% to 40%. During pregnancy, the increase in blood volume occurred over a 6-month period, so the heart had time to adjust to this change gradually. After birth, the increase in pressure takes place within 5 minutes, so the heart must make a rapid and major adjustment (Easterling & Stout, 2012). This is a critical period for women and they must be monitored carefully.

If a woman has severe congestive heart failure after birth, she needs a program of decreased activity and possibly anticoagulant and digoxin therapy until her circulation stabilises. Antiembolic stockings and ambulation may be needed to increase venous return from the legs. If prophylactic antibiotics had not been started prior to birth, they must be started immediately after birth to discourage subacute bacterial endocarditis caused by introduction of microorganisms through the placental site.

After discharge, additional rest and monitoring is required to evaluate cardiac function. Follow-up appointments are necessary for maternity and cardiac care.

Artificial valve prosthesis

Once, women with heart valve prostheses were advised not to become pregnant for fear the increased blood volume gained during pregnancy would overwhelm the artificial valve. Today, women with a valve prosthesis can complete pregnancy safely (Suri et al., 2011). One potential problem involves the use of oral anticoagulants that a woman takes to prevent the formation of clots at the valve site. Because sodium warfarin (Coumadin) may increase the risk of congenital anomalies in infants (pregnancy risk category D), women are usually placed on low-molecular-weight heparin therapy for conception and pregnancy to reduce this risk. Heparin does not cross the placenta and so does not interfere with fetal development or fetal coagulation (pregnancy risk category C). Subclinical bleeding from the anticoagulant in the mother can cause placental dislodgement. Observe a woman who is taking an anticoagulant for signs such as bleeding gums, petechiae, excessive bruising, epistaxis and signs of premature separation of the placenta during pregnancy and labour.

Chronic hypertension

Women with chronic hypertensive disease come into pregnancy with an elevated blood pressure (140/90 mmHg or above). Hypertension of this kind is usually associated with arteriosclerosis or renal disease, making it more common with advanced maternal age. Chronic hypertension places both the woman and fetus at high risk because fetal wellbeing can be compromised by poor heart, kidney, and/or placental perfusion (Gelson et al., 2011). Antihypertensive agents such as methyldopa (Aldomet) and calcium antagonists such as nifedipine, hydrazaline or labetolol are used to manage hypertension. Some antihypertensives are contraindicated in pregnancy as they may cause intrauterine growth restriction (IUGR), oligohydramnious, renal damage or hypotension.

Thromboembolic disease

Thrombophilias are a group of hypercoagulation abnormalities which predispose to venous thrombosis and may be acquired or inherited (Schub & March, 2015). Thromboembolic disease resulting in deep venous thrombosis and pulmonary embolism complicates 1 in 1000 to 1 in 2000 pregnancies and is a serious cause of maternal mortality. The incidence of venous thromboembolic disease increases during pregnancy because of a combination of risk factors present to some extent in all pregnancies: venous stasis, vascular damage and hypercoagulability due to elevated oestrogen. The likelihood of **deep vein thrombosis** (DVT) or pulmonary embolism (PE) leading to pulmonary emboli increases for women over 30 years of age (Sorensen et al., 2011). Genetic conditions such as factor V Lieden, hyperhomocysteinemia, antithrombin III deficiency, prothrombin G20210A deficiencies, activated protein C resistance, protein C and protein S deficiencies and antiphospholipid antibody syndrome increase the risk of thrombus formation (Schub & March, 2015). A family history of DVT or PE may indicate a genetic component. Women with antiphospholipid antibodies (aPLA) are at increased risk of thrombus formation, spontaneous miscarriage and hypertension (Danza, Ruiz-Irastorza & Khamashta, 2012). These antibodies probably represent an autoimmune process and women who are aPLA positive may be started on a prophylactic program of low dose aspirin and/or subcutaneous heparin during pregnancy. A DVT often presents with pain, redness and warmth which may be present in the calf or groin. Homan's sign (pain with dorsiflexion of the foot) may be present. DVT is diagnosed by history and Duplex Doppler ultrasonography or impedance plethysmography. Once diagnosed, a DVT is treated with subcutaneous low molecular weight heparin such as enoxaparin, for the duration of the pregnancy. It is generally recommended the lower abdomen be used for subcutaneous heparin administration.

The chief danger of thrombosis is pulmonary embolism or a clot lodging in the pulmonary artery and blocking circulation to the lungs and heart. Symptoms of pulmonary embolism include:

- Chest pain
- Sudden onset of dyspnoea
- Cough with haemoptysis
- Tachycardia or missed beats

- Severe dizziness or fainting from lowered blood pressure.

Pulmonary embolism needs to be recognised rapidly, as it is an emergency. It is essential for women to be aware of these symptoms and know they need to seek emergency care.

Women taking heparin may be instructed to reduce their heparin dose or discontinue heparin when contractions begin. Around 50% of thromboses occur in the postpartum period. Heparin is safe for breastfeeding as it has large molecules that do not cross into breast milk in significant amounts. Sodium warfarin (Coumadin) does cross into breast milk at very low levels. With dosage less than 12 mg daily, breastfeeding is considered safe. No adverse reactions have occurred in infants from maternal warfarin, even at higher doses, and it is considered to pose minimal risk to the breastfed infant (UpToDate, 2015).

CASE STUDY QUESTION

3. Suppose Angelina develops a deep vein thrombosis while in the hospital on bed rest and is prescribed heparin. Which of the following would be important in planning care for her?
   a. Showing her how to self-administer the drug as a rectal suppository.
   b. Cautioning her that her haemoglobin level will be closely monitored during therapy.
   c. Allowing her to choose a subcutaneous site for the injection.
   d. Monitoring her white blood cell count daily for decreased coagulation.

HAEMATOLOGICAL DISORDERS

Haematological disorders during pregnancy involve either blood formation or coagulation disorders.

Anaemia and pregnancy

Because the blood volume expands during pregnancy slightly ahead of the red cell count, most women have a normal physiological anaemia of pregnancy. True anaemia is present when a woman's haemoglobin concentration is less than 110 g/L (haematocrit, 33%) in the first or third trimester of pregnancy or haemoglobin concentration is less than 105 g/L (haematocrit, 32%) in the second trimester (Samuels, 2012).

Iron-deficiency anaemia

Iron-deficiency anaemia is the most common anaemia of pregnancy, occurring in 12% of all pregnancies in Australia, however, prevalence is higher in Indigenous communities. In non-western countries iron deficiency anaemia occurs in as many as 15% to 25% of pregnancies (Imdad & Bhutta, 2012). A deficiency of iron stores may result from a diet low in iron, heavy menstrual periods or unwise weight-reducing programs. Iron stores are apt to be low in women who were pregnant less than 2 years before the current pregnancy or those from low socioeconomic levels who have iron-poor diets. The World Health Organization (WHO) defines anaemia as an HB concentration below 110 g/L in pregnancy. An iron deficiency is suspected and is confirmed by a corresponding low serum iron level and an increased iron-binding capacity. Iron is made available to the body by absorption from the duodenum into the bloodstream after it is ingested. In the bloodstream, it is bound to transferrin for transport to the liver, spleen and bone marrow. At these sites, it is incorporated into haemoglobin or stored as ferritin.

Iron-deficiency anaemia is characteristically a microcytic (small red blood cell), hypochromic (less haemoglobin than the average red cell) anaemia, because when an inadequate supply of iron is ingested, iron is unavailable for incorporation into red blood cells. Pathological anaemia is treated by an iron supplement of 60–110 mg of elemental iron daily, in the form of ferrous sulphate or ferrous gluconate, and a diet high in iron and vitamins (green leafy vegetables, meat, legumes, fruit).

Iron is best absorbed from an acid medium. Therefore, advise women to take iron supplements with orange juice or a vitamin C supplement, which supplies ascorbic acid. When women begin to take a prescribed iron supplement, new red blood cells should begin to increase, or their reticulocyte counts should rise from a normal range 0.5% to 1.5%, to 3% to 4% in 2 weeks. Some women report constipation or gastric irritation when taking oral iron supplements. Increasing fibre in the diet and always taking the pills with food help reduce these symptoms. Ferrous sulphate turns stools black so caution women about this to prevent them worrying that they are bleeding internally. If iron-deficiency anaemia is severe and a woman has difficulty with oral iron therapy, intramuscular or iron polymaltose (Ferrosig) injection can be prescribed.

In Australia and New Zealand routine iron supplementation is not recommended, with iron supplementation based on individual assessment. Iron supplementation can have adverse effects in women who do not have pathological anaemia. A high haemoglobin increases the risk of preeclampsia, hypertension, gestational diabetes, liver and kidney damage, and IUGR. Iron supplementation in women without anaemia failed to improve pregnancy outcomes and has the potential to harm both mother and baby (Gaillard et al., 2014). Early high iron levels in pregnancy may be related to abnormal placentation and insufficient plasma volume expansion; low haemoglobin has been associated with a decreased risk of gestational hypertension and preeclampsia, improved fetal growth and longer pregnancy duration (Gaillard et al., 2014).

Folic acid-deficiency anaemia

Folic acid, or folacin, one of the B vitamins, is necessary for the normal formation of red blood cells in the mother as well as being associated with preventing neural tube defects and abdominal wall defects in the fetus. Folic acid-deficiency anaemia occurs most often in multiple pregnancies because of the increased fetal demand; in women with a secondary haemolytic illness in which there is rapid destruction and production of new red blood cells; in women who are taking hydantoin, an anticonvulsant agent that interferes with folate absorption; in women who have been taking oral contraceptives; and in women who have had a gastric bypass for morbid obesity (Greenberg et al., 2011). The anaemia that develops is a **megaloblastic anaemia** (enlarged red blood cells). The mean corpuscular volume will be elevated (due to the enlarged red blood cells) in contrast to the lowered level seen with iron-deficiency anaemia. The deficiency may take several weeks to develop, so it often becomes most apparent during the second trimester of pregnancy. It may be a contributory factor in early miscarriage or premature separation of the placenta.

Because the fetal effects of deficiency occur in the first few weeks of fetal development, women expecting to become pregnant are advised to begin a supplement of 400 mcg/0.4 mg of folic acid daily in addition to eating folacin-rich foods (green leafy vegetables, oranges, dried beans). During pregnancy, the folic acid requirement increases to 600 mcg per day. Women who develop folic acid-deficiency anaemia are prescribed even higher or therapeutic levels of folic acid (Clark, Thomson & Greer, 2012).

Sickle cell anaemia

Sickle cell anaemia is a recessively inherited haemolytic anaemia caused by an abnormal amino acid in the beta chain of haemoglobin. If the abnormal amino acid replaces the amino acid valine, sickle haemoglobin (HbS) results. If it is substituted for the amino acid lysine, non-sickling haemoglobin (HbC) results. An individual who is heterozygous (has only one gene in which the abnormal substitution has occurred) has the sickle cell trait (HbAS). If the person is homozygous (has two genes in which the substitution has occurred), sickle cell disease (HbSS) results (Rote & McCance, 2012).

With the disease, the majority of red blood cells are irregular or sickle-shaped so they cannot carry as much haemoglobin as normally-shaped red blood cells. When oxygen tension becomes reduced, as occurs at high altitudes, or blood becomes more viscid than usual, as occurs with dehydration, the cells tend to clump because of the irregular shape. This clumping can result in vessel blockage with reduced blood flow to organs. The cells then will haemolyse, reducing the number available, causing a severe anaemia. If a woman has an infection with a fever this may cause more perspiration leading to dehydration (Howard & Oteng-Ntim, 2012).

Although the sickle cell trait does not appear to influence the course of pregnancy, rates of prematurity, miscarriage or perinatal mortality may be higher for women with the homozygous disease. At any time in life, sickle cell anaemia is a threat to life if vital blood vessels such as those to the liver, kidneys, heart, lungs or brain become blocked. In pregnancy, blockage to the placental circulation can directly compromise the fetus, causing low birth weight and possibly fetal death. Fetal surveillance to assess for intrauterine growth restriction includes weekly CTG and ultrasound monitoring of blood flow velocity beginning at around 30 weeks' gestation. Normal birth is preferable to a caesarean section.

Thalassaemia

The thalassaemias are a group of autosomal recessively inherited blood disorders that lead to poor haemoglobin formation and severe anaemia. They occur most frequently in Mediterranean, African and Asian populations (Leung & Lao, 2012). Symptoms first appear in childhood. Treatment focuses on combating anaemia through such measures as folic acid supplementation and perhaps blood transfusion to infuse haemoglobin-rich red blood cells. Women do not usually take an iron supplement during pregnancy or they could receive an iron overload because of the iron also infused by blood transfusions.

Malaria

In Australia during 2011–2012 there were no notifications of locally-acquired malaria (Knope et al., 2014). Malaria is a protozoan infection that is transmitted to humans by Anopheles mosquitoes (Fried, Muehlenbachs & Duffy, 2012). Malaria causes red blood cells to stick to the surface of capillaries causing obstruction of these vessels leading to end-organ anoxia and poor organ perfusion. Treatment consists of antimalarial drugs which stop the disease and help reduce the incidence of low birth weight and preterm birth. Sulfadoxine/pyrimethamine is safe in the third trimester of pregnancy. Chloroquine is safe throughout pregnancy and is the drug of choice (Irvine, Einarson & Bozzo, 2011).

Coagulation disorders

Von Willebrand's disease is a coagulation disorder inherited as an autosomal dominant trait (Shahbazi, et al., 2012). There is often a history of menorrhagia or frequent episodes of epistaxis. If these symptoms are not severe the condition may go undiagnosed until pregnancy, when a spontaneous miscarriage or postpartum haemorrhage may occur. Women with the disorder have normal platelet counts, but bleeding time is prolonged. Levels of factor VIII-related antigen (VIII-R) and factor VIII coagulation activity (VIII-C) are both reduced. Replacement of these factors by infusion of cryoprecipitate or fresh-frozen plasma may be necessary before labour to prevent excessive bleeding. Although Von Willebrand factor levels often increase in pregnancy the risk of postpartum haemorrhage is about double that for women without bleeding disorders (ACOG, 2012).

Haemophilia B (Christmas disease, factor IX deficiency) is a sex-linked disorder, so the actual disease occurs only in males. However, female carriers may have only 33% of the normal level of factor IX. This can result in spontaneous miscarriage or haemorrhage with labour. Carriers of the disorder need to be identified before pregnancy. Restoration of factor IX levels can be done by infusion of factor IX concentrate or fresh-frozen plasma.

Idiopathic thrombocytopenic purpura (ITP), a decreased number of platelets, can occur at any time in life and occasionally occurs during pregnancy. The cause of the condition is unknown, but because symptoms usually occur shortly after a viral infection it is assumed to be an autoimmune illness (an antiplatelet antibody that destroys platelets is released) (Gasim, 2011). Laboratory studies reveal a marked thrombocytopenia (platelet count may be as low as 20,000 mm^3 from a usual count of 150,000 mm^3). Without an adequate level of platelets, minute petechiae or large ecchymoses appear on a woman's body and frequent nosebleeds may occur.

The illness typically runs a 1- to 3-month limited course. A platelet transfusion or plasmapheresis may be administered to temporarily increase the platelet count; oral prednisone is also effective. Women with ITP need to be identified during pregnancy because the decreased platelet count can lead to increased bleeding at birth. In addition, the antiplatelet factor can cross the placenta and cause accompanying platelet destruction in the newborn or allow a newborn to be born with ITP.

RENAL AND URINARY DISORDERS

Adequate kidney function is important to a successful pregnancy outcome because a woman is excreting waste products not only for herself but also for the fetus. This dual function makes any condition that interferes with kidney or urinary function potentially serious.

Urinary tract infection

During pregnancy progesterone dilates the ureters and relaxes the smooth muscle of the bladder promoting stasis of urine. Minimal glucosuria also occurs allowing more than the usual number of organisms to grow. In combination these factors cause asymptomatic urinary tract infections (UTIs) in as many as 10% to 15% of pregnant women (Trautner, 2012). Asymptomatic UTI's are potentially dangerous because they can progress to pyelonephritis (infection of the pelvis of the kidney) and are associated with preterm labour and premature rupture of membranes. Women with known vesicoureteral reflux (backflow of urine into the ureters) tend to develop UTIs or pyelonephritis more often than others. The organism most commonly responsible for UTI is *Escherichia coli* from an ascending infection. A UTI can also occur as a descending infection, or begin in the kidneys, from the filtration of organisms present from other body infections. If the infectious organism is determined to be *Streptococcus B*, vaginal cultures should be obtained because *streptococcal B* infection of the genital tract is associated with pneumonia in newborns.

A UTI is typically manifested by frequency and pain on urination, with pyelonephritis pain in the lumbar region (usually on the right side) that radiates downwards and the area feels tender to palpation. Accompanying nausea and vomiting, malaise, pain and frequency of urination may occur. Temperature may be elevated only slightly or may be as high as 39°C to 40°C. The infection usually occurs on the right side because there is greater compression and urinary stasis on the right ureter from the uterus being pushed right by the large bulk of the intestine on the left side. A clean catch urine culture with over 100,000 organisms per millilitre of urine is diagnostic of infection. A culture and sensitivity will determine the appropriate antibiotic.

Amoxicillin, ampicillin and cephalosporins are effective against most organisms causing UTIs and are safe antibiotics during pregnancy. The sulfonamides can be used early in pregnancy but not near term because they can interfere with protein binding of bilirubin, which then leads to hyperbilirubinaemia in the newborn. Tetracyclines are contraindicated in pregnancy as they cause retardation of bone growth and staining of the fetal teeth (McKenna & Mirkov, 2014).

UTI prevention

All women during pregnancy can be reminded of common measures to prevent UTIs, such as:

- Drink adequate fluids (6–8 glasses/day)
- Wipe front to back after voiding and bowel movements
- Wear cotton not synthetic fibre underwear
- Void before and after sexual intercourse
- Avoid strong soaps, sprays and powders
- Report early signs of a UTI
- Complete the prescribed course of antibiotics
- Avoid foods high in sugar.

Pyelonephritis occurs as an extension of a urinary tract infection or infection that originated in or spread to the kidney (Schneeberger et al., 2012). If this develops, a woman may be hospitalised for 24 to 48 hours while she is treated with intravenous antibiotics. After this acute episode, she will be maintained on a medication such as oral nitrofurantoin (Macrodantin) for the remainder of the pregnancy.

After birth, a woman who developed more than one UTI may have an intravenous pyelogram or ultrasound scheduled to help detect any urinary tract abnormality that might be present, such as vesicoureteral reflux, to help prevent future infections.

CASE STUDY QUESTION

4. It has been noted that a high number of pregnant women seen in the antenatal clinic, including Angelina, have developed UTIs during their pregnancies. The midwife or medical practitioner should emphasise which response to this issue?

a. Ensure that the cleaning department is adequately cleaning the toilets.
b. Suggest all women be prescribed a prophylactic antibiotic during their first trimester.
c. Educate women on the need for sound perineal care during pregnancy.
d. Urge women to restrict fluid to keep their urine acidic and concentrated.

Chronic renal disease

In the past, women with chronic renal disease did not reach childbearing age or were advised not to have children because of their high-risk status during pregnancy. Today, with conscientious prenatal care, most women with chronic renal disease and even women who have had renal transplants can expect to have healthy pregnancies and healthy children (Fontana et al., 2012). Women with chronic renal disease may develop severe anaemia during pregnancy because their kidneys do not produce erythropoietin, which is necessary for red cell formation. Fortunately, synthetic erythropoietin is now available and is safe to take during pregnancy (Jelkmann, 2011).

Because the glomerular filtration rate normally increases during pregnancy, a woman's serum creatinine level (a measure of kidney function that elevates when kidneys are under stress) may be actually slightly below normal during pregnancy. A normal serum creatinine level is 61 μmol/L (range 45–90 μmol/L); during pregnancy, it falls to about 44 μmol/L. Women with kidney disease who normally have a serum creatinine level of more than 176 μmol/L may be advised not to undertake a pregnancy in case the increased strain on already damaged kidneys leads to kidney failure.

Many women with renal disease routinely take a corticosteroid such as oral prednisone at a maintenance level. This medication therapy is typically continued throughout pregnancy. Although animal studies have shown an increased incidence of cleft palate from corticosteroid use during pregnancy, this does not appear to be true in humans. The infant may be hyperglycaemic at birth because of the suppression of insulin activity by the corticosteroid.

Although successful pregnancy in women with kidney transplants is to be expected, women should be considered individually to determine whether they will be able to carry a pregnancy to term before a pregnancy is initiated (Lopez et al., 2011). Criteria to be evaluated include:

- General health and the time since the transplant (preferably >2 years)
- Serum creatinine level
- The presence of **proteinuria** or hypertension or signs of graft rejection
- Medications taken to reduce graft rejection.

It is helpful if the medications a woman is taking are limited to prednisone and azathioprine (an antimetabolite [Imuran], but with no reports of fetal compromise from its use).

Women with severe renal disease may require dialysis to aid kidney function during pregnancy (Piccoli et al., 2010). Dialysis increases the risk of preterm labour, perhaps because progesterone is removed with the dialysis. To prevent this complication, progesterone may be administered intramuscularly before the procedure. If haemodialysis is used, it should be scheduled frequently and for short durations to avoid acute fluid shifts. The heparin administered with haemodialysis is safe in pregnancy because it does not cross the placenta. Peritoneal dialysis is preferred to haemodialysis during pregnancy because it normally causes less drastic fluid shifts. This can be accomplished using continuous ambulatory peritoneal dialysis.

Women with renal disease may need nutrition counselling during pregnancy to avoid a build-up of potassium and ensure a healthy diet; see Box 20.3.

BOX 20.3 Assessment * Assessing a pregnant woman with renal disease

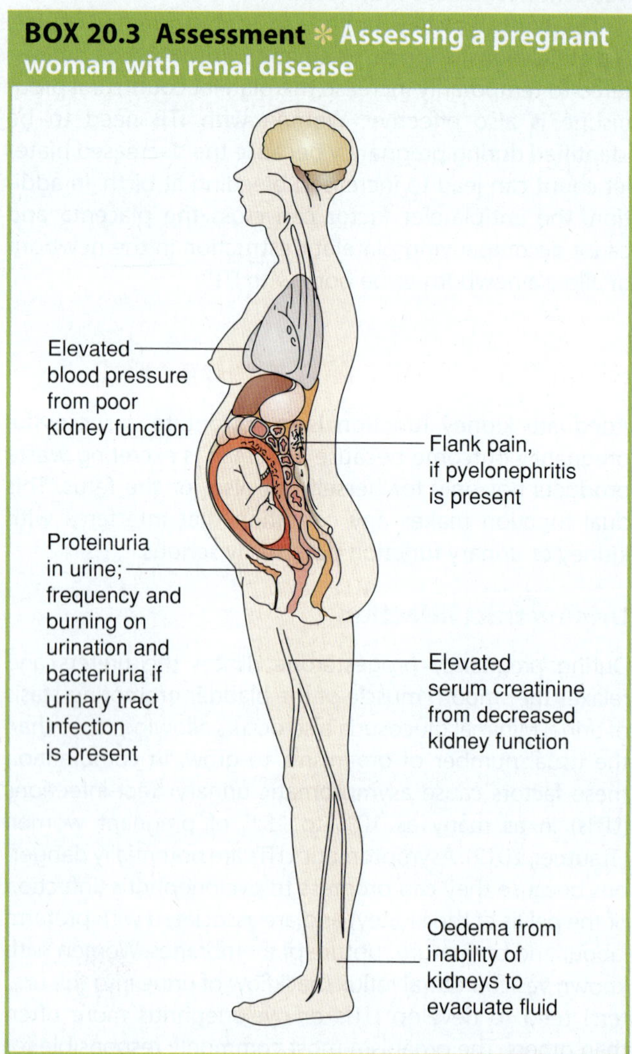

RESPIRATORY DISORDERS

Respiratory diseases range from mild (the common cold) to severe (pneumonia) to chronic (tuberculosis or chronic obstructive pulmonary disease [COPD]). Any respiratory condition can worsen in pregnancy because the rising uterus compresses the diaphragm, reducing the size of the thoracic cavity and available lung space. Any respiratory disorder can pose serious hazards to the fetus if allowed to progress to the point where the mother's oxygen-carbon dioxide exchange is altered or the mother or fetus cannot receive enough oxygen.

Acute nasopharyngitis

Acute nasopharyngitis (common cold) tends to be more severe during pregnancy than at other times because during pregnancy, oestrogen stimulation normally causes some degree of nasal congestion. This means that even with a minor cold, a woman can find it difficult to breathe. Aspirin should be avoided as a cold remedy during pregnancy because of possible interference with blood clotting in both mother and fetus and the possibility of prolonged pregnancy at term (McKenna & Mirkov, 2014). Because common colds are invariably caused by a virus, antibiotic therapy is unnecessary except to prevent a secondary infection. Although most simple cough syrups contain no ingredients that would make them unsafe for use during pregnancy, women should check with their healthcare provider before taking any over-the-counter medication for a cold (see Box 20.4).

BOX 20.4 * Focus on family teaching

Relieving upper respiratory symptoms during pregnancy

Q. Angelina tells you, "I get a lot of colds. What should I do to keep symptoms under control during pregnancy?"

A. Use the following guidelines to help combat common cold symptoms during pregnancy:

- Be sure to get extra rest and sleep and eat a diet high in vitamin C (orange juice and fruit) to help boost the immune system.
- If you experience any aches and pains, take paracetamol every 4 hours. Do not take acetylsalicylic acid (aspirin) during pregnancy.
- Use a room humidifier, especially at night, to moisten nasal secretions and help mucus drain.
- Use only over-the-counter cough drops or syrups that contain natural ingredients such as honey and lemon to help reduce coughing.
- Apply a medicated vapour rub to your chest, if you prefer, to help relieve nasal congestion.
- Use cool or warm compresses to relieve sinus headaches.
- Check with your healthcare provider regarding the use of over-the-counter cough drops, syrups or decongestants to be certain that any medication you take is safe during pregnancy.

Influenza

Influenza pandemics, such as the 2009 H1N1, have occurred in recent years and present a serious health risk to pregnant women who have higher infection rates. Seasonal and pandemic influenza increases risks for mother and fetus and have been associated with a fivefold increase in perinatal mortality and a threefold increase in prematurity and low birth weight (Memoli et al., 2013). Prevention strategies to limit pregnant women's exposure, such as avoiding infected people and infection control precautions are important. Influenza is a viral illness which spreads in epidemic form and is accompanied by high fever, extreme prostration, aching pains in the back and extremities, and often a sore, raw throat. Influenza infection has not been clearly correlated with congenital anomalies in children although it can be a cause of preterm labour. For unknown reasons, some studies have shown a link between influenza during pregnancy and schizophrenia in children born of that pregnancy (Moreno et al., 2011). Treatment includes an antipyretic, such as paracetamol, to control fever. The risk for a woman of not taking oseltamivir (TamiFlu), an oral antiviral medication that is category C, is greater than if it is not taken. It should therefore be prescribed and begun immediately during pregnancy (Donner et al., 2010). Because influenza vaccines are made from inert viruses, women may be immunised safely against influenza during pregnancy (Gorman et al., 2012).

Pneumonia

Pneumonia is the bacterial or viral invasion of lung parenchyma; the most common bacteria is *Streptococcus pneumoniae*, other bacteria are *Haemophilus influenzae*, *Mycoplasma pneumoniae* and *Legionella spp.* Viruses include influenza, varicella-zoster and measles. After the invasion, an acute inflammatory response occurs in the lung alveoli with exudate of red blood cells, fibrin and polymorphonuclear leucocytes into the alveoli. This process confines the bacteria or virus within segments of the lobes of the lungs but also fills the alveoli with fluid, blocking off breathing space. If the collection of fluid is extreme, it can limit the oxygen available to the woman and fetus. Serious complications can occur such as fetal loss, fetal malformations, fetal growth restriction, preterm birth, low infant birth weight and postnatal infection with most adverse outcomes occurring with comorbidities such as chronic respiratory disease (Buckley & Grose, 2013). Pneumonia tends to be both more severe and more difficult to treat in pregnancy (Buckley & Grose, 2013). Therapy involves the use of an appropriate antibiotic, oxygen administration if hypoxia is present, chest percussion and suction to help remove sputum and IV therapy. With severe disease, ventilatory support may be necessary. Pneumonia during pregnancy is associated with fetal growth restriction and preterm birth because of the oxygen deficit (Chen et al., 2012). If pneumonia is present during labour, oxygen should be administered so the fetus has adequate oxygen resources during contractions.

Asthma

Asthma is a common chronic disease with an incidence between 8–13% in Australia (Sawicki et al., 2011). Asthma is a disorder marked by reversible airflow obstruction, airway hyper-reactivity and airway inflammation. Symptoms are often triggered by an inhaled allergen such as pollen or cigarette smoke. With inhalation of the allergen, there is an immediate release of bioactive mediators such as histamine and leukotrienes from an immunoglobulin interaction. This results in constriction of the bronchial smooth muscle, marked mucosal inflammation and swelling, and the production of thick bronchial secretions. These three processes reduce the size of the lumen of air passages. This causes difficulty inhaling and exhaling; on exhalation, a high-pitched whistling sound (bronchial wheezing) occurs from air being pushed past the bronchial narrowing. The increase in free cortisol levels during pregnancy may make women less responsive to inflammatory triggers such as pollution and pollen (Goldie & Brightling, 2013). The increased progesterone of pregnancy relaxes the oesophageal sphincter and increases the frequency of gastro-oesophageal reflux which increases the risk for bronchospasm leading to a strong association between asthma and gastro-oesophageal reflux (Rance & O'Laughlen, 2013).

Maternal asthma can potentially reduce the oxygen supply to the fetus. Poorly controlled asthma is associated with increased risk for preeclampsia, gestational diabetes, premature contractions, premature rupture of membranes, prematurity, low birth weight, small for gestational age, placental abruption and increased caesarean section rates (Rejno et al., 2014), During pregnancy asthma becomes worse in about one-third of women, improves In one-third, and remains the same in one-third (Goldie & Brightling, 2013).

Inhaled short acting beta agonists (salbutamol and terbutaline) and inhaled corticosteroids such as budesonide are safe during pregnancy and breastfeeding (Lim, Hussainy & Abramson, 2013). Oral corticosteroids at the normal dosage used to prevent asthma exacerbations have not been related to significant risk for mother or fetus (Lim, Hussainy & Abramson, 2013). Women with asthma should continue medications to control their asthma because it is safer for them and their fetus to use asthma medications than to have poorly controlled asthma and exacerbations. Inhaled corticosteroid use during pregnancy has been associated with less risk of low birth weight babies and a reduction in asthma exacerbations; however high doses (>1000 micrograms daily in the first trimester) increase the risk of a baby with congenital malformations (Lim, Hussainy & Abramson, 2013). β-adrenergic agonists such as terbutaline and albuterol have the potential to reduce labour contractions; the dosage may be tapered close to term if possible (Mendola et al., 2013). During labour less than one fifth of women have an asthma attack. The first few months postpartum carry no increased risk of asthma exacerbations and women usually return to pre-pregnancy asthma patterns. Non-steroidal anti-inflammatory drugs (NSAIDs) are generally contraindicated as they may cause bronchospasm (some women with asthma can tolerate NSAIDs). Asthma triggers should be avoided, they include medications such as aspirin and β-blockers and food additives such as monosodium glutamate and tartrazine (Goldie & Brightling, 2013).

During lactation, asthma control continues to be important. Short-acting beta agonists at normal maintenance doses present negligible exposure to breastfed infants. Prednisolone at recommended doses is believed to be safe as low levels are excreted in human milk. Breastfeeding can be delayed for 4 hours after taking prednisolone to reduce the infants' exposure (Lim, Hussainy & Abramson, 2013).

Tuberculosis

Tuberculosis is a notifiable disease in Australia, which has one of the lowest rates of notification in the world, at 5–6 cases per 100,000 population (Lumb et al., 2009). New Zealand also has low rates of tuberculosis. However, worldwide, it is still one of the leading causes of death. With tuberculosis, lung tissue is invaded by *Mycobacterium tuberculosis*, an acid-fast bacillus. Symptoms of tuberculosis include:

- Chronic cough
- Weight loss
- Haemoptysis (coughing blood)
- Night sweats
- Low-grade fever
- Chronic fatigue.

Women with active tuberculosis need treatment during pregnancy (Nhan-Chang & Jones, 2010). Isoniazid (INH) and ethambutol hydrochloride (Myambutol), the medications of choice for tuberculosis, may be given without apparent teratogenic effects. INH may result in a peripheral neuritis if a woman does not take supplemental pyridoxine (vitamin B_6).

It is advisable to wait 1 to 2 years after the infection becomes inactive before attempting to conceive, as pressure on the diaphragm from the enlarging uterus changes the shape of the lung and can break open recently calcified pockets more readily than a well-calcified lesion. Pushing during labour may increase intrapulmonary pressure and cause the same phenomenon. Recent inactive tuberculosis may also become active during the postpartum period as the lung suddenly returns to its more vertical pre-pregnant position following birth, allowing calcium deposits to break open.

Although tuberculosis can be spread by the placenta to the fetus, it is usually spread to the infant after birth by the mother's coughing. Obtaining a negative sputum culture after birth rules out active tuberculosis. Woman should continue taking tuberculosis medications as prescribed during breastfeeding as only small amounts are secreted in breast milk and are safe for her infant.

Cystic fibrosis

Cystic fibrosis is a recessively-inherited disease resulting in generalised dysfunction of the exocrine glands (Thorpe-Beeston et al., 2013). This dysfunction leads to mucus secretions, particularly in the pancreas and lungs, becoming so viscid or thick that normal lung and pancreatic function is compromised.

Fertility may be lessened in women with cystic fibrosis because sperm cannot migrate through viscid cervical mucus. Reproductive technologies such as artificial insemination or in vitro fertilisation may be necessary for conception so sperm are not obstructed by cervical mucus. Typical symptoms of cystic fibrosis are chronic respiratory infection and over-inflation of the lungs from thickened mucus as well as an inability to digest fat and protein because the pancreas cannot release amylase. During pregnancy poor pulmonary function results in an inadequate oxygen supply to the fetus and increased risk of preterm labour and perinatal death. All babies who have a parent with cystic fibrosis will be carriers and all babies will be screened for cystic fibrosis with the newborn screen.

Therapy for cystic fibrosis consists of pancrelipase (Pancrease) to supplement pancreatic enzymes. Although pancrelipase is a pregnancy risk category C medication (teratogenic effects are unknown), it does not appear to affect the fetus and should be continued during pregnancy. Women are often also prescribed a bronchodilator or antibiotic to reduce pulmonary symptoms. In addition to pharmacological measures, women with cystic fibrosis must perform chest physiotherapy daily to reduce the build-up of lung secretions. As women with the disorder excrete a higher level of sodium in perspiration than others, they need to be carefully monitored during labour to be certain they do not become dehydrated. Although pregnancy is a strain on an already stressed respiratory system, pregnancy does not appear to shorten the life span of women with the disorder.

Because pancrelipase may interfere with iron absorption, a woman is at greater risk of iron-deficiency anaemia during pregnancy. Therefore, an iron supplement is usually prescribed. Women with cystic fibrosis have an increased incidence of gestational diabetes mellitus because of pancreatic involvement; therefore, women need close monitoring of serum glucose levels to detect the development of gestational diabetes.

Chest physiotherapy becomes difficult late in pregnancy because the process is exhausting. Moving to new positions is difficult and lying prone, a position used frequently in postural drainage, is contraindicated in late pregnancy. A woman may need to plan more frequent and shorter sessions in modified positions (other than prone) to prevent exhaustion (see Fig. 20.2). Fetal health will be monitored by ultrasound and cardiotocograph to identify intrauterine growth restriction.

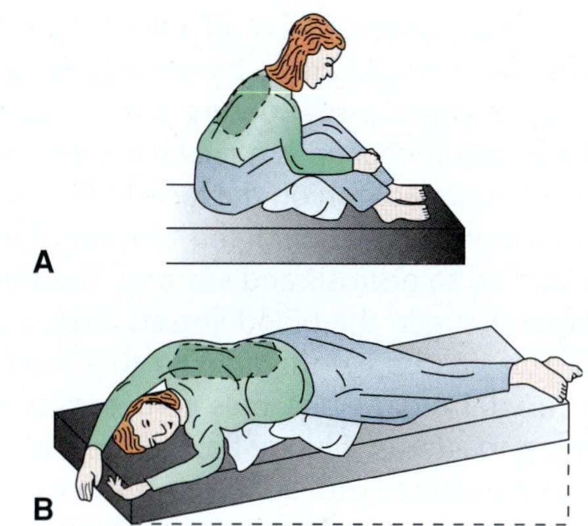

FIGURE 20.2 Modified positions for chest physiotherapy during pregnancy: (**A**) chest physiotherapy for the upper lobes; (**B**) chest physiotherapy for the lower lobes.

After birth extra rest may be required. Women with cystic fibrosis may breastfeed, however, they need to ensure they have an adequate calorie intake, their medications are safe for breastfeeding and the baby is growing appropriately. If not, formula supplementation may be recommended by the paediatrician.

RHEUMATIC DISORDERS

Careful history taking, assessment and planning improves pregnancy outcomes. Women with rheumatic disorders experience pain and discomfort during pregnancy and it may be difficult to achieve a pain-free pregnancy. Care needs to focus on keeping pain tolerable so women can enjoy their pregnancy and prepare for motherhood.

Rheumatoid arthritis

Rheumatic arthritis is a chronic autoimmune disease involving synovial membrane destruction, inflammation, swelling, erythema and painful joint motion tissue damage (Guthrie et al., 2010). The estimated prevalence is 0.5–1% (Orellana et al., 2014). Women with juvenile rheumatoid arthritis (JRA) frequently take corticosteroids, hydroxychloroquine and NSAIDs to prevent joint pain and loss of mobility. A number of women also take low-dose methotrexate (pregnancy risk category X) pre-pregnancy but this must be discontinued during pregnancy because of the danger of fetal defects.

Symptoms of rheumatoid arthritis improve in pregnancy for 48–66% of women, however postpartum flares occur in the first 4 months for most women as corticosteroid levels fall to the pre-pregnancy level (Ateka-Barrutia & Nelson-Piercy, 2013).

SYSTEMIC LUPUS ERYTHEMATOSUS

Systemic lupus erythematosus (SLE) is a multisystem chronic disease of connective tissue that occurs most frequently in women 20 to 40 years of age (Lateef & Petri,

2012). Widespread degeneration of connective tissue (especially of the heart, kidneys, blood vessels, spleen, skin and retroperitoneal tissue) occurs with onset of the illness. A marked skin change is a characteristic, erythematous butterfly-shaped rash on the face. In the kidneys, fibrin deposits develop, plugging and blocking the glomeruli and leading to necrosis and scarring. The thickening of collagen tissue in the blood vessels causes vessel obstruction. This can be life-threatening to a woman, if blood flow to vital organs becomes compromised, and life-threatening to a fetus, if blood flow to the placenta is obstructed. Many women with SLE have antiphospholipid antibodies, which increase the tendency for thrombi to form (Baer & Petri, 2011). In contrast, marked thrombocytopenia (decreased platelet count) is present, so clotting may be deficient.

A woman may be taking NSAIDs, heparin, salicylates hydroxychloroquine, low-dose prednisone, or azathioprine (an immunosuppressant) to reduce disease symptoms. These may be continued during pregnancy but salicylates may be reduced 2 weeks prior to labour to prevent bleeding in the newborn. The naturally increased circulation of corticosteroids during pregnancy may lessen symptoms in some women. In others, the chief complication of the disorder—acute nephritis with glomerular destruction—may occur for the first time during pregnancy. Nephritis leads to increased blood pressure, haematuria, decreased urine output, proteinuria and oedema. It is difficult to differentiate these symptoms from the symptoms of pregnancy-induced hypertension, except that with pregnancy-induced hypertension there is no haematuria. Frequent monitoring of serum creatinine levels is necessary to assess kidney function. If the creatinine level is over 132 μmol/L in combination with proteinuria and a decreased creatinine clearance, dialysis, to remove excess creatinine or plasmapheresis, to replace platelets, may be necessary to guard against haemorrhage in the woman at birth.

During the postpartum period, there may be an acute exacerbation of symptoms in a woman as corticosteroid levels fall to normal. Women with SLE have increased risk of preeclampsia, thrombosis, preterm birth and fetal growth restriction (Ateka-Barrutia & Nelson-Piercy, 2013).

Neonatal lupus syndrome can result from maternal antibodies crossing the placenta, causing symptoms in the fetus and neonate. The cutaneous form causes a lupus-like rash which usually disappears in 3–6 months. Congenital heart block is the most severe form and develops in utero between 16 and 30 weeks. The risk of perinatal death is 10–20% and most infants who survive require a pacemaker (Ateka-Barrutia & Nelson-Piercy, 2013).

GASTROINTESTINAL DISORDERS

Although minor gastrointestinal discomforts (such as nausea, heartburn, constipation) are common during pregnancy, acute abdominal pain and protracted vomiting are causes for concern. Abdominal pain may be associated with conditions completely unrelated to the pregnancy such as ulcerative colitis, hepatitis, hiatal hernia or cholecystitis. These conditions may be known to a woman before she becomes pregnant, or they may develop or be discovered during her pregnancy. Women who have colostomies can complete pregnancy without difficulty. Even a previous liver transplant is not a contraindication to pregnancy (Parhar, Gibson & Coffin, 2012).

Appendicitis

Appendicitis is inflammation of the appendix. Its incidence is high in young adults and so occurs as frequently as 1 in 1500 to 2000 pregnancies (Miloudi et al., 2012). A thorough history is important. Appendicitis usually begins with a few hours of nausea, and then an hour or two of generalised abdominal discomfort and vomiting followed by the typical sharp, peristaltic, lower right quadrant pain of acute appendicitis.

The pain associated with appendicitis is different from the pain that occurs suddenly from an overstretched round ligament during pregnancy. Pain from an overstretched ligament may cause sharp lower quadrant pain if a woman stands up suddenly, but the pain fades again almost instantly. Appendicitis pain continues and grows more intense. Appendicitis pain is also different from that of ectopic pregnancy. With ectopic pregnancy, a woman may have morning sickness because she is pregnant; the nausea and vomiting of appendicitis is much more intense. The pain of ectopic pregnancy may be either diffuse or sharp. In the non-pregnant woman, the pain of appendicitis becomes sharp and localised. In the pregnant woman, the appendix is often displaced higher in the abdomen so the localised pain may resemble the pain of gallbladder disease. A complete blood count will reveal leucocytosis (often normal in pregnancy). Elevated temperature and ketones in urine are common. An ultrasound will reveal the inflamed appendix. Once appendicitis it suspected it is important to prevent eating or drinking as increasing peristalsis could cause an inflamed appendix to rupture.

If a woman is near term (past 37 weeks) and the fetus is believed to be mature, a caesarean birth and appendectomy may be performed at the same time. If appendicitis occurs early in pregnancy, the inflamed appendix is removed by laparoscopy.

If the appendix ruptures before surgery, the risk to both mother and fetus increases dramatically. This is because with rupture, infected faecal material escapes into the peritoneum and could spread by the fallopian tubes to the fetus. Also generalised peritonitis is such an overwhelming infection that it is difficult for a woman's body to combat it effectively and also maintain the pregnancy.

Gastro-oesophageal reflux disease and hiatal hernia

Heartburn and acid reflux are common in pregnancy and are related to relaxation of the GI tract related to pregnancy hormones which reduce gastric motility and tone, and delay gastric emptying. Gastro-oesophageal reflux disease (GORD) refers to the reflux of acid stomach secretions into the oesophagus (Fill Malfertheiner et al., 2012). Hiatal hernia is a condition in which a portion of the stomach extends and protrudes up through the diaphragm into the oesophagus, trapping stomach acid and causing it to reflux into the oesophagus. Although these conditions can be present constantly, symptoms most often occur only sporadically after increased peristaltic action. Both conditions may generate symptoms for the first time during pregnancy as the uterus pushes the stomach up against the oesophageal valve and increases the reflux of acid or the extent of the hernia. Symptoms include:

- Heartburn, which is particularly extreme when lying supine after a full meal
- Gastric regurgitation
- Dysphagia (difficulty swallowing)
- Possible weight loss because of the inability to eat
- Haematemesis (vomiting of blood) if extreme oesophageal irritation occurs from the reflux of hydrochloric acid from the stomach.

In most women, antacids and lifestyle changes such as reducing caffeine, avoiding hypoglycaemia and stress, and sleeping with the head elevated will relieve pain. A histamine receptor antagonist, such as ranitidine, can be prescribed to inhibit gastric acid production and help minimise pain. The proton-pump inhibitor, omeprazole, is safe during pregnancy, but other proton-pump inhibitors are not recommended in pregnancy due to teratogenicity in animal studies. After pregnancy, as the uterine pressure is decreased, the symptoms generally become less noticeable or disappear.

Cholecystitis and cholelithiasis

Cholecystitis (gallbladder inflammation) and cholelithiasis (gallstone formation) are most frequently associated with women >40 years, obesity, multiparity and ingestion of a high-fat diet. Symptoms include constant aching and pressure in the right epigastrium, perhaps accompanied by jaundice. Gallstones are formed from cholesterol. It is debated whether the hypercholesterolemia that naturally occurs during pregnancy leads to an increased incidence of cholecystitis or cholelithiasis, but both these conditions are seen with pregnancy.

Medical therapy for both conditions is to lower fat intake. A woman should eat a low-fat but not a fat-free diet during pregnancy because of the importance of linoleic acid for fetal brain growth. Cholecystitis can be diagnosed by ultrasound. If an acute episode occurs during pregnancy, it can generally be managed by temporarily halting oral intake to rest the gastrointestinal tract, administering intravenous fluids to provide fluid and nutrients as well as analgesics for pain. Surgery for gallbladder removal by laparoscopic technique may be done during pregnancy if a woman's symptoms cannot be controlled by conservative management (Othman et al., 2012).

Inflammatory bowel disease

Crohn's disease (inflammation of the terminal ileus) and ulcerative colitis (inflammation of the distal colon) occur most often between ages 12 and 30 years and are therefore seen in pregnancy. The cause of these diseases is unknown, but an autoimmune process is thought to be responsible. They are associated with passive and active smoking (van der Heide et al., 2010). In both diseases, the bowel develops shallow ulcers. A woman experiences chronic diarrhoea, weight loss, occult blood in stool, nausea and vomiting. If extreme, obstruction and fistula formation with peritonitis can occur. With Crohn's disease, malabsorption, particularly of vitamin B (a substance whose absorption occurs almost entirely in the ileum), occurs. Because of the potential difficulty with absorbing nutrients, women with both disorders need careful monitoring for weight gain during pregnancy.

These diseases have the potential for interfering with fetal growth if extreme malabsorption occurs. Sulfasalazine (Azulfidine) an anti-inflammatory is a mainstay of therapy and may be continued during pregnancy. It poses a slight risk of haemolysis in the infant, and close to birth, the dosage is reduced because it may interfere with bilirubin binding sites and cause neonatal jaundice (McKenna & Mirkov, 2014).

EPILEPSY

Epilepsy is the most common neurological complication of pregnancy with an incidence of 0.3 to 0.7% (Ruth & Barnett, 2013). Epilepsy, and the medications used for its control, increase the risk of adverse fetal outcomes and the risk of congenital anomalies. Seizure prevention is important as severe seizures could result in fetal oxygen deprivation. However, 90% of infants born to women suffering from epilepsy will be healthy with appropriate management and monitoring (Jordan, 2010).

Preconception counselling provides information to women on their risk. Women should be informed to commence 4 mg of folic acid daily (antiepileptic medications interfere with folic acid metabolism) and to change medications if necessary, with monotherapy at the lowest dose being ideal (Ruth & Barnett, 2013). Seizure medications are mildly teratogenic but they must be continued during pregnancy (Burakgazi, Pollard & Harden, 2011). The risk of adverse maternal or fetal outcomes from seizures during pregnancy is greater than the risk of teratogenicity from anticonvulsant drugs (McKenna & Mirkov, 2014). All women should have an evaluation of serum medication levels before pregnancy or early in pregnancy to establish that their medication is being prescribed at a therapeutic level (Ruth & Barnett, 2013). As blood volume increases with pregnancy, some women may need their dosage increased or their serum level will be diluted. Common medications prescribed to control seizures are:

- Carbamazepine
- Sodium valproate
- Phenytoin
- Lamotrigine
- Levetiracetam.

Phenytoin sodium (Dilantin) can cause a syndrome involving fetal cognitive impairment and facial characteristics similar to fetal alcohol syndrome. This may occur because of competition for folic acid binding sites. Some infants have an increased danger of neural tube disorders as a result of this folic acid displacement. An ultrasound can rule out this possibility.

Infants are also prone to haemorrhagic disease of the newborn because of decreased levels of vitamin K coagulation factors at birth from phenytoin. To counteract this, women may be prescribed vitamin K during labour or in the last 4 weeks of gestation. Women who have been taking phenytoin (Dilantin) may have developed chronic hypertension. For these women, a baseline blood pressure should be established early in pregnancy so that changes can be interpreted correctly.

A normal birth is recommended with caesarean section for obstetric indications only. Medications should be continued during labour. If a general anaesthetic is necessary, the anaesthetist must be aware of the condition, otherwise, during anaesthesia induction, a seizure could occur. Breastfeeding is considered safe, however, there is a lack of studies on the effect of antiepileptic medications on infants.

MULTIPLE SCLEROSIS

Multiple sclerosis (MS) occurs predominantly in women of childbearing age, usually between 20 and 45 (McMurty, Baird & Dalton, 2013). Multiple sclerosis results from an autoimmune response which causes chronic inflammation that damages the myelin sheath around neurons resulting in acute and chronic lesions that alter the conduction of electrical impulses to muscles. Women develop symptoms of fatigue, weakness, numbness, blurred vision and loss of coordination. Pregnancy down-regulates the immune system so MS tends to improve during pregnancy; however, in the 3–6 months after birth the relapse rate increases significantly (McMurty, Baird & Dalton, 2013). If women experience worsening MS during pregnancy they may need corticosteroids. The side effects of corticosteroids include hyperglycaemia, hypertension, psychosis and poor wound healing. Corticosteroids also cross the placenta increasing risks for the fetus (McMurty, Baird & Dalton, 2013).

Many medications used to manage MS are not safe in pregnancy so medications should be adjusted prior to conception. Medications such as Interferon-β and glatiramer acetate do not increase teratogenic risk. Cyclophosphamide is a category D medication and is not considered safe in pregnancy. Existing bowel and bladder problems may be exacerbated, and risk of urinary tract infections increases. Women with MS are at increased risk of falls because of spasticity and weakness which is worsened by the changing centre of gravity of pregnancy. In labour, women with MS may not feel their contractions and may need to be shown how to palpate contractions so they are aware of the onset of labour.

Breastfeeding may be promoted if medications that are safe during breastfeeding are used. Additional help may be required for caring for the newborn and ensuring adequate rest for the mother.

ENDOCRINE DISORDERS

Diabetes mellitus is the most common endocrine disorder; the next most common is thyroid dysfunction. Endocrine disorders have the potential to be serious complications during pregnancy because enzymes and hormones control many specific body functions (Amin, Robinson & Teoh, 2011).

Thyroid dysfunction

The pregnancy hormones, human chorionic gonadotropin (hCG) and oestrogen increase thyroid hormone levels. The thyroid gland enlarges (hypertrophies) slightly because of increased vascularity and blood flow. Thyroid hormones are responsible for energy levels, body temperature regulation and assist organs to function. Adequate levels of thyroid hormones are important for fetal development.

Hypothyroidism

Worldwide, iodine deficiency is the most common cause of hypothyroidism. Iodine deficiency during pregnancy is associated with maternal goitre and decreased thyroid hormones. In Australia and New Zealand the most common cause of hypothyroidism in pregnancy is Hashimoto's disease, also known as chronic thyroiditis. This occurs when a woman's own antibodies attack the thyroid gland. Overall overt hypothyroidism occurs in 0.3–0.5% of pregnancies with subclinical hypothyroidism in 2–3% of pregnancies (Granfors et al., 2013). Overt hypothyroidism is symptomatic and marked by low free thyroxine hormone and elevated thyroid stimulating hormone (TSH). Subclinical hypothyroidism refers to thyroid hormone deficiency (normal free thyroxine but elevated TSH in women without clinical symptoms) (Reid et al., 2013). The symptoms of hypothyroidism include dry skin, difficulty concentrating, fatigue, hair loss, intolerance to cold, joint and muscle pain and weight gain, however women may also be asymptomatic.

Untreated hypothyroidism is associated with anovulatory cycles and difficulty conceiving. The complications of hypothyroidism during pregnancy include an increased risk of miscarriage, gestational hypertension and preeclampsia, placental abruption, anaemia and postpartum haemorrhage. Fetal complications include prematurity, IUGR, developmental delay, neonatal respiratory distress, increased rates of perinatal mortality and morbidity, and congenital hypothyroidism.

The treatment of choice for hypothyroidism is levothyroxine (Oroxine or Eutroxsig). International guidelines recommend treatment when the TSH level is above 2.5 mIU/L (Granfors et al., 2013). In the first trimester levothyroxine dosage will need to be increased to 30 to 50% above the preconception dose by 4–6 weeks of gestation to simulate the increase that would normally occur in pregnancy (De Groot et al., 2012). When hypothyroidism is diagnosed antenatally thyroid function tests should be normalised as quickly as possible. Thyroid function will need to be monitored every 4–6 weeks throughout pregnancy. Women should separate thyroxine ingestion from any preparations containing iron, aluminium, calcium sucrafate, proton pump inhibitors or soy products by about 4 hours because these substances can reduce absorption (McKenna & Mirkov, 2014). Women with hypothyroidism may be more sensitive to opioids and a normal dosage may cause excessive sedation (Jordan, 2010).

Postnatally the dose of levothyroxine prescribed for pregnancy is usually tapered; however, breastfeeding women may require more than their pre-pregnancy dosage (Juan, Adele, Rachel & Terry, 2010). Levothyroxine (T4) is a normal component of human milk and does not have adverse effects on infants. For breastfeeding mothers a daily intake of 250 μg iodine is recommended because breastfed infants are dependent on maternal iodine (De Groot et al., 2012).

Hyperthyroidism

Hyperthyroidism is an excessive production of thyroid hormones caused by both immune and non-immune factors. Thyroid disease occurs in approximately 0.1–0.4% of pregnancies and in 85–95% of cases is due to Graves' disease. In Graves' disease, the thyroid-stimulating immunoglobulin antibody (also called TSH receptor antibody) mimics TSH and stimulates the thyroid to overproduce thyroid hormone, eventually resulting in a hyperthyroid state (Vandana et al., 2014). Gestational transient hyperthyroidism is related to hyperemesis and is marked by an elevated serum fT4 and a low serum TSH with no detectable thyroid autoimmunity. Gestational transient thyrotoxicosis has not been linked with poor pregnancy outcomes (Vandana et al., 2014).

If a low serum TSH is detected during pregnancy, it must be differentiated from normal pregnancy changes and gestational thyrotoxicosis. Clinically hyperthyroidism can be confused with pregnancy changes such as nervousness, heat intolerance and palpitations, enlarged thyroid and weight loss (Vandana et al., 2014). Hyperthyroidism during pregnancy increases the risk of preterm birth, IUGR, preeclampsia, congestive heart failure and fetal death. Maternal overtreatment can cause iatrogenic fetal hyperthyroidism and under treatment can cause congenital hypothyroidism (De Groot et al., 2012). Untreated hyperthyroidism in pregnancy can result in severe thyrotoxicosis (thyroid storm), an acute life-threatening condition which presents with fever, tachycardia, tremor, nausea, vomiting, diarrhoea, dehydration and delirium or coma, and may lead to thyrotoxic heart failure (Vandana et al., 2014).

The preferred treatment for hyperthyroidism in the first trimester is propylthiouracil (PTU) because methimazole (MMI) taken during the period of organogenesis is associated with congenital abnormalities. In the second trimester MMI is recommended because, on rare occasions, PTU has been associated with liver toxicity (De Groot et al., 2012). Radioactive iodine is contraindicated in pregnancy and subtotal thyroidectomy is only considered if a woman has a serious reaction to antithyroid drug therapy, requires high doses or has uncontrolled hyperthyroidism; the optimal time for surgery is the second trimester (De Groot et al., 2012).

Fetal and neonatal hyperthyroidism leading to increased morbidity and mortality occurs in 1–5% of pregnancies complicated by Graves' disease (Vandana et al., 2014). Serial ultrasounds can be used to monitor fetal wellbeing. Newborns of mothers with Graves' disease should be evaluated at birth.

Thyroid receptor antibodies cross the placenta and may stimulate the fetal thyroid; evidence of fetal thyroid dysfunction includes enlarged thyroid, IUGR, hydrops, goitre, tachycardia or cardiac failure. Fetal goitre can obstruct the airway and make resuscitation difficult for the infant at birth. If hyperthyroidism is not regulated during pregnancy, an infant may be born with symptoms of hyperthyroidism because of the excess stimulation received in utero. The infant may appear jittery, and tachypnoea and tachycardia may be present. An assay of fetal cord blood will reveal the level of T4 and thyroid-stimulating hormone and the need for therapy in the infant.

Previously propylthiouracil (PTU) was considered the preferred antithyroid drug during lactation; however the association with liver toxicity may result in more use of methimazole (liver damage has not been reported in breastfeeding infants). Only small amounts of PTU are present in breastmilk and PTU dosages of 300 mg daily in divided doses are considered safe for breastfeeding mothers (Fumarola et al., 2011). To minimise infant exposure, PTU can be taken immediately after breastfeeding and then wait 3 to 4 hours before breastfeeding again.

Diabetes mellitus

Diabetes mellitus is a complex metabolic disorder with hyperglycaemia occurring as a result of defective insulin secretion and/or action. Insufficient insulin secretion and decreased tissue responses to insulin lead to deficient insulin action on the target tissues which in turns causes abnormalities of carbohydrate, fat and protein metabolism (Craig et al., 2014). According to the Australian Institute of Health and Welfare (AIHW), the prevalence of diabetes (excluding gestational diabetes mellitus) in Australia has more than doubled in the last 20 years from 1.5% to 4.2%. In 2011–2012 approximately 999,000 Australians were diagnosed as having diabetes (11.9% with type 1 and 84.9% with type 2), with Aboriginal and Torres Strait Islander peoples having three times the rate of non-Indigenous Australians (AIWH, 2013). The number of women of reproductive age with obesity, type 2 diabetes and gestational diabetes is increasing.

Before insulin was produced synthetically in 1921, women with type 1 diabetes died before reaching child-bearing age, were infertile or had spontaneous miscarriages early in pregnancy. Now that both type 1 and type 2 diabetes can be well managed, new challenges have developed:

- How to manage type 1 and type 2 diabetes during pregnancy to achieve a healthy glucose/insulin balance
- How to protect an infant in utero from the adverse effects of increased glucose levels
- How to care for the infant in the first 24 hours after birth until the infant's insulin-glucose regulatory mechanism stabilises.

Reproductive planning may be a fourth concern as both the oestrogen and progesterone in oral contraceptives increases insulin resistance (De Leo et al., 2013).

The primary problem of any woman with diabetes is controlling the balance between insulin and blood glucose levels to prevent hyperglycaemia or hypoglycaemia. If a woman's insulin level is insufficient, glucose cannot be used by body cells. The cells register their need for glucose and the liver quickly converts stored glycogen to glucose to increase the serum glucose level. Because of the insulin insufficiency, however, the body cells still cannot use the glucose, so the serum glucose levels continue to rise (hyperglycaemia). When the level of blood glucose rises the kidneys begin to excrete quantities of glucose in the urine (glycosuria) in an attempt to lower the level. Because of osmotic action, the increased amount of glucose in the urine reduces fluid absorption in the kidney and large quantities of fluid are lost in urine (polyuria). Normally this occurs with a blood glucose reading above 9–10 mmol/L; during pregnancy this may occur at a much lower blood glucose level.

As dehydration begins to occur, the blood serum becomes concentrated and the total blood volume decreases. With the reduced blood flow, cells do not receive adequate oxygen, and anaerobic metabolism reactions cause large stores of lactic acid to pour out of the muscles into the bloodstream. To replace needed glucose, fat is mobilised from fat stores and metabolised for energy, pouring large amounts of acidic ketone bodies into the bloodstream.

As the process continues, protein stores are tapped in a final attempt to find a source of energy. Utilising protein for energy reduces the supply of protein to body cells. As cells die, they release potassium and sodium, which is lost through extensive polyuria. The combination of these factors creates an immediate severe metabolic acidosis. Long-term effects are vascular narrowing that leads to kidney, heart and retinal dysfunction.

Diabetes during pregnancy

Pregnancy may be complicated by type 1, type 2 and gestational diabetes. Women with type 1 or type 2 diabetes who successfully regulated glucose and insulin metabolism before pregnancy may develop less-than-optimal control during pregnancy, because of changes in the glucose-insulin regulatory system as pregnancy progresses. In normal pregnancy, maternal glucose metabolism alters in order to meet the energy needs of the mother and her growing fetus, making pregnancy a diabetogenic state. Reduced insulin sensitivity occurs by 12–14 weeks gestation and continues to decline over the second and third trimesters (Lowe & Karban, 2014). The placenta and pregnancy hormones been implicated in the increased insulin resistance of normal pregnancy (human placental lactogen and high levels of cortisol, oestrogen, progesterone and catecholamines). Insulin secretion increases during pregnancy (to about double the pre-pregnancy levels) by the third trimester (Lowe & Karban, 2014). Fasting glucose levels typically decrease in pregnancy, stabilising at around 28 weeks' gestation, however in obese women this decrease does not occur (Lowe & Karban, 2014). Metabolomics is a new technology being used to examine insulin resistance and hyperglycaemia during pregnancy. Metabolites provide information on environmental exposures including physical activity, lifestyle, diet and underlying genetic factors (Low & Karban, 2014).

Placental insulinase may cause increased breakdown or degradation of insulin. This resistance to, or destruction of, insulin is helpful in a normal pregnancy because it prevents the blood glucose from falling to dangerous limits, despite the increased insulin secretion that occurs. It causes difficulty for a pregnant woman with diabetes, however, in that she must increase her insulin dosage, beginning at about week 24 of pregnancy, to prevent hyperglycaemia. At the same time, the continued use of glucose by the fetus may lead to **hypoglycaemia** (lowered serum glucose levels) for the mother between meals; this is most apt to occur overnight. A low maternal level of glucogenic amino acids (used by the liver to produce glucose) compounds this. A woman may become ketoacidotic from the breakdown of stored fat between meals, most likely during the second and third trimesters. An increase in the amount of amniotic fluid occurs in at least 25% of diabetic women, probably because of hyperglycaemia in the fetus that causes increased urine production.

If this becomes extreme, amniocentesis may need to be carried out, to decrease the level of amniotic fluid. Unfortunately, this exposes a woman to infection and possible preterm labour and is only a temporary measure because amniotic fluid is continually produced.

Glomerular filtration of glucose is increased (the glomerular excretion threshold is lowered), causing slight glycosuria. If a woman has pre-existing kidney disease (revealed by proteinuria, decreased creatinine clearance and hypertension), the risk of fetal growth restriction, asphyxia, stillbirth and maternal pregnancy-induced hypertension rises markedly (Negrato, Mattar & Gomes, 2012).

Infants of women with poorly-controlled diabetes tend to be large because maternal hyperglycaemia adds subcutaneous fat deposits. To counteract the overload of glucose the fetus produces more insulin, which acts as a growth stimulant, further increasing fetal growth (Tieu et al., 2014). A macrosomic infant (over 4000 grams) may create problems related to shoulder dystocia or cephalopelvic disproportion. When glucose regulation is poor, the risk of pregnancy-induced hypertension and infection (particularly monilial infection) increases. Infants of women with poorly-controlled diabetes tend to be large (over 4500 grams). At birth, the neonates are more prone to hypoglycaemia, respiratory distress syndrome, hypocalcaemia and hyperbilirubinaemia. Exposure to hyperglycaemia during pregnancy increases a child's risk of developing obesity and type 2 diabetes. A study on the long-term outcomes of children born to women with diabetes indicates a possible increased susceptibility to malignant neoplasms and circulatory system diseases related to maternal hyperglycaemia (Wu et al., 2012).

Diabetes classification

Type 1 diabetes mellitus is defined as an absolute deficiency of insulin resulting from chronic immune-mediated destruction of β-cells in the pancreas leading to insulin deficiency (Lung et al., 2013). The presence of diabetes-associated autoantibodies confirms the diagnosis of type 1 diabetes (Craig et al., 2014).

Type 2 diabetes mellitus results mainly from a relative insulin deficiency with an inadequate compensatory insulin secretory response, with or without insulin resistance (Craig et al., 2014). Monogenic diabetes is a milder, non-ketotic diabetes occurring in young people. It was originally named maturity-onset diabetes of the young (MODY), but is now considered as a group of heterozygous genetic mutations related to the development of β cells (Craig et al., 2014). There is significant overlap in the presentation of type 1, type 2 and monogenic diabetes. Type 2 diabetes is higher in all migrant groups when compared with Australian-born reference groups, with high rates for those born in Oceania, Southern and Central Asia, Northern Africa and the Middle East (Abouzeid et al., 2015).

Gestational diabetes mellitus (GDM) refers to glucose intolerance of variable severity, with an onset or first recognition during pregnancy (Nankervis et al., 2013). Higher rates of GDM occur in women from Chinese, Asian, Indian, Maori, Pacific Island and Aboriginal and Torres Strait Islander peoples. GDM usually occurs after the mid-point of pregnancy when insulin resistance becomes most noticeable. The incidence of gestational diabetes in a first pregnancy is 3.7% and the recurrence rate in a second consecutive pregnancy is 41.2% and in a third consecutive pregnancy 60.1% (Khambalia et al., 2013). Newly identified risk factors for recurrence include pregnancy hypertension, previous preterm birth and wide inter-pregnancy interval (Khambalia et al., 2013). GDM symptoms resolve at the completion of pregnancy, but the risk of developing type 2 diabetes later in life is increased. Risk factors for gestational diabetes are divided into moderate and high risk factors:

- Moderate risk factors:
  - Ethnicity: Asian, Indian subcontinent, Aboriginal, Torres Strait Islander, Pacific Islander, Māori, Middle Eastern, non-white African
  - BMI 25–35 kg/m^2
- High risk factors:
  - Previous GDM
  - Previously elevated blood glucose level
  - Maternal age ≥40 years
  - Family history of diabetes mellitus (1st-degree relative with diabetes or a sister with GDM)
  - BMI ≥35 kg/m^2
  - Previous macrosomia (baby with birth weight >4500 g or >90th percentile)
  - Polycystic ovarian syndrome
  - Medications: corticosteroids, antipsychotics.

Women in the high risk group for GDM (one high risk factor or two moderate risk factors) should have a 75-g POGTT with fasting, and one hour and two hour venous plasma samples once they are pregnant. Other risk factors may include a sedentary lifestyle, unexplained fetal or perinatal loss and congenital anomalies in previous pregnancies.

Assessment

The Hypertension and Adverse Pregnancy Outcome Study (HAPO) found a strong correlation between hyperglycaemia, obesity and poor maternal and fetal outcomes. The Australasian Diabetes in Pregnancy Society (ADIPS) introduced new Australian testing protocols for diabetes in pregnancy in 2014 and the new diagnostic criteria is scheduled for introduction in January 2015 (Wilkinson et al., 2014). The new diagnostic criteria will increase gestational diabetes mellitus (GDM) prevalence to around 13% (Nankervis et al., 2013). Diabetes can be a serious complication in pregnancy, therefore, the ADIPS consensus guidelines for the testing and diagnosis of gestational diabetes mellitus recommend all women should be screened for gestational diabetes. These recommendations were formulated in consultation with the International Association of Diabetes and Pregnancy Study

Groups (IADPSG) and are in line with current WHO recommendations:

1. Hyperglycaemia first detected at any time during pregnancy should be classified as either:
   (a) diabetes mellitus in pregnancy or
   (b) gestational diabetes mellitus
2. Diabetes mellitus in pregnancy should be diagnosed if one or more of the following criteria are met:
   (a) fasting plasma glucose is ≥7.0 mmol/L
   (b) 2-hour plasma glucose ≥11.1 mmol/L following a 75-g oral glucose load
   (c) a random plasma glucose ≥11.1 mmol/L in the presence of diabetes symptoms
3. The diagnosis of gestational diabetes mellitus at any time during pregnancy should be based on any of the following values:
   (a) Fasting plasma glucose 5.1–6.9 mmol/L
   (b) 1-hour post 75-g oral glucose load ≥ 10.0 mmol/L*
   (c) 2-hour post 75-g oral glucose load 8.5–11.0 mmol/L.

Monitoring a woman with diabetes

Women with type 1 or 2 diabetes should meet with an obstetrician or endocrinologist prior to conception because careful blood glucose control and prevention of hyperglycaemia can reduce the rate of congenital anomalies. The first trimester of pregnancy is the most important time for fetal development; if hyperglycaemia is minimised during this time, the chances of a congenital anomaly are greatly lessened. The **glycosylated haemoglobin** (HbA1c) should be maintained at <1% above the normal range which is generally <7%. A 1% increase in HbA1C increases the odds of poor pregnancy outcomes by 5–6%; however, preconception pregnancy care reduces the rates of congenital malformations and perinatal mortality (Wahabi, Alzeidan & Esmaeil, 2012). The rate of congenital cardiac abnormalities detected by ultrasound in women with diabetes was three times that found in women without diabetes (Newham et al., 2013).

The Australasian Diabetes in Pregnancy Society (ADIPS) recommends strict control of blood glucose levels prior to conception with HbA1c kept as close to normal as possible. A daily dose of 5 mg of folic acid should be commenced prior to conception for prevention of neural tube defects. Oral hypoglycaemic agents should be ceased prior to conception and screening for complications should be undertaken. General preconception advice should include the following: cessation of smoking; reduction of alcohol intake to safe levels; review of medications to ensure they are safe during pregnancy; assessment of immune status; and screening for infection, weight management and exercise. Pregnancy specific information and discussion should include: optimal glucose control to reduce risk of miscarriage, congenital malformation and perinatal mortality. Ideally, diabetes complications screening should be undertaken prior to pregnancy.

Nutrition

A healthy diet that provides optimum nutrition while maintaining normal blood glucose levels is recommended. Women who develop gestational diabetes are advised to begin a diabetic diet complemented by an exercise program as soon as they are diagnosed. Dietary control, or maintaining an adequate glucose intake so hypoglycaemia does not occur, may be extremely difficult early in pregnancy because of nausea and vomiting. Eating every 3–4 hours helps to keep the serum glucose level constant. Dietary recommendations vary but saturated fats should be reduced. Increasing fibre decreases postprandial hyperglycaemia and so lowers insulin requirements. Of dietary kilocalories, 20% should be from protein, 40% to 50% from carbohydrate and up to 30% from fat (Dornhorst & Williamson, 2012).

If vomiting, nausea or heartburn prevent eating and drinking, temporary intravenous fluid supplementation may be required. Women are extremely vulnerable to hypoglycaemia at night during pregnancy because of the continuous fetal use of glucose during the time they sleep. Eating a late evening snack containing protein and complex carbohydrate allows slow digestion during the night and will help prevent early morning hypoglycaemia.

Exercise during pregnancy

Exercise is another mechanism that lowers the serum glucose level and thereby the need for insulin. With exercise, the blood glucose level decreases because the muscles increase their need for glucose. This effect lasts for at least 12 hours after exercise. If the arm in which a woman injected insulin is actively exercised, the insulin is released so quickly that it can cause hypoglycaemia. To avoid this phenomenon, a woman should eat a snack consisting of protein or complex carbohydrate before exercise and should maintain a consistent exercise program (she should not do aerobic exercises one day and then none the next, but rather 30 minutes of walking every day). In a woman with poor blood glucose control, extreme exercise will cause hyperglycaemia and ketoacidosis as the liver both releases glucose and breaks down fatty acids in an attempt to supply enough energy for the exercise (yet the body cannot use them because of inadequate insulin) so exercise should be consistent day to day.

Therapeutic management

During pregnancy, management should be by a multidisciplinary team with experience in managing diabetes during pregnancy. Blood glucose monitoring during pregnancy and screening for diabetes complications is vital. An ophthalmic examination should be done once during pregnancy for a woman with gestational diabetes and at each trimester for women with known diabetes.

*There are no established criteria for the diagnosis of diabetes based on the 1-hour post-load value.

Background retinal changes, such as increased exudate, dot haemorrhage and macular oedema, can progress or originate during pregnancy. If proliferation retinopathy was present before pregnancy, this also progresses and can lead to blindness. Laser therapy to halt these changes can be carried out during pregnancy without risk to the fetus. A urine culture may be done each trimester to detect asymptomatic UTI as the increased glucose concentration in urine leads to increased infection. Screening for nephropathy should be done by an overnight 24-hour urine sample to note the albumin excretion rate, or an albumin/creatinine ratio from an early morning urine sample. If microalbuminuria is present the risk of preeclampsia is increased. Women with type 1 diabetes mellitus should have their thyroid function checked.

Monitoring of glucose levels is essential because maintaining blood glucose levels near normal helps minimise the risk of maternal and fetal complications. No studies have defined optimal glycaemic targets during pregnancy. The Australasian Diabetes in Pregnancy Society Consensus Guidelines Position Statement recognises the need for further research in this area and recommends the following, based on two standard deviations above the mean values for pregnant women without known risk factors:

- Fasting capillary blood glucose: ≤5.0 mmol/L
- 1-hour blood glucose after commencing meal: ≤7.4 mmol/L
- 2-hour blood glucose after commencing meal: ≤6.7 mmol/L.

The HbA1c should be monitored every 4–8 weeks and kept as close to the normal range as possible. Women with all categories of diabetes require more frequent antenatal visits than usual to ensure close monitoring of their condition and that of the fetus.

Insulin

Early in pregnancy, a woman with diabetes may need less insulin than before pregnancy because the fetus is using so much glucose for rapid cell growth. Later in pregnancy, she will need an increased amount because her metabolic rate increases. Women with gestational diabetes will be started on insulin therapy if diet alone is unsuccessful in regulating glucose values.

The type of insulin chosen is usually a short-acting insulin (regular) combined with an intermediate type. Two thirds of the total amount of the day's insulin is given in the morning; the other third is given in the evening. This is self-administered 30 minutes before breakfast in a ratio of 2:1 (intermediate to regular) and again just before dinner in a ratio of 1:1. Use of a very-short-acting insulin such as Lispro or aspart, which have a 1-hour peak time, can lead to more fluctuations in blood glucose levels than regular insulin but are ideal for some women. Women should eat almost immediately after injecting these short-acting insulins to prevent hypoglycaemia before mealtimes. Oral hypoglycaemia agents are not used for regulation during pregnancy because, unlike insulin, they cross the placenta.

A woman should be helped to plan her day based on the time interval her insulin takes to reach its peak. For example, an intermediate insulin given before breakfast reaches its peak after lunch or late in the afternoon, just before dinner. Regular insulin, given before breakfast, reaches its peak just after breakfast. An intermediate insulin, given in the evening, reaches its peak the next day before breakfast; the evening regular insulin injection peaks after dinner or at bedtime. Knowing when insulin reaches its peak level makes serum glucose monitoring meaningful and alerts women to the time of the day when they are most apt to be hypoglycaemic (see Chapter 48).

Blood glucose monitoring

Women with diabetes need to carry out blood glucose monitoring to determine whether hyperglycaemia or hypoglycaemia exists. For this, a woman typically uses a fingerstick technique, using one of her fingertips as the site of lancet puncture. She places a drop of blood on a test strip. The strip is then inserted into a glucose meter that determines the glucose level. If hypoglycaemia is present some form of sustained carbohydrate, such as a glass of milk and some crackers, should be ingested followed by a complex carbohydrate to help prevent rebound hypoglycaemia.

If hyperglycaemia is present urine should be tested for ketones. A healthcare provider should be notified if ketones are detected. Acidosis during pregnancy must be prevented because maternal acidosis leads to fetal anoxia due to fetal inability to use oxygen when body cells are acidotic. The most common time during pregnancy for hypoglycaemia is the second and third months, before insulin resistance peaks; for hyperglycaemia, it is the sixth month, or the time insulin resistance is becoming most pronounced.

Insulin pump therapy (continuous subcutaneous insulin infusion)

An effective method to keep serum glucose constant during pregnancy is to administer insulin by a continuous pump (de Valk & Visser, 2011). An insulin pump is a small, automatic device. A syringe of regular insulin is placed in the pump chamber and a small-gauge needle is attached to a length of thin polyethylene tubing and implanted into the subcutaneous tissue of the abdomen or thigh (see Fig. 20.3). The pump infuses a set rate of insulin per hour into the subcutaneous tissue. Bolus doses of insulin can be dialled in and administered.

Tests for placental function and fetal wellbeing

Monitoring of fetal wellbeing is individualised depending on the woman's overall health. Women with diabetes tend to have infants with a higher-than-normal incidence of

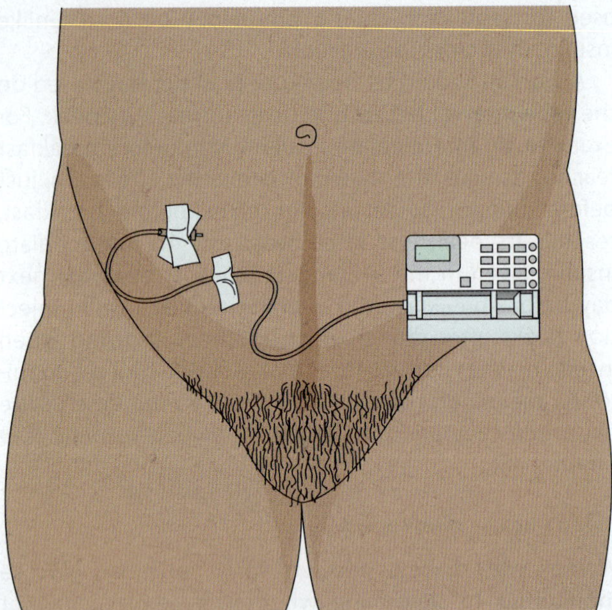

FIGURE 20.3 Using an insulin pump during pregnancy is the best assurance that insulin levels will remain constant.

birth anomalies, so screening tests are offered. The Australasian Diabetes in Pregnancy Society Position Statement (2005) recommends offering a first trimester nuchal translucency and first trimester biochemical screening with PAPP-A and B-hCG; a fetal morphology scan at 18–20 weeks with cardiac views at 24 weeks if required; and fetal growth at 28–30 weeks and 34–36 weeks. A creatinine clearance test may be ordered each trimester. A normal creatinine clearance rate suggests a woman's vascular system is intact because kidney function is normal. This implies uterine perfusion is also adequate. Placental functioning may also be assessed by a weekly non-stress test or biophysical profile during the last trimester with good glycaemic control or a daily non-stress test if glucose regulation is poor.

A woman may be asked to self-monitor fetal wellbeing by recording how many movements occur an hour. The healthy fetus makes approximately 10 movements per hour (see Chapter 9). Ultrasounds may be performed at week 28 and then again at weeks 36 to 38 to determine fetal growth, amniotic fluid volume, placental location and biparietal diameter. Oligohydramnios (a small amount of amniotic fluid) may indicate fetal growth restriction or fetal renal abnormality, whereas polyhydramnios (an excessive amount of amniotic fluid) may indicate gastrointestinal malformation or poorly controlled disease. With good glycaemic control and no additional complications there is no indication to induce labour before the pregnancy is full term.

Corticosteroids are given if a premature birth is anticipated but may lead to significant hyperglycaemia and an increased risk of ketoacidosis. Fetal lung maturity tends to occur later because synthesis of phosphatidylglycerol, the compound that stabilises surfactant, is delayed in a diabetes-complicated pregnancy. This increases the risk of infant respiratory distress syndrome (IRDS). During labour a woman with pre-existing diabetes needs to have her blood glucose monitored every 1–2 hours and maintained within 4–7 mmol/L. Management protocols vary between an insulin infusion, subcutaneous insulin injections or an insulin pump.

Regulating the glucose level carefully during labour reduces the possibility of rebound hypoglycaemia in the newborn. Interventions such as induction of labour and operative delivery should follow obstetric indications. Level 3 neonatal facilities may be necessary if birth occurs prior to 36 weeks or if there has been poor glycaemic control.

Postpartum management

Postpartum management of type 1 diabetes is important, as in the immediate postpartum period insulin requirements decrease rapidly. Close monitoring and adjustment of insulin therapy is required to avoid hypoglycaemia, particularly nocturnal hypoglycaemia and hypogloycaemia related to breastfeeding. Women with type 2 diabetes may maintain good glycaemic control postnatally with diet alone. Blood glucose levels should be monitored to ascertain the need for continued treatment with insulin.

A woman with gestational diabetes usually demonstrates normal glucose values by 24 hours after birth and needs no further diet or insulin therapy. During the immediate postpartum period the risk of haemorrhage may be increased due to poor uterine contractions related to hydramnios. Women with diabetes may breastfeed because insulin is one of the few substances that does not pass into breast milk from the bloodstream (de Valk & Visser, 2011).

A woman who had gestational diabetes is at risk of developing type 2 diabetes. Women with GDM should have a 75-g 2-hour OGTT, at 6–12 weeks postpartum. Women who desire another pregnancy should have an annual OGTT. Ongoing monitoring for the development of type 2 diabetes mellitus should be done every 1–2 years depending on the level of risk. For all women contraception options should be discussed; there is no evidence indicating any method of contraception is contraindicated.

MENTAL ILLNESS

Mental illness may precede or occur with pregnancy. Schizophrenia tends to have its highest incidence in adolescents and young adults and so may occur in young pregnant women. Depression occurs almost four times more commonly in women than in men and often in young adults. It is the most common mental illness seen in pregnant women.

Even normal levels of stress make it difficult to use effective coping mechanisms so pregnancy or childbirth may be the additional stress that reveals mental illness for the first time. Therefore, a woman with a psychiatric disorder should be cared for by both a psychiatric care team and an antenatal care group to ensure that the stress of pregnancy is not exacerbating the mental illness. Any psychotropic medication taken by a pregnant woman should be evaluated for possible fetal harm (Galbally, Snellen & Lewis, 2011). For example, lithium, a mainstay of therapy for mood disorders such as bipolar disorder (manic depression) and the serotonin-reuptake inhibitors used to counteract depression, are potentially teratogenic (McKenna & Mirkov, 2014).

Mental illness may also occur in the postpartum period (postpartum depression or psychosis; see Chapter 25).

Key points for review

- A high-risk pregnancy is one in which a concurrent disorder, pregnancy-related complication or external factor, jeopardises the health of the mother, the fetus, or both.
- Pregnancy is a stress to any family because it involves financial expenses plus changes in family roles. If a complication of pregnancy develops, this stress is almost automatically intensified. Families need support to be able to cope with the increased burden.
- When women with a pre-existing disease become pregnant, a thorough history and physical examination are crucial to obtain at the first antenatal visit to establish a baseline of information on the condition. Documentation of any medication being taken for a secondary condition is important to protect against adverse drug interactions and the possibility of teratogenic action on the fetus.
- Teaching is an important intervention because a woman with a pre-existing illness must make modifications in her usual therapy to adjust to pregnancy.
- Women who have a complication early in pregnancy may continue to worry about the health of their fetus all through pregnancy. They need to be assured (appropriately) that the episode was temporary and that, with continued monitoring, their fetus should not suffer harm.
- Because blood volume increases by as much as 50% during pregnancy, cardiac function may become inadequate if cardiovascular disease is present.
- Various forms of anaemia can cause complications of pregnancy; iron-deficiency anaemia, sickle cell anaemia and folic acid-deficiency anaemia are examples. All anaemias can result in fetal distress because of inadequate oxygen transport.
- Urinary tract disorders (UTIs) can lead to pregnancy complications because pregnancy increases the workload of the kidneys. UTIs and chronic renal disease are two disorders that may lead to early pregnancy loss.
- Acute nasopharyngitis, asthma, pneumonia and influenza are common respiratory disorders seen in pregnancy.
- Systemic lupus erythematosus is a rheumatic disorder seen in pregnancy. These disorders generally require large doses of NSAIDs for therapy. Women taking salicylates are advised to decrease use 2 weeks before birth to avoid bleeding disorders in the newborn.
- Some gastrointestinal illnesses that occur with pregnancy are hiatal hernia, cholecystitis, inflammatory bowel disease and appendicitis. If surgery is necessary for conditions such as cholecystitis or appendicitis, it can be performed by laparoscopic technique during pregnancy, but this may result in preterm labour.
- Recurrent seizures are the most frequently seen neurological condition during pregnancy. Many medications used to control seizures are teratogenic; women need to have their medical regimen carefully monitored during pregnancy.
- The major endocrine disorder seen during pregnancy is diabetes mellitus. Gestational diabetes is diabetes that occurs during pregnancy and resolves after birth.

CASE STUDY QUESTIONS

5. Angelina has developed congestive heart failure. She works at a job where she is on her feet almost all day. What suggestions could you make to help her incorporate some rest periods into her day?
6. Angelina has also developed gestational diabetes. She's resistant to learning about her condition, because she knows her symptoms are only temporary and will fade at the end of pregnancy. What type of teaching plan would you devise to help her learn in the face of this attitude?
7. Angelina is prone to urinary tract infections during pregnancy because of her gestational diabetes. What are common measures you can suggest to women to help avoid UTIs during pregnancy?
8. Examine the National Health Goals related to complications of pregnancy. Most government-sponsored money for nursing research is allocated based on these goals. What would be a possible research topic to explore pertinent to these goals that would be applicable to the Little family and also advance evidence-based practice?

Resources

For an extensive range of additional resources to enhance teaching and learning and to facilitate understanding of this chapter, please see the text's accompanying website located on thePoint at http://thepoint.lww.com.

References

Abouzeid, M., Versace, V. L., Janus, E. D., Davey, M. A., Philpot, B., Oats, J. & Dunbar, J. A. (2015). Socio-cultural disparities in GDM burden differ by maternal age at first delivery. *PLoS ONE, 10*(2), 1–11.

American Congress of Obstetricians and Gynecologists. (2012). ACOG Committee Opinion No. 486: Update on carrier screening for cystic fibrosis. *Obstetrics & Gynecology, 117*(4), 1028–1031.

Amin, A., Robinson, S. & Teoh, T. G. (2011). Endocrine problems in pregnancy. *Postgraduate Medical Journal, 87*(1024), 116–124.

Ateka-Barrutia, O. & Nelson-Piercy, C. (2013). Connective tissue disease in pregnancy. *Clinical Medicine, 13*(6), 580–584.

Australasian Diabetes in Pregnancy Society. (2005). Consensus guidelines for the management of patients with Type 1 and Type 2 diabetes in relation to pregnancy, accessed 31 March 2015 <http://adips.org/downloads/adips_pregdm_guidelines.pdf>.

Australasian Diabetes in Pregnancy Society. (2013). ADIPS consensus guidelines for the testing and diagnosis of gestational diabetes mellitus in Australia (2nd version), accessed 23 February 2015, <http://adips.org/downloads/ADIPSConsensusGuidelinesGDM-03.05.13VersionACCEPTEDFINAL.pdf>.

Australian Institute of Health and Welfare (AIHW). (2013). How common is diabetes? Accessed 31 March 2015, <www.aihw.gov.au/how-common-is-diabetes/#source>.

Australian Resuscitation Council (2015). Guidelines, accessed 31 March 2015, <http://resus.org.au/guidelines/>.

Baer, A. N. & Petri, M. (2011). Lupus and pregnancy. *Obstetrics and Gynecology Survey, 66*(10), 639–653.

Brushers, V. L. (2012). Alterations of pulmonary function. In S. E. Huether & K. L. McCance (Eds), *Understanding Pathophysiology* (5th ed.), pp. 678–706. St Louis: Elsevier Mosby.

Buckley, L. L. & Grose, S. (2013). Pneumonia in pregnancy. In D. Pravikoff & D. Pravikoff (Eds). Glendale, CA: Cinahl Information Systems.

Burakgazi, E. P., Pollard, J. & Harden, C. (2011). The effect of pregnancy on seizure control and antiepileptic drugs in women with epilepsy. *Reviews in Neurological Diseases, 8*(1–2), 16–22.

Chen, Y. H., Keller, J., Wang, I. T., et al. (2012). Pneumonia and pregnancy outcomes: A nationwide population-based study. *American Journal of Obstetrics & Gynecology, 207*(4), 288.e1–288.e7.

Clark, P., Thomson, A. J. & Greer, I. A. (2012). Haematological problems in pregnancy. In D. K. Edmonds (Ed), *Dewhurst's Textbook of Obstetrics & Gynaecology* (8th ed.), pp. 151–172. Oxford: John Wiley & Son.

Craig, M. E., Jefferies, C., Dabelea, D., Balde, N., Seth, A. & Donaghue, K. C. (2014). Definition, epidemiology, and classification of diabetes in children and adolescents. *Pediatric Diabetes, 15*(S20), 4–17.

Criteria Committee of the New York Heart Association. (1994). *Nomenclature and Criteria for Diagnosis of Diseases of the Heart and Great Vessels* (9th ed.). Boston: Little, Brown & Co.

Curry, R. A., Gelson, E., Swan, L., Dob, D., Babu-Narayan, S. V., Gatzoulis, M. A., Steer, P. J. & Johnson, M. R. (2014). Marfan syndrome and pregnancy: Maternal and neonatal outcomes. *BJOG, 121*, 610–617.

Danza, A., Ruiz-Irastorza, G. & Khamashta, M. (2012). Antiphospholipid syndrome in obstetrics. *Best Practice & Research in Clinical Obstetrics & Gynecology, 26*(1), 65–76.

De Groot, L., Abalovich, M., Alexander, E. K., et al. (2012). Management of thyroid dysfunction during pregnancy and postpartum: An Endocrine Society clinical practice guideline. *The Journal of Clinical Endocrinology and Metabolism, 97*(8), 2543–2565.

De Leo, V., Fruzzetti, F., Musacchio, M. C., Scolaro, V., Di Sabatino, A. & Morgante, G. (2013). Effect of a new oral contraceptive with estradiol valerate/dienogest on carbohydrate metabolism. *Contraception, 88*(3), 364–368.

de Valk, H. W. & Visser, G. H. (2011). Insulin during pregnancy, labour and delivery. *Best Practice & Research in Clinical Obstetrics and Gynaecology, 25*(1), 65–76.

Donner, B. N., Niranjan, V. & Hoffmann, G. (2010). Safety of oseltamivir in pregnancy: A review of preclinical and clinical data. *Drug Safety, 33*(8), 631–642.

Dornhorst, A. & Williamson, C. (2012). Diabetes & endocrine disease in pregnancy. In D. K. Edmonds (Ed.), *Dewhurst's Textbook of Obstetrics & Gynaecology* (6th ed., pp. 121–136). Oxford, UK: John Wiley & Son.

Easterling, T. R. & Stout, K. (2012). Heart disease. In S. G. Gabbe, J. R. Niebyl, J. L. Simpson, et al. (Eds), *Obstetrics: Normal and Problem Pregnancies* (8th ed.), pp. 825–850. Philadelphia: Elsevier/Saunders.

Fill Malfertheiner, S., Malfertheiner, M. V., Mönkemüller, K., et al. (2012). A prospective longitudinal cohort study: Evolution of GERD symptoms during the course of pregnancy. *BMC Gastroenterology, 12*(9), 131.

Fontana, I., Santori, G., Fazio, F., et al. (2012). The pregnancy rate and live birth rate after kidney transplantation: A single-center experience. *Transplantation Proceedings, 44*(7), 1910–1911.

Fried, M., Muehlenbachs, A. & Duffy, P. E. (2012). Diagnosing malaria in pregnancy: An update. *Expert Review of Anti-Infective Therapy, 10*(10), 1177–1187.

Fumarola, A., Di Fiore, A., Dainelli, M., Grani, G., Carbotta, G. & Calvanese, A. (2011). Therapy of hyperthyroidism in pregnancy and breastfeeding. *Obstetrical & Gynecological Survey, 66*(6), 378–389.

Gaillard, R., Eilers, P.H.C., Yassine, S., Hofman, A., Steegers, E.A.P. & Jaddoe, V.W.V. (2014). Risk factors and consequences of maternal anaemia and elevated haemoglobin levels during pregnancy: A population-based prospective cohort study. *Paediatric and Perinatal Epidemiology, 28*(3), 213–226.

Galbally, M., Snellen, M. & Lewis, A. J. (2011). A review of the use of psychotropic medication in pregnancy. *Current Opinion in Obstetrics & Gynecology, 23*(6), 408–414.

Gasim, T. (2011). Immune thrombocytopenic purpura in pregnancy: A reappraisal of obstetric management and outcome. *Journal of Reproductive Medicine, 56*(3–4), 163–168.

Gelson, E., Curry, R., Gatzoulis, M. A., et al. (2011). Effect of maternal heart disease on fetal growth. *Obstetrics and Gynecology, 117*(4), 886–891.

Gilbert, E. S. (2011). Cardiac disease. In E. S. Gilbert (Ed), *Manual of High Risk Pregnancy & Delivery* (5th ed.), pp. 243–257. St Louis: Mosby/Elsevier.

Goldie, M. H. & Brightling, C. E. (2013). Asthma in pregnancy. *Obstetrician & Gynaecologist, 15*(4), 241–245.

Gorman, J. R., Brewer, N. T., Wang, J. B., et al. (2012). Theory-based predictors of influenza vaccination among pregnant women. *Vaccine, 31*(1), 213–218.

Granfors, M., Akerud, H., Berglund, A., Skogö, J., Sundström-Poromaa, I. & Wikström, A. K. (2013). Thyroid testing and management of hypothyroidism during pregnancy: A population-based study. *Journal of Clinical Endocrinology & Metabolism, 98*(7), 2687–2692.

Greenberg, J. A., Bell, S. J., Guan, Y., et al. (2011). Folic acid supplementation and pregnancy: More than just neural tube defect prevention. *Reviews in Obstetrics & Gynecology, 4*(2), 52–59.

Guthrie, K. A., Dugowson, C. E., Voigt, L. F., et al. (2010). Does pregnancy provide vaccine-like protection against rheumatoid arthritis? *Arthritis & Rheumatism, 62*(7), 1842–1848.

Howard, J. & Oteng-Ntim, E. (2012). Management of sickle-cell disease. *Best Practice & Research: Clinical Obstetrics & Gynaecology, 26*(1), 25–36.

Humphreys, R. A., Wong, H. H., Milner, R., et al. (2012). Pregnancy outcomes among solid organ transplant recipients in British Columbia. *Journal of Obstetrics & Gynecology Canada, 34*(5), 416–424.

Imdad, A. & Bhutta, Z. A. (2012). Routine iron/folate supplementation during pregnancy: Effect on maternal anaemia and birth outcomes. *Paediatric & Perinatal Epidemiology, 26*(Suppl. 1), 168–177.

Irvine, M. H., Einarson, A. & Bozzo, P. (2011). Prophylactic use of antimalarials during pregnancy. *Canadian Family Physician, 57*(11), 1279–1281.

Jelkmann, W. (2011). Regulation of erythropoietin production. *Journal of Physiology, 589*(6), 1251–1258.

Johnson, S., Bonello, M. R., Li, Z., Hilder, L. & Sullivan, E. A. (2014). *Maternal Deaths in Australia 2006–2010.* Maternal deaths series no. 4. Cat. No. PER 61. Canberra: AIHW.

Jordan, S. (2010). *Pharmacology for Midwives: The Evidence Base for Safe Practice*. Basingstoke: Palgrave Macmillan.

Khambalia, A. Z., Ford, J. B., Nassar, N., Shand, A. W., McElduff, A. & Roberts, C. L. (2013). Occurrence and recurrence of diabetes in pregnancy. *Diabetic Medicine, 30*(4), 452–456.

Knope, K. E., Doggett, S. L., Kurucz, N., et al. (2014). Arboviral diseases and malaria in Australia, 2011-12: Annual report of the National

Arbovirus and Malaria Advisory Committee. *Communicable Diseases Intelligence Quarterly Report, 38*(2), E122–142.

Lam, W. W. (2012). Heart Disease and Pregnancy. *Texas Heart Institute Journal, 39*(2), 237–239.

Lateef, A. & Petri, M. (2012). Management of pregnancy in systemic lupus erythematosus. *Nature Reviews Rheumatology, 8*(12), 710–718.

Leung, T. Y. & Lao, T. T. (2012). Thalassaemia in pregnancy. *Best Practice & Research in Clinical Obstetrics & Gynaecology, 26*(1), 37–51.

Lewey, J. & Haythe, J. (2014). Cardiomyopathy in pregnancy. *Seminars in Perinatology, 38*(5), 309–317.

Lim, A., Hussainy, S. Y. & Abramson, M. J. (2013). Asthma drugs in pregnancy and lactation. *Australian Prescriber, 36*(5), 150–153.

Lopez, V., Martinez, D., Vinolo, C., et al. (2011). Pregnancy in kidney transplant recipients: Effects on mother and newborn. *Transplantation Proceedings, 43*(6), 2177–2178.

Lowe, W. L. & Karban, J. (2014). Genetics, genomics and metabolomics: New insights into maternal metabolism during pregnancy. *Diabetic Medicine, 31*(3), 254–262.

Lumb, R., Bastian, I., Carter, R., Jelfs, P., Keehner, T. & Sievers, A. (2009). Tuberculosis in Australia: Bacteriologically confirmed cases and drug resistance, 2007. *CDI, 33*(3), 298–303.

Lung, T.W.C., Clarke, P. M., Hayes, A. J., Stevens, R. J. & Farmer, A. (2013). Simulating lifetime outcomes associated with complications for people with type 1 diabetes. *PharmacoEconomics, 31*(6), 509–518.

McKenna, L. & Mirkov, S. (2014). *McKenna's Drug Handbook for Nursing & Midwifery* (7th ed.). Sydney: Lippincott Williams & Wilkins.

McMurty Baird, S. & Dalton, J. (2013). Multiple sclerosis in pregnancy. *Journal of Perinatal & Neonatal Nursing, 27*(3), 232–241.

Memoli, M. J., Harvey, H., Morens, D. M. & Taubenberger, J. K. (2013). Influenza in pregnancy. *Influenza & Other Respiratory Viruses, 7*(6), 1033–1039.

Mendola, P., Laughon, S. K., Männistö, T. I., et al. (2013). Obstetric complications among U.S. women with asthma. *American Journal of Obstetrics & Gynecology, 208*(2), 127.e1–127.e8.

Miloudi, N., Brahem, M., Ben Abid, S., et al. (2012). Acute appendicitis in pregnancy: Specific features of diagnosis and treatment. *Journal of Visceral Surgery, 149*(4), e275–279.

Mohan, A. R. & Nelson-Piercy, C. (2014). Drugs and therapeutics, including contraception, for women with heart disease. *Best Practice & Research Clinical Obstetrics and Gynaecology, 28*, 471–482.

Moreno, J. L., Kurita, M., Holloway, T., et al. (2011). Maternal influenza viral infection causes schizophrenia-like alterations of 5-HT. *Journal of Neuroscience, 31*(5), 1863–1872.

Nankervis, A., McIntyre, H. D., Moses, R. G., Ross, G. P. & Callaway, L. K. (2013). Testing for gestational diabetes mellitus in Australia. *Diabetes Care, 36*(5), e64–e64.

Negrato, C. A., Mattar, R. & Gomes, M. B. (2012). Adverse pregnancy outcomes in women with diabetes. *Diabetology & Metabolic Syndrome, 4*(1), 41.

Newham, J. J., Glinianaia, S. V., Tennant, P. W. G., Rankin, J. & Bell, R. (2013). Improved antenatal detection of congenital anomalies in women with pre-gestational diabetes: Population-based cohort study. *Diabetic Medicine, 30*(12), 1442–1448.

Ngô, C., Kayem, G., Habibi, A., Benachi, A., Goffinet, F., Galactéros, F. & Haddad, B. (2010). Pregnancy in sickle cell disease: Maternal and fetal outcomes in a population receiving prophylactic partial exchange transfusions. *European Journal of Obstetrics & Gynecology and Reproductive Biology, 152*(2), 138–142.

Nhan-Chang, C. L. & Jones, T. B. (2010). Tuberculosis in pregnancy. *Clinical Obstetrics & Gynecology, 53*(2), 311–321.

Orellana, C., Wedrén, S., Källberg, H., Holmqvist, M., Karlson, E. W., Alfredsson, L. & Bengtsson, C. (2014). Parity and the risk of developing rheumatoid arthritis: Results from the Swedish Epidemiological Investigation of Rheumatoid Arthritis study. *Annals of the Rheumatic Diseases, 73*(4), 752–755.

Othman, M. O., Stone, E., Hashimi, M., et al. (2012). Conservative management of cholelithiasis and its complications in pregnancy is associated with recurrent symptoms and more emergency department visits. *Gastrointestinal Endoscopy, 760*(3), 564–569.

Parhar, K. S., Gibson, P. S. & Coffin, C. S. (2012). Pregnancy following liver transplantation: Review of outcomes and recommendations for management. *Canadian Journal of Gastroenterology, 26*(9), 621–626.

Piccoli, G. B., Conijn, A., Consiglio, V., et al. (2010). Pregnancy in dialysis patients: Is the evidence strong enough to lead us to change our counseling policy? *Clinical Journal of The American Society of Nephrology, 5*(1), 62–71.

Rance, K. & O'Laughlen, M. C. (2013). Managing asthma during pregnancy. *Journal of the American Association of Nurse Practitioners, 25*(10), 513–521.

Reid, S. M., Middleton, P., Cossich, M. C., Crowther, C. A. & Bain, E. (2013). Interventions for clinical and subclinical hypothyroidism pre-pregnancy and during pregnancy. *Cochrane Database of Systematic Reviews* (5).

Rejnö, G., Lundholm, C., Gong, T., Larsson, K., Saltvedt, S. & Almqvist, C. (2014). Asthma during pregnancy in a population-based study - pregnancy complications and adverse perinatal outcomes. *PLoS ONE, 9*(8), 1–9.

Rote, N. S. & McCance, K. L. (2012). Structure and function of the hematologic system. In S. E. Huether & K. L. McCance, *Understanding Pathophysiology* (5th ed.), pp. 481–507. New York: Elsevier.

Ruth, D. J. & Barnett, J. (2013). Epilepsy in pregnancy. *Journal of Perinatal & Neonatal Nursing, 27*(3), 217–224.

Ruys, T. P., Roos-Hesselink, J. W., Hall, R., Subirana-Domenech, M. T., Grando-Ting, J., Estensen, M., Crepaz, R., Fesslova, V., Gurvitz, M., De Backer, J., Johnson, M. R. & Pieper, P. G. (2014). Heart failure in pregnant women with cardiac disease: Data from the ROPAC. *Heart, 100*, 231–238.

Samuels, P. (2012). Hematologic complications of pregnancy. In S. G. Gabbe, J. R. Niebyl, J. L. Simpson, et al. (Eds), *Obstetrics: Normal and Problem Pregnancies* (6th ed.), pp. 659–672. Philadelphia: Elsevier/Saunders.

Sawicki, E., Stewart, K., Wong, S., Leung, L., Paul, E. & George, J. (2011). Medication use for chronic health conditions by pregnant women attending an Australian maternity hospital. *Australian and New Zealand Journal of Obstetrics and Gynaecology, 51*(4), 333–338.

Schneeberger, C., Geerlings, S. E., Middleton, P., et al. (2012). Interventions for preventing recurrent urinary tract infection during pregnancy. *Cochrane Database of Systematic Reviews, 11* (CD009279).

Schub, T. & March, P. (2015). *Thrombophilia in pregnancy*. In D. Pravikoff & D. Pravikoff (Eds), p. 2. Glendale, CA: Cinahl Information Systems.

Shahbazi, S., Moghaddam-Banaem, L., Ekhtesari, F., et al. (2012). Impact of inherited bleeding disorders on pregnancy and postpartum hemorrhage. *Blood Coagulation & Fibrinolysis, 23*(7), 603–607.

Sorensen, H. T., Horvath-Puho, E., Lash, T. L., et al. (2011). Heart disease may be a risk factor for pulmonary embolism without peripheral deep venous thrombosis. *Circulation, 124*(13), 1435–1441.

Suri, V., Keepanasseril, A., Aggarwal, N., et al. (2011). Mechanical valve prosthesis and anticoagulation regimens in pregnancy: A tertiary center experience. *European Journal of Obstetrics & Gynecology and Reproductive Biology, 159*(2), 320–323.

Swan, L. (2014). Congenital heart disease in pregnancy. *Best Practice & Research Clinical Obstetrics and Gynaecology, 28*, 495–506.

Thorpe-Beeston, J., Madge, S., Gyi, K., et al. (2013). The outcome of pregnancies in women with cystic fibrosis-single centre experience 1998–2011. *BJOG: International Journal of Obstetrics & Gynaecology, 120*(3), 354–361.

Tieu, J., McPhee, A. J., Crowther, C. A. & Middleton, P. (2014). Screening and subsequent management for gestational diabetes for improving maternal and infant health. *Cochrane Database of Systematic Reviews, 2014*(2), (CD007222).

Traill, T. A. (2012). Valvular heart disease and pregnancy. *Cardiology Clinics, 30*(3), 369–381.

Trautner, B. W. (2012). Asymptomatic bacteriuria: When the treatment is worse than the disease. *Nature Reviews Urology, 9*(2), 85–89.

UpToDate. (2015). Patient information: Warfarin (Coumadin) (beyond the basics), accessed 31 March 2015, <www.uptodate.com/contents/warfarin-coumadin-beyond-the-basics>.

van der Heide, F., Nolte, I. M., Kleibeuker, J. H., et al. (2010). Differences in genetic background between active smokers, passive smokers, and non-smokers with Crohn's disease. *American Journal of Gastroenterology*, *105*(5), 1165–1172.

Vandana, Kumar, A., Khatuja, R. & Mehta, S. (2014). Thyroid dysfunction during pregnancy and in postpartum period: Treatment and latest recommendations. *Archives of Gynecology & Obstetrics*, *289*(5), 1137–1144.

Vause, S. & Clarke, B. (2014). Risk stratification and hierarchy of antenatal care. *Best Practice & Research: Clinical Obstetrics & Gynaecology*, *28*(4), 483–494.

Wahabi, H. A., Alzeidan, R. A. & Esmaeil, S. A. (2012). Pre-pregnancy care for women with pre-gestational diabetes mellitus: A systematic review and meta-analysis. *BMC Public Health*, *12*(1), 1–12.

Wilkinson, S. A., Lim, S. S., Upham, S., Pennington, A., et al., (2014). Who's responsible for the care of women during and after a pregnancy affected by gestational diabetes? *Medical Journal of Australia*, *201*(3 Suppl), S78–81.

Wolff, G. A. & Weitzel, N. S. (2011). Management of acquired cardiac disease in the obstetric patient. *Seminars in Cardiothoracic and Vascular Anesthesia*, *15*(3), 85–97.

Wu, C. S., Nohr, E. A., Bech, B. H., Vestergaard, M. & Olsen, J. (2012). Long-term health outcomes in children born to mothers with diabetes: A population-based cohort study. *PLoS ONE*, *7*(5), 1–7.

Suggested readings

Abayomi, J., Wood, L., Spelman, S., Morrison, G. & Purewal, T. (2013). The multidisciplinary management of type 2 and gestational diabetes in pregnancy. *British Journal of Midwifery*, *21*(4), 236–242.

Australian Diabetes Society. (2014). Life after gestational diabetes (GDM), accessed 23 February 2015, <https://diabetessociety.com.au/downloads/Life%20after%20gestational%20diabetes%20mellitus.pdf>.

Chamberlain, C., McLean, A., Oats, J., Oldenburg, B., Eades, S., Sinha, A. & Wolfe, R. (2015). Low rates of postpartum glucose screening among Indigenous and non-Indigenous women in Australia with gestational diabetes. *Maternal & Child Health Journal*, *19*(3), 651–663.

Chawla, R., Rankin, K. & Collins, J. (2014). The relation of a woman's impaired in utero growth and association of diabetes during pregnancy. *Maternal & Child Health Journal*, *18*(8), 2013–2019.

Diabetes Australia: <www.diabetesaustralia.com.au>.

Hayes, S. (2014). Using motivational interviewing to encourage women with gestational diabetes mellitus to breastfeed as a method of reducing their risk of type 2 diabetes mellitus. *Australian Nursing & Midwifery Journal*, *21*(10), 32–35.

Heart Foundation Australia: <www.heartfoundation.org.au>.

Heart Foundation New Zealand: <www.heartfoundation.org.nz>.

Poth, M. & Carolan, M. (2013). Pregnant women's knowledge about the prevention of gestational diabetes mellitus: A qualitative study. *British Journal of Midwifery*, *21*(10), 692–700.

Chapter 21

Sudden pregnancy complications

Previous chapters described normal pregnancy and pre-existing and newly acquired conditions that can complicate pregnancy. This chapter adds knowledge about complications directly related to the pregnancy. Such complications can cause as much concern and worry for women as illnesses brought into a pregnancy.

LEARNING OBJECTIVES

After mastering the contents of this chapter, you should be able to:

1. Describe complications of pregnancy that place a pregnant woman and her fetus at high risk.
2. Use critical thinking to analyse ways pregnancy complications can be prevented.
3. Assess a woman who is experiencing a complication of pregnancy.
4. Identify expected outcomes to minimise the risks to a pregnant woman and her fetus when a complication of pregnancy occurs.
5. Implement care specific to a woman who has developed a complication of pregnancy such as teaching her how to recognise the symptoms of preterm labour.
6. Evaluate expected outcomes for effectiveness and achievement of care.
7. Identify areas related to high-risk pregnancy that could benefit from additional research or the application of evidence-based practice.

KEY TERMS

- abortion
- ankle clonus
- cervical cerclage
- chorioamnionitis
- Couvelaire uterus
- early pregnancy failure
- eclampsia
- ectopic pregnancy
- erythroblastosis fetalis
- gestational trophoblastic disease
- HELLP syndrome
- hydramnios
- isoimmunisation
- miscarriage
- oligohydramnios
- placenta praevia
- post-term pregnancy
- preeclampsia
- premature cervical dilation
- premature separation of the placenta
- preterm labour
- preterm premature rupture of membranes
- recurrent pregnancy loss
- Rh incompatibility
- tocolytics

CASE STUDY

Belinda Muzuki is a 20 year-old, gravida 2, para 0, 30 weeks' pregnant woman who you see in an antenatal clinic. She has had symptoms of a urinary tract infection for the past few days but did not call the clinic because she knew she had an appointment today and thought getting some help for it could wait until she came in. Yesterday she noticed some mild abdominal pain but thought it was irritation from the bladder infection. During the night, she woke twice because of a nagging backache. This morning, she has intermittent sharp uterine contractions. "Why am I starting labour so early?" she asks you. "I didn't do anything wrong."

CASE STUDY QUESTIONS

1. Were Belinda's actions as informed as they could have been?
2. What additional health teaching might have prevented her from commencing labour so early?

CARE OF A WOMAN WHO DEVELOPS A COMPLICATION OF PREGNANCY

The majority of women who enter pregnancy in good health expect to complete pregnancy and birth without complications. In a few women, however, for reasons that usually are unclear, unexpected deviations or complications from the course of normal pregnancy occur. When this happens, it places a severe burden on the woman and her family as well as her healthcare providers. All families benefit from the support and skill of a midwife who helps them work through the stages of pregnancy and prepares them to become new parents. This provides essential support for families who, in addition to the usual tasks of pregnancy, must take special care to ensure the continuation of the pregnancy. The leading complications related directly to the pregnancy are thromboembolism, haemorrhage, infection, hypertension of pregnancy and ectopic pregnancy (Mehta & Sokol, 2013). All of these have the potential to threaten the life of the mother and the fetus.

BLEEDING DURING PREGNANCY

Vaginal bleeding is a common first-trimester complication occurring in approximately 25% of all pregnancies with 50% occurring in viable intrauterine pregnancies at <20 weeks' gestation (Walker, Dexter & Dadig, 2013). Pregnancy loss occurs in 30–50% of women presenting with vaginal bleeding prior to 20 weeks' gestation, the most common cause is chromosomal anomalies (Walker, Dexter & Dadig, 2013). Spotting and light bleeding for 1–2 days or less is not associated with increased risk of miscarriage, but heavy bleeding, especially if associated with pain, increases the risk of miscarriage (Murtaza et al., 2013). The primary causes of bleeding during pregnancy are summarised in Table 21.1.

TABLE 21.1 Summary of primary causes of bleeding during pregnancy

Time	Type	Cause	Assessment	Cautions
First trimester	Threatened miscarriage (early—under 16 weeks; late—16 to 24 weeks)	Unknown; possibly chromosomal, uterine abnormalities	Vaginal spotting, perhaps slight cramping	
	Imminent (inevitable) miscarriage		Vaginal spotting, cramping, cervical dilation	
	Missed miscarriage		Vaginal spotting, perhaps slight cramping; no apparent loss of pregnancy	Disseminated intravascular coagulation associated with missed miscarriage
	Incomplete miscarriage		Vaginal spotting, cramping, cervical dilation, but incomplete expulsion of uterine contents	
	Complete miscarriage		Vaginal spotting, cramping cervical dilation and complete expulsion of uterine contents	
	Ectopic (tubal) pregnancy	Implantation of zygote at site other than in uterus; tubal constricture, adhesions associated	Sudden unilateral lower abdominal quadrant pain; minimal vaginal bleeding, possible signs of shock or haemorrhage	May have repeat ectopic pregnancy in future if tubal scarring is bilateral
Second trimester	Hydatidiform mole (gestational trophoblastic disease)	Abnormal proliferation of trophoblast cells; fertilisation or division defect	Overgrowth of uterus; highly positive human chorionic gonadotropin (hCG) test; no fetus present on ultrasound; bleeding from vagina of old or fresh blood accompanied by cyst formation	Retained trophoblast tissue may become malignant (choriocarcinoma); follow for 6 months to 1 year with hCG testing
	Premature cervical dilation	Cervix begins to dilate and pregnancy is lost at about 20 weeks; unknown cause, but cervical trauma from dilation and curettage (D&C) may be associated	Painless bleeding leading to expulsion of fetus	Can have cervical sutures placed to ensure a second pregnancy
Third trimester	Placenta praevia	Low implantation of placenta possibly because of uterine abnormality	Painless bleeding at beginning of cervical dilation	No vaginal examinations to minimise placental trauma
	Premature separation of the placenta (abruptio placentae)	Unknown cause; associated with hypertension; placenta separates from uterus	Sharp abdominal pain followed by uterine tenderness; vaginal bleeding; signs of maternal shock, fetal distress	Disseminated intravascular coagulation associated with condition
	Preterm labour	Many possible etiological factors such as trauma, substance abuse, pregnancy-induced hypertension or cervicitis; increased chance in multiple gestation, maternal illness	Show (pink-stained vaginal discharge) accompanied by uterine contractions becoming regular and effective	Preterm labour may be halted if the cervix is less than 4 cm dilated and the membranes are intact. Corticosteroids are administered to aid fetal lung maturity.

Any woman with vaginal bleeding requires evaluation beginning with the history which should include: the woman's age; previous pregnancies; menstrual history, including cycle length and regularity and the last normal menstrual period; prior confirmation of pregnancy; current medications; drugs; and contraception, including the presence of an intrauterine device (IUD). If an IUD is present it should be removed, as left in situ the risk of spontaneous abortion is 50–60%. A woman should then be asked about the present complaint, including when the bleeding commenced, the amount, colour and consistency of the blood and the presence of clots. Precipitating factors such as sexual intercourse, heavy lifting, falls, accidents, domestic violence and vomiting should be considered.

A detailed assessment should be performed including vital signs and examination of the abdominal/pelvic area which includes presence of abdominal tenderness, distension, character and severity of pain, cramping or backache. Women with heavy bleeding, passage of tissue, pain or fever should be evaluated immediately and women who are haemodynamically unstable will require an IV (Walker, Dexter & Dadig, 2013). Traditionally a speculum or bimanual examination has been part of diagnosis of early pregnancy bleeding; however, a study in Australia indicates a speculum or bimanual examination does not improve diagnosis when women present with early pregnancy bleeding and ultrasound is available (Johnstone, 2013). Almost all first trimester vaginal bleeding during pregnancy can be evaluated safely and accurately through clinical assessment, serum β-hCG assay and ultrasound (Lane & Wong-You-Cheong, 2014). Women who present with vaginal bleeding and a positive pregnancy test will be anxious about the bleeding and its implications for their pregnancy. They need to talk with a sympathetic, supportive person about how they feel. Both early and late pregnancy bleeding may constitute a potential emergency. Causes of late pregnancy bleeding include placental praevia, placental abruption and preterm labour.

Miscarriage

Abortion is the medical term for any interruption of a pregnancy before a fetus is viable (able to survive outside the uterus if born at that time). A viable fetus is usually defined as a fetus of more than 20 weeks' gestation. Elective abortion (discussed in Chapter 6) is the planned medical termination of a pregnancy. When the loss of pregnancy prior to viability occurs spontaneously, it is clearer to refer to it as a **miscarriage**. Spontaneous miscarriage occurs in 15–20% of all clinically diagnosed pregnancies and arises from natural causes (Wahabi et al., 2011). A spontaneous miscarriage is an early miscarriage if it occurs before 12 weeks of pregnancy and a late miscarriage between 12 and 20 weeks. Medical complications of miscarriage include infection, haemorrhage, embolism and complications of anaesthesia (Nanda et al., 2012).

Spontaneous miscarriage

Spontaneous miscarriage affects 1% of all women and often occurs before the pregnancy is clinically recognised. Around 30% of miscarriage occurs between implantation and the sixth week of pregnancy (Jeve & Davies, 2014). Approximately 57% of fetuses that spontaneously miscarry have chromosomal abnormalities and this has remained constant over several decades (Jenderny, 2014). Other contributing factors are advanced maternal age, first pregnancy, history of early pregnancy loss, exposure to toxins (e.g. alcohol, tobacco); immunological factors may be present or rejection of the embryo through an immune response may occur. Another common cause of early miscarriage involves implantation abnormalities, as up to 50% of zygotes probably never implant securely because of inadequate endometrial formation or from an inappropriate site of implantation. Paternal age >35 years is significantly related to spontaneous first trimester miscarriage; other paternal factors such as toxic environmental exposures, smoking, infection, alcohol and drug abuse may influence sperm quality and contribute to embryo loss (Jaleel & Khan, 2013).

Miscarriage may also occur if the corpus luteum on the ovary fails to produce enough progesterone to maintain the decidua basalis. Therefore both oestrogen and progesterone supplementation have been postulated as a way of preventing miscarriage. A Cochrane review found no evidence that combined oestrogen and progestogens prevents miscarriage (Lim et al., 2013). Other risk factors are maternal infection including genital herpes simplex, group B streptococci and human immunodeficiency virus-1 (Nigro et al., 2011). Systemic infection such as rubella, syphilis, poliomyelitis, cytomegalovirus and toxoplasmosis cross the placenta and may also contribute. Urinary tract infections may be a cause but are more strongly associated with preterm birth. With an infection, if the fetus fails to grow, oestrogen and progesterone production by the placenta falls. This leads to endometrial sloughing. With the sloughing, prostaglandins are released, leading to uterine contractions and cervical dilation along with expulsion of the products of the pregnancy.

Some miscarriages may be prevented by modification of multiple risk factors with the most important being maternal age (<30) and alcohol ingestion during the first and second trimester. Other factors include being obese or underweight, lifting more than 20 kg and working night shift (Feodor Nilsson et al., 2014). Miscarriage can occur from many causes and often the cause cannot be determined with an early miscarriage, therefore couples may have difficulty understanding why it happened to them (see Box 21.1).

BOX 21.1 * Focus on family teaching

Coping with a spontaneous miscarriage

Q. Belinda Muzuki tells you, "I had a miscarriage when I was younger, but my doctor called it an abortion. What is the difference?"

A. *Abortion* is the medical term for any pregnancy loss before a fetus is mature enough to live outside the uterus. Think of the word as interchangeable with *miscarriage*.

Q. Did I do something wrong to cause the miscarriage?

A. Early miscarriage is largely not preventable, because it is caused by such things as abnormal chromosome formation or poor uterine implantation—things over which you have no control. Eating a nutritious diet, so you enter a pregnancy in good health, and avoiding cigarette smoking or drinking alcohol are sensible recommendations to reduce your risk of miscarriage. If you had extensive blood loss with your miscarriage, be certain to eat iron-rich foods (such as meat and green vegetables) to help restore red blood cells for a second pregnancy.

The presenting symptom of spontaneous miscarriage is almost always vaginal spotting. At the first indication of this, a woman should telephone her healthcare provider and describe what is happening. Assessment of vaginal bleeding during pregnancy needs to be carried out quickly (see Table 21.2).

Threatened miscarriage

Symptoms of a *threatened miscarriage* begin as vaginal bleeding, initially only scant and usually bright red. A woman may notice cramping, lower back pain, abdominal pain, nausea and vomiting. No cervical dilation is present on vaginal examination. Although miscarriage is defined as threatened, inevitable, incomplete, complete and missed abortion, it often presents as a continuum and a woman may present at any stage (Murtaza et al., 2013). A woman with vaginal bleeding and pain will be asked to come to the clinic or office to have fetal heart sounds assessed or an ultrasound performed to evaluate the viability of the fetus. A quantitative serum human chorionic gonadotropin hormone (B-hCG) may be drawn at the start of bleeding and again in 48 hours. If the placenta is still intact, the level in the bloodstream should double in this time. If it does not double, poor placental function is suspected. An abnormally low serum progesterone also predicts pregnancy failure.

Most women are disappointed to learn that there is no way to prevent miscarriage. As many as 50% of women with a threatened miscarriage continue the pregnancy; for the other 50%, unfortunately, the threatened miscarriage changes to imminent or inevitable miscarriage.

Inevitable (imminent) miscarriage

A threatened miscarriage becomes an inevitable miscarriage if uterine contractions and cervical dilation occur. With cervical dilation, the loss of the products of conception cannot be halted. The woman should save any tissue fragments she has passed and bring them with her so they can be examined. If no fetal heart sounds are detected and an ultrasound reveals an empty uterus or non-viable fetus a doctor may perform a vacuum extraction (dilation and evacuation [D&E]) to ensure that all the products of conception are removed (Gilbert, 2011) or expectant management can be used to allow the miscarriage to occur without any intervention. Without treatment 83% of women will have a complete miscarriage within 7 days (Murtaza et al., 2013). Women should be aware they need to monitor vaginal bleeding by recording the number of pads used. Saturating more than one pad per hour is abnormally heavy bleeding and if this occurs she should contact her healthcare provider.

TABLE 21.2 Immediate assessment of vaginal bleeding during pregnancy

Assessment factor	Specific questions to ask
Confirmation of pregnancy	Does the woman know for certain that she is pregnant (positive pregnancy test or doctor/nurse-midwife confirmation)? A woman who has been pregnant before and states that she is sure she is pregnant is probably right, even if she has not yet had this confirmed.
Pregnancy length	What is the length of the pregnancy in weeks?
Duration	How long did the bleeding episode last? Is it continuing?
Intensity	How much bleeding occurred? (Ask the woman to compare it to a common measure [e.g., a tablespoon, a cup].)
Description	Was blood mixed with amniotic fluid or mucus? Was it bright red (fresh blood) or dark (old blood)? Was it accompanied by tissue fragments? Was it odorous?
Frequency	Steady spotting? A single episode?
Associated symptoms	Cramping? Sharp pain? Dull pain? Has she ever had cervical surgery?
Action	What was happening when the bleeding started? What has she done (if anything) to control bleeding?
Blood type	Does she know this? (Rh-negative women will need Rh immune globulin to prevent Rh isoimmunisation.)

Complete miscarriage

In a complete miscarriage, the entire products of conception (fetus, membranes and placenta) are expelled spontaneously without any assistance. The bleeding usually slows within 2 hours and then ceases within a few days after passage of the products of conception. Because the process is complete no other interventions are required except advising a woman to report heavy bleeding. Following a miscarriage a woman who is Rh negative should be administered Rh immune globulin even though there is not well established evidence that antibody development occurs in the first trimester.

Incomplete miscarriage

In an incomplete miscarriage, part of the conceptus (usually the fetus) is expelled, but fetal and/or placental tissue is retained in the uterus. The term "incomplete" can be confusing for women. They may interpret it to mean that because the miscarriage is incomplete, the pregnancy will continue. Be careful not to encourage false hope by also misinterpreting this term. With an incomplete miscarriage, there is a danger of maternal haemorrhage as long as part of the conceptus is retained in the uterus because the uterus cannot contract effectively. It can be difficult to determine if a miscarriage is complete or incomplete, ultrasound in early pregnancy might not detect visual retained products of conception. The doctor will usually perform a dilation and curettage (D&C) or suction curettage to evacuate the remainder of the pregnancy from the uterus. It is important for women to know the pregnancy is already lost and that this procedure is being done only to protect her from haemorrhage and infection, not to end the pregnancy.

Missed miscarriage

In a missed miscarriage, also commonly referred to as an **early pregnancy failure**, the fetus dies in utero but is not expelled. Women may also find this term misleading because it suggests that if a miscarriage is "missed", then the pregnancy can continue. A missed miscarriage is usually discovered at an antenatal examination when the fundal height is measured and no increase in size can be demonstrated or when previously heard fetal heart sounds cannot be heard. A woman may have had symptoms of a threatened miscarriage (painless vaginal bleeding) or she may have had no prior clinical symptoms.

An ultrasound can establish whether the fetus has died. Often the embryo actually died 4–6 weeks before the onset of miscarriage symptoms or failure of growth was noted. In the past D & C has been the general method of managing miscarriage in the first trimester, but expectant management (waiting 7–14 days) and medical management are now recognised as safe and effective options which avoid the risks of surgery (Borrell & Stergiotou, 2013). After 14 weeks' gestation, labour may be induced using a prostaglandin such as Prostin gel or Cervadil or misoprostol (Cytotec) to dilate the cervix, followed by oxytocin administration; a D&C can also be performed. Ideally, follow-up should include a urine pregnancy test in 6 weeks and a serum hCG if abnormal bleeding persists and to rule out gestational trophoblastic disease (Petersen et al., 2013).

If the pregnancy is not actively ended, miscarriage usually occurs spontaneously within 2 weeks. There is a danger of allowing this normal course to happen, however, because disseminated intravascular coagulation (DIC), a coagulation defect, may develop if the dead (and possibly toxic) fetus remains too long in utero (Zheng, 2012b).

Recurrent miscarriage

Recurrent miscarriage is classically described as a history of three or more miscarriages, many researchers are now considering two or more pregnancy losses as recurrent miscarriage. The risk of miscarriage in subsequent pregnancies increases to 17–25% after 2 consecutive losses and 25–46% after 3 consecutive losses (Jeve & Davies, 2014).

It is important that a thorough investigation is carried out to discover the cause of recurrent miscarriage and help ensure the outcome of a future pregnancy. **Recurrent pregnancy loss** occurs in about 1% of women desiring pregnancy. Established causes include Antiphospholipid antibody syndrome (most important treatable cause), embryonic aneuploidy and uterine anomalies (Sugiura-Ogasawara, Ozaki & Suzumori, 2014). Possible causes include parental chromosomal anomalies, haematological abnormalities, endocrinological abnormalities such as polycystic ovarian syndrome (Li et al., 2013); insulin resistance and thyroid disorders (Jeve & Davies, 2014); inherited thrombophilias such as factor V Leiden, prothrombin gene mutation, protein C and protein S deficiencies and antithrombin. Women with recurrent miscarriage have significantly lower positive HPV DNA tests. A suggested reason is that a greater immune response occurs in some women with recurrent miscarriage (Ticconi et al., 2013). Lower basal serum prolactin levels and increased maternal age have been associated with an increased risk of miscarriage (Li et al., 2013). The role of prolactin is controversial, it may be related to continued corpus luteum function and progesterone secretion (Li et al., 2013); chorioamnionitis or uterine infection and resistance to uterine artery blood flow (Tsokos, 2011).

Treating women with antiphospholipid antibody syndrome with low molecular weight heparin (LMWH) and low dose aspirin decreases the miscarriage rate by 54% (Jeve & Davies, 2014). Therapies that provide immunological treatments to women with a history of recurrent miscarriage have not provided significant benefits when compared to placebo and do not lower the risk of recurrent miscarriage (Wong, Porter & Scott, 2014). Although some causes of recurrent miscarriage have been identified in approximately 40–50% of cases the cause is unknown (Ticconi et al., 2013).

Psychological support is important as stress is a risk factor in recurrent miscarriage. Jeve and Davies (2014) discuss the following treatments for unexplained recurrent miscarriage: 75 mg of aspirin daily may improve uterine perfusion (routine use is not recommended as strong evidence is absent); progesterone has not been shown to be effective for most women; low molecular weight heparin (LMWH) is not recommended unless antiphospholipid syndrome is present; human chorionic gonadotropin (hCG) is not recommended; prednisolone therapy may assist women with diagnosed connective tissue disorders; immunoglobulins and IV intralipid solution are not recommended until more research has been undertaken.

Antiphospholipid antibody syndrome

Antiphospholipid antibody syndrome (APS) is an autoimmune disease where abnormal proteins (antiphospholipid antibodies) initiate coagulation and lead to clotting in arteries and veins. If this occurs in placental vessels, it can block placenta growth, and thrombi can loosen the placenta and interfere with oxygen and nutrient exchange. This results in recurrent miscarriage and hypertension of pregnancy; postpartally, it can lead to deep vein thrombosis. Clotting episodes increase with reduced activity such as bed rest, smoking, obesity and use of oestrogen-based birth control pills (Mehta & Sokol, 2013).

Collaborative care

Ideally women can directly access an early pregnancy assessment service where management of women with pain or bleeding in early pregnancy can be rapidly assessed and managed by a supportive multidisciplinary team of healthcare providers. In most cases of spontaneous miscarriage women will pass the products of conception and the bleeding will cease. With an incomplete miscarriage expectant management may be used where the woman waits for the products of conception to be passed. Medical management entails the use of medications to promote the expulsion of the remaining products of conception. Uterotonic medications such as oxytocin, misoprostol or prostaglandin F2 alpha can be used. The final option is surgical D&C of the uterus. Women may need support in accepting the reality of the situation. A follow-up should be carried out after a miscarriage to check women are well physically and coping emotionally. Women need to be informed that grief is normal following a miscarriage. With late miscarriages lactation may occur and women need to be aware of this. Wearing a firm bra and avoiding breast stimulation may aid lactation suppression. Normal menstruation usually recurs after 4–6 weeks. Be certain to convey concerned assurance that miscarriages happen spontaneously not because of anything a woman did. Women with miscarriages look for reasons why this could have happened, such as running up a flight of stairs or forgetting to take an iron tablet. Being told that none of these events causes miscarriage can help to minimise the guilt that many women feel. Women may experience anxiety, grief and depression following miscarriage (Murphy, Lipp & Powles, 2012).

Complications of miscarriage

As with full-term childbirth, haemorrhage and infection are two complications which may occur after miscarriage. The risk of Rh isoimmunisation needs to be considered. All women who are Rh-negative should receive 250 IU Rh immune globulin intrauterine adhesions. Asherman syndrome may also complicate a miscarriage and D&C of the uterus (Hooker et al., 2014). Women with a history of miscarriage have increased risks of stress, anxiety and depression in subsequent pregnancies (Bicking Kinsey, 2014).

Haemorrhage

With a complete spontaneous miscarriage, serious or fatal haemorrhage is rare. With an incomplete miscarriage or in a woman who develops an accompanying coagulation defect (usually DIC), major haemorrhage is a possibility. Monitor vital signs for changes to detect possible hypovolaemic shock. If excessive vaginal bleeding is occurring, immediately lay the woman flat and massage the uterine fundus to try to aid contraction. This may be impossible with an early pregnancy because the small uterus is not palpable above the symphysis pubis (see Chapter 17). A woman may need a D&C or suction curettage to empty the uterus of the material that is preventing it from contracting and achieving haemostasis. A transfusion may be necessary to replace blood loss. Direct replacement of fibrinogen or another clotting factor may be used to increase coagulation ability. Applying pneumatic anti-shock garments can help maintain blood pressure (Kausar et al., 2012).

After a self-limiting complete miscarriage, a woman needs clear instructions on how much bleeding is abnormal (more than one sanitary pad per hour is excessive); what colour changes she should expect in bleeding (gradually changing to a dark colour and then to the colour of serous fluid as it does with the postpartum woman); and that any unusual odour or passing of large clots is also abnormal.

Infection

The possibility of infection is minimal when pregnancy loss occurs over a short time, bleeding is self-limiting and instrumentation is limited. However, there is always a possibility it may occur. Infection tends to develop in women who have lost appreciable amounts of blood. Such women need close observation to rule out this second and possibly fatal complication.

After a miscarriage women need to know the danger signs of infection, such as fever, abdominal pain or tenderness, and a foul smelling vaginal discharge. Usually fever is the most important sign of infection, but it can be a transient reaction to a period of decreased fluid intake that preceded the miscarriage. In other instances, the fever may be a systemic reaction to the miscarriage process. All temperatures higher than 38.0°C require careful evaluation to avoid overlooking the possibility that infection is developing.

The organism responsible for infection after miscarriage is usually *Escherichia coli* (spread from the rectum forwards into the vagina) or group A streptococcus (Rimawi, Soper & Eschenbach, 2012). Caution a woman to wipe her perineal area from front to back after voiding and particularly after defaecation to prevent the spread of bacteria from the rectal area. Tampons should be avoided because stasis of any body fluid increases the risk of infection.

Infection usually involves the inner uterine lining (endometritis), but it may be more extensive and lead to parametritis, peritonitis, thrombophlebitis or septicaemia. The management of these infections is the same as if they were occurring after the safe birth of a child (see Chapter 25).

Septic abortion

A septic abortion is an abortion that is complicated by infection (Barton & Sibai, 2012). Infection can occur after a spontaneous miscarriage, but more frequently it occurs in countries where termination of pregnancy is illegal and an abortion has been performed using a non-sterile technique. Because the uterus is a warm, moist, dark cavity, infectious organisms, once introduced, grow rapidly, particularly if products of conception such as necrotic membranes are still present.

The woman will have symptoms of fever and crampy abdominal pain; her uterus feels tender to palpation. Left untreated, such an infection can lead to toxic shock syndrome, septicaemia, kidney failure and death (Cappiello, Beal & Simmonds, 2011). Women with septic abortion need immediate, intensive assessment and treatment. Septic abortion may lead to pelvic inflammatory disease (PID) which can result in infertility because of uterine scarring or fibrotic scarring of the fallopian tubes.

Isoimmunisation

At any point in pregnancy the placenta may be dislodged resulting in some blood from the placental villi (the fetal blood) entering the maternal circulation. If the fetus is Rh positive and the woman is Rh negative, enough Rh-positive fetal blood may enter the maternal circulation to cause **isoimmunisation**—the production of antibodies against Rh-positive blood. If the woman's next child should have Rh-positive blood, these antibodies would attempt to destroy the red blood cells of this infant during the months it is in utero (Crowther, Middleton & McBain, 2013).

After a miscarriage, because the blood type of the conceptus is unknown, all women with Rh-negative blood should receive 250 IU Rh (D antigen) immune globulin (RhIG) to prevent antibody formation in the event the conceptus was Rh positive.

CASE STUDY QUESTION

3. Belinda had a miscarriage when she was younger. What would be the best advice to give a woman who tells you she is miscarrying?

a. Lie down and do not move for 24 hours to stop the bleeding
b. Do not do anything special; early miscarriages happen all the time
c. Save any clots or material passed for your healthcare provider
d. Use a tight tampon to put pressure on your cervix and stop the bleeding

Ectopic pregnancy

An **ectopic pregnancy** is one in which implantation occurs outside the uterine cavity. The most common site (in approximately 95% of such pregnancies) is in the fallopian tube (see Fig. 21.1). With ectopic pregnancy, fertilisation occurs as usual in the distal third of the fallopian tube. Immediately after the union of ovum and spermatozoon, the zygote begins to divide and grow. Unfortunately, because an obstruction is present, such as an adhesion of the fallopian tube from a previous infection, congenital malformations, scars from tubal surgery, or a uterine tumour, the zygote cannot travel the length of the tube. It lodges at a strictured site along the tube and implants there instead of in the uterus.

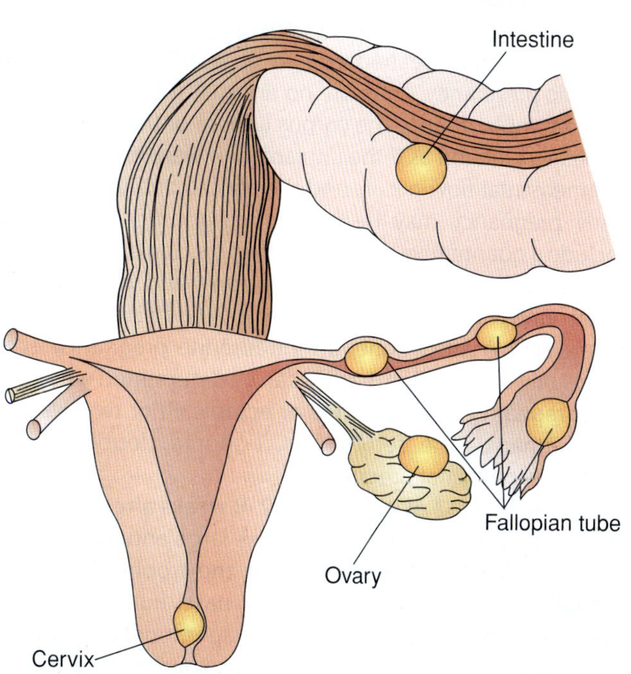

FIGURE 21.1 Sites at which an ectopic pregnancy may occur.

Ectopic pregnancy occurs in approximately 1–2% of pregnancies (Sherieh, Cottrell & Mancuso, 2014); it is the second most frequent cause of bleeding early in pregnancy. The incidence of ectopic pregnancies has increased and is partly attributed to increased rates of tubal infection resulting in scarring of the fallopian tubes and increased use of infertility treatments (Sherieh, Cottrell & Mancuso, 2014).

Genital infections such as *Chlamydia trachomatis* can result in permanent scarring of the fallopian tube. Ectopic pregnancy occurs more frequently in women who smoke compared with those who do not. There is some evidence that intrauterine devices (IUDs) used for contraception may slow the transport of the zygote and lead to an increased incidence of tubal or ovarian implantation. The incidence increases to around 5% following in vitro fertilisation (Murtaza et al., 2013). Women who have one ectopic pregnancy have a 10–20% chance that a subsequent pregnancy will also be ectopic. This is because salpingitis, which leaves scarring, is usually bilateral. For unknown reasons, oral contraceptives used before pregnancy, reduce the incidence of ectopic pregnancy (Abatangelo et al., 2010).

Assessment

It is essential to assess for ectopic pregnancy because the haemorrhage associated with tubal rupture can be life-threatening. The number of fatalities has decreased due to improved diagnosis; however, ectopic pregnancy continues to be the most common cause of maternal death and morbidity in early pregnancy (Murtaza et al., 2013). Approximately 6% of pregnancy-related maternal deaths are due to ectopic pregnancy (Sherieh, Cottrell & Mancuso, 2014). Many women are asymptomatic prior to tubal rupture and may be unaware they are pregnant (a urine pregnancy test may be negative in early pregnancy). With ectopic pregnancy, there are no unusual symptoms at the time of implantation. The corpus luteum of the ovary continues to function as if the implantation were in the uterus. No menstrual flow occurs and the nausea and vomiting of early pregnancy may be present. Diagnostic procedures include a quantitative serum β-human chorionic gonadotropin (β-HCG) level, serum progesterone and transvaginal ultrasound (TVUS). When the serum β-hCG is ≥1500 mIU/mL (the discriminatory zone) an intrauterine pregnancy can be visualised using TVUS and it can be determined whether the pregnancy is intrauterine or ectopic. Prior to 8 weeks of pregnancy the serum β-hCG should double every 48 hours in normal pregnancy.

By weeks 6–12 of pregnancy (2–8 weeks after a missed menstrual period), the zygote grows large enough to rupture the slender fallopian tube or the trophoblast cells actually break through the narrow base. Rupture of the fallopian tube can cause severe intraperitoneal bleeding. With tubal rupture a woman usually experiences a sharp, stabbing pain in one of her lower abdominal quadrants at the time of rupture, followed by vaginal spotting. The amount of vaginal bleeding from a ruptured ectopic pregnancy may not reflect the actual amount because the products of conception and blood from the ruptured tube may be expelled into the pelvic cavity. With placental dislodgment, progesterone secretion stops and the uterine decidua begins to slough, causing additional bleeding. Around 40–50% of women present with vaginal bleeding; other common signs are pain and abdominal tenderness (Sherieh, Cottrell & Mancuso, 2014).

Any woman with sharp abdominal pain and vaginal spotting needs to be evaluated to rule out the possibility of ectopic pregnancy. By the time a woman with a ruptured ectopic pregnancy arrives for evaluation she may already be in shock, as evidenced by a rapid, thready pulse, rapid respirations and orthostatic hypotension. A falling β-hCG or serum progesterone level suggests the pregnancy has ended, however, ultrasonography alone usually reveals a clear-cut diagnostic picture (Hsu & Euerle, 2012).

If a woman waits before seeking help, gradually her abdomen becomes rigid from peritoneal irritation. Her umbilicus may develop a bluish tinge (Cullen's sign) and continuing extensive or dull vaginal and abdominal pain may be present; movement of the cervix on pelvic examination may cause excruciating pain. There may be shoulder tip pain from blood in the peritoneal cavity causing irritation to the phrenic nerve. A tender mass is usually palpable in Douglas' cul-de-sac on vaginal examination.

Therapeutic management

When an ectopic pregnancy is revealed by an early ultrasound it can be treated with expectant management allowing natural reabsorption, if the woman is asymptomatic and has a low first serum B-HCG <200 mIU/mL and can be monitored closely with a serum B-HCG every 24–48 hours (Murtaza et al., 2013). Medical management with methotrexate is suitable for approximately 40% of women diagnosed with an ectopic pregnancy and 90% of these women can avoid surgery. Methotrexate is a folic acid antagonist chemotherapeutic agent, which targets fast-growing cells such as the trophoblast and decreases the growth of the ectopic pregnancy. The highest success is achieved when the initial serum B-HCG is <5000 mIU/mL and the ectopic area is <3.5 cm with no cardiac activity evident (Murtaza et al., 2013). Women are treated until a negative B-HCG titre is achieved. Methotrexate is contraindicated if women are breastfeeding or have immunodeficiency, alcoholism, liver disease, blood dyscrasia, haematological dysfunction, anaemia, active pulmonary disease, peptic ulcer and hepatic or renal disorders (Sherieh, Cottrell & Mancuso, 2014). After administration of methotrexate women should avoid alcohol, NSAIDs, folic acid, excessive exposure to sunlight and sexual intercourse. The use of a single intramuscular injection of 40 mg/m^2 (body surface area) of methotrexate has been reported to be safe and effective for ectopic pregnancy and ectopic pregnancies of unknown location (Wu et al., 2014). In some centres a single dose regimen may be 50 mg/m^2 (Sherieh, Cottrell & Mancuso, 2014).

If a ruptured ectopic pregnancy is suspected or diagnosed surgery needs to be performed immediately. A laparotomy or laproscopic approach can be used. During a salphingostomy, products of conception are flushed out of the fallopian tube through an incision, this preserves future fertility. With a salpingectomy the fallopian tube with the ectopic pregnancy is partially or completely excised. Intravenous fluid, using a large-gauge catheter to restore intravascular volume, is commenced and blood products can be administered if necessary. As with miscarriage, women with Rh-negative blood should receive Rh(D) immune globulin (RhIG) after an ectopic pregnancy to prevent isoimmunisation. The rate of successful intrauterine pregnancy and the risk of future ectopic pregnancies is similar in the surgically managed and medically managed groups (Murtaza et al., 2013).

A woman who has had an ectopic pregnancy not only has stages of grief to work through but also may have problems of diminished self-image and a sense of powerlessness to resolve if surgery included removal of a fallopian tube.

CASE STUDY QUESTION

4. Suppose Belinda was discovered to have an ectopic pregnancy. What advice would you give her?
   a. Most ectopic pregnancies go to completion, although the newborn is small
   b. If she must have a fallopian tube removed, she will be sterile afterwards
   c. She will have a continuous nagging pain through the rest of pregnancy
   d. Ectopic pregnancy can be either medically or surgically treated

Abdominal pregnancy

An abdominal pregnancy is a rare life-threatening event occurring in approximately 1 in 10,000 pregnancies with a maternal mortality rate around 90 times that of a normal pregnancy. The perinatal mortality rate is 40–95% (Whitney, Jones & Baker, 2014). There are two mechanisms causing an abdominal pregnancy. In a primary abdominal pregnancy the embryo implants in the peritoneal cavity and the fallopian tube and ovary are intact. A secondary abdominal pregnancy occurs when an already existing tubal pregnancy ruptures, with the embryo reimplanting in the peritoneal cavity (Whitney, Jones & Baker, 2014).

Diagnosis is through ultrasound or MRI. On examination the fetal outline is usually easy to palpate because it is directly below the abdominal wall. The danger of an abdominal pregnancy is the placenta infiltrating and eroding a major abdominal blood vessel leading to haemorrhage, bowel perforation, leaking of intestinal contents and peritonitis. The infant is delivered through a laparotomy. The placenta may be difficult to remove and may be left in place to absorb spontaneously over several months.

Gestational trophoblastic disease (hydatidiform mole)

Gestational trophoblastic disease is abnormal proliferation and then degeneration of the trophoblastic villi (Fu et al., 2012). As the cells degenerate, they become filled with fluid and appear as clear fluid-filled, grape-sized vesicles. The embryo fails to develop beyond a primitive start. Abnormal trophoblast cells must be identified because they are associated with choriocarcinoma, a rapidly metastasising malignancy (see Fig. 21.2).

The incidence of gestational trophoblastic disease is approximately 1 in every 1500 pregnancies. Two types of molar growth can be identified by chromosome analysis. With a *complete mole,* all trophoblastic villi swell and become cystic. If an embryo forms, it dies early at only 1 to 2 mm in size, with no fetal blood present in the villi. On chromosomal analysis, although the karyotype is a normal 46XX or 46XY, this chromosome component was contributed only by the father or an "empty ovum" was fertilised and the chromosome material was duplicated (see Fig. 21.3A).

With a *partial mole,* some of the villi form normally. The syncytiotrophoblastic layer of villi, however, is swollen and misshapen. A macerated embryo of approximately 9 weeks' gestation may be present and fetal blood may be present in the villi. In a complete molar pregnancy all of the chromosomes come from the father as the ovum has inactivated or missing chromosomes and the father's chromosomes are duplicated. In a partial molar pregnancy there are 69 chromosomes (a triploid formation in which

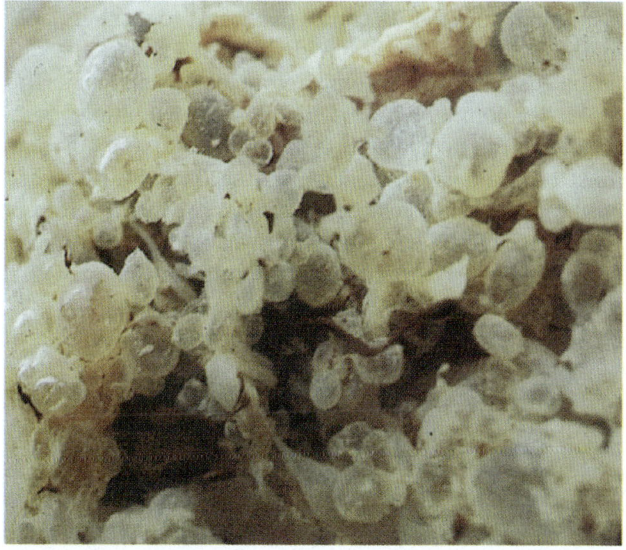

FIGURE 21.2 Gestational trophoblastic disease (hydatidiform mole). (From Rubin, E. & Farber, J. L. (1994). *Pathology* (2nd ed.). Philadelphia: JB Lippincott.)

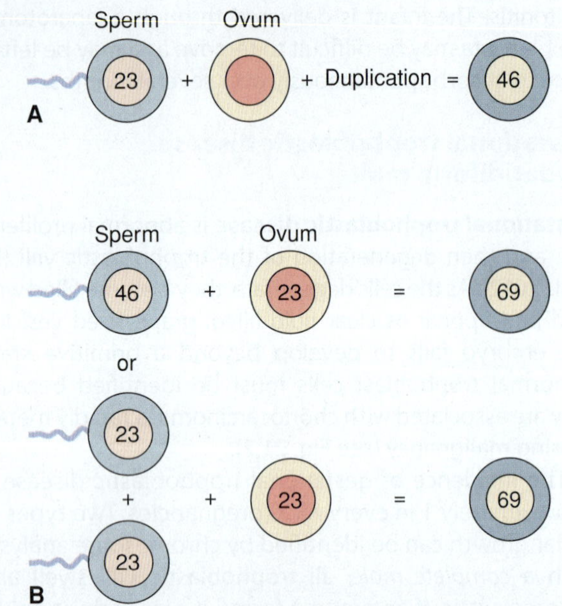

FIGURE 21.3 Formation of gestational trophoblastic disease (hydatidiform mole). (**A**) Complete mole. (**B**) Partial mole.

there are three chromosomes instead of two for every pair). This occurs when the ovum has normal chromosomes but has been fertilised by a sperm containing 46 chromosomes (a duplication) or when one ovum is fertilised by two sperm (see Fig. 21.3B).

In contrast to complete moles, partial moles rarely lead to choriocarcinoma. Although still above average, β-hCG titres are lower in partial than in complete moles; titres also return to normal faster after gestational trophoblast evacuation (Savage & Seckl, 2012).

Assessment

Because proliferation of the trophoblast cells occurs so rapidly with this condition, the uterus tends to expand faster than normal. This causes the uterus to reach its landmarks (just over the symphysis brim at 12 weeks, at the umbilicus at 20–24 weeks) before the usual time. This rapid development is also diagnostic of multiple pregnancy or a miscalculated due date, however, so the finding must be evaluated carefully. Because β-hCG is produced by the trophoblast cells that are overgrowing, a serum or urine test of β-hCG for pregnancy will be strongly positive (1 to 2 million IU compared with a normal pregnancy level of 400,000 IU).

Results continue to be strongly positive after day 100 of pregnancy, when the level of β-hCG would normally begin to decline. This fact must also be evaluated carefully, however, because highly positive test results can be characteristic of multiple pregnancies. The nausea and vomiting of early pregnancy is usually marked, probably because of the high β-hCG level present. Symptoms of pregnancy-induced hypertension such as elevated blood pressure, oedema and proteinuria may occur prior to 20 weeks of pregnancy. An ultrasound will show dense growth (typically a snowflake pattern) but no fetal growth in the uterus. No fetal heart sounds are heard because there is no viable fetus.

At approximately week 16 of pregnancy, if the structure was not identified earlier by ultrasound, it will identify itself with vaginal bleeding. This may begin as spotting of dark-brown blood or as a profuse fresh flow. As the bleeding progresses, it is accompanied by discharge of the clear fluid-filled vesicles. This is why it is important for any woman who begins to miscarry at home to bring any clots or tissue passed to the hospital with her. The presence of clear fluid-filled cysts changes the diagnosis from miscarriage to gestational trophoblastic disease.

Therapeutic management

Therapy for gestational trophoblastic disease is suction curettage to evacuate the abnormal trophoblast cells. Following extraction, women should have a baseline pelvic examination, a chest radiograph and a serum test for the beta subunit of β-hCG. The serum β-hCG levels are assessed every month for the next 6–12 months. Gradually declining β-hCG titres suggest no complication is developing. Levels that plateau or increase suggest that a malignant transformation is occurring. A woman should use a reliable contraceptive method, such as an oral contraceptive agent, for 12 months so that a positive pregnancy test (the presence of β-hCG) resulting from a new pregnancy will not be confused with increasing levels and a developing malignancy. After 6 months, if β-hCG levels are still negative, a woman is theoretically free of the risk of a malignancy developing. By 12 months, she could plan a second pregnancy. Following a molar pregnancy or gestational trophoblastic neoplasia (GTN) women can expect to have a pregnancy with outcomes similar to the general population; however, women who received chemotherapy for GTN have a slightly increased risk of stillbirth in future pregnancies (Vargas, Barroilhet, Esselen, Diver, et al., 2014). If gestational trophoblastic neoplasia occurs it is treated with a methotrexate regime, such as 30–50 mg/m^2 intramuscularly every week (Hasanzadeh et al., 2014).

> ***What if...***
>
> Belinda told you, after having had a gestational trophoblastic disorder, that she did not believe in birth control so she did not intend to take the oral contraceptives prescribed following evacuation of the gestational trophoblastic disease? How would you advise her?

Premature cervical dilation

Premature cervical dilation or cervical insufficiency, previously called an *incompetent cervix,* refers to a cervix that dilates prematurely and therefore cannot hold a fetus until term (Roman, 2013). It occurs in about 1% of women. The dilation is usually painless. Often the first symptom is

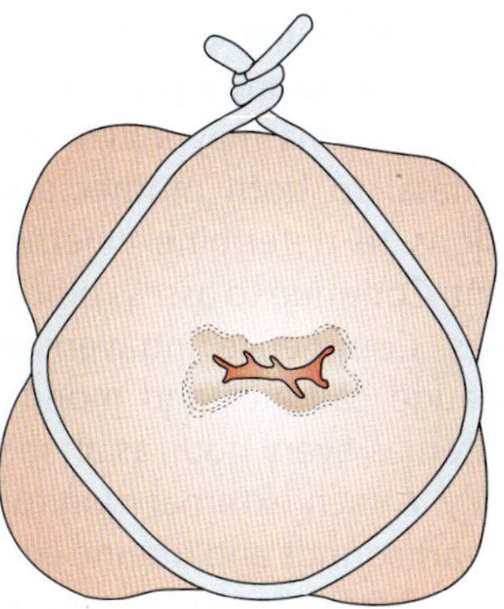

FIGURE 21.4 Shirodkar suture for cervical cerclage.

show (a pink-stained vaginal discharge) or increased pelvic pressure, which may be followed by rupture of the membranes and discharge of the amniotic fluid. Uterine contractions begin and after a short labour, the fetus is born. Unfortunately, this commonly occurs at approximately week 20 of pregnancy, when the fetus is still too immature to survive.

It is often difficult to explain in a particular instance what causes premature dilation. It is associated with increased maternal age, congenital structural defects and trauma to the cervix, such as might have occurred with a cone biopsy or repeated D&Cs. Although it may be diagnosed by an early ultrasound before symptoms occur, it is usually diagnosed only after the pregnancy is lost.

After the loss of one child because of premature cervical dilation, a surgical operation, termed **cervical cerclage**, can be performed to prevent this from happening in a second pregnancy (Alfirevic et al., 2012). As soon as an ultrasound confirms that the fetus of a second pregnancy is healthy, at approximately weeks 12 to 14, purse-string sutures are placed in the cervix by the vaginal route under regional anaesthesia. This procedure is called a McDonald or a Shirodkar procedure, after the surgeons who perfected the technique. The sutures serve to strengthen the cervix and prevent it from dilating early (see Fig. 21.4).

At weeks 37 to 38 of pregnancy the sutures are removed so the fetus can be born vaginally. Women who are discovered to have cervical dilation but with membranes still intact at an antenatal visit, may have emergent cerclage sutures placed in the cervix even at that point, as prophylaxis against preterm birth. The success of this procedure is lower than a prophylactic cerclage. Women need to report painless vaginal bleeding, as this is the symptom of a spontaneous miscarriage. Currently, the prognosis for a successful pregnancy after cervical cerclage is very favourable with an 80–90% success rate (McNair & Altman, 2011). An alternative to a cervical cerclage is to take repeated measurements of the length of the cervix using transvaginal ultrasound, as cervical length has been shown to shorten progressively prior to the onset of preterm labour.

Placenta praevia

Placenta praevia occur when the placenta is implanted abnormally in the lower uterine segment over or close to the internal os of the cervix (see Fig. 21.5). This results in inevitable placental separation and haemorrhage and is the most common cause of painless bleeding in the second half of pregnancy (Buckley & Schub, 2013). It occurs in four degrees: implantation in the lower rather than in the upper portion of the uterus (low-lying placenta); marginal implantation (the placenta edge approaches that of the cervical os); implantation that occludes a portion of the cervical os (partial placenta praevia); and implantation that totally obstructs the cervical os (total placenta praevia). The degree to which the placenta covers the internal cervical os is generally estimated in percentages: 100%, 75%, 30% and so forth.

Placenta praevia occurs in 0.3–0.5% of pregnancies. Risk factors include a previous history of placenta praevia, increased parity, maternal age >30 years, past caesarean births, past uterine curettage, multiple gestation, closely spaced pregnancies, endometriosis, erythroblastosis, smoking, poor vascularisation of the decidua and low

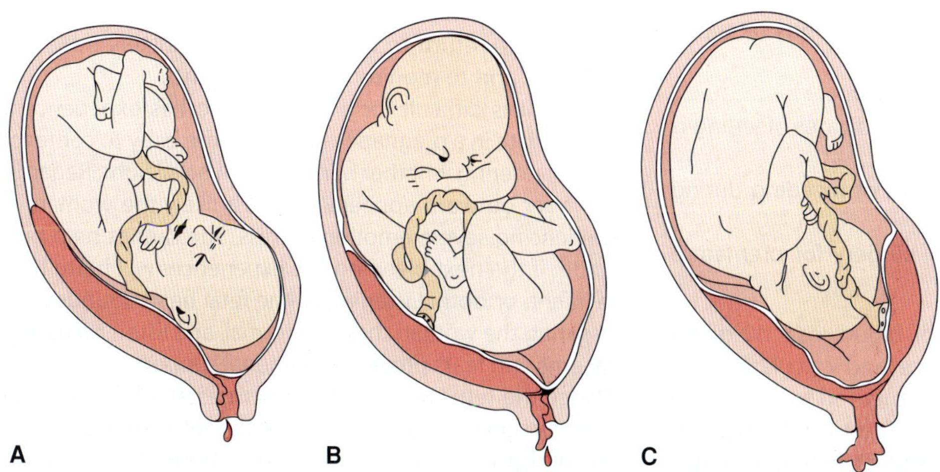

FIGURE 21.5 Degrees of placenta praevia: (**A**) low implantation; (**B**) partial placenta praevia; (**C**) total placenta praevia.

socioeconomic status (Buckley & Schub, 2013). Placenta praevia appears to be more common with a male fetus and has been linked with neurodevelopmental delay and sudden infant death syndrome (Buckley & Schub, 2013).

Assessment

The majority of cases of placenta praevia are diagnosed at the 20-week fetal anomaly scan. A low-lying placenta is frequently detected on early ultrasounds but most placentas will migrate upwards to a non-cervical position as the uterus grows. Bleeding with placenta praevia begins when the lower uterine segment starts to differentiate from the upper segment late in pregnancy (approximately week 30) and the cervix begins to dilate. The bleeding results from the placenta's inability to stretch to accommodate the differing shape of the lower uterine segment or the cervix. The bleeding that occurs is usually abrupt, painless, bright red and sudden enough to frighten a woman. It is not associated with increased activity or participation in sports. It may stop as abruptly as it began, so that by the time a woman is seen at the healthcare site she is no longer bleeding, or it may slow after the initial haemorrhage but continue as spotting. Fetal malpresentation is common.

Therapeutic management

Often the first bleed that occurs with placenta praevia is not excessive and does not require rapid birth. However, the bleeding can be acute and present an emergency situation. The site of bleeding, the open vessels of the uterine decidua (maternal blood), places the mother at risk of haemorrhage. The fetal oxygen supply may be compromised and the fetus is also at risk of preterm birth.

Immediate care measures

To ensure an adequate blood supply to a woman and fetus, place the woman immediately on bed rest in a side-lying position. Be sure to assess:

- The duration of the pregnancy
- The time the bleeding began
- A woman's estimation of the amount of blood—ask her to estimate in terms of cups or tablespoons (a cup is 240 mL; a tablespoon is 15 mL)
- Whether there was accompanying pain
- The colour of the blood (red blood indicates bleeding is fresh or is continuing)
- Whether there were prior episodes of bleeding during the pregnancy
- Whether she had prior cervical surgery for premature cervical dilation.

Assess the amount and rate of blood loss. Weighing perineal pads before and after use and calculating the difference by subtraction is a good method to determine vaginal blood loss. A Kleihauer-Betke test can be used to detect whether the blood is of fetal or maternal origin. *Never* attempt a pelvic examination with painless bleeding late in pregnancy, because any agitation of the cervix when there is a placenta praevia may initiate massive haemorrhage, possibly fatal to both mother and child. Obtain baseline vital signs to determine whether symptoms of shock are present. Continue to assess blood pressure every 5 to 15 minutes. Commence intravenous fluid therapy using a large-gauge catheter and monitor urine output frequently, as often as every hour, as an indicator of blood volume adequacy. Attach external monitoring equipment to record fetal heart sounds and uterine contractions. Internal monitoring is contraindicated. Haemoglobin, haematocrit, prothrombin time, partial thromboplastin time, fibrinogen, platelet count, type and cross-match, and antibody screen will be assessed to establish baselines, detect a possible clotting disorder and prepare blood for replacement if necessary. Vaginal birth is always safest for an infant. If the praevia is under 30% by ultrasound, it may be possible for the fetus to have a vaginal birth, however, theatre staff must be available and the mother and fetus require careful monitoring. If the praevia is over 30%, and the fetus is mature, the safest birth method for both mother and baby is a caesarean birth (Bedoya-Ronga & Currie, 2012). Staff trained in neonatal resuscitation should attend the birth.

Continuing care measures

The point at which a diagnosis of placenta praevia is made and the age of the gestation dictate the final management. If labour has begun, bleeding is continuing or the fetus is being compromised, birth must be accomplished regardless of gestational age. If the bleeding has stopped, the fetus is not compromised as evident by a reactive CTG, and if the fetus is not yet 36 weeks of age, a woman is usually managed by expectant watching. As many as half of all women with bleeding from placenta praevia are managed this way.

A woman is generally observed in hospital following an acute episode of bleeding. If the bleeding stops, she may be sent home but this needs to be assessed on an individual basis and may not be appropriate in remote and rural areas. Corticosteroids may be administered to hasten fetal lung maturity if the fetus is less than 34 weeks' gestation (see Box 21.2). If sent home, the woman needs to be instructed to return to the hospital immediately if bleeding occurs and to monitor fetal movements.

Often it is difficult for a woman who has experienced bleeding late in a pregnancy to wait for the baby to come to term, wondering whether her infant will be all right. Regardless of her outward appearance, most likely the woman is experiencing severe emotional stress. She cannot help but wonder if the next bleeding she experiences will harm her, the infant, or both. Listening to the fetal heart sounds and reassuring the woman they are normal, and listening to her concerns and fears provides emotional support.

Once the fetus reaches 38 weeks' gestation and bleeding occurs again, labour begins or the fetus shows symptoms of distress, the fetus needs to be born. On the day of

BOX 21.2 ✻ Focus on pharmacology

Betamethasone

Action: Betamethasone is a corticosteroid that acts as an anti-inflammatory and immunosuppressive agent. It is given to pregnant women 12 to 24 hours before birth to hasten fetal lung maturity if a fetus is less than 34 weeks' gestation and help prevent respiratory distress syndrome in the newborn (McKenna & Mirkov, 2014).

Pregnancy risk category: C

Dosage: 12–12.5 mg IM initially; may be repeated in 24 hours

Possible adverse effects: Burning, itching and irritation at the injection site; swelling, tachycardia, headache, dizziness, weight gain, sodium and fluid retention; increased risk of infection if used long term

birth, a woman needs a great deal of support. She may be as frightened as she was when her bleeding first began. If the pregnancy is past 36 weeks at the time of the initial bleeding, a decision to proceed with a caesarean section is one of the considered options for birthing.

Any woman who has had a placenta praevia is more prone than normal to postpartum haemorrhage because the placental site is in the lower uterine segment, which does not contract as efficiently as the upper segment. Also, because the uterine blood supply is less in the lower segment, the placenta tends to grow larger than it would normally, leaving a larger denuded surface area when it is removed. As a third complication, a woman is more likely to develop endometritis because the placental site is close to the cervix, the portal of entry for pathogens.

Premature separation of the placenta (abruptio placentae)

Premature separation of the placenta (abruptio placentae) is the premature separation of a normally situated placenta either partially or totally (see Fig. 21.6). Placental abruption occurs in 0.4–1% of pregnancies and is an obstetric emergency (Boisramé et al., 2014). The separation generally occurs late in pregnancy and may occur during an otherwise normal labour.

The primary cause of premature separation is unknown, but predisposing factors have been identified, including high parity, advanced maternal age, a short umbilical cord, chronic hypertensive disease, gestational hypertension, direct trauma (as from a motor vehicle accident or intimate partner abuse), vasoconstriction from cocaine or cigarette use, PPROM, previous placental abruption and thrombophilitic conditions that lead to thrombosis such as autoimmune antibodies, protein C and factor V Leiden (Ananth, Nath & Philipp, 2010). It may be caused by **chorioamnionitis**, which is an infection of the fetal membranes and amniotic fluid (Matsuda et al., 2011).

Premature separation of the placenta may also follow a rapid decrease in uterine volume, such as occurs with sudden release of amniotic fluid. Usually the fetal head is low enough in the pelvis that it prevents loss of the total volume of the amniotic fluid at one time, so normally a rapid reduction in amniotic fluid does not occur when membranes rupture.

Assessment

A placental abruption is characterised by pain and dark vaginal blood loss. The pain is often experienced as a sharp, stabbing pain high in the uterine fundus as the initial separation occurs, or as mild to severe cramping and lower back pain. If labour begins with the separation, each contraction will be accompanied by pain over and above the pain of the contraction. The uterus will be tender on palpation.

Heavy bleeding usually accompanies premature separation of the placenta although it may be concealed. There will be external bleeding only if the placenta separates first at the edges and blood escapes freely from the cervix. If the centre of the placenta separates first, blood can pool under the placenta, and although bleeding is intense, it is hidden from view. Whether blood is evident or not, signs of shock usually follow quickly because of the blood loss. The uterus becomes tense and feels rigid to the touch. If blood infiltrates the uterine musculature, the uterus becomes hard or board like. This is called a **Couvelaire uterus**. As bleeding continues, clotting factors may be

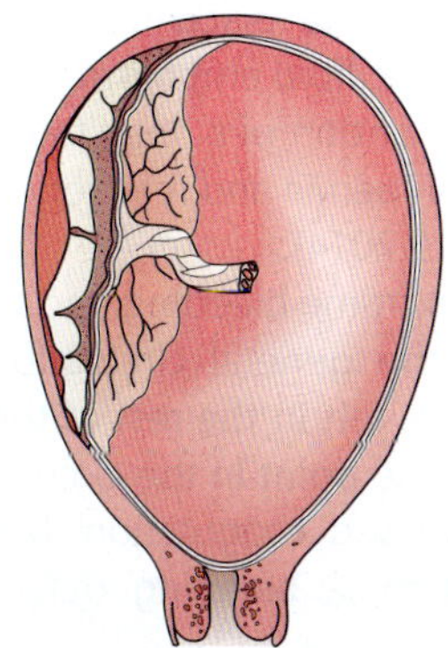
Partial separation (concealed haemorrhage)

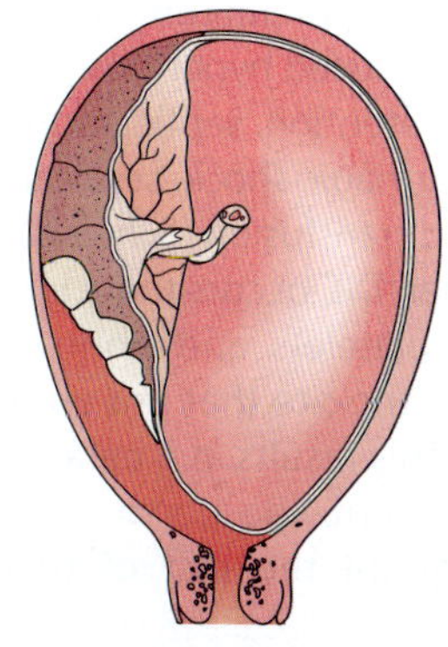
Partial separation (apparent haemorrhage)

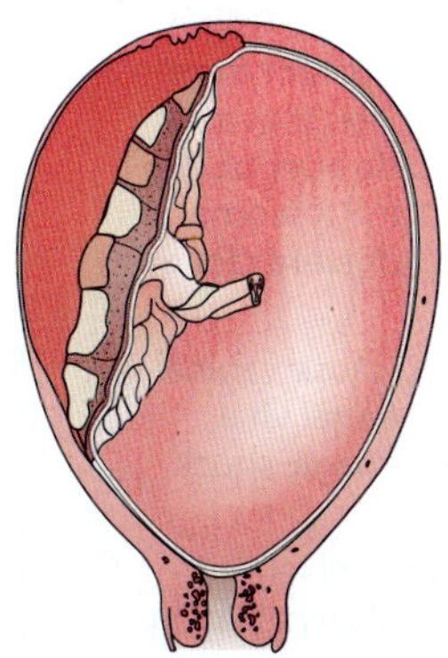
Complete separation (concealed haemorrhage)

FIGURE 21.6 Premature separation of the placenta.

used up in an attempt to accomplish effective clot formation and DIC can occur.

At initial assessment note the time the bleeding began, whether pain accompanied it, the amount and kind of bleeding and the woman's actions, in order to detect if trauma could have led to the placental separation. Initial blood tests should include haemoglobin level, typing and cross-matching, a fibrinogen level and detecting fibrin breakdown products to detect DIC.

Therapeutic management

Management of placental abruption is determined by fetal factors and maternal condition. If the fetus is alive an emergency caesarean should be performed unless birth is imminent. If the fetus has died a vaginal birth is preferable. A woman needs a large-gauge intravenous catheter inserted for fluid replacement and oxygen by mask to limit fetal anoxia. Monitor fetal heart sounds externally and record maternal vital signs every 5 to 15 minutes to establish baselines and observe progress. The baseline fibrinogen determination is followed by additional determinations up to the time of birth. Keep a woman in a lateral, not supine, position to prevent pressure on the vena cava and additional interference with fetal circulation. It is important not to disturb the injured placenta any further; therefore, do not perform any abdominal, vaginal or pelvic examination on a woman with a diagnosed or suspected placental separation.

For better prediction of fetal and maternal outcome, the degrees of placental separation can be graded (see Table 21.3). Unless the separation is minimal (grades 0 and 1), the pregnancy must be terminated because the fetus cannot obtain adequate oxygen and nutrients. If vaginal birth does not seem imminent, caesarean birth is the birth method of choice.

Maternal complications include clotting disorders, haemorrhagic shock and on rare occasions death. The major fetal complications are prematurity, intrauterine growth restriction and perinatal death in 15% of cases (Boisramé et al., 2014). A serious complication is the development of disseminated intravascular coagulation. If DIC has developed, caesarean surgery may pose a grave risk because of the possibility of haemorrhage during the surgery and later from the surgical incision. Intravenous administration of fibrinogen or cryoprecipitate (which contains fibrinogen) may be used to elevate a woman's fibrinogen level prior to, and concurrent with, surgery. With the worst outcome, a hysterectomy might be necessary to prevent exsanguination.

TABLE 21.3 Premature separation of the placenta: degrees of separation

Grade	Criteria
0	No symptoms of separation were apparent from maternal or fetal signs; the diagnosis that a slight separation did occur is made after birth, when the placenta is examined and a segment of the placenta shows a recent adherent clot on the maternal surface.
1	Minimal separation, but enough to cause vaginal bleeding and changes in the maternal vital signs; no fetal distress or haemorrhagic shock occurs, however.
2	Moderate separation; there is evidence of fetal distress; the uterus is tense and painful on palpation.
3	Extreme separation; without immediate interventions, maternal shock and fetal death will result.

Fetal prognosis depends on the extent of the placental separation, the degree of fetal hypoxia and the gestational age of the fetus. Maternal prognosis depends on how promptly treatment can be instituted. Death can occur from massive haemorrhage leading to shock and circulatory collapse or renal failure from the circulatory collapse. These factors cause premature separation of the placenta to be a significant cause of both maternal and fetal mortality.

Any woman who has had bleeding before birth is more prone to infection after birth than the average woman. A woman with a history of premature separation of the placenta, therefore, needs to be observed closely for the development of infection in the postpartum period.

Disseminated intravascular coagulation

Disseminated intravascular coagulation is a life-threatening disorder where thrombosis and haemorrhage occurs secondary to a disruption of the normal clotting cascade. During pregnancy the blood clots more easily to protect women from haemorrhage. DIC occurs in pregnancy when endothelial cells and/or platelets are damaged due to obstetric conditions and the ability to regulate coagulation is overwhelmed resulting in platelet aggregation and consumption of coagulation factors (Schub & Spears, 2014). Fibrinolysis commences, resulting in ischaemic damage from fibrin being deposited in small blood vessels and organs, which can result in shock, organ failure and maternal death (Schub & Spears, 2014).

Causes include a history of coagulopathy, preeclampsia, HELLP syndrome, placental abruption, retained placenta, amniotic fluid embolism, septic abortion, acute fatty liver of pregnancy, premature separation of the placenta, pregnancy-induced hypertension, amniotic fluid embolism, placental retention, septic abortion, retention of a dead fetus, haemorrhagic shock, septicaemia, viraemia and reaction to a blood transfusion (Schub & Spears, 2014).

When DIC occurs there is such extreme bleeding and so many platelets and fibrin from the general circulation rush to the site that not enough are left in the rest of the body. This results in a paradox: at one point in the circulatory system, the person has increased coagulation, but throughout the rest of the system, a bleeding defect exists.

The signs of DIC include profound haemorrhage; straw-coloured blood; blood that does not clot; bleeding from multiple body sites including nose, gums and cannula sites; petechiae; haematomas; signs of shock; pain; and abdominal distension. Tachycardia, hypotension, fever, acrocyanosis, decreased urine output and confusion may be present. To stop the process of DIC, the underlying cause must be treated, for example, after premature separation of the placenta with profuse bleeding the baby and placenta need to be born. Laboratory tests include CBC and coagulation studies. Pregnancy related DIC usually resolves within 12 hours of birth (Schub & Spears, 2014).

With active bleeding, blood components are administered, which may include warmed packed red blood cells and fresh frozen plasma using a one-to-one ratio. Coagulation factors such as platelets, fibrinogen, cryoprecipitates, antithrombin III, vitamin K and tissue factor pathway are given to replace lost clotting components (Schub & Spears, 2014). The use of low dose heparin to prevent thrombosis has been debated (Levi, 2014). An international DIC scoring system can be used to evaluate the results of blood tests and aid in diagnosis (Levi, 2014).

PRETERM LABOUR

Preterm labour is labour that occurs after 20 weeks and before 37 completed weeks of gestation. At a global level around 15 million premature babies are born annually with around 1 million dying from complications of prematurity (Bick, 2012). In Australia in 2010, 8.3% of babies were preterm and, overall, 6.2% of liveborn babies were low birthweight (<2500 grams) with a rate of almost double (11%) in mothers who smoked during pregnancy (Li et al., 2012). In the same year, the Australian Institute of Health and Welfare report shows that 0.9% of births occurred between 20 and 27 weeks; 0.8% between 28 and 31 weeks; and 6.6% between 32 and 36 weeks (these are the WHO gestational age classifications). A much higher rate of premature birth (13.5%) was recorded for Aboriginal and Torres Strait Islander women. Preterm birth occurred in 56.7% of twins and 97.3% of higher order multiple births (Li et al., 2012). Prematurity is the cause of 82% of stillbirths in Australia. The Perinatal Society of Australia and New Zealand Perinatal Death Classification (PSANZ_PDC) guidelines are generally used to classify perinatal death. The reasons for preterm birth appear to be complex and multifactorial, including genetic, pre-existing medical conditions, pregnancy complications and sociodemographic factors (Hammond et al., 2013).

Spontaneous preterm birth is associated with a higher risk of adverse neonatal outcomes and is the cause of perinatal death in around one quarter of births. The mortality and morbidity have decreased due to advances in neonatal care; however, it remains a substantial issue with 84% of mortality and most morbidity occurring under 32 weeks' gestation (Watson, Rayner & Forster, 2013). Infant morbidity includes physical or intellectual disability, hearing or visual impairment and cardiovascular problems (Bick, 2012).

It is important to understand the risk factors for preterm birth. Risk factors include lower education levels, previous medical conditions and/or new health problems developing during pregnancy, primigravidas, and multigravidas with previous miscarriage or abortion (Heaman et al., 2013). Domestic violence is significantly associated with preterm labour (Jamshidimanesh et al., 2013). A study on risk factors for very preterm birth (<32 weeks) in Australia found the risks factors were prior preterm birth, prior miscarriage or termination, primigravidity, prior caesarean section, treatment of precancerous cervical changes, endometriosis, fibroids, uterine abnormalities, being rhesus negative, assisted reproductive technology, bleeding in a prior pregnancy and being born outside Australia (Watson, Rayner & Forster, 2013).

Pre-existing maternal health risk factors for birth before 32 weeks were gastrointestinal tract problems, chronic hypertension, blood clotting disorders, diabetes, autoimmune diseases and chronic fatigue syndrome (Watson, Rayner & Forster, 2013). The pregnancy-related factors were vaginal bleeding, antepartum haemorrhage, preeclampsia, and threatened premature labour (Watson, Rayner & Forster, 2013). Factors which posed a high individual risk, but had a low impact on public health were constipation, infection exposure, cervical incompetence and gestational hypertension (Watson, Rayner & Forster, 2013).

Genetic variations have been implicated in spontaneous preterm birth with transcription regulators possibly related to the aetiology of spontaneous preterm birth and PPROM (Capece et al., 2014). Shortening of the cervix and effacement of the uterine cervix causes premature birth in some women. Early cervical shortening may indicate previous damage from surgery. During the second trimester cervical incompetence is the major cause of a shortened cervix (Guimarães Filho et al., 2013). New techniques to determine cervical distensibility and measure of cervical collagen content are being developed to understand the predictive value of these techniques (Khan, 2013).

Cervical mucus is more permeable and has different viscoelastic properties in women at high risk for preterm birth. The difference in cervical mucus may be associated with an increased incidence of microbial invasion but further studies are needed to determine the significance of these findings (Critchfield et al., 2013) (see Figs 21.7 and 21.8).

Epidemiological and biological studies indicate a pro-inflammatory process related to infections may increase the risk of prematurity. Infections include periodontal, urogenital, sexually transmitted infections, pneumonia and influenza and these may be targeted by prevention strategies (Webb, Mathew & Culhane, 2014). Emotional distress was not found to be associated with the risk of preterm birth (Lukasse et al., 2014). Other factors such as domestic violence may be another cause; however a percentage of women who develop preterm labour have no risk factors.

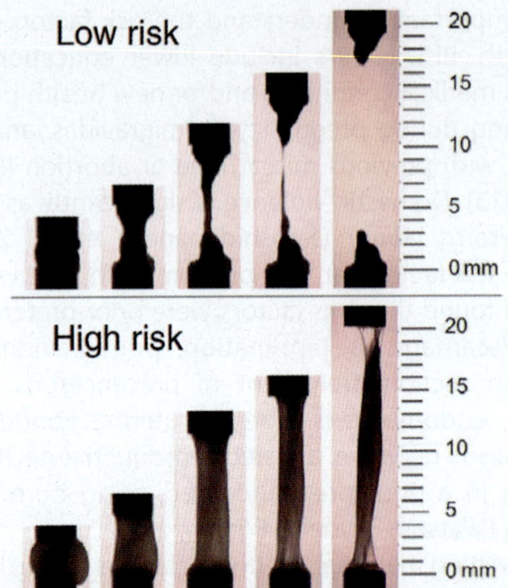

FIGURE 21.7 Example time series of spinnbarkeit test at 2, 5, 10, 15 and 20 mm in low-risk and high-risk cervical mucus samples. Almost all high-risk samples could be stretched to at least 20 mm without breaking (exhibiting spinnbarkeit). In contrast, mucus from low-risk patients had an average break length of 13.862.4 mm. (Critchfield, A. S., Yao, G., Jaishankar, A., Friedlander, R. S., Lieleg, O., Doyle, P. S., Ribbeck, K. et al. [2013]. Cervical mucus properties stratify risk for preterm birth. *PLoS ONE, 8*(8), 1–7.)

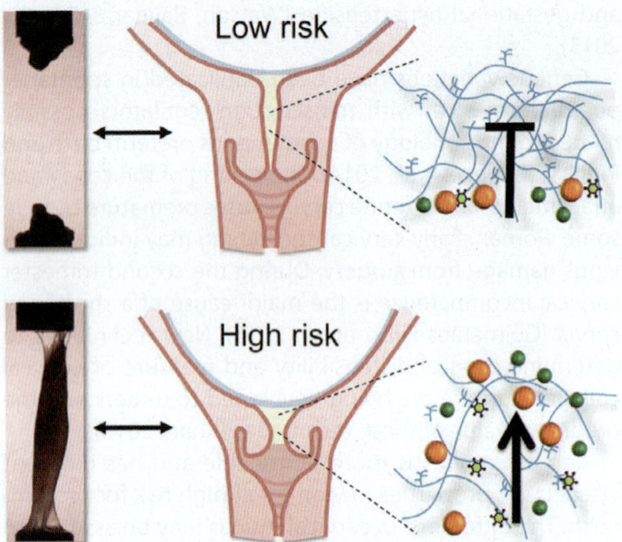

FIGURE 21.8 In women at high risk of preterm birth (with a short and dilated cervix), we find that the cervical mucus does display spinnbarkeit, is more weakly cross-linked and is a less effective barrier. (Critchfield, A. S., Yao, G., Jaishankar, A., Friedlander, R. S., Lieleg, O., Doyle, P. S., Ribbeck, K. et al. [2013]. Cervical mucus properties stratify risk for preterm birth. *PLoS ONE, 8*(8), 1–7.)

Assessment

Preterm labour may be difficult to diagnose. Common symptoms of early preterm labour include: a persistent, dull, low backache; vaginal spotting; a feeling of pelvic pressure or abdominal tightening; menstrual-like cramping; increased vaginal discharge; uterine contractions; intestinal cramping and diarrhoea. Women need to be aware of the signs and symptoms of preterm labour because they are often subtle and are best recognised by the woman herself. Any woman having persistent uterine contractions (4 every 20 minutes) should be considered to be in labour. A woman is documented as being in labour if she is having uterine contractions and cervical changes.

A woman with suspected preterm labour can be assessed using:

- a transvaginal ultrasound to see if the cervix is shortened or dilated and a cervical stress test to see how fundal pressure or maternal straining effect the cervix
- vaginal or cervical swabs and a clean-catch urine to check for infection
- a fetal fibronectin swab to determine if membranes are intact or ruptured (speculum exam, nitrazene or Amnisure test)
- a CTG to assess uterine contractions and the status of the fetus
- ultrasound fetal surveillance to determine fetal size, amniotic fluid volume, the presence of fetal anomalies, biophysical profile, Doppler studies and position and status of the placenta
- a complete blood count to assess for possible contributing factors.

A newer approach combining fFN and cervical length screening results in a higher sensitivity and positive predictive value for preterm birth risk while maintaining high negative predictive value (DeFranco, Lewis & Odibo, 2013).

Therapeutic management

If the cervical length is <25 mm, treatment may be initiated, There is a strong association between a shortened cervix and preterm labour (Alfirevic et al., 2013). A shortened cervix can be treated with expectant management, a cervical cerclage, progesterone (vaginal, rectal or IM), an Arabin cervical pessary, or sometimes a combination of therapies is used (Sharp & Alfirevic, 2014). Presently there is insufficient evidence to recommend routine transvaginal ultrasound screening of asymptomatic or symptomatic pregnant women because there is a non-significant association between being aware of the cervical length and a decreased incidence of preterm birth at less than 37 weeks in symptomatic women (Berghella, Baxter & Hendrix, 2013). The management of women at risk of preterm labour is variable and there is a lack of consensus on the cervical length measurement below which treatment should be instituted and a lack of consensus on the efficacy of progesterone and cerclage.

Treatment for genital tract infections such as bacterial vaginosis, chlamydia, trichomonas, gonorrhea, syphilis and HIV (but not candida) may reduce preterm births (Sangkomkamhang et al., 2009). If bacterial vaginosis is diagnosed treatment options include vaginal clindamycin, oral clindamycin, metronidazole or no treatment. Women may be advised to restrict physical activity, avoid sexual intercourse, stop/reduce work, improve nutrition (Sharp & Alfirevic, 2014), avoid smoking (Khader et al., 2011) and remain well hydrated (Chawanpaiboon, Pimol & Sirisomboon, 2011).

An Arabin pessary has been used in singleton pregnancies at high risk for preterm birth. It has been noted that the uterocervical angle is significantly less acute and the cervical length shorter than in low-risk patients. It may have a mechanical effect, by displacing the internal os towards the spine and altering the effect of gravity, perhaps by inducing cervical oedema. Further studies are required on its effectiveness (Cannie, et al., 2013; Arabin & Alfirevic, 2013).

Medication administration

Medical attempts can be made to stop labour if the fetal membranes are intact, fetal distress is absent and there is no evidence that bleeding is occurring and the cervix is not dilated.

Tocolytics are used to inhibit uterine contractions in order to delay labour so corticosteroids can be given and a woman in premature labour can be safely transferred to a tertiary care centre. If the pregnancy is under 34 weeks, the corticosteroid betamethasone is given to hasten fetal lung maturity (two doses of 12 mg of betamethasone given intramuscularly 12–24 hours apart). Betamethasone is used as it leads to lower rates of respiratory distress syndrome or bronchopulmonary dysplasia in newborns (Riley, Boozer & King, 2011). Corticosteroids interfere with glucose regulation by reducing uptake of glucose by cells, resulting in increased plasma glucose so women with diabetes must be monitored. It takes around 24 hours for betamethasone to have an effect, so tocolytics are given to delay labour.

Use of a tocolytic medication is associated with prolongation of pregnancy for up to 7 days but with no significant effect on preterm birth and no clear effect on perinatal or neonatal morbidity. Tocolysis may be considered for women with suspected preterm labour who have had an otherwise uncomplicated pregnancy. It is also reasonable not to use any tocolytic. Women most likely to benefit from a tocolytic are those who are in very preterm labour, those needing transfer to a hospital which can provide neonatal intensive care and those who have not yet completed a full course of corticosteroids.

Using multiple tocolytics is associated with an increased risk of adverse effects and therefore multiple tocolytic therapy should be avoided (Royal College of Obstetricians & Gynaecologists, 2011). Tocolytics should not be used when there are contraindications to prolonging pregnancy such as severe preeclampsia/eclampsia, intrauterine infection, fetal death, placental praevia, placental abruption, antepartum haemorrhage, fetal growth restriction and abnormal CTG.

Selective β_2 agonists

Selective β_2 agonists are ritodrine and terbutaline. Terbutaline is more frequently used. β_2 agonists cause blood vessels and bronchi to relax along with the uterine muscle causing side effects such as tachycardia, palpitations, tremor, headaches, nausea/vomiting, nasal stuffiness, dyspnoea and chest pains. Hypokalaemia may also occur from a shift of potassium into cells (Hubinont & Debrieve, 2011). Although selective β_2 agonists help to delay birth they are significantly associated with withdrawal from treatment due to adverse effects, some of which are serious (Neilson, West & Dowswell, 2014). Terbutaline should be used cautiously in women with diabetes mellitus because it causes hyperglycaemia. In a woman predisposed to develop gestational diabetes, terbutaline can raise her blood glucose enough to result in overt diabetes. Terbutaline can be given subcutaneously, intravenously or orally. It increases the maternal heart rate by 20–40 beats per minute and also causes fetal tachycardia. Although selective β_2 agonists delay birth this has not be shown to result in any improvements in neonatal outcomes or to reduce perinatal deaths or respiratory distress syndrome (Neilson, West & Dowswell, 2014).

Calcium channel blockers

Calcium channel blockers decrease the intracellular free calcium concentration and relax the myometrium. Nifedipine is usually the first-line tocolytic and is given orally (Jordan, 2010). Side effects of nifedipine include headaches, flushing, palpitations and hypotension.

Oxytocin receptor antagonists

Oxytocin receptor antagonists (atosiban) compete with myometrial and decidual oxytocin receptors and block calcium release associated with contractions. Atosiban has a low incidence of side effects (mainly nausea) and provides effective tocolysis. Atosiban is contraindicated with severe preeclampsia (Saleh, Al-Ramahi & Al Kazaleh, 2013).

Atosiban and nifedipine are effective in delaying delivery for 7 days or more in women presenting with pre-term labour. They have the same efficacy and associated minor side-effects; however, flushing, palpitation and hypotension are higher with nifedipine. Compared with beta-agonists, nifedipine is associated with improvement in neonatal outcome, although long-term data is not available (Royal College of Obstetricians & Gynaecologists, 2011). A recent study found no differences in efficacy or maternal safety when comparing nifedipine and indomethacin for acute tocolysis between 24 to 32 weeks' gestation (Klauser et al., 2014).

Cyclooxygenase (COX) inhibitors (prostaglandin-synthase inhibitors), such as indomethacin, block the action of prostaglandins which are uterine contraction inducers. Indomethacin can be administered rectally or orally. Indomethacin should be used for short duration and only prior to 32 weeks' gestation as it may cause closure of the fetal ductus arteriosis and decreased urine production leading to oligohydramnious. Maternal side effects include gastric ulcer or recurrence of asthma.

Nitric oxide donor

Nitric oxide donor nitroglycerine (transdermal nitroclycerine) has been used in a limited number of cases and showed effective tocolysis, but evidence from large studies is not available so it is not used routinely.

Progesterone

Progesterone and 17-α-hydroxyprogesterone caproate cause uterine quiescence. They can be given vaginally or intramuscularly, their side effects include sleepiness and headaches. They are more appropriate for previous preterm birth or short cervix than for preterm labour. There is limited evidence to suggest co-treatment with progesterone reduces preterm birth at less than 37 weeks' gestation but insufficient evidence to use progesterone as a tocolytic for preterm labour (Su, Samuel & Chong, 2014).

Magnesium sulfate

Magnesium sulfate has been evaluated in multiple trials and there is no clear evidence that it reduces the risk of preterm birth but it has been shown to reduce the risk of cerebral palsy (Merrill, 2013). Cerebral palsy effects approximately 40% of premature infants (The Australian Cerebral Palsy Register, 2009). The 2010 Australian National Clinical Practice Guidelines, endorsed by the National Health and Medical Research Council (NHMRC) recommend the use of magnesium sulfate for 24 hours or until birth when the gestational age is less than 30 weeks and the delivery of the infant is planned or expected to occur soon. Magnesium sulfate is given intravenously and is generally commenced with a 4-gram loading dose administered over 20 to 30 minutes followed by a maintenance dose of 1 gram per hour.

Fetal assessment

In addition to tocolytic therapy it is important to assess overall fetal welfare in a woman trying to delay preterm labour. A woman may have CTG monitoring and be instructed to use a daily fetal movement count or "count to 10" test. The typical fetus moves 10 times in an hour. To evaluate fetal movement, a woman lies down on her left side and notes the number of minutes it takes for her to feel 10 fetal movements (about an hour) or counts the number of fetal movements she feels in 1 hour (the average is 10 to 12). If the time it takes to feel 10 fetal movements is twice what it was the day before or if she feels fewer than 5 movements during an hour (half of what she should feel), she monitors again for a second hour. If at the end of this second hour fetal activity is still under 10 per hour, she should report it immediately.

Labour that cannot be halted

In some women, preterm labour is too far advanced when they are first seen in a healthcare facility for it to be halted. Usually, if membranes have ruptured or the cervix is more than 50% effaced and more than 3 to 4 cm dilated, it is unlikely labour can be halted. The rupturing of membranes, especially, can be thought of as a "point of no return" in stopping or delaying labour because of the increased risk of infection that begins from that point. If intensive neonatal care is not available and the fetus is less than 34 weeks' gestation the mother should be transported to hospital, if possible, as this has been shown to decrease neonatal mortality. If a woman is group B streptococcus positive or her status is unknown, prophylactic antibiotics should be given.

A woman in preterm labour is undergoing an extreme crisis situation and will need frequent and continued reassurance. The optimum method of birth for infants between 24 to 36 weeks' gestation has been controversial. In severely premature infants born between 25 to 32 weeks' gestation the risk of adverse perinatal outcome does not appear to be related to the mode of delivery; however, maternal complications were significantly increased following a caesarean section (Kok et al., 2014). Although many measures are available to help the preterm baby adjust to birth, a baby born preterm will be at risk of a variety of health problems, especially difficulty with respiration (see Chapter 26).

PRETERM PRELABOUR RUPTURE OF MEMBRANES (PPROM)

Preterm premature rupture of membranes (PPROM) is defined as rupture of the chorioamniotic membranes before the onset of labour prior to 37 weeks of gestation. PPROM is further classified by gestational age: mid-trimester (<24 weeks), early (24–34 weeks) and near-term (34–37 weeks). The causes of PPROM are unknown but appear to be multifactorial and are associated with smoking, lower socioeconomic status, sexually transmitted infections, vaginal bleeding and uterine distension; these associations may be related to choriodecidual infection/inflammation, decreased membrane collagen content and collagen degradation (Mackeen et al., 2014). PPROM can also result from invasive procedures such as amniocentesis, cordocentesis, chorionic villus sampling (CVS) and cerclage. Approximately 25–30% of premature labour results from preterm rupture of membranes and once the membranes rupture prematurely 50% of women will commence labour within 24–48 hours and 70–90% within 7 days (Kenyon, Boulvain & Neilson, 2013). Approximately 1–5% of pregnancies are complicated by PPROM.

If membrane rupture occurs early in pregnancy, it poses a major threat to the fetus because the seal to the fetus is lost and uterine and fetal infection may occur. Loss of amniotic fluid leads to oligohydramnious defined as an amniotic fluid Index of <5 cm on ultrasound. Lung development (especially from 16 to 26 weeks' gestation) depends on an adequate amount of amniotic fluid. Early oligohydramnios results in pulmonary hypoplasia which is adequate lung development with decreased alveoli and reduced functional lung capacity (Van Teeffelen et al., 2013). Pulmonary hypoplasia can cause severe respiratory failure, pulmonary haemorrhage, bronchopulmonary dysplasia and acute lung disease and has a perinatal mortality rate of around 70% (van Teeffelen et al., 2014). Early PROM may increase pressure on the umbilical cord (inhibiting fetal nutrition and oxygen). Preterm labour and birth often follow rupture of the membranes. Very early PROM (<25 weeks) is associated with high rates of severe neonatal morbidity and childhood outcomes at 2 years of age are poor compared with infants born after PROM at 25–31.9 weeks (Manuck & Varner, 2014).

Assessment

Diagnosis of rupture of the membranes is made from the maternal history, physical examination and ultrasound. A woman usually describes a sudden gush of clear fluid from her vagina, with continued leakage. Occasionally, a woman mistakes urinary incontinence for rupture of membranes. A women should be asked the time her membranes ruptured, the type, colour and amount of fluid and if there was any offensive smelling discharge. Baseline vital signs should be taken, and the fetal heart recorded and a CTG performed. Examination includes checking for uterine tenderness, fever and fetal tachycardia. A digital vaginal examination increases the risk of infection once the membranes have ruptured and should be avoided unless a woman is labouring and birth seems imminent. A sterile vaginal speculum examination is performed to observe for pooling of amniotic fluid. If the fluid is tested with Nitrazine paper, amniotic fluid causes an alkaline reaction on the paper (appears blue) and urine causes an acidic reaction (remains yellow). A positive AmniSure test indicates the presence of amniotic fluid. The fluid can also be tested for ferning, or the typical appearance of a high-oestrogen fluid on microscopic examination (amniotic fluid shows this; urine does not). Because PPROM is associated with vaginal infection a low vaginal swab is collected and an anorectal swab for Group B Streptococcus screening. If antenatal screening for sexually transmitted infections (STI) has not been done screening for chlamydia and other STI's can be offered. Blood is drawn for a full blood count and C-reactive protein, which increases with membrane rupture. A mid-stream urine (MSU) should be collected. An ultrasound should be arranged to confirm gestational age, fetal wellbeing, fetal growth and the amniotic fluid index (AFI).

Therapeutic management

Therapeutic management is influenced by the gestational age of the fetus, evidence of infection, fetal compromise or labour. With PPROM, routine treatment with maternal antibiotic therapy is associated with prolongation of pregnancy and improvements in a number of short-term neonatal morbidities, but no significant reduction in perinatal mortality. Antibiotic treatment significantly reduces chorioamnionitis; the number of babies born within 48 hours; neonatal infection; surfactant use; and abnormal cerebral ultrasounds. Short-term improvements in neonatal mortality are evident, therefore antibiotics are recommended; however, amoxicillin/Clavulanate should be avoided due to increased risk of neonatal necrotising enterocolitis (Kenyon, Boulvain & Neilson, 2013).

Routine treatment with antibiotics is not recommended with prelabour rupture of the membranes (PROM) at or near term (≥36 weeks) unless maternal infection has been confirmed. Rupture of membranes increases the risk of infection, however, in this group the rate of infection in women not treated with antibiotics is low and there is no convincing evidence that mothers or neonates benefit from the routine use of antibiotics for PROM at or near term (Wojcieszek, Stock & Flenady, 2014). Antibiotics have potential adverse side effects, and increase potential for antibiotic resistance, hence routine antibiotic treatment for PROM at or near term should be avoided (Wojcieszek, Stock & Flenady, 2014). Women positive for Streptococcus B need intravenous administration of penicillin to reduce the possibility of this infection in the newborn.

Antenatal corticosteroids should be administered to hasten fetal lung maturity between 23–34 weeks' gestation. A woman with no signs of infection may be administered a tocolytic agent to allow time for the corticosteroids to take effect and allow transfer to a tertiary centre; however, the use of tocolysis is controversial. Currently there is insufficient evidence to support tocolytic therapy for women with PPROM because delaying birth increases the risk of maternal chorioamnionitis. Using tocolytics to delay birth does not reduce the incidence of perinatal death, but increases neonatal morbidity (Mackeen et al., 2014). Evidence suggests that amnioinfusion (fluid inserted into the uterus through the cervix or transabdominally) following PPROM may benefit preterm infants by reducing infection and lung damage, however, insufficient evidence is available to recommend routine amnioinfusion for PPROM (Hofmeyr, Eke & Lawrie, 2014). Abdominal amnioinfusion at gestation less than 26 weeks has been proposed and two randomised controlled trials are underway but the data has not yet been published.

Ongoing management

Infection can have serious consequences for mother and fetus; therefore, women need to be observed for signs of infection such as elevated temperature, abdominal pain or tenderness, and offensive vaginal discharge. Women are advised to avoid vaginal intercourse, tampons, baths, swimming and to monitor fetal movements. Women need to report signs of threatened premature labour, vaginal bleeding, and abdominal pain or tenderness. Women with no signs of infection, preterm labour, fetal compromise and no risk factors may be considered for home care. A Cochrane review suggests that outcomes are very similar between women cared for at home and women who are hospitalised (Abou et al., 2014).

HYPERTENSIVE DISORDERS OF PREGNANCY

Hypertensive disorders affect approximately 10% of pregnancies in Australia. Preeclampsia and **eclampsia** are the most serious manifestations of hypertensive disorders in pregnancy. Risk factors for preeclampsia include nulliparity, age greater than 40 years, twin pregnancy, family history of preeclampsia, diabetes mellitus, angiotensin gene T235, hypertension, nephropathy, antiphospholipid syndrome, and vascular and connective tissue disorders.

In normal pregnancy blood pressure (BP) tends to fall in the first trimester and rises towards pre-conception levels in the third trimester. The Society of Obstetric Medicine in Australia and New Zealand (SOMANZ) has guidelines for the management of hypertensive disorders in pregnancy (2014) and use the following definitions of hypertension. *Hypertension in pregnancy* is defined as a systolic BP ≥140 mmHg and a diastolic BP ≥90 mmHg. *Severe hypertension in pregnancy* is defined as a systolic BP ≥170 mmHg and a diastolic BP ≥110 mmHg. Severe hypertension in pregnancy needs to be lowered promptly but carefully to prevent serious events such as cerebral haemorrhage and hypertensive encephalopathy. A rise in blood pressure of >30/15 mmHg has previously been considered useful but evidence suggests this is not associated with an increase in adverse outcomes but close observation is warranted particularly in the presence of hyperuricaemia proteinuria or poor fetal growth.

Pathophysiological events

The symptoms of pregnancy induced hypertension (PIH) affect almost all organs. Vasospasm occurs in small and large arteries and may be caused by the increased cardiac output that occurs with pregnancy. It injures the endothelial cells of the arteries and reduces the action of prostacyclin (a prostaglandin vasodilator) and increases production of thromboxane (a prostaglandin vasoconstrictor and stimulant of platelet aggregation). Usually during pregnancy blood vessels are resistant to the effects of pressor substances such as angiotensin and noradrenaline, so even with the increased blood supply, blood pressure remains normal during pregnancy. With gestational hypertension, this reduced responsiveness to blood pressure changes appears to be lost because of the prostaglandin release. Vasoconstriction occurs and blood pressure increases dramatically.

Beginning about the 20th week of pregnancy, almost all body systems begin to be affected. The cardiac system can easily become overwhelmed because the heart is forced to pump against rising peripheral resistance. This reduces the blood supply to organs, most markedly the kidney, pancreas, liver, brain and placenta. Poor placental perfusion may reduce the fetal nutrient and oxygen supply. Ischaemia in the pancreas may result in epigastric pain and an elevated amylase-creatinine ratio. Spasm of the arteries in the retina leads to vision changes. Vasospasm in the kidney increases blood flow resistance. Degenerative changes develop in kidney glomeruli because of back pressure. This leads to increased permeability of the glomerular membrane, allowing the serum proteins albumin and globulin to escape into the urine (proteinuria). The degenerative changes also result in

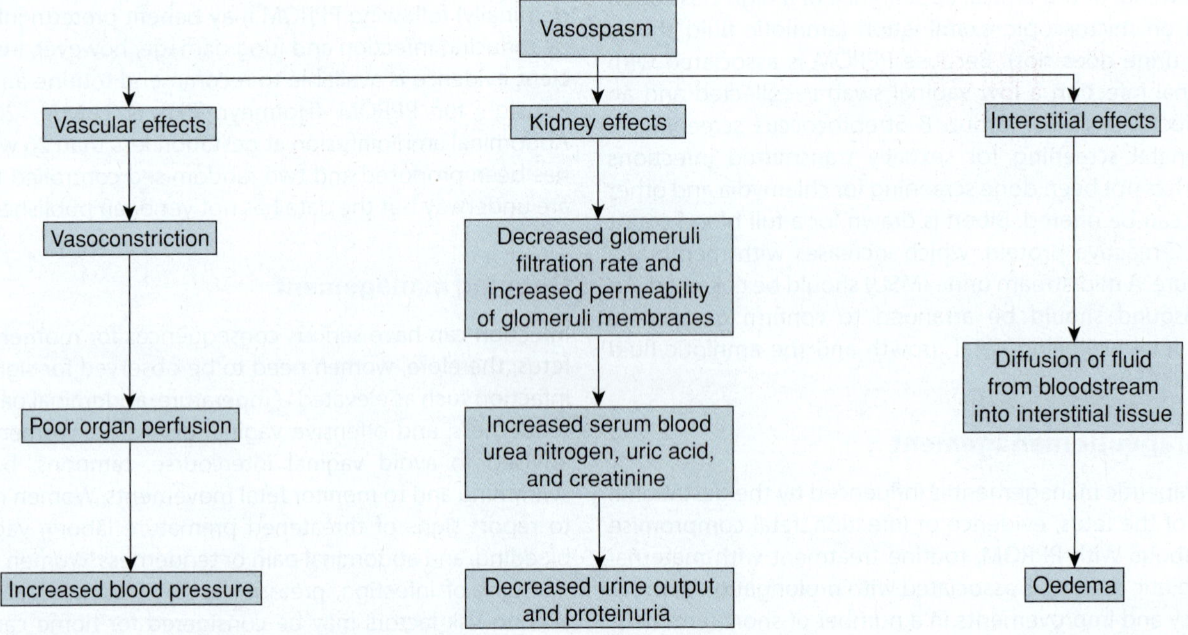

FIGURE 21.9 Physiological changes with gestational hypertension.

decreased glomerular filtration, so there is lowered urine output and clearance of creatinine. Increased kidney tubular reabsorption of sodium occurs and because sodium retains fluid, oedema results. Oedema is further increased because as more protein is lost, the osmotic pressure of the circulating blood falls and fluid diffuses from the circulatory system into the denser interstitial spaces to equalise the pressure (see Fig. 21.9). Extreme oedema can lead to cerebral and pulmonary oedema and seizures **(eclampsia)**.

Another effect is arterial spasm which causes the bulk of the blood volume in the maternal circulation to be pooled in the venous circulation, so a woman has a deceptively low arterial intravascular volume. In addition, thrombocytopenia or a lowered platelet count occurs as platelets cluster at the sites of endothelial damage. Measuring haematocrit levels helps to assess the extent of plasma loss to the interstitial space or the extent of the oedema (the higher the haematocrit, the more is being lost). A haematocrit level above 40% suggests significant fluid loss into interstitial spaces.

Assessment

Any woman with a high risk of preeclampsia should be observed carefully for symptoms at antenatal visits. Oedema frequently occurs in normal pregnancy and preeclampsia may present without oedema. However, rapidly developing generalised oedema should trigger screening for preeclampsia (see Box 21.3). It is important for women to be aware of symptoms to watch for so she can alert her doctor if additional symptoms occur between visits. It is important to assess blood pressure accurately. A manual sphygmomanometer is more accurate than an automated device which tends to record lower systolic pressures. The BP cuff should be the appropriate size and cover 80% of the arm circumference. The woman should sit comfortably with her feet touching the floor. The systolic blood pressure is taken from the first sound heard (Korotkoff 1) to the diastolic represented by the complete disappearance of the sound (Korotkoff 5).

BOX 21.3 Assessment ✻ Assessing the woman with preeclampsia

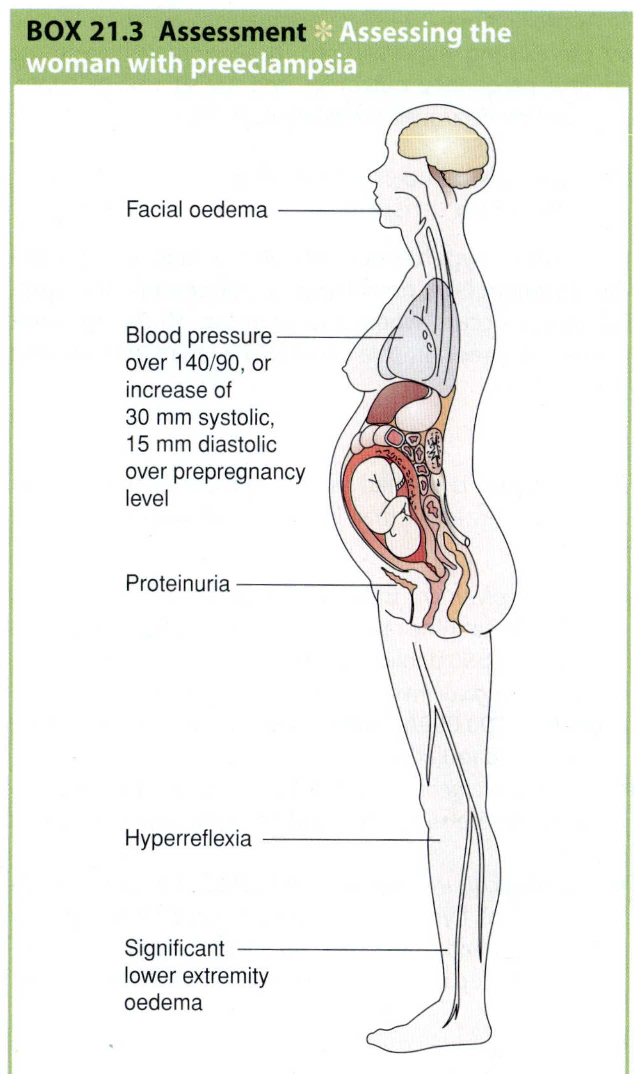

Gestational hypertension

Gestational hypertension is the new onset of elevated blood pressure after 20 weeks' gestation but with no maternal or fetal features that would suggest preeclampsia followed by a return to normal by 3 months' postpartum (Lowe et al., 2014). Gestational hypertension may develop into preeclampsia and if it persists beyond 3 months would be classified as chronic hypertension. Gestational hypertension occurring close to term has little effect on pregnancy outcomes, however, the earlier it presents the more likely it is to progress to preeclampsia or to cause adverse pregnancy outcomes. When gestational hypertension occurs near term there is little increase in the risk of poor outcomes.

Chronic hypertension

This category includes essential hypertension and secondary hypertension. Essential hypertension is defined as a blood pressure ≥140/90 mmHg that is confirmed prior to 20 weeks of completed gestation with no evident reason for the hypertension. *Secondary hypertension* is elevated blood pressure resulting from a known pre-existing medical condition such as chronic renal disease (e.g. glomerulonephritis, adult polycystic kidney disease), endocrine disorders (e.g. Cushing's syndrome, phaeochromocytoma, primary hyperaldosteronism) or systemic disease with renal involvement (e.g. diabetes mellitus, systemic lupus erythematosus). Most women with chronic hypertension (95%) will have essential hypertension. *White coat hypertension* is elevated blood pressure that occurs in the presence of a medical person. White coat hypertension can be evaluated by 24-hour ambulatory blood pressure monitoring prior to 20 weeks (it is less effective after 20 weeks). Approximately 50% of women with white coat hypertension will develop hypertension (Lowe et al., 2014).

Approximately 0.2–5% of pregnancies are complicated by pre-existing hypertension. These women have more adverse pregnancy outcomes and are at risk of superimposed preeclampsia (Lowe et al., 2014).

Preeclampsia superimposed on chronic hypertension

Pre-existing hypertension presents a high risk for the development of preeclampsia. Superimposed preeclampisa occurs when one or more of the systemic features of preeclampsia occur in a woman with chronic hypertension.

Preeclampsia

Preeclampsia is defined as hypertension occurring after 20 weeks' gestation that is associated with one of the following:

- *Renal involvement* indicated by proteinuria spot urine protein/creatinine ratio ≥30 mg/mmol; serum or plasma creatinine >90 µ; oliguria <80 mL/4 hours
- *Haematological involvement* indicated by thrombocytopenia <100,000/µ; haemolyis; disseminated intravascular coagulation
- *Liver involvement* indicated by raised serum transaminases; severe epigastric and/or right upper quadrant pain
- *Neurological involvement* indicated by convulsions (eclampsia), hyperreflexia with sustained clonus, persistent new headache, persistent visual disturbances (scotoma, photopsia, cortical blindness, retinal vasospasm); stroke
- *Pulmonary oedema*
- *Fetal growth restriction.*

The fetal mortality rate of preeclampsia is approximately 10%.

HELLP syndrome

HELLP syndrome (haemolysis, elevated liver enzymes and low platelets) is a variation of preeclampsia named for the common symptoms that occur: haemolysis that leads to anaemia; elevated liver enzymes that lead to epigastric pain; and low platelets that lead to abnormal bleeding/clotting and petechia (Abildgaard & Heimdal, 2013). HELLP syndrome is believed to be related to an autoimmune reaction leading to aggregation of platelets, endothelial malfunction and inborn errors of fatty acid oxidative metabolism. It is characterised by high mortality and morbidity rates leading to possibly life-threatening complications regarding both the mother and the fetus. Delivery is indicated if HELLP syndrome occurs after 34 gestational weeks or the fetal and/or maternal conditions deteriorate. Vaginal delivery is preferable. The syndrome occurs in 4–12% of patients with preeclampsia. It is a serious syndrome because it results in a maternal mortality rate as high as 24% and an infant mortality rate as high as 35%.

Why some women with severe preeclampsia also develop the HELLP syndrome is unknown. It occurs in both primigravidas and multigravidas. It may be associated with antiphospholipid syndrome or the presence of antiphospholipid antibodies (Mine & Shaul, 2011). In addition to proteinuria, oedema and increased blood pressure, additional symptoms of nausea, epigastric pain, general malaise and right upper quadrant tenderness from liver inflammation occur. Laboratory studies reveal haemolysis of red blood cells (they appear fragmented on a peripheral blood smear), thrombocytopenia (a platelet count, 100,000/mm^3), and elevated liver enzyme levels (alanine aminotransferase [ALT] and serum aspartate aminotransferase [AST]). The liver enzyme levels are elevated from haemorrhage and necrosis of the liver. Because of the low platelet count, women with the HELLP syndrome need close observation for bleeding, in addition to the observations necessary for preeclampsia and are therefore often cared for in the intensive care unit. Complications associated with the syndrome are subcapsular liver haematoma, hyponatraemia, renal failure and hypoglycaemia from poor liver function. Mothers are at risk of cerebral haemorrhages, aspiration pneumonia and hypoxic encephalopathy. Fetal complications can include growth restriction and preterm birth. Risk factors associated with HELLP include age >35 years, nulliparous, history of previous gestational hypertension and multiple pregnancy (Fitzpatrick et al., 2014).

With HELLP syndrome expectant management carries a 6.3% incidence of maternal death and an increased risk of placental abruption; therefore birth should be planned as soon as possible if the fetus is over 34 weeks' gestation (Aloizos et al., 2013). The infant is born as soon as feasible by either vaginal or caesarean birth. Maternal haemorrhage may occur at birth because of poor clotting ability. Epidural anaesthesia may not be possible because of the low platelet count and the high possibility of bleeding at the epidural site. Laboratory results return to normal after birth, and preeclamptic symptoms generally fade, but the experience of developing a HELLP syndrome is frightening. Women need assurance afterwards that symptoms were pregnancy related so will completely fade.

Eclampsia

Preeclampsia has progressed to eclampsia if one or more seizures have occurred. In Australia eclampsia is rare occurring in about 0.1%of births (Lowe et al., 2014). A European study found approximately 43% of women with eclampsia have had preeclampsia diagnosed and 70% have a history of hypertension in pregnancy (Schaap et al., 2014). Eclampsia is the most severe classification of preeclampsia and presents an obstetric emergency. A woman has passed into this stage when cerebral oedema is so acute that a grand-mal seizure (tonic–clonic) or coma occurs. With eclampsia, the maternal mortality rate is as high as 12% from causes such as cerebral haemorrhage, circulatory collapse, renal failure or pulmonary oedema

(Qureshi, Zaheer & Channa, 2014). The fetal prognosis with eclampsia is also poor because of hypoxia and consequent fetal acidosis. If premature separation of the placenta from vasospasm occurs, the fetal prognosis is even graver. If a fetus must be born before term, all the risks of immaturity will be faced.

Preeclampsia superimposed on chronic hypertension

The diagnosis of superimposed preeclampsia occurs when there is pre-existing hypertension and one or more features of preeclampsia develop after 20 weeks' gestation. When pre-existing hypertension exists the risk of development of preeclampsia is greatly increased. If hypertension and proteinuria are increasing in a women with pre-existing hypertension preeclampsia should be suspected.

Management of hypertensive disorders in pregnancy

Any woman with a new onset of hypertension after 20 weeks should be assessed for preeclampsia according to the 2014 SOMNAZ guidelines, which are as follows: spot urine PCR, full blood count, creatinine, electrolytes, urate, liver function tests, ultrasound assessment of fetal growth, amniotic fluid volume and umbilical artery Doppler assessment (Lowe et al., 2014). Blood test results should be interpreted with pregnancy-specific ranges and if symptoms of preeclampsia are present the following investigations should be undertaken: urinalysis for protein and urine microscopy from a mid-stream urine sample. If thrombocytopenia or a dropping haemoglobin is evident coagulation studies are warranted to investigate for DIC and haemolysis (Lowe et al., 2014).

Ongoing care

Preeclampsia generally continues to worsen as pregnancy advances. Birth of the baby is the definitive management and resolution of preeclampsia will follow usually in a few days. All women with preeclampsia should be monitored by an obstetrician. Women who are very preterm (<32 weeks) may require transfer to a tertiary institution. At each visit women should have their blood pressure checked and be assessed for proteinuria, if indicated preeclampsia bloods (FBC, electrolytes and creatinine, and liver function tests) plus coagulation studies if indicated (Lowe et al., 2014).

A woman has passed from mild to severe preeclampsia when her blood pressure rises to 160 mmHg systolic and 110 mmHg diastolic or above on at least two occasions, 6 hours apart, at bed rest (the position in which blood pressure is lowest) or her diastolic pressure is 30 mmHg above her pre-pregnancy level and there is marked proteinuria and extensive oedema.

Some women have severe epigastric pain, nausea and vomiting, possibly because of abdominal oedema or ischaemia to the pancreas and liver. If pulmonary oedema develops, a woman may report feeling short of breath. If cerebral oedema occurs, reports may be voiced of visual disturbances such as blurred vision or seeing spots before the eyes. Cerebral oedema also produces symptoms of severe headache and marked hyperreflexia and perhaps **ankle clonus** (a continued motion of the foot).

Women with beginning signs of hypertension will be seen approximately weekly or more frequently for the remainder of pregnancy. The seriousness of the condition can escalate rapidly. Therefore, women need to be aware of reporting any worsening of symptoms immediately. Preeclampsia will get worse as pregnancy progresses. The only way to halt its progression is to deliver the fetus. Continuing the pregnancy in the presence of preeclampsia has no benefit for the mother. Therefore, if the fetus is mature birth should be expedited. If the fetus is preterm then birth may be delayed, if the mother's condition permits, so corticosteroids can be given to aid fetal lung maturation. Women with preeclampsia should be cared for in hospitals with appropriate expertise.

Bed rest has not been shown to provide significant maternal or fetal benefit, however, women with severe preeclampsia require supervision in hospital. A woman needs a diet moderate to high in protein and moderate in sodium to compensate for the protein she is losing in urine. Stringent salt restriction to reduce oedema is not advised because sodium restriction may activate the renin-angiotensin-aldosterone system and result in increased blood pressure, compounding the problem.

An intravenous fluid line is usually initiated and maintained to serve as an emergency route for medication administration as well as to administer fluid to reduce haemoconcentration and hypovolaemia.

Maternal wellbeing

In monitoring a woman, take her blood pressure frequently (at least every 4 hours) or with a continuous monitoring device to detect any increase, which is a warning that her condition is worsening. Obtain blood studies such as a complete blood count, platelet count, liver function, blood urea nitrogen, and creatinine and fibrin degradation products as ordered to assess renal and liver function and the development of DIC, which often accompanies severe vasospasm. Because a woman is at high risk of premature separation of the placenta and resulting haemorrhage, a blood sample for type and cross-match is usually obtained.

Haematocrit levels are used to monitor blood concentration. This level will rise if increased fluid is leaving the bloodstream for interstitial tissue (oedema). An indwelling urinary catheter may be inserted to allow accurate recording of output and comparison with intake. Urinary output should be more than 600 mL per 24 hours (more than 30 mL per hour); an output lower than this suggests oliguria. Urinary proteins and specific gravity are measured and

TABLE 21.4 Antihypertensive medications used in pregnancy

Medication	Dose	Action	Contraindications	Practice points
Magesium sulfate	Loading dose: 4–6 grams in 100 mL infusion followed by continuous infusion of 1–3 grams per hour	Slows neuromuscular conduction, depression of CNS irritability	Pre-existing heart block, cardiac disease Myasthenia gravis	Given by IV infusion over 15–20 minutes
Labetalol	100–400 mg tds	Beta-blocker with mild alpha vasodilator effect	Asthma, chronic airways limitation	Bradycardia, bronchospasm, headache, nausea, scalp tingling
Hydralazine	25–50 mg tds	Vasodilation	Avoid 1st and 2nd trimester	Headache, flushing
Nifedipine	20 mg bd 60 mg SR bd	Ca channel antagonist	Aortic stenosis	Tachycardia, severe headache
Methyldopa	250–750 mg tds	Central	Depression	Onset occurs over 24 hours. Dry mouth, depression, sedation, blurred vision.
Calcium gluconate	1 gm (10% calcium gluconate in 10 mL) given IV slowly over 3–5 minutes	Antidote for magnesium sulfate toxicity		Have prepared at bedside for emergency administration when administering magnesium sulfate

recorded with voiding, or hourly if an indwelling catheter is present. A 24-hour urine sample may be collected for protein and creatinine clearance determinations to evaluate kidney function. A woman with mild preeclampsia spills between 0.5 grams and 1 gram of protein every 24 hours; a woman with severe preeclampsia spills approximately 5 grams per 24 hours.

Fetal wellbeing

In monitoring the fetus, generally single Doppler auscultation at approximately 4-hour intervals is sufficient. However, the fetal heart rate may be assessed continuously with an external fetal monitor. A woman may have a CTG or biophysical profile carried out daily to assess uteroplacental sufficiency (see Chapter 9).

Timing of birth

The timing of birth is related to the gestational age and the severity of preeclampsia. According to the SOMANZ (2014) guidelines, birth is indicated by the presence of: a severely growth restricted fetus; non-reassuring fetal status; gestational age ≥37 weeks; hypertension which cannot be controlled; a deteriorating platelet count; intravascular haemolysis; deteriorating liver or renal function; persistent neurological symptoms, epigastric pain, nausea or vomiting associated with abnormal liver function tests and pulmonary oedema.

Medications to prevent eclampsia

An antihypertensive medication such as hydralazine, labetalol or nifedipine may be prescribed to reduce hypertension (see Table 21.4). For acute control of severe hypertension 20–80 mg of labetalol may be given as an intravenous bolus over 2 minutes and repeated every 10 minutes as required (Lowe et al., 2014). These medications act to lower blood pressure by peripheral dilation and therefore do not interfere with placental circulation. They can cause maternal bradycardia. Therefore, assess pulse and blood pressure before and after administration. Diastolic pressure should not be lowered below 80 to 90 mmHg or inadequate placental perfusion could occur. Magnesium sulfate is the medication of choice to prevent an eclamptic seizure (Jordan, 2010).

Magnesium sulfate is first given intravenously in a loading or bolus dose of 4–6 grams over 15–20 minutes. The medication acts almost immediately although unfortunately the effect lasts only 30 to 60 minutes, so administration must be continuous. For magnesium sulfate to act as an anticonvulsant, blood serum levels must be maintained at a therapeutic level between 1.8 and 3 mmol/L (Jordan, 2010). If the blood serum level rises above this, respiratory depression, cardiac arrhythmias and cardiac arrest can occur. The importance of different serum levels is shown in Box 21.4.

The most evident symptoms of overdose from magnesium sulfate administration include decreased urine output, depressed respirations, reduced consciousness and decreased deep tendon reflexes (Jordan, 2010). Because magnesium is excreted from the body almost entirely through the urine, urine output must be monitored closely to ensure adequate elimination. Severe oliguria (less than 100 mL in 4 hours), can result in excessively high serum levels of magnesium. Therefore, before administering further magnesium sulfate, ensure that urine output is above 25 to 30 mL/hour, with a specific gravity of 1.010 or lower.

BOX 21.4 ✻ Focus on pharmacology

Magnesium sulfate

Action: Magnesium sulfate is a central nervous system depressant that acts to block neuromuscular transmission of acetylcholine to halt convulsions. It also halts premature labour, as it relaxes smooth muscle (McKenna & Mirkov, 2014).

Pregnancy risk category: A

Dosage: Initially, 4–6 grams mixed in 100 mL, given IV over 15–20 minutes. Followed with continuous infusion at 1–3 grams per hour to maintain therapeutic serum levels.

- Therapeutic range: 1.8–3 mmol/L
- Depression of deep tendon reflexes 2.5–3.5 mmol/L
- Somulence, loss of deep tendon reflexes, warning signs of toxicity 3.5–5 mmol/L
- Respiratory depression, ECG changes, toxicity 5 mmol/L
- Respiratory paralysis, complete heart block, extreme bradycardia, collapse 6–7.5 mmol/L
- Cardiac asystole 12.5 (range 4–15).

Possible adverse effects: Flushing, thirst with toxicity, absence of deep tendon reflexes, respiratory depression, cardiac arrhythmias, cardiac arrest and decreased urine output

Cautions for use

- Administer continuous infusion piggybacked into a main IV line so it can be discontinued immediately without interfering with fluid administration.
- Always use an infusion control device to maintain a regular flow rate.
- Assess maternal blood pressure and fetal heart rate continuously with bolus IV administration.
- Assess deep tendon reflexes every 1–4 hours during continuous infusion. Use patellar reflex. If patient has received epidural anaesthesia, use biceps reflex.
- Monitor intake and output every hour during continuous infusion. Urine output should be 30 mL/hr or greater.
- Assess client's level of consciousness, including ability to respond to questions, every hour.
- Obtain serum magnesium levels as indicated, usually every 6 to 8 hours.
- Keep calcium gluconate, the antidote for toxicity, readily available at the bedside.
- Maintain serum blood levels (for anticonvulsant use) at 5–8 mg/100 mL. If blood serum levels rise above this, respiratory depression, cardiac arrhythmias and cardiac arrest can occur.
- Do not administer additional doses and stop infusion if deep tendon reflexes are absent or if respiratory rate is less than 14 or urine output is less than 30 mL/hr.
- This drug may cause respiratory depression in the newborn if administered close to birth. Alert neonatal care personnel about this possibility.
- Magnesium sulfate may cause osteoporosis in the mother if given over a long time. Supplemental calcium can prevent this outcome.

Respirations should be above 12 per minute, a woman should be able to answer questions asked of her such as her name or address, and deep tendon reflexes should be present. Make these assessments every hour if a continuous intravenous infusion is being used. The easiest deep tendon reflex to assess is the patellar reflex (knee jerk). If an epidural block has been given for labour anaesthesia, assess the biceps or triceps reflex.

In addition to making the above assessments when magnesium sulfate is being given, a solution of 10 mL of a 10% calcium gluconate solution (1 gram) should be kept ready nearby for immediate intravenous administration should a woman develop signs and symptoms of magnesium toxicity, as calcium is the specific antidote for magnesium toxicity. Severe oliguria may be treated by the intravenous infusion of salt-poor albumin. This high-colloid solution will call fluid into the bloodstream from interstitial tissue by osmotic pressure; the kidneys will then excrete the extra fluid along with magnesium sulfate levels.

On the planned day of birth, a paediatrician should be alerted that the woman has been receiving magnesium sulfate. This is because magnesium sulfate given intravenously within 2 hours of a baby's birth, can cause respiratory depression because the medication crosses the placenta. A fetal heart rate monitor may show loss of variability of heartbeat immediately after magnesium therapy; an ultrasound may reveal reduced fetal breathing movements. Observe carefully for other signs of fetal effects, such as late deceleration with labour contractions. Magnesium sulfate is continued for 12 to 24 hours after birth in the woman to prevent eclampsia during this period. The dose is then tapered and discontinued. Breastfeeding usually is delayed until the medication is discontinued. A long-term effect of magnesium sulfate therapy is osteoporosis. A woman may be started on a course of calcium postpartum to address this problem.

Degeneration of a woman's condition from severe pre-eclampsia to eclampsia occurs when cerebral irritation from increasing cerebral oedema becomes so acute that a seizure occurs. This usually happens late in pregnancy but can happen up to 48 hours after childbirth. Immediately before a seizure, a woman's blood pressure rises suddenly from additional vasospasm. Her temperature rises sharply to 39.4°–40°C from increased cerebral pressure. She notices blurring of vision or severe headache (from the increased cerebral oedema) and her reflexes become hyperactive. She may experience a premonition that "something is happening". Vascular congestion of the liver or pancreas can lead to severe epigastric pain and nausea. Urinary output may decrease abruptly to less than 30 mL per hour. Eclampsia has actually occurred, however, only when a woman experiences a seizure.

Monitoring blood pressure and maternal status postpartum is important as eclampsia may occur after birth, usually in the first 24–72 hours, but sometimes later. Gestational hypertension normally resolves after birth. Women with pre-existing hypertension or preeclampsia may have hypertension or unstable blood pressure following birth. They require careful monitoring and may need to continue antihypertensive medication or to have the dosage adjusted. Blood pressure needs to be evaluated at the six week postpartum check to ensure it has returned to normal. If hypertension persists ongoing care needs to be initiated.

CASE STUDY QUESTION

5. If Belinda had developed severe preeclampsia, what would be the medication you would expect to administer?
   a. Magnesium sulfate
   b. Ranitidine (Zantac)
   c. A non-steroidal anti-inflammatory agent
   d. A loop diuretic

MULTIPLE PREGNANCY

Multiple gestation is considered a complication of pregnancy because a woman's body must adjust to the effects of more than one fetus. The incidence of multiple births has increased dramatically because of the use of in vitro fertilisation but still only occurs in 2–3% of all births. Twin births occur in about 1 in 80 births; triplets, 1 in 8000 (Bush & Pernoll, 2012).

Identical (monozygotic) twins begin with a single ovum and spermatozoon. In the process of fusion, or in one of the first cell divisions, the zygote divides into two identical individuals. Single-ovum twins usually have one placenta, one chorion, two amnions and two umbilical cords. The twins are always of the same sex. Two-thirds of twins are fraternal (dizygotic, non-identical), the result of the fertilisation of two separate ova by two separate spermatozoa. Dizygotic twins have two placentas, two chorions, two amnions and two umbilical cords. The twins may be of the same or different sex (see Fig. 21.10). It is sometimes difficult to determine by ultrasound or at birth whether twins are identical or fraternal because the two fraternal placentas may fuse and appear as one large placenta.

The higher a woman's parity and age, the more likely she is to have a multiple gestation. Inheritance appears to play a role in natural dizygotic twinning; this has a familial maternal pattern of occurrence.

Assessment

Multiple gestation is suspected early in pregnancy, when the uterus begins to increase in size at a rate faster than usual. Alpha-fetoprotein levels are elevated. At the time of quickening, a woman may report flurries of action at different portions of her abdomen rather than at one consistent spot (where the feet are located). On auscultation of the abdomen, multiple sets of fetal heart sounds are heard, but if one or more fetus has his or her back positioned towards a woman's back, only one fetal heart sound may be heard.

An ultrasound can reveal multiple gestation sacs early in pregnancy. In some instances, early ultrasound examinations reveal multiple amniotic sacs but then later in pregnancy, in as many as 30% of women, only one fetus remains (vanishing twin syndrome) (Sankaran et al., 2011). Women may grieve for a vanished twin as much as if the baby had died at birth, a feeling that could disrupt bonding in pregnancy.

Therapeutic management

Women with a multiple gestation are more susceptible to complications of pregnancy such as preeclampsia, polyhydramnios, placenta praevia, preterm labour and anaemia than are women carrying one fetus. They are also

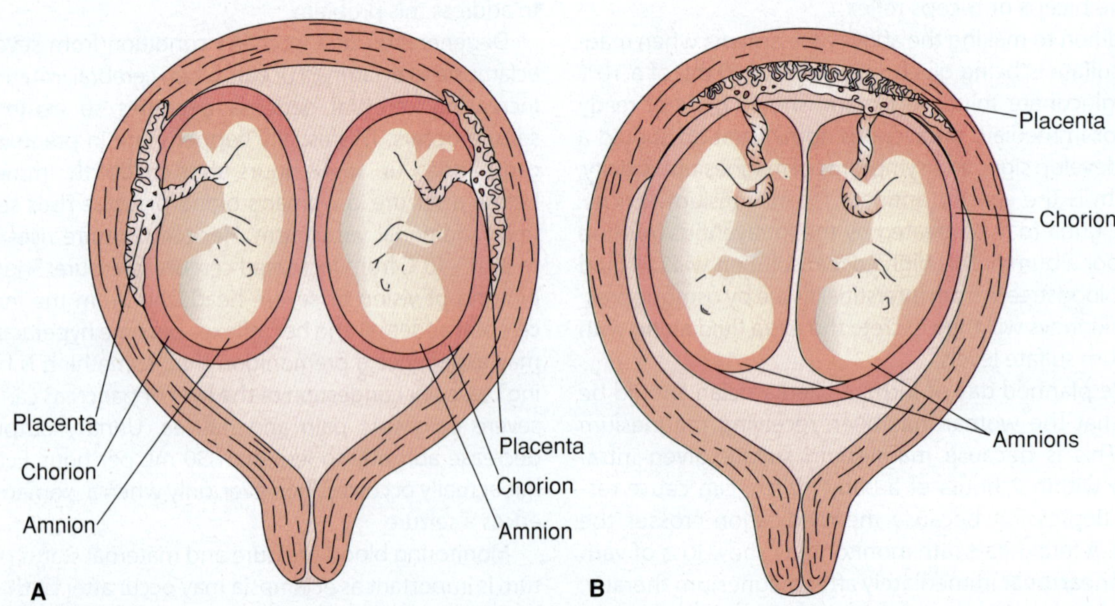

FIGURE 21.10 Multiple gestations. (**A**) Dizygotic twins showing two placentas, two chorions and two amnions. (**B**) Monozygotic twins with one placenta, one chorion and two amnions.

more prone to postpartum bleeding because of the additional uterine stretching that must occur. Because a multiple pregnancy usually ends before the normal term, 25% of low-birth-weight babies are from multiple pregnancies. There is a higher risk of congenital anomalies in twins, such as spinal cord defect, than with single births. There is a higher incidence of velamentous cord insertion (the cord inserted into the fetal membranes) with twins than with single births, so the risk of bleeding at the time of birth from a torn cord is increased. With monozygotic twins, the fetuses can share vascular communication, possibly leading to overgrowth of one fetus and undergrowth of the second (a twin-to-twin transfusion), resulting in discordant infants (Corsello & Piro, 2010) (see Chapter 26). If a single amnion is present, there can be knotting and twisting of umbilical cords, causing fetal distress or difficulty with birth. Because of the possibility of these complications, a woman with a twin pregnancy needs closer antenatal supervision than a woman with a single gestation, to detect these problems as early as possible. A woman carrying more than two fetuses is at greatest risk (Bush & Pernoll, 2012).

Because a woman is carrying a double weight during pregnancy, she may notice fatigue and backache and require more rest periods. Although there is little evidence that strict bed rest helps prolong multiple pregnancies (Hobbins, 2013), there is a need for extra rest, especially in a side-lying position during the day, to increase placental perfusion. As the growing uterus compresses her stomach, she may find her appetite decreasing and her intake falling. To compensate and maintain nutrition, a woman may need to eat six small meals a day rather than three large ones. She requires an adequate intake of iron and folic acid. Ambulation becomes increasingly difficult in late pregnancy and her abdomen may become so stretched that she feels as if she is going to burst.

Prematurity is increased in multiple pregnancy and the risk to the last-born infant is more hazardous. Nursing care at the birth of multiple infants is discussed in Chapter 23.

CASE STUDY QUESTION

6. If a patient developed a HELLP syndrome, what symptoms would be most important to assess for?
    a. Rapid, anxious breathing
    b. Ecchymosis or petechiae
    c. Blink reflex
    d. Enlarged thyroid

POLYHYDRAMNIOS

Usually the amniotic fluid volume during pregnancy is 500 to 1000 mL at term. Excess fluid more than 2000 mL or an amniotic fluid index above 24 cm is considered **hydramnios** (Juang & Snyder, 2012). Too much amniotic fluid can cause fetal malpresentation because the additional uterine space can allow the fetus to turn to a transverse lie. It can also lead to premature rupture of the membranes from the increased pressure with possible prostaglandin release. Preterm rupture of the membranes adds the additional risks of infection, prolapsed cord and preterm birth.

Assessment

Amniotic fluid is formed by a combination of the cells of the amniotic membrane and from fetal urine. It is evacuated by being swallowed by the fetus, absorbed across the intestinal membrane into the fetal bloodstream and transferred across the placenta. Although polyhydramnios can occur separately from fetal involvement, accumulation of amniotic fluid suggests difficulty with the fetus's ability to swallow or absorb, or excessive urine production. Inability to swallow occurs in infants who are anencephalic or who have tracheo-oesophageal fistula with stenosis or intestinal obstruction (Bishop, 2011). Excessive urine output occurs in the fetuses of diabetic women (hyperglycaemia in the fetus causes increased urine production).

The first sign of polyhydramnios may be unusually rapid enlargement of the uterus. The small parts of the fetus are difficult to palpate because the uterus is unusually tense. Auscultating the fetal heart rate is difficult because of the increased amount of fluid surrounding the fetus.

A woman may begin to notice extreme shortness of breath as the overly distended uterus pushes up against her diaphragm. She may develop lower extremity varicosities and haemorrhoids because of poor venous return from the extensive uterine pressure. She will have increased weight gain. Generally, an ultrasound is ordered to document the presence of polyhydramnios and to see if there is any reason evident.

Therapeutic management

Increased rest helps to increase uteroplacental circulation and reduces pressure on the cervix, which may help prevent preterm labour. Women should be aware of signs of ruptured membranes or uterine contractions. Constipation should be avoided by eating a high-fibre diet. Amniocentesis can be performed to remove some of the extra amniotic fluid, but because amniotic fluid is rapidly replaced it may need to be repeated. Polyhydramnious can lead to placental separation or rupture of membranes (Zheng, 2012a). Amniocentesis can be performed to remove some of the extra amniotic fluid, because amniotic fluid is replaced rapidly. If contractions begin, tocolysis may be begun to prevent or halt preterm labour.

After birth, the infant must be assessed carefully for factors that may have interfered with the ability to swallow in utero. Inability to swallow occurs in infants who are anencephalic, have tracheo-oesophageal fistula with stenosis or intestinal obstruction (Bishop, 2011).

OLIGOHYDRAMNIOS

Oligohydramnios refers to a pregnancy with less than the average amount of amniotic fluid (Kumar, 2012). Multiple definitions exist. Generally it is considered as an amniotic fluid index (AFI) less than 5 centimetres, but because amniotic fluid volume varies with gestational age a more sensitive definition may be an AFI less than the fifth percentile. Part of the amniotic fluid is formed by fetal urine, therefore renal or bladder disorders that interfere with voiding may be related to oligohydramnios. Oligohydramnios can occur from severe growth restriction. The condition is suspected during pregnancy when the uterus fails to meet its expected growth rate and is confirmed by ultrasound. Infants need careful inspection at birth to rule out kidney disease and compromised lung development.

POST-TERM PREGNANCY

A term pregnancy is 38 to 42 weeks long. A pregnancy that exceeds 42 weeks is called prolonged, **post-term**, *postmature* or a *postdates pregnancy*. The infant is considered postmature or dysmature, if there is evidence that placental insufficiency has interfered with fetal growth. Post-term pregnancy occurs in 3% to 12% of all pregnancies (Gulmezoglu, Crowther, Middleton, et al., 2012). Included in this group are some pregnancies that appear to extend beyond the due date set for them because of a faulty due date. Women who have long menstrual cycles (40 to 45 days, for example) do not ovulate on day 14 as in a typical menstrual cycle. Because they ovulate 14 days from the end of their cycle, or on day 26 or 31, their children will be "late" by 12 to 17 days. In other instances, the pregnancy is truly overdue. For some reason, the trigger that initiates labour did not turn on. Prolonged pregnancy can occur in a woman receiving a high dose of salicylates (for severe sinus headaches or rheumatoid arthritis) because salicylate interferes with the synthesis of prostaglandins, which may be responsible for the initiation of labour.

Remaining in utero for longer than 2 weeks beyond term creates a danger to a fetus for several reasons. Meconium aspiration is more apt to occur as fetal intestinal contents are more likely to reach the rectum. If the fetus continues to grow, macrosomia could create a birth problem. However, the usual effect of being post term is lack of growth. A placenta seems to have adequate functioning ability for only 40 to 42 weeks. After that time, it acquires calcium deposits which exposes a fetus to decreased blood perfusion. Such a fetus may suffer from a lack of oxygen, fluid and nutrients (Halloran et al., 2012). Oligohydramnios (a decreased amount of amniotic fluid from lessened urine production in the fetus) can lead to variable decelerations from cord compression.

If labour has not begun by 41 completed weeks of gestation, induction is considered after discussion with the woman and consideration of her opinion. Women should be aware that most labours occur spontaneously by 42 weeks. Care of the post-term infant at birth is discussed in Chapter 26.

ISOIMMUNISATION (Rh INCOMPATIBILITY)

According to the Australian Red Cross Blood Service approximately 17% of Caucasian women are missing the Rh (D) factor in their blood or have an Rh-negative blood type. The New Zealand Blood Service states 18% of the New Zealand population have an Rh-negative blood type. The percentage of Rh-negative women varies across ethnic groups. **Rh incompatibility** occurs when an Rh-negative mother (one negative for a *D* antigen or one with a *dd* genotype) carries a fetus with an Rh-positive blood type (*DD* or *Dd* genotype). For such a situation to occur, the father of the child must either be homozygous (*DD*) or heterozygous (*Dd*) Rh-positive. If the father of the child is homozygous (*DD*) for the factor, 100% of the couple's children will be Rh-positive (*Dd*). If the father is heterozygous for the trait, 50% of their children can be expected to be Rh-positive (*Dd*). Although this is basically a problem that affects the fetus, it causes such concern and apprehension in a woman during pregnancy that it becomes a maternal problem as well.

Because people who have Rh-positive blood have a protein factor (the *D* antigen) that Rh-negative people do not, when an Rh-positive fetus begins to grow inside an Rh-negative mother who is sensitised, it is as though her body is being invaded by a foreign agent. Her body reacts by forming antibodies against the invading substance. The Rh factor exists as a portion of the red blood cell, so these maternal antibodies cross the placenta and cause red blood cell destruction (haemolysis) of fetal red blood cells (see Fig. 21.11). A fetus can become so deficient in red blood cells that sufficient oxygen transport to body cells cannot be maintained. This condition is termed haemolytic disease of the newborn or **erythroblastosis fetalis**. Management of the infant born with this condition is discussed in Chapter 26.

Theoretically, there is no connection between fetal blood and maternal blood during pregnancy, so the mother should not be exposed to fetal blood. It is well documented, however, that an occasional villus ruptures, allowing a drop or two of fetal blood to enter the maternal circulation. Procedures such as amniocentesis or percutaneous umbilical blood sampling can also cause this. During a first pregnancy this effect is small. As the placenta separates after birth of the first child, there is an active exchange of fetal and maternal blood from damaged villi. Therefore, most of the maternal antibodies formed against the Rh-positive blood are not formed during pregnancy but in the first 72 hours after birth, making them a threat to a second pregnancy.

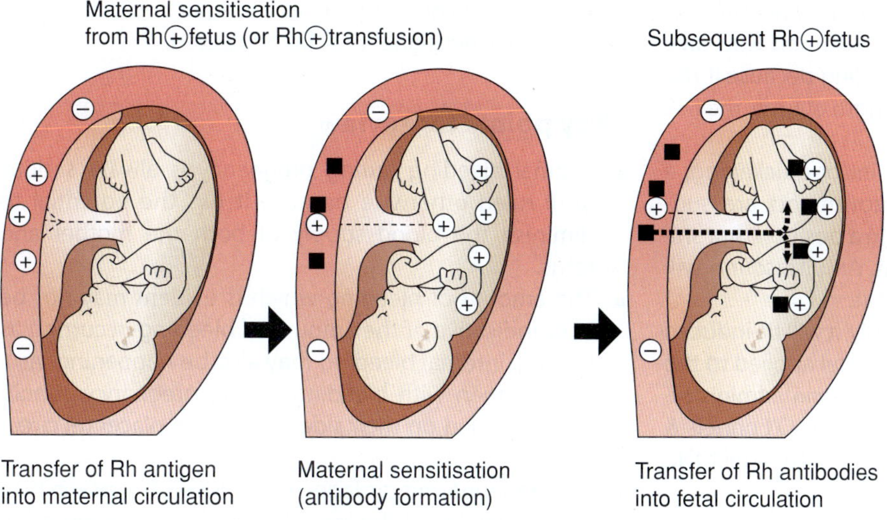

FIGURE 21.11 Maternal antibody formation against the Rh antigen.

Assessment

All women with Rh-negative blood should have an anti-D antibody titre performed at a first pregnancy visit. If the results are normal or the titre is minimal (normal is 0; a ratio below 1:8 is minimal), the test will be repeated at week 28 of pregnancy. If a woman's anti-D antibody titre is elevated at a first assessment (1:16 or greater), showing Rh sensitisation, the wellbeing of the fetus in this potentially toxic environment will be monitored every 2 weeks (or more often) by Doppler velocity of the fetal middle cerebral artery, a technique that can predict when anaemia is present or fetal red cells are being destroyed (Moise & Argoti, 2012).

Therapeutic management

The Royal Australian and New Zealand College of Obstetricians and Gynaecologists (RANZCOG), the National Blood Authority (Australia) and the New Zealand Blood Service recommend that Rh (D) immunoglobulin 250 IU (50 ug) should be given following any sensitising event in the first trimester of pregnancy. When a sensitising event occurs after the first trimester every Rh(D) negative woman should be given Rh (D) immunoglobulin 625 IU (125 ug). In Australia and New Zealand antenatal prophylaxis using 625 IU (125 ug) is given to all Rh (D) negative women at 28 and 34 weeks' gestation. Rh (D) immunoglobulin is given to Rh (D) negative women to reduce the number of maternal Rh (D) antibodies being formed. Postpartum every Rh (D) negative women with an Rh positive infant is administered 625 IU (125 ug) Rh (D) immunoglobulin in the first 72 hours after birth. After birth, the infant's blood type will be determined from a sample of the cord blood. If it is Rh-positive—Coombs' negative, indicating that a large number of antibodies are not present in the mother—the mother will receive the Rh (D) immunoglobulin injection. If the newborn's blood type is Rh-negative, no antibodies have been formed in the mother's circulation during pregnancy and none will form, so passive antibody injection is unnecessary.

In all cases where Rh (D) immunoglobulin is administered the woman should have no preformed anti-D antibodies and blood should be taken for an Rh antibody titre prior to administration of Rh (D) immunoglobulin (also known as anti-D).

Any woman who does not receive Rh (D) immunoglobulin injection after an induced abortion, miscarriage, ectopic pregnancy or amniocentesis can also have antibody formation.

CASE STUDY QUESTION

7. Suppose Belinda is Rh negative. Under what circumstance would she be eligible for Rh (D) immune globulin following her child's birth?
   a. If she had a multiple pregnancy
   b. If her fetus was found to be Rh negative
   c. If her fetus's heartbeat was tachycardic
   d. If her fetus's blood type was Rh positive

PREGNANCY LOSS

One of the most feared complications of pregnancy is fetal death. The most likely causes include chromosomal abnormalities, congenital malformations, and infections such as hepatitis B, immunological causes and complications of maternal disease. If fetal death occurs before the time of quickening, a woman will not be aware the fetus has died because she is not able to feel fetal movements. This type of fetal death may be discovered at a routine antenatal visit when no fetal heartbeat can be heard. A real-time ultrasound will reveal no fetal heartbeat is present.

When a fetus has died early in intrauterine life the loss may first be revealed by the natural miscarriage that occurs. A woman begins painless spotting, gradually accompanied by uterine contractions with cervical effacement and dilation. Carefully observe all women who give birth to a stillborn baby for excess bleeding because if the fetus has been dead in utero for any length of time, the risk of the development of DIC increases.

If a fetus dies in utero past the point of quickening, a woman becomes aware that fetal movements are suddenly absent. She may lie down or sit in a position that she knows usually causes fetal movement. An ultrasound will confirm the absence of a fetal heartbeat.

If labour does not begin spontaneously, it will be induced through a combination of prostaglandin gel applied to the cervix to effect cervical ripening and oxytocin administration to begin uterine contractions (Rattray, O'Connell & Baskett, 2012). Blood for coagulation studies to detect DIC should be obtained.

Going through labour knowing a fetus is dead is incredibly difficult. A woman grieves for both her dead child and her inability to carry a pregnancy to term. She may wonder what she could have done to cause this or may worry she is not as good a woman as others. It is important to listen to women and reassure them that their reactions are normal in the circumstances.

Ask a couple about their desire for clergy or religious rites, such as baptism. Encourage a support person to remain with a woman during labour, but remember the support person is grieving too. Although this is a difficult time, expressing grief makes the birth real, ends the pregnancy and allows the couple to begin rebuilding their life.

Many parents find it helpful to see their baby, so present their baby swaddled as normal. Point out particularly endearing features of the baby and similarities with the parent that may provide a focus for memories. Mementos such as a lock of hair, footprints, ID bracelet, a birth certificate and photographs will help validate their baby's life. Naming the baby as well as considerate respectful care will help parents begin the process of grieving.

If the child has a congenital anomaly that led to the death, prepare them for this before bringing the child to them, and explain how the anomaly affected the child. Explain hospital procedures such as when the body will be released or what additional permission for autopsy is needed.

Prepare the couple for the possibility that they may feel sad on the day the infant would have been born if the pregnancy had been carried to term, or if they visit a friend's child of the age their child would have been. Be certain before a woman is discharged from the hospital that she has a support person she can rely on during the following weeks and months, when the full impact of the fetal loss registers. With pregnancy loss for any reason it is important to assess a woman's adjustment and discuss feelings of powerlessness or anxiety, therefore a return appointment is necessary to evaluate her physiological and psychological health. Sadness and grief over the loss or a feeling that a woman has lost control of her life is to be expected. Do not forget to assess a partner's feelings as well, as a partner's grief may be neglected.

Key points for review

- Vaginal bleeding during pregnancy is always serious until ruled otherwise because it has the potential to diminish the blood supply of both the mother and fetus.
- The amount of bleeding which is evident may not be truly indicative of the amount of bleeding occurring as hidden, internal bleeding may also be happening. As a rule, women with bleeding during pregnancy should be positioned on their side to improve placental circulation.
- Spontaneous miscarriage is the loss of a pregnancy before viability of the fetus (20 weeks). The majority of these early pregnancy losses are attributed to chromosomal abnormalities. Miscarriages are classified as threatened, imminent, complete, incomplete, missed or recurrent pregnancy loss. Women who have a spontaneous miscarriage at home should bring any tissue passed to the hospital for an analysis for gestational trophoblastic disease.
- Ectopic pregnancy is pregnancy implantation outside the uterus, usually in a fallopian tube. If discovered before the tube ruptures, methotrexate or mifepristone can be administered to cause the conceptus to be reabsorbed. If not discovered early, sharp lower quadrant pain occurs at about 6 to 12 weeks as the tube ruptures. Surgery is performed to remove the conceptus and repair the tube to halt bleeding.
- Gestational trophoblastic disease is abnormal overgrowth of trophoblast cells. If not discovered by an ultrasound early in pregnancy, bleeding and expulsion of the abnormal growth occur at about the 16th week of pregnancy. Women need close follow-up after this because it can lead to choriocarcinoma, a malignancy.
- Premature cervical dilation occurs when the cervix dilates early in pregnancy, before viability of the fetus. Sutures (cervical cerclage) can be placed to prevent the cervix from dilating prematurely this way again in a second pregnancy.
- Placenta praevia is low implantation of the placenta so that it crosses the cervical os. If this is not discovered before labour, cervical dilation may cause the placenta to tear, causing severe blood loss. Women who have symptoms of placenta praevia (painless vaginal bleeding in the third trimester) should not have vaginal examinations carried out to prevent disruption of the low-implanted placenta.
- Premature separation of the placenta (abruptio placentae), placental separation from the uterus before the fetus is born, usually occurs late in pregnancy. This separation immediately cuts off blood supply to the fetus. Women with increased parity, those with previous uterine surgery and those who use cocaine are at

highest risk of this. Often it is manifested by sudden, sharp fundal pain, then a continuing pain and vaginal bleeding.

- Disseminated intravascular coagulation is a blood disorder that may occur with any trauma, so it can accompany such conditions as premature separation of the placenta and pregnancy-induced hypertension. Blood coagulation is so extreme at one point in the circulatory system that clotting factors are used up, resulting in their absence in the remainder of the system. Beginning symptoms of this include easy bruising, petechiae and oozing from intravenous sites. Heparin is used to stop the local coagulation and free up clotting factors for systemic use.
- Preterm labour is labour that occurs after 20 weeks and before the end of the 37th week of pregnancy. A woman is said to be in preterm labour when she has had uterine contractions every 10 minutes for 1 hour and cervical dilation begins. Common tocolytics, medications that can halt labour, are beta-sympathomimetic agents such as terbutaline.
- Preterm rupture of the membranes is tearing of the fetal membranes with loss of amniotic fluid before the pregnancy is at term. After rupture, there is a high risk of fetal and uterine infection (chorioamnionitis) and preterm birth.
- Pregnancy-induced hypertension is a unique disorder that occurs with pregnancy with three classic symptoms: hypertension, oedema and proteinuria. It is categorised as preeclampsia or eclampsia. If mild (blood pressure not over 140/90), treatment is bed rest and perhaps low-dose aspirin. If severe (blood pressure over 160/110), bed rest plus administration of magnesium sulfate is necessary. If a seizure occurs, the condition becomes eclampsia. Helping prevent the disease from progressing to this stage is an important nursing responsibility.
- The HELLP syndrome is a unique form of pregnancy-induced hypertension marked by haemolysis of red blood cells, elevated liver enzymes and a low platelet count.
- Multiple gestation puts an additional strain on a woman's physical resources and may lead to preterm birth with immaturity of her infants. Helping a woman plan adequate nutrition and rest during pregnancy are nursing responsibilities.
- Post term pregnancy is pregnancy that extends beyond 42 weeks. As the placenta deteriorates at this time, it can cause a fetus to receive decreased nutrients.
- Polydramnios is overproduction of amniotic fluid (above 2000 mL), a condition that can lead to ruptured membranes and premature birth because of increased intrauterine pressure. Oligohydramnios is the lessened amount of fluid and suggests a renal disorder exists in the fetus.
- Isoimmunisation (Rh incompatibility) is a possibility when a woman who is Rh negative is sensitised and carries a fetus who is Rh positive. Maternal antibodies form and destroy fetal red blood cells, leading to anaemia, oedema and jaundice in the newborn. Being certain women are screened for blood type and antibody titre early in pregnancy is a nursing responsibility.

CASE STUDY QUESTIONS

8. Belinda was in preterm labour at 30 weeks of pregnancy. She discounted the symptoms she was having because she did not think they could be early labour. What are the signs of early labour that you would have liked her to have been more aware of?
9. Suppose Belinda is bleeding because of placenta praevia; everyone else on the unit is at lunch, and you are alone. You know you should not do a pelvic examination with a placenta praevia. How would you estimate the amount of blood she has lost? How would you determine that blood loss was not affecting the fetus?
10. Suppose Belinda is placed on home care after preterm rupture of membranes at 30 weeks of pregnancy. What assessments would you want to do to ensure she is not developing chorioamnionitis?

Resources

For an extensive range of additional resources to enhance teaching and learning and to facilitate understanding of this chapter, please see the text's accompanying website located on thePoint at http://thepoint.lww.com.

References

Abatangelo, L., Okereke, L., Parham-Foster, C., et al. (2010). If pelvic inflammatory disease is suspected empiric treatment should be initiated. *Journal of American Nurse Practitioner*, *22*(2), 117–122.

Abildgaard, U. & Heimdal, K. (2013). Pathogenesis of the syndrome of hemolysis, elevated liver enzymes, and low platelet count (HELLP): A review. *European Journal of Obstetrics, Gynecology & Reproductive Biology*, *166*(2), 117–123.

Abou, E. Senoun, G., Dowswell, T. & Mousa, H. A. (2014). Planned home versus hospital care for preterm prelabour rupture of the membranes (PPROM) prior to 37 weeks' gestation. *Cochrane Database of Systematic Reviews*, (4), (CD008053).

Alfirevic, Z., Owen, J., Carreras Moratonas, E., Sharp, A. N., Szychowski, J. M., & Goya, M. (2013). Vaginal progesterone, cerclage or cervical pessary for preventing preterm birth in asymptomatic singleton pregnant women with a history of preterm birth and a sonographic short cervix. *Ultrasound in Obstetrics & Gynecology*, *41*(2), 146–151.

Alfirevic, Z., Stampalija, T., Roberts, D. & Jorgensen, A.L. (2012). Cervical stitch (cerclage) for preventing preterm birth in singleton pregnancy. *Cochrane Database of Systematic Reviews*, (4), (CD008991).

Aloizos, S., Seretis, C., Liakos, N., Aravosita, P., Mystakelli, C., Kanna, E. & Gourgiotis, S. (2013). HELLP syndrome: Understanding and management of a pregnancy-specific disease. *Journal of Obstetrics & Gynaecology*, *33*(4), 331–337.

Ananth, C., Nath, C. & Philipp, C. (2010). The normal anticoagulant system and risk of placental abruption: Protein C, protein S and resistance to activated protein C. *Fetal Neonatal Medicine*, *23*(12), 1377–1383.

Arabin, B. & Alfirevic, Z. (2013). Cervical pessaries for prevention of spontaneous preterm birth: Past, present and future. *Ultrasound in Obstetrics & Gynecology*, *42*(4), 390–399.

Australian Cerebral Palsy Register (ACPR) Group. (2009). *Report of the Australian Cerebral Palsy Register, Birth Years 1993–2003*. Sydney: ACPR Group.

Barton, J. R. & Sibai, B. M. (2012). Severe sepsis and septic shock in pregnancy. *Obstetrics & Gynecology, 120*(3), 689–706.

Bedoya-Ronga, A. & Currie, I. (2012). Which patients should be offered caesarean section? *Practitioner, 256*(1749), 16–18.

Berghella, V., Baxter, J. K. & Hendrix, N. W. (2013). Cervical assessment by ultrasound for preventing preterm delivery. *Cochrane Database of Systematic Reviews*, (1), (CD007235).

Bick, D. (2012). Born too soon: The global issue of preterm birth. *Midwifery, 28*(4), 401–402.

Bicking Kinsey, C. (2014). *Effect of prior perinatal loss on maternal depressive symptoms and maternal-infant bonding.* (Ph.D.), Pennsylvania State University. Retrieved from http://ezproxy.csu.edu.au/login?url=http://search.ebscohost.com/login.aspx?direct=true&db=rzh&AN=2012782679&site=ehost-live. Available from EBSCOhost rzh database.

Bishop, W. P. (2011). The digestive system. In K. J. Marcdante, R. M. Kliegman, H. B. Jenson, et al. (Eds.), *Nelson Essentials of Pediatrics* (6th ed.), pp. 463–498. Philadelphia: Saunders/Elsevier.

Boisramé, T., Sananès, N., Fritz, G., Boudier, E., Aissi, G., Favre, R. & Langer, B. (2014). Placental abruption: Risk factors, management and maternal-fetal prognosis. Cohort study over 10 years. *European Journal of Obstetrics & Gynecology & Reproductive Biology, 179*, 100–104.

Borrell, A. & Stergiotou, I. (2013). Miscarriage in contemporary maternal-fetal medicine: Targeting clinical dilemmas. *Ultrasound in Obstetrics & Gynecology, 42*(5), 491–497.

Buckley, L. L. & Schub, T. (2013). Placenta previa. In D. Pravikoff & D. Pravikoff (Eds), pp. 2p. Glendale, CA: Cinahl Information Systems.

Bush, M. C. & Pernoll, M. L. (2012). Multiple gestation. In D. K. Edmonds (Ed), *Dewhurst's Textbook of Obstetrics & Gynaecology* (8th ed.), pp. 301–309. Oxford, UK: John Wiley & Son.

Cannie, M. M., Dobrescu, O., Gucciardo, L., Strizek, B., Ziane, S., Sakkas, E., Jani, J. C., et al. (2013). Arabin cervical pessary in women at high risk of preterm birth: A magnetic resonance imaging observational follow-up study. *Ultrasound in Obstetrics & Gynecology, 42*(4), 426–433.

Capece, A., Vasieva, O., Meher, S., Alfirevic, Z. & Alfirevic, A. (2014). Pathway analysis of genetic factors associated with spontaneous preterm birth and pre-labor preterm rupture of membranes. *PLoS ONE, 9*(9), 1–11.

Cappiello, J., Beal, M. & Simmonds, K. (2011). Clinical issues in postabortion care. *Nurse Practitioner, 36*(5), 35–40.

Chawanpaiboon, S., Pimol, K. & Sirisomboon, R. (2011). Comparison of success rate of nifedipine, progesterone, and bed rest for inhibiting uterine contraction in threatened preterm labor. *Journal of Obstetrics & Gynaecology Research, 37*(7), 787–791.

Corsello, G. & Piro, E. (2010). The world of twins: An update. *Journal of Maternal–Fetal & Neonatal Medicine, 23*(Suppl. 3), 59–62.

Critchfield, A. S., Yao, G., Jaishankar, A., Friedlander, R. S., Lieleg, O., Doyle, P. S., Ribbeck, K., et al. (2013). Cervical mucus properties stratify risk for preterm birth. *PLoS ONE, 8*(8), 1–7.

Crowther, C. A., Middleton, P. & McBain, R. D. (2013). Anti-D administration in pregnancy for preventing Rhesus alloimmunisation. *Cochrane Database of Systematic Reviews* (2).

DeFranco, E. A., Lewis, D. F. & Odibo, A. O. (2013). Improving the screening accuracy for preterm labor: Is the combination of fetal fibronectin and cervical length in symptomatic patients a useful predictor of preterm birth? A systematic review. *American Journal of Obstetrics & Gynecology, 208*(3), 233.e231–233.e236.

Feodor Nilsson, S., Andersen, P. K., Strandberg-Larsen, K. & Nybo Andersen, A. M. (2014). Risk factors for miscarriage from a prevention perspective: A nationwide follow-up study. *BJOG: An International Journal of Obstetrics & Gynaecology, 121*(11), 1375–1385.

Fitzpatrick, K. E., Hinshaw, K., Kurinczuk, J. J. & Knight, M. (2014). Risk factors, management, and outcomes of hemolysis, elevated liver enzymes, and low platelets syndrome and elevated liver enzymes, low platelets syndrome. *Obstetrics & Gynecology, 123*(3), 618–627.

Fu, J., Fang, F., Xie, L., et al. (2012). Prophylactic chemotherapy for hydatidiform mole to prevent gestational trophoblastic neoplasia. *Cochrane Database of Systematic Reviews*, (10), CD007289.

Gilbert, E. S. (2011). *Spontaneous abortion. In manual of high risk pregnancy & delivery* (5th ed.), pp. 311–330. St Louis, MO: Mosby Elsevier.

Guimarães Filho, H., Araujo Júnior, E., Pires, C., Nardozza, L. & Moron, A. (2013). Short cervix syndrome: Current knowledge from etiology to the control. *Archives of gynecology and obstetrics, 287*(4), 621–628.

Gulmezoglu, A., Crowther, C., Middleton, P. & Heatley, E. (2012). Induction of labour for improving birth outcomes for women at or beyond term. *Cochrane Database of Systematic Reviews*, (6).

Halloran, D. R., Cheng, Y. W., Wall, T. C., et al. (2012). Effect of maternal weight on postterm delivery. *Journal of Perinatology, 32*(2), 85–90.

Hammond, G., Langridge, A., Leonard, H., Hagan, R., Jacoby, P., DeKlerk, N. & Stanley, F. (2013). Changes in risk factors for preterm birth in Western Australia 1984–2006. *BJOG: An International Journal of Obstetrics & Gynaecology, 120*(9), 1051–1060.

Hasanzadeh, M., Tabari, A., Homae, F., Shakeri, M., Bakhshandeh, T. & MadaniSani, F. (2014). Evaluation of weekly intramuscular methotrexate in the treatment of low risk gestational trophoblastic neoplasia. *Journal of Cancer Research & Therapeutics, 10*(3), 646–650.

Heaman, M., Kingston, D., Chalmers, B., Sauve, R., Lee, L. & Young, D. (2013). Risk factors for preterm birth and small-for-gestational-age births among Canadian women. *Paediatric & Perinatal Epidemiology, 27*(1), 54–61.

Hobbins, J. C. (2013). Preventing Preterm Birth in Twins. *OB/GYN Clinical Alert, 30*(6), 41–43.

Hofmeyr, G. J., Eke, A. C. & Lawrie, T. A. (2014). Amnioinfusion for third trimester preterm premature rupture of membranes. *Cochrane Database of Systematic Reviews*, (3), (CD000942).

Hooker, A. B., Lemmers, M., Thurkow, A. L., Heymans, M. W., Opmeer, B. C., Brölmann, H.A.M., Huirne, J. A. F. et al. (2014). Systematic review and meta-analysis of intrauterine adhesions after miscarriage: Prevalence, risk factors and long-term reproductive outcome. *Human Reproduction Update, 20*(2), 262–278.

Hsu, S. & Euerle, B. D. (2012). Ultrasound in pregnancy. *Emergency Medicine Clinics of North America, 30*(4), 849–867.

Hubinont, C. & Debrieve, F. (2011). Prevention of preterm labour: 2011 update on tocolysis. *Journal of Pregnancy, 2011*.

Jaleel, R. & Khan, A. (2013). Paternal factors in spontaneous first trimester miscarriage. *Pakistan Journal of Medical Sciences, 29*(3), 748–752.

Jamshidimanesh, M., Soleymani, M., Ebrahimi, E. & Hosseini, F. (2013). Domestic violence against pregnant women in Iran. *Journal of Family & Reproductive Health, 7*(1), 7–10.

Jenderny, J. (2014). Chromosome aberrations in a large series of spontaneous miscarriages in the German population and review of the literature. *Molecular Cytogenetics (17558166), 7*(1), 2–16.

Jeve, Y. B. & Davies, W. (2014). Evidence-based management of recurrent miscarriages. *Journal of Human Reproductive Sciences, 7*(3), 159–169.

Johnstone, C. (2013). Vaginal examination does not improve diagnostic accuracy in early pregnancy bleeding. *Emergency Medicine Australasia, 25*(3), 219–221.

Jordan, S. (2010). *Pharmacology for Midwives: The Evidence Base for Safe Practice* (2nd ed.), Basingstoke: Palgrave Macmillan.

Juang, D. & Snyder, C. L. (2012). Neonatal bowel obstruction. *Surgical Clinics of North America, 92*(3), 685–711.

Kausar, F., Morris, J. L., Fathalla, M., et al. (2012). Nurses in low resource settings save mothers' lives with non-pneumatic anti-shock garment. *MCN: American Journal of Maternal Child Nursing, 37*(5), 308–316.

Kenyon, S., Boulvain, M. & Neilson, J. P. (2013). Antibiotics for preterm rupture of membranes. *Cochrane Database of Systematic Reviews*, (12), (CD001058).

Khader, Y., Al-Akour, N., Alzubi, I., et al. (2011). The association between second hand smoke and low birth weight and preterm delivery. *Maternal & Child Health Journal*, *15*(4), 453–459.

Khan, A. N. (2013). Cervical incompetence imaging, accessed 15 January 2015, <http://emedicine.medscape.com/article/402598-overview>.

Klauser, C. K., Briery, C. M., Martin, R. W., Langston, L., Magann, E. F. & Morrison, J. C. (2014). A comparison of three tocolytics for preterm labor: A randomized clinical trial. *Journal of Maternal-Fetal & Neonatal Medicine*, *27*(8), 801–806.

Kok, N., Ruiter, L., Hof, M., Ravelli, A., Mol, B. W., Pajkrt, E. & Kazemier, B. (2014). Risk of maternal and neonatal complications in subsequent pregnancy after planned caesarean section in a first birth, compared with emergency caesarean section: a nationwide comparative cohort study. *BJOG: An International Journal of Obstetrics & Gynaecology*, *121*(2), 216-223.

Kumar, S. (2012). Fetal anomalies. In D. K. Edmonds (Ed), *Dewhurst's Textbook of Obstetrics & Gynaecology* (8th ed.), pp. 219–229. Oxford, UK: John Wiley & Son.

Lane, B. F. & Wong-You-Cheong, J. J. (2014). Imaging of vaginal bleeding in early pregnancy. *Applied Radiology*, *43*(9), 8–16.

Levi, M. (2014). Diagnosis and treatment of disseminated intravascular coagulation. *International Journal of Laboratory Hematology*, *36*(3), 228–236.

Li, W., Ma, N., Laird, S. M., Ledger, W. L. & Li, T. C. (2013). The relationship between serum prolactin concentration and pregnancy outcome in women with unexplained recurrent miscarriage. *Journal of Obstetrics & Gynaecology*, *33*(3), 285–288.

Li, Z., Zeki, R., Hilder, L. & Sullivan, E. A. (2012). *Australia's Mothers and Babies 2010*. Perinatal statistics series no. 27. Cat. no. PER 57. Canberra: AIHW National Perinatal Epidemiology and Statistics Unit.

Lim, C., Ho. K. W., Cheng, N. & Wong, F. W. (2013). Combined use of oestrogen and progesterone for preventing miscarriage. *Cochrane Database of Systematic Review*, *9*, (CD009278).

Lowe, S. A., Bowyer, L., Lust, K., McMahon, L. P., Morton, M. R., North, R. A., Said, J. M., et al. (2014). The SOMANZ Guidelines for the management of hypertensive disorders of pregnancy 2014. *Australian & New Zealand Journal of Obstetrics & Gynaecology*, *55*(1), 11–16.

Lukasse, M., Helbig, A., Benth, J. Š. & Eberhard-Gran, M. (2014). Antenatal maternal emotional distress and duration of pregnancy. *PLoS ONE*, *9*(7), 1–8.

Mackeen, A. D., Seibel-Seamon, J., Muhammad, J., Baxter, J. K. & Berghella, V. (2014). Tocolytics for preterm premature rupture of membranes. *Cochrane Database of Systematic Reviews*, (2), (CD007062).

McKenna, L. & Mirkov, S. (2014). *McKenna's Drug Handbook for Nursing and Midwifery* (7th ed.). Sydney: Lippincott Williams & Wilkins.

McNair, T. & Altman, K. (2011). Miscarriage and recurrent pregnancy loss. In K. J. Hurt, M. W. Guile, J. L. Bienstock, et al. (Eds), *The Johns Hopkins Manual of Gynecology and Obstetrics* (4th ed.), pp. 438–447. Philadelphia, PA: Lippincott Williams & Wilkins.

Manuck, T. A. & Varner, M. W. (2014). Neonatal and early childhood outcomes following early vs later preterm premature rupture of membranes. *American Journal of Obstetrics and Gynecology*, *211*(3), 308.

Matsuda, Y., Hayashi, K., Shiozaki, A., et al. (2011). Comparison of risk factors for placental abruption and placenta previa: Case-cohort study. *Journal of Obstetrics & Gynaecology Research*, *37*(6), 538–546.

Mehta, S. H. & Sokol, R. J. (2013). Assessment of high-risk pregnancy. In A. H. DeCherney, L. Nathan, T. M. Goodwin, et al. (Eds), *Current Diagnosis and Treatment: Obstetrics and Gynecology* (11th ed.), pp. 223–233, Columbus, OH; McGraw-Hill/Lange.

Merrill, L. (2013). Magnesium sulfate during anticipated preterm birth for infant neuroprotection. *Nursing for Women's Health*, *17*(1), 42–51.

Mine, C. & Shaul, P. W. (2011). New insights into the molecular basis of the antiphospholipid syndrome. *Drug Discovery Today: Disease Mechanisms*, *8*(1–2), e47–e52.

Moise, K. J. Jr. & Argoti, P. S. (2012). Management and prevention of red cell alloimmunization in pregnancy: A systematic review. *Obstetrics & Gynecology*, *120*(5), 1132–1139.

Murphy, F. A., Lipp, A. & Powles, D. L. (2012). Follow-up for improving psychological well being for women after a miscarriage. *Cochrane Database Systematic Review*, (3), (CD008679).

Murtaza, U. I., Ortmann, M. J., Mando-Vandrick, J. & Lee, A.S.D. (2013). Management of first-trimester complications in the emergency department. *American Journal of Health-System Pharmacy*, *70*(2), 99–111.

Nanda, K., Lopez, L. M., Grimes, D. A., Peloggia, A. & Nanda, G. (2012). Expectant care versus surgical treatment for miscarriage. *Cochrane Database of Systematic Reviews*, *14*(3).

Neilson, J. P., West, H. M. & Dowswell, T. (2014). Betamimetics for inhibiting preterm labour. *Cochrane Database of Systematic Reviews*, (2), (CD004352).

Nigro, G., Mazzocco, M., Mattia, E., Di Renzo, G., Carta, G. & Anceschi, M. (2011). Role of the infections in recurrent spontaneous abortion. *Journal of Maternal Fetal Neonatal Medicine*, *24*(8), 983–989.

Petersen, S. G., Perkins, A. R., Gibbons, K. S., Bertolone, J. I. & Mahomed, K. (2013). The medical management of missed miscarriage: Outcomes from a prospective, single-centre, Australian cohort. *Medical Journal of Australia*, *199*(5), 341–346.

Qureshi, S. R., Zaheer, S. & Channa, S. R. (2014). Eclampsia; maternal morbidity and mode of delivery in the management. *Professional Medical Journal*, *21*(4), 628–632.

Rattray, D. D., O'Connell, C. M. & Baskett, T. F. (2012). Acute disseminated intravascular coagulation in obstetrics: A tertiary centre population review. *Journal of Obstetrics & Gynaecology Canada*, *34*(4), 341–347.

Riley, C., Boozer, K. & King, T. (2011). Antenatal corticosteroids at the beginning of the 21st century. *Journal of Midwifery & Women's Health*, *56*(6), 591–597.

Rimawi, B. H., Soper, D. E. & Eschenbach, D. A. (2012). Group A streptococcal infections in obstetrics and gynecology. *Clinical Obstetrics & Gynecology*, *55*(4), 864–874.

Roman, A. S. (2013). Late pregnancy complications. In A. H. DeCherney, L. Nathan, T. M. Goodwin, et al. (Eds), *Current Diagnosis and Treatment: Obstetrics and Gynecology* (11th ed.), pp. 250–266. Columbus, OH: McGraw-Hill/Lange.

Royal College of Obstetricians & Gynaecologists (2011). Tocolysis for women in preterm labour. Green top guideline no. Ib, accessed 1 April 2015, <www.rcog.org.uk/globalassets/documents/guidelines/gtg_1b.pdf>.

Saleh, S. S., Al-Ramahi, M. Q. & Al Kazaleh, F. A. (2013). Atosiban and nifedipine in the suppression of pre-term labour: A comparative study. *Journal of Obstetrics & Gynaecology*, *33*(1), 43–45.

Sangkomkamhang, U. S., Lumbiganon, P., Prasertcharoensook, W. & Laopaiboon, M. (2009). Antenatal lower genital tract infection screening and treatment programs for preventing preterm delivery. *Cochrane Database of Systematic Reviews*, (2), (CD006178).

Sankaran, S., Rozette, C., Dean, J., et al. (2011). Screening in the presence of a vanished twin: Nuchal translucency or combined screening test? *Prenatal Diagnosis*, *31*(6), 600–601.

Savage, P. & Seckl, M. (2012). Gestational trophoblast tumours. In D. K. Edmonds (Ed), *Dewhurst's Textbook of Obstetrics & Gynaecology* (8th ed.), pp. 88–100. Oxford, UK: John Wiley & Son.

Schaap, T. P., Knight, M., Zwart, J. J., Kurinczuk, J. J., Brocklehurst, P., van Roosmalen, J. & Bloemenkamp, K.W.M. (2014). Eclampsia, a comparison within the International Network of Obstetric Survey Systems. *BJOG: An International Journal of Obstetrics & Gynaecology*, *121*(12), 1521–1528.

Schub, T. & Spears, T. L. (2014). Disseminated intravascular coagulation in pregnancy. In D. Pravikoff & D. Pravikoff (Eds), p. 2p. Glendale, California: Cinahl Information Systems.

Sharp, A. N., & Alfirevic, Z. (2014). Provision and practice of specialist preterm labour clinics: A UK survey of practice. *BJOG: An International Journal of Obstetrics & Gynaecology*, *121*(4), 417–421.

Sherieh, M., Cottrell, D. B. & Mancuso, P. (2014). Medical management of ectopic pregnancy. *Clinician Reviews*, *24*(7), 29–38.

Su, L.L., Samuel, M. & Chong, Y. S. (2014). Progestational agents for treating threatened or established preterm labour. *Cochrane Database of Systematic Reviews*, (1), (CD006770).

Sugiura-Ogasawara, M., Ozaki, Y. & Suzumori, N. (2014). Management of recurrent miscarriage. *Journal of Obstetrics & Gynaecology Research*, *40*(5), 1174–1179.

Ticconi, C., Pietropolli, A., Fabbri, G., Capogna, M. V., Perno, C. F. & Piccione, E. (2013). Recurrent miscarriage and cervical human papillomavirus infection. *American Journal of Reproductive Immunology*, *70*(5), 343–346.

Tsokos, G. C. (2011). Systemic lupus erythematosus. *New England Journal of Medicine*, *365*(22), 2110–2121.

van Teeffelen, A.S.P., van der Ham, D. P., Willekes, C., Al Nasiry, S., Nijhuis, J. G., van Kuijk, S., Pajkrt, E., et al. (2014). Midtrimester preterm prelabour rupture of membranes (PPROM): Expectant management or amnioinfusion for improving perinatal outcomes (PPROMEXIL – III trial). *BMC Pregnancy & Childbirth*, *14*(1), 1–12.

van Teeffelen, S., Pajkrt, E., Willekes, C., Van Kuijk, S.M.J. & Mol, B.W.J. (2013). Transabdominal amnioinfusion for improving fetal outcomes after oligohydramnios secondary to preterm prelabour rupture of membranes before 26 weeks. *Cochrane Database of Systematic Reviews*, (8), (CD009952).

Vargas, R., Barroilhet, L. M., Esselen, K., Diver, E., Bernstein, M., Goldstein, D. P. & Berkowitz, R. S. (2014). Subsequent pregnancy outcomes after complete and partial molar pregnancy, recurrent molar pregnancy, and gestational trophoblastic neoplasia: An update from the New England Trophoblastic Disease Center. *Journal of Reproductive Medicine*, *59*(5–6), 188–194.

Wahabi, H. A., Fayed, A. A., Esmaeil, S. A. & Al Zeidan, R. A. (2011). Progestogen for treating threatened miscarriage. *Cochrane Database of Systematic Review*, *7*(12).

Walker, K. D., Dexter, K. & Dadig, B. A. (2013). Vaginal bleeding in the early stages of pregnancy. *Clinical Advisor*, *16*(4), 41–47.

Watson, L. F., Rayner, J. A. & Forster, D. (2013). Identifying risk factors for very preterm birth: A reference for clinicians. *Midwifery*, *29*(5), 434–439.

Webb, D. A., Mathew, L. & Culhane, J. F. (2014). Lessons learned from the Philadelphia Collaborative Preterm Prevention Project: The prevalence of risk factors and program participation rates among women in the intervention group. *BMC Pregnancy & Childbirth*, *14*(1), 1–18.

Whitney, E. C., Jones, K. & Baker, A. L. (2014). Against the odds: Ectopic abdominal pregnancy. *Journal of Diagnostic Medical Sonography*, *30*(5), 268–271.

Wojcieszek, A. M., Stock, O. M. & Flenady, V. (2014). Antibiotics for prelabour rupture of membranes at or near term. *Cochrane Database of Systematic Reviews*, (10), (CD001807).

Wong, L. F., Porter, T. F. & Scott, J. R. (2014). Immunotherapy for recurrent miscarriage. *Cochrane Database of Systematic Reviews*, (10), (CD0001121).

Wu, J., Ludlow, J. P., De Vries, B., Black, K. & Beale, P. (2014). Single-dose methotrexate treatment for ectopic pregnancy and pregnancy of unknown location and progesterone as a predictor of success. *Australian and New Zealand Journal of Obstetrics and Gynaecology*, *54*(5), 469–474.

Zheng, T. (2012a). Antepartum testing. In T. Zheng (Ed), *Comprehensive Handbook of Obstetrics & Gynecology* (2nd ed.), pp. 92–95. Paradise Valley, AZ: Phoenix Medical Press.

Zheng, T. (2012b). Spontaneous abortion. In T. Zheng (Ed), *Comprehensive Handbook of Obstetrics & Gynecology* (2nd ed.), pp. 230–233. Paradise Valley, AZ: Phoenix Medical Press.

Suggested readings

Hurrell, K. (2014). Anti-D: Getting it right. *Midwives*, *17*(6), 46–47.

Rh-Negative Blood Type and Pregnancy. (2013). *Journal of Midwifery & Women's Health*, *58*(6), 725-726.

Townsend, N. S. & Drummond, S. B. (2012). Preeclampsia: Pathophysiology and implications for care. *Journal of Perinatal & Neonatal Nursing*, *25*(3), 245–252.

Chapter 22

Care of a pregnant family with special needs

Previous chapters discussed high-risk pregnancies for women who are ill when they become pregnant and for those who develop an illness while pregnant. This chapter presents information about women who do not fit the description of the average pregnant woman—a well young adult who maintains a healthy lifestyle. Representative of such women are very young adolescents, women who have waited until midlife to have their first child, those who are physically or cognitively challenged, those who are accidentally injured and those who are drug dependent.

LEARNING OBJECTIVES

After mastering the contents of this chapter, you should be able to:

1. Identify the characteristics and the risks of pregnancy of a pregnant woman who has special needs, such as one who has been injured, an adolescent, a woman over the age of 40, one who is physically or cognitively challenged, or a woman who is drug dependent.
2. Use critical thinking to analyse ways that nursing care of a pregnant woman with a special need can be optimally family-centred.
3. Assess a woman with special needs during pregnancy.
4. Identify expected outcomes for a pregnant woman with special needs.
5. Plan care to address the special needs of women at the extremes of the childbearing spectrum who have a physical or cognitive challenge, have been injured or are substance dependent.
6. Develop an understanding of care for a woman with special needs.
7. Evaluate outcomes for effectiveness and achievement of care.
8. Identify areas related to care of a pregnant woman with special needs that would benefit from additional research or application of evidence-based practice.
9. Integrate knowledge of the risks of pregnancy for women with special needs to achieve quality child and family health nursing care.

KEY TERMS

- autonomic dysreflexia
- emancipated minor
- substance dependent

CASE STUDY

Mandy Carson, who is 16 years old and 15 weeks' pregnant, was in a motor vehicle accident on her way into her antenatal clinic this morning. She received a 10-cm laceration on one leg. The father of Mandy's baby is a university student. He does not want Mandy to keep her baby after the birth because he does not want to get married until he graduates. Mandy insists she is old enough to be a parent and wants to keep her baby. Mandy's mother accuses the father of sharing methamphetamines with Mandy. She is worried Mandy has been working as a sex worker to support her drug habit. Mandy turns to you and asks you what you would recommend she do.

CASE STUDY QUESTIONS

1. What type of immediate assessment does Mandy need?
2. Is she old enough to be a parent?
3. What qualities would you look for in her to decide if she is ready to parent?

Nationally, in 2013, Australia had a birth rate of 14.6 babies per 1000 women aged 15–19 years. The rate varies substantially between the states and territories, with the ACT recording the lowest rate of teenage births at 8.2 babies per 1000 women and the Northern Territory recording the highest at 40.5 babies per 1000 women (ABS, 2014). The overall birth rate for teenage Aboriginal and Torres Strait Islander women was much higher, at 62.7 babies per 1000 women. The median age of birth in Australia has increased from 29.8 years in 2000 to 30.8 years in 2013. The rate of adolescent pregnancy is much lower than in the United States, where the live birth rate for women aged 15–19 years is 34.3 per 1000 women (2010)—more than double the rate in Australia.

There is some concern in New Zealand that the birth rate for teenage girls has remained much the same since the 1980s. The birth rate for women aged 15–19 years increased from 54 per 1000 in 1962, to 69 per 1000 in 1972, before dropping to 30 per 1000 in 1984. It has hovered around 31 per 1000 ever since and was 29 per 1000 in 2010 (Statistics New Zealand, 2015). Demographic trends show that children born to Māori mothers tend to be of more than one ethnicity. In 2010, the median age of Māori mothers was 26 years, four years younger than for the total population (30 years). Māori women had a total fertility rate of 2.8 births per woman in 2010 and Māori women aged 20–24 had the highest fertility rate (156 births per 1000 women) (Statistics New Zealand, 2015).

Adolescents who have disabilities have an increased likelihood of pregnancy compared to adolescents without disabilities. Adolescents with disabilities may lack opportunities for sexual health education and information (Linton & Rueda, 2014). The students with disabilities at one school received assistance with sexuality decisions and struggled with cognitive impairment, emotional issues, the desire to fit in with other adolescent, histories of sexual abuse, communication problems, self-esteem and low impulse control (Linton & Rueda, 2014).

The following websites provide further information on the support of teenage pregnancy in Australia and New Zealand:

- Australian Institute of Family Studies, Child Family Community Australia; Supporting young parents <https://www3.aifs.gov.au/cfca/publications/supporting-young-parents>
- Department of Education and Early Childhood Development <www.education.vic.gov.au/healthwellbeing/childyouth/catalogue/adolescent/teenpregnancy-ind1.htm>
- Families Commission <www.nzfamilies.org.nz/research/parenting/teenage-pregnancy-and-parenting>
- Family and Community Services, a service of the Ministry of Social Development <www.familyservices.govt.nz/my-family/everyday-family-life/family-relationship/teen-pregnancy.html>
- Healthdirect Australia <www.healthdirect.org.au/about-us/about-healthdirect-australia>
- Kiwi Families for passionate parents <www.kiwi families.co.nz/articles/teen-parent-overview>.

The pregnancy rate is increasing among women who are physically or cognitively challenged, including those with conditions such as cerebral palsy that might have precluded pregnancy a few years ago. Physical and cognitive conditions present a challenge to childbearing and childrearing but do not necessarily prevent women from establishing their own families. Supportive nursing care that considers the limitations imposed by a particular disability, while focusing on the normal aspects of childbearing and childrearing, and a woman's strengths, help to make these pregnancies successful.

Women who are drug dependent or who are injured are further categories of high-risk women who require a great deal of nursing support and care. Ideally, a woman would give up substance abuse for the health of a fetus, but that may not be possible. When this does not happen, every effort must be made to provide enough antenatal care and attention to protect the fetus in other ways. Women who are injured in motor vehicle accidents or from intimate partner abuse can have substantial blood loss that threatens the health of the fetus. They need rapid emergency department assessment and care to be certain that fetal health is protected.

CARE OF A PREGNANT WOMAN WITH SPECIAL NEEDS

Assessment

Assessing the challenges individual women face is always crucial to establish an accurate diagnosis and realistic outcomes, as well as planning effective care. When a woman has special needs, assessment becomes even more important. Establishing a thorough database early in pregnancy helps to predict the risks a woman may be exposed to when pregnancy is affected by age extremes, physical or cognitive challenges, an accidental injury or an unhealthy lifestyle.

Planning and interventions

When caring for a woman who is physically challenged, be aware that physical disabilities occur in degrees; therefore, first establish the impact of the disability on a woman's lifestyle before offering any guidance for care measures during pregnancy. The capacity of a woman with special needs to adapt to pregnancy depends both on her physical capabilities, her ability to overcome obstacles and her social support. It is important to assess physical strengths as well as limitations and psychosocial strengths as well as challenges. A woman with a spinal cord injury, for example, is likely to have developed ways of coping in daily life that may never occur to someone who has not experienced that disability.

For some drug-dependent women, pregnancy may be the impetus they need to break a drug habit, whereas for others all that they can accomplish is to reduce their drug use. In both instances, encourage the woman to keep coming for antenatal care. As long as a woman feels comfortable with you during regular visits, you may be able to establish a trusting relationship that will eventually provide her with the confidence to try a healthier pattern of living. Be especially careful to establish realistic outcomes given a woman's particular condition or situation. A woman who is visually challenged may not be able to read a digital display on a glucometer or use a wall clock to time contractions, no matter how much she would like to.

Often, a pregnant woman with a special need already has significant stressors to deal with in her life. Adolescence, for example, is a period of growth and change that can be stressful for both the teenager and her family. The physically challenged woman constantly copes with a condition that must be considered in all activities, even if she has adjusted completely to the limitations the disability imposes. The drug-dependent woman is confined by a life-threatening habit. A woman who has been injured in an accident may have to temporarily restructure her life to accommodate a hospital admission.

Pregnancy brings with it a whole new set of stressors that can be overwhelming if a woman has no outside support. Planning for a pregnant woman with a special need, therefore, often involves identifying support people to help with this added stress. This support can come from family, friends, a professional organisation, or healthcare providers. If a woman is not totally independent in her care, some planning may be required with her support person, who may be the person who actually carries out the proposed action. At the same time, be sure not to ignore a woman and plan around her. Only if she approves of the plan can pregnancy be the enjoyable experience she had planned it would be. This principle applies to any woman, but especially to one with special needs.

Plans should include ways to strengthen confidence and self-esteem, crucial attributes for a new mother. These are also areas in which a woman with a special need may be affected, especially one who perceives herself as too young or too old or who has experienced physical dysfunction. Drug dependence may also be related to feelings of lowered self-worth, which may have been intensified if the drug-dependent woman has tried unsuccessfully to limit her drug intake in the past.

Being certain that plans are established in a wide range of areas helps to ensure that planning is comprehensive. Remember to include safe care of the newborn in plans as well, as once an infant is born, it may be too late to make these plans in a comprehensive manner.

Interventions for the high-risk pregnant woman include promoting a healthy pregnancy and preventing pregnancy complications. Care focuses on facilitating a woman with any special need to determine how best to manage her pregnancy according to her particular situation.

Most adolescents do not plan to become pregnant, so finding out they are pregnant can be frightening. They are concerned about the reaction of their parents and may feel scared, vulnerable and guilty. A high proportion of adolescents do not seek antenatal care early in pregnancy because they deny they are pregnant or they are fearful and overwhelmed. Others may not feel comfortable in a healthcare facility at which mainly adults are seen. The same may be true of a woman with a drug dependency who fears reprimands from healthcare providers regarding her drug use. An ultrasound following an injury may first reveal that a woman is pregnant. She needs to be scheduled for antenatal care. A non-judgemental, welcoming attitude that focuses on the pregnancy and the baby, while avoiding recriminations about a woman's youth or circumstances, is essential to attracting such women to antenatal care and keeping them coming for regular visits. If they hear from a friend that the staff members at the clinic are helpful, not judgemental, they may then take the first step into the facility.

For women who are physically challenged, modifications may be necessary for some interventions associated with typical pregnancy-related procedures. For example, it may be necessary to modify a pelvic examination when a woman cannot place her legs in table stirrups. Modifying procedures promotes individualised care for all women.

THE PREGNANT ADOLESCENT

Adolescent pregnancy is not a new phenomenon. Historically, it was common for women to marry as early as the age of 12 or 13 and have their first baby at the age of 15. In today's society, however, marriage and childbearing are life situations that are thought of as belonging to later years. Teenage pregnancies still continue, however. Reasons for the high number of teenage pregnancies include:

- Earlier age of menarche (the average age is 12.4 years; menstruation often commences as early as 10 years and ovulating and conception can occur by the age of 11 years)
- Increase in the rate of sexual activity among teenagers
- Lack of knowledge about contraceptives
- Desire to have a child.

Having an equally young sexual partner can contribute to pregnancy incidence, as in this situation neither partner may be well versed in contraceptive options. In addition, some adolescents become pregnant as the result of rape or incest (Young et al., 2011).

Failure of adolescents to obtain adequate knowledge of contraceptive measures is an issue that can be addressed by healthcare providers. Access to emergency contraception is not associated with increased rates of unprotected intercourse or with higher rates of pregnancy or sexually-transmitted infections (Wilkinson et al., 2012). Unfortunately, providing this type of information does not always resolve the problem because adolescents may lack money to purchase protection such as birth control pills. In addition, the egocentric phenomenon of adolescence makes a sexually-active teenager believe she will not become pregnant: "It won't happen to me." Conversely some adolescents believe being pregnant will free them from an intolerable school or home situation and give them someone to love and someone to love them. This puts a tremendous responsibility on a newborn to furnish love and change an adolescent's life, and child abuse can occur when the newborn cannot meet such expectations (Valentino et al., 2012).

At one time, pregnant unmarried adolescents were sent to a "secret" home or shelter where they would stay throughout their pregnancy, give birth, place the child for adoption and return home as if nothing had happened to them. Today, pregnant teenagers remain at home and attend antenatal clinics just as older women do. The majority of teenage mothers keep their babies (Martin et al., 2011) (see Fig. 22.1). Despite more accepting attitudes of teenage mothers they often, however, remain economically and socially disadvantaged.

Developmental tasks of adolescence

Adolescence is a vulnerable time for pregnancy because the developmental tasks of pregnancy are superimposed

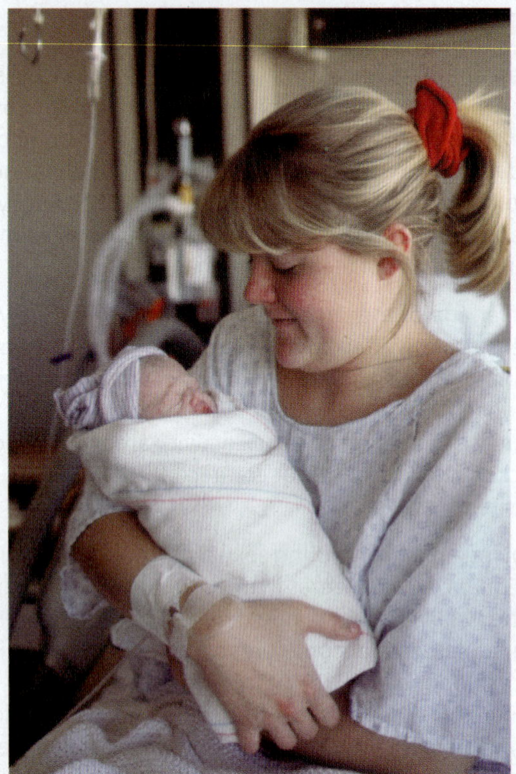

FIGURE 22.1 A new adolescent mother begins to bond with her infant. (© Photo Network/Alamy)

on those of adolescence. The developmental tasks of the average adolescent are fourfold: to establish a sense of self-worth or a value system, to emancipate from parents, to adjust to a new body image and to choose a vocation (Erikson, 1963). An adolescent in the process of separating from her parents may be devastated by the reality of someone else being dependent on her. She may need her parents' financial help more than ever to obtain antenatal care and buy clothing for her new baby. Helping adolescents to make their own healthcare decisions helps to foster a sense of independence in the middle of this forced dependency.

Parents may have difficulty allowing a daughter to make her own healthcare decisions. You may need to remind them that a pregnant adolescent is regarded as an **emancipated minor** or a *mature minor*—a person capable of making healthcare decisions—and so may sign consent for her own care. Soon she will be caring for an infant, so she needs this practice in independence and responsibility.

Pregnancy may interfere with the development of a healthy sexual relationship and cause difficulty in establishing future intimate relationships. Frequently pregnant adolescents are abandoned by the father of their baby and often paternity is denied. Establishing a value system or sense of identity can be difficult if healthcare personnel treat a pregnant adolescent as though she is irresponsible. Pregnant teenagers and teenage mothers report that they are often met by judgemental attitudes and disapproval. Evidence indicates pregnant teenagers are subject to psychosocial stress factors, social trauma and social disruption. Risk factors for adverse outcomes for pregnant teenagers include childhood trauma, such as living with parents who are emotionally or physically abusive. Living in a home where there is domestic violence, substance abuse or mental illness is associated with risk-taking behaviours such as unprotected intercourse. Adolescent parenthood is a risk factor for the neglect and abuse of children and these vulnerable families must be supported.

Antenatal assessment

In 2010–2011 the World Health Organization (WHO) conducted a multi-country survey including 29 countries. Findings indicated the main factors complicating adolescent pregnancy are preterm birth, eclampsia, postpartum endometriosis, systemic infections, low birthweight infants and severe neonatal conditions (WHO, 2011). The WHO defines adolescent pregnancy as from 10 to 19 years of age (Ganchimeg et al., 2014).

In older teenagers obstetric risk is not increased by their age. In some aspects teenage mothers have better outcomes; they have less obstetric interventions and caesarean sections, less maternal and perinatal morbidity and a higher rate of normal vaginal births. The incidence of poor outcomes increase with mothers younger than 15 years and those who have been menstruating for 2 years or less. Preterm birth is associated with poorer outcomes and the incidence of idiopathic preterm birth is associated with poverty and lower socioeconomic status. In Australia the adolescent pregnancy rate is almost 8 times higher in the most socially disadvantaged areas (AIHW, 2015). Many adolescents are subject to social deprivation, social isolation, mental health issues, family violence or intimate partner violence, smoking, alcohol and illicit drug use, poor nutrition and inadequate weight gain, genitourinary infection, social stresses such as low income, unemployment, poor housing or homelessness (Allen et al., 2013).

Adolescent pregnancies are classified as high risk because of their increased risk of complications such as preterm birth. These risks, however, are minimised by good antenatal care and a careful history, including any childhood trauma and personal difficulties along with evaluation of the family situation. Early and consistent antenatal care is important for adolescent women. Unfortunately, many adolescents do not seek antenatal care until late in their pregnancies and attend less appointments. Both of these factors are associated with poor perinatal outcomes. Contributing factors include:

- Denial that the adolescent is pregnant
- Lack of knowledge of the importance of antenatal care
- Dependence on others for transportation
- Feeling awkward in an antenatal setting (an adult setting)
- Fear of a first pelvic examination
- Difficulty relating to authority figures.

A continuity of care approach that minimises the number of healthcare providers a teenager is exposed to may be the most effective method of providing care during the antenatal period. Some adolescents do well in group antenatal care because it allows them to interact with a peer group. If a community does not have a facility designed especially for adolescents, all settings should accommodate adolescents' needs, eliminating this reason for poor antenatal care.

Health history

Take a detailed health history at the first antenatal visit of an adolescent to establish individual risks. This is best done without the adolescent's parents present. This provides an opportunity to be responsible for her own health and helps prevent her fabricating an answer to please a parent. Many adolescents want to keep their world totally separate from the adult world and, to keep it separate, they do not voluntarily share information with adults. When interviewing adolescents, be certain to press for the responses needed to assess safety. Do not accept statements such as, "I eat okay" as a nutrition history or, "I'm a very active person" as a history of rest and activity. Ask for details.

If a parent does accompany the adolescent, ask the parent separately what, if any, concerns he or she wishes to discuss. A young adolescent is still a daughter and a parent may be as concerned about her health during this pregnancy as the parent was at health visits for a cold or a sports injury.

A baby's father may accompany a pregnant adolescent into the clinic to have the pregnancy diagnosis established. If he is not married to her, he does not have a legal right to participate in her decision concerning pregnancy, abortion or adoption. If he is an adolescent, he may feel sorrow that because of his age he cannot provide adequate support. If a complication occurs, he may feel genuine grief. Allowing him to offer support in the current pregnancy helps him to learn more about himself and better define his role.

Pregnant adolescents need to be aware of common pregnancy symptoms such as urinary frequency, fatigue and breast tenderness. Asking what symptoms an adolescent is having and reassuring her they are part of a normal pregnancy can alleviate worry and help prevent her from attempting to treat them with potentially dangerous over-the-counter medications.

As pregnancy progresses, listen for signs of "nest-building" behaviour. An adolescent may not have the financial resources to buy clothing or a bed for the baby. She may reveal nest-building feelings by asking an increasing number of questions about newborns. Some adolescents have difficulty telling their parents about the pregnancy. Role-playing or simulation may be an effective technique to help them prepare to do this. Some pregnant adolescents report on a second visit that their parents were not nearly as angry as they had anticipated. Instead, their parents reacted as if they had been waiting to hear this news, having accepted it as inevitable months before.

Family profile

Adolescents may leave home if their family disapproves of their pregnancy, joining the ranks of homeless or adolescent runaways. Others do not leave home but separate themselves emotionally from their family. Trying to manage by themselves leaves adolescents with a tremendous financial strain and a devastating sense of loneliness. Be sure to ask where a pregnant adolescent is living, the source of her income and who she would call if she suddenly became ill.

Asking about home life may reveal a dysfunctional family or an incestuous relationship as the cause of the pregnancy. If the she is under legal age, incest is considered child abuse and must be reported. Because of family relationship problems, a girl may need help in making arrangements for the next few months of her pregnancy and for childcare afterwards. Family and social supports for pregnant adolescents have been shown to be important influences on the maintenance of a healthy pregnancy lifestyle and to help prevent low birth weight in their children (Hodnett, Fredericks, & Weston, 2010; Jutte, Roos & Brownell, 2010). If adolescents believe their pregnancy will negatively impact on their life they have increased symptoms of depression; however, this effect is "buffered" by social support (Kirven, 2014). Adolescents who feel well supported by their mother and partner have a protective buffer against poor adjustment to pregnancy and depression (Kirven, 2014).

History

Ask about nutritional practices, sleep, daily activity, use of drugs and whether she has friends who can support her through this experience. Note medication history, including over-the-counter medications. Some adolescents take acne medication that is potentially teratogenic, such as tetracycline or isotretinoin (Roaccutane) (McKenna & Mirkov, 2014). Some take frequent doses of over-the-counter cold remedies or herbal supplements. Impress upon adolescents the importance of not taking any medication—even non-prescription—without prior approval from their doctor or healthcare providers during pregnancy. Pregnancy can become an important growth experience if it provides the motivation some adolescents need to withdraw from recreational drug use.

Physical examination

Physical examination procedures with pertinent adolescent findings are discussed in Chapter 34. Explain procedures as you carry out the examination. Use a Doppler technique to obtain fetal heart tones, if possible, because hearing the fetal heart helps an adolescent acknowledge the reality of her pregnancy. Assessment of fundal height will reassure her that the baby is growing well. Be certain she knows a healthy weight gain is important for fetal growth and that this weight can be lost after the pregnancy.

CASE STUDY QUESTION

4. Mandy is still an adolescent. What is a task of adolescence, according to Erikson, that she needs to complete to be ready to become a mother?
   a. Establish a value system
   b. Grow to her final height
   c. Prepare clothes for the baby
   d. Finish her education

Pregnancy education

Once an adolescent's pregnancy is confirmed, the expectant mother and, if possible, father need health education on antenatal care and positive parenting. The stresses of pregnancy add increased complexity to adolescents and their relationships and may lead to unhealthy practices, depression, anxiety and overeating (East, Chien & Barber, 2012). They are also often unwilling to follow healthcare advice that makes them different in any way from their peers. On the other hand, adolescents often do not have well-established health practices, so they are adaptable. Health professionals can promote pregnancy, birth and breastfeeding as normal healthy processes and encourage adolescents' confidence and adjustment and support life skill development to help adolescents reduce their levels of anxiety and become successful parents (Kirven, 2014).

Adolescents also need instructions about possible discomforts and changes associated with pregnancy and measures to relieve them. (See Chapter 12 for a complete discussion.) Adolescents may also develop many striae across the sides of their abdomens because so much stretching of the abdominal skin occurs. Assure them again that, because of skin elasticity, these marks will fade after pregnancy. Chloasma, excess pigment deposition on the face and neck, appears at the same rate in adolescents as in older women. Adolescents, however, may be more conscious of this pigment because overall they are more conscious and concerned about their facial appearance. Offering reassurance that the pigmentation will fade after pregnancy can help.

Nutrition

Good nutrition can be a major problem during an adolescent pregnancy because many girls enter pregnancy with poor nutritional stores from years of eating a less-than-optimal diet. Lack of good nutrition can result in preterm birth and low-birth-weight newborns. The younger an adolescent the more likely she is to have a low-birth-weight infant. To prevent these complications, a sufficient diet is necessary to allow for the growth of a fetus and also provide for the needs of her own growing body. Otherwise, protein, iron, folic acid, and vitamin A and C deficiencies may become acute. She may need to gain more weight than does the mature woman, to supply adequate nutrients.

As more and more youth are obese today than ever before because of overeating and lack of exercise, many adolescents enter pregnancy overweight or obese. This can lead to macrosomia or overgrowth in a fetus, a situation that leads to an increase in the number of caesarean births (Alexandra et al., 2011). Such adolescents should not actively restrict nutrients during pregnancy, however, because although they are obese, their body may be deficient in protein and vitamins. Many adolescents eat poorly during pregnancy because they simply do not know what constitutes good nutrition. Some have little choice in what foods are prepared at home. Besides eating the right amount of food, a pregnant adolescent should be sure to eat healthy foods.

What if...

Mandy tells you her daily nutrition consists of a liquid diet beverage for breakfast and lunch and then she has pizza for dinner? Will this typical teenage diet be adequate for her during pregnancy?

Physiological changes

A young adolescent may have distorted beliefs about her body. All pregnant adolescents need substantial education about the physiological changes that occur during pregnancy. In addition, specific information about labour and birth is essential to counteract all the "scare stories" she may be hearing from her peers. Gaining this type of knowledge is another way that pregnancy can be a growth experience. At the end of the pregnancy, this adolescent will know a great deal more about her body and her ability to monitor her health than her average classmate.

Childbirth preparation

Adolescents have a strong need for peer companionship. When they become pregnant, they are often cut off from fellow adolescents. This makes them "ripe", therefore, to join a class of adolescents in preparation for childbirth. Adolescents are often excellent students because being a student is age-appropriate for them. They have enough childish magical belief operating that they are not sceptical about whether prepared childbirth will work. In fact, believing that prepared childbirth will work is an important component in a successful prepared childbirth experience, so this becomes a self-fulfilling prophecy.

Plans for the baby

Adolescents may need additional time at antenatal visits to talk to a good listener about how they feel about being pregnant and becoming a mother. Be certain they know all the options available to them: keeping the baby, placing the baby in a temporary foster home or adoption.

Adolescents, like all women, should be encouraged to breastfeed (Grassley, 2010). Breast tissue matures with pregnancy, so even the very young adolescent is physically capable of breastfeeding.

Complications of adolescent pregnancy

Adolescent pregnancy carries an increased incidence of iron-deficiency anaemia and preterm labour. Fortunately, with conscientious antenatal care, these complications can be minimised.

Pregnancy-induced hypertension

Historically, very young adolescents and nulliparas have been considered at higher risk of preeclampsia; however some studies indicate the risk of preeclampsia in teenage women is not increased. Because preeclampsia remains a major cause of maternal and fetal morbidity and mortality it is important to monitor all women carefully and to ensure a baseline blood pressure is taken and that the young woman is aware of her normal baseline blood pressure (see Chapter 21).

Iron-deficiency anaemia

Many adolescents are deficient in iron because their low protein intake cannot make up the amount of iron lost with menstrual flows. Deficiency is revealed by chronic fatigue, pallor, pale mucous membranes, dizziness, feeling cold and a haemoglobin level less than 110 grams per litre. If necessary, iron and folate studies should be taken. A pregnancy compounds iron-deficiency anaemia because if an adolescent is still growing she must now supply enough iron for fetal growth and her increasing blood volume. Provide information on iron-rich foods and a referral to a dietician, if necessary.

Preterm labour

Adolescents are at high risk of preterm labour. Possible reasons include infection and psychosocial stresses such as isolation, homelessness and exposure to violence (Kirven, 2014). Teenagers should be screened and treated for possible asymptomatic genitourinary infections, as teenage-specific antenatal clinics have found a high level of positive cultures on screening. They also found a reduction in the rate of preterm birth with teenage-specific antenatal care which they believe was partly the result of prevention and treatment of ascending genital tract infection and holistic teen-specific care.

Review the signs of labour with a pregnant adolescent by the third month of pregnancy. Stress that labour contractions begin as only a sweeping contraction, no more intense than menstrual cramps and that any vaginal bleeding is suspicious of labour and should be reported. Adolescents may have gained much of their knowledge of labour from television (where a woman suddenly announces she is in labour and within 15 minutes gives birth), therefore, they may dismiss light contractions as simple discomfort, not realising they might be the start of labour. Adolescents who recognise labour contractions early can seek care to have premature labour halted.

Complications of adolescent labour, birth and the postpartum period

Teenagers are less likely to initiate breastfeeding and like many women discontinue breastfeeding soon after discharge from hospital. Breastfeeding needs to be encouraged and supported. A caseload model of midwifery, where a known midwife provides care antenatally, at birth, and postnatally is ideal for providing ongoing support and continuity of care. Teenagers should be informed about contraception and be assisted with obtaining the contraception of their choice.

CASE STUDY QUESTION

5. Mandy was placed on an iron supplement because her haemoglobin level was below normal. What is a common test to demonstrate a need for an iron supplement?

a. Assessing if her skin appears darker/lighter
b. Assessing her blood reticulocyte count
c. Analysing her urine for iron deposits
d. Measuring if she has grown in height

THE PREGNANT WOMAN OVER AGE 40

In Australia the overall birth rate is falling, however this trend is reversed in women aged between 40 and 44 years and the fertility rate in this group continues to increase. Over the last 3 decades the birth rate for women over 40 has almost tripled (ABS, 2014). The incidence of women delaying their first pregnancy until their late 30s or early 40s is increasing. In Australia 25% of births occur in women over 35 years of age (ABS, 2014). In 2011 women over 40 years of age accounted for 4.3% of births in Australia and 0.2% of women were over 45 (AIHW, 2015). In the past, it was assumed a woman of this age was past the optimal age for childbearing and was at risk of many complications. There is some debate regarding the age where increased risk begins, with some believing the risk is only clinically significant over 40 years of age (Mills & Lavender, 2010). Today, with the exception of a greater incidence of chromosomal abnormality, most women over 40 have healthy pregnancies. However, advanced maternal age has been associated with increased morbidity and mortality for mother and baby.

A woman over the age of 40 has an increased risk of previously diagnosed conditions such as hypertension, diabetes and varicosities. Women older than 45 years have higher risk of death, transfusion, myocardial infarction/ischaemia, acute heart failure, pulmonary embolism, deep venous thrombosis, acute renal failure, caesarean birth, gestational diabetes, fetal demise, fetal anomaly and placenta praevia when compared to women under 35 years (Grotegut et al., 2014).

Antenatal assessment

A woman over 40 years who is pregnant may begin to feel ambivalent during pregnancy, because she may want to continue with her normal activities, yet also wants to concentrate on her pregnancy and the growing fetus.

Women who have a child after the age of 40 fall into one of two groups: those who are having their final child and those who have delayed childbearing because of education or a career and are having their first child. Many adults over the age of 40 care for ageing parents. This additional responsibility may make it difficult for a woman to cope with the psychological effect of pregnancy. It also may create extra strain on her finances and time (creates a "sandwich generation", or one pressured by responsibilities for both older and younger family members). Worries also include having enough energy, arranging for childcare and financial strain. Women who are over 40 also have many advantages, including greater life experience. They are more likely to have a tertiary education, a better financial situation, a healthy lifestyle and positive feelings about their pregnancy (Mills & Lavender, 2010).

A woman over 40 years of age, like all women, should begin antenatal care early in pregnancy. Fortunately, most women of this age group are well-informed about the advisability of early antenatal care.

Health history and physical examination

Ask women in this age group about their present symptoms of pregnancy, how they feel about the pregnancy, and how it fits into their lifestyle. If a woman did not realise she was pregnant, she may have self-medicated. Ask if she has been taking any medication or herbal remedies to relieve reported symptoms, such as nausea or fatigue. Review dietary intake including calcium such as milk, cheese and yoghurt to ensure it is adequate.

Some women over the age of 40 who are pregnant for the first time have recently changed their life pattern (have married or become involved in a long-term sexual relationship) or have decided to have a child, perhaps through in vitro fertilisation, without a spouse before they are no longer able to conceive. Whereas a younger woman often waits a while after marrying to become pregnant, a woman over the age 40 often plans to become pregnant immediately after marriage because she senses her reproductive time clock ticking. Because of this, she may find herself making many adjustments at once (not only to a new life partner, house or apartment, and perhaps community, but also to a pregnancy).

Take a thorough history including previous and pre-existing conditions as the incidence increases with age, as well as a physical examination. Note type of work, activity level, major stressors as well as support people. Establish her general health to identify any problems, such as hypertension, diabetes or circulatory disturbances such as varicose veins. Obtain a urine specimen and test it for specific gravity, glucose and protein to evaluate overall renal function and the possibility of gestational or type 2 diabetes, because older women are more prone than younger women to develop these conditions.

Assess a woman's breasts for any abnormalities, as women over the age of 40 are in a higher-risk group for breast cancer than younger women. In addition, assess for fetal heart sounds and fetal movement at antenatal visits because gestational trophoblastic disease (hydatidiform mole) is also more common in women over the age of 40 (see Chapter 21).

Women who are over 45 have higher risks of the following pre-existing conditions when compared to women under 35: cardiomyopathy, valvular heart disease, history of myocardial infarction/chronic ischemia, asthma, diabetes mellitus, thyroid disorders, systemic lupus erythematous (SLE), rheumatoid arthritis/collagen vascular disorders, thrombophilia/anti-phospholipid antibody syndrome, thrombocytopenia, chronic hypertension and chronic renal failure (Grotegut et al., 2014).

Chromosomal assessment

Increases in average maternal age have increased the number of pregnancies affected by trisomies (Loane et al., 2013). First trimester chromosomal screening includes: nuchal translucency (NT); crown-rump length (CRL) and maternal age; Pregnancy Associated Placental Protein-A (PAPP-A) and free β-hCG. Second trimester chromosomal screening includes: alpha fetoprotein (AFP); free β-hCG; unconjugated oestriol (μE3) and may also include inhibin A. If this test is positive, an amniocentesis will be scheduled at the 16th week of pregnancy. Women should be aware that false-positive results can occur with AFP testing, which is why amniocentesis is important. Many women of this age group do not begin nest-building until these tests confirm that their child will be healthy.

Complications of pregnancy for a woman over age 40

In the United Kingdom the incidence of maternal death has been noted to increase with age, with 12.4 maternal deaths per 100,000 in women 25–29 years rising to 29.4 deaths per 100,000 in women over 40 years of age. The complications of pregnancy most likely to occur in a woman over the age of 35 are hypertension of pregnancy (preeclampsia), diabetes, placenta praevia, leiomyomata, preterm or post-term birth and caesarean birth. Possible reasons include ageing factors such as decreased myometrial efficiency and decreased pliability of pelvic joints, malpresentations related to uterine fibroids and multiparity.

Pregnancy-induced hypertension

A woman over the age of 40 may have a higher incidence of pregnancy-induced hypertension than a younger woman. This is possibly related to blood vessel inelasticity or because hypertension tends to occur more frequently in nulliparas than in multiparas as well as those with already elevated blood pressure (Gaillard et al., 2011).

Complications of labour, birth and the postpartum period for a woman over age 40

Failure to progress in labour

Labour in an older primipara may be prolonged because cervical dilation may not occur as spontaneously as in a younger woman. Graphing labour progress is a good method to use to determine when labour is becoming prolonged and interventions such as an instrumental or caesarean birth are indicated. Encourage a woman to verbalise how she is feeling about her progress throughout labour to allow for reassurance and prompt intervention should problems arise. All women benefit from a support person who is present during their labour and birth.

Difficulty accepting the event

Most women have some feelings of ambivalence about their pregnancy and women over the age of 40 may begin to have second thoughts about childbearing this late in life as the reality of a new baby registers with them during the intrapartal and postpartum periods. Although they may have read a great deal about babies during pregnancy, they may wish they had read more or were as confident with this phase of their life as they are about other areas, such as their home, office or classroom. Review plans for childcare and postpartum rest, with an emphasis on helping women learn to balance their lives, especially if they are planning on returning to work soon after the birth. They might appreciate help making childcare arrangements. You can assure them that daycare for preschool children has positive socialisation results (Goldfield et al., 2012).

Postpartum haemorrhage

Just as the cervix may not dilate as readily during labour, the uterus may not contract as readily in the postpartum period. Therefore, a woman over 40 may be at higher risk for postpartum haemorrhage (Yogev, Melamed, Bardin, et al., 2010). She may also be more prone to perineal–anal tears because her perineum is less pliable (Lyndon et al., 2012).

✔ *Checkpoint question 22.1*

Women over 40 are at increased risk of developing pregnancy-induced hypertension. The reason for this is:

a. Many are overweight before they enter pregnancy
b. They drink more fluids daily than younger women
c. They do not exercise much, so oedema fluid accumulates
d. Their blood vessels are not as elastic as those of younger women

THE PREGNANT WOMAN WHO IS PHYSICALLY OR COGNITIVELY CHALLENGED

The global population report estimates one billion people (15% of the world's population) have some kind of disability with an estimated prevalence of 10% among women of childbearing age (WHO, 2011). Disabilities can be physical, mental, neurological, sensory, cognitive, recent or long-term, progressive or stable (Redshaw et al., 2013). In the past, women with disabilities were often sheltered by their families and unable to meet potential sexual or marriage partners and so did not become pregnant. In addition, most people believed people with disabilities should not have children. Today, women with varying degrees of disability attend public schools, work in offices, join community organisations, establish sexual relationships, marry and plan pregnancies just like everyone else. However, women with disabilities often have poorer health, less education, more unemployment and may face difficulties accessing health facilities and accessing care providers (Redshaw et al., 2013).

It is desirable for women with a physical or cognitive disability or illness to arrange preconception care so medicines they are taking can be evaluated and careful planning for safe pregnancy care can be started early (Signore, Spong & Krotoski, 2011). Women with recurrent seizures, for example, may need to have their dose of antiseizure medication reduced during pregnancy because these may be teratogenic (Burakgazi, Pollard & Harden, 2011).

Care for women with disabilities (and sometimes their support persons) who wish to negotiate the challenges of their condition and care during pregnancy successfully must be designed so the needs of the woman and her family can be addressed and met (Walsh-Gallagher, Sinclair & McConkey, 2012). Health professionals may have experience caring for women with intellectual or physical disabilities but may have received very little training in this area. A study in Sweden found midwives felt unsure about how to adapt care and advice for women with intellectual disabilities (Höglund, Lindgren & Larsson, 2013). Health service providers need to ensure their knowledge is current and evidence-based so they can provide supportive care (Höglund, Lindgren & Larsson, 2013).

Table 22.1 lists general areas of care that are important in planning for the physically or cognitively-challenged woman who is pregnant.

Rights of the physically or cognitively challenged person

In Australia people with disabilities must be given equal opportunity and access to services and it is unlawful to discriminate against people with disabilities. The *Disability Discrimination Act 1992* protects people with a disability from direct or indirect discrimination in public life including employment, education and access to premises. The

TABLE 22.1 Areas of planning with physically or cognitively challenged women during pregnancy

Area	Assessment and planning guidelines
Transport	Ask if a woman has transport for antenatal care and for emergencies.
Pregnancy counselling	Assess the special modifications of care that will need to be made depending on a woman's special challenge. Use additional visual or auditory aids to make your teaching points clear.
Support person	Determine who is the woman's support person. In some instances, a woman's condition requires so much assistance during pregnancy that one support person will not be enough. If necessary, contact community agencies to lend additional support, with her consent.
Health	Do not lose track of a woman's primary health problem. For example, a woman with cerebral palsy may need to continue an active muscle exercise program during pregnancy for her primary illness.
Work	Assess whether a woman works outside her home and, if work is discontinued during pregnancy, what she could substitute for a social contact activity. Women with physical or cognitive challenges may be lonely because they do not have a wide range of friends or social contacts.
Recreation	Assess whether her level of activity is adequate and make concrete suggestions within her limitations for increasing it. Many women with a physically challenging condition lead a rather sedentary life (partly because they do not have many social contacts).
Self-esteem	Assess a woman's level of self-esteem: it may be low because of repeated failures in her life. Give praise at antenatal visits and help her make pregnancy a growth experience.

Australian Human Rights Commission is responsible for implementation of this Act and also has significant responsibilities through the International Convention on the Rights of Persons with Disabilities (Australian Human Rights Commission, 2012). A woman with a disability has full rights to her child, so the baby cannot be taken from her at birth without her full consent. Likewise, she cannot be forced to terminate a pregnancy or undergo sterilisation unless that is her informed decision.

Modifications for pregnancy

Explore with women at a first antenatal visit the exact nature of their disability and their general self-image to identify what modifications of care they may need during pregnancy. Some women who are physically or cognitively challenged maintain high self-esteem despite severe limitations and are able to modify, grow and learn with a pregnancy, whereas others have a poor sense of self-esteem that will make this particularly difficult for them. For many of them, pregnancy will become a special event, a 9 month announcement to everyone that, despite their seeming limitations, they are equal to other women and capable of participating in one of life's miracles. Research evidence indicates many women with disabilities find their maternity care needs are ignored, they feel invisible to the healthcare system and their social and political concerns are not addressed because health carers focus more on issues such as physical accessibility (Redshaw et al., 2013).

Safety and emergency contacts

Safety is a key area of concern when caring for a pregnant woman who is physically or cognitively challenged. It is important for women to plan for their individual needs, such as mobility, transport, elimination, and possible emergencies such as an autonomic response. Assist women to develop an emergency plan so they can contact someone in case of a pregnancy-related emergency. Ensure she knows how to activate the emergency medical system (000 in Australia; 111 in New Zealand). If a woman's speech is not clear, evaluate whether she will be understood while using a telephone to call for help in an emergency. Some women with limited mobility, such as those with spinal cord injury or cerebral palsy, have a specially designed telephone contact system in their home that connects to a paramedic or hospital emergency service through a beeper system. Women who are hearing challenged use a specially equipped telephone (a TDD device) that prints out messages for them.

Transport

Assess the woman's ability to come for antenatal care. If a woman depends on a support person for transport to a healthcare facility, appointments may have to be arranged according to that person's schedule to prevent missed appointments. If a woman does not drive, someone should be available to transport her if a pregnancy-related emergency should occur. Women with cognitive or vision challenges, for example, may not qualify for a driver's licence and so may need someone, such as a family member or friend, to drive. Women with spinal cord injury may have difficulty transferring into the specially equipped, hand-controlled car they usually drive as pregnancy progresses.

Mobility

All women who use wheelchairs are taught to press with their hands against the armrests and lift their buttocks up off the wheelchair seat for 5 seconds every hour. This prevents the formation of pressure ulcers on the buttocks and posterior thighs. Encourage a pregnant woman to continue to perform this manoeuvre during pregnancy as the increased weight of a fetus increases her risk for pressure

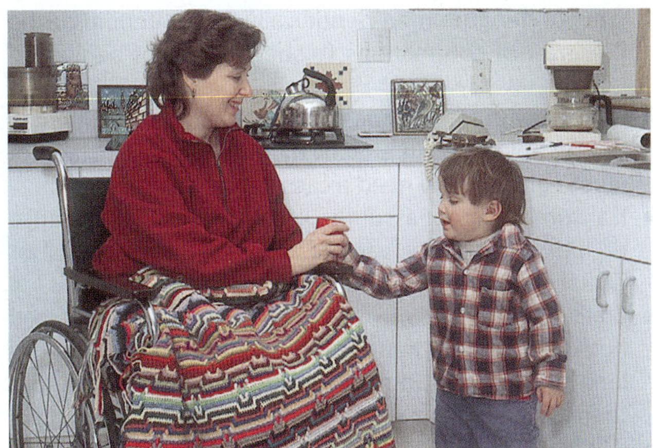

FIGURE 22.2 During pregnancy, a woman who is physically challenged may need to use a wheelchair to help safeguard herself against injury. Assure her that she may still enjoy her independence and daily activities, such as caring for an older child. (© Keith/Custom Medical Stock Photograph.)

ulcer formation from compression. In addition, severe hip flexion from sitting in a wheelchair limits venous return from the lower extremities. For at least one hour every morning and afternoon, encourage women who ambulate by wheelchair to decrease the sharp bend at their knees that results from sitting in the chair, to promote venous return and help prevent varicosities and thrombi formation. Adjusting the footrests of the wheelchair so a woman's legs are not sharply bent at the knees accomplishes this.

If balance is a problem, a woman may need re-evaluation at the midpoint of pregnancy as the weight of her abdomen increases. She may need to use crutches if she did not use them before, or use a wheelchair if she was ambulatory with crutches or a walker before pregnancy. Keep in mind that a woman who is physically challenged achieved the degree of ambulation that she first presents with usually after years of physical therapy and strengthening of leg and arm muscles. Help her to see that reducing her degree of independence during pregnancy is not a step backwards for her but a step forwards, allowing her to have a safe pregnancy without the danger of falling (see Fig. 22.2).

Elimination

When mobility is an effort, a woman may not drink as much as usual or use a toilet as frequently as she would if those actions were effortless. Encourage a high fluid intake and frequent voiding, however, to prevent urinary tract infections. Women with spinal cord injury who use an indwelling catheter are at especially high risk of contracting urinary tract infections during pregnancy. Women who perform self-catheterisation or change their own indwelling catheter may be unable to continue to do this late in pregnancy because the increasing size of their abdomen interferes with their ability to see or reach their perineum comfortably. If this happens, it may be necessary for a woman to arrange for a support person, a home care nurse or a home health aide to do this for her.

Autonomic responses

In a woman who has a high spinal cord injury (cervical or high thoracic), observe for **autonomic dysreflexia** during pregnancy, labour and the immediate postpartum period. This is an exaggerated autonomic response to stimuli. Any irritating condition, such as a distended bladder, increasing uterine size, labour contractions or breastfeeding, may initiate the response (Rabchevsky & Kitzman, 2011). Without upper motor neuron control to reverse the phenomenon, extreme symptoms such as severe hypertension (300/160 mmHg), throbbing headache, flushing of the skin and profuse diaphoresis above the level of the spinal lesion, nausea and bradycardia may occur. Immediate action is necessary to protect against cerebrovascular accident or intraocular damage. Elevate a woman's head to reduce cerebral pressure and locate the irritating stimulus (usually a distended bladder or bowel). If bladder distension is the cause, the woman needs bladder pressure relieved by catheterisation, if an indwelling catheter is not in place. If a catheter is in place, check to see why it is not draining, then encourage it to drain by unkinking or flushing it to allow urine to flow freely again. Anticipate the need for an antihypertensive agent to alleviate the extreme hypertension, although as soon as the source of irritation is removed, symptoms typically fade quickly.

Antenatal care modifications to meet specific needs

Physical examination may need to be modified depending on individual circumstances for women with disabilities (Bates, Carroll, & Potter, 2011; Sudduth & Linton, 2011). Although women with disabilities may have been followed by a healthcare provider most of their life, they may never have had a pelvic examination before and so need clear instructions about why it is needed and what it will consist of. Many obstetric examining tables are built for the comfort of the examiner and are too high for a woman to transfer to from a wheelchair by simply sliding onto the table. To help a woman move to the table, a ramp from the physical therapy department may be necessary so the wheelchair can be elevated to the level of the table. Women with spinal cord injury or cerebral palsy may be unable to maintain their legs in a lithotomy position because of either hip flexion contracture or laxness of leg support. This means a dorsal recumbent, rather than a lithotomy position may be required for a pelvic examination.

When interviewing or teaching visually challenged women, do not to use your hands to illustrate points ("I'll need a urine sample of at least this much urine [measured with your fingers]"). Do not use colours as descriptions of objects ("put on the blue gown"). Use demonstration aids that allow a woman to feel or touch instead. When helping with or performing physical assessment, let a woman know you are closing the door or drawing a curtain to ensure privacy. Always alert a woman when you are going to touch her, so as not to startle her. If a woman is hearing impaired, she may not be able to see the examiner's face during a pelvic examination. This means any question asked of her during this time will not be understood because she cannot see the examiner's lips to lip read (Middleton et al., 2010).

Pregnancy education

Modify health teaching to meet each woman's specific needs. For a woman who is cognitively challenged, for example, instructions about pregnancy may need to be limited to those few items crucial for safety, such as "do not drink alcohol or take any medicine". If a woman and her support person are both visually challenged, pamphlets about pregnancy care will not be useful. If the support person can see, offer the pamphlets to him or her, suggesting the support person read them to the pregnant woman as a shared activity. This will not only be helpful to her but also make the partner a more-informed support person.

Nutritional education is another area that should be designed based on each client's specific challenges and usual routine. A visually challenged woman or one who ambulates by wheelchair, for example, may prepare her own breakfast and lunch, meals that do not require a stove. The one hot meal a woman eats is one a support person cooks in the evening. Nutrition counselling for two meals daily, therefore, needs to centre on foods that can be prepared without cooking.

Activity and exercise, important for any pregnant woman, are crucial for a woman who is physically challenged. If mobility is a concern, exercise can be planned and modified with the assistance of a physiotherapist. In this case, be sure a woman understands that walking around her home or apartment can provide the same level of exercise as if she were walking around the block or exercising at a health club.

Although labour and her child's birth may be modified somewhat because of a woman's physical condition, gaining general knowledge about labour and birth and participating in a shared experience with her partner are still valuable. Urge women to attend childbirth preparation classes if at all possible. If a woman is not working outside her home, she may have more time than others to practise breathing exercises and may enter labour more adept at using such a method to control pain in labour than other women. More time may be required at antenatal visits to allow for factors such as an interpreter. If an interpreter is present speak to the woman directly, not her interpreter.

Modifications for labour and birth

Women who are physically or cognitively challenged will need adaptations in preparation for labour and birth. Helpful suggestions are:

- A woman with spinal cord injury may not be able to feel uterine contractions. Late in pregnancy she will need to palpate her abdomen periodically for tightening or the presence of contractions so she is aware of beginning labour.
- Women with muscle spasticity or spinal cord injury may not be able to push effectively for the second stage of labour and so may need a caesarean or forceps birth.
- If a woman cannot assume a lithotomy position because of hip contracture, vaginal delivery from a Sims' or dorsal recumbent position is best.
- Braille watches used by visually challenged persons may not have second hands. They may need to time the length of contractions by counting rather than timing them by a watch.
- During labour, the hearing-challenged woman cannot hear information on how she is progressing if you are not directly facing her. If she needs to communicate with her support person in sign language, act as an advocate to keep her hands unencumbered by equipment such as intravenous lines. Remember she cannot hear her infant cry at birth. Hand the infant to her as soon as possible after birth so she can see and feel the baby is crying and breathing well.
- Be certain to identify the usual sounds of birthing rooms (the beeping of a monitor, the swish of a central supply system and so forth) for the visually challenged woman. Hearing sounds and not being able to identify them can be frightening.

Modifications for postpartum care

After birth, be sure to assess and teach:

- Whether a woman desires contraceptive information
- Whether she needs additional support to be successful at breastfeeding
- Whether she has a return appointment for both herself and her infant for follow-up care and that the arrangements are within her capabilities, transportation and understanding.

Women with disabilities generally feel a need to space pregnancies, so be certain they receive information on their contraceptive choices as these may be different than for women without disabilities (Grover, 2011). A woman with poor hand control, for example, might not be able to effectively insert a diaphragm; a woman who is cognitively challenged might not understand the importance of taking an oral contraceptive every day.

Planning childcare

Allow for extra time during the first days after birth for mother–child interaction. For example, after birth, a woman who is cognitively challenged may need extra time to understand the transition from "being pregnant" to "having a baby". She may have difficulty learning to judge when her infant is hungry. She may need extra supervision to be certain she does not leave the baby unprotected on a bed. A woman with a spinal cord disability may be particularly interested in inspecting her baby's back. A visually challenged woman will probably want to reassure herself her baby can see. Be sure to give her baby to her as soon as possible after birth so she can touch the baby and feel for intact body parts.

Breastfeeding has special advantages for women who are physically or cognitively challenged because it is the method of feeding that is not only best for the baby, but also requires the least preparation and effort on the mother's part. For a woman who is visually challenged and unable to read printed instructions, breastfeeding eliminates formula errors. For a woman who uses a wheelchair, breastfeeding eliminates trips to the refrigerator. However, breastfeeding may not be possible for a woman with muscle spasticity because the let-down reflex, which depends on muscle relaxation, may not occur. Be certain that women who are cognitively challenged understand they need to feed until the infant is satisfied, not until they are tired of feeding.

Equipment modifications are available such as cot rails which lower by pressure on a foot pedal. An occupational therapist will be able to assist with home modifications and the woman will be the expert on capabilities and needs. Women using wheelchairs may find an anterior baby sling effective. Many adaptations are available for hearing-impaired women such as vibration pads that indicate the baby is crying.

It is important to work in partnership with women and their families to formulate collaborative, innovative, flexible and individualised plans for pregnancy, birth and the postpartum period. A relationship of mutual trust and honesty needs to be established and the woman's strengths and desires recognised. Women with a disability may feel frightened and vulnerable and it is important to communicate and explain procedures and processes. Such women have the right to make informed choices about their care and have their wishes respected. Carers need to be aware of non-verbal communication and should have excellent interpersonal skills.

✔ *Checkpoint question 22.2*

Women with high thoracic spinal cord injury can develop autonomic dysreflexia during labour. The best action to take for this would be:

a. Ask her to lie flat and take deep breaths
b. Elevate her legs to restore her blood pressure
c. Give a prescribed hypotensive medicine
d. Talk to her calmly to reduce her anxiety

A WOMAN WHO IS SUBSTANCE DEPENDENT

Substance dependence is a growing health problem in women of childbearing age, so its incidence during pregnancy is increasing. The Illicit Drug Data Report (IDDR) 2012–2013 produced by the Australian Crime Commission reports that the number of illicit drug arrests is now the highest on record with illegal substances including amphetamine-type stimulants, cannabis, heroin, cocaine and steroids (Australian Crime Commission, 2014). The Australian Drug Foundation indicates that the non-medical use of pharmaceutical drugs is increasing with 4.7% of Australians misusing pharmaceutical drugs in 2013 (up from 3.7% in 2007) (Australian Drug Foundation, 2015). Adolescents have an increased rate of inhalant abuse and binge drinking.

Substance abuse is defined as the inability to meet major role obligations, an increase in legal problems or risk-taking behaviour, or exposure to hazardous situations because of an addicting substance. A person is **substance dependent** when he or she has withdrawal symptoms following discontinuation of the substance, combined with abandonment of important activities, spending increased time in activities related to substance use, using substances for a longer time than planned, or continued use despite worsening problems because of substance use.

Typically, substance-dependent women are thought to be in the younger age group, as the overall incidence of drug use is highest in this group, however, any woman may be substance dependent so all pregnant women need to be assessed for this possibility.

A woman with substance abuse problems often comes late in the pregnancy for antenatal care because of fear that her drug use will be discovered and she will be reported to authorities. If she is using a drug that sustains her for only a few hours, she will not be able to wait long at a healthcare facility to be seen for an appointment. She may have difficulty following antenatal instructions for proper nutrition because although she may desire to eat well, she may lack sufficient money to buy both drugs and nutritious food and choosing drugs over food makes her nutrition inadequate. She may not have money for supplemental vitamins or iron preparations for the same reason.

Illicit drugs tend to be of small molecular weight, so they readily cross the placenta. As a result, a fetus of an addicted mother has a drug concentration of about 50% that of the mother. Because this can lead to fetal effects, drug abuse can account for fetal abnormalities or preterm birth (Sithisarn, Granger, & Bada, 2011). If a woman uses injected drugs, the risk of hepatitis B, hepatitis C or human immunodeficiency virus (HIV) infection increases. Women with substance abuse problems expect to be stigmatised and treated with hostility. Such women have frequently been poorly parented and have a history of emotional, physical and sexual abuse as well as depression and other psychiatric illnesses.

Women who are substance dependent need anticipatory guidance and support during pregnancy to maintain the healthiest possible lifestyle. Often, women who abuse substances have few effective support people to discuss their problems or concerns with or who can answer their questions about pregnancy. Because of their numerous needs, they require a multidisciplinary team approach, not only from pregnancy healthcare providers but substance abuse treatment providers as well. Fortunately, with good support and active participation in a treatment program, pregnancy can become a stimulus for drug withdrawal and a maturing and growth experience for a woman.

If a woman is still abusing a drug by the time she begins labour, her infant may experience drug withdrawal symptoms after birth (usually nervousness, irritability or lethargy and possibly seizures; see Chapter 26). Many women use multiple drugs such as cannabis, amphetamines, cocaine and heroin. Prescription medications may also be abused. Cannabis is often seen as a soft drug. However, its active components are excreted in breast milk and there are concerns it may affect the infant's nervous system development and muscle tone; therefore cannabis use should be avoided or minimised by breastfeeding mothers. Infants should not be exposed to the inhalation of cannabis. Cocaine exposure through breastmilk can result in irritability, agitation, tachycardia, tremulousness and seizures in the newborn (Cressman et al., 2012). The decision to breastfeed must be balanced with the risk to the infant, and women who choose to breastfeed and continue intermittent cocaine use should abstain from breastfeeding for 24 hours after usage to allow drug elimination (Cressman et al., 2012). Women receiving methadone as part of the treatment for opiate addiction can safely breastfeed as only a small amount of this drug is excreted in breast milk (Prasad, 2014). In fact, breastfeeding is beneficial to women on methadone as it helps break the cycle of abuse by increasing bonding with the infant and decreasing maternal stress (Prasad, 2014). However, women who abuse any drugs are at risk for adverse outcomes due to poor judgment, impaired decision making, increased risk of domestic violence, infectious diseases, sexually transmitted Infections and mental health disorders (Worley, 2014).

What if...

Mandy tells you she is not using drugs during her pregnancy, but when she opens her handbag you notice several packets of white powder inside? What would you do?

Common substances abused during pregnancy

Recreational drugs commonly used in pregnancy are those commonly used by women in their childbearing years: cocaine, amphetamines, marijuana, inhalants, opiates and alcohol. The number of women who are pregnant and abusing prescription drugs is increasing and is estimated to range from 5% to 20%; the main categories abused are opiates, benzodiazepines and stimulants (Worley, 2014). A wide variety of substances are abused during pregnancy including heroin, methadone, and oxycodone. Substance abuse during pregnancy carries risks of adverse outcomes. Urine toxicology will identify opiate metabolites (morphine, codeine, methadone) for 1 to 3 days after use, but screening should occur with maternal consent and education (Prasad, 2014).

Cocaine

Cocaine is derived from *Erythroxylum coca,* a plant grown almost exclusively in South America. Cocaine is absorbed across the mucous membranes and results in sudden vasoconstriction leading to a rapid increase in heart rate and blood pressure. Cocaine has become one of the most frequently abused drugs during pregnancy. Its use is exceptionally harmful during pregnancy because the extreme vasoconstriction that occurs can severely compromise placental circulation, leading to premature separation of the placenta, which then results in preterm labour or fetal death (see Box 22.1). Infants born to cocaine-dependent women may suffer the immediate effects of intracranial haemorrhage and a withdrawal syndrome of tremulousness, irritability and muscle rigidity. Long-term effects are not well documented, but learning defects are suspected (Accornero et al., 2011).

Counselling women to discontinue cocaine use during pregnancy often results in disappointment. The effects of the drug are so intense that it is difficult for addicted women to withdraw. Cocaine use can be detected by urinalysis because the metabolites of cocaine can be detected in urine up to one week after use.

Amphetamines

Methamphetamine (speed) has a pharmacological effect similar to cocaine. Its use is becoming more common because it is easily and cheaply manufactured (Oei et al., 2012). Ice, a rock type of methamphetamine that is smoked, can produce high concentrations of the drug in the maternal circulation. Newborns, whose mothers used the drug, show jitteriness and poor feeding at birth and may be growth-restricted (Terplan & Wright, 2011).

Marijuana and hashish

Both marijuana and hashish are obtained from the hemp plant, cannabis. When smoked, they produce tachycardia and a sense of wellbeing. These drugs are frequently part of polydrug abuse, so their effects on fetal development are not well-documented (Minnes et al., 2011). They are associated with loss of short-term memory and an increased incidence of respiratory infection in adults. A frequent user may not be able to breastfeed because of reduced milk production and the risk to the newborn from excretion of the drug in the milk.

Phencyclidine

Phencyclidine (PCP) is an animal tranquiliser that is a frequently used street drug in polydrug abuse. It causes increased cardiac output and a sense of euphoria. It has the potential for causing long-term hallucinations

BOX 22.1 Assessment ✻ Assessing the effects of cocaine in the pregnant woman

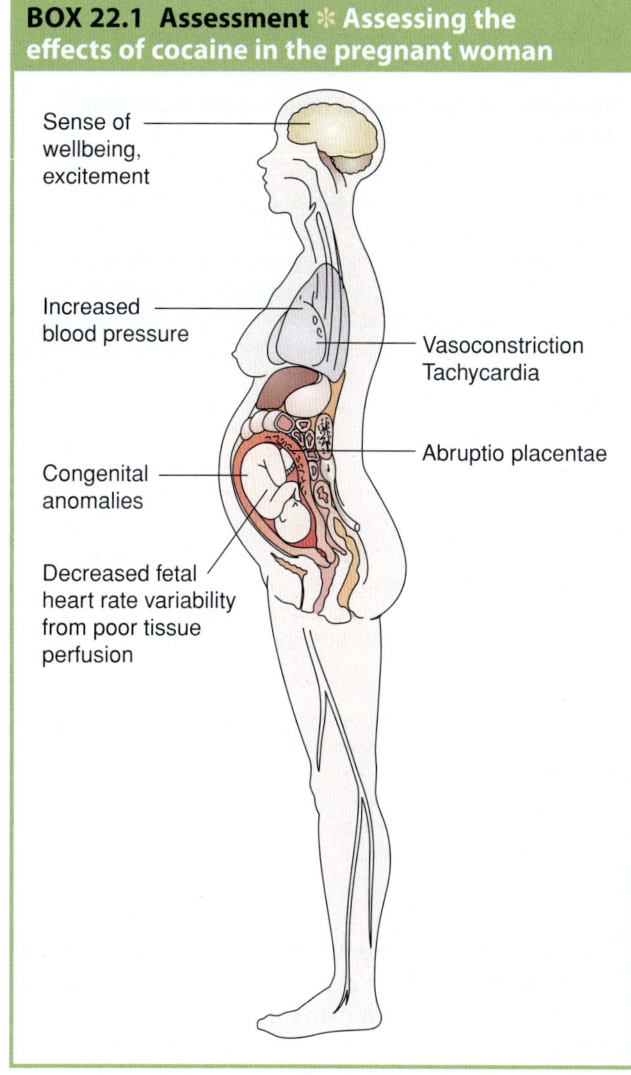

(flashback episodes). PCP tends to leave the maternal circulation and concentrate in fetal cells, so it may be particularly injurious to a fetus.

Narcotic agonists

Narcotic agonists, used for the treatment of pain (e.g. morphine or pethidine and cough suppressant, codeine), are also widely abused because of their potent analgesic and euphoric effect. Heroin, a raw opiate, is the main opiate used recreationally to the point of dependence and its use is increasing in incidence in young adults. A short-acting narcotic, heroin is inactive until it crosses the blood-brain barrier (which it does more quickly than morphine). It may be administered intradermally ("skin popping"), through inhalation ("snorting"), or intravenously ("shooting"). It produces an immediate and short-lived feeling of euphoria followed by sedation. Pregnancy complications related to its use include pregnancy-induced hypertension and, because narcotics are often injected with shared needles, phlebitis, subacute bacterial endocarditis, and hepatitis B and HIV infections.

Withdrawal symptoms include nausea, vomiting, diarrhoea, abdominal pain, hypertension, restlessness, shivering, insomnia, body aches and muscle jerks. Withdrawal symptoms may begin as soon as 6 hours after the last drug dose and can continue for several days. Their severity and duration depend on the amount of drug used daily and the length of the dependence period.

Heroin abuse in the pregnant woman can result in fetal opiate dependence and severe withdrawal symptoms in the infant after birth. Infants of opiate-abusing women tend to be small for gestational age and have an increased incidence of fetal distress and meconium aspiration. They will have the same withdrawal symptoms after birth as the mother would have if she abruptly stopped taking the drug.

Because the fetus is exposed to drugs that must be processed by the liver during pregnancy, the fetal liver is forced to mature faster than normal. For this reason, newborns of substance-abusing women seem better able to cope with bilirubin at birth than other babies; hyperbilirubinaemia is therefore rarely a problem. Fetal lung tissue also appears to mature more rapidly than usual, apparently from the stress of the intrauterine drug exposure. Therefore, although an infant is born preterm, the chance that he or she will develop a condition such as respiratory distress syndrome is less than average.

If possible, an opiate-dependent woman should be enrolled in a methadone maintenance program during pregnancy (Nosyk et al., 2010). Infants of women taking methadone do not escape withdrawal symptoms at birth and some infants appear to have more severe reactions to methadone withdrawal than to heroin withdrawal. Because a woman is being provided an oral drug legally, a fetus is at least ensured better nutrition, better antenatal care and less exposure to pathogens such as hepatitis B and HIV (Devarajah et al., 2012). Drug withdrawal symptoms in the newborn and accompanying nursing care are discussed in Chapter 26.

Inhalants

Inhalant abuse refers to the "sniffing" or "huffing" of aerosol drugs. Frequently abused substances include model aeroplane glue, cooking sprays and computer keyboard cleaner. Most of these substances contain freon as a propellant and can lead to severe respiratory and cardiac irregularities. The effect of these drugs during pregnancy is not well-documented, but they appear to have effects similar to alcohol abuse (Reid et al., 2011). The respiratory depression they can cause could be enough to limit the fetal oxygen supply to a serious level.

Alcohol

Although alcohol can be legally purchased and is served generously at social functions, it is just as detrimental to fetal growth as illegal drugs. There is little documentation regarding how much alcohol must be ingested before fetal alcohol syndrome, a syndrome with significant facial features, possible cognitive challenges and memory deficits, occurs, so women are advised to drink no alcohol during pregnancy (Feldman et al., 2011). When discussing alcohol ingestion with young adults, discuss binge drinking (five or more alcoholic drinks on one occasion) to be certain a woman knows this is unsafe during pregnancy.

CASE STUDY QUESTION

6. Mandy tells you she takes methamphetamines almost daily. The fetus of a drug-addicted mother receives approximately what percentage of the mother's drug concentration?
   a. 20%
   b. 50%
   c. 70%
   d. 100%

TRAUMA AND PREGNANCY

Trauma (injury by force) is a phenomenon that seems remote from pregnancy because pregnant women usually take extra safety precautions to protect their body. However, trauma in women occurs at a high incidence during the childbearing years because, for this age group, motor vehicle accidents, homicide and suicide are among the leading causes of death. A high incidence occurs during the last trimester because of poor balance and fainting from hyperventilation. Orthopaedic injuries such as broken wrists or sprained ankles occur because a pregnant woman's sense of balance is altered (see Box 22.2). In a motor vehicle accident, a pregnant woman is often the front-seat passenger and this is the passenger who often receives the most severe injuries. Other women seen in emergency departments have suffered intimate partner abuse (Rodrigues, Rocha & Barros, 2008).

BOX 22.2 * Focus on evidence-based practice

The most common types of injuries seen in pregnant women

Women become high risk for tripping and falling in late pregnancy because their balance becomes unstable. They may also be so busy thinking about pregnancy tasks that they are responsible for motor vehicle accidents. To investigate the common types of injuries which occur, nursing researchers analysed the records of 100,051 women seen for injuries during pregnancy. Overall, of these women, one in seven sought hospital care for pregnancy-associated injuries at some point in pregnancy, and rates were as high as one in four for some subgroups. Most women (91%) were seen in emergency departments.

More than 4% of women had a motor vehicle collision, the leading cause of injury. The risk of injury was significantly higher among women who were adolescents, black non-Hispanic or had less than a high school education than for other groups. The researchers recommend that preparation for childbirth classes include information on accident prevention.

Would the above study be helpful to mention when discussing accident prevention with pregnant women?

Source: Nannini, A., et al. (2008). Injury: a major cause of pregnancy-associated morbidity in Massachusetts. *Journal of Midwifery and Women's Health, 53*(1), 3–10.

Preventing accidents

Accidents occur more frequently in people under stress than in those with little stress in their lives because, under stress, people concentrate on the stressor, not their immediate surroundings. Because pregnancy is an event that may cause stress in a family's life, a woman and her family should take extra precautions for safety during this time. Pregnancy counselling should include education about ways to avoid accidents and trauma, such as motor vehicle seat belt use (Motozawa et al., 2010).

Physiological changes in pregnancy that affect trauma care

In an emergency situation for physical assessment to be meaningful you must consider the physiological changes that normally occur with pregnancy. A primary rule to remember is that after a traumatic injury, a woman's body will maintain her own homeostasis at the expense of the fetus. To maintain blood pressure in the face of haemorrhage, for example, a woman's body will use peripheral vasoconstriction. As the uterus is a peripheral organ in a shock response, the blood supply to the uterus can be greatly diminished and the nutrient supply to the fetus greatly compromised.

A woman's total plasma volume increases during pregnancy from approximately 2600 mL to 4000 mL at term. This increase serves as a safeguard to a woman if trauma with bleeding should occur, because a woman can lose more blood than normal (up to 30% of her blood volume) before hypovolaemia is clinically evident. This also means, however, that fluid replacement volume will undoubtedly have to be higher because a pregnant woman needs more fluid than a non-pregnant woman to restore her circulatory volume.

The bladder of a pregnant woman is extremely susceptible to rupture because it is the most anterior organ and is elevated abnormally (see Box 22.3). After abdominal trauma, an indwelling bladder catheter is often inserted to assess for blood in the urine.

Psychosocial considerations

After an accident, pregnant women are apt to be apprehensive and frightened about their safety and the safety of the baby. Under stress, information is not processed

BOX 22.3 Assessment ✻ Assessing the effects of trauma in the pregnant woman

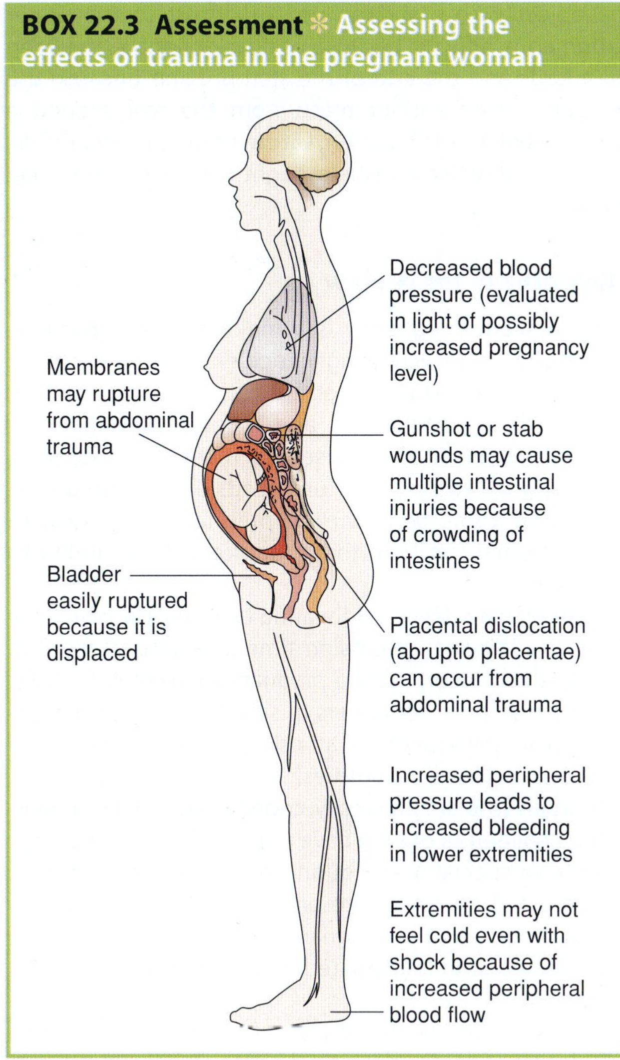

as well and may not be remembered correctly. Always try to review information with a woman before discharge from an emergency department to be certain she has the facts of her injury and understands the follow-up care necessary.

Assessment

Assessment of an injured pregnant woman must be done quickly yet thoroughly and should include both her psychological and physical status. A pregnant woman may be so concerned with her fetus' health that she does not realise she is injured. Another woman might not even consider the possibility that her fetus could be injured until someone asks if she has felt the fetus move since the accident (not realising that a loss of blood from her leg would affect uterine blood flow). Assessment, therefore, should be done concurrently with supportive reassurance ("Your blood pressure is low, but the fetal heartbeat sounds good") to try to relieve her fear of fetal damage. Use a Doppler, if possible, to assess fetal heart tones to demonstrate to a woman, as well as yourself, that the fetus still appears to be well. External monitoring of fetal heart rate and uterine contractions best rules out fetal distress and preterm labour.

In an emergency situation a woman needs her support people around her. Locate them as necessary and also assess their reaction to the trauma.

Health history

Take a brief pregnancy history as well as a trauma history (i.e. length of pregnancy or any complications). Ask specifically if fetal heart tones have been heard by an examiner during the pregnancy, if the woman has felt the fetus move since the accident, if she has any sensation of tightening or pain in her abdomen or back that could be uterine contractions, and if she knows what her pre-pregnancy and pregnancy blood pressures have been to help evaluate the extent of blood loss from the trauma. Document the circumstances of the trauma: what happened, the time of the injury, signs and symptoms of the injury she is experiencing, and actions she has taken to counteract these.

As a final measure, evaluate whether a woman's degree of injury is in proportion to the history. Injuries out of proportion to the history (a woman states she tripped on her front steps, but you notice all her extremities are ecchymotic and her jaw is broken) suggest intimate partner abuse rather than a simple accident (Brownridge et al., 2011). It is important to identify such women as they can have an increased incidence of postpartum depression and perhaps an increased risk of self-harm (Cerulli et al., 2011). (See Chapter 55 for care of an abused woman.) Also analyse whether a woman seems to be using a sensible degree of caution for the circumstances. In rare situations, this may reveal a woman who self-inflicted an injury in an attempt to end an unwanted pregnancy. Likewise, depression or other mental health issues may have resulted in a suicide attempt.

Physical examination

Accidents become fatal when lung, heart, kidney or brain function becomes inadequate; fetal health is in jeopardy when uteroplacental function is impaired. Following trauma, therefore, it is important to evaluate these body systems first. All women who receive a blow to their abdomen need to be evaluated for complications, such as premature separation of the placenta, although the incidence of this occurring is actually small (Mirza, Devine & Gaddipati, 2010; Petrone et al., 2011).

With multiple trauma, a nasogastric tube is usually inserted to empty the stomach. A Foley catheter is inserted to assess urine output and to rule out a ruptured bladder (blood would return or urine would be blood-tinged if bleeding were occurring).

To prevent supine hypotension syndrome, be certain a woman does not lie supine for an examination. If she must lie on her back, manually displace the uterus from the vena cava by placing a rolled towel or blanket under her right side to tip her body approximately 15 degrees to the side. If surgery is necessary, the operating table can be tipped to achieve this same effect.

CASE STUDY QUESTION

7. Mandy received a laceration on her leg from a motor vehicle accident. Why are lacerations of lower extremities potentially more serious in pregnant women than in others?
   a. A woman is less able to keep the laceration clean because of her fatigue
   b. Increased bleeding can occur from uterine pressure on lower extremity veins
   c. Lacerations can provoke allergic responses because of gonadotropic hormones
   d. Healing is limited during pregnancy, so these will not heal until after birth

Therapeutic management

If respirations are not present or are ineffective, commence cardiopulmonary resuscitation (CPR). Women who are less than 20 weeks gestation do not require interventions specific to pregnancy so the guidelines for adult resuscitation in Australia and New Zealand should be followed (see Chapter 20). After 20 weeks' gestation the gravid uterus can reduce maternal cardiac return by 30% and decrease perfusion to the uterus and placenta, so to prevent this the woman should be placed in a left lateral tilt of 15–30 degrees. Although an enlarged uterus puts considerable pressure on the diaphragm and consequently the lungs, only normal pressure is necessary to inflate the lungs fully in a resuscitation attempt. If the woman fails to respond to talking and touch or is unconscious, CPR must be commenced with a ratio of 30 compressions to two breaths. A defibrillator or monitor should be attached and cardioversion carried out according to the usual agency protocol.

After assessment of the level of consciousness and cardiovascular and respiratory status, if there has been blood loss, a central line may be inserted and Hartman's solution or another isotonic solution infused to restore fluid volume or provide an open line for emergency medication. If hypotension is present, it must be corrected quickly to maintain a pressure gradient across the placenta. However, any antihypotensive agent that achieves increased blood pressure by causing peripheral vasoconstriction is contraindicated (vessels in the uterus would constrict and cut off the fetal blood supply). After emergency intervention, care depends on the specific injury or trauma present.

Choking

If a pregnant woman chokes on a piece of meat or any foreign object blocks her airway, attempting to dislodge the object with a sudden upward thrust to the upper abdomen is difficult because of a lack of space between the uterus and the end of the sternum and because the average person cannot reach from the rear around a woman's enlarged abdomen. Late in pregnancy, therefore, a person administering help might use successive chest thrusts instead.

Key points for review

- Adolescent pregnancy is a major concern, because although it is decreasing in incidence, it still occurs at a high rate and can interfere with the development of both an adolescent and a fetus. Nursing care needs to be individualised to meet the antenatal, intrapartal and postpartum needs of this age group. Helping adolescents view a pregnancy as a growth experience can help them mature in their ability to parent.
- Women who delay childbearing until the age of 40 may need additional discussion time at antenatal visits to help them incorporate a pregnancy into their lifestyle. They may need reminders to save time during the day for rest, particularly if at risk of pregnancy-induced hypertension or varicosities.
- Women who are physically, cognitively, visually or hearing challenged or who have a spinal cord injury are apt to have special needs during pregnancy that must be addressed by healthcare providers. Providing time for discussion early in pregnancy so these needs can be identified and anticipated is an important role for nurses.
- Women who are physically or cognitively challenged may need help in adjusting their usual regimen to pregnancy. Be certain they are aware of how to contact help in an emergency. Ensure that all medications they are taking for their primary disorder are safe for use during pregnancy.
- A woman who is substance dependent presents a unique challenge during pregnancy. Encouraging her to decrease or halt her drug intake to safeguard the health of a fetus is a short-term goal. Addressing her need to decrease drug intake for the remainder of her life so she can be a quality parent is a long-term goal.
- A fetus of a woman who is substance dependent is at high risk because of the direct effects of the drug and the indirect effects of an unhealthy lifestyle. Women should be encouraged to join drug reduction maintenance programs if possible to reduce fetal risk.
- Trauma in pregnancy results from sources such as violence, motor vehicle accidents and falls. Women with traumatic injuries need to be carefully assessed to determine if intimate partner abuse was the cause of the trauma.

CASE STUDY QUESTIONS

8. Mandy tells you she is old enough to be a responsible parent and plans to keep her baby. What clues would you look for to see if her self-evaluation is correct?
9. Mandy makes friends with Clare, a 44-year-old woman, at the antenatal clinic. Clare works at a desk job as a stockbroker. She eats most of her meals at restaurants. Mandy lives at home and attends school. Both have inactive lifestyles. Mandy "experiments" with methamphetamine. Clare takes no drugs but acetaminophen (Tylenol). How would what you teach to prevent pregnancy complications differ for these two women?
10. Mandy was seen in an emergency department after a motor vehicle accident. Following a severe injury of this kind, what body systems would you assess first?
11. What would be a possible research topic to explore pertinent to these goals that would be applicable to the Carson family and also advance evidence-based practice?

Resources

For an extensive range of additional resources to enhance teaching and learning and to facilitate understanding of this chapter, please see the text's accompanying website located on thePoint at http://thepoint.lww.com.

References

Accornero, V. H., Anthony, J. C., Morrow, C. E., et al. (2011). Estimated effect of prenatal cocaine exposure on examiner-rated behavior at age 7 years. *Neurotoxicology & Teratology, 33*(3), 370–378.

Alexandra, P., Vassilios, B., Alexandra, V., et al. (2011). Population-based trends of pregnancy outcome in obese mothers. What has changed over 15 years? *Obesity, 19*(9), 1861–1865.

Allen, J., Stapleton, H., Tracy, S. & Kildea, S. (2013). Is a randomised controlled trial of a maternity care intervention for pregnant adolescents possible: An Australian feasibility study, *BMC Medical Research Methodology, 13*(1), 138.

Australian Bureau of Statistics (ABS) (2014). *Births, Australia 2013.* Accessed 7 April 2015, <www.abs.gov.au/ausstats/abs@.nsf/mf/3301.0>.

Australian Crime Commission. (2014). *Illicit drug data report 2012–13.* Accessed 7 April 2015, <www.crimecommission.gov.au//publications/intelligence-products/illicit-drug-data-report/illicit-drug-data-report-2012-13>.

Australian Drug Foundation. (2015). Druginfo: Facts and resources about alcohol and drugs. Accessed 7 April 2015, <www.druginfo.adf.org.au/topics/statistical-trends>.

Australian Human Rights Commission (2012). About us. Accessed 7 April 2015, <www.humanrights.gov.au/sites/default/files/content/about/publications/brochure/about-us.pdf>.

Australian Institute of Health and Welfare (AIHW). (2015). *Child health, development & wellbeing.* Accessed 7 April 2015, <www.aihw.gov.au/child-health/risk-factors/>

Bates, C. K., Carroll, N. & Potter, J. (2011). The challenging pelvic examination. *Journal of General Internal Medicine, 26*(6), 651–657.

Boardman, F. K. (2014). The expressivist objection to prenatal testing: The experiences of families living with genetic disease. *Social Science & Medicine, 107*(0), 18–25.

Brownridge, D. A., Taillieu, T. L., Tyler, K., et al. (2011). Pregnancy and intimate partner violence: Risk factors, severity, and health effects. *Violence Against Women, 17*(7), 858–881.

Burakgazi, E., Pollard, J. & Harden, C. (2011). The effect of pregnancy on seizure control and antiepileptic drugs in women with epilepsy. *Reviews in Neurological Diseases, 8*(1–2), 16–22.

Cerulli, C., Talbot, N. L., Tang, W., et al. (2011). Co-occurring intimate partner violence and mental health diagnoses in perinatal women. *Journal of Women's Health, 20*(12), 1797–1803.

Cressman, A. M., Koren, G., Pupco, A., Kim, E., Shinya Ito, S. & Bozzo, P. (2012). Maternal cocaine use during breastfeeding, *Canadian Family Physician, 58*(11), 1218–1219.

Devarajah, S., Sullivan, J. V., Purcell, A., et al. (2012). Methadone use in pregnancy: Evidence of progression in the severity of addiction. *Journal of Obstetrics & Gynaecology, 32*(8), 753–755.

East, P. L., Chien, N. C. & Barber, J. S. (2012). Adolescents' pregnancy intentions, wantedness and regret: Cross-lagged relations with mental health and harsh parenting. *Journal of Marriage and Family, 74*(1), 167–185.

Erikson, E. (1963). *Childhood and Society*. New York: Norton.

Feldman, H. S., Jones, K. L., Lindsay, S., et al. (2011). Patterns of prenatal alcohol exposure and associated non-characteristic minor structural malformations: A prospective study. *American Journal of Medical Genetics, 155*(12), 2949–2955.

Gaillard, R., Bakker, R., Steegers, E. A., et al. (2011). Maternal age during pregnancy is associated with third trimester blood pressure level: The generation R study. *American Journal of Hypertension, 24*(9), 1046–1053.

Ganchimeg, T., Ota, E., Morisaki, N., Laopaiboon, M., Lumbiganon, P., Zhang, J. & Mori, R. (2014). Pregnancy and childbirth outcomes among adolescent mothers: A World Health Organization multicountry study. *BJOG: An International Journal of Obstetrics & Gynaecology, 121*, 40–48.

Gardner, S. (2014). Caring for women with a disability. *British Journal of Midwifery, 22*(3), 156–156.

Goldfield, G. S., Harvey, A., Grattan, K. & Adamo, K. B. (2012). Physical activity promotion in the preschool years: A critical period to intervene, *Int J Environ Res Public Health, 9*(4), 1326–1342.

Grassley, J. (2010). Adolescent mothers' breastfeeding social support needs. *Journal of Obstetric, Gynecologic, & Neonatal Nursing, 39*(6), 713–722.

Grotegut, C. A. Chisholm, C. A., Johnson, L.N.C., Brown, H. L., Heine, R. P. & James, A. H. (2014). Medical conditions present at time of delivery in hospital discharges among women age 35–44 and age 45 and older compared to women under age 35, *Nationwide Inpatient Sample years 2008–2010.* Table_2.xls. PLOS ONE. 10.1371/journal.pone.0096237.t002.

Grover, S. R. (2011). Gynaecological issues in adolescents with disability. *Journal of Pediatrics & Child Health, 47*(9), 610–613.

Guedes, M. & Canavarro, M. C. (2014). Risk knowledge and psychological distress during pregnancy among primiparous women of advanced age and their partners. *Journal of Midwifery & Women's Health, 59*(5), 483–493.

Hodnett, E. D., Fredericks, S. & Weston, J. (2010). Support during pregnancy for women at increased risk of low birthweight babies. *Cochrane Database of Systematic Reviews,* (6), CD000198.

Höglund, B. & Larsson, M. (2013). Struggling for motherhood with an intellectual disability—A qualitative study of women's experiences in Sweden. *Midwifery, 29*(6), 698–704.

Höglund, B., Lindgren, P. & Larsson, M. (2013). Midwives' knowledge of, attitudes towards and experiences of caring for women with intellectual disability during pregnancy and childbirth: A cross-sectional study in Sweden. *Midwifery, 29*(8), 950–955.

Jutte, D., Roos, N., Brownell, M., et al. (2010). The ripples of adolescent motherhood: Social, educational, and medical outcomes for children of teen and prior teen mothers. *Academic Pediatrics, 10*(5), 293–301.

Kirven, J. (2014). Maintaining their future after teen pregnancy: Strategies for staying physically and mentally fit. *International Journal of Childbirth Education, 29*(1), 57–61.

Linton, K. F. & Rueda, H. A. (2014). Experiences with pregnancy of adolescents with disabilities from the perspectives of the school social workers who serve them, *Health and Social Work, 39*(2), 92–100.

Loane, M., Morris, J. K., Addor, M. C., Arriola, L., Budd, J., Doray, B. & Salvador, J. (2013). Twenty-year trends in the prevalence of Down syndrome and other trisomies in Europe: Impact of maternal age and prenatal screening. *European Journal of Human Genetics, 21*(1), 27–33.

Lyndon, A., Lee, H. C., Gilbert, W. M., et al. (2012). Maternal morbidity during childbirth hospitalization in California. *Journal of Maternal-Fetal & Neonatal Medicine, 25*(12), 2529–2535.

McKenna, L. & Mirkov, S. (2014). *McKenna's Drug Handbook for Nursing & Midwifery* (7th ed.). Sydney: Lippincott Williams & Wilkins.

Martin, J., Hamilton, B., Ventura, S., et al. (2011). Births: Final data for 2009. *National Vital Statistics Reports, 60*(1), 1–4.

Middleton, A., Turner, G. H., Bitner-Glindzicz, M., et al. (2010). Preferences for communication in clinic from deaf people: A cross-sectional study. *Journal of Evaluation in Clinical Practice, 16*(4), 811–817.

Mills, T. A. & Lavender, T. (2010). Advanced Maternal Age. *Obstetrics, Gynaecology and Reproductive Medicine, 21*(4), 107–111.

Minnes, S., Lang, A. & Singer, L. (2011). Prenatal tobacco, marijuana, stimulant, and opiate exposure: Outcomes and practice implications. *Addiction Science & Clinical Practice, 6*(1), 57–70.

Mirza, F. G., Devine, P. C. & Gaddipati, S. (2010). Trauma in pregnancy: A systematic approach. *American Journal of Perinatology, 27*(7), 579–586.

Motozawa, Y., Hitosugi, M., Abe, T., et al. (2010). Effects of seat belts worn by pregnant drivers during low-impact collisions. *American Journal of Obstetrics & Gynecology, 203*(1), e1–e8.

Nosyk, B., Marsh, D. C., Sun, H., et al. (2010). Trends in methadone maintenance treatment participation, retention, and compliance to dosing guidelines in British Columbia, Canada: 1996–2006. *Journal of Substance Abuse & Treatment, 39*(1), 22–31.

Oei, J. L., Kingsbury, A., Dhawan, A., et al. (2012). Amphetamines, the pregnant woman and her children: A review. *Journal of Perinatology, 32*(10), 737–747.

Pebdani, R., Johnson, K. & Amtmann, D. (2014). Personal experiences of pregnancy and fertility in individuals with spinal cord injury. *Sexuality & Disability, 32*(1), 65–74.

Petrone, P., Talving, P., Browder, T., et al. (2011). Abdominal injuries in pregnancy: A 155-month study at two level 1 trauma centers. *Injury, 42*(1), 47–49.

Pires, R., Araújo-Pedrosa, A. & Canavarro, M. (2014). Examining the links between perceived impact of pregnancy, depressive symptoms, and quality of life during adolescent pregnancy: The buffering role of social support. *Maternal & Child Health Journal, 18*(4), 789–800.

Prasad, M. (2014). When opiate abuse complicates pregnancy. *Contemporary OB/GYN, 59*(2), 28–38.

Rabchevsky, A. G. & Kitzman, P. H. (2011). Latest approaches for the treatment of spasticity and autonomic dysreflexia in chronic spinal cord injury. *Neurotherapeutics, 8*(2), 274–282.

Rahman, M. & Berenson, A. B. (2013). Pregnancy test taking is a correlate of unsafe sex, contraceptive nonadherence, pregnancy, and sexually transmitted infections in adolescent and young adult women. *Journal of Women's Health (15409996), 22*(4), 339–343.

Redshaw, M., Malouf, R., Gao, H. & Gray, R. (2013). Women with disability: The experience of maternity care during pregnancy, labour and birth and the postnatal period. *BMC Pregnancy & Childbirth, 13*(1), 1–14.

Reid, A., Glass, D. C., Bailey, H. D., et al. (2011). Parental occupational exposure to exhausts, solvents, glues and paints, and risk of childhood leukemia. *Cancer Causes & Control, 22*(11), 1575–1585.

Rodrigues, T., Rocha, L. & Barros, H. (2008). Physical abuse during pregnancy and preterm delivery. *American Journal of Obstetrics & Gynecology, 198*(2), 171.e1–6.

Signore, C., Spong, C. Y., Krotoski, D., et al. (2011). Pregnancy in women with physical disabilities. *Obstetrics and Gynecology, 117*(4), 935–947.

Sithisarn, T., Granger, D. T. & Bada, H. S. (2011). Consequences of prenatal substance use. *International Journal of Adolescent Medicine & Health, 24*(2), 105–112.

Statistics New Zealand. (2015). Births and Deaths: Year ended December 2014, accessed 9 June 2015 at <www.stats.govt.nz/browse_for_stats/population/births/BirthsAndDeaths_HOTPYeDec14.aspx>.

Sudduth, A. & Linton, D. (2011). Gynecologic care of women with disabilities: Implications for nurses. *Nursing for Women's Health, 15*(2), 138–147.

Terplan, M. & Wright, T. (2011). The effects of cocaine and amphetamine use during pregnancy on the newborn: Myth versus reality. *Journal of Addictive Diseases, 30*(1), 1–5.

Valentino, K., Nuttall, A. K., Comas, M., et al. (2012). Intergenerational continuity of child abuse among adolescent mothers. *Child Maltreatment, 17*(2), 72–181.

Walsh-Gallagher, D., McConkey, R., Sinclair, M. & Clarke, R. (2013). Normalising birth for women with a disability: The challenges facing practitioners. *Midwifery, 29*(4), 294–299.

Walsh-Gallagher, D., Sinclair, M. & McConkey, R. (2012). The ambiguity of disabled women's experiences of pregnancy, childbirth and motherhood: A phenomenological understanding. *Midwifery, 28*(2), 156–162.

Wilkinson, T., Fahey, N., Suther, E., et al. (2012). Access to emergency contraception for adolescents. *Journal of the American Medical Association, 307*(4), 362–363.

Woodhead, J. (2013). All those women. *Overland, 211*, 22–27.

World Health Organization (WHO). (2011). *Disabilities and rehabilitation*. Accessed 7 April 2015, <www.who.int/disabilities/world_report/2011/en/>.

Worley, J. (2014). Identification and management of prescription drug abuse in pregnancy. *Journal of Perinatal & Neonatal Nursing, 28*(3), 196–203.

Yogev, Y., Melamed, N., Bardin, R., et al. (2010). Pregnancy outcome at extremely advanced maternal age. *American Journal of Obstetrics & Gynecology, 203*(6), e1–e7.

Young, M., Deardorff, J., Ozer, E., et al. (2011). Sexual abuse in childhood and adolescence and the risk of early pregnancy among women aged 18–22. *Journal of Adolescent Health, 49*(3), 287–293.

Suggested readings

Dixon, V. (2014). Teenage pregnancy: Identifying young people aspiring or ambivalent to parenthood. *British Journal of School Nursing, 9*(1), 38–44.

Malouf, R., Redshaw, M., Kurinczuk, J. J. & Gray, R. (2014). Systematic review of heath care interventions to improve outcomes for women with disability and their family during pregnancy, birth and postnatal period. *BMC Pregnancy & Childbirth, 14*(1), 1–24.

Redshaw, M., Malouf, R., Gao, H. & Gray, R. (2013). Women with disability: The experience of maternity care during pregnancy, labour and birth and the postnatal period. *BMC Pregnancy & Childbirth, 13*(1), 1–14.

Turnage, B. F. & Pharris, A. D. (2013). Supporting the pregnant adolescent. *International Journal of Childbirth Education, 28*(4), 72–76.

Wu, M., Lagasse, L., Wouldes, T., Arria, A., Wilcox, T., Derauf, C., Lester, B., et al. (2013). Predictors of inadequate prenatal care in methamphetamine-using mothers in New Zealand and the United States. *Maternal & Child Health Journal, 17*(3), 566–575.

Chapter 23

Care of a family experiencing a complication of labour or birth

Previous chapters discussed pregnancy and normal labour and birth. This chapter adds information about what happens when complications of labour occur. Midwives play a vital role in making labour safe. Recognising disturbances in the rhythm of labour provides an opportunity for interventions that support normal labour. If a complication is recognised early it provides the best opportunity to correct the situation and protect both fetal and maternal health.

LEARNING OBJECTIVES

After mastering the contents of this chapter, you should be able to:

1. Define the term dystocia and consider factors leading to labour dystocia such as emotional distress, deviations in the power (force of labour), the passage or the passenger.
2. Use critical thinking to analyse ways to maintain family-centred care when deviations from the normal in labour or birth occur.
3. Assess a woman in labour and during birth for deviations from the normal labour process.
4. Formulate diagnoses related to deviations from normal in labour and birth.
5. Identify expected outcomes associated with deviations from normal labour and birth and resultant complications.
6. Plan interventions to help the family meet expected outcomes when complications of labour occur.
7. Implement care related to complications of labour or birth such as preparing the family for a caesarean birth.
8. Evaluate expected outcomes for achievement and effectiveness of care.
9. Identify areas related to complications of labour that could benefit from additional research or application of evidence-based practice.
10. Integrate the knowledge of deviations of normal in labour and birth to achieve quality child and family healthcare.

KEY TERMS

- amniotic fluid embolism
- augmentation of labour
- battledore placenta
- external cephalic version
- forceps birth
- hypertonic uterine contractions
- hypotonic uterine contractions
- induction of labour
- labour dystocia
- oxytocin
- pathological retraction ring
- placenta accreta
- placenta circumvallata
- placenta marginata
- placenta succenturiata
- precipitate labour
- umbilical cord prolapse
- uterine inversion
- vacuum extraction

CASE STUDY

Rachel Bigalow, a 28-year-old woman about to give birth to her first baby, is admitted to a birthing room. Her contractions have been 5 minutes apart for 10 hours. She feels more pain in her back than in her abdomen, "like my spine is tearing apart". A contraction monitor shows contractions are hypotonic. On palpation the fetus feels large and is in an occipitoposterior position. Her husband asks you if the reason Rachel's labour is taking so long is because she's overweight.

CASE STUDY QUESTION

1. How would you answer Mr Bigalow?

Although labour often proceeds without any deviation from the normal, complications can occur. A difficult labour (dystocia) or a prolonged labour can arise from any of the four main components of the labour process: (a) the power, or the force that propels the fetus (uterine contractions), (b) the passenger (the fetus), (c) the passageway (the birth canal) or (d) the psyche (the woman's and family's perception of the event). The earlier in labour that a complication is recognised, the better is the chance that it can be resolved (Lanni & Seeds, 2013).

Continuous support in labour helps women feel in control of their labour and avoids fear and anxiety, which may interfere with the progress of labour. If a complication arises a woman needs someone who is knowledgeable about the deviation and its treatment, as well as a person who understands her feelings of helplessness and provides skilled physical and emotional care (Anderson & Kilpatrick, 2012). Women-centred care focuses on women's experiences and the factors important to women such as kind, considerate care in a pleasant calming environment (Begley et al., 2014).

VARIATIONS IN THE RHYTHM OF LABOUR

Disturbances to the rhythm of **labour** can occur at any stage of labour, but it is generally classified as primary (occurring at the onset of labour) or secondary (occurring later in labour). Prolonged labour increases the risk of obstructed labour, ruptured uterus, maternal infection, operative interventions, haemorrhage and psychological trauma. Prolonged labour increases infant morbidity and mortality because the fetus is at higher risk of intrauterine hypoxia and acidosis. It is the midwife's role to assess for and recognise complications during labour (Le Ray et al., 2011).

Prolonged labour appears to result from several factors: cephalopelvic disproportion (the diameters of the fetus are larger than the diameters of the birth canal); abnormal presentations (increased fetal diameters); fetal macrosomia (fetus >90th percentile); cervical dystocia; and maternal obesity. One of the most common causes of prolonged labour is an occipitoposterior position of the fetus. Other less common causes are fetal abnormalities such as hydrocephalus or reproductive tract masses which decrease pelvic diameters. Problems with the strength or frequency of contractions may also prolong labour.

Incoordinate uterine contractions

Uterine contractions are the basic force moving the fetus through the birth canal. They occur because of the interplay of the contractile enzyme adenosine triphosphate and the influence of major electrolytes such as calcium, sodium and potassium, specific contractile proteins (actin and myosin), adrenaline and noradrenaline, **oxytocin** (a posterior pituitary hormone), oestrogen, progesterone and prostaglandins. In most labours, contractions become longer and stronger and are accompanied by effacement and dilation of the cervix. When contractions become abnormal or ineffective, labour may be prolonged (Kish, 2013).

Hypotonic contractions

Figure 23.1(A) illustrates the appearance of normal uterine contractions. **Hypotonic uterine contractions** are mild or infrequent (see Fig. 23.1(B)). Hypotonic contractions are related to a poorly-fitting presenting part or with cephalopelvic disproportion. Hypotonic contractions are most likely to occur during the active phase of labour. They may occur after the administration of narcotic analgesia or an epidural, especially if the cervix is not dilated to 3–4 cm or if bowel or bladder distension prevents descent or firm engagement. They may occur in a uterus that is overstretched by a multiple gestation, a larger-than-usual single fetus, polyhydramnios or in a uterus that is lax from grand multiparity.

Hypotonic contractions increase the length of labour, because more of them are necessary to achieve cervical dilation. This can cause the uterus to not contract as effectively during the postpartum period because of exhaustion, increasing a woman's chance of postpartum haemorrhage. In the first hour after birth, following a labour of hypotonic contractions, palpate the uterus and assess lochia every 15 minutes to ensure that postpartum contractions are not also hypotonic and therefore inadequate to halt bleeding.

Hypertonic contractions

Hypertonic uterine contractions may occur with a precipitate labour or with overuse of IV oxytocin or prostaglandin (see Fig. 23.1(C)). Hypertonic contractions are most often seen in the latent phase of labour. They may occur because more than one pacemaker is stimulating contractions. They tend to be more painful than usual, because the myometrium becomes tender from constant lack of relaxation and the anoxia of uterine cells that results.

A danger of hypertonic contractions is that the lack of relaxation between contractions may not allow optimal uterine artery filling; this could lead to fetal anoxia early in the latent phase of labour.

To help identify the difference, hypotonic and hypertonic contractions are compared in Table 23.1.

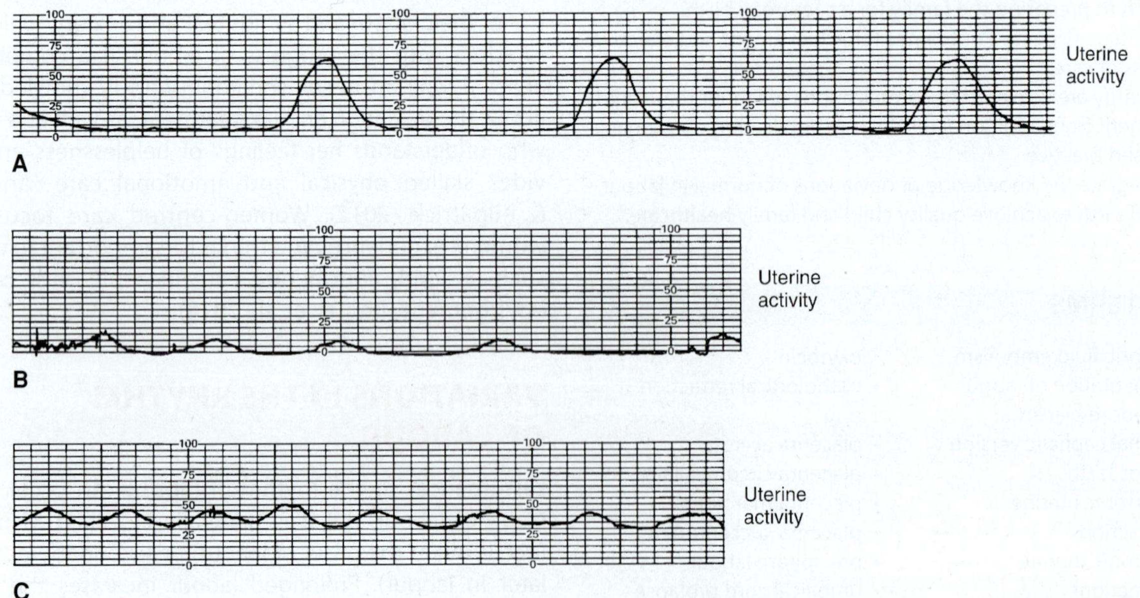

FIGURE 23.1 (**A**) Normal uterine contractions. (**B**) Hypotonic contractions; notice rise in pressure no more than 10 mmHg. (**C**) Hypertonic contractions; notice the high resting pressure (35–40 mmHg).

TABLE 23.1 Comparison of hypotonic and hypertonic contractions

Criteria	Hypertonic	Hypotonic
Phase of labour	Latent	Active
Symptoms	Painful	Limited pain
Medications used:		
Oxytocin	Unfavourable reaction	Favourable reaction
Sedation	Helpful	Little value

Incoordinate uterine action

Normally, all contractions are initiated at one pacemaker point high in the uterus. A contraction sweeps down over the organ, encircling it; repolarisation occurs; relaxation or a low resting tone is achieved; and another pacemaker-activated contraction begins. With uncoordinated contractions, more than one pacemaker may be initiating contractions, or receptor points in the myometrium may be acting independently of the pacemaker. Uncoordinated contractions may occur erratically such as a long period without a contraction and then one on top of another, which may make it difficult for a woman to rest between contractions.

Dystocia and associated stages of labour

Labour dystocia may be defined as difficult labour or abnormally slow progress of labour. For a graphic illustration of the most frequent times labour dystocia is likely to occur, see Figure 23.2. Regardless of when labour dystocia occurs, the effect on the woman and her support person will be the same: anxiety, fear or discouragement. The woman needs a good explanation of what is happening; see Box 23.1.

Disturbances during the first stage of labour

Prolonged latent phase

The latent phase of first stage labour is the time period up to 4 cm. This period is characterised by irregular contractions

BOX 23.1 Common causes of labour dystocia

- Inappropriate use of analgesia (excessive or too early administration)
- Pelvic bone contraction that has narrowed the pelvic diameter so that a fetus cannot pass such as could occur in a woman with rickets
- Poor fetal position (posterior rather than anterior position)
- Extension rather than flexion of the fetal head
- Overdistension of the uterus, as with multiple pregnancy, polyhydramnios or an excessively oversized fetus
- Cervical rigidity (unripe)
- Presence of a full rectum or urinary bladder that impedes fetal descent
- Woman becoming exhausted from labour
- Primigravida status

and occurs prior to active labour which is generally considered to commence when the cervix is 4 cm dilated. A prolonged latent phase, as defined by Friedman (1978), is a latent phase that is longer than 20 hours in a nullipara or 14 hours in a multipara. This may occur if the cervix is not "ripe" at the beginning of labour and time must be spent getting truly ready for labour. Women who are admitted to hospital during the latent phase of labour are more likely to undergo interventions. For example they may be given analgesic early in labour which slows or stops their contractions. A Swedish study compared the use of expectant management versus induction in nulliparous women with a prolonged latent phase and found no significant differences in birth or neonatal outcomes; however, both groups had a high risk of caesarean section (Bräne, Olsson & Andolf, 2014).

Prolonged active phase

A prolonged active phase is associated with being a primi gravida, fetal malposition (such as occiptioposterior, brow or face presentation) or cephalopelvic disproportion.

The partograph

Friedman (1978) defined prolonged labour in the active phase of first stage as cervical dilation of less than 1.2 cm per hour in nulliparous women and 1.5 cm per

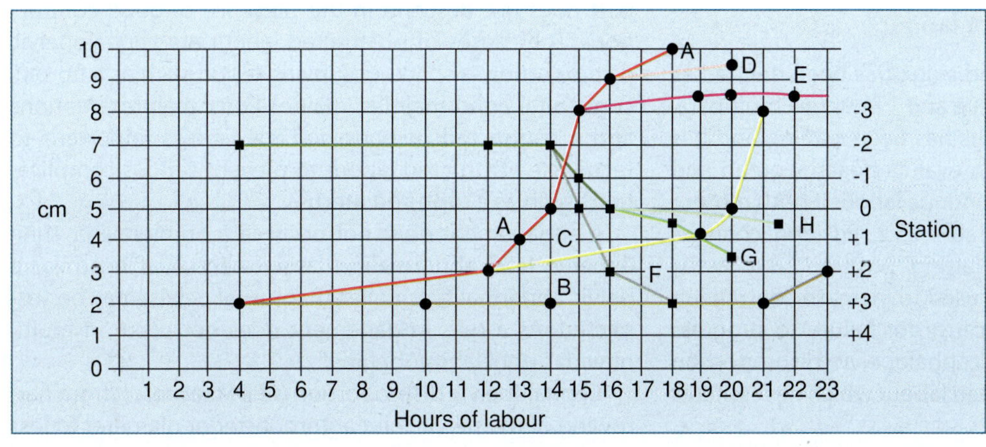

FIGURE 23.2 Graph showing types of prolonged labour. (A) Normal labour curve. (B) Prolonged latent phase. I Protracted active-phase dilation. (D) Prolonged deceleration phase. (E) Secondary arrest of dilation. (F) Normal descent. (G) Prolonged descent. (H) Arrest of descent.

BOX 23.2 * Focus on family teaching

Understanding augmentation of labour

Q. Rachel Bigalow says to you, "My doctor said she's going to augment my labour. What did she mean by that?"

A. Augmentation of labour is used when labour contractions are ineffective. It can shorten labour and avoid the necessity of caesarean birth. The drug used is oxytocin, a synthetic form of the hormone naturally released by your body during labour. It is administered intravenously. Once labour contractions begin by this method, they are the same as naturally occurring contractions. You will be able to use your prepared breathing exercises with them.

TABLE 23.2 Lengths of phases and stages of normal labour in hours

	Primipara		Multipara	
Phase	**Average**	**Upper normal**	**Average**	**Upper normal**
Latent phase	8.6	20.0	5.3	14.0
Active phase	5.8	12.0	2.5	6.0
Second stage	1	1.5	0.25	—*

*There is no limit to the length of the second stage as long as progress is being made and fetal distress is not present.

hour in multigravid women. This heralded the introduction of the partogram and monitoring to see if women fitted the 'normal' labour pattern. Not all women progress at the same rate and dilation of 0.3–0.5 cm is normal for some women although they would be identified as 'abnormal' using the partogram and be subject to interventions such as artificial rupture of the membranes and augmentation. A 2013 Cochrane review found there was no evidence partogram use reduced caesarean section rates or affected labour care and concluded that partogram use cannot be recommended as standard labour management (Lavender, Hart & Smyth, 2013). However in resource poor countries such as Africa, partograph use may reduce the caesarean section rate by using early interventions when prolonged labour is detected (Lavender, Hart & Smyth, 2013).

It is often hard to define exactly what constitutes a prolonged labour. If labour appears to be progressing slowly the midwife can assist with midwifery interventions that may help labour progress. Midwifery interventions include: supportive one-to-one care; using warm water for comfort/pain relief; assisting with mobility and position change; and adequate fluid and nutrition. Other interventions are: amniotomy (artificial rupture of the membranes) and augmentation with oxytocin. Augmentation with oxytocin has been shown to shorten labour (Begley et al., 2014): see Box 23.2.

Prolonged second stage of labour

Historically, prolonged second stage has been defined as more than 2 hours in a nullipara and 1 hour in a multipara. Adherence to these time limits has been waning and it is now considered important to evaluate each woman and her labour individually and continue labour if both mother and fetus are healthy; see Table 23.2. Position changes such as an upright or squatting position may assist descent, or oxytocin may be used to increase contraction strength. The most serious cause for failure to progress during the second stage is cephalopelvic disproportion which can lead to an obstructed labour which necessitates a caesarean birth.

CASE STUDY QUESTION

2. Rachel has prolonged labour. What is the most serious cause for arrest of descent during the second stage of labour?
   a. Cephalopelvic disproportion
   b. Maternal calcium deficiency
   c. The fetus is asleep during labour
   d. The maternal outlet is narrow

Labour requires a large amount of energy and can deplete a woman's glucose stores, so fluids and light snacks should be available. Although the effect of emotion on labour is difficult to document, it seems that the cervix dilates more rapidly and labour is shortened if a woman is neither tense nor frightened. Assist women to be as comfortable as possible, respond to any concerns and offer explanations of all procedures. Help the support person feel just as welcome and comfortable as the woman herself, empower and respect the couple's choices. A full bladder prevents descent of the fetus and may impede uterine contractions so it is helpful if women can void every 2 hours to keep the bladder empty to aid progress.

Obstructed labour

Obstructed labour occurs when the passage of the fetus through the pelvis is obstructed and the fetal presenting part does not descend in the presence of good contractions. The causes of obstructed labour are cephalopelvic disproportion, a space-occupying lesion such as a fibroid, congenital abnormalities, malpositions, malpresentations and a contracted or narrowed pelvis. It is important to recognise obstructed labour to prevent serious complications such as a ruptured uterus.

If engagement does not occur in a primigravida, then either a fetal abnormality (larger-than-usual head) or a pelvic abnormality (smaller-than-usual pelvis) may be suspected. As a rule, engagement does not occur in multigravidas until labour begins.

Cephalopelvic disproportion (CPD) may result from narrowing of the pelvic inlet anteroposterior diameter to less than 11 cm or of the transverse diameter to 12 cm or less. It usually is caused by rickets in early life or by an inherited small pelvis. Rickets is rare in developed countries but can occur among immigrants who were raised in an undeveloped country where milk supplies were not plentiful. With cephalopelvic disproportion, because the fetus does not engage but remains "floating", a malposition may occur, further complicating an already difficult situation. CPD may also result from outlet contraction which occurs when the transverse diameter at the outlet is less than 11 cm. This is the distance between the ischial tuberosities, a measurement that is easy to make during a prenatal visit, so the narrow diameter can be anticipated before labour begins. It is also easily reassessed during labour.

During obstructed labour, in an attempt to birth the baby, uterine contractions may become tonic and eventually the uterus will not be able to contract effectively. Maternal temperature increases, tachycardia is present and maternal distress is evident. In advanced obstructed labour, a **pathological retraction ring** (Bandl's ring) may form. A Bandl's ring is a hard band that forms across the uterus at the junction of the upper and lower uterine segments and interferes with fetal descent. It is a warning sign that severe labour dystocia is occurring as it is formed by excessive retraction of the upper uterine segment; the uterine myometrium is much thicker above the ring and below the ring the lower segment is dangerously thin (see Fig. 23.3). Administration of IV morphine sulfate or the inhalation of amyl nitrite may relieve a retraction ring. A tocolytic can also be administered to halt contractions. If the situation is not relieved, uterine rupture and neurological damage to the fetus may occur.

Precipitate labour

Precipitate labour and birth occur when uterine contractions are so strong and frequent that a woman gives birth rapidly. A precipitate labour is defined as a labour that takes less than 2 hours in total. *Precipitate dilation* is cervical dilation that occurs at a rate of 5 cm or more per hour in a primipara or 10 cm or more per hour in a multipara (Silver & Sabatino, 2012). Such rapid labour is likely to occur with grand multiparity, or it may occur after induction of labour by oxytocin or amniotomy. Contractions can be so forceful that they lead to premature separation of the placenta, placing the woman at risk of haemorrhage (Melamed et al., 2013). Rapid labour also poses a risk to the fetus because subdural haemorrhage may result from the rapid release of pressure on the head. A woman may sustain lacerations of the birth canal from the forceful birth. She may also feel overwhelmed by the speed of labour.

What if...

Rachel tells you that her sister was in labour for only 1 hour when she had her baby, but Rachel is planning to spend the last days of this pregnancy in a rural retreat 120 km from the hospital? What would you do?

Induction and augmentation of labour

Induction of labour means that labour is started artificially with oxytocin and/or an amniotomy (artificial rupture of the membranes). **Augmentation of labour** refers

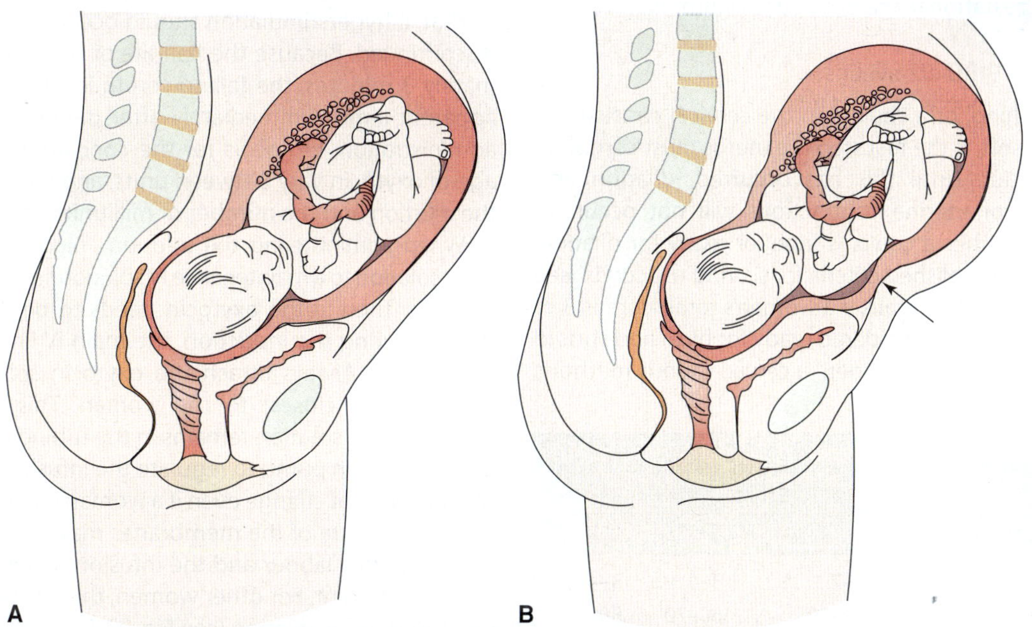

FIGURE 23.3 Pathological retraction ring. (**A**) Uterus in the normal second stage of labour. Notice how the upper uterine segment is becoming thicker and the lower uterine segment is thinning. A physiological retraction ring is normally formed at the division of the upper and lower uterine segments. (**B**) Uterus with a pathological retraction ring (Bandl's ring). The wall below the ring is thin and the abdomen shows an indentation. This constriction is caused by obstructed labour and is a warning sign that if the obstruction is not relieved, the lower segment may rupture.

to assisting labour that has started spontaneously but is not effective and oxytocin and or amniotomy are used to strengthen the already existing contractions (Mozurkewich et al., 2011). Induction may be necessary to initiate labour before it occurs spontaneously because a fetus is in danger or because labour has not commenced and the fetus is post-dates. The primary reasons for inducing labour include: the presence of pre-eclampsia; eclampsia; severe hypertension; diabetes; Rh sensitisation; prolonged rupture of the membranes; intrauterine growth restriction; and postmaturity (also called post-dates and refers to a pregnancy lasting beyond 42 weeks)—all situations that increase the risk to a fetus of remaining in utero. Augmentation of labour or assistance to make uterine contractions stronger may be necessary if the contractions are hypotonic or too weak or infrequent to be effective.

Because augmentation or initiation of labour carries a risk of uterine rupture, decrease in the fetal blood supply from poor cotyledon filling or premature separation of the placenta, it is used cautiously with women with a multiple gestation, polyhydramnios, grand parity, maternal age older than 40 years or previous uterine scars. Induction of labour is associated with higher rates of intervention including caesarean section and should be carefully considered.

Before induction of labour is begun, the following conditions should be present:

- The fetus is in a longitudinal lie
- The cervix is ripe or ready for birth
- A presenting part is engaged
- There is no cephalopelvic disproportion
- The fetal gestational age has been confirmed.

Cervical ripening

Cervical ripening, or a change in the cervical consistency from firm to soft, is the first step the uterus must complete in early labour. Until this has occurred, dilation and coordination of uterine contractions will not occur. To determine whether a cervix is "ripe" or ready for dilation, Bishop (1964) established criteria for scoring the cervix (see Table 23.3). Using this scale, if a woman's total score is 8 or greater, the cervix is considered ready for birth and should respond to induction. To "ripen" a cervix, various methods can be instituted. One is known as "stripping the membranes", or separating the membranes from the lower uterine segment manually, using a gloved finger in the cervix. Possible complications of this mechanical method include bleeding from an undetected low-lying placenta, inadvertent rupture of membranes and the possibility of infection if membranes should rupture.

A more commonly used method of speeding cervical ripening is the application of a prostaglandin gel, such as Prostin, which is inserted into the posterior fornix of the cervix. Additional doses may be applied every 6 hours. Two or three doses are usually adequate to cause ripening. Women should remain in bed in a side-lying position to prevent leakage of the medication and the fetal heart rate (FHR) should be monitored continuously for at least 30 minutes after each dose. Side effects are vomiting, fever, diarrhoea and hypertension, so these should also be monitored. Oxytocin induction may be started 6 to 12 hours after the last prostaglandin dose (beginning it sooner might lead to hyperstimulation of the uterus) (McKenna & Mirkov, 2014). Even with their side effects, prostaglandins are well accepted by women (Taher et al., 2011). As a rule, they should be used with caution in women with asthma, renal or cardiovascular disease, or glaucoma. They are contraindicated for women who have had past caesarean births (McKenna & Mirkov, 2014).

TABLE 23.3 Bishop's score

	Score			
Scoring factor	**0**	**1**	**2**	**3**
Dilation (cm)	0	1–2	3–4	3–4
Effacement (%)	0–30	40–50	60–70	80
Station	−3	−2	−1–0	+1–+2
Consistency	Firm	Medium	Soft	
Position	Posterior	Mid-position	Anterior	

Adapted with permission from Bishop, E. H. (1964). Pelvic scoring for elective induction. *Obstetrics and Gynecology, 24*(2), 266.

Induction of labour by oxytocin

Intravenous oxytocin is administered to initiate contractions in a uterus at pregnancy term (Zheng, 2012) (see Box 23.3). Oxytocin is always administered intravenously, so that, if hyperstimulation should occur, it can be quickly discontinued. Because the half-life of oxytocin is approximately 3 minutes, the falling serum level and effects are apparent almost immediately after discontinuation of IV administration. Protocols for the concentration and dosage of oxytocin vary between units, and it is vital to know the dilution and the number of milliunits per millilitre.

When administering the infusion, "piggyback" the oxytocin solution to a maintenance IV solution such as Hartman's solution. Then, if the oxytocin needs to be discontinued quickly during the induction, the main IV line can still be maintained. Always attach the oxytocin solution to the infusion port closest to the woman. This way, if it is stopped, little solution remains in the tubing to still infuse. Use an infusion pump to regulate the infusion rate, so that the rate will not change even if a woman changes position. Artificial rupture of the membranes may be performed to further induce labour and the infusion may be discontinued at that point. For other women, the infusion is continued through full dilation (see Fig. 23.4).

Peripheral vessel dilation, a side effect of oxytocin, may cause extreme hypotension. To ensure safe induction, take the woman's pulse and blood pressure every 15–30 minutes. Monitor uterine contractions and FHR conscientiously. Contractions should occur no more

BOX 23.3 ✻ Focus on pharmacology

Oxytocin for labour induction

Classification: Oxytocin is a synthetic form of the naturally occurring posterior pituitary hormone.

Action: Used to initiate uterine contractions in a term pregnancy

Pregnancy risk category: C

Dosage: Initially 1 to 2 mU/min by intravenous (IV) infusion, increased at a rate no more than 1 to 2 U/min at 15–30 min intervals until a contraction pattern similar to normal labour is achieved

Possible adverse effects: Nausea, vomiting, cardiac arrhythmias, uterine hypertonicity, tetanic contractions, uterine rupture (with excessive dosages), severe water intoxication and fetal bradycardia

Implications

- Use an infusion pump to ensure accurate control of infusion rate.
- Regulate infusion rate to establish uterine contractions similar to a normal labour pattern.
- Monitor frequency, duration and strength of contractions.
- Assess maternal pulse and blood pressure, and watch for possible hypertension. If hypertension occurs, discontinue drug and notify doctor.
- Continuously monitor fetal heart rate for signs of fetal distress.
- Monitor intake and output and watch for signs of possible water intoxication, such as headache or vomiting. Limit IV fluids to 150 mL/hr.
- Prepare the woman for birth (McKenna & Mirkov, 2014)

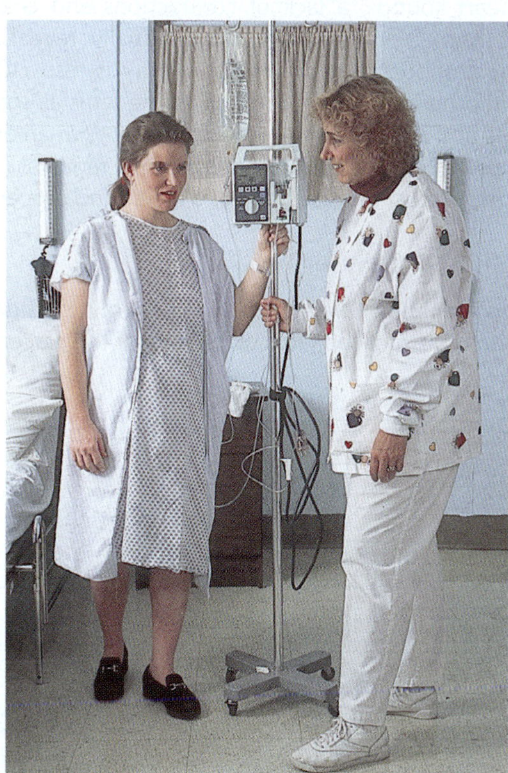

FIGURE 23.4 If intravenous fluid is used for women in labour, it does not need to limit mobility.

often than every 2 minutes and should not last longer than 70 seconds. If contractions become more frequent or longer in duration than these safe limits, or if signs of fetal distress occur, stop the IV infusion and seek help immediately. Oxygen may be administered at 10 L/min. Excessive stimulation of the uterus by oxytocin may lead to tonic uterine contractions with fetal death or rupture of the uterus.

If stopping the oxytocin infusion does not stop the hyperstimulation, the beta-adrenergic receptor medication terbutaline 250 mg can be given subcutaneously, or IV nitroglycerine 50–200 mg, or 1–2 metered doses of sublingual nitroglycerine spray (400–800 mg) to decrease myometrial activity.

Oxytocin has an antidiuretic side effect that can result in decreased urine flow, possibly leading to water intoxication. Water intoxication is first manifested by headache and vomiting. If you observe these danger signs in a woman during induction of labour, report them immediately and halt the infusion (see Box 23.4). Water intoxication in its most severe form can lead to seizures, coma and death

BOX 23.4 Assessment ✻ Assessing the pregnant woman for danger signs of oxytocin administration

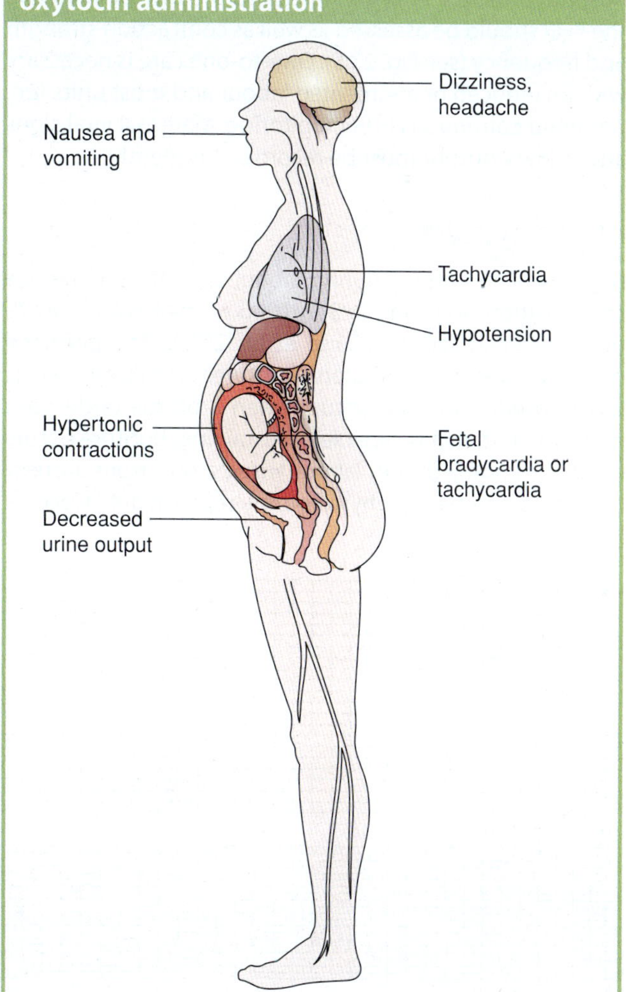

because of the large shift in interstitial tissue fluid. Keep an accurate intake and output record, and test and record urine specific gravity throughout oxytocin administration to detect fluid retention. Limit the amount of IV fluid being given to 150 mL/hr by ensuring that the main IV fluid line is infusing at a rate not greater than 2.5 mL/min.

Women may worry that induced labour will be more painful or "different" from normal labour or that it will progress so fast it will be harmful to the fetus. Induced labours do tend to have a slightly shorter first stage than the average unassisted labour. Induction of labour with oxytocin can predispose a newborn to hyperbilirubinaemia (jaundice) therefore the infant should be observed closely for the first few days of life.

Augmentation by oxytocin

Augmentation of labour is required if labour contractions begin spontaneously but then become so weak, irregular or ineffective (hypotonic) that assistance is needed to strengthen them. Precautions regarding oxytocin augmentation are the same as for primary induction of labour. A uterus may be very responsive or respond very effectively to oxytocin used as augmentation. The oxytocin rate should be increased in small increments according to the hospital protocol. Prior to increasing the rate of oxytocin, the FHR should be assessed as well as contraction strength and frequency (see Fig. 23.5). One-to-one care is necessary with an induced or augmented labour and most units recommend continuous FHR monitoring. Maternal vital signs and urinary output must be recorded frequently.

Uterine rupture

Rupture of the uterus during labour is a rare but serious complication occurring in 3 in 1000 women with a previous caesarean section (Guise et al., 2010). The perinatal mortality rate when the uterus ruptures is 6% (Guise et al., 2010). Uterine rupture occurs when a uterus undergoes more strain than it is capable of sustaining. Rupture occurs most commonly during labour when a scar from a previous caesarean birth or hysterotomy repair tears (it occurs in less than 1% of women who have a caesarean scar from a previous pregnancy) (Smith et al., 2015). Contributing factors may include prolonged labour, abnormal presentation, multiple gestation, unwise use of oxytocin, obstructed labour and traumatic manoeuvres, forceps or traction. When uterine rupture occurs, fetal death will follow unless immediate caesarean birth can be accomplished.

Impending rupture may be preceded by a pathological retraction ring (see earlier discussion) and by strong uterine contractions without any cervical dilation. To prevent rupture when these symptoms are present, anticipate the need for an immediate caesarean birth. If a uterus should rupture, the woman experiences a sudden, severe pain during a strong labour contraction, which she may report as a "tearing" sensation. Rupture can be complete, going through the endometrium, myometrium and peritoneum layers, or incomplete, leaving the peritoneum intact. With a complete rupture, uterine contractions will immediately stop. Two distinct swellings will be visible on the woman's abdomen: the retracted uterus and the extrauterine fetus. Haemorrhage from the torn uterine arteries floods into the abdominal cavity and possibly into the vagina. Signs of shock begin, including rapid, weak pulse; falling blood pressure; cold and clammy skin; and dilation of the nostrils from air hunger. Fetal heart sounds fade and then are absent (see Box 23.5).

If the rupture is incomplete, the signs of rupture are less evident. With an incomplete rupture, a woman may experience only a localised tenderness and a persistent aching pain over the area of the lower uterine segment. However, fetal heart sounds, a lack of contractions and changes in the woman's vital signs will gradually reveal fetal and maternal distress. The initial priority is resuscitation of the mother and surgery to deliver the fetus as soon as possible and control uterine haemorrhage. With an extensive rupture of the uterus a hysterectomy (removal of the damaged uterus) may be done as a life-saving procedure.

Inversion of the uterus

Uterine inversion refers to the uterus turning inside out with either birth of the fetus or delivery of the placenta. It

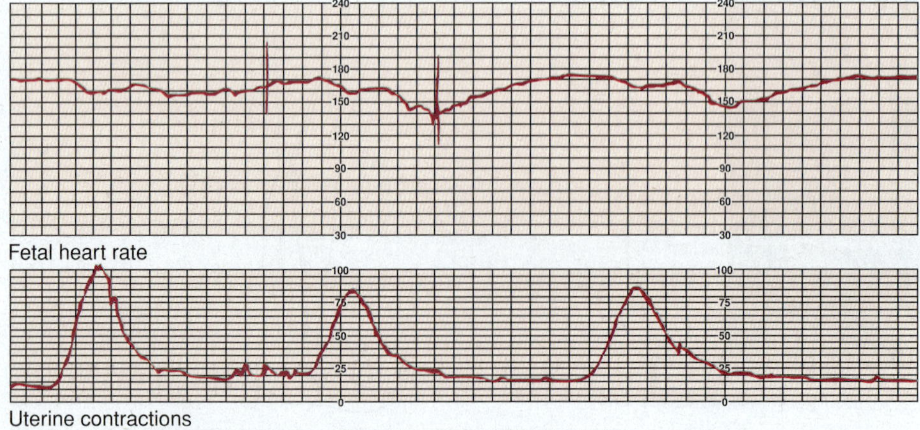

FIGURE 23.5 Hypertonic uterine contractions caused by an oxytocin infusion. Contractions are as high as 100 mmHg in intensity. Late decelerations and an FHR of 170 beats per minute baseline are present.

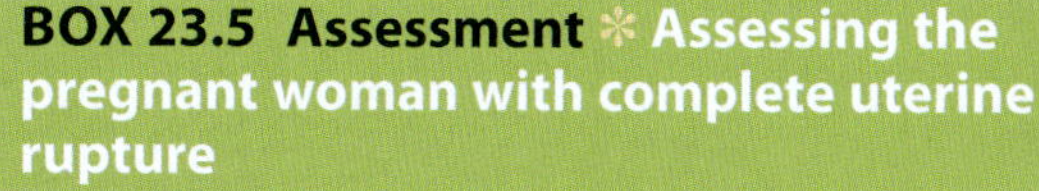

BOX 23.5 Assessment * Assessing the pregnant woman with complete uterine rupture

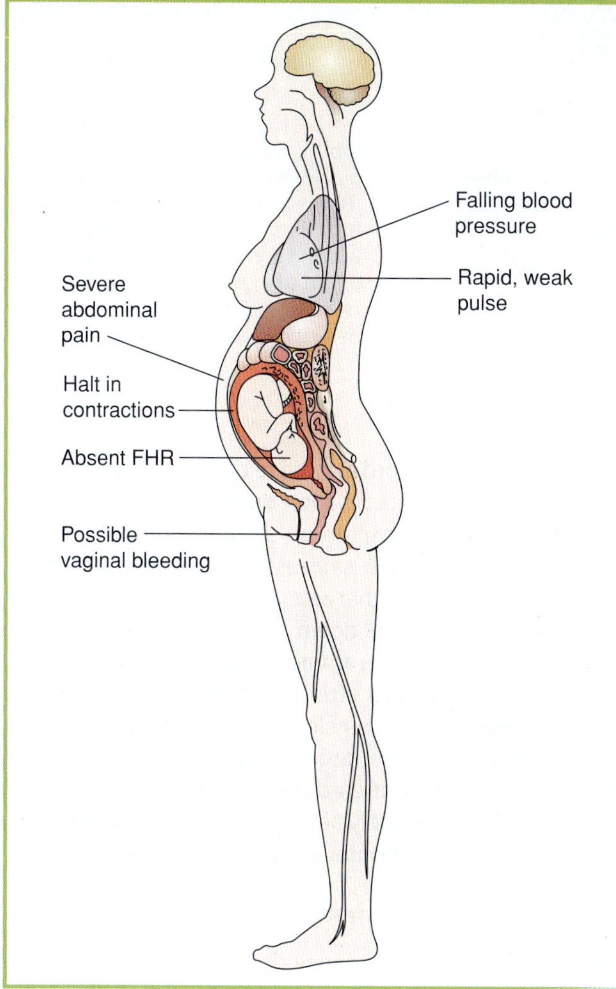

is a rare phenomenon, occurring in about 1 in 20,000 births (Stevens & Wittich, 2011). It may occur if excessive traction is applied to the umbilical cord to remove the placenta or if pressure is applied to the uterine fundus when the uterus is not contracted. It may also occur if the placenta is attached at the fundus so that, during birth, the passage of the fetus pulls the fundus downwards (Purcell & Bienstock, 2012).

Inversion occurs in various degrees with the inverted fundus remaining within the uterine cavity or it may protrude from the vagina. When an inversion occurs, a large amount of blood suddenly gushes from the vagina. The fundus is not palpable in the abdomen and the uterus may appear as a bluish-grey mass protruding from the vagina. If the loss of blood continues unchecked for longer than a few minutes, the woman will show signs of blood loss: hypotension, dizziness, paleness or diaphoresis. Neurogenic and hypovolaemic shock may. In about 50% of cases the placenta is still adhered to the uterus and no attempt should be made to remove it as this may cause a life-threatening haemorrhage. The uterus can be replaced immediately by an obstetrician putting three or four fingers in the centre of the fundus and pushing up until the uterus reverts. Tocolytics may be given to aid reinversion of the uterus and resuscitation measures are required with shock and haemorrhage. If the uterus can be successfully reverted, oxytocin, ergometrine or prostaglandins are given to maintain uterine tone. If the uterus cannot be reverted, immediate transfer to the operating theatre is necessary.

CASE STUDY QUESTION

3. During Rachel's prolonged labour the midwife expresses concern about the risk of uterine rupture. What is uterine rupture?
   a. A rare but serious complication
   b. It more often occurs in women who have previously had a caesarean section
   c. It occurs when the uterus undergoes more strain than it can sustain
   d. All of the above

Amniotic fluid embolism (anaphylactoid syndrome of pregnancy)

Amniotic fluid embolism (AFE) is possibly an acute anaphylactic-like response that occurs when amniotic fluid is forced into an open maternal uterine blood sinus through some defect in the membranes or after membrane rupture or partial premature separation of the placenta (Sahni, 2012). AFE may occur during labour or in the postpartum period. The incidence is about 1 in 20,000 births and it has a high mortality and morbidity rate (Knight et al., 2010). The mortality rate reported in older studies is more than 50%, however recent studies report a rate between 13 and 35% (Benson, 2014). AFE is not preventable because it cannot be predicted. Possible risk factors include uterine hyperstimulation with oxytocin administration, abruptio placentae polyhydramnios, intrauterine fetal demise and instrumental or caesarean section.

The clinical picture is sudden and dramatic with sudden dyspnoea, acute hypotension, cardiopulmonary collapse and disseminating intravascular (Kramer et al., 2013). CPR must be initiated immediately but may be ineffective, because these procedures (inflating the lungs and massaging the heart) do not relieve the pulmonary constriction. Therefore, blood still cannot circulate to the lungs. Death may occur within minutes and intensive care is required with endotracheal intubation to maintain pulmonary function and therapy with fibrinogen to counteract DIC. A caesarean section is undertaken as quickly as possible in an effort to save the fetus and to enable effective maternal resuscitation.

Prolapse of the umbilical cord

In **umbilical cord prolapse,** a loop of the umbilical cord slips down in front of the presenting fetal part

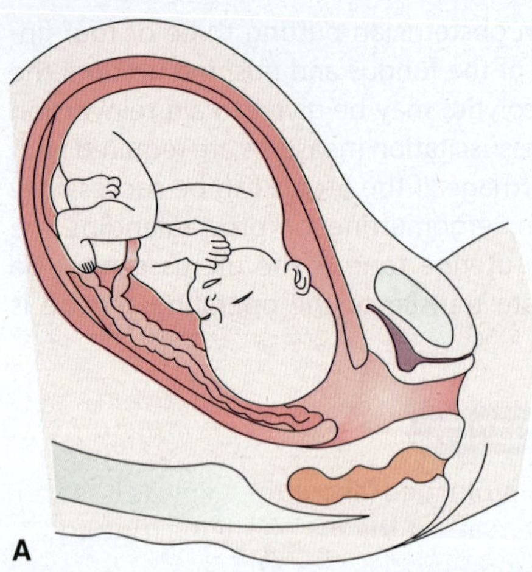

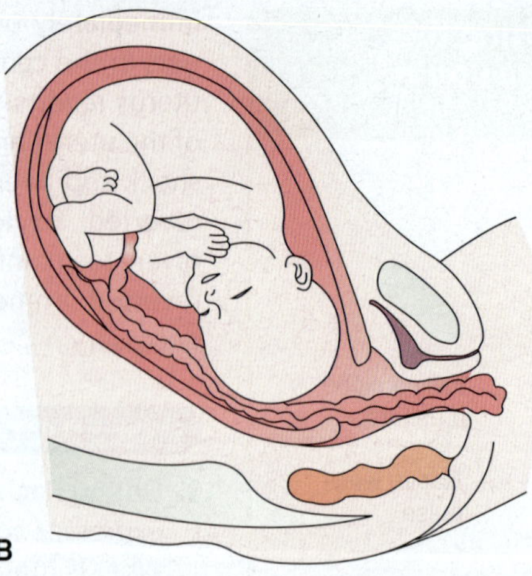

FIGURE 23.6 Prolapse of the umbilical cord. (**A**) The cord is prolapsed but still within the uterus. (**B**) The cord is visible at the vulva. In both instances the fetal nutrient supply is being compromised, although only a cord such as that shown in B would be visible. Both prolapses could be detected by fetal monitoring.

(see Fig. 23.6). Prolapse may occur at any time after the membranes rupture if the presenting fetal part is not fitted firmly into the cervix. Umbilical cord prolapse is an obstetric emergency requiring rapid action. It tends to occur most often with:

- Premature rupture of membranes
- Fetal presentation other than cephalic
- Placenta praevia
- Intrauterine tumours preventing the presenting part from engaging
- A small fetus (prematurity, IUGR, SGA)
- Cephalopelvic disproportion preventing firm engagement
- Polyhydramnios
- Multiple gestation
- Cord abnormalities
- Fetal anomalies
- Grand multiparity.

According to Holbrook & Phelan (2013), around 50% of cord prolapses result from iatrogenic causes which include:

- Amniotomy
- Placement of a fetal scalp electrode
- Amnioinfusion
- Attempted rotation of the fetal head
- Placement of a cervical ripening balloon catheter
- External cephalic version.

The incidence of cord prolapse has decreased and the perinatal survival rate increased from 46% to 94% over the last 70 years (Gibbons, O'Herlihy & Murphy, 2014). Factors influencing the changes in cord prolapse are less grandmultiparas giving birth (historically 75% of cord prolapse occurred in grandmultiparas) and management using caesarean section (Gibbons, O'Herlihy & Murphy, 2014). Other possible factors decreasing the rate of cord prolapse are less or later amniotomy, the use of prostaglandins to ripen the cervix and the birth of footling breech presentations by caesarean section (Silver, 2014). Current incidence is estimated at between 1.4 and 6.2 per 1000 pregnancies (Holbrook & Phelan, 2013).

Assessment

In rare instances, the cord may be felt as the presenting part on an initial vaginal examination during labour. It may also be identified in this position on an ultrasound. When this happens, caesarean birth is necessary before rupture of the membranes occurs. Otherwise, membrane rupture will cause the cord to slide down into the vagina from the pressure exerted by the amniotic fluid. Mostly cord prolapse is first discovered after the membranes have ruptured. Severe variable decelerations or bradycardia may occur after membrane rupture or the cord may be visible at the vulva. To rule out cord prolapse, always assess fetal heart sounds immediately after rupture of the membranes whether this occurs spontaneously or by amniotomy.

Therapeutic management

Cord prolapse is an emergency situation because the fetal presenting part presses against the cord at the pelvic brim leading to cord compression and decreased fetal oxygenation. Prompt caesarean section improves outcomes and this should be arranged rapidly (Holbrook & Phelan, 2013). Management is aimed at relieving cord compression and the resulting fetal anoxia. This may be done by placing a gloved hand in the vagina and manually elevating the fetal head off the cord, or by placing the woman in a knee–chest or Trendelenburg position, which causes the fetal head to fall back from the cord. Administering oxygen at 10 L/min by face mask to the woman is also helpful to improve oxygenation to the fetus.

As an adjunct a tocolytic agent such as terbutaline 250 mcg given subcutaneously to reduce uterine activity and pressure on the fetus. If caesarean section is not available, bladder filling (Vago's method) can be used to allow time for transport to a centre where caesarean is available. A Foley catheter is inserted into the bladder and filled with 500–750 mL of urine and clamped so the bladder provides upward pressure on the fetus relieving cord compression (Holbrook & Phelan, 2013). The efficacy of tocolysis and bladder filling are less certain management techniques (Silver, 2014).

If the cord has prolapsed to the extent that it is exposed to room air, drying will begin, leading to atrophy of the umbilical vessels. Avoid touching the cord, do not attempt to push any exposed cord back into the vagina. This may add to the compression by causing knotting, kinking or spasm. Instead, cover any exposed portion with warm wet saline packs.

If the cervix is fully dilated at the time of the prolapse, the obstetrician may choose to deliver the infant quickly, possibly with forceps, to prevent fetal anoxia. If dilation is incomplete, the birth method of choice is upward pressure on the presenting part, applied by a practitioner's hand in the woman's vagina, to keep pressure off the cord until the baby can be born by caesarean. Prolapsed cord is always an emergency situation, because the reduced blood flow to the fetus can quickly cause fetal harm. With quick recognition and emergency caesarean section, short- and long-term neurological impairment following cord prolapse are now rare (Gibbons, O'Herlihy & Murphy, 2014).

Multiple gestation

Multiple gestations have increased substantially partly due to the role of in vitro fertilisation (Tiitinen, 2012). Additional personnel capable of neonatal resuscitation are required and there should be one for each infant. In the middle of all the preparatory activity, it is easy to forget that a woman having a multiple birth may be more frightened than excited. Be sure to focus on her needs as well as those of her babies. Twins may be born vaginally if the presenting twin is cephalic, but by caesarean otherwise. With a multiple pregnancy with three or more infants a caesarean section is usually performed, because of the increased incidence of cord entanglement and premature separation of the placenta (Tul et al., 2012).

Anaemia and pregnancy-induced hypertension occur at higher-than-usual incidences during multiple gestations. To detect these, be certain to assess the woman's haematocrit level and blood pressure closely.

If a woman with a multiple gestation will be giving birth vaginally, she is usually instructed to come to the hospital early in labour. The first stage of labour does not differ greatly from that of a woman with a single-gestation pregnancy.

If possible, monitor each FHR by a separate fetal monitor during labour. Because the babies are usually small, firm head engagement may not occur, increasing the risk of cord prolapse after rupture of the membranes. Because of the multiple fetuses, abnormal fetal presentation may occur. Uterine dysfunction from a long labour, an overstretched uterus, unusual presentation and premature separation of the placenta after the birth of the first child may also be more common.

Most twin pregnancies present with both twins vertex. This is followed in frequency by vertex and breech, breech and vertex, and then breech and breech (see Fig. 23.7). Multiple gestations of three or more fetuses have extremely

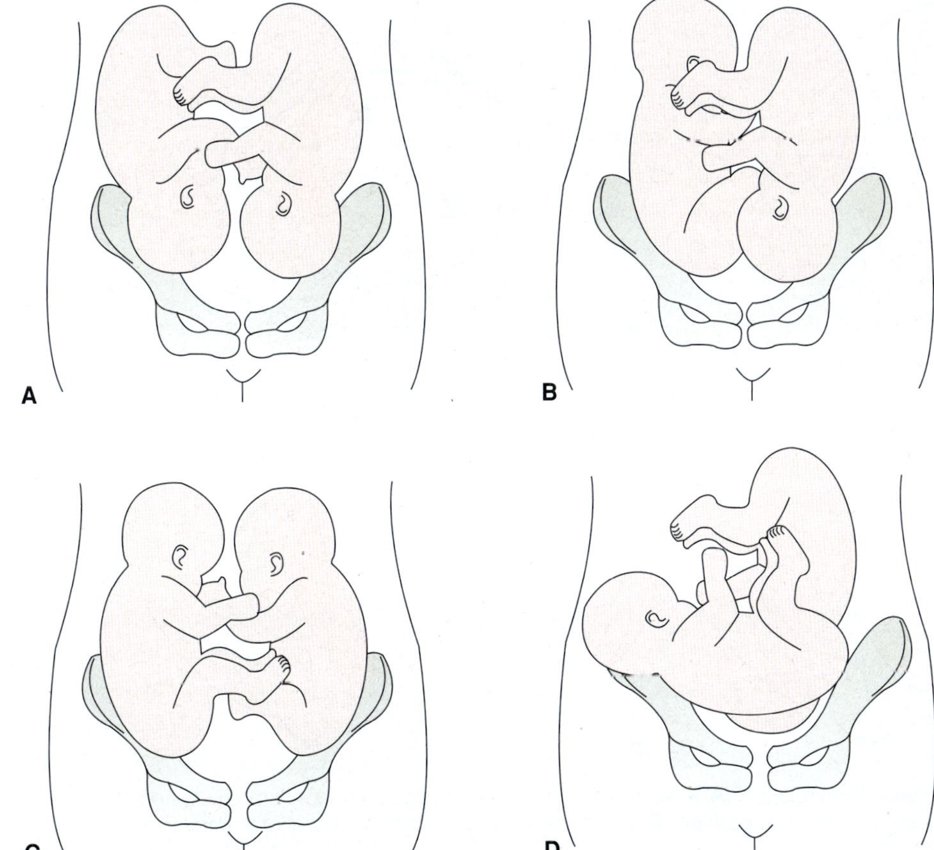

FIGURE 23.7 Four different twin presentations. (**A**) Both infants vertex. (**B**) One infant vertex and one breech. (**C**) Both infants breech. (**D**) One infant vertex and one in a transverse lie.

varied presentations. After the first infant is born the umbilical cord is clamped. This prevents haemorrhage through an open cord end if additional infants have shared the placenta. The first infant is identified as *Twin A* and newborn care is started. In singleton pregnancies oxytocin is usually given immediately to contract the uterus and minimise bleeding after an infant is born; with this woman, however, it will not be given, to avoid compromising the circulation of the infants not yet born.

After the birth of the first child, the lie of the second fetus is determined by external abdominal palpation or ultrasound. If the presentation is not vertex, external version may be attempted and sublingual nitroglycerine may be given to help relax the uterus (Hofmeyr & Kulier, 2012). If this is not successful, a decision for a breech birth or caesarean birth must be made (Hehir et al., 2012).

Parents usually want to inspect multiple-gestation infants thoroughly after birth. The time allowed for this inspection depends on the infants' weights and conditions. Some parents worry that the hospital will confuse their infants through improper identification. Review with them the measures used to ensure correct identification.

Even though women have known for months that they are having multiple infants, many have difficulty believing that this has really happened. They feel a need to recount over and over their surprise and to view all their infants together to prove to themselves that it is true. If parents are unable to inspect their infants thoroughly immediately after birth because of the infants' low birth weights and the danger of chilling, they need the opportunity to do so as soon as possible, to dispel any fears they had throughout pregnancy that the babies would be born less than perfect.

Assess the woman carefully in the immediate postpartum period, because the uterus that has been overly distended owing to the multiple gestation may have more difficulty contracting than usual, placing her at risk of haemorrhage from uterine atony (lacking normal tone). In addition, the risk of uterine infection increases if labour or birth was prolonged. The infants need careful assessment to determine their true gestational age and whether a phenomenon such as twin-to-twin transfusion has occurred.

Malpostions and malpresentations

Occipitoposterior position

Occiputoposterior (OP) position occurs during first stage in around 25% of labours, around 15% during second stage and 5% persist at the time of birth (Carseldine et al., 2013). This indicates that for 95% of women the OP fetus will rotate prior to birth. An OP position is associated with prolonged labour, instrumental birth, caesarean section, severe perineal trauma, post-partum haemorrhage and fetal distress (Guittier et al., 2014).

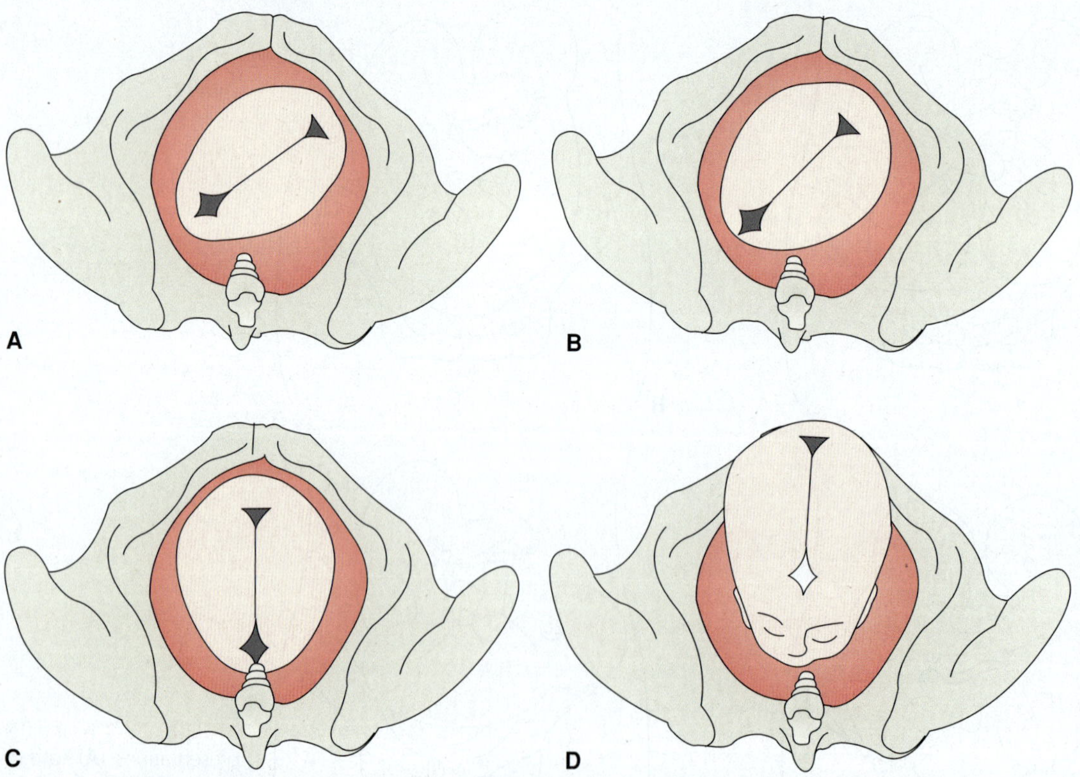

FIGURE 23.8 Left occipitoanterior (LOA) rotation. (**A**) A fetus in a cephalic presentation, LOA position. View is from the outlet. The fetus rotates 90 degrees from this position. (**B**) Descent and flexion. (**C**) Internal rotation complete. (**D**) Extension; the face and chin are born.

A study in New South Wales noted that an OP position in the early second stage of labour was strongly associated with operative delivery, larger babies and a longer second stage; a mean 2 hours 59 minutes in the OP group and 1 hour 54 minutes in the OA group (Carseldine et al., 2013). The study also found the other independent risk factors for operative delivery were nulliparity, abnormal second stage cardiotocograph and epidural analgesia (Carseldine et al., 2013). Operative and instrumental births increase birth trauma making women subject to all the increased risks associated with an instrumental or operative birth.

In an OP position the occiput of a vertex presentation is directed diagonally and posteriorly, either to the right (ROP) or to the left (LOP). A fetus in the OP position often has a deflexed head which increases the presenting diameter to as much as 12.5 cm. During internal rotation, the fetal head must rotate, not through a 90° arc, but through an arc of approximately 135° (see Figs. 23.8 and 23.9). Rotation from a posterior position can be aided by having the woman assume a hands and knees position, squatting or lying on her side (on her left side if the fetus is ROP; on her right side if the fetus is LOP). Theoretically, shifting the weight from right to left or "lunging" or swinging her body right to left while elevating her left foot on a chair widens the pelvic path and makes fetal rotation easier.

The position of the fetus is determined by abdominal palpation and auscultation (the fetal heart sounds are heard laterally or in the centre of the abdomen) and vaginal examination. The abdomen may look flattened

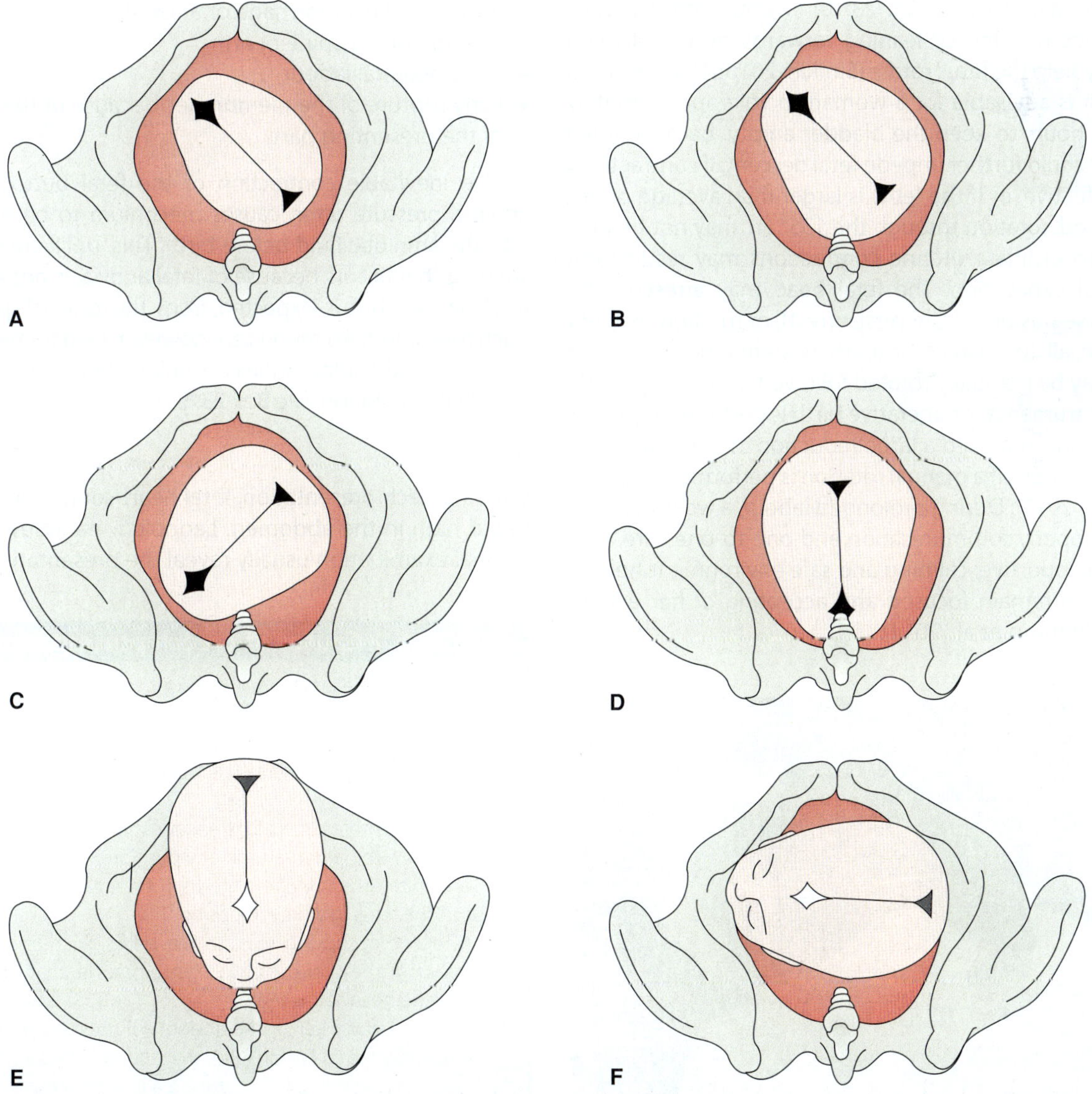

FIGURE 23.9 Left occipitoposterior (LOP) rotation. (**A**) Fetus in a cephalic presentation, LOP position. View is from outlet. The fetus rotates 135 degrees from this position. (**B**) Descent and flexion. (**C**) Internal rotation beginning. Because of the posterior position, the head will rotate in a longer arc than if it were in an anterior position. (**D**) Internal rotation complete. (**E**) Extension; the face and chin are born. (**F**) External rotation; the fetus rotates to place the shoulders in an anteroposterior position.

and the head is often high. The majority of fetuses presenting in posterior positions, of average size with good flexion and aided by forceful uterine contractions, rotate through the large arc, arrive at a good birth position for the pelvic outlet and are born satisfactorily with only increased moulding and caput formation. Because the arc of rotation is greater, it is usual for the labour to be prolonged (Gilbert, 2011) often with a prolonged active phase and slow descent. Epidural anaesthesia may predispose the fetus to an occiptioposterior position (Jackson, 2013).

Because the fetal head rotates against the sacrum, a woman may experience pressure and pain in her lower back owing to sacral nerve compression. These sensations may be so intense that the intense back pressure and pain is more difficult than contractions. Midwifery interventions include: applying counter-pressure on the sacrum; massage; applying heat or cold, whichever feels best, and position changes (see Fig. 23.10). Maintaining a hands-and-knees position or leaning forwards over a birthing ball may help the fetus rotate (Simkin, 2010). During a long labour it is advisable for a woman to void approximately every 2 hours to keep the bladder empty, because a full bladder could further impede fetal descent. If contractions are ineffective, or if the fetus is larger than average or not well flexed, rotation through the 135° arc may not be possible. Incoordinate uterine contractions may result from maternal exhaustion. The fetal head may arrest in the transverse position (transverse arrest), or rotation may not occur at all (persistent occipito posterior position). The fetus may be manually rotated followed by a normal birth, or an instrumental or operative birth is performed. Various studies have reported a large reduction in operative birth for OP positions if a manual rotation is performed (Carseldine et al., 2013). During prolonged labour, a woman needs good support, communication and one-to-one care. Creating a supportive, calming and safe environment helps a woman to remain focused and accepting of her experience (Whitburn et al., 2014).

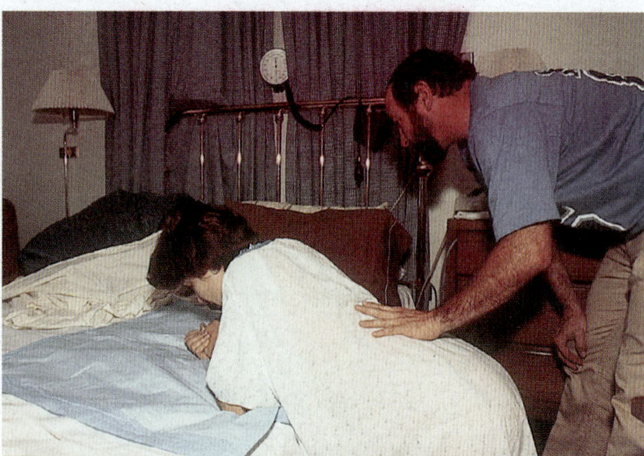

FIGURE 23.10 With a posterior fetal position, a woman may feel extensive back pressure. Pressure on her lower back by her support person may help relieve this problem. (© Kathy Sloane.)

Breech presentation

Most fetuses are in a breech presentation early in pregnancy. However, by week 38, a fetus normally turns to a cephalic presentation (see Fig. 23.11(A)). Although the fetal head is the widest single diameter, the fetus's buttocks (breech), plus the legs, actually take up more space. The fact that the fundus is the largest part of the uterus is probably the reason why, in approximately 97% of all pregnancies, the fetus turns so that the buttocks and lower extremities are in the fundus; leaving 3–4% in the breech position at term (see Fig. 23.11(B)). There are several types of breech presentation: complete, frank and footling (see Fig. 23.12) (see Chapter 15). Breech presentation is more hazardous to a fetus than a cephalic presentation, because there is a higher risk of:

- Anoxia from a prolapsed cord
- Traumatic injury to the after coming head (possibility of intracranial haemorrhage or anoxia)
- Fracture of the spine or arm
- Dysfunctional labour
- Early rupture of the membranes because of the poor fit of the presenting part.

The inevitable contraction of the fetal buttocks from cervical pressure often causes meconium to be extruded into the amniotic fluid before birth. This, unlike meconium staining that occurs because of fetal anoxia, is not a sign of fetal distress but is expected from the buttock pressure. Such meconium excretion can, however, lead to meconium aspiration if the infant inhales amniotic fluid. For causes of breech presentation, see Box 23.6.

Assessment

With a breech presentation, fetal heart sounds are usually heard high in the abdomen. Leopold's manoeuvre and a vaginal examination usually reveal the presentation. If the

BOX 23.6 ✻ Causes of breech presentation

- Gestational age less than 40 weeks
- Abnormality in a fetus, such as anencephaly, hydrocephalus or meningocele. (In a fetus with hydrocephalus, the widest fetal diameter is the head, so it retains the most "comfortable" position)
- Hydramnios that allows for free fetal movement, so that the fetus fits within the uterus in any position
- Congenital anomaly of the uterus, such as a midseptum, that traps the fetus in a breech position
- Any space-occupying mass in the pelvis, such as a fibroid tumour of the uterus or a placenta praevia, that does not allow the head to present
- Pendulous abdomen. If the abdominal muscles are lax, the uterus may fall so far forwards that the fetal head comes to lie outside the pelvic brim, causing a breech presentation
- Multiple gestation. The presenting infant cannot turn to a vertex position
- Unknown factors

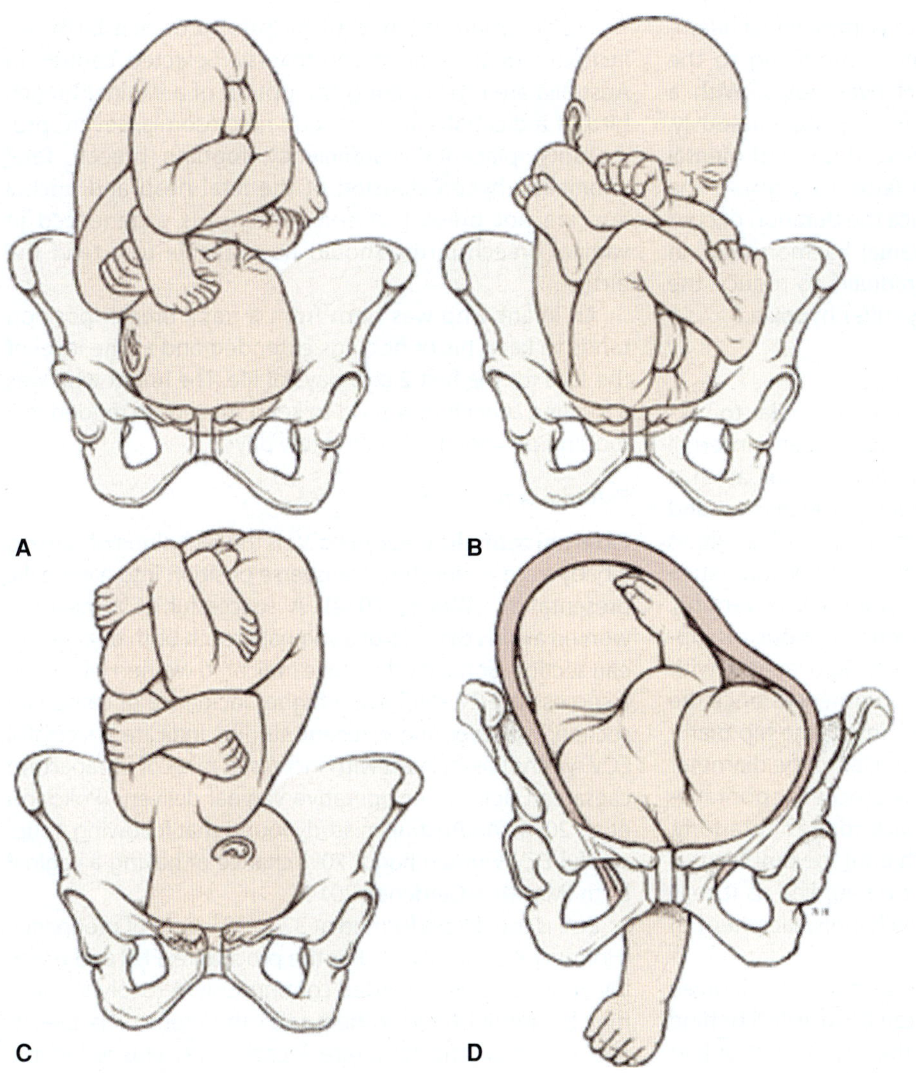

FIGURE 23.11 Fetal presentations. (**A**) Cephalic; (**B**) Breech; (**C**); Face; (**D**) Transverse. (Nettina, S. M. (2013). *Lippincott Manual of Nursing Practice*. Philadelphia, PA: Lippincott Williams & Wilkins.)

breech is complete and firmly engaged, the tightly stretched gluteal muscles of the fetus may be mistaken on vaginal examination for a head; the cleft between the buttocks may be mistaken for the sagittal suture line. If the presentation is unclear, ultrasound clearly confirms a breech presentation. Such a study also gives information on pelvic diameters, fetal skull diameters and evidence of possible placenta praevia causing the breech presentation.

Birth of the head is the most hazardous part of a breech birth. Because the umbilicus precedes the head, a loop of cord passes down alongside the head. The pressure of the head against the pelvic brim automatically compresses this loop of cord.

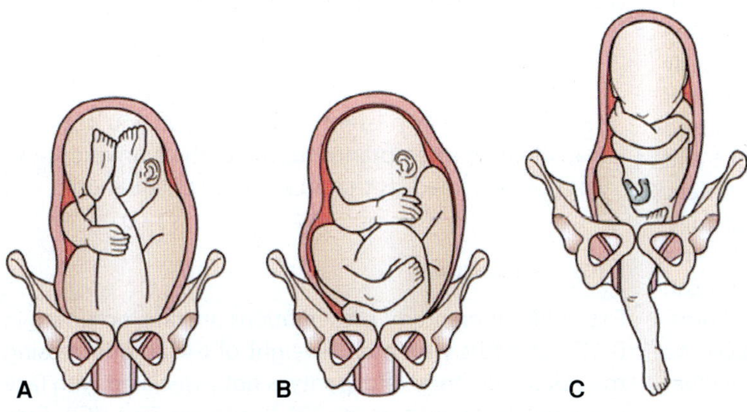

FIGURE 23.12 Types of breech presentations. **A:** Frank breech—the lower extremities of the fetus are flexed at the hips and extended at the knees. **B:** Complete breech—both the hips and knees of the fetus are flexed. **C:** Incomplete breech—one or both of the lower extremities of the fetus are extended at the hips. (Reproduced with permission from Evans, A.T. (2007). *Manual of Obstetrics* (7th ed.). Philadelphia, PA: Lippincott Williams & Wilkins.)

A second danger of a breech birth is intracranial haemorrhage. With a cephalic presentation, moulding to the confines of the birth canal occurs over hours. With a breech birth, pressure changes occur instantaneously. Tentorial tears, which can cause gross motor and mental incapacity or lethal damage to the fetus, may result. The infant who is born suddenly to reduce the duration of cord compression may suffer an intracranial haemorrhage. In contrast, the infant who is born gradually to reduce the possibility of intracranial injury may suffer hypoxia.

Physiological breech birth

In a breech birth the first stage of labour is similar to normal labour. The same stages of flexion, descent, internal rotation, expulsion and external rotation occur as in a vertex birth. Continuous FHR monitoring is recommended and progress should be carefully monitored. This allows early detection of fetal distress from a complication such as prolapsed cord and allows for prompt intervention. Once full dilation is present an all-fours, upright or supported squatting position aids gravity and assists with descent of the fetus. Active pushing commences once the buttocks distend the vulva. In a term infant the hip diameter with flexed or extended legs is similar to the diameter of the fetal head. The birth generally proceeds spontaneously. As the torso descends the back rotates anteriorly, hands should be kept off the breech until the umbilicus is at the introitus. Traction should not be applied as it may cause extension of the head and nuchal displacement of the arms.

Normally the legs will spring out spontaneously if given time, if they do not an index finger can be inserted behind the thigh flexing and abducting the leg. The shoulder blades appear next and the arms usually slip out unassisted and the shoulders are born in the anteroposterior diameter of the pelvis. If the arms are not born readily, the arm of the posterior shoulder may be drawn down by passing two fingers over the infant's shoulder and down the arm to the elbow, then sweeping the flexed arm across the infant's face and chest and out. The other arm is delivered in the same way. The infant's torso is born and the fetal back should be kept uppermost.

To aid in the birth of the head the modified Mauriceau Smellie Veit (MSV) manoeuvre is used. With this manoeuvre the trunk of the infant is usually straddled over one forearm with a finger placed on each maxillae to apply pressure on the lower face and promote flexion. The other hand is placed above the fetus with one finger inserted into the woman's vagina and placed on the occiput and the other two fingers are placed on the fetal shoulders. Pressure is applied to the occiput to flex the head fully. Gentle traction applied to the shoulders (upwards and outwards) delivers the head. An experienced assistant can follow the head abdominally and apply subrapubic pressure to flex the head as it passes through the pelvis. An aftercoming head may also be delivered by the aid of Piper forceps to control flexion and the rate of descent.

The optimum method of birth for a breech birth has incited a great deal of controversy. Selected centres in Australia are now offering the option of a vaginal breech birth if indications such as fetal macrosomia, severe prematurity, placental insufficiency, footling breech, fetal anomalies, hyperextension of the fetal head and nuchal arm are not present. A clinician who is experienced in vaginal breech births should be available to attend the birth.

An infant who was born from a frank breech position tends to keep his or her legs extended and at the level of the face for the first 2 or 3 days of life. The infant who was a footling breech may tend to keep the legs extended in a footling position for the first few days.

External cephalic version

External cephalic version (ECV) is the technique of turning a baby from a breech or transverse position into a cephalic presentation (Walker, 2014). A successful ECV means a women avoids the risks of a vaginal breech birth or a caesarean section. Some studies have indicated women who have a successful ECV still have a higher incidence of caesarean section; however, more recent studies indicate successful ECV was not associated with increased rates of intrapartum caesarean delivery or operative vaginal delivery (Policiano et al., 2014). An Australian study found that following a successful ECV women had a 70% chance of having a vaginal birth (Mowat & Gardener, 2014).

ECV is usually performed at 37 to 38 weeks of pregnancy (Hofmeyr & Kulier, 2012). For the procedure, FHR and possibly ultrasound are recorded continuously. A tocolytic agent may be administered to help relax the uterus. The breech and vertex of the fetus are located and grasped transabdominally by the practitioner's hands on the woman's abdomen. Gentle pressure is then exerted to rotate the fetus in a forward direction to a cephalic lie (see Fig. 23.13). Contraindications to the procedure include multiple gestation, severe oligohydramnios, contraindications to vaginal birth, a cord that wraps around the fetal neck and unexplained third-trimester bleeding, which might be a placenta praevia. External version can be uncomfortable for a woman because of the feeling of pressure. Women who are Rh negative should receive Rh immunoglobulin after the procedure in case minimal bleeding occurs.

> ***What if...***
>
> Rachel's baby was presenting breech and you noticed that when her membranes ruptured, the amniotic fluid was green-stained? Is this an emergency situation?

Face presentation

Face (chin or mentum) presentations are rare, occurring in 0.14% of births with a birthweight of ≥4000 g increasing the risk almost threefold; parity is not associated with face presentation (Tapisiz et al., 2014) (see Fig. 23.11(C)). Face

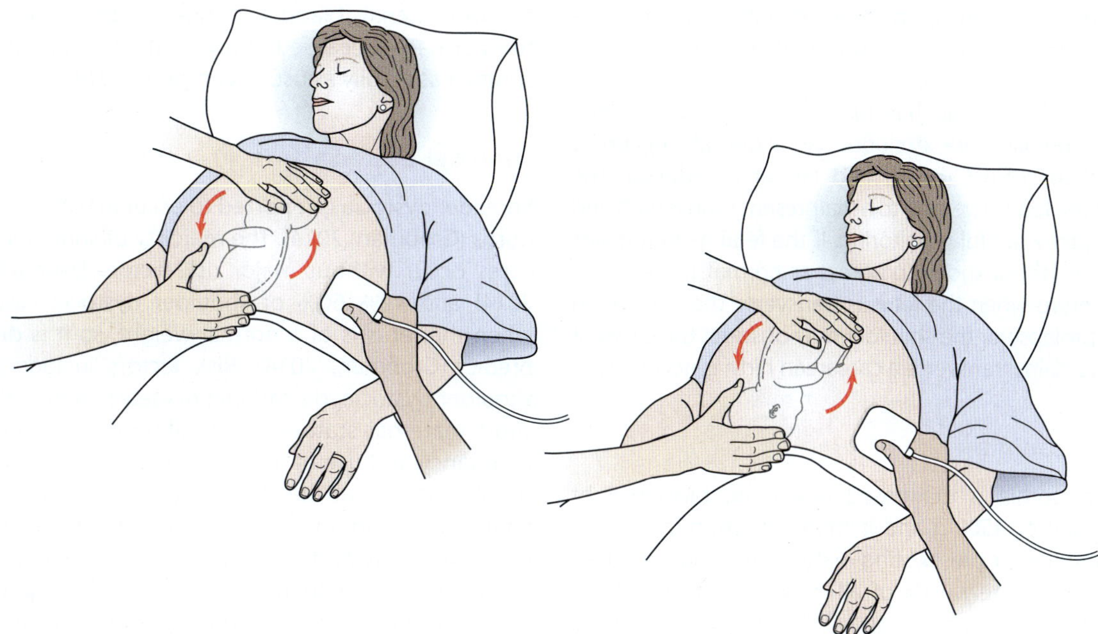

FIGURE 23.13 External cephalic version. The fetus is rotated by external pressure to a cephalic lie. An ultrasound helps guide a safe result.

presentation is not easily diagnosed with only 70% noted from examination (Tapisiz et al, 2014). The fetal head feels more prominently than normal, with no engagement apparent on manoeuvres. The head and back are both felt on the same side of the uterus with Leopold's manoeuvres suggesting a face presentation. The back is difficult to outline in this presentation because it is concave. If the back is extremely concave, fetal heart tones may be transmitted to the forward-thrust chest and be heard on the side of the fetus where feet and arms can be palpated. A face presentation is confirmed by vaginal examination when the nose, mouth or chin can be felt as the presenting part. It can also be confirmed by ultrasound.

The causes of face presentation according to Tapisiz et al. (2014) are related to factors that favour extension of the fetal head and they include:

- Congenital malformations (especially anencephaly)
- High parity
- Pendulous abdomen
- Very large fetus
- Contracted pelvis or cephalopelvic disproportion
- Marked enlargement of the neck or coils of cord about the neck (rare).

It is vital to determine the position of the chin as only an anterior face presentation can be born vaginally. A persistent posterior face presentation will result in obstructed labour. Babies born after a face presentation have a great deal of facial oedema and may be purple from ecchymotic bruising. Observe the infant closely for a patent airway. In some infants, lip oedema is so severe that they are unable to suck for a day or two.

Brow presentation

A brow presentation is the rarest of the presentations occurring in approximately 1 in 500 to one in 1400 births. It occurs in a multipara or a woman with relaxed abdominal muscles. It almost invariably results in obstructed labour, because the head becomes jammed in the brim of the pelvis as the large 13.5-cm occipitomental diameter presents. The causes of a brow presentation are cephalopelvic disproportion, a premature fetus and multiparity. Unless the presentation spontaneously corrects, caesarean birth will be necessary to deliver the infant safely. Brow presentations also leave an infant with extreme ecchymotic bruising on the face. On seeing this bruising over the same area as the anterior fontanelle or "soft spot", parents may need additional reassurance that the child is well after birth.

Transverse lie

Transverse lie (shoulder presentation) occurs in 0.3% of women (see Fig. 23.11(D)). Common causes are a lax or pendulous abdomen, uterine fibroid tumours that obstruct the lower uterine segment, contraction of the pelvic brim, congenital abnormalities of the uterus, placenta praevia, or polyhydramnios. It may occur in infants with hydrocephalus or another abnormality that prevents the head from engaging. It may also occur with prematurity if the infant has room for free movement, in multiple gestation (particularly in a second twin) or if there is a short umbilical cord.

A transverse lie is usually obvious on inspection, because the ovoid shape of the uterus is found to be more horizontal than vertical. The abnormal presentation can be confirmed by Leopold's manoeuvre. An ultrasound may be taken to further confirm the abnormal lie and to provide information on pelvic size.

If contraindications such as placenta praevia and uterine or fetal anomalies are excluded an external version is attempted to correct the lie and labour is induced. The chance of the fetus reverting to a malpresentation is high and labour requires careful monitoring. If the fetal head remains in the pelvis labour should progress as normal. If the membranes rupture when the fetus is transverse the cord or an arm may prolapse or the shoulder may obstruct the cervix. If the fetus remains transverse a caesarean birth is necessary.

Fetal macrosomia

Fetal macrosomia is diagnosed when the birth weight exceeds 4000 or 4500 g and is more common in women with gestational or pre-existing diabetes (Ouzounian et al., 2011). Approximately 10% of all newborns have a birth weight >4000 g and 1.5% weigh >4500 g (Bamberg, Hinkson & Henrich, 2013).The current trend is to define fetal macrosomia as >4500 g or above the 97th gestational age percentile. Macrosomia has a poor predictive value as 70%–90% of macrosomic fetuses are born without sequelae (Mehta & Sokol, 2014).

Large babies are associated with multiparity, because each infant born to a woman tends to be slightly heavier and larger than the previous infant. Woman who are ≤155 cm in height with a macrosomic fetus ≥4500 g are at higher risk of having an infant with a birth injury. Recently the Hart formula has been developed to estimate fetal macrosomia with ultrasound. Although the formula appears to improve accuracy, detection of macrosomia is limited by factors such as unfavourable fetal position and maternal obesity and can be incorrect by 25% (Bamberg, Hinkson & Henrich, 2013).

Induction of labour is considered a contraindication with fetal macrosomia as it increases the rate of shoulder dystocia (Campbell, 2014). Performing a caesarean section would require 3700 women to have an elective caesarean section to prevent one case of permanent brachial plexus injury (Rouse et al., 1996).

An oversized infant may cause incoordinate uterine contractions during labour or at birth because of overstretching of the fibres of the myometrium. The wide shoulders may pose a problem at birth because they can cause fetal pelvic disproportion or even uterine rupture from obstruction. A macrosomic fetus may be more difficult to detect when maternal obesity is present because the fetal contours are difficult to palpate.

The perinatal mortality rate of macrosomic infants is substantially increased to about 15%, compared with the normal 4%. In addition, a large infant born vaginally has increased risk of cervical nerve palsy, diaphragmatic nerve injury or fractured clavicle because of shoulder dystocia. The mother is at increased risk of emergency caesarean section, instrumental delivery, shoulder dystocia and trauma to the birth canal, bladder, perineum and anal sphincter haemorrhage, because the over-distended uterus may not contract as readily as usual (Campbell, 2014).

Shoulder dystocia

Shoulder dystocia is reported to occur in 0.2%–3% of newborns (Grobman, 2014). The majority of shoulder dystocia cases occur without major risk factors (Mehta & Sokol, 2014) and 40%–60% of shoulder dystocia cases occur when the fetus is of a normal weight, so it is difficult to predict (Grobman, 2014). Risk factors include previous shoulder dystocia, gestational diabetes, maternal obesity, short maternal stature, pelvic abnormalities, post-dates pregnancy and use of a vacuum extractor or forceps. The problem occurs at the second stage of labour, when the fetal head is born but the shoulders are impacted against the maternal symphysis pubis because the fetal shoulder diameter is larger than the diameter of the pelvic inlet. This is hazardous to the woman because it can result in vaginal, cervical or perineal tears, postpartum haemorrhage, development of a rectovaginal fistula, uterine rupture or symphyseal separation. It is hazardous to the fetus if the cord is compressed between the fetal body and the bony pelvis which may result in fetal hypoxia, permanent neurological damage or fetal death. The most common fetal injury is a fractured clavicle or a brachial plexus injury. Neonatal brachial plexus injury (flaccid paresis of either arm) related to injury of the brachial plexus, when cranial nerves C5 and C6 are effected it is known as Erb's palsy (Chauhan, Blackwell & Ananth, 2014).

Shoulder dystocia is not usually diagnosed until the head has already been born and the wide anterior shoulder locks beneath the symphysis pubis. The condition may be suspected earlier if the second stage of labour is prolonged, if there is arrest of descent, or if, when the head appears on the perineum (crowning), it retracts instead of protruding with each contraction (a turtle sign).

Management of shoulder dystocia includes asking a woman to flex her thighs sharply on her abdomen (the McRobert's manoeuvre) and apply suprapubic pressure which helps to widen the pelvic outlet (see Fig. 23.14). Rolling the woman onto all fours (the Gaskin manoeuvre) may also increase the pelvic diameter and the movement may dislodge the shoulder (see Fig. 23.15). These two maternal manoeuvres will resolve shoulder dystocia in 40–60% of cases (Grobman, 2014).

Internal rotation can be used to rotate the anterior shoulder under the maternal symphysis pubis. The woodscrew manoeuvre attempts to disimpact the anterior shoulder. The reverse woodscrew manoeuvre attempts to rotate the fetal shoulder in the opposite direction. If this is not successful, the posterior arm can be removed by using two fingers to flex the posterior arm and sweep the arm across the chest.

Shoulder dystocia is an obstetric emergency and staff need to be well versed in their response. Stimulation team

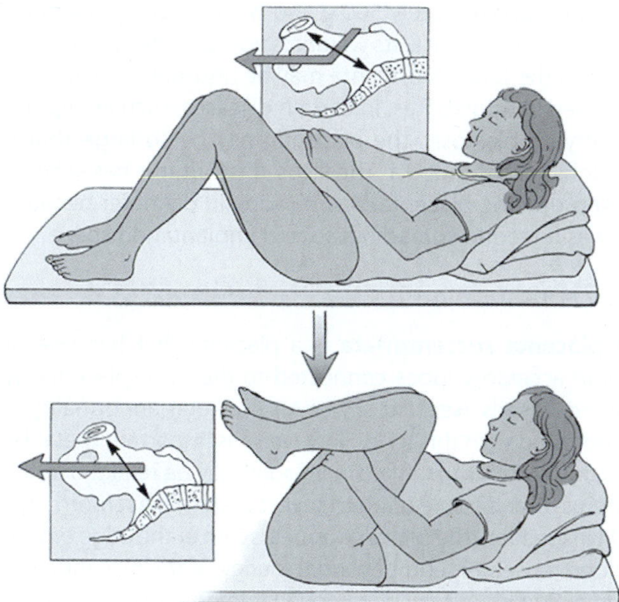

FIGURE 23.14 Shoulder dystocia technique: The McRobert's manoeuvre. (Gala, R. B. & Diallo, A. (2010). *Obstetrics and Gynecology Work-Up*. Philadelphia, PA: Lippincott Williams & Wilkins.)

practice has been shown to improve manoeuvres, communication and general performance (Grobman, 2014).

Fetal anomalies

Fetal anomalies affecting the head such as hydrocephalus (fluid-filled ventricles) or anencephaly (absence of the cranium) can also complicate birth because the fetal presenting part does not engage the cervix well (see Chapter 27 for a discussion of these).

Forceps birth

Obstetrical forceps are steel instruments constructed of two blades that slide together at their shaft to form a handle. One blade is slipped into the woman's vagina next to the fetal head and then the other is slipped into place on the other side of the head. Next, the shafts of the instrument are brought together in the midline to form the handle. The practitioner then applies pressure on the handle to extract the fetus from the birth canal manually.

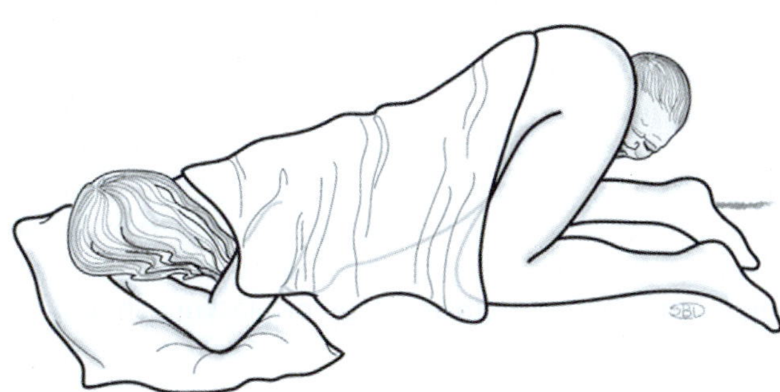

FIGURE 23.15 The Gaskin manoeuvre is used when shoulder dystocia is seen during delivery. One re-positions the mother in the knee-chest position. (Simon, R. R., Ross, C., Bowman, S. H. & Wakim, P. E. (2012). *Cook County Manual of Emergency Procedures*. Philadelphia, PA: Lippincott Williams & Wilkins.)

In years past, babies were routinely born with forceps. Today, the technique is rarely used (about 4% to 8% of births) because it can lead to rectal sphincter tears in the woman which lead to dyspareunia, anal incontinence or increased urinary stress incontinence in women (Murphy et al., 2011). Forceps may be used when the following conditions occur:

- Inability to push with contractions, regional anaesthesia or a spinal cord injury.
- Cessation of descent in the second stage of labour.
- Maternal illness such as cardiac or intracranial disease.
- A fetus is in an abnormal position or is immature.
- A fetus is in distress from a complication such as a prolapsed cord.

Although forceps appear as if they would put forceful pressure on the fetal head, the pressure registers on the steel blades rather than the head so they actually reduce pressure. Reducing pressure in this way can avoid subdural haemorrhage in a fetus as the fetal head reaches the perineum, which is why forceps may be used with preterm birth (Werner et al., 2011).

A **forceps birth** is a forceps outlet procedure in which the forceps are applied after the fetal head reaches the perineum. The term *low forceps birth* may be used to indicate that the fetal head is at +2 12 station or more. If the fetal head is engaged at +1 or +2 12 station, the procedure is called a *midforceps birth*. This type of forceps extraction is rarely justified, because it has been associated with birth trauma to both the woman and the fetus, and caesarean birth involves less risk. A high forceps is never appropriate. Some anaesthesia, at least a pudendal block, is necessary for forceps application to achieve pelvic relaxation and reduce pain. An episiotomy may be performed to prevent perineal tearing due to pressure on the perineum.

Before forceps are applied:

- Consent must be given.
- There is adequate anaesthesia.
- Membranes must be ruptured.
- Cephalopelvic disproportion must not be present.
- The cervix must be fully dilated.
- The fetal head must be engaged in the pelvis.
- Fetal station, presentation and position of the fetal head are known.
- The bladder must be empty.

Record the FHR before application of the forceps. Because there is a danger that the cord could be compressed between the forceps blade and the fetal head, assess the FHR again immediately after application. The woman's cervix needs to be carefully assessed after a forceps birth to be certain that no laceration has occurred. To rule out bladder injury, record the time and amount of the first voiding. In addition, assess the newborn to be certain that no facial palsy or subdural haematoma exists.

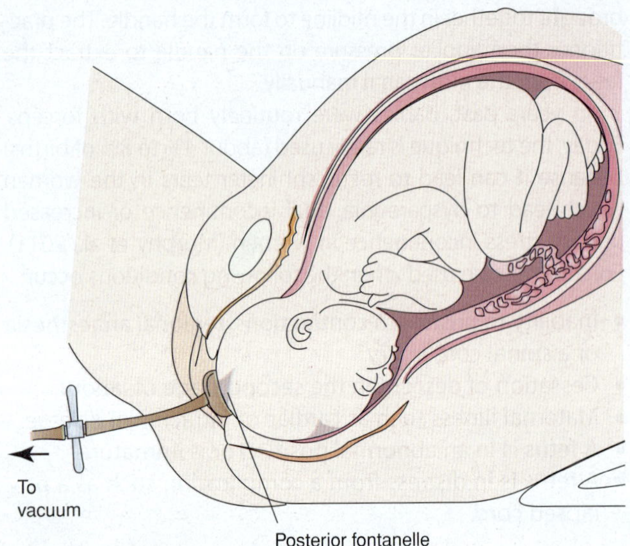

FIGURE 23.16 Vacuum extraction.

A forceps birth may leave a transient erythematous mark on the newborn's cheek (see Chapter 18). This mark will fade in 1 to 2 days with no long-term effects.

Vacuum extraction

A fetus, if positioned far enough down the birth canal, may be born by **vacuum extraction** (Schuller et al., 2012). With the fetal head at the perineum, a disk-shaped cup is pressed against the fetal scalp, over the posterior fontanelle. When vacuum pressure is applied, air beneath the cup is suctioned out and the cup then adheres so tightly to the fetal scalp that traction on the cord leading to the cup extracts the fetus (see Fig. 23.16).

Vacuum extraction has advantages over forceps birth in that less anaesthesia is necessary (leaving the fetus with less respiratory depression at birth) (Melamed et al., 2013). However, women are often given insufficient pain relief and the incidence of vaginal and perineal lacerations is increased (Ahlberg, Saltvedt & Ekéus, 2013). Its major disadvantage is that it causes a marked caput on the newborn head that may be noticeable as long as 7 days after birth. Tentorial tears from extreme pressure may have also occurred. A woman may need reassurance that the caput swelling is harmless to her infant and will decrease rapidly. Vacuum extraction should not be used as a method of birth if fetal scalp blood sampling was used, because the suction pressure can cause severe bleeding at the sampling site. Moreover, vacuum extraction is not used for infants of less than 34 weeks' gestation because of the softness of the premature skull.

ANOMALIES OF THE PLACENTA AND CORD

Anomalies of the placenta

The placenta and cord are always examined for the presence of anomalies after birth. The normal placenta weighs approximately 500 g and is 15–20 cm in diameter and 1.5–3.0 cm thick. Its weight is approximately one-sixth that of the fetus. A placenta may be unusually enlarged in women with diabetes. In certain diseases, such as syphilis or erythroblastosis, the placenta may be so large that it weighs half as much as the fetus. If the uterus has scars or a septum, the placenta may be wide in diameter because it was forced to spread out to find implantation space.

Placenta succenturiata

A **placenta succenturiata** is a placenta that has one or more accessory lobes connected to the main placenta by blood vessels (see Fig. 23.17(A)). No fetal abnormality is associated with this type. However, it is important that it be recognised, because the small lobes may be retained in the uterus after birth, leading to severe maternal haemorrhage. On inspection, the placenta appears torn at the edge or torn blood vessels extend beyond the edge of the placenta. The remaining lobes may be removed from the uterus manually to prevent maternal haemorrhage from poor uterine contraction with no adverse maternal effects.

Placenta circumvallata

Ordinarily, the chorion membrane begins at the edge of the placenta and spreads to envelop the fetus; no chorion covers the fetal side of the placenta. In **placenta circumvallata**, the fetal side of the placenta is covered to some extent with chorion (see Fig. 23.17(B)). The umbilical cord enters the placenta at the usual midpoint and large vessels spread out from there. They end abruptly however, at the point where the chorion folds back onto the surface. (In **placenta marginata**, the fold of chorion reaches just to the edge of the placenta.) Although no abnormalities are associated with this type of placenta, its presence should be noted.

Battledore placenta

In a **battledore placenta**, the cord is inserted marginally rather than centrally (see Fig. 23.17(C)). This anomaly is rare and has no known clinical significance.

Velamentous insertion of the cord

Velamentous insertion of the cord is a situation in which the cord, instead of entering the placenta directly, separates into small vessels that reach the placenta by spreading across a fold of amnion (see Fig. 23.17(D)). This form of cord insertion is most frequently found with multiple gestation. Because it may be associated with fetal anomalies, an infant born with this type of placenta should be examined carefully.

Vasa praevia

In vasa praevia, the umbilical vessels of a velamentous cord insertion cross the cervical os and therefore deliver before the fetus (Robinson & Grobman, 2011). The vessels

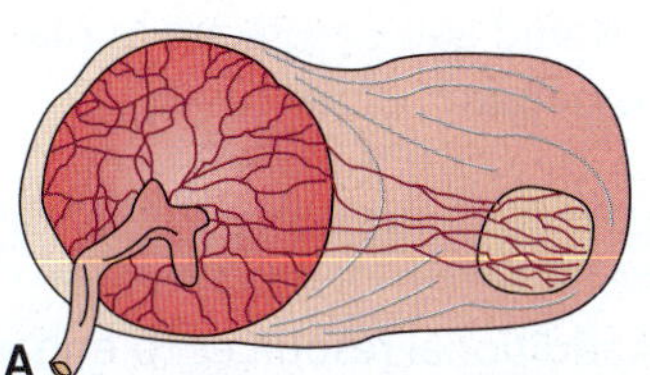

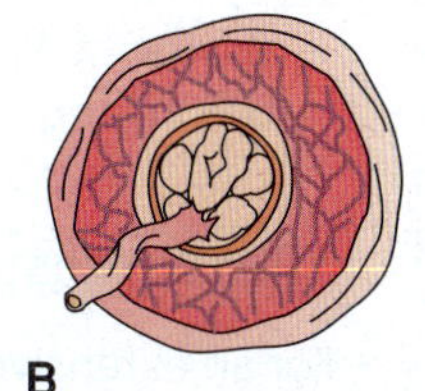

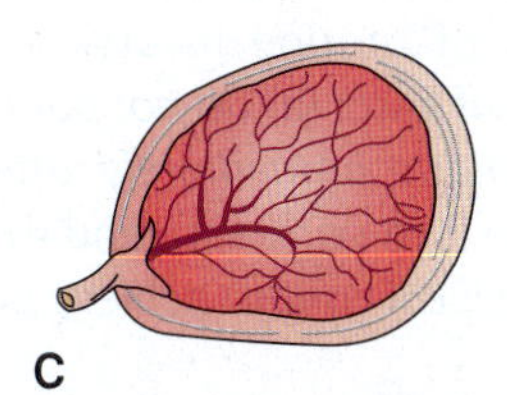

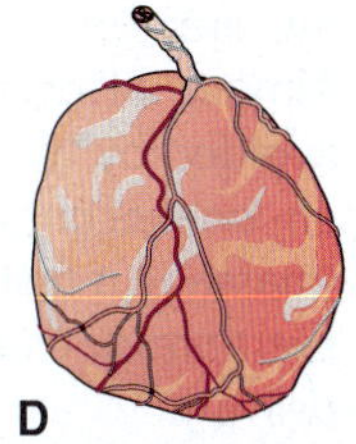

FIGURE 23.17 Abnormal placental formation. (**A**) Placenta succenturiata. (**B**) Placenta circumvallata. (**C**) Battledore placenta. (**D**) Velamentous cord insertion.

may tear with cervical dilation, just as a placenta praevia may tear. Before inserting any instrument such as an internal fetal monitor, be certain to identify structures to prevent accidental tearing of a vasa praevia as tearing would result in sudden fetal blood loss. If sudden, painless bleeding occurs with the beginning of cervical dilation, either placenta praevia or vasa praevia is suspected. It can be confirmed by ultrasound. If vasa praevia is identified, the infant needs to be born by caesarean.

Placenta accreta

Placenta accreta is an unusually deep attachment of the placenta to the uterine myometrium so deeply that the placenta will not loosen and deliver (Kazandi, 2010). Attempts to remove it manually may lead to extreme haemorrhage because of the deep attachment. Hysterectomy or treatment with methotrexate to destroy the still-attached tissue may be necessary.

Anomalies of the cord

Two-vessel cord

A normal cord contains one vein and two arteries. The absence of one of the umbilical arteries is associated with congenital heart and kidney anomalies, because the insult that caused the loss of the vessel may have affected other mesoderm germ layer structures as well. Inspection of the cord as to how many vessels are present must be made immediately after birth, before the cord begins to dry, because drying distorts the appearance of the vessels. Document the number of vessels present conscientiously. An infant with only two vessels needs to be observed carefully for other anomalies during the newborn period.

> **BOX 23.7 Focus on evidence-based practice**
>
> **Human papillomavirus (HPV)**
>
> It is well-documented that HPV is associated with the development of cervical cancer. To analyse whether it could also be responsible for some preterm births, researchers examined links between cervical cytology, placental pathology and preterm birth. The study found a positive HPV DNA test was associated with abnormal placental findings and preterm birth.
>
> *Would the above study suggest another reason to advise adolescent girls to have an HPV vaccine (Gardasil)?*
>
> Zhuang, Z., Goel, S. & Carter, J. E. (2011). Association of cervical cytology and HPV DNA status during pregnancy with placental abnormalities and preterm birth. *American Journal of Clinical Pathology, 136*(2), 260–265.

Unusual cord length

Although the length of the umbilical cord rarely varies, some abnormal lengths may occur. An unusually short umbilical cord can result in premature separation of the placenta or an abnormal fetal lie. An unusually long cord may be easily compromised because of its tendency to twist or knot. Occasionally, a cord actually forms a knot, but the natural pulsations of the blood through the vessels and the muscular vessel walls usually keep the blood flow adequate. Nuchal cords occur in 15–34% of births and are not associated with poor outcomes even in the 6% classified as "tight" (Henry, Andres & Christensen, 2013).

CASE STUDY QUESTION

4. Oxytocin is administered to Rachel to augment labour. What are the first symptoms of water intoxication to observe for during this procedure?
   a. A high, choking voice
   b. Headache and vomiting
   c. A swollen, tender tongue
   d. Abdominal bloating and pain

Key points for review

- Complications of labour can arise from problems with the force of labour, the passage, the passenger or the woman's reaction to the experience (the psyche). Hypotonic, hypertonic and uncoordinated contractions can all occur, resulting in ineffective first or second stages of labour.
- Precipitate labour is birth that is completed in less than 2 hours. It can be responsible for subdural haemorrhage in the fetus and cervical lacerations in the woman.
- Uterine rupture, although rare, is usually preceded by a pathological retraction ring (shown by an indentation across the abdomen over the uterus).
- Uterine inversion is a grave complication. If the situation is not immediately corrected, emergency

hysterectomy is necessary to save the woman's life. Almost all occurrences of uterine inversion can be avoided by two axioms of care: (a) *do not put pressure on an uncontracted fundus immediately after birth* (massage it first to cause it to contract); and (b) *do not exert pressure on an umbilical cord to achieve placental delivery.*

- Amniotic fluid embolism occurs when amniotic fluid is forced into an open maternal uterine blood sinus. A woman has chest pain and dyspnoea and deteriorates rapidly and resuscitation and an emergency team response is required.
- Prolapse of the umbilical cord is an emergency situation that requires prompt action. Position a woman quickly into either a Trendelenburg or a knee-chest position to relieve cord compression, or apply manual pressure vaginally to lift the fetal head away from the cord and request emergency assistance.
- Multiple gestation can complicate birth. Many infants of multiple gestations are born by caesarean birth.
- Abnormal position, presentation or size of the fetus (such as occipitoposterior position; breech, face or brow presentation; transverse lie), as well as problems of the passage such as inlet and outlet contraction, can lead to labour complications.
- Be certain a woman meets the criteria for labour induction before preparing an oxytocin solution. These criteria include engagement of the fetal head, a "ripe" cervix and absence of cephalopelvic disproportion. Question an order if these criteria are not met.
- Always prepare oxytocin as a "piggyback" solution, being extremely careful of the dosage used. Both a uterine monitor and a FHR monitor should be used continuously during labour induction. Observe that contractions occur no less than 2 minutes apart and are no longer than 70 seconds in duration.
- Vacuum extraction and forceps are methods to assist birth. The woman as well as the infant needs special observation after these procedures to detect head trauma or cervical or vaginal tearing.
- Anomalies of the placenta and cord (such as placenta succenturiata, velamentous cord insertion, vasa praevia and two-vessel cord) can lead to birth complications.

CASE STUDY QUESTIONS

5. Rachel's fetus is in a posterior position and she has severe back pain. What actions could her husband take to help relieve his wife's pain caused by this posterior fetal position?
6. Suppose that, after rupture of Rachel's membranes, the fetal monitor shows variable decelerations. On inspection, you are able to see the umbilical cord at the vaginal opening. You are aware that this is a fetal emergency. In order of priority, what would be your best actions?
7. Rachel is scheduled for augmentation of labour with oxytocin. What factors would you ensure are in place before augmentation is begun?

Resources

For an extensive range of additional resources to enhance teaching and learning and to facilitate understanding of this chapter, please see the text's accompanying website located on thePoint at http://thepoint.lww.com.

References

Ahlberg, M., Saltvedt, S. & Ekéus, C. (2013). Insufficient pain relief in vacuum extraction deliveries: A population-based study. *Acta Obstetricia et Gynecologica Scandinavica, 92*(3), 306–311.

Anderson, C. J. & Kilpatrick, C. (2012). Supporting patients' birth plans: Theories, strategies & implications for nurses. *Nursing & Women's Health, 16*(3), 210–218.

Bamberg, C., Hinkson, L. & Henrich, W. (2013). Prenatal detection and consequences of fetal macrosomia. *Fetal Diagnosis and Therapy, 33*(3), 143–148.

Begley, C. M., Gross, M. M., Dencker, A., Benstoem, C., Berg, M. & Devane, D. (2014). Outcome measures in studies on the use of oxytocin for the treatment of delay in labour: A systematic review. *Midwifery, 30*(9), 975–982.

Benson, M. D. (2014). Amniotic fluid embolism: The known and not known. *Obstetric Medicine (1753-495X), 7*(1), 17–21.

Bishop, E. H. (1964). Pelvic scoring for elective induction. *Obstetrics and Gynecology, 24*(2), 266.

Bräne, E., Olsson, A. & Andolf, E. (2014). A randomized controlled trial on early induction compared to expectant management of nulliparous women with prolonged latent phases. *Acta Obstetricia et Gynecologica Scandinavica, 93*(10), 1042–1049.

Campbell, S. (2014). Fetal macrosomia: A problem in need of a policy. *Ultrasound in Obstetrics & Gynecology, 43*(1), 3–10.

Carseldine, W. J., Phipps, H., Zawada, S. F., Campbell, N. T., Ludlow, J. P., Krishnan, S. Y. & De Vries, B. S. (2013). Does occiput posterior position in the second stage of labour increase the operative delivery rate? *Australian & New Zealand Journal of Obstetrics & Gynaecology, 53*(3), 265–270.

Çayır, G. & Şendir, M. (2014). Uterine rupture complication in women vaginal birth after caesarean: A systematic review. *Sezaryen sonrası vajinal doğum yapan kadınlarda uterus rüptür komplikasyonu: Bir sistematik inceleme, 11*(2), 176–189.

Champion, P. (2013). Review: Effect of partogram use on outcomes for women in spontaneous labour at term. *Essentially MIDIRS, 4*(1), 27–30.

Chauhan, S. P., Blackwell, S. B. & Ananth, C. V. (2014). Neonatal brachial plexus palsy: Incidence, prevalence, and temporal trends. *Seminars in Perinatology, 38*(4), 210–218.

Friedman, E. (1978). *Labor, Clinical Evaluation and Management* (2nd ed.). New York: Appleton-Century-Crofts.

Gibbons, C., O'Herlihy, C. & Murphy, J. F. (2014). Umbilical cord prolapse—changing patterns and improved outcomes: A retrospective cohort study. *BJOG: An International Journal of Obstetrics & Gynaecology, 121*(13), 1705–1708.

Gilbert, E. S. (2011). Dysfunctional labor. In E. S. Gilbert (Ed), *Manual of High Risk Pregnancy & Delivery* (5th ed.), pp. 610–659. St Louis, MO: Mosby Elsevier.

Grobman, W. A. (2014). Shoulder dystocia: Simulation and a team-centered protocol. *Seminars in Perinatology, 38*(4), 205–209.

Guise, J. M., Denman, M. A., Emeis, C., Marshall, N., Walker, M., Fu, R., et al. (2010). Vaginal birth after cesarean: New insights on maternal and neonatal outcomes. *Obstetrics & Gynecology, 115*(6), 1267–1278.

Guittier, M. J., Othenin-Girard, V., Irion, O. & Boulvain, M. (2014). Maternal positioning to correct occipito-posterior fetal position in labour: A randomised controlled trial. *BMC Pregnancy & Childbirth, 14*(1), 1–14.

Hehir, M. P., O'Connor, H. D., Kent, E. M., et al. (2012). Changes in vaginal breech delivery rates in a single large metropolitan area. *American Journal of Obstetrics & Gynecology, 206*(6), 498.e1–498.e4.

Henry, E., Andres, R. L. & Christensen, R. D. (2013). Neonatal outcomes following a tight nuchal cord. *Journal of Perinatology, 33*(3), 231–234.

Hofmeyr, G. J. & Kulier, R. (2012). External cephalic version for breech presentation at term. *Cochrane Database of Systematic Reviews*, (10), CD000083.

Holbrook, B. D. & Phelan, S. T. (2013). Umbilical cord prolapse: A plan for an ob emergency. *Contemporary OB/GYN, 58*(9), 28–36.

Jackson, R. (2013). Can midwives promote normality in an occipito-posterior labour through autonomous practice? *Practising Midwife, 16*(11), 14–16.

Jansen, L., Gibson, M., Carlson Bowles, B. & Leach, J. (2013). First do no harm: Interventions during childbirth. *Journal of Perinatal Education, 22*(2), 83–92.

Kanayama, N. & Tamura, N. (2014). Amniotic fluid embolism: Pathophysiology and new strategies for management. *Journal of Obstetrics and Gynaecology Research, 40*(6), 1507–1517.

Kazandi, M. (2010). Conservative and surgical treatment of abnormal placentation: Report of five cases and review of the literature. *Clinical & Experimental Obstetrics & Gynecology, 37*(4), 310–312.

Khvorostukhina, N. F., Kozlova, T. U., Novichkov, D. A. & Bebeshko, O. I. (2014). Analysis of effectiveness and safety of assisted delivery. (English). *Saratov Journal of Medical Scientific Research / Saratovskii Nauchno-Meditsinskii Zhurnal, 10*(2), 346–349.

Kish, K. (2013). Malpresentation & cord prolapse. In A. H. DeCherney, L. Nathan, N. Laufer, et al. (Eds), *Current Diagnosis and Treatment: Obstetrics and Gynecology* (11th ed.), pp. 317–333. Columbus, OH: McGraw-Hill/Lange.

Knight, M., Tuffnell, D., Brocklehurst, P., et al. (2010). Incidence and risk factors for amniotic-fluid embolism. *Obstetrics & Gynecology, 115*(5), 910–917.

Kramer, M. S., Abenhaim, H., Dahhou, M., Rouleau, J. & Berg, C. (2013). Incidence, risk factors, and consequences of amniotic fluid embolism. *Paediatric & Perinatal Epidemiology, 27*(5), 436–441.

Lanni, S. M. & Seeds, G. W. (2013). Malpresentations and shoulder dystocia. In S. G. Gabbe, J. R. Niebyl, J. L. Simpson, et al. (Eds), *Obstetrics: Normal and Problem Pregnancies* (6th ed.), pp. 388–414. Philadelphia, PA: Elsevier/Saunders.

Lavender, T., Hart, A. & Smyth, R. M. (2013). Effect of partogram use on outcomes for women in spontaneous labour at term. *Cochrane Database Systematic Review, 10*(7), CD005461.

Le Ray, C., Fraser, W., Rozenberg, P., et al. (2011). Duration of passive and active phases of the second stage of labour and risk of severe postpartum haemorrhage in low-risk nulliparous women. *European Journal of Obstetrics, Gynecology & Reproductive Biology, 15*(2), 167–172.

McKenna, L. & Mirkov, S. (2014). *McKenna's Drug Handbook for Nursing & Midwifery* (7th ed.). Sydney: Lippincott Williams & Wilkins.

Madhudar, C., Ghori, A., Khurshid, F., Ali Shah, S. Z. & Devrajani, T. (2013). Uterine rupture. *Professional Medical Journal, 20*(5), 726–730.

Mehta, S. H. & Sokol, R. J. (2014). Should dystocia: Risk factors, predictability, and preventability. *Semin Perinatol, 38*(4), 189–193.

Melamed, N., Gavish, O., Eisner, M., et al. (2013). Third- and fourth degree perineal tears—Incidence and risk factors. *Journal of Maternal-Fetal & Neonatal Medicine, 26*(7), 660–664.

Mowat, A. & Gardener, G. (2014). Predictors of successful external cephalic version in an Australian maternity hospital. *Australian and New Zealand Journal of Obstetrics and Gynaecology, 54*(1), 59–63.

Mozurkewich, E. L., Chilimigras, J. L., Berman, D. R., et al. (2011). Methods of induction of labour, a systematic review. *Obstetrics and Gynecology, 24*(2), 266.

Murphy, D. J., Macleod, M., Bahl, R., et al. (2011). A cohort study of maternal and neonatal morbidity in relation to use of sequential instruments at operative vaginal delivery. *European Journal of Obstetrics, Gynecology, and Reproductive Biology, 156*(1), 41–45.

Ouzounian, J. G., Hernandez, G. D., Korst, L. M., et al. (2011). Pre-pregnancy weight and excess weight gain are risk factors for macrosomia in women with gestational diabetes. *Journal of Perinatology, 31*(11), 717–721.

Policiano, C., Costa, A., Valentim-Lourenço, A., Clode, N. & Graça, L. M. (2014). Route of delivery following successful external cephalic version. *International Journal of Gynecology & Obstetrics, 126*(3), 272–274.

Purcell, E. & Bienstock, J. L. (2011). Complications of labor & delivery. In K. J. Hurt, M. W. Guile, J. L. Bienstock, et al. (Eds), *The Johns Hopkins Manual of Gynecology and Obstetrics* (4th ed.), pp. 99–109. Philadelphia, PA: Lippincott Williams & Wilkins.

Reid, E. W., McNeill, J. A., Holmes, V. A. & Alderdice, F. A. (2014). Women's perceptions and experiences of fetal macrosomia. *Midwifery, 30*(4), 456–463.

Robinson, B. K. & Grobman, W. A. (2011). Effectiveness of timing strategies for delivery of individuals with vasa previa. *Obstetrics & Gynecology, 117*(3), 542–549.

Rouse, D. J., Owen, J., Goldenberg, R. L. & Cliver, S. P. (1996). The effectiveness and costs of elective cesarean delivery for fetal macrosomia diagnosed by ultrasound. *JAMA, 276*(18), 1480–1486.

Sahni, G. (2012). Chest pain syndromes in pregnancy. *Cardiology Clinics, 30*(3), 343–367.

Schuller, C., Känel, N., Müller, O., et al. (2012). Stress and pain response of neonates after spontaneous birth and vacuum-assisted and cesarean delivery. *American Journal of Obstetrics & Gynecology, 207*(5), 416.e1–416.e6.

Silver, D. W. & Sabatino, F. (2012). Precipitous and difficult deliveries. *Emergency Medical Clinics of North America, 30*(4), 961–975.

Silver, R. M. (2014). Umbilical cord prolapse—progress! *BJOG: An International Journal of Obstetrics & Gynaecology, 121*(13), 1709.

Simkin, P. (2010). The fetal occiput posterior position, state of the science and a new perspective. *Birth, 3*(1), 61–71.

Smith, D., Stringer, E., Vladutiu, C. J., Zink, A. H. & Strauss, R. (2015). Risk of uterine rupture among women attempting vaginal birth after caesarean with an unknown uterine scar, accessed 8 April 2015, <www.ajog.org/article/S0002-9378(15)00112-X/abstract>.

Stevens, J. R. & Wittich, A. C. (2011). A rare case of occult uterine inversion at an army community hospital, a case report. *Military Medicine, 176*(12), 1450–1452.

Taher, S. E., Inder, J. W., Soltan, S. A., et al. (2011). Prostaglandin E2 vaginal gel or tablets for the induction of labour at term, a randomised controlled trial. *International Journal of Obstetrics and Gynecology, 118*(6), 719–725.

Tapisiz, O. L., Aytan, H., Kiykac Altinbas, S., Arman, F., Tuncay, G., Besli, M. & Danışman, N. (2014). Face presentation at term: A forgotten issue. *Journal of Obstetrics and Gynaecology Research, 40*(6), 1573–1577.

Tiitinen, A. (2012). Prevention of multiple pregnancies in infertility treatment. *Best Practice & Research: Clinical Obstetrics & Gynaecology, 26*(6), 829–840.

Tul, N., Verdenik, I., Trojner-Bregar, A., et al. (2012). Correlates of the trend of cesarean section rates in twin pregnancies. *Journal of Perinatal Medicine, 40*(3), 241–243.

Vendittelli, F., Rivière, O. & Bréart, G. (2012). Is prenatal identification of fetal macrosomia useful? *European Journal of Obstetrics & Gynecology and Reproductive Biology, 161*(2), 170–176.

Walker, S. (2014). To ECV or not to ECV? The current evidence base concerning external cephalic version. *The Practising Midwife, 17*(9), 30–33.

Werner, E. F., Janevic, T. M., Illuzzi, J., et al. (2011). Mode of delivery in nulliparous women and neonatal intracranial injury. *Obstetrics and Gynecology, 118*(6), 1239–1246.

Whitburn, L. Y., Jones, L. E., Davey, M. A. & Small, R. (2014). Women's experiences of labour pain and the role of the mind: An exploratory study. *Midwifery, 30*(9), 1029–1035.

Zeb, L. & Bibi, S. (2013). Trends in frequency and causes of uterine rupture in a tertiary care center between year 2001 and 2011. *JPMI: Journal of Postgraduate Medical Institute, 27*(3), 317–321.

Zheng, T. (2012). Labor & delivery. In T. Zheng, *Comprehensive Handbook of Obstetrics and Gynecology* (2nd ed.), pp. 16–58. Phoenix, AZ: Phoenix Medical Press.

Zhuang, Z., Goel, S. & Carter, J. E. (2011). Association of cervical cytology and HPV DNA status during pregnancy with placental abnormalities and preterm birth. *American Journal of Clinical Pathology, 136*(2), 260–265.

Suggested readings

Ampt, A. J., Ford, J. B., Roberts, C. L. & Morris, J. M. (2013). Trends in obstetric anal sphincter injuries and associated risk factors for vaginal singleton term births in New South Wales 2001-2009. *Australian & New Zealand Journal of Obstetrics & Gynaecology, 53*(1), 9–16.

Barger, M. K., Nannini, A., DeJoy, S., Wisner, K. & Markenson, G. (2013). Maternal and newborn outcomes following uterine rupture among women without versus those with a prior cesarean. *Journal of Maternal-Fetal & Neonatal Medicine, 26*(2), 183–187.

Fong, A., Wu, E., Pan, D., Chung, J. H. & Ogunyemi, D. A. (2014). Temporal trends and morbidities of vacuum, forceps, and combined use of both. *Journal of Maternal-Fetal & Neonatal Medicine, 27*(18), 1886–1891.

Ito, F., Akasaka, J., Koike, N., Uekuri, C., Shigemitsu, A. & Kobayashi, H. (2014). Incidence, diagnosis and pathophysiology of amniotic fluid embolism. *Journal of Obstetrics & Gynaecology, 34*(7), 580–584.

Jackson, R. (2013). Can midwives promote normality in an occipito-posterior labour through autonomous practice? *Practising Midwife, 16*(11), 14–16.

Neal, J. L., Lowe, N. K., Patrick, T. E., Cabbage, L. A. & Corwin, E. J. (2010). What is the slowest-yet-normal cervical dilation rate among nulliparous women with spontaneous labor onset? *JOGNN: Journal of Obstetric, Gynecologic & Neonatal Nursing, 39*(4), 361–369.

Shallow, H. (2013). Deviant mothers and midwives: Supporting VBAC with women as real partners in decision making. *Essentially MIDIRS, 4*(1), 17–21.

Stock, S. J., Ferguson, E., Duffy, A., Ford, I., Chalmers, J. & Norman, J. E. (2013). Outcomes of induction of labour in women with previous caesarean delivery: A retrospective cohort study using a population database. *PLoS ONE, 8*(4), 1–7.

Chapter 24

Care of a family during caesarean birth

Previous chapters described the physiology of labour and the sequence of usual birth. This chapter adds information about caesarean birth for those women who choose to have a caesarean birth or must have a caesarean birth to ensure a safe outcome for themselves or their child.

LEARNING OBJECTIVES

After mastering the contents of this chapter, you should be able to:

1. Describe the usual indications for caesarean birth.
2. Use critical thinking to analyse how to keep the birth family-centred when a caesarean birth is scheduled.
3. Assess a woman scheduled for caesarean birth for effective preoperative, intraoperative and postoperative needs.
4. Formulate diagnoses related to the family experiencing a caesarean birth.
5. Establish outcomes that meet the needs of a woman requiring a caesarean birth.
6. Plan appropriate care for the family experiencing a caesarean birth.
7. Implement common preoperative and postoperative care measures for caesarean birth.
8. Evaluate expected outcomes for achievement and effectiveness of care.
9. Identify areas related to caesarean birth that could benefit from additional research or application of evidence-based practice.
10. Integrate knowledge of caesarean birth to achieve quality child and family health nursing care.

KEY TERMS

- caesarean birth
- classic caesarean incision
- low segment incision

CASE STUDY

Katrina Hamma is a 29-year-old woman pregnant with her first baby. Her labour began with ruptured membranes and dark green meconium-stained amniotic fluid. Katrina called her midwife, who asked her to come to the hospital immediately. Katrina drove herself and arrived in 20 minutes. The fetal heart rate was 100 beats per minute. An obstetrician was consulted, and she scheduled Katrina for an immediate caesarean birth. Katrina reacted calmly to the news that she needed surgery until she realised her boyfriend would not be able to get to the hospital until her surgery was over. At that point she refused to sign for permission, saying, "I can't. I just can't go through this alone."

CASE STUDY QUESTIONS

1. Is Katrina's response typical of a woman who is told she needs a surgical procedure for the birth of her baby?
2. What would be your best action to help her accept this procedure?

Caesarean birth, or birth accomplished through an abdominal incision into the uterus, is one of the oldest types of surgical procedures known. It is always slightly more hazardous than vaginal birth, but compared with other surgical procedures, it is one of the safest types of surgery and has few complications (Speichinger & Holschneider, 2013). The word "caesarean" is derived from the Latin word *caedore,* which means "to cut". At one time, there was a popular belief that Julius Caesar was born by a caesarean birth and the procedure was named after him. However, because Caesar was born before antibiotics and sterile surgical technique, it seems unlikely that his mother (who is known to have been alive in his adult years) would have survived such a procedure. The term *caesarean birth,* rather than *caesarean delivery,* is used to accentuate that this is a birth more than a surgical procedure.

A WOMAN HAVING A CAESAREAN BIRTH

The same important outcomes apply to a woman giving birth by caesarean as a woman giving birth vaginally: a healthy mother and a healthy child. Because caesarean birth decisions can be made suddenly, planning can be limited to only a few minutes. This means you have only a very short time to organise pre-surgical steps such as gastrointestinal or anaesthesia preparation (and run through the pre-surgical checklist when it is an emergency). Plans must include discharge instructions and home care, because a woman will remain in the healthcare facility only 2 or 3 days.

Every woman is aware that childbirth poses some risk to her health. When major surgery is superimposed on top of this, it is imperative that a woman and her support person feel confidence in the healthcare personnel who will care for them. Otherwise, they could have difficulty coping with the additional insult of surgery. When giving care to any woman during labour, be certain to establish a supportive relationship with both the woman and her support person early on. These relationships become especially advantageous should the birth method need to be altered.

An important intervention includes coordination of healthcare team members such as an anaesthetist, surgeon, paediatrician or neonatologist, and recovery room or nursery personnel. This is particularly important if the surgery will be performed in a hospital surgical department rather than in a labour and birthing suite, or if the infant will be transferred to an intensive care nursery or a distant site for intensive care after the birth.

Many interventions focus on teaching and support, because the more a woman understands about what is happening, the more she can accept and cooperate with procedures. During surgery, sterile technique is essential. A postpartum infection can be devastating to a woman who has already made many other physical adaptations. After surgery, be sure to provide adequate "talk time" to allow a woman time to review what has happened and integrate it into what she and her partner expected.

CAESAREAN BIRTH

In Australia there has been concern with rising caesarean section (CS) rates which have increased from 21.8% in 1999 to 31.6% in 2010 (Li et al., 2012; Gardner et al., 2014). The rates of CS have continued to rise throughout the developed world despite the fact that evidence indicates CS rates >15% do not improve outcomes. In the United States in 2011, 32.8% of women had a CS, which equates to around 1.3 million women annually (Shorten, Shorten & Kennedy, 2014). Mexico has reported one of the highest CS rates in the world at 43.9% and the Netherlands has the lowest at 13.9% (Niino, 2011). Women with private insurance, private obstetrician care and who are from a higher socioeconomic background have an increased rate of CS (Niino, 2011).

The global increase in CS results from a combination of factors including the use of electronic fetal monitoring, epidural anaesthesia, increased number of inductions, obesity (Mantakas & Farrell, 2010), fear of professional negligence litigation, repeat CS, doctor convenience and prevention of potential urinary or anal incontinence later in life (Gyhagen et al., 2012; Lavender et al., 2012). The Term Breech Trial in 2000 indicated CS was safer than a vaginal breech birth and this almost instantaneously changed international practice as CS became the preferred method of birth for breech presentation (Borbolla Foster et al., 2014). A trial in Australia found women who elected a planned vaginal breech birth had a 58% success rate with low mortality rates (Borbolla Foster et al., 2014). There has been an increased perception that more women are requesting elective CS and this may be because many women believe a CS is safer for their baby and are unaware of the risks a CS presents to them (Thompson, 2010).

As a rule, midwifery birthing services have a lower incidence of caesarean births than hospital services because of the higher incidence of low-risk women in these settings (Liva et al., 2012). Continuous support during labour also appears to decrease the incidence of CS (Hodnett et al., 2012).

A CS entails major surgery that increases morbidity for women and has implications for future pregnancies. The risks of CS include maternal death, emergency hysterectomy, haemorrhage, stroke, blood clots, bowel obstruction, injuries from surgery, infection, antibiotic resistance, pelvic pain, poor bonding, depression and psychological trauma (Niino, 2011). For the neonate, risks include an increase in preterm infants and increased neonatal respiratory morbidity (Dickinson, 2014). Other serious long-term iatrogenic complications include caesarean scar, ectopic pregnancy, placenta praevia and placenta accreta (Dickinson, 2014). It is significant that new research indicates placenta accreta and its variants are frequently associated with implantation on a uterine scar (Timor-Tritsch et al., 2014).

Scheduled caesarean birth

Currently, caesarean birth is used most often as a prophylactic measure, to alleviate problems such as cephalopelvic disproportion or failure to progress in labour. There are two types of caesarean birth: scheduled and emergency. In the first instance, there is time for thorough preparation for the experience throughout the antepartal period. With emergency caesarean birth, preparation must be done much more rapidly but with the same concern for fully informing a woman and her support person about what circumstances created the need for a caesarean birth and how the birth will proceed. Caesarean birth is mentioned in most childbirth classes, so any woman who has taken such a class may at least understand that caesarean births are sometimes necessary.

Although many caesarean births are done because the woman had a past caesarean birth, with new surgical techniques, particularly the use of a low cervical incision, "once a caesarean, always a caesarean" no longer applies. Most women who have had a caesarean birth within the past 10 years are eligible to give birth vaginally in subsequent pregnancies if the circumstances are otherwise appropriate for vaginal birth (Eden et al., 2012). In Australia, the women who elected to have a vaginal birth after a previous caesarean birth (VBAC) increased from 17.2% (2006) to 27.0% in (2010) with a success rate of 64.4% in a metropolitan hospital providing a next birth after caesarean clinic (Gardner et al., 2014). For more information on VBAC, see Chapter 15.

Caesarean birth is mandatory when there is a physical indication such as a transverse presentation, active genital herpes or cephalopelvic disproportion. Caesarean birth may reduce the transfer of the human immunodeficiency

BOX 24.1 ✻ Selected indications for caesarean birth

Maternal factors
Active genital herpes or perhaps human papillomavirus
AIDS or HIV-positive status
Cephalopelvic disproportion
Cervical cerclage
Disabling conditions, such as severe hypertension of pregnancy, that prevent pushing to accomplish the pelvic division of labour
Failed induction or failure to progress in labour
Obstructive benign or malignant tumour
Previous caesarean birth by classic incision
Elective—no indicated risks

Placenta factors
Placenta praevia
Premature separation of the placenta
Umbilical cord prolapse

Fetal factors
Compound conditions such as macrosomic fetus in a breech lie
Extreme low birth weight
Fetal distress
Major fetal anomalies, such as hydrocephalus
Multigestation or conjoined twins
Transverse fetal lie

virus (HIV), hepatitis C or herpes type 2 from mother to newborn, so it is recommended for women who have these infections (Tita, 2012). It may be advantageous for a preterm birth to avoid pressure on the fetal head (Zeitlin et al., 2010). It is generally contraindicated when there is a documented fetus demise (labour can be induced to avoid a surgical procedure).

Emergency caesarean birth

Emergency caesarean births are done for reasons such as placenta praevia, premature separation of the placenta, fetal distress or failure to progress in labour (see Box 24.1). An emergency caesarean birth carries with it the risk of any emergency surgery: the woman may not be a prime candidate for anaesthesia and is psychologically unprepared for the experience. In addition, the woman may have a fluid and electrolyte imbalance and be both physically and emotionally exhausted from a long labour.

EFFECTS OF SURGERY ON A WOMAN

Like any surgical procedure, caesarean birth has systemic effects.

Stress response

Whenever the body is subjected to stress, either physical or psychosocial, it responds with measures to preserve the function of major body systems. This results in release of adrenaline and noradrenaline from the adrenal medulla. Adrenaline causes an increased heart rate, bronchial dilation and elevation of the blood glucose level. It also leads to peripheral vasoconstriction, which forces blood to the central circulation and increases blood pressure. These normally positive responses (the person is tensed or ready for action with good heart and lung function and glucose for energy) may antagonise anaesthetic action, which is aimed at minimising body activity. In the pregnant woman, such responses may minimise blood supply to the lower extremities. The woman is already prone to thrombophlebitis from stasis of blood flow, so these responses compound or greatly increase the risk of thrombophlebitis. Combined with interferences to major body systems, these effects can add to the risks of surgery.

Interference with body defences

The skin serves as the primary line of defence against bacterial invasion. When skin is incised for a surgical procedure, this important line of defence is lost. Strict adherence to aseptic technique during surgery, and in the days following the procedure, is necessary to compensate for this impaired defence. If caesarean birth is performed hours after the membranes ruptured, a woman's risk of infection will be higher than if the membranes were intact. Many women receive prophylactic antibiotics, such as ampicillin or a cephalosporin to ensure protection against postsurgical endometritis, even if the membranes were intact (Alfirevic, Gyte & Dou, 2010).

Interference with circulatory function

Although vessels that must be cut for surgery are immediately clamped and ligated, some blood loss always occurs with surgery. Extensive blood loss can lead to hypovolaemia and lowered blood pressure. This could lead to ineffective perfusion of all body tissues if the problem is not quickly recognised and corrected. The amount of blood lost in caesarean birth is comparatively high, because pelvic vessels are congested with blood waiting to supply the placenta. During a vaginal birth, a woman loses 300 to 500 mL of blood. This loss increases to 500 to 1000 mL with a caesarean birth (Arulkumaran, 2012).

Interference with body organ function

When any body organ is handled, cut or repaired in surgery, it may respond with a temporary disruption in function. Pressure from oedema or inflammation as fluid moves into the injured area further impairs function of the primary organ involved, as well as that of surrounding organs. If blood vessels become compressed as a result of oedema, distant organs may be deprived of blood flow, leading to reduced function in those organs. Postoperatively, close assessment, not only of the primary organ involved but of total body function, is necessary, therefore, to determine the total degree of disruption.

Because the uterus is handled during caesarean birth, it may not contract well afterwards, which can lead to postpartum haemorrhage. For a surgeon to reach the uterus, the bladder must be displaced anteriorly. As a result of this handling, the bladder may not sense filling as well as usual after the procedure (Gungorduk et al., 2010). During surgery, pressure is also felt by the intestine, so a paralytic ileus or halting of intestinal function may occur (Harma et al., 2011). Thrombopheblitis from impaired lower extremity blood flow is yet another possibility. After a caesarean birth, therefore, uterine, bladder, intestinal and lower extremity circulatory function must all be carefully assessed.

Interference with self-image or self-esteem

Surgery always leaves an incisional scar that will be noticeable to some extent afterwards. Fortunately, the scar resulting from caesarean birth (a horizontal one across the lower abdomen) is not overly noticeable, but its appearance may cause a woman to feel self-conscious. Although most women accept caesarean birth well, a woman may feel a loss of self-esteem if she believes it marks her as a woman less than others because she was unable to have a vaginal birth (Barbadoro et al., 2012).

CASE STUDY QUESTION

3. Katrina is concerned she may lose an excessive amount of blood with caesarean surgery. What is the usual amount of blood lost with caesarean birth?

   a. 100–220 mL
   b. 250–350 mL
   c. 300–500 mL
   d. 500–1000 mL

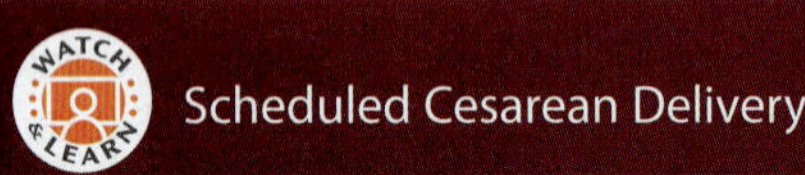

Scheduled Cesarean Delivery

CARE OF A WOMAN ANTICIPATING A CAESAREAN BIRTH

A woman who is admitted to the hospital for an anticipated caesarean birth may be more worried about the procedure, because she has had more time to worry, than a woman who is told during labour that an emergency caesarean is necessary. After the woman is admitted to the healthcare facility, allow her time to talk about any fears she has. Encourage her to do as much as possible for herself preoperatively, to help her feel in control and diminish her fear (Wang et al., 2010).

A woman undergoing surgery cannot begin to relax as long as her support person is nervous and worried. Make a point of including this person in all explanations and admission routines, to keep his or her anxiety under control as well.

Preoperative interview

Both the surgeon and the anaesthetist will interview a woman preoperatively to obtain a health history and make an assessment and decision for safe use of anaesthesia. Be sure to ask about any past surgeries, secondary illnesses, allergies to foods or medications, reactions to anaesthesia, bleeding problems and current medications to help establish surgical risk. Also ask if a woman has any piercing that needs to be removed because of the use of the bovie or arterial cauterising machine. In addition, include questions to discover:

- The woman's knowledge about the procedure
- The length of hospitalisation anticipated
- If she knows about any postsurgical equipment to be used, such as an indwelling catheter or intravenous fluid line
- Any special precautions that will be necessary for her infant.

Operative risk for a woman

For any surgery to be performed safely, a woman must be in the best possible physical and psychological state. Women who are in less than optimal physical or psychological health are at risk of a complicated surgical outcome unless the risk factor is identified and special precautions are taken.

Altered general health

A woman who has a secondary illness such as cardiac disease, diabetes mellitus, anaemia, or kidney or liver disease is at greater than usual surgical risk, depending on the extent of disease, because the pathology from the secondary illness may interfere with her ability to adjust physically to the demands of surgery. A woman with a secondary illness may also have an accompanying nutritional or electrolyte imbalance caused by her primary illness. Therefore, asking about any secondary illnesses is an essential component of a preoperative history.

A general medication history is also important, because some medications increase surgical risk by interfering with the effect of an anaesthetic or with healing of tissue. Examples of medications that pregnant women might be taking and their potential complications are shown in Table 24.1.

Fear

Women who are extremely worried need a very detailed explanation of the procedure before they can enter surgery without intense fear. Most caesarean births are currently performed under epidural anaesthesia, so they are less frightening for women than when general anaesthesia is used.

Operative risk to the newborn

Caesarean birth places a newborn at a greater risk than does a vaginal birth for a number of reasons. When a fetus

TABLE 24.1 Medications that may result in complications of surgery

Type of drug	Action
Antibiotics	Specific antibiotics may predispose to renal insufficiency or increase neuromuscular blockage; can lead to opportunistic infections
Anticoagulants	May cause haemorrhage due to lack of haemostasis during surgery
Anticonvulsants	May increase liver action and metabolism of anaesthetic agent
Antihypertensives	May result in hypotension after anaesthesia
Corticosteroids	May block body's response to shock and lead to lack of adrenal function
Insulin	May lead to hypoglycaemia during labour or hyperglycaemia if a dextrose solution is administered
Antianxiety agents	May cause hypotension after anaesthesia

is pushed through the birth canal, pressure on the chest helps to rid the newborn's lungs of fluid. This makes respirations more likely to be adequate at birth than if a fetus had not been subjected to this pressure. For this reason, more infants born by caesarean birth develop some degree of respiratory difficulty for a day or two after birth than those born vaginally (Abenhaim & Benjamin, 2011; Patel & Jain, 2010). See Chapter 26 for a discussion of this condition, which is often referred to as transient tachypnoea of the newborn.

Preoperative diagnostic procedures

Preoperative diagnostic procedures for a woman who is to have a caesarean birth include assessments of circulatory and renal function and fetal heart rate including:

- Vital sign determination
- Urinalysis
- Complete blood count
- Coagulation profile (prothrombin time [PT], partial thromboplastin time [PTT])
- Serum electrolytes and pH
- Blood typing and cross-matching
- Ultrasound to determine fetal presentation and maturity.

During pregnancy, a woman, and particularly one who was in prolonged labour, may have an elevated leucocyte count (up to 20,000/mm^3), so this finding is not as helpful an indicator for the presence of infection in the pregnant woman as it is in others.

Preoperative teaching

Fear of the unknown is one of the hardest fears to conquer. Preoperative teaching is aimed at acquainting a woman with caesarean procedure and any special equipment to be used, to make her as informed as possible. Explain the preoperative measures that will be necessary, such as surgical skin preparation, fasting prior to surgery, premedication and method of transport to surgery. Review the necessity for an indwelling catheter, intravenous fluid administration, placement of an epidural catheter, and the advantage of early ambulation afterwards.

Teaching to prevent complications

Women who practise exercises to maintain good respiratory and circulatory function postoperatively will tend to experience fewer postoperative respiratory and circulatory complications than those who do not. These preventive exercises are best taught during the preoperative period, when the woman is free of pain and can concentrate on learning. Such teaching also gives a woman a positive outlook about surgery and a sense of control over her situation.

Deep breathing

Periodic deep breathing exercises fully aerate the lungs and help to prevent the stasis of lung mucus from the prolonged time spent in the supine position during surgery. Because stasis always has the potential to cause infection, preventing this helps prevent lung infections such as pneumonia. A typical exercise is to take 5 to 10 deep breaths every hour. Teach a woman to do this simply by inhaling as deeply as possible, holding her breath for a second or two, and then exhaling as deeply as possible. Be certain she inhales and exhales fully. Otherwise, she might experience light-headedness from hyperventilation.

Incentive spirometry

A common device used postoperatively to encourage deep breathing is an incentive spirometer. These devices which cause a small ping-pong-like ball to rise in a narrow tube or cause lights to flash, are not only easy and fun to operate but give a woman a sense of reward for her effort. The initial impression is that the device works by blowing into it. Because its purpose is to fully aerate lung spaces, though, most models are triggered by *inhalation*, not exhalation.

Ambulation

The most effective way to stimulate lower-extremity circulation after a caesarean birth is by early ambulation. For this reason, most surgeons prefer a woman to be out of bed and walking within hours after surgery (as soon as the effect of the epidural anaesthesia has worn off). Helping a woman ambulate this early can be difficult, because she is both fatigued and in pain. Help her to understand that ambulation is extremely important after caesarean birth,

Patient concerns		Completed
Skin preparation		______
Identification in place		______
Temperature, pulse, respiration	______	______
Blood pressure	______	______
Height ______	Weight ______	______
Voided ______ Time ______	Amount ______	______
NPO after	______	______
Hospital gown		______
Hairpins removed		______
Nail polish removed		______
Jewellery removed		______
Preoperative medication	______	______
Dentures removed ______	In place ______	______
Contact lenses removed	______	______
Prosthetic devices removed	______	______
Abdominal piercing removed	______	______
Chart concerns		
Addressograph plate attached		______
Operative permit obtained		______
Urinalysis		______
Haematocrit or CBC		______
Blood order of	______	______
	Signature ______	R.N.

FIGURE 24.1 Preoperative checklist for caesarean birth. Checklists vary from hospital to hospital.

because the oedema of the low pelvic surgery compresses circulation to the lower extremities, increasing the risk for lower-extremity circulatory stasis. Antiembolic stockings (TEDS) are used to support and encourage venous return in addition to ambulation.

Immediate preoperative care measures

A number of measures must be taken immediately before surgery to ensure a safe outcome (see Fig. 24.1). Informed consent is required and women will need to go through the normal preoperative preparation. The surgical checklist must be completed prior to transfer to surgery. Prior to a caesarean birth women require an oral antacid such as sodium citrate which neutralises acid stomach secretions. This precaution is necessary to minimise damage if oesophageal reflux or aspiration occur.

To reduce bladder size and keep the bladder away from the surgical field, an indwelling urinary catheter may be prescribed before transport for surgery or after arrival in the surgical suite. After catheter insertion, be certain that urine is draining freely, because fetal pressure on the urethra may reduce the flow of urine considerably. During transport, keep the drainage bag below the level of the woman's bladder, to prevent urine backflow and the possible introduction of microorganisms into the bladder.

If catheterisation is difficult before surgery, do not traumatise the urethra by repeated attempts. Catheterisation can be done in the birthing room after the anaesthetic agent is given. If there is a delay between the catheter insertion time and surgery, mark the drainage bag just before surgery with the amount in the bag, or empty it, so that pre-surgery urine output can be differentiated from post-surgery urine output. One of the gravest dangers of any surgical procedure is kidney failure from the physiological stress of surgery or lack of blood flow to the kidneys due to decreased blood pressure. All reproductive tract surgery puts ureter flow as well as kidney function at risk, because oedema that collects in the surgery area can press on the ureters.

Most women have an intravenous fluid line begun before surgery with a fluid such as lactated Hartman's solution. Doing so helps to ensure that a woman is fully hydrated and will not experience hypotension from epidural anaesthesia administration, temporary use of a supine position, or blood loss at birth. Be certain that this line is started in the woman's non-dominant hand, so that she can hold her newborn after surgery without interference (see Fig. 24.2). Use a large-size catheter (18 or 20 gauge), so that blood replacement therapy can be administered, if needed, by the same line.

Role of the support person

In most instances, a woman's family can be as involved in a caesarean birth as they would be in a vaginal birth. A support person may need more encouragement to watch a caesarean birth because they may believe it will be much bloodier than it actually is.

✔ *Checkpoint question 24.1*

How can you reduce the size of the bladder and keep it away from the surgical field during a caesarean birth?

a. Restrict fluids in the woman for 4 hours before surgery
b. Insert a urinary catheter to drain the bladder and decrease its size
c. Administer an oxytocic to contract the bladder
d. Give a diuretic to reduce the bladder to its smallest size

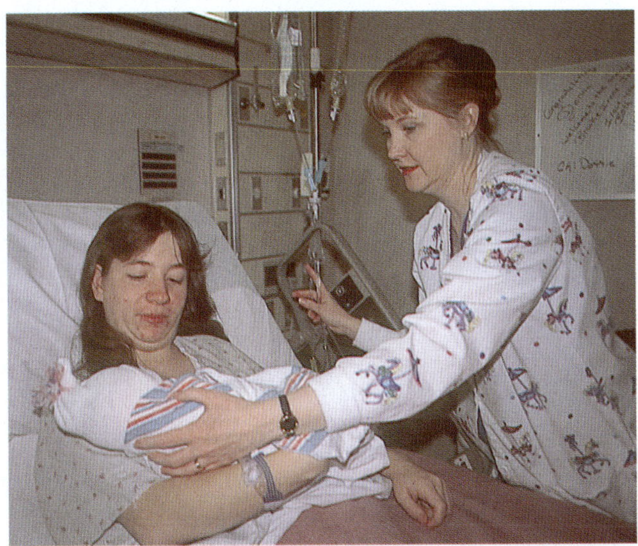

FIGURE 24.2 Assisting with holding the newborn and positioning the equipment so that the intravenous line does not interfere with mother–child interactions. (© Caroline Brown, RNC, MS, DEd.)

CARE OF A WOMAN HAVING AN EMERGENCY CAESAREAN BIRTH

Many women who will have a caesarean birth have no warning during pregnancy that this will be necessary. Suddenly, during labour, they develop a complication such as prolapsed cord or fetal distress, and it becomes necessary. A woman who was having severe pain with labour and is told an emergency procedure is necessary actually may be relieved that surgery has been suggested, because the surgery will alleviate the pain. In contrast, another woman might feel great disappointment when told her baby must be born by caesarean birth. In many women, both emotions are present.

Surgical risk in an emergency situation is determined from the baseline history and physical examination information previously obtained at the beginning of labour. Preoperative preparation measures such as vital signs, urinalysis and blood tests have also been obtained. Immediate preparation concerns such as informed consent, application of elastic stockings (if appropriate), gastrointestinal tract preparation, bladder catheterisation and establishment of an intravenous line will be the same. Because most caesarean births are completed within 30 minutes of the time one is documented to be necessary, teaching about postoperative measures needs to be delayed until after surgery (Lipman et al., 2013).

Available time must be spent explaining the immediate procedures to the woman such as transfer, abdominal preparation and anaesthesia. Document carefully what was discussed, so that the nurse caring for the woman postoperatively will be aware of the need for additional teaching. At birth, at least one person whose sole responsibility is neonatal resuscitation should be present to care for the baby. Approximately 10% of babies born by caesarean birth need assistance to begin breathing at birth; about 1% of babies need extensive resuscitation to survive (Gilbert, 2011).

Most women appreciate that caesarean births are done to prevent their infant from being harmed. Others interpret a caesarean birth as being done because the harm has already occurred. Some women interpret a caesarean birth as an indication they are somehow not as competent as other women. Still others are relieved that labour is being interrupted. Be certain to ask enough questions so that you can learn the importance or meaning of the event to an individual woman.

INTRAOPERATIVE CARE MEASURES

Caesarean birth is most similar to vaginal birth if the woman is awake during the surgery; therefore, after discussion with a woman, the anaesthesia of choice is usually a regional block.

Administration of anaesthesia

A surgical nurse will assist a woman to move from the transport stretcher or bed to the operating room table and will remain with her while anaesthesia is administered. If the woman has an epidural catheter in place from labour, be careful not to dislodge it while she is being moved. During transport or in surgery, encourage the woman to remain on her side, or insert a pillow under her right hip to keep her body slightly tilted to the side, to prevent supine hypotension syndrome. Spinal or epidural anaesthetic will be administered by the anaesthetist who will want the woman sitting up or lying on her side.

Surgical incision

After anaesthetic administration, a woman is positioned with a towel under her right hip to move abdominal contents away from the surgical field and to lift her uterus off the vena cava. A screen may be placed at her shoulder level and covered with a sterile drape to block the flow of bacteria from her respiratory tract to the incision site. This also helps block the woman's and support person's lines of vision, preventing additional anxiety caused by the sight of the incision. Be sure the support person is positioned at the woman's head to provide support.

The incision area and the woman's abdomen are prepped with an antiseptic such as iodine, and draped, leaving only a small area of skin exposed. Watching a caesarean birth is usually the first time a father or support person has ever witnessed surgery. Because of this, the person may be too overwhelmed by and interested in the procedure to be of optimum support. He or she may become concerned about the amount of manipulation and cutting that occurs before the uterus itself is cut (assuming fetal distress is not extreme).

Prepare the woman and support person for the sights they might see, or help talk them through them as they occur (see Fig. 24.3).

Types of caesarean incision

There are two types of caesarean incision (see Fig. 24.4). The type chosen depends on the presentation of the fetus and the speed with which the procedure will be performed.

In a **classic caesarean incision**, the incision is made vertically through both the abdominal skin and the uterus. It is made high on the uterus so that it can be used with a placenta praevia, to avoid cutting the placenta. A disadvantage of this type of incision is that it leaves a wide skin scar and also runs through the active contractile portion of the uterus. Because this type of scar could rupture during labour, it is likely, if this type of incision is used, that

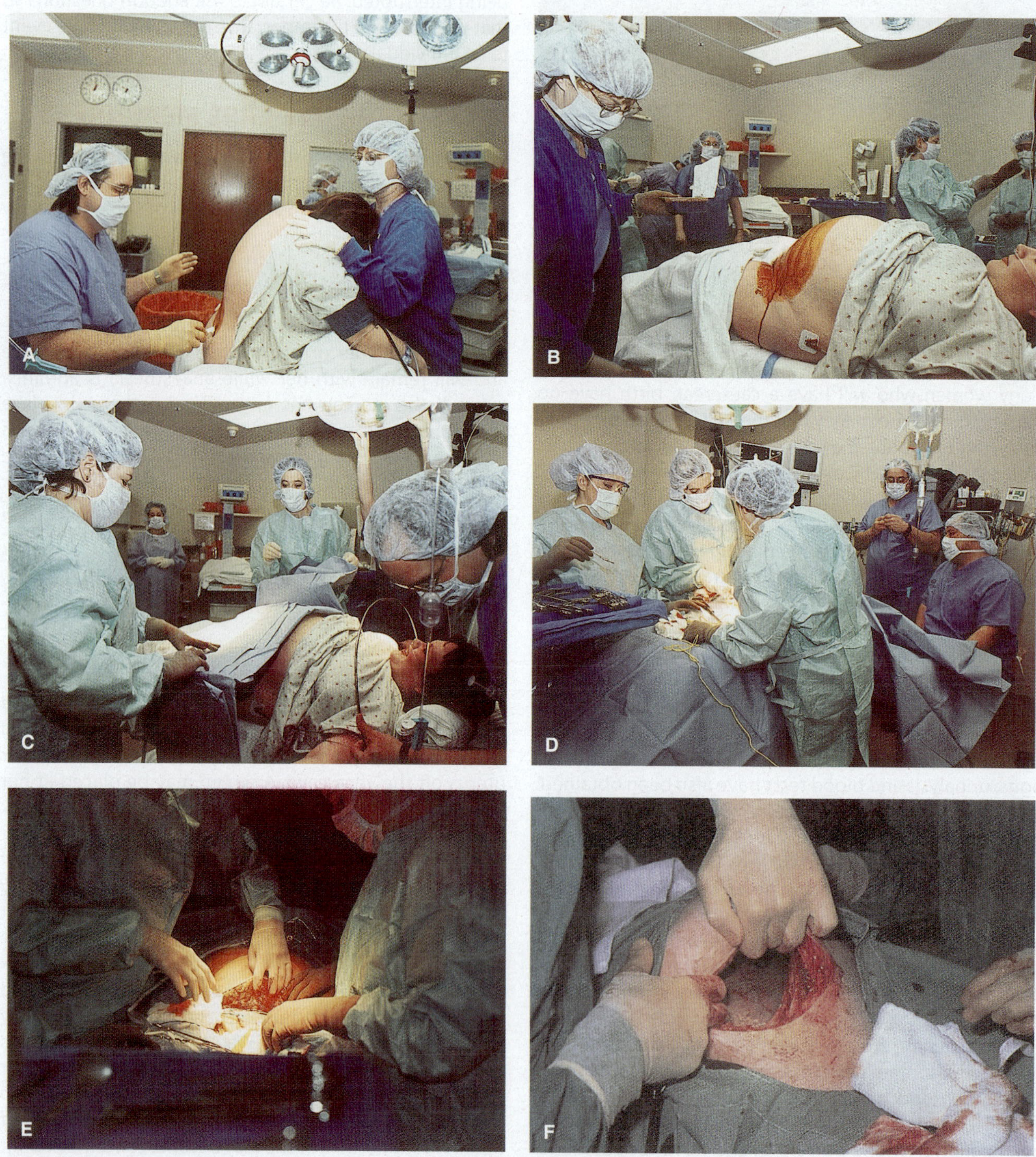

FIGURE 24.3 Caesarean birth. (**A**) Preparation for anaesthesia. (**B**) Abdominal skin preparation. (**C**) Draping of operative site. (**D**) Preparation for initial incision. (**E**) Initial incision. (**F**) Opening of the peritoneum.

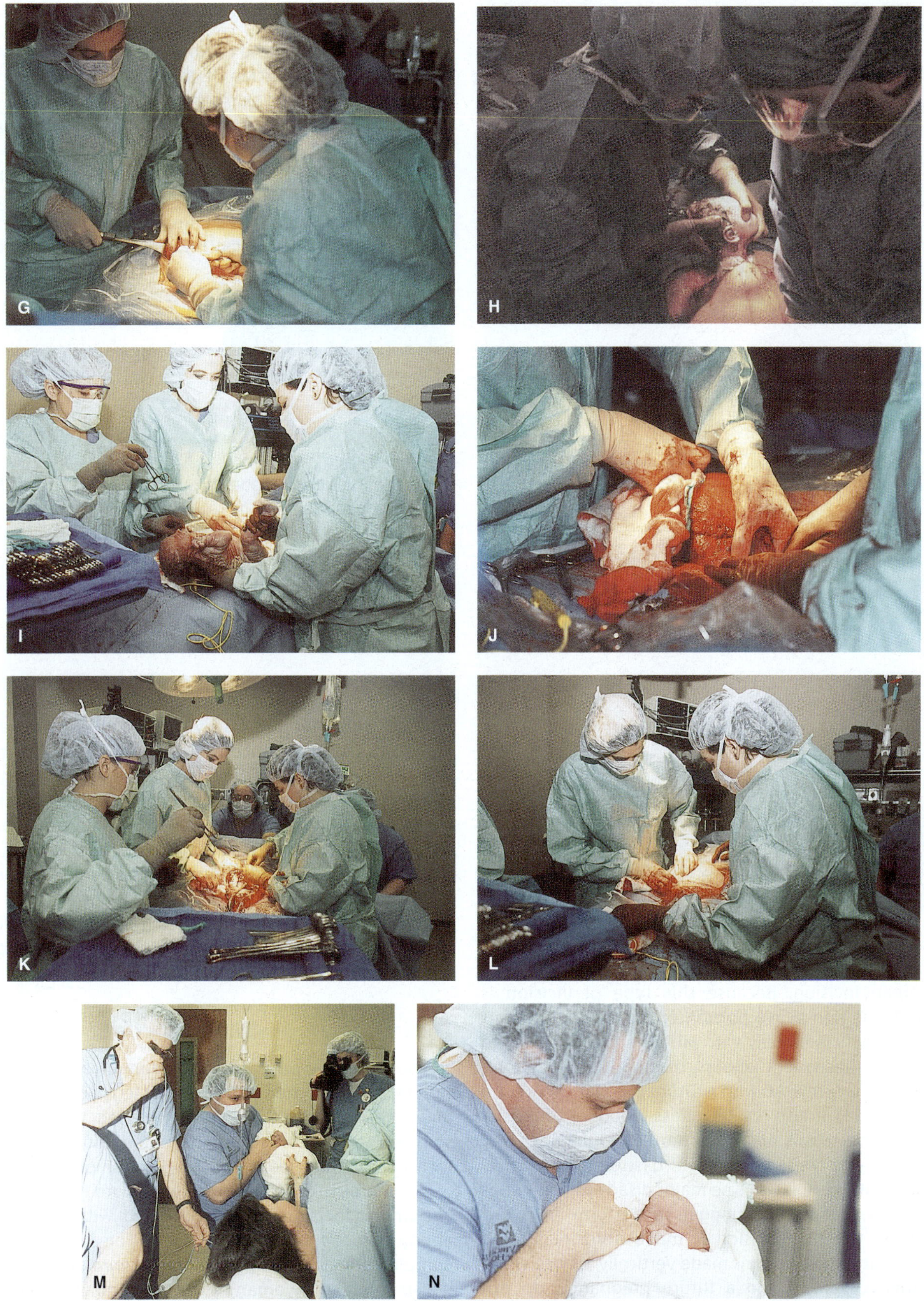

FIGURE 24.3 (*Continued*) (**G**) Retractors in place. (**H**) Birth of head and posterior shoulder. (**I**) Infant born. (**J**) Suturing of uterus complete. (**K**) Suturing of abdominal layers. (**L**) Skin closure. (**M**) Family bonding with mother's first touch. (**N**) Father bonding with newborn. (© Caroline Brown, RNC, MS, DEd.)

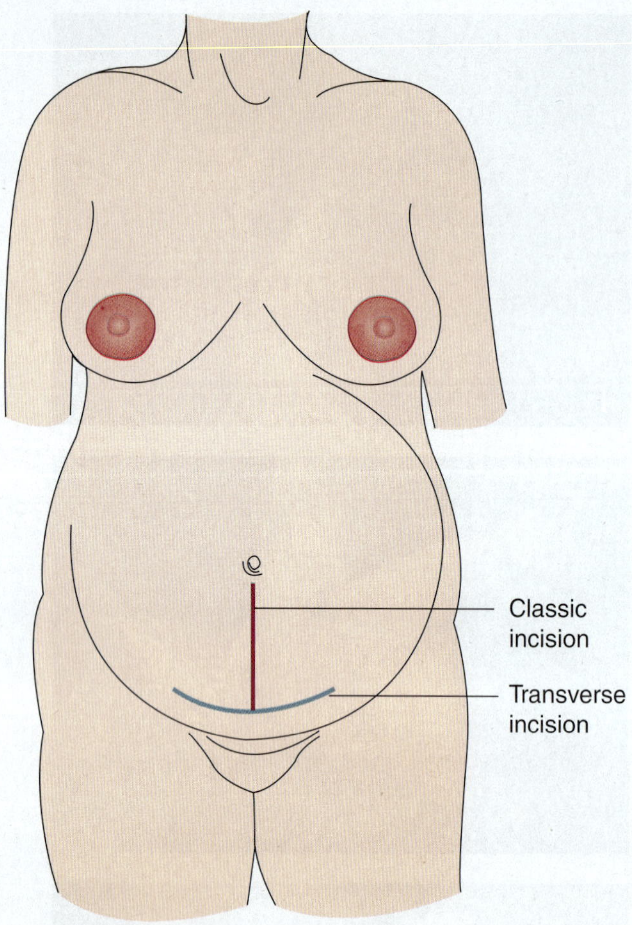

FIGURE 24.4 Types of caesarean incisions.

a woman will not be able to have a subsequent vaginal birth.

A **low segment incision** is also referred to as a low transverse incision, bikini line or Pfannestein incision and is made horizontally across the abdomen just over the symphysis pubis and horizontally across the uterus just over the cervix. This is the most common type of caesarean incision. Because this type of incision is through the non-active portion of the uterus (the part that contracts minimally with labour), it is less likely to rupture in subsequent labours, making it possible for a woman to have a VBAC with a future pregnancy (Aguirre & Chou, 2011). It also results in less blood loss, is easier to suture, decreases postpartum uterine infections and is less likely to cause postpartum gastrointestinal complications (Gilbert, 2011). The major disadvantage of this incision is that it takes longer to perform. In a few instances, the skin incision is made horizontally and then the uterine incision is made vertically, or vice versa. For this reason, during a future pregnancy, do not assume that a woman who has a transverse skin incision also has had a transverse rather than a vertical uterine incision. If the woman wishes to have a tubal ligation, it can be done during the caesarean section.

The newborn

The midwife receives the newborn in a sterile baby blanket from the obstetrician. If the newborn is breathing spontaneously skin-to-skin contact can be facilitated and may assist bonding, breastfeeding outcomes and maternal satisfaction (Stevens et al., 2014). The mother and her support person will need the assistance of staff and preplanning will need to take place. Seeing, touching and holding the newborn is an important foundation for bonding. Breastfeeding can be initiated in the recovery room.

CASE STUDY QUESTION

4. Katrina asks you how big her scar will be after caesarean birth. Your best answer would be:
   a. The incision is big and runs vertically across your abdomen
   b. The incision is made through the vagina so it does not leave a scar
   c. Most caesarean birth incisions are so low they do not show over a bikini
   d. It is so large that it will always show, but think of it as a mark of pride

POSTPARTUM CARE MEASURES

Women who have infants by caesarean birth develop an additional care concern in the immediate postpartum period because they are not only postpartum patients but postsurgical ones as well. Due to the strain of the unexpected procedure, they may have increased difficulty bonding with their new infant. They have postsurgical pain in additional to afterpains. The postpartum phase for a woman who has her child by caesarean birth can be divided into an immediate recovery period (the so-called fourth stage of labour) and an extended postpartum period.

The immediate postpartum period

To avoid blood clots women have pneumatic compression devices attached to their lower legs during surgery and in the immediate postpartum period; the compression device is later replaced with antiembolic stockings. In the past, pain control was a major problem after caesarean birth. Pain was so intense from the uterine or abdominal incision that it interfered with a woman's ability to move and breathe deeply. This led to surgical complications such as pneumonia or thrombophlebitis. It also impaired a woman's ability to bond with her newborn, because holding her infant was so painful. Today, a number of effective types of pain management are available. Use a pain rating scale to allow a woman to rate her pain.

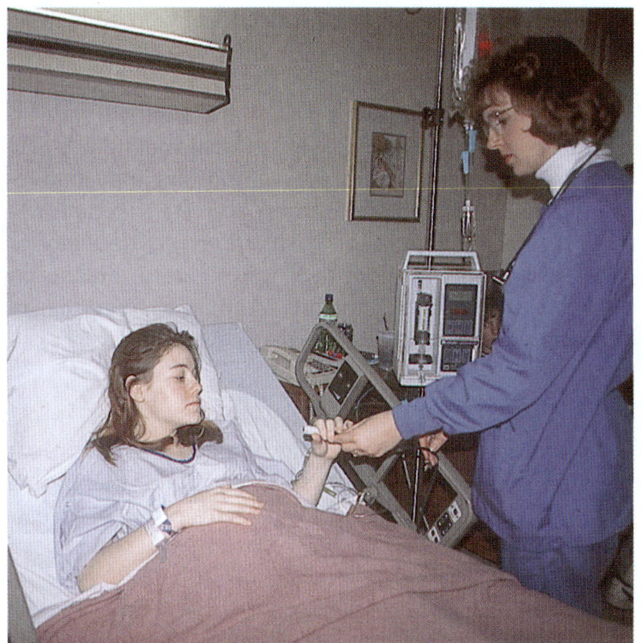

FIGURE 24.5 Patient-controlled analgesia (PCA) pump. By pushing the button, she delivers a bolus of narcotic to herself. (© Caroline Brown, RNC, MS, DEd.)

A woman who is concerned about her infant may experience more pain than a woman who feels confident that her infant is doing well, because anxiety and fear heighten a pain response, and a tense body posture causes pressure on sutures. Be certain a woman understands that her infant has survived the surgical birth well (assuming this is true) or what steps are being taken to make the infant well.

Women who had a long-acting morphine epidural for labour have good pain relief up to 24 hours. Patient-controlled analgesia (PCA) or continued epidural injections give maximum pain relief. No matter what system of pain relief is used, when administering analgesics after surgery, be sure to supplement them with other comfort measures, such as change of position or straightening of bed linen. Always ask a woman what type of pain she is experiencing before administering a new dose of analgesia, to be certain that she is describing incisional or uterine pain and not pain in a leg or some other body part that would suggest a complication of surgery. Check for abdominal distension, which suggests the pain may be caused by intestinal gas rather than incision pain. If so, ambulation is often the most effective method to relieve this type of pain.

Adequate analgesia both in hospital and at home helps women to ambulate, breastfeed and enjoy holding their infant. Be certain she understands not to use acetylsalicylic acid (aspirin), because this can interfere with blood clotting and healing. Many women who are breastfeeding are reluctant to accept any type of analgesic, especially just before breastfeeding, for fear that it will pass in breast milk to the infant. Although it is true that most analgesics do pass in breast milk, the infant takes such a small amount of breast milk (mainly colostrum) during the first days after surgery that the amount of analgesia received would be negligible. Placing a pillow over her lap while she feeds, or using the football hold can deflect the weight of the infant from her suture line and lessen pain.

Patient-controlled analgesia

Patient-controlled analgesia is a method of pain control in which women administer doses of intravenous narcotic analgesia such as morphine to themselves as needed. Although the technique may be used during labour, it is most frequently used to control postsurgical pain. The pump has a "lock-out" setting that prevents a woman from administering a larger dose or doses more frequently than would be safe, such as every 8 minutes. With PCA, a fairly constant level of pain relief can be maintained, and the pain and fear of injections are eliminated. PCA works well with post-caesarean women because they feel well enough to be interested in self-care and self-administration of analgesia. Overall, women tend to use less analgesia with a PCA system than they would with intramuscular injections (see Fig. 24.5).

Epidural analgesia

Although epidural analgesia provides effective pain relief after caesarean birth, side effects of epidural morphine administration, such as intense itching, and nausea and vomiting, can occur. An antihistamine such as promethazine hydrochloride (phenergan) may be given to reduce pruritus; an antiemetic such as metoclopramide (Maxalon) may be administered to counteract nausea. The use of fentanyl reduces the risk of these side effects. Even with these annoying side effects, however, epidural analgesia with morphine can be a very effective means of pain control after caesarean birth (Woods et al., 2012).

What if...

Katrina refuses to allow you to assess her fundal height after her caesarean birth because she is in so much pain? How would you approach this situation?

Fluid volume

The potential always exists for deficient fluid volume because of blood loss from surgery until all blood vessels that were cut and ligated during surgery have thrombosed, sclerosed and permanently sealed closed. The risk of heavy bleeding doubles for the postpartum woman, because she may haemorrhage vaginally from an uncontracted uterus as well as internally from blood vessels that were not securely ligated. This danger is most acute during the first hour after surgery, but it remains an acute problem for the first 24 hours.

To detect the earliest signs of bleeding, monitor blood pressure, pulse and respiratory rate approximately every 15 minutes for the first hour after surgery, every 30 minutes for the next 2 hours, every hour for the next 4 hours, or as specifically ordered. Signs indicative of possible haemorrhage include:

- Falling blood pressure (more than 20 mmHg), a systolic blood pressure less than 80 mmHg or a drop of 5 to 10 mmHg over several readings
- A change in pulse rate (greater than 110 beats per minute or less than 60 beats per minute)
- Rapid respirations
- Restlessness and a sense of thirst.

Inspect the dressing over the surgical incision for blood staining each time vital signs are assessed. Observe the perineal pad for lochia flow and palpate the fundal height each time as well. Lochial discharge may be decreased in a woman after a caesarean birth because the uterus was cleaned during surgery, but some lochia will always be present, and it follows a typical rubra, serosa, alba pattern. Be certain to help a woman turn so you can look under her body for bleeding. Blood oozing from a surgical wound or vaginally can pool considerably under a woman before it is visible.

Oxytocin may be ordered to be added to the first 1 or 2 litres of intravenous fluid after surgery to ensure firm uterine contraction. If the rate of fluid administration gets behind, be careful about "catch-up" administration. Oxytocin can elevate blood pressure by causing vasoconstriction. It may be safer to allow the fluid to remain behind for a time, rather than risk causing blood pressure to elevate. Be aware that a woman is very prone to haemorrhage at the point the oxytocin is discontinued, because this is the first time her uterus is being asked to maintain contraction on its own. Notify her care provider of any changes in vital signs that might indicate haemorrhage, so that prompt action can be taken. Remember that a minimal but continued change in vital signs (pulse steadily increasing, blood pressure steadily declining) is as ominous a sign of haemorrhage as a sudden alteration in these measurements.

Palpate the uterus gently to prevent increased pain but thoroughly enough to determine uterine consistency. At the same time you assess a woman's uterus for firmness, assess the remainder of her abdomen for softness. A hard, "guarded" abdomen is one of the first signs of peritonitis (peritoneal infection), a complication that may occur with any abdominal surgical procedure.

The average woman whose child is born by caesarean birth remains in the hospital from 48 hours to 4 days. During this period and until she returns to have her sutures or staples removed, several interventions are necessary to promote healing, prevent postoperative complications and help the woman and her family establish bonding with the new child. Common concerns of women include pain, fatigue, interference with gastrointestinal function and reduced activity level.

Adequate fluid intake is important after surgery, to replace blood loss from surgery and to maintain blood pressure and renal function. It is important that intravenous fluids be infused post-surgery at a rate that does not lead to cardiac overload or at an amount inadequate for circulatory compensation. Keep an accurate intake and output record for at least the first 24 hours, to be certain an adequate fluid balance has been achieved.

Bowel movements

Because the bowel is not actually handled, there is probably little reason to withhold food and fluid (Mangesi & Hofmeyr, 2009). Each hospital will have a protocol for eating and drinking post caesarean birth. Bowel sounds can be auscultated to ensure intestinal function has returned. Passage of flatus is another indication that intestinal function is again active. Note carefully the time of a woman's first bowel movement after surgery. If there has been no bowel movement by the time of hospital discharge, her doctor may order a stool softener, a suppository or an enema to facilitate stool evacuation. Reassure a woman who is not receiving much food yet that it is normal not to have bowel movements for 3 or 4 days postoperatively.

Advise women to eat a diet high in roughage and fluid and to attempt to move their bowels at least every other day to avoid constipation after they return home. Some women need a stool softener prescribed, because incisional pain interferes with their ability to use their abdominal muscles effectively. Caution them not to strain to pass stools, because this puts pressure on their incision. Keep their water jug full to remind them to drink fluids.

Urinary elimination

Voiding after surgery provides evidence of adequate renal and circulatory function, because the kidneys must have adequate blood flow through them to function. Because the bladder was handled and displaced during surgery, its tone or ability to sense filling may be inadequate to initiate voiding. For this reason, the indwelling catheter placed before surgery is usually left in place for 4 to 24 hours to ensure good urine drainage. Assess that the catheter is draining (a postpartum woman has a urine output of 3000 to 5000 mL per 24 hours). Bladder distension will occur rapidly if the catheter becomes blocked.

Before catheter removal, a urine culture may be ordered to check for the possibility of a urinary tract infection. After removal of the catheter, the average woman voids in 4 to 8 hours. Assessing for bladder filling can be done using a bladder scanner or by palpation, pressing lightly over the symphysis pubis to assess fullness, and by percussion (see Fig. 24.6). On percussion, an empty bladder sounds dull; a full bladder, resonant; and an extended bladder, hyperresonant. If a bladder has filled to capacity but cannot

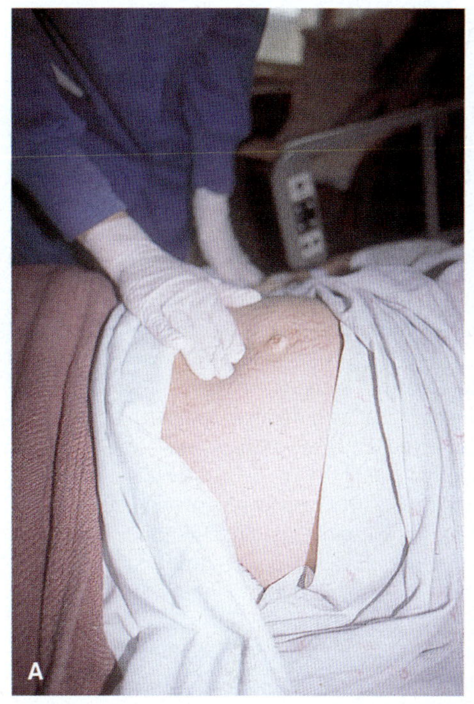

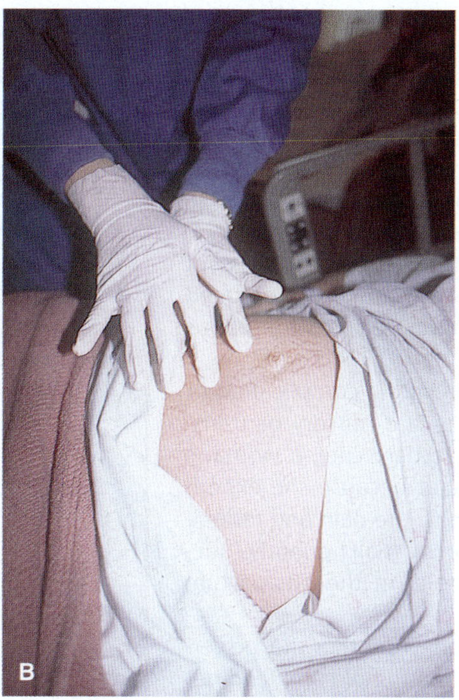

FIGURE 24.6 (**A**) Assessing bladder filling by palpation. (**B**) Assessing bladder filling by percussion. (© Caroline Brown, RNC, MS, DEd.)

empty properly, the woman may have "retention with overflow", or voiding 30 to 60 mL of urine every 15 to 20 minutes.

Teach women to continue to drink adequate fluid (at least five to six glasses daily) to ensure an adequate fluid output and help prevent urinary tract infection after they return home. Be certain they know to telephone their primary care provider if they should develop symptoms of a urinary tract infection.

Mobility

Because a woman's abdominal muscles are lax from the stretching that occurred during pregnancy, abdominal contents tend to shift forwards and put pressure on the suture line when she is sitting or standing, causing pain and an uncomfortable feeling often described as "everything falling out". A woman may feel more comfortable turning and sitting up if she supports her abdomen with one hand or splints the incision with a pillow.

Leg exercises such as flexing and extending her knees and early ambulation are a woman's best safeguards against lower-extremity circulatory problems. Antiembolic stockings are used to help promote venous return and prevent venous stasis. Teach a woman to apply these before arising, while she is supine and venous distension is minimal. Always allow her to sit on the edge of the bed for a few minutes before helping her to a standing position, to prevent orthostatic hypotension (sudden low blood pressure that occurs with sudden position changes). Assessing blood pressure before a woman gets out of bed for the first time is an additional safeguard. Before ambulation, also assess the lower extremities for pain in the calf on dorsiflexion of the foot (Homans' sign—which may or may not be reliable) or for pain, oedema, warmth or redness in the calf, to detect the possibility of a thrombus. It is dangerous for a woman to ambulate if signs of a thrombus are present. A thrombus could shift, becoming an embolus, a potentially lethal situation.

Often, it is difficult for women to understand the importance of turning and ambulating as soon as possible after surgery. Still experiencing the "taking in" postpartum phase, a woman may prefer to spend the first days after surgery just resting quietly in bed. Providing adequate analgesia enables her to move and ambulate with the least amount of pain. Reinforce the need for continued activity balanced with rest after discharge. Be certain she understands the signs and symptoms of complications, such as thrombophlebitis (see Fig. 24.7).

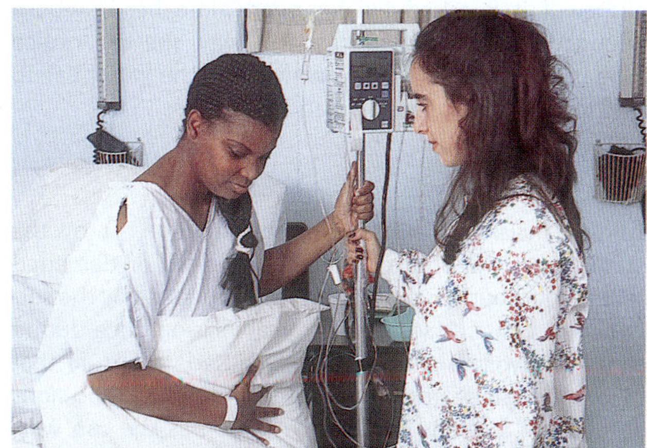

FIGURE 24.7 Encouraging women to be out of bed will help prevent complications from a caesarean birth. It is important to splint the incision area while getting up and ambulating. (© Barbara Proud.)

Parenting

When a caesarean birth is unscheduled, a woman does not have much time preoperatively to think about how she will feel after surgery. Most women are surprised to realise how well they feel overall but also how quickly they become fatigued and how painful a simple surgical incision can be. Being reassured they are recovering well but that surgery is a physiological shock to their system helps them to accept temporary discomforts. Encourage women to breastfeed even if this causes temporary uterine pain as the uterus contracts with breastfeeding.

If the woman's baby was born with a complication or has been placed in an intensive care nursery or transferred to a distant hospital for tertiary care, a woman's postpartum course can be difficult because she experiences a sense of loss in addition to the pain and fatigue of surgery. Depression, which can slow all her body functions and her ability to "take hold" in the postpartum period, can occur.

Unless her baby was transferred to another site, be certain to provide her with ample time to hold and feed her child if possible. Most women can breastfeed satisfactorily after caesarean birth. She may have some reason to think her baby is not quite perfect—after all, the baby was not born "perfectly"—so she may need additional time to inspect her baby and feel comfortable with him or her.

Fatigue

Although a woman needs activity and movement after surgery, she also needs adequate rest. Many women attempt to handle their own and their newborn's needs immediately after surgery, because their excitement about their baby and their new role makes them unaware of their underlying fatigue. Extreme fatigue interferes with healing. Explore her plans for care at home to be certain that her plans for rest seem realistic for a postsurgical-postpartum woman.

Once a woman returns home, rest is often best accomplished if it is scheduled for every time her newborn sleeps. Without adequate rest this way, she can notice increased uterine bleeding, which has the potential to lead to excessive loss of fluid and iron stores.

Skin integrity

Surgical incisions heal by primary intention, or by the gradual removal and replacement of dead or damaged cells at the wound site with new cells produced by the surrounding tissue. Assess the surgical incision once during each shift while a woman is hospitalised, to ensure that the wound edges are approximated and there are no signs of infection, such as erythema. As soon as she can walk steadily, a woman can have a shower (after first removing the dressing), because warm, clean water on the incision is soothing. After this point, she can make a decision about whether to continue to wear a dressing. Lack of a dressing prevents moisture accumulation at the incision site and decreases the possibility of infection.

Teach women to continue to observe their incision daily at home. Instruct them in signs and symptoms of possible infection, including redness or the presence of a discharge, and to report any of these signs to their primary care provider. Women with diabetes or obesity are at increased risk of delayed wound healing. Wound infections delay healing, cause pain and can lead to wound dehiscence and in extreme circumstances sepsis (Nobbs & Crozier, 2011). With a caesarean birth, healing will be adequate enough by day 3 that skin sutures or clamps can be removed, although many are left in place until the woman returns for a follow-up appointment.

BOX 24.2 ✻ Focus on family teaching

Measures to regain energy after a caesarean birth

Q. Katrina tells you, "I feel so tired after my caesarean. What can I do to feel stronger again?"

A. After a caesarean birth, women usually regain energy rapidly. This is because, unlike most people who have had surgery, you did not have it because you were ill, but because it was an alternative method to have a healthy baby. Good suggestions to help regain your energy rapidly are:

- Drink adequate fluid daily (at least six glasses). This helps prevent a urinary tract infection and also supplies all the cells in your body with adequate fluid.
- Rest twice a day for at least one-half hour each time. This helps because your baby will probably wake you at least once during the night.
- Do not hesitate to accept help from family and friends for tasks such as house cleaning or grocery shopping.
- Limit the number of stairs that you climb daily to one flight once a day. Also limit the amount of weight you lift to the weight of your new baby.
- Do not attempt to be the "perfect" new mum. Relax and enjoy your new baby.

Discharge planning

A woman being discharged after caesarean birth takes home not only her new baby but a fair amount of pain and discomfort. Be certain to discuss home care arrangements, emphasising the need for adequate help with her newborn and other responsibilities at home, before discharge (see Box 24.2). Be sure a woman is aware of any restrictions on exercise or activity that she needs to follow (common restrictions are not to lift any object heavier than 5 kg or walk upstairs more than once a day for the first two weeks). Also teach her to recognise signs of possible complications directly related to the surgery, such as:

- Redness or drainage at the incision line.
- Lochia heavier than a normal menstrual period.
- Abdominal pain (other than suture line or afterpain discomfort).
- Temperature greater than 38°C.
- Frequency or burning on urination.

As with a vaginal birth a woman can plan on resuming coitus as soon as the incision has healed and she feels comfortable and ready. Caesarean birth does not interfere with future fertility so be sure that she has contraceptive information, if desired (Baldwin, Rodriguez & Edelman, 2012). Also ensure that she has an appointment for a return visit with her healthcare provider (usually in 2 weeks), for both herself and her newborn and organise a home visit by the midwife if this is available.

Unless the reason for the caesarean birth was cephalopelvic disproportion, a woman can probably have her next child vaginally (see Chapter 15). Being certain the woman is aware of this not only makes her an informed consumer of healthcare but also can influence whether she plans an additional child. In Australia the Birthrites website <www. birthrites.org> is dedicated to supporting women who have had a previous caesarean birth and provides information on what to expect with a caesarean birth. In New Zealand information on VBAC is available from the Kiwifamilies website <www.kiwifamilies.co.nz>. The New Zealand College of Midwives also has a consensus statement supporting VBAC as a safe option for women.

CASE STUDY QUESTION

5. Katrina wonders if she can breastfeed following a caesarean birth. Your best answer would be:
   a. You do not recommend she try to breastfeed because she will feel so ill
   b. It is difficult for a woman with an abdominal incision to hold a newborn
   c. She will need too much analgesia postoperatively to make breastfeeding safe
   d. Women can breastfeed without difficulty following a caesarean birth

Key points for review

- The term *caesarean birth* is preferred to *caesarean section* or *delivery*, because it puts the focus on the childbirth rather than surgical elements of the procedure.
- Caesarean birth may be either a scheduled or an emergency procedure. Because it carries more risk for the woman and infant than does vaginal birth, it is usually undertaken only when medically necessary.
- Establishing surgical risk includes assessment of nutritional status, age, general health, fluid and electrolyte balance, and psychological condition.
- Assessment measures before surgery usually include vital sign determination; urinalysis; blood studies such as complete blood count, electrolytes, blood typing and cross-matching; and ultrasound.
- The skin incision may be vertical (a classic incision), although it is usually a horizontal one just above the pubic hair. The internal incision into the uterus is also usually a horizontal incision into the lower uterine segment.
- The old saying, "Once a caesarean, always a caesarean" is no longer true, as long as cephalopelvic disproportion does not exist and the previous incision was a low transverse incision.
- Support people can lose a great deal of their ability to support if they feel intimidated and out of place in an operating room; offer them support as needed to make this a positive experience for them as well.
- Caesarean birth is one of the safest types of surgery performed. To keep a woman safe after the procedure, remember that she is both a postsurgical and a postpartum patient. Make assessments to ensure that neither postpartum nor postsurgical complications occur.
- Adequate pain management is important to allow a woman a sense of control and comfort and bonding with her newborn.
- Women are physically exhausted after caesarean birth and may be psychologically exhausted because of the emergency nature of the experience. Provide rest time to relieve the physical strain and a chance to verbalise the experience to help relieve the psychological strain.
- A major intervention after caesarean birth is early ambulation to prevent complications. Incisional pain may make this difficult, so strong nursing support and adequate pain management are necessary.

CASE STUDY QUESTIONS

6. Katrina was afraid to have a caesarean birth because she did not want to be alone. What actions could you take to make her situation easier to accept?
7. Suppose Katrina is receiving PCA after her caesarean birth. She tells you that she is not interested in PCA and would rather have injections for pain. Describe and explain the action you might take. Would you advocate for use of PCA or advocate with her doctor for a changed order?
8. Katrina's boyfriend tells you that he cannot possibly stay with her in the operating room while she has a caesarean birth. He's sure he'll feel nauseated and probably faint. How would you intervene to promote family-centred care and meet the couple's needs?

Resources

For an extensive range of additional resources to enhance teaching and learning and to facilitate understanding of this chapter, please see the text's accompanying website located on thePoint at http://thepoint.lww.com.

References

Abenhaim, H. A. & Benjamin, A. (2011). Effect of prior cesarean delivery on neonatal outcomes. *Journal of Perinatal Medicine*, *39*(3), 241–244.

Aguirre, F. & Chou, B. (2011). Normal labor & delivery, operative delivery & malpresentations. In K. J. Hurt, M. W. Guile, J. L. Bienstock, et al. (Eds.),

The Johns Hopkins Manual of Gynecology and Obstetrics (4th ed.), pp. 73–89. Philadelphia, PA: Lippincott Williams & Wilkins.

Alfirevic, Z., Gyte, G. M. & Dou, L. (2010). Different classes of antibiotics given to women routinely for preventing infection at caesarean section. *Cochrane Database of Systematic Reviews*, (10), CD008726.

Arulkumaran, S. (2012). Malpresentation, malposition, cephalopelvic disproportion & obstetric procedures. In D. K. Edmonds (Ed), *Dewhurst's Textbook of Obstetrics & Gynaecology* (8th ed.), pp. 311–325. Oxford, UK: John Wiley & Sons.

Baldwin, M. K., Rodriguez, M. I. & Edelman, A. B. (2012). Lack of insurance and parity influence choice between long-acting reversible contraception and sterilization in women postpregnancy. *Contraception, 86*(1), 42–47.

Barbadoro, P., Cotichelli, G., Chiatti, C., et al. (2012). Socio-economic determinants and self-reported depressive symptoms during postpartum period. *Women & Health, 52*(4), 352–368.

Borbolla Foster, A., Bagust, A., Bisits, A., Holland, M. & Welsh, A. (2014). Lessons to be learnt in managing the breech presentation at term: An 11-year single-centre retrospective study. *Australian and New Zealand Journal of Obstetrics and Gynaecology, 54*(4), 333–339.

Dickinson, J. E. (2014). Caesarean delivery: Truths and consequences. *Australian and New Zealand Journal of Obstetrics and Gynaecology, 54*(4), 295–297.

Eden, K. B., Denman, M. A., Emeis, C. L., et al. (2012). Trial of labor and vaginal delivery rates in women with a prior cesarean. *Journal of Obstetric, Gynecology & Neonatal Nursing, 41*(5), 583–598.

Gardner, K., Henry, A., Thou, S., Davis, G. & Miller, T. (2014). Improving VBAC rates: The combined impact of two management strategies. *Australian and New Zealand Journal of Obstetrics and Gynaecology, 54*(4), 327–332.

Gilbert, E. S. (2011). *Manual of High Risk Pregnancy & Delivery* (5th ed.). St Louis, MO: Mosby Elsevier.

Gungorduk, K., Asicioglu, O., Celikkol, O., et al. (2010). Iatrogenic bladder injuries during caesarean delivery: A case control study. *Journal of Obstetrics and Gynaecology, 30*(7), 667.

Gyhagen, M., Bullarbo, M., Nielsen, T., et al. (2012). The prevalence of urinary incontinence 20 years after childbirth: A national cohort study in singleton primiparae after vaginal or caesarean delivery. *BJOG: International Journal of Obstetrics and Gynaecology, 119*(12), 1471–1782.

Harma, M., Harma, M. I., Karadeniz, G., et al. (2011). Idiopathic ileoileal invagination two days after cesarean section. *Journal of Obstetric & Gynaecology Research, 37*(2), 160–162.

Hodnett, E. D., Gates, S., Hofmeyr, G. J., et al. (2012). Continuous support for women during childbirth. *Cochrane Database of Systematic Reviews*, (2), CD003766.

Lavender, T., Hofmeyr, G. J., Neilson, J. P., et al. (2012). Caesarean section for non-medical reasons at term. *Cochrane Database of Systematic Reviews*, (3), CD004660.

Li, Z., Zeki, R., Hilder, L. & Sullivan, E.A. (2012). *Australia's Mothers and Babies 2010*. Perinatal statistics series no. 27. Cat. No. Canberra: AIHW National Perinatal Epidemiology and Statistics Unit, 2012.

Lipman, S. S., Carvalho, B., Cohen, S. E., et al. (2013). Response times for emergency cesarean delivery: Use of simulation drills to assess and improve obstetric team performance. *Journal of Perinatology, 33*(4), 259–263.

Liva, S. J., Hall, W. A., Klein, M. C., et al. (2012). Factors associated with differences in Canadian perinatal nurses' attitudes toward birth practices. *Journal of Obstetric, Gynecology & Neonatal Nursing, 41*(6), 761–773.

Mangesi, L. & Hofmeyr, G. J. (2009). Early compared with delayed oral fluids and food after caesarean section. *Cochrane Database of Systematic Reviews, 2009*(1), CD003516.

Mantakas, A. & Farrell, T. (2010). The influence of increasing BMI in nulliparous women on pregnancy outcome. *European Journal of Obstetrics, Gynecology & Reproductive Biology, 153*(1), 43–46.

Niino, Y. (2011). The increasing cesarean rate globally and what we can do about it. *BioScience Trends, 5*(4), 139–150.

Nobbs, S. & Crozier, K. (2011). Wound management in obese women following caesarean section. *British Journal of Midwifery, 19*(3), 150–156.

Patel, R. M. & Jain, L. (2010). Delivery after previous cesarean: Short-term perinatal outcomes. *Seminars in Perinatology, 34*(4), 272–280.

Shorten, A., Shorten, B. & Kennedy, H. P. (2014). Complexities of choice after prior cesarean: A narrative analysis. *Birth, 41*(2), 178–184.

Speichinger, E. & Holschneider, C. H. (2013). Surgical disorders in pregnancy. In A. H. DeCherney, L. Nathan, T. M. Goodwin, et al. (Eds.), *Current Diagnosis and Treatment: Obstetrics and Gynecology* (11th ed), pp. 433–453. Columbus, OH: McGraw-Hill/Lange.

Stevens, J., Schmied, V., Burns, E. & Dahlen, H. (2014). Immediate or early skin-to-skin contact after a Caesarean section: A review of the literature. *Maternal & Child Nutrition, 10*(4), 456–473.

Thompson, H. (2010). Caesarean section at maternal request: A literature review. *British Journal of Midwifery, 18*(8), 484–491.

Timor-Tritsch, I. E., Monteagudo, A., Cali, G., Vintzileos, A., Viscarello, R., Al-Khan, A., Zamudio, S., Mayberry, P., M. Cordoba, M. M. & Dar, P. (2014). Cesarean scar pregnancy is a precursor of morbidly adherent placenta. *Ultrasound Obstet Gynecol, 44*, 346–353.

Tita, A. T. (2012). When is primary cesarean appropriate: Maternal and obstetrical indications. *Seminars in Perinatology, 36*(5), 324–327.

Wang, B. S., Zhou, L. F., Coulte, D., et al. (2010). Effects of caesarean section on maternal health in low risk nulliparous women. *BMC Pregnancy and Childbirth, 10*(12), 78.

Woods, A. B., Crist, B., Kowalewski, S., et al. (2012). A cross-sectional analysis of the effect of patient-controlled epidural analgesia versus patient controlled analgesia on postcesarean pain and breastfeeding. *Journal of Obstetric, Gynecology & Neonatal Nursing, 41*(3), 339–346.

Zeitlin, J., Di Lallo, D., Blondel, B., et al. (2010). Variability in caesarean section rates for very preterm births at 28–31 weeks of gestation in 10 European regions. *European Journal of Obstetrics, Gynecology & Reproductive Biology, 149*(2), 147–152.

Suggested readings

Beddall, H. (2015). Placenta praevia: Diagnosis and management. *British Journal of Midwifery, 23*(2), 88–94.

Brocklehurst, P. (2013). CORONIS: International study of caesarean section surgical techniques: The follow-up study. *BMC Pregnancy & Childbirth, 13*(1), 1–22.

Dryden, M., Goddard, C., Madadi, A., Heard, M., Saeed, K. & Cooke, J. (2014). Using antimicrobial Surgihoney to prevent caesarean wound infection. *British Journal of Midwifery, 22*(2), 111–115.

Laws, P., Li, A. & Sullivan, E. A. (2010). *Australia's Mothers and Babies 2008*. Perinatal statistics series no. 24. Cat. No. PER 50, Canberra: AIHW.

McLaurin, R. & Geraghty, S. (2013). Placenta praevia, placental abruption and amphetamine use in pregnancy: A case study. *Women & Birth, 26*(2), 138–142.

Prosser, S. J., Miller, Y. D., Thompson, R. & Redshaw, M. (2014). Why 'down under' is a cut above: A comparison of rates of and reasons for caesarean section in England and Australia. *BMC Pregnancy & Childbirth, 14*(1), 1–26.

Roberts, C. L., Algert, C. S., Todd, A. L. & Morris, J. M. (2013). Reducing caesarean section rates—No easy task. *Australian & New Zealand Journal of Obstetrics & Gynaecology, 53*(3), 310–313.

Sholapurkar, S. L. (2013). Increased incidence of placenta praevia and accreta with previous caesareans. A hypothesis for causation. *Journal of Obstetrics & Gynaecology, 33*(8), 806–809.

Simpson, K. R. (2007). Surgical safety: Minimizing risk of retained foreign bodies during caesarean birth. *MCN: The American Journal of Maternal/Child Nursing, 32*(3), 200.

Chapter 25

Care of a family experiencing a postpartum complication

In an earlier chapter, you learned about caring for a woman during the usual postpartum period. This chapter adds information about how to care for a woman and her family when there is a complication during this time. Conscientious care is important when a postpartum complication develops because it plays a major role in protecting the health of both women and their families.

LEARNING OBJECTIVES

After studying this chapter, you should be able to:

1. Describe common deviations from the normal that can occur during the puerperium.
2. Use critical thinking to analyse ways that promote family-centred care when a postpartum complication occurs.
3. Assess a woman and her family for deviations from the normal during the puerperium.
4. Identify expected outcomes for a postpartum woman experiencing a complication.
5. Plan interventions that meet the special needs of a family with a postpartum complication, such as planning for an extended hospitalisation.
6. Implement care when a postpartum complication such as haemorrhage, infection, pregnancy-induced hypertension or postpartum psychosis develops.
7. Evaluate expected outcomes for achievement and effectiveness of care.
8. Identify areas related to care of women with postpartum complications that could benefit from additional research or application of evidence-based practice.
9. Integrate knowledge of postpartum complications with the nursing process to achieve quality child and family health nursing care.

KEY TERMS

- endometritis
- mastitis
- peritonitis
- postpartum depression
- postpartum psychosis
- thrombophlebitis

CASE STUDY

Mary Blackhawk is a 30-year-old woman who had a "textbook-perfect" pregnancy. You enter her room 4 hours after she gave birth to a 3.6-kg girl, but, because she is sleeping and appears comfortable, you hesitate to wake her. When you observe her more closely, however, you realise she appears abnormally pale. You obtain her vital signs and document her pulse as 90 beats per minute and her blood pressure as 96/50 mmHg. When you fold back her bedclothes, you discover her bed is soaked with blood. You suspect she is experiencing one of the most serious complications of pregnancy: postpartum haemorrhage. Yet because she was sleeping, she was totally unaware of it.

CASE STUDY QUESTIONS

1. What immediate measures does Ms Blackhawk need?
2. What would be your first action?

Although the puerperium is usually a period of health, complications can occur. It is important to be knowledgeable about predisposing factors and clinical manifestations of postpartum complications to ensure the prompt initiation of corrective measures in order to prevent long-term consequences for a woman and her family (Furuta, Sandall & Bick, 2012). Postpartum morbidities include: postpartum haemorrhage, fever and infection, abdominal and back pain, abnormal discharge, thromboembolism, urinary tract complications as well as psychological and mental health problems such as postnatal depression (Yonemoto, Dowswell, Nagai & Mori, 2013).

Postpartum complications are potentially serious because they can impact on so many people. A complication may be so serious it could cause a personal injury, leave a woman with her future fertility impaired or even result in death. Any complication that affects the health of the mother can also affect her interactions with her newborn, such as causing her to discontinue breastfeeding (Brown & Jordan, 2012). Her family can also be disrupted because of an extended hospital stay that prevents her from performing her normal family responsibilities. In addition, financial difficulties may arise because of her inability to maintain employment as well as the need for additional child and healthcare. Fortunately, most postpartum complications are preventable, and if they do occur, the majority can be treated effectively without long-term complications if they are detected. Australia currently lacks consistent guidelines for health professionals on what constitutes a routine postpartum visit and services have been described as fragmented and inconsistent (Brodribb, Zadoroznyj & Dane, 2013). Ideally

TABLE 25.1 Antenatal and intrapartum risk factors for PPH

Maternity - Prevention, early recognition and management of postpartum haemorrhage (PPH)

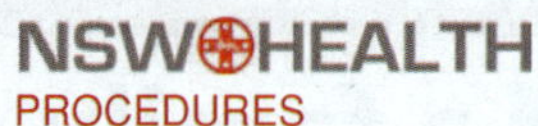

Cause	Aetiology	Clinical Risk Factors
Abnormalities of uterine contraction (Tone) **70%**	• Atonic uterus	• Physiological management of the third stage • Prolonged third stage (>30 mins)
	• Over distended uterus	• Polyhydramnios • Multiple pregnancy • Macrosomia
	• Uterine muscle exhaustion	• Rapid or incoordinate labour • Prolonged labour (1st or 2nd stage) • Labour dystocia • High parity • Labour augmented with oxytocin
	• Intra-amniotic infection	• Pyrexia • Prolonged ruptured membranes (>24 hours)
	• Drug-induced uterine hypotonia	• Magnesium sulphate, nifedipine, salbutamol • General anaesthesia
	• Functional or anatomic distortion of the uterus	• Fibroid uterus • Uterine anomalies
Genital tract trauma (Trauma) **20%**	• Episiotomy or lacerations (cervix, vagina or perineum)	• Induced labour • Augmented labour • Abnormal labour (dystocia) • Malposition • Precipitous birth • Instrumental birth (forceps or vacuum)
	• Extensions / lacerations at caesarean section	• Malposition • Deep engagement
	• Uterine rupture	• Previous uterine surgery
	• Uterine inversion	• Strong cord traction in 3rd stage (especially with fundal placenta) • Short umbilical cord • High parity • Uterine relaxation • Placenta accreta (especially with fundal placenta) • Congenital uterine anomalies or weakness • Antepartum use of magnesium sulphate or oxytocin
Retained pregnancy tissue (Tissue) **10%**	• Retained products • Abnormal placenta • Retained cotyledon or succenturiate lobe	• Incomplete placenta at birth • Placenta accreta • Previous uterine surgery • High parity • Abnormal placenta on ultrasound
Abnormalities of coagulation (Thrombin) **1%**	• Retained blood clots	• Atonic uterus
	• Coagulation disorders acquired during pregnancy • Idiopathic thrombocytopenic purpura (ITP) • Von Willebrand's disease • Haemophilia • Thrombocytopenia with pre-eclampsia • Disseminated intravascular coagulation (DIC) • Pre-eclampsia • Retained dead fetus • Severe infection • Placental abruption • Amniotic fluid embolism	• Bruising • Elevated blood pressure • Fetal death • Fever • Antepartum haemorrhage • Sudden collapse
	• Therapeutic anticoagulation	• History of thrombo-embolism

Source: Maternity—Prevention, early recognition and management of postpartum haemorrhage (PPH). (Reproduced by permission, NSW Ministry of Health © 2015.)

continuity of care with a known midwife should be available for women and midwives are ideally placed to recognise complications during the puerperium and to provide care and referral as needed.

A WOMAN EXPERIENCING A POSTPARTUM COMPLICATION

Assessment

The postpartum period brings significant physical, emotional and social changes which some women feel ill-equipped to deal with including; exhaustion, stress, poor body image and marital discord. Women have also described themselves as unprepared for symptoms such as urinary incontinence, headaches, hair loss and back pain (Martin et al., 2014). Even symptoms they knew might occur postpartum were a surprise because they were different to previous experiences, for example postpartum lochia is very different to menstrual bleeding. Many women are unaware of the impact postpartum changes will have on their lives and how they function (Martin et al., 2014). It can thus be difficult for women to discern between what is normal postpartum and what is a complication they should consult a healthcare professional about. Around 70% of women have a physical problem during the 12 months after childbirth, for 25% this is a moderately severe problem and for 20% a severe problem (Haran et al., 2014). When health professionals focus mainly on care of the infant, breastfeeding mothers can feel as if there is a lack of continuity of care and a disconnect between them and their health providers (Martin et al., 2014).

Assessment findings associated with a postpartum complication may be extremely subtle, such as tenderness in the calf of a leg, a slight increase in uterine or perineal pain, a slight elevation in temperature or a slight increase in the amount of lochia flow. Because the average woman usually has no postpartum complications and the length of stay in a hospital is short, it is easy to overlook these subtle signs. It is important to be alert to any findings that are "different from usual", because they may be the beginning of a problem. Interventions for a woman with a postpartum complication should include instruction for both self-care and childcare (if appropriate), emphasising the transitory nature of the complication.

Postpartum haemorrhage

Postpartum haemorrhage (PPH) is one of the most important causes of maternal mortality in Australia and New Zealand. The incidence of PPH in Australia is 5–15%. Although many cases of PPH cause minimal morbidity, it remains a leading cause of maternal death in Australia and New Zealand as well as globally (RANZCOG, 2015). Traditionally, PPH has been defined as any blood loss from the uterus greater than 500 mL during and after childbirth (Poggi, 2012). It is defined as a primary PPH if it occurs within the first 24 hours following birth and a secondary PPH if it occurs between 24 hours and 6 weeks postpartum. A severe PPH is defined as blood loss of 1000 mL or more or any amount of blood loss that results in haemodynamic compromise (NSW Health, 2010). The greatest danger of haemorrhage is in the first 24 hours because of the denuded and unprotected uterine area left after detachment of the placenta.

The incidence of PPH may be underestimated by 50% because of the difficulty in estimating postpartum blood loss. One perineal pad contains between 25–50 mL of blood. Counting the number of perineal pads provides a rough estimate of blood loss. Five pads saturated in half an hour is a very different situation from five pads saturated in 8 hours. In either situation a woman will have lost approximately 250 mL of blood and should be assessed. Weighing perineal pads before and after use and subtracting the difference is an accurate way to measure vaginal blood loss. One gram of weight is comparable to 1 mL of blood volume. Ensure that a thorough inspection is undertaken when inspecting for blood loss as a large amount of blood may be pooled underneath. The main causes of PPH are known as the 'four T's (see Table 25.1 and Fig. 25.1).

1. Tone—related to uterine atony or a relaxed uterus
2. Trauma—related to genital tract trauma such as lacerations to the genital tract or episiotomy; this includes uterine rupture and uterine inversion (uterine inversion is discussed in Chapter 23)
3. Tissue—related to retained products of conception such as a retained cotyledon or succenturiate lobe
4. Thrombin—abnormalities of coagulation such as pre-existing coagulation disorders or disseminated intravascular coagulopathy (DIC).

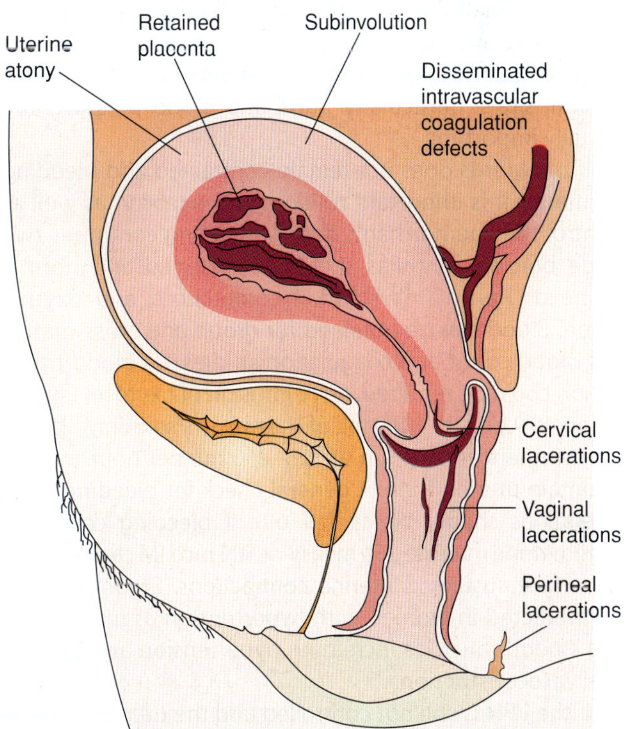

FIGURE 25.1 Common causes of postpartum haemorrhage.

Therapeutic management

Uterine atony, or relaxation of the uterus, is the most frequent cause of PPH (Bryant et al., 2012). The uterus must remain in a contracted state after birth to keep the open vessels at the placental site from bleeding. If the uterus suddenly relaxes, there will be an abrupt gush of blood vaginally from the placental site. If the vaginal bleeding is extremely copious, a woman will exhibit symptoms of shock and blood loss. This can occur immediately after birth or more gradually, over the first postpartum hour, as the uterus slowly relaxes. When the vaginal bleeding occurs gradually, it results in seepage, not a gush of blood. Over a period of hours, however, continued seepage can be as serious as a sudden release of blood. If uterine atony is identified, the first step in controlling haemorrhage is to attempt uterine massage to encourage uterine contraction. Unless the uterus is extremely lacking in tone, this procedure is usually effective in causing a contraction, and, after a few seconds, the uterus assumes its healthy, grapefruit-like feel. (See Box 25.1 for fundal massage.)

With uterine atony, even if the uterus responds well to massage, the problem may not be completely resolved. After you remove your hand from the fundus the uterus may relax and bleeding may begin again. Therefore, remain with the woman after massaging her fundus, to be certain the uterus is not relaxing again. Observe carefully, including fundal height and consistency as well as lochia, for the next 4 hours.

Palpate a woman's fundus at frequent intervals postnatally to be certain that her uterus is well-contracted. This is the best measure for preventing early haemorrhage. When palpating a uterine fundus, if you are unsure whether you have located it, the uterus is probably relaxed. Under normal circumstances, a well-contracted uterus is firm and easily recognised. Frequent assessments of lochia, as well as vital signs, particularly pulse and blood pressure, are equally important.

If the uterus does not remain contracted and bleeding continues it is important to identify the reason as well as control the haemorrhage. If brisk bleeding continues two large bore IV cannulas should be inserted and normal saline or Hartmann's solution commenced and oxygen given. Blood can be obtained for group and cross-match, full blood count and coagulation studies if a blood transfusion could be required. An IV infusion of oxytocin (syntocinon 40 IU/mL in 1000 mL of Hartmann's solution) should be commenced and run at 125–250 mL per hour to help maintain uterine tone. A general check for bleeding from lacerations should be carried out. If bleeding continues ergometrine maleate 250 mcg IV or 500 mcg IM can be given to induce sustained uterine contractions. Ergometrine is contradicted in women with hypertension as it contracts the smooth muscles increasing hypertension and peripheral vasoconstriction.

If the PPH is still not controlled and the uterus is atonic Prostaglandin F2 alpha (Dinoprost) is given intramyometrially. The dosage of Prostaglandin F2 alpha is 250 mcg which can be repeated at the doctor's discretion if the uterus remains atonic, the maximum dose is 3 mL (6 mL of prepared solution). The dose is prepared as follows: 1 mL of 5 mg/mL solutions is mixed with 9 mL of normal saline, 1 mL (0.5 mcg) is then injected into each side of the uterine fundus (NSW Health, 2010). Prostaglandin F2 alpha can be lifesaving in cases of haemorrhage that fails to resolve with other measures. However, it should be used cautiously in women with asthma, hypertension or renal, liver or pulmonary disease. The side effects include pyrexia, nausea, vomiting, diarrhoea, hypertension and headache. In New Zealand carboprost (Hemabate) is used for treatment of PPH if uterine massage and oxytocics have failed. An initial dose of 250 mcg is given as a deep IM injection and can be repeated every 15–90 minutes but the amount should not exceed 2 mL (8 doses). Misoprostol (Cytotec®) a prostaglandin E1 analogue is no longer recommended to control PPH as it is less effective than oxytocin.

Additional measures that can be helpful include:

- Ensure voiding at least every 4 hours to be certain her bladder is empty. A full bladder pushes an uncontracted uterus into an even more uncontracted state. If a PPH is occurring a urinary catheter should be inserted and uterine output monitored with the aim of achieving urine output >30 mL per hour.
- If a woman is experiencing respiratory distress from decreasing blood volume, administer oxygen by face mask at a rate of about 6–8 L per minute. Position her supine to allow adequate blood flow to her brain and kidneys.
- Obtain vital signs frequently and make sure to interpret them accurately, looking for trends. For example, a continuously rising pulse rate is an ominous pattern.

If a woman is losing enough blood to affect her systemic circulation, she will develop signs of shock such as: an increased, thready and weak pulse; decreased blood pressure; increased and shallow respirations; pale, clammy skin; and increasing anxiety.

In the event of slow bleeding, there is little change in pulse and blood pressure at first because of circulatory compensation. Suddenly, however, the system can compensate no more and then the pulse rate rises rapidly. The pulse becomes weak and thready and the blood pressure drops abruptly. The woman's skin becomes cold and clammy and she shows obvious signs of shock. Consistent frequent assessments of uterine tone and vital signs and laboratory assessments such as haemoglobin and haematocrit levels help to detect blood loss before this point is ever reached.

Bimanual compression

If fundal massage and administration of oxytocin or prostaglandins are not effective in stopping uterine bleeding, bimanual compression of the uterus can be used. With this

BOX 25.1 Nursing procedure ✻ Fundal massage

Purpose: The purpose of fundal massage is to stimulate uterine contraction, promote uterine tone and consistency, and minimise the risk of haemorrhage.

Procedure	Principle
1. Explain the procedure to the woman and provide privacy.	**1.** Explanations help to decrease anxiety; providing privacy enhances self-esteem.
2. Ask the woman to void (unless bleeding is extensive and more rapid action seems necessary).	**2.** An empty bladder prevents displacement of the uterus and ensures accurate assessment of uterine tone.
3. Place the woman supine with her knees flexed and feet together.	**3.** Proper positioning enhances visualisation and effectiveness of procedure.
4. a. Put on gloves. Place one hand on the abdomen just above the symphysis pubis.	**4. a.** This location anchors the lower uterine segment.
b. Place the other hand around the top of the fundus (see Fig. A).	**b.** This location helps to assess and locate the fundus and determine height.
5. Rotate the upper hand to massage the uterus until it is firm, being careful not to over-massage (see Fig. B).	**5.** Massage should be done only when uterus is not firm; otherwise muscle fatigue and uterine relaxation may occur. Aggressive massage may lead to partial or complete uterine prolapse.
6. When the uterus is firm, gently press the fundus between the hands using slight downward pressure against the lower hand.	**6.** Gently squeezing with downward pressure helps to expel blood or clots collected in the uterine cavity.
7. Remove the perineal pad. Observe the perineum for passage of clots and amount of bleeding.	**7.** This helps to assess the degree of bleeding.
8. When the uterus is again firm, cleanse the perineum and apply a clean perineal pad. Discard gloves and soiled pads.	**8.** This helps to promote comfort and hygiene while reducing the risk of infection.
9. Document results of procedure. Continue to assess fundus and lochia. Notify doctor or nurse-midwife if fundus does not remain firm or bleeding continues.	**9.** Documentation provides a means of evaluation. Continued assessment allows for early identification and prompt intervention with additional measures, such as oxytocin, to prevent haemorrhage.

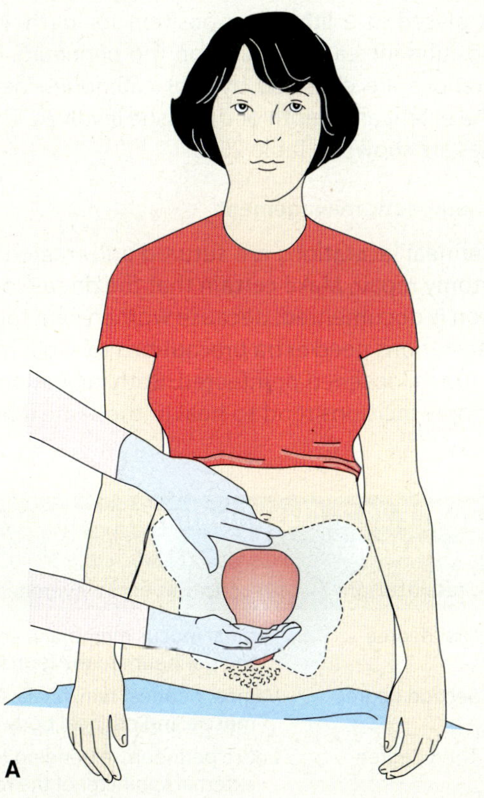

A

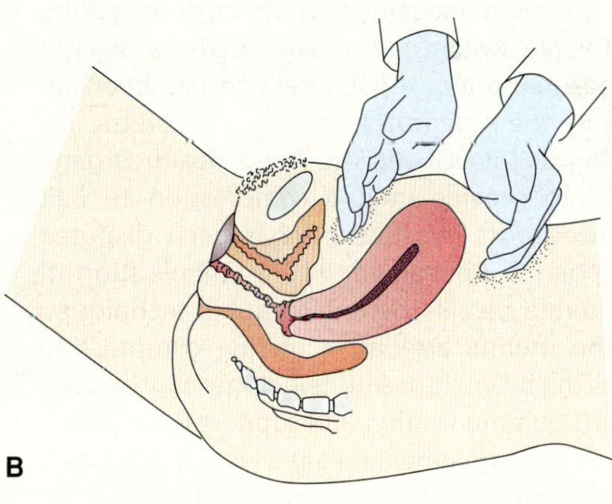

B

procedure, one hand is inserted into a woman's vagina while pushing against the fundus through the abdominal wall with the other hand. The woman may be taken to the operating theatre to so that her uterine cavity can be explored manually by the attending doctor and adequate analgesia can be provided. Uterine packing may be inserted during this procedure to help halt bleeding. If uterine packing is used, be certain this is documented in a woman's chart so it can be removed when the bleeding has resolved. Retained packing serves as a growth medium for microorganism invasion that could lead to a postpartum infection (Laas et al., 2012).

Blood replacement

Blood transfusion to replace blood loss with PPH may be necessary. Make certain that blood typing and cross-matching were done when the woman was admitted and that blood is available. Some women donate blood during pregnancy so that they can be autotransfused if haemorrhage should occur postpartum.

Extensive blood loss is one of the precursors of postpartum infection because of the general debilitation that results. For any woman who has experienced more than a normal loss of blood, observe for changes in lochia and monitor temperature to detect infection. Make certain the woman knows how to check for normal lochia and temperature once she has been discharged.

Tamponade, hysterectomy or suturing

Usually, therapeutic management is effective in halting bleeding. In the rare instance of extreme uterine atony not responding to uterotonics a Bakri balloon has been recommended by the American Congress of Obstetricians and Gynegologists (ACOG) and the World Health Organization (WHO) to provide uterine compression to halt bleeding; however, its effectiveness has been disputed (Wright, Chauhan & Abuhamad, 2014). Embolisation of pelvic and uterine vessels by angiographic techniques; ligation of the uterine arteries; a uterine compression suture such as the B-Lynch; or a hysterectomy may be used as a last resort. Communication and support is necessary in this situation if the treatment means a woman has unexpectedly lost her ability to have any more children.

Lacerations

Small lacerations or tears of the birth canal are common and may be considered a normal consequence of childbearing. Large lacerations, however, can cause complications. They occur most often:

- With difficult or precipitate births
- In primigravidas
- With the birth of a large infant (4 kilograms)
- With the use of a lithotomy position and instruments.

Either cervical, vaginal or perineal lacerations may occur. After birth, any time a uterus feels firm but bleeding persists, suspect a laceration of one of these three sites.

Cervical lacerations

Lacerations of the cervix are usually found on the sides of the cervix, near the branches of the uterine artery. Repair of a cervical laceration is difficult, because the bleeding can be so intense that it obstructs visualisation of the area and regional anaesthetic may be required.

Vaginal lacerations

Vaginal lacerations are easier to locate and assess than cervical lacerations, because they are easier to view.

Therapeutic management

Unfortunately, vaginal tissue is friable making vaginal lacerations difficult to suture. A balloon tamponade similar to the type used with a uterine haemorrhage may be effective if suturing does not achieve haemostasis (Ghirardina, Alboni & Mabrouk, 2012). Some oozing often occurs after a repair, so the vagina may be packed to maintain pressure on the suture line. An indwelling urinary catheter (Foley catheter) may be placed at the same time, because the packing causes pressure on the urethra and can interfere with voiding. If packing is inserted, document in a woman's chart when and where it was placed, so you can be certain it will be removed after 24 to 48 hours or before discharge.

Perineal lacerations

Lacerations of the perineum usually occur when a woman is placed in a lithotomy position for birth, because this position increases tension on the perineum. Perineal lacerations are classified by four categories, depending on the extent and depth of the tissue involved. These categories are shown in Table 25.2.

Therapeutic management

Perineal lacerations are sutured and treated as an episiotomy repair. Make certain that the degree of the laceration is documented, because women with fourth-degree lacerations need extra precautions to avoid having repair sutures loosened or infected. Both lacerations and episiotomy incisions tend to heal in the same length of time.

TABLE 25.2 Classification of perineal lacerations

Classification	Description of involvement
First degree	Vaginal mucus membrane and skin of the perineum to the fourchette
Second degree	Vagina, perineal skin, fascia, levator ani muscle and perineal body
Third degree	Entire perineum, extending to reach the external sphincter of the rectum
Fourth degree	Entire perineum, rectal sphincter, and some of the mucus membrane of the rectum

A diet high in fluid and a stool softener may be prescribed for the first week after birth to prevent constipation and hard stools. Any woman who has a third- or fourth-degree laceration should not have an enema or a rectal suppository prescribed. Although fourth-degree lacerations can lead to dyspareunia, rectal incontinence or sexual dissatisfaction, they usually heal without further complications.

Retained placental fragments

Occasionally, a placenta does not deliver in its entirety; fragments of it separate and are left behind. Because the portion retained keeps the uterus from contracting fully, uterine bleeding occurs. Although this is most likely to happen with a succenturiate placenta—a placenta with an accessory lobe (see Chapter 23)—it can happen in any instance. Placenta accreta—a placenta that fuses with the myometrium because of an abnormal decidua basalis layer—may also be retained. This is associated with previous caesarean birth and in vitro fertilisation and occurs at occurs at an incidence of about 1 in 3000 births; it can be identified by an ultrasound during pregnancy. Removing such a deeply embedded placenta can lead to severe PPH (Balayla & Bondarenko, 2012). To identify the complication of retained placenta, every placenta should be inspected carefully after birth to see that it is complete. Retained placental fragments may also be detected by ultrasound. A blood serum sample that contains human chorionic gonadotropin hormone (hCG) also reveals that part of a placenta is still present.

Assessment

If an undetected retained fragment is large, bleeding will be apparent in the immediate postpartum period, because the uterus cannot contract with the fragment in place. If the fragment is small, bleeding may not be detected until postpartum day 6 to 10, when the woman notices an abrupt discharge and a large amount of vaginal bleeding. On examination, the uterus is usually not fully contracted.

Therapeutic management

Removal of the retained placental fragment is necessary to stop the bleeding. Usually, a dilatation and curettage (D&C) is performed to remove the placental fragment. If it cannot be removed, methotrexate may be prescribed to destroy the retained fragment. Because the haemorrhage from retained fragments may be delayed until after a woman is at home, ensure women know to continue to observe the colour of lochia and to report any tendency for the discharge to change from lochia serosa or alba back to rubra. In some instances, placenta accreta is so deeply attached that balloon occlusion and embolisation of the internal Iliac arteries may be necessary to minimise blood loss, sometimes a hysterectomy must be performed (ACOG, 2012).

CASE STUDY QUESTION

3. Suppose Mary has a retained placental fragment that is causing extensive postpartum bleeding. What hormone test would you anticipate being ordered to detect whether any placenta is still present?

   a. Placental and cord blood oestrogen
   b. Progesterone from the placenta
   c. Human chorionic gonadotropin hormone
   d. Systemic prolactin (a pituitary hormone)

Subinvolution

Subinvolution is incomplete return of the uterus to its prepregnant size and shape. With subinvolution, at a 4–6 week postpartum visit, the uterus is still enlarged and soft. Lochial discharge usually is still present. Subinvolution may result from a small retained placental fragment, a mild **endometritis** (infection of the endometrium), or an accompanying problem such as a uterine myoma that is interfering with complete contraction.

Therapeutic management

If the uterus is tender to palpation, suggesting endometritis, an oral antibiotic will be prescribed. Ensure women are able to recognise the normal process of involution and lochial discharge so they are able to identify subinvolution and seek early healthcare if it occurs. A chronic loss of blood from subinvolution will result in infection or anaemia and lack of energy, conditions that could possibly interfere with infant bonding.

Perineal haematomas

A perineal haematoma is a collection of blood in the subcutaneous layer of tissue of the perineum. The overlying skin, as a rule, is intact with no noticeable trauma. Such blood collections can be caused by injury to blood vessels in the perineum during birth. They are most likely to occur after rapid, spontaneous births and in women who have perineal varicosities. They may occur at the site of an episiotomy or laceration repair if a vein was punctured during suturing. They can cause acute discomfort, however bleeding is usually minor.

Assessment

Perineal sutures almost always give a postpartum woman some discomfort. If a woman reports severe pain in the perineal area or a feeling of pressure, inspect the perineal area for a haematoma. If one is present, it appears as an area of purplish discolouration with obvious swelling. It may be as small as 2 cm or as large as 8 cm in diameter. The area is tender to palpation. At first it may feel fluctuant, but as seepage into the area continues and tissue is drawn taut, it palpates as a firm globe (see Fig. 25.2).

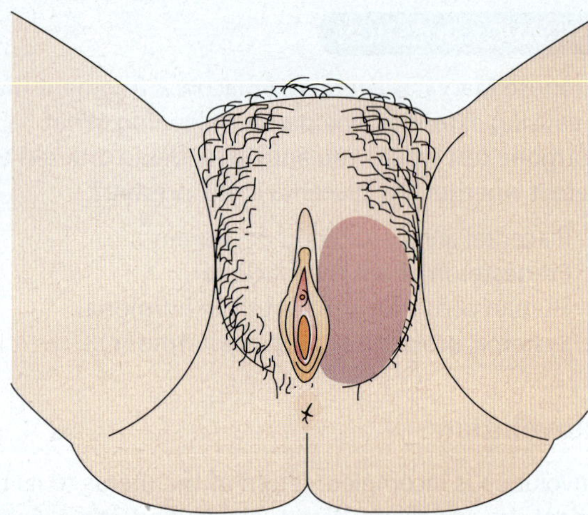

FIGURE 25.2 Appearance of a perineal haematoma from a bleeding subcutaneous vessel.

Therapeutic management

Report the presence of a haematoma, its size and the degree of the woman's discomfort to her primary care provider. Assess the size by measuring it in centimetres with each inspection. Administer analgesia as ordered for pain relief. Applying an ice pack (covered to prevent thermal injury to the skin) may prevent further bleeding. Usually the haematoma is absorbed over the next 3 or 4 days. If the haematoma is large when discovered or continues to increase in size, the woman may have to have the site incised and the bleeding vessel ligated under local anaesthesia. In most women, haematomas absorb over the next 6 weeks, causing no further difficulty.

POSTPARTUM INFECTION

Infection of the reproductive tract is another leading cause of maternal mortality (Edmonds, 2012). When caring for a woman who has any of the conditions described in Box 25.2, be aware that the risk of postpartum infection is greatly increased. Postpartum or puerperal genital infections disrupt recovery from childbirth, bonding and breastfeeding.

Theoretically, the uterus is sterile during pregnancy and until the membranes rupture. After rupture, pathogens can invade. The risk of infection is even greater if tissue oedema and trauma are present. If infection occurs, the prognosis for complete recovery depends on:

- Virulence of the invading organism
- The woman's general health
- Portal of entry
- Degree of uterine involution at the time of the microorganism invasion
- Presence of lacerations in the reproductive tract.

If a postpartum infection is not recognised and treated promptly it can infiltrate other sites through venous lymphatic pathways and increase the risk of serious sepsis (Karsnitz, 2013). A localised infection is able to spread to involve the peritoneum **(peritonitis)** or the circulatory system (septicaemia). These conditions can be fatal to a woman whose body is already stressed from childbirth. Many postpartum infections commence after a woman is discharged so maternal education of danger signs such as temperature over 38°C orally or offensive smelling lochia are important (Karsnitz, 2013).

BOX 25.2 ✻ Conditions that increase a woman's risk of postpartum infection

1. Rupture of the membranes more than 24 hours before birth (bacteria may have started to invade the uterus while the fetus was still in utero)
2. Placental fragments retained within the uterus (the tissue necroses and serves as an excellent bed for bacterial growth)
3. Postpartum haemorrhage (the woman's general condition is weakened)
4. Pre-existing anaemia (the body's defence against infection is lowered)
5. Prolonged and difficult labour, particularly instrument births (trauma to the tissue may leave lacerations or fissures for easy portals of entry for infection)
6. Internal fetal heart monitoring (contamination may have been introduced with placement of the scalp electrode)
7. Local vaginal infection was present at the time of birth (direct spread of infection has occurred)
8. The uterus was explored after birth for a retained placenta or abnormal bleeding site (infection was introduced with exploration)

Management for postpartum infection focuses on the use of an appropriate antibiotic after culture and sensitivity testing of the isolated organism. Organisms commonly cultured postpartum include group B streptococci and aerobic gram-negative bacilli such as *Escherichia coli*. Staphylococcal infections also are becoming more common. Staphylococcal infections are the cause of toxic shock syndrome, an infection similar to puerperal infection in its ability to cause death and morbidity (see Chapter 47).

Instruct a postpartum woman in proper perineal care, including wiping from front to back so that she does not bring *E. coli* organisms forwards from the rectum. Use good handwashing technique before, during and after any care to prevent cross-contamination. When administering perineal care, both wash your hands and wear gloves.

Intravenous antibiotics are usually prescribed for a postpartum infection. Frequently used antibiotics include ampicillin, gentamicin and third-generation cephalosporins such as cefotaxime. If the woman will be continuing medication at home, stress that she must take the full course to prevent the infection from recurring. Be certain that women who are breastfeeding are not prescribed antibiotics incompatible with breastfeeding. Alert them to observe for problems in their infant, such as white plaques or thrush (oral *Candida*) in their infant's mouth. This occurs because a portion of the maternal antibiotic passes into breast milk and can cause an overgrowth of fungal organisms (opportunistic infection) in the infant. The infant should also be assessed for easy bruising. A decrease of microorganisms in the bowel caused by an antibiotic passed in breast milk may lead to insufficient vitamin K formation and, consequently, decreased blood-clotting ability.

Endometritis

Endometritis is an infection of the endometrium, the lining of the uterus (Jones & Henderson, 2011). Bacteria gain access to the uterus through the vagina and enter the uterus either at the time of birth or during the postpartum period. This may occur with any birth, but the infection is usually associated with chorioamnionitis and caesarean birth (Black, Hinson & Duff, 2012).

Assessment

A benign temperature elevation may occur on the first postpartum day, particularly if a woman is not drinking enough fluid. The fever of endometritis usually manifests within 2 to 4 days postpartum, suggesting that much of the invasion occurred during labour or birth (consistent with the time it takes for infectious organisms to grow). Endometritis can also present up to 6 weeks postpartum. Normally, the white blood cell count of a postpartum woman is increased to 20,000 to 30,000 cells/mm^3. Because of this increase, the conventional method of detecting infection (elevated white blood cell count) is not of great value in the puerperium.

Infection should be suspected in all postpartum women with a temperature >38°C. Other signs and symptoms include uterine tenderness, purulent discharge and subinvolution; however, the symptoms may be vague and indistinct (Karsnitz, 2013). Because many women are at home when elevated temperatures occur, any woman who feels as if she has an increased temperature should measure her temperature to be certain.

Depending on the severity of the infection, a woman may have accompanying chills, loss of appetite and general malaise. Her uterus usually is not well-contracted and is painful to the touch. She may feel strong afterpains. Lochia usually is dark brown and has a foul odour. It may be increased in amount because of poor uterine involution, but if the infection is accompanied by high fever, lochia may be scant or absent. Ultrasound may be ordered to confirm the presence of placental fragments that are a possible cause of the infection.

Therapeutic management

Treatment of endometritis consists of the administration of an appropriate antibiotic, such as clindamycin as determined by a culture of the lochia. Be sure to obtain the culture from the vagina, using a sterile swab, rather than from a perineal pad, to ensure that you are culturing the endometrial infectious organism and not an unrelated one from the pad. An oxytocic agent such as ergometrine may be prescribed to encourage uterine contraction. Additional fluid is required to combat fever and analgesics for strong afterpains.

As with any infection, endometritis can be best controlled if it is discovered early. If you can interpret the normal colour, quantity and odour of lochia discharge and the size, consistency and tenderness of a normal postpartum uterus, you may be the first person to recognise that infection is present. Because a woman may be at home when signs of infection occur, teaching about the signs and symptoms of endometritis is essential.

If the infection is limited to the endometrium, the course of infection is about 7 to 10 days. Endometritis can lead to tubal scarring and interference with future fertility. At a future time, if the woman desires more children, she may need a fertility assessment; with mild endometritis this is usually not a problem.

What if...

Mary tells you she has developed chills and a fever of 41.6°C on her second postpartum day? Her lochia is dark brown and foul smelling. On palpation, you notice her abdomen is very tender. What should you do next?

Infection of the perineum

If a woman has a suture line on her perineum from an episiotomy or a laceration repair, a portal of entry exists for bacterial invasion.

Assessment

Infections of the perineum usually remain localised. They are revealed by symptoms similar to those of any suture-line infection, such as pain, heat and a feeling of pressure. The woman may or may not have an elevated temperature, depending on the systemic effect and spread of the infection. Inspection of the suture line reveals the inflammation. One or two stitches may be sloughed away, or an area of the suture line may be open with purulent drainage present (see Fig. 25.3). Notify the woman's doctor or midwife of the localised symptoms and culture the discharge using a sterile cotton-tipped applicator touched to the secretions.

Therapeutic management

Typically, a systemic or topical antibiotic is ordered even before the culture report is returned. An analgesic may be prescribed to alleviate discomfort. It may be necessary to remove perineal sutures, to open the area and allow for drainage. Packing may be placed in the open lesion to keep it open and allow drainage. Sitz baths or moist warm

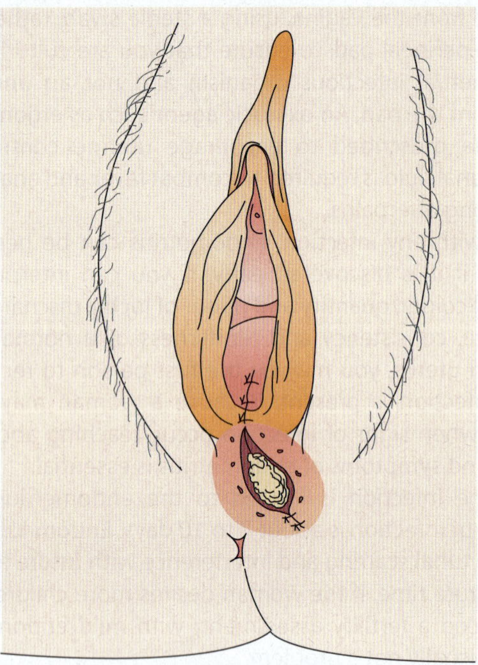

FIGURE 25.3 An infected suture line appears reddened and oedematous and often contains infected secretions.

compresses may be ordered to hasten drainage and cleanse the area. Remind the woman to change perineal pads frequently, because they are contaminated by drainage. If they are left in place too long, they might cause vaginal contamination or reinfection. Be certain a woman wipes from front to back after a bowel movement, to prevent bringing faeces forwards onto the healing area.

Puerperal sepsis (obstetric sepsis)

Puerperal sepsis is defined as genital tract infection occurring in the 42 days postpartum and accompanied by fever >38°C lasting more than 24 hours accompanied by one or more of the following signs: pelvic pain; abnormal vaginal discharge; abnormal odour; or delay in involution (Karsnitz, 2013). The symptoms of puerperal sepsis normally appear 24 or more hours after birth. Puerperal sepsis often commences with endometritis which has extend into the peritoneal cavity and cause parametritis (infection of the pelvic peritoneum) which causes peritonitis (infection of the peritoneal cavity) and septicaemia (infection of the blood). It is one of the gravest complications of childbearing and is a major cause of death from puerperal infection. The infection spreads through the lymphatic system or directly through the fallopian tubes or uterine wall to the peritoneal cavity. An abscess may form in the cul-de-sac of Douglas, because this is the lowest point of the peritoneal cavity and gravity causes infected material to localise there.

A New Zealand study found obstetric sepsis was one of the three most common reasons for women to be admitted to hospital with severe acute maternal morbidity. In many cases the illness could potentially have been less serious if carers had recognised the serious and complex nature of the condition and acted promptly (Sadler et al., 2013). Puerperal sepsis is a serious infection and if the causative organism is Group A streptococcus (GAS), *Streptococcus pyogenes*, the rates of morbidity and mortality are high; if sepsis occurs (streptococcal toxic shock syndrome) the mortality rate approaches 30–50% (Anderson, 2014).

Assessment

Symptoms of peritonitis are the same as those of a surgical patient in whom a peritoneal infection develops: rigid abdomen, abdominal pain, high fever, rapid pulse, vomiting and the appearance of being acutely ill. A rigid abdomen (guarding) is one of the first symptoms of peritonitis. Symptoms of sepsis are a low systolic blood pressure, tachycardia, fever, altered mental status and oliguria; women with septicaemia may progress to septic shock (Miller, 2014).

Therapeutic management

Peritonitis is often accompanied by paralytic ileus (blockage of inflamed intestines). This requires insertion of a nasogastric tube to prevent vomiting and rest the bowel. Intravenous fluid or total parenteral nutrition may be necessary. A woman will need analgesics for pain relief. Large doses of antibiotics will be administered to treat the infection. With effective antibiotic therapy, the outcome is usually good, however peritonitis can result in infertility through scarring and adhesions in the peritoneum. Septicaemia is treated by broad spectrum antibiotics, fluid resuscitation and vasopressors to treat hypotension (Miller, 2014).

THROMBOPHLEBITIS

Phlebitis is inflammation of the lining of a blood vessel. **Thrombophlebitis** is inflammation with the formation of blood clots. Thrombophlebitis is classified as superficial vein disease (SVD) or deep vein thrombosis (DVT). When thrombophlebitis occurs in the postpartum period, it tends to occur with the following:

- A woman's fibrinogen level is still elevated from pregnancy, leading to increased blood clotting
- Dilatation of lower extremity veins is still present as a result of pressure of the fetal head during pregnancy and birth
- The relative inactivity of the period or a prolonged time spent in delivery or birthing room stirrups leads to pooling, stasis and clotting of blood in the lower extremities
- Obesity from increased weight before pregnancy and pregnancy weight gain can lead to relative inactivity and lack of exercise
- Cigarette smoking (nicotine causes vasoconstriction and reduces blood flow)
- Pre-existing varicose veins

BOX 25.3 * Focus on family teaching

Preventing thrombophlebitis

Q. Mary Blackhawk tells you, "My sister got thrombophlebitis after the birth of her first baby. How can I prevent that from happening to me?"

A. Here are a few helpful hints for preventing thrombophlebitis:

- Ask your primary care provider if you can use a side-lying or back-lying (supine recumbent) position for birth, rather than a lithotomy position (lithotomy position can increase the tendency for pooling of blood in the lower extremities).
- If you will be using a lithotomy position, ask for padding on the stirrups to prevent calf pressure.
- Drink adequate fluids to be certain you're not dehydrated (6–8 glasses of fluid/day).
- Do not sit with your knees bent sharply and avoid wearing constricting clothing such as knee-high stockings.
- Ambulate as soon after birth as you are able. Early ambulation is the best preventive measure. When resting in bed, wiggle your toes or do leg lifts to improve venous return.
- Ask your primary care provider if they recommend support stockings in the immediate postpartal period. Be certain to put these on before ambulating in the morning, before leg veins fill.
- Quit smoking as this is associated with the development of thrombophlebitis.

- Postpartum infection
- History of previous thrombophlebvitis
- Age greater than 35 years or increased parity
- High incidence of thrombophlebitis in the family medical history.

Venous stasis should be avoided. If a woman had varicose veins during pregnancy, wearing support stockings for the first 2 weeks after birth can help increase venous circulation. (For further information on preventing thrombophlebitis see Box 25.3.)

Femoral thrombophlebitis

Femoral thrombophlebitis involves the femoral, saphenous or popliteal veins. Although the inflammation site in thrombophlebitis is a vein, an accompanying arterial spasm often occurs, diminishing arterial circulation to a leg as well. This decreased circulation, along with oedema, gives the leg a white or drained appearance.

If femoral thrombophlebitis develops, temperature is elevated and chills, pain, redness and swelling occur in the affected leg about 10 days after birth. Homans' sign (pain in the calf of the leg on dorsiflexion of the foot) may be positive; however, a negative Homans' sign does not rule out obstruction. The diameter of the leg at thigh or calf level may be increased compared with the other leg. Doppler ultrasound or contrast venography is usually ordered to confirm the diagnosis (O'Connor et al., 2011).

Therapeutic management

Treatment consists of bed rest with the affected leg elevated, administration of anticoagulants and application of moist heat (to decrease inflammation). Never massage the skin over the clot; this could loosen the clot, causing a pulmonary or cerebral embolism. Heat supplied by a moist, warm compress can help decrease inflammation.

The pain of thrombophlebitis is usually severe enough to require administration of an analgesic. An appropriate antibiotic to reduce the initial infection is prescribed. Often, an anticoagulant (coumarin derivative or heparin) or a thrombolytic agent such as streptokinase or urokinase is prescribed to dissolve the clot through the activation of fibrinolytic precursors and prevent further clot formation. Blood coagulation levels to determine the effectiveness of the medication are measured daily before administration of the anticoagulant. Depending on the medication prescribed, a baseline activated partial thromboplastin time (aPTT) or prothrombin time (PT) is obtained.

Heparin, an anticoagulant, can be administered by continuous intravenous infusion or intermittently by intravenous or subcutaneous injection. If a woman will be discharged on subcutaneous therapy, be certain she has demonstrated good injection technique before discharge and understands the importance of required blood tests (coagulation studies) so that she schedules these appropriately. Protamine sulfate, the antagonist for heparin, should be readily available any time heparin is administered. (For further information on heparin see Box 25.4.)

A woman can continue to breastfeed while receiving heparin because due to its high molecular weight it is not excreted in the breast milk. Warfarin is also safe during breastfeeding because very little medication crosses into the breast milk. If warfarin is continued postpartum close monitoring through an anticoagulant clinic is warranted. Lochia is usually increased in a woman who is receiving anticoagulants and will need to be monitored.

Pulmonary embolus

During pregnancy and the postpartum period women are at increased risk of thrombosis due to hypercoagulability (Morris, Algert & Roberts, 2010). A pulmonary embolus is obstruction of the pulmonary artery by a blood clot; it usually occurs as a complication of thrombophelebitis when a blood clots moves from a leg vein to the pulmonary artery (Henzler et al., 2012). The signs of pulmonary embolus are: sudden, sharp chest pain; tachypnoea; tachycardia; orthopnoea (inability to breathe except in an upright position); and cyanosis (the blood clot is obstructing the pulmonary artery, blocking blood flow to the lungs and return to the heart). It is an emergency. A woman needs oxygen administered immediately and is at high risk of cardiopulmonary arrest. Because of the seriousness of this condition, a woman with a pulmonary embolism is commonly transferred to an intensive care unit for continuing care. Her condition requires careful monitoring until the

BOX 25.4 ✻ Focus on pharmacology

Heparin calcium injection (calciparin) or enoxaparin (low-molecular-weight heparin)

Classification: Heparin is an anticoagulant.

Action: Heparin blocks the conversion of prothrombin to thrombin and of fibrinogen to fibrin, decreasing clotting ability and resulting in the inhibition of thrombus and clot formation. It is used to prevent and treat thrombosis and pulmonary embolism (McKenna & Mirkov, 2014).

Pregnancy risk category: B

Dosage: Dosage is dependent on coagulation studies. Dosage is considered therapeutic when the activated partial thromboplastin time (aPTT) is 1.5 to 3 times the control value. The medication can be given by continuous intravenous (IV) infusion or by intermittent direct IV or subcutaneous injection.

Possible adverse effects: haemorrhage, bruising, thrombocytopenia, urticaria

Nursing implications

- Obtain baseline coagulation studies as ordered.
- Continue to monitor aPTT results and adjust dosage as ordered. Obtain aPTT results 30 minutes before intermittent dosage administration or every 4 hours for continuous IV infusion.
- Anticipate use of an intermittent infusion device to minimise the number of intravenous injections.
- Avoid any intramuscular injection of other medications, because a haematoma may form at injection site.
- When administering an IV infusion, do not add heparin to existing IV solutions or piggyback other medications into a heparin infusion. Use an infusion pump.
- When administering heparin subcutaneously, inject deeply and rotate injection sites. Do not aspirate for blood return or massage the injection site afterwards. Apply direct pressure to the injection site after administration. Inspect the injection site for signs of haematoma formation.
- Assess for signs and symptoms of bleeding, such as oozing from the gums, nosebleeds, haematuria, or frank or occult blood in stool.
- Closely monitor lochia, including amount and colour. Assess pad count to determine extent of vaginal bleeding.
- Keep protamine sulfate, the antidote, readily available in case of overdose.
- Instruct about antibleeding precautions such as using a soft toothbrush to minimise the risk of gum bleeding.

clot is lysed or adheres to the pulmonary artery wall and is reabsorbed.

MASTITIS

Mastitis (infection of the breast) may occur as early as the seventh postpartum day or not until the baby is weeks or months old (Crepinsek et al., 2012). The organism causing the infection usually enters through cracked and fissured nipples. Therefore, measures that prevent cracked and fissured nipples also help prevent mastitis. These measures include:

- Making certain the baby is positioned correctly and latching, includes both nipple and areola
- Releasing a baby's grasp on the nipple before removing the baby from the breast
- Washing hands between handling perineal pads and touching the breasts
- Exposing nipples to air for at least part of every day
- If a woman has one cracked and one well nipple, encourage her to begin breastfeeding (when the infant sucks most forcefully) on the unaffected nipple.

Assessment

Mastitis is usually unilateral, the affected breast is painful, swollen and reddened. Fever accompanies these first symptoms within hours.

Therapeutic management

Treatment consists of antibiotics effective against penicillin-resistant staphylococci such as dicloxacillin or a cephalosporin (Summers, 2011). Breastfeeding is continued, because keeping the breast emptied of milk helps to prevent growth of bacteria. Some women find an infected breast too painful to allow their infant to suck and prefer to express milk manually from the affected breast until their antibiotic has taken effect and the mastitis has diminished (about 3 days). Cold or ice compresses and a good supportive bra help with pain relief until the condition improves. Warm, wet compresses may be ordered to reduce inflammation and oedema.

If therapy is started as soon as symptoms are apparent, the condition runs a short course of about 2 or 3 days. If left untreated, a breast infection can become a localised abscess. This may involve a large portion of the breast and rupture through the skin, with thick, purulent drainage, necessitating incision and drainage of the abscess. If an abscess forms, breastmilk is expressed from that breast and breastfeeding ceased until the abscess has resolved. Some women find that the infected breast is too tender to do this. They can be reassured that formula feeding is an acceptable alternative for their child.

Neither mastitis nor breast abscess leave any permanent breast disease. A woman can be assured that such an incident is not associated with development of breast cancer and does not interfere with future breastfeeding potential.

URINARY SYSTEM DISORDERS

Because a woman's bladder is compressed by the infant's head during birth, several urinary tract disorders can occur.

Urinary retention

Urinary retention occurs when the bladder is unable to empty completely (Mulder et al., 2012). After childbirth, bladder sensation for voiding is decreased because of bladder oedema caused by the pressure of birth. Unable to empty, the bladder fills to over-distension. When the woman does void, instead of emptying completely, the bladder empties only a small portion of its contents (retention with overflow). As a result, it becomes over-distended again. Bladder over-distension is potentially serious. If it is allowed to continue, permanent damage may occur from loss of bladder tone, leading to permanent incontinence (Humburg et al., 2011).

Assessment

Urinary retention is associated with the use of anaesthesia, especially epidural anaesthesia (Mulder et al., 2012). In a postpartum woman, urinary retention with overflow may be more difficult to detect than primary or simple over-distension. With primary over-distension a woman does not void at all. A longer-than-usual time (8 hours) passes after the birth or between voids. Assessment by percussion, palpation or a bladder scanner reveals bladder distension. With urinary retention and overflow a woman is able to void. Voiding is very frequent, however, and in small amounts; her overall output is inadequate. Always measure the amount of a woman's first voiding after birth. As a rule, if this voiding is less than 100 mL, suspect urinary retention.

Urinary retention is confirmed by catheterising a woman immediately after she voids. If residual urine is greater than 100 mL, the woman has retention of more than the normal amount. An indwelling catheter may be required. This can be difficult in the early postpartum period due to pain and oedema. More than 800 mL should not be removed from the bladder at any one time. Often after 24 hours the indwelling catheter is clamped for a short time and then removed. Voiding should occur within 4 to 6 hours.

Urinary tract infection

A woman who is catheterised at the time of childbirth or during the postpartum period is prone to development of a urinary tract infection, because bacteria may be introduced into the bladder at the time of catheterisation.

Assessment

If a urinary tract infection develops, a woman notices symptoms of burning on urination, possibly blood in the urine (haematuria) and a feeling of frequency or that she always has to void. The pain is so sharp on voiding that she may resist voiding, further compounding the problem of urinary stasis. She may also have a low-grade fever and discomfort from lower abdominal pain. Obtain a clean-catch urine specimen from any woman with symptoms of urinary tract infection. Avoid contamination of the urine with lochia if possible by covering the vaginal area.

Therapeutic management

Although sulfa drugs are normally prescribed for urinary tract infection, they are contraindicated for breastfeeding women because they can cause neonatal jaundice. Typically, therefore, a broad-spectrum antibiotic such as amoxicillin or ampicillin will be prescribed to treat postpartum urinary tract infections. An antibiotic compatible with breastfeeding should be prescribed.

Encourage a woman to drink large amounts of fluid (a glass every hour) to help flush the infection from her bladder. She may need an oral analgesic, such as paracetamol to reduce the pain of urination for the next few times she voids until the antibiotic begins to have an effect and the burning sensation disappears.

Although symptoms of urinary tract infection decrease quickly, be certain a woman understands the importance of continuing to take the prescribed antibiotic for the full 5 to 7 days to eradicate the infection completely. Be certain she is aware of common methods all women should use to prevent urinary tract infections.

> ***What if...***
>
> It has been approximately 7 hours since Mary Blackhawk gave birth and she still has not voided? What should you do next?

REPRODUCTIVE SYSTEM DISORDERS

Pregnancy may leave reproductive system organs weakened or displaced, especially in women with grand multiparity or an instrumental birth.

Reproductive tract displacement

If the support systems of the uterus are weakened because of pregnancy, the ligaments may no longer be able to maintain the uterus in its usual position or level after pregnancy. Problems of retroflexion, anteflexion, retroversion and anteversion or prolapse of the uterus may occur. These uterine displacement disorders may interfere with future childbearing and fertility and may cause continued pain or a feeling of lower abdominal heaviness or discomfort.

If the walls of the vagina are weakened, a cystocoele (outpouching of the bladder into the vaginal wall) or a rectocoele (outpouching of the rectum into the vaginal wall) may occur. These are identified on pelvic exam or by ultrasound (Chantarasorn & Dietz, 2012). These problems tend to develop most frequently in women with a high parity and after a forceps birth. Surgery to repair such conditions may be necessary. If stress incontinence (involuntary voiding on exertion) occurs, Kegel exercises to strengthen perineal muscles, injections of bulking agents, or Botox may be helpful (Elser, 2012).

Separation of the symphysis pubis

During pregnancy many women feel some discomfort at the symphysis pubis because of relaxation of the joint preparatory to birth. If a fetus is unusually large or fetal position is not optimal, the ligaments of the symphysis pubis may be so stretched by birth that they actually tear. After birth, the woman experiences acute pain on turning or walking; her legs tend to rotate externally, giving her a waddling gait. A defect over the symphysis pubis can be palpated; the area is swollen and tender to touch (Nitsche & Howell, 2011).

Bed rest and the application of a snug pelvic binder to immobilise the joint are necessary to relieve pain and allow healing. As with all ligament injuries, a 4–6-week period is necessary for healing to take place. During this time, a woman may need to arrange for a person to help her with childcare at home. She should avoid heavy lifting for an extended period, until healing in the pubic ligaments is complete. She may be advised to consider caesarean birth for any future pregnancy.

EMOTIONAL AND PSYCHOLOGICAL COMPLICATIONS OF THE POSTPARTUM PERIOD

Any woman who is extremely stressed or who gives birth to an infant who in any way does not meet her expectations such as being the wrong sex, being physically or cognitively challenged, or being ill may have difficulty bonding with her infant. Inability to bond is a postpartum complication with far-reaching implications, possibly affecting the future health of the entire family.

A woman whose child is born with an illness or is physically challenged

If possible, it is important for the parents to care for the child during the postpartum period, so that they have an opportunity to touch, relate to and bond with the infant. Many women wait until their support person is present to visit an intensive care nursery, so that visiting their newborn is a family activity. Open lines of communication between the parents and the hospital staff that allow for free discussion of feelings and fears will do much to strengthen parent–child relationship and prepare for future hospitalisations or care of the child.

A woman whose newborn has died

A woman whose newborn dies at birth always has questions about what happened. She is likely to feel bewildered, perhaps bitter and resentful that the hospital staff could not save her child. "Why me? Of all the women here, why did my baby die?" She needs concerned support from healthcare personnel to help her through the crisis initiated by such a devastating loss.

Most women wish to see their baby and this may assist the beginning of the grieving process. Wrap the baby and let the parents have time with the infant. Photographs should be taken and kept for the parents. Be familiar with the forms the mother or father have to sign when a baby dies or is stillborn. Most parents wish to name their baby and a box of mementoes including footprints, a lock of hair and a birth card should be made and presented to parents as well as written information about what to expect. A private room is required where family can visit freely. The process of grieving and the support a woman requires at this time is further discussed in Chapter 56.

Postpartum depression

Many women notice changes in their feelings and mood following birth. The common and transient baby blues affect around 80% of women and generally last from 1–2 days. The baby blues are characterised by weepiness or laughing for no apparent reason, feeling anxious and difficulty sleeping. This is probably a normal response related to hormonal shifts as the levels of oestrogen, progesterone and gonadotropin-releasing hormone in her body change.

In as many as 20% of women, these normal feelings continue beyond the immediate postpartum period and may even be present for longer than 1 year. The sensations of overwhelming sadness can interfere with breastfeeding, childcare and returning to work (see Box 25.5). In addition to an overall feeling of sadness, a woman may notice extreme fatigue, an inability to stop crying, increased anxiety about her own or her infant's health, insecurity (unwillingness to be left alone or inability to make decisions), psychosomatic symptoms (nausea and vomiting, diarrhoea) and either depressive or manic mood fluctuations. Depression of this kind is termed **postpartum depression** and reflects a more serious problem than normal baby blues (Table 25.3). Risk factors for postpartum depression include a history of depression, a troubled childhood, low self-esteem, stress in the home or

BOX 25.5 ✻ Focus on evidence-based practice

Postpartum depression

To investigate the effect of intention to breastfeed on postpartum depression researchers analysed Edinburgh Postnatal Depression Scale responses and intention to breastfeed during pregnancy. The outcomes of women who intended to breastfeed were compared with those of women who did not intend to breastfeed. The study found most mothers who had no symptoms of depression before birth and who breastfed as intended had a decreased risk of postpartum depression; but women who planned to breastfeed and did not breastfeed were more depressed. Maternal-infant bonding can be compromised by postnatal depression.

What interventions could you use with postpartum women who had expressed an intention to breastfeed during their pregnancy to help them feel confident about breastfeeding?

Source: Borra, C., Iacovou, M. & Sevilla, A. (2015). New evidence on breastfeeding and postpartum depression: The importance of understanding women's intentions. *Maternal & Child Health Journal*, *19*(4), 897–907.

TABLE 25.3 Comparing postpartum blues, depression and psychosis

	Postpartum blues	Postpartum depression	Postpartum psychosis
Onset	1–10 days after birth	1–12 months after birth	Within first year after birth
Symptoms	Sadness, tears	Anxiety, feeling of loss, sadness	Delusions or hallucinations of harming infant or self
Incidence	70% of all births	10% of all births	1%–2% of all births
Aetiology (possible)	Probable hormonal changes, stress of life changes	History of previous depression, hormonal response, lack of social support	Possible activation of previous mental illness, hormonal changes, family history of bipolar disorder
Therapy	Support, empathy	Counselling, drug therapy	Psychotherapy, drug therapy
Nursing role	Offer compassion and understanding	Refer to counselling	Refer to psychiatric care, safeguarding mother from injury to self or to newborn

at work and lack of effective support people. Different expectations between partners (if a woman wants a child and her partner does not) or disappointment in the child (a boy instead of a girl) could also play a role.

A number of depression scales to help detect postpartum depression are available but conscientious observation and discussion with women can reveal symptoms as well. A woman may need counselling and possibly antidepressant therapy to integrate the experience of childbirth into her life (Kurzweil, 2012). This is crucial to development of a healthy maternal-infant bond, to the health of any other children in the family and to overall family functioning. Ask at postpartum return visits and well-child visits about symptoms that would suggest depression and recommend an appropriate referral. Support is available from:

- beyondblue <www.beyondblue.org.au>,
- Post and Antenatal Depression Association Inc. (PANDA) <www.panda.org.au>
- SANE <www.sane.org>.

BOX 25.6 ✻ Focus on family teaching

Q. Mary asks you, "How can I avoid becoming depressed after I return home with my new baby?"

A. Some helpful guidelines are:

- Plan a balanced program of nutrition, exercise and sleep. Plan meals that are easy to prepare; sleep whenever your baby sleeps; begin a program of walking daily with your baby.
- Share your feelings with a support person. Many communities have postpartum support groups to help with this.
- Take some time every day to do something for yourself (work on a scrapbook, go shopping so you have a break from baby care.
- Do not try to be perfect. Analyse what are the important things to do and get them done. Let unimportant things go for another day.
- Do not let yourself be isolated by baby care. Use the internet or telephone to keep in contact with your friends so you are not lonely.

Almost all women experience some fatigue after childbirth. As many as 70% experience a temporary feeling of sadness (baby blues). About 10%, however, develop depression severe enough to need therapy. Be sure to ask enough questions to be certain that a woman's crying is not something more serious than simple baby blues before she is discharged from the healthcare facility. In this way, a woman who has more serious problems can be referred to the proper professionals for help and support. (For more information on preventing postpartum depression see Box 25.6.)

Postpartum psychosis

Postpartum psychosis is rare, occurring in 1–2 women per 1000 and involves a loss of touch with reality, which may present as hallucinations, delusions, illogical thoughts, anxiety and agitation. The majority of these women have had symptoms of mental illness before pregnancy. A woman with a postpartum psychosis may deny that she has had a child and, when the child is brought to her, insist that she was never pregnant. She may voice thoughts of infanticide or that her infant is possessed. Postpartum psychosis requires immediate assessment. Treatment includes medication, counselling and support.

CASE STUDY QUESTION

4. Which statement by Mary is most suggestive of a woman developing postpartum psychosis?
   a. "I wish my baby had more hair."
   b. "My baby has the devil's eyes."
   c. "I feel exhausted since birth."
   d. "Breastfeeding is harder than I thought."

Key points for review

- Establishing a strong family–newborn relationship may be difficult when a woman has a postpartum complication. Investigate ways that will allow a woman to care for her baby or offer necessary support to family members so that they can fulfil this role.

- Haemorrhage (defined as a loss of blood greater than 500 mL within a 24-hour period) is a major potential danger in the immediate postpartum period. The most frequent cause of postpartum haemorrhage is uterine atony. Continuous limited blood loss can be as important over time as sudden, intense bleeding. With haemorrhage, administration of oxytocin may be necessary to initiate uterine contraction and halt the bleeding.
- Other causes of haemorrhage include lacerations (vaginal, cervical or perineal) and retained placental fragments. Lacerations are most apt to occur with forceps birth or with the birth of a large infant. Disseminated intravascular coagulation can also cause postpartum haemorrhage.
- Postpartum infection (a temperature greater than 38°C) is a potential complication after any birth until the denuded placental surface has healed. Retained placental fragments and the use of internal fetal heart monitoring leads are potential sources of infection.
- Thrombophlebitis, an inflammation of the lining of a blood vessel, occurs most often as an extension of an endometrial infection. Therapy includes bed rest with moist heat applications and anticoagulant therapy. Never massage the leg of a woman with thrombophlebitis; doing so can cause the clot to move and become a pulmonary embolus, a possibly fatal complication.
- Mastitis is infection of the breast. The symptoms include pain, swelling and redness. Antibiotic medication is necessary.
- Urinary retention resulting in an over-distended bladder requires monitoring and treatment to avoid complications including infection. A bladder scanner is useful to assess bladder distension. If a urinary tract infection occurs women should increase fluid intake, complete prescribed antibiotics and take measures to prevent reinfection.
- Perineal exercises should be encouraged to prevent and treat stress incontinence. Instrumental birth may stretch ligaments and result in cystocoele or rectocele.
- A woman whose child is born with a physical or cognitive challenge needs special consideration after birth. This is obviously a time of stress and a woman needs supportive nursing care.
- Postpartum "blues" are a normal accompaniment to birth. Postpartum depression (a feeling of extreme sadness) and postpartum psychosis (an actual separation from reality) are not normal and need accurate assessment so a woman can receive adequate therapy for these conditions.

CASE STUDY QUESTIONS

5. Mary was having heavy vaginal bleeding at 4 hours after birth. Because she was sleeping, however, she was totally unaware of it. What action on your part would have prevented so much blood loss? What action would be most appropriate now?
6. Eight hours after birth, Mary tells you that she has frequency and burning on urination. She had a urinary tract infection during pregnancy, so she recognises the symptoms. She has some medicine left from pregnancy and tells you that she will take it to cure the infection. What advice would you give her?
7. When Mary returns for a postpartum check-up, you notice red streaks on both legs along the course of her veins and she has pain on dorsiflexion of her foot. You are concerned that she is developing thrombophlebitis. Describe a plan of care that could have reduced this risk during labour and in the immediate postpartum period.

Resources

For an extensive range of additional resources to enhance teaching and learning and to facilitate understanding of this chapter, please see the text's accompanying website located on thePoint at http://thepoint.lww.com.

References

American Congress of Obstetricians & Gynecologists [ACOG]: Committee on Obstetric Practice. (2012). Committee opinion no. 529: Placenta accreta. *Obstetrics & Gynecology, 120*(1), 207–211.

Anderson, B. L. (2014). Puerperal Group A Streptococcal Infection. *Obstetrics & Gynecology, 123*(4), 874–882.

Balayla, J. & Bondarenko, H. D. (2012). Placenta accreta and the risk of adverse maternal and neonatal outcomes. *Journal of Perinatal Medicine, 15*(12), 1–9.

Black, L. P., Hinson, L. & Duff, P. (2012). Limited course of antibiotic treatment for chorioamnionitis. *Obstetrics & Gynecology, 119*(6), 1102–1105.

Brodribb, W., Zadoroznyj, M. & Dane, A. (2013). The views of mothers and GPs about postpartum care in Australian general practice. *BMC Family Practice, 14*(1), 1–9.

Brown, A. & Jordan, S. (2012). Impact of birth complications on breastfeeding duration: An internet survey. *Journal of Advanced Nursing, 69*(4), 828–839.

Bryant, A., Mhyre, J. M., Leffert, L. R., et al. (2012). The association of maternal race and ethnicity and the risk of postpartum hemorrhage. *Anesthesia & Analgesia, 115*(5), 1127–1136.

Chantarasorn, V. & Dietz, H. P. (2012). Diagnosis of cystocele type by clinical examination and pelvic floor ultrasound. *Ultrasound in Obstetrics & Gynecology, 39*(6), 710–714.

Crepinsek, M. A., Crowe, L., Michener, K., et al. (2012). Interventions for preventing mastitis after childbirth. *Cochrane Database of Systemic Reviews*, (10), CD007239.

Edmonds, D. K. (2012). Puerperium and lactation. In D. K. Edmonds (Ed), *Dewhurst's Textbook of Obstetrics & Gynaecology* (8th ed.), pp. 365–376. Oxford: John Wiley & Son.

Elser, D. M. (2012). Stress urinary incontinence and overactive bladder syndrome: Current options and new targets for management. *Postgraduate Medicine, 124*(3), 42–49.

Furuta, M., Sandall, J. & Bick, D. (2012). A systematic review of the relationship between severe maternal morbidity and post-traumatic stress disorder. *BMC Pregnancy & Childbirth, 12*(1), 125.

Ghirardini, G., Alboni, C. & Mabrouk, M. (2012). Use of balloon tamponade in management of severe vaginal postpartum hemorrhage and vaginal hematoma: A case series. *Gynecology & Obstetric Investigation, 74*(4), 320–323.

Haran, C., Van Driel, M., Mitchell, B. L. & Brodribb, W. E. (2014). Clinical guidelines for postpartum women and infants in primary care—a systematic review. *BMC Pregnancy & Childbirth, 14*(1), 1–19.

Henzler, T., Schoenberg, S. O., Schoepf, U. J., et al. (2012). Diagnosing acute pulmonary embolism: Systematic review of evidence base and cost-effectiveness of imaging tests. *Journal of Thoracic Imaging, 27*(5), 304–314.

Humburg, J., Troeger, C., Holzgreve, W., et al. (2011). Risk factors in prolonged postpartum urinary retention. *Archives of Gynecology & Obstetrics, 283*(2), 179–183.

Jones, V. A. & Henderson, J. (2011). Gestational complications. In K. J. Hurt, M. W. Guile, J. L. Bienstock, et al. (Eds.). *The Johns Hopkins Manual of Gynecology and Obstetrics* (4th ed.), pp. 110–121. Philadelphia: Lippincott Williams & Wilkins.

Karsnitz, D. B. (2013). Puerperal infections of the genital tract: A clinical review. *Journal of Midwifery & Women's Health, 58*(6), 632–642.

Kurzweil, S. (2012). Psychodynamic therapy for depression in women with infants and young children. *American Journal of Psychotherapy, 66*(2), 181–199.

Laas, E., Bui, C., Popowski, T., et al. (2012). Trends in the rate of invasive procedures after the addition of the intrauterine tamponade test to a protocol for management of severe postpartum hemorrhage. *American Journal of Obstetrics & Gynecology, 207*(4), 281.e1–281.e7.

Martin, A., Horowitz, C., Balbierz, A. & Howell, E. (2014). Views of women and clinicians on postpartum preparation and recovery. *Maternal and Child Health Journal, 18*(3), 707–713.

McKenna, L. & Mirkov, S. (2014). *McKenna's Drug Handbook for Nursing and Midwifery* (7th ed.). Sydney: Lippincott Williams & Wilkins.

Miller, J. (2014). Surviving sepsis: A review of the latest guidelines. *Nursing, 44*(4), 24–31.

Morris, J. M., Algert, C. S. & Roberts, C. L. (2010). Incidence and risk factors for pulmonary embolism in the postpartum period. *Journal of Thrombosis & Haemostasis, 8*(5), 998–1003.

Mulder, F. E., Schoffelmeer, M. A., Hakvoort, R. A., et al. (2012). Risk factors for postpartum urinary retention: A systematic review and meta-analysis. *BJOG: International Journal of Obstetrics & Gynaecology, 119*(12), 1440–1446.

NSW Health. (2010). *Maternity – Prevention, Early Recognition & Management of Postpartum Haemorrhage (PPH)*, Policy Directive, accessed 19 January 2015, <www.health.nsw.gov.au/policies/pd/2010/pdf/PD2010_064.pdf>.

Nitsche, J. F. & Howell, T. (2011). Peripartum pubic symphysis separation: A case report and review of the literature. *Obstetrics & Gynecology Survey, 66*(3), 153–158.

O'Connor, D. J., Scher, L. A., Gargiulo, N. J. 3rd, et al. (2011). Incidence and characteristics of venous thromboembolic disease during pregnancy and the postnatal period: A contemporary series. *Annals of Vascular Surgery, 25*(1), 9–14.

Poggi, S. B. H. (2012). Postpartum hemorrhage & the abnormal puerperium. In A. H. DeCherney, L. Nathan, T. M. Goodwin, et al., (Eds.). *Current Diagnosis and Treatment: Obstetrics and Gynecology* (11th ed.), pp. 349–368. Columbus, OH: McGraw-Hill/Lange.

Royal Australian and New Zealand College of Obstetricians and Gynaecologists (RANZCOG) (2015). *Guidelines on Management of Postpartum Haemorrhage (PPH)*. Last updated May 2015; accessed 12 June 2015 from <www.ranzcog.edu.au/college-statements-guidelines.html>.

Sadler, L. C., Austin, D. M., Masson, V. L., McArthur, C. J., McLintock, C., Rhodes, S. P. & Farquhar, C. M. (2013). Review of contributory factors in maternity admissions to intensive care at a New Zealand tertiary hospital. *American Journal of Obstetrics and Gynecology, 209*(6), 549.e541–549.e547.

Summers, A. (2011). Managing mastitis in the emergency department. *Emergency Nurse, 19*(6), 22–25.

Wright, C. E., Chauhan, S. P. & Abuhamad, A. Z. (2014). Bakri Balloon in the Management of Postpartum Hemorrhage: A Review. *American Journal of Perinatology, 31*(11), 957–963.

Yonemoto, N., Dowswell, T., Nagai, S. & Mori, R. (2013). Schedules for home visits in the early postpartum period. *Cochrane Database of Systematic Reviews*, (7), CD009326.

Suggested readings

Alzahrani, H. A. A. (2014). Does episiotomy prevent perineal trauma? *MIDIRS Midwifery Digest, 24*(4), 478–483.

Cortet, M., Maucort-Boulch, D., Deneux-Tharaux, C., Dupont, C., Rudigoz, R. C., Roy, P. & Huissoud, C. (2015). Severity of post-partum hemorrhage after vaginal delivery is not predictable from clinical variables available at the time post-partum hemorrhage is diagnosed. *Journal of Obstetrics & Gynaecology Research, 41*(2), 199–206.

Faulkner, Z., English, H. & Gray, H. (2014). Breastfeeding: A focus on conditions which may affect breastfeeding in either mother or baby. *Essentially MIDIRS, 5*(7), 24–29.

Krishnan, D., Ongso, Y. & Leknys, M. (2014). Misoprostol for post-partum haemorrhage in the Australian bush. *Australian Family Physician, 43*(8), 569–570.

Lutomski, J. E., Murphy, M., Devane, D., Meaney, S. & Greene, R. A. (2014). Private health care coverage and increased risk of obstetric intervention. *BMC Pregnancy & Childbirth, 14*(1), 1–18.

Mitra, M., Iezzoni, L., Zhng, J., Long-Bellil, L., Smeltzer, S. & Barton, B. (2015). Prevalence and risk factors for postpartum depression symptoms among women with disabilities. *Maternal & Child Health Journal, 19*(2), 362–372.

Rafferty, L. (2013). Well informed midwives can help: Perinatal mental health. *Practising Midwife, 16*(6), 35 37.

Rikard-Bell, J., Iyer, J. & Rane, A. (2014). Perineal outcome and the risk of pelvic floor dysfunction: A cohort study of primiparous women. *Australian & New Zealand Journal of Obstetrics & Gynaecology, 54*(4), 371–376.

Thompson, R. & Miller, Y. D. (2014). Birth control: To what extent do women report being informed and involved in decisions about pregnancy and birth procedures? *BMC Pregnancy & Childbirth, 14*(1), 1–17.

Zietlow, A. L., Schlüter, M., Nonnenmacher, N., Müller, M. & Reck, C. (2014). Maternal self-confidence postpartum and at pre-school age: The role of depression, anxiety disorders, maternal attachment insecurity. *Maternal & Child Health Journal, 18*(8), 1873–1880.

Chapter 26

Nursing care of a family with a high-risk newborn

Previous chapters described the birth and care of well newborns. This chapter adds information on care of newborns who are ill or have a significant variation in gestational age or weight. Learning to recognise these infants at birth and organising care for them can be instrumental in helping protect both their present and future health.

LEARNING OBJECTIVES

After mastering the contents of this chapter, you should be able to:

1. Define the following terms—small-for-gestational-age infant, term infant, large-for-gestational-age infant, preterm infant and postterm infant
2. Describe common illnesses that occur in these and other high-risk newborns.
3. Use critical thinking to analyse the special crisis imposed on families when alterations of newborn development or neonatal illness occur to make nursing family-centred.
4. Assess a high-risk newborn to determine whether safe transition to extrauterine life has occurred.
5. Discuss expected outcomes for a high-risk newborn and family.
6. Discuss nursing care focused on priorities to stabilise a high-risk newborn's body systems.
7. Discuss implementation of nursing care for a high-risk newborn such as monitoring body temperature.
8. Discuss expected outcomes for achievement and effectiveness of care.
9. Identify areas related to the care of high-risk newborns that could benefit from additional nursing research or application of evidence-based practice.
10. Integrate knowledge of the needs of a high-risk newborn with nursing process to achieve quality child and family health nursing care.

KEY TERMS

- apnoea
- brown fat
- fetal alcohol syndrome
- gestational age
- hyperbilirubinaemia
- intrauterine growth restriction (IUGR)
- large for gestational age (LGA)
- low-birth-weight infants
- preterm infants
- small for gestational age (SGA)
- sudden infant death syndrome (SIDS)
- vitamin K deficiency bleeding (VKDB)

CASE STUDY

Karen and Tom Atkins are the parents of a 34-week-gestation, 1-kg baby boy born last night after a short, 4-hour labour. Their baby took a few gasping breaths at birth but then stopped breathing. He was resuscitated and transported to the neonatal intensive care unit (NICU). Tom was not present for the birth because he was out of town on business. You notice that Karen has not visited the NICU to see her son. Karen feels confused and distraught and is aware that her husband is also not coping well. Tom stated to his wife that he is reluctant to visit the baby as he does not want to get too attached knowing that his son may not live much longer.

CASE STUDY QUESTION

1. What type of help do the Atkins need to better accept what has happened to them?

During pregnancy, screening women for risk factors that could lead to illness in a newborn is essential to identify infants who may need greater than usual care at birth (Pinheiro, 2009). Risk factors that could potentially be identified include: younger or older than average maternal age; concurrent disease conditions such as diabetes or human immunodeficiency virus (HIV) infection; pregnancy complications such as placenta praevia; and an unhealthy maternal lifestyle such as drug abuse. Unfortunately, not all instances of high risk can be predicted. Even a newborn from a normal pregnancy may require specialised care or develop a problem over the first few days of life necessitating special intervention. Any infant who is born before term or postterm, or who is underweight or overweight for gestational age is also at risk of complications at birth or in the first few days of life. Parents need thorough education about their baby's health because these problems may require re-hospitalisation or additional follow-up at home. Being able to predict an infant who is at high risk allows for advanced preparation so that specialised, skilled healthcare personnel can be present at the child's birth to perform necessary interventions, including resuscitating a newborn who has difficulty establishing respiration. Immediate, skilled handling of any problems that occur may help to save the newborn's life and also prevent future problems, such as neurological disorders (Kattwinkel, 2011).

FAMILY OF A HIGH-RISK NEWBORN

Assessment

All infants need to be assessed at birth for obvious congenital anomalies and **gestational age** (number of weeks they remained in utero). Both determinations can be done by the midwife who first examines an infant. For high-risk infants who require admission to the NICU continuing assessment involves cardiorespiratory monitoring, oxygen saturations and temperature. However, no matter how many monitors are used, instruments never replace the role of frequent, close, common-sense observation.

Nursing considerations

It is important to be aware of the normal assessment parameters of newborns. Nursing considerations generally centre on the following eight priority areas of care for any newborn:

- Airway clearance
- Cardiovascular tissue perfusion
- Fluid volume maintenance
- Thermoregulation
- Nutritional requirements
- Infection risk—related to lowered immune response
- Bonding difficulties
- Limited stimulation.

A goal that implies complete recovery from a major illness, for example, may be unrealistic for one newborn but completely appropriate for another. Care is planned that is individualised considering a newborn's developmental as well as physiological strengths, weaknesses and needs. This helps to ensure that parents as well as the healthcare team understand the newborn's particular care priorities and potential. Many families of high-risk newborns will need continued support to care for their infants at home. Helpful Internet sites to use for referring parents include:

- Austprem <www.austprem.com>
- National Premmies Foundation <www.prembaby.org.au>
- The Neonatal Trust New Zealand <www.neonataltrust.co.nz>
- SiDS New Zealand <www.sids.org.nz>
- sids and kids <www.sidsandkids.org>.

Care for any high-risk newborn should focus on conserving the baby's energy and providing a thermoneutral environment to prevent exhaustion and chilling. Painful procedures should be kept to a minimum to help the infant achieve a sense of comfort and balance. Assisting parents to participate in care such as skin-to-skin care, bathing or feeding their infant may help start the bonding process.

High-risk newborns need long-term follow-up so any consequences of their birth status, such as minimal neurological injury, can be identified and arrangements for special schooling or counselling can be made. Positive outcomes for an "at high risk" newborn would be:

- Infant maintains a patent airway
- Infant tolerates all procedures without accompanying apnoea
- Infant's growth and development is appropriate for gestational age, birth weight and condition
- Infant maintains body temperature at 37.0°C in an open cot with one added blanket
- Parents are supported and encouraged to make regular visits or contact with the NICU
- Parents are supported to develop positive coping skills and behaviours in response to the newborn's condition.

NEWBORN PRIORITIES IN THE FIRST DAYS OF LIFE

All newborns have eight priority needs in the first few days of life:

1. Initiation and maintenance of respiration
2. Establishment of extrauterine circulation
3. Control of body temperature
4. Intake of adequate nourishment
5. Establishment of waste elimination
6. Prevention of infection
7. Establishment of an infant–parent relationship
8. Developmental care, or care that balances physiological needs and stimulation for best development.

These are also the priority needs of high-risk newborns. Because of small size, immaturity or illness, fulfilling these needs may require special equipment or care measures. Not all newborns will be able to achieve full wellness because of extreme health disabilities at birth or difficulty adjusting to extrauterine life. Indications that a newborn is having difficulty making the transition from intrauterine to extrauterine life may be apparent during the intrapartum period, at birth, or at initial assessment because of a low Apgar score (see Chapter 18).

Initiating and maintaining respiration

Ultimately, the prognosis of a high-risk newborn depends primarily on how the first moments of life are managed. Most deaths occurring during the first 48 hours after birth result from the newborn's inability to establish or maintain adequate respiration. Australia and New Zealand have both experienced a drop in infant mortality rates in the last decade. In 2002, New Zealand's infant mortality rate was around 4 per 1000 live births, compared with 3.4 per 1000 in Australia. In 2011 in Australia and in 2013 in New Zealand around 2.7 per 1000 babies died in the neonatal period (ABS, 2014; New Zealand Government, 2014).

An infant who has difficulty accomplishing effective respiratory action in the first hours of life and yet survives may experience residual neurological difficulties because of cerebral hypoxia. Prompt, thorough care is necessary for effective intervention. Most infants are born with some degree of respiratory acidosis. However, this is rapidly corrected by the spontaneous onset of respiration. If respiratory activity does not begin immediately, respiratory acidosis will increase. The blood pH and bicarbonate buffer system will fail. Newborn defence mechanisms are inadequate to reverse the process. Therefore, the effort to establish respirations must be started

BOX 26.1 * Factors predisposing infants to respiratory difficulty in the first few days of life

Low birth weight
Maternal history of diabetes
Premature rupture of membranes
Maternal use of barbiturates or narcotics close to birth
Meconium-stained liquor
Irregularities detected by fetal heart monitor during labour
Cord prolapse
Lowered Apgar score (<7) at 1 or 5 minutes
Postmaturity
Small for gestational age
Breech birth
Multiple birth
Chest, heart or respiratory tract anomalies

immediately after birth. By 2 minutes, the development of severe acidosis is already well under way (Thilo & Rosenberg, 2008). Any infant who sustains some degree of asphyxia in utero, such as could occur from cord compression, maternal anaesthesia, placenta praevia, or preterm separation of the placenta, may already be experiencing acidosis at birth and may have difficulty before the first 2 minutes of life.

Resuscitation

Factors that commonly predispose infants to respiratory difficulty and so may require resuscitation are shown in Box 26.1. If breathing is ineffective, blood flow to the pulmonary system remains low causing persistent fetal circulation where circulatory shunts, particularly the ductus arteriosus, can fail to close. Struggling to breathe and circulate blood, an infant uses available serum glucose quickly and may become hypoglycaemic, compounding the initial problem. For all these reasons, resuscitation becomes important for infants who fail to take a first breath or have difficulty maintaining adequate respiratory movements on their own. Resuscitation follows an organised process: (a) establish and maintain an airway; (b) expand the lungs; and (c) initiate and maintain effective ventilation. If respiratory depression becomes severe, a newborn's heart will fail.

Airway

Babies born premature, or who are not breathing and floppy at birth will require resuscitative measures and will be placed under a radiant warmer for assessment and initiation of resuscitation. The midwife or nurse will suction the baby's oropharynx and nose to clear the airway and position the baby with the head slightly extended in the sniffing position to align the larynx, pharynx and trachea. Concurrently the baby will be dried thoroughly to provide stimulation and prevent heat loss. Other forms of stimulation such as rubbing the baby's back or flicking the soles of the feet are not recommended as time is wasted that may be used in implementing further resuscitation. It

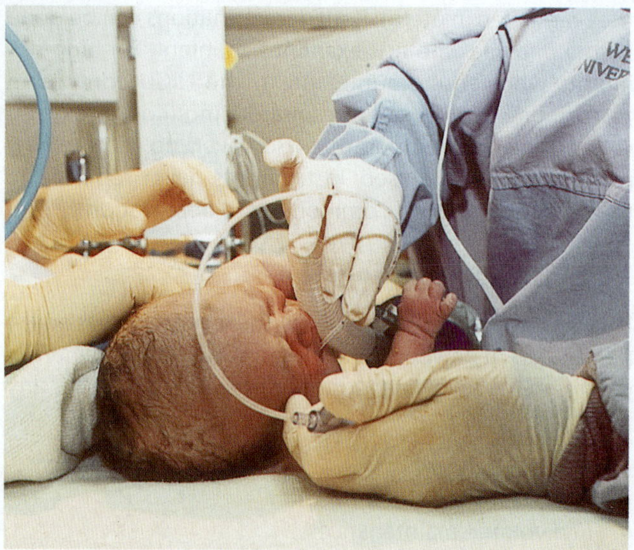

FIGURE 26.1 Suctioning a newborn with mechanical suction controlled by a finger valve. The suction is applied as the catheter is withdrawn. If the catheter is rotated as it is withdrawn, the risk of traumatising the membrane is reduced.

is important to keep the baby warm. Newborns cannot shiver and need to increase their internal metabolism to increase their temperature. This uses up glucose and oxygen which will make resuscitation more difficult. For babies born through meconium-stained liquor who are in need of resuscitation, stimulation is withheld until the trachea is suctioned of meconium by personnel experienced in intubation (see Fig. 26.1).

In the presence of severe hypoxia the baby will go through a period of rapid breathing before experiencing a primary apnoea accompanied by bradycardia. After a few minutes, if resuscitative measures are not instigated the baby will then experience a period of irregular gasping before a secondary apnoea which is accompanied by a further drop in the heart rate and significant hypotension. At the point of secondary apnoea, stimulation will not be effective in establishing respiration and positive pressure ventilation is required. Although usually a phenomenon that occurs after birth, both types of apnoea may occur in utero. It is important that every birth is attended by personnel trained in neonatal resuscitation with high-risk births requiring personnel with advanced skills such as intubation and intravenous access. (Australian Resuscitation Council, 2010; Kattwinkel, 2011).

Lung expansion

Once an airway has been established, a newborn's lungs need to be expanded. Well newborns inflate their lungs adequately with a first breath. The sound of the baby crying is proof that lung expansion is good because the vocal sounds are produced by a free flow of air over the vocal cords. Babies who do not initiate spontaneous respirations at birth, who breathe spontaneously but then cannot sustain effective respiration, or who have a heart rate below 100 beats per minute will require intermittent positive pressure ventilation. Studies over the last few decades have discovered that newborns resuscitated using air (21% oxygen) have better mortality rates and establish respiration earlier than those resuscitated in 100% oxygen. There is evidence that babies resuscitated in 100% oxygen may experience harm (Australian Resuscitation Council, 2010; Kattwinkel et al., 2010). Internationally, neonatal resuscitation guidelines recommend using air initially for babies requiring intermittent positive pressure ventilation, with oxygen use reserved for those babies who show no improvement after 60–90 seconds of ventilation in air.

Intermittent positive pressure ventilation can be delivered via bag and mask, T-piece resuscitator or intubation. When using bag and mask or a T-piece resuscitator the mask should cover both the mouth and the nose to be effective but should not cover the eyes, because it can cause eye injury mechanically from the mask or drying of the cornea from the flow. Ventilation should be commenced at 40–60 breaths per minute continuously. As noted above, babies who show little improvement through resuscitation in air will require 100% oxygen. If resuscitation and stabilisation is prolonged oxygen should be administered both warmed (between 32° and 34°C) and humidified (60–80%) to prevent cooling of the baby and drying of the airway.

Care must be taken not to overinflate the baby's lungs which can result in a pneumothorax. Although a bag and mask has a "pop-off" valve for prevention of pneumothorax the bag should only be squeezed enough to result in chest rise. When using a T-piece resuscitator the pressure can be set to ensure the lungs are not overinflated. To be certain that ventilation is effective it is recommended to monitor the newborn's oxygen saturation level with pulse oximetry in addition to auscultating the chest for the sound of breathing (Australian Resuscitation Council, 2010). The use of a pulse oximeter will also aid in monitoring the heart rate. An improvement in the heart rate is the best indicator that ventilation is effective because it demonstrates that the cardiac muscle is being re-oxygenated which results in improved cardiac output (Kattwinkel, 2011).

Establishing extrauterine circulation

Although establishing respiration is the priority during resuscitation, lack of cardiac function may be present concurrently or may develop if respiratory function cannot be quickly initiated and maintained. If, after effective ventilation in air for at least 30 seconds, an infant has no audible heartbeat, or if the cardiac rate is below 60 beats per minute, closed-chest massage should be started. Hold an infant with fingers supporting the back and depress the sternum with two fingers. Depress the sternum approximately one third of its depth (1 or 2 cm) at a rate of 90 times per minute (Australian Resuscitation Council, 2010). Lung ventilation at a rate of 30 times per minute should be continued and interspersed with the cardiac massage at a ratio of 1:3. The nurse should continue to monitor transcutaneous oxygen or pulse oximetry to evaluate respiratory function and cardiac efficiency.

Maintaining fluid and electrolyte balance

After an initial resuscitation attempt, hypoglycaemia (decreased blood glucose) may result from the effort the newborn has expended to begin breathing. Dehydration may also result from increased insensible water loss from rapid respirations. Infants with hypoglycaemia are treated with a 10% dextrose infusion at 4–6 mg/kg/min to ensure blood glucose levels remain above 2.5 mmol/L (Australian Resuscitation Council, 2010). For the treatment of dehydration 10% dextrose is generally used at a rate of 60 mL/kg/day (State Government of Victoria, 2014). Electrolytes (particularly sodium and potassium) are added as necessary, depending on electrolyte analysis.

The rate of fluid administration must be carefully monitored because a high fluid intake can lead to patent ductus arteriosus or heart failure. When using a radiant warmer, there is an increase in water loss from convection and radiation. A newborn on a warmer, therefore, will require more fluid than if they were placed in a double-walled humidicrib.

Dehydration may be monitored by urine output and urine specific gravity measures. An output less than 2 mL/kg/hr or a specific gravity greater than 1.015 to 1.020 suggests inadequate fluid intake. Elevated specific gravity may also be caused by inappropriate antidiuretic hormone secretion or kidney failure because of a primary illness.

Regulating temperature

All high-risk infants may have difficulty maintaining a normal temperature. This is because, in addition to stress from an illness or immaturity, the infant's body is often exposed during procedures such as resuscitation and blood drawing. It is important to keep newborns in a neutral-temperature environment, one that is neither too hot nor too cold, placing less demand on them to maintain a minimal metabolic rate necessary for effective body functioning (see Fig. 26.2). If the environment is too hot, they must decrease metabolism to cool their body. If it is too cold, they must increase metabolism to warm body cells. The increased metabolism requires calls for increased oxygen; without this oxygen available, body cells become hypoxic. To save oxygen for essential body functions, vasoconstriction of blood vessels occurs. If this process continues for too long, pulmonary vessels become affected and pulmonary perfusion becomes decreased. An infant's Po_2 level falls and Pco_2 increases. The decreased Po_2 level may open fetal right-to-left shunts again. Surfactant production may halt, which may further interfere with lung function. To supply glucose to maintain increased metabolism, an infant begins anaerobic glycolysis, which pours acid into the bloodstream. An infant becomes acidotic, and with acidosis comes the increased risk of kernicterus (invasion of

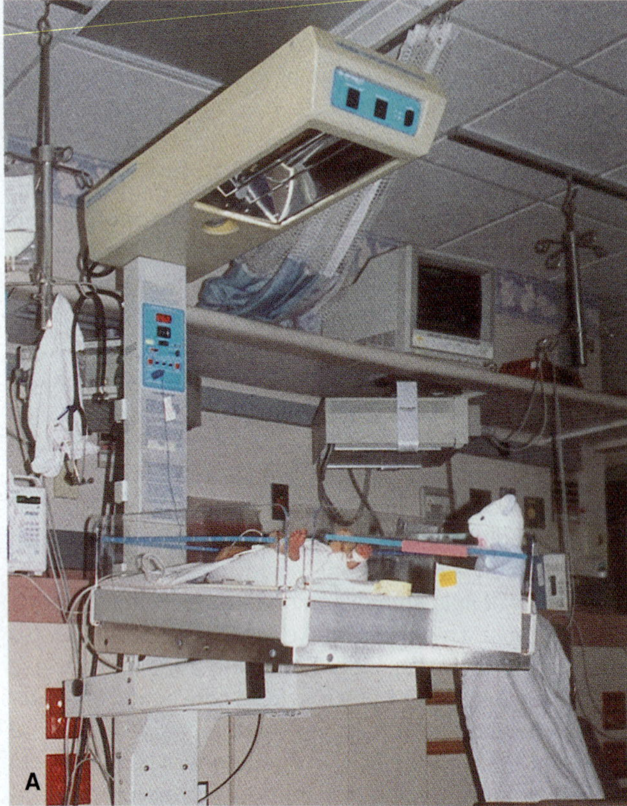

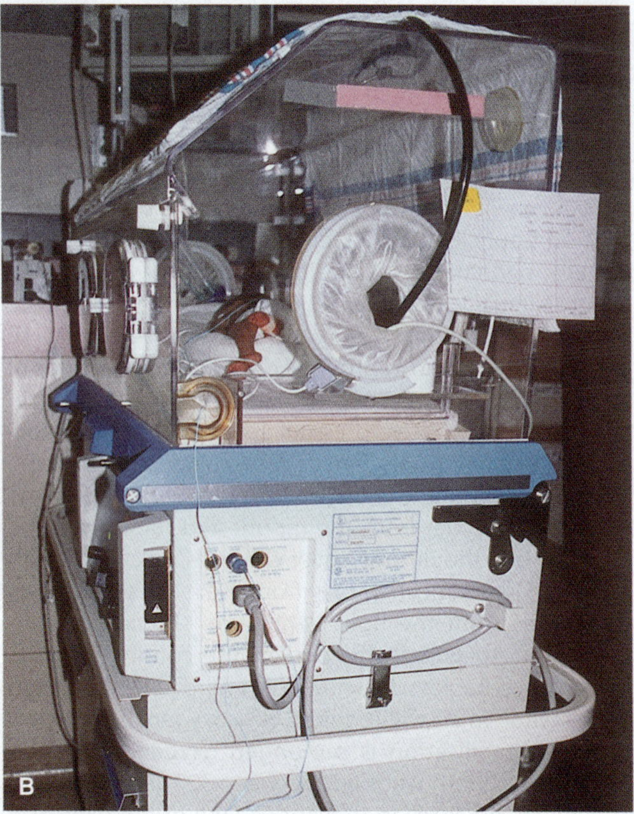

FIGURE 26.2 Neutral thermal environment. (**A**) A neonate in the intensive care bed with overhead radiant warmer can be examined periodically with ease. (**B**) Use of an incubator allows maintenance of a neutral thermal environment for neonates not requiring minute-to-minute intervention.

brain cells with unconjugated bilirubin) as more bilirubin-binding sites are lost and more bilirubin is free to pass out of the bloodstream into brain cells. In short, because of becoming chilled, heart action, breathing and electrolytic balance are all affected.

Well babies are able to regulate their own temperature if they are dried and placed skin-to-skin with their mother. For high-risk newborns who require extra care, prevent chilling after birth by wiping them dry, covering the head with a cap and placing them immediately under a pre-warmed radiant warmer, in a warmed humidicrib or skin-to-skin against the mother if they are stable (see Box 26.2). Additional measures are the use of plastic wrap, plastic shields, or warmed mattresses. Air, humidicrib, or radiant warmer temperatures should be kept regulated to maintain an infant's axillary temperature between 36.5 and 37.2°C. Be certain that during procedures an infant is placed on a radiant heat warmer and not placed directly on cool x-ray tables, scales, or an unheated radiant warmer in order to prevent heat loss.

Radiant heat sources

Radiant heat warmers are open beds that have an overhead radiant heat source. Such units have servocontrol probes, which when placed on an infant's skin continually monitor their temperature. Abdominal skin temperature, when measured this way, should be 36.0° to 36.5°C (Brown & Landers, 2011). If an infant's temperature falls below this level, an alarm will sound. Be certain to tape the probe or disk onto the infant's abdomen between the umbilicus and the xiphoid process. Do not tape it under an infant or it will

BOX 26.2 ✻ Focus on evidence-based practice

Guarding against hypothermia

It is critical to guard against hypothermia in low-birth-weight infants because they are prone to heat loss through their large surface area to body weight ratio and they have difficulty increasing their metabolic rate to warm themselves again. To investigate whether the simple act of covering the infant's head with a cap prevents enough evaporation and heat loss to prevent hypothermia, researchers reviewed six studies with a total of 304 infants comparing different methods of guarding against newborn cooling. Conclusions of this meta-analysis revealed that plastic wraps or bags, skin-to-skin care and warmed mattresses all keep preterm infants warmer, leading to higher temperatures on admission to neonatal units.

Based on this study, at the birth of a low-birth-weight infant, would you omit a cap or use it in addition to other measures?

Source: McCall, E. M., et al. (2009). Interventions to prevent hypothermia at birth in preterm and/or low birth weight infants. *Cochrane Database of Systematic Reviews, 2009*(1), (CD004210).

register a falsely high reading. Be sure it is not over the rib cage, where the thin subcutaneous tissue will not allow an accurate reading. Also do not place it over the liver, because increased metabolism may lead to false high readings. A plastic bridge or shield placed over the child will better preserve heat by reducing convection and radiation losses; plastic wrap placed over an infant will produce this same effect. When performing care or leaning over an infant, be careful not to block the heat from an overhead source. An additional warming pad placed under an infant may be necessary for very preterm infants or for lengthy procedures to maintain body heat.

Humidicribs

After an initial resuscitation attempt, newborns may be cared for in humidicribs. The temperature of humidicribs varies with the amount of time portholes remain open and the temperature of the area in which the humidicrib is placed. Placing it in direct sunlight or near a warm radiator can increase the internal temperature markedly. For this reason, a newborn's temperature must be checked at frequent intervals when in a humidicrib to be certain the temperature level designated is being maintained. Use of an additional acrylic shield inside the humidicrib helps prevent radiation and convection heat loss when portholes are opened for care.

Skin-to-skin care

Originally referred to as "kangaroo care", skin-to-skin care is the use of skin-to-skin contact to maintain body heat. Provide a quiet setting with lights dimmed. Undress the infant except for a nappy and perhaps a cap. Assist the parent to sit comfortably in a chair and hold the infant snugly against their chest, skin-to-skin. Place a blanket over the infant for added warmth. In addition, studies have shown that babies receiving skin-to-skin care experience a range of benefits including greater weight gain, more successful establishment of breastfeeding, better brain functioning and improved parent–child bonding (Ludington-Hoe, 2011).

Establishing adequate nutritional intake

Infants who experienced severe asphyxia at birth usually receive intravenous fluids so they do not become exhausted from sucking or until necrotising enterocolitis (NEC) has been ruled out, as this could result from the temporary reduction in oxygen to the bowel (see Chapter 45 for a discussion of NEC). If an infant's respiratory rate remains rapid and NEC has been ruled out, nasogastric tube feeding may be introduced. Preterm infants should receive breast milk either through breastfeeding or via the nasogastric tube because of the immune protection and digestive benefits this offers (see Fig. 26.3). If breastfeeding is not possible because the infant is too immature to suck effectively, a mother can manually express breast milk or use a breast pump to initiate and continue her milk supply until the infant is mature enough or otherwise ready for effective sucking. Preterm infants reveal hunger by the same signs as term infants, such as rooting and crying and sucking motions.

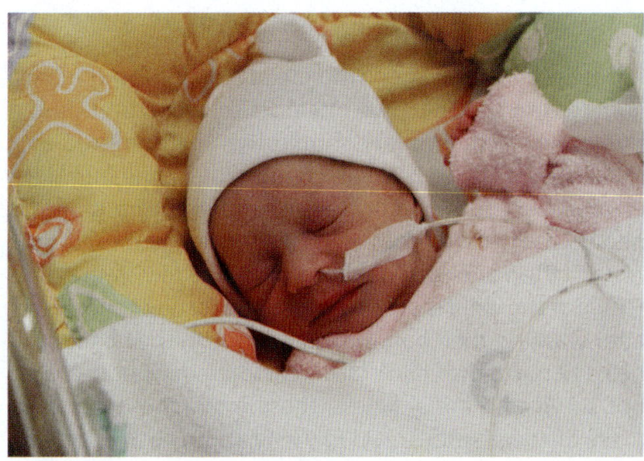

FIGURE 26.3 Infants who are ill at birth often need supplemental feedings by nasogastric or gastrostomy tube. (© Lauren Kidziak.)

Establishing waste elimination

Although most immature infants void within 24 hours of birth, they may void later than term newborns because, as a result of all the procedures that may be necessary for resuscitation, their blood pressure may not be adequate to optimally supply their kidneys. Carefully document any voids that occur during resuscitation. This is proof that hypotension is improving and the kidneys are being perfused. Immature infants also may pass stool later than the term infant because meconium has not yet reached the end of the intestine at birth.

Preventing infection

Contracting an infection could drastically complicate a high-risk newborn's ability to adjust to extrauterine life. Infection, like chilling, increases metabolic oxygen demands, which the high-risk newborn may not be able to meet. In addition, infection stresses the immature immune system and already strained defence mechanisms of a high-risk newborn. Infections may have antenatal, perinatal or postnatal causes. All babies with risk factors for infection should be carefully monitored.

Common viruses that affect infants in utero are cytomegalovirus and toxoplasmosis virus. An infant with either of these infections may be born with congenital anomalies from the virus invasion (see Chapter 12). The most prevalent perinatal infections are those contracted from the vagina during birth. Early-onset sepsis is most commonly caused by group B streptococcus, *E. coli*, *Kelbsiella* and *Listeria monocytogenes*. Late-onset, or nosocomial, infections are more commonly caused by *Staphylococcus aureus*, *Enterobacter* and *Candida*. These late-onset infections are probably most commonly spread to newborns from healthcare personnel.

Establishing parent–infant bonding

It is helpful if all women who are at risk of having a baby admitted to the NICU are offered a tour of a unit during pregnancy. If their infant should then be admitted to a NICU, they will thus be more comfortable in the high-tech environment. Be certain that the parents of a high-risk newborn are kept informed of what is happening during resuscitation at birth. They should be able to visit the NICU to which the child is admitted as often as they choose and, after washing their hands, hold and touch their child. This helps to make the child's birth real to them. Should a child not survive an initial illness, these interactions can help make the death more real. Only when both birth and death seem real can parents begin to work through their feelings and accept these events.

If an infant dies despite newborn resuscitation attempts, parents need to see their baby without a myriad of equipment around. This is a time for parents to reassure themselves that their newborn was a perfect baby in every other way except for whatever was the infant's fatal disorder. Thinking this way can give them confidence to plan for other children or simply to continue their lives after such a stressful experience.

High-risk infants and child abuse

When a child is ill or born preterm, we would expect parents to want to protect the child even more than a well or term baby so no further harm can result. In reality however, particularly with reference to preterm children, the opposite may occur. Preterm children can be at high risk for abuse. This is possibly because of the separation of the child from the family at birth, which can interfere with bonding. Child abuse is discussed in Chapter 55.

> ***What if...***
>
> Karen is about to visit her preterm newborn for the first time and states, "I'm so scared. He's so tiny and frail. How can I even hold him?" How should you respond to this new mother to make her visit easier?

THE NEWBORN AT RISK BECAUSE OF ALTERED GESTATIONAL AGE OR BIRTH WEIGHT

Infants need to be evaluated as soon as possible after birth to determine their weight and gestational age. Classification by growth charts and gestational history is important to determine immediate healthcare needs and to help anticipate possible problems. Birth weight is normally plotted on a growth chart. Infants born after the beginning of week 38 and before week 42 of pregnancy are classified as *term infants*. Approximately 90% of all live births are term. Infants born before term (less than 37 completed weeks of pregnancy) account for approximately 7% to 19% of all births and are classified as **preterm infants**, regardless of their birth weight. Infants born after the onset of week 43 of pregnancy are classified as *postterm*.

Normally, birth weight varies for each gestational week of age. Infants who fall between the 10th and 90th percentiles of weight for their age regardless of gestational age are considered appropriate for gestational age. Infants who fall below the 10th percentile of weight for their age are considered **small for gestational age (SGA)**. Those who fall above the 90th percentile in weight are considered **large for gestational age (LGA)**. Infants weighing under 2500 g are **low-birth-weight infants**. All such infants have immediate needs that are different from, or more pronounced than, the needs of term newborns. Each of these categories carries its own set of potential risks.

The small-for-gestational-age infant

An infant is SGA if the birth weight is below the 10th percentile on an intrauterine growth curve for that age. SGA infants may be born preterm (before week 38 of gestation), term (between weeks 38 and 42), or postterm (past 42 weeks). SGA infants are small for their age because they have experienced **intrauterine growth restriction (IUGR)** or failed to grow at the expected rate in utero (Volpi-Wise & Waller, 2010). This characteristic makes them distinctly different from infants whose weight is low but who are average for gestational age (see also Table 26.1).

Aetiology

A woman's nutrition during pregnancy plays a major role in fetal growth, so lack of adequate nutrition may be a major contributor to IUGR. However, the most common cause of IUGR is a placental anomaly: either the placenta did not obtain sufficient nutrients from the uterine arteries or it was inefficient at transporting nutrients to the fetus. Placental damage, such as partial placental separation with bleeding, limits placental function because the area of placenta that separated becomes infarcted and fibrosed, reducing the placental surface available for nutrient exchange. A developmental defect in the placenta can also prevent it from functioning properly. Women with systemic diseases that decrease blood flow to the placenta, such as severe diabetes mellitus or pre-eclampsia (both are diseases in which blood vessel lumens are narrowed), are at higher risk of having SGA babies than others. Women who smoke heavily or use narcotics also tend to have SGA infants (Volpi-Wise & Waller, 2010).

Appearance

Generally, an infant who suffers nutritional deprivation early in pregnancy, when fetal growth consists primarily of an increase in the number of body cells, is below average in weight, length and head circumference. An infant who suffers deprivation late in pregnancy, when growth consists primarily of an increase in cell size, may have only a reduction in weight. Regardless of when deprivation occurs, an SGA infant tends to have an overall wasted appearance. The child may have a small liver, which can cause difficulty regulating glucose, protein and bilirubin levels after birth. The infant also may have poor skin turgor and generally appear to have a large head because the rest of the body is so small. Skull sutures may be widely separated from lack of normal bone growth. Hair may be dull and lustreless. The abdomen may be sunken. The umbilical cord often appears dry and may be stained yellow.

In contrast, because an infant's age is more advanced than the weight implies, a child may have better-developed neurological responses, sole creases and ear cartilage than expected for a baby of that weight. The skull may be firmer, and the infant may seem unusually alert and active for that weight. The SGA infant needs careful assessment for possible congenital anomalies occurring as a result of the poor nutritional intrauterine environment.

Nursing considerations

Compromised respiratory effort

Newborns should maintain respiration at a rate of 30 to 60 breaths per minute after resuscitation at birth. Birth asphyxia is a common problem for SGA infants, both because they have underdeveloped chest muscles and because they are at risk of developing meconium aspiration syndrome as a result of hypoxia during labour. Fetal hypoxia causes a reflex relaxation of the anal sphincter and increased intestinal movement. When gasping for breath in utero, the fetus draws meconium that was discharged from the intestine into the amniotic fluid down into the trachea and bronchi. Acting as a foreign substance, this blocks airflow into the alveoli, leading to hypoxaemia, acidosis and hypercapnia. For this reason, many SGA infants require resuscitation at birth. Closely observe both respiratory rate and character in the first few hours of life. Underdeveloped chest muscles can make SGA infants unable to sustain the rapid respiratory rate of a normal newborn.

Ineffective thermoregulation

A newborn's temperature is maintained at 36.5–37.2°C axillary. SGA infants are less able to control body temperature than other newborns because they lack subcutaneous fat. A carefully controlled environment is essential to keep the infant's body temperature in a neutral zone (see Chapter 18).

✔ *Checkpoint question* 26.1

Why are SGA newborns at risk of difficulty maintaining body temperature?

a. They are preterm so they are born relatively small in size
b. They are more active than usual so they throw off covers
c. They do not have as much fat stores as do other infants
d. Their skin is more susceptible to conduction of cold

The large-for-gestational-age infant

An infant is LGA (*macrosomic*) if the birth weight is above the 90th percentile on an intrauterine growth chart for that gestational age. Such a baby appears deceptively healthy at birth because of the weight, but a gestational age examination will reveal immature development. It is important that LGA infants be identified immediately so that they can be given care appropriate to their gestational age rather than being treated as term newborns (Lawrence, 2007).

Aetiology

Infants who are LGA have been subjected to an overproduction of growth hormone in utero. This happens most often to infants of women with diabetes mellitus or women who are obese (Volpi-Wise & Waller, 2010). Extreme macrosomia occurs in fetuses of diabetic women whose symptoms are poorly controlled; these fetuses are exposed to high glucose levels. Multiparous women are also prone to having large babies because with each succeeding pregnancy, babies tend to grow larger. Other conditions associated with LGA infants include transposition of the great vessels, Beckwith syndrome (a rare condition characterised by overgrowth) and congenital anomalies such as omphalocele.

Appearance

At birth, LGA infants may show immature reflexes and low scores on gestational age examinations in relation to their size. They may have extensive bruising or a birth injury such as a broken clavicle or Erb-Duchenne paralysis from trauma to the cervical nerves if they were born vaginally. Because the head is large, it may have been exposed to more than the usual amount of pressure during birth, causing a prominent caput succedaneum, cephalhaematoma or moulding.

Hypoglycaemia

LGA infants also need to be carefully assessed for hypoglycaemia in the early hours of life because infants require large amounts of nutritional stores to sustain their weight. If the mother had diabetes that was poorly controlled, the infant will have had an increased blood glucose level in utero causing production of elevated levels of insulin. After birth, these increased insulin levels will continue for up to 24 hours of life, possibly causing rebound hypoglycaemia.

Nursing considerations

Compromised respiratory rate

Some LGA infants have difficulty establishing respiration at birth because of birth trauma. Increased intracranial pressure from birth of the larger-than-usual head could have led to pressure on the respiratory centre. This, in turn, can cause a decrease in respiratory function. A diaphragmatic paralysis may occur because of cervical nerve trauma as the head is bent sideways to allow for birth of the large shoulders. This prevents active lung motion on the affected side. If an infant was born by caesarean, transient fluid can remain in the lungs and interfere with effective gas exchange. Careful observation is needed to detect these conditions. Care of an infant with transient lung fluid is discussed later in this chapter.

As a rule, an LGA infant needs to be breastfed immediately to prevent hypoglycaemia. The infant may need supplemental formula feedings after breastfeeding to supply enough fluid and glucose for their larger-than-normal size for the first few days. Newborns who are offered bottles often have more difficulty than do others learning to breastfeed. Offer both the mother and baby support to overcome this hurdle. Do not overestimate LGA infants' ability to suck effectively at birth. Such infants may seem as if they should be able to suck well because they appear older. However, the infant is an inexperienced newborn, so sucking may not be effective enough to obtain the larger-than-usual amount of milk needed.

The preterm infant

A preterm infant is traditionally defined as a live-born infant born before the end of week 37 of gestation. In 2011 in Australia, 13.8% of all preterm births occurred in Indigenous mothers. This was almost double the rate of preterm births among non-Indigenous mothers (8.1%) in the same period (AIHW, 2014).When a preterm infant is recognised by a gestational age assessment, observe closely for the specific problems of prematurity, such as respiratory distress syndrome, hypoglycaemia and intracranial haemorrhage. The maturity of a newborn is determined by physical findings such as sole creases, skull firmness, ear cartilage and neurological findings that reveal gestational age, as well as the mother's report of the date of her last menstrual period and ultrasound estimations of gestational age.

BOX 26.3 ✻ Common factors associated with preterm birth

- Low socioeconomic level
- Poor nutritional status
- Lack of antenatal care
- Multiple pregnancy
- Previous early birth
- Race (non-Caucasians have a higher incidence of prematurity than Caucasians)
- Cigarette smoking
- Age of the mother (highest incidence is in mothers younger than aged 20)
- Order of birth (preterm birth is highest in first pregnancies and in those beyond the fourth pregnancy)
- Closely spaced pregnancies
- Abnormalities of the mother's reproductive system, such as intrauterine septum
- Infections (especially urinary tract infections)
- Obstetric complications, such as premature rupture of membranes or premature separation of the placenta
- Early induction of labour for medical indications
- Elective caesarean birth for medical indications

All preterm infants need intensive care from the moment of birth to give them their best chance of survival without neurological after-effects. A lack of lung surfactant makes them extremely vulnerable to respiratory distress syndrome (Gardner, Enzman-Hines & Dickey, 2011).

Preterm babies, regardless of their weight, need to be differentiated at birth from SGA babies (who also may have a low birth weight). The two conditions result from different situations and therefore will cause different problems in adjustment to extrauterine life (see Box 26.3 and Table 26.1). A preterm infant is immature and small but well proportioned for age. Unlike the SGA infant, this baby appears to have been doing well in utero. For an unexplained reason,

TABLE 26.1 Differences between small-for-gestational-age and preterm infants

Characteristic	Small-for-gestational-age infant	Preterm infant
Gestational age	24–44 weeks	<37 weeks
Birth weight	<10th percentile	Normal for age
Congenital malformations	Strong possibility	Possibility
Pulmonary problems	Meconium aspiration, pulmonary haemorrhage, pneumothorax	Respiratory distress syndrome
Hyperbilirubinaemia	Possibility	Very strong possibility
Hypoglycaemia	Very strong possibility	Possibility
Intracranial haemorrhage	Strong possibility	Possibility
Apnoea episodes	Possibility	Very strong possibility
Feeding problems	Most likely because of accompanying problem such as hypoglycaemia	Small stomach capacity; immature sucking reflex
Weight gain in nursery	Rapid	Slow
Future restricted growth	Possibly always be <10th percentile because of poor organ development	Not likely to be restricted in growth as "catch-up" growth occurs

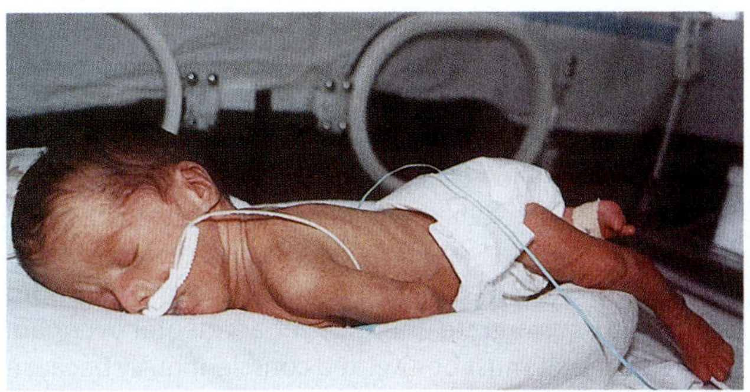

FIGURE 26.4 An immature infant. Notice the lax position of limbs because of immature muscle development.

however, the trigger that initiates labour was activated too early and birth resulted, even though the baby is immature. However, preterm infants are invariably also low-birth-weight infants (see Fig. 26.4).

Aetiology

Perinatal death statistics include all fetal deaths (at least 20 weeks' gestation or at least 400 grams birth weight) and neonatal deaths (all live born babies who die within 28 completed days of birth, regardless of gestation or birth weight) (ABS, 2014). The neonatal mortality rate has greatly reduced due to improved medical care and technology, such as developments in neonatal intensive care, and a major reduction in the number of deaths from **sudden infant death syndrome (SIDS)** (ABS, 2010). Infant mortality could be further reduced dramatically if the causes of preterm birth could be discovered and corrected and all pregnancies brought to term. However, the exact cause of premature labour and early birth is not known.

There is a high correlation between low socioeconomic levels and preterm birth. A study by Joseph and colleagues (2014) found that spontaneous preterm birth was more likely in women of lower socioeconomic status and the risk increased for women with either high or low BMI.

Iatrogenic (healthcare-caused) issues, such as elective caesarean birth and inducing labour for medical reasons, also result in preterm births. Risk factors for spontaneous and iatrogenic preterm birth include chronic illness, smoking, previous low-birth-weight baby, pregnancy-related complications such as placenta praevia and hypertension (Joseph et al., 2014; see Box 26.3). The increasing use of assisted fertility methods such as in vitro fertilisation, resulting in more multiple births, has also contributed to an increased preterm rate; more multiple pregnancies result in preterm birth than term pregnancies (McDonald et al., 2010).

Anaemia of prematurity

Many preterm infants develop a normochromic, normocytic anaemia (normal cells, just few in number). The reticulocyte count is low because the bone marrow does not increase its production until approximately 32 weeks. The infant will appear pale and may be lethargic and anorectic. The problem appears to be due to immaturity of the haematopoietic system combined with destruction of red blood cells because of low levels of vitamin E, which normally protects red blood cells against oxidation.

Kernicterus

Kernicterus (or chronic bilirubin encephalopthy) occurs when bilirubin infiltrates the brain causing damage (Shapiro, 2010). This invasion results from the high concentration of indirect bilirubin in the blood caused by excessive breakdown of red blood cells. Preterm infants are more prone to the condition than term infants because, with the acidosis that occurs from poor respiratory exchange, brain cells are more susceptible to the effect of indirect bilirubin than usual. Preterm infants also have less serum albumin available to bind indirect bilirubin and inactivate its effect. Because of this, kernicterus may occur at lower levels than for term infants. If jaundice occurs, phototherapy or exchange transfusion can be initiated to prevent excessively high indirect bilirubin levels.

Persistent patent ductus arteriosus

Because preterm infants lack surfactant, their lungs are non-compliant. Thus it is more difficult for them to move blood from the pulmonary artery into the lungs. This condition leads to pulmonary artery hypertension, which may interfere with closure of the ductus arteriosus. Administer intravenous therapy cautiously to preterm infants to avoid increasing blood pressure and further compounding this problem. Either indomethacin or ibuprofen may be administered to close the patent ductus arteriosus. A side effect of indomethacin is oliguria, so urine output needs to be monitored closely if this is used.

Periventricular/intraventricular haemorrhage

Preterm infants are prone to periventricular haemorrhage (bleeding into the tissue surrounding the ventricles) or intraventricular haemorrhage (bleeding into the ventricles); these conditions occur in as many as 30% of infants of very low birth weight (between 401 and 1500 g) (Kenet et al., 2011). It occurs because preterm infants have both fragile capillaries and immature cerebral vascular development. When there is a rapid change in cerebral blood pressure, such as with hypoxia, intravenous infusion, ventilation or pneumothorax, capillaries rupture. An infant experiences brain anoxia distal to the rupture. Hydrocephalus may occur from bleeding into the aqueduct of Sylvius with resulting clotting and obstruction of the aqueduct. Preterm infants often have a cranial ultrasound performed after the first few days of life to detect if a haemorrhage has occurred. An infant's prognosis is guarded until it can be shown that development is progressing normally after an intracranial bleed.

Other potential complications

Preterm infants are particularly susceptible to several illnesses in the early postnatal period, including respiratory distress syndrome, apnoea, retinopathy of prematurity and NEC (discussed in Chapter 45). Because a preterm infant has few body resources, both physiological and psychological stress must be reduced as much as possible and interventions initiated gently to prevent depletion of resources. Close observation and analysis of findings are essential to manage problems quickly.

Nursing considerations

Impaired gas exchange

Many preterm babies, particularly those under 32 weeks of age, have an irregular respiratory pattern (a few quick breaths, a period of 5 to 10 seconds without respiratory effort, a few quick breaths again, and so on). There is no bradycardia with this irregular pattern (sometimes termed periodic respiration). Although the pattern is seen in term infants as well, it seems to be intensified by immaturity. With true apnoea, the pause in respiration is more than 20 seconds and bradycardia does occur. True apnoea is discussed in more detail later in this chapter.

Preterm infants have great difficulty initiating respiration at birth because pulmonary capillaries are still so immature. Lung surfactant does not form in adequate amounts until about the 34th to 35th week of pregnancy. Inadequate lung surfactant leads to alveolar collapse with each expiration. This condition forces an infant to use maximum strength to inflate lung alveoli each time. It is very difficult for infants to maintain effective expirations under these conditions. In addition, because a fetus usually turns to a vertex presentation late in pregnancy, a preterm infant may still be in a breech position at birth. Breech-born infants are apt to expel meconium into the amniotic fluid. If the fetus aspirates either vaginal secretions or meconium, the respiratory problem can be aggravated by inflammation or pneumonia.

Giving 100% oxygen to preterm infants during resuscitation or to maintain respiration presents two additional dangers: pulmonary oedema and retinopathy of prematurity (blindness of prematurity) may develop. The development of both of these conditions depends on saturation of the blood with oxygen (Po_2 of more than 100 mmHg, which usually occurs when oxygen is administered at a concentration over 70%). Although a newborn's oxygen saturation level should be continually monitored, as long as an infant is cyanotic, the blood saturation level of oxygen is likely to be low or well beneath this level.

Deficient fluid volume

A preterm newborn experiences a high insensible water loss because of a large body surface relative to total body weight. Preterm infants also cannot concentrate urine well because of immature kidney function. Because of this, a high proportion of body fluid is excreted. All these factors make it important for a preterm baby to receive up to 160 to 200 mL of fluid per kilogram of body weight daily (higher than the term infant).

Intravenous fluid administration typically begins within hours after birth to fulfil this fluid requirement and provide glucose to prevent hypoglycaemia. Intravenous fluid should be given via a continuous infusion pump to ensure a constant infusion rate and prevent accidental overload. Intravenous sites must be checked conscientiously because if infiltration should occur, the lack of subcutaneous tissue places a preterm newborn at risk of damaged tissue. Specially designed 27-gauge needles are available for use on small veins. Many preterm infants lack adequately sized peripheral veins for even this small a needle. Therefore, they need to receive intravenous fluid by an umbilical venous catheter.

Monitor the baby's weight, urine output and specific gravity, and serum electrolytes to ensure adequate fluid intake. Too little fluid and calories can lead to dehydration and starvation, acidosis and weight loss. Overhydration may lead to non-nutritional weight gain, pulmonary oedema and heart failure. Most preterm infants void and pass meconium within 24 hours after birth, although this is delayed in very small infants. Measure urine output by weighing nappies rather than using urine collection bags; disposable collection bags can lead to skin irritation and breakdown from frequent changing and leaking. The amount of urine output for the first few days of life in preterm babies is high in comparison with that of the term baby because of poor urine concentration: 40 to 100 mL per kilogram per 24 hours, compared with 10 to 20 mL per kilogram per 24 hours. The specific gravity is low, rarely more than 1.012 (normal term babies may concentrate urine up to 1.030). Also, test urine for glucose and ketones.

Imbalanced nutrition

Nutrition problems can arise with a preterm infant as the infant's body attempts to continue to maintain the rapid rate of intrauterine growth. Because of this, a preterm newborn requires a larger amount of nutrients than the mature infant. If these nutrients are not supplied, an infant can develop hypocalcaemia (decreased serum calcium) or azotaemia (low protein level in blood). Delayed feeding and a resultant decrease in intestinal motility may also add to hyperbilirubinaemia, a problem an infant already is at high risk of developing when fetal red blood cells begin to be destroyed.

Digestion and absorption of nutrients in a preterm infant's stomach and intestine may be immature. Nutrition problems are further compounded by a preterm infant's immature reflexes, which make swallowing and sucking difficult. Increased activity that occurs from ineffective sucking may increase the metabolic rate and oxygen requirements. This increases the kilojoule requirements even more. In addition, the preterm infant's stomach capacity is small, possibly limiting adequate intake. If a small stomach is distended from a full feeding, this puts pressure on the diaphragm and can lead to respiratory distress. An immature cardiac sphincter (between the stomach and oesophagus) allows regurgitation to occur readily. The lack of a cough reflex may lead an infant to aspirate regurgitated formula.

Feeding schedule

With the early administration of intravenous fluid to prevent hypoglycaemia and supply fluid, feedings may be safely delayed until an infant has stabilised their respiratory effort from birth. Preterm infants may be fed by total parenteral nutrition until they are stable enough for other means. Breast, nasogastric tube feeding or bottle feedings are begun as soon as an infant is able to tolerate them to prevent deterioration of the intestinal villi. Most preterm infants have a chest radiograph taken before a first feeding. Because preterm infants have a smaller stomach capacity than term neonates, they cannot take large feedings and so must be fed more frequently with smaller amounts. Feedings may be as small as 1 or 2 mL every 2 to 3 hours.

Nasogastric tube feeding

A gag reflex is not intact until 32 weeks' gestation. Although a sucking reflex is present earlier, the ability to coordinate sucking and swallowing is inconsistent until approximately 34 weeks' gestation. Infants who are born before 32 to 34 weeks' gestation and those who are ill or experiencing respiratory distress are usually started on nasogastric tube feeding. Bottle feeding or breastfeeding is gradually introduced as the infant matures and begins to demonstrate feeding behaviours such as being awake, moving or fussing as if hungry. To avoid tiring the neonate, preterm teats that are softer than regular teats should be used.

Thermoregulation

Preterm newborns have a great deal of difficulty maintaining body temperature because they have a relatively large surface area per kilogram of body weight. In addition, because they do not flex their body well but remain in an extended position, rapid cooling from evaporation is more likely to occur (Brown & Landers, 2011). A preterm infant has little subcutaneous fat for insulation and poor muscular development and so cannot move as actively as an older infant to produce body heat. A preterm infant also has a limited amount of **brown fat**, the special tissue present in newborns to maintain body temperature. Preterm infants also cannot shiver, a useful mechanism to increase body temperature; at the same time, they cannot sweat and thereby reduce body temperature because of an immature central nervous system and hypothalamic control. This makes preterm infants dependent on the environmental temperature provided to keep warm. In a birthing room preterm infants should be kept under radiant heat warmers or warmed by skin-to-skin contact. A 1500-g infant exposed to a low temperature loses 1°C of body heat every 3 minutes if left unprotected. Be certain that a radiant heat warmer is warmed before the infant is born. Unless there are obvious abnormalities noted when the child is born, physical assessment of a preterm infant, even weighing, can be delayed until the infant can be placed in the warmth of a humidicrib or under a radiant warmer with a servocontrol.

Risk of infection

The skin of a preterm baby is easily traumatised and therefore offers less resistance to infection than the skin and mucus membranes of a mature baby. In addition, preterm infants have a lowered resistance to infection. They have difficulty producing phagocytes to localise infection and they have a deficiency of IgM antibodies because of insufficient production. To help prevent infection, linen and equipment used with preterm infants must not be shared with other infants. Staff members must be free of infection; handwashing regulations should be strictly enforced.

Bonding and the preterm infant

In a preterm infant, the first and second periods of reactivity normally observed in newborns at 1 hour and 4 hours of life (see Chapter 18) may be delayed. In some infants, no period of increased activity or tachycardia may appear until 12 to 18 hours after birth. If the purpose of a period of reactivity is to stimulate respiratory function, this places a preterm infant at an even greater threat of respiratory failure. A second consequence of a delayed period of reactivity is the loss of an opportunity for interaction between parents and the newborn in the early postpartum period.

Although it is extremely important to conserve a preterm infant's strength by reducing sensory stimulation as much as possible and handling them gently, it is now recognised that preterm infants need as much loving attention as term newborns. Current evidence strongly shows that preterm infants have better outcomes and improved parental bonding where skin-to-skin care is practised (Bailey, 2012). Skin-to-skin care should therefore be integrated into all aspects of care for a premature infant where possible. If an infant cannot be removed from a humidicrib or a radiant heat warmer, parents can still handle and stroke them in the humidicrib or warmer. Because parents may not be psychologically ready for birth when a preterm baby is born, it may be more difficult for them to believe they have a child. Encourage the mother to express breast milk for her infant if the child is too young to breastfeed. If a woman decides not to breastfeed, encourage her to come to the hospital and hold the baby before and after nasogastric tube feedings or to give bottle feedings. By feeding her baby or expressing milk for the feedings, she is directly participating in the care and taking on responsibility for the infant's welfare.

If the baby is transferred to a regional centre, make sure the parents have an opportunity to see the baby before the transfer. A photograph of the baby for them to keep is

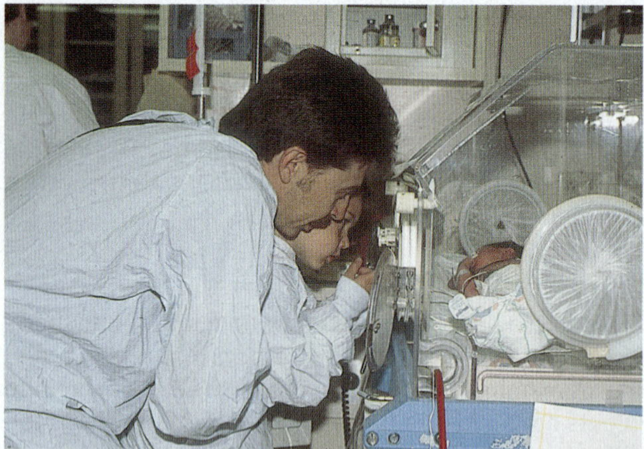

FIGURE 26.5 Encourage families to visit with immature infants to establish bonding. (© Caroline Brown, RNC, MS, DEd.)

helpful in making the birth more real. Encourage them to visit the distant site as often as possible. Parents visiting a NICU often need a great deal of support from nursing personnel. Remember that although radiant warmers, humidicribs, ventilators and monitors are familiar equipment to nurses, they are unusual and frightening to parents. Because preterm infants are hospitalised for long periods, parents can become confused, receiving information from different healthcare professionals every time they visit. Making the baby's siblings welcome in the NICU is yet another major role for a nurse of high-risk infants (see Fig. 26.5).

Preterm infants need rest to conserve energy for growth and respiratory function, to combat hypoglycaemia and infection, to stabilise temperature, and to develop inner balance and attentiveness. To allow for this, procedures should be organised to maximise the amount of rest available to an infant. If this is not appropriately coordinated, an infant may be awakened constantly for procedures. In addition, preterm infants may have more difficulty blocking out stimuli than term infants do because their nervous systems are immature. They may react negatively and exhibit such behaviours as gagging, crying, splaying fingers and toes, or going limp when exposed to bright lights, noise, or overly strenuous handling. Because these infants have little strength to move away from an unwanted stimulus, it is a carer's responsibility to be sensitive to these cues and move the object or noise away from the infant. The infant may need to be shielded from noise and light as much as possible until ready to take in stimuli. Likewise, pain should be kept to a minimum.

At the same time as a preterm infant needs rest, they also need planned periods of pleasing sensory stimulation. Like all newborns, preterm infants respond best to stimulation that appeals to their senses—sight, sound and touch. A passive face, picture, or design may be appealing for only short periods.

The view into the humidicrib can be distorted by the acrylic dome. Most people view an infant in a humidicrib from the side. This means an infant's face is rarely in the same line of vision as the adult's (an "en face" position). It is important to look directly at an infant in the straightforward position so they are provided with the stimulation of a human face. As infants mature, they should have mobiles (perhaps black and white) or bright objects placed in view. As an infant's position is changed from side to stomach to opposite side, the object should be moved to be in line with the child's vision. Infants in closed humidicribs may be able to hear nothing but the sound of the humidicrib motor. They may see people looking or nodding at them and may see their mouths moving, but they cannot benefit from the sound of their voices because this is obscured by the continuous hum of the motor. Provide some "talk time"—words spoken softly but clearly to an infant's ear—during each nursing shift to offer normal contact.

Parental education requirements

Discharge from an NICU is a major transition for parents as well as their infant. Before discharge, the parents of a preterm infant need to learn and practise any special methods of care necessary for their infant and any interventions required to help maximise their child's development. Some parents tend to be overprotective of preterm infants, such as not allowing visitors or not taking them outside. Let parents know their concern is normal, but overprotectiveness is not necessary.

Ongoing health maintenance of a preterm infant follows the usual pattern of well-child care. Basic immunisations are given according to the chronological age of an infant. However, a preterm infant can be expected to meet first-year milestones not at the chronological age but at the corrected age.

To evaluate the parents' transition to having so small an infant at home, ask at health promotion visits if the parents are:

- Beginning to feel more comfortable with their infant
- Able to allow the child to stay with a babysitter or another family member
- Beginning to incorporate their infant normally into their family life
- Making plans for the infant beyond the immediate newborn period.

The postterm infant

A postterm infant is one born after the 42nd week of a pregnancy. Often labour is induced between 41 and 42 weeks of gestation to avoid postterm births. However, when gestational age has been miscalculated or if for some other reason labour is not induced until week 43 of pregnancy or after, the pregnancy may result in a postterm infant.

An infant who stays in utero past week 42 of pregnancy is at special risk because a placenta appears to function effectively for only 40 weeks. After that time, it seems to lose its ability to carry nutrients effectively to the fetus. A fetus who remains in utero with a failing placenta may die or develop postterm syndrome. Infants with this syndrome have many of the characteristics of the SGA infant: dry, cracked, almost leather-like skin from lack of fluid and absence of vernix. They may be lightweight from recent weight loss that occurred because of poor placental function. The amount of amniotic fluid may be less at birth than normal and it may be meconium-stained. Fingernails will have grown well beyond the end of the fingertips. Such infants may demonstrate an alertness much more like a 2-week-old baby than a newborn.

Any woman is anxious when she does not have her baby around her due date. During discussions about the risks of stillbirth, neonatal morbidity and mortality for postterm babies, women and families may become very worried. It is important to ensure they are well informed about the care of their postterm baby with the underlying care rationale clearly explained.

ILLNESS IN THE NEWBORN

A number of illnesses occur specifically in newborns. These automatically cause the infant to become high risk.

Respiratory distress syndrome

Respiratory distress syndrome (RDS) of the newborn, formerly termed *hyaline membrane disease*, occurs most often in preterm infants, infants of diabetic mothers, infants born by caesarean birth, or those who for any reason have decreased blood perfusion of the lungs, such as occurs with meconium aspiration (Gardner et al., 2011). The pathological feature of RDS is a hyaline-like (fibrous) membrane formed from an exudate of an infant's blood that begins to line the terminal bronchioles, alveolar ducts and alveoli. This membrane prevents exchange of oxygen and carbon dioxide at the alveolar–capillary membrane. The cause of RDS is a low level or absence of surfactant, the phospholipid that normally lines the alveoli and reduces surface tension to keep the alveoli from collapsing on expiration. Because surfactant does not form until the 34th week of gestation, as many as 30% of low-birth-weight infants and as many as 50% of very-low-birth-weight infants are susceptible to this complication.

An infant with RDS must be kept warm because cooling increases acidosis in all newborns and for the newborn with RDS it may increase to lethal levels. Keeping an infant warm also reduces the metabolic oxygen demand. Provide hydration and nutrition with intravenous fluids, glucose or nasogastric tube feeding because the respiratory effort makes an infant too exhausted to suck.

Transient tachypnoea of the newborn

Transient tachypnoea of the newborn (TTN), otherwise known as wet lung syndrome or RDS Type 2, is caused by delayed reabsorption of fetal lung fluid at birth, where fluid is retained in the peribronchiolar lymphatics and the bronchovascular spaces (Gardner et al., 2011). Symptoms include a rapid rate of respiration greater than 60 breaths per minute, rib recession, grunting and nasal flaring. Feeding is difficult because the child cannot suck and breathe this rapidly at the same time. A chest x-ray will reveal a "wet silhouette" and fluid in a horizontal pattern (Edwards et al., 2013).

Transient tachypnoea may reflect a slight decrease in production of phosphatidyl glycerol or mature surfactant but is a direct result of retained lung fluid. Retained lung fluid limits the amount of alveolar surface that is available for oxygen exchange. This limitation requires an infant to increase respiratory rate and depth of respiration to better use the surface available. Transient tachypnoea occurs more often in infants who are born by caesarean birth, in infants whose mothers received extensive fluid administration during labour and in preterm infants. Infants born by caesarean are probably more prone to develop this form of respiratory distress because the thoracic cavity is not compressed as it is in vaginal birth, so less lung fluid is expelled than normally.

Close observation of such a newborn is a priority. Watch carefully to be certain the increased effort is not tiring. Also watch for beginning signs of a more serious disorder, because a rapid respiratory rate is often the first sign of respiratory obstruction. Oxygen administration may be necessary. Transient tachypnoea of the newborn peaks in intensity at approximately 36 hours of life and then begins to fade. Typically, by 72 hours of life, it spontaneously fades as the lung fluid is absorbed and respiratory activity becomes effective.

Meconium aspiration syndrome

Meconium is present in the fetal bowel as early as 10 weeks' gestation. If hypoxia occurs, a vagal reflex is stimulated, resulting in relaxation of the rectal sphincter. This releases meconium into the amniotic fluid. Babies born breech may expel meconium into the amniotic fluid from pressure on the buttocks. In both instances, the appearance of the fluid at birth is green to greenish black from the staining. Meconium staining occurs in approximately 8–19% of all pregnancies; in 2–33% of these pregnancies, infants will aspirate the meconium (Gardner et al., 2011). Meconium aspiration does not tend to occur in extremely-low-birth-weight infants because the substance has not passed far enough in the bowel for it to be at the rectum.

An infant may aspirate meconium either in utero or with the first breath at birth. Meconium can cause severe respiratory distress in three ways: it causes inflammation of bronchioles because it is a foreign substance; it can block small bronchioles by mechanical plugging; and it can cause a decrease in surfactant production through lung trauma. Hypoxaemia, carbon dioxide retention, and intrapulmonary and extrapulmonary shunting occur. A secondary infection of injured tissue may lead to pneumonia.

Apnoea

Apnoea is a pause in respiration longer than 20 seconds with accompanying bradycardia. Beginning cyanosis also may be present. Many preterm infants have periods of apnoea as a result of fatigue or the immaturity of their respiratory mechanisms. Babies with secondary stresses, such as infection, hyperbilirubinaemia, hypoglycaemia or hypothermia, tend to have a high incidence of apnoea (Gardner et al., 2011). Gently shaking an infant or flicking the sole of the foot often stimulates the baby to breathe again, almost as if the child needed to be reminded to maintain this function. If an infant does not respond to these simple measures, resuscitation is necessary.

Closely observe all newborns, but especially preterm ones, to detect these apnoeic episodes. Apnoea monitors that record respiratory movements are invaluable tools to detect failing respiration and sound a warning when an infant needs attention. Infants with frequent or difficult-to-correct episodes may be placed on ventilators to provide respiratory coordination until they are more mature. Infants who have had an apnoeic episode severe enough to require resuscitation are at a high risk for sudden infant death syndrome (SIDS). Such infants may be discharged home with a monitoring device to be used for 2–6 months.

Sudden infant death syndrome

Sudden infant death syndrome (SIDS) is sudden unexplained death in infancy (SUDI). It tends to occur at a higher-than-usual rate in infants of adolescent mothers, infants of closely spaced pregnancies, and underweight and preterm infants. Also prone to SIDS are infants with bronchopulmonary dysplasia, twins and infants of narcotic-dependent mothers. The peak age of incidence is 2 to 4 months of age (Gelfer & Tatum, 2014). Although the cause of SIDS is unknown, in addition to prolonged but unexplained apnoea, other possible contributing factors include:

- Viral respiratory infection
- Pulmonary oedema
- Brain stem abnormalities
- Neurotransmitter deficiencies
- Heart rate abnormalities
- Distorted familial breathing patterns
- Decreased arousal responses
- Possible lack of surfactant in alveoli
- Sleeping prone
- Sleeping in a room without moving air currents (the infant re-breathes expired carbon dioxide).

Typically, affected infants are well nourished. Parents report that an infant may have had a slight head cold. After being put to bed at night or for a nap, the infant is found dead a few hours later. Infants who die this way do not appear to make any sound as they die, which indicates they die with laryngospasm. Although many infants are found with blood-flecked sputum or vomitus in their mouths or on the bedclothes, this seems to occur as the result of death, not as its cause. An autopsy often reveals petechiae in the lungs and mild inflammation and congestion in the respiratory tract. However, these symptoms are not severe enough to cause sudden death. It is clear these children do not suffocate from bedclothes or choke from overfeeding, underfeeding or crying. Both Australia and New Zealand have well developed SIDS organisations that are active in health education and fundraising for research to reduce the incidence of sudden infant death syndrome. Their websites provide current research into the possible causes of SIDS as well as bereavement support services for families: see <www.sids.org.nz> and <www.sids andkids.org>.

Parents have a difficult time accepting the death of any child. This can be especially difficult when it happens so suddenly. In discussing the child, they often use both the past and present tenses as if they are not yet aware of the death. Many parents experience a period of somatic symptoms that occur with acute grief, such as nausea, stomach pain or vertigo. Parents should be counselled by a nurse or someone else trained in counselling at the time of the infant's death; it helps if they can talk to this same person periodically for however long it takes to resolve their grief.

When another child is born, parents can be expected to become extremely frightened at any sign of illness. They need support to see them through the first few months of the second child's life, particularly past the point at which the first child died. Some parents may need support to view a second child as an individual child and not as a replacement for the one who died. Often a new baby born to a family in which a SIDS infant died is screened using a sleep assessment as a precaution within the first 2 weeks of life. Depending on the parents' level of anxiety, the new baby may receive this screening before hospital discharge. The baby may then be placed on continuous apnoea monitoring pending the results of the sleep assessment.

Haemolytic disease of the newborn

The term "haemolytic" is derived from the Latin word for "destruction" (lysis) of red blood cells. Lysis of red blood cells in the newborn leads to **hyperbilirubinaemia** (an elevated level of bilirubin in the blood). This can result from destruction of red blood cells by a normal physiological process (see Chapter 18). When abnormal destruction of red blood cells occurs, it is termed haemolytic disease. In the past, haemolytic disease of the newborn was most often caused by an Rh blood type incompatibility. Because prevention of Rh antibody formation has been available for almost 40 years, the disorder is now most often caused by an ABO incompatibility. In both instances, the mother builds antibodies against an infant's red blood cells, leading to haemolysis (destruction) of the cells. The destruction of red blood cells causes severe anaemia and hyperbilirubinaemia. Prevention of the condition begins in pregnancy, as discussed in Chapter 21.

Rh incompatibility

Theoretically, no direct connection exists between the fetal and maternal circulation, so no fetal blood cells should enter the maternal circulation. In actuality, occasional placental villi break and a drop or two of fetal blood can enter the maternal circulation. If the mother's blood type is Rh (D) negative and the fetal blood type is Rh positive (contains the D antigen), the introduction of fetal blood causes sensitisation to occur, and the woman begins to form antibodies against the D antigen. Few antibodies form this way, however. Most form in the woman's bloodstream in the first 72 hours after birth because there is an active exchange of fetal–maternal blood as placental villi loosen and the placenta is delivered. After this sensitisation, in a second pregnancy there will be a high level of antibody D circulating in the woman's bloodstream, which will then act to destroy the fetal red blood cells early in the pregnancy if the new fetus is Rh positive. By the end of pregnancy, a fetus can be severely compromised by the action of these antibodies crossing the placenta and destroying red blood cells. Some infants require intrauterine transfusions to combat red cell destruction.

ABO incompatibility

In most instances of ABO incompatibility, the maternal blood type is O and the fetal blood type is A; it may also occur when the fetus has type B or AB blood. A reaction in an infant with type B blood is often the most serious.

Haemolysis can become a problem with a first pregnancy in which there is an ABO incompatibility as the antibodies to A and B cell types are naturally occurring antibodies or are present from birth in individuals whose red cells lack these antigens. Unlike the antibodies formed against the Rh D factor, these antibodies are of the large (IgM) class and do not cross the placenta. An infant of an ABO incompatibility, therefore, is not born anaemic, as is the Rh-sensitised child. Haemolysis of the blood begins with birth, when blood and antibodies are exchanged during the mixing of maternal and fetal blood as the placenta is loosened; destruction of red cells may continue up to 2 weeks of age. Interestingly, preterm infants do not seem to be affected by ABO incompatibility. This may be because the receptor sites for anti-A or anti-B antibodies do not appear on red cells until late in fetal life. Even in the mature newborn, a direct antibody test may be only weakly positive because of the few anti-A or anti-B sites present. The reticulocyte count (immature or newly formed red blood cells) is usually elevated as the infant attempts to replace destroyed cells.

Initiation of early feeding

Bilirubin is removed from the body by being incorporated into faeces. Therefore, the sooner bowel elimination begins, the sooner bilirubin removal begins. Early feeding therefore stimulates bowel peristalsis and accomplishes this. Colostrum is particularly useful as it contains properties that initiate the movement of meconium.

Phototherapy

Phototherapy is used for the treatment of hyperbilirubinaemia. An infant's liver processes little bilirubin in utero because the mother's circulation does this for an infant. With birth, exposure to light apparently triggers the liver to assume this function. Additional light supplied by phototherapy appears to speed the conversion potential of the liver. In phototherapy, an infant is continuously exposed to specialised light such as quartz halogen, cool white daylight or special blue fluorescent light. The lights are placed 30–75 cm above the newborn's bed or humidicrib. Specialised fibreoptic light systems incorporated into a fibreoptic blanket have also been developed and are ideal for home care. The infant is undressed except for a nappy so as much skin surface as possible is exposed to the light. Term newborns are generally scheduled for phototherapy when the total serum bilirubin level rises at 24 hours of age; preterm infants may have treatment begun at levels lower than this (Symons & Mahoney, 2008).

Continuous exposure to bright lights this way may be harmful to a newborn's retina, so the infant's eyes must always be covered while under phototherapy lights. Eye dressings or cotton balls can be firmly secured in place by an infant mask. Check the dressings frequently to be certain they have not slipped or are causing corneal irritation. A constant concern is that suffocation from eye patches could occur (see Fig. 26.6).

The stools of an infant under phototherapy lights are often bright green because of the excessive bilirubin that is excreted as a result of the therapy. They are also frequently loose and may be irritating to skin. Urine may be dark-coloured from urobilinogen formation. Monitor axillary temperature to prevent an infant from overheating under the bright lights. Assess skin turgor and intake and output to ensure that dehydration is not occurring from the warm environment.

Infants receiving phototherapy should be removed from under the lights for feeding so that they continue to

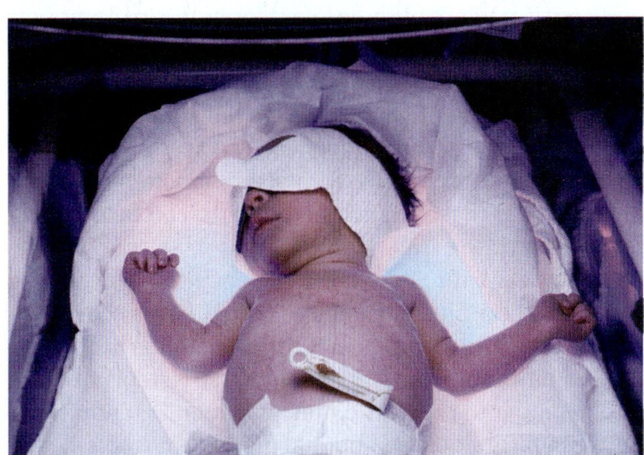

FIGURE 26.6 A newborn receiving phototherapy is undressed except for a nappy so she receives maximum exposure to the lights. Her eyes are covered snugly to protect them from the bright light. (© Lauren Kidziak.)

have interaction with their mother. Remove the eye patches while the infant is with the mother to give them a period of visual stimulation. To prevent a lengthy hospital stay, infants may be discharged and continue therapy at home.

Exchange transfusion

Intensive phototherapy in conjunction with hydration and close monitoring of serum bilirubin levels is the preferred method of treatment of neonatal jaundice. Despite these measures, if bilirubin levels continue to rise, exchange transfusion may be necessary. Before the procedure, the baby's stomach is aspirated to minimise the risk of aspiration from the manipulation involved. The umbilical vein is catheterised as the site for transfusion. The procedure involves alternatively withdrawing small amounts (2–10 mL) of the infant's blood and then replacing it with equal amounts of donor blood. The blood is exchanged slowly this way to prevent alternating hypovolaemia and hypervolaemia. This can make an exchange transfusion a lengthy procedure of 1 to 3 hours. Automatic pumps are helpful to perform the exhausting repeated ritual. At the end of the procedure, using the last specimen of blood withdrawn, haematocrit, bilirubin, electrolytes (especially calcium), glucose determination, and blood cultures are taken. Exchange transfusions may need to be repeated because additional unconjugated bilirubin from tissue moves into the circulation after the exchange.

Vitamin K deficiency bleeding

Vitamin K deficiency bleeding (VKDB), formerly known as haemorrhagic disease of the newborn, results from a deficiency of vitamin K dependant clotting factors in the newborn (Volpi-Wise & Waller, 2010) Vitamin K is essential for the formation of prothrombin by the liver. Lack of it causes decreased prothrombin function and impaired blood coagulation. Vitamin K is formed by the action of bacteria in the intestine. Because the intestinal tract of a newborn is sterile at birth, an infant forms minimal amounts of vitamin K until normal intestinal tract flora are established at about 24 hours of age. Babies born to women receiving anticonvulsive medication are at high risk of the condition because many of these medications interfere with vitamin K formation. Administering vitamin K intramuscularly to these women before birth can help to protect the newborn.

Newborns with vitamin K deficiency show petechiae from superficial bleeding into the skin. They may have conjunctival, mucus membrane or retinal haemorrhage. They may vomit fresh blood or pass black, tarry stools because of bleeding into the gastrointestinal tract. Distinguishing between tarry stools and normal meconium stools can be difficult in the first 1 or 2 days of life by simple observation. However, if an infant's stool does not change as it should from greenish-black (meconium) to the yellow colour of a bottle-fed or breastfed baby, or if the stool colour changes normally and then becomes black again, gastrointestinal bleeding should be suspected. Vitamin K deficiency bleeding usually occurs on day 2 to day 5 of life, when the available prothrombin is at its lowest level. The prothrombin time will be prolonged; the coagulation time may be normal or prolonged. VKDB can be prevented by the intramuscular administration of 1 mg of vitamin K to all newborns immediately after birth.

Group B streptococcal infection

The major cause of infection in newborns is the β-haemolytic, group B streptococcal organism (GBS). This gram-positive bacterium is a natural inhabitant of the female genital tract and is present in the vagina in 10–30% of births. Between 40% and 50% of infants born to colonised mothers will become colonised (Homer et al., 2014). It may be spread from baby to baby if good handwashing technique is not used in handling newborns. If a woman is found to be positive for GBS during late pregnancy, Benzyl penicillin is administered intravenously during labour to reduce the possibility of newborn exposure.

Ophthalmia neonatorum

Also called neonatal conjunctivitis, this condition is an eye infection that occurs at birth or during the first month (Matejcek & Goldman, 2013). The most common causative organisms are *Neisseria gonorrhoeae* and *Chlamydia trachomatis*. An infant contracts the organism during birth, from vaginal secretions. *N. gonorrhoeae* infection is an extremely serious form of conjunctivitis because, if left untreated, the infection progresses to corneal ulceration and destruction, resulting in opacity of the cornea and severe vision impairment.

Hepatitis B virus infection

Hepatitis B virus (HBV) can be transmitted to the newborn through contact with infected vaginal blood at birth when the mother is positive for the virus (HBsAg or HBeAg). Up to 25% of children who develop chronic hepatitis B infection during the peripartum period will later die of the disease (Isaacs & Wood, 2012).

To reduce the possibility of HBsAg being spread to newborns in the future, infants are now routinely vaccinated at birth (Isaacs & Wood, 2012). If the mother is identified as HBsAg1, an infant is also administered immune serum globulin (HBIG) within 12 hours of birth to decrease the possibility of infection. The infant should be bathed as soon as possible after birth to remove HBV-infected blood and secretions. Gentle suctioning is necessary to avoid trauma to the mucus membrane, which could allow HBV invasion. Although the virus is transmitted in breast milk, once immune globulin has been administered, women may breastfeed without risk to an infant. Hepatitis B is further discussed in Chapter 45, because it also occurs in older children.

An infant of a woman who has diabetes mellitus

An infant of a woman who has diabetes mellitus, whose illness was poorly controlled during pregnancy, is typically longer and weighs more than other babies (macrosomia). The baby also has a greater chance of having a congenital anomaly such as a cardiac anomaly, being born prematurely, and experiencing birth trauma due to their large size. Caudal regression syndrome (hypoplasia of the lower extremities) is a syndrome that occurs almost exclusively in such infants (Negrato et al., 2012).

Most of these babies have a cushingoid (fat and puffy) appearance. They tend to be lethargic or limp in the first days of life as a result of hyperglycaemia. The macrosomia results from overstimulation of pituitary growth hormone and extra fat deposits created by high levels of insulin during pregnancy. The infant's large size is deceptive, however: such babies are often immature. RDS occurs frequently in these infants because they may be born preterm or, even at term, lecithin pathways may not mature as rapidly in them. High fetal insulin secretion during pregnancy to counteract the hyperglycaemia may interfere with cortisol release.

In Australia, Indigenous women experience pre-existing diabetes in pregnancy at a rate of three to four times that of non-Indigenous women, and gestational diabetes at a rate of twice that of non-Indigenous women (AIHW, 2010).

An infant of a drug-dependent mother

Infants of drug-dependent women tend to be SGA. If the woman is dependent on a drug, an infant will show withdrawal symptoms (neonatal abstinence syndrome) shortly after birth. These include such signs as:

- Irritability
- Disturbed sleep pattern
- Constant movement, possibly leading to abrasions on the elbows, knees or nose
- Tremors
- Frequent sneezing
- Shrill, high-pitched cry
- Possible hyperreflexia and clonus (neuromuscular irritability)
- Convulsions
- Tachypnoea (rapid respiration), possibly so severe that it leads to hyperventilation and alkalosis
- Vomiting and diarrhoea, leading to large fluid losses and secondary dehydration.

Specific neonatal abstinence scoring tools may be used to quantify and assess an infant's status (see Box 26.4). In newborns experiencing opiate withdrawal, signs usually begin 24–48 hours after birth, but in some infants they may not appear for up to 10 days. Generally signs last approximately 2 weeks, but mild signs may appear for up to 6 months. In heroin-addicted neonates, the signs begin within the first 2 weeks of life, with an average onset of approximately 72 hours. The signs may last 8–16 weeks or longer. In methadone-addicted newborns, withdrawal begins later and lasts longer than heroin withdrawal. The onset varies. A newborn may exhibit signs beginning at 24–28 hours, or these early signs may improve, then reappear at 2–4 weeks of age. Other newborns exhibit no signs until they are 2–3 weeks old.

Infants of drug-dependent women usually seem most comfortable when firmly swaddled. Keep them in an environment free from excessive stimuli (a small isolation nursery, not a large, noisy one). Many infants of heroin-addicted women suck vigorously and continuously and seem to find comfort and quiet if given a dummy. Infants of methadone- and cocaine-addicted women may have extremely poor sucking ability and may have difficulty achieving sufficient fluid intake unless nasogastric tube-fed.

Specific therapy for an infant is individualised according to the nature and severity of the signs. Maintenance of electrolyte and fluid balance is essential. If an infant has vomiting or diarrhoea, intravenous administration of fluid may be indicated. Once an infant has been identified as having been exposed to drugs in utero, the mother needs treatment for withdrawal symptoms and follow-up care as much as the infant. In addition, infants who are exposed to drugs in utero may have long-term neurological problems (Oei et al., 2012). Social services follow-up for babies of drug addicted mothers should be commenced in the antenatal period to allow for planning and management of child safety.

BOX 26.4 Assessment ✻ Assessing the newborn of a drug-addicted mother

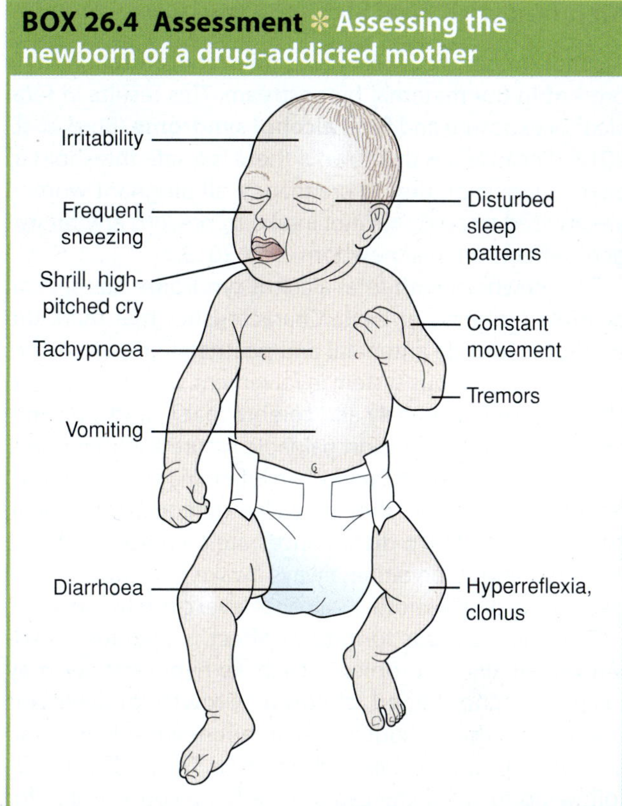

An infant with fetal alcohol exposure

Alcohol crosses the placenta in similar concentrations as is present in the maternal bloodstream. This results in fetal alcohol exposure and **fetal alcohol syndrome** (Burd et al., 2012). Because it is unknown if there is a safe threshold of alcohol ingestion during pregnancy, all pregnant women are advised to avoid alcohol intake to prevent any teratogenic effects on their newborn (Day, 2012).

The newborn with fetal alcohol syndrome has several possible problems at birth. Characteristics that mark the syndrome include antenatal and postnatal growth restriction; central nervous system involvement such as cognitive challenge, microcephaly and cerebral palsy; and a distinctive facial feature of a short palpable fissure and thin upper lip. During the neonatal period, an infant may be tremulous, fidgety and irritable: they may also demonstrate a weak sucking reflex. Sleep disturbances are common, with the baby tending to be either always awake or always asleep, depending on the mother's alcohol level close to birth.

The most serious long-term effect is cognitive challenge. Behaviour problems such as hyperactivity may occur in school-aged children. Growth deficiencies may remain throughout life. An infant needs follow-up so any future problems can be discovered. The mother needs follow-up to see if she can reduce her alcohol intake for better overall health. Salman (2008) in a New Zealand study on the awareness of the effect of alcohol use during pregnancy showed that more than 50% of women believed that if a pregnant woman wanted to drink, some alcohol was safe in pregnancy. Nearly 20% of all women had binged on at least one occasion in pregnancy, most having done so before they realised they were pregnant.

Australian data suggest the prevalence of fetal alcohol syndrome is increasing. In Victoria, data showed a prevalence of 0.01–0.03 per 1000 live births, none of whom were Indigenous. In South Australia data examined between 1986 and 2005 showed a prevalence of 0.03 per 1000 live births; while in Western Australia the prevalence based on data collected from 1980–2003 was 0.4 per 1000 births. The highest prevalence is in the Northern Territory with 0.68 per 1000 live births, all of whom were Indigenous (Burns et al., 2013). You can find further information about this condition on the following websites:

- Nofasard <www.nofasard.org>
- Alcohol Advisory Council of New Zealand <www.alcohol.org.nz>
- Fetal Alcohol Network <www.fan.org.nz>.

✔ *Checkpoint question* 26.2

Why is it important for infants of diabetic women to be fed early?

a. Their stomachs are empty at birth
b. To help prevent hypoglycaemia
c. Their mothers could not eat during labour
d. To clear mucus from their intestinal tracts

Key points for review

- Priorities for infants born with special needs, such as preterm or postterm infants, are the same as for term infants: initiation and maintenance of respiration, establishment of extrauterine circulation, control of body temperature, intake of adequate nourishment, establishment of waste elimination, establishment of an infant–parent relationship, prevention of infection, and provision of developmental care for mental and social development.
- Many high-risk infants need resuscitation at birth. Prompt action with such measures as warmth, oxygen, intubation and suctioning are needed.
- A small-for-gestational-age (SGA) infant is one whose birth weight is below the 10th percentile on an intrauterine growth curve for that age. An infant could be preterm, term or postterm.
- SGA infants have difficulty maintaining body warmth because of low fat stores and may develop hypoglycaemia from low glucose stores.
- A large-for-gestational-age (LGA) infant is one whose birth weight is above the 90th percentile on an intrauterine growth chart for that gestational age. The infant could be born preterm, term or postterm.
- LGA infants tend to be infants of diabetic women; they are particularly prone to hypoglycaemia or birth trauma.
- A preterm infant is one born before 37 weeks of gestation. Preterm infants have particular problems with respiratory function, anaemia, jaundice, persistent patent ductus arteriosus and intracranial haemorrhage. Infants who are born weighing 1500 to 2500 g are also termed low-birth-weight infants; those born weighing 1000 to 1500 g are very-low-birth-weight infants; those born weighing between 500 and 1000 g are extremely very-low-birth-weight infants. All such infants need intensive care from the moment of birth to give them their best chance of survival without neurological after-effects caused by their being so close to the age of viability.
- A postterm infant is one who has remained in utero past week 42 of pregnancy. Postterm infants have particular problems with establishing respiration, meconium aspiration, hypoglycaemia, temperature regulation and polycythaemia.
- Respiratory distress syndrome (RDS) commonly occurs in preterm infants from a deficiency or lack of surfactant in the alveoli. Without surfactant, the alveoli collapse on expiration and require extreme force for reinflation.
- Transient tachypnoea of the newborn is a temporary condition caused by slow absorption of lung fluid at birth. Close observation of the infant is necessary until the fluid is absorbed and breathing slows to a normal rate.
- Meconium aspiration syndrome occurs when an infant aspirates meconium-stained amniotic fluid before or

during birth. Meconium is irritating to the airway and leads to both airway spasm and pneumonia. Infants need oxygen, ventilatory support and possibly an antibiotic until the effects of the insult to the airway subside. Infants should be suctioned before oxygen administration under pressure to prevent meconium from being forced further into their lungs.

- Apnoea is a pause in respiration longer than 20 seconds, with accompanying bradycardia. It tends to occur in preterm infants who have secondary stresses such as infection, hyperbilirubinaemia, hypoglycaemia or hypothermia. Apnoea monitors are used to detect this and infants who are at high risk of apnoea may be discharged home on a home monitoring program.
- Sudden infant death syndrome (SIDS) is the sudden, unexplained death of an infant. It is associated with infants sleeping on their stomachs (prone) and preterm birth. An important preventive measure is advising parents to position their infant on the back for sleeping.
- Hyperbilirubinaemia results from the destruction of red blood cells, owing either to a normal physiological response or an abnormal destruction of red blood cells. Haemolytic disease of the newborn is destruction of red blood cells from Rh or ABO incompatibility. The administration of RHIG (Rh antibodies) to Rh-negative mothers during pregnancy and after the birth of an Rh-positive infant to an Rh-negative mother has greatly reduced the incidence of the condition. Affected infants are jaundiced from release of bilirubin from injured red blood cells. Phototherapy and exchange transfusion are used to prevent kernicterus (deposition of bilirubin in brain cells, causing destruction of the cells).
- Haemorrhagic disease of the newborn is a lack of clotting ability resulting from a deficiency of vitamin K at birth. This disorder is prevented by administering vitamin K to infants at birth.
- Severe infections acquired at birth that may be seen in newborns include streptococcal group B pneumonia, hepatitis B infection, ophthalmia neonatorum (gonococcal and chlamydial conjunctivitis), and herpes virus infection. Assessing newborns for symptoms of these infections is an important nursing responsibility.
- Infants of women with diabetes and those of drug abusing women are at high risk at birth for further complications. Both need careful assessment for respiratory distress and hypoglycaemia.

CASE STUDY QUESTIONS

2. Karen was confused and distraught and had not visited her new baby. How would you advise her?
3. Infants who are cared for in neonatal intensive care units may need either reduced stimulation because they tire so easily or increased stimulation because their stay in the nursery will be so extended. What are examples of developmental care you might use with Baby Atkins?

Resources

For an extensive range of additional resources to enhance teaching and learning and to facilitate understanding of this chapter, please see the text's accompanying website located on thePoint at http://thepoint.lww.com.

References

Australian Bureau of Statistics. (2010). The health and welfare of Australia's Aboriginal and Torres Strait Islander peoples, 2008, accessed 9 February 2015, <www.abs.gov.au/AUSSTATS/abs@.nsf/39433889d406eeb9ca2570610019e9a5/B2AB19063526127FCA2574390014B1FA>.

Australian Bureau of Statistics. (ABS) (2014), accessed 9 February 2015, <www.abs.gov.au/ausstats/abs@.nsf/Lookup/3303.0Chapter392011>.

Australian Institute of Health and Welfare (AIHW). (2010). Diabetes in pregnancy: Its impact on Australian women and their babies, accessed 9 February 2015, <www.aihw.gov.au/publication-detail/?id=6442472448>.

Australian Institute of Health and Welfare (AIHW). (2014). Australia's mothers and babies 2011, accessed 9 February 2015 <www.aihw.gov.au/WorkArea/DownloadAsset.aspx?id=60129545698>.

Australian Resuscitation Council (2010). Section 13 Neonatal guidelines, accessed 9 February 2015 <www.resus.org.au/policy/guidelines/>.

Bailey, S. (2012). Kangaroo mother care: Review. *British Journal of Hospital Medicine*, *73*(5), 278–281.

Brown, V. & Landers, S. (2011). Heat balance. In S. Gardner, B. Carter, M. Enzman-Hines & J. Hernandez (Eds.). *Merenstein & Gardner's Handbook of Neonatal Intensive Care* (7th ed.). St Louis: Mosby Elsevier.

Burd, L., Blair, J. & Dropps, K. (2012). Prenatal alcohol exposure, blood alcohol concentrations and alcohol elimination rates for the mother, fetus and newborn, *Journal of Perinatology*, *32*(9), 652.

Burns, L., Breen, C., Bower, C., O'Leary, C. & Elliot, E. (2013). Counting fetal alcohol spectrum disorder in Australia: The evidence and the challenges. *Drug and Alcohol Review*, *32*(5), 461–467.

Day, S. (2012). Alcohol consumption during pregnancy: The growing evidence, *Developmental Medicine and Child Neurology*, *54*(3), 200.

Edwards, M., Kotecha, S.J. & Kotecha, S. (2013). Respiratory distress in the term infant. *Paediatric Respiratory Reviews*, *14*(1). 29–37.

Gardner, S., Enzman-Hines, M. & Dickey, L. (2011). Respiratory diseases. In S. Gardner, B. Carter, M. Enzman-Hines & J. Hernandez (Eds.). *Merenstein & Gardner's Handbook of Neonatal Intensive Care* (7th ed.). St Louis: Mosby Elsevier.

Gelfer, P. & Tatum, M. (2014). Sudden infant death syndrome. *Journal of Pediatric Health Care*, *28*(5), 470–474.

Homer, C., Scarf, V., Catling, C. & Davis, D. (2014). Culture based versus risk based screening for prevention of group B streptococcal disease in newborns: A review of national guidelines. *Women and Birth*, *27*(1), 46–51.

Isaacs, D. & Wood, N. (2012). Hepatitis B vaccination in pregnancy. Expert Review of Vaccines, 11(2), 125.

Joseph, K., Fahey, J., Shankardass, K., Allen, V., O'Campo, P., Dodds, L., Liston, R. & Allen, A. (2014). Effects of socioeconomic position and clinical risk factors on spontaneous and iatrogenic preterm birth. *BMC Pregnancy and Childbirth*, *14*, 117.

Kattwinkel, J. (Ed). (2011). *Neonatal Resuscitation Textbook* (6th ed.). American Heart Association and American Academy of Pediatrics.

Kattwinkel, J., Perlman, J., Aziz, K., Colby, C., Fairchild, K., Gallagher, J., Hazinski, M., Halamek, L., Kumar, P., Little, G., McGowan, J., Nightengale, B., Ramirez, M., Ringer, S., Simon, W., Weiner, G., Wyckoff, M. & Zaichkin, J. (2010). Neonatal resuscitation: 2010 American heart association guidelines for cardiopulmonary resuscitation and emergency cardiovascular care. *Pediatrics*, *126*(5), e1400–e1413.

Kenet, G., Kuperman, A., Strauss, T. & Brenner, B. (2011). Neonatal IVH: Mechanisms and management. *Thrombosis Research*, *127*(3), S120–S122.

Knobel, R. & Holditch-Davis, D. (2007). Thermoregulation and heat loss prevention after birth and during neonatal intensive-care unit stabilization of extremely low-birth weight infants. *JOGNN: Journal of Obstetric, Gynecologic, and Neonatal Nursing, 36*(3), 280–287.

Lawrence, E. J. (2007). A matter of size: Evaluating the large-for-gestational-age neonate. *Advances in Neonatal Care, 7*(4), 187–197.

Ludington-Hoe, S. (2011). Thirty years of kangaroo care: Science and practice. *Neonatal Network, 30*(5), 357–362.

McCall, E. M., et al. (2009). Interventions to prevent hypothermia at birth in preterm and/or low birth weight infants. *Cochrane Database of Systematic Reviews, 2009*(1), CD004210.

McDonald, S., Han, Z., Mulla, S., Ohlsson, A., Beyene, J. & Murphy, K. (2010). Preterm birth and low birth weight among in vitro fertilization twins: A systematic review and meta analyses. *European Journal of Obstetrics and Gynecology, 148*(2), 105–113.

McKenna, L. & Mirkov, S. (2014). McKenna's Drug Handbook for Nursing and Midwifery (7th ed.). Sydney: Lippincott Williams & Wilkins.

Matejcek, A. & Goldman, R. (2013). Treatment and prevention of opthalmia neonatorum. *Canadian Family Physician, 59*, 1187–1189.

Negrato, C., Mattar, R. & Gomes, M. (2012). Adverse pregnancy outcomes in women with diabetes. *Diabetology & Metabolic Syndrome, 4*(41).

New Zealand Government. (2014). Statistics New Zealand, births and deaths, accessed 9 February 2015, <www.stats.govt.nz/browse_for_stats/population/births/BirthsAndDeaths_HOTPYeDec13.aspx>.

Oei, J., Kingsbury, A., Burns, L., Feller, J. & Clews, S. (2012). Amphetamines, the pregnant woman and her children: A review. *Journal of Perinatology, 32*(10), 737.

Pinheiro, J. M. (2009). The Apgar cycle: a new view of a familiar scoring system. *Archives of Disease in Childhood Fetal & Neonatal Edition, 94*(1), F70–72.

Salman, J. (2008). Fetal alcohol spectrum disorder: New Zealand birth mothers' experiences. *Canadian Journal of Clinical Pharmacology, 15*(2), e191–213.

Shapiro, S. (2010). Chronic bilirubin encephalopathy: Diagnosis and outcome. *Seminars in Fetal and Neonatal Medicine, 15*(3), 157–163.

State Government of Victoria. (2014). Neonatal eHandbook, accessed 9 February 2015, <www.health.vic.gov.au/neonatalhandbook/procedures/iv-infusion-for-scn-admissions.htm>.

Symons, A. B. & Mahoney, M. C. (2008). Neonatal hyperbilirubinemia. In J. E. South-Paul, S. C. Matheny, & E. L. Lewis. (Eds). *Current Diagnosis and Treatment in Family Medicine* (2nd ed.). Columbus, OH: McGraw-Hill.

Thilo, E. H. & Rosenberg, A. A. (2008). The newborn. In W. W. Hay et al. (Eds). *Current pediatric diagnosis and treatment* (18th ed.). Columbus, OH: McGraw-Hill.

Volpi-Wise, M. & Waller, N. (2010). Complications of the newborn. In S. Pairman, S. Tracy, C. Thorogood & J. Pincombe (Eds.). *Midwifery: Preparation for Practice* (2nd ed). Sydney: Churchill Livingstone Elsevier.

Suggested readings

Ahrabi, A. & Schanler, R. (2013). Human milk is the only milk for premmies in the NICU. *Early Human Development, 89*(2), S51–S53.

Axelin, A., Lehtonen, L., Pelander, T., et al. (2010). Mothers' different styles of involvement in preterm infant pain care. *Journal of Obstetrics, Gynecologic & Neonatal Nursing, 39*(4), 415–424.

Campbell, M., Johnston, C., Benoit, B., Latimer, M., Vincer, M. & Walker, C. (2013). Trial of repeated analgesia with kangaroo mother care (TRAKC Trial). *BMC Pediatrics, 13*(1), 182.

Fenton, T. & Kim, J. (2013). A systematic review and meta-analysis to revise the Fenton growth chart for preterm infants. *BMC Pediatrics, 13*(1), 59.

Fink, A. M. (2011). Early hospital discharge in maternal and newborn care. *Journal of Obstetrics, Gynecologic & Neonatal Nursing, 40*(2), 149–156.

Harris, G. (2014). Family-centred rounds in the neonatal intensive care unit. *Nursing for Women's Health, 18*(1), 18–27.

Moore, T. A., Berger, A. M., & Wilson, M. E. (2012). A new way of thinking about complications of prematurity. *Biologic Research for Nursing*. Advance online publication.

Chapter 27

Care of the child born with a physical or developmental challenge

Previous chapters described the importance of assessing all infants at birth. This chapter adds information about common congenital challenges or structural disturbances that may occur in newborns. This information can serve as a basis for newborn assessment and for health teaching for parents.

LEARNING OBJECTIVES

After studying the contents of this chapter, you should be able to:

1. Describe common physical and developmental birth disorders.
2. Use critical thinking to analyse the effect of a physical or developmental challenge on the child and family and propose ways to make care more family-centred.
3. Assess a child who is born with a physical or developmental challenge.
4. Formulate nursing considerations for children born with a physical or developmental challenge.
5. Establish expected outcomes to meet the needs of a child with a physical or developmental abnormality.
6. Plan nursing care to meet the needs of a child born with a physical or developmental abnormality.
7. Implement nursing interventions for care of children born with a physical or developmental challenge.
8. Evaluate expected outcomes to determine achievement and effectiveness of care.
9. Identify areas related to physically- or developmentally-challenged infants that could benefit by additional nursing research or application of evidence-based practice.
10. Integrate knowledge of congenital physical or developmental challenge with nursing interventions to achieve quality child and family health nursing care.

KEY TERMS

- ankyloglossia
- atresia
- cleft lip
- cleft palate
- congenital hip dysplasia (CHD)
- fistula
- frenulum
- hydrocephalus
- meconium plug
- omphalocele
- polydactyly
- spina bifida
- stenosis
- syndactyly
- transillumination
- volvulus

CASE STUDY

Caitlin Jones is a newborn admitted to the Special Care Nursery (SCN) post-birth with a neural tube disorder and congenital hip dysplasia. Caitlin's parents, Emma and Brad, are in attendance, with Emma being obviously visibly upset over the diagnosis. She says, "What did I do wrong during the pregnancy to cause this to happen?"

CASE STUDY QUESTIONS

1. How would you answer Emma?
2. What type of advice would be most helpful to her?

When a child is born with an apparent physical or developmental challenge, nurses must play a major role in supporting and educating the parents to help them move forwards from this point. Some congenital disorders require surgery but the prognosis is good, so this is only a temporary concern. Other disorders, however, represent serious, even life-threatening concerns for infants and financially-draining long-term responsibilities for parents. This chapter covers the physical congenital disorders that are apparent at birth or soon after. Such disorders primarily involve the gastrointestinal, neurological and skeletal systems. Congenital disorders of the cardiovascular system, which also represent life-threatening problems for an infant, are addressed in Chapter 41.

CARE OF THE CHILD BORN WITH A PHYSICAL OR DEVELOPMENTAL CHALLENGE

Assessment

Nursing assessment of a newborn with a physical or developmental challenge focuses on determining an infant's immediate physiological needs required to sustain life, and the parents' immediate emotional needs to promote bonding between the child and parents. The parents' response to the diagnosis of a congenital challenge must also be assessed. Anomalies that affect a child's appearance may have the most immediate effect on the parents' ability to establish a positive feeling about their child. It is important, however, not to jump to conclusions about parents' responses. Assessment of the family's verbal and non-verbal responses may reveal parents are ready to meet this infant's special needs.

Nurses play an important role in providing care to high-risk infants at birth and guarding their health until a childcare team arrives to transport the infant to a high-risk unit. When establishing expected outcomes and planning care, be certain to consider both the short- and long-term needs of the newborn and how these needs may affect the family. Also consider the family's resources, both emotional and financial, and devise a plan of care with these in mind. Parents with supportive family members nearby may be able to accept the limits of a child's challenge and turn their attention to the planned treatment regimen or care priorities sooner than those without close friends or relatives to whom they can turn for comfort and support. For the latter, you may need to act not only as a source of information and support but also as a sounding board and advocate until the parents can begin to develop positive coping mechanisms that will help them come to terms with this unexpected event. Referrals to support groups may be beneficial, allowing parents to learn they are not alone in this situation. The following organisations can be helpful sources of support for parents:

- Australasian Cleft Lip & Palate Association Inc. <www.cleft.org.au>
- CCS Disability Action <www.ccsdisabilityaction.org.nz>
- Cleft New Zealand <www.faceit.org.nz>
- Down Syndrome Australia <www.downsyndrome.org.au>
- Hydrocephalus Support Association <www.hydrocephalus.org.au>
- NZ Down Syndrome Association <www.nzdsa.org.nz>
- Pierre Robin Australia <www.pierrerobin.org.au>
- Spina Bifida Foundation Victoria <www.sbfv.org.au>.

Nursing considerations

Nursing considerations for a baby born with a physical challenge include immediate life-sustaining measures such as providing for adequate intake of nutrients when a disorder prevents the infant from sucking. Educating the parents about pretreatment and post-treatment procedures and encouraging them to hold, touch and talk with their baby are especially important to the future emotional well-being of the child and family.

Parents may suffer a loss of self-esteem with the child's birth, feeling as if the baby is proof that something in the combination of their genes or the prenatal environment they provided was inadequate. They may need to hear positive comments about themselves and be given support until they can realise that by caring for the child they are accomplishing more, not less, than other couples. You can expect parents to move through the same stages of grief as those whose child has died at birth. Chapter 56 describes those stages and helpful nursing interventions in more detail.

Parents are acutely aware of what people think of their child. They watch closely how nurses and other healthcare providers handle their baby to see if they are giving as much attention to their baby as to other babies. To encourage parents to accept the child, be certain to treat the child in the same manner as any other—for example, rocking the baby after feeding or cooing and talking to the baby as much as with other babies. Otherwise, parents may think that if a professional finds their child distasteful, how will they dare show the child to their family and friends? If you are able to look past the challenge to the whole child, however, they will begin to do so, too. Through positive role modelling, you can set the stage for healthy parent–child interaction every time you handle an infant born with a physical or developmental challenge.

Evaluation should focus on expected outcomes established for a child's physical health and developmental needs, as well as the family's ability to cope with whatever special care and growth needs the child may have in the future. Be sure parents have appropriate health professionals with contact details to call for questions, follow-up care and support.

IMMEDIATE CARE AT THE BIRTH OF AN INFANT BORN PHYSICALLY OR DEVELOPMENTALLY CHALLENGED

Most doctors, nurses and midwives believe that relating the news of congenital physical or developmental anomalies to parents is their responsibility. However, because the doctor or nurse/midwife must deliver the placenta and suture the perineum if an episiotomy was used for birth, if a neonatal specialist is not immediately available, many minutes may pass before this person is ready to make a second inspection of the baby, assess the extent of the disorder from the physical symptoms present, and tell the parents about the baby's condition and prognosis. This delay affects the parents in two ways: it leaves them either believing they have just given birth to a perfect, normal child among people who do not share their enthusiasm, or they have just given birth to a child so deformed all the professionals in the room find it too horrible to even talk to them. Because parents are aware of the atmosphere in a birthing room, the second response is by far more likely. In terms of parent–child interaction, this response is unhealthy. Parents may begin anticipatory grieving for what they believe is a severely deformed child. Even when they are told later the disorder is not extensive and is easily correctable, and that as soon as the correction is made the child will be fine, the anticipatory grief reaction may be hard to stop. They may continue to distance themselves emotionally from their child.

For this reason, nurses need to be familiar with the most frequently encountered physical or developmental anomalies so that as the person who at that moment in the birth process is most available for parent education, they can explain the problem to parents. In other instances, nurses must be ready to serve as back-up informants to answer parents' questions after they have been told by a primary care provider (obstetrician, midwife, paediatrician) that their child has been born less than perfect.

The causes of most congenital anomalies are unknown, although they are thought to arise from a combination of environmental and genetic factors. Still, many cultures persist in believing that infants with congenital anomalies are born to people less deserving than others or to those who have sinned or have been looked on by someone with envy during pregnancy. That eating raisins during pregnancy causes brown spots, and that strawberries cause haemangiomas, are common beliefs still prevalent in some cultures.

New parents need an explanation of their child's anomaly and a chance to talk about why they believe it occurred, to relieve their guilt that they were the cause and to allow them to regain sufficient self-esteem to be able to raise a child with a congenital disorder.

It is probably best to explain to parents what the disorder consists of and what the usual prognosis is before showing the baby to them. Parents may find it hard to look at an infant with a cleft lip or palate or exposed abdominal contents, for example, and also listen. Their minds are so consumed with the sight, so unlike the child they had imagined, that they cannot hear. A typical explanation would be: "Your baby's upper lip isn't completely formed. That's called a cleft lip. Your doctor will call one of the plastic surgeons here to look at your baby. This is a problem that can be repaired so well surgically you'll barely be able to tell your baby had this problem. I'll bring the baby over so you can meet her. Remember when you look at her this can be repaired. She seems perfect in every other way."

These are the sort of statements that define and limit the problem for the parents. They also give them direction about where and how they should proceed in beginning to seek help for their child. As most congenital abnormalities involve surgery, be certain to plan for adequate pain assessment and management postoperatively to make the experience of surgery this early in life not an unbearable procedure for a neonate (Harrison et al., 2010).

PHYSICAL AND DEVELOPMENTAL DISORDERS OF THE GASTROINTESTINAL SYSTEM

Many of the most common congenital anomalies involve the gastrointestinal system because the gastrointestinal tract forms first as a solid tube, then undergoes canalisation. If this canalisation does not occur, a partial or complete blockage or obstruction can occur. Other disorders of the tract, such as cleft lip and cleft palate, are the result of midline closure failure extremely early in intrauterine life. All of these disorders can interfere with an infant's ability to take in nourishment at birth. Breastfeeding can be difficult or may not be possible to begin with. You may need to reinforce a mother's resolve to breastfeed as appropriate to aid in her success with this method of feeding when possible. Mothers wishing to breastfeed should be encouraged and supported to express breast milk, which can be given to their baby via tube feeds until breastfeeding can later be established.

Ankyloglossia (tongue-tie)

Ankyloglossia is an abnormal restriction of the tongue caused by an abnormally tight lingual **frenulum**, the membrane attached to the lower anterior tip of the tongue (Kline, 2014). Normally, in newborns, the frenulum appears short and is positioned near the tip of the tongue. As the anterior portion of the infant's tongue grows, the frenulum becomes located farther back. In most instances, therefore, an infant suspected of being tongue-tied has a normal tongue at birth; it just seems short to parents who are unaware of a newborn's appearance. In the past, the frenulum under the tongue was routinely divided in babies or children with tongue-tie. Today, doctors are more inclined to wait and see what happens to the frenulum with growth. This condition rarely causes speech difficulty or destructive pressure on gingival tissue. If it does, then surgical release can be performed, following assessment by a paediatric surgeon or maxillofacial surgeon experienced in performing the procedure. For babies having difficulty establishing breastfeeding, an assessment for tongue tie should be made. A shortened tight frenulum may interfere with the ability to "latch on" correctly. In this instance a referral should be made to the paediatric surgeon for further assessment and management as soon as possible so as to not further impede the establishment of breastfeeding. The presence of a tongue tie does not appear to have such an impact on babies feeding from a bottle.

Thyroglossal cyst

A thyroglossal cyst arises from an embryogenic fault that leaves a cyst formed at the base of the tongue, which then drains through a **fistula** (opening) to the anterior surface of the neck (D. Lee et al., 2011). This condition may occur as a dominantly inherited trait. The cyst may involve the hyoid bone (the bone at the anterior surface of the neck at the root of the tongue) or may contain aberrant thyroid gland tissue. As the cyst fills with fluid, swelling and obstruction can lead to respiratory difficulty from pressure on the trachea. If infected, the cyst appears swollen and reddened, with drainage of mucus or pus from the anterior neck.

The cyst is surgically removed to avoid future infection of the space or, if thyroid tissue is present, the possibility of developing thyroid carcinoma later in life. Observe infants closely in the immediate postoperative period for respiratory distress, because the operative area will develop some oedema from surgical trauma. Position infants on their side so secretions drain freely from their mouths. Intravenous fluid therapy is given after surgery until the oedema at the incision recedes somewhat and swallowing is safe once more (approximately 24 hours). If the mother is breastfeeding but the infant is NBM, encourage her to express her milk manually to preserve her milk supply. Observe infants closely the first time they take fluid orally to be certain they do not aspirate. Be certain parents feed their infant before the infant is discharged from the surgical unit so they can see that the infant is swallowing safely. This is important to help them develop confidence in themselves as parents and their ability to feed the infant at home in a relaxed and comfortable way.

Cleft lip and palate

The maxillary and median nasal processes normally fuse between weeks 5 and 8 of intrauterine life. In infants with **cleft lip**, the fusion fails to occur in varying degrees, causing this disorder to range from a small notch in the upper lip to total separation of the lip and facial structure up into the floor of the nose, with even the upper teeth and gingiva absent. The deviation may be unilateral or bilateral. The nose is generally flattened because the incomplete fusion of the upper lip has allowed it to expand in a horizontal dimension. Cleft lip appears to be caused by the transmission of multiple genes aided by teratogenic factors present during weeks 5 to 8 of intrauterine life, such as a viral infection, certain seizure medicines such as phenytoin, maternal smoking or binge drinking, hyperthermia, stress and maternal obesity (Bishop, 2011; Dixon, Marazita & Beaty et al., 2011). Folic acid deficiency may also be associated with incomplete anterior midline closures (Kelly, O'Dowd & Reulbach, 2012).

The palatal process closes at approximately weeks 9 to 12 of intrauterine life. A **cleft palate**, an opening of the palate, is usually on the midline and may involve the anterior hard palate, the posterior soft palate, or both (see Fig. 27.1). It may be a separate anomaly, but as a rule it occurs in conjunction with a cleft lip. As a single entity, it tends to occur more frequently in girls than boys. Like cleft lip, it appears to be the result of polygenic inheritance or environmental influences. In connection with cleft lip, the incidence is approximately 1 in every 1000 births. As a single entity, it occurs in approximately 1 in every 2000 births (Hoffman, 2008).

Assessment

Cleft lip may be detected by ultrasound while an infant is in utero. If not detected then, it is readily apparent on inspection at birth. Cleft palate can be determined by depressing the newborn's tongue with a tongue blade. This reveals the total palate and the extent of any cleft present. Be sure to have good lighting to visualise the palate clearly. Because cleft palate is a component of many syndromes, a child with a cleft palate must be assessed for other congenital anomalies.

Parents of a child with a cleft lip should be referred for genetic counselling to ensure they understand that they have about a 4% chance of having another child with a cleft lip or palate and future children are at a greater risk than usual for this problem.

Therapeutic management

A cleft lip is generally repaired surgically at 3–4 months of age, however different hospitals and surgeons may have slightly different timeframes. Some infants may have a nasal mould apparatus applied before surgery to shape a better nostril (Garfinkle et al., 2011). Early repair helps infants experience the pleasure of sucking as soon as possible. It is equally important from a psychological standpoint that these disorders be repaired early. Parents can find it extremely difficult to bond with an infant whose face is deformed in this way. This is not a sign of a "bad" parent, but it is a reality and a problem that requires intervention. Because facial contours change as a child grows, a revision of the original repair or a nasal rhinoplasty to straighten a deviated nasal septum may be necessary when the child reaches 4 to 6 years of age.

The optimal time for repair of cleft palate is controversial as early repair increases speech development but may result in a necessary second-stage repair as the child's palate arch grows. A two-stage palate repair, with soft palate repair at 3 to 6 months of age and hard palate repair at 15 to 18 months of age, may be recommended (van Aalst et al., 2008). Because palate repair narrows the upper

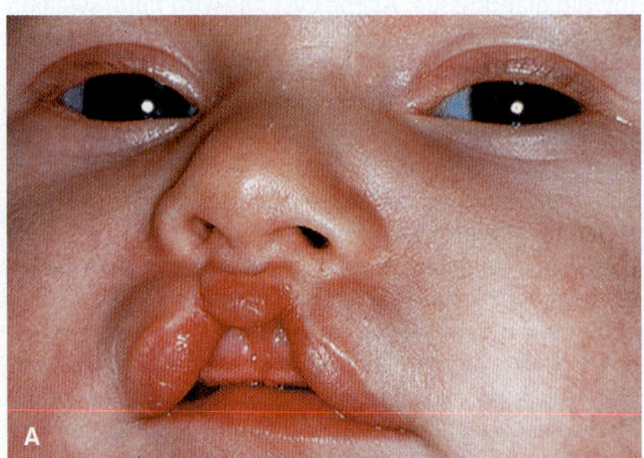

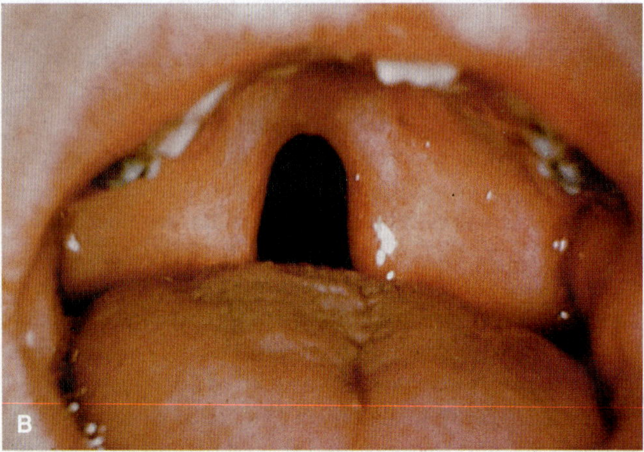

FIGURE 27.1 Appearance of (**A**) a cleft lip and (**B**) a cleft palate. (From Lippincott Williams & Wilkins' *Comprehensive Dental Assisting*, 2011).

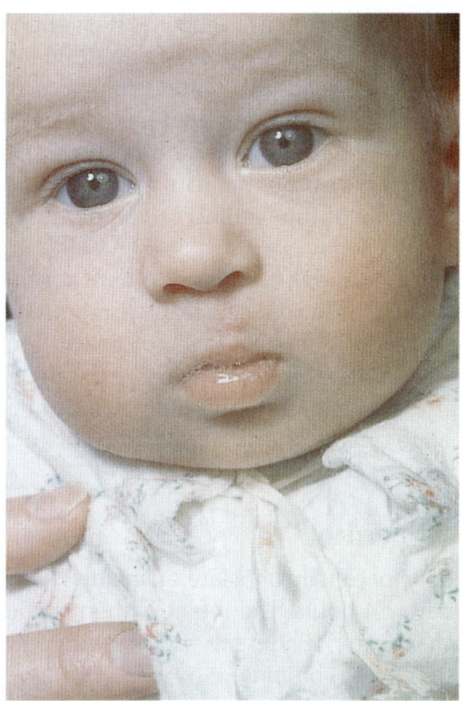

FIGURE 27.2 Infant showing surgical repair of cleft lip. Parents can be encouraged that the results of cleft lip repair are generally excellent. (Photo Researchers, Inc.)

dental arch, there may be less space in the upper jaw for the eruption of teeth, causing poor teeth alignment. All children born with a cleft palate need follow-up treatment by a paediatric dentist/orthodontist, or a dentist skilled in children's dental problems, so that as the child grows, extractions or realignment of teeth can be done as indicated. They also need follow-up to detect if speech or hearing difficulty occurs.

Currently, the results of surgical repair of cleft lip and cleft palate are excellent (see Fig. 27.2). It is helpful to show parents photographs of babies post-repair to assure them that their child's outcome can also be this successful.

Nursing considerations

To promote bonding, parents need to hold and interact with their infant during both the preoperative and postoperative periods. Caution them that the incision line will appear swollen in the immediate postoperative period. Reassure them this appearance will improve over time. As soon as the child's sutures have been removed, the infant may be bottle fed (with an ordinary bottle) or breastfed. Caution both the breastfeeding mother (who has been maintaining her milk supply through expression) and the formula-feeding mother that because the infant has never sucked before, time will be needed to learn, just as does a newborn.

Notice whether the parents look at their baby's face while feeding. Help them to understand that any negative feelings directed towards the child or themselves, such as sadness or anger their baby was born this way, are normal. This does not instantly make them feel better about what has happened, but the knowledge that what they are experiencing is normal can help them begin to deal with such emotions. Many communities have support groups for parents of children born with a cleft lip or palate. Referral to these groups can be helpful.

If a scar remains after cleft lip surgery, children may need some help adjusting to it until a cosmetic repair can be completed later in life. Reinforce children's positive attributes, stressing that the scar is only one small aspect of who they are. As children reach adolescence, you may need to review a familial inheritance pattern of cleft lip so they are informed of the possible risk of transmission to their own children.

Infants with a cleft palate will begin to make speech sounds at the normal time (aged 2 months), although their speech may be guttural and harsh. By 9 months, when other infants begin to say meaningful words ("bye-bye," "mama," "dada"), assuming the cleft palate is still unrepaired, speech sounds will be unclear. Some parents try to discourage their baby from talking, thinking if the child does not talk until after the cleft palate repair is made, a speech impediment will not develop. Speech occurs at a specified developmental time, however, and despite the unfused palate it should be encouraged at these age-appropriate times. A child with a cleft palate can enunciate vowel sounds with the most clarity, so these are the sounds a parent should encourage the child to voice. Words such as "me," "they," "no," "mumma," "home," "moon," "rain," "yell," and "row" are words consisting largely of vowel sounds and can be enunciated most clearly by the child before a cleft palate repair.

Depending on the age of the child when the cleft palate is repaired, some children will continue to have accompanying speech difficulty because the soft palate must function for the child to pronounce "p" and "b" sounds (Mildinhall, 2012). If cleft palate surgery is going to be delayed much past the age of 2 years (as might happen if the child has other congenital anomalies, such as heart disease), a plastic prosthesis to cover the incomplete palate may be prescribed. This allows the child to articulate more normally.

Children do not spontaneously outgrow faulty speech patterns, so training by a speech therapist may be necessary. Commonly used exercises children are asked to perform include blowing games, such as blowing a feather or a table tennis ball, as a blowing motion is what is required to pronounce "p" and "b".

Nutrition

Preoperative period

Before a cleft lip or palate is repaired, feeding the infant is a problem because the infant has difficulty maintaining suction. In addition, it is important that the child does not aspirate. It may be possible for an infant with a cleft lip to breastfeed because the bulk of the mother's breast tends

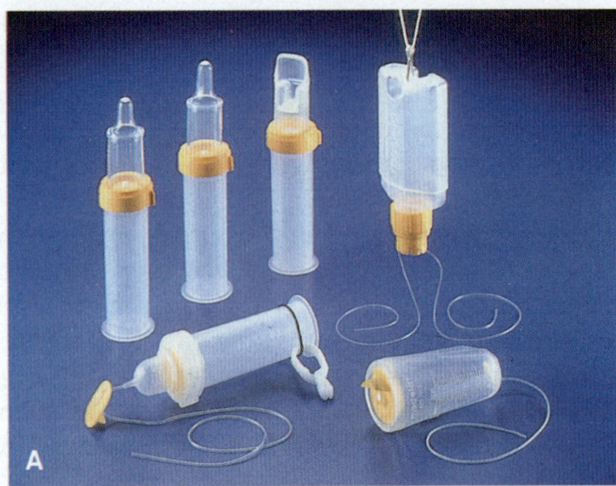

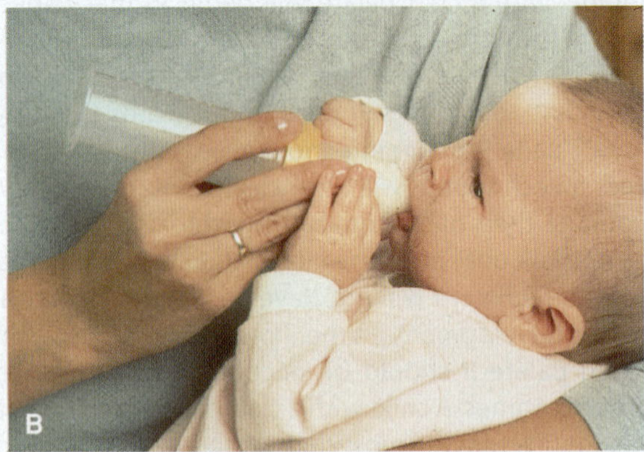

FIGURE 27.3 (**A**) Specialty feeding devices used for infants with cleft lip and cleft palate. (**B**) An infant uses a Haberman Feeder™.

to form a seal against the incomplete upper lip. Although the baby needs the enjoyment of sucking, some surgeons do not want a baby to breastfeed or suck on a nipple before surgical correction of the disorder to avoid any local bruising of tissue. Therefore, the best feeding method for the child with cleft lip may be to support the baby in an upright position and feed the infant gently using a commercial cleft lip nipple. A Breck feeder, an apparatus similar to a bulb syringe, or a Haberman feeder may also be used (see Fig. 27.3). If the surgical repair will be done immediately, the mother will be able to breastfeed as early as 7 to 10 days after surgery. Teach her how to pump or manually express breast milk to maintain a milk supply for this time. If surgery will be delayed for 1 month, she will need to decide whether she wants to continue to express milk for this long a period; continuing support from the nursing staff could be important to encourage her to do this.

Be certain an infant with cleft lip is burped well after feeding because of a tendency to swallow air caused by the inability to grasp a nipple or syringe edge securely with the mouth. If a cleft extends to the nares, an infant will breathe through the mouth, causing the oral mucus membranes and lips to become dry.

Infants with cleft palate cannot suck effectively either, because pressing their tongue or a nipple against the roof of their mouth would force milk up into their pharynx, leading to aspiration. The most successful method for feeding this infant, like the child with cleft lip, therefore, is to use a commercial cleft palate nipple that has an extra flange of rubber to close the roof of the mouth. The nipple can be used with a plastic bottle that can be squeezed gently to increase the flow of the feeding to compensate for poor sucking.

If surgery is delayed beyond 6 months of age or the time solid food would be introduced, teach parents to be certain any food offered is soft. Particles of coarse food could invade the nasopharynx and cause aspiration. Infants whose surgery is delayed to this point can be fitted with a plastic palate guard to form a synthetic palate and help prevent this.

Postoperative period

After surgery for cleft lip or palate, an infant is kept NBM for approximately 4 hours. The infant is then introduced to liquids (plain water). Begin the process with only a small amount to prevent vomiting.

It is important that no tension is placed on a lip suture line; avoiding tension helps keep the sutures from pulling apart and leaving a large scar. During this immediate postoperative period, the infant is usually fed using a specialised feeder because this causes less suture-line tension than bottle feeding or breastfeeding.

After palate surgery, liquids are generally continued for the first 3 or 4 days, and then a soft diet is followed until healing is complete. Ask parents what fluids the child prefers so they can be available after surgery.

After a cleft palate repair, when children begin eating soft food, they should not use a spoon, because they will invariably push it against the roof of the mouth and possibly disrupt sutures. It is better to leave a child on a liquid diet until the sutures are removed if being fed rather than being allowed to self-feed evokes an intense reaction. Be certain milk is not included in the first fluids offered because milk curds tend to adhere to the suture line. After a feeding, offer the child clear water to rinse the suture line and keep it as clean as possible.

Respiratory difficulty

Because of the local oedema that occurs after cleft lip or palate surgery, observe children closely in the immediate postoperative period for respiratory distress. Before surgery, the infant with a cleft lip breathed through the mouth. After surgery, the infant now has to learn to breathe through the nose, possibly adding to respiratory difficulty. Generally, however, this is not a problem because newborns are normally strict nose-breathers.

Infants may need suction to remove mucus, blood and unswallowed saliva. When performing suctioning, be gentle and do not touch the suture line with the catheter. After cleft lip surgery, place infants on their side to allow mouth secretions to drain. Support them well so they do

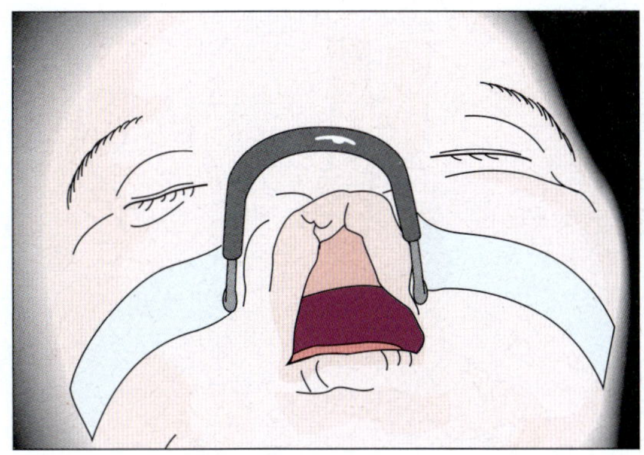

FIGURE 27.4 A Logan bar is an apparatus that may be used to protect the surgical incision for a cleft lip repair.

not turn onto their abdomen, as this could put pressure on the suture line, possibly tearing it. Placing them in an infant rocker chair is another possibility.

Postoperative care generally

After cleft lip surgery, the suture line is held in close approximation by a Logan bar (a wire bow taped to both cheeks; see Fig. 27.4) or an adhesive bandage, such as a Band-Aid, simulating a bar that brings together the incision line but does not cover the incision. Assess the Logan bar or Band-Aid–simulated bar after each feeding or cleaning of the suture line to be certain it is secure and continues to protect the suture line from tension. Furnish adequate pain relief so, if possible, the infant does not cry, because crying increases tension on the sutures. To help avoid crying, try to anticipate the infant's needs. Have formula ready to feed on demand—do not wait until after the infant is awake and crying. Help the parents use whatever measures, such as rocking, carrying or holding, that are necessary to make the infant feel secure and comfortable. The baby also will need to be burped well after a feed because there is a tendency to swallow more air than the average infant.

Nothing hard or sharp must come into contact with a recent cleft suture line. Observe infants after palate repair carefully to be certain they do not put toys with sharp edges into their mouths. They should not use a straw to drink, nor should they brush their own teeth—they will certainly brush the suture line accidentally. Keep elbow restraints in place as necessary when no one is with them so they do not put their fingers in their mouth and poke or pull at the sutures. Most children run their tongue over their sutures because of the odd feeling in the roof of their mouth, and most children this age do not respond to a caution not to do this. Because this often occurs when children have nothing to think about, help the parents provide diversional activities such as reading or singing to the child.

If parents will be continuing to give an analgesic such as paracetamol after they return home, be certain they are aware of the correct dosage and time schedule for administration. Be sure they can demonstrate measures to protect the suture line at home until healing is complete.

Risk of infection

Infection, and subsequent scarring, may result if crusts from serous drainage are allowed to form on a cleft lip suture line. Most surgeons prescribe cleaning the suture line with sterile water or sterile saline or with sterile, cotton-tipped applicators after every feed or whenever the normal serum that forms on suture lines accumulates. Use a smooth, gentle, rolling motion to apply the solution. Do not rub, because this can loosen sutures. Gently dry the suture line with a dry, sterile cotton-tipped applicator. Remember that an infant has sutures on the inside of the lip that need the same meticulous care as those visible on the outside.

Changing the contour of the palate when it is repaired also changes the slope of the eustachian tube to the middle ear. This can lead to a high incidence of middle ear infection (otitis media) because organisms are more readily able to reach this area from the oral cavity. Review the signs of infection such as fever, pain, pulling on the ear or discharge from the ear with parents. Also remind them of the importance of reporting pharyngeal infection to their primary care provider promptly so it can be treated before the infection spreads to the middle ear. Because the eustachian tube may remain partially closed because of its changed position, serous otitis media (accumulation of fluid in the middle ear) also tends to occur more frequently in these children than in others. If this happens, myringotomy (grommets) tubes may be inserted to drain middle ear fluid and help protect hearing (see Chapter 50). Be certain that parents understand the need for routine screening for hearing loss during childhood, because this is a common early sign of serous otitis media.

Pierre Robin sequence

The Pierre Robin sequence (PRS) is a triad of micrognathia (small mandible), cleft palate and glossoptosis (a tongue malpositioned downwards). It is an example of cleft palate occurring as only one part of a syndrome (Hoffman, 2008). It is rare, occurring only once in every 8500 births (Lidsky et al., 2008). Children may have associated disorders of congenital glaucoma, cataracts or cardiac disorders. They need thorough physical and genetic assessments to be certain that none of these associated disorders are present.

Observe all infants with Pierre Robin sequence carefully to be certain they are not developing an airway obstruction. They may need frequent nasopharyngeal suctioning to remove unswallowed saliva. Beginning at birth, children with this syndrome are apt to have episodes in which they have difficulty breathing because, as a result of their small jaws, their tongues are too large for their mouths. This discrepancy causes the tongue to drop backwards and obstruct the airway. Obstruction is most likely to occur when the child is in a supine position. Unlike well infants, no infant with this syndrome should be placed in a supine position to sleep; they are in grave danger of anoxia if left in this position. Use a side-lying position instead. Occasionally,

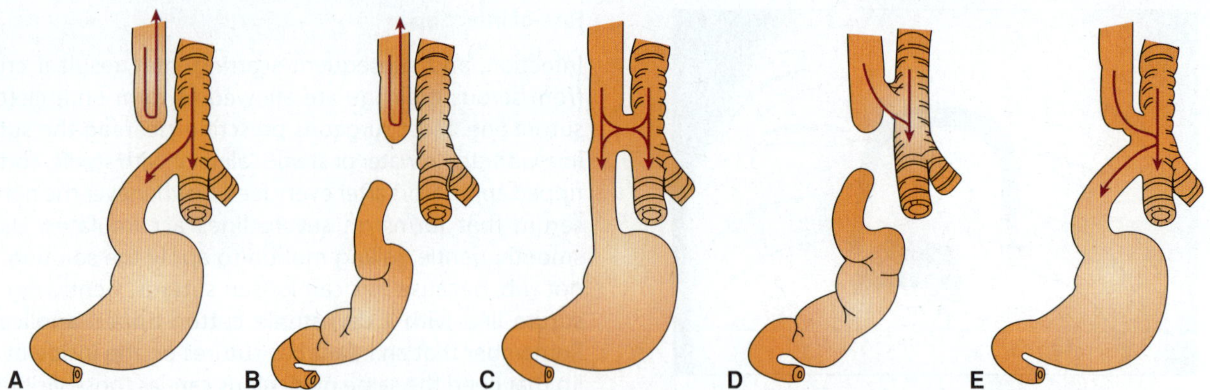

FIGURE 27.5 Oesophageal atresia and tracheo-oesophageal fistula. (**A**) In the most common type of oesophageal atresia, the oesophagus ends in a blind pouch. The trachea communicates by a fistula with the lower oesophagus and stomach (approximately 90% of infants with the defect have this type). (**B**) Both upper and lower segments end in blind pouches (5%–8% of infants with the defect have this type). (**C**) Both upper and lower segments communicate with the trachea (2%–3% of infants with the defect have this type). (**D**) Very rarely, the upper segment ends in a blind pouch and communicates by a fistula to the trachea, or (**E**) a fistula connects to both upper and lower segments of the oesophagus.

infants have such extensive airway obstruction that attaching a suture to the anterior aspect of the tongue and pulling it forwards is used to provide relief. The suture is attached to the mucus membrane of the lower lip, creating an artificial tongue-tied condition.

Parents need instructions in order to feed these infants with the same care and concern given all children with cleft palate. A gastrostomy tube or button may be inserted to relieve feeding difficulty (see Chapter 37). As the child grows older, the jaw will grow somewhat, although the mandible will always be small. Growth, coupled with a repair of the cleft palate, will decrease the respiratory problems.

Parents of the child with Pierre Robin sequence take on a great deal of responsibility when they assume their infant's care. Be certain they have the name and number of a healthcare provider they can call when they have questions. Many of these parents grow exhausted during the first few weeks of their child's life, afraid they may fall soundly asleep at night and miss their child having respiratory difficulty. Using a respiratory apnoea monitor at night can be helpful to give assurance that the infant is breathing. Encouraging parents to attend paediatric life support classes is strongly encouraged. Some healthcare facilities may provide this prior to discharge. As parents' confidence grows in their ability to provide care, this problem lessens, but it may be months or even years before a high level of confidence is achieved.

Tracheo-oesophageal atresia and fistula

Between weeks 4 and 8 of intrauterine life, the laryngo tracheal groove develops into the larynx, trachea, and beginning lung tissue. The oesophageal lumen forms parallel to this. A number of anomalies may occur if the trachea and oesophagus are affected by some teratogen that does not allow the two organs to separate but remain connected.

Oesophageal atresia is obstruction of the oesophagus. Often a fistula (opening) occurs between the closed oesophagus and the trachea. The five usual types of oesophageal atresia that occur are:

1. The oesophagus ends in a blind pouch; there is a tracheo-oesophageal fistula between the distal part of the oesophagus and the trachea (see Fig. 27.5A).
2. The oesophagus ends in a blind pouch; there is no connection to the trachea (see Fig. 27.5B).
3. A fistula is present between an otherwise normal oesophagus and trachea (see Fig. 27.5C).
4. The oesophagus ends in a blind pouch. A fistula connects the blind pouch of the proximal oesophagus to the trachea (see Fig. 27.5D).
5. There is a blind end portion of the oesophagus. Fistulas are present between both widely spaced segments of the oesophagus and the trachea (see Fig. 27.5E).

These are all serious disorders because during a feeding, milk can fill the blind oesophagus and overflow into the trachea, or a fistula can allow milk to enter the trachea, resulting in aspiration. The incidence of tracheo-oesophageal fistula is approximately 1 in 3000 live births (Fowler & Lee, 2008).

Assessment

Tracheo-oesophageal atresia must be ruled out in any infant born to a woman with hydramnios (excessive amniotic fluid). Hydramnios occurs because normally a fetus swallows amniotic fluid during intrauterine life. A fetus with a tracheo-oesophageal atresia cannot swallow, so the amount of amniotic fluid can grow abnormally large. Many infants with tracheo-oesophageal fistula are born preterm because of the accompanying hydramnios, compounding their original problem with immaturity. The infant needs to be examined carefully for other congenital anomalies that could have occurred from the teratogenic effect at the same week in gestation, such as *v*ertebral, *a*nal, *c*ardiac, *t*racheo-oesophageal, *r*enal, and *l*imb anomalies (a VACTERL syndrome) (Bartels et al., 2012).

If not diagnosed in utero, diagnosing a newborn who has a tracheo-oesophageal fistula before the infant is first fed is important. Otherwise, the infant will cough, become cyanotic, and have obvious difficulty breathing as fluid is aspirated. Newborns who have so much mucus in their mouths that they appear to be blowing bubbles should be suspected of having tracheo-oesophageal fistula. The condition can be diagnosed with certainty if a catheter cannot be passed through the infant's oesophagus to the stomach or the stomach contents cannot be aspirated. If doing this, use a firm catheter because a soft one will curl in a blind-end oesophagus and appear to have passed. If a radiopaque catheter is used, it can be demonstrated coiled in the blind end of the oesophagus on x-ray. A flat-plate x-ray of the abdomen or ultrasound also may reveal a stomach distended with the air that is passing from the trachea into the oesophagus and stomach. Either a barium swallow or a bronchial endoscopy examination can also reveal the blind-end oesophagus and fistula.

Therapeutic management

Emergency surgery for the infant with tracheo-oesophageal fistula is essential to prevent the development of pneumonia from leakage of stomach secretions into the lungs, dehydration or an electrolyte imbalance from lack of oral intake. Antibiotics may be prescribed to help prevent infection. A gastrostomy may be performed and the tube allowed to drain by gravity to keep the stomach empty of secretions and prevent reflux into the lungs. Upper right lobe pneumonia from aspiration is one of the major complications of this disorder.

Surgery consists of closing the fistula and anastomosing the oesophageal segments. It may be necessary to complete the surgery in different stages and to use a portion of the colon to complete the anastomosis if the oesophageal segments are far apart from each other. Observe infants closely at postoperative days 7 to 10, when sutures dissolve, because leaks occurring at anastomosis sites can occur at this time. If this occurs, fluid and air leak out into the chest cavity, and pneumothorax (collapse of the lung) can occur.

In some infants, some stenosis or stricture at the anastomosis site remains. If this occurs, oesophageal dilation at periodic intervals to keep the repaired oesophagus fully patent may be necessary. Gastro-oesophageal reflux may also occur after a repair, especially if the oesophagus is left shorter than usual; this can lead to recurrent fistula formation and irritation from the presence of stomach acid in the oesophagus (Catalano et al., 2011).

The ultimate prognosis for children with this disorder will depend on the extent of the repair necessary, the condition of the child at the time of surgery, and the presence or absence of other congenital anomalies. If the defect is a simple fistula, it can be repaired by endoscopic technique and application of fibrin glue to seal the fistula. Even with larger disorders, if surgery can be performed before pneumonia develops, the prognosis is good. However, the mortality rate for the condition remains high because of the presence of other congenital disorders and low birth weight that often accompanies the tracheal abnormality.

Nursing considerations

Outcomes established for the child with tracheo-oesophageal fistula must be realistic in terms of the extent of the disorder, the timing of anticipated surgery, and the stage of grief or readiness for decision making and planning the parents have reached.

Before surgery, because oral fluid cannot be given until the oesophagus is repaired, intravenous therapy or total parenteral nutrition can supply fluid and kilojoules. This is continued for a time after surgery until the possibility of vomiting from the anaesthetic is decreased. Then the infant may be fed orally, may be continued on total parenteral nutrition, or may be started on gastrostomy feedings, depending on whether the surgery could be completed in one stage or not. Early introduction of oral fluid may help to ensure patency of the oesophagus because it helps to decrease adhesion formation at the anastomosis site and also allows the infant the enjoyment and practice of sucking. If formula is given by gastrostomy feedings, introduce it into the tube slowly and allow it to run by gravity pressure only to prevent fluid from entering the oesophagus and putting pressure on the suture line. After the feeding, the end of the tube should be elevated, covered by sterile gauze, and kept in the elevated position. Do not clamp it closed. In this way, any air introduced during the feeding will bubble from the tube and not enter the oesophagus and pass the fresh suture line. This also helps to ensure that if the infant should vomit, the vomitus will be projected into the gastrostomy tube and will not contaminate the fresh sutures. Most newborns enjoy sucking a dummy during gastrostomy feedings for sucking pleasure. If a mother wishes to breastfeed, she can manually express breast milk for the gastrostomy feedings.

If the child is to return home to await a second-stage operation, the gastrostomy tube will be left in place for a month or two. Therefore, parents must learn how to do gastrostomy feedings. Be certain they know to continue usual infant care, such as holding or talking to the infant in the face of this different feeding method.

Preoperative care

Before surgery, position the infant upright in an infant chair or on the right side to prevent gastric fluid from entering the lungs from the fistula. Because the infant cannot swallow mucus, frequent oropharyngeal suctioning is necessary. A catheter may be passed into the blind-end oesophagus and attached to low continuous or intermittent suction to keep this segment of the oesophagus from filling with swallowed saliva and causing aspiration from overflow. Irrigation of the catheter may be necessary to keep it patent, because mucus tends to dry and plug it.

Keeping the infant under a radiant heat warmer with a high-humidity oxygen source helps to maintain body heat and liquefy bronchial secretions while awaiting surgery. Try to keep the infant from crying; with crying, air enters the stomach from the trachea, distending the stomach and possibly causing vomiting with aspiration into the lungs. A dummy may help relax a baby and also satisfy a sucking need.

Postoperative care

After surgery, the infant will have one or two chest tubes in place because the chest cavity was entered for the repair. The posterior tube drains collecting fluid; the anterior tube allows air to leave the chest space, re-expanding the lungs. Care of the child with chest tubes is discussed in Chapter 41.

In the first few days after surgery, observe the infant closely for respiratory distress. Continue to suction saliva from the mouth as ordered because mucus tends to accumulate in the pharynx from surgical trauma. Suctioning must be done only shallowly, however, to prevent the suction catheter from touching the suture line in the oesophagus. Turn the child frequently to discourage fluid from accumulating in the lungs. Humidified oxygen helps to keep respiratory secretions moist. Keep an infant laryngoscope and endotracheal tube readily available at the bedside in case extreme oedema develops, increasing the infant's risk of airway obstruction.

Abdominal wall defects

Abdominal wall defects, with the exception of umbilical hernia, are potentially serious disorders because they directly affect the gastrointestinal system and infant nutrition.

Omphalocele

An **omphalocele** is a protrusion of abdominal contents through the abdominal wall at the point of the junction of the umbilical cord and abdomen (see Fig. 27.6). The herniated organs are usually the intestines, but they may include stomach and liver. They are usually covered and contained by a thin transparent layer of amnion and chorion with the umbilical cord protruding from the exposed sac. When the defect is less than 4 cm, it is termed a hernia of the umbilical cord; when greater than 10 cm, it is a true omphalocele. This condition occurs because at approximately weeks 6 to 8 of intrauterine life, the fetal abdominal contents, growing faster than the fetal abdomen, are extruded from the abdomen into the base of the umbilical cord. At 7 to 10 weeks, when the abdomen has enlarged sufficiently, the intestine returns to the abdomen. Omphalocele occurs when the abdominal contents fail to return in the usual way. The occurrence is associated with chromosomal aberrations.

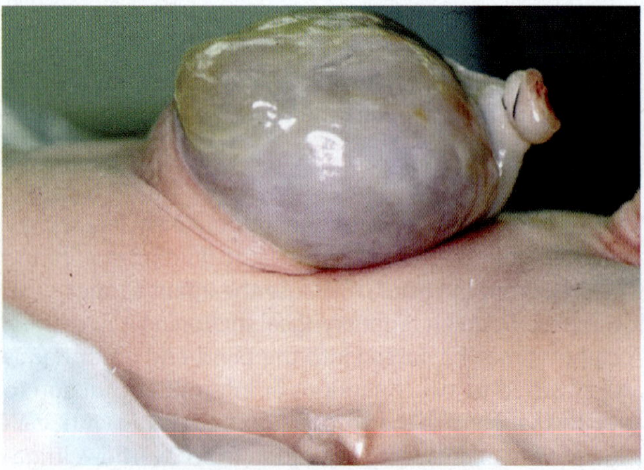

FIGURE 27.6 An omphalocele with a membrane sac covering the organs.

The incidence of omphalocele is about 1 in 5000 live births. Many omphaloceles are diagnosed by prenatal ultrasound. It may also be revealed by an elevated maternal serum a-fetoprotein (MSAFP) examination during pregnancy (Smith & Henderson, 2007). If not, the presence of an omphalocele is obvious on inspection at birth. When an omphalocele is identified in utero, caesarean birth may be performed to protect the exposed intestine. If this is the only disorder identified, however, vaginal birth can be allowed to proceed. Be sure to document the omphalocele's general appearance and its size in centimetres at birth.

Therapeutic management

Most infants will have surgery within 24 hours to replace the bowel before the thin membrane surrounding it ruptures or becomes infected. It is often difficult to replace the entire bowel with immediate surgery because the infant's abdomen, which did not need to grow to accommodate the abdominal contents, is smaller than usual. If the total bowel were replaced into this small abdomen, respiratory distress could result from the pressure of the visceral bulk on the diaphragm and lungs. Also, the bowel might not have room for effective peristalsis. If the omphalocele is small, a one-stage repair may be possible (van Eijck et al., 2008). If large, one surgical approach is the use of a prosthetic patch repair that bridges the unformed gap on the abdomen with a synthetic material with the skin drawn tight and closed over the patch. A second approach is to replace only a portion of the bowel. The remainder is contained by a Silastic pouch, termed a "silo", suspended over the infant's bed. Over the next 5 to 7 days, bowel is gradually returned to the abdomen. During this time, the infant can be fed by total parenteral nutrition to supply nutrients and keep the bowel from filling with air or stool.

Nursing considerations

Outcomes established for the infant with omphalocele must be realistic in terms of the extent of the disorder, the timing of anticipated surgery, and the stage of grief or readiness for decision making and planning that the parents have reached. Omphalocele is a shock to parents; it is a condition that is obviously severe yet one that is generally unknown.

Preoperative care. Before surgery, it is important that the lining of peritoneum covering the omphalocele not be ruptured or allowed to dry out and crack; if this happens, infection and malrotation of the uncontained intestine can occur, complicating the surgical repair. Exposure of intestine to air also causes a rapid loss of body heat. Therefore, immediately place the baby in a warmed incubator. Do not leave the infant under a radiant heat source because this will quickly dry the exposed bowel. To keep the sac moist, cover it with either sterile saline-soaked gauze or a sterile plastic bowel bag until surgery. Because of the large amount of exposed intestinal surface, the saline used must be at body temperature to prevent lowering body temperature. If the omphalocele is large, infants may be prescribed a topical application of a solution such as silver sulfadiazine to prevent infection of the sac.

The prognosis for a final successful surgical repair is good. Except for a large abdominal scar, the child who had an omphalocele will be the child originally envisioned by parents. If the size of the scar is a problem for the child in later life, cosmetic surgery can reduce its appearance.

Nutrition. A nasogastric tube is inserted at birth to prevent intestinal distension, which would enlarge the bowel lumen, making it even more difficult to replace. Do not feed the infant orally or allow the infant to suck on a dummy until the bowel repair is complete, as doing so would distend the exposed bowel with food or air and also make its return to the abdomen more difficult. Some infants have an accompanying volvulus (a twisting of the bowel causing obstruction), which is another reason to omit oral feedings. After surgery, the infant is maintained on total parenteral nutrition. Once the final stage of bowel repair is completed, a normal infant diet can be introduced gradually. Observe infants carefully for signs of obstruction such as abdominal distension, constipation, diarrhoea or vomiting when they begin oral feedings.

Infants with omphalocele can be hospitalised or receive home care for a long time (a minimum of 1 or 2 months) while waiting for a second-stage or even a third-stage operation, depending on the extent of bowel involved. If the infant is hospitalised, encourage parents to visit frequently. Be sure the infant has age-appropriate toys available for stimulation.

Parents can become distressed that their child's operation is being done in such small stages. Offer support to help them accept that this treatment method is the best way to manage this type of intestinal disorder.

Gastroschisis

Gastroschisis is a condition similar to omphalocele, except that the abdominal wall disorder is a distance from the umbilicus, usually to the right, and abdominal organs are not contained by a membrane but rather spill freely from the abdomen (Thilo & Rosenberg, 2008). Also, a greater amount of intestinal content tends to herniate, increasing the potential for volvulus and obstruction. The condition occurs because of ischaemia to blood vessels that supply the abdominal wall during the first trimester of pregnancy. For unknown reasons, it is increasing in incidence from about 2 in 10,000 births to 4.5 per 10,000 births, particularly in young mothers (Lund, Bauer & Berrios, 2007). The care and surgical procedure are the same as those for omphalocele. Children with gastroschisis often have decreased bowel motility, and even after surgical correction may have difficulty with absorption of nutrients and passage of stool. Long-term follow-up may be necessary to ensure that nutrition and elimination are adequate (Holland, Walker, & Badawi, 2010).

✔ Checkpoint question 27.1

What is the most important consideration in the care of the child with an omphalocele at birth?

a. Position the infant on their stomach to contain the intestine
b. Wrap the omphalocele in cold icy gauze to prevent fever
c. Keep the infant seated upright under a radiant warmer
d. Contain the intestine in a sterile saline-lined bowel bag

Intestinal obstruction

If canalisation of the intestine does not occur in utero at some point in the bowel, an **atresia** (complete closure) or **stenosis** (narrowing) of the fetal bowel can develop. The most common site of this occurrence is in the duodenum.

Obstruction may occur because the mesentery of the bowel twisted as the bowel re-entered the abdomen (after being contained in the base of the umbilical cord early in intrauterine life) or from looseness of the intestine in the abdomen after it has returned (Juang & Snyder, 2012). This twisting pattern is termed a **volvulus** and continues to be a problem for the first 6 months of life until the infant develops firmer intestinal supports. Obstruction also can occur because of thicker-than-usual meconium formation, blocking the lumen (meconium plug or meconium ileus).

Assessment

Intestinal obstruction may be anticipated if the mother had hydramnios during pregnancy (swallowed amniotic fluid could not be absorbed effectively by the fetus) or if more than 30 mL of stomach contents can be aspirated from the newborn stomach by catheter and syringe at birth (fluid is not passing freely through the tract). If the obstruction is not revealed by either of these findings, then symptoms of intestinal obstruction in the neonate are the same as at any other time in life: the infant passes no meconium or may pass one stool (meconium that formed below the obstruction) and then not pass any more; the abdomen becomes distended and tender. As the effect of the obstruction progresses, the infant will vomit. Remember that many neonates spit up feedings when burped. This rapid ejection of milk smells barely sour. True vomiting is usually sour-smelling (stomach acid has acted on it) and occurs spontaneously without coughing or back-patting.

Obstructions are rare above the ampulla of Vater, the junction of the bile duct with the duodenum, so vomitus is more likely be bile stained (greenish). Because meconium is black, vomitus may also be dark. Bowel sounds increase with obstruction because of the increase in peristaltic action that occurs as the intestine attempts to push stool past the point of obstruction. Waves of peristalsis may be apparent across the abdomen. The infant may evidence pain by crying—hard, forceful, indignant crying—and by pulling the legs up against the abdomen. The child's respiratory rate will increase as the intestine fills and the diaphragm is pushed up against the lungs and lung capacity decreases. An abdominal flat-plate x-ray or ultrasound will reveal no air below the level of obstruction in the intestines. A barium swallow or barium enema x-ray film may be used to reveal the position of the obstruction.

Therapeutic management

When bowel obstruction is confirmed, an orogastric or a nasogastric tube is inserted and left to drain freely to prevent further gastrointestinal distension from swallowed air (see Chapter 37). Intravenous therapy is necessary to restore fluid, and immediate surgery is scheduled because bowel obstruction is an emergency that must be treated before dehydration, electrolyte imbalance or aspiration of vomitus occurs (Ingoe & Lange, 2007).

Repair of the obstruction (with the exception of meconium plug syndrome) is accomplished by laparoscopy or through an abdominal incision. The area of stenosis or atresia is removed, and the bowel is anastomosed. If the repair is anatomically difficult or the infant has other anomalies that interfere with overall health, a temporary colostomy may be constructed and the infant discharged to home care, with surgery rescheduled at about 3 to 6 months of age. Care of the child with a colostomy is discussed in Chapter 37. A final surgical procedure will restore the child to full health unless a large portion of the bowel had to be removed, which would have an impact on nutrient absorption (short bowel syndrome).

Nursing considerations

Once an obstruction is suspected, keep an infant NBM to prevent the bowel from filling and compounding the problem, and to prevent vomiting and aspiration. Vomiting in neonates is always serious, not only because aspiration may occur but also because infants lose fluid rapidly, which results in dehydration. They also lose chloride (a component of the hydrochloric acid found in stomach contents), and this leads to metabolic alkalosis. The body attempts to compensate for the loss of chloride by excreting potassium, which can cause infants to become hypokalaemic quickly. Keeping an infant NBM, restoring fluid by intravenous therapy, and monitoring laboratory values for electrolyte balance until surgery can be scheduled are crucial.

Meconium plug syndrome

A **meconium plug** is an extremely hard portion of meconium that has completely blocked the intestinal lumen, causing bowel obstruction. The cause is unknown but probably reflects normal variations of meconium consistency. Meconium plugs usually form in the lower end of the bowel because this meconium formed early in intrauterine life and is most likely to become dry and obstruct the bowel lumen. It may be associated with Hirschsprung's disease and is strongly associated with cystic fibrosis (Balfour-Lynn, 2008).

Assessment

Because the obstruction is low in the intestinal tract, signs of obstruction such as abdominal distension and vomiting may not occur for at least 24 hours. Typically, the infant will be identified first as an infant who has had no meconium passage and is past 24 hours of age. A gentle rectal examination may reveal the presence of hardened stool, although the plug may be too high up in the bowel to be palpated. An x-ray or ultrasound may reveal distended air-filled loops of bowel up to the point of obstruction. A slightly hypertonic water-soluble contrast agent enema not only may reveal the level of obstruction but also may be therapeutic in loosening the plug.

Therapeutic management

The administration of normal saline (0.9%) enemas administered in small volumes may cause enough peristalsis to expel the plug. Instillation of acetylcystiene rectally under fluoroscopy may also be prescribed to dissolve the plug.

Once the thickened portion of meconium has been passed, the infant should have no further difficulty and, over the next several hours, may pass a great amount of stool. Observe the infant for further passage of meconium (should occur at least once daily) over the next 3 days, however, to be certain that additional plugs do not exist farther up in the bowel. If an infant is going to be discharged before this time, instruct parents on the importance of observing for meconium and also about phoning their primary care provider should the infant have no further bowel movements while at home.

Occasionally, a neonate passes a small plug of hardened meconium—hard enough to have caused an obstruction except that it is so small—in the first 1 or 2 days of life. Be certain to record and report such a finding, because the infant will need close observation for continued defecation, the same as for the infant who actually had an obstruction, to be certain that there is not a larger and truly obstructing plug higher in the bowel.

Assess the family history of a newborn who has a meconium plug for cystic fibrosis, a recessively inherited disorder (see Chapter 40), or aganglionic megacolon (Hirschsprung's disease), a polygenic inherited disorder (see Chapter 45), as these disorders may be the cause of the hardened meconium. Hypothyroidism is yet another disorder that may present with constipation or hardened stool in newborns. Additional signs of hypothyroidism include a large protruding tongue, lethargy and subnormal body temperature. Both hypothyroid and cystic fibrosis screening is done along with phenylketonuria screening at 3–5 days of age. Be certain this blood test is obtained in any newborn with a meconium plug.

Meconium ileus

Meconium ileus (obstruction of the intestinal lumen by hardened meconium) is a specific phenomenon that occurs almost exclusively in infants with cystic fibrosis and reflects extreme meconium plugging (Efrati et al., 2010). With cystic fibrosis, a genetically recessive disease, the enzyme that moistens and makes all body fluids free-flowing is absent. All body fluids are therefore thick and tenacious. Cystic fibrosis (see Chapter 40) is most often thought of as a lung disorder, because the most severe manifestation of tenacious secretions is in the lung; tenacious lung fluid leads to stasis and infection, and alveolar obstruction that reduces air exchange. Intestinal and pancreatic secretions are affected also, however, and this may be signalled at birth by hardened obstructive meconium at the ileus level from lack of pancreatic trypsin secretion (meconium ileus). This will lead to the usual symptoms of bowel obstruction: no meconium passage, abdominal distension and vomiting of bile-stained fluid. If the obstruction is too high for enemas to reduce it, the bowel must be incised and the hardened meconium removed by laparotomy. The infant must be further assessed for cystic fibrosis in the following weeks.

Diaphragmatic hernia

A diaphragmatic hernia is a protrusion of an abdominal organ (usually the stomach or intestine) through a defect in the diaphragm into the chest cavity. This usually occurs on the left side, causing cardiac displacement to the right side of the chest and collapse of the left lung. It occurs in approximately 1 in 2000 to 4000 live births, with a slightly increased frequency in boys (Tovar, 2012). It occurs because early in intrauterine life, the chest and abdominal cavity are one; at approximately week 8 of growth, the diaphragm forms to divide them. If the diaphragm does not form completely, the intestines can herniate through the diaphragm opening into the chest cavity (see Fig. 27.7).

Assessment

Diaphragmatic hernia is occasionally detected in utero by an ultrasound. If extreme, surgery to remove the bowel from the chest can be attempted by fetoscopy while the fetus is still in utero. More often, however, the condition is diagnosed at birth. Newborns with a diaphragmatic hernia

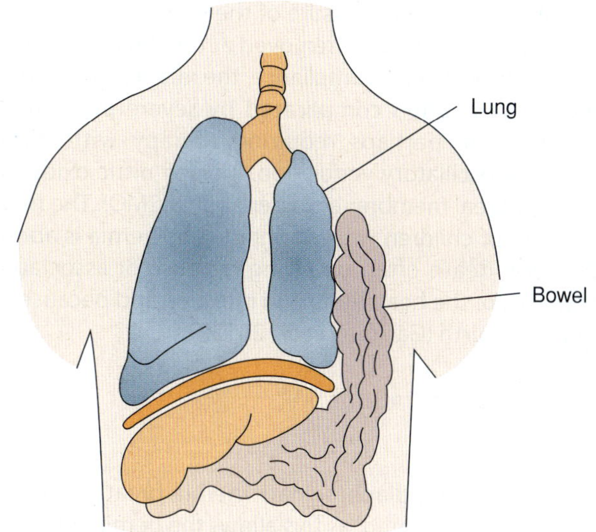

FIGURE 27.7 Diaphragmatic hernia. The bowel loop in the chest compresses the heart and lung on that side.

will have respiratory difficulty from the moment of birth, because at least one of the lobes of their lungs cannot expand completely (and may not have fully formed). Their abdomen generally appears sunken because it is not as filled with intestine as in the normal newborn. Breath sounds will be absent on the affected side of the chest cavity. There may be cyanosis and intercostal or subcostal retractions. These infants have a potential for developing persistent pulmonary hypertension because blood cannot perfuse readily through the unexpanded lung. This leads to right-to-left shunting through the foramen ovale in the heart and also causes the ductus arteriosis to remain patent. One condition, then, has led to another, and heart involvement complicates an already complicated lung picture. The mechanics of right-to-left heart shunts are further discussed in Chapter 41.

Therapeutic management

Although surgical repair may be delayed until an infant is better stabilised, treatment is usually an emergency surgical repair of the diaphragm and replacement of the herniated intestine back into the abdomen (Moyer et al., 2009). A surgical repair can be accomplished by laparoscopy, a helpful technique for newborns as it requires less anaesthesia and cold exposure (Harres, 2007). Difficult repairs may require a thoracic incision and the placement of chest tubes. If the disorder of the diaphragm is large, an insoluble polymer (Teflon) patch may be used in reconstruction. The repair is complicated if there is not enough room in the abdomen for the intestine to be returned. In these infants, the abdominal incision may not be closed but left open to allow the intestine to protrude abdominally. It is covered by silicone elastomer (Silastic) and left to be closed at a later date after the abdomen has grown.

Over the next week, the compressed lung (if it is normal) will gradually expand and begin to function. If it is hypoplastic from the pressure of the intestine in utero, it will not expand; it will be removed at the time of surgery. Because of poor lung compliance, the infant's postoperative course is often complicated by severe pulmonary hypertension, perhaps requiring therapy with high-frequency oscillatory ventilation, inhaled nitric oxide, or extracorporeal membrane oxygenation (ECMO). The mortality rate of children with diaphragmatic hernia is about 40%, with death often occurring because of associated anomalies of the heart, lung and intestine and because of premature birth (Garriboli et al., 2012).

Nursing considerations

Respiratory

The infant with a diaphragmatic hernia breathes better with the head elevated, as this allows the herniated intestine to fall back as far as possible into the abdomen, providing a maximum amount of respiratory space in the chest. Positioning the infant so the compressed lung is down also allows the unaffected lung to expand most completely. A nasogastric tube or a gastrostomy tube is inserted immediately to prevent distension of the herniated intestine, which would cause further respiratory difficulty. Be certain only low intermittent suction is used to avoid injuring the lining of the stomach. Keep the infant NBM, again, to prevent the bowel from filling and becoming distended.

After surgery, continue to maintain the infant in a semi-Fowler's position in an infant chair to keep the pressure of the replaced intestine off the repaired diaphragm. Keep the infant in a warmed humidified environment to encourage lung fluid drainage from the now uncompromised lungs. Suction the airway as necessary. Chest physiotherapy may be ordered to ensure that lung secretions do not pool and to prevent pneumonia. Positive-pressure ventilation may be ordered to increase lung expansion, although this pressure is kept to a minimum to prevent tearing the undeveloped or previously unopened lung tissue. Maintaining arterial oxygen (Po2) at a high level of 100 mmHg and the Pco2 at a low level of 30 to 35 mmHg may help to prevent arterial vasoconstriction of the hypoplastic lung, thereby improving lung function.

Nutrition

After surgery, to prevent pressure on the suture line in the diaphragm by a full stomach and bowel, nutrition will be supplied intravenously, such as with total parenteral nutrition. When starting oral feeds, be certain to burp the infant well after feeding to reduce the amount of swallowed air and limit bowel pressure against the diaphragm.

Umbilical hernia

An umbilical hernia is a protrusion of a portion of the intestine through the umbilical ring, muscle, and fascia surrounding the umbilical cord (Wiler, 2012). This creates a bulging protrusion under the skin at the umbilicus. It is rarely noticeable at birth while the cord is still present but becomes increasingly noticeable at healthcare visits during the first year.

Umbilical hernias are common in the neonatal period with 90% requiring no treatment and closing by 2 years of age. The structure is generally 1–2 cm in diameter but may be as large as an orange when children cry or strain. The size of the protruding mass is not as important as the size of the fascial ring through which the intestine protrudes. If this fascial ring is less than 2 cm, closure will usually occur spontaneously and no repair of the disorder will be necessary. If the disorder is more than 2 cm wide, surgery for repair will generally be indicated to prevent herniation and intestinal obstruction or bowel strangulation. This usually is done when the child is 1 to 2 years of age, or sooner if required.

Some parents believe that holding an umbilical hernia in place by using "belly bands" or taping a silver coin over the area will help to reduce the hernia. These actions can actually lead to bowel strangulation and should be avoided.

Surgery is generally accomplished as a day-surgery procedure. The child returns from surgery with a pressure dressing, which remains in place until the sutures are well healed. Remind parents to sponge-bathe the child until they return for a postoperative visit and the dressing is removed.

Imperforate anus

Imperforate anus (see Fig. 27.8) is stricture of the anus (Gourlay, 2013). In week 7 of intrauterine life, the upper bowel elongates to pouch and combine with a pouch invaginating from the perineum. These two sections of bowel meet, the membranes between them are absorbed, and the bowel is then patent to the outside. If this motion towards each other does not occur or if the membrane

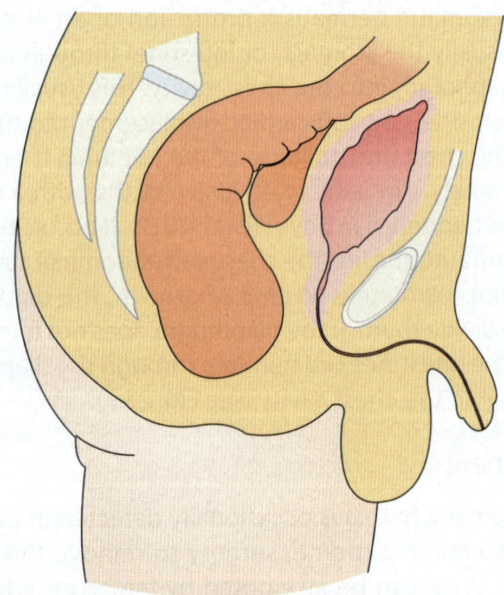

FIGURE 27.8 Imperforate anus. The lower bowel ends in a blind pouch.

between the two surfaces does not dissolve, imperforate anus occurs. The disorder can be relatively minor, requiring just surgical incision of the persistent membrane, or much more severe, involving sections of the bowel that are many inches apart with no anus. There may be an accompanying fistula to the bladder in boys and to the vagina in girls, further complicating a surgical repair. The problem occurs in approximately 1 in 5000 live births, more commonly in boys than in girls. Imperforate anus may occur as an additional complication of spinal cord disorders, because both the external anal canal and the spinal cord arise from the same germ tissue layer.

Assessment

The condition may be detected by a prenatal ultrasound. It is definitely discovered at birth when inspection of a newborn's anal region reveals that no anus is present, although this observation may not be helpful, because the anus can appear normal and the condition can still exist far inside, so that it is missed on simple inspection. Occasionally, the condition may be revealed because a membrane filled with black meconium can be seen protruding from the anus. A "wink" reflex (touching the skin near the rectum should make it contract) will not be present if sensory nerve endings in the rectum are not intact. If these methods fail to detect the condition, it can be discovered in a newborn by the inability to insert a rubber catheter into the rectum. No stool will be passed and abdominal distension will become evident.

Formerly, when all newborns stayed in the hospital for 3 to 4 days after birth, imperforate anus was always discovered. When infants failed to pass stools after the first 24 hours, the reason was investigated. Currently, because newborns are discharged at 2 or 3 days or even a few hours after birth, possibly no-one will notice that an infant has not passed a stool in that time. For an infant born in a birth centre or at home, follow-up, therefore, must include assessment of whether the infant is defecating. Collect a urine specimen from infants with imperforate anus so it can be examined for the presence of meconium to help determine whether the child has a rectal–bladder fistula. Placing a urine collector bag over the vagina in girls may reveal a meconium-stained discharge or a rectovaginal fistula.

Therapeutic management

The degree of difficulty in repairing an imperforate anus depends on the extent of the problem. If the rectum ends close to the perineum (below or at the level of the levator ani muscle) and the anal sphincter is formed, repair involves simple anastomosis of the separated bowel segments. The repair becomes complicated if the end of the rectum is at a distance from the perineum (above the levator ani muscle) or the anal sphincter exists only in an underdeveloped form. All repairs are complicated if a fistula to the bladder or vagina is present. If the repair will be extensive, the surgeon may create a temporary colostomy, anticipating final repair when the infant is somewhat older (6–12 months). For a successful repair, it is unnecessary for an internal rectal sphincter to be present as long as the subrectal muscle is judged to be intact.

Nursing considerations

Nutrition

Before surgery, keep the infant NBM to avoid further bowel distension. A nasogastric tube allowed to drain freely will be inserted to relieve vomiting and prevent pressure on other abdominal organs or the diaphragm from the distended intestine. Intravenous therapy or total parenteral nutrition will be started to maintain fluid and electrolyte balance.

The newborn will return from surgery with a nasogastric tube still in place. When bowel sounds are present and the nasogastric tube is removed, small oral feedings of glucose water, formula or breast milk can be begin.

Some infants, who are scheduled for repair in a second-stage operation and who have a temporary colostomy, are not permitted high-residue foods to lessen the bulk of stools. Although this is rarely a problem with infants because their diet naturally is a low-residue one, do not assume that parents know what low residue means. Examples include rice cereal and strained fruits and vegetables. They should avoid unrefined rice and grains, vegetables with fibres, or fruits with peels.

Postoperative care

If a rectal repair was completed, remember there is a fresh suture line at the rectum. Infants should also have no enemas, suppositories or any other intrusive rectal procedures, including rectal temperature measurement. Infants may be given a stool softener daily to keep the stool from becoming hard and tearing the healing suture line. Clean the suture line well after bowel movements by irrigating it with normal saline. Placing a nappy under, not on, the infant may be helpful so bowel movements can be cleansed away as soon as they occur. Do not place the infant on the abdomen because, in this position, newborns tend to pull their knees under them, causing tension in the perineal area. A side-lying position is best.

An infant may need rectal dilation done once or twice a day for a few months after surgery to ensure proper patency of the rectal sphincter. Review this technique with the parents and document that they are able to perform this procedure before the child is discharged. Be certain they also understand the importance of the procedure. The best surgical repair could end in failure if constriction occurs because the parents do not follow up with this procedure. If infants are to be discharged with a prescription for a daily stool softener, be certain parents understand why this is also important and have a plan for remembering the correct times and dosage.

An imperforate anus may be a difficult challenge for a parent to accept because it deals with a body area that they may not feel comfortable discussing. If it involves a temporary (or permanent) colostomy, learning to care for their infant may be difficult. For these reasons, parents need a great deal of support following the diagnosis. If a final surgical repair can be completed, they can be assured their child will have normal bowel function thereafter. If a final repair cannot be surgically achieved, they have the even harder task of caring for a child with a permanent ostomy. They can be assured that children who have ostomies accept these well as they grow older because they have never known any other method of defecation (see Chapter 37 for a discussion of care priorities for the child with an ostomy).

✔ Checkpoint question 27.2

What is an important nursing measure for a newborn with a diaphragmatic hernia?

a. Feed the infant immediately to decrease air in the intestine
b. Keep the infant positioned head down so the intestine can expand
c. Wrap the infant's abdomen tightly to better contain the intestine
d. Position the infant in an infant chair to contain the intestine in the abdomen

PHYSICAL AND DEVELOPMENTAL DISORDERS OF THE NERVOUS SYSTEM

The most common developmental disorders of the nervous system at birth include abnormal accumulation of cerebrospinal fluid (CSF) (hydrocephalus), which has several causes, and abnormalities associated with neural tube closure (meningocele or spinal dysraphism). All these are the result of multifactoral inheritance as well as nutritional deficits (Donahue, 2008).

Hydrocephalus

CSF is formed in the first and second ventricles of the brain and then passes through the aqueduct of Sylvius and the fourth ventricle to empty into the subarachnoid space of the spinal cord, where it is absorbed. **Hydrocephalus** is an excess of CSF in the ventricles or the subarachnoid space (Lewis, 2011). In the infant whose cranial sutures are not firmly knitted, this excess fluid causes enlargement of the skull. If fluid can reach the spinal cord, the disorder is called communicating hydrocephalus or extraventricular hydrocephalus. If there is a block to such passage of fluid, the disorder is an obstructive hydrocephalus or intraventricular non-communicating hydrocephalus. Hydrocephalus is also classified regarding whether it occurs at birth (congenital) or from an incident later in life (acquired). The cause of congenital hydrocephalus is unknown, although maternal infection such as toxoplasmosis or infant meningitis may be factors (Smith & Henderson, 2007).

An excess of CSF in the newborn occurs for one of three main reasons:

- Overproduction of fluid by a choroid plexus in the first or second ventricle, as could occur from a growing tumour (rare).
- Obstruction of the passage of fluid in the narrow aqueduct of Sylvius (the most common cause). Other common sites of obstruction include the foramina of Magendie and Luschka, the openings that allow fluid to leave the fourth ventricle. Obstruction occurs because infections such as meningitis or encephalitis may leave adhesions behind that block fluid flow. Haemorrhage from trauma or a growing tumour also may obstruct the passage of CSF. An Arnold-Chiari disorder (elongation of the lower brain stem and displacement of the fourth ventricle into the upper cervical canal) is yet another cause.
- An interference with the absorption of CSF from the subarachnoid space if a portion of the subarachnoid membrane is removed, as occurs with surgery for meningocele, or after extensive subarachnoid haemorrhage, when portions of the membrane absorption surface become obscured.

Assessment

Hydrocephalus occurs in approximately 3 to 4 per 1000 live births (Sinha et al., 2012). With an obstruction present, excessive fluid accumulates and dilates the system above the point of obstruction. If hydrocephalus is present prenatally, it can sometimes be detected on a prenatal ultrasound and can even be shunted in utero. The condition is generally not evident during pregnancy or even at birth, however, because of the effect of intrauterine pressure. It becomes evident in the first few weeks or months of life. The infant's fontanelles widen and appear tense, the suture lines on the skull separate, and the head diameter enlarges. As the fluid accumulation continues, the scalp becomes shiny and scalp veins become prominent. The brow bulges forwards (bossing) and the eyes become "sunset eyes" (the sclera shows above the iris because of upper lid retraction). Infants show symptoms of increased intracranial pressure, such as decreased pulse and respirations, increased temperature and blood pressure, hyperactive reflexes, strabismus and optic atrophy. They may become either irritable or lethargic, and they fail to thrive. They may have a typical shrill, high-pitched cry (see Box 27.1).

Treatment is most effective when the disorder is recognised early, because once intracranial pressure becomes so acute that brain tissue is damaged and motor or mental deterioration results, even the best shunting procedure cannot replace and repair this damage to the brain cells. Assisting with detection of hydrocephalus is an important role for nurses in ambulatory child health settings. All children under the age of 2 years should have their head circumference recorded and plotted on an

BOX 27.1 Assessment ✻ Assessing an infant with hydrocephalus

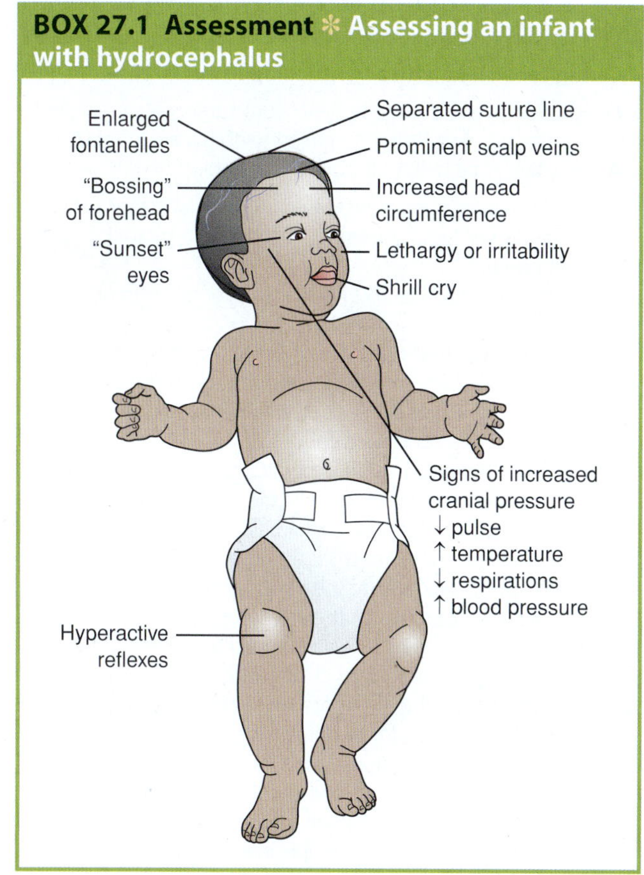

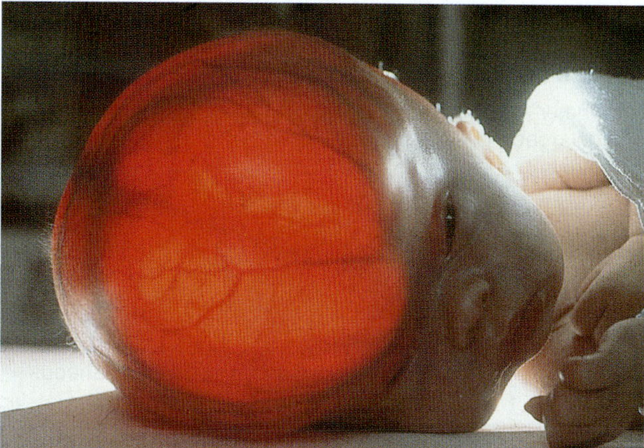

FIGURE 27.9 An infant with hydrocephalus. Transillumination reveals a fluid-filled skull. (Southern Illinois University/Photo Researchers, Inc.)

appropriate growth chart at health centre visits, so a child whose head is growing abnormally can be detected (Zahl & Wester, 2008).

Measure the head circumference of all infants within an hour of birth and again before discharge from the healthcare facility to establish a baseline. Older children who have suffered head trauma severe enough to be seen in a medical facility should have their head circumference noted at the time of the accident; then, if other symptoms of increased intracranial pressure appear, this head circumference measurement may be a meaningful part of the store of information available concerning the child's condition.

In addition to the general enlargement of the head, note any asymmetry that is occurring, because this may suggest the point of obstruction. The infant's motor function becomes impaired as the head enlarges, because of both neurological impairment and atrophy caused by the inability to move such a heavy head. However, as long as a child has more than 1 cm of cerebral tissue present, motor function often is not impaired. Even with an extremely enlarged head, children's intelligence may remain normal, although fine motor development may be affected.

That hydrocephalus is present can be demonstrated by ultrasound, computed tomography (CT), or magnetic resonance imaging (MRI). A skull x-ray film will reveal the separating sutures and thinning of the skull. **Transillumination** (holding a bright light such as a torch or a specialised light against the skull with the child in a darkened room) will reveal the skull is filled with fluid rather than solid brain (see Fig. 27.9). If the hydrocephalus is a non-communicating type, dye inserted into a ventricle through the anterior fontanelle will not appear in CSF obtained from a lumbar puncture.

Therapeutic management

The treatment of hydrocephalus depends on its cause and extent. If it is caused by overproduction of fluid, acetazolamide (Diamox), a diuretic, may be prescribed to promote the excretion of this excess fluid. Hydrocephalus is usually caused by obstruction so the treatment usually involves laser surgery to reopen the route of flow or bypassing the point of obstruction by shunting the fluid to another point of absorption.

As ventricular endoscopy is perfected and obstructions in the third or fourth ventricle can be relieved, the next generation of children with hydrocephalus may not need artificial shunting. Children today may still undergo a shunting procedure, however, and you may care for many older children or adults who have shunts in place (Komolafe et al., 2008). A shunting procedure involves threading a thin polyethylene catheter under the skin from the ventricles to the peritoneum (see Fig. 27.10). Fluid drains via this route into the peritoneum and is absorbed across the peritoneal membrane into the body circulation. This type of shunt usually has to be replaced as the child grows or it will become too short. As another complication, it could become enclosed in a fold of peritoneum and become obstructed or it could become infected.

The ultimate prognosis for a child with hydrocephalus depends on whether brain damage occurred before shunting and, if a shunt is in place, whether the parents can recognise when it needs to be replaced to prevent increased intracranial pressure.

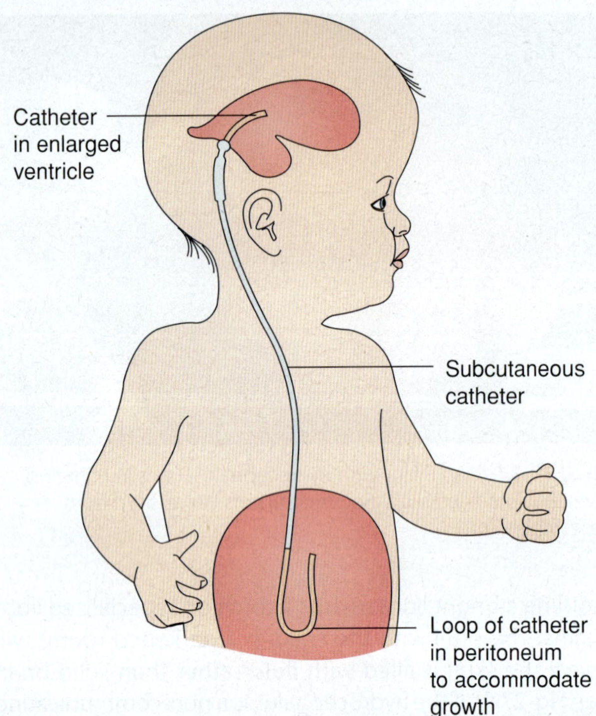

FIGURE 27.10 A ventriculoperitoneal shunt removes excessive cerebrospinal fluid from the ventricles and shunts it to the peritoneum. A one-way valve is present in the tubing behind the ear.

Nursing considerations

Nutrition and parent–child bonding are two major concerns for the infant with hydrocephalus, as is the risk of ineffective cerebral tissue perfusion related to increased intracranial pressure.

Postoperative care

After a shunt is inserted, the infant's bed is usually left flat or raised only about 30° so the child's head remains level with the body. This is because if the child's head is raised excessively, CSF may flow too rapidly and decompression can then occur too rapidly, leading to possible tearing of cerebral arteries.

A one-way valve is inserted in the shunt that opens when CSF has accumulated to the extent that pressure has increased. It closes when enough fluid has drained to reduce the pressure. The surgeon who performs the shunting procedure writes specific orders about how often the infant is to be turned and to what side after surgery. Often infants are not turned to lie on the side with the shunt to prevent putting pressure on the valve, which might cause it to open and rapidly decompress CSF.

Assess for signs of increased intracranial pressure after surgery such as tense fontanelles, increasing head circumference, irritability or lethargy, decreased level of consciousness, poor sucking ability, vomiting, an increase in blood pressure, increasing temperature, and a decrease in pulse and respiratory rates (see Chapter 49 for tips on a complete neurological assessment). Also assess for symptoms of infection such as increased temperature, increased pulse rate, general malaise, and signs of meningitis such as a stiff neck and marked irritability (see Box 27.2). Be certain a child receives adequate pain management, because crying elevates CSF pressure.

Home care

Caring for a child with a shunt in place is an ongoing responsibility for parents. If parents do not seem to be asking many questions about the child's care after surgery, do not assume this is because they are taking the child's care in their stride. They may be too frightened or not understand neuroanatomy enough to know what questions to ask. An opening such as, "Most parents are a little nervous when they think about taking a child home with a shunt in place; do you feel that way?" gives them an opportunity to admit how they feel. Talking about how nervous they feel about the responsibility will not immediately make them more comfortable with the child's care. However, it can provide them with a starting point to bring their anxiety down to a manageable size. Assure them that the healthcare providers caring for their child are interested in helping and supporting them.

BOX 27.2 ✻ Focus on family teaching

Caring for a child with a ventriculoperitoneal shunt

Q. Following ventriculoperitoneal shunt surgery, Baby Caitlin's mother asks you, "What do I need to do to care for her?"

A. Here are some helpful things to remember:

- Observe for signs of increased intracranial pressure, such as drowsiness, vomiting, headache, irritability and anorexia.
- Observe the valve /pump site daily for any sign of swelling or redness.
- Have your child sleep with her head slightly elevated at night to help ensure fluid flow through the tube. Do not allow your child to fall asleep with her head hanging over the side of a couch or bed.
- Do not allow your child to become constipated, because hard stool might press against the shunt in the abdomen and obstruct the flow of fluid. Encourage fruit, vegetables, cereal and a generous amount of fluid in her diet.
- Do not call attention to the pump behind your child's ear; teach her not to touch the valve/pump
- Be certain your child wears a helmet for tricycle and bicycle riding (as should all children) to avoid injury to the shunt. Otherwise, there are no special precautions that need to be taken for normal play.
- If your child develops signs of infection such as an increased temperature, phone your primary care provider. Also remind the person that your child has a shunt in place. This is probably a simple infection of childhood but could indicate an infected shunt.
- Be certain to keep your regularly scheduled health assessment visits. As your child grows taller, the shunt will eventually need to be replaced for proper functioning.

If a valve has been inserted in the shunt, it can be palpated underneath the skin just behind the ear. Remind parents to stress to their child that this strange object is not to be felt continually. A child nervously fidgeting with a pressure pump can inadvertently evacuate CSF from the ventricles at a dangerously rapid rate.

Before an infant is discharged after surgery, be certain the parents have ample opportunity to feed and provide care so they can be comfortable and feel they "know" their infant. Because irritability, lethargy, vomiting and a change in the baby's cry are signs of increased intracranial pressure, be certain parents know to report these immediately to their primary care provider. Before parents can report a change in the infant's disposition in this way, they must know the infant well, which is why it is important that they give care while their infant is hospitalised. A referral for home care follow-up may be appropriate to offer further support.

Growth and development

Like all children, children with hydrocephalus need intellectual and emotional stimulation: they need to be talked to, smiled at and played with. If the child's head is enlarged, turning it to look at things can be difficult. It may be necessary to reposition mobiles or pictures so the child receives adequate visual stimulation. Role-model talking and singing to the child to help parents include these actions in their care.

At the time of hospital discharge, be certain parents have the telephone number of the person they should call if they have a question or concern about their child's condition or care, and a referral for home care follow-up, if appropriate. They also need an appointment for the child's first check-up. Be sure they understand that infection of the shunt is a possibility and a severe complication because it can lead to meningitis. If this should occur, the infant will show signs of increased intracranial pressure as well as an increased temperature. In addition to being hospitalised, receiving the usual treatment for meningitis (see Chapter 49), and receiving intravenous antibiotics, the child may have an extraventricular shunt placed to promote drainage during this time. This allows antibiotics to be administered directly to the CSF and ensures that infected CSF is not draining to the peritoneal cavity, where it could cause peritonitis.

✔ *Checkpoint question 27.3*

What vital sign changes occur with increasing intracranial pressure?

a. Decreased temperature; increased blood pressure
b. Increased respirations; decreased pulse rate
c. Increased temperature; decreased pulse rate
d. Decreased blood pressure; increased temperature

Neural tube defects

Because the neural tube forms in utero first as a flat plate and then moulds to form the brain and spinal cord, it is susceptible to malformation. The term **spina bifida** (Latin for "divided spine") is most often used as a collective term for all spinal cord disorders, but there are well-defined degrees of spina bifida involvement, and not all neural tube defects involve the spinal cord. All of these defects, however, occur because of lack of fusion of the posterior surface of the embryo in early intrauterine life. They can be compared with cleft palate or cleft lip—these are also midline closure disorders.

The incidence of neural tube defects has fallen dramatically in recent years, from 3 to 0.6 per 1000. Such disorders may occur as a polygenic inheritance pattern, but poor nutrition, especially a diet deficient in folic acid, appears to be a major contributing factor (Lumley et al., 2009). As a result, pregnant women are advised to ingest 600 mg of folic acid daily to help prevent these disorders. The risk of bearing a second child with a neural tube disorder once one child is born with such a disorder increases to as much as 1 in 20. For this reason, women who have had one child with a neural tube defect are advised to have a maternal serum assay or amniocentesis for AFP levels to determine if such a defect is present in a second pregnancy (levels will be abnormally increased if there is an open spinal lesion). Serum assessment of MSAFP is done at week 15 of pregnancy, when AFP reaches its peak concentration. If the result is elevated, an amniocentesis is then done to assess the level of AFP in amniotic fluid. A prenatal sonogram is also helpful to determine the presence of the disorder (see Chapter 11 for further discussion of these prenatal assessments).

Types of defects

Anencephaly

Anencephaly is absence of the cerebral hemispheres. It occurs when the upper end of the neural tube fails to close in early intrauterine life. It is revealed by an elevated level of AFP in the maternal serum or on amniocentesis and confirmed by a prenatal sonogram.

Infants with anencephaly may have difficulty in labour because the underdeveloped head does not engage the cervix well. Many such infants present in a breech position. On visual inspection at birth, the disorder is obvious (see Fig. 27.11). Children cannot survive with this disorder because they have no cerebral function. Because the respiratory and cardiac centres are located in the intact medulla, however, they may survive for several days after birth. Babies born with this condition will require thoughtful and sensitive palliation.

When the condition is discovered prenatally, parents are offered the option of terminating the pregnancy on medical grounds, and should receive qualified genetic counselling and support regardless of their decision regarding progress of the pregnancy.

Nurses and midwives need to think through their personal thoughts and feelings about caring for such infants, because it can be emotionally and ethically difficult to give

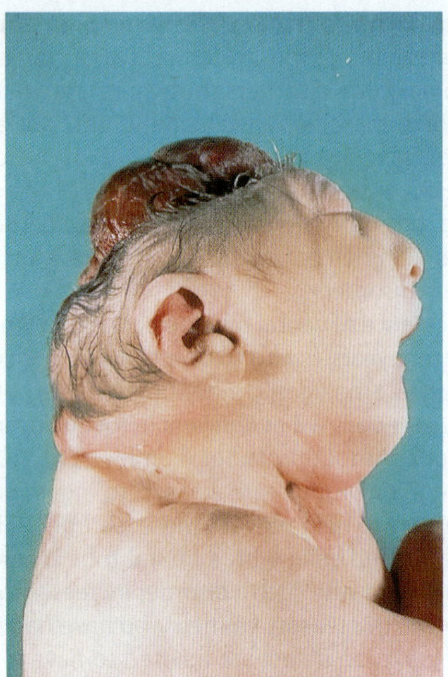

FIGURE 27.11 An infant with anencephaly. (Joseph R. Siebert, PhD/Custom Medical Stock Photograph.)

care to an infant who will most likely die as a result of their condition, when the condition is not compatible with life. Support for healthcare professionals in such circumstances is also of vital importance

Microcephaly

Microcephaly is a disorder in which brain growth is so slow that it falls more than three standard deviations below normal on growth charts. The cause might be a disorder in brain development associated with an intrauterine infection such as rubella, cytomegalovirus or toxoplasmosis. Microcephaly may also result from severe malnutrition or anoxia in early infancy.

The prognosis for a normal life is guarded in children with microcephaly and depends on the extent of restriction of brain growth and on the cause. Generally the infant is cognitively challenged because of the lack of functioning brain tissue. True microcephaly must be differentiated from *craniosynostosis* (normal brain growth but premature fusion of the cranial sutures), which also causes decreased head circumference. Infants with craniosynostosis have abnormally closed fontanelles and often show bossing of the forehead and signs of increased intracranial pressure similar to infants with hydrocephalus. With surgery, craniosynostosis can be relieved and brain growth will be normal.

Spina bifida occulta

Spina bifida occulta occurs when the posterior laminae of the vertebrae fail to fuse. This occurs most commonly at the fifth lumbar or first sacral level but may occur at any point along the spinal canal. The normal spinal cord is shown in Figure 27.12A. Spina bifida occulta may be noticeable as a dimpling at the point of poor fusion; abnormal tufts of hair or discoloured skin may be present (Sponseller, 2007). Simple spina bifida occulta is a benign disorder; it occurs as frequently as in one of every four children (see Fig. 27.12B).

The term "spina bifida" is often used to denote all spinal cord anomalies. Because of this usage, parents, when told that their child has a spina bifida occulta, may interpret this as meaning their child has an extremely serious disorder. Help clarify the degree of defect for them.

Meningocele

If the meninges covering the spinal cord herniate through unformed vertebrae, a meningocele occurs. The anomaly appears as a protruding mass, usually approximately the size of an orange, at the centre of the back (see Fig. 27.12C). It generally occurs in the lumbar region, although it might be present anywhere along the spinal canal. The protrusion may be covered by a layer of skin or only the clear dura mater.

Myelomeningocele

In a myelomeningocele, the spinal cord and the meninges protrude through the vertebrae the same as with a meningocele. The difference is that the spinal cord ends at the point, so motor and sensory function is absent beyond this point (see Fig. 27.12D). Because this results in lower

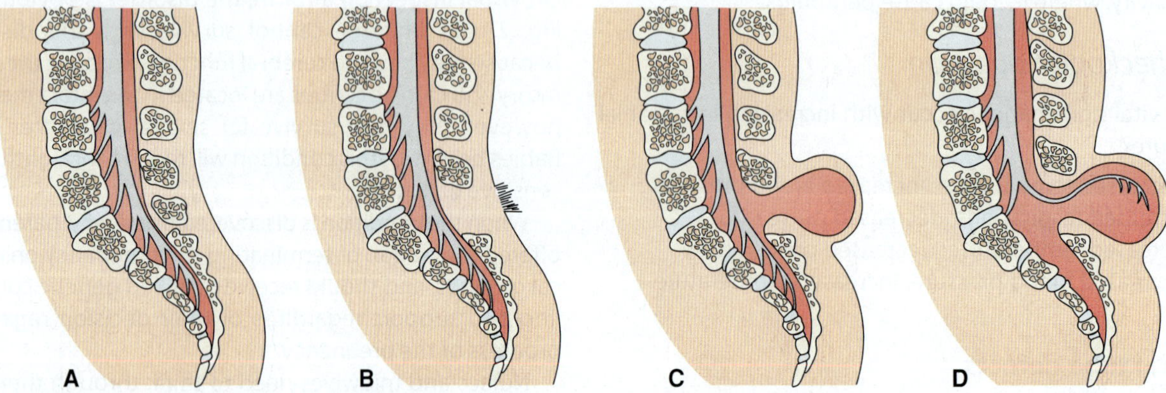

FIGURE 27.12 Degrees of spinal cord anomalies. (**A**) Normal spinal cord. (**B**) Spina bifida occulta. (**C**) Meningocele. (**D**) Myelomeningocele.

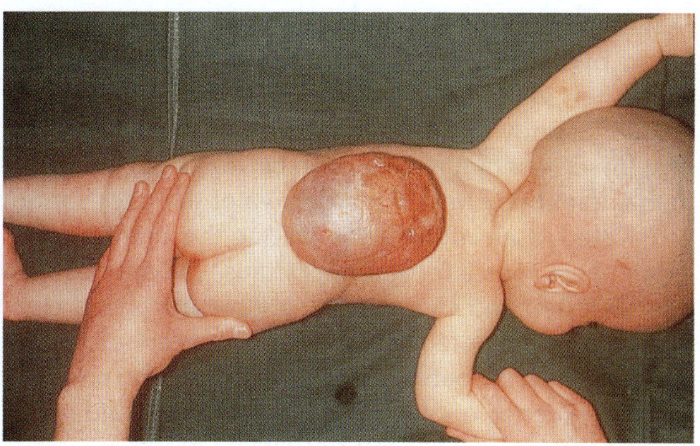

FIGURE 27.13 A myelomeningocele. The infant also has hydrocephaly and a subluxated hip. (NMSB/Custom Medical Stock Photograph.)

motor neuron damage, the child will have flaccidity and lack of sensation of the lower extremities and loss of bowel and bladder control. Infants' legs are lax, and they do not move them; urine and stools continually dribble because of lack of sphincter control. Children often have accompanying talipes (clubfoot) disorders and developmental hip dysplasia. Hydrocephalus accompanies myelomeningocele in as many as 80% of infants because of the lack of an adequate subarachnoid membrane for CSF absorption; the higher the myelomeningocele occurs on the cord, the more likely it is that hydrocephalus will accompany it. It is generally difficult to tell from visual appearance whether the disorder is myelomeningocele or the simpler meningocele (see Fig. 27.13). A CT, ultrasound scan or MRI will reveal this.

Encephalocele

An encephalocele is a cranial meningocele or myelomeningocele. The disorder occurs most often in the occipital area of the skull but may occur as a nasal or nasopharyngeal disorder. Encephaloceles generally are covered fully by skin, but they may be open or covered only by the dura. It is difficult to tell from the size of the encephalocele if only CSF is trapped in the protruding meninges or whether brain tissue could also be involved. Transillumination of the sac will reveal solid substance or fluid in the sac. CT, MRI or ultrasound will reveal the size of the skull disorder.

Assessment

Neural tube disorders may be discovered during intrauterine life by prenatal ultrasound, fetoscopy, amniocentesis (discovery of increased AFP in amniotic fluid), or analysis of AFP in the maternal serum. If the condition is discovered in utero, it may be possible to close the lesion by fetoscopic surgery. Infants may be born by caesarean birth to avoid pressure and injury to the spinal cord. Observe and record whether an infant born with a neural tube disorder has spontaneous movement of the lower extremities to assess if the child has lower motor function.

Therapeutic management

Children with spina bifida occulta need no immediate surgical correction. The parents should be made aware of the defect, however, so they are not surprised if it is revealed on a spinal x-ray taken for some reason later in life. Some children may eventually need surgery to prevent vertebral deterioration because of the unbalanced spinal column.

Treatment for a meningocele, myelomeningocele or encephalocele involves immediate surgery to replace the contents that are replaceable and to close the skin disorder to prevent infection. Currently, it is done as soon after birth as possible (usually within 24 to 48 hours) so infection through the exposed meninges does not occur.

Surgery for repair of a meningocele or myelomeningocele is not without risk, and brain disorders accompanying an encephalocele may limit the child's cognitive potential. The loss of meninges removed by surgery may limit the rate of absorption of CSF. This may lead to a build-up of CSF, resulting in hydrocephalus. Parents need a great deal of support to care for a child with a myelomeningocele because their child has multiple challenges. The child with a myelomeningocele will continue to have paralysis of the lower extremities and loss of bowel and bladder function after surgery because the absent lower cord cannot be replaced. Table 27.1 provides a classification of motor function ability according to the location of spinal cord disruptions.

TABLE 27.1 Motor function ability in children with myelomeningocele

Spinal cord lesion	Resultant effects
T6–12	Complete flaccid paralysis of the lower extremities; weakened abdominal and trunk musculature in higher lesions; kyphosis and scoliosis common; ambulation with maximal support
L1–2	Hip flexion present; paraplegia, ambulation with maximal support
L3–4	Hip flexion, adduction and knee extension present; hip dislocation common; some control of hip and knee movement possible; ambulation with moderate support
L5	Hip flexion, adduction and varying degrees of abduction; knee extension and weak knee flexion; paralysis of the lower legs and feet; ambulation with moderate support
S1–2	As above, with preservation of some foot and ankle movement; ambulation with minimal support
S3	Mild loss of intrinsic foot muscular function possible; ambulation without support

Nursing considerations: Immediate concerns

Although parents of an infant with a myelomeningocele are told before surgery that their child's spinal disorder is a type that means motor and sensory function are absent in the child's lower extremities, they may not necessarily "hear" this information. Only after surgery may they begin to comprehend the extent of the condition. When the child is discharged from the hospital, be certain the parents understand what the next step they need to follow for further care is. This prevents them from feeling deserted when they most need support—the time when they first begin to appreciate what this problem will mean to them in the coming years, and what it will mean to their child throughout life.

Infection risk

If the exposed meningeal sac is allowed to dry, it can crack, allowing CSF to drain and microorganisms to enter. Pressure on the protruding mass is a prime reason why the sac ruptures, leading to quick decompression of the CSF (which can lead to herniation of the brainstem into the spinal cord and interference with respiratory and cardiac centres) and possibly to infection (meningitis). Such pressure may also force CSF from the sac into the spinal column, increasing intracranial pressure. Therefore, it is crucial to prevent drying of and pressure on the exposed membrane.

Preoperative positioning. Before surgery, use sterile gloves and sterile linens when caring for the infant. Position infants carefully to prevent pressure on the exposed meninges, either in a prone position or supported on their side. When they are on their side, use a rolled blanket or cloth nappy placed behind their upper back (above the disorder) and a separate one behind their lower back (below the disorder). This way, no pressure will be exerted on the lesion, and the infant will be protected from rolling backwards onto it. Placing infants on their abdomen has the added advantage of keeping the flow of faeces and urine away from the spinal defect as well as keeping it free from pressure. A folded towel under the abdomen helps to flex the infant's hips, reduces pressure on the sac, and ensures good leg position. If an infant is lying on a side, putting a folded nappy between the legs prevents skin surfaces from touching and rubbing (and also helps to keep the hips from internally rotating). Always notice the position of the infant's legs. If they are paralysed because of lack of motor control, the infant cannot move and straighten them to a more comfortable position.

Placing a piece of plastic or sturdy plastic wrap below the meningocele on the child's back like an apron and taping it in place is another method of preventing faeces from touching the open lesion. A sterile wet compress of normal saline (0.9%) over the lesion may be used to keep the sac moist. Rather than remove this to wet it again and risk rupturing the sac, merely add additional fluid.

Although no pressure should be exerted on the open lesion by a top sheet, make certain that the child is adequately warmed. The presence of the sac adds to the amount of body surface area exposed, thereby increasing heat loss. The infant may need to be kept in an incubator to maintain body heat if a large area of the back cannot be covered. Use caution when placing the infant under a radiant heat source for warmth because radiant heat can dry the lesion and cause cracking. Any seepage of clear fluid from the defect should be reported promptly, because this is probably escaping CSF. Checking any leakage for evidence of glucose will confirm the fluid is CSF (urine or mucus will not test positive for glucose).

Postoperative care. After surgery, a child is again placed on the abdomen until the skin incision has healed (about 7 days). The same careful precautions against allowing urine or faeces to touch the incision area are necessary.

Nutrition

To maintain nutrition, help parents hold the infant in as normal a feeding position as possible. Make certain that a supporting arm does not press against the lesion. Remind parents that when burping the infant, they should not pat the back over the defect. If the defect is large and the risk in picking up the infant is too great, the infant may be fed while lying on the side in bed or prone on a specialised bed frame. Raise the infant's head slightly by slipping a folded nappy under it. Stroke the head, arms or upper back while the infant sucks to give the child the same comfort and assurance at feeding time as a baby receives while being held. Infants may enjoy a dummy after feeding, because they do not experience the same enjoyment of sucking while feeding that would be experienced if they could be held and cuddled. All new parents have some difficulty getting comfortable with feeding an infant. Parents who must feed their child in an unusual position or with an infant on a support frame will have even more difficulty. Role-model a warm, comforting parental role so parents can begin to form a positive parent–child interaction.

Children with increased intracranial pressure tend to suck poorly. If this complication develops after surgery, breastfeeding may be difficult. Parents need a realistic explanation of the treatment planned for the child so they can decide whether to continue breastfeeding. If it is necessary to forgo breastfeeding for this child, you can assure parents that the child will thrive on commercial formula.

Increased intracranial pressure

Preoperative care. Increasing head size from poor absorption of CSF (hydrocephalus) is a common complication of neural tube disorders. To detect increased head size (development of hydrocephalus), measure head circumference once daily (or more frequently if ordered) in the preoperative period. Head circumference measurements are accurate only if the tape measure is placed on the same points of the child's head each time. Placing small marks with permanent marker on the forehead just above the eyebrows and at the most prominent point of the occiput allows different people to measure the head during the day and yet be sure that they all measure at the same point.

Postoperative care. Children may develop hydrocephalus after surgery as well, probably because of interference with subarachnoid absorption of CSF. Observe the child frequently for signs of increased intracranial pressure such as changes in vital signs, neurological signs such as pupillary changes, or an increase in head circumference or bulging fontanelles, as well as behavioural changes such as irritability or lethargy to help detect if this is happening.

Skin care

Preserving skin integrity is a major problem before surgery because the constant prone position puts pressure on the infant's knees and elbows. Laying the infant on a synthetic sheepskin helps reduce friction; after surgery, use paper tape or stockinette for dressing changes or place protective dressings such as Stomahesive on the skin under the area where the tape will touch. Change nappies frequently to prevent excessive contact of acid urine with skin. If hydrocephalus has developed, the head will be heavy and pressure areas at the temples can occur if the head is not repositioned about every 2 hours.

Nursing considerations: Long-term concerns

Mobility

Help parents begin to plan stimulation activities their infant can accomplish with limited mobility. Encourage them to take the infant to the places children normally accompany parents—relatives' homes, shopping, the zoo, and so forth as encouraging children to be independent helps them lead as active a life as possible (O'Mahar et al., 2010; see Fig. 27.14).

Parents will need to perform passive exercises to prevent muscle atrophy and formation of contractures if a child has impaired lower extremity motor control. The child may need leg braces to help maintain good alignment and enable walking with crutches. Parents are generally anxious to do something for their child and follow routines of passive exercises well if they are given sufficient support for their accomplishments at healthcare visits. As the child grows older, tendon transplants or osteotomy may be necessary to prevent contractures and poor bone alignment. Because children with myelomeningocele have no sensation in their lower extremities, parents should make a routine of inspecting the child's lower extremities and buttocks daily for any area of irritation or possible infection. Teach children as they grow older to do this themselves.

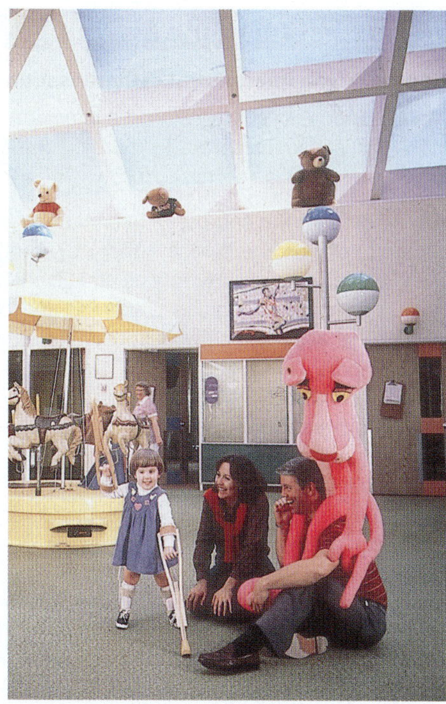

FIGURE 27.14 A child born with a neural tube disorder demonstrates her ability to walk using braces and a crutch. (Alexander Tsiara/Photo Researchers, Inc.)

Elimination

To ensure bladder emptying, an intermittent clean urinary catheterisation technique may be taught to parents (inserting a clean catheter through the urethra into the bladder every 4 hours to drain urine from the bladder; see Box 27.3). As children reach early school-age, they can learn this technique for themselves. Prescription of a drug such as oxybutynin hydrochloride (Ditropan) may improve bladder capacity and mean less frequent catheterisation is necessary (see Box 27.4) (McKenna and Mirkov, 2014). It is possible to place artificial bladder sphincters in some children to help establish continence. In some children, a continent urinary reservoir or ureterosigmoidostomy is constructed to bypass the non-functioning bladder. Children who are begun on intermittent clean catheterisation from birth require fewer bladder augmentation procedures as they grow older.

PHYSICAL AND DEVELOPMENTAL DISORDERS OF THE SKELETAL SYSTEM

Either genetic or environmental factors can compromise fetal physical growth to such an extent that they result in skeletal disorders in the newborn.

Absent or malformed extremities

Congenital skeletal disorders may result from reasons such as maternal drug ingestion, virus invasion during pregnancy or amniotic band formation in utero. In most

BOX 27.3 ✻ Focus on family teaching

Instructions for clean intermittent catheterisation

Q. Baby Caitlin's mother needs to learn clean intermittent catheterisation for her daughter. She asks you, "How do I do this?"

A. Here are some helpful guidelines to follow:

1. Remember that the purpose of intermittent catheterisation is to keep the bladder empty by using clean technique and frequent emptying so microorganisms do not have time to grow in urine in the bladder. Always use clean equipment and catheterise at least every 4 hours.
2. Always carry catheterisation equipment with you when away from home (a plastic bag containing a clean catheter and water-soluble lubricant). This enables you to stay longer away from home if you wish. If you will be using a public toilet, you might want to include a presoaped washcloth rather than have to use rough paper towels.
3. To begin catheterisation, wash your hands in warm, soapy water. This reduces the chance you will introduce germs from your hands into your child's bladder.
4. Next wash around your child's urinary meatus with a clean washcloth or paper towel and warm, soapy water. Rinse the washcloth and wash again with clear water. This reduces the chance that germs on the child's skin will be pushed into the bladder.
5. Coat the tip of a clean catheter with water-soluble lubricant. This reduces friction and makes the catheter slide into the bladder easily.
6. Quickly but gently insert the catheter into the urinary meatus approximately 8 cm. Urine should begin to flow immediately through the catheter. Let this drain into a collecting basin.
7. When urine stops flowing, gently remove the catheter and dispose of appropriately.
8. Be certain that on special days such as family celebrations or holidays you do not forget the importance of catheterisation.
9. As your child reaches school age, you can teach her how to do this herself. She will need to insert the catheter about 15 cm. Be certain she will be able to have access to a school bathroom every 4 hours during the day.
10. Phone your healthcare provider if urine is blood-tinged, smells foul, or is cloudy rather than clear or if your child appears to have pain in her abdomen or lower back or has an elevated temperature. These may be symptoms of a urinary tract infection.

instances, however, the cause of the anomaly cannot be established. Children born without an extremity or with a malformed extremity can be fitted with a prosthesis early in life. In most instances, children will have better function if the malformed portion of an extremity is amputated before a prosthesis is fitted. This is a difficult decision for parents to make, however, because it is one that they cannot undo later. They need assurance that hands with malformed fingers, for example, will not later grow to become normal. A well-fitted prosthesis that a child learns to use at

BOX 27.4 ✻ Focus on pharmacology

Oxybutynin hydrochloride (Ditropan)

Classification: Oxybutynin is an anticholinergic, urinary antispasmodic.

Action: Relaxes smooth muscle to relieve symptoms of bladder instability associated with neurogenic bladder (McKenna & Mirkov, 2014).

Pregnancy risk category: B1

Dosage: 5 mg orally twice daily

Possible adverse effects: Drowsiness, dizziness, blurred vision, decreased sweating

Nursing considerations

- Advise the parents to give or have the child take the medication exactly as prescribed.
- Alert the parents about the need for frequent bladder examinations during treatment to document the drug's effect.
- Ask the child to report drowsiness or blurred vision. Caution the child not to attempt activities that require balance while taking the drug.
- Caution the child and parents that with decreased sweating, body temperature can rise. Encourage the parents to keep the child's environment cool and avoid high temperatures.

an early age will provide more function and allow a more normal childhood and adult life than if the original disorder is left unchanged (see Fig. 27.15). Lower extremity prostheses are fitted as early as the age of 6 months (so an infant will learn to stand at the normal time). Upper extremity prostheses are fitted this early also, so an infant can handle and explore objects readily.

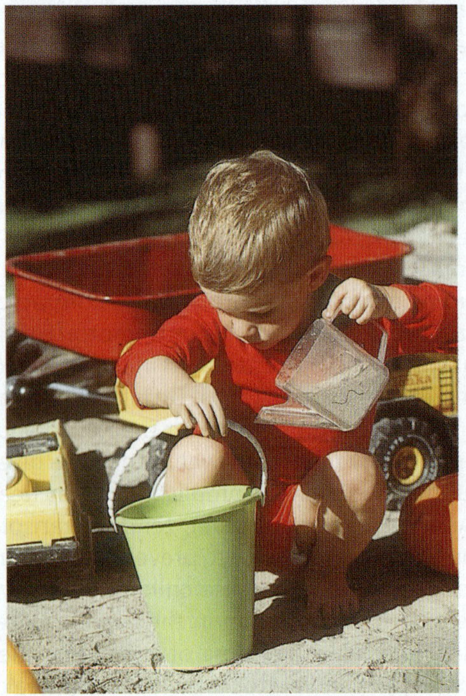

FIGURE 27.15 A young child learns to use a hand prosthesis during play. (M. Grecco/Stock Boston.)

Introducing a prosthesis early also prevents a child from adjusting to a missing extremity, such as writing with the feet or sliding across a floor rather than walking. Children can become so proficient at these adjustments that later in life they do not see the advantage of a prosthesis and refuse to use one. Although these self-adjustments may be cute in infants, in the long run they greatly limit a child's potential.

Learning to use a hand prosthesis takes weeks to months. Help parents think of interesting activities when introducing the prosthesis so the child can see immediately how useful it will be to use. Gait training for use of lower extremity prostheses begins with the use of parallel bars and proceeds to independent walking and mastery of steps.

Children who are born with an absent extremity may need help in mastering not only the use of a prosthesis but also a positive body image of themselves as whole. If possible, in the newborn period, introduce parents to the rehabilitation team who will be following their child. Further steps then will be outlined for them to help them move past the helplessness they may feel to more positive action. Visiting a child who uses a prosthesis well can be a great help in convincing parents that their child can lead a normal life. Children with a congenital extremity loss do not grieve over the lost extremity as do adults or older children, which means they are often better prepared to move on quickly to rehabilitation.

Finger and toe conditions

Finger or hand deformities occur in about 3% of all births. **Polydactyly** is the presence of one or more additional fingers or toes. When an entire extra finger or toe forms, the supernumerary digit is usually amputated in infancy or early childhood. These extra fingers are often just cartilage or skin tags, and removal is simple and cosmetically sound. In **syndactyly** (two fingers or toes are fused), the fusion is usually caused by a simple webbing (see Fig. 27.16); separation of the digits into two sound and cosmetically appealing ones is usually successful. In other instances, the bones of the fingers or toes are also fused, and cosmetic appearance and function cannot be fully reconstructed.

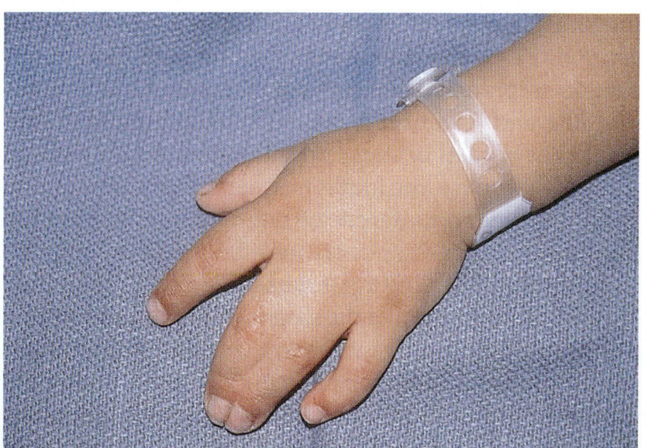

FIGURE 27.16 Syndactyly. (JPD/Custom Medical Stock Photograph.)

These hand anomalies are always upsetting to parents (one of the first things that new parents do is count the fingers and toes of newborns). They may need time to air their feelings and concerns. They may need reassurance at health maintenance visits throughout their child's development that the child is normal in other ways so they can accept and help the child develop self-esteem. Children need this same type of assurance so they can think of themselves as well people.

Torticollis (wry neck)

Torticollis is a term derived from *tortus* (twisted) and *collum* (neck). Torticollis (wry neck) occurs as a congenital anomaly when the sternocleidomastoid muscle is injured and bleeds during birth (S. J. Lee et al., 2011). This tends to occur in newborns with wide shoulders when pressure is exerted on the head to deliver the shoulder. The infant holds the head tilted to the side of the muscle involved; the chin rotates to the opposite side. The injury may not be noticeable in the newborn and may become evident only as the original haemorrhage recedes and fibrous contraction occurs at 1 to 2 months of age. A thick mass over the muscle can usually be palpated at this time.

To relieve torticollis, parents need to begin a program of passive stretching exercises, lying the infant on a flat surface and rotating the head through a full range of motion. In addition, parents should always encourage the infant to look in the direction of the affected muscle. They can encourage this by holding the child to feed in such a position that the child must look in the desired direction. Placing a mobile on the child's crib to encourage the child to look towards the affected side also is helpful. Speaking to and handing the child objects from the affected side to make the child look that way are also helpful exercises.

If manual stretching is begun early and consistently by the parents, further treatment usually is not necessary. Help parents understand that these actions are important therapy and not just games. Otherwise, the exercises seem so simple parents may not take them seriously. In the few instances in which simple exercises are not effective and the condition still exists at 1 year of age, surgical correction followed by a neck immobiliser will be necessary. If extreme injury to the muscle occurred, torticollis can lead to the continued elevation of one shoulder. Although a rare complication, this has the potential to lead to scoliosis later in life.

✔ Checkpoint question 27.4

What is an important care measure to teach parents of a child with torticollis?

a. Encourage the infant to turn his head to stretch the neck
b. Wrap the infant's neck in a warm towel twice daily
c. Massage the infant's shoulders and torso at bedtime
d. Administer ibuprofen daily

Craniosynostosis (craniostenosis)

Craniosynostosis is premature closure of the sutures of the skull. This may occur in utero or early in infancy because of rickets or irregularities of calcium or phosphate metabolism; it also occurs as a dominantly inherited trait. It occurs more often in boys than in girls (Roder, 2010).

This condition needs to be detected early because premature closure of the suture line will seal the skull closed and compromise brain growth. When the sagittal suture line closes prematurely, the child's head tends to grow anteriorly and posteriorly. If the coronal suture line fuses early, the orbits of the eyes become misshapen, and the increased intracranial pressure may lead to exophthalmos, nystagmus, papilloedema, strabismus and atrophy of the optic nerve with consequent loss of vision. Premature closure of the coronal suture line is associated with syndactyly. Therefore, closely observe all infants with syndactyly for head circumference. Conversely, assess all infants with craniosynostosis for syndactyly. Cardiac anomalies, choanal atresias or disorders of elbows and knee joints are also associated with craniosynostosis.

Measure head circumference on all children 2 years or younger at health maintenance visits and compare these measurements with normal head circumference charts. The posterior fontanelle normally closes at 2 months of age, the anterior fontanelle at 12 to 18 months. Children whose fontanelles close before these typical times need continued assessment to ensure that craniosynostosis is not developing.

Craniosynostosis is diagnosed by x-ray or ultrasound, which reveals the fused suture line. If the suture line is the sagittal one, treatment may involve only careful observation; if the coronal suture line is involved, it will need to be surgically opened to prevent brain compression and an abnormally shaped head by 9 to 12 months (Okada & Gosain, 2012).

Achondroplasia

Achondroplasia (chondrodystrophia) is a failure of bone growth inherited as a dominant trait. It causes a disorder in cartilage production in utero. The epiphyseal plate of long bones cannot produce adequate cartilage for longitudinal bone growth, which results in both arms and legs becoming stunted.

Because the bones of the cranium are of membranous origin, they continue to grow normally. Heads of children with achondroplasia will therefore appear unusually large in contrast to their extremities. The forehead is prominent and the bridge of the nose is flattened. Because this is a cartilage, not a brain, problem, intelligence proceeds normally. Children's trunks are of near-normal size, but a thoracic kyphosis (outward curve) and lumbar lordosis (inward curve) of the spine may develop.

Achondroplasia can be diagnosed in utero or at birth by comparing the length of extremities with the normal length (in the average child, the arms can be extended to the distance of the mid thigh) or by x-ray, which will reveal characteristic abnormally flaring epiphyseal lines. People with achondroplasia rarely reach a height of more than 140 cm. Women with this condition will have difficulty with childbearing because of a small pelvis, generally necessitating a caesarean birth.

Children with achondroplasia become aware of their appearance as early as the preschool years. They are apt to become acutely aware of their appearance during school age, when they realise they look different from other children. Children may be prescribed growth hormone to increase their ultimate height or, although controversial, leg lengthening may be possible (Singh et al., 2010). Ideally, such children have parents who have adjusted well to their own short stature and therefore have developed good self-esteem and can implant these qualities in their child.

Children should be informed that, as with all dominantly inherited disorders, there is a high probability that their children will inherit the disorder. Adolescence may be a particularly difficult time for these children as they realise that occupational and reproductive options may be limited for them. Continued guidance or counselling can help them to emerge from this period with feelings of high self-esteem in themselves as adults.

Talipes disorders

Talipes is a word formed from the Latin words *talus* ("ankle") and *pes* ("foot"). The talipes deformities are ankle–foot disorders. Current orthopaedic correction techniques should leave the child with normal foot position. However, depending on the extent of the original deformity, shoe size may vary as much as two shoe sizes, and the child may have asymmetry of leg length.

Approximately 1 in every 1000 children is born with a talipes disorder, occurring more often in boys than in girls. It probably is inherited as a polygenic pattern. It usually occurs as a unilateral problem (Eilert, 2008).

Some newborns have a pseudo-talipes disorder that has developed because of their intrauterine position. In these infants, the foot looks to be turned in but can be brought into a straight position by manipulation. In a true disorder, the foot cannot be properly aligned without further intervention. Be certain to demonstrate to parents that if a pseudo-disorder is present, the foot can easily be brought into line and is not deformed. Otherwise, the first time parents fit booties or shoes on the infant, they will notice this and worry that the foot is misshapen.

A true talipes disorder can be one of four separate types: plantar flexion (an equinus or "horsefoot" position, with the forefoot lower than the heel); dorsiflexion (the heel is held lower than the forefoot or the anterior foot is flexed towards the anterior leg); varus deviation (the foot turns in); or valgus deviation (the foot turns out). Most children with talipes deformities have a combination of these conditions or have an equinovarus (see Fig. 27.17A) or a calcaneovalgus disorder (a child walks on the heel with the foot everted).

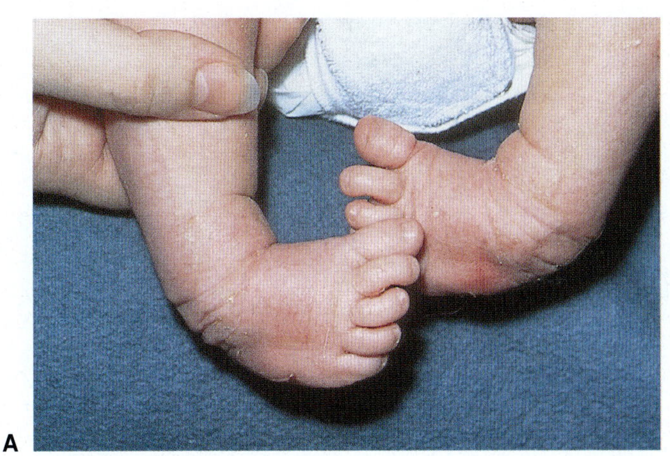
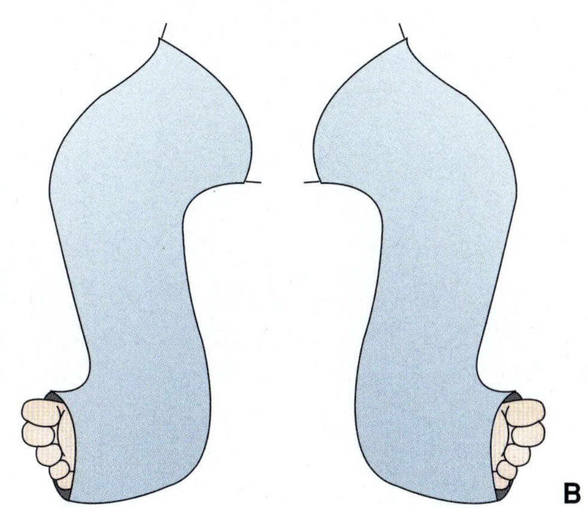

FIGURE 27.17 (**A**) Talipes equinovarus. (SPL/Photo Researchers, Inc.) (**B**) Casts for bilateral equinovarus.

Assessment

The earlier a true disorder is recognised, the better will be the correction. Make a habit of straightening all newborn feet to the midline as part of initial assessment to detect this disorder.

Therapeutic management

Correction is achieved best if it is begun in the newborn period. A cast is applied while the foot is placed in an overcorrected position. Although the disorder involves the ankle, the cast extends above the knee to ensure firm correction (see Fig. 27.17B). (Care of the child in a cast is discussed in Chapter 51.) Because talipes casts are high on the leg, change nappies frequently to prevent a wet nappy from touching the cast and causing it to become soaked with urine or meconium/faeces. Review with parents how to check the infant's toes for coldness or blueness and how to blanch a toenail bed and watch it turn pink to assess for good circulation. Because a newborn cannot report pain except by generalised crying, crying episodes in the infant must be evaluated carefully.

Infants grow so rapidly in the neonatal period that casts for talipes deformities must be changed almost every 1 or 2 weeks. Be certain that the family knows to make arrangements to bring the infant to the hospital for cast changes.

After approximately 6 weeks (the time varies depending on the extent of the problem), the final cast is removed. After this, parents may need to perform passive foot exercises such as putting the infant's foot and ankle through a full range of motion several times a day for several months. These seem like simple manoeuvres, so be sure to stress their importance to the parents; otherwise, they are easy exercises to omit when people's lives are busy. The infant may have to sleep in splints or shoes attached to a metal bar to maintain position or high-top shoes at night for a few more months.

Although a successful correction cannot be guaranteed, the prognosis for a full correction is good. For children who do not achieve correction by casting, surgery is yet another option to achieve a final correction.

Congenital hip dysplasia

Congenital hip dysplasia (CHD) is improper formation and function of the hip socket. The disorder occurs in 1 in 1000 births. It may be evident as subluxation or dislocation of the head of the femur (see Fig. 27.18).

With this disorder, the acetabulum of the pelvis is flattened or shallow. This prevents the head of the femur from remaining in the acetabulum and rotating adequately. In a subluxated hip, the femur "rides up" because of the flat acetabulum; in a dislocated hip, the femur rides so far up that it actually leaves the acetabulum. Why the disorder occurs is unknown, but it may be from a polygenic inheritance pattern. It may also occur from a uterine position that causes less-than-usual pressure of the femur head on the acetabulum.

Congenital hip dysplasia occurs most often in children of Mediterranean ancestry. It is found six times more frequently in girls than in boys, possibly because the hips are normally more flaring in females and possibly because the maternal hormone relaxin causes the pelvic ligaments to be more relaxed. Therefore, the femur does not press as effectively into the acetabulum during intrauterine life, deepening the space. Involvement usually is unilateral.

Assessment

Detecting congenital hip dysplasia in the newborn is important because the longer the condition goes undetected, the more difficult it is to correct. Sometimes the affected leg may appear slightly shorter than the other one because the femur head rides so high in the socket. This is most noticeable when the child is lying supine and the thighs are flexed to a 90° angle towards the abdomen. One knee will appear to be lower than the other (a Galeazzi sign (see Fig. 27.19A)). An unequal number of skin folds may be present on the posterior thighs (see Fig. 27.19B). This finding is unreliable, however, because some infants with

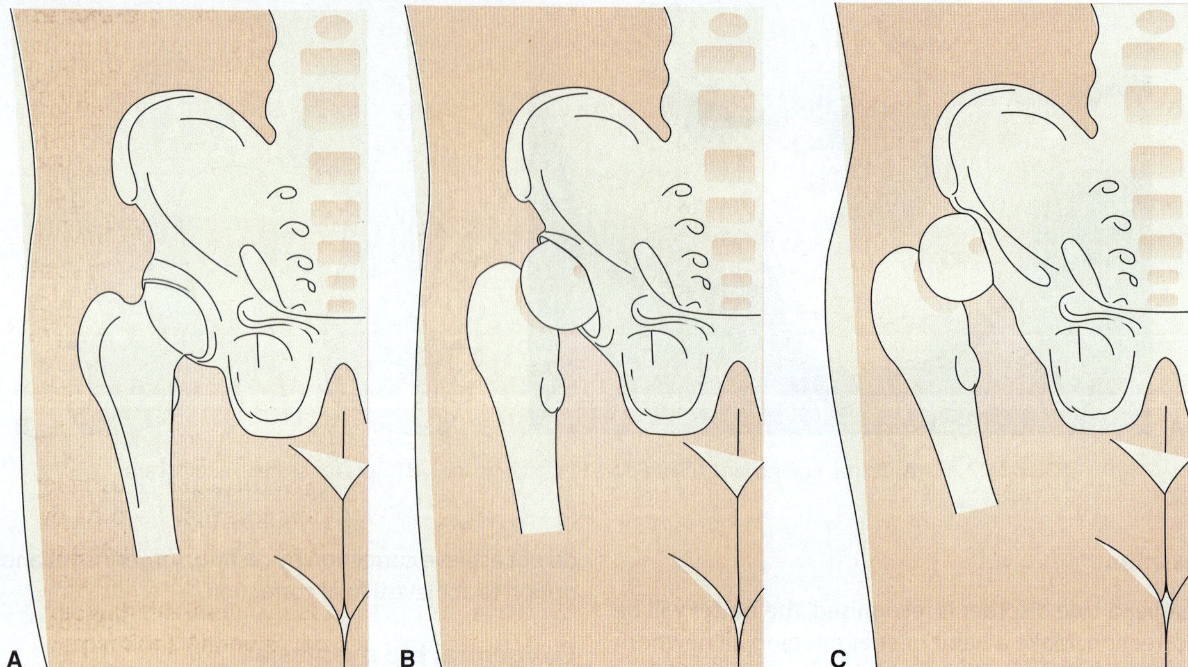

FIGURE 27.18 Hip dysplasia. (**A**) A normal femur head and acetabulum. (**B**) A subluxated hip. The femur head is "riding high" in the shallow acetabulum. (**C**) A dislocated hip. The femur head is not engaged in the shallow acetabulum.

normal hips have an uneven number of posterior thigh skin folds. Subluxated or dislocated hips are best assessed by noting whether the hips abduct (see Box 27.5).

In some infants, the hip abducts properly at a newborn assessment, but at the time of a health maintenance visit at 4 to 6 weeks, a secondary shortening of the adductor muscles will have occurred, and the disorder will be evident. Hip dysplasia is difficult to detect at birth in an infant who was born from a footling or frank breech presentation because the knees are stiff and do not flex readily. Always assess hip function in these infants at each health maintenance visit. Tight adductor muscles occur in children with cerebral palsy, so this disorder must be ruled out. X-ray, ultrasound or MRI will reveal the shallow acetabulum and a more lateral placement of the femur head than is ordinarily seen.

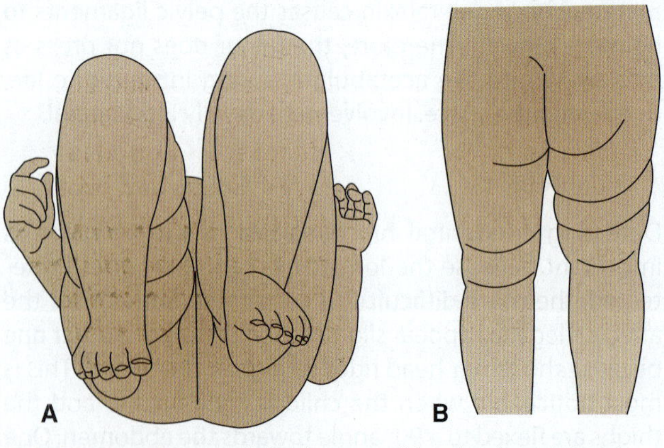

FIGURE 27.19 Signs of developmental hip dysplasia. (**A**) With child in a supine position, the right knee on the side of the subluxation appears lower than the left because of malposition of the femur head. (**B**) Asymmetry of skin folds and prominence of the trochanter on the right side.

Therapeutic management

Correction of subluxated and dislocated hips involves positioning the hip into a flexed, abducted (externally rotated) position to press the femur head against the acetabulum and cause it to deepen its contour by the pressure. Splints, halters or casts may be used. The small number of children who do not achieve correction by these methods will have surgery and a pin inserted to stabilise the hip.

Splints

Splint correction (to hold the legs in a frog-leg, or abducted, externally rotated position) often begins during the newborn's initial hospital stay.

Pavlik harness

A Pavlik harness is an adjustable chest halter that abducts the legs. It is the method of choice for long-term therapy because it reduces the time interval for therapy to 3 to 4 weeks and simplifies care (see Fig. 27.20A). Soft plastic stirrups (booties) with quick-fastening closures such as Velcro attach to leg extension straps and hold the hips flexed, abducted and externally rotated. It is common for infants to wear the harness continuously for the first month. Following review they may have short periods of up to one hour per day without the harness. The harness is then worn continually except for bathing. Advise parents to assess the skin under the straps daily for irritation or redness.

A Pavlik harness does not show under a shirt and long trousers and promotes gentle reduction of the hip. However,

BOX 27.5 Nursing procedure ✻ Assessing Ortolani's and Barlow's signs

Purpose: To assist in detecting developmental hip dysplasia.

Procedure	Principle
1. Lay the infant supine and flex the knees to 90° at the hips.	**1.** Proper positioning ensures accurate results.
2. Place your middle fingers over the greater tro chanter of the femur and your thumb on the internal side of the thigh over the lesser trochanter (see Fig. A).	**2.** Placing your fingers in this way allows for abduction of the hips.
3. Abduct the hips while applying upward pressure over the greater trochanter, and listen for a clicking sound.	**3.** Normally, no sound is heard. A clicking or clunking sound is a positive Ortolani's sign and occurs when the femoral head re-enters the acetabulum.
4. Next, with your fingers in the same position, and holding the hips and knees at 90° flexion, apply a backward pressure (down and laterally) and adduct the hips (see Fig. B). Note any feeling of the femoral head slipping.	**4.** Normally, the hip joint is stable. A feeling of the femur head slipping out of the socket posterolaterally is a positive Barlow's sign indicative of hip instability associated with developmental hip dysplasia.

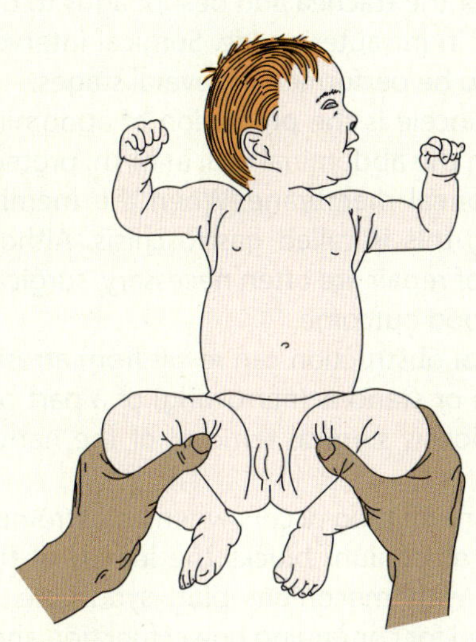

FIGURE A

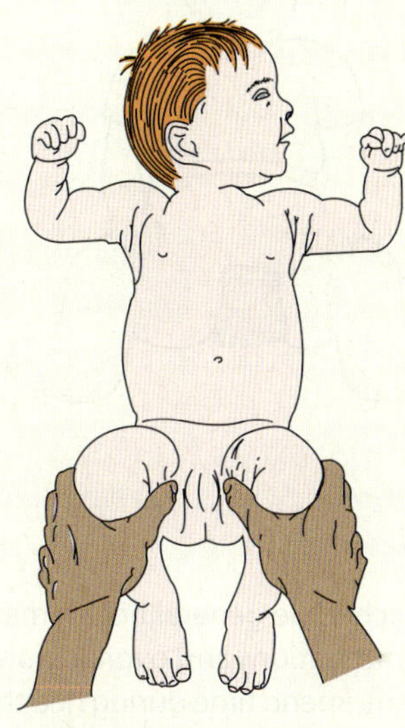

FIGURE B

if a hip is completely dislocated, a Pavlik harness may not be firm enough to hold the hips in the proper position. In addition, the harness will be ineffective if parents remove it too frequently.

Spica cast

If a hip is fully dislocated or the subluxation is severe, an infant may be placed immediately in a frog-leg, A-line cast or a spica (hip spica) cast to maintain an externally rotated hip position (see Fig. 27.20B). These casts are heavy and are so wide that dressing infants or sitting them in an infant car seat or bassinet can be difficult. Be certain parents have a car seat that can be modified to accommodate a large cast. Newborns are unable to report that a cast is causing circulatory constriction, so they need to be assessed hourly for circulation to the extremities for the first 24 hours the cast is in place and daily thereafter. Teach parents how to do this type of neurovascular assessment (check temperature and circulation in toes) before they take an infant home from the hospital so they can prevent circulatory compression from a rapidly growing leg outgrowing a cast. Casts will be changed periodically but maintained for 6 to 9 months. If a reduction manoeuvre for congenital dislocated hip was forceful, causing tension in the soft tissues around the hip, the resulting compression of the joint may cause transient blockage of the blood supply to the femoral head or avascular necrosis. In its severest form, this can lead to femoral head death and loss of future growth at the proximal growth plate causing unequal leg lengths.

General care guidelines

No matter what type of therapy is used—harness or cast—surgery may still be necessary for a final correction. Making parents aware of this from the start prevents them from thinking their child's condition is so serious that the usual methods of treatment failed. It helps them from becoming discouraged or dissatisfied with healthcare. It also helps them to accept from the beginning that this condition will be a long-term care concern. Some children will be 2 years old before the final cast or harness is removed.

The child and parents will have to visit a paediatric orthopaedic surgeon frequently during these early years. Ensure

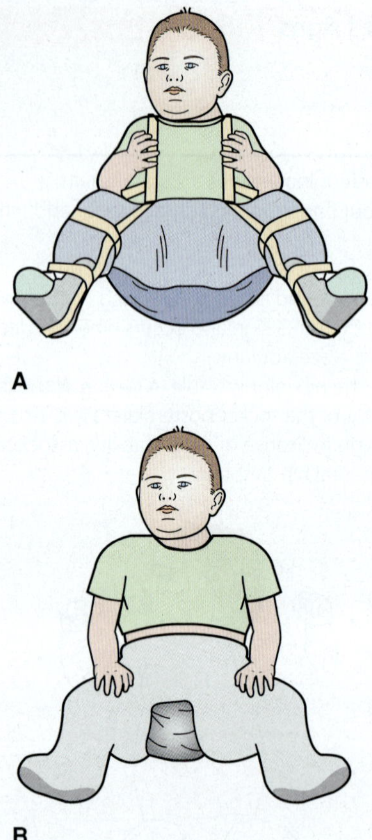

FIGURE 27.20 (**A**) A Pavlik harness. (**B**) A hip abduction cast for correction of subluxation of the hip.

that parents also schedule general health maintenance visits for routine immunisations and overall growth and development assessment. Spend time during health maintenance visits talking with them about infant stimulation. Because the child is not fully mobile, special adaptations are necessary. Teach parents to hold their child for feeding and to rock and cuddle the infant, even though a large cast or a brace may be bulky and awkward. They need to bring experiences to the infant because the child cannot crawl and walk towards interesting objects in the environment. A child's wagon/trolley can supply convenient and fun transportation. The child may also be able to lie prone and move about on a large skateboard. Many parents worry that the child who is still in a large cast at the normal age for walking (12 months) will never learn to walk. They can be assured that this is not a problem; when the cast is removed, the child will quickly catch up with this developmental step.

✔ Checkpoint question 27.5

Children with developmental hip dysplasia have a Pavlik harness prescribed. You would advise the parents of a child with this type of therapy that their child:

a. Will be anaesthetised to have the harness applied
b. Will experience dull pain all the time it is in place
c. Will need to wear this for only 1 or 2 weeks
d. Should wear it continuously until reviewed

Key points for review

- Learning about the way a child will be physically challenged immediately after birth helps parents adjust most easily. Advocate for parents by helping them obtain as much information as they need about their child's condition.
- Parent–infant bonding can be difficult to establish when a child is hospitalised at birth. Assess family relationships at health maintenance visits to see that bonding is occurring.
- Cleft lip and palate result from the failure of the maxillary process to fuse in intrauterine life. Surgical repair is possible early in life, with a good prognosis for both these conditions.
- Tracheo-oesophageal atresia and fistula occur from failure of the trachea and oesophagus to divide appropriately in intrauterine life. Surgical intervention often needs to be performed in several stages.
- Omphalocele is the protrusion of abdominal contents through the abdominal wall at birth, protected only by a peritoneal membrane. When the membrane is not present, this is called gastroschisis. Although several stages of repair are often necessary, surgical correction has a good outcome.
- Intestinal obstruction can result from atresia (complete closure) or stenosis (narrowing) of a part of the bowel. Correction is surgical removal of the narrowed bowel portion.
- A meconium plug occurs when an extremely hard portion of meconium blocks the lumen of the intestine. Infants with meconium plug syndrome need to be observed for continuing bowel function and need to be assessed for cystic fibrosis, because a meconium plug is often a symptom of this.
- Diaphragmatic hernia occurs when the abdominal organs protrude through a defect in the diaphragm into the chest cavity. This prevents the lungs from fully expanding at birth. These infants are critically ill at birth and need extensive surgical correction.
- Imperforate anus is stricture of the anus, resulting in inability to pass stool. The infant may have a temporary colostomy created before a final surgical correction can be completed.
- Physical developmental disorders of the nervous system include hydrocephalus (excess cerebrospinal fluid in the ventricles) and spina bifida (incomplete closure of the spinal cord). Infants with hydrocephalus need surgery to relieve a ventricular obstruction or have a shunt implanted from their ventricles to the peritoneal cavity to remove excess cerebrospinal fluid. Children with myelomeningocele, the most severe form of neural cord disorder, face permanent loss of lower neuron function and require continued rehabilitation.
- Absent or malformed extremities may range from absence of a finger to absence of an entire limb. Children may need physical therapy and teaching about

how to use a prosthesis to gain full mobility and function.

- Congenital hip dysplasia is the improper formation and function of the hip socket; talipes deformities are foot and ankle deformities. Children may need extensive bracing and casting to correct these disorders.

CASE STUDY QUESTIONS

3. Baby Caitlin has congenital hip dysplasia and will be placed in a Pavlik harness. What suggestions could you make to Emma and Brad to help instil a strong sense of trust in their child? A sense of autonomy?
4. You notice that Emma is obviously upset at her child's appearance. She does not want to feed the baby and voices the thought of placing her for adoption. In contrast, Brad handles the baby warmly and asks questions about surgery. No grandparents visit. What interventions would you want to begin with this family?

Resources

For an extensive range of additional resources to enhance teaching and learning and to facilitate understanding of this chapter, please see the text's accompanying website located on thePoint at http://thepoint.lww.com.

References

Balfour-Lynn, I. M. (2008). Newborn screening for cystic fibrosis: evidence for benefit. *Archives of Disease in Childhood, 93*(1), 7–10.

Bartels, E., Jenetzky, E., Solomon, B. D., et al. (2012). Inheritance of the VATER/VACTERL association. *Pediatric Surgery International, 28*(7), 681–685.

Bishop, W. P. (2011). Oral cavity. In K. J. Marcdante, R. M. Kliegman, H. B. Jenson, et al. (Eds.), *Nelson Essentials of Pediatrics* (6th ed., pp. 475–476). Philadelphia: Saunders/Elsevier.

Brunnegard, K. & Lohmander, A. (2007). A cross-sectional study of speech in 10-year-old children with cleft palate: Results and issues of rater reliability. *Cleft Palate-Craniofacial Journal, 44*(1), 33–44.

Catalano, P., Di Pace, M. R., Caruso, A. M., et al. (2011). Gastroesophageal reflux in young children treated for esophageal atresia. *Journal of Pediatric Gastroenterology & Nutrition, 52*(6), 686–690.

Dixon, M. J., Marazita, M. L., & Beaty, T. H. et al. (2011). Cleft lip and palate: Understanding genetic and environmental influences, *Nature Review Genetics, 12*(3), 167–178.

Donahue, D. (2008). Meningomyelocele. In F. J. Domino (Ed). *The 5-minute Clinical Consult*. Philadelphia: Lippincott Williams & Wilkins.

Efrati, O., Nir, J., Fraser, D., et al. (2010). Meconium ileus in patients with cystic fibrosis is not a risk factor for clinical deterioration and survival. *Journal of Pediatric Gastroenterology and Nutrition, 50*(2), 173–178.

Eilert, R. E. (2008). Orthopedics. In W. W. Hay, et al. (Eds) *Current Pediatric Diagnosis and Treatment* (18th ed.). Columbus, OH: McGraw-Hill.

Fowler, S. F. & Lee, H. (2008). Congenital disorders of the trachea and esophagus. In A. K. Lalwani (Ed). *Current Diagnosis and Treatment in Otolaryngology—Head and Neck Surgery* (2nd ed.). Columbus, OH: McGraw-Hill.

Garfinkle, J. S., King, T. W., Grayson, B. H., et al. (2011) A 21-year anthropometric evaluation of the nose in bilateral cleft lip-cleft palate patients following nasoalveolar molding and cutting bilateral cleft lip and nose reconstruction. *Plastic and Reconstructive Surgery, 127*(4), 1659–1667.

Garriboli, M., Duess, J. W., Ruttenstock, E., et al. (2012). Trends in the treatment and outcome of congenital diaphragmatic hernia over the last decade. *Pediatric Surgery International, 28*(12), 1177–1181.

Gourlay, D. M. (2013). Colorectal considerations in pediatric patients. *Surgical Clinics of North America, 93*(1), 251–272.

Harres, A. E. (2007). Minimally invasive neonatal surgery. *Journal of Perinatal and Neonatal Nursing, 21*(1), 39–49.

Harrison, D., Yamada, J. & Stevens, B. (2010). Strategies for the prevention and management of neonatal and infant pain. *Current Pain and Headache Reports, 14*(2), 113–123.

Hoffman, W. Y. (2008). Cleft lip and palate. In A. K. Lalwani (Ed). *Current Diagnosis and Treatment in Otolaryngology—Head and Neck Surgery* (2nd ed.). Columbus, OH: McGraw-Hill.

Holland, A. J. A., Walker, K., & Badawi, N. (2010). Gastroschisis: An update. *Pediatric Surgery International, 26* (9), 871–878.

Ingoe, R. & Lange, P. (2007). The Ladd's procedure for correction of intestinal malrotation with volvulus in children. *AORN: Association of Perioperative Registered Nurses Journal, 85*(2), 300–312.

Juang, D. & Snyder, C. L. (2012). Neonatal bowel obstruction. *Surgical Clinics of North America, 92*(3), 685–711.

Kelly, D., O'Dowd, T. & Reulbach, U. (2012). Use of folic acid supplements and risk of cleft lip and palate in infants: A population-based cohort study. *British Journal of General Practice, 62*(600), e466–e472.

Kline, U. (2014). Oral medicine & dentistry. In W. Hay, M. Levin, R. Deterding, et al. (Eds.), *Current Diagnosis & Treatment Pediatrics* (22nd ed., pp. 470–471). New York: McGraw-Hill/Lange.

Komolafe, E. O., Adeolu, A. A. & Komolafe, M. A. (2008). Treatment of cerebrospinal fluid shunting complications in a Nigerian neurosurgery programme. *Pediatric Neurosurgery, 44*(1), 36–42.

Lee, D., Lim, S. & Lee, J. K. (2011). Thyroglossal duct cyst presenting with airway obstruction in a neonate. *Otolaryngology: Head and Neck Surgery, 144*(1), 127–128.

Lee, S. J., Han, J. D., Lee, H. B., et al. (2011). Comparison of clinical severity of congenital muscular torticollis based on the method of child birth. *Annals of Rehabilitation Medicine, 35*(5), 641–647.

Lewis, D. W. (2011). Neurology. In K. J. Marcdante, R. M. Kliegman, H. B. Jenson, et al. (Eds.), *Nelson Essentials of Pediatrics* (6th ed., pp. 671–712). Philadelphia: Saunders/Elsevier.

Lidsky, M. E., Lander, T. A. & Sidman, J. D. (2008). Resolving feeding difficulties with early airway intervention in Pierre Robin sequence. *Laryngoscope, 118*(1), 120–123.

Louik, C., et al. (2007). First-trimester use of selective serotonin-reuptake inhibitors and the risk of birth defects. *New England Journal of Medicine, 356*(26), 2675–2683.

Lumley, J., et al. (2009). Periconceptional supplementation with folate and/or multivitamins for preventing neural tube defects. *Cochrane Database of Systematic Reviews,* (1), CD001056.

Lund, C. H., Bauer, K. & Berrios, M. (2007). Gastroschisis: Incidence, complications, and clinical management in the neonatal intensive care unit. *Journal of Perinatal and Neonatal Nursing, 21*(1), 63–68.

McKenna, L. & Mirkov, S. (2014). *McKenna's Drug Handbook for Nursing and Midwifery* (7th ed.). Sydney: Lippincott Williams & Wilkins.

Mildinhall, S. (2012). Speech and language in the patient with cleft palate. In M. T. Cobourne (Ed.), *Cleft Lip and Palate: Epidemiology, Aetiology and Treatment*. Unionville, CT: Karger.

Moyer, V., et al. (2009). Late versus early surgical correction for congenital diaphragmatic hernia in newborn infants. *Cochrane Database of Systematic Reviews, 2009*(1), CD001695.

Okada, H. & Gosain, A. K. (2012). Current approaches to management of nonsyndromic craniosynostosis. *Current Opinion in Otolaryngology & Head Neck Surgery, 20*(4), 310–317.

O'Mahar, K., Holmbeck, G. N., Jandasek, B., et al. (2010). A camp-based intervention targeting independence among individuals with spina bifida. *Journal of Pediatric Psychology, 35*(8), 848–856.

Roder, M. (2010). A primer on craniosynostosis. *Midwifery Today with International Midwife, 2010–2011 Winter* (96), 43–45.

Singh, S., Song, H. R., Venkatesh, K. P., et al. (2010). Analysis of callus pattern of tibia lengthening in achondroplasia and a novel method of regeneration assessment using pixel values. *Skeletal Radiology, 39*(3), 261–266.

Sinha, S. K., Dhua, A., Mathur, M. K., et al. (2012). Neural tube defect repair and ventriculoperitoneal shunting: Indications and outcome. *Journal of Neonatal Surgery, 1*(2), 21.

Smith, M. H. & Henderson, J. L. (2007). Congenital anomalies. In K. B. Fortner et al. (Eds). *The Johns Hopkins Manual of Gynecology and Obstetrics*. Philadelphia: Lippincott Williams & Wilkins.

Sponseller, P. D. (2007). Spina bifida. In F. J. Frassica, P. D. Sponseller & J. H. Wilckens (Eds). *5-minute Orthopaedic Consult*. Philadelphia: Lippincott Williams & Wilkins.

Thilo, E. H. & Rosenberg, A. A. (2008). The newborn. In W. W. Hay et al. (Eds). *Current Pediatric Diagnosis and Treatment* (18th ed.). Columbus, OH: McGraw-Hill.

Tovar, J. A. (2012). Congenital diaphragmatic hernia. *Orphanet Journal of Rare Diseases, 7*(1), 1–17.

van Aalst, J. A., Kolappa, K. K. & Sadove, M. (2008). Nonsyndromic cleft palate. *Plastic and Reconstructive Surgery, 121*(1 Suppl), 1–14.

van Eijck, F. C., et al. (2008). Closure of giant omphaloceles by the abdominal wall component separation technique in infants. *Journal of Pediatric Surgery, 43*(1), 246–250.

Wiler, J. L. (2012). Symptoms: Hernia with acute pain and swelling. *Emergency Medicine News, 34*(1), 18–21.

Zahl, S. M. & Wester, K. (2008). Routine measurement of head circumference as a tool for detecting intracranial expansion in infants: What is the gain? *Pediatrics, 121*(3), e416–e420.

Suggested readings

Australasian Cleft Lip & Palate Association Inc. <www.cleft.org.au>.

CCS Disability Action <www.ccsdisabilityaction.org.nz>.

Cleft New Zealand <www.faceit.org.nz>.

Down Syndrome Association <www.downsyndromevictoria.org.au>.

Habich, M., Wilson, D., Thielk, D., et al. (2012). Evaluating the effectiveness of pediatric pain management guidelines. *Journal of Pediatric Nursing, 27*(4), 336–345.

Hydrocephalus Support Association <www.hydrocephalus.org.au>.

Moore, K. N., Fader, M. & Getliffe, K. (2009). Long-term bladder management by intermittent catheterisation in adults and children. *Cochrane Database of Systematic Reviews, 2009*(1), CD006008.

NZ Down Syndrome Association <www.nzdsa.org.nz>.

Pierre Robin Australia <www.pierrerobin.org.au>.

Spina Bifida Foundation Victoria <www.sbfv.org.au>.

Unit 5

The nursing role in health promotion for a childrearing family

Chapter 28

Principles of growth and development

Nurses are directly responsible for assessing the growth and development of children in many healthcare settings. Previous chapters discussed childbearing and the significant first weeks of a child's life after birth. This chapter provides information about growth and development that is important for all the continuing years of a child's life.

LEARNING OBJECTIVES

After mastering the contents of this chapter, you should be able to:

1. Describe principles of growth and development and developmental stages according to major theorists.
2. Use critical thinking to analyse ways that paths to achieving a new developmental stage remain family-centred.
3. Assess a child to determine the stage of development that has been achieved.
4. Formulate nursing considerations that address wellness as well as both a potential for and an actual delay in growth and development.
5. Plan nursing interventions to assist a child in achieving and maintaining normal growth and development.
6. Integrate knowledge of growth and development with nursing process to achieve quality child and family health nursing care.

KEY TERMS

- abstract thought
- accommodation
- autonomy versus shame or doubt
- centring
- cognitive development
- conservation
- development
- developmental milestones
- developmental task
- egocentrism
- growth
- identity versus role confusion
- industry versus inferiority
- initiative versus guilt
- integrity versus despair
- intimacy versus isolation
- permanence
- reversibility
- role fantasy
- schemas
- sensorimotor stage
- temperament
- trust versus mistrust

CASE STUDY

John Olson is a 6-year-old boy you see in the emergency department because he has a broken leg from a bicycle accident. At 4 months of age, John was taken away from his mother because she was not caring for him adequately. He was then moved back and forth among 12 different foster homes until he was finally adopted at the age of 3. His adoptive parents have 3-year-old twins of their own. They tell you although John has lived with them for 3 years, they find him cold and unloving. They ask you what they can do to change this.

CASE STUDY QUESTIONS

1. How has John's background contributed to his behaviour?
2. What stage of psychosocial development does he not seem to have achieved?
3. How could his adoptive parents help him at this point?

All children pass through predictable stages of growth and development as they mature. Parents often ask what to expect from their children regarding their developmental progress at healthcare visits. Such visits provide opportunities for you not only to assess present growth and development but also to provide assistance and support to the parents in providing care for their child.

For these reasons, including growth and development is essential in the establishment of complete and effective nursing care plans for children. This chapter addresses the most important factors to assess for each age group. Later chapters supply detailed descriptions of individual age groups.

PROMOTION OF NORMAL GROWTH AND DEVELOPMENT

Assessment

Measurement and plotting height and weight on a standard growth chart for children at all healthcare visits to document growth is necessary to ensure a child's growth

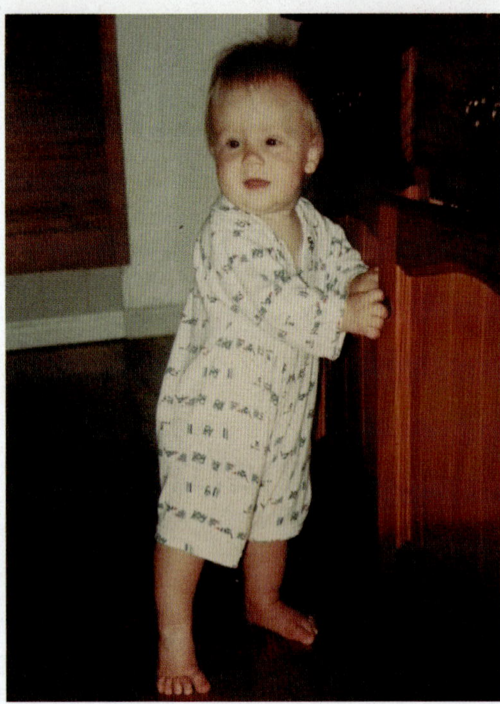

FIGURE 28.1 This 12-month-old demonstrates mastery of well-coordinated and intentional hand movements. (© Caroline Hunter.)

remains within a constant percentile. It is important to take a health history from both parents if possible and the child and observe what specific activities the child can accomplish to establish whether **developmental milestones** (major markers of normal development) are being met (see Fig. 28.1). Documentation of a 24-hour recall history for nutritional intake, sleep and a description of school and play behaviours is necessary, in as much detail as possible. For the most accurate assessments, also ask about time of illness, difficulty with sleep, if any, fatigue or "bad days".

Nursing considerations

When assessment is completed, a child profile can be devised and needs and problems identified. Examples of nursing considerations applicable to this area include:

- Delayed growth and development related to prolonged illness
- Imbalanced nutrition, less than body requirements, related to parental knowledge deficit regarding child's protein needs
- Deficient knowledge related to potential long-term effects of obesity in school-age child.

To provide holistic nursing care, consider all aspects of a child's health (physical, emotional, cultural, cognitive, spiritual, nutritional and social), remembering that each child's developmental progress is unique. Children cannot be forced to achieve milestones faster than their own timetable will allow. However, through family assistance agencies and information providers, children and families can be encouraged to reach maximum developmental potential. Nurses can play important roles in suggesting expected outcomes and guidance to both a child and family on ways to encourage child development and preparing children for new experiences.

GROWTH AND DEVELOPMENT AND THE ROLE OF THE NURSE

Information about growth and development is important in all phases of childcare.

Health promotion and illness prevention

Determining a child's developmental stage is often the primary focus of a health interview. For instance, during her child's 24-month check-up, a mother might ask if it is normal that her child cannot yet pedal a tricycle. Parenting style and competence are major influences on the behavioural and mental health of children (Barton & Kirtley, 2012). In addition to reassurance that their child is doing well, parents also need periodic anticipatory guidance regarding their child's development. For example, it would be important to discuss additional home safety with a parent when a child is approaching the age for crawling. Parents of a child who is almost 1 year old will appreciate being cautioned that their child's appetite may decrease during the coming year; armed with this knowledge, they will not interpret a child's rejection of food as the beginning of a feeding problem but will see it as a usual step in development.

How does the nurse best improve growth and development? This cannot be done alone. Through preventive health measures and care optimal growth and development can be achieved. Information may be given during the pre- and post-natal periods, maternal and health visits, and through improvements in the education programs provided. The parents' awareness and knowledge of their child's needs is increased as is their receptivity to information about health and development and so they increase in parental confidence. These programs for improving health in early life should aim to:

- Increase the general level of education and provide equal opportunity of access to education
- Improve the health of mothers, families and babies in the long run
- Provide good nutrition, health, education and health and preventive care facilities, and adequate social and economic resources, before first pregnancies, during pregnancy and in infancy, to improve growth and development before birth and throughout infancy, and reduce the risk of disease and malnutrition in infancy
- Ensure that the parent-child bonds are supported from birth, ideally through home visiting and the encouragement of good parental relations with schools, to increase

parental knowledge of children's emotional and cognitive needs to stimulate cognitive development and social behaviour in the child, and to prevent further complications between parent and child.

Health restoration and maintenance

It is equally essential to consider developmental stages when caring for a sick child or one having surgery. Preparing a 5-year-old child for surgery, for example, would be ineffective unless you know how much a 5-year-old child can be expected to comprehend. You would need to assess if a child will understand, for example, an anaesthetic is a gas, what a surgeon does, what stitches are for etc. It is just as important to keep developmental stages in mind when teaching parents; for example, you need to evaluate whether an oral form of medicine is appropriate for a child or if a child is too young to coordinate tongue and throat muscles. Physical growth is another important factor to consider because disease affects children differently at various stages of growth.

PRINCIPLES OF GROWTH AND DEVELOPMENT

Growing up is a complex phenomenon because of the many interrelated facets involved. Children do not merely grow taller and heavier as they get older; maturing also involves growth in their ability to perform skills, to think, to relate to people, and to trust or have confidence in themselves.

The terms "growth" and "development" are occasionally used interchangeably, but they are different. **Growth** is generally used to denote an increase in physical size or a quantitative change. Growth in weight is measured in kilograms; growth in height is measured in centimetres. **Development** is used to indicate an increase in skill or the ability to function (a qualitative change). Development can be measured by observing a child's ability to perform specific tasks such as how well a child picks up small objects such as raisins, by recording the parent's description of a child's progress, or by using standardised age-appropriate physical and psychosocial assessments.

Psychosexual development is a specific type of development that refers to developing instincts or sensual pleasure (Freudian theory). Psychosocial development refers to Erikson's stages of personality development. Moral development is the ability to know right from wrong and to apply these to real-life situations. Kohlberg is a theorist who studied this throughout childhood and adolescents. Moral development grows with the child. At this early stage the child is only at the beginner level and still relies on adults and significant others to assist with moral judgement.

Cognitive development refers to the ability to learn or understand from experience, to acquire and retain knowledge, to respond to a new situation, and to solve problems (see the section below on Piaget's theory of cognitive development). It is measured by intelligence tests and by observing children's ability to function effectively in their environment.

Neither physical growth nor aspects of maturation occur haphazardly but in typical patterns governed by several principles (see Box 28.1).

CASE STUDY QUESTION

4. John is 6 years old. What body system is reaching its peak point of development at this time?
   a. Neurological system
   b. Lymphatic system
   c. Reproductive system
   d. Musculoskeletal system

FACTORS INFLUENCING GROWTH AND DEVELOPMENT

Several factors impact on growth and development. WHO defines the social determinants of health (SDoH) as: "the conditions in which people are born, grow, live, work and age, including the health system. These circumstances are shaped by the distribution of money, power and resources at global, national and local levels, which are themselves influenced by policy choices. The social determinants of health are mostly responsible for health inequities—the unfair and avoidable differences in health status seen within and between countries." The risks to the developing child are significantly greater among those in poor socio-economic circumstances. The foundations of adult health are laid in early childhood and before birth. Slow growth and poor emotional support raise the lifetime risk of poor physical health and reduce physical, cognitive and emotional functioning in adulthood. An infant's experience is important to later health because of the continued malleability of biological systems. As cognitive, emotional and sensory inputs program the brain's responses, insecure emotional attachment and poor stimulation can lead to reduced readiness for school, low education attainment, problem behaviour, and the risk of social marginalisation in adulthood.

Slow or disrupted physical growth in infancy is associated with reduced cardiovascular, respiratory, pancreatic and kidney development and function and this leads to increased risk of illness in adulthood. We need to remember not only the SDoH but the next factors also when assessing a young child and family's health. When assessing the growth and development of children we must also look at other cultures, in particular Indigenous cultures. "Indigenous peoples remain on the margins of society: they are poorer, less educated, die at a younger age, are much more likely to commit suicide, and are generally in worse health than the rest of the population" (IWGIA, 2006, p. 10). When working with Indigenous people you must

BOX 28.1 ✻ Principles of growth and development

Growth and development are continuous processes from conception until death. Although there are highs and lows in terms of the rate at which growth and development proceed, at all times a child is growing new cells and learning new skills. An example of how the rate of growth changes is a comparison between that of the first year and later in life. An infant triples birth weight and increases height by 50% during the first year of life. If this tremendous growth rate were to continue, the 5-year-old child, ready to begin school, would weigh 725 kg and be 4 m tall.

Growth and development proceed in an orderly sequence. Growth in height occurs in only one sequence—from smaller to larger. Development also proceeds in a predictable order. For example, the majority of children sit before they crawl, crawl before they stand, stand before they walk, and walk before they run. Occasionally, a child will skip a stage (or pass through it so quickly that the parents do not observe the stage). Occasionally, a child will progress in a different order, but most children follow a predictable sequence of growth and development.

Different children pass through the predictable stages at different rates. All stages of development have a range of time rather than a certain point at which they are usually accomplished. Two children may pass through the motor sequence at such different rates, for example, that one begins walking at 9 months, another only at 14 months. Both are developing normally. They are both following the predictable sequence; they are merely developing at different rates.

All body systems do not develop at the same rate. Certain body tissues mature more rapidly than others. For example, neurological tissue experiences its peak growth during the first year of life, whereas genital tissue grows little until puberty.

Development is cephalocaudal. *Cephalo* is a Greek word meaning "head"; *caudal* means "tail". Development proceeds from head to tail. Newborns can lift only their head off the bed when they lie in a prone position. By age 2 months, infants can lift both the head and chest off the bed; by 4 months, the head, chest and part of the abdomen; by 5 months, infants have enough control to turn over; by 9 months, they can control legs enough to crawl; and by 1 year, children can stand upright and perhaps walk. Motor development has proceeded in a cephalocaudal order—from the head to the lower extremities.

Development proceeds from proximal to distal body parts. This principle is closely related to cephalocaudal development. It can best be illustrated by tracing the progress of upper extremity development. A newborn makes little use of the arms or hands. Any movement, except to put a thumb in the mouth, is a flailing motion. By age 3 or 4 months, the infant has enough arm control to support the upper body weight on the forearms, and the infant can coordinate the hand to scoop up objects. By 10 months, the infant can coordinate the arm and thumb and index fingers sufficiently well to use a pincer-like grasp or be able to pick up an object as fine as a piece of breakfast cereal on a highchair tray.

Development proceeds from gross to refined skills. This principle parallels the preceding one. Once children are able to control distal body parts such as fingers, they are able to perform fine motor skills (a 3-year-old colours best with a large crayon; a 12-year-old can write with a fine pen).

There is an optimum time for initiation of experiences or learning. Children cannot learn tasks until their nervous system is mature enough to allow that particular learning. A child cannot learn to sit, for example, no matter how much the child's parents have him or her practice, until the nervous system has matured enough to allow back control. Children who are not given the opportunity to learn developmental tasks at the appropriate or "target" times for that task may have more difficulty than the usual child learning the task later on. A child who is confined to a body cast at 12 months, the time the child would normally learn to walk, may take a long time to learn this skill once free of the cast at, say, age 2 years. The child has passed the time of optimal learning for that particular skill.

Neonatal reflexes must be lost before development can proceed. An infant cannot grasp with skill until the grasp reflex has faded nor stand steadily until the walking reflex has faded. Neonatal reflexes are replaced by purposeful movements.

A great deal of skill and behaviour is learned by practice. Infants practise over and over taking a first step before they accomplish this securely. If children fall behind in growth and development because of illness they are capable of "catch-up" growth to bring them equal again with their age group.

take into account their definition of health. Health is defined in WHO's Constitution as "a state of complete physical, mental and social wellbeing and not merely the absence of disease or infirmity". This definition extends beyond the traditional Western biomedical paradigm which treats body, mind and society as separate entities and reflects a more holistic understanding of health. Indigenous peoples have a similar understanding of health, as wellbeing is about the harmony that exists between individuals, communities and the universe (Hampton & Toombs, 2013).

Genetic inheritance, or whether a child receives healthy genes or genes that will lead to an illness, and environmental influences, such as whether the family a child is born into has sufficient funds to supply adequate food, are two primary factors that determine a child's pattern of growth and development. Temperament (the typical way a child reacts to situations) is an example of genetic influence. A unique combination of these factors determines how each child grows and matures (Pike, Jane Pillow & Lucas, 2012).

Genetics

From the moment of conception when a sperm and ovum fuse, the basic genetic makeup of an individual is cast. Although each child is unique, certain gender-related characteristics will influence growth and development. In addition to physical characteristics such as eye colour and height potential, inheritance determines other characteristics such as learning style and temperament. An individual may also inherit a genetic abnormality, which could result in disability or illness at birth or later in life.

Gender

On average, girls are born lighter (by 30–50 grams) and shorter (by 3–5 cm) than boys. Boys tend to keep this height and weight advantage until pre-puberty, at which time girls surge ahead because they begin their puberty growth spurt 6 months to 1 year earlier than boys. By the end of puberty (14 to 16 years), boys again tend to be taller and heavier than girls (see Appendix B; Pastor & Reuben, 2011).

Health

A child who inherits a genetically transmitted disease may not grow as rapidly or develop as fully as a healthy child, depending on the type of illness and the therapy or care available for the disease (Dea, 2011; Morgan, 2012).

Intelligence

Children with high intelligence do not generally grow faster physically than other children, but they do tend to advance faster in skills. Occasionally, children of high intelligence fall behind in physical skills because they spend their time with books or mental games rather than with games that develop motor skills and so do not receive practice in these areas.

Temperament

Temperament is the usual reaction pattern of an individual, or an individual's characteristic manner of thinking, behaving, or reacting to stimuli in the environment (Johnston et al, 2012). Unlike cognitive or moral development, temperament is not developed by stages but is an inborn characteristic set at birth. Understanding that children are not all alike—some adapt quickly to new situations and others adapt slowly, and some react intensely and some passively—can help parents better understand why their children are different from each other and help them care for each child more constructively (Carr-Gregg, 2014).

Reaction patterns

Chess and Thomas (1995) identified nine separate characteristics that define temperament or how children react to situations. Each child's pattern is made up of a combination of these individual elements.

Activity level

The level of activity among children differs widely. Some babies are constantly on the go and rarely quiet. They wiggle and squirm in their cot as early as 2 weeks of age. Parents put such children to sleep at one end of a cot and find them at the other end an hour later; such children will not stay seated in bathtubs and refuse to be confined in playpens. Other babies, by contrast, move little, stay where they are placed, and appear to take in their environment in a quieter, more docile way. Both patterns are normal.

Rhythmicity

A child who has *rhythmicity* manifests a regular rhythm in physiological functions. Even as infants, such children tend to wake up at the same time each morning, are hungry at regular 4-hour periods, nap at the same time every day, and have a bowel movement at the same time every day. They are predictable and easy to care for because their parents learn early on what to expect from them. On the other end of the scale are infants with an irregular rhythmicity. They rarely awaken at the same time 2 days in a row. They may go a long time without eating one day and the next day appear hungry almost immediately after a feeding. Such children may be more difficult to care for because it is difficult to plan a schedule for them. Parents must constantly adapt their own routine to the child's routine.

Approach

Approach refers to a child's response on initial contact with a new stimulus. Some children approach new situations in an unruffled manner. They smile and "talk" to strangers and accept a first feeding or a new food without vomiting or fussing. They explore new toys without apprehension. Other children demonstrate withdrawal rather than approach to new situations. They cry at the sight of strangers, new toys and new foods; they fuss the first time they are placed in a bath.

Adaptability

Adaptability is the ability to change one's reaction to stimuli over time. Infants who are adaptable can change their first reaction to a situation without exhibiting extreme distress. The first time such children are placed in a bathtub they might protest loudly, for example, but by the third time they sit splashing happily. This is in contrast to infants who cry for months whenever they are put into a bathtub or who cannot seem to accustom themselves to a new bed, new car seat or new carer.

Intensity of reaction

Some children react to situations with their whole being. They cry loudly, thrash their arms and begin temper tantrums when their nappies are wet, when they are hungry and when their parents leave them. Others rarely demonstrate such overt symptoms of anger or have a mild or low-intensity *reaction to stress.*

Distractibility

Children who are easily distracted or who can easily shift their attention to a new situation (*distractibility*) are easy to care for. If they are crying over the loss of a toy, they can be appeased by the offer of a different one. Other children cannot be distracted in this way; their parents may describe them as stubborn, wilful or unwilling to compromise because they persistently return to an activity or refuse to adapt or change.

Attention span and persistence

Attention span is the ability to remain interested in a project or activity. Like other aspects of temperament, this varies among children. Some play by themselves with one toy for an hour; others spend no more than 1 or 2 minutes with each toy. The degree of *persistence* also varies. Some infants keep trying to perform an activity even when they fail time after time; others stop trying after one unsuccessful attempt.

Threshold of response

The *threshold of response* is the intensity level of stimulation that is necessary to evoke a reaction. Children with a low threshold need little stimulation; those with a high threshold need intense stimulation before they become upset over a situation.

Mood quality

A child who is always happy and laughing has a positive *mood quality*. Obviously, this can make a major difference to the parents' enjoyment of a child. Parents are bound to spend more time with a child who is always happy than with a child who has a negative mood quality.

Nursing considerations regarding temperament

Noticing children's temperamental characteristics as they are admitted to a hospital can help you anticipate children's probable reactions to procedures or pain. For example, a child with a mild reactivity pattern may not show a great deal of response to even acute pain, but a child with an intense pattern may react as strongly to minor discomfort as to major pain, making it difficult to evaluate the true level of pain the child is experiencing (Hudson et al., 2011).

Environment

Although children cannot grow taller than their genetically programmed height potential allows, their adult height may be considerably less than their genetic potential if their environment hinders their growth in some way. For example, a child could receive inadequate nutrition because of a family's low socioeconomic status; a parent could lack childcare skills or not give a child enough attention; or a child could have a chronic illness (Rossow & Moan, 2012). Environmental influences, however, are not always detrimental (Rossow & Moan, 2012). For example, children with phenylketonuria, an inherited metabolic disease, can achieve normal growth and development in spite of their genetic makeup if their diet (a part of the environment) is properly regulated. The following environmental influences are those most likely to affect growth and development.

Socioeconomic level

Because healthcare and good nutrition both cost money, children born into families of low socioeconomic means may not receive adequate health supervision or good nutrition. Poor health supervision can leave them without immunisation against measles or other childhood illnesses and therefore vulnerable to diseases that could cause permanent neurological damage if complications occur (Mulholland et al., 2012). Poor nutrition can also leave them vulnerable to disease as antibody formation depends on a good protein intake (Whitney & Rolfes, 2012).

Parent–child relationship

Cultural norms within a family play a role in determining when a child is expected to achieve particular developmental milestones. Children who are loved thrive better than those who are not. Either parent or a non-parent carer may serve as the primary carer or form a primary parent–child love relationship. It is the quality of time spent with children, not the amount of time that is important. Loss of love from a primary carer, as might occur with the death of a parent, or interruption of parental contact through hospitalisation, imprisonment, divorce or inadequate parental love, can interfere with a child's desire to eat, improve and advance. Helping parents feel involved in their child's care is important in both healthcare and childcare settings (Feigelman, 2012; Vicedo, 2011).

Ordinal position in the family

The position of a child in the family (first-born child, middle child, youngest child, only child) and the size of the family have some bearing on a child's growth and development. An only child or the oldest child in a family, for example, generally excels in language development because conversations are mainly with adults. Youngest children may develop language more slowly, especially if older children talk "baby talk" with them. Children learn by watching other children, however, so a youngest child who has many examples to watch may excel in other skills, such as toilet training at an early age.

Health

Diseases that come from environmental sources can have as strong an influence on growth and development as genetically inherited diseases. Infants cared for in neonatal intensive care units, for example, may develop some decrease in hearing because of the overstimulation of sound, an example of health being directly influenced by the environment (Matook et al., 2010). Children who have residual heart impairment as a result of contracting rheumatic fever might be limited in their ability to play an active sport. The eventual degree of disability will depend not only on the damage caused by the actual disease but also on the attitudes of the people around the child—how disabled they believe the child to be (Russell et al., 2012).

Nutrition

The quality of a child's nutrition during the growing years (including prenatally) has a major influence on health and stature (Whitney & Rolfes, 2012). Poor maternal nutrition may limit the growth and intelligence potential of a child from the moment of birth. Children whose diets lack essential nutrients show inadequate physical growth. A lack of energy and stamina prevents children from learning at their best intellectual level. Children who eat too many carbohydrates and become obese may develop motor skills more slowly than other children because physical movement is more tiring for them.

Nutrition plays a vital role in the body's susceptibility to disease because poor nutrition limits the body's ability to resist infection. Poor nutrition also plays a major role in the development of chronic illness. Of the eight leading causes of death in adults, six have been linked to dietary excesses: heart disease, cancer, cerebrovascular disease, diabetes mellitus, cirrhosis and arteriosclerosis. It is clear, too, that dietary habits have a cumulative effect; for instance, although heart disease is not one of the top causes of death in children, the arterial changes that cause cardiovascular disease begin in childhood (Sizer & Whitney, 2014). Establishing healthy eating patterns early in life, therefore, can contribute to better health in adult years <www.nutritionaustralia.org>.

Guidelines for a healthy diet

Good nutrition in children should follow a number of healthy eating guidelines, including the following:

- **Eat a variety of foods.** Choices from all food pyramid groups—dairy, meat and poultry, fruits, vegetables, cereals and grains—should be included in meals every day (vegetarians omit meat and poultry but supplement this with vegetable protein). It is also important to vary choices within each food group, as not all foods within a group are nutritionally equivalent.
- **Balance the food you eat with physical activity—maintain or improve your weight.** Although the tendency for obesity may be inherited, being overweight in early life also appears to play a role. Urge parents to be certain their infants receive all the nutrients they need for the substantial growth they are undergoing (including a percentage of fat because this is important for myelination of nerves); at the same time, it is important that infants not be overfed so they do not become obese.
- **Choose a diet with plenty of grain products, vegetables and fruits.** Foods with starch and fibre are more beneficial for gastrointestinal function than more processed foods. Fibre, in particular, has been linked to the lowered incidence of a variety of illnesses such as constipation and perhaps colon cancer in later life. Fibre can be included as early as during preschool years in the form of whole-grain cereals and raw fruits such as apples.
- **Choose a diet low in fat, saturated fat and cholesterol.** For children, fat intake does not need to be restricted for the first 2 years of life. Thereafter, fat intake can be tailored to meet the guidelines of 30% total intake for both children and adults.
- **Choose a diet moderate in sugars.** Too much sugar in a diet can contribute to both dental caries and obesity. In addition, refined sugar such as that used in soft drinks, prepared foods, lollies and chocolate represents "empty" kilojoules: it is high in kilojoules yet provides no essential nutrients. Although children need adequate carbohydrates for energy, parents can give their children a good start by preventing excessive sugar intake.
- **Choose a diet moderate in salt and sodium.** The taste for salt is acquired. If unsalted or only lightly salted solid food is offered to infants, they do not develop a desire for heavily salted foods. It is helpful to assess the diet of school-age children and check whether they are eating a diet heavier in salt than necessary because of many salty after-school snacks <www.nutritionaustralia.org>.

Components of a healthy diet

Eating a variety of foods from all five pyramid food groups in moderation is a way of guaranteeing the intake of a balanced diet of proteins, carbohydrates, fats, vitamins and minerals (see Table 28.1 and Appendix E).

- **Protein.** Protein is the major component of bones, skin, hair and muscle and is responsible for a wide variety of essential functions in the body. Because it is essential for growth, protein intake is crucial for children.
- **Carbohydrate.** Carbohydrates are the main and preferred fuel of the body to supply energy, so they are essential to the functioning of most body systems, the neurological system in particular. This is why carbohydrates are so important to infants and toddlers, whose brain cells are actively growing. Sugar supplies an immediate but short-term source of energy; starches, as a rule, supply sustained energy.
- **Fat.** Dietary fat is also a source of energy to the body. It can be an immediate energy source or can be stored if not used, then released when energy is required. Some fat deposits also serve as insulating material for subcutaneous tissues; in infants, fats are necessary to ensure myelination of nerve fibres.
- **Vitamins.** Vitamins are organic compounds that are essential for specific metabolic actions in cells. They do not produce energy but are needed by cells to produce energy. For children, fat-soluble vitamins (A, D, K and E) are mainly supplied by fortified dairy products, fortified cereals, and plant oils or fish oils. Such vitamins can leave the gastrointestinal tract and be used by the body only by being absorbed along with fat molecules. Once absorbed, they are used by the cells for growth and function or are stored in the liver and fat cells for later use. Because fat-soluble vitamins can be stored by the body, an infant or child can ingest too many of them, although overdosing usually occurs from supplements rather than dietary sources.

TABLE 28.1 Recommended number of serves for children, adolescents and toddlers

Recommended average daily number or serves from each of the five food groups*						Additional serves for more active, taller or older children and adolesoents
	Vegetables and legumes/ beans	Fruit	Grain (cereal) foods, mostly wholegrain	Lean meat and poultry, fish, eggs, nuts and seeds, and legumes/beans	Milk, yoghurt, cheese and/or alternatives (mostly reduced fat)	Approx. number of additional serves from the five food groups or discretionary choices
Toddlers**						
1–2	2–3	½	4	1	1–1 ½	
Boys						
2–3	2 ½	1	4	1	1 ½	0–1
4–8	4 ½	1 ½	4	1 ½	2	0–2 ½
9–11	5	2	5	2 ½	2 ½	0–3
12–13	5 ½	2	6	2 ½	3 ½	0–3
14–18	6 ½	2	7	2 ½	3 ½	0–5
Girls						
2–3	2 ½	1	4	1	1 ½	0–1
4–8	4 ½	1 ½	4	1 ½	1 ½	0–1
9–11	5	2	4	2 ½	3	0–3
12–13	5	2	5	2 ½	3 ½	0–2 ½
14–18	5	2	7	2 ½	3 ½	0–2 ½
Pregnant	5	2	8	3 ½	3 ½	0–3
Breastfeeding	5 ½	2	9	2 ½	4	0–3

*Includes an allowance for unsaturated spreads or oils, nuts or seeds (½ serve [4.5g] per day for children 2–3 years of age, 1 serve [7–10 g] per day for children 3–12 years of age; 1½ serve [11–15 g] per day for children 12–13 years, and 2 serves [14–20 g] per day for adolescents 14–18 years of age and for pregnant and breastfeeding girls).

**An allowance for unsaturated spreads or oils, nuts/seed paste of 1 serve (7–10 g) per day is included. Whole nuts and seeds are not recommended for children of this age because of the potential choking risk.

Source: National Health and Medical Research Council, under a Creative Commons Attribution 3.0 Australia licence.

- **Minerals.** Minerals are necessary to build new cells and regulate body processes such as fluid and electrolyte balance, nerve transmission and muscle contraction, so they are vital to the health of a growing infant or child. Deficiency in a mineral such as potassium can lead to poor heart function and childhood growth <www.nsa.asn.au>.

Promoting adequate nutritional intake in vegetarian diets

Increasing numbers of adults of childrearing age are vegetarians; therefore, many women during pregnancy and children during their years of most rapid growth eat such diets. Although a balanced vegetarian diet can be sufficient during childhood, careful assessment and family education are necessary to ensure that it is adequate for growth. Nurses are in a prime position to assist parents to become knowledgeable about good nutrition so they are aware of ways to include essential nutrients for growing children in vegetarian diets, particularly if their children participate in active sports.

For most healthy children, a vegetarian diet can provide a nutritious alternative to a diet that includes meat. However, special care needs to be taken with children on all vegetarian diets, especially vegan diets. Strict vegan diets are generally not recommended for very young children. There are different types of vegetarians, determined by the types of foods a person does not eat. Vegetarians can be classified into the following groups:

- Lacto-ovo vegetarians—exclude red meat, offal, fish and poultry. Obtain protein from dairy products, eggs, beans, legumes, pulses and nuts
- Lacto-vegetarians—exclude red meat, offal, fish, poultry and eggs. Obtain protein from dairy products, beans, legumes, pulses and nuts
- Vegans—exclude red meat, offal, poultry, fish, eggs and dairy products. Obtain protein from beans, legumes, pulses, nuts and soy products like tofu.

The type of vegetarian diet most commonly associated with significant nutritional problems in children is the vegan diet. To make sure your child gets enough of all the nutrients needed for a growing child, their vegetarian diet must include:

- Protein alternatives such as nuts, eggs, legumes and tofu
- Energy for growth and development
- Iron to prevent anaemia

- Vitamin B_{12}
- Vitamin D and calcium to prevent bone disease
- Suitable fats from non-meat sources
- Food in the correct form and combination to make sure nutrients can be digested and absorbed.

Breast milk or formula will remain an important food for babies up until 12 months. Talk to your child and maternal health nurse about the introduction of solids.

What if...

John's mother tells you she cannot afford to buy meat, explaining she can get more food for the family if she purchases mostly pasta and cereals? How would you help her plan meals that are low in cost but high in nutritional value?

THEORIES OF DEVELOPMENT

A *theory* is a systematic statement of principles that provides a framework for explaining some phenomenon. Developmental theories provide road maps for explaining human development. A **developmental task** is a skill or a growth responsibility arising at a particular time in an individual's life, the achievement of which will provide a foundation for the accomplishment of future tasks. It is not so much chronological age as the completion of developmental tasks that defines whether a child has passed from one developmental stage of childhood to another. For example, children are not toddlers just because they are 1 year plus 1 day old; they become toddlers when they have passed through the developmental stage of infancy. For reference, however, childhood is generally divided into the age periods shown in Table 28.2.

Freud's psychoanalytic theory

Sigmund Freud (1856–1939), an Austrian neurologist and the founder of psychoanalysis, offered the first real theory of personality development. Freud based his theory on his observations of mentally disturbed adults. He described adult behaviour as being the result of instinctual drives that have a primarily sexual nature (*libido*) that arise from within the person and the conflicts that develop between these instincts (represented in the individual as the *id*), reality (the *ego*) and society (the *superego*). He described child development as being a series of psychosexual stages in which a child's sexual gratification becomes focused on a particular body part. Freud's stages of childhood are summarised in Table 28.3.

TABLE 28.2 Basic divisions of childhood

Stage	Age period
Neonate	First 28 days of life
Infant	1 month–1 year
Toddler	1–3 years
Preschooler	3–5 years
School-aged child	6–12 years
Adolescent	13–21 years

The infant

Freud termed the infant period the "oral phase" because infants are so interested in oral stimulation or pleasure during this time. According to this theory, infants suck for enjoyment or relief of tension, as well as for nourishment.

The toddler

Freud described the toddler period as an "anal phase" because during this time, children's interests focus on the anal region as they begin toilet training. Elimination takes on new importance for them. Children find pleasure in both the retention of faeces and defecation. This anal interest is part of toddlers' self-discovery, a way of exerting independence and probably accounts for some of the difficulties parents may experience in toilet training children of this age.

The preschooler

During the preschool period, children's pleasure zone appears to shift from the anal to the genital area. Freud called this period the "phallic phase". Masturbation is common during this phase. Children may also show exhibitionism, suggesting they hope this will lead to increased knowledge of the two sexes.

The school-aged child

Freud saw the school-age period as a "latent phase", a time in which children's libido appears to be diverted into concrete thinking. He saw no developments as obvious as those in earlier periods appearing during this time.

The adolescent

Freud termed the adolescent period the "genital phase". Freudian theory considers the main events of this period to be the establishment of new sexual aims and the finding of new love objects.

Criticisms of Freud's theory

To construct his theory, Freud relied on his knowledge of people with mental illness or looked at circumstances that led to mental illness. This "looking at illness" rather than "looking at wellness" perspective limits the applicability of the theory as a health promotion measure, although the behaviours he discussed are as observable as ever.

Erikson's theory of psychosocial development

Erik Erikson (1902–1996) was trained in psychoanalytic theory but later developed his own theory of psychosocial development, a theory that stresses the importance of culture and society in development of the personality

TABLE 28.3 Summary of Freud's and Erikson's theories of personality development

	Freud's stages of childhood		Erikson's stages of childhood	
	Psychosexual stage	**Nursing considerations**	**Developmental task**	**Nursing considerations**
Infant	Oral stage: Child explores the world by using mouth, especially the tongue.	Provide oral stimulation by giving dummies; do not discourage thumb-sucking. Breastfeeding may provide more stimulation than formula-feeding because it requires the infant to expend more energy.	Developmental task is to form a sense of trust versus mistrust. Child learns to love and be loved.	Provide a primary carer. Provide experiences that add to security, such as soft sounds and touch. Provide visual stimulation for active child involvement.
Toddler	Anal stage: Child learns to control urination and defecation.	Help children achieve bowel and bladder control without undue emphasis on its importance. If at all possible, continue bowel and bladder training while child is hospitalised.	Developmental task is to form a sense of autonomy versus shame. Child learns to be independent and make decisions for self.	Provide opportunities for decision making, such as offering choices of clothes to wear or toys to play with. Praise for ability to make decisions rather than judging correctness of any one decision.
Preschooler	Phallic stage: Child learns sexual identity through awareness of genital area.	Accept children's sexual interest, such as fondling their own genitals, as a normal area of exploration. Help parents answer child's questions about birth or sexual differences.	Developmental task is to form a sense of initiative versus guilt. Child learns how to do things (basic problem solving) and that doing things is desirable.	Provide opportunities for exploring new places or activities. Allow play to include activities involving water, clay (for modelling) or finger paint.
School-age child	Latent stage: Child's personality development appears to be non-active or dormant.	Help children have positive experiences with learning so their self-esteem continues to grow and they can prepare for the conflicts of adolescence.	Developmental task is to form a sense of industry versus inferiority. Child learns how to do things well.	Provide opportunities such as allowing child to assemble and complete a short project so that child feels rewarded for accomplishment.
Adolescent	Genital stage: Adolescent develops sexual maturity and learns to establish satisfactory relationships with the opposite sex.	Provide appropriate opportunities for the child to relate with opposite sex; allow child to verbalise feelings about new relationships.	Developmental task is to form a sense of identity versus role confusion. Adolescents learn who they are and what kind of person they will be by adjusting to a new body image, seeking emancipation from parents, choosing a vocation, and determining a value system.	Provide opportunities for an adolescent to discuss feelings about events important to him or her. Offer support and praise for decision making.

Adapted from Erikson, E. H. (1993). *Childhood and society.* New York: W. W. Norton; and Freud, S. (1962). *Three essays on the theory of sexuality.* New York: Hearst Corporation, with permission.

(Erikson, 1993). One of the main tenets of his theory, that a person's social view of self is more important than instinctual drives in determining behaviour, allows for a more optimistic view of the possibilities for human growth. While Freud looked at ways mental illness develops, Erikson looked at actions that lead to mental health. Erikson describes eight developmental stages covering the entire life span. At each stage, there is a conflict between two opposing forces. The resolution of each conflict, or accomplishment of the developmental task of that stage, allows the individual to go on to the next phase of development. Table 28.3 shows Erikson's and Freud's developmental stages through adolescence.

The infant

According to Erikson, the developmental task for infants is learning **trust versus mistrust** (other terms are "learning confidence" or "learning to love"). Infants whose needs are met when those needs arise, whose discomforts are quickly removed, who are cuddled, played with and talked to, come to view the world as a safe place and people as helpful and dependable. However, when their care is inconsistent, inadequate or rejecting, this fosters a basic mistrust: infants become fearful and suspicious of the world and of people. Like a burned child who avoids fire, emotionally-burned children may shun the potential pain of further emotional involvement and carry this attitude through later stages of development. Such children can be "stuck" emotionally at this stage, although they continue to grow and develop in other ways.

Fortunately, because not all children achieve developmental tasks readily, each task need not be resolved once and for all the first time it arises. The problem of trust versus mistrust, for example, is not resolved forever during the first year of life but arises again at each successive stage of development. Children who enter school with a sense of mistrust may come to trust a teacher with whom they form a close relationship; given this second chance, children may overcome early mistrust. On the other hand, children who come through infancy with a vital sense of trust intact may still have a sense of mistrust activated at a later stage if their parents are divorced or separate under unpleasant circumstances.

The toddler

Erikson defines the developmental task of the toddler age as learning **autonomy versus shame or doubt**. Autonomy (self-government or independence) builds on children's new motor and mental abilities. Children take pride in new accomplishments and want to do everything independently, whether it is pulling the wrapper off a lolly, selecting a vitamin tablet out of the bottle, flushing the toilet, or replying, "No!" If parents recognise toddlers need to do what they are capable of doing, at their own pace and in their own time, then children develop a sense of being able to control their muscles and impulses during this time. When carers are impatient and do everything for them, this enforces a sense of shame and doubt. If children are never allowed to do things they want to do, they will eventually doubt their ability to do them; they will stop trying and cannot do them. If children leave this stage with less autonomy than shame or doubt, they can be disabled in their attempts to achieve independence and may lack confidence in their abilities to achieve well into adolescence and adulthood (see Fig. 28.2).

The preschooler

The developmental task of the preschool period is learning **initiative versus guilt**. Learning initiative is learning how to do things. Children can initiate motor activities of various sorts on their own and no longer merely respond to or imitate the actions of other children or of their parents. The same is true for language and fantasy activities.

Whether children leave this stage with a sense of initiative outweighing a sense of guilt depends largely on how parents respond to self-initiated activities. When children are given much freedom and opportunity to initiate motor play such as running, bike riding, sliding, and wrestling or are exposed to such play materials as finger paints, sand,

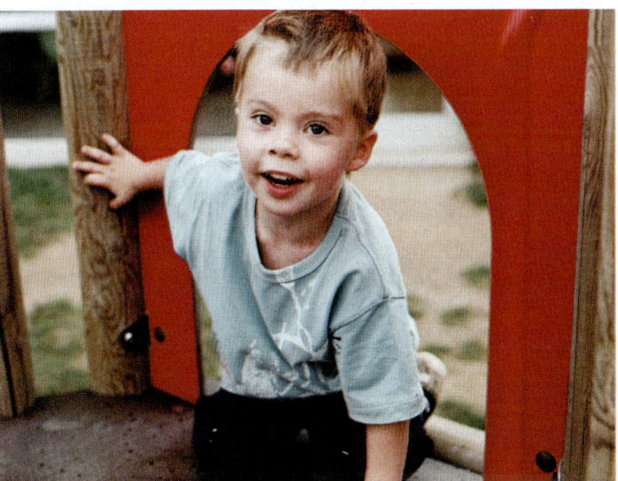

FIGURE 28.2 A toddler enjoys active, independent exploration as part of building a sense of autonomy. Here, a boy plays outdoors on playground equipment, a setting that allows for independent decision making.

water, and modelling clay, their sense of initiative is reinforced. Initiative is also encouraged when parents answer a child's questions (intellectual initiative) and do not inhibit fantasy or play activity. If children are made to feel their motor activity is bad (perhaps in a small apartment or a hospital), their questions are a nuisance, or their play is silly and stupid, they may develop a sense of guilt over self-initiated activities that will persist in later life. Those who do not develop initiative may later have limited brainstorming and problem-solving skills; they wait for clues or guidance from others before acting.

> ***What if...***
>
> John's father does not allow his preschool twins to play freely because he demands an orderly household? They begin to show signs of poor initiative. How would you counsel this parent?

The school-aged child

Erikson viewed the developmental task of the school-age period as developing **industry versus inferiority**, or accomplishment rather than inferiority. During the preschool period, children learned initiative—how to do something. During the school stage, children learn how to do things *well*. A school-aged child, while doing a project will ask, "Am I doing a good job? Am I doing this right?" When they are encouraged in their efforts to do practical tasks or make practical things and are praised and rewarded for the finished results, their sense of industry grows (see Fig. 28.3). Parents who see their children's efforts at making and doing things as merely "busy work" or who do not show appreciation for their children's efforts may cause them to develop a sense of inferiority rather than pride and accomplishment.

During the primary school years, a child's world grows to include the school and community environment, and

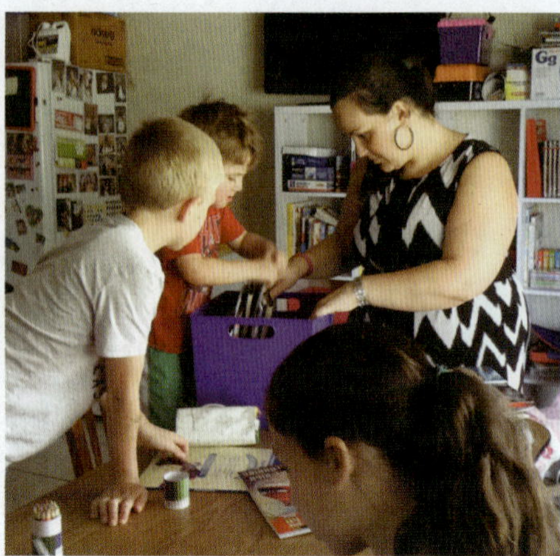

FIGURE 28.3 School-aged children develop a sense of industry by working on projects that result in a feeling of accomplishment. (© Lisa Speedie.)

success or failure in those settings can have a lasting impact. Children with an intelligence quotient of 80 or 90 (slightly below normal), for example, may have a particularly traumatic school experience, even when their sense of industry is rewarded and encouraged at home. Their learning style may be so different from the average child's they have difficulty competing with children of average ability; this causes repeated failures in their efforts to learn, reinforcing their sense of inferiority. On the other hand, children whose sense of industry has not been supported at home may have it revitalised at school through the efforts of a committed teacher. A nurse during a hospitalisation could also fulfil this role. The important role of nurses during the hospitalisation of children will be discussed in more detail in Chapter 36.

The adolescent

Erikson believed the new interpersonal dimension that emerges during adolescence is a sense of **identity versus role confusion**. To achieve this, adolescents must bring together everything they have learned about themselves as a son or daughter, an athlete, a friend, a fast-food cook, a student, a garage band musician and so on, and integrate these different images into a whole that makes sense. If adolescents cannot do so, they are left with role confusion; that is, they are left unsure of what kind of person they are and are uncertain what they can do or what kind of person they can become. Some adolescents seek a negative identity: being identified as a drug abuser or runaway may be preferable to having no identity at all. Body piercing and tattooing can help establish identity as they are outward expressions of who adolescents think they are.

The young adult

The developmental crisis of the young adult is achieving a sense of **intimacy versus isolation**. Intimacy is the ability to relate well with other people, not only with members of the opposite sex but also with one's own sex to form long-lasting friendships. A sense of intimacy grows out of earlier developmental tasks because people need a strong sense of identity before they can reach out fully and offer deep friendship or love. As there is always the risk of being rejected or hurt when offering love or friendship, individuals cannot offer it if they do not have confidence they can cope with rejection, or if they did not develop a sense of trust as an infant.

The middle-aged adult

The developmental task of middle age is to establish a sense of generativity versus stagnation. People extend their concern from just themselves and their families to the community and the world. They may become politically active, work to solve environmental problems, or participate in far-reaching community or world-based decisions. People with a sense of generativity are self-confident and better able to juggle their various lives (mother, soccer coach, church member, teacher, political party chairperson, gourmet cook). People without this sense become stagnated or self-absorbed.

The older adult

Older adults play a role in childrearing today because many of them provide childcare to young children while parents work. The developmental task of older adults is **integrity versus despair**. Older adults with integrity feel good about the life choices they have made; those with a feeling of despair wish life could begin again so that things could turn out differently (Newman & Newman, 2011).

Criticism of Erikson's theory

Erikson's main contribution to human development was the creation of stages so that development can be broken down into separate phases for study. A criticism of his theory is that life does not occur in easily divided stages, and trying to divide it that way can create superficial divisions.

CASE STUDY QUESTION

5. John is a school-aged child. What must he learn, according to Erikson, to complete the developmental task of this period?

a. How to be creative
b. How to think abstractly
c. How to trust others
d. How to do things well.

Piaget's theory of cognitive development

Jean Piaget (1896–1980), a Swiss psychologist, introduced concepts of **cognitive development**, or the way children learn and think, that have roots similar to those of both Freud and Erikson and yet separate from each (Wadsworth, 2003). Piaget defined four stages of cognitive development; within each stage are finer units or **schemas**. Each period is an advance over the previous one. To progress from one period to the next, children reorganise their thinking processes to

TABLE 28.4 Piaget's stages of cognitive development

Stage of development	Age span	Nursing implications
Sensorimotor		
Neonatal reflex	1 month/s	Stimuli are assimilated into beginning mental images. Behaviour entirely reflexive.
Primary circular reaction	1–4 month/s	Hand–mouth and ear–eye coordination develop. Infant spends much time looking at objects and separating self from them. Beginning intention of behaviour is present (the infant brings thumb to mouth for a purpose: to suck it). Enjoyable activity for this period: a rattle or tape of parent's voice.
Secondary circular reaction	4–8 month/s	Infant learns to initiate, recognise, and repeat pleasurable experiences from environment. Memory traces are present; infant anticipates familiar events (a parent coming near him will pick him up). Good toy for this period: mirror; good game: peek-a-boo.
Coordination of secondary reactions	8–12 month/s	Infant can plan activities to attain specific goals. Perceives that others can cause activity and that activities of own body are separate from activity of objects. Can search for and retrieve toy that disappears from view. Recognises shapes and sizes of familiar objects. Because of increased sense of separateness, infant experiences separation anxiety when primary caregiver leaves. Good toy for this period: nesting toys (i.e. coloured boxes).
Tertiary circular reaction	12–18 month/s	Child is able to experiment to discover new properties of objects and events. Capable of space perception and time perception as well as permanence. Objects outside self are understood as causes of actions. Good game for this period: throw and retrieve.
Invention of new means through mental combinations	18–24 month/s	Transitional phase to the preoperational thought period. Uses memory and imitation to act. Can solve basic problems, foresee manoeuvres that will succeed or fail. Good toys for this period: those with several uses, such as blocks, coloured plastic rings.
Preoperational thought	2–7 year	Thought becomes more symbolic; can arrive at answers mentally instead of through physical attempt. Comprehends simple abstractions but thinking is basically concrete and literal. Child is egocentric (unable to see the viewpoint of another). Displays static thinking (inability to remember what they started to talk about so that at the end of a sentence children are talking about another topic). Concept of time is now, and concept of distance is only as far as they can see. Centring or focusing on a single aspect of an object causes distorted reasoning. No awareness of reversibility (for every action there is an opposite action) is present. Unable to state cause–effect relationships, categories, or abstractions. Good toy for this period: items that require imagination, such as modelling clay.
Concrete operational thought	7–12 year	Concrete operations includes systematic reasoning. Uses memory to learn broad concepts (fruit) and subgroups of concepts (apples, oranges). Classifications involve sorting objects according to attributes such as colour; seriation, in which objects are ordered according to increasing or decreasing measures such as weight; multiplication, in which objects are simultaneously classified and seriated using weight. Child is aware of reversibility, an opposite operation or continuation of reasoning back to a starting point (follows a route through a maze and then reverses steps). Understands conservation, sees constancy despite transformation (mass or quantity remains the same even if it changes shape or position). Good activity for this period: collecting and classifying natural objects such as native plants, sea shells, etc. Expose child to other viewpoints by asking questions such as, "How do you think you'd feel if you were a nurse and had to tell a boy to stay in bed?"
Formal operational thought	12 year	Can solve hypothetical problems with scientific reasoning; understands causality and can deal with the past, present and future. Adult or mature thought. Good activity for this period: "talk time" to sort through attitudes and opinions.

From Piaget, J. (1961). *The growth of logical thinking from childhood to adolescence.* New York: Basic Books, with permission.

bring them closer to adult thinking. These stages of cognitive development are summarised in Table 28.4.

The infant

Piaget referred to the infant stage as the **sensorimotor stage**. Sensorimotor intelligence is practical intelligence, because words and symbols for thinking and problem solving are not yet available at this early age. At the beginning of infancy, babies relate to the world through their senses, using only reflex behaviour. As infants progress through this stage (which includes the schemas of primary and secondary circular reactions and coordination of secondary reactions, as defined in Table 28.4), they learn the basic concept that people are entities separate from objects. Piaget used the term "primary" to refer to activities related to a child's own body and the term "circulatory reaction" to show that repetition of behaviour occurs (infants accidentally bring their thumb to their mouth, enjoy the sensation of sucking, and so repeat it).

The term "secondary" refers to activities that are separate from a child's body. An example of secondary schema learning is when a baby hits a mobile, notices that this makes it move, and so hits it again. During this secondary schema, infants also learn that objects in the environment—bottle, blocks, bed or even a parent—are permanent and continue to exist even though they are out of sight or changed in some way. For example:

- Infants will search for a block hidden by a blanket, knowing the block still exists
- Infants can recognise that a parent remains the same person whether dressed in a robe and slippers or pants and a T-shirt
- Infants play peek-a-boo because they realise the person playing with them exists behind his or her hands
- Infants learn they are a separate entity from objects. They learn where their body stops and their bed, playthings or parent begins.

A great deal of the mouthing and handling of objects by infants and the delight of watching a carer appear is part of primary and secondary schemas and discovering **permanence**. The world begins to make sense and the developmental task of achieving trust falls into place when the concept of permanence has been learned (infants know their parents exist and will return to them). Gaining a concept of permanence also contributes to "eighth-month anxiety," a stage in which infants continue to cry for their parents because they know their parents still exist even when out of sight.

During the final phase of the infant year (coordination of secondary reactions), infants begin to demonstrate goal-directed behaviour. After noticing that hitting a mobile makes it move, infants then reach for and hit a music box nearby, in this way actively seeking new experiences. It is important for infants to have stimulating objects around for exploring in this way so that experimenting and learning can proceed.

The toddler

The toddler period is one of transition as children complete the final stages of the sensorimotor period (defined in Table 28.4 as tertiary circular reaction and invention of new means) and begin to develop some cognitive skills of the preoperative period, such as symbolic thought and egocentric thinking. In the tertiary circular reaction schema, children use trial and error to discover new characteristics of objects and events. A toddler sitting in a high chair who keeps dropping objects over the edge of the tray is exploring both permanence and the different actions of toys. During the schema of "invention of new means", children become able to think through actions or mentally project the solution to a problem. Toddlers following a ball that has rolled under a coffee table no longer have to follow the ball's path to retrieve it but can project where it will have rolled and walk around the coffee table to find it again.

During the period of *preoperational thought*, children relearn on a conceptual level some of the lessons they mastered as infants at the sensorimotor level, before having language. Now, children are able to use symbols to represent objects. They may have difficulty viewing one object as being different from another, however. On a walk through a department store decorated with teddy bears, for example, children are not sure whether they are seeing a succession of bears or if the same bear keeps reappearing as if it is following them, asking to be taken home.

Toddlers draw conclusions only from obvious facts they see: Daddy is shaving; therefore he must be going to work, because he went to work after he shaved yesterday. This type of faulty reasoning (prelogical reasoning) can lead children to wrong conclusions and faulty judgement.

How children think has many implications for nursing. If you made John's bed yesterday and then he went to surgery, he may cry at the sight of you approaching with clean sheets today, thinking he will have to go to surgery again.

The preschooler

Piaget saw preschool children as moving on to a substage of preoperational thought termed *intuitive thought*. During this time, children tend to look at an object and see only one of its characteristics (referred to as **centring**). For example, they see that a banana is yellow but do not notice it is also long. Centring is noticeable when children are learning about medicine (they observe it tastes bitter but cannot understand it is also good for them).

Centring contributes to the preschooler's lack of **conservation** (the ability to discern truth, even though physical properties change) or **reversibility** (ability to retrace steps). For example, if preschoolers see water being poured from one glass into another glass that is taller and thinner than the first one, they will notice only one changing characteristic. They might say that there is now more water in the second glass (because the level has risen), or there is less water (because the second glass is narrower), even when told that no water has been added or removed. When the water is poured back into the first glass, they still will not understand that the amount of water is unchanged. This immature perception leads children, as it did during the toddler period, to make faulty conclusions. It takes more years of development for children to learn that when thought processes such as knowing that the amount of water did not change and perceptions conflict, thought processes are more trustworthy.

Preschool thinking is also influenced by **role fantasy**, or how children would like something to turn out. Children use assimilation (taking in information and changing it to fit their existing ideas) as a part of this. For example, because a child wants to go outside and play, he says the outside is calling him to come and play. Children believe their wishes are as real as facts, and dreams are as real as daytime happenings during this stage. They perceive animals and even inanimate objects as being capable of thought and feeling (they say a dog took their doll because the dog was feeling sad; they say a footstool meant to trip them). This is often called "magical thinking." Later, children learn **accommodation** (they change their ideas to fit reality rather than the reverse).

Egocentrism, or perceiving that one's thoughts and needs are better or more important than those of others, is also strong during this period. Preschoolers cannot believe that not everyone knows facts they know; if asked, "What is your name?" they may reply, "Don't you know my name?" As a part of this, children define objects mainly in relation to themselves, so that a spoon is "what I eat with," not just a curved metal object.

The school-aged child

Piaget viewed school age as a period during which *concrete operational thought* begins as school-age children can discover concrete solutions to everyday problems and recognise cause-and-effect relationships. A child who understands water does not change in amount just because it is poured from one glass to another has grasped the concept of conservation. Conservation of numbers is learned as early as age 7 years, conservation of quantity at age 7 or 8 years, conservation of weight at age 9 years and conservation of volume at age 11 years. Reasoning during school age tends to be inductive, proceeding from specific to general: school-age children tend to reason that a toy they are holding is broken, the toy is made of plastic, so all plastic toys break easily.

The adolescent

Piaget saw adolescence as the time when cognition achieves its final form, that of formal operational thought. When this stage is reached, adolescents are capable of thinking in terms of possibility—what could be **(abstract thought)**—rather than being limited to thinking about what already is (concrete thought). This makes it possible for adolescents to use scientific reasoning or also understand deductive reasoning, or reasoning that proceeds from the general to the specific (plastic toys break easily, the toy they are holding is plastic; it will break easily).

Criticism of Piaget's theory

Piaget has been criticised because he used only a small sample of subjects (his own children) to develop his theory. Because children today begin activities to learn reading much earlier than they did at the time the theory was devised, the age groups and "norms" may no longer be accurate. Learning computer skills at an early age may be changing both the rate and type of children's cognitive development.

Kohlberg's theory of moral development

Lawrence Kohlberg (1927–1987), a psychologist, studied the reasoning ability of boys and, based on Piaget's development stages, developed a theory on the way children gain knowledge of right and wrong, or moral reasoning. These stages, as described by Kohlberg (1984), are summarised in Table 28.5.

Recognising where a child is at according to these stages can help identify how children may feel about an illness, such as whether children think it is fair that they are

TABLE 28.5 Kohlberg's stages of moral development

Age (year)	Stage	Description	Nursing considerations
Preconventional (Level I)			
2–3	1	Punishment/obedience orientation ("heteronymous morality"). Child does right because a parent tells him or her to and to avoid punishment.	Child needs help to determine what are right actions. Give clear instructions to avoid confusion.
4–7	2	Individualism. Instrumental purpose and exchange. Carries out actions to satisfy own needs rather than society's. Will do something for another if that person does something for the child.	Child is unable to recognise that like situations require like actions. Unable to take responsibility for self-care because meeting own needs interferes with this.
Conventional (Level II)			
7–10	3	Orientation to interpersonal relations of mutuality. Child follows rules because of a need to be a "good" person in own eyes and eyes of others.	Child enjoys helping others because this is "nice" behaviour. Allow child to help with bed making and other like activities. Praise for desired behaviour such as sharing.
10–12	4	Maintenance of social order, fixed rules, and authority. Child finds following rules satisfying. Follows rules of authority figures as well as parents in an effort to keep the "system" working.	Child often asks what are the rules and is something "right." May have difficulty modifying a procedure because one method may not be "right." Follows selfcare measures only if someone is there to enforce them.
Postconventional (Level III)			
Older than 12	5	Social contract, utilitarian law-making perspectives. Follows standards of society for the good of all people.	Adolescents can be responsible for self-care because they view this as a standard of adult behaviour.
	6	Universal ethical principle orientation. Follows internalised standards of conduct.	Many adults do not reach this level of moral development.

From Kohlberg, L. (1984). *The psychology of moral development*. New York: Harper & Row, with permission.

ill. Recognising moral reasoning also helps determine whether children can be depended on to carry out self-care activities such as administering their own medicine or whether children have internalised standards of conduct so they do not "cheat" when away from external control. Moral stages closely approximate cognitive stages of development because children must be able to think abstractly (be able to conceptualise an idea without a concrete picture) before being able to understand how rules apply even when no one is there to enforce them (Juujärvi, Pesso & Myyry, 2011).

The infant

The infant period is a *pre-religious stage*. Infants have little concept of any motivating force beyond that of their parents. Infants learn that when they do certain actions, parents give affection and approval; for other actions, parents scold and label the behaviour "bad." To support this stage of development, it is important for carers to praise infants for doing what they have been asked to do. Carers should also know the average infant is trying hard to please; if an infant falls short of doing this, it is probably because of immature development rather than any effort to displease.

The toddler

Toddlers begin to formulate a sense of right and wrong, but their reason for doing right is centred most strongly in "mother or father says so" rather than in any spiritual or societal motivation. Kohlberg referred to this as a "punishment obedience orientation" (a child is good because a parent says a child must be good, not because it is "right" to be good). Toddlers may not obey requests from people other than their parents because they do not view their authority as being at the same level as their parents' authority. This means that while providing nursing care, it might be necessary to ask a parent to reinforce instructions to be certain a toddler will follow them.

The preschooler

Preschoolers tend to do good out of self-interest rather than out of true intent to do good or because of a strong spiritual motivation. When asked why it is wrong to steal from a neighbour, for example, a preschooler might answer, "Because my mother won't like me anymore." Because of egocentrism, a preschooler may do things for others only in return for things done for him or her. This means it may be necessary to remind children of actions taken on their behalf or trade off actions such as, "Lie still now for me while I change your dressing and I'll read you a story when I'm through."

Children at this age also imitate what they see, so if they see less-than-perfect role models, they may copy those wrong actions, assuming those actions are correct. Preschoolers have great difficulty knowing what rules apply to new situations because they cannot judge whether a previously learned principle of right or wrong can be applied to this new situation (does not recognise that stealing money in a hospital setting is the same as stealing it at home).

The school-aged child

School-aged children enter a stage of moral development termed *conventional development*, a level at which many adults continue to function. Young school-aged children adhere to a phase of development termed the "nice girl, nice boy" stage. Children engage in actions that are "nice" or "fair" rather than necessarily right. Sharing, for example, is "nice". Taking turns is "fair". Stealing is not. Young school-aged children may lie about their actions to disguise that they have been involved in an action that is not "nice". When asked why it is wrong to steal from a neighbour, the school-aged child most often answers, "Because it's not nice or fair".

Later in the school-age period, as children learn about community resources, they become aware that community laws are enforced by police. They may have difficulty following self-care measures reliably when out of a nurse's or parent's sight during this time because they feel it is necessary to obey rules only when the rules can be clearly enforced. At this point, they might answer the question about stealing from a neighbour with, "You shouldn't steal because the police will put you in gaol."

The adolescent

As adolescents become capable of abstract thought, they can internalise standards of conduct (they do what they think is right regardless of whether anyone is watching). This is termed *postconventional development* and is the mature form of moral reasoning. In this stage, if asked why it is wrong to steal from a neighbour, adolescents may answer, "Because it deprives my neighbours of possessions they have earned." Adolescents can carry out self-care measures even when someone else is not present when they enter this stage because they can understand not only the importance of the measures to themselves but also the principle that certain things should be done simply because they are right to do. Many adolescents do not enter this phase of development, however, and as adults they continue at a school-age level, doing right things only when obvious authority or set rules are present.

Criticism of Kohlberg's theory

Kohlberg's theory is frequently challenged as being male-oriented because his original research was conducted entirely with boys. Carol Gilligan (1993), a sociologist, has suggested that girls may not score well on Kohlberg's scale because, being more concerned with relationships than boys, they make moral decisions based on individual circumstances, a different criterion for decision making.

CASE STUDY QUESTION

6. Suppose John tells you his broken leg wants to get better. What type of thinking is he using?

   a. Magical thinking
   b. Deductive reasoning
   c. Concrete operational thinking
   d. Sensorial thought

Key points for review

- Knowledge of growth and development is important in health promotion and illness prevention because it lays the basis for assessment and anticipatory guidance.
- Genetic factors that influence growth and development are gender, ethnicity, intelligence, and health.
- Environmental influences include quality of nutrition, socioeconomic level, parent–child relationship, ordinal position in the family, and environmental health.
- To meet growth and development milestones, children need to follow basic guidelines for a healthy diet, such as eating a variety of foods; maintaining ideal weight; avoiding extreme levels of saturated fat and cholesterol; eating foods with adequate starch and fibre; and avoiding too much sugar, the same as adults.
- Temperament is a child's characteristic manner of thinking, behaving or reacting. Helping parents understand the effect of temperament is a nursing role.
- Common theories of development are Freud's psychoanalytic theory and Erikson's theory of psychosocial development. Both of these theories describe specific tasks children must complete at each stage of development to become a well-adapted adult.
- Piaget's theory of cognitive development describes ways that children learn. Kohlberg advanced a theory of moral development, or how children use moral reasoning to solve problems they face.
- Although growth and development occur in known patterns, their rate varies from child to child. Caution parents not to be concerned because two siblings are very different as long as they both fit within usual parameters.

CASE STUDY QUESTIONS

7. John lived in many foster homes before he was adopted. His parents state that they find him cold and unloving. What developmental task was John unable to complete because of these frequent moves at such a young age? What actions could his new parents take to try to strengthen this developmental task at this point?
8. John's mother describes her 3-year-old twins as "totally different" from each other. One is shy, quiet and agreeable; the other is aggressive and persistent. What characteristic is she describing? Which child does she probably view as easier to care for? What anticipatory guidance could you give her to help her better understand these differences in her children?
9. Children who are hospitalised for long periods may fall behind in development. What specific measures could you take to promote developmental growth and encourage a sense of autonomy if John were a hospitalised 2-year-old?

Resources

For an extensive range of additional resources to enhance teaching and learning and to facilitate understanding of this chapter, please see the text's accompanying website located on thePoint at http://thepoint.lww.com.

References

Barton, A. L. & Kirtley, M. S. (2012). Gender differences in the relationships among parenting styles and college student mental health. *Journal of American College Health*, *60*(1), 21–26.

Carr-Gregg, M. (2014). *Strictly Parenting. Everything you Need to Know about Raising School-age Kids*. Penguin Australia.

Chess, S. & Thomas, A. (1995). *Temperament in Clinical Practice*. New York: Guilford Publications.

Dea, T. L. (2011). Pediatric obesity & type 2 diabetes. *MCN: American Journal of Maternal Child Nursing*, *36*(1), 42–48.

Erikson, E. H. (1993). *Childhood and Society*. New York: W. W. Norton.

Feigelman, S. (2012). Overview and assessment of variability. In R. M. Kliegman, B. F. Stanton, J. W. St Geme, N. Schor & R. E. Behrman (Eds.). (2011). *Nelson Textbook of Pediatrics: Expert Consult Premium Edition* (19th ed.) pp. 192–212. Philadelphia: Elsevier/Saunders.

Freud, S. (1962). *Three Essays on the Theory of Sexuality*. New York: Hearst Corporation.

Gilligan, C. (1993). *In a Different Voice: Psychological Theory and Women's Development*. Cambridge, MA: Harvard University Press.

Hampton, R. & Toombs, M. (Eds). (2013). *Indigenous Australians and Health: The Wombat in the Room*. Melbourne: Oxford University Press.

Hudson, J. L., Dodd, H. F., Lyneham, H. J., Bovopoulous, N. (2011). Temperament and family environment in the development of anxiety disorder: Two year follow-up. *Journal of the American Academy of Child & Adolescent Psychiatry*, *50*(12), 1255–1264.

International Working Group on Indigenous Affairs (IWGIA). (2006). *The Indigenous World 2006, ECOSOC Consultative Status*. Copenhagen: IWGIA.

Johnston, M., Landers, S., Noble, L., Szucs, K. & Viehmann, L. (2012). Breastfeeding and the use of human milk. *Pediatrics*, *129*(3), e827–e841.

Juujärvi, S., Pesso, K. & Myyry, L. (2011). Care-based ethical reasoning among first year nursing and social services students. *Journal of Advanced Nursing*, *67*(2), 418–427.

Kohlberg, L. (1984). *The Psychology of Moral Development*. New York: Harper & Row.

Matook, S. A., Sullivan, M. C., Salisbury, A., Miller, R. J. & Lester, B. M. (2010). Variations of NICU sound by location and time of day. *Neonatal Network*, *29*(2), 87–95.

Morgan, A. R. (2012). Determining genetic risk factors for pediatric type 2 diabetes. *Current Diabetes Reports*, *12*(1), 88–92.

Mulholland, E. K., Griffiths, U. K. & Biellik, R. (2012). Measles in the 21st century. *New England Journal of Medicine*, *366*(19), 1755–1757.

Newman, B. M. & Newman, P. R. (2011). Later adulthood. In B. M. Newman & P. R. Newman. *Development Through Life: A Psychosocial Approach*. (pp. 526–559). Belmont, CA: Cengage Learning.

Pastor, P. N. & Reuben, C. A. (2011). Emotional/behavioral difficulties and adolescent obesity: Effect of sex and Hispanic origin/race. *International Journal of Pediatric Obesity*, *6*(5–6), 462–466.

Piaget, J. (1958). *The Growth of Logical Thinking from Childhood to Adolescence*. New York: Basic Books.

Pike, K., Jane Pillow, J. & Lucas, J. S. (2012). Long term respiratory consequences of intrauterine growth restriction. *Seminars in Fetal & Neonatal Medicine*, *17*(2), 92–98.

Rossow, I. & Moan, I. S. (2012). Parental intoxication and adolescent suicidal behavior. *Archives of Suicide Research, 16*(1), 73–84.

Russell, S. T., Sinclair, K. O., Poteat, V. P., et al. (2012). Adolescent health and harassment based on discriminatory bias. *American Journal of Public Health, 102*(3), 493–495.

Sizer, F. & Whitney, E. (2014). The vitamins. In F. Sizer & E. Whitney (Eds.). *Nutrition: Concepts & Controversies* (13th ed.). Belmont, CA: Cengage Learning.

Vicedo, M. (2011). The social nature of the mother's tie to her child: John Bowlby's theory of attachment in post-war America. *British Journal for the History of Science, 44*(162, Pt 3), 401–426.

Wadsworth, B. J. (2003). *Piaget's Theory of Cognitive and Affective Development: Foundations of Constructivism* (5th ed.). New York: Longman.

Whitney, E. N. & Rolfes, S. R. (2012). Life cycle nutrition: Pregnancy and lactation. In *Understanding Nutrition*. Belmont, CA: Wadsworth Publishing. (pp. 492–527)

World Health Organization. (2006). Constitution of the World Health Organization, accessed 26 February 2015, <www.who.int/governance/eb/who_constitution_en.pdf>.

Suggested readings

Australian Dietary Guidelines, <www.eatforhealth.gov.au>.

Coren, E. & Barlow, J. (2009). Individual and group-based parenting programmes for improving psychosocial outcomes for teenage parents and their children. *Cochrane Database of Systematic Reviews*, (1), CD002964.

Demicheli, V., Rivetti, A., Debalini, M. G. & Di Pietrantonj, C. (2012). Vaccines for measles, mumps and rubella in children. *Cochrane Database of Systematic Reviews*, (1), CD004407.

Eat Well Australia: An Agenda for Action in Public Health Nutrition 2000–2010, available at <www.health.vic.gov.au/archive/archive2014/nphp>.

Krebs, N. F. & Primak, L. E. (2015). Pediatric nutrition and nutritional disorders. In K. J. Marcdante & R. M. Kleigman (Eds.). *Nelson Essentials of Pediatrics* (7th ed.). Philadelphia: Elsevier/Saunders. (pp. 103–122).

Kristjansson, E. A., Petticrew, M., MacDonald, B., Krasevec, J., Janzen, L., Greenhalgh, T., Wells, G. A., MacGowan, J., Farmer, A. P., Shea, B., Mayhew, A., Tugwell, P. & Welch, V. (2009). School feeding for improving the physical and psychosocial health of disadvantaged students. *Cochrane Database of Systematic Reviews*, (1), CD004676.

New Zealand Ministry of Health. *Food and Nutrition Guidelines*. Accessed 11 February 2015 <www.health.govt.nz/our-work/preventative-health-wellness/nutrition/food-and-nutrition-guidelines>.

Pak, L., &Allen, P. J. (2012). The impact of maternal depression on children with asthma. *Pediatric Nursing, 38*(1), 11–19.

Rolfes, S. R., Pinna, K. & Whitney, E. N. (2011). *Understanding Normal and Clinical Nutrition*. New York: Cengage Learning.

Ting, W. H., Huang, C. Y., Tu, Y. K. & Chien, K. L. (2012). Association between weight status and depressive symptoms in adolescents: Role of weight perception, weight concern, and dietary restraint. *European Journal of Pediatrics, 171*(8), 1247–1255.

Chapter 29

Nursing care of a family with an infant

Previous chapters described the newborn and the capabilities with which children are born. This chapter adds information about the dramatic changes, both physical and psychosocial, that occur during the first year. Such information can build a base for care and health teaching for the age group.

LEARNING OBJECTIVES

After studying the contents of this chapter, you should be able to:

1. Describe normal infant growth and development and associated parental concerns.
2. Assess an infant for normal growth and developmental milestones.
3. Formulate nursing considerations related to infant growth and development and associated parental concerns.
4. Plan nursing care to meet an infant's growth and developmental needs such as teaching parents to childproof their home.
5. Implement nursing care related to normal growth and development of an infant such as encouraging eye/hand coordination.
6. Integrate knowledge of infant growth and development with nursing process to achieve quality child and family health nursing care.

KEY TERMS

- baby-bottle syndrome
- binocular vision
- deciduous teeth
- eighth-month anxiety
- extrusion reflex
- hand regard
- natal teeth
- neck-righting reflex
- neonatal teeth
- object permanence
- pincer grasp
- seborrhoea
- social smile
- thumb opposition

CASE STUDY

You meet Anne Simpson, 19, at a paediatric clinic when she brings in her 2-month-old son, Kai. She looks tired. She tells you she is exhausted because her baby is "awake all night, crying constantly". She stopped breastfeeding and changed him to formula to see if that would help. It didn't. She tells you his bowel movements are normal. When you weigh Kai, you find he has gained weight well. When you talk to him, he demonstrates a social smile.

CASE STUDY QUESTION

1. What areas are important for the nurse to discuss with Anne at her first interview and assessment of her baby?

Traditionally, infancy is designated as the period of time from 1 month to 1 year of age. In these important months, an infant undergoes such rapid development that parents sometimes believe their baby looks different and demonstrates new abilities every day. During this time, an infant triples their birth weight and increases their length by 50%. Infant's reflexes develop and senses sharpen and, with the process of attachment to primary carers, they form a first social relationship. Because of the growth and learning potential that occurs, this first year is a crucial one. Without proper nutrition a baby will not grow and physically thrive and without proper stimulation and nurturing care by consistent carers an infant may not develop a healthy interest in life or a feeling of security essential for future development.

Although infant healthcare visits are scheduled less frequently than formerly, a standard schedule is for 2-week, 2-month, 4-month, 6-month and 12-month visits. These visits are as important for the parents as they are for an infant because they provide an opportunity for parents to ask questions about their child's growth pattern and developmental progress. They also provide opportunities for healthcare providers to assess for potential problems.

HEALTHY DEVELOPMENT OF AN INFANT

Assessment

Nursing assessment of an infant begins with an interview with the primary carer. Important areas to discuss include nutrition, growth patterns and development. An infant's height, weight and head circumference are important indicators of growth, so they should be measured and plotted on standard growth charts (Parsons et al., 2011). These charts represent average growth and can determine if the baby's growth remains within the same relative percentile at each check-up.

Physical assessment of an infant must be done quickly yet thoroughly because a baby can tire or become hungry, making it difficult to judge overall behaviour and temperament.

The primary carer should be present to make a child feel comfortable. Using a calm approach helps the infant remain calm as well.

Nursing considerations

Much of your assessment of an infant and family will focus on basic needs such as sleep, nutrition and activity and the parents' adjustment to their new role. Examples of nursing considerations are:

- Ineffective breastfeeding related to maternal fatigue
- Disturbed sleep pattern (maternal) related to baby's need to nurse every 2 hours
- Deficient knowledge related to normal infant growth and development
- Imbalanced nutrition, less than body requirements, related to infant's difficulty sucking
- Health-seeking behaviours related to adjusting to parenthood
- Delayed growth and development related to lack of stimulating environment
- Risk for impaired parenting related to long hospitalisation of infant
- Readiness for enhanced family coping related to increased financial pressure
- Social isolation (maternal) related to lack of adequate social support
- Ineffective role performance related to new responsibilities within the family.

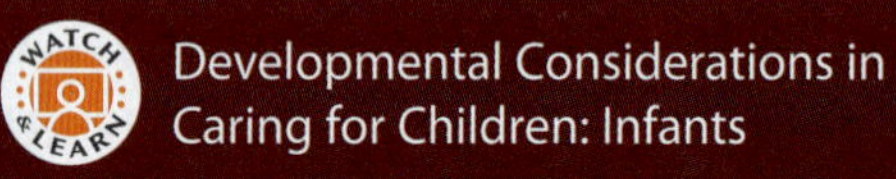

Developmental Considerations in Caring for Children: Infants

GROWTH AND DEVELOPMENT OF AN INFANT

Infants grow rapidly both in size and in their ability to perform tasks. Although development follows set patterns, some of it is dependent on cultural factors. One difference is in the way mothers carry their infants. Many mothers tend to carry infants in their arms, while other women carry their infant in a shoulder sling or on their hip or even in a forward-facing harness, positions that allow a woman to continue to work or walk while holding an infant close.

The amount of infant bathing that is done is also inconsistent across cultures. In colder climates or countries where clean water is not readily available, infant bathing is more limited. The use of nappies varies also. In hot climate countries, infants are often not made to wear a nappy. In Australia, both cloth and disposable nappies are used singularly and together. Being aware of these cultural differences leads to better understanding of the reasons for an individual woman's particular method of childrearing (Families NSW, 2015).

An excellent resource for nurses when doing assessments is the Victorian Government Department of Education and Early Childhood Development Maternal and Child Health Service (MCHS) <www.education.vic.gov.au/childhood/professionals/health/Pages/maternalchildhealth.aspx>. This website contains several fact sheets and booklets and assessments relating to 0–5 years of age.

When performing assessments and using guidelines and other documents provided by the MCHS it is important to be mindful that these are guidelines only and that cultural adaptations have not been taken into consideration. These may include things such as: height, weight and age of milestones. If referral to a paediatrician is required, a clear picture of clinical signs of concern and in-depth history are valuable tools.

Physical growth

The physiological changes that occur in the infant years reflect both increasing maturity and the growth of body organs. The following sections will discuss the changes that are typically seen in the first year of life.

Weight

Infants will lose weight initially after birth and are expected to regain this weight within 2–3 weeks. As a rule, most infants double their birth weight by 6 months of age and triple it by 1 year. During the first 6 months, infants typically average a weight gain of 1.2 kg per month. During the second 6 months, weight gain is approximately 600 g per month. The average 1-year-old boy weighs 10 kg; the average girl weighs 9.5 kg. An infant's weight, however, is relevant only when plotted on a standard growth chart and compared to that child's own growth curve (see Appendix B). Measure an infant's weight on an appropriately-sized beam scale with non-detectable weights. Weigh an infant naked and lying or sitting on a scale that measures to the nearest 10 g (see Fig. 29.1). Plot the weight measurement on an age- and gender-appropriate growth chart.

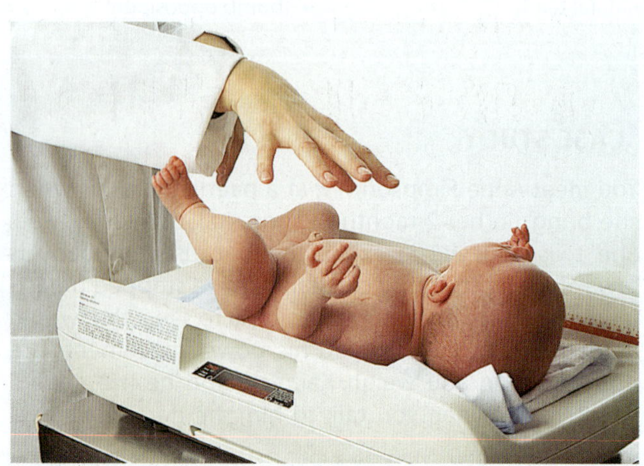

FIGURE 29.1 Weighing an infant. (© B. Proud)

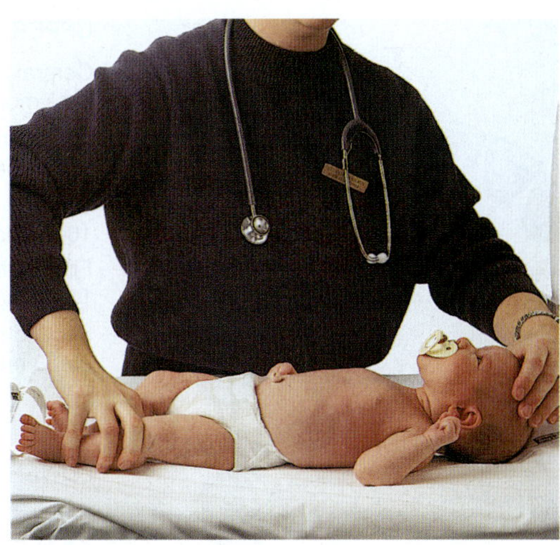

FIGURE 29.2 Positioning for measuring an infant's height.

Height

An infant increases in height during the first year by 50% or grows from an average birth length of 50.8 to 76.2 cm. Height, like weight, is best assessed if it is plotted on a standard growth chart. Determine height by measuring the recumbent length. Fully extend the body, holding the head in midline and gently grasping the knees and pushing them downwards until the legs are fully extended and touching the table. Using a measuring board, place the head at the top of the board and the heels firmly at the bottom, then measure the distance between the two points (see Fig. 29.2). Plot the height measurement on an age- and gender-appropriate growth chart.

Infant growth is most apparent in the trunk during the early months. During the second half of the first year, it becomes more apparent as lengthening of the legs. At the end of the first year, the child's legs may still appear disproportionately short and bowed.

Head circumference

By the end of the first year, the brain has already reached two-thirds of its adult size. Head circumference increases rapidly during the infant period to reflect that rapid brain growth. Measure head circumference (HC) or occipital frontal circumference (OFC) at every physical examination for infants and toddlers younger than 2 years and older children when conditions warrant (see Fig. 29.3). Plot the measurement on standardised growth charts specific for gender from birth to 36 months.

Some infants' heads appear asymmetrical until the second half of the first year. This may occur from always being placed in one sleeping position, causing the skull bones to flatten on that side. Suggest to parents that they place the infant on the back to sleep and prone when playing, to prevent this. This early head distortion gradually corrects itself as the child sleeps less and spends more time with the head in an erect position. Persistence of asymmetry may suggest that an infant is not receiving enough stimulation or is spending the majority of time lying in bed.

Body proportion

Body proportion changes during the first year from that of a newborn to a more typical infant appearance. The mandible becomes more prominent as bone grows. By the end of the infant period, the lower jaw is prominent and remains that way throughout life. The circumference of the chest is generally less than that of the head at birth by about 2 cm. It is even with the head circumference in some infants as early as 6 months and in most by 12 months. The abdomen remains protuberant until the child has been walking well for some time, generally well into the toddler period. Cervical, thoracic and lumbar vertebral curves develop as infants hold up their head, sit and walk. Lengthening of the lower extremities during the last 6 months of infancy readies the child for walking and often changes the appearance from "baby-like" to "toddler-like".

Body systems

In the cardiovascular system, heart rate slows from 120–160 bpm to 100–120 bpm by the end of the first year. The heart continues to occupy a little over half the width of the chest. Pulse rate may begin to slow with inhalation (sinus arrhythmia), but this does not become marked until preschool age. The respiratory rate of an infant slows from 30 to 60 breaths per minute to 20 to 30 breaths per minute by the end of the first year. Because the lumen (tubal cavity) of the respiratory tract remains small and mucus production by the tract to clear invading microorganisms is still inefficient, upper respiratory infections occur readily and tend to be more severe than in adults.

At birth, the gastrointestinal tract is immature in its ability to digest food and mechanically move it along. These functions mature gradually during the infant year. The liver

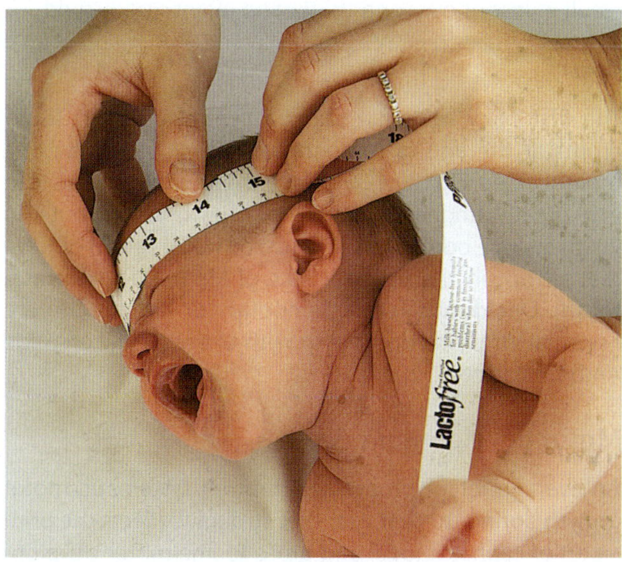

FIGURE 29.3 Measuring head circumference. (© B. Proud)

of an infant remains immature, possibly causing inadequate conjugation of medications (if a medicine is necessary for treatment of illness) and inefficient formation of carbohydrate, protein and vitamins for storage. Until the age of 3 or 4 months, an **extrusion reflex** (food placed on an infant's tongue is thrust forwards and out of the mouth) prevents some infants from eating effectively.

The kidneys remain immature and not as efficient at eliminating body wastes as in an adult. The infant is also unable to concentrate urine as much as an adult, which causes them to be more prone to dehydration. The endocrine system remains particularly immature in response to pituitary stimulation, such as adrenocorticotropic hormone or insulin production from the pancreas. Without these hormones functioning effectively, an infant may not be able to respond to stress effectively.

An infant's immune system becomes functional by at least 2 months of age; an infant can actively produce both IgG and IgM antibodies by 1 year. The levels of other immunoglobulins (IgA, IgE and IgD) are not plentiful until preschool age, which is the reason infants continue to need protection from infection (Goldson & Reynolds, 2014).

The ability to adjust to cold is mature by the age of 6 months. By this age, an infant can shiver in response to cold (which increases muscle activity and provides warmth) and has developed additional adipose tissue to serve as insulation. The amount of brown fat, which protected the newborn from cold, decreases during the first year.

Although the fluid in body compartments shifts to some extent, extracellular fluid accounts for approximately 35% of an infant's body weight, with intracellular fluid accounting for approximately 40% by the end of the first year, by contrast with adult proportions of 20% and 40%, respectively. This proportional difference increases an infant's susceptibility to dehydration from illnesses such as diarrhoea, because loss of extracellular fluid could result in loss of over one-third of an infant's body fluid.

Teeth

The first baby tooth (typically a central incisor) usually erupts at the age of 6 months, followed by a new one monthly (see Fig. 29.4). However, teething patterns can vary greatly among children. Some newborns (about 1 in 2000) may be born with teeth (called **natal teeth**) or have teeth erupt in the first 4 weeks of life (called **neonatal teeth**). **Deciduous teeth** (temporary or baby teeth) are essential for protecting the growth of the dental arch (de Amorim Lde et al., 2011).

Motor development

An average infant progresses through systematic motor growth during the first year that strongly reflects the principles of cephalocaudal and gross to fine motor development. Control proceeds from head to trunk to lower extremities in a progressive, predictable sequence. Different infants show individual variations in accomplishing different tasks; the ages given here are averages.

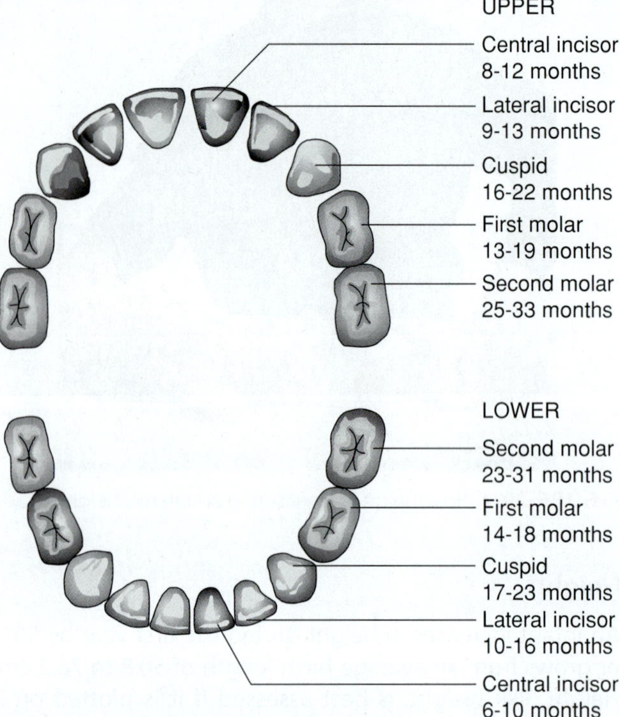

FIGURE 29.4 Eruption pattern of deciduous teeth.

Gross motor development

To assess gross motor development, an infant is observed in four positions: ventral suspension, prone, sitting and standing.

Ventral suspension position

Ventral suspension refers to an infant's appearance when held in mid-air on a horizontal plane, supported by a hand under the abdomen (see Fig. 29.5A). In this position, the newborn allows the head to hang down with little effort at control. A 1-month-old child lifts the head momentarily, then drops it again. Two-month-old children hold their heads in the same plane as the rest of their body, a major advance in muscle control. A 3-month-old child lifts and maintains the head well above the plane of the rest of the body in ventral suspension.

A *Landau reflex* develops at 3 months. When held in ventral suspension, an infant's head, legs and spine extend. When the head is depressed, the hips, knees and elbows flex. This reflex continues to be present in most infants during the second 6 months of life, but then it becomes increasingly difficult to demonstrate. A child with motor weakness, cerebral palsy or other neuromuscular defect will not be able to demonstrate the reflex.

At 6 to 9 months, an infant also demonstrates a *parachute reaction* from a ventral suspension position. When infants are suddenly lowered towards an examination

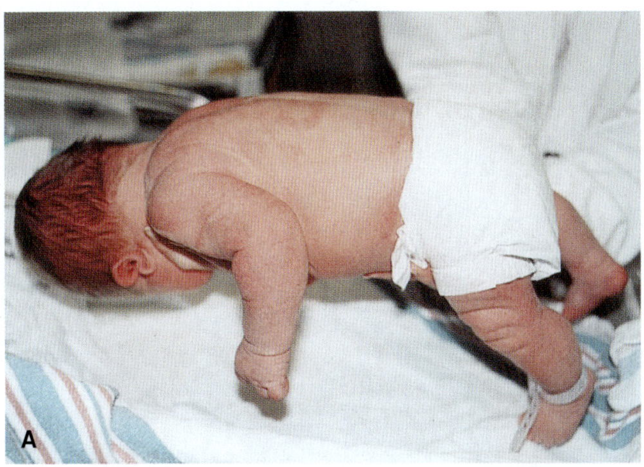

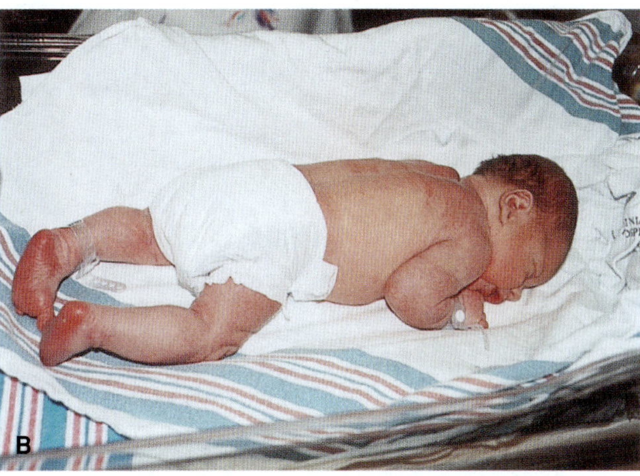

FIGURE 29.5 (**A**) Ventral suspension position. (**B**) Prone position.

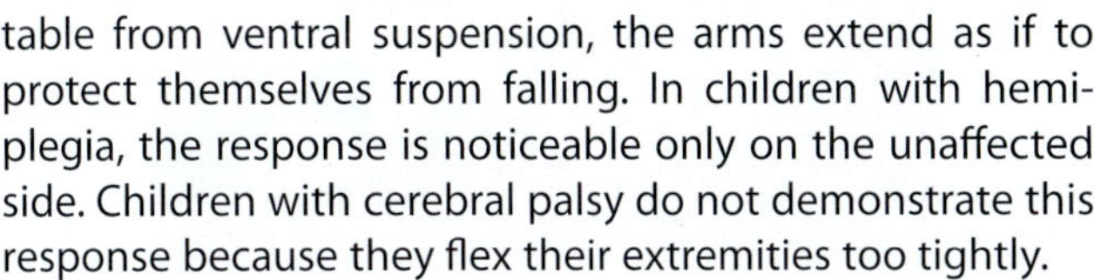

table from ventral suspension, the arms extend as if to protect themselves from falling. In children with hemiplegia, the response is noticeable only on the unaffected side. Children with cerebral palsy do not demonstrate this response because they flex their extremities too tightly.

Prone position

When lying on their stomach, newborns can turn their heads to move them out of a position where breathing is impaired, but they cannot hold them raised (see Fig. 29.5B). By 1 month of age, infants lift their heads and turn them easily to the side. They still tend to keep their knees tucked under the abdomen as they did as a newborn. Two-month-old infants can raise their heads and maintain the position, but they cannot yet raise their chests high enough to look around. Their head is still held facing downwards.

A 3-month-old child lifts the head and shoulders well off the table and looks around when prone (see Fig. 29.6). The pelvis is flat on the table, no longer elevated. Some children can turn from a prone to a side-lying position at this age.

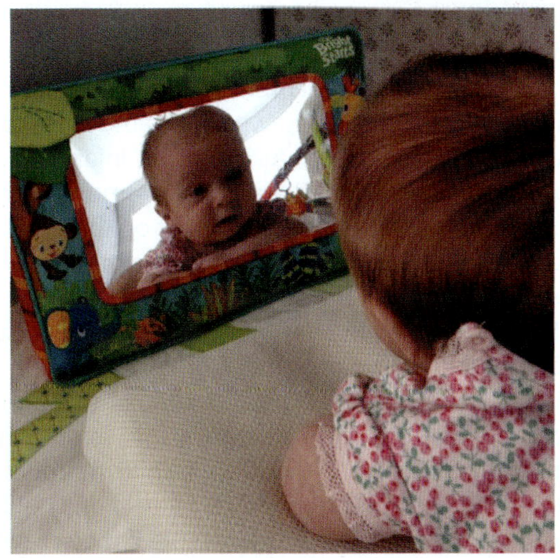

FIGURE 29.6 This 3-month-old can lift her head and shoulders well and is very interested in the world around her. (© Lauren Kidziak.)

Four-month-old children lift their chests off the bed and look around actively, turning their heads from side to side. They can turn from front to back. The first time, this tends to occur as an extension of lifting the chest combined with a **neck-righting reflex**, which begins at this age. When an infant turns the head to the side, the shoulders, trunk and pelvis turn in that direction, too. This reflex causes babies to lose their balance and roll sideways when lifting the head up. The baby is frightened by the sudden feeling of rolling free and probably cries. After this happens a few more times, however, a baby begins to delight in this new accomplishment. Most babies turn from front to back first and then, 1 month later, from back to front.

Five-month-old children rest weight on their forearms when prone. They can turn completely over, from front to back and from back to front. At 6 months, infants rest their weight on their hands with extended arms. They can raise their chests and the upper part of their abdomens off the table.

By 9 months, a child can crawl from the prone position. Crawling is a new skill, advanced from hitching (in which infants slide along the floor) that they may have been doing. Crawling means the child has the abdomen off the floor and moves one hand and one leg and then the other hand and leg, using the knees on the floor to locomote (see Fig. 29.7).

Sitting position

When placed on the back and then pulled to a sitting position, a 1-month-old child has gross head lag as in the first days of life. In a sitting position, the back appears rounded and an infant demonstrates only momentary head control. Two-month-olds can hold their head fairly steady when sitting up, although it does tend to bob forwards. An infant at this age still has head lag when pulled to a sitting position.

A 3-month-old child has only slight head lag when pulled to a sitting position. A 4-month-old child reaches an important milestone by no longer demonstrating head lag when pulled to a sitting position. A 5-month-old infant

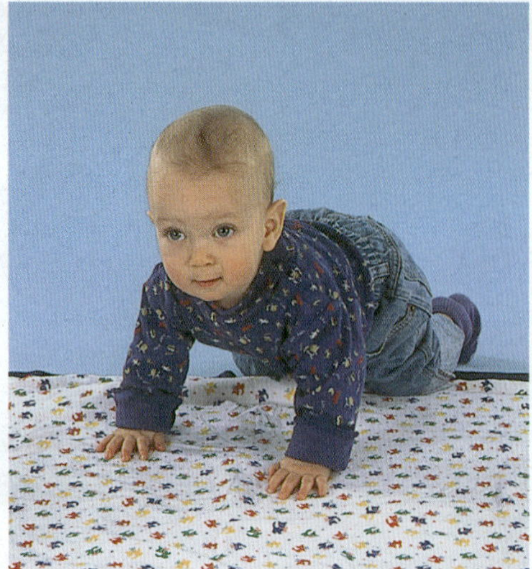

FIGURE 29.7 Crawling. The older infant moves forwards, carrying his torso above and parallel to the floor.

can be seen to straighten the back when held or propped in a sitting position. By 6 months, children sit momentarily without support. They anticipate being picked up and reach up with their hands from this position. Some parents expect a child of this age to sit securely and are worried because their sitting posture is still extremely shaky. However, it is more common for a 6-month-old child to have only a limited ability to sit independently (see Fig. 29.8). Six-month-old children often sit with their legs spread and their arms stiffened between them, hands on the floor, as a prop. Infants are capable of movement by hitching or sliding backwards from this position. Alert parents that an infant this young is capable of moving from one spot to another in this way, so they are prepared for this and can prevent accidents.

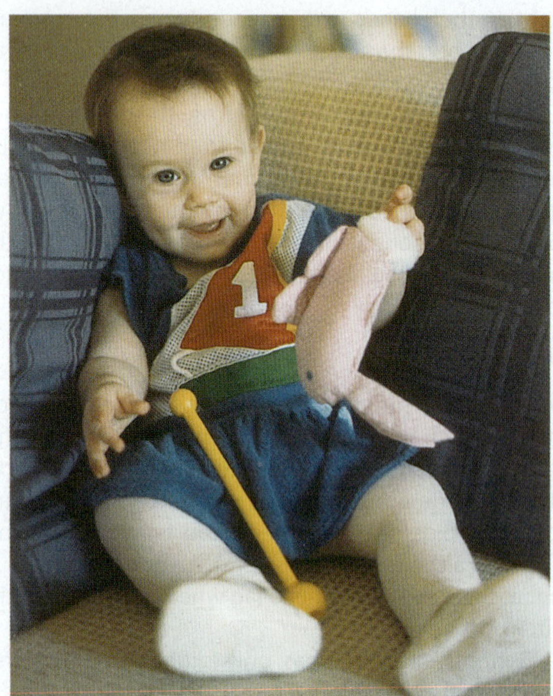

FIGURE 29.8 A 6-month-old infant sitting. Notice how she is propped with pillows to maintain the position.

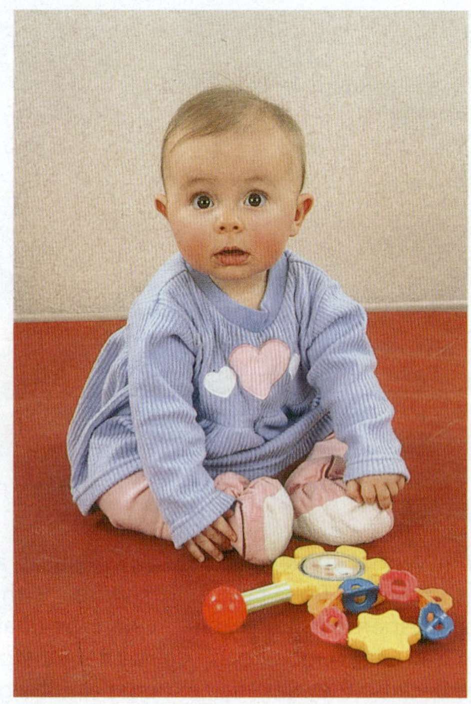

FIGURE 29.9 At 8 months an infant sits independently.

A 7-month-old child sits alone, but only when the hands are held forwards for balance. An 8-month-old child can sit securely without any additional support (see Fig. 29.9). This is a major milestone in development that should always be considered in assessment. Children with delayed cognitive or motor development may not accomplish this step at this time. At 9 months, infants sit so steadily that they can lean forwards and regain their balance. They may still lose their balance if they lean sideways, a skill not achieved for another month.

Standing position

A newborn stepping reflex can still be demonstrated at 1 month of age. In a standing position, an infant's knees and hips flex rather than support more than momentary weight. Two-month-old children, when held in a standing position, hold their heads up with the same show of support as in a sitting position. At 3 months, infants begin to try to support part of their weight. At 4 months, infants begin to be able to support their weight on their legs. They are successful at doing this because the stepping reflex has faded.

A 5-month-old child continues the ability to sustain a portion of weight. The tonic neck reflex should be extinguished and the Moro (startle) reflex is fading. By 6 months, infants support nearly their full weight when in a standing position. A 7-month-old child bounces with enjoyment in a standing position. Nine-month-old children can stand holding onto a low table if they are placed in that position. Some 9-month-old children can pull up to that position. Ten-month-old children can pull themselves

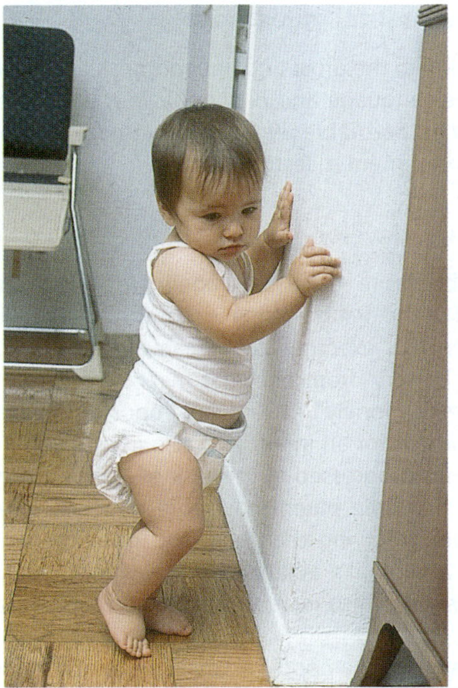

FIGURE 29.10 An 11-month-old child cruising along the walls. Further childproofing of the house will be necessary to keep her safe. (From Photo Researchers, Inc.)

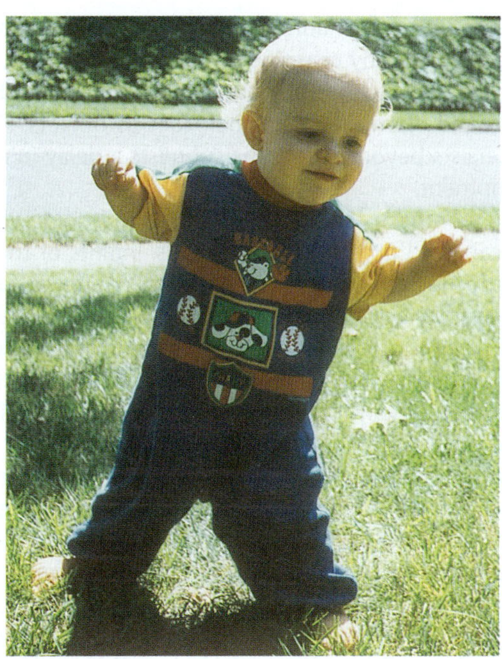

FIGURE 29.11 There is a wide variation in the age at which children take a first step, typically ranging from 8 to 15 months. Here a child has mastered walking by 1 year.

to a standing position by holding onto the side of a playpen or a low table, but they cannot let themselves down again as yet.

At around 11 months, a child learns to "cruise" or move about the cot or room by holding onto objects such as cot rails, chairs, walls and low tables (see Fig. 29.10). At 12 months, children stand alone at least momentarily. Some parents expect children to walk at this age and are disappointed to see they are merely standing. A child has until about 22 months of age to walk and still be within the normal limit, however (see Fig. 29.11).

CASE STUDY QUESTION

2. Kai is 2 months old. At what age would you expect him to sit securely?

   a. 2½ months
   b. 6 months
   c. 8 months
   d. 12 months

Fine motor development

One-month-old infants still have a strong grasp reflex and they hold their hands in fists so tightly it is difficult to extend the fingers. As the grasp reflex begins to fade, a 2-month-old child will hold an object for a few minutes before dropping it. The hands are held open, not closed in fists.

At 3 months, infants reach for attractive objects in front of them. Their grasp is unpractised, however, so they usually miss them. Assure parents this is part of normal development. Otherwise, they may think their child is nearsighted or farsighted or has poor coordination.

By 4 months, infants bring their hands together and pull at their clothes. They will shake a rattle placed in their hand. **Thumb opposition** (ability to bring the thumb and fingers together) is beginning, but the motion is a scooping or raking one, not a picking-up one, and is not very accurate. An infant is limited to handling large objects (see Fig. 29.12). Palmar and plantar grasp reflexes have disappeared.

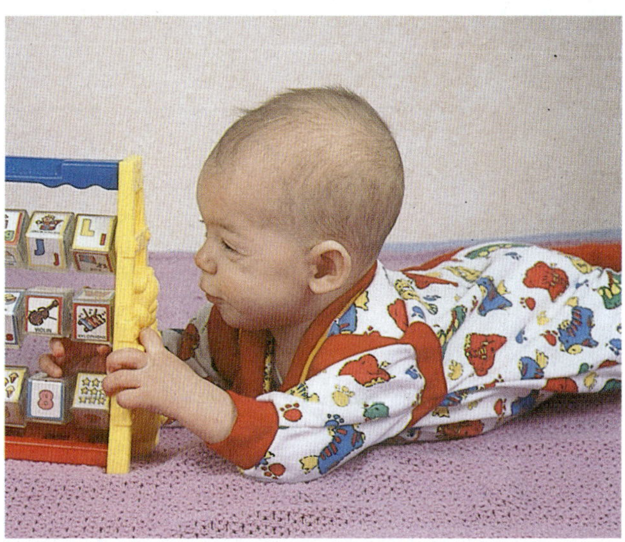

FIGURE 29.12 By the age of 4 months, an infant is able to manipulate large objects.

Five-month-old children can accept objects that are handed to them by grasping with the whole hand. They can reach and pick up objects without the object being offered and often play with their toes as objects. Fisting that persists beyond 5 months suggests a delay in motor development.

By 6 months, grasping has advanced to a point where a child can hold objects in both hands. Infants of this age will drop one toy when a second one is offered for the same hand. They can hold a spoon and start to feed themselves (with much spilling). Moro, palmar grasp and the tonic neck reflex have completely faded. A Moro reflex that persists beyond this point should arouse suspicion of neurological disease.

Seven-month-old children can transfer toys from one hand to the other. They hold a first object when a second one is offered. By 8 months, random reaching and ineffective grasping have disappeared as a result of advanced eye-hand coordination.

A major milestone of 10 months is the ability to bring the thumb and first finger together in a **pincer grasp** (see Fig. 29.13). This enables children to pick up small objects such as crumbs or pieces of cereal from a highchair tray. They use one finger to point to objects. They offer toys to people but then cannot release them.

At 12 months, infants can draw a semi-straight line with a crayon. They enjoy putting objects such as small blocks in containers and taking them out again. They can hold a cup and spoon to feed themselves fairly well (if they have been allowed to practise) and can take off socks and push their hands into sleeves (again, if they have been allowed to practise). They can offer toys and release them.

What if...

Kai learns to pick up very small articles such as marbles by 10 months? How would being able to do this affect his safety?

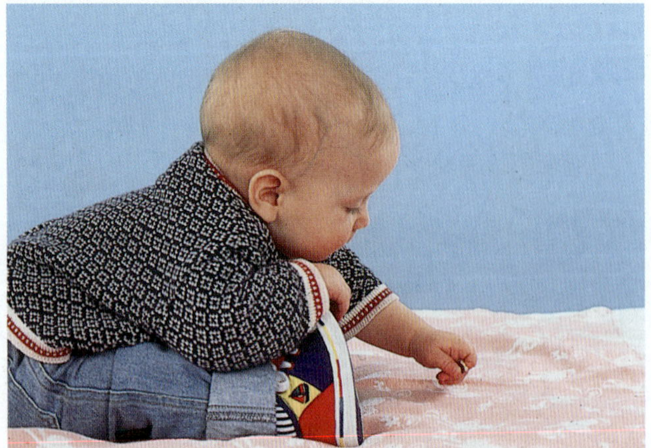

FIGURE 29.13 An infant almost ready to demonstrate a pincer grasp.

Developmental milestones

In addition to the gross and fine motor skills developing at this time, language and play behaviour also reach major milestones. See Table 29.1 for a summary of the growth and development milestones.

Language development

A child begins to make small, cooing (dovelike) sounds by the end of the first month. A 2-month-old child differentiates a cry. For example, carers can distinguish a cry that means "hungry" from one that means "wet" or from one that means "lonely". This is an important milestone in development for an infant and also in marking how far a parent has progressed in the task of learning the infant's cues. A first-time parent has more difficulty making the distinction in crying than one who has experienced this before. An infant's ability to make throaty, gurgling or cooing sounds also increases at this time (Mesman et al., 2012).

In response to a nodding, smiling face or a friendly tone of voice, a 3-month-old child will squeal with pleasure. This is an important step in development because it makes a baby even more fun to be with. Parents spend increased time with infants at this age, not just to care for them but because they enjoy their company. By 4 months, infants are very "talkative", cooing, babbling and gurgling when spoken to. They definitely laugh out loud. By 5 months, an infant says some simple vowel sounds (for example, "goo-goo" and "gah-gah"). At 6 months, infants learn the art of imitating. They may imitate a parent's cough, for example, or say "Oh!" as a way of attracting attention.

The amount of talking infants do increases at 7 months. They can imitate vowel sounds well (for example, "oh-oh", "ah-ah" and "oo-oo"). By 9 months, an infant usually speaks a first word: "da-da" or "ba-ba". Occasionally a mother may need reassurance that "da-da" for daddy is an easier syllable to pronounce than "ma-ma" for mummy. German mothers report the first word their babies say is "here", as that is "da" in German. By 10 months, an infant masters another word such as "bye-bye" or "no". By 12 months, infants can generally say two words besides "ma-ma" and "da-da"; they use those two words with meaning.

Play

Parents often ask what toys their infant would enjoy. Because 1-month-olds can fix their eyes on an object, they are interested in watching a mobile hung over their cot or playpen. Mobiles are best if they are black and white or brightly coloured and light enough in weight so they move when someone walks past. They should face down towards the infant, not towards an adult standing beside the cot. Musical mobiles provide extra stimulation. One-month-old children also spend a great deal of time watching their parent's face, appearing to enjoy this activity so much a face may become their favourite "toy". Help

TABLE 29.1 Summary of infant growth and developmental milestones

Month	Motor development	Fine motor development	Socialization and language	Time reflexes fade	Play
0–1	Largely reflex actions	Keeps hands fisted; able to follow object to midline with eyes			Enjoys watching face of primary carer; needs play time in prone position
2	Holds head up when prone	Demonstrates social smile	Makes cooing sounds; differentiates cry	Grasp reflex fading	Enjoys bright-colored mobiles
3	Holds head and chest up when prone	Follows object past midline with eyes	Laughs out loud	Landau reflex is strong	Spends time looking at hands (hand regard); "tummy time" important during the day
4	Turns back to front; no longer has head lag; bears partial weight on feet			Stepping, tonic neck, extrusion reflexes are fading	Needs space to practise turning
5	Should turn readily front to back and back to front			Tonic neck reflex fading	Handles rattles well
6	Beginning to show ability to sit	Uses palmar grasp	May say vowel sounds (*oh-oh*)	Moro & tonic neck reflex have faded	Enjoys bathtub toys, rubber ring for teething
7	Reaches out to be picked up; first tooth (central incisor) erupts	Transfers objects hand to hand	Shows beginning fear of strangers		Likes objects that are good size for transferring
8	Sits securely without support		Fear of strangers peaks		Enjoys manipulation, rattles, and toys of different textures
9	Creeps or crawls (abdomen off floor)		Says first word (*da-da*)		Needs safe space for creeping
10	Pulls self to standing	Uses pincer grasp (thumb and finger) to pick up small objects			Plays games like patty-cake and peek-a-boo
11	"Cruises" (walks with support)				"Cruising" can be main activity
12	Stands alone; some infants take first step	Holds cup and spoon well; helps to dress (pushes arm into sleeve)	Says two words plus *ma-ma* and *da-da*	Landau reflex fades	Likes toys that fit inside each other (pots and pans); nursery rhymes; will like pull toys as soon as walking

parents to understand that they are not spoiling infants by sitting and holding them for long periods of time in their early months. Parents will enjoy recalling such calm moments later, when they are stacking blocks, winding up toys or playing board games with their growing child.

Hearing is a second sense that is a source of pleasure for children in early infancy. Even newborns "listen" to the sound of a music box or a musical rattle. They stir and seem apprehensive at the sound of a raucous rattle. Two-month-old infants will hold light, small rattles for a short period of time but then drop them. They are very attuned to mobiles or cradle gyms strung across their cot. They continue to spend a great deal of time just watching the people around them.

Three-month-old children can handle small blocks or small rattles. Four-month-old children need a playpen or a sheet spread on the floor so they have an opportunity to exercise their new skill of rolling over. Rolling over is so intriguing it may serve as a "toy" for the entire month.

Five-month-old infants are ready for a variety of objects to handle, such as plastic rings, blocks, squeeze toys, rattles and plastic keys. All these should be small enough so an infant can lift them with one hand, yet big enough so the baby cannot possibly swallow them. A 6-month-old child can sit steadily enough to be ready for bath toys such as rubber ducks or plastic boats. Because they are starting to teethe, infants enjoy a teething ring to chew on at this time.

Because 7-month-old children can transfer toys, they are interested in items such as blocks, rattles or plastic keys that are small enough to be used for this. As their mobility increases, they begin to be more interested in brightly coloured balls or toys that previously rolled out of reach. Eight-month-old children are sensitive to differences in texture. They enjoy having toys that have different feels to them, such as velvet, fur, fuzzy, smooth or rough items.

The 9-month-old infant needs the experience of crawling. This means time out of a cot or playpen so there is room to manoeuvre. Many 9-month-olds begin to enjoy toys that go inside one another, such as a nest of blocks or rings of assorted sizes that fit on a centre post. Some are more interested in pots and pans that stack rather than toys.

By 10 months, infants are ready for peek-a-boo and will spend a long time playing the game with their hands or with a cloth over their head that they can reach and remove. They can clap and are also ready to play patty-cake. These games have a positive value, just as laughing out loud did for the 3-month-old child. They make a baby feel like an active part of the household. A family feeling begins to grow as the baby can participate in active games. At 11 months, children have learned to cruise or walk along low tables by holding on. They often find this so absorbing they spend little time doing anything else during the month.

Twelve-month-old infants enjoy putting things into and taking things out of containers. They like little boxes that fit inside one another or dropping small blocks into a cardboard box. As soon as they can walk, they will be interested in pulltoys. A lot of time may be spent listening to someone saying nursery rhymes or listening to music.

✔ Checkpoint question 29.1

How many words does a typical 12-month-old infant use?

a. Two, plus "ma-ma" and "da-da"
b. About 12 words
c. Twenty or more words
d. About 50 words

Development of senses

Like other facets of development, maturation of the senses proceeds step-by-step during the infant year.

Vision

One-month-old infants regard an object in the midline of their vision (something directly in front) as soon as it is brought in as close as about 46 cm. They follow it a short distance, but not across the midline as yet. They study or regard a human face with a fixed stare. Two-month-old infants focus well (from about age 6 weeks) and follow objects with the eyes (although still not past the midline). Ability to follow and focus in this way is a major milestone in development, indicating an infant has achieved **binocular vision**, or the ability to fuse two images into one (see Fig. 29.14). Teach parents to make a point of initiating eye-to-eye contact with newborns right from the beginning as a method of stimulating vision as well as promoting socialisation.

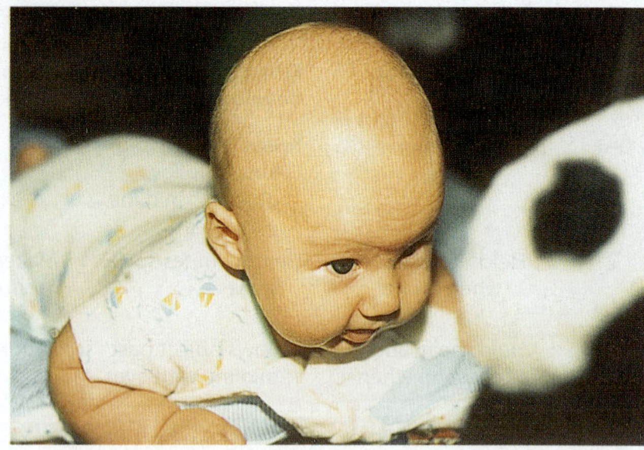

FIGURE 29.14 A 2-month-old infant focuses steadily and lifts her head up while prone. Note her interest in the stuffed bear.

Three-month-old infants can follow an object across their midline. They typically hold their hands in front of their face and study their fingers for long periods of time (**hand regard**). Blind children also demonstrate this phenomenon, however, so it may not be so much a test of vision as of cognitive or exploratory development. Up until 6 months of age, infants may experience difficulty in establishing eye coordination. After 3 months, however, an infant whose eyes still "cross" should be examined by a doctor.

Four-month-old infants recognise familiar objects, such as a frequently-seen bottle, rattle or toy animal. They follow their parents' movements with their eyes eagerly. At 6 months, infants are capable of organised depth perception. This increases the accuracy of their reach for objects as they begin to perceive distances accurately.

Seven-month-old children pat their image in a mirror. Their depth perception has matured to the extent that they can perform such tasks as transferring toys from hand to hand. By 10 months, an infant looks under a towel or around a corner for a concealed object (beginning of object permanence).

Most parents are aware that infants enjoy mobiles and a cot mirror (see Fig. 29.15). Occasionally they supply so many of these they can overdo the amount of visual stimulation, overwhelming their infant with too many patterns and objects dangling above the cot. Ask parents to consider how all these trappings must appear from an infant's view.

In a hospital environment, assess that an infant is receiving visual stimulation. Add or reduce objects as appropriate. If a child's movement is restricted in any way, move the position of the mobile from time to time. Photographs of family members brought from home or pictures drawn by older brothers or sisters can be posted near an infant's cot. Ask the parents if there are any items from home an infant would normally see during the course of the day while being fed, changed or bathed. It may be possible to bring those items into the hospital for visual stimulation.

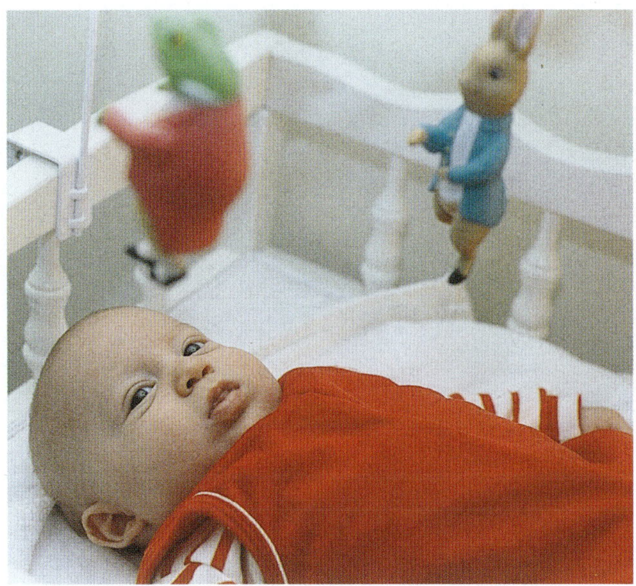

FIGURE 29.15 A 2-month-old infant enjoys watching a simple mobile.

Hearing

Hearing is demonstrated by the 1-month-old child who settles momentarily at a distinctive sound such as a bell or a squeaky rubber toy. Hearing awareness becomes so acute by 2 months of age that infants will stop an activity at the sound of spoken words. Many 3-month-old infants turn their heads in an attempt to locate a sound. At 4 months of age, when infants hear a distinctive sound, they turn and look in that direction.

By 5 months of age, infants demonstrate that they can localise sounds downwards and to the side, by turning their head and looking down. Six-month-olds have progressed to being able to locate sounds made above them. By 10 months, infants can recognise their name and listen acutely when spoken to. By 12 months, infants can easily locate sound in any direction and turn towards it. A vocabulary of two words plus "ma-ma" and "da-da" also demonstrates that an infant can hear.

Infants appear to enjoy soft, musical sounds or soft, cooing voices; they are startled by harsh, raucous rattles or loud bangs. Urge parents to choose for an infant's first toys ones that make these types of welcoming sounds. Tape-recordings of maternal heart sounds can be soothing to very young infants. For the hospitalised infant, a recording of family voices might be a soothing reminder of their existence. Encourage parents to read to their child daily from the beginning of life through the early school-age years, not only because the sound of the parent's voice is comforting but also because this increases language development dramatically.

Touch

An infant needs to be touched to experience skin-to-skin contact. Clothes should feel comfortable and soft rather than rough; nappies should be dry rather than wet. Teach parents to handle infants with assurance and gentleness. Because premature infants need to be kept warm while being held, parents are often advised to cuddle an infant next to their bare chest ("skin-to-skin contact"). This is also effective with term infants as a way of promoting close physical contact.

Taste

Infants demonstrate that they have an acute sense of taste by turning away from or spitting out a taste they do not enjoy. Urge parents to make mealtime a time for fostering trust as well as supplying nutrition by being certain feedings are done at an infant's pace and the amount offered fits the child's needs and not the parent's idea of how much should be eaten.

Smell

Infants can smell accurately within 1 or 2 hours of birth. They respond to an irritating smell by drawing back from it. They appear to enjoy pleasant odours and learn early in life to identify the familiar smell of breast milk. Teach parents to be alert to substances that cause sneezing when sprayed into the air, such as room deodorisers or cleaning compounds, and to keep irritating odours out of the child's environment.

Emotional development

Socialisation, or learning how to interact with others, is an extensive phenomenon. One-month-old infants show they can differentiate between faces and other objects by studying a face or the picture of a face longer than other objects. They settle best and eat best for the person who has been their primary carer.

When an interested person nods and smiles at a 6-week-old infant, the infant smiles in return. This is a **social smile** and is a definite response to the interaction, not the faint, quick "smile" that younger infants, even newborns, demonstrate. By 3 months, infants demonstrate increased social awareness by readily smiling at the sight of a parent's face (see Fig. 29.16). Three-month-old infants laugh out loud at the sight of a funny face.

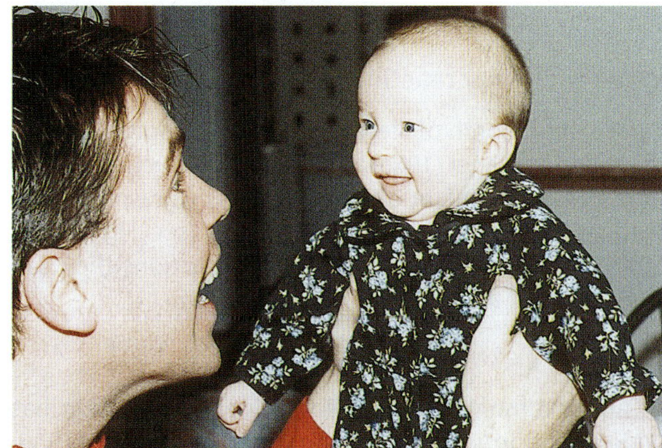

FIGURE 29.16 A 3-month-old smiles delightedly at her father's happy face. This indicates increased social awareness.

By 4 months, when a person who has been playing with and entertaining an infant leaves, an infant is likely to cry to show how enjoyable this type of interaction has been. Infants of this age recognise their primary carer and prefer that person's presence to others. By 5 months, infants may show displeasure when an object is taken away from them. This is a step beyond showing displeasure when a person leaves.

By 6 months, infants are increasingly aware of the difference between people who regularly care for them and strangers. They may begin to draw back from unfamiliar people. Seven-month-old infants begin to show obvious fear of strangers. They may cry when taken from their parent, attempt to cling to the parent and reach out to be taken back. Parents may view this as a bad trait or a regression in socialisation. Help them appreciate it is actually a big step forwards, because it shows their infant can differentiate between persons and recognises the difference between persons to trust and others.

Fear of strangers reaches its height during the eighth month, so much so that this phenomenon is often termed **eighth-month anxiety** or stranger anxiety (Levine, 2011). An infant at the height of this phase will not go willingly from a parent's arms to a nurse's. Taking a few minutes to talk to the child and parent first is time well-spent.

Nine-month-old infants are very aware of changes in tone of voice. They will cry when scolded, not because they understand what is being said but because they can sense their parent's displeasure. By 12 months, most children have overcome their fear of strangers and are alert and responsive again when approached. They like to play interactive nursery rhymes and rhythm games and "dance" with others. They like being at the table for meals and joining in family activities.

Cognitive development

In the first month of life, an infant mainly uses simple reflex activity. There is little evidence that infants at this age see themselves as separate from their environment. However, this does not mean they cannot respond actively or interact with people. They tend to enjoy people and faces more than they do objects.

Primary circular reaction

By the third month of life, a child enters a cognitive stage identified by Piaget (1966) as *primary circular reaction*. During this time, an infant explores objects by grasping them with the hands or by mouthing them (see Fig. 29.17). Infants appear to be unaware of what actions they can cause or what actions occur independently.

Secondary circular reaction

At about 6 months of age (cognitive development has wide variation), infants pass into a stage Piaget (1966) called *secondary circular reaction*. During this time, infants can grasp the idea that their actions can initiate pleasurable sensations. Now when infants reach for a mobile above the cot, hit it and watch it move, they realise that it was their hand that initiated the motion and so hit it again.

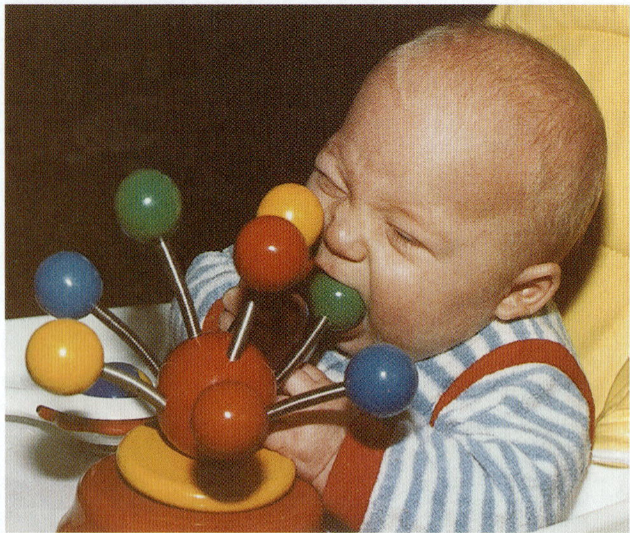

FIGURE 29.17 Infants explore the world by mouthing objects or fingering them. This also helps them separate self from environment.

Infants are still unaware of the permanence of objects by the end of this stage. For example, if an object is hidden from vision (a baby drops it from her hand or it is hidden by a blanket), an infant will not search for it: gone is gone. If any part of the object is exposed, the infant can visualise the whole object and will reach to obtain it.

Coordination of secondary schema

Infants of 10 months discover **object permanence** or become aware that an object out of sight still exists. Infants are ready for peek-a-boo once they have gained the concept of permanence. They know their parent still exists even when hiding behind a hand or blanket and wait excitedly for the parent to reappear. Piaget (1966) called this stage of cognitive development *coordination of secondary schema*.

As infants reach 1 year of age, they are capable of reproducing interesting events (they deliberately hit a mobile once; it moves; they hit it again) and producing new events. They drop objects from a highchair or playpen and watch where they fall or roll. This is a frustrating activity for carers because it involves a great deal of reaching and picking up.

✔ *Checkpoint question 29.2*

Which action would show that an infant has developed object permanence?

a. He looks for a toy that falls off his highchair tray
b. He cries when he is either hungry or lonely
c. He prefers a large yellow ball to a small red one
d. He smiles when the mobile on his cot jingles

HEALTH PROMOTION FOR AN INFANT AND FAMILY

A large part of providing health promotion to both the family and the child involves promoting a comprehensive, coordinated family-centred service system. This system needs to be able to respond to the emerging and changing needs of children and their families in a local community setting.

In 2007 the Commonwealth government set out a comprehensive plan to make the early years a national priority. This plan involves reforms to early childhood education and care, and a greater focus on early childhood development. Two major initiatives have been agreed to:

- The National Early Childhood Development Strategy—Investing in the Early Years
- National Partnership Agreement of Indigenous Early Childhood Development.

The National Early Childhood Development Strategy contains an outcomes framework and outlines characteristics of effective early childhood services. It identifies a number of specific reform priorities:

- Strengthen universal maternal, child and family health services
- Support vulnerable children
- Improve early childhood infrastructure
- Build parent and community understanding of the importance of early childhood development
- Strengthen the workforce across early childhood development and family support services
- Build better information and a solid evidence base.

The National Partnership Agreement of Indigenous Early Childhood Development brings together three key strategies to improve services and outcomes for Indigenous children and their families:

- Integration of early childhood services through the development of children and family centres
- Increased access to antenatal care, pre-pregnancy and teenage sexual and reproductive health
- Increased access to and use of MCH services by Indigenous families (Victorian Government Department of Education and Early Childhood Development, 2014).

In Victoria, the Maternal Child Health (MCH) Service is part of the broader service system that builds on the identification of individual, family and community needs at a local level. It involves cooperation between general practitioners, kindergarten and childcare services, Indigenous organisations, early childhood intervention services, parenting and family services, school nursing services, child protection services, and specialist services such as those addressing disability, drug and alcohol abuse, mental illness and family violence issues.

Dardee Boorai: the Victorian Charter of Safety and Wellbeing for Aboriginal Children and Young People (Dardee Boorai), is just one of the many things MCH is responsible for. Dardee Boorai offers a commitment to an equitable, culturally competent service system and affirms the strength and resilience of Victoria's Indigenous culture, communities and families (Victorian Government Department of Education and Early Childhood Development, 2014).

Within New Zealand there is the Lead Maternity Carer (LMC), a program that meets all needs of pregnancy. The LMC works with women throughout pregnancy and the early weeks following the birth, involving partners and whānau in all aspects of care <www.health.govt.nz/your-health/services-and-support/health-care-services/maternity-services/your-lead-maternity-carer>. He Korowai Oranga: Māori Health Strategy sets the framework for the government and the health and disability sector to achieve the best health outcomes for Māori <www.health.govt.nz/our-work/populations/maori-health/he-korowai-oranga>. This model looks at treating the whole family and community to improve child and family health. It has recently been updated and expanded from whānau ora to pae ora—healthy futures:

- Mauri ora—healthy individuals
- Whānau ora—healthy families
- Wai ora—healthy environments.

The nursing role with infants is wide-ranging because infants are so dependent on their carers for safety, learning and emotional development.

Promoting achievement of developmental task: Trust versus mistrust

Erikson (1993) proposed that the developmental task of the infant period is to form a sense of trust. When an infant is hungry, a parent feeds and makes the infant comfortable again. When an infant is wet, a parent changes a nappy and the infant is dry again. When an infant is cold, a parent holds the baby closely. By this process, infants learn to trust that when they have a need or are in distress, a person will come and meet that need.

A synonym for trust in this connotation is love. By the way infants are handled, fed, talked to and held, they learn to love and recognise they are loved. Infants who have numerous carers, who may be fed one day on a rigid schedule and the next only when they are hungry, who sometimes are treated roughly and sometimes gently, can have difficulty learning to trust. If infants cannot trust, they cannot enjoy deeply satisfying interactions with others and can have difficulty trusting themselves or experiencing high self-esteem (see Fig. 29.18). They may have difficulty establishing close relationships as adults.

It is important for infants to establish the ability to love or trust in this way, early in life, because development is sequential. If a first developmental step is inadequate, this inadequacy can pervade all future steps. With reference to

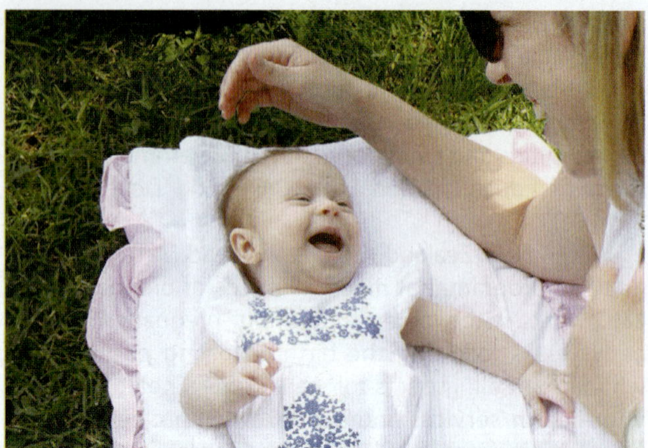

FIGURE 29.18 An infant's sense of trust develops through warm interpersonal relationships. Here a mother and baby share a "together" moment. (© Lauren Kidziak.)

trust, the end result could be an adult who is unable to instil a sense of trust in a child, perpetuating the inadequacy from generation to generation.

How do parents (or a nurse) encourage a sense of trust in an infant? Trust arises primarily from a sense of confidence that one can predict what is coming next. This does not mean parents should set up a rigid schedule of care for a child. It does imply establishing some schedule—for example, breakfast, bath, playtime, nap, lunch, walk outside, quiet playtime, dinner, story and bedtime. This gentle rhythm of care gives infants a sense of being able to predict what is going to happen and gives life some consistency. Infants thrive on routine, such as the same story read over and over again at bedtime or the same spoon every day for lunch. Infancy is not too early for children to learn family traditions, such as decorating for a traditional event, that will help them feel secure in the world as they grow.

Promoting infant safety

Accidents are a leading cause of death in children from 1 month through to 24 months of age. Most accidents in infancy occur because parents either underestimate or overestimate a child's ability. Nursing considerations that help parents become sensitive to their infant's developmental progress not only help establish sound parent–child relationships but also guard infant safety.

Aspiration prevention

Aspiration is a potential threat to infants throughout the first year. Round, cylindrical objects are more dangerous than square or flexible objects. A 3.2-cm cylinder, such as a carrot or hot dog, is particularly dangerous because it can totally obstruct an infant's airway. A deflated balloon can be sucked into the mouth, obstructing the airway in the same way. Educate parents who feed their infant formula not to prop bottles. Children under about 5 years of age should not be offered popcorn or peanuts because of the danger of aspiration. As infants become more adept at handling toys, parents need to reassess toys for loose pieces or parts.

Falls prevention

Falls are a second major cause of infant accidents. As a preventive measure, no infant, beginning with a newborn, should be left unattended on a raised surface. Normal wriggling can bring a baby to the edge of a bed, couch or table top, resulting in a fall.

Teach parents to be prepared for their infant to roll over by 2 months of age. From that time on, they must be especially vigilant not to leave the baby unattended on a changing table or counter. If the child sleeps in a cot, the mattress should be lowered to its bottom position so the height of the side rails increases; rails should meet Australian or New Zealand Safety Standards. Two months is about the maximum length of time infants can safely sleep in a bassinet; they need the protection of a cot and high side rails before they turn over.

All of these safety precautions apply to the hospital environment as well as to the home. Be sure cot sides are raised and secure before anyone walks away from the cot, even for just a moment. Also ensure that the space between the mattress and headboard is small enough so that an infant's head could not become trapped.

Car safety

Teaching car safety for infants (as well as for the whole family) is a vital preventive health measure. The use of car seats for newborns is discussed in Chapter 18. Car seats should continue to be used without interruption as per Australian and New Zealand Safety Standards.

Safety with siblings

As infants become more fun to play with at about 3 months, older brothers and sisters grow more interested in interacting with them. You may need to remind parents that children under 5 years of age, as a group, are not responsible enough or knowledgeable enough about infants to be left unattended with them. They might introduce an unsafe toy or engage in play that is too rough for an infant. Some preschoolers may be so jealous of a new baby that they will physically harm an infant if left alone.

Bathing and swimming safety

As babies begin to develop good back support, many parents begin to bathe them in an adult bath. Caution parents never to leave an infant unattended in a tub, even when propped up out of the water or sitting in a bath ring or bath seat. Normal wriggling can easily cause a baby to slip down under the water. This applies to a hospital setting as well.

Many communities offer infant swimming programs for babies as young as 6 months. If their child is enrolled in one of these programs, parents may become overconfident about their infant's ability to operate safely in water. Because children can dog-paddle momentarily in a swimming pool does not mean they can sustain that position for any length of time in a bathtub or pool. Being able to swim momentarily may also cause children to lose their instinctive fear of water and so be in more danger when around water than children who are still naturally more cautious. Such programs may also cause hypothermia and spread microorganisms, because infants of this age are not yet toilet-trained. Exposure to chlorinated water can damage lung epithelium that may be a precursor to childhood asthma (Klootwijk & Krul, 2011).

Pet safety

As many people have pets before or after a child enters the family, it is important that families become aware of pet safety. Consult with the family vet in relation to pet and child interactions as well as what needs to be considered for baby and child safety.

Childproofing

When infants begin teething at 5 to 6 months, they chew on any object within reach to lessen gum-line pain. Remind parents to check for possible sources of lead paint, such as painted cots, playpen rails or windowsills. If an infant is going to be allowed to play on the floor, parents should move furniture in front of electrical fixtures or buy protective caps for outlets. Infants are especially fascinated by the holes and will probe them with (often wet) fingers. Parents may need to install safety gates at the top and bottom of stairways as other safety measures.

Urge parents to move all potentially poisonous substances from bottom cupboards and store them well out of their infant's reach. Infants of any age should not be left unattended in prams, highchairs, grocery shopping trolleys or strollers. Baby walkers are extremely dangerous because infants can manoeuvre them near stairways and fall the length of the stairs.

When infants begin crawling remind parents to recheck bottom cupboards and stairways for safety. When the child begins to walk, higher areas, such as low tables, need to be cleared of dangerous items. By 10 months, achievement of a pincer grasp makes infants able to pick up very small objects. Remind parents to check play areas or areas such as table tops for pins or other sharp objects that could be swallowed. Children who can walk may venture into the street or a swimming pool if not carefully supervised (see Fig. 29.19). Although they seem very independent and able to take care of themselves, their judgement about what is dangerous is immature (Ibrahim et al., 2011).

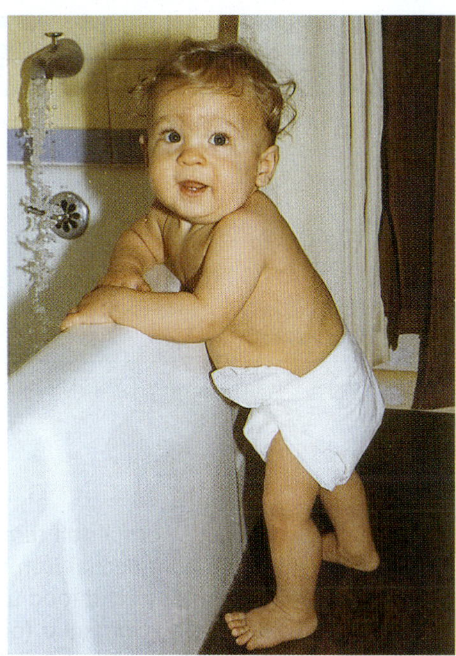

FIGURE 29.19 Once walking begins, the extended range of activities brings an infant in contact with potentially dangerous places or objects unless the house is childproofed. The bathroom is an important place to begin.

CASE STUDY QUESTION

3. You review infant safety with Kai's mother. What are two of the most common types of accidents in infants?
   a. Drowning and murder
   b. Poisoning and burns
   c. Falls and motor vehicle accidents
   d. Aspiration and falls

Promoting nutritional health of an infant

The first choice for feeding an infant during the first 12 months of life is breast milk (see Chapter 19). All the necessary nutrients, vitamins, minerals and water are provided by human milk for the first 6 months of life, with the exception of vitamin K (1 mg intramuscularly is administered at birth) (Whitney & Rolfes, 2012; Townsend & Prichford, 2012). How long mothers continue to breastfeed is an individual choice, although it is recommended throughout the entire first year (MCaFHNA, 2012).

For infants whose mothers choose not to or are unable to breastfeed, a commercial iron-fortified formula will supply adequate nutrition (Krebs & Primak, 2011). Infants who are changed to cow's milk before 1 year of age (a practice that is not recommended because the protein in cow's milk is difficult for an infant to digest, possibly leading to such intestinal irritation that slight but continuous gastrointestinal bleeding occurs, resulting in anaemia) should receive a supplementary form of vitamin C and iron to make up for the deficiency of these in cow's milk.

TABLE 29.2 Suggested schedule for introduction of solid foods

Age (mo)	Food to introduce*	Rationale
5–6	Iron-fortified infant cereal mixed with breast milk, orange juice or formula	Aids in preventing iron-deficiency anaemia; the least allergenic type of food; an easily digested food
7	Vegetables	Good source of vitamin A; adds new texture and flavours to diet
8	Fruit	Best source of vitamin C, good source of vitamin A; adds new texture and flavours to diet
9	Meat	Good source of protein, iron and B vitamins
10	Egg yolk	Good source of iron

*Wheat, tomatoes, oranges, fish and egg whites should be omitted if there are allergies in the family, because these foods are most likely to cause allergies.

Introduction of solid food

From a nutritional standpoint, a normal full-term infant can thrive on breast milk or a commercial iron-fortified formula without the addition of any solid food until 4 to 6 months (Conti et al., 2011). Delaying solid food until this time helps prevent overwhelming an infant's kidneys with a heavy solute load that can occur when protein is ingested. Although difficult to document, it also may delay the development of food allergies in susceptible infants and be another way to help prevent future obesity (Gaffney et al., 2012).

Most parents are eager to begin feeding their infant solid food, hoping this will help their child sleep through the night. Some parents do begin solid food before 6 months without apparent ill effects, possibly because much of the food is not processed by the gastrointestinal tract, passing through undigested, because of the immaturity of the digestive system and decreased amylase and lipase secretion (van Dijk et al., 2012). See Table 29.2 for a suggested schedule for the introduction of solid foods.

Generally speaking, infants are physiologically ready for solid food when they are nursing vigorously every 3 to 4 hours and do not seem satisfied or are taking more than 960 mL of formula a day and do not seem satisfied. Infants are not ready to digest complex starches until amylase is present in saliva at approximately 2 to 3 months. Biting movements begin at approximately 3 months. Chewing movements do not begin until 7 to 9 months. Therefore, foods that require chewing should not be given until this age. To begin, give one food at a time to assess for any allergy or reactions such as significant loose bowel actions, allergies, such as rash or vomiting.

Loss of extrusion reflex

When anything is placed on the anterior third of a newborn's tongue, it is automatically extruded or thrust out of the mouth by the tongue. This is a life-saving reflex because it prevents infants from swallowing or aspirating foreign objects that touch the mouth. Infants extrude food when a spoonful of it is placed on the tongue in the same way. The reflex fades at 3 to 4 months. Until this time, it may be difficult to get an infant to eat solid food.

Cereal

The first food generally given to infants is infant cereal fortified with B vitamins and iron. These are precooked, fine dry powders to which expressed breast milk or infant formula is added. The first cereal introduced is usually rice cereal, because fewer children are allergic to rice products than to wheat and corn products. Usually, it is offered twice a day, morning and evening. Once the child has taken rice cereal for 1 week, parents can try another kind. Infant cereal is so rich in iron that parents should continue feeding it at least throughout the first year. Ideally, children should eat infant cereal until the age of 3 or 4 years, as few popularly advertised products can match the nutrients of fortified infant cereal.

Vegetables and fruit

Because their iron content is generally higher than that of fruits, vegetables are usually the second food added to the diet (at 5–7 months of age). Parents who have a blender, strainer or grinder can prepare their own. They simply cook a vegetable and then blend or strain it so it does not have to be chewed. Caution parents not to add butter or salt to the preparation, because infants have difficulty digesting fats until almost the end of the first year and the added salt is unnecessary. When vegetables are added to the diet, they are usually offered at lunch. Remind parents to offer both green and yellow vegetables. Help them to remember that their own dislike of a particular vegetable does not mean their child will feel the same way about it.

Fruit is usually offered 1 month after beginning vegetables (at 6–8 months). It can be given in addition to cereal for breakfast and dinner. As with vegetables, parents should offer a selection so an infant is exposed to different tastes and textures.

Meat and eggs

Meat is usually introduced at 9 months. Parents can grind a portion of the meat they have prepared for their own meal so it is tender or they can use commercially prepared products. Chicken has the advantage of being low in cholesterol, but this is not a priority with infants. Beef and pork have more iron than chicken, so encourage parents to offer these more frequently than chicken.

Egg yolks are offered by 10 months of age. Egg yolks contain the bulk of the iron content of eggs; the white contains the bulk of protein. Egg yolk alone should be given at first, because the protein of the egg white can lead to allergy or can be difficult for an infant to digest. Eggs may be prepared by hard-boiling (then adding a little formula or breast milk to the mashed yolk to make it more liquid) or purchased as commercial baby food. Soft-boiling or poaching is not usually recommended, because salmonella, the chief offending microorganism that may be in eggs, may not be killed by these methods. Also, thorough cooking makes protein easier to digest.

Table food

With the introduction of solid food, encourage parents to establish a three-meals-a-day pattern, if that is the family's lifestyle, and to have the infant join the family at the table. Generally, encourage parents to use homemade foods rather than relying on commercially prepared infant foods, although commercial foods are now prepared without excessive additives and are convenient for parents who have little preparation time.

Remind parents that highchairs are one of the most dangerous pieces of baby equipment they own. Urge them always to fasten the restraint and never leave an infant unattended in a highchair, because even a 6-month-old can squirm out of a chair with little effort. Nurses must also keep this in mind when feeding infants in a hospital setting.

Establishment of healthy eating patterns

Some parents may need to be reminded that although rules for infant feeding are designed to promote healthy nutrition, they should individualise their approach according to the cues their child is giving them for readiness. A child who adapts poorly to change may have difficulty accepting the first solid food, for example, and may have difficulty with each new food. Parents may need support to remember a child is not conducting this struggle out of a desire for conflict but because this is a characteristic of temperament. Giving food to others is interpreted by many as giving love, so refusing food is equated with refusing love. Help parents understand that this is not what is happening. Refusing a teaspoonful of carrots is refusing a teaspoonful of carrots, nothing more. An infant who is fatigued or overstimulated may not eat well. Providing a quiet environment away from older brothers or sisters before mealtime may solve this problem.

Encourage parents not to force infants to eat if they do not seem hungry. Healthy, happy infants will be hungry at mealtime and will eat. Those who refuse a meal may be tired, distracted or perhaps ill. Forcing only leads to regurgitation or, if they are ill, vomiting. It also can result in feeding problems or a situation in which infants refuse to eat altogether. Infants who are eating and not thriving or not eating and therefore not thriving should be examined to determine if a cause such as a metabolic disorder or failure to thrive exists (see Chapter 48).

Weaning

Infants are capable of approximating their lips to a cup so they can drink effectively from one at about 9 months of age. The sucking reflex begins to diminish in intensity between ages 6 and 9 months, which makes this the time to consider weaning. To wean from formula or breast milk, the mother chooses one feeding a day and then begins offering fluid by the new method at that feeding. She should choose a time of day that is not an infant's fussy period; other than that, the time is immaterial. After 3 days to 1 week, when an infant has adjusted to the one change, the mother changes a second feeding. Should an illness such as an upper respiratory infection occur or the child have teething discomfort, there will be setbacks, so no set number of weeks should be prescribed to complete weaning. Infants usually need more fluid during hot weather than cold weather because of increased perspiration. This may make it more difficult to begin weaning during the summer.

Self-feeding

At approximately 6 months of age, infants become interested in handling a spoon and beginning to feed themselves. Their coordination, unfortunately, has not developed enough for them to use a spoon without a great deal of spilling, so they are much more adept at feeding themselves with their fingers (see Fig. 29.20). When an infant becomes fatigued or frustrated at attempts at self-feeding, a parent can then quietly help without making an issue of it. Parents who insist on continuing to spoon-feed past the time infants want to feed themselves can cause infants to balk at eating. Often a compromise is helpful. If a parent gives the infant a spoon, the child can poke at a cereal dish with it while the parent continues to offer bites from a

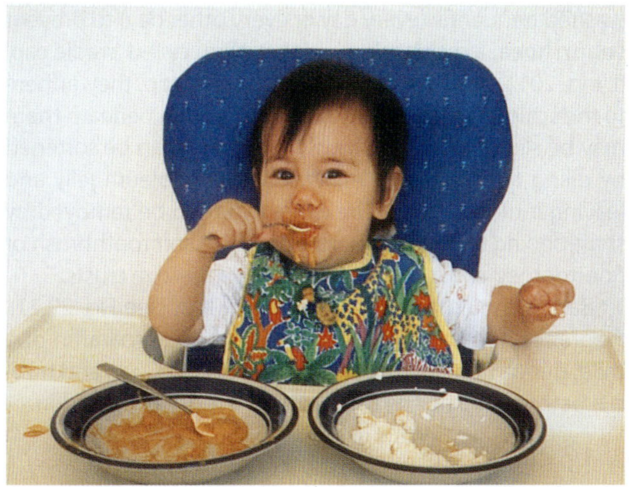

FIGURE 29.20 Self-feeding is not always a neat process for an infant.

second spoon. In this way, a child is "in charge" of the feeding yet receptive to taking food from the parent.

Adequate intake with a vegetarian diet

An infant eating a vegetarian diet should continue to be breastfed or ingest an iron-fortified, balanced commercial formula for the entire first year. If a milk allergy is present, a soy-based formula can be used. When solid foods are added at 6 months, an assortment of foods should be provided, including: vegetables such as avocados, potatoes and broccoli; fruits such as apples, prunes (high in iron) and bananas; infant cereal; tofu; wheatgerm; legumes; brewer's yeast; and synthetic vitamin D. Feeding fortified cereal throughout the first year will ensure that iron stores are built. If the diet is to include dairy products, these can be added towards the end of the first year as usual (Conti et al., 2011). Because vegetarian diets are high in fibre, infants who eat them may have more frequent and looser-than-normal bowel movements.

Promoting infant development in daily activities

In the first year, caring for an infant—feeding, bathing, dressing and so forth—occupies what may seem like nearly all of the parents' waking hours. Worrying about their infant's sleep patterns may take up the rest of their time, often because the parents are not getting enough sleep themselves. All of these basic care-related activities provide important opportunities for carers and infants to get to know one another and to become used to each other's personalities and patterns. Nurses can play a key role in teaching parents about these activities and stressing their importance.

Bathing

Except in very hot weather, an infant does not need a bath every day. If a parent is tired and would not enjoy bath time or if some days are just too rushed, a complete bath can be omitted, with only an infant's face, hands and nappy area being washed. Some infants do need their head and scalp washed frequently (every day or every other day) to prevent **seborrhoea**, a scaly scalp condition often called "cradle cap" (Lyon, 2011). If seborrhoea lesions do develop, they adhere to the scalp in yellow, crusty patches. The skin beneath them may be slightly erythematous. The patches can be softened by oiling the scalp with mineral oil or petroleum jelly and leaving it on overnight. The crusts can then be removed by shampooing the hair the next morning. A soft toothbrush or fine-toothed comb can be used to help remove crusts.

Babies should be bathed in warm water (see Fig. 29.21). Fragrance-free bath oil containing light liquid paraffin or a mild, gentle non-soap cleanser may be used. Soap and bubble bath should not be used as they will dry out the skin.

Nappy area care

The most effective means of promoting good nappy area hygiene is to change nappies frequently, about every 2 to 4 hours. However, it is rarely good practice to interrupt the child's sleep to change nappies. If an infant develops a rash from sleeping in a wet nappy, air drying or sleeping without a nappy may be a solution.

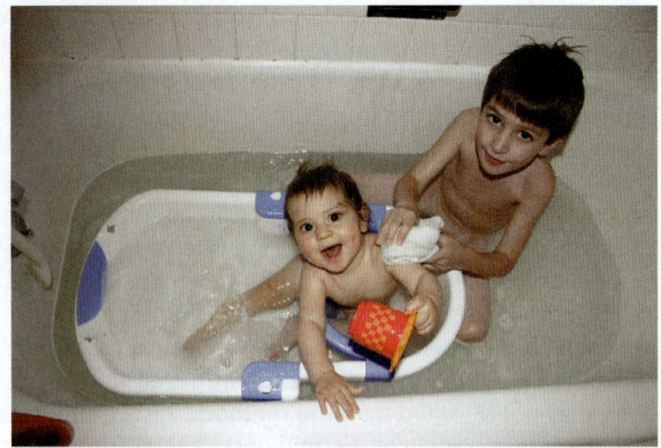

FIGURE 29.21 An infant enjoys bath time with his big brother. Parents should always watch carefully while infants and toddlers are in the bath.

The nappy area is exposed to constant moisture, occlusion and rubbing and this may irritate and damage the skin and cause nappy rash. To prevent this, nappies should be changed frequently and babies should be allowed as much time as possible without a nappy. At each nappy change, the parents should wash the skin with clear water or with a commercial alcohol-free nappy wipe (and perfume-free if an infant has sensitive skin), then pat or allow to air dry. A thick layer of nappy rash cream should then be applied; talcum powder is not necessary.

Skin care

Babies' skin is thinner, more fragile and more sensitive than adult skin. It can also be easily irritated as it is less resistant to bacteria and harmful substances in the environment. Advise new parents to take the following steps to look after and protect their baby's skin. Applying a good-quality moisturiser to baby's skin immediately after the bath can increase skin hydration. Thicker creams and ointments are more effective than lotions. If the baby's skin often seems dry, moisturiser may need to be applied two to four times a day.

Care of teeth

It is well accepted that exposing developing teeth to fluoride is one of the most effective ways to promote healthy tooth formation and prevent tooth decay. The most important time for children to receive fluoride is between 6 months and 12 years of age. In communities where the water supply does not provide enough fluoride, the use of an oral fluoride supplement beginning at 6 months or the use of fluoride toothpaste or rinses after tooth eruption is recommended.

Teach parents to begin "brushing" even before teeth erupt by rubbing a soft washcloth over the gum pads. This eliminates plaque and reduces the presence of bacteria, creating a clean environment for the arrival of the first teeth. Once teeth erupt, all surfaces should be brushed with a soft brush or washcloth once or twice a day. Children lack the coordination to brush effectively until they are school-age, so parents must be responsible for this activity well past infancy. Toothpaste is not necessary for an infant, because it is the scrubbing that removes the plaque (Milgrom & Chi, 2011). The initial dental check-up should be made by 1 year of age; check-ups should continue at 6-monthly intervals until adulthood.

Sleep

Sleep needs and habits vary greatly among infants, but most infants require 10 to 12 hours of sleep at night and one or several naps during the day. Parents are usually advised to let a baby sleep in a separate space rather than in their bed so they do not awaken at every toss and squeak. Doing so allows infants to learn to settle themselves and go back to sleep should they awaken briefly. This may help prevent sleep problems such as night waking in the future. Other parents prefer to have infants sleep with them in a family bed, as they believe this practice promotes a feeling of security (Scollan-Koliopoulos & Koliopoulos, 2010). Bed sharing also promotes breastfeeding but has the danger of accidental suffocation. Caution parents not to place pillows in an infant's bed to avoid suffocation. Always place infants on their back to sleep because this position markedly reduces the incidence of sudden infant death syndrome (SIDS). See Chapter 26 for a further discussion of SIDS.

Exercise

Infants benefit from outings in a pram or stroller because sunlight provides a natural source of vitamin D. In hot weather, caution parents to protect an infant from sunburn by exposing the child to the sun for only very short periods, beginning with 3 to 5 minutes the first day, a little more the next day and so on up to 15 to 20 minutes at a time.

Towards the end of the first year, infants need space to crawl and then to walk, such as in an enclosed outdoor play space. In addition to providing fresh air, going for leisurely walks while pointing out the sights of the world—trees, birds, dogs, houses, neighbours—helps children develop language. When outdoors in warm weather babies should wear light clothing, hats and have sunshades on prams. Shade is the best protection against UV. Older infants can have a broad-spectrum sunscreen of SPF 30 applied to exposed areas of skin.

Parental concerns and problems related to normal infant development

Some of the difficulties parents are apt to have in evaluating the health of infants are shown in Table 29.3. New parents may need reassurance and answers to questions about childcare procedures or health during the infant period because they have not yet learned their child's

TABLE 29.3 Common difficulties parents experience in evaluating the health of infants

Difficulty	Suggestions for improving assessment
Evaluating pain	Infants manifest pain by fussiness. They can reveal arm and leg pain by immobility of the body part; ear pain by brushing or tugging at the ear; stomach pain by pulling up the legs against the abdomen.
Evaluating degree of reduced activity	Lack of interest in smiling or interaction is an important observation. Increased sleeping or lying supine with legs non-flexed (frog-legged) as if exhausted is important.
Evaluating infant temperature	All parents should learn how to take an axillary or tympanic temperature so they can report a specific degree of fever rather than a subjective finding, such as "feels hot".
Evaluating amount of vomiting or diarrhoea	Knowing the number of times vomiting and/or diarrhoea has occurred is important. Estimating amount in comparison with what the child has eaten is helpful as well as estimating an amount (a cupful, etc.). Knowing whether nappies are "soaked" or "stained" with stools is important in estimating amount. Caution parents that vomiting and diarrhoea are always serious in infants.

cues. However, the need for reassurance may be just as great in experienced parents. The unique characteristics of each child require some adjustment from parents.

Teething

Most infants have little difficulty with teething, but some appear very distressed. Generally, the gums are sore and tender before a new tooth breaks the surface. As soon as the tooth is through, the tenderness passes. Because of this pain, infants can be resistant to chewing for a day or two and be slightly cranky, possibly because they are hungry from not eating as much as usual. High fever, seizures, vomiting or diarrhoea and earache are never normal signs of teething. An infant with any of these symptoms has an underlying infection or disease process requiring further evaluation (Kiran et al., 2011).

Thumb-sucking

Sucking is a surprisingly strong need: antenatal ultrasounds even demonstrate fetal thumb-sucking in utero. Many infants begin to suck a thumb or finger at about 3 months of age and continue the habit through the first few years of life. The sucking reflex peaks at 6 to 9 months, whereas thumb-sucking peaks at about 18 months. Parents can be assured that thumb-sucking is normal and does not deform the jaw line as long as it stops by school-age. It does not cause "baby talk" or any of the other symptoms commonly attributed to it. The best approach is to be certain an infant has adequate sucking pleasure and then to ignore thumb-sucking. Making an issue of it rarely causes a child to stop; if anything, it usually intensifies and prolongs it (Montaldo et al., 2011).

Use of dummies

Whether to use dummies is a question parents must settle for themselves, depending on how they feel about them and their infant's needs. Infants rarely have such a need for sucking that they must have a dummy in their mouth constantly. Discussing a few pros and cons with the parents clarifies the subject. Use of a dummy at bedtime may reduce the risk of SIDS as, with a dummy, a baby rouses periodically from sleep to suck and so does not continue for an extended time in deep phases of sleep.

A major drawback of dummies is the problem of cleanliness. If used at times other than bedtime, they tend to fall on the floor or footpath and are then put back into an infant's mouth. If not well constructed, they may come apart and be aspirated. Hanging a dummy on a string around an infant's neck could cause strangulation. Parents should attempt to wean a child from a dummy any time after 3 months of age and certainly during the time the sucking reflex is fading at 6 to 9 months. Weaning after this age is difficult because a dummy becomes a comfort mechanism, like a warm blanket or fuzzy toy to which a child may cling (Nelson, 2012).

Head banging

Some infants rhythmically bang their heads against the bars of a cot for a period of time before falling asleep. This is distressing behaviour for parents. Head banging in this limited fashion—beginning during the second half of the first year of life and continuing through to the preschool period, associated with naptime or bedtime and lasting under 15 minutes—can be considered normal. Children use this measure to relax and fall asleep. Investigating stress factors operating in the house may be helpful. If some of them can be relieved such as parents' overestimation of the child's development, marital discord or illness in another family member, the head banging may decrease or it may have already become such a strong habit that it will persist for months or even years (Carr-Greg, 2012; Singer, 2011).

Sleep problems

Sleep problems develop in early infancy because of colic or because an otherwise healthy infant takes longer than usual to adjust to sleeping through the night. Breastfed babies tend to wake more often than those who are formula-fed because breast milk is more easily digested, so infants become hungry sooner. In late infancy, the problem of waking at night and remaining awake for an hour or more becomes common. Although an infant may be content and not cry during this time, parents are reluctant to sleep while the child is awake, so they may become extremely fatigued. This is an increasing concern because more and more families today consist of two wage-earning parents; there is no time for parents to nap during the day to make up for sleep lost at night. Suggestions for eliminating or at least coping with night waking are: (a) delay bedtime by 1 hour; (b) shorten an afternoon sleep period; (c) do not respond immediately to infants at night so they can have time to fall back to sleep on their own; and (d) provide soft toys or music to allow infants to play quietly alone during this wakeful time. Reassuring parents that infants take varying lengths of time to adjust to night sleeping is helpful in assuring them their child is normal. Suggesting that parents use the time they are awake at night to do such things as solve a problem at work, watch a late television program or plan a shopping list may help them view the situation as a constructive time rather than a problem (Price et al., 2012).

There are several agencies that can assist with sleep and settling issues. In Australia, Tresillian has a 24-hour help line and many other online services and information. Most states do have some similar but a good starting point of contact is Tresillian <www.tresillian.net>. In New Zealand Plunket offer a toll-free parent helpline and advice service available to all families, whānau and carers 24 hours a day, seven days a week as well as online information and other services <www.plunket.org.nz>.

Constipation

Breastfed infants are rarely constipated because their stools tend to be loose. Constipation may occur in formula-fed infants if their diet is deficient in fluid. This can be corrected simply with the addition of more fluid. Some parents misinterpret the normal pushing movements of a newborn as constipation. When infants defecate, their faces do turn red and they grimace and grunt. As long as stools are not hard and contain no evidence of fresh blood (as might occur with a rectal fissure), this is normal infant behaviour. If constipation persists beyond 5 or 6 months of age, encourage parents to check with the infant's healthcare provider about measures to relieve this.

All infants with a history of constipation for more than 1 week should be examined for an anal fissure or tight anal sphincter. Softening stools and thereby relieving the pain of defecation often solves the problem and helps the fissure to heal. Chronic constipation also may occur in children with congenital hypothyroidism (decreased functioning of the thyroid gland). Therefore, an infant with constipation should also be carefully observed for characteristic signs of hypothyroidism, such as lethargy, protruding tongue and failure to meet developmental milestones (see Chapter 48). Infants with either Hirschsprung's disease or hypothyroidism need therapy to correct the disorder.

Loose stools

Many new parents are unfamiliar with the consistency or colour of normal newborn stools, so they mistakenly report normal stools as diarrhoea. Stools of breastfed infants are generally softer than those of formula-fed infants. If a mother takes a laxative while breastfeeding, an infant's stools may be very loose. An infant who is formula-fed can have loose stools if the formula is not diluted properly. Occasionally, loose stools may begin with the introduction of solid food, such as fruit. Malabsorption syndrome (coeliac disease), or an inability to digest fat, may manifest themselves first by loose stools and a distended abdomen and deficiency of fat-soluble vitamins (see Chapter 45).

When talking to a parent about loose stools, ask about the duration of the loose stools, the number of stools per day, their colour and consistency, and whether there is any mucus or blood in them. Is there associated fever, cramping or vomiting? Infants with associated signs and symptoms such as fever, cramping, vomiting, loss of appetite, a decrease in voiding and weight loss should be examined by their healthcare provider because this suggests an infectious process. Dehydration occurs rapidly in a small infant who is not eating and is losing body fluid through loose stools (Mehal et al., 2012).

Colic

Colic is paroxysmal abdominal pain that generally occurs in infants under 3 months of age and is marked by loud, intense crying (Shergill-Bonner, 2010). An infant cries loudly and pulls the legs up against the abdomen. The infant's face becomes red and flushed, the fists clench and the abdomen becomes tense. If offered a bottle, the infant will suck vigorously for a few minutes as if starved, then stop, as another wave of intestinal pain occurs.

The cause of colic is unclear. It may occur in susceptible infants from overfeeding or from swallowing too much air while drinking. Formula-fed babies are more likely to have colic than breastfed babies, possibly because they swallow more air while drinking or because formula is harder to digest. Although infants continue to thrive despite colic, the condition should not be dismissed as unimportant. It is a distressing and frightening problem for parents not only because an infant appears to be in acute pain, but also because the distress persists for hours, usually into the middle of the night, so no-one in the family gets adequate rest.

Take a thorough history of an infant with signs of colic because intestinal obstruction or infection may mimic an attack of colic and be misinterpreted by the casual interviewer. Ask parents about the duration of the problem and its frequency (it usually lasts up to 3 hours a day and occurs at least 3 days every week). Ask what happens just before the attack (colic usually occurs at a time removed from a feeding) and ask the parent to describe the attack itself and associated symptoms. Document the number and type of bowel movements the infant has, because bowel movements are not abnormal with colic. Constipation; narrow, ribbonlike stools; and the presence of blood or mucus in the stool all suggest other problems. A family medical history is important to obtain because an allergy to milk may simulate colic.

Determine the baby's feeding pattern (breastfed or bottle fed). If bottle fed, ask about the type of formula and how it is prepared. Ask parents if they are holding the baby upright so air bubbles can rise and whether they burp the infant adequately after feeding (Gahagan, 2011; Iacovou et al., 2011; Thomas & Greer, 2010).

Some parents try placing a hot water bottle on their infant's stomach for comfort, but this should be discouraged. A basic rule for any abdominal discomfort is to avoid heat in case appendicitis is developing. This is highly unlikely in so young an infant, but parents will remember they once used heat and may use it again when the child is older. Hot water bottles and heating pads might also burn the delicate skin of infants.

It is important to think of colic as a family problem or else a vicious circle may begin. An infant cries and the parents become tense and unsure. An infant senses the tension and develops more colic. Help parents plan away time from infant care to relieve their stress levels and prevent this cycle. In most infants, colic disappears almost magically at 3 months of age, probably because it becomes easier to digest food and an infant maintains a more upright position by this time, which allows less gas to form.

Vomiting

Almost all infants vomit, although formula-fed babies appear to do it more than breastfed babies. A baby who vomits a mouthful of milk (rolling down the chin) two or three times a day (or sometimes after every meal) is experiencing normal, early-infancy spitting up. Associated signs such as diarrhoea, abdominal cramps, fever, cough, cold or loss of activity suggest illness. If an infant is vomiting so forcefully that milk is projected a metre away, it may be the beginning of pyloric stenosis (an abnormally tight valve between the stomach and duodenum), which requires surgical intervention. If the vomiting is a large amount with each feeding, parents may be describing gastroesophageal reflux, in which a lax cardiac sphincter from the stomach into the oesophagus allows regurgitation of gastric contents into the oesophagus. This also requires medical attention (see Chapter 45). Burping a baby thoroughly after a feeding often limits vomiting. Parents may try sitting an infant in an infant chair for half an hour after feeding. Changing formulas generally is of little value.

Miliaria

Miliaria, or prickly heat rash, occurs most often in warm weather or when babies are overdressed or sleep in overheated rooms. Clusters of pinpoint, reddened papules with occasional vesicles and pustules surrounded by erythema usually appear on the neck first and may spread upwards to around the ears and onto the face or downwards onto the trunk.

Bathing an infant twice a day during hot weather, particularly if a small amount of baking soda is added to the bath water, may improve the rash. Eliminating sweating by reducing the amount of clothing on an infant or lowering the room temperature should bring almost immediate improvement and prevent further eruptions.

Baby-bottle syndrome

Putting an infant to bed with a bottle of formula, breast milk, orange juice or glucose water can result in aspiration. It can also lead to decay of all the upper teeth and the lower posterior teeth (see Fig. 29.22; Bishop, 2011). Decay occurs because while an infant sleeps, liquid from the propped bottle continuously soaks the upper front teeth and lower back teeth (the lower front teeth are protected by the tongue). The problem, called **baby-bottle syndrome**, occurs because the carbohydrate in solutions such as formula or glucose water ferments to organic acids that demineralise the tooth enamel until it decays.

To prevent this problem, advise parents never to put their baby to bed with a bottle. If parents insist a bottle is necessary to allow a baby to fall asleep, encourage them to fill it with water and use a teat with a smaller hole to prevent the baby from receiving a large amount of fluid.

Obesity in infants

Obesity in infants is defined as a weight greater than the 90th to 95th percentile on a standardised height/weight chart. Obesity occurs when there is an increase in the number of fat cells because of excessive kilojoule intake. Preventing obesity in infants is important because the extra fat cells formed at this time are likely to remain throughout childhood and even into adulthood. If a child becomes obese because of over ingestion of milk, iron-deficiency anaemia may also be present because of the low iron content of both breast and commercial milk. Once infant obesity begins, it is difficult to reverse, so prevention is the key (Taylor et al., 2011).

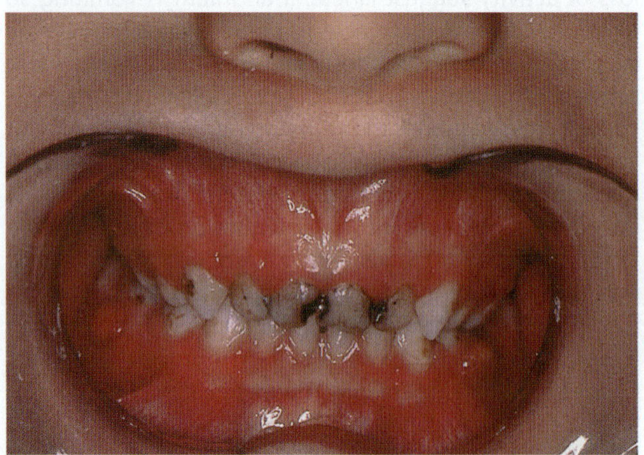

FIGURE 29.22 Baby-bottle syndrome. Notice the extensive decay in the upper teeth. (From K. L. Boyd, DDS/Custom Medical Stock Photograph.)

Overfeeding in infancy often occurs because parents were taught to eat everything on their plate and they continue to instil this concept in their children. This occurs most often with formula-fed infants whose parents urge them to empty their bottle or finish a cereal serving. It can occur any time parents automatically feed an infant when the child cries, rather than investigating what the cry might really mean. As a general rule, an infant should take no more than 650 to 750 mL of formula daily.

Another way to help prevent obesity is to add a source of fibre, such as wholegrain cereal and raw fruit, to an infant's diet. These prolong the stomach-emptying time, so they can help reduce food intake. Caution parents about giving obese infants foods with high amounts of refined sugars, such as pudding, cake, biscuits and lollies. Encourage parents to learn more about balanced nutrition and to provide this for their entire family.

Concerns of the family with a cognitively or physically challenged or chronically ill infant

An infant born with a cognitive or physical challenge or an illness is usually hospitalised immediately after birth for diagnosis and treatment. This can result in delayed bonding because the newborn is separated from the parents during this time. Encourage parents to visit an intensive care unit regularly to help form a strong parent-child attachment. If parents cannot visit, urge them to call the hospital as frequently as they can to inquire about their child. In addition, nurses can supply digital photographs of an infant for parents to take home.

Many of the developmental events of the infant year (social smile, laughing out loud, reaching for an object, uttering the first word, sitting, talking) are activities that encourage parent-child interaction because they make an infant fun to be with and naturally make a parent want to spend more time with the child. Children who are cognitively challenged may not reach these milestones. Children who are physically challenged may be unable to achieve them as well if they cannot reach up and pat a parent's face or hold out their arms to be picked up by a parent. If children cannot interact with parents in these ways, parents may find themselves equally unable to interact with their children. If infants leave the hospital with a cast or other equipment such as a ventilator for care, parents may be so concerned with these items that they cannot initiate normal singing and playing activities with their children.

To encourage a good parent-child relationship, point out the positive things an infant can do. Perhaps the child's facial expression says, "Pick me up", even though he does not reach up with his hands; perhaps her eyes follow her mother's actions even though she cannot yet call out.

Helping parents to interact more fully with their infants helps to build a sense of trust in an infant. Without a sense of trust, children have difficulty expressing themselves to others; they may not believe they are lovable or that people want to interact with them. Physically challenged individuals, no matter what their ages, need people around them to give them help at whatever point they cannot meet their own needs. It is unfortunate when physically challenged children cannot reach out for help because they do not have a sense of trust (Stevens et al., 2011).

Infants who are cognitively or physically challenged or chronically ill experience the same health and growth problems as other infants. Parents may be reluctant to bring up these concerns at healthcare visits because they believe such problems pale in comparison with the primary illness or condition. When taking the health histories of children with chronic or longstanding medical problems, ask parents about secondary concerns. "What about everyday things? Any problems there?" Treat these concerns seriously, so parents can feel confident about bringing them to your attention at future healthcare visits. Also mention that they are part of normal infant development so parents can begin to view their child apart from the primary illness.

Nutrition and the cognitively or physically challenged infant

Nutrition is often a concern for infants who are born physically challenged or are ill at birth. Infants who have fevers because of illness have increased metabolic needs and require more kilojoules than normal. To compound the problem, ill children may become too fatigued to take adequate feeding. If any degree of neurological involvement exists, sucking and swallowing reflexes may not be coordinated. With gastrointestinal involvement, feeding may be impossible.

To ensure adequate kilojoule and protein intake, infants may need to be maintained on nasogastric tube or gastrostomy feedings, or total parenteral nutrition. These methods limit the amount of sucking that is possible. Because sucking provides pleasure as well as satisfying thirst, this is a major loss. Provide an infant with non-nutritive sucking experiences if possible to fill this need (Wilken, 2012).

Infants who are ill for a long time may not eat solid foods eagerly once they are introduced because they are not hungry enough to be interested in a new eating method. Help parents to experiment with different foods to find a taste that does appeal to ill children or teach them to limit foods to only those the child appears to like most from all five food groups to ensure the infant receives adequate nutrition.

Family-centred care

Being the parent of a newborn infant requires large amounts of energy and good humour. Sometimes this is difficult if parents are feeling tired and overwhelmed by their new responsibilities. Parents who are feeling anxious should be reassured that there are many positive aspects to being a new parent, including many rewards and precious moments as they watch their baby grow and develop. It may also be helpful to discuss with them the points in Box 29.1.

BOX 29.1 * Important points for new parents to remember

Here are some important points to discuss with new parents:

- Parenting is a learnt skill—most parents learn on the job
- Be kind to yourselves:
  - Take time out to do something you enjoy—this may be a walk in the park, swimming or reading a book for 30 minutes
  - Try to limit the amount of housework you need to do (especially in the early weeks of parenthood)
  - Learn some quick relaxation techniques to use when things get difficult
  - Try to sleep or rest when your baby is asleep
  - Take care of your physical needs by eating well and exercising regularly
  - Join a new parents' group—this allows you to meet other new families in your community
  - Arrange regular childcare by a grandparent, friend or childcare centre
  - Plan time together as a couple
  - Arrange a night out—including baby sitting
  - If a night out isn't possible, think of activities that you can do as a family
  - Find time to have a conversation together about your feelings, relationship and needs
- Start each day afresh even if the day before things have been difficult
- Think positively, be practical and stay in touch with the outside world
- Try to retain your sense of humour
- Be efficient when cooking—make extra meals that can be frozen for times when you are feeling too tired to prepare a meal
- Talk about your feelings or concerns with a sympathetic listener—this may be a friend, parent or health professional
- If you are feeling lonely or isolated, ask your child and family health nurse to arrange a volunteer home visitor to come on a regular basis

Key points for review

- The infant period is from 1 month to 12 months. Children typically double their birth weight at 4 to 6 months and triple it at 1 year.
- Infants develop their first tooth at about 6 months; by 12 months, they have six to eight teeth.
- Important gross motor milestones during the infant year are lifting the chest off a bed at 2 months, sitting at 6 to 8 months, crawling at 9 months, "cruising" at 10 to 11 months and walking at 12 months.
- Important fine motor accomplishments are the ability to pass an object from one hand to the other (7 months) and a pincer grasp (10 months).
- Important milestones of language development during the first year are differentiating a cry (2 months),

making simple vowel sounds (5 to 6 months) and saying two words besides "ma-ma" and "da-da" (12 months). The more infants are spoken to, the easier it is for them to acquire language.

- Providing infants with proper toys for play helps development. All infant toys need to be checked to be certain they are too large to be aspirated.
- Important milestones of vision development are the ability to follow a moving object past the midline (3 months) and ability to focus securely without eyes crossing (3 months).
- According to Erikson, the developmental task of the infant year is the development of a sense of trust versus mistrust.
- Safety is important. Infants must be protected from falls and aspiration of small objects. A skill an infant cannot accomplish one day, such as crawling, may be accomplished the next.
- Solid food is generally introduced into an infant's diet at 4 to 6 months of age. Before infants can eat solid food, they must lose their extrusion reflex.
- Common concerns related to infant development include teething, thumb-sucking, use of dummies, sleep problems, constipation, colic, nappy dermatitis, baby-bottle syndrome (decayed teeth from sucking on a bottle of formula while they sleep) and obesity. Nurses play a key role in teaching parents about these problems and measures to deal with them.
- Remember that parent-infant attachment is critical to mental health. Urge parents to continue to give as much care as possible to sick infants to maintain this important relationship.

CASE STUDY QUESTIONS

4. Kai was diagnosed with colic. What are common suggestions you could make to his parents to help reduce his discomfort and crying?
5. Kai's mother wants to "childproof" her house. What questions would you ask to assess whether the infant's house is safe for him?
6. Kai's father tells you that he has difficulty feeding Kai solid food because Kai "spits out" everything he tries to get him to eat. How could you help this father?

Resources

For an extensive range of additional resources to enhance teaching and learning and to facilitate understanding of this chapter, please see the text's accompanying website located on thePoint at http://thepoint.lww.com.

References

Australian Association of Maternal Child and Family Health Nurses (AAMCFHN) see Maternal, Child and Family Health Nurses Australia (MCaFHNA).

Bernard, A., et al. (2007). Infant swimming practice, pulmonary epithelium integrity, and the risk of allergic and respiratory diseases later in childhood. *Pediatrics, 119*(6), 1095–1103.

Bishop, W. P. (2011). Oral cavity. In K. J. Marcdante, R. M. Kliegman, H. B. Jenson, et al. (Eds.), *Nelson Essentials of Pediatrics* (6th ed., pp. 475–476). Philadelphia: Saunders/Elsevier.

Bolte, R. (2007). The crying child: Potential causes. What are they trying to tell us? *Contemporary Pediatrics, 24*(5), 74–81.

Carr-Gregg, M. (2014). *Strictly Parenting. Everything you Need to Know about Raising School-age Kids*. Melbourne: Penguin Australia.

Conti, T. D., Patel, M. & Bhat, S. (2011). Breast-feeding and infant nutrition. In J. E. South-Paul, S. C. Matheny & E. L. Lewis (Eds.), *Current Diagnosis & Treatment in Family Medicine* (3rd ed., pp. 28–35). Columbus, OH: McGraw-Hill.

de Amorim Lde, F., Estrela, C., & da Costa, L. R. (2011). Effects of traumatic dental injuries to primary teeth on permanent teeth. *Dental Traumatology, 27*(2), 117–121.

Erikson, E. (1993). *Childhood and Society* (3rd ed.). New York: Norton.

Families New South Wales (2015), accessed 23 February 2015, <www.families.nsw.gov.au>.

Gaffney, K. F., Kitsantas, P. & Cheema, J. (2012). Clinical practice guidelines for feeding behaviors and weight-for-age at 12 months. *Worldviews on Evidence Based Nursing, 9*(4), 234–242.

Gahagan, S. (2011). Crying and colic. In K. J. Marcdante, R. M. Kliegman, H. B. Jenson, et al. (Eds.), *Nelson Essentials of Pediatrics* (6th ed., pp. 45–47). Philadelphia: Saunders/Elsevier.

Goldson, E. & Reynolds, A. (2014). Child development and behavior. In Hay, W. W., et al. (Eds). *Current Pediatric Diagnosis and Treatment* (22nd ed.). Columbus, OH: McGraw-Hill.

Iacovou, M., Ralston, R. A., Muir, J., et al. (2011). Dietary management of infantile colic: A systematic review. *Maternal Child Health Journal, 16*(6), 1319–1331.

Ibrahim, N. G., Wood, J., Margulies, S. S., et al. (2011). Influence of age and fall type on head injuries in infants and toddlers. *International Journal of Development & Neuroscience, 30*(3), 201–206.

Kiran, K., Swati, T., Kamala, B. K., et al. (2011). Prevalence of systemic and local disturbances in infants during primary teeth eruption. *European Journal of Paediatric Dentistry, 12*(4), 249–252.

Klootwijk, T. & Krul, M. (2011). Some concerns remain about the proposed association between swimming and asthma. *American Journal of Respiratory Critical Care Medicine, 184*(12), 1419–1420.

Krebs, N. F. & Primak, L. E. (2011). Pediatric nutrition and nutritional disorders. In K. J. Marcdante, R. M. Kliegman, H. B. Jenson, et al. (Eds.), *Nelson Essentials of Pediatrics* (6th ed., pp. 103–107). Philadelphia: Saunders/Elsevier.

Levine, D. A. (2011). Normal development. In K. J. Marcdante, R. M. Kliegman, H. B. Jenson, et al. (Eds.), *Nelson Essentials of Pediatrics* (6th ed., pp. 16–18). Philadelphia: Saunders/Elsevier.

Lyon, V. B. (2011). Dermatology. In K. J. Marcdante, R. M. Kliegman, H. B. Jenson, et al. (Eds.), *Nelson Essentials of Pediatrics* (6th ed., pp. 713–734). Philadelphia: Saunders/Elsevier.

Maternal, Child and Family Health Nurses Australia (MCaFHNA), (2012), Breastfeeding position statement, accessed 23 February 2015, <www.mcafhna.org.au/Portals/0/PositionStmt-PDF/AAMCFHN%20Breastfeeding%20Position%20Statement.pdf>.

Mehal, J. M., Esposito, D. H., Holman, R. C., et al. (2012). Risk factors for diarrhea-associated infant mortality in the United States, 2005–2007. *Pediatric Infectious Disease Journal, 31*(7), 717–721.

Mesman, J., Oster, H. & Camras, L. (2012). Parental sensitivity to infant distress: What do discrete negative emotions have to do with it? *Attachment & Human Development, 14*(4), 337–348.

Milgrom, P. & Chi, D. L. (2011). Prevention-centered caries management strategies during critical periods in early childhood. *Journal of the California Dental Association, 39*(10), 735–741.

Montaldo, L., Montaldo, P., Cuccaro, P., et al. (2011). Effects of feeding on non-nutritive sucking habits and implications on occlusion in mixed dentition. *International Journal of Paediatric Dentistry, 21*(1), 68–73.

Nelson, A. M. (2012). A comprehensive review of evidence and current recommendations related to pacifier usage. *Journal of Pediatric Nursing, 27*(6), 690–699.

Parsons, H. G., George, M. A. & Innis, S. M. (2011). Growth assessment in clinical practice: Whose growth curve? *Current Gastroenterology Reports, 13*(3), 286–292.

Piaget, J. (1966). *The Origins of Intelligence in Children.* New York: International University Press.

Price, A. M., Wake, M., Ukoumunne, O. C., et al. (2012). Outcomes at six years of age for children with infant sleep problems: Longitudinal community-based study. *Sleep Medicine, 13*(8), 991–998.

Scollan-Koliopoulos, M. & Koliopoulos, J. S. (2010). Evaluation and management of apparent life-threatening events in infants. *Pediatric Nursing, 36*(2), 77–79.

Shergill-Bonner, R. (2010). Infantile colic: Practicalities of management, including dietary aspects. *Journal of Family Health Care, 20*(6), 206–209.

Singer, H. S. (2011). Stereotypic movement disorders. *Handbook of Clinical Neurology, 100*(1), 631–639.

Stevens, B. J., Abbott, L. K., Yamada, J., et al. (2011). Epidemiology and management of painful procedures in children in Canadian hospitals. *Canadian Medical Association Journal, 183*(7), E403–E410.

Taylor, B. J., Heath, A. L., Galland, B. C., et al. (2001), Prevention of Overweight in Infancy (POI.nz) study: A randomised controlled trial of sleep, food and activity interventions for preventing overweight from birth, *BMC Public Health, 11*(1), 942.

Thomas, D. W. & Greer, F. R. (2010). Probiotics and prebiotics in pediatrics. *Pediatrics, 126*(6), 1217–1231.

Townsend, E. & Pitchford, N. J. (2012). Baby knows best? The impact of weaning style on food preferences and body mass index in early childhood in a case-controlled sample. *British Medical Journal, 2*(1), e000298.

van Dijk, M., Hunnius, S. & van Geert, P. (2012). The dynamics of feeding during the introduction to solid food. *Infant Behavior & Development, 35*(2), 226–239.

Victorian Government Department of Education and Early Childhood Development, (2014), *Maternal and child health service guidelines*, accessed 23 February 2015, <www.education.vic.gov.au/Documents/childhood/professionals/health/mchsguidelines.pdf>.

Whitney, E. N. & Rolfes, S. R. (2012). Life cycle nutrition: Infant, childhood & adolescence. In E. N. Whitney & S. R. Rolfes, *Understanding Nutrition* (pp. 528–573). Belmont, CA: Wadsworth Publishing.

Wilken, M. (2012). The impact of child tube feeding on maternal emotional state and identity: A qualitative meta-analysis. *Journal of Pediatric Nursing, 27*(3), 248–255.

Suggested readings

Kramer, M. S. & Kakuma, R. (2009). Optimal duration of exclusive breastfeeding. *Cochrane Database of Systematic Reviews,* (1), CD003517.

Morin, K. H. (2008). Oral health: Getting off to a good start. *MCN: The American Journal of Maternal/Child Nursing, 33*(1), 58.

Plunket <www.plunket.org.nz/>.

Tresillian <www.tresillian.net>.

Underdown, A., et al. (2009). Massage intervention for promoting mental and physical health in infants aged under six months. *Cochrane Database of Systematic Reviews,* (1), CD005038.

Chapter 30

Nursing care of a family with a toddler

The previous chapter discussed the growth and development of infants and abilities infants develop in the first year. This chapter adds information about the dramatic changes, both physical and psychosocial, that occur during the toddler years. These changes form the basis for care and health teaching for this age group.

LEARNING OBJECTIVES

After studying the contents of this chapter, you should be able to:

1. Describe and assess normal growth and development of a toddler as well as common parental concerns.
2. Use critical thinking to analyse methods of care for toddlers to be certain care is family-centred.
3. Formulate nursing considerations related to toddler growth and development or parental concerns regarding growth and development.
4. Identify expected outcomes for nursing care of a toddler.
5. Plan nursing care to meet a toddler's growth and development needs, such as anticipatory guidance to prevent problems such as sleep disturbances.
6. Implement nursing care to promote normal growth and development of a toddler, such as discussing toddler developmental milestones with parents.
7. Evaluate expected outcomes for achievement and effectiveness of care.
8. Identify areas related to care of a toddler that could benefit from additional nursing research or application of evidence-based practice.
9. Integrate knowledge of toddler growth and development with nursing process to achieve quality child and family health nursing care.

KEY TERMS

- autonomy
- discipline
- lordosis
- parallel play
- punishment

CASE STUDY

Angus is a 2½-year-old boy you see at a paediatric clinic. His parents, Chris and Ella, tell you he has changed completely in the past 6 months from an easy-to-care-for baby into a "monster" who refuses to do anything they ask. The only word he says anymore is "no". He has a tantrum every night at dinner over some type of food. They tell you this has changed parenting from "fun" to "a real chore".

CASE STUDY QUESTION

1. What advice could you give Angus' parents to help them regain a positive view of parenting?

During the toddler period (ages 1 to 3 years), vast changes take place in a child and, consequently, in a family. During this period, children accomplish a wide array of developmental tasks and change from largely immobile and preverbal infants who are dependent on carers for the fulfilment of most needs to walking, talking young children with a growing sense of **autonomy** (independence). To match this growth, parents must also change during this period. Healthy children and families are constantly being challenged by the process of normal development, therefore parents often have questions about how to guide their child in different situations and how to cope with special needs and concerns relevant to this age.

HEALTHY DEVELOPMENT OF A TODDLER

Assessment

Assessment of the toddler involves completing a health history and performing a physical and developmental evaluation (refer to Chapter 34 for details). Asking parents about a toddler's ability to carry out activities of daily living offers not only assessment information on the child's developmental progress but also important clues about the child–parent relationship. Parents see their children daily and are the best source of information when a child seems to be acting "out of sorts" or "different" (a typical sign a child may not be feeling well).

Acknowledging parents' expertise facilitates a partnership approach to nursing practice (Davis, 2010). To improve outcomes for children and families, nurses should incorporate additional partnership qualities such as shared decision making and responsibility, mutual trust and respect, open communication and negotiation (Davis, 2010; Hopwood et al., 2013). Refer to Chapter 1 for details on this strengths-based approach and Chapter 35 for information on effective communication strategies for children and families. Cultural considerations are discussed in Chapter 2.

During the assessment, the toddler's weight, height and head circumference are assessed according to standard growth charts (see Appendix B and Chapter 34 for details). It is essential to note that these growth charts are based on averages of Caucasian Australian or New Zealand children and may not reflect normal growth in other ethnic backgrounds.

Nursing considerations

Nursing considerations for toddlers are often related to normal growth and development or safety issues. Examples are:

- Health-seeking behaviours related to normal toddler development
- Methods of toilet training
- Risk of injury related to impulsiveness of the toddler
- Interrupted family process related to the need for close supervision of toddlers
- Family coping related to parents' ability to adjust to new needs of the toddler
- Awareness of poison prevention
- Disturbed sleep pattern related to lack of bedtime routine.

Support parents with concerns during the toddler period using a partnership approach. Assist parents to establish realistic goals and outcomes so they can meet the rapidly-changing needs of their toddler and learn to cope with typical toddler behaviours. Parents may expect too much of a toddler and become frustrated, instead of enjoying being a parent of a child this age. Helpful parent websites about growth and development, including multicultural resources are: the Raising Children Network <http://raisingchildren.net.au/>; BabyCenter Australia <www.babycenter.com.au>; Kidspot Australia <www.kidspot.com.au>; Well Child <www.wellchild.org.nz>; and Kids Health NZ <www.kidshealth.org.nz>. When teaching parents about typical toddler behaviour, a good rule is to think of a toddler as a visitor from a foreign land who wants to participate in everything the family is doing but does not know the customs or the language. Parents need to help their toddler learn these, the same way that they would for a stranger.

Assist parents with current problems but also discuss methods for resolving similar situations that may arise in the future. It is important for parents to learn methods that can be applied throughout their child's growing years, as they may "win battles but lose wars". For instance, parents may find that promising children a treat when they are in the middle of a tantrum will stop the tantrum, but it will not prevent other tantrums from occurring in the future (and, in fact, may encourage them). Help parents to explore healthy coping techniques and model effective communication skills when interacting with their toddler.

Expected outcomes must be evaluated frequently during the toddler period because children change so much and learn so many new skills during this time that their abilities and associated parental concerns can change from day to day. Examples of expected outcomes are:

- Parents state child maintains a consistent bedtime routine within the next 2 weeks.
- Parents state they have childproofed their home by putting a lock on kitchen cupboards by the next clinic visit.

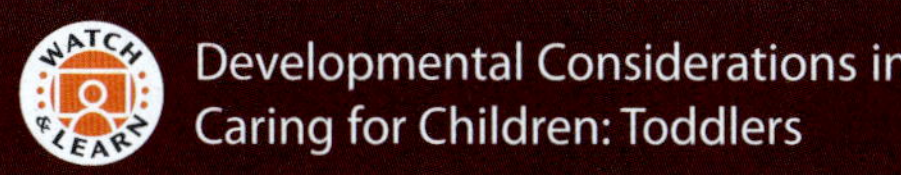

Developmental Considerations in Caring for Children: Toddlers

GROWTH AND DEVELOPMENT OF A TODDLER

Assessing the growth and development of toddlers includes evaluating physical, developmental, emotional and cognitive aspects.

Physical growth

The toddler's weight, height and head circumference are documented on a standard growth chart at each health-care visit to determine if progress is normal for that particular child (see Appendix B). Although toddlers are making great strides developmentally during this stage, their physical growth begins to slow. Height and weight increase in a step-like manner rather than a linear progression that reflects the growth spurts and lags common in toddlerhood (Lewis & Foley, 2014).

A change in body contour is evident, as toddlers tend to have a prominent abdomen (see Fig. 30.1A). Although they are walking well, their abdominal muscles are not yet strong enough to support abdominal contents as well as they will later. They also have a forward curve of the spine at the sacral area (**lordosis**). As they become more experienced at walking, this will correct itself naturally. In addition, many toddlers waddle or walk with a wide stance. This stance seems to increase the lordotic curve, but it keeps them on their feet (see Fig. 30.1B).

Weight, height, head circumference

A toddler gains about 2.5 kg and grows approximately 12 cm a year, which is much less than the rate of infant growth. As subcutaneous tissue, or baby fat, begins to disappear towards the end of the second year, the child changes from a plump baby into a leaner, more muscular little girl or boy (see Box 30.1). Head circumference increases by about 2 cm during the second year and between the ages of 12 and 18 months the anterior fontanel closes and skull growth begins to slow.

Body systems

During the toddler years the cardiopulmonary system stabilises; the heart and respiratory rates slow and blood pressure increases (Crisp et al., 2012). Typical vital signs for a toddler can be found in Appendix G.

Teeth

Eight new teeth (the canines and the first molars) erupt during the second year. Lower teeth usually erupt before the upper teeth and females often develop earlier than males (Dental Health Services Victoria, 2010). A full set of deciduous (baby) teeth is usually present by 3 years of age

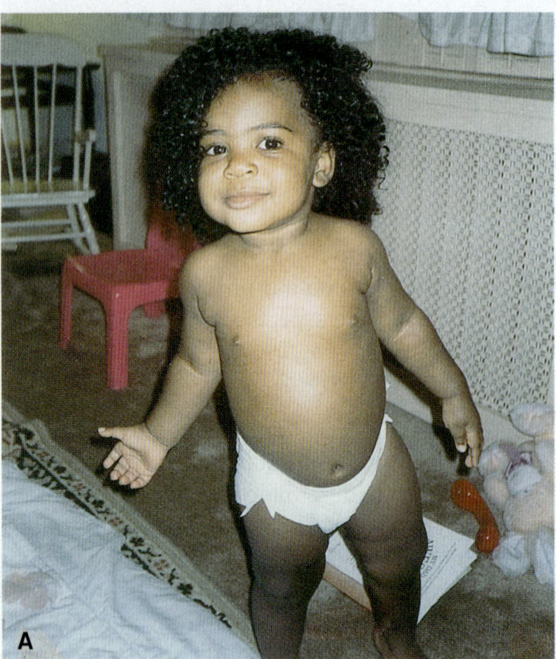

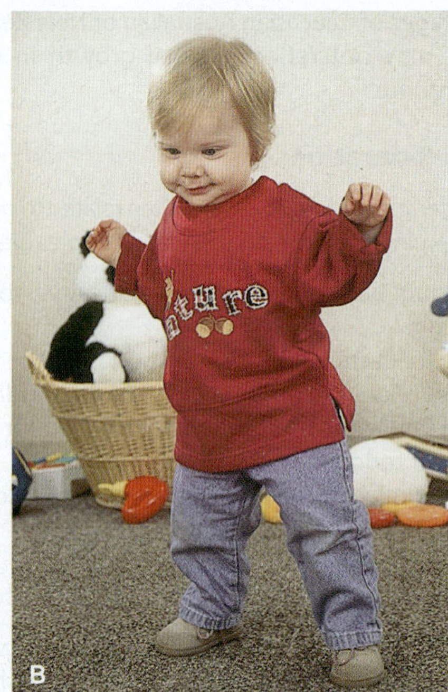

FIGURE 30.1 Physical characteristics of toddlers. (**A**) Toddlers typically have a prominent abdomen. (**B**) Toddlers typically walk with an unsteady gait for better stability.

(Dental Health Services Victoria, 2010). Dental care will be discussed later in this chapter.

Developmental milestones

The developmental milestones of the toddler years are less numerous but no less dramatic than those of the infant year, because this is a period of slow and steady, not sudden, growth. Toddler development is influenced to some extent by the amount of social contact and the number of opportunities children have to explore and experience new degrees of independence. Differences are observed between the sexes and different cultures (Onis, 2006). It is also strongly influenced by individual readiness for a new skill. Table 30.1 highlights growth and developmental milestones of gross and fine motor, language and play development of the toddler years. The Denver Developmental Screening Test (Appendix C) is a useful tool to assess developmental milestones.

> **BOX 30.1 Assessment ✻ Assessing the average toddler**
>
> Speaks in two-word sentences
>
> 20 deciduous teeth present at 2.5 years
>
> Heart rate: 90 to 110 bpm
>
> "Pouchy" abdomen from weak abdominal muscles
>
> Chest cirumference becomes bigger than head circumference at 2 years
>
> Noticeable lordosis
>
> "Baby fat" begins to disappear
>
> Wide-based gait

Language development

Toddlerhood is a critical time for language development, although even this varies among children, because to master language, children need to practise. A child who is 2 years old and does not talk in two-word, noun–verb simple sentences needs a careful assessment to determine the cause. However, a delay in language may only be a temporary setback in development.

A word that is used frequently by toddlers and is a manifestation of their developing autonomy is "no". Toddlers may use the word to mean they are refusing a task, or they do not understand it, or they may only be practising a sound that they have noticed has potent effects on those around them. To learn other words, children need exposure to conversation and need to be read to often. Language develops most quickly if parents respect what toddlers have to say so children grasp the use and purpose of language.

Urge parents to encourage language development by naming objects as they play with their child ("ball", "block",

TABLE 30.1 Milestones of toddler growth and development

Age (months)	Fine motor	Gross motor	Language	Play
15	Puts small pellets into small bottles. Scribbles voluntarily with a pencil or crayon. Holds a spoon well but may still turn it upside down on the way to mouth	Walks alone well; can seat self in chair; can crawl upstairs	4–6 words	Can stack 2 blocks; enjoys being read to; drops toys for adult to recover (exploring sense of permanence)
18	No longer rotates a spoon to bring it to mouth	Can run and jump in place. Can walk up and down stairs holding onto a person's hand or railing. Typically places both feet on one step before advancing	7–20 words, uses jargoning; names 1 body part	Imitates household chores, dusting, etc.; begins parallel play (playing beside not with another child)
24	Can open doors by turning doorknobs, unscrews lids	Walks up stairs alone still using both feet on same step at same time	50 words, 2-word sentences (noun-pronoun and verb), such as "Daddy go", "me come"	Parallel play evident
30	Makes simple lines or strokes for crosses with a pencil	Can jump down from chairs	Verbal language increasing steadily. Knows full name; can name one colour and holds up fingers to show age	Spends time playing house, imitating parents' actions; play is "rough-housing" or active

"music box", "doll") or when they give their toddler something ("Here is your drink of water", "Let's put on these pyjamas" and so on). This helps children grasp the fact that words are not meaningless sounds; they apply to people and objects and have uses. Always answering a child's questions is another good way to do this. Be sure answers for toddlers are simple and brief because they have such a short attention span.

Some toddlers do not develop language readily because they are not called on to use it. When they point at an object, someone hands it to them; when they climb into their highchair, someone places a meal in front of them. In other families, an older child may speak for a younger one. Children should not be made to name an object before they can have it (because their vocabulary is so limited, the objects they could have would be restricted to 10 or fewer), but parents can reinforce language by rewording a question; for example, "Would you like the ball?" Reading aloud strengthens vocabulary in the same way. Reading the exact words in a book is not as important to toddlers as pointing to the pictures that accompany them. For example, Jane threw the ball ("See Jane throwing the ball?").

Children who are very active may use fewer words than children who are less active. Active children are too busy doing things to describe what they are doing or too busy obtaining objects to need to ask for many things. Such children probably have a large unexpressed vocabulary, however, or understand more words (comprehensive vocabulary) than can be expressed (expressive vocabulary).

Because children learn language from imitating what they hear, they will speak like those around them. If they are spoken to in baby talk, their enunciation of words can be poor; if they hear examples of bad grammar, they will not use good grammar. Remind parents that pronouns are difficult for children to use correctly; many children are 3½ or 4 years of age before they can separate the different uses of "I", "me", "him" and "her". Bilingual children interchange words from both languages. If language development is not progressing as expected, an assessment can be conducted to detect speech and hearing problems (refer to Chapter 34).

✔ *Checkpoint question 30.1*

Kathy is concerned about her daughter Lilly. Her husband only speaks to Lilly in Japanese, while Kathy speaks English. Kathy is worried that Lilly will become confused. How would you respond to Kathy's concerns?

Emotional development

Children change a great deal in their ability to understand the world and how they relate to people during the toddler years.

Autonomy

The developmental task of the toddler years according to Erikson (1993) is the development of a sense of autonomy versus shame or doubt. Children who have learned to trust themselves and others during the infant year are better prepared to do this than those who cannot trust themselves or others.

To develop a sense of autonomy is to develop a sense of independence. A healthy level of autonomy is achieved when parents are able to encourage independence while still maintaining consistently sound rules for safety. Children who are constantly told not to try things because they will hurt themselves may be left with a stronger sense of doubt than confidence at the end of the toddler period. Children who are made to feel it is wrong to be independent may leave the toddler period with a stronger sense of shame than autonomy.

Infants appear to have difficulty differentiating between their bodies and those of others; they think of their bodies as extensions of their parents' or their primary carers'. When infants approach toddlerhood, they begin to make the differentiation. As they recognise they are separate individuals, they also realise they do not always have to do what others want them to do. From this realisation comes the reputation toddlers have for being negative, obstinate and difficult to manage. A toddler's refusal to accept help putting on shoes may be seen as disobedience, whereas children may view this as insisting on performing a task they can do independently—a positive expression of autonomy.

Socialisation

Once toddlers are walking well, they become resistant to sitting in laps and being cuddled. This is not lack of a desire for socialisation but a function of being independent. At 15 months, children are still enthusiastic about interacting with people, provided those people are willing to follow them where they want to go. By 18 months, toddlers imitate the things they see a parent doing, such as "study" or "sweep", so they seek out parents to observe and initiate interactions. By 2 or more years, children become aware of gender differences and may point to other children and identify them as "boy" or "girl".

Play behaviour

During the toddler period, children play beside other children, next to them, not with them. This side-by-side play (called **parallel play**) is not unfriendly but is a normal developmental sequence that occurs during the toddler period (see Fig. 30.2). Toddlers who have an aggressive personality probably have the most difficulty adapting to play groups.

The toys toddlers enjoy most are those they can play with by themselves and that require action. Trucks they can make go, squeaky frogs they can squeeze, waddling ducks they can pull, rocking horses they can ride, pegs they can pound, blocks they can stack and a toy telephone they can talk into are all favourites. These are toys children can control, giving them a sense of power in manipulation, an expression of autonomy. At 15 months, children are still in a put-in, take-out stage, so they continue to enjoy stacks of boxes or balls that fit inside each other (see Fig. 30.3). They enjoy throwing toys out of a playpen or from a highchair tray as long as someone will pick them up and return them again and again.

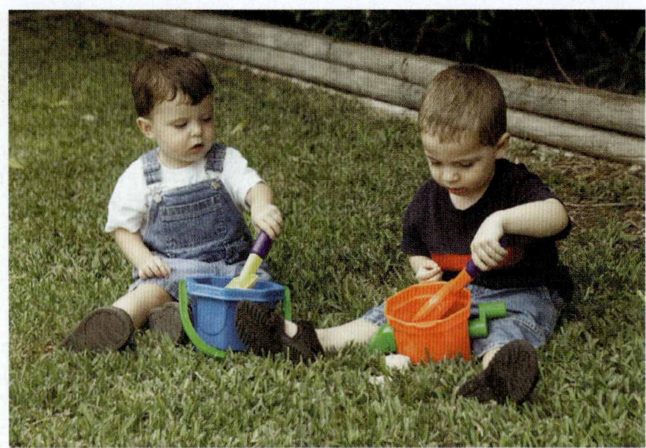

FIGURE 30.2 Parallel play. The toddler usually plays alongside another child rather than cooperatively. (Lewis, P. & Foley, D. (2014). *Health Assessment in Nursing*. Sydney: Lippincott Williams & Wilkins.)

The 18-month-old child is walking securely enough to enjoy pull toys. Toys should be strong enough to take a great deal of abuse, because there are many things in the world toddlers do not recognise or know about and so often toddlers use toys differently to the way they were intended to be used. For example, a toddler picks a stuffed toy up by the tail and swings it, or pulls at it. There is no need for parents to correct children about the way they are using a toy as long as it appears to give satisfaction. If toddlers find a toy frustrating because they are holding or using it incorrectly, showing them the right way will ease frustration.

By the age of 2, when toddlers begin to spend time imitating adult actions in their play such as wrapping a doll and putting it to bed, "setting the table" or "driving the car", they begin to use fewer toys than before. The act of imitating has become their play. By the end of the toddler period, both boys and girls begin to like rough-housing and spend at least part of every day in this very active, stimulating type of play.

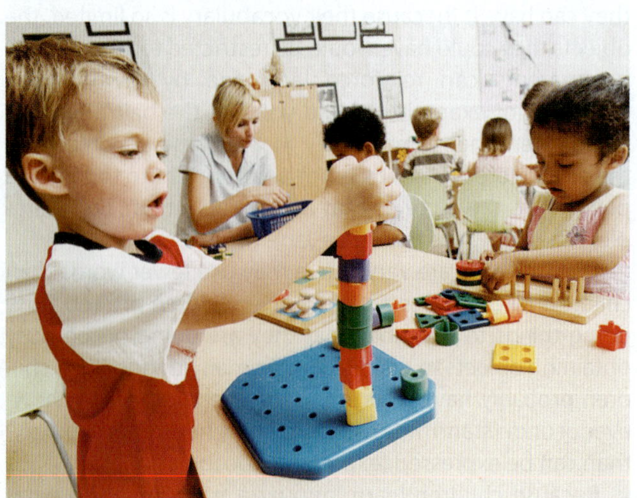

FIGURE 30.3 Toddlers enjoy toys that they can manipulate.

BOX 30.2 ✻ Focus on evidence-based practice

Structured task versus free play

A US study explored parenting quality, children's engagement, play behaviours and parent–child language. Comparisons were made between mothers and fathers, and structured tasks versus free play. Sixty, predominately middle-class, two-parent families with toddlers participated in the study. Families were observed and video recorded during two 15-minute sessions including mother–child and father–child interaction (5 minutes free play, 5 minutes structured play and 5 minutes clean-up time). Analysis of these interactions revealed that free play rather than structured play was associated with increased engagement in child–parent interactions, play and language use. During free play, both parents used higher levels of cognition, less negative parenting and more complex language when interacting with their toddler. In conclusion, supportive, responsive adult–child interactions increase engagement and should be included in early childhood settings.

How could you apply this research to your nursing practice?

Source: Kwon, K., Bingham, G., Lewsader, J., Jeon, H. & Elicker, J. (2013). Structured Task Versus Free Play: The Influence of Social Context on Parenting Quality, Toddlers' Engagement with Parents and Play Behaviors, and Parent–Toddler Language Use. *Child Youth Care Forum, 42,* 207–224.

Researchers have highlighted the importance of father–child relationships and rough and tumble play for cognitive, social and emotional development of children (Fletcher, St George & Freeman, 2012; see also Box 30.2 and Fig. 30.4). Encouraging parents to schedule this type of play outdoors, where vases or other prized possessions cannot be broken, makes it more acceptable. A child who feels a need for active play is unable to sit down and eat, fall asleep or play quiet games so may be described as "trouble". Because of this rough activity, most toddlers have at least one bruise on their legs at all times from tripping over their feet while trying to run too fast or jumping or bumping into a chair.

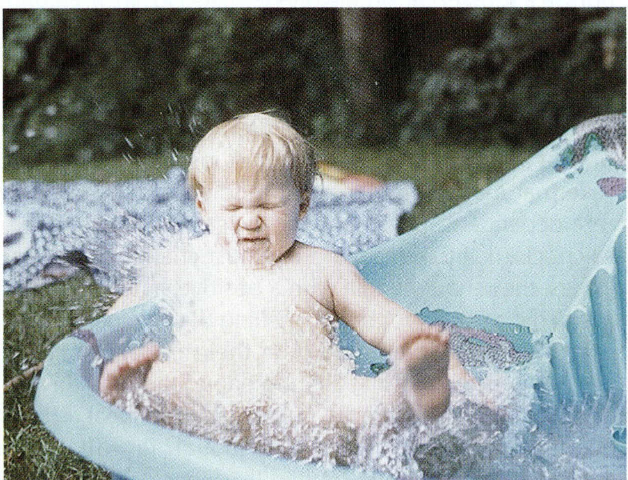

FIGURE 30.4 Toddlers usually enjoy rough-and-tumble play.

✔ Checkpoint question 30.2

Stacy says she doesn't like her husband wrestling with her 2-year-old-son, Toby, as it seems to make him more energetic and difficult to settle. How would you respond to her concerns?

HEALTH PROMOTION FOR A TODDLER AND FAMILY

Toddlers tend to develop many upper respiratory and ear infections but otherwise come to healthcare facilities most often for immunisations (refer to Chapter 34 for the immunisation schedule). These visits allow you to focus on health promotion and early detection of growth and developmental delays. It also provides the opportunity to support parents through the normal crises of the toddler period.

Promoting toddler safety

Accidents are the major cause of death in children of all ages. Accidental ingestions (poisoning) are the type of accident that occurs most frequently in toddlers (AIHW: Pointer, 2014). Although poisoning can involve medicine such as paracetamol, it most often occurs from ingestion of cleaning products. Aspiration or ingestion of small objects such as watch or hearing aid batteries, pencil erasers or crayons is also a major danger for children of this age (AIHW: Pointer, 2014). Urge parents to childproof their home by putting all poisonous products, medications and small objects out of reach by the time their infant is crawling and certainly by the time their infant is walking (Kidsafe: Child Accident Prevention Foundation, 2013).

Other accidents that occur frequently in toddlers include motor vehicle accidents, burns, falls, drowning and playground injuries. These occur because toddlers' motor ability develops ahead of their judgement. To prevent serious injury, a toddler must be supervised at all times. Toddlers can walk fast enough so that if they are left outside to play, they can very quickly travel a block away. Due to lack of judgement concerning moving vehicles, they walk across streets with no regard for oncoming cars. Backyard pools need to be securely fenced as per Australian state government legislation (check state government websites) or in New Zealand by the Fencing of Swimming Pools Act 1987 (New Zealand Government, 1987).

All states of Australia and New Zealand require babies, toddlers and children to be in an age-weight- and height-appropriate child restraint until the age of 7 when travelling in motor vehicles (check state government websites and the New Zealand government website for details). Helmets are required by law for bike or tricycle riding both in Australia and New Zealand. New Zealand has a national law for helmets, whereas helmets are legislated state-by-state in Australia.

As soon as babies and toddlers start to climb out of their cot, consider moving them to a bed to prevent falls. A safety gate on the door of the room is another way to keep a toddler contained and safe. As the child reaches 2 years of age and begins to imitate housework or repairing a car, parents must be sure the child does not use real cleaning compounds or sharp tools. Refer to Box 30.3 for suggested safety measures to prevent injuries.

CASE STUDY QUESTION

2. Angus' parents are having problems with his behaviour while in the car. He often refuses to let them fasten his car seat and screams and kicks for long periods of time. Yesterday he unfastened his car seat while they were driving. How would you approach this safety issue with his parents?

Promoting nutritional health of a toddler

Growth slows abruptly after the first year of life, therefore a toddler's appetite is smaller than an infant's. Children who ate hungrily 2 months earlier may sit and play with their food. If feeding problems begin at this time, it is often because parents are unaware that their toddler's appetite has decreased and food consumption will be less. The amount of food eaten daily varies from one child to another. A suggestion for parents is to place a small amount of food on the plate and allow their child to eat it and ask for more, rather than serve a large portion that the child cannot finish. It is important to educate parents that this decline in food intake will occur, so they will not be concerned when it happens.

Allowing self-feeding is a major way to strengthen independence in a toddler. Toddlers often want to feed themselves and generally will resist eating if a parent insists on feeding them. Nutritious finger foods that toddlers enjoy include pieces of chicken, slices of banana, pieces of cheese and crackers. Many toddlers prefer to eat the same type of food over and over again because of the sense of security this offers. However, it is important to offer new foods to provide a variety of nutrients in the diet (National Health and Medical Research Council, 2013). Toddlers typically need three small main meals a day and small healthy snacks in between (National Health and Medical Research Council, 2013; Ministry of Health, 2013). Encourage parents to offer fruit or protein foods for snacks rather than high-carbohydrate items such as biscuits, not only for the nutrition involved but also because protein snacks help prevent dental caries more than sugar snacks, by limiting exposure of the child's teeth to carbohydrates. Toddlers may not like food that is "mixed up" such as casseroles (except maybe spaghetti); they often prefer that different foods do not touch one another on their plate. Frequently they eat all of one item before going on to another.

Toddler nutrition

Parents may become frustrated when trying to provide adequate nutrition for their toddler due to their varying and unpredictable appetite and food preferences. Although a toddler's daily food consumption may vary greatly, energy needs are generally met when sufficient food is supplied in a positive environment.

Healthy eating guidelines can be found at the following web links:

- <www.eatforhealth.gov.au/sites/default/files/files/the_guidelines/n55_australian_dietary_guidelines.pdf>
- <www.nutritionfoundation.org.nz/nutrition-facts/healthy-eating-for-all-ages>
- <www.health.govt.nz/our-work/preventative-health-wellness/nutrition/food-and-nutrition-guidelines>.

Refer to Chapter 2 for nutritional cultural considerations. See also Appendices E and F for serving sizes and healthy eating guidelines for children.

Promoting toddler development in daily activities

A toddler's new independence and developing abilities in self-care, such as dressing, eating and, to a limited extent, hygiene, present special challenges for parents. Learning how to promote autonomy yet maintain a safe, healthy environment should be a major goal for the family.

Dressing

By the end of the toddler period, most children can put on their own socks, underpants and singlet. Some may also be able to pull on trousers, jumpers (the sleeves of a shirt often confuse a toddler) or simple dresses (see Fig. 30.5). Parents may be reluctant to encourage toddlers to dress themselves, as it is often easier and quicker to put their clothes on for them. Encourage parents to support the child's developing sense of autonomy. If children end up with underpants or a shirt on backwards in most instances it does not make that much difference and toddlers are not likely to feel independent and confident if their attempts at dressing are criticised. If parents feel they must change the child's clothes, they should begin with a positive statement, such as "you did a good job", before making the change.

As soon as children are up on their feet and walking, they need shoe soles that are firm enough to provide protection from rough surfaces. Sneakers are an ideal toddler shoe because the soles are hard enough for rough surfaces and arch support is limited (to allow for developing toddler arches).

BOX 30.3 * Focus on family teaching

Common safety measures to prevent accidents during the toddler years

Q. Angus' parents tell you, "Our toddler is constantly on the go. How can we keep him safe?"

A. Accident prevention must be ongoing while your child is a toddler. Try the following precautions:

Potential accident	Prevention measure
Motor vehicles	Maintain child in car seat; do not be distracted from safe driving by a child in the car. Do not allow child to play outside unsupervised. Do not allow child to operate electronic garage doors. Supervise toddler who is too young to be left alone on a tricycle. Teach safety with pedalling toys (look before crossing driveways; do not cross streets) but do not expect that toddler will obey these rules at all times (in other words, stay close by).
Falls	Keep house windows closed or keep secure screens in place. Place gates at top and bottom of stairs. Supervise at playgrounds. Do not allow child to walk with sharp object in hand or mouth. Raise cot rails and check to make sure they are locked before walking away from cot.
Aspiration	Examine toys for small parts that could be aspirated; remove toys that appear dangerous. Do not feed toddler popcorn, peanuts etc.; urge children not to eat while running. Do not leave toddler alone with a balloon.
Drowning	Do not leave toddler alone in a bath or near water (including buckets of cleaning water and washing machines).
Animal bites	Do not allow toddler to approach strange dogs. Supervise child's play with family pets.
Poisoning	Never present medication as lollies. Buy medications with childproof caps; put away immediately after use. Never take medication in front of child. Place all medications and poisons in locked cabinets or overhead shelves where child cannot reach them. Never leave medication in a bag or pocket, where child can reach it. Always store foods and substances in their original containers. Know the names of house plants and find out if they are poisonous. (Call state or national poisons information centre.) Hang plants or set them on high surfaces beyond toddler's grasp. Be certain that small batteries or magnets are out of reach. Post telephone number of the local poison information centre by the telephone (13 11 26 in Australia; 0800 764 766 in New Zealand). Inspect toys to be certain they are free of lead-based paint.
Burns	Buy flame-retardant clothing. Cook on the back burners of the stove if possible and turn handles of pots towards back of stove to prevent toddler from reaching up and pulling them down. Use cool-mist vaporiser rather than steam vaporiser or remain in room when vaporiser is operating so child is not tempted to play with it. Keep screen in front of fireplace or heater. Monitor toddlers carefully when they are near lit candles. Do not leave toddlers unsupervised near hot-water taps. Check temperature setting for hot-water heater and turn down thermostat if it is over 52°C. Do not leave coffee/tea cups on a table where child can reach them. Never drink hot beverages when a child is sitting on your lap or playing within reach. Do not allow toddlers to blow out matches (teach that fire is not fun); store matches out of reach. Keep electric wires and cords out of toddler's reach; cover electrical outlets with safety plugs.
General	Know whereabouts of toddlers at all times. Toddlers can climb onto chairs, stools etc. they could not manage before; can turn door knobs and go places they could not go before. Be aware that the frequency of accidents increases when the family is under stress and therefore less attentive to children. Special precautions must be taken at these times. Be aware some children are more active, curious and impulsive and therefore more vulnerable to accidents than others.

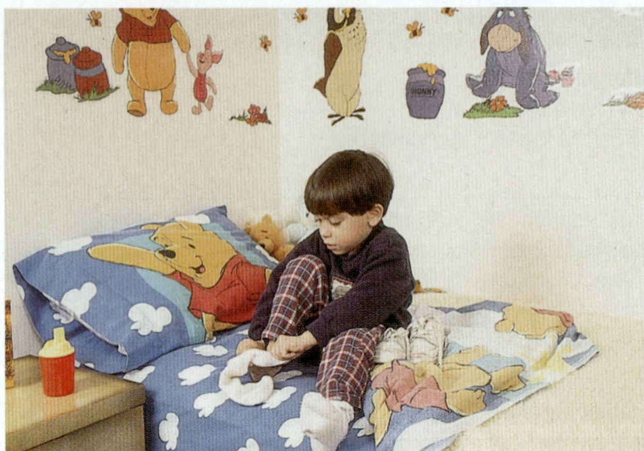

FIGURE 30.5 Getting dressed by himself is a fun morning activity for this older toddler.

Sleep

The amount of sleep children need gradually decreases as they grow older (Teng et al., 2012). They may begin the toddler period napping twice a day and sleeping 12 hours each night and end it with one nap a day and only 8 hours' sleep at night. Parents who are not aware that the need for sleep declines at this time may view a child's disinterest in sleeping as a problem. If a child cannot fall asleep at night, it may be time to omit or shorten an afternoon nap. If a child is so short-tempered at dinnertime that eating is impossible, perhaps the child needs two naps a day. Some common sleeping problems for toddlers include separation anxiety and nightmares (Tresillian, 2014). Helpful resources can be found at <www.tresillian.net>.

Toddlers may resist naptime due to their developing independence. Parents might minimise this by including a nap as part of a lunchtime routine, not as a separate activity: the child always goes from the table directly to bed. The parent can state simply, "It's naptime now" and then give a secondary choice: "Do you want to sleep with your teddy bear or your rag doll?" Towards the end of the toddler period, when children are ready to omit their afternoon naps, they may still be agreeable to a "shoes-off" or quiet-play period until they begin to attend school full-time.

As with any other activity in this period, a toddler loves a bedtime routine: bath, pyjamas, a story, brushing teeth, being tucked into bed, having a drink of water, choosing a toy to sleep with and turning out the lights. Parents must be careful, however, not to let a child manoeuvre them into such a long procedure that sleep is delayed considerably past the time initially set.

Many toddlers are ready to be moved out of a cot into a bed by the end of the toddler period. Remind parents to stress that sleeping in a regular bed does not give children the right to get in and out of bed as they choose. Some toddlers do well if they are allowed to sleep in a regular bed and a safety gate is placed across the door to their room. This arrangement gives them a feeling of independence but still keeps them safe. When first moved to a bed without side rails, many children are found sleeping on the floor of the room in the morning. There is no harm in this unless it is cold or drafty. Dressing the child in warm pyjamas or putting a blanket on the floor might be solutions to help parents accept this.

Bathing

The time for a toddler's bath should depend on the parents' and the child's wishes and schedule. Some parents prefer to bathe a toddler before the evening meal because it has a quieting effect and prepares a child for eating; others prefer to give it at bedtime because it has a relaxing effect and helps a child sleep. The time, however, is not as important as the attempt to establish a sense of routine, a sense that life has order. Learning to be independent is sometimes frightening and there is security in knowing certain events are predictable.

Toddlers usually enjoy bath time and parents should make an effort to make it fun by providing a toy, such as a rubber duck, boat or plastic fish. Bath time is usually so enjoyable for toddlers that parents can use it as a recreational activity or something to do on a rainy day when they can find nothing else to interest their child. Remind parents that although toddlers can sit well in a bath, it is still not safe to leave them alone unsupervised due to risk of drowning or burns.

Care of teeth

Parents should brush their toddler's teeth using a small, soft toothbrush and add low-fluoride (400–550 ppm) toothpaste from the age of 18 months (Dental Health Services Victoria, 2010). Towards the end of the toddler period, children can begin to do the brushing themselves under supervision (all children need some supervision until about the age of 8). In addition, children should drink fluoridated water, if it is available, to prevent tooth decay (Rugg-Gunn & Do, 2012). Calcium-rich foods such as milk, cheese and yoghurt are also important for the development of strong teeth and are good snack choices.

Early exposure, at approximately 2 years of age, to an oral health professional is important to prevent oral disease and encourage a positive view of dental health (Dental Health Services Victoria, 2010). Parents can prepare their child by reading a story about a dentist visit, sitting the child on their knee while the dentist checks the toddler's teeth and answering their child's questions honestly without going into too much detail. Children rarely have cavities at this age, therefore the visit is usually painless and sets a positive stage for future dental appointments. The Australian Dental Association website <www.babyteeth.com.au> has useful information sheets for parents.

Some dental issues that may arise for parents during this stage include thumb sucking or dummy use, transitioning from a bottle to a cup and nutrition. Thumb sucking often stops before the age of 4 years and does not usually cause long-term dental problems (Dental Health Services Victoria, 2010). Dummies should not be dipped in any foods or liquids and use should be gradually decreased (Dental Health Services Victoria, 2010). Toddlers should be encouraged to drink from a cup rather than a bottle. Water should be given as the preferred drink and avoidance of regular high-sugar or acidic foods is encouraged to prevent dental caries (Dental Health Services Victoria, 2010).

✔ *Checkpoint question 30.3*

Steven and Susan usually give their 2-year-old daughter a bottle of milk when they put her to bed, as it is the only way she will fall asleep. Would this practice have implications for dental health?

Promoting healthy family functioning

Learning self-reliance is the primary goal of a child during the toddler period. Parents who enjoyed caring for their child as an infant may find it difficult to have their authority challenged by a toddler. Assist parents to understand that their responses to these attempts at independence are crucial to the healthy development of their child. Although the child still needs firm limits to feel secure, a child must be given some room to make independent decisions in areas that the parents feel they do not need to control. An outside person, such as a nurse, can provide an important perspective on this issue.

If parents punish children excessively at each move towards independence, children will not fight them indefinitely. Instead, they will begin to feel guilty for wanting to do things independently. Adults without a sense of autonomy feel this way about independent thought. They may follow orders well, but when the job calls for a new program or function, they cannot reach into unknown areas without a great deal of consultation and help.

You may need to caution some parents not to begin to function at the same level as their toddler. An easy reaction to a toddler's refusal to allow a parent to help is, "You won't let me help you with this, so I won't do anything for you". This is a defence mechanism that prevents parents from feeling rejected. Explain to parents that refusing to accept help is not refusing to accept love. Refusing to let mother put on a shoe is an instance of refusing to let mother put on a shoe, nothing more.

At bedtime, naptime or anytime they are tired, toddlers may become much more like their old selves, wanting to sit on a parent's lap and be rocked or picked up and carried. This does not signal babyish behaviour or regression in a toddler; it is a natural transition between infant and preschool ages.

Parental concerns associated with the toddler period

Parental concerns during the toddler period often arise because of conflict over autonomy. The Parents' Evaluation of Developmental Status (PEDS) screening tool (see Appendix D) provides practitioners with a platform to discuss parental concerns about toddler behaviour and development. It can be used as a developmental screen with children from birth to 8 years. The tool comprises four components: a Brief Administration and Scoring Guide, a Response Form, a Score Form and an Interpretation Form. The parent completes the 10-item questionnaire Response Form and this is then scored and interpreted by the practitioner using the Score and Interpretation Forms. Using the PEDS tool it is possible to identify concerns that may predict problems at a particular time in a child's development. Thus, skilful application of the tool supports the early detection of developmental and behavioural concerns in babies and children. More information can be found at <www.peds.org.au>.

Toilet training

Toilet training is an important aspect of toddler development and is an individualised task for each child. It should begin and be completed according to a child's ability to accomplish it, not according to a set schedule (see Fig. 30.6). Box 30.4 has parental information on toilet training.

In Australia and New Zealand, toilet training is usually introduced during the toddler period. Like so many other aspects of childrearing, the time parents begin these activities is culturally determined. Praise is used in Australia and New Zealand as a common means of encouraging toddlers to learn new tasks; other small rewards such as a sticker on a chart or in a book may also be appropriate.

Before children can begin toilet training, they must have reached three important developmental levels, one physiological and two cognitive:

- They must have control of rectal and urethral sphincters, usually achieved at the time they walk well.

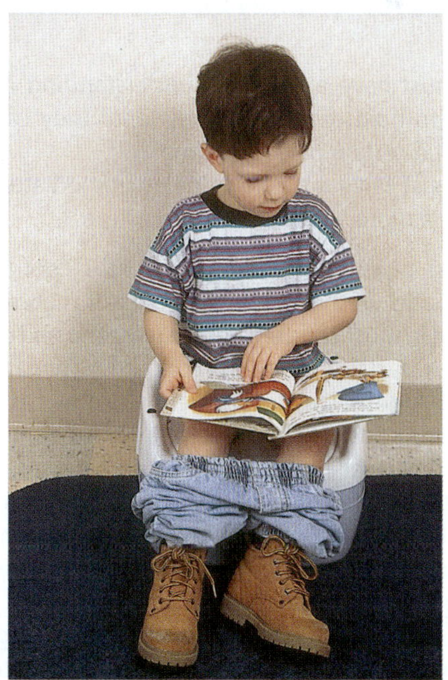

FIGURE 30.6 Toddlers are interested in toilet training as an expression of autonomy.

BOX 30.4 ✻ Focus on family teaching

How to toilet train a toddler

Q. Zach's parents ask you, "How can we tell if our 2-year-old is ready for toilet training? And if he is, how do we start?"

A. Try the following suggestions:

1. Children are physically ready for toilet training when they walk securely. Plan 1 or 2 weeks of psychological "readiness" activities, which will help your child realise the task of toilet training is a step towards growing up. If your child feels toilet training is something only toddlers do, he may react with extreme negativism. Readiness activities may include showing your child that other family members use the toilet; making it clear that bigger people customarily leave urine and faeces in the toilet, without suggesting that these materials are dirty or distasteful; and introducing training pants and showing your child that bigger people wear underpants too.
2. Check that training pants pull down readily and that trousers are free of complicated buttons or grippers; otherwise, your child will have accidents because he cannot undress quickly enough.
3. Purchase either a potty chair that sits on the floor or an infant seat that is placed on the regular toilet. The potty is low and potentially less frightening to a child, but it must be emptied and cleaned after each use. If you choose an infant seat, place a footstool in front of the toilet so your child has some support for his feet.
4. Put your child on the chair or toilet at regular intervals (e.g. when the child wakes up in the morning, after breakfast, during midmorning, before lunch, after lunch).
5. Praise your child if he does urinate or defecate. Remind him to wash his hands.
6. Be careful not to flush the toilet while the child is sitting on it. Two-year-old children are unable to realise they will not be flushed away and may become frightened. Encourage your child to flush the toilet independently after you have helped him get re-dressed.
7. Do not allow a child to remain on a potty chair for much longer than 10 minutes (less than that if he is resistant). Also, do not allow your child to use the potty to eat or as a play table, so he does not become confused regarding its purpose.
8. If your child is not ready or does not successfully use the potty on a day-to-day basis, have him return to nappies for a short period. Be careful not to make him feel as if this represents failure. Be careful not to equate "good" with being dry and "bad" with being wet. Continue with readiness activities. Reintroduce training pants and attempt toilet training again when your child seems more ready.
9. When boys have mastered defecation, it is time to include urination. Boys enjoy standing to urinate and aiming at objects in a toilet bowl, such as several pieces of breakfast cereal.
10. Some toddlers have difficulty remaining dry at night until they are 3 to 4 years old. Do not pressure your child to accomplish night-time dryness, but assume that he is doing the best he can do. Put him into training pants for the night by explaining (not punitively) that it is hard to keep dry while he sleeps. After your child has been dry during the night for about 1 month, he has probably mastered night-time dryness.
11. Do not wake your child during the night and carry him to the bathroom to void. This system may keep him dry during the night, but it does not help him stay dry for long periods. It may even prolong night-time wetness, because it conditions him to void every 4 hours or so instead of retaining urine for 12 hours while he sleeps.

- They must have a cognitive understanding of what it means to hold urine and stools until they can release them at a certain place and time.
- They must have a desire to delay immediate gratification for a more socially-accepted action.

Because physiological development is cephalocaudal, the rectal and urethral sphincters are not mature enough for control in most children until at least the end of the first year, when tracts of the spinal cord are myelinated to the anal level. A good way for a parent to know that a child's development has reached this point is to wait until the child can walk well independently.

Toilet training need not start this early, however, because cognitively and socially, many children do not understand what is being asked of them until they are 2 or even 3 years old. The markers of readiness are subtle, but as a rule children are ready for toilet training when they begin to be uncomfortable in wet nappies. They demonstrate this by pulling or tugging at a dirty nappy; they may bring a parent a clean nappy after they have soiled so they can be changed.

Teach parents not to underestimate the difficulty of the task they are expecting their child to achieve. Toddlers live by a pleasure principle: they want what they want when they want it. Before they can complete toilet training, they must be able to give up an immediate pleasure—relieving themselves whenever they have the urge—to gain other pleasure later on—improved physical comfort and another step in growing up.

Most children will be continent of urine during the day by the age of 3 years and at night by the age of 5 years. Some children, however, continue to experience night-time incontinence after the age of 5 years. Studies have shown a strong genetic link to bedwetting and a higher prevalence in males (Kiddoo, 2012). Useful information for parents can be found at <http://raisingchildren.net.au/articles/bedwetting_(cyh).html> and <www.kidshealth.org.nz/bedwetting>.

Ritualistic behaviour

Although toddlers spend a great deal of time every day investigating new ways to do things and doing things they have never done before, they also enjoy ritualistic patterns. They may use only "their" spoon at mealtime, only "their" washcloth at bathtime. They may not go outside unless their mother or father locates their favourite cap. This is normal behaviour. The child who seems to need an excessive number of objects to cling to or an excessive number of routines, however, may be trying to say, "I need more guidelines, more rules. Don't let me be quite so independent".

✔ *Checkpoint question 30.4*

Three-year-old Callum will go to sleep only if he has his favourite teddy bear. Callum's father is concerned that his wife continues to give into this demand and thinks Callum should be able to sleep without it. How would you approach this issue?

Negativism

As part of establishing their identities as separate individuals, toddlers typically go through a period of extreme negativism. They do not want to do anything a parent wants them to do. Their reply to every request is a very definite "no". It is easy for parents to believe their authority is being questioned when this happens and to worry that their child is becoming so disrespectful they will have difficulty getting along in the world. They can be baffled by the extreme change from happy, cooperative infant who lived to please them to irritating, uncooperative toddler. Explain to parents that this a normal phenomenon of toddlerhood and a positive stage in development. This change indicates that toddlers have learned they are separate individuals with separate needs. It is important that toddlers do this if they are to grow up to be persons who are independent and able to take care of their own needs and desires.

Once it runs its course, extreme negativism passes. In the meantime, the more parents try to make children obey them, the more children are likely to resist. Some long-term parent–child interaction problems begin during this period because parents insist on being obeyed totally or are inconsistent in their approach. A toddler's "no" can best be eliminated by limiting the number of questions asked of the child. A father does not really mean, for example, "Are you ready for dinner?" He means, "Come to the table. It's dinnertime". When a mother asks, "Will you come take a bath now?" She means, "It's time for your bath". Making a statement instead of asking a question can avoid a great many negative responses.

A toddler needs experience in making choices, however. To provide the opportunity to do this, a parent could give a secondary choice. "No" is not allowed for the major task, so the parent states, "It's bathtime now" but then says, "Do you want to take your duck or your toy boat into the bath with you?" Another example is: "It's lunchtime. Do you want to use a big or little plate?" Although this solution is simple, it is one that parents may not arrive at by themselves because finding a solution is always more difficult for a person in the middle of a problem than for an objective observer. Parents usually find this approach helpful in smoothing out the friction caused by the negativism of the toddler period (see Box 30.5).

Discipline

Some parents ask during the last part of the infant year or the early toddler period when they should start to discipline their child or when toddlers are old enough to be punished. Remind parents that "discipline" and "punishment" are not interchangeable terms**. Discipline** means setting rules or "road signs" so children know what is expected of them. **Punishment** is a consequence that results from a breakdown in discipline, from the child's disregard of the rules that were learned.

Parents should begin to instil some sense of discipline early in life because part of it involves setting safety limits and protecting others or property: for example, a child must stay away from the fireplace or heater; she must not go into the street; she must not hit other children. Enforcing limits, however, arises out of the day-to-day interaction with the child, out of the rhythm of childcare, not out of a set procedure such as, "Today, I'm going to teach discipline". Two general rules to follow are: (a) parents need to be consistent and (b) rules are learned best if correct behaviour is praised rather than wrong behaviour punished.

"Timeout" is a technique to help children learn that actions have consequences. To use "timeout" effectively, parents first need to be certain their child understands the rule they are trying to enforce: for instance, "If you hit your brother, you'll have timeout". Parents should give one warning. If the child repeats the behaviour, parents select an area that is non-stimulating, such as a corner of a room or a hallway. The child is directed to go immediately to the "timeout" space. The child then sits there for a specified period of time. If the child cries or shows any other disruptive behaviour, the timeout period does not begin until there is quiet. When the specified time period has passed, the child can return to the family. A guide regarding how long children should remain in their "timeout" space is 1 minute per year of age. Using a timer that rings when time is up lets children know when they can return to the family.

Useful parent resources can be found at Raising Children Network <http://raisingchildren.net.au/discipline/toddlers_discipline.html> and Kids Health <www.kidshealth.org.nz/parenting-positively websites>.

Separation anxiety

As discussed in Chapter 29, fear of being separated from parents begins at about 6 months of age and persists throughout the preschool period. This universal fear of this age group is known as separation anxiety. For this reason, toddlers have difficulty accepting being separated from

BOX 30.5 * Focus on communication

Jenny Matthis has brought her 2-year-old son, Jason, to the clinic for a health check. Jason is boisterous and uncooperative. Jenny is obviously frustrated.

Less effective communication

Nurse: Come on, Jason, sit quietly so I can hear your heartbeat.
Jason: No!
Jenny: Jason, listen to the nurse.
Jason: No!
Nurse: If you promise to sit still, I'll let you play with the stethoscope.
Jason: Okay.
Jason plays with the stethoscope.
Jenny: Jason, now it's time to give the stethoscope back to the nurse.
Jason: No.
Nurse: There are other children waiting to see me. I really must listen to your heart now.
Jenny takes the stethoscope from Jason. Jason starts crying.
Jenny: Jason, if you stop crying and sit still, I'll buy you an ice cream on our way home.
Jason (whimpering a bit): Okay.
Jenny: Sometimes he can be so difficult.
Nurse: Oh, those terrible twos!

More effective communication

Nurse: Jason, I need to listen to your heart so you must be very quiet. Would you rather sit quietly on the chair or the table?
Jason: The table.
Nurse: All right, Jason, jump up.
Jason climbs onto the table and starts to fidget.
Jenny: Jason, sit still for the nurse.
Jason: No!
Nurse: If you'd like, you can play with the stethoscope for a few seconds. Do you want to listen to your mum's heart or my heart?
Jason: Mum's.
Nurse: Great, now we will both be very quiet so you can hear.
Jason listens to his mother's heart.
Nurse: Good, now it's my turn.
Jason: Okay. (Jason hands back the stethoscope.)
Jenny: How did you get him to listen so well? At home he never listens. It can be so frustrating.
Nurse: Yes, this can be a frustrating period. By giving Jason choices, you can help him feel more in control without having to directly challenge your authority.

Toddlerhood can be a challenging and frustrating time for parents. You can teach parents effective communication skills to help toddlers assert their independence, while allowing parents to maintain discipline. It is important that parents offer choices rather than bribes as it is a far more effective and long-lasting method of modifying a toddler's behaviour. In the first scenario, the nurse and mother both bribe Jason. Jason finally does what they want, but the situation is still frustrating and his behaviour change will not be long-lasting. In the second scenario, the nurse demonstrates how to better communicate by offering choices. The situation is much more enjoyable for everyone.

their primary carer to spend the day at a day-care centre or if they or their primary carer is hospitalised. Chapter 36 discusses nursing responsibility for care of toddlers in the hospital as well as the reactions of toddlers to the separation caused by hospitalisation and the methods used to minimise these reactions.

Parents may ask what they can do about separation anxiety when leaving their child with a babysitter or at day care. Most toddlers react best to separation if a regular babysitter is employed or the day-care centre is one with consistent carers. Many are more comfortable if they are cared for in their own home. It helps if they have fair warning that they will have a babysitter. For example, they could be told, "Mummy is making dinner early because Mummy and Daddy are going to visit some friends tonight. Marsha is going to come and babysit for you. She'll put you to bed. When you wake up in the morning, Mummy and Daddy will be here again".

No matter how well prepared toddlers are, they may cry when the babysitter actually appears or may greet the babysitter warmly only to cry when the parents reach for their coats. It helps if parents say goodbye firmly, repeat the explanation that they will be there when the child wakes in the morning and then leave. Prolonged goodbyes only lead to more crying. Sneaking out prevents crying and may ease the parents' guilt, but it can strengthen fear of abandonment so should be discouraged. This applies to hospital visits as well.

TABLE 30.2 Differentiating between tantrums, breath holding and seizures

Assessment	Tantrums	Breath holding	Seizures
Provocation	Usually provoked—parent can state a reason for it (she asked toddler to come to dinner, toddler wanted to finish an activity)	Usually provoked; child very angry; child breathes out and forgets to breathe in	Not provoked
Appearance of cyanosis	Child holds breath, becomes cyanotic, then slumps to floor	Child breathes out, becomes cyanotic, then slumps to floor	Child slumps to floor first, then becomes cyanotic

Tantrums

Almost every toddler has a tantrum at one time or another. The child may kick, scream, stamp feet, shout "No, no, no", lie on the floor, flail arms and legs, and bang their head against the floor. Children may even hold their breath until they become cyanotic. When a child is breath holding, the chest becomes distended (a halt after inspiration), with air-filled cheeks and increasing distress as the child's body registers the need for oxygen. This is harmless breath holding; ignoring it will make it ineffective and the child will stop. True breath holding is a neurological problem in which children, under stress, appear to "forget" to breathe in or halt breathing after expiration, usually at the peak of anger. They become so short of breath that they slump to the floor. Breath holding can be mistaken for seizures because of the fall to the floor (see Chapter 49 and Table 30.2). Toddlers should be medically assessed to differentiate whether the breath holding is harmless or caused by a neurological disorder.

Tantrums are common during the toddler stage of development. They occur because toddlers are independent enough to know what they want, but they do not have the vocabulary or the wisdom to express their feelings in a more socially acceptable way. For example, tantrums occur most often when children are tired, just before naptime or bedtime or during a long shopping trip or visit.

Probably the best approach is for parents to tell a child simply that they disapprove of the tantrum and then ignore it. They might say, "I'll be in the bedroom. When you're done kicking, you can come into the bedroom too". Children who are left alone in a room this way will not usually continue a tantrum but will stop after 1 or 2 minutes and rejoin their parents. Parents should then accept the child warmly and proceed as if the tantrum had not occurred. This same approach works well for nurses caring for hospitalised toddlers.

Toddlers with physical limitations or a chronic illness

It may be difficult for children with physical limitations or chronic illness to achieve a sense of autonomy or independence because they may never be totally independent. It is important for these children to develop as strong a sense of autonomy as possible, so they see themselves as independent and can work to become increasingly self-sufficient as they grow older. Nursing actions designed to help children with physical limitations or chronic illness develop a sense of autonomy are outlined in Table 30.3. Most important are actions that allow toddlers to do as much for themselves as possible. For example, toddlers who have physical limitations may be unable to explore freely or pound and manipulate toys; however they may have the ability to work at a project while they sit in a chair at a table.

A toddler who has a long-term illness or physical limitations can be expected to exhibit usual toddler behaviours, such as tantrums and negativism. Tantrums in children with coordination issues or neurological disease may be mistaken for seizure activity. Investigate such activity carefully and explain to parents the difference between the two. Parents may also mistake toddler's insistence on having their own way as a manifestation of illness. Explore this issue with parents, as often the behaviour is an indication of age and development rather than of illness.

Toilet training is difficult for a child who is hospitalised at periodic intervals, as success usually requires a consistent carer; in addition, hospitalisation can result in regressive behaviours. If a chronically ill child has difficulty with ambulation, soiling accidents may occur beyond the usual age because of inability to reach a bathroom easily.

Parents tend to protect and shelter children who survive a long-term illness and may need a reminder that even though chronically ill, a toddler will demand independence and has the right to explore. A child who uses a lower-extremity prosthesis, for example, might prefer to crawl somewhere rather than wait for help to put the prosthesis in place. Although this degree of independence is good, parents may have to limit how it is expressed so the child will learn how to use the prosthesis (for example, they could make a rule the child must use the prosthesis to walk but can choose whether to use a spoon when eating).

Nutrition for toddlers with physical limitations or a chronic illness

Toddlers need to experience feeding themselves if at all possible. Explain to parents that accidents may occur with self-feeding, particularly if the child has difficulty with coordination; and suggest finger foods if possible. If on a special diet, children may not be allowed to eat finger foods; if they are tube-fed, they receive no experience with finger foods at all. For these toddlers, parents should try to provide other, comparable experiences in independence, such as letting them choose what toy to take to bed. They should also provide different play experiences such as play dough or a basin with cooked, cold wet pasta for tactile sensations that the child is not receiving through feeding.

TABLE 30.3 Nursing interventions to help a child who has a physical limitation or chronic illness develop a sense of autonomy

Area	Nursing action
Nutrition	A special diet may limit typical finger foods. Use imagination to offer other foods not usually eaten this way as finger foods. Allow child to help pour liquid diet for a tube feeding. Toddlers are frightened by vomiting because they have no control over it. Check for possibility of nausea; toddlers have no way to express this other than by not eating.
Dressing changes	A child can hold pieces of tape or put tape in place to maintain sense of control. The child can remove an old bandage if it is not contaminated. Allow children to view their incisions and watch dressing changes; explaining each step of a procedure as you perform it helps a child maintain control. Restrain only those body parts necessary during a procedure to allow a child a sense of control. Remove all supplies after a procedure, or the child may "redo" the dressing.
Medication	Allow children no choice regarding whether a medicine will be taken. Do allow a child to choose a "chaser", such as milk or juice, after oral medicine. Do not ask a toddler to indicate a choice of site for an injection or intravenous insertion; this is too advanced a decision for a toddler to handle.
Rest	Locate or create a ritual for bedtime (e.g. put child into bed, tuck him in, say, "Goodnight, Bobby." Tuck in bear. Say, "Goodnight, Bear"). Allow a choice of toy or cover but not a choice of bedtime or naptime hour.
Hygiene	Allow a child a choice of bathtub toy or clothing. Allow a child to wash face and hands to gain control of the situation. Allow the child to put toothpaste on a brush, but you should brush or "touch up" teeth afterwards to ensure that all plaque has been removed.
Pain	Encourage a child to express pain ("Say 'ouch' when I pull off the tape"). Help channel a child's self-expression to what is acceptable (e.g. the child may shout but may not kick).
Stimulation	Provide a toddler with a toy that can be manipulated, such as boxes that fit inside one another and can be taken out again, trucks that can be pushed and pegs that can be pounded. In a healthcare setting, items can usually be found that fit together (boxes or plastic vials from the pharmacy). Another action toy: buy a non-latex balloon and tie it to the cot side to be used as a punching bag; another one tied to the foot of the cot can serve as a leg exerciser.
Elimination	A child who is toilet trained needs to be encouraged to use a potty or toilet during an illness. Help children with ureter or bowel stomas to help with changing bags so they are as independent in bowel function as possible.

Key points for review

- Erikson's developmental task for the toddler period is to form a sense of autonomy or independence versus shame or doubt.
- Toddlers make great strides forward in development, but their physical growth slows.
- A critical milestone of toddler development is being able to form two-word sentences (a noun and a verb) by 2 years of age.
- Important aspects of care are promoting toddler safety; promoting toddler development, such as promoting daily activities; and healthy family functioning.
- Toddler appetites decrease from those of the infant, so children eat proportionally less than they did as infants.
- Common concerns of parents during the toddler period are toilet training, ritualistic behaviour, negativism, tantrums, discipline and separation anxiety.
- Promoting autonomy in the child who has physical limitations or a chronic illness calls for creative planning, because there may be tasks that must be done for the child to be certain they are done safely.

CASE STUDY QUESTIONS

3. Angus is cared for by his grandmother, Rhonda, 3 days a week while Chris and Ella work. Ella says that Rhonda doesn't allow Angus to feed himself as he makes too much mess. How would you respond to Ella?
4. Chris and Ella are in disagreement on how to manage Angus' tantrums in public. Yesterday they were at the supermarket and he started screaming when he wasn't given a toy that he wanted. Chris said he was embarrassed, so he gave him the toy to stop him screaming. Ella doesn't think that was an appropriate solution. How could you assist this family to find a suitable approach?

Resources

For an extensive range of additional resources to enhance teaching and learning and to facilitate understanding of this chapter, please see the text's accompanying website located on thePoint at http://thepoint.lww.com.

References

AIHW: Pointer, S. (2014). Hospitalised injury in children and young people 2011–12. *Injury Research and Statistics Series no. 91*. Cat. no. INJCAT 167. Canberra: AIHW.

Crisp, J., Taylor, C., Douglas, C. & Rebeiro, G. (2012). *Potter & Perry's Fundamentals of Nursing* (4th ed.), Mosby: St Louis.

Davis, H. (2010). *Working in Partnership: The Family Partnership Model.* London: Pearson.

Dental Health Services Victoria. (2010). Teeth: Oral health information for maternal and child health nurses. Accessed 19 January 2014, <www.dhsv.org.au/__data/assets/pdf_file/0011/3989/teeth-oral-health-information-for-maternal-and-child-health-nurses-manual.pdf>.

Erikson, E. H. (1993). *Childhood and Society*. New York: W. W. Norton.

Fletcher, R., St George, J. & Freeman, E. (2013). Rough and tumble play quality: Theoretical foundations for a new measure of father–child interaction, *Early Child Development and Care*, *183*(6), 746–759.

Hopwood, N., Fowler, C., Lee, A., Rossiter, C. & Bigsby, M. (2013). Understanding partnership practice in child and family nursing through the concept of practice architectures. *Nursing Inquiry*, *20*(3), 199–210.

Kiddoo, D. A. (2012). Nocturnal enuresis. *Canadian Medical Association Journal*, *184*(8), 908–911.

Kidsafe: Child Accident Prevention Foundation. (2013). Poisoning prevention. Accessed 19 January 2015, <www.kidsafensw.org/imagesDB/wysiwyg/PoisoningPrevention2013_5.pdf>.

Lewis, P. & Foley, D. (2014). *Health Assessment in Nursing* (2nd ed.). Sydney: Lippincott Williams & Wilkins.

Ministry of Health. (2013). Eating for health: Babies and toddlers. Accessed 19 January 2015, <www.healthed.govt.nz/resource/eating-healthy-babies-and-toddlersngā-kai-tōtika-mō-te-hunga-kōhungahunga>.

National Health and Medical Research Council. (2013). Australian Dietary Guidelines. Canberra: National Health and Medical Research Council.

New Zealand Government. (1987). Fencing of Swimming Pools Act 1987. Accessed 19 January 2015, <www.legislation.govt.nz/act/public/1987/0178/latest/DLM124442.html>.

Onis, M. (2006). Assessment of sex differences and heterogeneity in motor milestone attainment among populations in the WHO Multicentre Growth Reference Study. *Acta Paediatrica*, *95*(S450), 66–75.

Rugg-Gunn, A. J. & Do, L. (2012). Effectiveness of water fluoridation in caries prevention. *Community Dentistry and Oral Epidemiology*, *40*(s2), 55–64.

Teng, A., Bartle, A., Sadeh, A. & Mindell, J. (2012). Infant and toddler sleep in Australia and New Zealand. *Journal of Paediatrics and Child Health*, *48*(3), 268–273.

Tresillian. (2014). Settling techniques: 12 months to toddlers. Accessed 19 January 2015, <www.tresillian.net/tresillian-tips/settling-techniques-12-months-to-toddlers.html>.

Suggested readings

ARACY <www.aracy.org.au>

BabyCenter Australia <www.babycenter.com.au>

Johnston, C. C., Rennick, J. E., Filion, F., et al. (2011). Maternal touch and talk for invasive procedures in infants and toddlers in the pediatric intensive care unit. *Journal of Pediatric Nursing*, *27*(2), 144–153.

Kidsafe NSW Inc <www.kidsafensw.org>

Kidshealth NZ <www.kidshealth.org.nz>

Kidspot Australia <www.kidspot.com.au>

Lutz, H. R., Patterson, B. J., & Klein, J. (2012). Coping with autism: A journey toward adaptation. *Journal of Pediatric Nursing*, *27*(3), 206–213.

Ministry of Health NZ <www.health.govt.nz>

Ministry of Social Development: Community Investment <www.familyservices.govt.nz>

Raising Children Network <http://raisingchildren.net.au>

Tresillian <www.tresillian.net>

Triple P <www.triplep.net/glo-en/home/>

Well Child <www.wellchild.org.nz>

Chapter 31

Nursing care of a family with a preschool child

The previous chapter described toddler growth and development and the abilities children develop during that period. This chapter adds information about the changes, both physical and psychosocial, that occur during the preschool years. Such information builds a base for care and health teaching for the age group.

LEARNING OBJECTIVES

After studying the contents of this chapter, you should be able to:

1. Describe normal growth and development as well as common parental concerns of the preschool period.
2. Use critical thinking to analyse methods of care for preschoolers to be certain care is family-centred.
3. Assess a preschooler for normal growth and developmental milestones.
4. Formulate nursing considerations related to preschool growth and development and common parental concerns.
5. Identify expected outcomes for nursing care of a preschooler.
6. Plan nursing care to meet a preschooler's growth and development needs, such as planning age-appropriate play activities.
7. Implement nursing care related to normal growth and development of a preschooler, such as preparing a preschooler for an invasive procedure.
8. Evaluate expected outcomes for achievement and effectiveness of care.
9. Integrate knowledge of preschool growth and development with nursing process to achieve quality child and family health nursing care.

KEY TERMS

- broken fluency
- bruxism
- conservation
- ectomorphic
- endomorphic
- intuitional thought
- secondary stuttering

CASE STUDY

Cathy Edwards is a 3-year-old girl. Her father Matt is her sole carer while her mother Jackie is hospitalised as a result of preterm labour for a second pregnancy. Matt tells you he is concerned because Cathy talks constantly with an imaginary friend named Emma. She makes up stories about events that cannot possibly be true. When corrected, Cathy stutters so badly no-one can understand her.

CASE STUDY QUESTION

1. Is Matt describing typical preschool behaviour or does Cathy need a referral to a child guidance counsellor?

The preschool period traditionally includes ages from 3 to 6 years. Although physical growth slows considerably during this period, personality and cognitive growth continue at a rapid rate. This is also an important period of growth for parents. They may be unsure about how much independence and responsibility for self-care they should allow their preschooler. Most children of this age want to do things for themselves—choose their own clothing and dress by themselves, feed themselves, wash their own hair and so forth. As a result, parents of a preschooler may find their child dressed in one red sock and one green sock, going to preschool with unwashed ears or trying to eat soup with a fork. They need reassurance that this behaviour is typical as it is the way that children adjust to new experiences. Parents may also need some guidance in separating those tasks a preschooler can accomplish independently from those that still require some adult supervision, so they can set sensible limits. Setting limits this way protects children from harming themselves or others while participating in all the interesting experiences available to them (Fergusson, Boden, & Horwood, 2013).

HEALTHY DEVELOPMENT OF THE PRESCHOOLER

Assessment

Regular assessment of a preschooler includes obtaining a health history and performing a developmental, cognitive and physical evaluation.

Preschoolers who find a health visit stressful may speak very little during the assessment; they may even revert to baby talk or babyish actions such as thumb-sucking. Alternatively, they may speak constantly during the assessment, with no link, however, to what you are asking them, to the assessment or to what their parent/s or carer may be saying. This will very much depend on the preschooler's social skills. For example, those with older siblings or those attending day care may have more confidence in speaking. Also much of the interaction within assessments will depend on the assessor's abilities and communication skills. Preschool children imitate moods as well as actions. An important nursing consideration, therefore, is role-playing a mood or attitude you would like a child to learn. To project an attitude that a health assessment is an enjoyable activity, you might suggest preschoolers participate by listening to their heart or colouring the table paper. A history that details their usual performance level is very important for accurate evaluation. Feedback from the child's preschool teacher, if they attend preschool, may also be of assistance for the assessment.

For the physical evaluation, assess a child's weight and height according to standard growth charts (see Appendix B). Keep in mind these charts are based on average weights and heights of Caucasian Australian or New Zealand children, so those for children from other ethnic or cultural backgrounds may not completely agree with these norms. (The growth charts will be discussed in further depth later in this chapter.) Also assess a child for general appearance.

For many parents, preschool is a difficult time because a child is at an in-between stage—no longer an infant, although not yet ready for formal school. Planning and establishing expected outcomes for care of children at this age often begins with establishing a schedule for discussing normal preschool development with the parents. Planning for unintentional injury prevention, such as how to cross streets safely, becomes increasingly important as children begin to enjoy experiences away from home. It is also important to plan opportunities for adventurous activities and interaction with other children.

Nursing considerations

Nursing considerations for preschoolers typically concern health promotion. Examples are:

- Health-seeking behaviours related to developmental expectations
- Readiness for enhanced parenting related to parents' pride in child.

Other nursing considerations include:

- Risk of injury related to increased independence outside the home
- Delayed growth and development related to frequent illness
- Risk of poisoning related to the developmental age of the child
- Parental anxiety related to lack of understanding of childhood development
- Imbalanced nutrition related to a child's food dislikes.

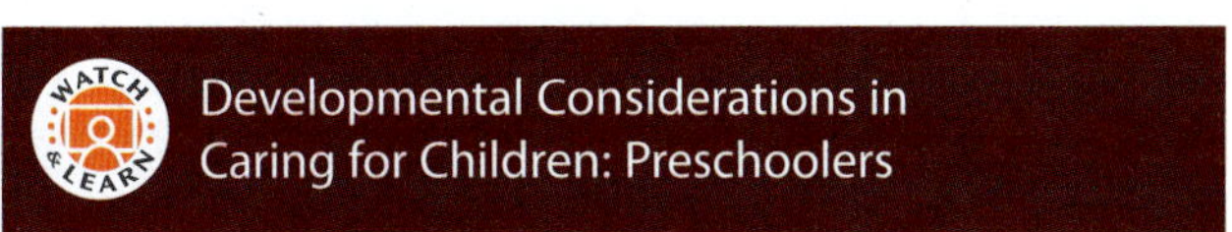

GROWTH AND DEVELOPMENT OF A PRESCHOOLER

Assessment of preschoolers needs to include physical, cognitive and developmental growth emotional, moral and spiritual development (see Box 31.1).

BOX 31.1 Assessment ❋ Assessing the average preschooler

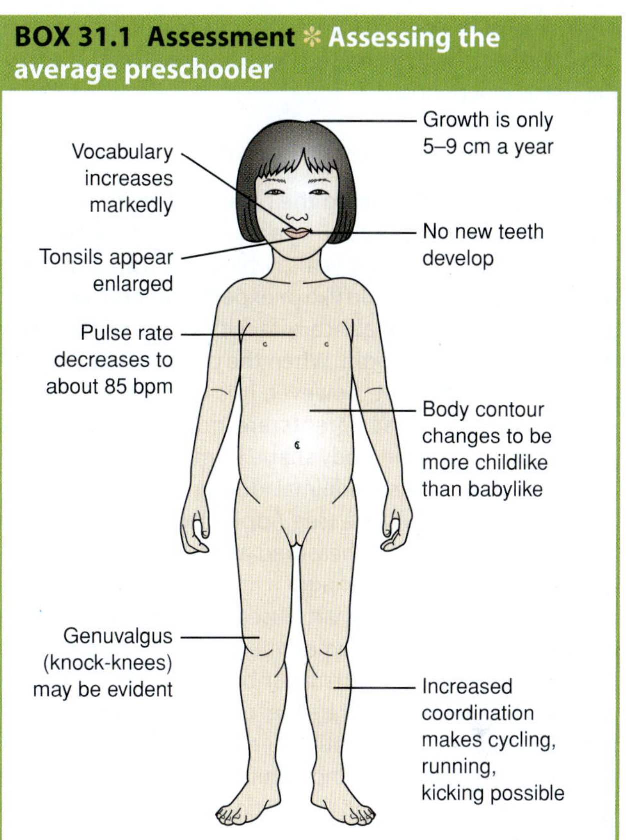

Physical growth

A definite change in body contour occurs during the preschool years. The wide-legged gait and large abdomen of the toddler changes to slimmer, taller and much more childlike proportions. Contour changes are so definite that future body type—**ectomorphic** (slim) or **endomorphic** (large)—becomes apparent. Handedness begins to be obvious. Lymphatic tissue begins to increase in size, particularly the tonsils; levels of immune globulin IgG and IgA antibodies increase. These changes tend to make preschool illnesses more localised (e.g. an upper respiratory infection remains localised to the nose with little systemic fever). Physiological splitting of heart sounds may be present for the first time on auscultation; innocent heart murmurs may also be heard for the first time. This type of murmur occurs because of the changing size of the heart in reference to the thorax because the anteroposterior and transverse diameters of the chest have not yet reached adult proportions. Pulse rate decreases to about 85 beats/min and blood pressure holds at about 100/60 mmHg.

The bladder is easily palpable above the symphysis pubis; voiding is frequent enough (9 or 10 times a day) that play must be interrupted and voiding accidents may occur if a child becomes absorbed in an activity.

A child who earlier in life had an indeterminate longitudinal arch in the foot generally demonstrates a well-formed arch now. Muscles are noticeably stronger, so activities such as gymnastics become possible. Many children at the beginning of the period exhibit genuvalgus (knock-knees); this disappears with increased skeletal growth at the end of the preschool period.

Weight, height and head circumference

Weight gain is slight during the preschool years: the average child gains only about 2 kg a year. Appetite remains as it was during the toddler years, which is considerably less than some parents would like or expect. Parents may bring a preschooler to a healthcare facility because they fear their child is losing weight. When the child's weight is plotted on a growth chart, however, it is evident the child is gaining weight; what parents are noticing is the age-appropriate change in body shape from rounded to slim.

Height gain is also minimal during this period: only 5–9 cm a year on average (see Appendix B). Head circumference is not routinely measured at physical assessments of children over 2 years of age.

The current growth charts used throughout Australia and New Zealand are based on the studies in 2000 to 2006 by WHO. The current charts must be used with the understanding that these charts are the "normal growth" expectations for children under optimal environmental conditions. In other words, describing how children *should* grow, rather than measuring how child populations *are* growing.

Teeth

Children generally have all 20 of their deciduous teeth by 3 years of age. Preserving these teeth is important as they hold the position for the permanent teeth as the child's jaw grows larger (de Amorim Lde, Estrela & de Costa, 2011).

Developmental milestones

Each year during the preschool period marks a major step forwards in gross motor, fine motor and language development. Play activities change focus as the preschooler learns new skills and understands more about the world (see Fig. 31.1). Table 31.1 summarises the major milestones of the period.

Language development

A 3-year-old child has a vocabulary of about 900 words. These are used to ask questions constantly, up to 400 a day, mostly "how" and "why" questions, such as "Why is

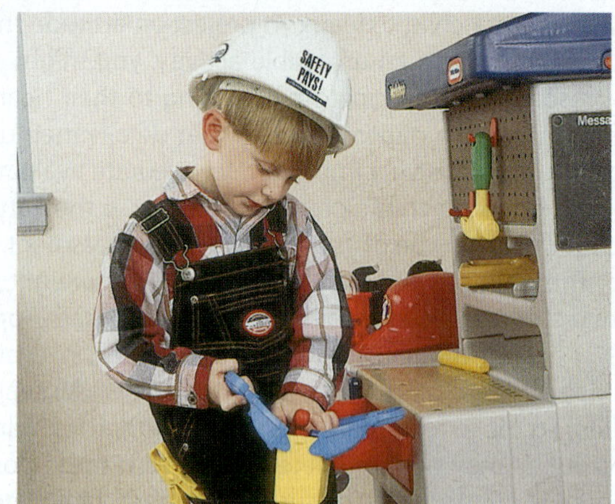

FIGURE 31.1 Preschoolers like to imitate the roles of adults, as they learn about the world around them.

snow cold?" "How do worms hear?" What does your tongue do?" A child needs simple answers to such questions so curiosity, vocabulary building and questioning are encouraged, and also because the depth of a child's understanding is often deceptive. For example, if a parent tells a child shoes should go on with the buckles on the outside, a child may seem to understand but may return in a few minutes to ask, "Why do I have to go outside to put on my shoes?" Words that sound alike but mean different things such as whether and weather can be truly confounding to children of this age.

Four- and five-year-old children continue to ask many questions. They enjoy participating in mealtime conversation and can describe something from their day in great detail. Preschoolers imitate language exactly, so if they hear less-than-perfect language, this is the language pattern they adopt. They may imitate and use vulgarities or crudities if not corrected because of the attention from adults this generates. Preschoolers are egocentric, so they define objects in relation to themselves (a key is not a metal object but "what I use to open a door" and a car is not a means of transportation but "what Mum uses to take me to school").

Whether children are allowed to ask questions is culturally determined and can make a difference in how much vocabulary a child uses. In a society in which children are expected to be seen and not heard, a preschool child may not have the same expressive vocabulary as a child who has been encouraged to ask questions. Recognition that

TABLE 31.1 Summary of preschool growth and development milestones

Age (years)	Fine motor	Gross motor	Language	Play
3	Undresses self; stacks tower of blocks; draws a cross	Runs; alternates feet on stairs; rides tricycle; stands on one foot	Vocabulary of 900 words	Able to take turns; very imaginative
4	Can do up simple buttons	Constantly in motion; jumps; skips	Vocabulary of 1500 words	Pretending is major activity
5	Draws a 6-part man; can lace shoes	Throws overhand	Vocabulary of 2100 words	Likes games with numbers or letters

differences among cultures can affect levels of development means that assessment must be individualised and meaningful in terms of the cultural milieu.

Play

Preschoolers do not need many toys. Their imaginations are keener than they will be at any other time in their lives so they enjoy games that use imagination such as pretending to be teachers, cowboys and firefighters. They imitate exactly what they see parents doing: eating meals, mowing the lawn, cleaning the house, arguing and so forth, so parents' actions directly influence their behaviour. Many preschoolers have imaginary friends as a normal part of having an active imagination. These often exist until children formally begin school. Four- and five-year-olds divide their time between rough and imaginative play. Five-year-olds are interested in group games or songs they have learned in kindergarten or preschool.

CASE STUDY QUESTION

2. Cathy asks constant questions. How many does a typical 3-year-old ask in a day?
   a. Less than 50
   b. 100–200
   c. 300–400
   d. 1200 or more

Emotional development

Children change a great deal in their ability to understand the world and how they relate to people during the preschool years.

Initiative

The developmental task of the preschool years, according to Erikson, is to form a sense of initiative versus guilt (Erikson, 1993). A child with a well-developed sense of initiative has discovered that learning new things is fun. Parents can be guided to a number of government sites that identify the development stages children will meet in the 3–5-year age group. It is important to inform parents that these are guides only and that children develop skills at varying ages depending on a number of factors; for example, gender, environment, health and genetic factors. A quick checklist guide can be found at the State Government of Victoria, Department of Education and Training website <www.education.vic.gov.au/childhood/parents/health/pages/preschoolers.aspx> for parents who may be concerned with the development of their child. This informative website also directs parents to numerous other sources where they can obtain further information. Online education has become a major source of information for parents in our current society. Readily available and current health information increases parents' ability to be active in promoting the health of children by early identification of potential developmental problems.

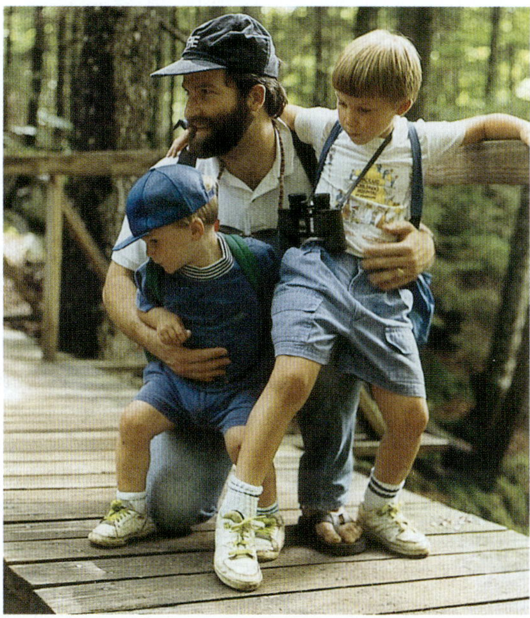

FIGURE 31.2 Preschoolers like exposure to new events and places. Here a 3-year-old is eager to explore the bush during a walk with the family.

If children are criticised or punished for attempts at initiative, they develop a sense of guilt for wanting to try new activities or have new experiences. Those who leave the preschool period with guilt may carry it with them into new situations, such as starting primary school. They may even have difficulty later in life making decisions about everything from changing jobs to choosing a home, because they cannot envision they are capable of solving associated problems.

To gain a sense of initiative, preschoolers need exposure to a wide variety of experiences and play materials so they can learn as much about how things work as possible. They are ready to explore outside their homes, such as enjoying a trip to the zoo or the park (see Fig. 31.2). They enjoy going with their family on holidays and trips. These types of experiences lead to increased vocabulary (e.g. at the zoo, words such as "elephant" and "bear" come alive, because they are transferred from abstract concepts to the actual animals). Preschoolers tend to have active imaginations and need little guidance to play or make things. What they make may not be recognisable; it is the enjoyment of feeling the material and how it manipulates that is the experience.

Imitation

Preschoolers need free rein to imitate the roles of the people around them. Again, role-playing should be fun and does not have to be accurate. If a boy is pretending to be a police officer and is busy putting out fires or a firefighter and is stopping playmates from speeding, the fact he is freely imitating a role is more important than getting the role absolutely correct. If a parent is concerned a child should separate these two roles accurately, it is usually best not to stop the play to do so. Rather, the next time they are driving past the fire station, the parent could explain this is where firefighters work and they put out fires or the police station is where police officers work and they make sure that people drive safely.

Fantasy

Toddlers cannot differentiate between fantasy and reality; they believe cartoon characters or children in books are real. Preschoolers begin to make this differentiation. They may become so engrossed in a fantasy role, however, they become afraid they have lost their own identity or have become "stuck" in their fantasies. Such intense involvement in play is part of "magical thinking" or believing thoughts and wishes can come true.

Parents sometimes strengthen this feeling without realising it: they (and you) need to be careful in this regard. A preschooler, for example, may be pretending she is a white rabbit. Her mother walks into the room, is aware of the game and decides to participate. She says, "That's strange, I don't see Cindy anywhere. All I see is a white rabbit". Then she leaves the room. Cindy can be frightened she has actually become a white rabbit. A better response for the mother would be to support the imitation—this is age-appropriate behaviour and a good way of exploring roles—while helping the child to maintain the difference between pretend and real. She might say, "What a nice white rabbit you're pretending to be", both supporting the fantasy and yet reassuring the child she is still herself. In a healthcare setting, it is particularly important that you let children know they are still recognisable. When examining the ears of a girl who tells you she is a rabbit, comment that her ears are all better again, rather than play to the make-believe with remarks about long, furry rabbit ears.

Gender roles

Preschoolers need exposure to an adult of the opposite gender so they can become familiar with opposite gender roles. Encourage single parents to plan opportunities for their children to spend some time with adults other than themselves, such as a grandparent, a friend or a relative of the opposite sex. A preschool teacher may serve as this person. Because most preschool teachers are women, a mother may have to look elsewhere to find an adult male role model. If a child is hospitalised during the preschool period, a male nurse could fill this role if a grandparent, other relative or family friend is not available.

Children's gender-typical actions are strengthened by parents, strangers, preschool teachers, other family members and other children. Many parents do not want their child to grow up as they did, with a fixed role as a result of gender stereotyping. Help them understand they reinforce such attitudes by their actions as well as by their words. For example, a father may tell his son it is important for both boys and girls to do housework, but if the father never does the dishes, he is teaching his son that housework is not a man's job.

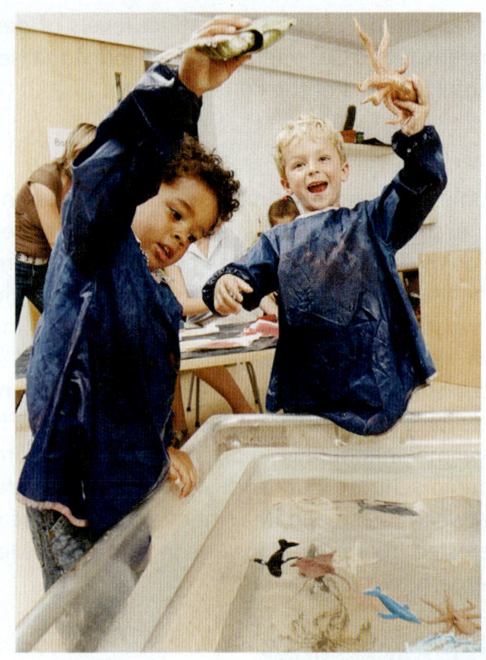

FIGURE 31.3 The preschool child begins to develop friendships.

Socialisation

Because 3-year-olds are capable of sharing, they play with other children their age much more agreeably than do toddlers, which is why the preschool period is a sensitive and critical time for socialisation. Children who are exposed to other playmates have an easier time learning to relate to people than those raised in an environment where they never see other children of the same age (Paulus & Moore, 2012; see Fig. 31.3).

Although 4-year-olds continue to enjoy playgroups, they may become involved in arguments more than they did at the age of 3, especially as they become more certain of their role in the group. This development, like so many others, may make parents worry a child is regressing. However, it is really forward movement, involving some testing and identification of their group role.

Five-year-olds begin to develop "best" friendships, perhaps on the basis of who they walk to school with or who lives closest to them. The elementary rule that an odd number of children will have difficulty playing well together pertains to children at this age: two or four will play, but three or five will quarrel.

Cognitive development

At the age of 3 years, cognitive development according to Piaget is still preoperational (Piaget, 1969). Although children during this period do enter a second phase called **intuitional thought**, they lack the insight to view themselves as others see them or put themselves in another's place (termed *centring*). Because preschoolers cannot make this kind of mental substitution, they feel that they are always right. This causes them to argue with a forcefulness that comes from believing they are 100% correct. This is an important point to remember when explaining procedures to preschoolers. They cannot see your side of the situation; they cannot hurry because you must have something done by 10 a.m.; they cannot hold still just because you want them to.

Also, preschoolers are not yet aware of the property of **conservation**. This means that if they have two balls of clay of equal size, but one is squashed flatter and wider than the other, preschoolers will insist the flatter one is bigger (because it is wider) or that the intact one is bigger (because it is taller). They cannot see that only the form, not the amount, has changed. This inability to appreciate conservation has implications for nursing care. Preschoolers are not able to comprehend that a procedure done two separate ways is the same procedure. Therefore, if the nurse before you told a child to turn on his right side and then his left side while his bed was made, you may have to allow him to turn those same ways.

Moral and spiritual development

Children of preschool age determine right from wrong based on their parents' rules. They have little understanding of the rationale for these rules or even whether the rules are consistent. If asked the question, "Why is it wrong to hit other children?" the average preschooler answers, "Because my mother says it's wrong". When pressed further, the preschooler justifies that conviction with, "It just is, that's all". Because preschoolers depend on their parents to supply rules for them, when faced with a new situation they may have difficulty seeing that the rules they know may also apply to the new situation.

Preschoolers begin to have an elemental concept of God if they have been provided with some form of religious education. Belief in an outside force aids in the development of conscience; however, preschoolers tend to do good out of self-interest rather than because of strong spiritual motivation (Kohlberg, 1984). Children this age enjoy the security of religious holidays and rituals, such as prayer and grace before meals, because these rituals offer them the same reassurance and security as a familiar nursery rhyme read over and over again.

> ***What if...***
>
> Cathy, 3 years old, understands the rule "Don't steal from shops"? Would she also understand "Don't steal from a hospital"?

HEALTH PROMOTION FOR A PRESCHOOLER AND FAMILY

Preschoolers are old enough to begin to take responsibility for their own actions. The preschooler's safety, nutritional health, daily activities and family functioning are all affected by this increased responsibility.

Promoting preschooler safety

As preschoolers broaden their horizons, safety issues increase. By the age of 4, children may project an attitude of independence and the ability to take care of their own needs. Part of this is pseudo-independence; they still need supervision to be certain they do not injure themselves or other children while playing and to ensure they do not stray too far from home. Their interest in learning adult roles may lead them to exploring the blades of a lawn mower or an electric saw or a neighbour's pool (Bowman, Aitken, Robbins, et al., 2012). They must be reminded repeatedly not to walk behind or in front of cars. Otherwise, a preschooler's thought "I want to play with Mary across the road" can be so quick and so intense a child will run into the middle of the road before remembering the rules "Watch out for cars" and "Don't cross the road".

Additional safety points for the preschool period are summarised in Box 31.2.

Keeping children safe, strong and free

The preschool years are not too early a time to educate children about the potential threat of harm from strangers or even how to address bullying behaviour from people (children or adults) they meet at preschool or at play. This includes:

- Warning a child never to talk with or accept a ride from a stranger
- Teaching a child how to call for help in an emergency (yelling or running to a designated neighbour's house if outside or dialling 000 in Australia and 111 in New Zealand if near a telephone)
- Describing what police officers look like and explaining that police officers can help in an emergency situation
- Explaining that if children or adults ask them to keep secrets about anything that has made them uncomfortable, they should tell their parents or another trusted adult, even if they have promised to keep the secret
- Explaining that bullying behaviour from other children is not to be tolerated and should be reported so they can receive help managing it.

It is often difficult for parents to impart this type of information to preschoolers because they cannot imagine their child will ever be in situations in which the information will be needed, nor do they want to terrify their child about the world. However, if the information is presented in a calm yet serious manner, children can begin to use it to build safe habits that will help them later when they are old enough to walk home from school alone or play with their friends, unsupervised, at a public playground.

Motor vehicle and bicycle safety

With more and more cars being equipped with front-seat air bags, make certain parents safely buckle preschoolers into car seats in the back seat as per Australian safety regulations. These regulations are in place because of child

BOX 31.2 ✻ Focus on family teaching

Common safety measures to prevent accidents during the preschool years

Q. Cathy's father says to you, "My preschooler is so active! How can I keep her safe?"

A. All of the safety measures that apply to toddlers also apply to preschoolers. In addition, try these tips:

Possible accident	Prevention measure
Motor vehicles	Teach safety with a bicycle or tricycle (look before crossing driveways; do not cross roads). Teach the child to wear a helmet when riding a bicycle. Teach the child to always hold hands with a grown-up before crossing the road. Teach carpark safety (hold hands with a grown-up; do not run behind cars that are reversing).
Falls	Supervise a preschooler in the playground. Remove drawstrings from hooded clothing. Help the child to judge safe distances for jumping or safe heights for climbing.
Drowning	Teach beginning swimming.
Animal bites	Do not allow the child to approach strange dogs. Supervise the child's play with family pets.
Poisoning	Never present medication as a lolly. Never take medication in front of a child. Never store foods or substances in containers other than their own. Post the telephone number of the local poison control centre by the telephone (13 11 26 in Australia; 0800 764 766 in New Zealand). Teach the child that medication is a serious substance and not for play.
Burns	Store matches in closed containers. Do not allow a preschooler to help light birthday candles, fireplaces, etc. (fire is not fun or a "treat").
Community safety	Teach a preschooler that not all people are friends ("Do not talk to strangers or take lollies from strangers"). Define a stranger as someone a child does not know, not as someone odd-looking. Teach the child to say "no" to people whose touching the child does not enjoy, including family members. (When a child is sexually abused, the offender is usually a family member or close family friend.)
General	Know the whereabouts of a preschooler at all times. Be aware that the frequency of accidents is increased when parents are under stress. Special precautions must be taken at these times. Be aware that some children are more active, curious and impulsive and therefore more vulnerable to accidents than others.

anatomy and risk of injury and death due to air bags and other safety features of cars. Parents should stress the important role of seatbelts in preventing injury in accidents and should make it a rule that the car does not move until seatbelts are fastened. See <www.safekids.org/Australia> and <www.safekids.org.nz>.

Preschool is also the right age to promote bicycle safety (Agarwal & Pruthi, 2010). Head injuries are a major cause of death and injury to preschoolers, and bicycle accidents are among the major causes of such injuries. Once children begin riding independently they definitely need a safety helmet approved for children of their age and size. Encourage parents who ride bicycles to demonstrate safe riding habits by wearing helmets as well. Seeing a parent routinely wearing a helmet may well be the most compelling reason for a preschooler to wear one.

What if...

Cathy tells you she knows not to leave preschool with anyone who is strange? Is that the same as knowing not to leave with a stranger?

Promoting nutritional health of the preschooler

Like the toddler period, the preschool years are not a time of fast growth, so preschool children are not likely to have ravenous appetites. Offering small servings of food is still a good idea, so a child is not overwhelmed by the amount on a plate and is allowed the successful feeling of cleaning a plate and asking for more. Parents need to check that children are not snacking at the expense of planned meals to be certain children receive a complete range of nutrients (Raman, 2011).

Most children are hungry after preschool and enjoy a snack when they arrive home. Sugary foods can dull a child's appetite for dinner and it is not too soon to begin measures to prevent childhood obesity. Urge parents to offer foods such as fruit, cheese or milk rather than biscuits; and water only, not sugar drinks, such as cordial, juice boxes or soft drinks (Bevan & Reilly, 2011). Teach parents to make mealtimes a happy and enjoyable part of the day for everyone. Some preschool children learn to eat as quickly as possible (and perhaps incompletely) to escape from the table before something unpleasant happens, such as an argument they can sense is brewing. See also Appendices E and F for advice on the amount and types of foods needed to stay healthy.

Recommended dietary reference intakes

As with all age groups, foods selected for preschoolers should be based on food pyramid groups and parents should make sure to offer variety. Preschoolers may not eat a great deal of meat because it can be hard to chew. Many parents ask whether their preschooler needs to take supplementary vitamins because they eat so little. As long as a child is eating foods from all pyramid food groups and meets the criteria for a healthy child, such as being alert and active with height and weight within normal averages, additional vitamins are probably unnecessary: see <www.nhmrc.gov.au/guidelines/publications/n29-n30-n31-n32-n33-n34>.

Promoting nutritional health with a vegetarian diet

A vegetarian diet is usually colourful and therefore appeals to preschoolers. Many vegetables, fruits and grains are also good snack foods and so are convenient for a child who eats frequently during the day. If vegetarian diets are deficient in any aspects, they usually lack calcium, vitamin B_{12} and vitamin D. Check to see a child is ingesting a variety of calcium sources (green leafy vegetables, milk products) as this is so important for bone growth. Vitamin D is found in fortified cereals and milk. Vitamin B_{12} is found almost exclusively in animal product, so a child may need a supplemental source of this (Whitney & Rolfes, 2013). See <www.eatforhealth.gov.au> for vegetarian and cultural adaptions.

Promoting development of the preschooler in daily activities

The preschooler has often mastered the basic skills needed for most self-care activities, including feeding, dressing, washing (with supervision) and brushing teeth (again, with supervision).

Dressing

Many 3-year-olds and most 4-year-olds can dress themselves except for difficult buttons, although there may be conflict over what a child will wear. Preschoolers prefer bright colours or prints and so may select items that do not match. As with other preschool activities, children need the experience of choosing their own clothes. If children insist on wearing mismatched clothes, parents should make no apologies for their appearance. A simple statement such as "Mark chose his own clothes today" explains the situation. Anyone who understands preschoolers appreciates that the experience children gain in being able to select their own clothing is worth more than a perfect appearance by adult standards.

Sleep

Many toddlers, going through a typical negative phase, resist taking naps no matter how tired they are. Preschoolers, on the other hand, are more aware of their needs; when they are tired, they often curl up on a couch or soft chair and fall asleep. Many, particularly those who attend afternoon childcare or preschool, give up afternoon naps. If they nap at a preschool, they may have some difficulty going to sleep at the usual bedtime established at home. Children may, however, refuse to go to sleep because of fear of the dark. Night waking from nightmares or night terrors reaches its peak in this age group (Byars et al., 2012). This means preschoolers may need a night light, even if they did not need one before. A helpful suggestion for parents is to screen out frightening stories or television watching just prior to bedtime and continue familiar bedtime routines.

Exercise

The preschool period is an active phase, so children receive a great deal of exercise. Rough-play is a good way of getting rid of tension and should be allowed as long as it does not become destructive. In addition, preschoolers love time-honoured games such as ring-around-the-rosy, leap frog or other more structured games they were not ready for as toddlers. Promoting this type of active game play and reducing television watching can help children develop motor skills as well as being a step towards preventing childhood obesity. The recommended time of play activity for preschool children is three periods of 20–30 minutes per day (Hodges et al., 2012; Mitka, 2012).

Hygiene

Preschoolers can wash and dry their hands adequately if the tap is regulated for them so they do not scald themselves with hot water. Preschoolers do not clean their fingernails very well, so these often need additional cleaning by a parent or older sibling. The child may also need the assistance of a parent or older sibling to clean their ears during bath time. Hair washing can be a problem as well. Although preschoolers may sit well in bathtubs, they should still not be left unsupervised at bath time. Caution parents about using bubble bath with preschoolers as some girls develop vulvar irritation (and perhaps bladder infections) from exposure to such products (Smith, 2011; Goldman, 2012).

Care of teeth

If independent tooth-brushing was not started as a daily practice during the infant or toddler years, it should be started during the preschool years. Preschoolers will still need help, however, to ensure that their teeth have been well cleaned, particularly the molars and inside surfaces. Age-appropriate toothbrush and toothpaste should be used. One good tooth-brushing period a day is often more effective than more frequent half-hearted brushing (Smith & Riedford, 2012). Tooth-brushing is generally well-accepted by preschoolers because it imitates adults. Encouraging children to eat apples, carrots, celery, chicken or cheese for snacks rather than lollies is yet another way to attempt to prevent tooth decay.

Children should have made a first visit to a dentist by 2 years of age for evaluation of tooth formation. Because this visit usually shows no cavities, this should have been a pain-free experience, so a child should not fear the dentist and the idea that dentists like to help rather than hurt should have been implanted. If parents did not take a child for this visit previously, it should be done during the preschool period. Deciduous teeth must be preserved to protect the dental arch. If teeth have to be extracted as a result of disease, the permanent teeth can drift out of position or the jaw may not grow enough to accommodate them (Tubert-Jeannin et al., 2011; Merlino & Gigli, 2012). For more information, see the publication *Oral Health Information for Maternal and Child Health Nurses* available at <www.dhsv.org.au/__data/assets/pdf_file/0011/3989/teeth-oral-health-information-for-maternal-and-child-health-nurses-manual.pdf>.

Night grinding

Bruxism, or grinding the teeth at night (usually during sleep), is a habit of many young children (Merlino & Gigli, 2012). Teeth grinding may be a way of "letting go", similar to body rocking, that children do for a short time each night to release tension and allow themselves to fall asleep. Children who grind their teeth extensively may have greater-than-average anxiety. Children with cerebral palsy may do it because of the spasticity of jaw muscles. If the grinding is extensive, the crowns of the teeth can become abraded. The condition can advance to such an extent that tooth nerves become exposed. If the problem seems to stem from anxiety, identifying and relieving the source of anxiety are essential for treatment. If some damage is evident, refer the family to a paediatric dentist so the teeth can be evaluated, repaired (capped) and conserved (www.betterhealth.vic.gov.au/bhcv2/bhcarticles.nsf/pages/dental_care).

Promoting healthy family functioning

Some parents who enjoyed maintaining a rhythm of care for an infant and allowed for ritualistic behaviour of a toddler may have difficulty being the parents of a preschooler because more flexibility and creativity are required. Others come into their own as the parents of a preschooler; they delight in encouraging imaginative games and play. A major parental role during this time is to encourage vocabulary development. One way to do this is to read aloud to a child; another is to answer questions so a child sees language as an organised system of communication. Answering a preschooler's questions can be difficult because the questions are frequently philosophical; for example, "Why is grass green?" A child may listen to an explanation of chlorophyll but then repeat the question, regardless of the clarity of the explanation, because the parent underestimated the extent of the question: the child did not want to know what makes grass green, but why, philosophically, it is not red or blue or yellow. The obvious answer is, "I don't know". Parents who are confident can give this answer without feeling threatened. Parents who are less sure of themselves may feel extremely uncomfortable when they realise they do not know the answers to a 4-year-old's questions.

Consequences

Preschoolers have definite opinions on things such as what they want to eat, where they want to go and what they want to wear. This may bring them into opposition with parents. A major parental responsibility when this happens is to guide a child through these struggles without discouraging the child's right to have an opinion. "Timeout" is a good technique to correct behaviour throughout the preschool years (see Chapter 30). This technique allows parents to discipline without using physical punishment and allows a child to learn a new way of behaviour without extreme stress.

Parental concerns associated with the preschool period

A number of common health problems and fears usually arise during the preschool years.

Common health problems

The mortality of children during the preschool years is low and becoming lower every year as more infectious diseases become preventable. However, the number of minor illnesses, such as colds, ear infections and flu symptoms, is high. Children who live in homes in which parents smoke have a higher incidence of ear (otitis media) and respiratory infections than others (Yilmaz, Caylan & Karacan, 2012). Children who attend childcare or preschool programs also have an increased incidence of gastrointestinal disturbances (such as vomiting and diarrhoea) from exposure to other children (Sun & Sundell, 2011).

Many parents find it extremely difficult to cope with the constant minor infections that occur, causing stress between parent and child. Children may demonstrate frequent whining or clinging behaviour because they do not feel completely well. Such constant illness can cause parents to perceive a child as sickly or not able to cope with everyday life. Parents who encouraged independence before may now begin to overprotect. Give reassurance that frequent, minor illnesses are common in preschoolers. As parents become more experienced in handling these conditions, their perception of whether an illness is a problem will change (see Table 31.2).

TABLE 31.2 Parental difficulties evaluating illness in a preschool child

Difficulty	Helpful suggestions for parents
Evaluating seriousness of illness or condition	Preschoolers are eager to please and tend to answer all questions such as, "Does your stomach hurt?" with a "yes". Observing the child for signs of illness—refusing to eat, holding an arm stiffly, having to go to the toilet frequently—is often more productive as an evaluation technique.
Evaluating bowel and bladder problems	Preschoolers are independent in toilet habits for the first time, so parents do not have nappy contents to evaluate. Frequent trips to the toilet, rubbing the abdomen and holding genitals are the usual signs of bowel or bladder dysfunction.
Evaluating nutritional intake	Preschoolers begin to eat away from home at friends' houses or at childcare, or to stay overnight with grandparents, so parents do not observe daily food intake as accurately as before. Observing whether a child is growing and active is better than monitoring any one day's food intake.
Evaluating bedwetting	Many preschoolers continue to have occasional enuresis at night until school age. If other signs are present—pain, low-grade fever, listlessness—a child should have a urine culture, as persistent bedwetting can indicate a low-grade urinary tract infection.
Evaluating activity vs. hyperactivity	Many lay magazines have articles on hyperactivity in children. Parents often wonder whether their active child is truly hyperactive. As a rule of thumb, if a child can sit through a meal (when he is hungry), watch a half-hour television show (that is his favourite) or sit still while his favourite story is read to him, he is not hyperactive.
Age-specific diseases to be aware of	Preschool age is a time for vision and hearing assessments. For the first time, a child is able to be tested by a standard chart or by audiometry. Urinary tract infections tend to occur with a high frequency in preschool-age girls. Language assessment should be done if a child is not able to make wants known by complete, articulated sentences by the age of 3 (exceptions are transposing "w" for "r" and broken fluency: "I want-want-want to go").

Common fears

Because preschoolers' imaginations are so active, this can lead to a number of fears. Fear of the dark, mutilation and separation or abandonment are all very real to a preschooler. These can rise in incidence when combined with the stress of an illness or hospitalisation (Kushnir & Sadeh, 2011). Although most of these fears can be handled by comforting from parents, in some children, fears are so intensified that they need therapy, such as desensitisation to the fear.

Fear of the dark

The tendency to fear the dark is an example of a fear heightened by a child's vivid imagination: a stuffed toy by daylight becomes a threatening monster at night. Children wake up screaming because of nightmares. They may be reluctant to go to bed or to go back to sleep by themselves.

If parents are prepared for this fear and understand it is a phase of growth, they are better able to cope with it. It is generally helpful if they monitor the stimuli their children are exposed to, especially around bedtime. This includes television, adult discussions and frightening stories. Parents are sometimes reluctant to leave a child's light on at night because they do not want to cater to the fear. Burning a dim night light, however, can solve the problem (see Fig. 31.4). Children who wake up terrified and screaming need reassurance they are safe. They may require an understanding adult to sit on their bed until they can fall back to sleep again. While most preschoolers do not remember in the morning that they had such a dream, they remember for a lifetime that they received comfort when they needed it.

If parents take sensible precautions against fear of the dark or nightmares and a child continues to have this kind of disturbance every night, it may be a reaction to undue stress. In these instances, the source of the stress needs to be investigated. Giving sleep medication to counteract the sleep disturbance does not help solve the basic problem, so this is rarely recommended. Fear of the dark can

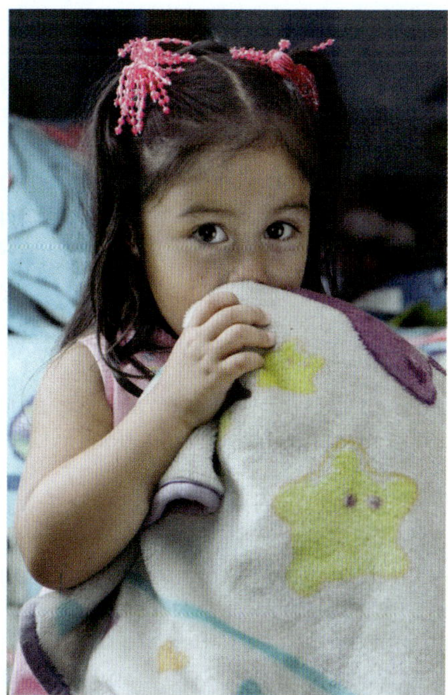

FIGURE 31.4 With a dim night light left on, this young child finds security and comfort in her favourite blanket. (Ricci, S. S., Kyle, T. & Carmen, S. (2012). *Maternity and Pediatric Nursing*. Philadelphia: Lippincott Williams & Wilkins.)

become intensified in a hospital setting and requires careful planning to relieve (Linder & Christian, 2011).

Fear of mutilation

Fear of mutilation is also significant during the preschool years, as revealed by the intense reaction of a preschooler to even a simple injury such as falling and scraping a knee or having a needle inserted for an immunisation. A child cries afterwards not only from the pain but also from the intrusiveness of the injury or procedure. Part of this fear arises because preschoolers do not know which body parts are essential and which ones—like a patch of scraped skin—can be easily replaced. Preschoolers can worry that if some blood is taken out of their bodies, all of their blood will leak out. They often lift a bandage to peek at an incision or cut to see if their body is still intact underneath. They dislike procedures such as injections, otoscopic examination or having a nasogastric tube passed into their stomach. They need good explanations of the limits of healthcare procedures such as a tympanic thermometer does not hurt and a finger prick heals quickly, or distraction techniques in order to feel safe (Erreich, 2011).

Fear of separation or abandonment

Fear of separation continues to be a major concern for preschoolers. For some children it intensifies because their keen imagination allows them to believe they have been deserted when they are safe. Their sense of time is still so distorted they cannot be comforted by assurances such as, "Mummy will pick you up from preschool at lunchtime". Their sense of distance is also limited, so making a statement such as "I work nearby" is not reassuring. Relating time and space to something a child knows, such as meals, television shows or a friend's house, is most effective. For example, stating, "Mummy will pick you up from preschool after you have had your snack" or showing a child the workplace might be more comforting. A hospital admission or going to a new school often brings a child's fear of separation to the forefront. Help parents thoroughly prepare preschoolers for these experiences so they can survive them in sound mental health (Chapter 36).

Behaviour variations

A combination of a keen imagination and immature reasoning results in common behaviour variations in preschoolers.

Telling tall tales

Stretching stories to make them seem more interesting is a phenomenon frequently encountered in this age group. After a trip to the zoo, for example, if you ask a child of this age, "What happened today?" the child perceives you want something exciting to have happened, so might answer, "A bear jumped out of his cage and ate up the boy next to me". This is not lying, but merely supplying an expected answer. Caution parents not to encourage this kind of storytelling, but instead help the child separate fact from fiction by saying, "That's a good story, but now tell me what really happened". This conveys the idea a child has not told the truth, yet does not squash imagination or initiative (Talwar & Crossman, 2011).

Imaginary friends

Many preschoolers have an imaginary friend who plays with them (Nielsen, 2012). They tell a parent to "wait for Eric" or "set a place at the table for Lucy". Parents can help their preschooler separate fact from fantasy about their imaginary friend by saying, "I know Eric isn't real, but if you want to pretend, I'll set a place for him". This response helps a child understand what is real and what is fantasy without restricting their imagination or creativity.

Although imaginary friends are a normal, creative part of the preschool years and can be invented by children who are surrounded by real friends as well as by those who have few, parents may find them disconcerting. If so, ask parents to make certain their child has exposure to real playmates. As long as imaginary friends do not take centre stage in children's lives or prevent them from socialising with other children, they should not pose a problem and often leave as quickly as they come. In the meantime, they can encourage language development and may provide an outlet for a child to express innermost feelings or serve as a handy scapegoat for behaviour about which a child has some conflict.

Difficulty sharing

Sharing is a concept that first comes to be understood around the age of 3 years. Before this, children engage in parallel play (two children need two toys and two spaces to play, because they cannot pass one toy back and forth or play together). Around 3 years of age, children begin to understand that some things are theirs, some belong to others and some can belong to both. For the first time they can stand in line to wait for a drink, take turns using a spade in a sandpit and share a packet of crayons. Sharing does not come easily, however; children who are ill or under stress have even greater difficulty with it than usual. Assure parents that sharing is a difficult concept to grasp and that, as with most skills, preschoolers need practice to understand and learn it.

Parents need to accompany sharing with experiences in learning property rights: "This is my private drawer and no one touches what is in it but me"; "That is your shelf and no one touches the things on it but you"; "This spade is ours and can be used by everyone playing in the sandpit". Defining limits and exposing children to these three categories (*mine, yours, ours*) helps them determine which objects belong to which category.

Regression

Some preschoolers, generally in relation to stress, revert to behaviour they previously outgrew, such as thumb-sucking, negativism, loss of bladder control and inability to separate from their parents. Although the stress that causes this may take many forms, it is usually the result of such things as a new baby in the family, a new school experience, seeing frightening and graphic television news, stress in the home from financial or other problems, marital difficulties or separation caused by hospitalisation.

Help parents understand that regression in these circumstances is normal and a child's thumb-sucking is similar to a parent's reaction to stress (smoking, nail biting, overeating, etc.). Obviously, removing the stress is the best way to help a child discontinue this behaviour. The stresses mentioned, however, are not easily removed. New babies cannot be returned, irreparable marriages cannot be patched together, frightening news happens every day and hospitalisations do occur.

Children undergoing less severe stress should be assured that although situations are changing, the important aspect of their life—someone still loves them and will continue to take care of them—is not. Thumb-sucking or other manifestations of stress are best ignored; calling them to a child's attention merely causes more stress, because it makes children aware they are not pleasing parents, in addition to experiencing the primary stress.

Sibling rivalry

Jealousy of a brother or sister may first become evident during the preschool period (Snowling, 2011). This occurs partly because this is the first time that children have enough vocabulary to express how they feel and partly because preschoolers are more aware of family roles and how responsibilities at home are divided.

A firstborn child is rarely allowed the privileges of a second child because the parents were untried, unsure of how far they should let a child venture or what level of responsibility a child could accept when the child was younger. Alternatively, the firstborn serves as the "trial run" for all children who come after. This phenomenon can lead to sibling rivalry, because children as young as preschool can sense that a younger sibling is being allowed behaviour that was not tolerated in them. They are little appeased by the explanation, "Your brother is just a baby". To help preschoolers feel secure and promote self-esteem, supplying them with a private drawer or box for their things, that parents or other children do not touch, can be helpful. This can help defend their possessions against younger children who do not appreciate their property rights.

Preparing for a new sibling

Introduction of a new sibling is such a major event that parents need to take special steps to be certain their preschooler will be prepared (see Fig. 31.5). There is no rule as to when this preparation should begin, but it should be before the time the child begins to feel the difference the new baby will make. This is perhaps when the mother first begins to look pregnant. It is certainly before parents begin to make physical preparations for the new child. It is always less frightening for a child of any age to understand why

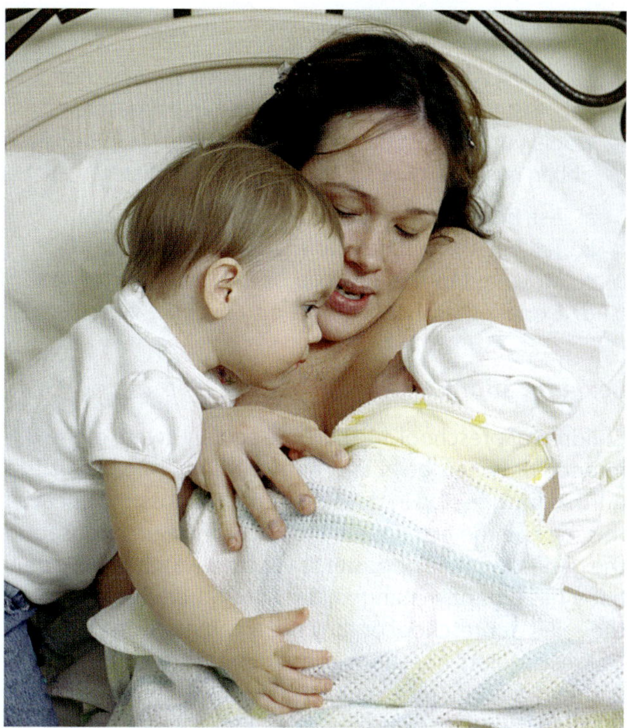

FIGURE 31.5 A toddler greets her new baby sister. (Ricci, S. S., Kyle, T. & Carmen, S. (2012). *Maternity and Pediatric Nursing*. Philadelphia: Lippincott Williams & Wilkins.)

things are happening, no matter how distasteful they may be, rather than hear people whispering or having parents obviously evading the issue. The unknown is always more fearful than a definite event that can be faced and conquered.

Help parents not to underestimate the significance of a bed to a preschool child. It is security, consistency and "home". If their preschooler is sleeping in the cot that is to be used for the new baby, it is usually best if the preschooler is moved to a bed about 3 months in advance of the birth. The parents might explain, "It's time to sleep in a new bed now because you're a big boy". The fact that he is growing up is a better reason for such a move than because a new brother or sister wants the old bed. The latter is a direct cause of sibling rivalry and jealousy.

If children are to start preschool or childcare, they should do so either before the new baby is born or 2 or 3 months afterwards, if possible. That way, children can perceive starting school as a result of maturity and not of being pushed out of the house by the new child.

If the mother will be hospitalised for the birth, she should be certain her child is prepared for this separation in advance. Encourage women to maintain contact with their preschooler during the short time they are hospitalised for the new birth. Some preschoolers may react very coldly to their mothers, turning their head away and refusing to come to them after even just a few days' separation. Allowing the child to visit in the hospital can help relieve this type of separation anxiety.

CASE STUDY QUESTION

3. Cathy will need to change to a new bed because her baby sister will need Cathy's old cot. What measure would you suggest that her parents take to help decrease sibling rivalry between Cathy and her new sister?
   a. Ask her to get her cot ready for the new baby
   b. Tell her she will have to share with the baby
   c. Move her to the new bed before the baby arrives
   d. Explain that sisters grow up to become best friends

Sex education

Children of preschool age become acutely aware of the difference between boys and girls, possibly because it is a normal progression in development and possibly because this may be the first time in their lives they are exposed to the genitalia of the opposite sex as they watch while a new baby has a nappy changed, they see other children using the toilet at preschool or they see a parent nude.

Preschoolers' questions about genital organs are simple and fact-finding; for example, "Why does James look like that?" or "How does Jasmine wee?" Explanations should be just as simple: "Boys look different from girls. The different part is called a penis". It is important for parents not to convey that these body parts are never to be talked about in order to leave an open line of communication for later sexual questions.

It is common for preschoolers to engage in masturbation while watching television or being read to or before they fall asleep at night. The frequency of this may increase under stress, as does thumb-sucking. If observing a child doing this bothers parents, suggest they explain that certain things are done in some places but not in others. Children can relate to this kind of direction without feeling inhibited, just as they can accept the fact that they use a toilet in private or eat only at the table. Calling unnecessary attention to the act can increase anxiety and the activity itself.

An important part of sex education for preschoolers is teaching them to avoid sexual abuse, such as not allowing anyone to touch their body unless they agree. Because children have been taught this, remember to ask permission before giving nursing care that involves touching (Pérez-Fuentes et al., 2012).

Because this may be the time a new brother or sister comes into the family, it is also the most likely time for questions such as, "Where do babies come from?" Parents usually find a simple, factual answer to this type of question is best: "Babies grow in a special place in a mother's body called a uterus". Saying "uterus" rather than "tummy" prevents children from envisioning babies and food all mixed together in their mother's stomach (see Fig. 31.6). Many new books for children explain where babies come from, including descriptions of sexual relations and orgasm. These are helpful for parents to read to a child to increase understanding. See also <www.betterhealth.vic.gov.au/bhcv2/bhcarticles.nsf/pages/sex_education_primary_school_children>.

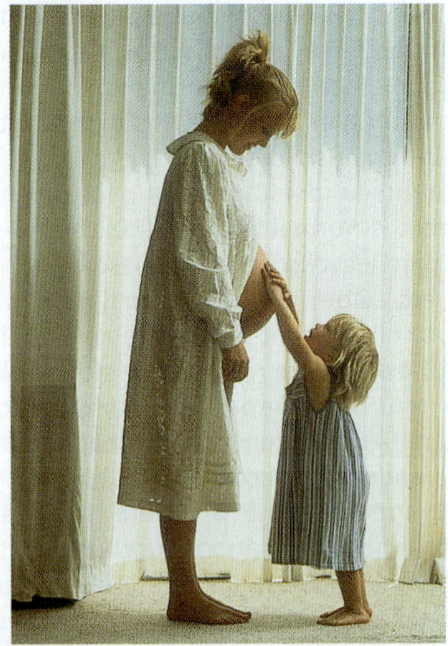

FIGURE 31.6 Preschool children are interested in learning where babies grow and have beginning sexual awareness. (From Taeke Henstra/Science Source/Photo Researchers, Inc.)

Choosing a preschool or childcare centre

A school or childcare experience is helpful for preschoolers, as peer exposure appears to have a positive effect on social development (Gubbels, Van Kann & Jansen, 2013). Children who have learned to be comfortable in a preschool group approach school comfortably, while children who have played only infrequently in groups during the preschool years are forced into learning to handle a new situation when they start school.

To continue to evaluate their child's school experience, urge parents to make a habit of asking children what happened at school, what they learned and the names of any new friends. For the remainder of the growing years, school will have important effects on their child's development. By taking an active role in education, parents influence what and how their child learns.

Preparing a child for school

At the end of the preschool period, children begin a formal school experience as they enter kindergarten or first year. As school involves a great deal of children's time and influences their future greatly, it is important for parents to take time to prepare preschoolers not only physically (being certain their immunisations are up-to-date) but emotionally as well.

Essential to this preparation is the parents' attitude. If school is always discussed as something to look forward to, as an adventure that will be satisfying and rewarding, a child comes to view it as a positive experience. If school is presented as a punishment ("Wait until you get into Year 1—your teacher will make you sit up and behave"), there can be little delight in anticipating it. If a child did not attend preschool, the parents may have to change their daily routine a few months in advance of beginning school to accustom the child to waking earlier or going to bed earlier.

Finally, going to school is a form of separation, especially if a child has not attended childcare or preschool, so parents must prepare for this. It might be good to arrange to have a child stay with another carer for part of a day. Staying at school can then be compared to that event.

These are minimum preparations parents can complete to ready their child for school. Caution both parents and children that no matter how hard they try, not everything can be anticipated; school will bring some new happenings that cannot be predicted. If a child has been led to believe that learning is fun and new experiences are enjoyable (creating a strong sense of initiative), these unpredictable instances can be accepted as fun. The concept that new experiences are enjoyable will prepare a child not only for a first day at school but for thousands of profitable days and experiences ahead.

Broken fluency

Developing language is such a complicated process that children from 2 to 6 years of age typically have some speech difficulty. A child may begin to repeat words or syllables, saying, "I-I-I want a n-n-new spoon-spoon-spoon". This is called **broken fluency** (repetition and prolongation of sounds, syllables and words). It is often referred to as **secondary stuttering** because the child began to speak without this problem and then, during the preschool years, developed it. Unlike the adult who stutters, children are unaware that they are not being fluent unless it is called to their attention. It is a part of normal development and, if accepted as such, will pass. It is associated with rapid speech patterns that may also be present in the parents (Nippold & Packman, 2012). A parent who knows a persistent stutterer or who was a persistent stutterer as a child may react to this normal broken fluency of the preschooler in a more emotional way than the problem deserves. If a child becomes conscious of a disrupted speech pattern, it is less likely the problem will correct itself (see Box 31.3).

BOX 31.3 * Focus on family teaching

Suggestions to reduce broken fluency in a preschool child

Do not discuss in the child's presence that they are having difficulty with speech because this can make the child conscious of speech patterns and compound the problem.

- Listen with patience rather than interrupt or ask the child to speak more slowly or to start over. These actions make the child aware speech is repetitious and broken fluency increases.
- Always talk to the child in a calm, simple way to role model slow speech. If adults talk quickly, the child imitates this pattern and has difficulty speaking clearly.
- Protect space for the child to talk if there are other children in the family. Rushing to say something before a second child interrupts is the same as rushing to conform to adult speech.
- Do not force a child to speak if they do not want to. Do not ask preschoolers to recite or sing for strangers.
- Do not reward a child for fluent speech or punish for non-fluent speech.

Broken fluency is a developmental stage in language formation, not an indication of regression or a chronic speech pattern.

Family with a physically challenged or chronically ill preschooler

Learning how to do things when you have physical limitations can be frustrating. Being unable to understand how to do things because of physical or mental limitations can be even more so. To learn problem solving, however, is part of developing a sense of initiative. A preschooler with a disability such as cerebral palsy has a greater need for problem-solving skills than the average child, because even simple procedures such as eating or getting dressed can be difficult if a physical challenge limits the options.

Physically challenged or chronically ill preschoolers should attend a preschool program if at all possible because of the socialisation benefits. Many of the learning activities that preschoolers enjoy, such as playing with paint, clay or soap bubbles, are messy. If a child must remain in bed, parents may be reluctant to offer these types of experiences. A large tray of dry oats or other breakfast cereal with spades or cars and trucks is a good substitute activity for such a child. Although not necessarily neat, these substances (which are available even in a hospital setting) can be swept away easily at the finish of play. Table 31.3 lists nursing actions that can aid a chronically challenged child to solve problems and develop a sense of initiative.

Experiences with eating help to reinforce a sense of initiative in preschoolers. Chronically ill preschoolers who are limited in the foods they can eat (perhaps they have to maintain a diet of soft foods) or in their ability to help with food preparation may miss this reinforcement. If their appetite is diminished because of illness to the point where they take little or nothing orally, it is still important they continue to join the family at meals. In most households, this is a time for socialisation and preschoolers are ripe for the learning that goes with this type of daily interaction. Encourage parents to include the ill child in family meals and other social occasions whenever possible.

CASE STUDY QUESTION

4. Cathy's parents want to know how to react to her when she begins to masturbate while watching television. What would you suggest?
   a. They give her "timeout" when this begins
   b. They refuse to allow her to watch television
   c. They remind her some activities are private
   d. They schedule a health check-up for vaginal disease

TABLE 31.3 Nursing actions that encourage a sense of initiative in a physically challenged or chronically ill preschooler

Consideration	Nursing actions
Nutrition	Serving toast or sandwiches cut into animal shapes with biscuit cutters, cereal in the form of alphabet characters, or food arranged on a plate to make a face appeals to the imagination and may make a preschooler more interested in food. Respect a child's food preferences.
Dressing changes	Allow a preschooler to measure and cut tape or draw a face on it. Allow child to see incision site. Explain steps of dressing change as you work to reduce unknowns and areas of fear. Provide extra bandages to put on a doll so child can see that bandages themselves are not to be feared.
Medicine	Allow a child to choose a chaser such as juice or milk after oral medicine. Choosing site for injection or intravenous line is too advanced for the preschooler; do not suggest such choices.
Rest	Provide a light in the room or bring the child's bed into the hallway so fear of the dark is reduced. Identify sounds the preschooler might hear in the hospital, such as an air conditioner turning on.
Hygiene	Allow a child to choose bathtime toys, clothing. Allow a child to wash own hands and face. Allow a child to splash in water as a play activity as well as for cleanliness.
Pain	Encourage a preschooler to express pain. Allow a child to handle syringe or suction catheter, and give "injections" or suction to a doll to alleviate anger or fear. Encourage a child to ask for analgesics if necessary.
Stimulation	Guessing games encourage a sense of initiative. Draw a dog or a house and ask the child to close his or her eyes while you add one more detail to the drawing, such as an ear or a chimney; ask the child to identify new item. Reverse the game and ask the child what you erased from the drawing or allow the child to do own drawing. Provide manipulative toys, such as finger paint, soapy water, clay or dry cereal to use as sand. Allow a preschooler to accompany you to other departments as a way of teaching more about the hospital. Use "Simon Says" games not only for socialisation but also to urge treatments, such as deep-breathing exercises. Encourage use of playroom for socialisation. Encourage a child to interact with family by drawing pictures for siblings or using the telephone to call home.

Key points for review

- Although preschoolers grow only slightly and gain just a little weight, they seem much taller than when they were toddlers because their contour changes to more childlike proportions.
- Erikson's developmental task for the preschool period is to gain a sense of initiative or learn how to do things. Play materials ideal for this age group are those that stimulate creativity, such as modelling clay or coloured pens and pencils.
- Promoting childhood safety is a major role because preschoolers' active imaginations can lead them into dangerous situations.
- Appetite is not large in this age group because this is not a rapid growth time. Preschoolers can be interested in helping with food preparation.
- Common parental concerns during the preschool period are broken fluency, imaginary friends, difficulty sharing and sibling rivalry.
- Preschool is often the time when a new sibling is born. Good preparation for this event is necessary to prevent intense sibling rivalry.
- Preschoolers may have a number of universal fears, including fear of the dark, mutilation and abandonment. All care provided for this age group should include active measures to reduce these fears as much as possible.
- Preschoolers are still operating at a cognitive level that prevents them from understanding conservation (objects have not changed substance although they have changed appearance). This means they need an explanation, for example, of how they will be the same person postoperatively as they were preoperatively.
- Preschoolers are self-centered (egocentric). This makes it difficult for them to share and view someone else's side of a problem. They need good explanations of how a procedure will benefit them before they can agree to it.
- Many preschoolers begin preschool programs or childcare. Late in the preschool period, they may be enrolled in kindergarten. Parents often appreciate guidance on how to prepare their children for these new experiences.
- Preschoolers who are physically challenged or who have chronic illnesses may have difficulty achieving a sense of initiative, because they may be limited in their ability to participate in activities that stimulate initiative. They may need special playtimes set aside for stimulation and learning.

CASE STUDY QUESTIONS

5. Cathy's father Matt is concerned because Cathy tells exaggerated stories about events at her preschool. How would you recommend her father handle this?

6. Because her family is moving, Cathy will be starting at a new preschool next week. What suggestions could you make to Matt about choosing a safe setting? How should he prepare Cathy for this experience?

7. Matt and Jackie tell you that Cathy keeps the entire family awake at night because she is so afraid of the dark. What suggestions could you make to help relieve this problem?

Resources

For an extensive range of additional resources to enhance teaching and learning and to facilitate understanding of this chapter, please see the text's accompanying website located on thePoint at http://thepoint.lww.com.

References

Agarwal, A. & Pruthi, M. (2010). Bicycle-spoke injuries of the foot in children. *Journal of Orthopedic Surgery*, *18*(3), 338–341.

Bevan, A. L. & Reilly, S. M. (2011). Mothers' efforts to promote healthy nutrition and physical activity for their preschool children. *Nursing*, *26*(5), 395–403.

Bowman, S. M., Aitken, M. E., Robbins, J. M., et al. (2012). Trends in US pediatric drowning hospitalizations, 1993–2008. *Pediatrics*, *129*(2), 275–281.

Byars, K. C., Yolton, K., Rausch, J., et al. (2012). Prevalence, patterns, and persistence of sleep problems in the first 3 years of life. *Pediatrics*, *129*(2), 276–284.

de Amorim Lde, F., Estrela, C. & da Costa, L. R. (2011). Effects of traumatic dental injuries to primary teeth on permanent teeth. *Dental Traumatology*, *27*(2), 117–121.

Erreich, A. (2011). More than enough guilt to go around: Oedipal guilt, survival guilt, separation guilt. *Journal of the American Psychoanalytical Association*, *59*(1), 131–151.

Erikson, E. H. (1993). *Childhood and Society*. New York: W. W. Norton.

Fergusson, D. M., Boden, J. M., & Horwood, L. J. (2013). Nine-year follow-up of a home-visitation program: A randomized trial. *Pediatrics*, *131*(2), 297–303.

Goldman, R. D. (2012). Cranberry juice for urinary tract infection in children. *Canadian Family Physician*, *58*(4), 398–401.

Gubbels, J. S., Van Kann, D. H. & Jansen, M. W. (2013). Play equipment, physical activity opportunities, and children's activity levels at childcare. *Journal of Environmental & Public Health*, 326520.

Hodges, E. A., Smith, C., Tidwell, S., et al. (2012). Promoting physical activity in preschoolers to prevent obesity. *Journal of Pediatric Nursing*, *28*(1), 3–19.

Kohlberg, L. (1984). *The Psychology of Moral Development*. New York: Harper & Row.

Kushnir, J. & Sadeh, A. (2011). Sleep of preschool children with nighttime fears. *Sleep Medicine*, *12*(9), 870–874.

Linder, L. A. & Christian, B. J. (2011). Characteristics of the nighttime hospital bedside care environment (sound, light, and temperature) for children with cancer. *Cancer Nursing*, *34*(3), 176–184.

Merlino, G. & Gigli, G. I. (2012). Sleep related movement disorders. *Neurological Sciences*, *33*(3), 491–513.

Mitka, M. (2012). Programs to reduce childhood obesity seem to work, say Cochrane reviewers. *Journal of the American Medical Association*, *307*(5), 444–445.

Nielsen, M. (2012). Imitation, pretend play, and childhood: Essential elements in the evolution of human culture? *Journal of Comparative Psychology*, *126*(2), 170–181.

Nippold, M. A. & Packman, A. (2012). Managing stuttering beyond the preschool years. *Language, Speech & Hearing Services in Schools*, *43*(3), 338–343.

Paulus, M. & Moore, C. (2012). Producing and understanding prosocial actions in early childhood. *Advances in Child Development & Behavior*, *42*(8), 271–305.

Pérez-Fuentes, G., Olfson, M., Villegas, L., et al. (2012). Prevalence and correlates of child sexual abuse: A national study. *Comprehensive Psychiatry*, *54*(1), 16–27.

Piaget, J. (1969). *The Theory of Stages in Cognitive Development*. New York: McGraw-Hill.

Raman, L. (2011). Why do we eat? Children's and adults' understanding of why we eat different meals. *Journal of Genetic Psychology*, *172*(4), 401–413.

Smith, G. A. & Riedford, K. (2012). Epidemiology of early childhood caries: Clinical application. *Journal of Pediatric Nursing*, *28*, 369–373.

Smith, S. (2011). Vulvovaginitis. In K. J. Marcdante, R. M. Kliegman, H. B. Jenson, et al. (Eds), *Nelson Essentials of Pediatrics* (6th ed.), pp. 415–416. Philadelphia: Saunders/Elsevier.

Snowling, M. J. (2011). Editorial: What's behind sibling rivalry: Checks and balances in the sibling relationship. *Journal of Child Psychology & Psychiatry & Allied Disciplines*, *52*(6), 629–630.

Sun, Y. & Sundell, J. (2011). Early daycare attendance increases the risk for respiratory infections and asthma of children. *Journal of Asthma*, *48*(8), 790–796.

Talwar, V. & Crossman, A. (2011). From little white lies to filthy liars: The evolution of honesty and deception in young children. *Advances in Child Development & Behavior*, *40*(4), 139–179.

Tubert-Jeannin, S., Auclair, C., Amsallem, E., et al. (2011). Fluoride supplements (tablets, drops, lozenges or chewing gums) for preventing dental caries in children. *Cochrane Database of Systematic Reviews*, (12), CD007592.

Whitney, E. N. & Rolfes, S. R. (2013). Life cycle nutrition: Infancy, childhood and adolescence. In E. N. Whitney & S. R. Rolfes, *Understanding Nutrition* (13th ed., pp. 504–550). New York: Wadsworth/Cengage Learning.

Yilmaz, G., Caylan, N. D. & Karacan, C. D. (2012). Effects of active and passive smoking on ear infections. *Current Infectious Disease Reports*. Accessed 23 March 2015, <www.ncbi.nlm.nih.gov/pubmed/22302576>.

Suggested readings

ARACY <www.aracy.org.au>

BabyCenter Australia <www.babycenter.com.au>

Kidsafe—Child Accident Prevention Foundation of Australia <www.kidsafe.com.au>

Kidshealth NZ <www.kidshealth.org.nz>

Kidspot Australia <www.kidspot.com.au>

Lemelin, L., Gallagher, F., & Haggerty, J. (2012). Supporting parents of preschool children in adopting a healthy lifestyle. *BMC Nursing*, *11*(1), 12.

Ministry of Health NZ <www.health.govt.nz>

Ministry of Social Development: Community Investment <www.familyservices.govt.nz>

Raising Children Network <http://raisingchildren.net.au>

Rosales, P. P., & Allen, P. L. (2012). Optimism bias and parental views on unintentional injuries and safety: Improving anticipatory guidance in early childhood. *Pediatric Nursing*, *38*(2), 73–79.

Safekids Aotearoa <www.safekids.org.nz>

Tresillian <www.tresillian.net>

Triple P <www.triplep.net/glo-en/home/>

Well Child <www.wellchild.org.nz>

Chapter 32

Nursing care of a family with a school-aged child

The previous chapter discussed the preschooler and the abilities children develop in those years. This chapter adds information about the dramatic changes, both physical and psychosocial, that occur during the school-aged years. Such information builds a base for care and health teaching for this age group.

LEARNING OBJECTIVES

After studying the contents of this chapter, you should be able to:

1. Describe the normal growth and development patterns and common parental concerns of the school-aged period.
2. Use critical thinking to analyse ways in which the care of school-aged children can be more family-centred.
3. Assess a school-aged child for normal growth and developmental milestones.
4. Formulate nursing considerations that speak to both school-aged children and their families.
5. Identify expected outcomes for nursing care of a school-aged child.
6. Plan anticipatory guidance to prevent problems of growth and development in a school-aged child such as teaching about normal puberty.
7. Implement nursing care to help achieve normal growth and development of a school-aged child.
8. Evaluate expected outcomes for achievement and effectiveness of care.
9. Integrate knowledge of school-aged growth and development with nursing process to achieve quality child and family health nursing care.

KEY TERMS

- accommodation
- cavities
- class inclusion
- conservation
- cottonwool children
- decentring

CASE STUDY

Susie Lewis is a 12-year-old girl who recently started high school. Her mother tells you that although Susie, who is overweight, says she likes school, she has developed a lot of nervous habits such as nail biting since school started. Her mother asks if this is normal.

CASE STUDY QUESTION

1. How would you advise Susie's mother?

The term "school-aged" commonly refers to children between the ages of 6 and 12 years. Although these years represent a time of slow physical growth, cognitive growth and development continue to proceed at rapid rates. Because of this, there are many differences among children at each year of this age group. For example, 7- and 10-year-old children have very different needs and outlooks than do 11- and 12-year-old children. Because of these big differences, always assess children as individuals to understand the particular developmental needs of each child based on what developmental status has been achieved, not on what stage you think the child should have reached (Lowe et al., 2013). Unlike the infant or toddler periods, when progress is marked by obvious new abilities and skills such as the ability to sit up or roll over or the ability to speak a full sentence, the development of a school-aged child is much more subtle and may be marked by irregular mood swings; what the child enjoys on one occasion may not be acceptable on the next. For instance, a child may ask his parents for a guitar and lessons, but then after the family invests in these, he may quickly lose interest in music and prefer soccer. School-aged children are also more influenced by the attitudes of their friends. They may choose not to do something that was previously enjoyable because no friends are interested in the activity.

The school-aged period is usually the first time children begin to make truly independent judgements. Because parents may not be prepared for this, additional conflicts may develop between parents and their children.

HEALTHY DEVELOPMENT OF A SCHOOL-AGED CHILD

Assessment

Use both history and physical examination to assess growth and development of a school-aged child. Include questions about school activities and progress. School-aged children are interested and able to contribute to their own health history; to allow for this, it is useful to interview children 10 years or older at least in part without their parents present. During the physical examination, show your respect for children's adult-level modesty by providing a gown. Explain all procedures to both the parents/carers and the child.

Parents of school-aged children often mention behavioural issues or conflicts during annual health visits. Some parents feel they are losing contact with their children during these years. This can cause them to misinterpret a normal change in behaviour, especially if they are not prepared. Other parents may consider children who behave differently from their siblings as "abnormal" when children are just expressing their own personality.

When problems are discussed in the healthcare setting, take the history from the parent/carer but also allow the child to express the problem. If the problem is related to a medical condition, the effect on the family should also be assessed, as the illness of a child can impact on the functioning of the entire family.

Nursing considerations

Common nursing considerations pertinent to growth and development during the school-aged period are:

- Health-seeking behaviours related to normal school-aged growth and development
- Anxiety related to slow growth pattern of child
- Risk of injury related to deficient parental knowledge about safety precautions for a school-aged child
- Imbalanced nutrition related to frequent consumption of snack foods
- Delayed growth and development related to speech, motor, psychosocial or cognitive concerns.

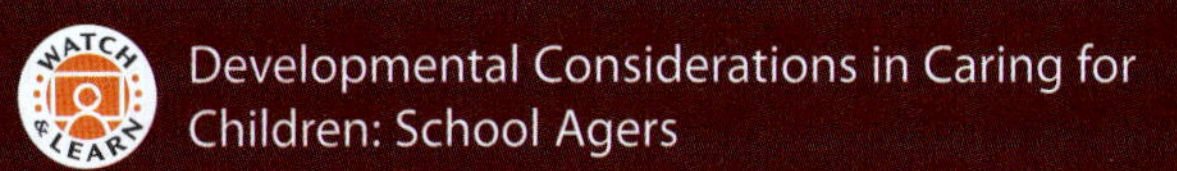

GROWTH AND DEVELOPMENT OF A SCHOOL-AGED CHILD

Growth and development of a school-aged child occur slowly and over a relatively long time span although children grow and develop extensively during this period.

Physical growth

School-aged children's annual average weight gain is approximately 1.3 to 2.2 kg; the increase in height is 2.5 to 5 cm. Children who did not lose the lordosis and knock-kneed appearance of toddlers during the preschool period lose these now. Posture becomes more erect. By 10 years of age, brain growth is complete, so fine motor coordination becomes refined. As the eye globe reaches its final shape at about this same time, an adult vision level is achieved. If the eruption of permanent teeth and growth of the jaw do not correlate with final head growth, *malocclusion* (a deviation from the normal) with teeth malalignment may be present (El-Dawlatly, Fayed & Mostafa, 2012).

The immune globulins IgG and IgA each reach adult levels, and lymphatic tissue continues to grow in size until about 9 years of age. The resulting abundance of tonsillar and adenoid tissue in young school children is often mistaken for disease because the tonsils seem to fill the entire back of the throat. This may also result in temporary conduction deafness from Eustachian tube obstruction until the tissue recedes normally. The appendix is also lined with lymphatic tissue, so swelling of this tissue in the narrow tube can lead to trapped faecal material and inflammation (appendicitis) in the early school-aged child (Bishop, 2011). Frontal sinuses develop at about 6 years of age, so sinus headaches become a possibility (before then, a headache in children is rarely caused by a sinus infection) (Smith, 2011).

The left ventricle of the heart enlarges to be strong enough to pump blood to the growing body. Innocent heart murmurs may become apparent due to this extra blood crossing heart valves. The pulse rate decreases to 70 to 80 beats/min; blood pressure rises to about 112/60 mmHg. Maturation of the respiratory system leads to increased oxygen–carbon dioxide exchange, which increases exertion ability and stamina. Scoliosis may become apparent for the first time in late childhood (Fletcher & Bruce, 2012). All school-aged children over 8 years should be screened for this at all health appraisals (see Chapter 51).

Sexual maturation

At a set point in brain maturity, the hypothalamus transmits an enzyme to the anterior pituitary gland to begin production of gonadotrophic hormones, which activate changes in testes and ovaries and produce puberty. Hormonal changes that occur with puberty are discussed in Chapter 5. Table 32.1 describes the usual order in which secondary sex characteristics develop.

Timing of the onset of puberty varies widely, between 10 and 14 years of age. The length of time it takes to pass through puberty to sexual maturity also varies. Sexual maturation in girls usually occurs between 12 and 18 years; in boys, between 14 and 20 years. However, puberty is occurring increasingly earlier and, in a class of 10-year-old students, it is not unusual to discover that more than half of the girls are already menstruating (Edmonds, 2012).

Sexual and physical concerns

The changes in physical appearance that come with puberty can lead to concerns for both children and parents. School age is a time for parents to discuss with children the physical changes that will occur and the sexual responsibility these changes dictate. This is also a time to reinforce previous teaching with children that their body is their own, to be used only in the way they choose (see Box 32.1 for strategies to help children avoid sexual abuse).

In both sexes, puberty brings changes in the sebaceous glands. Under the influence of androgen, glands become more active, setting the stage for acne (see Chapter 33). Vasomotor instability commonly leads to blushing; perspiration also increases (Daley, 2011).

Concerns of girls. Prepubertal girls are usually taller, by about 5 cm or more, than pre-adolescent boys because their typical growth spurt begins earlier. In a culture in

TABLE 32.1 Chronological development of secondary sex characteristics

Age (years)	Boys	Girls
9–11	Prepubertal weight gain occurs.	Breasts: elevation of papilla with breast bud formation; areolar diameter enlarges.
11–12	Sparse growth of straight, downy, slightly pigmented hair at base of penis. Scrotum becoming textured; growth of penis and testes begins. Sebaceous gland secretion increases. Perspiration increases.	Straight hair along the labia. Vaginal epithelium becomes cornified. pH of vaginal secretions becomes acidic; slight mucous vaginal discharge present. Sebaceous gland secretion increases. Perspiration increases. Dramatic growth spurt.
12–13	Pubic hair present across pubis. Penis lengthens. Dramatic linear growth spurt. Breast enlargement may occur.	Pubic hair grows darker; spreads over entire pubis. Breasts enlarge, still no protrusion of nipples. Axillary hair present. Menarche occurs.

which boys are expected to be taller than girls, this can cause concern. Sometimes a girl notices the change in her pelvic contour when she tries on a skirt or dress from the year before and realises her hips are becoming broader. She may misinterpret this finding as a gain in weight and attempt a crash diet. She can be reassured that broad bone structure of the hips is part of an adult female profile.

Girls are usually conscious of breast development and whether they are overdeveloped or underdeveloped. Also, breast development is not always symmetrical, so it is not unusual for a girl to have breasts of slightly different sizes. After the condition has been checked during a physical examination, she can be reassured that this development is normal. Supernumerary (additional) nipples may darken or increase in size at puberty. Be sure girls understand that a supernumerary nipple is affected by the hormones in her body in the same way as other breast tissue, so she understands these changes are normal.

BOX 32.1 * Focus on family teaching

Teaching points to help children avoid sexual abuse

Q. Susie's mother wants to protect her daughter from sexual abuse. She asks you, "What are good rules to teach children without scaring them?"

A. A number of common rules are:

1. Your body is your property and you can decide who looks at it or touches it.
2. Secrets are fun things to keep. If a person asks you not to tell about something that was done to you that you did not like, it is not a secret. It is all right to tell about it.
3. Do not go anywhere with a stranger (a stranger is someone you do not know, not someone "strange"). Do not be fooled by people asking you to give them directions or to go with them because your mother is sick or hurt or they have lost a pet.
4. Being touched by someone you like is a good feeling. You do not have to allow anyone to touch you in a way you do not like. Do not allow yourself to be left alone with a person you are uncomfortable with because that person touches you in a way you do not like.
5. A "private part" is the part of you a swimming costume touches. If anyone asks you to show them a private part or touches a private part, tell them to stop and tell someone else.
6. If the person you tell does not believe you, keep telling people until someone does believe you.

Early preparation for menstruation is important for the girl's concept of herself as a woman (Marván & Molina-Abolnik, 2012). In addition to an explanation of the reason for menstrual flow, girls need an explanation of good hygiene and reassurance they can bathe, shower and swim during their periods. They can use either sanitary napkins or tampons; if they choose tampons, they must take precautions to avoid toxic shock syndrome (see Chapter 47).

The average age at which menarche (the first menstrual period) occurs is 12.4 years (Horne & Critchley, 2012). Most girls have some menstrual irregularity during the first year or two after menarche. This occurs primarily because a girl's cycles are anovulatory at first. With maturity and the onset of ovulation, cycles become more regular. A pre-adolescent who is experiencing consistent irregularities in her period should be assessed for malnourishment and obesity as possible influences. Emotions can also cause irregularity. If irregularity continues beyond the first year, a careful history of the girl's school, social life, nutritional intake, level of exercise and home adjustment should be taken. Dysmenorrhoea, or painful menstruation, is discussed in Chapter 47.

Girls also need to know that vaginal secretions will begin to be present. If this is not explained, a girl may fear needlessly that she has contracted an infection. Explain that any secretions that cause vulvar irritation should be checked at a healthcare facility because this does suggest infection.

Concerns of boys. Boys who are not prepared for the physical changes of puberty are equally as concerned about them as girls. Just as girls are keenly aware of breast development, boys are aware of increasing genital size. If they do not know that testicular development precedes penis growth, they can worry that their growth will be inadequate. As seminal fluid is produced, boys begin to notice ejaculation

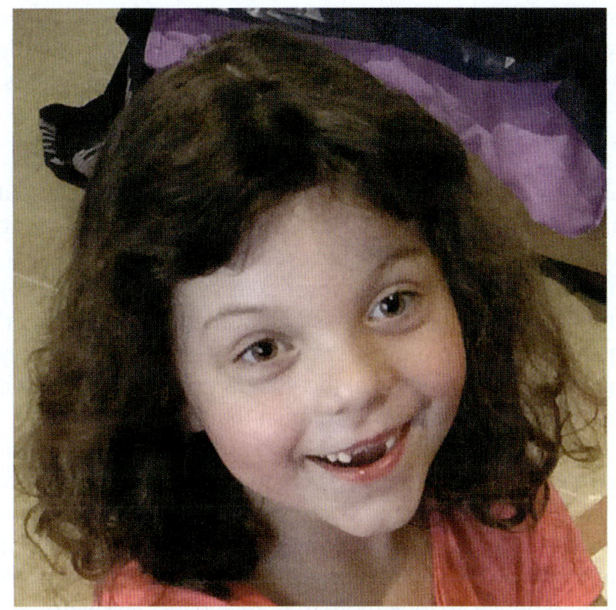

FIGURE 32.1 Younger school-aged children typically have a missing upper incisor as deciduous teeth are replaced by permanent teeth. (© Lisa Speedie.)

during sleep, termed *nocturnal emissions* (Widaman & Helm, 2012).

Boys should also be informed that hypertrophy of breast tissue (gynaecomastia) can occur in prepuberty (most often in stocky or obese boys) and that this is a transitory phenomenon. Although it may cause self-conscious reactions, it will fade as soon as the male hormones become more mature and active. Some boys also become concerned because, although they have pubic hair, they cannot yet grow a beard or do not have chest hair—outward, easily recognised signs of maturity. You can assure them that pubic hair normally appears first and that chest and facial hair may not grow until several years later.

Teeth

Deciduous teeth are lost and permanent teeth erupt during the school-aged period (see Fig. 32.1). The average child gains 28 teeth between 6 and 12 years of age: the central and lateral incisors; first, second and third cuspids; and first and second molars (see Fig. 32.2). Teeth and dental care will be discussed further later in this chapter.

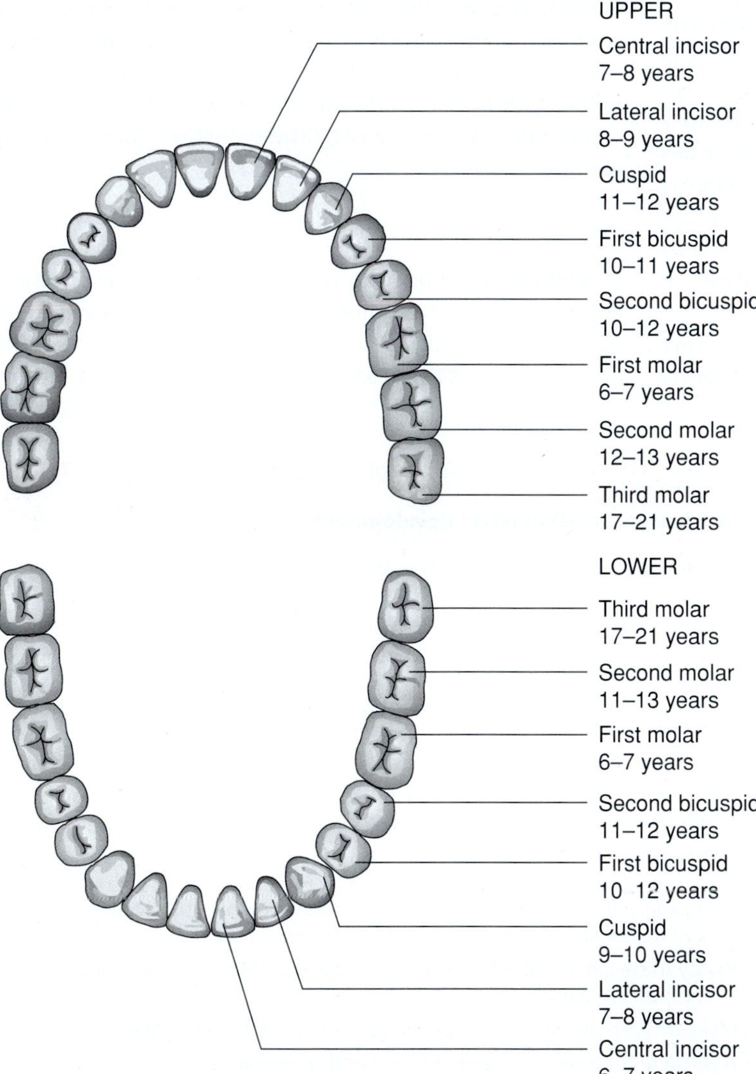

FIGURE 32.2 Eruption pattern of permanent teeth.

Developmental milestones

As with all ages, you can measure school-aged children's progress by whether they meet typical developmental milestones.

Gross motor development

School-aged development milestones are summarised in Table 32.2. At the beginning of the school-aged period (age 6), children endlessly jump, tumble, skip and hop. They have enough coordination to walk in a straight line. Many can ride a bicycle. A 7-year-old appears quiet compared with a rough-and-tumble 6-year-old. Gender differences usually begin to manifest in play: there are "girl games", such as dressing dolls and "boy games", such as pretending to be pirates.

The movements of 8-year-olds are more graceful than those of younger children, although as their arms and legs grow, they may stumble on furniture or spill milk and food. They ride a bicycle well and enjoy sports such as gymnastics, soccer and hockey.

Nine-year-olds are on the go constantly, as if they always have a deadline to meet. They have enough eye–hand coordination to enjoy baseball, basketball and volleyball. By 10 years of age, they are more interested in perfecting their athletics skills than they were previously.

At the age of 11, many children feel awkward because of their growth spurt and drop out of sports activities rather than look ungainly. They may channel their energy into constant motion instead: drumming fingers and tapping pencils or feet. This fall in sports participation may concern parents who see sport as the key to popularity or self-esteem.

Twelve-year-olds plunge into activities with intensity and concentration. They often enjoy participating in sports events for charities, such as walk-a-thons. They may be refreshingly cooperative around the house, able to handle a great deal of responsibility and to complete given tasks.

Fine motor development

Six-year-olds can easily tie their shoelaces. They can cut and paste well and draw a person in detail. They can print, although they may routinely reverse letters. Seven-year-olds concentrate on fine motor skills even more than they did the year before. This has been called the "eraser year" because children are never quite content with what they have done. They set too high a standard for themselves and then have difficulty performing at that level.

By 8 years of age, children's eyes are developed enough to read regular-sized type. This can make reading a greater pleasure and school more enjoyable. Eight-year-olds learn to write script rather than print. They enjoy showing off this new skill in cards, letters or projects. By the age of 9, their writing begins to look more mature and less awkward.

Older school-aged children begin to evaluate their teachers' ability and may perform at varying levels, depending on each teacher's expectations. The school curriculum involves more complex science and mathematics courses than previously as well as more challenging literature. This may be a child's first exposure to reading as a fulfilling and worthwhile experience rather than just as an assignment: it may be the time a child is "turned on" to reading.

Play

Play continues to be rough at the age of 6. However, when children discover reading as an enjoyable activity that opens doors to other worlds, they may begin to spend quiet time with books. Many children spend hours

TABLE 32.2 Summary of school-aged development milestones

Age (years)	Physical development	Psychosocial and cognitive development
6	A year of constant motion; skipping is a new skill; first molars erupt.	Primary school teacher becomes authority figure; adjustment to all-day school may be difficult and lead to nervous manifestations of fingernail biting, etc. Defines words by their use: a key is to unlock a door, not a metal object.
7	Central incisors erupt; difference between sexes becomes apparent in play (e.g. pirate games vs. dolls); spends time in quiet play.	A quiet year; striving for perfection leads to this year being called an "eraser year." Conservation (water poured from tall container to a wide, flat one is the same amount of water) is learned; can tell time; can make simple change.
8	Coordination definitely improved; playing with gang becomes important; eyes become fully developed.	"Best friends" develop; whispering and giggling begin; can write as well as print; understands concepts of past, present and future.
9	All activities done with gang.	Gang age; a 9-year-old club is formed to spite someone, has secret codes, is all boy or all girl; gangs disband and reform quickly.
10	Coordination improves.	Ready to stay away from home; collecting age; likes rules; ready for competitive games.
11	Active, but awkward and ungainly.	Insecure with members of opposite sex; repeats off-colour jokes.
12	Coordination improves.	A sense of humour is present; is social and cooperative.

playing increasingly difficult video games, an activity that can either foster a healthy sense of competition or create isolation from others. The playing and use of computer games and other electronic games should be monitored due to short- and long-term negative effects. The Australian Government has published several fact sheets regarding recommendations around age-appropriate games and playing times for all ages, which can assist parents to make healthy choices for their children; see <www.mychild.gov.au/sites/mychild/families-and-carers/pages/health-wellbeing>.

Around 7 years of age, children require more props for play, which indicates the start of a decline in imaginative play; this may continue unless a child receives adequate encouragement to use imagination. Children also begin to develop an interest in collecting items such as rugby cards, dolls, rocks or marbles. The type of item may not be as important as the quantity.

By the age of 8, collections may become increasingly structured as children develop skills for sorting and cataloguing. Most girls and boys of this age also enjoy helping in the kitchen with jobs such as making biscuits and salads or icing cakes. They start to be more involved in simple science projects and experiments. Eight-year-olds also like table games but hate to lose, so they tend to avoid competitive games. They may change the rules in the middle of a game to keep from losing.

Nine-year-olds play hard. They wake in the morning, squeeze in some activity before school and plan something the moment they arrive home again (see Fig. 32.3). They may have difficulty going to bed at night because they want to play just one more game. Play is rough; children are not as interested in perfecting their skills as they will be in another year. Conflict may arise when parents or coaches expect children of this age to be more interested in perfecting their skills.

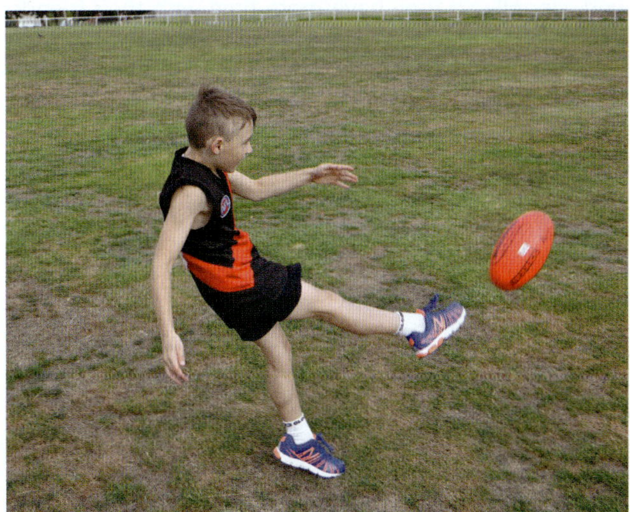

FIGURE 32.3 A young male plays football after a full day at school. (© Lisa Speedie.)

Nine years of age is also a time for discovering the Internet. Not yet wise enough to recognise the dangers associated with talking to strangers online, this is an activity parents need to supervise (Briggs, Simon & Simonsen, 2011). Box 32.3 later in the chapter provides strategies for online safety.

At about 10 years of age, children become very interested in rules and fairness in competitive play situations. Music and artistic expression also become important during this time. Many schools begin music lessons for children at this age. Children do well if others in their group are taking similar lessons. Talent for music or art becomes evident and children respond with new interest in school or wherever they are exposed to these arts.

During preteen years, listening to music and learning popular dances take the place of earlier simple games. They are accommodating enough again to be able to play with younger siblings who need the rules modified to their advantage. Time with friends is often spent just talking. If older school-aged children use their bedroom as a place to meet with friends, they become more interested in keeping it tidy. Twelve-year-olds typically like to do jobs such as raking leaves or babysitting for money. Both boys and girls seem to feel they are on the verge of something great and anxiously wait to turn 13 years old and become teenagers.

Language development

Six-year-olds talk in full sentences, using language easily and with meaning. They no longer sound as though talking is an experiment but appear to have incorporated language permanently. They still define objects by their use: a key is to unlock a door while a fork is to eat with.

Most 7-year-olds can tell the time in hours, but they may have trouble with concepts such as "half past" and "quarter to", especially with the prevalence of digital clocks and watches. They know the months of the year and can name the months in which holidays fall. They can add and subtract and make simple calculations (if they have had experience), so they can go to the shop and make basic purchases. Much of children's talk is concerned with these concepts as they practise them and show them off to family or friends.

As children discover "dirty" jokes at about the age of 9, they like to tell them to friends or try to understand those told by adults. They use swear words to express anger or just to show other children they are growing up. They may have a short period of intense fascination with vulgarity as they did during preschool years. As before, if parents want to discourage this, they should make it clear they find such language unacceptable and refrain from using it themselves in their child's presence. By 12 years of age, a sense of humour is apparent. Twelve-year-olds can carry on an adult conversation, although stories are limited because of their lack of experience.

Emotional development

Ideally, children enter the school-aged period with the ability to trust others and a sense of respect for their own worth. They can accomplish small tasks independently because they have gained a sense of autonomy. They should have practised or mimicked adult roles and had the opportunity to explore at preschool or other social environments. They should have learned to share, to have discovered that learning is fun and an adventure, and that doing things is more important and more rewarding than watching things being done (a sense of initiative).

Developmental task: industry versus inferiority

During the early school years, children attempt to master yet another developmental step: learning a sense of industry or accomplishment (Erikson, 1993). If gaining a sense of initiative can be defined as learning how to do things, then gaining a sense of industry is learning how to do things well.

If children are prevented from achieving a sense of industry or do not receive rewards for accomplishment, they can develop a feeling of inferiority or become convinced they cannot do things they actually can do. These children will have difficulty tackling new situations later in life (new job, new school, new responsibility) because they cannot envision how they could be successful. This can result in frustration with school or work activities.

The questions a preschool child asks reflect curiosity, such as "how", "why" and "what". During the early school years, children concentrate their questions on the "how" of tasks: "Is this the right way to do this?", "Am I making this right?", "Is this good?" Often school-aged children will comment, "I can't do anything right" because their craft project does not look perfect or falls short of expectations. School-aged children need reassurance they are doing things correctly and this reassurance is best if it comes frequently.

In relation to reading, the most preferred type of book for school-aged children has many short chapters; children feel a sense of accomplishment when they finish each chapter. Hobbies and projects are also enjoyed best if they are small and can be finished within a short time (see Fig. 32.4). Most school-aged children, for example, prefer putting together two or three fairly simple model kits to assembling one extremely complicated kit. The multiple kits offer multiple rewards; the involved one delays the reward so long the child may become bored and never complete it. With adolescence will come more respect for quality. Children will realise if they want the better model, they will have to spend the extra energy and attention—quality products involve quality work.

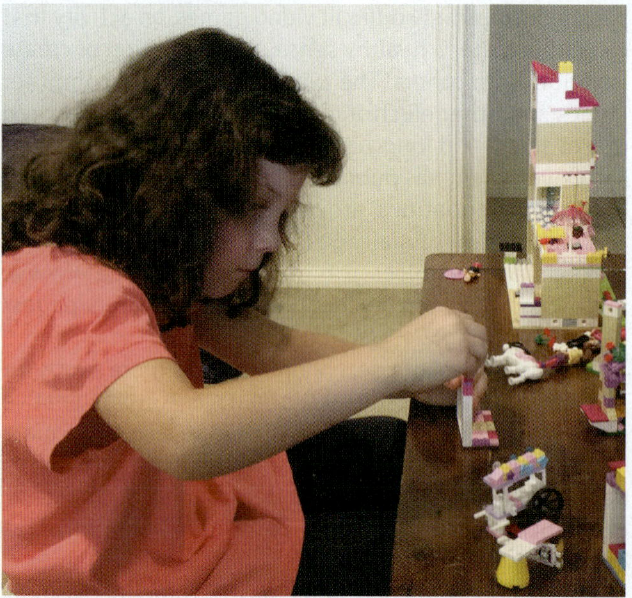

FIGURE 32.4 Assembling toys such as Lego in a short time helps a school-aged child to gain a sense of industry. (© Lisa Speedie.)

Home as a setting to learn industry

Parents of a school-aged child need to take a step forwards in development along with their child. For the first time, they realise their child looks to role models other than themselves. Parents who enjoyed fostering imagination in a preschooler may feel frustrated when a school-aged child begins to conform to rules and insists on the "right way" to do things. They may feel they have failed to encourage the child's creativity, but conformity is vital to children of this age. It is how they learn more about their world's rules.

Eight- or nine-year-olds begin to spend more and more time with their peers and less time with their family. They forget to do household chores they once enjoyed, such as setting the table or mowing the lawn, or they may do the work sloppily so they have more time with their friends. Although this may seem like a regression in behaviour, it is actually a step of independence away from the parents and into the larger world, a developmental task that will help them become emotionally mature. This is an example of a new role the child is trying out, one of many that will be tried in the process of reaching maturity, when an eventual "right-fit" is found.

School as a setting to learn industry

Adjusting to and achieving in school are two of the major tasks for this age group. Ideally, a child's teacher will think of learning as fun and will encourage a child to plunge into new experiences. Schools are increasingly assuming responsibility for education about sex, safety, avoidance of substances of abuse and preparation for family living. These discussions are generally superficial, however, and if the classes are large, they may raise more questions than they answer. Although learning these skills with peers helps children learn other people's opinions in these areas, such classes should not replace parental teaching.

Structured activities

Youth groups, Scouts and Girl Guides are respected school-aged activities. If the local organisations are well run by leaders who understand children's needs, they can provide hours of constructive activity and strengthen a sense of industry. As with school activities, parents should determine the suitability of each organisation for their individual child.

Urge parents to evaluate competitive sports programs as well. Before children can compete successfully, they must be able to lose a game without feeling devastated—in other words, to be able to say, "I lost because I played badly", not "I lost because I am a bad person". Children do not usually develop sufficient ego strength to do this until they are about 10 years old. Another problem to consider with organised contact sports is the possibility of athletics injuries. Encourage parents to consider their child's maturity and the risk of injury (see Chapter 51) before they decide whether team competition is right for their child (Theisen et al., 2013).

Problem solving

An important part of developing a sense of industry is learning how to solve problems. Parents and teachers can help children develop this skill by encouraging practice. When a child asks, "Is this the right way to do this?" a parent can encourage problem solving by saying, "Let's talk about possible ways of doing it" rather than offering a quick solution.

The world depends on machinery, so mishaps and breakdowns (and therefore sudden changes) do occur. A child who can create an indoor playhouse with a card table and blanket when it is too wet or cold to use an outdoor playhouse will be able to problem solve with creative solutions as an adult. This attitude of optimism rather than pessimism towards problem solving produces adults who rarely say, "It can't be done". Just as importantly, it leaves these adults with confidence and a sense of pride.

Learning to live with others

School-aged children are sometimes so interested in tasks and in accomplishing physical projects that they forget they must work with other people to achieve these goals. A good time to urge children to learn compassion and thoughtfulness towards others is during the early school years. Writing thank-you letters and helping elderly neighbours are activities that can help children develop empathy towards others. Learning to give a present without receiving one in return or doing a favour without expecting a reward is also a part of this process and can be taught by example. Children should see their parents doing such things with an attitude not of "What will I get?" but "What can I contribute?"

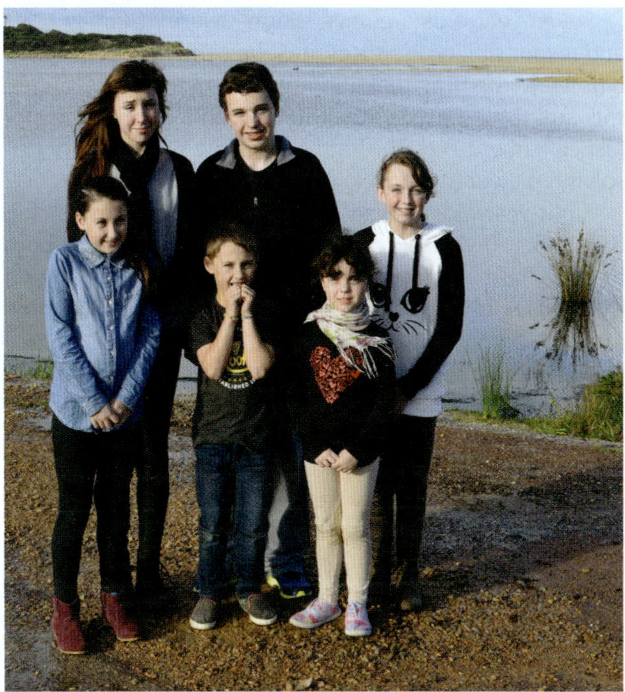

FIGURE 32.5 Blended families can add challenges to learning to live with others within families. (© Lisa Speedie.)

Another learning experience in living with others is with blended families; learning to live with step parents and siblings. Many young people struggle with this until they become comfortable with others and what is expected of them. Blended families can have children of varying ages (see Fig. 32.5) and this may cause added difficulty for the young people. Parents must lead by example and show fairness and love to all children.

Children may show empathy towards others as early as 20 months, but cognitively they cannot relate others' experiences to their own until about 6 years of age. Therefore, it is usually ineffective to lecture a child by saying, "It was cruel to call Mary names". The child may feel she had every right to do so. A better technique is to ask children to put themselves in Mary's place for a minute and imagine how they would feel if they were Mary.

Socialisation

Six-year-old children play in groups, but when they are tired or under added stress, they prefer one-to-one contact. In an infants' classroom, students can compete actively for a few minutes of special time with their teacher. At the end of the day, they then enjoy time spent individually with parents. You may have to remind parents this is not babyish behaviour but that of a typical 6-year-old.

Seven-year-olds are increasingly aware of family roles and responsibility. Promises must be kept, because 7-year-olds view them as definite, firm commitments. Children this age tattle because they have such a strong sense of justice (Loke, 2011). This tattling has the side effect of dissolving play groups quickly.

Eight-year-olds actively seek the company of other children. Most 8-year-old girls have a close girl friend; boys have a close boy friend. Girls begin to whisper among themselves as they share secrets with close friends, annoying both parents and teachers.

Nine-year-olds take the values of their peer group very seriously. They are much more interested in how other children dress than in what their parents want them to wear. This is typically the friend, gang or club age because children form groups, usually "spite clubs". This means if there are four girls who live on the same street, three form a club and exclude the fourth. The reason for exclusion is often unclear; it might be that the fourth child has a chronic disease, she has more or less money than the others, she was at the dentist's the day the club was formed, or simply that the club cannot exist unless there is someone to exclude. Such clubs typically have a secret password and secret meeting place. Membership is generally all girls or all boys.

If an excluded child does not react badly to being shut out, the club will probably disband after a few days because its purpose is lost. The next day, the excluded member may meet with two others and snub a different child. Parents need to use caution deciding whether to intervene with this type of play because loyalties shift quickly: the child who is club president today may be the excluded one tomorrow.

Because they are so ready for social interaction, 9-year-olds enjoy activities away from home, such as a school camp. They can take care of their own needs and are mature enough to be separated from their parents for periods of time. Although 10-year-olds enjoy groups, they also enjoy privacy. They like having their own bedroom or at least their own cupboard, where they can store a collection and know it is free from parents' or siblings' eyes. One of the best gifts for a 10-year-old is a box that locks.

Girls become increasingly interested in boys and vice versa by 11 years of age. Favourite activities are mixed-sex rather than single-sex ones. Children of this age are particularly insecure, however, and girls tend to dance with girls while boys talk together in corners. Better socialisation patterns need not be rushed. Just as infants crawl before they walk, so 11-year-olds must attempt many awkward and uncomfortable social experiences before they become comfortable forming relationships with the opposite sex.

Twelve-year-olds feel more comfortable in social situations than they did the year before. Boys experience erections on small provocation so may feel uncomfortable being pushed into boy–girl situations until they know how to control their body better. As some children develop faster than others, every group has some members who are almost adolescent and some who are still children, making social interactions sometimes difficult.

CASE STUDY QUESTION

2. Susie has belonged to a series of clubs for 9-year-olds. A usual characteristic of clubs for this aged child is:
   a. The club has formal rules and regulations
   b. It is designed to help shy children socialise
   c. It is designed to spite or exclude another child
   d. Clubs include both boys and girls

Cognitive development

The period from 5 to 7 years of age is a transitional stage where children undergo a shift from the pre-operational thought they used as preschoolers to concrete operational thought or the ability to reason through any problem they can actually visualise (Piaget, 1969; see Fig. 32.6).

Children can use concrete operational thought because they learn several new concepts, such as:

- **Decentring**, the ability to project oneself into other people's situations and see the world from their viewpoint rather than focusing only on their own view.
- **Accommodation**, the ability to adapt thought processes to fit what is perceived, such as understanding that there can be more than one reason for other people's actions. A preschooler might expect to see the same nurse in the morning who was there the evening before; a school-aged child can understand that different nurses work different shifts.
- **Conservation**, the ability to appreciate that a change in shape does not necessarily mean a change in size. If you pour 30 mL of cough medicine from a thin glass into a wide one, the preschooler will say that one glass holds

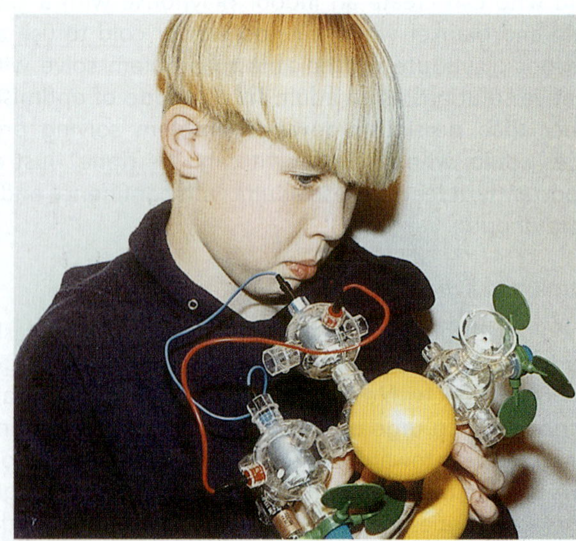

FIGURE 32.6 School-aged children learn concrete operational thought or concentrate on phenomena they can actually see occurring.

more than the other; a school-aged child will say both glasses hold an equal amount.

- **Class inclusion**, the ability to understand that objects can belong to more than one classification. A preschooler can categorise items in only one way, for example, such as stones and shells are found at the beach; a school-aged child can categorise them in many ways such as stones and shells are both found at the beach but are made of different materials, are different in size etc.

These cognitive developments lead to some of the typical changes and characteristics of the school-aged period. Decentring enables a school-aged child to feel compassion for others, which was not possible in younger years. Because understanding conservation is possible, a school-aged child is not fooled by perceptions as often as before; because of this, sibling arguments over food (your piece of pie is bigger than mine, his glass of juice is bigger than mine) decrease during the school-aged years. The ability to classify objects leads to the collecting activities of the school-aged period. Class inclusion is also necessary for learning mathematics and reading, systems that categorise numbers and words.

> ***What if...***
>
> You make a child's hospital bed one day and then give him an injection? What if the next day the child starts to cry while you're making the bed? The lack of what cognitive process led him to believe your action would be the same the second day?

Moral and spiritual development

School-aged children begin to mature in terms of moral development as they enter a stage of *preconventional reasoning*, sometimes as early as 5 years of age (Kohlberg, 1984). During this stage, if asked, "Why is it wrong to steal from your neighbour?" school-aged children will answer, "The police say it's wrong" or "Because if you do, you'll go to gaol". They concentrate on "niceness" or "fairness" and cannot see yet that stealing hurts their neighbour, the highest level of moral reasoning.

School-aged children begin to learn about the rituals and meaning behind their religious practices, so the distinction between right and wrong becomes more significant to them than it was when they were preschoolers. Parent role modelling is also important. Because they are still limited in their ability to understand others' views, they may interpret something as being right because it is good for them, not because it is right for humanity as a whole.

> ***What if...***
>
> Susie understands stealing from a neighbour is wrong? Will she also understand that stealing from a shopping centre or taking things from a health clinic is wrong?

HEALTH PROMOTION FOR A SCHOOL-AGED CHILD AND FAMILY

Because of still limited judgement, school-aged children need guidelines with reference to safety, nutrition and daily care. These are always excellent topics for discussion at healthcare visits.

Promoting school-aged safety

School-aged children are ready for time on their own without direct adult supervision. Many children as young as 8 or 9 stay by themselves after school. Children are generally ready for this type of experience if they can reliably follow instructions (don't use the fireplace; don't open the door) and can occupy themselves for an hour's time. Australian recommendations are no more than 2–3 hours alone at this age. In New Zealand it is an offence to leave children under the age of 14 for any period of time. Be certain school-aged children know to use seatbelts in cars and bicycle safety around cars (see Box 32.2). As with adults, accidents tend to occur when children are under stress.

School age is not too early for parents to look at the effect of carrying heavy backpacks on children's posture. A backpack that weighs more than 10% of the child's body weight is enough to cause a child to have to lean forwards to bear the weight. This can lead to chronic back pain (Kistner, Fiebert & Roach, 2012).

Sexual abuse is an unfortunate and all-too-common hazard for school-aged children (see Chapter 55). For strategies to help children avoid sexual abuse, see Box 32.1.

Today, with the growth in telecommunications and widespread Internet use, people's contact with others can easily extend beyond the local environment to other suburbs and regions of the world. Research suggests that there are a number of benefits associated with Internet usage. Bond University's School of Communication and Media for the Interactive Games and Entertainment Association (2012) cites a number of examples within Australian society where parents identified the use of online games as a positive parental experience and interaction. The research found that games and parenting are intertwined more than ever: Eighty-three percent of parents reported playing video games and of those 88% played them with their children. However, the virtual community can pose threats to children and young people when communication with unknown adults occurs without parental knowledge. Box 32.3 lists some strategies that parents and carers can follow to keep children safe online.

Promoting nutritional health of a school-aged child

Most school-aged children have good appetites, although any meal is influenced by the day's activity. If children have had a full day of activities, they may come to the dinner table ready to eat anything. If a day was filled with frustration—a

BOX 32.2 * Focus on family teaching

Common safety measures to prevent accidents during the school years

Q. Susie's mother tells you, "My school-aged child is constantly on the go. How can I keep her free from accidents when I'm not always with her?"

A. Putting preventive steps in place is the key.

Accident	Preventive measure
Motor vehicle accidents	Insist children use seatbelts in a car; role model their use. Teach street-crossing safety; stress that streets/roads are no place for rough play, pushing or shoving. Teach bicycle safety, including advice not to take "passengers" on a bicycle and to use a helmet. Teach carpark and bus safety (do not walk behind parked cars, wait for pedestrian crossing supervisor, etc.).
Community	Warn children to avoid unsafe areas, such as train yards, grain silos, back streets. Caution children not to go with strangers (parents can establish a code word with the child; the child does not leave school with anyone who does not know the word). Children should say "no" to anyone who touches them if they do not wish it, including family members (most sexual abuse is by a family member, not a stranger). For older school-age, teach rules of safer sex (use of condoms; inspecting partner, etc.).
Burns	Teach safety with candles, matches, campfires—fire is not "fun". Teach safety with beginning cooking skills (remember to include microwave oven safety, such as closing firmly before turning on oven; not using metal containers). Teach safety with sun exposure—use sun block, hats, etc. Warn children not to climb electrical poles.
Falls	Teach that rough play on fences, climbing on roofs, etc., is hazardous. Teach skateboard, scooter and skating safety.
Sports injuries	Teach that wearing appropriate equipment (face mask for hockey; mouthguard for football; helmet for cycling, skateboarding or in-line skating; batting helmet for baseball/cricket) is not babyish but smart. Stress not to play to a point of exhaustion or in a sport beyond physical capability. Warn children to use trampolines only with adult supervision to avoid serious injury.
Drowning	Teach children how to swim and explain that dares and rough play when diving or swimming are not appropriate. Warn children not to swim beyond the limits of their capabilities. Warn children never to swim alone, particularly in rivers and dams; and not to swim in rivers or dams if no swimming experience. Provide river and dam safety education to young children also.
Drugs	Help the child to avoid all recreational drugs and caution them to take prescription medicine only as directed. Educate the child to avoid tobacco and alcohol.
General	School-aged children should keep adults informed about where they are and what they are doing. Be aware that the frequency of accidents increases when parents are under stress and therefore less attentive. Special precautions must be taken at these times. Some children are more active, curious and impulsive, therefore they are more vulnerable to accidents than others.

child received a poor mark in school, had an argument with a friend or has a big game to think about—they may only pick at food. This is no different from the way adults feel at times, so should be respected.

Establishing healthy eating patterns

School-aged children need breakfast to provide enough energy to get them through active mornings at school. They eat best if parents get up in the morning and eat some breakfast themselves. Children react badly to the instruction, "Do as I say, not as I do".

If children take a packed lunch to school, urge parents to allow them to have some say in the meal because packed lunches become tedious for everyone after a while. Whether they take lunch or buy it at school, school-aged children should know some elementary facts of nutrition so they do not swap a sandwich for cake. Healthcare professionals should play an active role in nutrition education at health maintenance visits. Most children are hungry after school and enjoy a snack when they arrive home. Because sugary foods may dull a child's appetite for dinner, urge parents to make the snack nutritious: fruit, cheese or milk, rather than biscuits and a soft drink (see Appendices E and F).

Early school-age is not too young to put in place preventive measures against cardiovascular changes later in life. Limiting salty foods, for example, can help prevent hypertension (Harika et al., 2011). Excessive saturated fat can lead to the formation of artery plaques and cardiovascular disease (Caprio, 2012). Teach parents to make mealtime a happy and enjoyable part of the day for everyone. Some school-aged children learn to eat as quickly as

BOX 32.3 ✻ Strategies for keeping children safe online

Parents can use the following strategies to ensure that their children are safe online:

- Know what your child is doing online.
- Agree on what is acceptable behaviour online and on which sites to visit.
- Use software to restrict sensitive personal information from being transmitted online, to limit the occasions when your child can go online and to block access to sites that you feel are inappropriate.
- Ensure your child knows the rules about giving out personal information and meeting with new online friends.
- Tell your child to exercise caution at all times regarding whom they accept as friends on social networking sites.
- Teach your child to consider the feelings of others when sending content by mobile phone or online.
- Teach your child how to determine whether online information comes from a credible source.
- If your child shows signs of being bullied online, listen to their concerns and work with them to take control of the situation.

Source: Kids Helpline (2012). Social networking safety. Available at <www.kidshelp.com.au/grownups/news-research/hot-topics/social-networking-safety.php>.

possible (and so incompletely) to escape from the table before something unpleasant happens, such as an argument they can sense is brewing.

Fostering industry

As a part of encouraging industry, school-aged children usually enjoy helping to plan meals. They may eat meals they have planned or prepared more willingly than ones that are just set in front of them. Most parents would like children to develop better table manners. Because they are in a hurry to finish eating, school-aged children tend to gulp their food. Many meals are interrupted by spilled drinks. As children become teenagers and are more aware of the impression they make on others, manners often improve dramatically. It is often comforting for parents to know that children typically display better table manners in other people's homes than in their own.

Recommended dietary reference intakes

Although parents may have less to say about what a school-aged child eats, it is important that the increasing energy requirements that come with this age (often in spurts) are met daily with foods of high nutritional value. During the late school years, the recommended dietary intakes for children begin to be separated into categories for girls and boys because boys require more kilojoules and other nutrients at this time. Because school-aged children typically dislike vegetables, their intake may be deficient in fibre. Both girls and boys require more iron in prepuberty than they did between the ages of 7 and 10. Adequate calcium and fluoride intake remains important to ensure good teeth and bone growth.

Promoting nutritional health with a vegetarian diet

School-aged children who are raised in vegetarian homes need to learn aspects of vegetarian nutrition if they are going to eat in a school canteen or other's homes. Unfortunately, many school canteen menus offer mainly milk and meat or cheese foods, such as sausage rolls, meat pies or pizza. This forces children who are vegetarians to carry packed lunches. Vegetarian lunches can be varied with foods such as cucumber or tomato sandwiches on whole-grain bread, hot soups, salads, vegetable sticks and fruit. When eating at a friend's house, children need to learn to notify the host that they eat a special diet or know how to choose correctly from foods they are offered.

A potential problem to assess with vegetarian school-aged children is whether they are obtaining enough protein and calcium to be prepared for the rapid growth spurt of puberty (Van Winckel et al., 2011). Foods high in calcium are green, leafy vegetables such as spinach prunes, nuts, enriched breads and cereals. Soybeans, legumes, nuts, grains and immature seeds like green beans, lima beans and corn are relatively high in protein. As with any individual on a vegetarian diet, children may need a vitamin B_{12} supplement. Encourage outside activities for sun exposure to increase vitamin D. Iron may need to be supplemented, especially in girls with heavy menstrual flows (Rolfes, Pinna & Whitney, 2012; Whitney & Rolfes, 2015).

Nutrition and the school-aged child with a challenge

Food preparation and washing the dishes are times for socialising in most households. A school-aged child who cannot be involved in these activities because of a physical challenge may need extra time during the day to make up for these lost socialising experiences, such as a specific hour set aside for talking or sharing a project that can be accomplished in one sitting.

When eating at school or a friend's home, children with special diets are usually tempted to select the same food as everyone else rather than limit what they choose. They may decline invitations rather than admit to requiring a special diet or needing help with eating. Ask at healthcare visits if any of these problems are present. Help children with special diets to plan ways they could be comfortable in social food-based settings, such as bringing a party snack that is appropriate and can be easily eaten, or how to politely decline particular foods. Help children who are hospitalised to select a diet that is enjoyable as well as nutritious.

Obesity

The number of overweight children in Australia and New Zealand has doubled in recent years. The impact of this is that now a quarter of children are considered overweight or obese. This rise in the number of overweight children is disturbing because obesity causes health complications, such as diabetes types 1 and 2 and can lead to social problems. Overweight children are more likely to be bullied by their peers or to develop low self-esteem or body image problems. Once children are overweight, it requires a lot of effort and commitment for them to return to a healthy weight (Krebs & Primak, 2011). Being overweight and obesity are among the most important risks to children's long- and short-term health. Overweight children are very likely to become overweight adults and have chronic health complaints and ongoing self-esteem issues.

Risk factors for childhood obesity

To maintain a healthy weight, you need to use ("burn") the energy from the foods you eat. If you eat more than you use, your body will store extra energy as fat. Factors that may cause children to become overweight and obese include:

- **Food choices**—choosing high-fat and sugary foods instead of healthier options
- **Lack of physical activity**—Australian and New Zealand children are less active than their parents and grandparents
- **Spending a lot of time on sedentary pursuits**—Australian and New Zealand children watch, on average, 2½ hours of television per day, as well as playing computer and other electronic games
- **Overweight parents**—a family's eating patterns and time management can have a major influence on whether a child maintains a healthy weight
- **Genetics**—some rare gene disorders cause severe childhood obesity. In other cases, particular genes acting together can increase the risk of some children being more susceptible to obesity. If there is a family tendency to become overweight, parents need to be more responsible in making healthy food choices for the whole family (Victorian Government, 2012).

Obese children begin to develop many of the same health problems as obese adults, such as hypertension, type 2 diabetes and an elevated total cholesterol level with possible atherosclerosis. They may also be ridiculed for their size and be unable to participate in team sports. This is strong evidence for the need for active measures to help preteens regulate their weight.

Those who become so obese that friends exclude them from activities or who cannot play sports because they tire so quickly may develop such a poor self-image that they have little motivation for self-improvement. A weight-reduction program aimed specifically for school-aged children and that emphasises long-term lifestyle changes is most successful in helping such children to lose weight (Victorian Government, 2012).

As a way of increasing daily activity, pre-adolescents do well with formal exercise classes because they enjoy the support of other children. In addition, encourage children to increase informal exercise, such as walking to and from school. Educate sports coaches to accept obese children as part of a team, not because the child will necessarily benefit the team, but because the exercise will benefit the child. Exercise burns up kilojoules and if children's daylight hours are filled with activities and friends, they have less time to eat (Schantz, 2012).

Lifestyle change is the ultimate goal for the entire family because obesity is usually a family problem. Rather than preparing special meals for just the obese child, the entire family probably needs to eat in a healthier manner. Because pre-adolescents do not generally prepare their own food, the person most responsible for meal preparation requires as much information on the planned weight loss as the child. Old concepts (such as "A clean plate is good"; "How can you leave food when people in other countries are starving?") may have to be changed so children and other family members reduce their intake appropriately. The importance of exercise should also be reflected in the home. Family members not only should encourage the obese child to exercise but also should partake in some form of daily activity themselves.

There may be some danger in pointing out to pre-adolescents that they are terribly overweight because some children become so obsessed with losing weight that they become bulimic or anorexic (Schantz, 2012) (see Chapter 54). Stressing that children can "become healthier" or "improve stamina" may be better advice than talking about dieting.

Promoting development of a school-aged child in daily activities

With life centred on school activities and friends, a school-aged child still needs parental guidance for most daily activities. The habits and lifestyle patterns gained during this period will form the basis for the patterns of living later in life. Along with nutritional needs, areas of concern for a school-aged child and family include dressing, sleep, exercise, hygiene and dental care.

Dress

Although school-aged children can fully dress themselves, they are not good at taking care of their clothes until later in the school-aged years. This is the right age, however (if not started already), to teach children the importance of caring for their own belongings. School-aged children have definite opinions about clothing styles, often based on the likes of their friends or a popular public figure rather than the preferences of their parents. Help parents be aware that a child who wears clothing different from their peers may become the object of exclusion from a school club or group.

Sleep

Sleep needs vary among individual children. Younger school-aged children typically require 10 to 12 hours of sleep each night and older ones require about 8 to 10 hours. Most 6-year-olds are too old for naps but do require a quiet time after school to get them through the remainder of the day. Night-time terrors may continue during the early school years and may actually increase during the first year as a child reacts to the stress of beginning school.

During early school years, many children enjoy a quiet talk or reading at bedtime. At about the age of 9, when friends become more important, children can be ready to give up pre-bedtime talks with parents, preferring to communicate with friends (Chahal et al., 2012). Children with television sets, electronic games or smartphones in their bedrooms not only have shorter sleep times at night but also are more likely to be obese (Chahal et al., 2012).

Exercise

School-aged children need daily exercise. Although they go to school all day, they do not automatically receive much exercise because school is basically a sit-down activity. Children who take public transport or are driven to school may therefore return home without having spent much time in active exercise.

Exercise need not involve organised sports. It can come from neighbourhood games, walking with parents or a dog, or bicycle riding. As children enter pre-adolescence, those with poor coordination may become reluctant to exercise. Urge them to participate in some daily exercise, or else obesity or osteoporosis later in life can result (Eagle et al., 2012; Gunter, Almstedt & Janz, 2012).

Hygiene

Children of 6 or 7 years of age still need help in regulating bath water temperature and in cleaning their ears and fingernails. By the age of 8, children are generally capable of bathing themselves but may not do it well because they are too busy to take the time or because they do not consider bathing important.

Both boys and girls become interested in showering as they approach their teens. This can be encouraged as perspiration increases with puberty, along with sebaceous gland activity. When girls begin to menstruate, they may be afraid to have baths or wash their hair during their period if they have heard this is not safe. They need information on the importance and safety of good hygiene during their menses. Boys who are uncircumcised may develop inflammation under the foreskin from increased secretions if they do not wash regularly (Meng & Tenagho, 2013).

Care of teeth

With proper dental care, the average child today can expect to grow up cavity free. To ensure this, school-aged children should visit a dentist at least twice yearly for a check-up, cleaning and possibly a fluoride treatment to strengthen and harden the tooth enamel (Tubert-Jeannin et al., 2011; see Fig. 32.7). Some children develop a fear of dentists and, if a dentist visit is painful, want to avoid going at all. The advantage of frequent visits is that if cavities are filled when they are small, the drilling required is minimal and little pain is involved. If cavities are not treated promptly, the treatment may be more invasive and painful, causing these children to refuse to go back to the dentist. More large cavities then develop and a vicious cycle develops.

School-aged children have to be reminded to brush their teeth twice daily. If brushing becomes an area of conflict, brushing well once a day may be more effective than brushing more often but doing an inadequate job. For effective brushing, a child should use a soft toothbrush, fluoride-based toothpaste and dental floss to clean between teeth to help remove plaque and food particles.

Not all bottled water is fluoridated so ensure that this is not their main source of drinking water. Snacks are best limited to high-protein foods such as chicken and cheese rather than lollies. Fruits, vegetables and cereals fortified with minerals and vitamins (not "empty kilojoule" ones) can all be fun after-school snacks for school-aged children. If the child does eat lollies, choose ones which can be

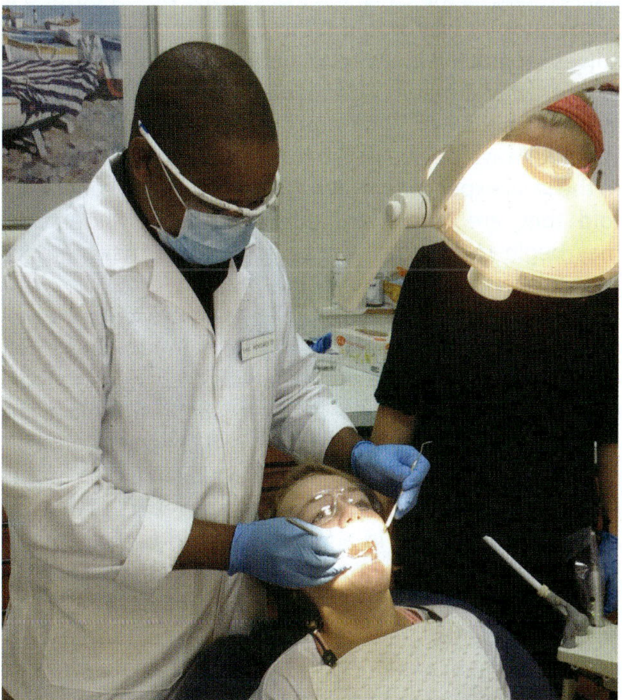

FIGURE 32.7 Dental cavities are the number one health problem in school-aged children. Teach children good dental health and encourage them to visit a dentist twice a year. (© Lisa Speedie.)

eaten quickly rather than slowly dissolving or sticky lollies which stay in contact with the teeth longer.

Promoting healthy family functioning

At 6 years of age, most children have passed through a preschool phase of attraction for the parent of the opposite sex and identify again with the parent of the same sex (Freud, 1962). Children from single-parent homes, or those with a parent who has difficulty being a good role model, may need help in finding a suitable adult to serve as this important person in their life.

To their parents' annoyance, many 6-year-olds often quote their teacher as the final authority on all subjects. This may be the first time the parents see someone surpassing them in their child's eyes and accepting the situation can be painful. Children also cite their friends as guides for behaviour: "Jane doesn't have to go to bed until 10 o'clock" or "Sean's mother lets him go to the movies every Saturday". Parents may need help to realise these remarks are a normal consequence of being exposed to other adults and children. A simple statement such as, "There are all kinds of ways to do things, but in our house, the rule is this", shows no criticism of Sean or Jane's families, yet conveys a special "our house" feeling and offers security to a child.

Parents often must be reminded that even the simplest tasks of everyday life require repeated practice before they can be accomplished well. The way parents correct children as they learn these tasks can influence children's opinions of themselves and their ability to continue learning. "Putting all the cutlery in a pile is one way of putting it away; another way would be to divide spoons, forks and knives separately" is always preferable to "What a silly way to put away cutlery!" Comments such as, "Can't you do anything right?" or "Why don't you ever do what I say?" should always be avoided because children will rise only to the level expected of them. Children who are constantly told they are stupid, thoughtless, bad or ill-behaved may begin to act that way to conform to their parents' expectations.

If parents have difficulty telling what a child's completed project is supposed to be, the time-honoured "Tell me about it" is preferable to "What is it?" It is good for parents to find a redeeming characteristic in a project, no matter how shakily put together it is: "I like the bright colour you painted it" or "That must have been fun to make". Displaying and using children's gifts are part of having school-aged children in a family. In talking to parents of school-aged children, good questions to ask to estimate the degree of interaction that occurs in the home and whether parents are strengthening a child's sense of accomplishment are:

- How do you correct John when he does something wrong?
- Do you display his school projects?
- Does he have chores that are his to accomplish?

Common health problems of the school-aged period

Children in their early school years have one of the lowest rates of death and serious illness of any age group. The two leading causes of death are accidents and cancer. Minor illnesses are largely because of dental cavities, gastrointestinal disturbances and upper respiratory infections (Australian Bureau of Statistics, 2006). Childhood immunisations are a major safeguard for children against common illnesses. (For the Australian and New Zealand immunisation schedules and for further information on childhood immunisation, see Chapter 34.)

Dental cavities

Cavities are progressive, destructive lesions or decalcification of the tooth enamel and dentin. The enamel on primary teeth is thinner than on permanent teeth, so primary teeth are even more susceptible to destruction than permanent teeth. The distance from the enamel to the pulp is shorter, too, so invasion of the tooth nerve can occur quickly. Neglected cavities result in poor chewing and therefore poor digestion, abscess and pain, and sometimes osteomyelitis (bone infection).

As stated earlier, dental cavities are largely preventable with proper brushing and use of fluoridated water or fluoride application. When cavities do occur, it is important they be treated quickly and the child's dental hygiene practices be evaluated and improved if necessary. Most importantly, children must believe that they have a stake in the health of their teeth, so even though they are cavity free, they willingly undertake the self-care measures necessary to ensure healthy teeth with parental support rather than parental command (Wen et al., 2012).

Malocclusion

The upper jaw in children matures rapidly in early childhood along with skull growth; the lower jaw forms more slowly, forcing teeth to make a prolonged series of changes until they reach their final adult alignment and position. Good tooth occlusion, in which the upper teeth overlap the lower teeth by a small amount and teeth are evenly spaced and in good alignment, is necessary for optimal formation of teeth, health of the supporting tissue, optimal speech development and what most people view as a pleasant physical appearance.

Malocclusion (a deviation of tooth position from the normal) may be congenital and related to conditions such as cleft palate, a small lower jaw or familial traits tending towards malocclusion. Malocclusion may be either crossbite (sideways), anterior or posterior. The condition can result later on from constant mouth breathing or abnormal tongue position (tongue thrusting). Thumb-sucking is still another possibility if it persists past the time of eruption of the permanent front teeth (6 to 7 years) (Sandler, Madahar & Murray, 2011). The loss of teeth due to extraction or an unintentional injury may lead to malocclusion if not properly treated so that alignment is maintained.

Children with a malocclusion should be evaluated by an orthodontist to see if orthodontic braces or other therapy is necessary. The time to begin correction varies with the extent of the malocclusion and jaw size. Braces are painful when they are first applied and at periodic visits when they are tightened to maintain pressure for further straightening. Some children develop mild, shallow ulcerations (canker sores) on the buccal membrane from friction of metal wires.

Rubbing the offending wire with dental wax dulls the surface and gives relief. Oral paracetamol or an analgesic agent such as Bonjela or SM33 (an over-the-counter drug) rubbed on the ulceration may also offer relief. All children who wear braces need to brush their teeth well and be assessed periodically to see that they are brushing properly around the braces (a Waterpik is often recommended for thorough cleaning). They should use dental floss to remove plaque from around wires. After the removal of braces, children usually wear retainers to maintain the correction the braces achieved.

There are also now many other options available besides braces. Of these options many involve retainers and other not-fixed braces. Although braces are wired into place, retainers are not. Loss of a retainer can be a problem if it must be removed when eating. The choice of product will depend on the dental alignment needed, but all will cause some level of discomfort and pain on commencement. Show appropriate sympathy and help children problem solve if they are bothered by the appearance of braces or the retainer. Once thought of as implements to be made fun of, teeth braces have become such a common feature of life for schoolchildren that most children who wear them find comfort in not being the only one to suffer this indignity and, once used to their own appliances, experience little reluctance in letting their classmates see them. Some even view them as a mark of pride or a status symbol (Hamdan, Singh & Rock, 2012).

CASE STUDY QUESTION

3. If Susie eats lollies, which type would cause fewer cavities?

a. Toffee
b. A chocolate bar
c. Chewy caramels
d. Hard lollies

Concerns and problems of the school-aged period

One of the most important disorders of the school-aged period is attention-deficit/hyperactivity disorder (ADHD) because it interferes so dramatically with school progress (see Chapter 54). Other problems parents need to be aware of are outlined in Table 32.3.

TABLE 32.3 Parental difficulties evaluating health problems in the school-aged child

Difficulty	Helpful suggestions for parents
Evaluating seriousness of illness	For the first time, a school-aged child may view illness as a way to avoid unpleasant activities (school, a coach who asks too much, household chores). Evaluating whether the child has symptoms when asked to do a favourite thing often reveals the difference between exaggeration and an ill child (e.g. too sick to eat spinach, not too sick to eat ice cream; too sick to go to school, not too sick to go skateboarding). If the child uses symptoms of illness as a means of avoiding situations, parents must evaluate what it is about the situation they could improve or see if some change should be made in their expectations.
Evaluating nutritional intake	Many school-aged children eat lunch at school and they may spend weekends away from home. As with all ages, noting whether they are growing and active is better than monitoring any one day's food intake.
Evaluating puberty changes	There is a wide variation in the time secondary sex characteristics occur. Children should be examined if and when they or their parents are concerned pubertal changes are delayed or appearing too early.
Age-specific diseases to be aware of	School age is a time to evaluate vision because vision changes occur with increased maturity of the eye globe. Squinting, rubbing the eyes or poor marks in school may be signs of poor vision. Streptococcal sore throats occur frequently in young school-aged children. Those with sore throats should be examined by a healthcare provider to prevent complications, such as glomerulonephritis or rheumatic fever, from developing. Girls, in particular, must be evaluated for scoliosis (curvature of the spine). Parents may detect this by noticing that a girl's skirt hangs unevenly or bra straps are uneven. Parents may need to be cautioned that vomiting or a headache in the morning that passes fairly quickly (at about the same time the school bus leaves) may be a symptom of school phobia, but a physical examination is in order because these are also symptoms of other conditions. Absence seizures, a neurological condition that typically arises in the school-aged years, can be confused with behaviour problems if observation is not thorough (see Chapter 49). Attention-deficit/hyperactivity disorder (ADHD) (see Chapter 54) can also lead to behaviour or inattention disorders.

Problems associated with language development

The common speech problem of the preschool years is broken fluency; the most common problem of a school-aged child is articulation. The child has difficulty pronouncing *s, z, th, l, r* and *w* or substitutes *w* for *r* ("wabbit" instead of "rabbit") or *r* for *l* ("radies room" instead of "ladies room"). This is most noticeable during infant school and usually disappears by primary age. Unless it persists, speech therapy for this normal developmental stage is not necessary.

Common fears and anxieties of a school-aged child

School-aged children are old enough to experience adult reactions to problems at home or school.

Anxiety related to beginning school

Adjusting to school is a big task for 6-year-olds. Even if they attended preschool, primary school is different: the rules are firmer. In Australia, the minimum school leaving age is 17 years (NSW Department of Education & Communities, 2014), a time span too long for a young child to even imagine.

Because school is an adjustment, a health assessment of all school-aged children should include an inquiry about progress in school. You can obtain information by asking a parent, "How is Susan doing in school?" followed by a second question, "How does her teacher say she is doing?" If there is a discrepancy between the answers, the situation bears study. The answer to the first question reveals the parent's attitude towards the child's progress. The answer to the second may indicate a child who is having trouble adjusting to a structured school environment. Some parents have to alter their expectations of how much their child should be achieving to conform to their child's actual ability. This can be difficult (Pass et al., 2012).

One of the biggest tasks of the first year of school is learning to read. It is best if parents have prepared children for this by reading to them since infancy, pointing to the words and pictures as they go along. This helps children realise sentences flow from left to right and the words, not the pictures, tell the story.

Many kindergarteners/first graders are capable of mature action at school but appear less mature when they return home. They may bite their fingernails, suck their thumb or talk "baby talk". Some develop tics (irregular movements of isolated muscle groups), such as wrinkling the forehead, shrugging the shoulders, clearing the throat or frequently blinking. Such movements may occasionally be confused with seizure activity. Tics, however, disappear during sleep and occur mainly when the child is subjected to stress or anxiety. Scolding, nagging, threatening or punishing does not stop either tics or nail biting and invariably makes these problems worse.

Methods such as using anti-biting nail polish and restraining the child's hands to prevent nail biting are also ineffective. These behaviours stop when the underlying stress is discovered and alleviated. Urge parents to spend some time with the child after school or in the evening so the child continues to feel secure in the family and does not feel excluded by being sent to school. If such behaviour manifestations persist despite attempts to eliminate their cause, the family might benefit from formal counselling, including temporary pharmacological support for the child (Pringsheim et al., 2012).

School refusal or phobia

School refusal is fear of attending school. It is a type of "social phobia" similar to agoraphobia (fear of going outside the home). Children who resist attending school may develop physical signs of illness, such as vomiting, diarrhoea, headache or abdominal pain on school days (Scheffer, 2011). This lasts until after the child is allowed to stay home for the day. The child may be reacting to a situation such as a harsh teacher or facing a class bully every day. In these instances, the child's fear may be well-grounded. Counselling may help the child manage the situation better. If not, parents should approach the school to notify them of their concerns and work together to resolve this situation.

School refusal may also result from fear of separation from parents. The child may be overly dependent on the parents or may be reluctant to leave home because of worry that younger siblings will usurp the parents' affection. The anxiety of separation may also result because the parent is overprotective of the child or is the one having difficulty separating.

Managing school refusal requires coordination between the school, parents and other appropriate services. A school nurse is, where possible, the ideal person to coordinate such efforts and to help parents allow the child some independence not only in going to school but also in other activities. A few children have such difficulty they require psychological intervention to resolve their difficulties (Scheffer, 2011).

Home schooling

A number of children are home schooled today (Anthony & Burroughs, 2010). It is important to identify these children at a healthcare visit because with less extensive peer exposure than other children, they may not be as comfortable with peer interaction. As their main contact has been with parents at home, their vocabulary may be advanced or can suggest they are older than their real age. They may be experts at computer searching but know less than other children about health prevention measures as they have not had contact with school nurses or health curriculum. When discussing home schooling with parents, assess if children do have peer experiences, perhaps through participation in community sports teams. Ask if they receive exposure to other cultures or families.

Children who spend time independently

Some schoolchildren have no adult supervision for part of each weekday and carry a key so they can let themselves into their home after school. A major concern about children staying alone is that they will develop an increased tendency towards accidents, delinquent behaviour, alcohol or drug abuse, or decreased school performance from lack of adult supervision. For children who feel safe in their community, however, a short period of independence every day may actually be beneficial; it encourages problem solving in self-care. If you have concerns about this issue make contact with community services for child safety and welfare in your state or territory (Mack, Dellinger & West, 2012).

Cottonwool children

Another area of concern is **cottonwool children**. Experts warn that anxious parents are raising a generation of children who are denied the independence, experience and education that comes from exploring the outdoor world. If children cannot get out and explore the natural world, we run the risk of raising children whose experiences are defined by websites and computer games. These children will also struggle with building their resilience and coping skills for life's difficulties (Atkins, 2010).

Sex education

It is important that school-aged children be educated about pubertal changes and responsible sexual practices. Also, preteens should have adults to whom they can turn for answers to questions about sex. Ideally, these should be their parents, but because sex is an emotionally charged topic, some parents may be extremely uncomfortable discussing it with their children. As a result, healthcare professionals often become an important resource. As a healthcare professional, answer questions openly and honestly and encourage the young person to ask questions without judgement.

It may be more common to hear parents talking about their children's first teeth and first steps than it is to hear about a child's sexual development. Although this is understandable, a lack of knowledge about what is "normal" sexual development can lead to unnecessary anxiety about a child's interest in nudity and sex. Parents need to understand the stages of sexual development that children are likely to go through and what they can do to help their child adjust to these changes. Box 32.4 outlines normal sexual development for a primary school child.

Many parents educate their children about sex when they talk about body parts and body functions, and when they prepare their child for puberty—teaching their child to care for, respect and protect their body. Choosing the right age to discuss a question such as 'Where do I come from?' is more about how comfortable parents feel talking about such topics, rather than there being a perfect time. Talking about such issues shows children that they can talk with trusted adults. Families lay the groundwork for children to feel okay about their bodies and to feel confident to ask questions or seek help. School programs are vital to support this process. If families and schools don't lead the way, children will turn to other sources of information that may not be reliable, such as friends or the Internet. Box 32.5 contains some general suggestions for encouraging parents to talk to their child about sexual issues.

BOX 32.4 * Normal sexual development of a primary school child

In the primary school years, typical behaviours include:

- Children become modest and/or embarrassed about being naked in front of their parents.
- Children gravitate towards same-sex friends and may complain about "girl germs" or "boy germs" when speaking of the opposite sex.
- Children may play games that include kissing and marriage role-play.
- Children are curious about gender differences, sexual intercourse and pregnancy, and may discuss these issues among themselves with varying degrees of accuracy.
- Children may continue with sex play that began in their earlier years, such as "playing doctor", because children of this age are interested in knowing more.

Source: Victorian Government. (2015). Sex education—primary school children. <www.betterhealth.vic.gov.au/bhcv2/bhcarticles.nsf/pages/Sex_education_primary_school_children?open>.

Stealing

Some younger school-aged children go through a period during which they steal loose change from their parents. This usually happens at around 7 years of age, when children first learn how to make calculations and also discover the importance of money. Stealing occurs because, although a child is gaining an appreciation for money, this appreciation is not yet balanced by strong moral principles. Some shoplifting occurs in young school-aged children, but the major problem with this arises during pre-adolescence.

As a rule, early-childhood stealing is best handled without a great deal of emotion. A parent should tell the child the money is missing. The importance of property rights should be reviewed: mother's and father's money is theirs; the child's money is the child's; they are not interchangeable. Youngsters who continue to steal past 9 years of age may require counselling because they should have progressed beyond this normal developmental step by this age (Sourander et al., 2012).

Parents should set good examples if they expect their child to be honest. If one parent takes money from the other without permission, neither should be surprised to find their child attempting to do the same. If a parent changes price tags or unwraps items and eats them without paying for them in the supermarket, they cannot expect a child to do otherwise.

Nurses have a role in educating adolescents to learn more about their moral beliefs and also role-modelling. Nurses often have the trust of the young person and the

BOX 32.5 ✻ General suggestions on talking to children about personal safety and sexual issues

If children ask questions about sex or sexual safety, don't dismiss them; encourage them to ask questions and then inform their parents/carers that the young person is asking questions. Suggest to the parents that they speak with their child, as, if ignored, the child may never ask again or be too shy to do so which may impact on their sexual safety, knowledge and skills.

Encourage parents to become knowledgeable about safety and sex education so they can have open conversations with their children and reassure their children they can talk to them about this "stuff". Encourage them to learn together; to seek out resources in this information in their community. Encourage parents to give their child options to discuss safety and sex. Use correct language when talking with parents and encourage them to do the same with their children. This helps to communicate more clearly body parts and their function and avoids confusion.

Begin the conversation with parents about teaching their children to say no and that it is safe to tell someone they trust if someone is touching them inappropriately. Teach parents to talk with their children, building their trust so they feel comfortable.

Educate parents about the age children may start to masturbate and that this is normal; that children just need to learn that this is something that is done in private. Let parents know that this is also a good time to begin talking with older school-aged children about where babies come from and conception.

Discuss with parents body changes and emotional changes and what this means for the child in mid to late primary school. Explain that some girls have their period before the end of primary school so safety and sex is important learning for them. Encourage parents to make use of online safety and sex resources for themselves and their children. The Thinkuknow website <www.thinkuknow.org.au> has an Internet safety program that provides advice for parents.

Source: Victorian Government. (2015). Sex education—primary school children. <www.betterhealth.vic.gov.au/bhcv2/bhcarticles.nsf/pages/Sex_education_primary_school_children?open>.

young person may divulge to them about stealing. Do not scold the young person or threaten to tell their parents. Discuss with them what they think they should do about the situation. Encourage them to talk with their parents or someone they trust further about the situation if you feel the behaviour may continue.

Violence or terrorism

Children basically view their world as safe, so it is a shock when violence enters their lives (Dowdell, 2012). Nurses are in a role where they can discuss with parents the violence and terrorism that can be viewed through social media and TV and the impact this may have on children. Inform parents of available information that will help guide them in deciding what their child can view. Common recommendations for parents to help children feel safe are:

- Assure children they are safe; the violence is isolated to another part of the world and they are out of danger
- Assure children their parents are actively involved in keeping them safe
- Observe for signs of stress such as sleep disturbance, fatigue, lack of pleasure in activities or signs of substance abuse
- Do not allow children or adolescents to view footage of traumatic events over and over again, as this decreases their ability to feel safe
- Watch news programs with children and explain that the situation portrayed is not nearby and that they are safe
- Explain that there are bad people in the world and bad people do bad things, but help children appreciate that not all people in a particular group or who look a particular way are bad; lashing out at people who resemble the bad people only causes more harm
- Prepare a family disaster plan, including such things as bottled water, blankets, toiletries, pet supplies, appropriate clothing, torches and information such as what immunisations the children have had (particularly tetanus)—if a child is ill, include a history of medical needs or care
- Designate a "rally point" where the family will meet if ever separated by a disaster or evacuation.

Some parents may be reluctant to talk to their children about a disaster plan for the family, believing that these preparations will frighten children unnecessarily, but such preparations should have the effect of increasing a feeling of safety, not decreasing it. Fear of the unknown is always more intense than fear of something tangible.

Bullying

A frequent reason school-aged children cite for feeling unhappy at school is ridicule or bullying (Cooper, Clements & Holt, 2012). Why do some children become bullies and some become victims? Traits commonly associated with school-aged bullies are:

- Advanced physical size and strength for their age
- Aggressive temperament (both male and female)
- Parents who are indifferent
- Parents who are permissive with an aggressive child
- Parents who typically resort to physical punishment
- Presence of a child who is a "natural victim" (underweight, small, anxious, insecure, cautious or sensitive, with low self-esteem).

Advise parents to discuss bullying with their school-aged child and tell them how it should be reported, so that adults can intervene. School bullying has long-term effects on mental health from the view of both the bully and the victim (Sourander et al., 2012).

Recreational drug use

Once considered a university or high school problem, illegal drugs such as marijuana are now available to children as early as primary school. Cocaine and amphetamines are also becoming increasingly easy for children to obtain (Blake & Davis, 2011; Young, Glover & Havens, 2012).

Cigarette smoking also begins in school-aged children. With the sure knowledge that cigarette smoking plays a large part in the development of lung cancer and other serious respiratory illnesses, many parents assume their children will know not to start. Smoking is considered by children to be an adult activity, however, so adopting the habit can be considered a giant step on the road to adulthood. Although the amount of cigarette advertising targeting young people as consumers has decreased, school-aged children should be taught to recognise advertising aimed at them. Caution children against experimenting with smokeless tobacco as this can lead to mouth and throat cancer (Baydala, 2010; Zhou et al., 2012).

Parents should suspect inhalant abuse or other recreational drug use if their child regularly appears irritable, inattentive or drowsy (Adegbite-Adeniyi et al., 2012). Inhalants, which are easily available to school-aged children for abuse, include aeroplane glue (toluene) and aerosol cooking oil. Children do not become physically addicted to glue but do become psychologically dependent on it. To achieve the desired effect, they drop quantities of the glue into a paper bag, then sniff the fumes to experience a feeling of exhilaration or giddiness. This may seem like a harmless procedure, but, in high concentrations, glue fumes can cause extensive liver damage or enough pulmonary oedema to be fatal. Cooking spray or computer keyboard cleaner give the same effect. Because these products contain CFCs and/or butane they can cause severe respiratory and cardiac irregularity (Baydala, 2010). Children who report being happy and are able to communicate with their family are less likely to be regular users than others (Farmer & Hanratty, 2012).

Androgenic steroids and human growth hormone to enhance sports performance are yet other drugs that preteen children may abuse. Counsel children against using these substances because abuse of steroids can lead to cardiovascular irregularities, uncontrollable aggressiveness and possible cancer in later life (Oberlander & Henderson, 2012).

Children of alcoholic parents

It has been estimated that roughly 13% of Australian children live in a home with at least one adult who misuses alcohol (Dawe et al., 2007; Australian Institute of Family Studies, 2015). Such children are at greater risk of having emotional problems because of the frequent disruption in their lives. Alcoholism may have a genetic cause, so children of alcoholics may be more likely to become alcoholics. They also can learn poor coping behaviour. The immediate problems that can occur with children of alcoholics are:

- A feeling of guilt that they are the cause of the parent's drinking
- Constant worry that the alcoholic parent will become sick or die, leaving the child; at the same time, fear of violence from the alcoholic parent and a wish the parent would leave
- A feeling of shame that prevents the child from inviting friends home or asking for help
- Decreased ability to trust adults because the parent has been unreliable so many times
- Concern because the alcoholic parent's behaviour is so erratic that no regular schedule exists
- Anger at the alcoholic parent for drinking and at the non-alcoholic parent for not doing more to change things
- Helplessness to change the situation.

Such fears may be revealed by failing marks in school, withdrawal from friends or social activities and delinquent behaviour such as stealing. With adolescence may come depression, suicidal thoughts or abuse of drugs or alcohol.

Concerns of the physically challenged or chronically ill school-aged child

One of the biggest problems facing school-aged children with long-term illness or physical challenges is time lost from school. Frequent absences threaten not only academic achievement but also children's relationships with their peers. Whether children are confined to the home or hospitalised, helping them to keep in contact with friends by telephone, email or text messaging can help foster the socialisation that is important for continued development. Encourage parents (or school friends) to obtain schoolwork and help these children with their homework so they can progress with learning at the usual pace and continue to build self-esteem.

Urge parents of children with physical or cognitive challenges to assign them household chores just like other children their age and allow them to participate in activities. It is important for such children to develop a sense of industry or accomplishment so they can persevere in measures that will help them to be as independent as possible (Singer, 2013; see Fig. 32.8).

When you are caring for a school-aged child who is chronically ill or physically challenged, choose short-term activities that can be completed independently. Conversely, be careful not to insult a child with tasks that are obviously not age-appropriate. Table 32.4 describes some nursing actions to help develop a sense of industry in children who are physically challenged or chronically ill.

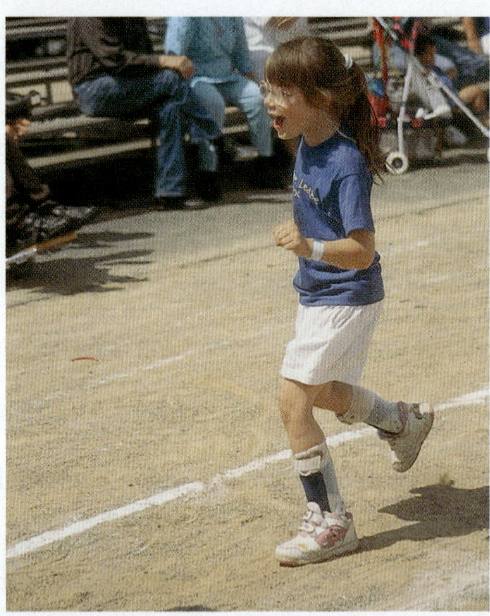

FIGURE 32.8 A school-aged child who is physically challenged is elated at the finish line. This accomplishment can go far towards her developing a sense of industry. (© Jose Carillo/Stock Boston.)

✔ *Checkpoint question 32.1*

School-aged children can begin drug abuse. What is a common household product frequently abused by school-aged children?

a. Grated orange peel
b. Laundry bleach
c. Aerosol cooking oil
d. Shredded cabbage

Key points for review

- School-aged children mature slowly but steadily.
- At about 10 years of age, children begin to develop secondary sex characteristics. Preparation for this helps them accept these changes positively.
- Deciduous teeth are lost and permanent teeth erupt during the school-aged period.
- Erikson's developmental task for the school-aged period is to gain a sense of industry or how to do things well.
- Common health problems during the school-aged period include minor respiratory and gastrointestinal infections as well as dental cavities and malocclusion.
- Common parental concerns during this period are language development, fears and anxieties, and behaviour problems such as stealing and recreational drug use.
- As many as 90% of parents of school-aged children are dual-income families. This means many school-aged children return home before their parents.
- Children in a concrete stage of operational thought are limited to understanding concepts they can actually see. When health teaching, use concrete examples (actually let them hold a syringe, do not just talk about it) to increase their understanding.
- School-aged children thrive on rules. It is confusing for them when rules are changed (medicine will now be taken four rather than three times a day) unless they have a clear explanation of why the change is occurring.
- School-aged children are looking for good adult role models; it is hard for them to feel confidence in an adult

TABLE 32.4 Nursing actions that encourage a sense of industry in a physically challenged or chronically ill school-aged child

Category	Actions
Nutrition	Allow choices of food and respect food preferences. Provide small food servings that child can finish, encouraging sense of accomplishment.
Medicine	Teach child name and action of medicine. Encourage child to keep track of medication times by clock or record. Child may feel more in control of injections or intravenous insertions if allowed to choose the site from among options offered. Allow child to choose oral medicine form (capsules or liquid) if possible.
Rest	Establish clear rules for rest periods (reading or watching television is alright but playing a game is not, etc.).
Hygiene	Respect modesty of school-aged child at an adult level. Allow as much choice as possible such as own clothing, timing of self-care.
Pain	Encourage child to express and rate pain. Encourage child to use distraction techniques, such as counting backwards from 100 or imagery, during episodes of pain. Explain source and cause of pain to give child sense of mastery. Ask for suggestions regarding how bulky the child wants dressing, where to apply tape.
Stimulation	Encourage school work. Encourage activity that ends in a product (putting together a picture puzzle rather than listening to a CD). Encourage paper-and-pencil games, such as connect the dots, tic tac toe. Card games provide social interaction and also encourage simple addition skills. Do not suggest competitive games for children less than 10 years of age. Encourage using playroom for socialisation. Encourage child to keep in contact with school friends by telephone, text messaging or email.

who is not honest with them or who fails to live up to their expectations by not following through on promises.

- School-aged children with a family tendency towards obesity may become overweight. Helping the family learn a healthier lifestyle is important.

CASE STUDY QUESTIONS

4. Susie's mother told you that Susie has developed many nervous habits since she started high school. She asks you if this is normal. How would you answer? What suggestions would you make to her mother regarding this?
5. Susie has become obese in the last year. School-aged children develop obesity because of excessive nutritional intake, lack of exercise and inheritance or family factors. What suggestions could you make to help prevent Susie from gaining more weight? What is a possible consequence of telling school-aged children that they are overweight?
6. Susie's best friend is a 12-year-old boy who is confined to a wheelchair because of muscular dystrophy. Why might developing a sense of industry be particularly difficult for him? What suggestions could you make to encourage this?

Resources

For an extensive range of additional resources to enhance teaching and learning and to facilitate understanding of this chapter, please see the text's accompanying website located on thePoint at http://thepoint.lww.com.

References

Adegbite-Adeniyi, C., Gron, B., Rowles, B. M., et al. (2012). An update on antidepressant use and suicidality in pediatric depression. *Expert Opinion on Pharmacotherapy*, *13*(15), 2119–2130.

Anthony, K. V. & Burroughs, S. (2010). Making the transition from traditional to home schooling: Home school family motivations. *Current Issues in Education*, *13*(4), 1–30.

Atkins, S. (2010). Cotton wool kids. Accessed 23 February 2015, <http://sueatkinsparentingcoach.com/cotton-wool-kids>.

Australian Bureau of Statistics. (2006). Children's injuries. Accessed 23 February 2015, <www.abs.gov.au/ausstats/abs@.nsf/Previousproducts/1301.0Feature%20Article152006?opendocument&tabname=Summary&prodno=1301.0&issue=2006&num=&view=>.

Australian Institute of Family Studies. (2015). An overview of alcohol misuse and parenting. Accessed 25 February 2015, <www3.aifs.gov.au/cfca/publications/overview-alcohol-misuse-and-parenting>.

Baydala, L. (2010). Inhalant abuse. *Paediatrics & Child Health*, *5*(7), 443–448.

Blake, K. & Davis, V. (2011). Substance abuse. In Marcdante, K. J. & Kliegman, R. M. (Eds.), *Nelson Essentials of Pediatrics* (7th ed., pp. 282–284). Philadelphia: Saunders/Elsevier.

Bishop, W. P. (2011). The digestive system. In Marcdante, K. J. & Kliegman, R. M. (Eds.), *Nelson Essentials of Pediatrics* (7th ed., pp. 463–498). Philadelphia: Saunders/Elsevier.

Briggs, P., Simon, W. T. & Simonsen, S. (2011). An exploratory study of Internet-initiated sexual offenses and the chat room sex offender: Has the internet enabled a new typology of sex offender? *Sexual Abuse*, *23*(1), 72–91.

Caprio, S. (2012). Calories from soft drinks—Do they matter? *New England Journal of Medicine*, *367*(15), 1462–1463.

Chahal, H., Fung, C., Kuhle, S. & Veugelers, P. J. (2012). Availability and night-time use of electronic entertainment and communication devices are associated with short sleep duration and obesity among Canadian children. *Pediatric Obesity*, *8*(1), 42–51.

Cooper, G. D., Clements, P. T. & Holt, K. E. (2012). Examining childhood bullying and adolescent suicide: Implications for school nurses. *Journal of School Nursing*, *28*(8), 275–283.

Daley, A. M. (2011). Providing adolescent-friendly HPV education. *Nurse Practitioner*, *36*(11), 35–40.

Dawe, S., Frye, S., Best, D., Moss, D., Atkinson, J., Evans, C., et al. (2007). *Drug Use in the Family: Impacts and Implications for Children.* Canberra, ACT: Australian National Council on Drugs.

Dowdell, E. B. (2012). Urban seventh grade students: A report of health risk behaviors and exposure to violence. *Journal of School Nursing*, *28*(2), 130–137.

Eagle, T. F., Sheetz, A., Gurm, R., et al. (2012). Understanding childhood obesity in America: Linkages between household income, community resources, and children's behaviors. *American Heart Journal*, *163*(5), 836–843.

Edmonds, D. K. (2012). Puberty and its disorders. In Edmonds, D. K. (Ed.), *Dewhurst's Textbook of Obstetrics & Gynaecology* (8th ed.). Oxford, UK: John Wiley & Son.

El-Dawlatly, M. M., Fayed, M. M. & Mostafa, Y. A. (2012). Deep overbite malocclusion: Analysis of the underlying components. *American Journal of Orthodontics & Dentofacial Orthopedics*, *142*(4), 473–480.

Erikson, E. H. (1993). *Childhood and Society*. New York: W. W. Norton & Company.

Farmer, S. & Hanratty, B. (2012). The relationship between subjective wellbeing, low income and substance use among schoolchildren in the north west of England: A cross-sectional study. *Journal of Public Health (Oxford)*, *34*(4), 512–522.

Fletcher, N. D. & Bruce, R. W. (2012). Early onset scoliosis: Current concepts and controversies. *Current Reviews in Musculoskeletal Medicine*, *5*(2), 102–110.

Freud, S. (1962). *Three Essays on the Theory of Sexuality*. New York: Hearst Corporation.

Gunter, K. B., Almstedt, H. C., & Janz, K. F. (2012). Physical activity in childhood may be the key to optimizing lifespan skeletal health. *Exercise & Sport Science Reviews*, *40*(1), 13–21.

Hamdan, A. M., Singh, V. & Rock., W. P. (2012). Assessment of the relationship between perceptions of dental aesthetics and demand for orthodontic treatment in 10–11 year old school children in Birmingham, UK. *Community Dental Health*, *29*(1), 124–128.

Harika, R. K., Cosgrove, M. C., Osendarp, S. J. & Zock, P. L. (2011). Fatty acid intakes of children and adolescents are not in line with the dietary intake recommendations for future cardiovascular health: A systematic review of dietary intake data from thirty countries. *British Journal of Nutrition*, *106*(3), 307–316.

Horne, A. W. & Critchley, H. O. D. (2012). Menstrual problems: Heavy menstrual bleeding and primary dysmenorrhoea. In Edmonds, D. K. (Ed.), *Dewhurst's Textbook of Obstetrics & Gynaecology* (8th ed.). Oxford, UK: John Wiley & Son.

Interactive Games & Entertainment Association (2012). Digital Australia 12. Brisbane: Bond University. Accessed 23 February 2015, <www.igea.net/wp-content/uploads/2011/10/DA12FinalLinkVideo.pdf>.

Kistner, F., Fiebert, I. & Roach, K. (2012). Effect of backpack load carriage on cervical posture in primary schoolchildren. *Work*, *41*(1), 99–108.

Kohlberg, L. (1984). *The Psychology of Moral Development.* New York: Harper & Row.

Krebs, N. F. & Primak, L. E. (2011). Pediatric nutrition and nutritional disorders. In Marcdante, K. J. & Kliegman, R. M. (Eds.), *Nelson Essentials of Pediatrics* (7th ed.). Philadelphia: Saunders/Elsevier.

Loke, I. C., Heyman, G. D., Forgie, J., McCarthy, A. & Lee, K. (2011). Children's moral evaluations of reporting the transgressions of peers: Age differences in evaluations of tattling. *Developmental Psychology*, *47*(6), 1757–1762.

Lowe, S. R., Godoy, L., Rhodes, J. E., et al. (2013). Predicting mothers' reports of children's mental health three years after hurricane Katrina. *Journal of Applied Developmental Psychology, 34*(1), 17–27.

Mack, K. A., Dellinger, A. & West, B. A. (2012). Adult opinions about the age at which children can be left home alone, bathe alone, or bike alone: Second Injury Control and Risk Survey (ICARIS-2). *Journal of Safety Research, 43*(3), 223–226.

Marván, M. L. & Molina-Abolnik, M. (2012). Mexican adolescents' experience of menarche and attitudes toward menstruation: Role of communication between mothers and daughters. *Journal of Pediatric & Adolescent Gynecology, 25*(6), 358–363.

Meng, M. V. & Tanagho, E. A. (2013). Physical examination of the genitourinary tract. In McAninch, J. & Lue, T. F. (Eds.), *Smith & Tanagho's General Urology* (18th ed.). New York: McGraw-Hill Publishing Company.

NSW Department of Education & Communities. (2014). The new school leaving age: A guide for parents. Accessed 23 February 2015, <www.schools.nsw.edu.au/leavingschool/schoolleaveage/index.php>.

Oberlander, J. G. & Henderson, L. P. (2012). The Sturm und Drang of anabolic steroid use: Angst, anxiety, and aggression. *Trends in Neurosciences, 35*(6), 382–392.

Pass, L., Arteche, A., Cooper, P., Cresswell, C. & Murray, L. (2012). Doll play narratives about starting school in children of socially anxious mothers, and their relation to subsequent child school-based anxiety. *Journal of Abnormal Child Psychology, 40*(8), 1375–1384.

Piaget, J. (1969). *The Theory of Stages in Cognitive Development. An Address by Jean Piaget to the CTB/McGraw-Hill Invitational Conference on Ordinal Scales of Cognitive Development.* New York: McGraw-Hill.

Pringsheim, T., Doja, A., Gorman, D., et al. (2012). Canadian guidelines for the evidence-based treatment of tic disorders: Pharmacotherapy. *Canadian Journal of Psychiatry, 57*(3), 133–143.

Rolfes, S. R., Pinna, K. & Whitney, E. N. (2012). *Understanding Normal and Clinical Nutrition* (9th ed.) New York: Wadsworth/Cengage Learning.

Sandler, P. J., Madahar, A. K. & Murray, A. (2011). Anterior open bite: Aetiology and management. *Dental Update, 38*(8), 522–524.

Schantz, S. (2012). Overweight and obesity in youth. *Journal of School Nursing, 28*(6), 167–168.

Scheffer, R. (2011). Anxiety and phobias. In Marcdante, K. J. & Kliegman, R. M. (Eds.), *Nelson Essentials of Pediatrics* (7th ed.). Philadelphia: Saunders/Elsevier.

Serec, M., Svab, I., Kolšek, M., Svab, V., Moesgen, D., Klein, M. (2012). Health-related lifestyle, physical and mental health in children of alcoholic parents. *Drug & Alcohol Review, 31*(7), 861–870.

Singer, B. (2013). Perceptions of school nurses in the care of students with disabilities. *Journal of School Nursing, 29*(5), 329–336.

Smith, S. (2011). Sinusitis. In Marcdante, K. J. & Kliegman, R. M. (Eds.), *Nelson Essentials of Pediatrics* (7th ed.). Philadelphia: Saunders/Elsevier.

Sourander, A., Fossum, S., Rønning, J. A., et al. (2012). What is the long-term outcome of boys who steal at age eight? Findings from the Finnish nationwide "From a Boy to a Man" birth control study. *Social Psychiatry & Psychiatric Epidemiology, 47*(9), 1391–1400.

Theisen, D., Frisch, A, Malisoux, L., et al. (2013). Injury risk is different in team and individual youth sport. *Journal of Science and Medicine in Sport, 16*(3), 200–204.

Tubert-Jeannin, S., Auclair, C., Amsallem, E., et al. (2011). Fluoride supplements (tablets, drops, lozenges or chewing gums) for preventing dental caries in children. *Cochrane Database of Systematic Reviews,* (12), CD007592.

Van Winckel, M., Vande Velde, S., De Bruyne, R., Van Biervliet, S. (2011). Clinical practice: Vegetarian infant and child nutrition. *European Journal of Pediatrics, 170*(12), 1489–1494.

Victorian Government. (2012). Obesity in children—causes. Accessed 25 February 2015, <www.betterhealth.vic.gov.au/bhcv2/bhcarticles.nsf/ pages/obesity_in_children>.

Wen, A., Goldberg, D., Marrs, C. F., et al. (2012). Caries resistance as a function of age in an initially caries-free population. *Journal of Dental Research, 91*(7), 671–675.

Whitney, E. N. & Rolfes, S. R. (2015). Life cycle nutrition: Infancy, childhood & adolescence. In *Understanding Nutrition* (13th ed.). Belmont, CA: Wadsworth Publishing.

Widaman, K. F. & Helm, J. L. (2012). Nocturnal emissions: A failure to replicate. *American Journal of Psychology, 125*(1), 39–50.

Young, A. M., Glover, N. & Havens, J. R. (2012). Nonmedical use of prescription medications among adolescents in the United States: A systematic review. *Journal of Adolescent Health, 51*(1), 6–17.

Zhou, J., Michaud, D. S., Langevin, S. M., et al. (2012). Smokeless tobacco and risk of head and neck cancer: Evidence from a case-control study in New England. *International Journal of Cancer, 132*(8), 1911–1917.

Suggested readings

ARACY <www.aracy.org.au>

Eagle, T. F., Sheetz, A., Gurm, R., et al. (2012). Understanding childhood obesity in America: Linkages between household income, community resources, and children's behaviors. *American Heart Journal, 163*(5), 836–843.

Gaither, M. (2008). Why homeschooling happened. *Educational Horizons, 86*(4), 226–237.

Kidsafe NSW Inc <www.kidsafensw.org>

Kidshealth NZ <www.kidshealth.org.nz>

Kidspot Australia <www.kidspot.com.au>

Ministry of Health NZ <www.health.govt.nz>

Ministry of Social Development: Community Investment <www.familyservices.govt.nz>

Oruche, U. M., Gerkensmeyer, J., Stephan, L., et al. (2012). The described experience of primary caregivers of children with mental health needs. *Archives of Psychiatric Nursing, 26*(5), 382–391.

Rabbitt, A. & Coyne, I. (2012). Childhood obesity: Nurses' role in addressing the epidemic. *British Journal of Nursing, 21*(12), 731–735.

Raising Children Network <http://raisingchildren.net.au>

Tresillian <www.tresillian.net>

Triple P <www.triplep.net/glo-en/home>

Well Child <www.wellchild.org.nz>

White, R. & Mason, R. (2011). Bullying and gangs. *International Journal of Adolescent Medicine & Health, 24*(1), 57–62.

Chapter 33

Nursing care of a family with an adolescent

The previous chapter discussed school-aged children and the capabilities they develop during that time period. This chapter adds information about the changes, both physical and psychosocial, that occur during adolescence. Such information builds a base for care and health teaching for this age group.

LEARNING OBJECTIVES

After studying the contents of this chapter, you should be able to:

1. Describe normal growth and development and common parental concerns of the adolescent period.
2. Use critical thinking to analyse ways in which care of an adolescent could be more family-centred.
3. Understand the issues involved in teaching adolescents to accept pubertal changes.
4. Discuss the nursing care related to the special needs of an adolescent.
5. Identify areas related to care of adolescents that could benefit from additional nursing research or application of evidence-based practice.
6. Understand the importance of applying sound theoretical knowledge of adolescent growth and development to clinical practice.

KEY TERMS

- adolescence
- formal operational thought
- glycogen loading
- identity
- puberty
- role confusion
- substance abuse

CASE STUDY

James is a 15-year-old teenager you see at a local doctor's surgery. His chief concern is a head cold. You notice he has numerous acne lesions on his forehead and cheeks. James' parents tell you that although James appeared to be depressed after his girlfriend broke up with him, he now seems happy again. While talking to James, he asks you how many pills it would take to kill someone, then jokes he was "just kidding". The GP in the clinic prescribes a decongestant for his head cold and suggests James return in 6 months.

CASE STUDY QUESTION

1. Did James have some needs that were not met by his clinic visit?

Adolescence is generally defined as the period between 13 and 18 or 20 years of age, a time that serves as a transition between childhood and young adulthood. It can be divided into an early period (13 to 14 years), a middle period (15 to 16 years) and a late period (17 to 20 years). During all periods, adolescence is defined not so much by chronological age as by physiological, psychological and sociological changes. The drastic changes in physical appearance and the change in expectations of others (especially parents) that occur during the period can lead to both emotional and physical health problems (Sass & Kaplan, 2013).

Adolescents invariably feel a sense of pressure throughout this period because they are mature in some respects but still young in others. For example, an adolescent's sexual interests are awakening, yet personal or parental pressures discourage sexual exploration. An adolescent may not feel mature enough to live away from home, yet parents and teachers may encourage the adolescent to apply to study at a tertiary institution that is far from home. This duality causes a major dilemma for an adolescent, leading to many of the growth and developmental concerns of the age (Ahern & Norris, 2011). Prior to developing an understanding of the emotional and physical health problems pertaining to the adolescent, it is important to review normal patterns of growth and development.

HEALTHY DEVELOPMENT OF AN ADOLESCENT

Assessment

Parents rarely bring adolescents for routine health maintenance visits the way they did when they were younger and adolescents generally don't come to healthcare facilities on their own unless they are ill. Until adolescents need a physical examination for athletic or some other clearance, therefore, they are often not seen for health assessments. When adolescents are accompanied by their parents at health visits, it is best to obtain a health history separately from the adolescent to promote independence and responsibility for self-care. When performing physical examinations on adolescents, be aware they may be very self-conscious of their body. They need assurance and appreciate comments such as "Your blood pressure is 120/70, which is within the normal range for your age" or "Your pulse rate is 68 and this is normal for your age" so they can learn more about their rapidly changing bodies.

Planning and interventions

When planning care with adolescents, respect the fact that they have a strong desire to exert independence or do things their own way. This means they are not likely to adhere to a plan of care that disrupts their lifestyle or makes them appear different from others their age if needed for medical or care reasons. Because of this, including them in planning is essential so the plan will be agreeable and accepted. Establishing a contract, such as asking an adolescent to agree to take medication daily, may be the most effective means to reach a mutual understanding. Remember that adolescents are very oriented to the present, so a program that provides immediate results will usually be carried out well. In contrast, a regimen oriented towards the future, with long-term goals such as preventing hypertension at middle age, may not be as successful. This does not mean it is not important to teach adolescents about the necessity of reducing future health risks—by eating well, not smoking and generally taking care of their bodies—but that information will be best accepted if geared as much as possible to specific, short-term benefits to their health, where immediate results can been seen.

Adolescents have little patience with adults who do not demonstrate the behaviour they are being asked to achieve; a parent or nurse who smokes and asks an adolescent not to smoke, for example, will probably not be successful. For best results, evaluate how an intervention appears from an adolescent's standpoint before beginning teaching.

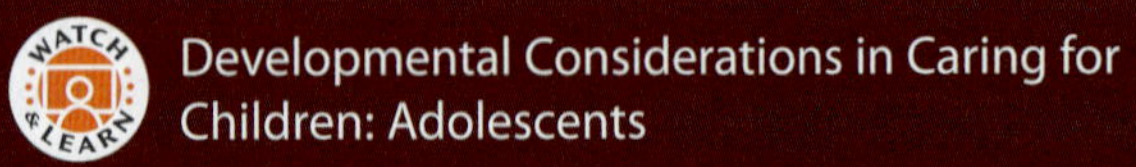

Developmental Considerations in Caring for Children: Adolescents

GROWTH AND DEVELOPMENT OF AN ADOLESCENT

Adolescents grow rapidly and mature dramatically. In developed countries such as Australia and New Zealand, adolescence covers a long time span. In contrast, in developing countries, adolescence tends to be much shorter because children must take full-time jobs early in life to help support their families. Socioeconomic factors definitely influence the length of adolescence across all cultures. Recognising that adolescents may have differing responsibilities and life experiences based on cultural expectations is important to consider when making an assessment.

Physical growth

The major milestones of development in the adolescent period are the onset of puberty at 9 to 12 years of age and the cessation of body growth at 16 to 20 years. Between these milestones, physiological growth and development of adult coordination occur. At first, the gain in physical growth is mostly in weight, leading to the stocky, slightly obese appearance of prepubescence; later comes the thin, gangly appearance of late adolescence.

Most girls are 2.4 to 5 cm taller than boys coming into adolescence but generally stop growing within 3 years of menarche. Those girls who started menstruating at 10 years of age, therefore, may reach their adult height by the age of 13. Boys grow about 10 to 30 cm in height and gain about 7 to 30 kg during adolescence. Girls grow 5 to 20 cm in height and gain 7 to 25 kg. Growth stops with closure of the epiphyseal lines of long bones. This occurs at about 16 or 17 years of age in females and about 18 to 20 years of age in males.

The increase in body size does not occur in all organ systems at the same rate. For example, adolescents' skeletal system grows faster than muscle and muscle mass increases more rapidly than heart size. These differences in growth rates make adolescents appear long-legged and awkward during a rapid growth spurt because their extremities elongate first, followed by trunk growth. Both sexes may lack coordination during these times. A 13-year-old child, for example, may reach to pick up a glass of milk at the dinner table and spill it, having reached beyond it because their arm is longer than they realise.

Because the heart and lungs increase in size more slowly than the rest of the body, blood flow and oxygen availability are reduced. This means adolescents may have insufficient energy and become fatigued trying to finish the various activities that interest them. Pulse rate and respiratory rate decrease slightly (to 70 beats per minute and 20 breaths per minute, respectively) and blood pressure increases slightly (to 120/70 mmHg), reaching adult levels by late adolescence. With adulthood, blood pressure becomes slightly higher in males than females because more force is necessary to distribute blood to the larger male body mass.

During adolescence, androgen stimulates sebaceous glands to extreme activity, sometimes resulting in acne, a common adolescent skin problem. Apocrine sweat glands (glands present in the axillae and genital area) form shortly after puberty. Apocrine sweat glands produce a strong odour in response to emotional stimulation. Therefore, adolescents begin to notice they must shower or bathe more frequently than when they were younger in order to be free of body odour.

Teeth

Adolescents gain their second molars at about 13 years of age and their third molars (wisdom teeth) between 18 and 21 years of age. Third molars may erupt as early as 14 to 15 years of age. The jaw, however, reaches adult size only towards the end of adolescence. As a result, adolescents whose third molars erupt before the lengthening of the jaw is complete may experience pain and may need these molars extracted because they do not fit their jaw line (Marciani, 2012).

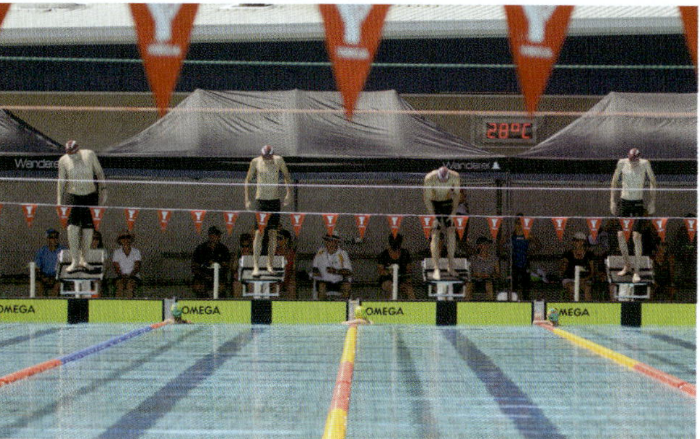

FIGURE 33.1 Older male adolescents build mateship and competitiveness when competing in sports. This builds self-esteem and resilience. (© Lisa Speedie.)

Puberty

Puberty is the time at which an individual first becomes capable of sexual reproduction. A girl has entered puberty when she begins to menstruate; a boy enters puberty when he begins to produce spermatozoa. These events usually occur between ages 11 and 14 years. The age of first menstruation in girls is gradually decreasing from a mean of 13 years to 12.4 years, which is probably related to more weight gain in girls (Ledger, 2012). Puberty creates many questions for early teenagers about what is normal and what is not (Marván & Molina-Abolink, 2012).

Secondary sex changes

Secondary sex characteristics such as body hair configuration and breast growth are those characteristics which distinguish the sexes from each other but play no direct part in reproduction. The secondary sex characteristics that began in the late school-age period (see Chapter 32) continue to develop during adolescence. Sexual maturity in males and females is classified according to Tanner stages, named after the pioneering researcher on sexual maturity (Tanner, 1962).

CASE STUDY QUESTION

2. James is concerned about developing body odour. What body glands are responsible for this?
   a. Adipose glands
   b. Apocrine glands
   c. Sebaceous glands
   d. Dermal pod glands

Developmental milestones

The same assessment categories of younger children apply to adolescents.

Play or recreation

Twelve to thirteen-year-old children change from school-age activities of games to more adult forms of recreation such as listening to music, texting or chatting, or following a sports team's wins and losses. Team (or school) loyalty becomes intense (see Figure 33.1). A coach's instructions can become mandatory, similar to the loyalty 6-year-old children showed towards their first-year teacher. Injuries from athletics occur in early adolescence until adolescents learn more about their limits and begin to respect the advice of adults on being well prepared and trained for sports. It becomes a learning process for adolescents to listen rather than just act.

Most adolescents spend a great deal of time just talking with peers as social interaction, either face to face or through electronic media. Conflict can arise if parents disapprove of the number of hours spent in this activity, afraid their children are wasting time. For an adolescent, however, talking is no more a waste of time than was imaginative play as a preschooler. It is a major way they learn about values and responsibilities. Beginning at age 16 years, most adolescents want part-time jobs to earn money. Such jobs can teach young people how to work with others, accept responsibility, and how to save and spend money wisely.

Emotional development

Developmental task: identity versus role confusion

According to Erikson (1993), the developmental task in early and mid-adolescence is to form a sense of **identity** or decide who they are and what kind of person they will be. In late adolescence, the task is to form a sense of intimacy or close relationships with persons of the opposite as well as the same sex (see Fig. 33.2). It is the concentration on these two tasks that leads to typical adolescent behaviour. The four main areas in which adolescents must make gains to achieve a sense of identity are:

1. Accepting their changed body image
2. Establishing a value system or what kind of person they want to be
3. Making a career decision
4. Becoming emancipated from their parents.

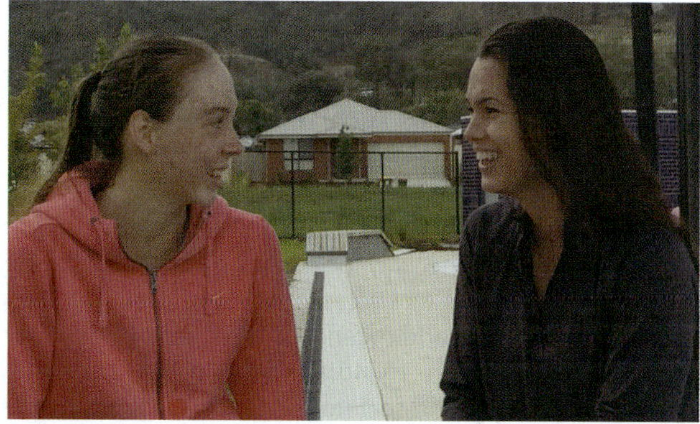

FIGURE 33.2 Late adolescents aged 17–20 years. Often closer relationships are formed in this period and changes in sharing and trust occur. (© Lisa Speedie.)

If young people do not achieve a sense of identity, they develop a sense of **role confusion** or can have little idea what kind of person they are (Erikson, 1993). This can lead to difficulty functioning effectively as adults, because they are unable, for example, to decide what stand to take on a particular issue or how to approach new challenges or situations. This can lead them to exhibit acting-out (attention-getting) behaviours because they may believe it is better to make a negative impression than none at all.

Body image

Adolescents who develop a strong sense of industry during their school-age years and learn to solve problems are best equipped to adjust to their new body image. Nurses can do much to educate adolescents about their bodies and help them to accept the changes that mark maturity.

Adolescents are usually their own worst critics, never pleased with any aspect of their bodies. Those with low self-esteem may need parental or healthcare provider support to understand that a person's worth is based on more than physical appearance. They may need help to realise that the characteristics that make someone creative, compassionate and fun to be with are the qualities on which lasting relationships are built.

Self-esteem

Like body image, self-esteem may undergo major changes during the adolescent years and can be challenged by *all* the changes that occur during adolescence. Garzon and Dunn (2013) identified the following events:

- Changes in one's body and physiological functioning
- Changes in feelings and emotional focus
- Changes in social relationships (including relationships with both family and friends)
- Changes in family and school expectations.

All of these factors can have an effect on adolescents' feelings about themselves, sometimes resulting in crisis. Help parents to understand how important it is for adolescents to have immediate successes, such as making the high school sports team or having a date for the first time. Parental comments such as "When you're older, these things won't be so important", are not likely to erase the hurt that comes from being 16 years old and not being included in such major events. Empathic understanding ("It's hard to be left out") is a better communication technique.

In recent years, a number of researchers have looked at the differences in the way boys and girls handle these emotional upheavals of adolescence. Several researchers have proposed that adolescence is a period of particular crisis for girls who are trying to find a place in a male-dominated society. The sociologist Carol Gilligan and her colleagues interviewed more than 500 girls between the ages of 7 and 16 years over a 5-year period and found many girls who, at age 11 years, were feisty, confident and eager to speak their minds became hesitant to voice their opinions by early adolescence, having pushed their earlier resistance "underground" (Gilligan, 1982). Gilligan tied this change to a growing realisation among girls that their forthrightness may not be appealing to boys. They begin to self-censor, hoping to become more popular. Girls also struggle with a tug of war between valuing academic (or athletic) success (i.e. men's values) over maintaining close friendships (i.e. women's values).

Although the turmoil of adolescence can be just as confusing to boys as it is to girls, Gilligan (1982) hypothesised boys may feel less pressure as they become adults because they learn more easily to be competitive, independent and separated from feelings. Girls, because they are encouraged to maintain their concern for people throughout their lives, are caught in a conflict between that and being independent and competitive. This places girls at risk of more conflicting feelings throughout adolescence. Long-term psychological problems, notably eating disorders, which occur in both boys and girls, may be one unfortunate result of repressing innate feelings in order to conform. Parents can help both girls and boys deal with these conflicts by encouraging them to maintain their honesty and forthrightness.

Value system

Adolescents develop values through talking to peers. In early adolescence, girls tend to band together with girls and boys with boys. They dress identically with other members of their group: jeans and jumpers, special jackets or whatever the fashion may be. On the surface, this makes adolescents appear to be losing their identities rather than finding them. Adolescents who are different for any reason, such as being overweight or from another socioeconomic, racial or cultural background are often excluded from groups. This behaviour may seem immature, but, like banding together, it is a necessary way for adolescents to establish a sense of identity. They know they are like the rest of the group because they dress, talk and think the same way and go to the same places. They know they are not like the excluded member. Knowing who they are *not* is one step in discovering who they are. Helping adolescents to appreciate that it is not fair to exclude others on the basis of superficial characteristics helps them move more quickly through this stage.

Parents may be concerned about an early adolescent's lack of interest in the opposite sex. They can worry about an intensely close girl–girl or boy–boy relationship. You can assure parents that adolescents must feel secure and pleased with their own sex before they can relate comfortably to the opposite sex. For other parents, because this is the time when gay or lesbian adolescents begin to demonstrate their sexual preferences, this may be the time to talk to their adolescent about their acceptance of all sexual orientations so sexual preference doesn't have to be repressed.

Emancipation from parents

Emancipation from parents may become a major issue during the middle and late adolescent years for two reasons. Some parents may not yet be ready for their child to be totally independent and some adolescents may not yet be sure they want to be on their own. They may fight bitterly for a right—for example, to stay out until midnight or later on a weekend—then never use the privilege once they have gained it. Winning the battle was more important than exercising the newly-won right.

In many instances, the closer the tie adolescents feel with their parents, the more severe can be their struggle. As long as parents are reasonable in their restrictions, the degree of protest being made may be proof the ties are strong and separation or emancipation is not easy. The adolescent feels safe to act out and trusts that the safety of their parents and family will remain (Carr-Greg, 2012). Encourage parents to give adolescents more freedom in areas such as choosing their own clothes or after-school activities; at the same time, help parents continue to place some restrictions on adolescent behaviour, such as age-appropriate times out on school nights. These are not unreasonable rules and actually help adolescents accept the responsibility that comes with independence.

Both parents and adolescents may need help to understand that emancipation does not mean severance but rather a change in a relationship. People who are independent of one another can have even better relationships than those who are dependent on one another. This step is actually no different from the one children accomplished when they grew from infants to toddlers, when they changed from wanting to be held and rocked to wanting to run. If parents can think of it in this light, they will gain a better perspective and may realise they will not lose their children because they become adults. By the time children are 18 years of age, they have survived leaving high school. They are at university or have found a first job and have begun to manage their own lives. Many 18-year-olds so enjoy their new independence they find it difficult to understand why adulthood is thought to be challenging. A little more maturity will help them realise that initial success as an independent young adult does not necessarily guarantee additional success, that beginning adult life may be far easier than continuing it in the years ahead.

Sense of intimacy

Once adolescents have achieved a sense of identity in early or mid-adolescence, they are ready to work on the second developmental task, that of achieving a sense of intimacy (Erikson, 1993). The ability to form intimate relationships is strongly correlated with the sense of trust, the first developmental task in infancy. Infants who are unable to form a sense of trust may be unable to relate to others on a deep enough level to form lasting and close relationships as adults. Conversely, adults unable to gain a sense of intimacy may be unable to foster a sense of trust in an infant. Those who do not develop a sense of intimacy are left feeling isolated; in a crisis situation, they have no one to whom they feel they can turn for help or support. A sense of intimacy is closely related to the sense of trust learned in the first year of life because, without the feeling that one can trust others, building a sense of intimacy is difficult.

Some adolescents require help from parents or other adults to differentiate between sound relationships and those that are based only on sexual attraction. Some parents may not be able to listen to their adolescent without interjecting their own opinions because they worry that relationships based on infatuation will lead to a sexual relationship. Parents should feel an obligation to inform their children of their feelings about early sexual relationships. At the same time, they have to be realistic that some adolescents will not follow their advice, as shown by the rising rates of teenage pregnancy and sexually transmitted diseases, including HIV.

Teenage pregnancy is a significant issue. In Australia around 30% of young women will become pregnant in their teenage years (Health Direct Australia, 2014). In New Zealand, for every 1000 teenage girls, approximately 50 will fall pregnant. Of these pregnancies, approximately half will result in abortion, meaning that there are more than 3800 babies born to teenage mothers in New Zealand every year (Kiwi Families, 2011). If parents suspect their adolescent is sexually active, they should counsel them to be sure they are knowledgeable about safer sex practices (State Government of Victoria, 2015). For further guidance, see Chapter 5 for guidelines regarding safer sex and Chapter 22 for a discussion of teenage pregnancy.

In our busy modern society in which adolescents engage in such a variety of activities, they may need help learning how to project themselves into another person's situation and to ask themselves how the world looks from that position. This concept, *empathy*, is the ability to understand the feelings of another, or, in other words, a developed sense of intimacy in its finest form. This is a time to start role modelling compassion and empathy to adolescents to help build their identity and understand healthy intimacy.

Socialisation

Younger teenagers may feel more self-doubt than self-confidence when they meet another adolescent with whom they would like to begin a lasting relationship. Both male and female early adolescents tend to be loud and boisterous, particularly when someone whose attention they would like to attract is nearby. They are impulsive and very much like 2-year-old children in that they want what they want immediately, not when it is convenient for others. Many 13-year-olds begin to experience "crushes" or infatuations with school mates. At this age, however, they may spend more time longing for someone than they do instituting an in-depth and rewarding relationship. They have too little experience with life and too limited a frame of reference yet to know how to offer a deep commitment to another or accept one from that person.

By 14 years of age, most teenagers have become quieter and more introspective. They are becoming used to their changing bodies, feel more confidence in themselves and have greater self-esteem. For those who have not achieved this state, this time can be full of low self-esteem and daily challenges.

Adolescents watch adults carefully during this period, searching for good role models with whom they can identify. They may form a friendship with an older adolescent, trying to imitate that person in everything from thoughts to clothing. If the older adolescent has dropped out of school or plays a particular sport, the younger person may express a wish to drop out or train for that sport too. This can be a challenging time for parents and the adolescent.

Most 15-year-olds fall "in love" several times a year. However, many of these relationships are based on attraction because of physical appearance, not because of inner qualities or characteristics that are compatible with their own. Because infatuation is fleeting, it can lead to extremely intense but brief attachments that fade once the two young people discover they have little in common. Beginning romantic attachments this often, however, does not mean their feelings are any less strong or that they feel any less pain when the relationship ends. By age 16 years, boys are becoming sexually mature (although they continue to grow taller until about 18 years of age). Both sexes are better able to trust their bodies than they were the year before. By age 17, they tend to have adult values and responses to events. They have left behind the childish behaviours they used in early adolescence—shoving and punching—to get the attention of others.

✔ Checkpoint question 33.1

A shy, quiet 14-year-old girl you care for in a hospital setting tells you she is concerned because she has not menstruated yet. This is making her feel "left out" at school. How would you counsel her? What if she were 16 and had the same concern?

Cognitive development

The final phase of cognitive development, the stage of **formal operational thought**, begins at the age of 12 or 13 years and grows in depth over the adolescent years (Piaget, 1969). This stage involves the ability to think in abstract terms and use the scientific method to arrive at conclusions. The problems that adolescents are asked to solve in school depend on this type of thought; for example, a boy rowing upstream at 10 km/h against a current of 4 km/h will go how far in 1 hour? Problem solving in any situation depends on the ability to think abstractly and logically.

With the ability to use scientific reasoning, adolescents can plan their future. They can create a hypothesis (What if I go to university? What if I don't go to university?) and think through the probable consequences. Thinking abstractly is what allows adolescents to project themselves into the minds of others and imagine how others view them or their actions (display compassion).

Moral and spiritual development

Because adolescents enlarge their thought processes to include formal reasoning, they are able to respond to the question, "Why is it wrong to steal from your neighbour's house?" with "It would hurt my neighbour by requiring him to spend money to replace what I stole", rather than with the immature response of the school-aged child, "The police will punish me". Some adolescents, however, may have difficulty envisioning a large shop or corporation as capable of suffering economic loss from stealing, a concept that can contribute to the frequent practice of petty shoplifting at this age.

Almost all adolescents question the existence of God and any religious practices they have been taught (Kohlberg, 1984). This questioning is a natural part of forming a sense of identity and establishing a value system at a time in life when they draw away from their families.

CASE STUDY QUESTION

3. James is entering the final stage of cognitive development. This stage is termed:

a. Formal operational thought
b. Cognitive attainment
c. Concrete operational thought
d. Scientific formulating

HEALTH PROMOTION FOR AN ADOLESCENT AND FAMILY

Because of still limited judgement, adolescents need guidelines with reference to safety, nutrition and daily care.

Promoting adolescent safety

In Australia and New Zealand, accidents, most commonly those involving motor vehicles, are the leading cause of death among the 17–25 years age group (Bureau of Infrastructure, Transport and Regional Economics, 2014). Although teenagers and young adults are at the peak of their physical and sensory motor functioning, their need to rebel against authority or to gain attention can lead them to take risks while driving, such as speeding or driving while intoxicated.

In the interest of an adolescent's safety and that of others, emotional maturity rather than age should be the qualification for obtaining a driver's licence. Additionally, encouraging adolescents to seek out a community-sponsored driving course, not only to learn the techniques of safe driving but also to learn a sense of responsibility towards others, is also beneficial (Vassallo, Lahausse & Edwards, 2013).

Equally dangerous for adolescents are motorbikes and motor scooters, which are appealing because of their low cost and convenience in parking. Both drivers and riders should wear safety helmets to prevent head injury; long pants to prevent leg burns from exhaust pipes; and full body covering to prevent abrasions in case of an accident. Advise adolescents who choose these forms of transport to be as familiar with safety rules as car drivers. They need to wait to drive motorcycles or scooters until they are emotionally mature enough to use sound driving judgement.

Although drowning tends to occur in younger children, it does occur in adolescence. It can happen when good swimmers go beyond their capabilities on dares or in hopes of impressing friends. It is offer related to alcohol intoxication. Teaching water safety, such as not swimming alone or when tired, is as important as teaching the mechanics of swimming.

Athletic injuries tend to increase in number during adolescence because of the vigorous level of competition that occurs in organised sports. These are often overuse injuries because of poor conditioning. Types of athletic injuries are discussed in Chapter 51. Other common causes of death in adolescents are homicide and self-harm (i.e. suicide) (Swahn et al., 2012).

Promoting nutritional health for an adolescent

Adolescents are experiencing so much growth they may always feel hungry. If adolescents' eating habits are unsupervised, they tend to eat faddish or quick snack foods rather than more nutritionally sound ones because of both hunger and peer pressure. Some adolescents turn away from the five pyramid food groups to eat great quantities of sweets, soft drinks or empty-kilojoule snacks so they are left poorly-nourished despite their large intake. This can lead to issues with weight (Wengle et al., 2012). One form of adolescent rebellion is to refuse to eat foods that parents stress are good for them. Parents who stock their kitchens with more nutritious foods, who always keep plenty of milk and healthy snacks such as fruit and vegetables on hand, and who are willing to meet their adolescents halfway in terms of food preferences, such as serving pizza once a week, can be more certain their child is eating nutritious foods during the day. Giving an adolescent some responsibility for food planning or meals, such as making dinner every Wednesday night, can teach some important lessons about nutrition without conflict.

Adolescents who are slightly obese because of prepubertal changes may begin low-kilojoule or starvation diets to lose excessive weight. Some develop eating disorders such as bulimia or anorexia nervosa (see Chapter 54). A weight-loss diet may be appropriate during adolescence but it must be supervised to ensure that an adolescent consumes sufficient kilojoules and nutrients for growth.

Recommended dietary reference intakes

An adolescent needs an increased number of kilojoules to support the rapid body growth that occurs. As shown in Appendix B, males grow more than females during this period. One of the most important things adolescents can learn is that just filling their stomachs will not provide adequate nutrition. Foods that supply the necessary carbohydrates, vitamins, proteins and minerals are essential.

The nutrients that are most likely to be deficient in both male and female adolescent diets are iron, calcium and zinc. Large amounts of iron are necessary to meet expanding blood volume requirements. Females require a high iron intake not only because of increasing blood volume but also because iron begins to be lost with menstruation. Girls with a heavy menstrual flow (menorrhagia) may need to take an additional iron supplement to prevent iron-deficiency anaemia (Fernandez-Gaxiola & De-Regil, 2011; McClung, 2012) (see Chapter 44). Increased calcium and physical exercise are necessary for rapid skeletal growth as well as to "stockpile" calcium to prevent osteoporosis later in life (Chouinard, Randall Simpson & Buchholz, 2012). Zinc is necessary for sexual maturation and body growth. Good sources of iron are meat and green vegetables; calcium is abundant in milk and dairy products; meat and milk are also high in zinc. See also Appendices E and F for advice on the amount and types of foods needed to stay healthy.

Promoting nutritional health with a varied diet

Vegetarian diets

Because vegetables generally contain fewer kilojoules than meat, adolescents need to consume large amounts to achieve an adequate kilojoule intake with a vegetarian diet. Textured vegetable protein such as tofu can be added to meals to increase the amount of protein supplied and to help meet adolescent growth needs (Whitney & Rolfes, 2015). Some adolescents may find it difficult to follow a vegetarian diet because it makes them different from their peers and limits the foods they can eat at parties or at school, such as pizza, meat pies or hot dogs. Whether to continue to follow this type of diet is a decision an adolescent must make as part of achieving a sense of identity. Well-balanced vegetarian diets can supply enough energy for an active athlete (Timko, Horrnes & Chubski, 2012). It is important to ascertain whether adolescent vegetarians are following a diet or are eating only fruit and vegetables as a method of losing weight.

Glycogen loading

Athletes need more carbohydrates or energy than people who do not engage in strenuous activity. The source of carbohydrate that best sustains athletes comes from the breakdown of glycogen because this supplies a slow and steady release of glucose. **Glycogen loading** is a procedure used to ensure there is adequate glycogen to sustain energy through an athletic event. Several days before a sports event, athletes lower their carbohydrate intake and exercise heavily to deplete muscle glycogen stores. They then switch to a diet high in carbohydrates. With the renewed carbohydrate intake, muscle glycogen is stored at approximately twice the usual level, ready to supply twice the glucose for sustained energy. Because the effects of frequent glycogen loading are unknown, the practice is not recommended for adolescents. As a rule, the goals of nutrition that are best for everyone, such as eating a well-balanced diet, are also the best for athletes, rather than diets that interfere with carbohydrate, fluid or fat intake (Bagnulo, 2012).

Promoting development of an adolescent in daily activities

Maintaining adequate nutrition to support rapid adolescent growth is essential to continued healthy development, as discussed earlier. Adequate sleep, hygiene and exercise are also important and should become an adolescent's responsibility rather than the parents'. Parents can, however, encourage adolescents to engage in healthy patterns of living—primarily through role modelling.

Care of teeth

Adolescents are generally very conscientious about teeth brushing because of a fear of developing bad breath. They should continue to use a fluoride paste rather than a brand advertised as promoting white teeth. They should continue to drink fluoridated water to ensure firm enamel growth (Armfield, 2010). Adolescents tend to snack a great deal so their teeth are always exposed to bacterial erosion. Some may develop cavities for the first time during this period. Teenagers with braces must be extremely conscientious about teeth brushing to prevent plaque build-up on hidden tooth surfaces.

Dress and hygiene

Adolescents are capable of total self-care and, because of their body awareness, may even be overly conscientious about personal hygiene and appearance. Both sexes try many types of shampoo, deodorant, breath fresheners and toothpaste. They may take seriously (without admitting it) the content of ads showing that toothpastes or deodorants can help win an attractive person or gain instant success. Remember that, when caring for hospitalised adolescents, providing time for self-care, such as shampooing hair, is important to include in the adolescent's nursing care plan.

Adolescents can be acutely aware of how their peers dress. When hospitalised, most teenagers seem to improve markedly when allowed to wear their own clothing rather than a hospital gown. Adolescents may also completely ignore dress and hygiene at this time due to low self-esteem, feelings of powerlessness and underlying trauma and mental health issues.

Sleep

Although it is widely believed that everyone needs 8 hours of sleep a night, some need more and others can adjust to considerably less. Because protein synthesis occurs most readily during sleep and adolescents are building so many new cells, adolescents need proportionately more sleep than any other age group. In addition, because this is a stressful period, adolescents may sleep restlessly as their mind reworks the day's tensions; even long periods of sleep, therefore, may not leave them feeling refreshed (Short et al., 2012).

Many adolescents attempt to get by with too little sleep because they are constantly busy and because staying up late is a symbol of being an adult. Frequent lack of sleep can lead to chronic fatigue or depression. This is why adolescents admitted to hospital for even a minor illness may sleep as if they are exhausted as they make up for a chronic lack of sleep (Frost & Burns, 2013).

Exercise

Just as with younger children, adolescents need exercise every day both to maintain muscle tone and to provide an outlet for tension. Unlike younger children, although they are constantly on the go, adolescents often receive little real exercise. They catch a bus to school, sit for classes, sit at a shopping centre after school and talk to friends and sit and watch television in the evening. They have put in a full day from 7 in the morning until 11 at night, yet they have had little exercise compared with the amount they used to get when they came home from school and played outside before dinner. Because of this, adolescents who have had an injury and must learn an activity such as crutch walking need to do muscle-strengthening exercises at first, just as adults must.

Adolescents who are involved in structured athletic activities receive daily exercise. If, however, they have not participated in competitive sports before, they may need advice on increasing exercise gradually so they do not overexercise and consequently develop muscle sprains or other overuse injuries (Hoang et al., 2012).

Sun exposure

Because some adolescents spend a great deal of time outdoors participating in athletics and social activities, it is a critical time for them to avoid excessive sun exposure so they don't develop skin cancer (i.e. melanoma) from ultraviolet rays. Encourage teenagers to use sunscreen, avoid tanning beds and report to their primary healthcare provider any skin mole that changes in shape or colour. Do this as creatively as possible because teenagers have difficulty looking to the future and imagining how drastically the development of melanoma could affect their lives (Cohen et al., 2013). Help support and educate around SunSmart behaviours and long-term dangers of sun exposure.

Common health problems of an adolescent

Hypertension

Hypertension is present if blood pressure is above the 95th percentile or 127/81 mmHg for 16-year-old girls and 131/81 for 16-year-old boys for two consecutive readings in different settings. Adolescents who are obese, who are of Indigenous or Torres Strait Islander origin, who eat a diet high in salt or who have a family history of hypertension are most susceptible to developing the condition (Australian Government Department of the Prime Minister and Cabinet, 2015). This is particularly important for adolescents because new medications plus education can help to greatly reduce the incidence of cardiovascular disease as they reach adulthood (Blake & Davis, 2011). Prevention and management of hypertension in children and adolescents are discussed in Chapter 41.

Poor posture

Many adolescents demonstrate poor posture, a tendency to round shoulders and a shambling, slouchy walk. This is due in part to the imbalance of growth that arises from the skeletal system growing a little more rapidly than the muscles attached to it. Poor posture particularly seems to develop in adolescents who reach adult height before their peers. They slouch to appear no taller than anyone around them. Girls especially may slouch so as not to appear taller than boys, in the belief that boys only like girls shorter than themselves. Girls may also slouch to diminish the appearance of their breast size if they are developing more rapidly than their friends. Slouching can also result from carrying heavy backpacks or school bags (Kistner, Fiebert & Roach, 2012). Assessment of posture is important to detect the difference between simple poor posture and the beginning of scoliosis (lateral curvature of the spine; see Chapters 34 and 51).

Body piercing and tattoos

Body piercing and tattoos are a strong mark of adolescence (Stein & Jordan, 2012). Both sexes have ears, lips, chins, navels and breasts pierced and filled with studs, or tattoos applied to arms, legs or their torso. These acts have become a way for adolescents to make a statement that they are different from their parents. Be certain they know the symptoms of infection at a piercing or tattoo site (redness, warmth, drainage, swelling, mild pain) and to report these to a healthcare provider if they occur because serious staphylococcal or streptococcal infections can occur at piercing sites. Caution adolescents that sharing needles for piercing or tattooing carries the same risk as sharing needles for intravenous drug use.

Fatigue

So many adolescents comment that they feel fatigued to some degree that this can be considered normal for the age group. However, because fatigue may be a beginning symptom of disease, it is important it is investigated as a legitimate concern and not underestimated. Assess an adolescent's diet, sleep patterns and activity schedules, because all can contribute greatly to fatigue. Note when the fatigue began. A short period of extreme tiredness is more likely to suggest disease than a long, ill-defined report of always feeling tired.

If an adolescent's sleep and diet appear to be adequate, the activity schedule is reasonable and physical assessment suggests no illness, then the fatigue may be of an emotional origin. It can be a means of avoiding school, conflict with parents or social situations. Those who are under-stimulated by school may develop fatigue as a sign of boredom.

Blood tests may be used to rule out anaemia and the infection that is so common in adolescents—infectious mononucleosis (see Chapter 43). Chronic fatigue syndrome may also need to be ruled out (Lloyd, Chalder & Rimes, 2012). If it is determined that teenagers do not have these conditions, they can be assured they are healthy and offered guidance to solve the problem with better diet, more sleep, fewer activities and development of better problem-solving techniques to relieve tensions.

Menstrual irregularities

Menstrual irregularities can be a major health concern of adolescent girls as they learn to adjust to their individual body cycles. Chapter 47 discusses these problems in detail.

Acne

Acne (see Fig. 33.3) is a self-limiting inflammatory disease that involves the sebaceous glands that empty into hair shafts (the pilosebaceous unit). It is the most common skin disorder of adolescence, occurring in as many as 80% to 95% of adolescents (Morelli & Prok, 2012). It occurs slightly more frequently in boys than in girls. The peak age for the lesions to occur in girls is 14–17 years; for boys, 16–19 years. Although not proved, genetic factors may play a part in their development.

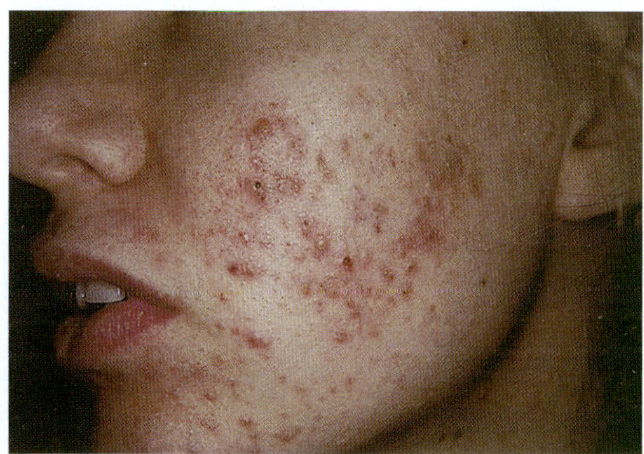

FIGURE 33.3 Facial acne in an adolescent.

Before the rapid increase in androgen secretion occurs with puberty, the sebaceous glands that enter into hair follicles are small and relatively inactive, so acne is non-existent. Changes associated with puberty cause acne to develop:

- As androgen levels rise in both sexes, sebaceous glands become active.
- Abnormal keratinisation (cell growth) of the lining of the ducts occurs; this overgrowth obstructs the ducts.
- The output of sebum increases. Sebum is largely composed of lipids, mainly triglycerides.
- If all of the material formed cannot be eliminated to the skin surface because of the narrow gland ducts, the glands enlarge and trapped sebum causes whiteheads or closed comedones.
- As trapped sebum darkens from accumulation of melanin and oxidation of the fatty acid component on exposure to air, blackheads or open comedones form.
- Bacteria (generally, *Propionibacterium acnes*) lodge and thrive in the retained secretions, forming papules.
- Leakage of free fatty acid causes a dermal inflammatory reaction.
- If glands rupture, sebum is extruded into adjacent skin, which produces reddened inflammatory cysts.

Acne is categorised as mild (comedones are present), moderate (papules and pustules are also present) or severe (cysts are present). The most common locations of acne lesions are the face, neck, back, upper arms and chest. Flare-ups are associated with emotional stress, menstrual periods or the use of greasy hair creams or makeup that can further plug gland ducts. Lesions are less noticeable in summer months, probably because of greater sun exposure, which increases epidermic peeling, or the reduction in stress as a result of being on holidays.

Assessment

Always ask adolescents at health assessments if they are troubled with acne and to what extent it interferes with their self-image as this can be a major cause of stress. Inspect for facial, chest and back lesions on physical examination.

Therapeutic management

The goal of therapy for acne is threefold: (a) decrease sebum formation; (b) prevent comedones; and (c) control bacterial proliferation. See Box 33.1.

External medication

Medications that are applied externally peel away the superficial skin layer to prevent sebum plugs forming and are sufficient if only comedones are present. The most frequently used over-the-counter medications contain benzoyl peroxide. A common prescription medication is tretinoin (Retin-A cream). This reduces keratin formation and plugging of ducts. Caution adolescents using a vitamin A cream to avoid prolonged sun exposure or to use a sun block of SPF 30 or higher, because the cream makes their skin more susceptible than usual to ultraviolet rays. Also warn them that, for the first week or two of therapy, peeling or oxidising may make the complexion actually appear worse. Topical antibiotic creams such as erythromycin may be prescribed to reduce the bacterial level on skin, but usually only after oxidising agents have not succeeded; these creams may

BOX 33.1 ✻ Focus on family teaching

Guidelines for the prevention and treatment of acne

Q. James says to you, "I've had acne for the last 3 months. How can I make this go away?"

A. Most adolescents have some acne. Try the following suggestions:

1. Do not pick or squeeze acne lesions, which ruptures glands and spreads sebum into the skin, increasing symptoms. The times you are most likely to do this are during periods of stress, such as when you are taking a test. When you find your hand on your face, distract yourself with some other motion, such as interlocking your fingers.
2. Makeup, greasy hair preparations or tight sweatbands can plug ducts of glands and increase comedone formation. Avoid these, if possible. Using medicated makeup both covers and helps lesions heal.
3. Topical acne preparations work by unplugging glands. You must use them consistently to make them effective. Plan enough time in the morning before school and a time in the evening to apply these. Post a chart by your bathroom mirror to remind yourself.
4. Washing daily to remove irritating fatty acids is helpful. Excessive washing is not necessary to prevent lesion formation. In fact, excessive washing can actually sabotage healing by rupturing glands.
5. If you are taking oral vitamin A (Roaccutane), do not take another source of vitamin A in tablet form. Roaccutane is very harmful to fetal growth. Girls taking Roaccutane should take measures to prevent pregnancy while taking the drug and for 1 month afterwards. If a girl does become pregnant while taking the drug, she should stop taking it immediately and notify her doctor.
6. Both topical and oral vitamin A make your skin very sensitive to sunlight. Avoid long exposures to sunlight or you will sunburn readily.
7. No acne medication works immediately. While you are waiting for lesions to heal, keep yourself occupied with a new activity (join a school club, try dancing lessons). When your skin is clear once more, these experiences will help make you an interesting person as well as one with clear skin.
8. Although diet does not influence the development of acne lesions, you should eat a healthy, well-balanced diet for good general health.

sensitise adolescents unnecessarily to antibiotics (McKenna & Mirkov, 2014; Simonart, 2012).

Systemic medication

Isotretinoin, a form of vitamin A, is an extremely effective oral drug for reducing sebum production and abnormal keratinisation of gland ducts (see Box 33.2). It is prescribed for cystic acne. In pustular and cystic acne, systemic (oral) antibiotics are also helpful. Tetracycline (500 mg twice daily the first week, then tapered to 250 mg daily for maintenance) is effective against the anaerobic bacteria that break down sebum to form irritating acids. Improvement is not generally seen for 2 weeks, so you may need to encourage adolescents to continue with the medication during the waiting period. Without noticeable improvement, adolescents have a tendency to continue taking the higher dose or even increase the dose, hoping to initiate a faster effect. Tetracycline is not prescribed for children under 12 years of age because it can cause permanent staining of teeth and possibly interfere with growth of long bones. Likewise, tetracycline should not be given to females who may be pregnant because it causes faulty bone growth in a fetus (McKenna & Mirkov, 2014). Because tetracycline may interfere with oral contraceptives, adolescent girls should use another method of birth control while taking the antibiotic.

Food impairs the absorption of tetracycline so the medication should be taken on an empty stomach (2 hours before or after eating). Adolescents must be certain of the date of expiration of the medication; outdated tetracycline breaks down into an extremely toxic composition. Females taking systemic antibiotics for long periods of time become susceptible to developing candidal vaginitis and need to be aware of the symptoms: a white, pruritic vaginal discharge.

BOX 33.2 * Focus on pharmacology

Isotretinoin

Classification: Isotretinoin is a vitamin A metabolite.
Action: Reduces sebum secretion
Pregnancy risk category: X
Dosage: 0.5–2 mg/kg PO per day for 15 to 20 weeks
Possible adverse effects: Nausea, vomiting, dry skin, pruritus, fatigue, headache, epistaxis, dry nose, dry mouth, eye irritation, elevated sedimentation rate, hypertriglycerdaemia, proteinuria, haematuria (McKenna & Mirkov, 2014)

Nursing implications

- Medication may be associated with an increased risk of suicide.
- Medication is highly teratogenic (destructive to fetal growth). Girls should have a pregnancy test before treatment and before prescription renewal to be certain they are not pregnant. Suggest girls use a form of birth control to prevent pregnancy while on the medication and for 1 month afterwards.
- Serum levels of both triglycerides and cholesterol and liver function studies should be obtained, both baseline and monitoring, because both triglycerides and cholesterol serum are raised by the medication.
- Medication is extremely drying to skin; caution adolescents to discontinue all other acne medications during therapy to reduce this effect.
- Advise adolescents to avoid sunlight or use a sunblock. If eyes become too dry, patient may need to discontinue the use of contact lenses.
- Recommend adolescents take medication with meals, to avoid gastric irritation.
- Adolescents with severe headache or visual disturbances should report these symptoms and the medication should be discontinued.
- Advise adolescents not to donate blood while taking the medication, because of potential damage to the fetus of a recipient.

Other treatment methods

If inflammatory reactions from acne are extreme, a corticosteroid such as prednisone or a non-steroidal anti-inflammatory drug (NSAID) may be prescribed. Steroids must be used with caution in growing adolescents because they can lead to stunted growth. Cortisone may be injected directly into cystic lesions to reduce inflammation. This type of injection may reduce keloid formation, which is why it is usually reserved for adolescents who are prone to this permanent form of scarring.

Oestrogen, alone or in combination with progesterone, suppresses sebaceous gland activity and is therefore a useful therapy in some girls. However, isotretinoin is more often prescribed instead of oestrogen for two reasons: (a) high oestrogen levels tend to close epiphyseal centres of long bones, causing bone growth to stop; and (b) long-term therapy has potential side effects, including embolism and thrombophlebitis and possibly breast and uterine cancer.

Some degree of scarring may result from acne lesions. Laser therapy is a follow-up possibility to reduce scarring.

Obesity

Most overweight adolescents have obese parents, suggesting that both inheritance and environment play a part in the development of adolescent obesity. It can be difficult for adolescents to learn to like themselves (achieve a sense of identity) if they do not like their reflection in a mirror. It is equally difficult if they are always excluded from groups because of their weight. This has led to the suicide rate for obese adolescents being higher than for non-obese adolescents (Zhang et al., 2013). Some adolescents may be unaware their food intake is excessive because they have been told they need excess nutrients for healthy adolescent growth and everyone in their family eats large portions. They may state that their friends are overweight but their own weight seems all right, even though they are considerably overweight. Health education needs to begin with a discussion of "normal" weight. If they do not begin this as adolescents, they will become obese adults.

A reducing diet of fewer than 5800 to 6700 kilojoules per day can rarely be tolerated by adolescents. Such a diet would not provide sufficient protein and could be deficient in vitamins. If adolescents eat a diet that is too low in protein for any length of time, they can develop a faulty nitrogen balance, which can lead to seriously impaired growth. They generally can adhere to a diet closer to 7500 kilojoules per day. In addition to reducing kilojoules consumed, encourage activities that expend kilojoules, such as swimming or participation in gym classes and other school activities (Loprinzi et al., 2012).

Adolescents who use overeating as their main reaction to stress may require psychological counselling rather than diet counselling if they are to develop a more mature emotional response. Behaviour modification is sometimes successful with adolescents as a means of helping them lose weight, but it is rarely recommended for obesity alone. If the obesity is causing serious body image problems, lowered self-esteem and depression, behaviour modification might be suggested (see Chapter 35). General measures to help adolescents reduce overeating include:

- Making a detailed log of the amount they eat, the time and the circumstances (including how they felt while they were eating) and then changing those circumstances
- Always eating in one place (the kitchen table) instead of while walking home from school or watching television
- Slowing the process of eating by counting mouthfuls, putting the fork down beside the plate between bites and being served food on smaller plates so helpings look larger.

These measures may be of little use, however, unless they are combined with a suitable diet and adequate exercise. Despite all these interventions, weight reduction may not always be effective with adolescents. For some, a more realistic goal might be to prevent additional weight gain until they reach adulthood.

Changes in eating habits and patterns

Young people may feel that being with friends is more important than having a meal with their family at home. This can be annoying for parents if they have already prepared a meal and their child heads out instead. Young people need to consider and respect others in the household. It can help to have rules in place, such as giving at least an hour's notice if they won't be dining at home.

Some young people may skip meals to lose weight. However, skipping meals does not help weight control: the key to maintaining a healthy weight is regular exercise and a healthy, balanced diet. For signs of problems with eating and food with young people, see Box 33.3.

BOX 33.3 * Signs of problems with eating and food

Emotional and social changes

- Not being as happy as usual
- Not wanting to mix with friends or family
- Being moody
- Being less confident
- Not wanting to do anything
- Doing poorly at school
- Excessive sleeping
- Being angry

Other changes

- Restricting the amount or types of food eaten
- Counting kilojoules or the fat content of food
- Devising rules about how to eat, e.g. eating food in a certain order or no food after 6 p.m.
- Playing with, rather than eating food
- Always saying they have just eaten or will eat later or will grab something when they are out
- Dieting
- Binge eating (eating very large amounts of food)
- Avoiding eating in public
- Frequently checking weight or looking in the mirror
- Comparing self to others
- Asking if they look fat
- Saying that they are fat even when weight is normal or low
- Exercising to extreme, even if injured or sick
- Vomiting after meals
- Using laxatives

What parents can do

- Build a strong relationship with your child to encourage open discussion.
- Know what triggers stress for them and talk about it. Let your child know you support the right to their own choices but you still have some "house rules" about meal times and healthy eating.
- Build a positive attitude to food and healthy eating in your family. Encourage healthy eating as a normal and enjoyable part of life.
- Let your child decide what they eat and the amount they need.
- Don't label foods as "good" or "bad" or link guilt with eating.
- Provide a range of healthy foods (every day foods). Foods such as chips, biscuits, lollies or soft drinks (sometime foods) are for special occasions.

Anorexia nervosa

Anorexia nervosa is a serious and potentially life threatening mental illness. The reasons underpinning this disorder differ from person to person, however, known causes include genetic predisposition and a combination of environmental, social and cultural factors. Restricting food and weight can be a way of imposing control over areas of life that feel out of control. Body image can come to define their entire sense of self-worth. It can also be a way of expressing emotions that may feel too complex or frightening such as pain, stress or anxiety.

Restrictive dieting and excessive exercise can be contributing factors to the onset of anorexia nervosa. Women and girls may use dieting behaviour in a bid to achieve a culturally constructed thin ideal whereas men may over-exercise and control what they eat to achieve a muscular body. While it is generally accepted that anorexia nervosa is more common in females across the ages (only 10% of sufferers are males), recent research suggests that the incidence is rising among teenage males.

Bulimia nervosa

Bulimia nervosa is a serious mental illness that requires treatment. The disorder is characterised by repeated episodes of binge eating followed by compensatory behaviours. During these times the young person feels a loss of control and may not be able to stop. Young people with bulimia nervosa place great importance on their body, shape and weight. This leads to the young person having difficulties with self-esteem and confidence (National Eating Disorders Collaboration, 2014).

Sexuality and sexual activity

Changing societal norms have meant that adolescents may engage in high-risk sexual behaviours exposing them to sexually-transmitted infections or conception. Because of this, as part of routine health assessment of adolescents and pre-adolescents, it is important to determine if they are sexually active or are concerned about risky sexual behaviours (Taylor & Joshi, 2012).

Adolescents are usually interested in discussing sexuality concerns with a healthcare provider because they are concerned they are exposing themselves to sexually-transmitted diseases and to pregnancy. At the same time, it is a difficult topic for them to discuss. Some adolescents may feel trapped into engaging in sex, even though they are unwilling because they perceive it as a way of having friends. For adolescents who want to have intercourse, the primary reasons given are sexual curiosity (50% of boys; 24% of girls) and affection for their partner (25% of boys; 48% of girls). For adolescents who agree to have intercourse but do not really want to, the primary reasons given are peer pressure (about 30%), curiosity (50% of boys; 25% of girls) and affection for their partner (>33%) (Katsufrakis & Nusbaum, 2011). Sometimes adolescents use a relatively minor health condition as a reason to come to a healthcare facility, where they hope that someone will stumble onto their real concern about sexual activity. This is why it is important to ascertain whether adolescents are sexually active and determine if they are interested in learning more about contraception and safe sex practices.

Adolescence is also the time when teenagers deal with the realisation they are gay or lesbian. Although this orientation is something they have been aware of for years, actually accepting it is another step—and for many families, a difficult one (Bregman et al., 2013).

Stalking

Stalking refers to repetitive, intrusive and unwanted actions such as constant and threatening pursuit directed at an individual to gain the individual's attention or to evoke fear. Stalking may mainly take place as Internet correspondence (i.e. cyberstalking), such as sending unwanted e-mails or text messages (Briggs, Simon & Simonsen, 2011). In some instances, the stalker goes so far as to attack a victim and even murder the victim. Stalking behaviour begins as early as adolescence. Although the usual stalker is a male who stalks a female who has rejected him, both males and females can become stalkers or victims (McNamara & Marsil, 2012). It is difficult to prevent stalking because no one can evaluate when they begin a relationship that it will end so badly. To avoid stalking, adolescents should be aware of and avoid situations where they will be vulnerable to being alone with a stalker and to report stalking to the police or someone they trust who can help, so they can obtain a restraining order to prevent the stalker from coming near them again.

Bullying and hazing

Bullying that began during the school years (see Chapter 32) can easily continue into adolescence and actually become more serious, because this can be the time the bullied child has the ability to retaliate through self-destructive behaviour or school violence. Hazing, a form of organised bullying, refers to demeaning or humiliating rituals that prospective members have to undergo to join sororities, fraternities, adolescent gangs or sports teams (Allan & Madden, 2011). Most rituals are secret and in the past were accepted as "rites of passage". In recent years, hazing has become so extreme the practice has moved out of the "just fun" category into activities that can cause physical and psychological harm, such as being forced to wear demeaning clothing or engaging in crude or lewd skits. It can be extended to such an extreme that adolescents may be punched or kicked, sodomised or forced to drink alcohol until they vomit, pass out or even die from alcohol intoxication.

Substance abuse

Substance abuse refers to the use of chemicals to improve a mental state or induce euphoria. Based on responses to the National Drug Strategy Household Survey (NDSHS), 38% of the Australian population aged 14 years and over have used an illicit drug at least once (Australian Institute of Health and Welfare, 2013). Similarly, in New Zealand, the mean age for first time use of alcohol, tobacco and cannabis is around 14 years of age (Benjet et al., 2012). Drug use occurs in adolescence from a desire to expand consciousness or to feel more confident and mature; it also can be a response to peer pressure or a form of adolescent rebellion.

Types of abused substances

Drugs that adolescents abuse are those they can obtain on limited budgets and through limited contacts.

Prescription and over-the-counter drugs

Adolescents may begin drug experimentation by taking sedatives, pain medication or cough syrup containing dextromethorphan. A small amount of dextromethorphan causes light-headedness. In larger doses, it can result in distortions of colour and sound, visual hallucinations or "out-of-body" experiences. This is called "pharming"; unaware of usual dosages, adolescents who use drugs this way can easily overdose (Young, Glover, Havens, 2012). Methylphenidate (Ritalin) is a drug frequently prescribed for attention-deficit/hyperactivity disorder. When oral Ritalin tablets are crushed and injected intravenously, they induce a feeling of giddiness and extreme well-being. Unfortunately, because they do not completely dissolve, the resultant small particles remaining in the bloodstream can result in pulmonary embolus or emphysema.

Inhalants and household items

Common inhalants, such as a spray-type oil for cooking, or gas, butane or lighter fluid, can be abused by adolescents. Screening for abuse of inhalants or readiness to abuse such substances is important, as inhalant abuse can lead to cardiac failure (Hadlock et al., 2011). Mephedrone, commonly called "bath salts", is a stimulant that creates an "enjoyable high" and is available online, so is easily obtained by adolescents. Consequences of use include reckless driving and unconsciousness (Baumann, Partilla & Lehner, 2013).

Tobacco

Although it is well documented that cigarette smoking leads to significant health issues, research demonstrates the problematic prevalence of smoking in young people aged 12 to 17 years. Involvement with smoking becomes more common as adolescents progress through secondary school (Department of Health and Ageing, 2012). Adolescents usually begin smoking because the habit conveys a stamp of maturity; smoking may be viewed as especially desirable by those who are having difficulty demonstrating maturity in other areas. One of the strongest determinants of whether adolescents will begin smoking is whether their friends smoke. Although at one time proportionately more males than females smoked, adolescent girls are now the population most likely to begin smoking.

It is well documented that adolescents are influenced to begin smoking by advertising (Widome et al., 2013). Most school curriculums initiate programs as early as kindergarten which caution children against cigarette smoking and advertising. Unfortunately, the ultimate danger of illness or death in middle age is not a strong threat to young persons who are interested only in the present. More effective, therefore, might be campaigns that point out that cigarette smoking causes foul-smelling hair, clothes and breath and this detracts from physical appearance. Helping adolescents find other methods to demonstrate their maturity, such as allowing them opportunities for increased decision making and emphasising that being able to *not* smoke is a sign of true maturity, may also be effective (Larzelere & Williams, 2012). Adolescents can be urged to quit cigarette smoking through enrolling in a formal cigarette withdrawal program. Nicotine gum and nicotine patches have both been successfully used with adolescents.

Alcohol

In Australia and New Zealand, experience with alcohol is high among secondary school students and use becomes more common with increasing age (Department of Health and Ageing, 2012). Alarmingly, 7 out of 10 (71.6%) secondary school students in New Zealand report having drunk alcohol, with almost half of current secondary school drinkers reporting consumption of five or more drinks in a casual drinking session (New Zealand Ministry of Health, 2010). Although its use is correlated with motor vehicle accidents and suicide in adolescents, alcohol has never carried the stigma of other drugs. Alcohol use cannot be taken lightly, however, because it is linked to diseases such as cirrhosis, cognitive impairment and destructive behaviours such as addiction and depression.

Environment has a definite role in the use of alcohol, but hereditary may play a part in whether an adolescent becomes addicted. Most adolescents will admit they use alcohol if asked two specific questions: (a) Do you think you have a drinking problem? and (b) When was your last drink? Adolescents who answer yes to the first and "within the last 24 hours" to the second are candidates for further assessment.

Marijuana

Marijuana is derived from the leaves and stems of the Indian hemp plant, *Cannabis sativa.* It is generally rolled into cigarettes and smoked, although it can be mixed with food or sniffed. Scraping the resin from the flowering leaves produces a much stronger substance called hashish. *Sinsemilla* is a seedless form that is even more potent.

Breakdown products of marijuana are not readily eliminated from the body but remain in the fatty cells of the brain. This residue results in synaptic gaps that can delay electrical brain waves and memory storage, especially for short-term memory. Physical and psychological effects of all forms of marijuana are euphoria and a sense of well-being, temporary impairment of coordination or motor activities, altered sensory perceptions, rapid mood swings, altered self-image, decreased attention span and loss of memory for recent events (up to 1 hour). Withdrawal symptoms include irritability, drowsiness and cravings for high-carbohydrate snacks. Long-term side effects can include disorders such as sinusitis, bronchitis, emphysema and perhaps lung cancer (these can develop after only 1 year of use compared with 20 years of use for cigarette smoking) and lack of sperm formation or testicular cancer in males (Fronczak, Kim & Barqawi, 2012).

Despite its known dangers, marijuana is a common illicit substance used by adolescents. It is important to educate adolescents that marijuana is more than an amusing leisure activity or a way to relieve stress so they can put its use into long-term perspective. Because it is used medically to relieve nausea and vomiting, adolescents may view it as harmless.

Amphetamines

The amphetamines are a group of drugs sometimes used in the treatment of hyperactivity and narcolepsy, among other central nervous system disorders. They are easily manufactured in "meth labs" in people's homes and so are readily available to adolescents. Amphetamines are called *uppers* or *speed* because they give the user a false sense of well-being, alertness or self-esteem (Auten et al., 2012). A newer, stronger form that produces intense symptoms is known as *ice*. Some of the side effects that can occur are aggressive or demanding behaviour, paranoia and extreme restlessness. Chronic methamphetamine abuse results in severe blackened, crumbling teeth. Because amphetamines suppress the appetite, adolescents may lose weight or eat only sporadically while taking them. Use without a prescription is illegal.

Cocaine

Cocaine is one of the most popular drugs of abuse for young adults and its use may begin in adolescence. The drug may be sniffed into the nose (snorted), smoked or injected intravenously. Occasionally it is combined with heroin and injected. A stronger form, called *crack,* is manufactured by heating cocaine powder with baking soda and water. This preparation process is dangerous in itself because it involves volatile solvents that can ignite or explode. The resulting drug, often called *freebase* or *rock,* is so strong it can cause immediate cardiac and respiratory arrhythmias (Paczynski & Gold, 2011).

Cocaine that is either inhaled or smoked is absorbed through the mucous membrane into the bloodstream. After absorption, blood levels rise rapidly for the first 20 minutes, peak at 60 minutes and then decline over the next 3 hours. Although a toxic dose of cocaine is usually considered to be 600 to 700 mg, toxicity has been reported with doses as low as 20 mg. Cocaine produces the physical effects of increased pulse and respiration rates, increased temperature, increased blood pressure and decreased appetite. Psychological effects produced are euphoria, excitement and restlessness, increased sociability and possible hallucinations.

Toxic symptoms include seizures, tachyarrhythmias, tachypnoea, hypertension, increased deep tendon reflexes, decreased response to stimuli, nausea and vomiting, abdominal pain, headaches and chills and fever. It is a major cause of cardiovascular arrest in young adults (Stoduto et al., 2012).

It is important to educate adolescents that although cocaine sniffing may be fascinating and offer temporary pleasure and relief from stress, it also causes psychological dependency and is potentially extremely dangerous because of its cardiac and respiratory effects. Chronic inhalation of cocaine can cause ulceration in the mucous membrane of the nose and injection of the substance exposes an adolescent to the risk of HIV/AIDS, hepatitis and other diseases contracted through contaminated equipment. Cocaine taken during pregnancy can cause separation of the placenta with potential fetal and maternal death (Mbah et al., 2012).

Hallucinogens

Examples of hallucinogenic drugs used by adolescents are lysergic acid diethylamide (LSD), dimethyltryptamine (DMT), 2,5-dimethoxy-4-methamphetamine (STP), phencyclidine hydrochloride (PCP), *Salvia divinorum*, mephedrone ("bath salts") and methaqualone (Quaalude). The use of LSD has substantially increased in popularity since the 1960s when it first became available because it can be manufactured in a "kitchen lab". Methylenedioxymethamphetamine (MDMA, also known as "ecstasy") was previously used by some psychotherapists to make patients more receptive to therapy. It is now illegal as chronic use destroys the serotonin system of the brain, causing progressive decline of immediate and delayed memory and alterations in mood (Hittner & Schachne, 2012).

All of these drugs cause bizarre mind reactions such as distortion in vision, smell or hearing. Adolescents report seeing colours more vividly than they have ever seen them before, hearing sounds so clear they cause physical pain or perceiving themselves as being totally impervious to harm leading to "good trips" or "bad trips". Recurrences or flashbacks of drug-induced experiences may, unfortunately, happen at unpredictable times and in unexpected places. Such flashbacks not only are disconcerting but also can be dangerous, especially if they occur while a person is driving a motor vehicle. They can be so frightening that some users believe they are becoming obsessed and experience high levels of paranoia and are dangerous to themselves and others.

Opiates

Opiates include drugs such as heroin, meperidine (Demerol) and morphine. At one time, these were not typically used by adolescents because they were expensive, but they are now gaining popularity among teens. Opiates can be extremely dangerous because of their tendency to decrease the respiratory rate. Addiction to them can cause such physiological cravings in adolescents, like adults, that they may steal, defraud and turn to prostitution to secure enough money to buy a day's supply. In addition to the direct danger of opiates, adolescents who use them risk the danger of contracting HIV/AIDS and hepatitis B if they share contaminated needles. "Snorting" heroin can lead to an acute cerebrovascular accident and death.

Methadone or levomethadyl acetate (LAAM) programs can be prescribed to help adolescents wean themselves from opiates (Eisendrath & Lichtmacher, 2013). Although methadone is a narcotic and its use may be associated with motor vehicle accidents, because adolescents do not have to pay for it, they no longer have to steal or prostitute themselves to obtain it. It allows them to stay in school or hold a job and become productive citizens (Bramness et al., 2012).

Assessment of substance abuse

If adolescents trust healthcare personnel, they will generally admit they have engaged in drug experimentation. Some common findings on health history that suggest an adolescent is abusing substance are:

- Demonstration of poor reasoning ability
- Decreased school attendance
- Frequent mood swings
- Deteriorating physical appearance
- Recent change in peer group
- Expressed negative perceptions of parents.

These are not necessarily diagnostic findings, however, because they can also be part of an adolescent's search for identity. Substance abuse can be strongly suspected in an adolescent who is hospitalised for hepatitis B or who is HIV positive, as well as one who appears overly anxious to leave a healthcare facility or who receives no benefit from usual analgesic agents. General physical symptoms that indicate drug abuse are summarised in Table 33.1.

Depression and attempted suicide

Suicide is deliberate self-injury with the intent to end one's life. In Australia and New Zealand suicide is a leading cause of death among young people, second only to motor vehicle accidents. Suicide rates among 15–24-year-old males trebled between 2011 and 2013 and in rural and regional areas of Australia, suicide rates for young males are nearly twice those of males living in capital cities. Suicide is rare in childhood but becomes more common during adolescence. Successful suicide occurs more frequently in males than in females, although more females apparently attempt suicide than males. Studies have found that between 23.5% and 49% of teenagers have thoughts of suicide at some time (Harrison, Moller & Bordeaux, 2011).

Incest, abuse, increased chemical dependency, marital instability in the family and poor problem-solving ability are reasons that may lead an adolescent to decide that death may be easier than coping with overwhelming problems. A wish to "get even" over some hurt or drug and alcohol use may contribute to suicide by further impairing judgement (Eaton et al., 2012).

Some degree of depression is present in most adolescents, because they are not only losing their parents at this time as they grow apart from them, but they are also losing their carefree childhood (Fried et al., 2013). If school failure or loss of a friend or losing a competition is superimposed on an existing depression, the pressure may be great enough to cause some adolescents to attempt suicide. Some other reasons for attempting suicide include anger with others and manipulation (psychological blackmail) as a way of having one's needs met. Loss of a parent, loss of a girlfriend or boyfriend, loss of a community and loss of self-esteem are all significant and can trigger a suicide. Because some adolescents may be unable to believe that a parent was at fault in the case of divorce or that the death of a parent could not have been prevented, they may believe, instead, they somehow caused the parent to leave or to die. The loss of a girlfriend or boyfriend is particularly significant because it involves two types of loss: friendship and self-esteem. Rejection from a peer group, sports team or school club may cause a similar loss of self-esteem.

Assessment

Adolescents need to have thorough physical examinations at health assessment visits to assure them they are in good physical health. Assess for signs of depression such as eating disorders, insomnia, excessive fatigue or weight loss. In younger adolescents, depression may be manifested by behavioural problems such as disobedience, temper tantrums, truancy and running away from home. Self-destructive behaviour or accident proneness may be noted. Difficulties at school; acting out with chemicals, alcohol or sexual promiscuity; or trouble with legal authorities may be further clues. Occasionally, depressed adolescents find it so hard to be alone they seek constant activity as a means of escape. In contrast, others may withdraw from contact with other persons and become completely isolated. Either behaviour can be detected through assessment of activity and interaction levels.

Adolescents who attempt suicide fall into no one category, although many tend to be loners or to have difficulty expressing their feelings to others and, therefore, do not

TABLE 33.1 Symptoms to help identify drug abusers

Drugs used	Symptoms of use	Dangers
Glue	Violence, drunken appearance, dreamy or blank expression Glue smears on clothing or fingers; tubes of glue, paper bags in possession	Lung, brain or liver damage; death through suffocation or choking; anaemia
Heroin, morphine, codeine	Stupor, drowsiness, needle marks on body, watery eyes, loss of appetite, bloodstains on shirt sleeve, runny nose Needle or hypodermic syringe, cotton, tourniquet string, burnt bottle caps or spoons, glassine envelopes in possession	Death from overdose; addiction; liver and other infections due to unsterile needles
Cough medicine containing codeine and opium	Drunken appearance, lack of coordination, confusion, excessive itching Empty bottle of cough medicine in possession	Addiction
Marijuana	Sleepiness, wandering mind, enlarged pupils, lack of coordination Strong odour of burnt leaves, small seeds in pocket lining, cigarette paper, discoloured fingers	Psychological dependence; possibly testicular cancer
Hallucinogens (LSD, DMT, PCP)	Severe hallucinations, feelings of detachment, incoherent speech, cold hands and feet, laughing and crying, vomiting Possession of cube sugar with discolouration in centre, strong body odour	Suicidal tendencies, unpredictable behaviour; chronic exposure may have neurological effects
Stimulants (methamphetamine, cocaine)	Aggressive behaviour, giggling, silliness, rapid speech, confused thinking, no appetite, extreme fatigue, black cavities, dry mouth, shakiness, insomnia. Pills or capsules of varying colours in possession; absence of nasal hair; possession of a glass pipe	Death from overdose; hallucinations; psychosis
Depressants (barbiturates, alcohol)	Drowsiness, stupor, dullness, slurred speech, drunken appearance, vomiting Pills or capsules of varying colours in possession; odour of alcohol on breath	Death or unconsciousness from overdose; addiction; seizures from withdrawal
Steroids	Aggressive behaviour; increase in muscle strength and mass	Violent actions; possibly tumour growth

receive emotional support from friends. Others are very good students. The stress of trying to achieve continually at this level, however, is the trigger that provokes suicide. Gay and lesbian youths appear to have higher levels of suicide than others, reflecting the level of stress they may be experiencing (Shields et al., 2012).

Because suicide usually reflects a problem in family interaction, family assessment is helpful. A thorough family history may reveal conflict with one or both parents. School friends may often be aware before the parents that an adolescent is contemplating suicide. Close to the chosen time of suicide, some adolescents may demonstrate characteristic behaviours that show they are making preparations to end their life (see Box 33.4). Crisis intervention for adolescents who are contemplating suicide includes trying to alleviate their pain and depression and counselling them in an effort to help them change their perspective on the value of life (Suicide Prevention Australia, 2011; New Zealand Ministry of Health, 2015).

For an adolescent's safety, a period of observation in a hospital setting is desirable after a suicide attempt to prevent the adolescent from inflicting personal injury again and to allow assessment in a neutral setting, away from the stress that precipitated the attempt. This can take place in an adolescent mental health service rather than a general mental health facility. For example, in Victoria, Orygen Youth Health (OYHCP) is a youth-focused mental health organisation that provides mental health assessment and treatment to 15-to-24-year-olds who live in the Western and North Western areas of Melbourne (Orygen Youth Health Clinical Program, n.d.).

Antidepressant medicine alone, a therapy used with depressed adults, may be of little value in treating depressed adolescents. Tricyclic antidepressants generally are ineffective and may cause serious adverse effects. Evidence of the effectiveness of selective serotonin reuptake inhibitors is limited. Fluoxetine is an example of a drug approved for the treatment of depression in children 8 to 17 years of age. All antidepressants have a warning

BOX 33.4 * Focus on family teaching

Suicide warning signs

Q. James' father says to you, "Our neighbour's son recently committed suicide. What are warning signs of this to look for in our son?"

A. The following are commonly seen clues:

- Giving away prized possessions
- Organ donation questions, such as, "How do you leave your body to a medical school?"
- Sudden, unexplained elevation of mood. Mood elevation may indicate that the individual has reached a decision about suicide and feels relief
- Accident proneness, carelessness and death wishes
- A statement such as, "This is the last time you will see me"
- Decrease in verbal communication
- Withdrawal from peer activities or previously enjoyed events
- Previous attempt (80% of all completed suicides have been preceded by a failed attempt)
- Preference for art, music and literature with themes of death
- Recent increase in interpersonal conflict with significant others
- Running away from home
- Recent experience of a friend or famous person committing suicide
- Inquiring about the hereafter
- Asking for information (supposedly for a friend) about suicide prevention and intervention
- Almost any sustained deviation from the normal pattern of behaviour.

because some have been associated with elevating the mood of depressed children enough to allow them to formulate a plan and commit suicide after taking them (Shields et al., 2012). Continuing evaluation by both history taking and physical examination is necessary, because the young person who has attempted suicide may attempt it again if support people and better problem-solving ability are not available in the future.

Runaways

A runaway is commonly defined as a child between the ages of 10 and 17 years who has been absent from home at least overnight without the permission of a parent or guardian. The frequency of running away for adolescents may be as high as 1 in 8. Fortunately, most do not go far or stay away long (less than 1 week) (Moskowitz, Stein & Lightfoot, 2013); however, about 1 in 20 adolescent runaways stay away as long as 1 year and some never return home. Runaway adolescents are most likely to be from low- or high-income families. Unemployment, alcoholism, sexual abuse, attempted suicide and poverty are frequent characteristics. They are slightly more likely to be male than female. Events they encounter may be so traumatic they develop a post-traumatic syndrome (Moskowitz, Stein & Lightfoot, 2013).

In 2013–2014, 10,000 young people accessed specialist homelessness services in NSW alone. This was an increase of 4 per cent compared to 2012–2013. The data collected has indicated that more young people under 16 have sought homelessness services due to domestic violence. The nurse needs to be aware of these statistics and aware of trauma and issues faced by young people and provide appropriate support and education if confronted with young people in these situations.

Assessment

Running away is usually preceded by an argument with parents that is often the last straw after a number of long-term disagreements. Other reasons may be personal concerns such as loneliness, pregnancy and problems with friends, school or the police. Incest can also be a precipitating cause, as can other forms of parental abuse. A school history often reveals frequent truancy, failing grades, possible drug use and runaway behaviour by friends.

Common health reasons for which runaway adolescents are seen at healthcare facilities are sexually-transmitted infections, including HIV/AIDS, rape, pregnancy, substance abuse, hepatitis and vaginitis. They also have a high incidence of suicide attempts (Palepu et al., 2012). When caring for adolescents with these concerns, it is important to secure a thorough history so the fact they are no longer living at home will not be missed. Ask if the adolescent wants to return home. Even though being homeless is highly stressful and many adolescent runaways want to take the first step back towards their parents, they may not know how to begin the process.

Unique concerns of the family with a physically challenged or chronically ill adolescent

Achieving a sense of identity may be difficult for adolescents who have a chronic illness or other challenge. It is vital, however, for such individuals to learn to look past their particular condition to their real selves. For example, a 16-year-old girl in a wheelchair must learn to perceive herself as a teenager who is normal intellectually, is a good conversationalist, has a good sense of humour, enjoys watching football and only incidentally uses a wheelchair to move about.

Some of the biggest problems of chronically ill adolescents are likely to be difficulties in being as independent as they would like to be, achieving in school and establishing intimate relationships. Those who cannot learn to drive when their friends are learning to do so, who are not invited to dances and parties because of a disability or

TABLE 33.2 Nursing actions that encourage a sense of identity in the physically challenged or chronically Ill adolescent

Category	Actions
Nutrition	If adolescent is on special diet, discuss role of food preferences with dietitian (meat pies, pizza, etc.). Respect food preferences.
Dressing change	Allow adolescent to order supplies. Ask for suggestions as to final appearance of dressing. If soaks are included, have adolescent time the treatment. Allow adolescent to choose time for dressing change.
Medicine	Offering the adolescent a choice of site for injection or intravenous insertion encourages a sense of control. Teach name, action and possible side effects of medicine.
Rest	Contract with adolescent for time and length of rest periods.
Hygiene	Respect modesty of the adolescent as being at adult level. Contract with adolescent for extent of self-care (will give own bath and make bed, not medicate self).
Pain	Encourage adolescent to express pain; teach distraction technique for sharp pain, such as deep breathing, counting backwards from 100. Encourage adolescent to ask for analgesics as needed.
Stimulation	Provide favourite music with headphones. Provide a radio for adolescent to listen to talk show to foster active involvement. Encourage school work and crossword puzzles (you may need to help adolescents divide school assignments into smaller tasks so they do not become overly fatigued and frustrated). Provide cards for games to increase socialisation (make or have the adolescent make a card deck from pieces of paper if one is not available). Encourage adolescents to network with one another. Encourage adolescents to keep in contact with friends by telephone, email or messaging.

who are too hesitant to ask someone to go with them, may feel acute loss of self-esteem. Moreover, the loss of many hours of school because of illness or frequent hospitalisation may result in the inability to pursue a desired career, at least without a delay. Adolescence may be the first time these children realise that certain occupations or opportunities, such as a military career, may be closed to them. As they prepare to leave the security of a familiar school system, it may be the first time they examine just how they will be able to function on their own. Some may come to realise they will never be able to do so with complete independence.

Chronic hospitalisation or the realisation they will never be free of symptoms can cause depression in adolescents, placing them at high risk of substance abuse or suicide. Helping these adolescents realise that even completely well people must compromise life decisions for other reasons, such as lack of money, lack of ability or qualifications or extra personal responsibilities can help them feel they are not so different from others. This type of guidance can be time-consuming but sometimes the fact that an adult is willing to make this time commitment is enough to give these adolescents the self-esteem they need to alter aspirations and plans and find a future role consistent with their capabilities (see Table 33.2).

Nutrition and the chronically ill adolescent

Adolescents who are not fully mobile must be aware of their total kilojoule intake or, as growth needs decline at the end of adolescence, they can become obese. They should also be knowledgeable about good nutrition, so they can participate in meal planning, an action that helps them feel a sense of control over this area of their life. Assess how often they have a chance to eat at fast-food restaurants; although this is not a source of excellent nutrition, eating there occasionally provides an important social experience and a chance to be like their peers.

Key points for review

- The major milestones of development in the adolescent period are the onset of puberty and the cessation of body growth. Between these milestones, physical growth is rapid, although the development of adult coordination and thought processes is slow.
- The development of secondary sex characteristics is completed during adolescence. These are rated according to Tanner stages.
- The developmental task of an adolescent according to Erikson is to establish independence from parents by gaining a sense of identity versus role confusion. Adolescents therefore usually respond best to health-care personnel who respect their attempts at independence and allow them as many choices as possible in care.
- Adolescents reach a point of cognitive development termed *formal operational thought*. With this, they are able to think in abstract terms and use the scientific method to arrive at conclusions.

- Adolescents need to consume adequate kilojoules and especially protein, iron, calcium and zinc to meet their increased growth needs.
- Being an adolescent is difficult in today's world. Be aware that to reduce stress some adolescents begin to use substances of abuse. Asking about an adolescent's drug experiences, if any, during a health assessment is not intruding on privacy; it is conducting safe health interviewing.
- Promoting adolescent safety is an important nursing role. Motor vehicle accidents and suicide are leading causes of death in this age group.
- Common health problems in an adolescent are sometimes minor and include poor posture, fatigue or acne, body piercing and tattoos, menstrual irregularities; they can also be serious, such as obesity, substance abuse and scoliosis. Identifying these problems and referring an adolescent for help are important nursing actions.

CASE STUDY QUESTIONS

4. James' parents tell you that James was depressed after the loss of a girlfriend but now is suddenly happy. He has been collecting rare model cars since he was 8 years old. Recently, he gave his collection away to a neighbourhood boy because "I won't need them where I'm going". Why might you be concerned about James? What additional questions might you ask him? If you learned he is about to leave to be an exchange student in England, how would this affect your assessment of the situation?
5. Suppose James tells you he does not smoke, but you smell cigarette smoke on his clothing. Although he says he does not use drugs, a number of blue-and-white capsules fall out of his shirt pocket when he unbuttons his shirt. What questions would you ask to determine if he is smoking cigarettes or using drugs? Describe your next action if he does admit he is not only heavily into drugs but does not intend to stop using them.

Resources

For an extensive range of additional resources to enhance teaching and learning and to facilitate understanding of this chapter, please see the text's accompanying website located on thePoint at http://thepoint.lww.com.

References

Ahern, N. R. & Norris, A. E. (2011). Examining factors that increase and decrease stress in adolescent community college students. *Journal of Pediatric Nursing*, *28*(6), 530–540.

Allan, E. J. & Madden, M. (2011). The nature and extent of college student hazing. *International Journal of Adolescent Medicine & Health*, *24*(1), 83–90.

Armfield, J. M. (2010). Community effectiveness of public water fluoridation in reducing children's dental disease. *Public Health Reports*, *125*(5), 655–664.

Australian Government Department of the Prime Minister and Cabinet. (2015). Closing the gap – the Prime Minister's report 2015, accessed 8 April 2015, <www.dpmc.gov.au/pmc-indigenous-affairs/publication/closing-gap-prime-ministers-report-2015>.

Australian Institute of Health and Welfare. (2013). *Statistics on Drug Use in Australia*. Drug Statistics Series No. 18. Cat. No. PHE 80. Canberra: AIHW.

Australian Institute of Health and Welfare (2014). *Specialist Homelessness Services 2013–14*. Cat. no. HOU 276. Canberra: AIHW.

Auten, J. D., Matteucci, M. J., Gaspary, M. J., et al. (2012). Psychiatric implications of adolescent methamphetamine exposures. *Pediatric Emergency Care*, *28*(1), 26–29.

Bagnulo, J. D. (2012). Carbohydrate. In Kohlstadt, I. (Ed), *Scientific Evidence for Musculoskeletal, Bariatric & Sports Nutrition*. Boca Raton, FL: Taylor & Francis.

Baumann, M. H., Partilla, J. S. & Lehner, K. R. (2013). Psychoactive "bath salts": Not so soothing. *European Journal of Pharmacology*, *698*(1–3), 1–5.

Benjet, C., Borges, G., Medina-Mora, M. E., et al. (2012). Chronic childhood adversity and stages of substance use involvement in adolescents. *Drug & Alcohol Dependence*. Advance online publication.

Blake, K. & Davis, V. (2011). Adolescent medicine. In K. J. Marcdante, R. M. Kliegman, H. B. Jenson, et al. (Eds), *Nelson Essentials of Paediatrics* (6th ed.). Philadelphia: Saunders/Elsevier.

Bramness, J. G., Skurtveit, S., Mørland, J., et al. (2012). An increased risk of motor vehicle accidents after prescription of methadone. *Addiction*, *107*(5), 967–972.

Bregman, H. R., Malik, N. M., Page, M. J., Makynen, E. & Lindahl, K. M. (2013). Identity profiles in lesbian, gay, and bisexual youth: The role of family influences. *Journal of Youth & Adolescence*, *42*(3), 417–430.

Briggs, P., Simon, W. T. & Simonsen, S. (2011). An exploratory study of Internet-initiated sexual offenses and the chat room sex offender: Has the Internet enabled a new typology of sex offender? *Sexual Abuse*, *23*(1), 72–91.

Bureau of Infrastructure, Transport and Regional Economics (BITRE) (2014). *Road Deaths Australia 2013: Statistical Summary*. Canberra: Department of Infrastructure and Regional Development.

Carr-Gregg, M. (2014). *Strictly Parenting. Everything You Need to Know about Raising School-age Kids*. Penguin: Australia.

Chouinard, L. E., Randall Simpson, J. & Buchholz, A. C. (2012). Predictors of bone mineral density in a convenience sample of young Caucasian adults living in southern Ontario. *Applied Physiology, Nutrition & Metabolism*, *37*(4), 706–714.

Cohen, L., Brown, J., Haukness, H., et al. (2013). Sun protection counselling by pediatricians has little effect on parent and child sun protection behavior. *Journal of Pediatrics*, *162*(2), 381–386.

Department of Health and Ageing (2012). *Australian Secondary School Students' Use of Tobacco, Alcohol and Over the Counter and Illicit Substances in 2011*. Drug Strategy Branch Report, prepared by White, V. & Bariola, E. Canberra: Department of Health and Ageing.

Eaton, D. K., Kann, L., Kinchen, S., Shanklin, S., Flint, K. H., Hawkins, J., Harris, W. A., Lowry, R., McManus, T., Chyen, D., Whittle, L., Lim, C. & Wechsler, H. (2012). Youth risk behavior surveillance—United States, 2011. *Surveillance Summaries*, *61*(SS04), 1–162.

Eisendrath, S. J. & Lichtmacher, J. E. (2013). Substance use disorders. In M. Papadakis & S. J. McPhee (Eds), *Current Medical Diagnosis & Treatment*, 2013 (52nd ed.). New York: McGraw-Hill/Lange.

Erikson, E. H. (1993). *Childhood and Society*. New York: W. W. Norton.

Fernández-Gaxiola, A. C. & De-Regil, L. M. (2011). Intermittent iron supplementation for reducing anaemia and its associated impairments in menstruating women. *Cochrane Database of Systematic Reviews*, *12*, (CD009218).

Fried, L. E., Williams, S., Cabral, H. & Hacker, K. (2013). Differences in risk factors for suicide attempts among 9th and 11th grade youth: A longitudinal perspective. *Journal of School Nursing*, *29*(2), 113–122.

Fronczak, C. M., Kim, E. D. & Barqawi, A. B. (2012). The insults of illicit drug use on male fertility. *Journal of Andrology*, *33*(4), 515–528.

Frost, L. A. & Burns, C. E. (2013). Sleep and rest. In Burns, C. E., Dunn, A. M., Brady, M. A., Barber Starr, N. & Blosser, C. G. (Eds), *Pediatric Primary Care* (5th ed.). Philadelphia: Elsevier/Saunders.

Garzon, D. L. & Dunn, A. M. (2013). Developmental management of adolescents. In Burns, C. E., Dunn, A. M., Brady, M. A., Barber Starr, N. & Blosser, C. G. (Eds), *Pediatric Primary Care* (5th ed.). Philadelphia: Elsevier/Saunders.

Gilligan, C. (1982). *In a Different Voice: Psychological Theory and Women's Development*. Cambridge, MA: Harvard University Press.

Hadlock, G. C., Webb, K. M., McFadden, L. M., et al. (2011). 4-Methylmethcathinone (mephedrone): Neuropharmacological effects of a designer stimulant of abuse. *Journal of Pharmacology & Experimental Therapeutics, 339*(2), 530–536.

Harrison, J., Moller, J. & Bordeaux, S. (2011). Youth suicide and self-injury Australia [Supplement to Issue 15]. Accessed 1 March 2015 <http://nisu.flinders.edu.au/pubs/bulletin15/bulletin15sup.html>.

Health Direct Australia. (2014). Teenage pregnancy. Accessed 1 March 2015, <www.cyh.com/HealthTopics/HealthTopicDetails.aspx?p=114&np=122&id=1617>.

Hittner, J. B. & Schachne, E. R. (2012). Meta-analysis of the association between ecstasy use and risky sexual behavior. *Addictive Behavior, 37*(7), 790–796.

Hoang, Q. B., Coel, R. A., Vidal, A., Wilson, P. E. & Pengel, B. (2012). Sports medicine. In Hay, W., Levin, M., Deterding, R., Azbug, M. J. & Sondheimer, J. M. (Eds), *Current Diagnosis & Treatment Pediatrics* (21st ed.). New York: McGraw-Hill/Lange.

Katsufrakis, P. J. & Nusbaum, M.R.H. (2011). Adolescent sexuality. In South-James, J. E., Matheny, S. C. & Lewis, E. L. (Eds), *Current Diagnosis & Treatment in Family Medicine* (3rd ed.). Columbus, OH: McGraw-Hill/Lange.

Kistner, F., Fiebert, I. & Roach, K. (2012). Effect of backpack load carriage on cervical posture in primary schoolchildren. *Work, 41*(1), 99–108.

Kiwi Families, (2011). Teen parent overview. Accessed 1 March 2015, <www.kiwifamilies.co.nz/Topics/Parenting/Teen-Parents-Corner/Teenage+Parent+Overview.html>.

Kohlberg, L. (1984). *The Psychology of Moral Development*. New York: Harper & Row.

Larzelere, M. M. & Williams, D. E. (2012). Promoting smoking cessation. *American Family Physician, 85*(6), 591–598.

Ledger, W. L. (2012). The menstrual cycle. In Edmonds, D. K. (Ed), *Dewhurst's Textbook of Obstetrics & Gynaecology* (8th ed.). Oxford: John Wiley & Son.

Lloyd, S., Chalder, T. & Rimes, K. A. (2012). Family-focused cognitive behaviour therapy versus psycho-education for adolescents with chronic fatigue syndrome: Long-term follow-up of an RCT. *Behavior Research & Therapy, 50*(11), 719–725.

Loprinzi, P. D., Cardinal, B. J., Loprinzi, K. L. & Lee, H. (2012). Benefits and environmental determinants of physical activity in children and adolescents. *Obesity Facts, 5*(4), 597–610.

Marciani, R. D. (2012). Complications of third molar surgery and their management. *Atlas of the Oral & Maxillofacial Surgery Clinics of North America, 20*(2), 233–251.

Marván, M. L. & Molina-Abolnik, M. (2012). Mexican adolescents' experience of menarche and attitudes toward menstruation. *Journal of Pediatric & Adolescent Gynecology, 25*(6), 358–363.

Mbah, A. K., Alio, A. P., Fombo, D. W., Bruder, K., Dagne, G. & Salihu, H. M. (2012). Association between cocaine abuse in pregnancy and placenta-associated syndromes using propensity score matching approach. *Early Human Development, 88*(6), 333–337.

McClung, J. P. (2012). Iron status and the female athlete. *Journal of Trace Elements in Medicine & Biology, 26*(2–3), 124–126.

McKenna, L. & Mirkov, S. (Eds). (2014). *McKenna's Drug Handbook for Nursing and Midwifery* (7th ed.). Sydney: Lippincott Williams & Wilkins.

McNamara, C. L. & Marsil, D. F. (2012). The prevalence of stalking among college students: The disparity between researcher and self-identified victimization. *Journal of American College Health, 60*(2), 168–174.

Morelli, J. G. & Prok, L. D. (2012). Acne. In Hay, W., Levin, M., Deterding, R., Azbug, M. J. & Sondheimer, J. M. (Eds), *Current Diagnosis & Treatment Pediatrics* (21st ed.). New York: McGraw-Hill/Lange.

Moskowitz, A., Stein, J. A. & Lightfoot, M. (2013). The mediating roles of stress and maladaptive behaviors on self-harm and suicide attempts among runaway and homeless youth. *Journal of Youth & Adolescence, 42*(7), 1015–1027.

National Eating Disorders Collaboration (NEDC) (2014). *Bulimia Nervosa – fact sheet*. Accessed 1 March 2015, <www.nedc.com.au/files/Resources/Bulimia%20Nervosa%20Fact%20Sheet.pdf>.

New Zealand Ministry of Health (NZMOH). (2010). Alcohol quick facts. Accessed 1 March 2015, <www.health.govt.nz/system/files/documents/publications/alcohol-factsheets.pdf>.

New Zealand Ministry of Health. (2015). Suicide prevention in New Zealand. Accessed 1 March 2015, <www.health.govt.nz/our-work/mental-health-and-addictions/working-prevent-suicide>.

Orygen Youth Health Clinical Program (OYHCP). Accessed 1 March 2015, <http://oyh.org.au/>.

Paczynski, R. P. & Gold, M. S. (2011). Cocaine and crack. In Ruiz, P. & Strain, E. (Eds), *Lowinson and Ruiz's Substance Abuse: A Comprehensive Textbook* (5th ed.). Philadelphia: Wolters Kluwer/Lippincott Williams & Wilkins.

Palepu, A., Hubley, A. M., Russell, L. B., Gadermann, A. M. & Chinni, M. (2012). Quality of life themes in Canadian adults and street youth who are homeless or hard-to-house: A multi-site focus group study. *Health & Quality of Life Outcomes, 10*(8), 93.

Piaget, J. (1969). *The Theory of Stages in Cognitive Development*. New York: McGraw-Hill.

Sass, A. E. & Kaplan, D. W. (2013). Adolescence. In Hay, W., Levin, M., Deterding, R., Azbug, M. J. & Sondheimer, J. M. (Eds), *Current Diagnosis & Treatment Pediatrics* (21st ed.). New York: McGraw-Hill/Lange.

Shields, J. P., Whitaker, K., Glassman, J., Franks, H. M. & Howard, K. (2012). Impact of victimization on risk of suicide among lesbian, gay, and bisexual high school students in San Francisco. *Journal of Adolescent Health, 50*(4), 418–420.

Short, M. A., Gradisar, M., Lack, L. C., Wright, H. R., Dewald, J. F., Wolfson, A. R. & Carskadon, M. A. (2012). A cross-cultural comparison of sleep duration between U.S. and Australian adolescents: The effect of school start time, parent-set bedtimes, and extracurricular load. *Health Education & Behavior, 40*(3), 323–330.

Simonart, T. (2012). Newer approaches to the treatment of acne vulgaris. *American Journal of Clinical Dermatology, 13*(6), 357–364.

State Government of Victoria. (2015). Sex education: Talking to young people. Accessed 1 March 2015, <www.betterhealth.vic.gov.au/bhcv2/bhcarticles.nsf/pages/Sex_education_talking_to_teenagers?open>.

Stein, T. & Jordan, J. D. (2012). Health considerations for oral piercing and the policies that influence them. *Texas Dental Journal, 129*(7), 687–693.

Stoduto, G., Mann, R. E., Ialomiteanu, A., Wickens, C. M. & Brands, B. (2012). Examining the link between collision involvement and cocaine use. *Drug & Alcohol Dependence, 123*(1–3), 260–263.

Suicide Prevention Australia. (2011). Youth suicide prevention position statement. Accessed 1 March 2015, <http://suicidepreventionaust.org/?statement=youth-suicide-prevention-in-australia>.

Swahn, M. H., Ali, B., Bossarte, R. M., et al. (2012). Self-harm and suicide attempts among high-risk, urban youth in the U.S.: Shared and unique risk and protective factors. *International Journal of Environmental Research & Public Health, 9*(1), 178–191.

Tanner, J. M. (1962). *Growth at Adolescence* (2nd ed.). Oxford, UK: Blackwell.

Taylor, M. & Joshi, A. (2012). Surveys assessing STI related health information needs of adolescent population. *Technology & Health Care, 20*(4), 247–261.

Timko, C. A., Hormes, J. M. & Chubski, J. (2012). Will the real vegetarian please stand up? An investigation of dietary restraint and eating disorder symptoms in vegetarians versus non-vegetarians. *Appetite, 58*(3), 982–990.

Vassallo, S., Lahausse, J. & Edwards, B. (2013). *Stability and Change in Risky Driving from the Late Teens to the Late Twenties* (Research Paper No. 51). Melbourne: Australian Institute of Family Studies.

Wengle, J. G., Hamilton, J. K., Manlhiot, C., et al., (2012). The 'Golden Keys' to health—A healthy lifestyle intervention with randomized individual mentorship for overweight and obesity in adolescents. *Paediatric & Child Health*, *6*(8), 473–478.

Whitney, E. N. & Rolfes, S. R. (2015). Life cycle nutrition: Infancy, childhood & adolescence. In Whitney, E. N. & Rolfes, S. R. (Eds), *Understanding Nutrition*. (13th ed.). Belmont, CA: Wadsworth Publishing.

Widome, R., Brock, B., Noble, P. & Forster, J. L. (2013). The relationship of neighborhood demographic characteristics to point-of-scale tobacco advertising and marketing. *Ethnicity & Health*, *18*(2), 136–151.

Young, A. M., Glover, N. & Havens, J. R. (2012). Nonmedical use of prescription medications among adolescents in the United States: A systematic review. *Journal of Adolescent Health*, *51*(1), 6–17.

Zhang, J., Yan, F., Li, Y. & McKeown, R. E. (2013). Body mass index and suicidal behaviors: A critical review of epidemiological evidence. *Journal of Affective Disorders*, *148*(2–3), 147–160.

Suggested readings

ARACY <www.aracy.org.au>.

Better Health Channel <www.betterhealth.vic.gov.au>

Chen, H., Cao, L. & Logan, D. B. (2012). Analysis of risk factors affecting the severity of intersection crashes by logistic regression. *Traffic Injury Prevention*, *13*(3), 300–307.

Gampetro, P., Wojciechowski, E. A. & Siarkowski Amer, E. (2012). Life concerns and perceptions of care in adolescents with mental health care needs: A qualitative study in a school-based health clinic. *Pediatric Nursing*, *38*(1), 23–30.

Headspace National Youth Mental Health Foundation <www.headspace.org.au>.

Homelessness Australia (HA) <www.homelessnessaustralia.org.au>.

Kaul, K. (2013). Adolescent substance abuse. In Hay, W., Levin, M., Deterding, R., Azbug, M. J. & Sondheimer, J. M. (Eds), *Current Diagnosis & Treatment Pediatrics* (21st ed.). New York: McGraw-Hill/Lange.

Kirby, T. & Barry, A. E. (2012). Alcohol as a gateway drug: A study of U.S. 12th graders. *Journal of School Health*, *82*(8), 371–379.

Ministry of Health NZ <www.health.govt.nz>.

Ministry of Social Development: Community Investment <www.familyservices.govt.nz>.

Morrison, S., Dashiff, C., Abdullatif, H., et al. (2012). Parental separation anxiety and diabetes self-management of older adolescents: A pilot study. *Pediatric Nursing*, *38*(2), 88–95.

National Eating Disorders Collaboration (NEDC) <www.nedc.com.au>.

Raising Children Network <http://raisingchildren.net.au>.

Safekids Aotearoa <www.safekids.org.nz>.

Tresillian <www.tresillian.net>.

Triple P <www.triplep.net/glo-en/home>.

Well Child <www.wellchild.org.nz>.

Chapter 34

Child health assessment

Previous chapters described the normal growth and development of children. This chapter adds information about techniques for assessing the health of children. This information builds a base for care and health teaching for differing age groups throughout childhood.

LEARNING OBJECTIVES

After studying the contents of this chapter, you should be able to:

1. State the purposes of health assessment in children of all ages.
2. Use critical thinking to analyse ways health assessment skills can be incorporated into nursing care procedures to maintain family-centred care.
3. Demonstrate an understanding of how to assess a child and family by health interview, physical examination and developmental screening.
4. Discuss expected outcomes based on health assessment findings.
5. Discuss nursing care based on health assessment findings such as informing parents of health deviations.
8. Demonstrate knowledge of child development when undertaking a health assessment.
9. Discuss the factors to consider when determining the capacity of a child/young person to give informed consent.
10. Demonstrate the ability to deliver culturally appropriate care.
11. Discuss specific cultural considerations when conducting health assessments and examinations.

KEY TERMS

- adolescent assessment
- auscultation
- capacity
- developmental assessment
- health assessment
- immunisation
- informed consent
- newborn assessment
- primary concern
- resilience
- stage of development

CASE STUDY

Maddie and Kristie Williams are sisters. Their single parent father, Dave, has brought both the girls for health assessments. Maddie is about to begin year 7 and Kristie will enter kindergarten at the same time. Their father is worried that Maddie does not see well because she always sits close to the TV. He is also worried that wearing glasses may stop Maddie from playing her favourite sports and she will become an inactive teenager. Maddie has indicated that she will never wear glasses as her friends will call her names. At the same time, Dave has noticed that Kristie has been turning the TV up quite loudly. Dave also appears worried that he is providing appropriate care as a single father and seems to be seeking positive guidance and reinforcement for his parenting skills.

CASE STUDY QUESTIONS

1. What questions would you want to ask Maddie?
2. What could you do to help her adjust to wearing glasses, if they are prescribed?
3. Identify questions you could ask Dave to explore his concerns about Kristie's possible hearing deficit.

Nursing assessment is a fundamental step in the nursing process as it provides the basis for an effective plan of care, or nursing intervention. Child **health assessment**, therefore, provides the nurse with an opportunity to empower the family by: sharing information, e.g. expected growth and development; and the promotion of family **resilience**, where parents have the necessary knowledge and skills to nurture and protect their children, e.g. immunisation, healthy nutrition.

Effective assessment of children and families requires the nurse to be familiar with health maintenance standards and the relevant clinical guidelines relating to child and family health. Most health screening is undertaken in ambulatory settings, such as well child centres, doctors' surgeries, schools or paediatric outpatient clinics (Sleeper, Ariza & Binns, 2009).

Prior to undertaking any examination, it is common courtesy to seek permission before touching or examining someone. Indeed, clearly explaining what will happen and why, is a fundamental element of **informed consent**. This is especially important when working with individuals or families from cultural groups where physical touch, without permission, is culturally inappropriate and even offensive (Aboriginal and Torres Strait Islander Cultural Practice Program, Queensland Health). In some cultures specific parts of the body have significance. For example, in New Zealand Māori culture the head is seen to be sacred (Tapu) and casual touching of a child's head should be avoided. It would also be inappropriate to place a pillow under the child's head that was used to sit on (Barnes & Rowe, 2013; Medical Council of New Zealand, 2008).

The nurse should also be aware of racial characteristics that can have an impact on a health assessment. For example, when examining for cyanosis in fair-skinned children the ear tips, lips and extremities can be used. However, this can be more difficult in dark-skinned children, where examination of the mucous membranes may be required. Height, weight and body mass (BMI) measurements use standardised scales based on middle-class Caucasian children. Consequently, measurements of children or young people from other ethnic groups may not comply with these standardised measurements, due to different body types. There is currently a debate on the accuracy of the Body Mass Index (BMI) as a measure of obesity in people of different ethnic groups. A study comparing Pacific with European populations in New Zealand, suggested that "ethnic-specific measures should ensure greater accuracy as they account for differences observed in body type (composition)" (Sundborn et al., 2010).

CASE STUDY QUESTION

4. When commencing the interview with Maddie and her family, it is important to:
   a. Develop a therapeutic relationship
   b. Explain the assessment procedure
   c. Seek permission to commence the assessment
   d. All of the above

HEALTH ASSESSMENT OF THE CHILD AND FAMILY

Assessment

Health assessment of children should be a positive experience for the child and an educational opportunity for the parents/carers. The nurse must take time to listen carefully to any concerns and answer any questions honestly. The nurse must be cognisant of the assessment environment. If the assessment is being conducted in a clinic, children should be given time to familiarise themselves with the space and the equipment that is to be used. Most clinics today have furniture, colour schemes and decoration that is child and family friendly. If the assessment is being undertaken in the family's home, the nurse must be aware of appropriate customs and practices, such as removing footwear before entering the house or accepting hospitality if it is offered.

Obtaining health histories and performing physical examinations can be done independently or as part of a total preventive healthcare program for a child. Health promotion and illness prevention are vital parts of outcome identification following health assessment. Helping parents plan for their child's next developmental stage or keeping them aware of important safety measures and other ways to keep children well are also important.

Nursing considerations

In 2008 the Royal Australasian College of Physicians (RACP), in partnership with other agencies, published National Standards for the care of children and adolescents in health services. RACP represents physicians in Australia and New Zealand and the purpose of these shared standards is to ensure that children and young people receive "quality health care in an environment that is safe and appropriate for their age and stage of development" (Royal Australasian College of Physicians, 2008).

Since 2001, the Adolescent Health Research Group (AHRG) at Auckland University has surveyed 28,000 young people across New Zealand to identify the risks and protective factors impacting on young people's lives (Adolescent Health Research Group, 2015). This series of surveys has provided a wealth of information that has influenced and guided youth health service development in New Zealand. In 2011, the Australian Institute of Health and Welfare (AIHW), published *Young Australians: Their Health and Wellbeing 2011*. This is the fourth in a series of reports that examine a range of information and indicators that provide a snapshot of young people's health. This latest report highlights areas where improvement seems to have been made (e.g. a decline in death rates, particularly relating to injuries) and areas requiring attention (e.g. a rise in diabetes and sexually transmitted infections [STIs]) (Australian Institute of Health and Welfare, 2011).

HEALTH HISTORY: ESTABLISHING A DATABASE

The assessment of a young child begins with an interview of the child's parents or legal guardians. An adolescent or preadolescent may choose to be interviewed without a parent present, although many preadolescents and adolescents still prefer to have a parent with them for support. Where a young person requests to be seen without their parents the nurse must take into consideration the young person's capacity to give informed consent and the nature of the health assessment. Before commencing the assessment or interview the nurse must ensure that the young person is aware of privacy and confidentiality arrangements, including situations where the nurse is legally required to report to other people, for example where abuse has occurred.

In some cultures it is common to have several family members attend with the child. This is often the case with Māori and Pacific Island families where the extended family is an important support network (Barnes & Rowe, 2013). This can sometimes prove problematic if the consulting room is small, however, good communication and listening to the family normally results in a culturally appropriate outcome.

The purpose of a health interview is to gather information that will direct physical or laboratory examinations to complete a thorough health evaluation. An extensive interview elicits facts such as parental problems in childrearing or detection of future health problems. It lays a foundation for health education and other nursing interventions. Important principles of child health interviewing include the interview setting, the type of questions asked and the type of information collected. The nurse must ensure that the structure and content of questions asked and information shared is at the appropriate level for the child's age and level of development.

Interview setting

An interview is best conducted in a private room with all parties seated comfortably; if not seated a healthcare provider appears rushed and cannot interact at eye level. The area should not be cluttered with furniture or other unnecessary items. At the same time it is best to avoid a sterile or medical environment that can be intimidating for children and their parents. Every effort should be made to provide an area with good lighting and flow of air.

Types of questions asked

The phrasing of questions varies depending on the type of answer desired. Closed-ended and open-ended questions are two types of effective questions; compound, expansive and leading questions, on the other hand, are three types of questions to avoid. During the interview, the healthcare provider should call the parents by their names. This lets them know their input and opinions about how their child is developing are valued. A question such as, "Does Kristie speak in sentences yet, Mr Williams?" is far more personal and a better form than, "Does your baby talk yet?" As children grow, they are able to answer questions directly.

Closed-ended questions

This simplest form of question asks directly for a fact: "Does Kristie walk yet?" "Did you take Kristie's temperature?" This is an effective type of question if particular information is being sought. It is limited in scope, however, because the response will usually be only a yes or no, with no further elaboration.

Open-ended questions

An open-ended question allows a parent to elaborate. In contrast to a closed-ended question like "Did you take Kristie's temperature?" the question "What did you do for Kristie?" is open-ended. The parent answers with a listing of all the things he did: took Kristie's temperature, had her lie on the couch, gave her extra fluid and so on. It is also important to ask open-ended questions with school-aged children and adolescents so they are encouraged to describe a problem fully. "Maddie, how do you feel about your dad's concerns with your eye sight?" "How would you feel if you had to wear glasses?" "Kristie, can you tell me about your friends?" These questions are important for not only assessing the health problems but in developing a therapeutic relationship between the nurse and the family.

Compound questions

Compound questions are confusing and should be avoided because the information they elicit is often inaccurate and must be followed by a clarifying question. An example is, "Did Kristie have nausea and vomiting?" The parent answers yes, but it still is not known whether Kristie had vomiting and nausea, just vomiting or just nausea. Another example is asking if Maddie does well at school and sport. Simplifying questions avoids any confusion when trying to ascertain if there is a particular health problem.

Expansive questions

This is an inappropriate open-ended question because it is too vague to answer. "What can you tell me about Maddie?" leaves a parent wondering where to start. "How has Maddie been since her last visit?" limits the question and makes it answerable.

Leading questions

A leading question supplies its own answer and so should be avoided. "Kristie has had all her immunisations, hasn't she?" implies that Kristie should have had them and perhaps the parent is a poor carer if they answer that question in any way but yes. The outcome for such an exchange could be a child left vulnerable to disease. Considering Dave's sole parental role, it is important to ensure that his efforts to care for his family are not undermined by ill-considered questioning.

Categories of a health interview

Data gathering for an initial health assessment can be divided into categories, which are all discussed below. At return visits, the categories used generally include only introduction and explanation, primary concern, family profile, current health history and daily living pattern.

Introduction and explanation

As a matter of courtesy, parents and children should be told to whom they are talking and what topics they will be discussing. "Hello Mr Williams, I'm Janet Dickson, a nurse here in the Community Health Centre and I'd like to talk to you about Maddie and Kristie" is an example of a suitable introduction. Because some families have never had the benefit of in-depth healthcare, it is also helpful to include a statement about the subjects that will be discussed during the interview. For example, "So that I can get a picture of Maddie's overall health, I'd like to ask you questions about why you've brought her here today, her mother's pregnancy with her, concerns you've had in the past and questions about your typical day," would be appropriate. Hearing that, parents begin to concentrate on those areas because they realise healthcare providers in this setting are interested not just in Maddie's health on this particular day but in her total health.

Demographic data

To begin collecting demographic data, obtain a child's name, address, gender and the name of the person who will be providing information. To provide culturally appropriate or congruent care and make provisions for special needs, a child's culture, ethnicity, place of birth, religious or spiritual practices, and primary and secondary languages should also be identified. Be certain to identify the child's primary carer. If the parents are divorced or deceased, it is especially important to identify who has custody of the child and who has the right to sign a consent form. If the child is being fostered or has some other sort of arrangement in place, it is essential the legal guardianship can be confirmed.

Primary concern

After gathering demographic data, begin data collection with the reason the parents have brought the child to the health facility: the **primary concern**. This is what parents are most anxious to discuss, so it is important they get this immediate concern off their minds early in the interview. An effective way to elicit this information is to ask an open-ended question such as, "Why did you bring Maddie and Kristie to the hospital today Mr Williams?" Such an opening allows the parent freedom to answer with a number of areas of concern: physical, emotional, nutritional and developmental. If asked, "How are Maddie and Kristie feeling today?" or "Is Kristie ill?" a parent is left to think only about physical aspects and may not voice the biggest concern: Kristie's teething difficulty or frequent temper tantrums. Record a primary concern in the child's record exactly as it is stated ("He has constant headaches" not "Headache") as the parent's description often reveals not only information about a condition but also the depth of the parent's concern about the symptom (Geller, 2007).

History of primary concern

Once a parent has voiced a primary concern, ask him or her to describe at least six aspects of the problem including duration, intensity, frequency, description, associated symptoms and actions taken. In discussing duration, determine when children were last well to establish when they became ill. For example, on Saturday morning, Kristie began having long crying periods. On Monday night, she developed a fever. On Tuesday afternoon, her father brought her into the hospital for a checkup. The parent states Kristie vomited three times Monday morning and thinks this was caused by teething. Unless the parent is asked when Kristie was last well, he may pinpoint Monday as the beginning of the illness (the vomiting) when actually it was Saturday (the crying).

Obtaining information about the primary concern also puts the parent's observations in proper perspective. In the previous example, the parent is probably not describing teething difficulty (teething does not cause vomiting); it is more likely that the child has a viral gastroenteritis. Unless the problem is investigated, it is easy to accept the parent's statement at face value as a teething problem without appreciating its full significance.

During this phase of the interview, it is also important to gather information about related or other health concerns. After the primary concern is documented, ask another open-ended question to elicit additional information: "Is there anything else that worries you about Kristie?" Now the parent might want to talk about Kristie's temper tantrums. Unless asked about a second problem, a parent can go home with the first problem cared for but the second one still not addressed. When the parent arrives home and Kristie begins stomping her feet in the car, unwilling to go into the house, the parent will feel that the healthcare Kristie received was less than adequate because he did not receive help with this concern.

Do not assume parents will always reveal their most important concern in the initial minute of an interview: discussing certain symptoms such as constipation can be embarrassing for parents (Bisanz, 2007). It also can be frightening to put a fear that a child has a serious illness into words. As long as a concern hangs as a nebulous thought in the mind, it is easy to tell oneself it may not be true. Only when a parent voices the thought ("Do you think Kristie is retarded?" "Do you think this is leukaemia?" "Could this be inherited?"), does the fear become real. Before parents dare to speak openly this way, they must trust healthcare providers not to treat their statement lightly. For this reason, it is helpful to repeat the question about a second concern once more, at the very end of the interview.

Health and family profile

Before pursuing the past history or development of a child, document the circumstances in which the child lives. A good introduction to a health and family profile is a sentence such as, "Before we talk about any past illnesses or happenings with Maddie and Kristie, let me ask you some questions about their health and your family as a whole." Important questions to ask concerning a child's current health status include:

- Who is the child's primary healthcare provider?
- Are the child's immunisations up-to-date?
- What is the child's general state of health? How does it compare to the child's health 1 and 5 years ago (if appropriate)?
- Does the child have any known allergies?
- Does the child have a chronic illness or disability?
- Is the child taking any prescription medications, over-the-counter medications or complementary therapies?
- Is the child undergoing any treatments?

Important information concerning the family includes family structure, for example siblings, extended family members and friends. Obtaining a health and family profile is sometimes delayed until the end of the interview, when, theoretically, a parent or child is more comfortable and will answer these personal questions more readily. However, by following a nursing model and obtaining the information earlier in the interview, the healthcare practitioner can better assess the child and evaluate data.

Daily living patterns

The child's current cognitive and motor skills, sleep patterns, hygiene practices, eating habits and interactions with the family can all be elicited by asking a parent to describe a typical day. Daily living patterns are fun to obtain because most parents are eager to describe their day with their child and information gained this way is surprisingly rich and pertinent, much more so than if parents are just asked how their child sleeps, eats or plays.

Begin by asking, "Was yesterday a fairly typical day for Kristie?" (The parent says yes, it was.) "Describe for me everything Kristie did yesterday, beginning with when she first woke up." Some parents offer this information in great detail; with others, it is necessary to backtrack for particular details: "What did she eat for breakfast? Does she use a fork and spoon? Does she sit in a high chair or on your lap?"

Play

Play, the work of children, reveals a great deal about the child's development and overall well-being. Important questions to ask about play include:

- What are Maddie and Kristie's favourite toys?
- Do they play active, chasing games or engage in quiet, pretending types of activities?
- Can you tell me about your daily interactions with your children?

Social

"Does Kristie go to daycare or childcare during the week?" "What is the report of activity from childcare employees?" Social behaviours can be indicative of cognitive functioning. Autism can be detected through lack of or inappropriate social engagement. "Does Maddie have a circle of friends with whom she mixes socially?" "How do you think Maddie will find high school?"

Sleep

Every child needs adequate rest for healthy growth and development. Poor sleep patterns can often reveal a psychosocial or physical health problem. Important questions regarding sleep include:

- When the child sleeps, how long does she sleep?
- Is falling asleep a problem?
- Where does she sleep? Does she have night terrors?
- Does she sleepwalk?
- Does she wet her bed? (Depending on whether the child is toilet-trained.)

Hygiene

Good hygiene practices promote healthy teeth, gums and skin, prevent infections and improve self-esteem. Poor hygiene may reflect neglect, depression, drug abuse or poor living conditions. Important questions regarding hygiene include:

- How much self-care does the child do?
- Does the child have baths or showers?
- Does the child brush her teeth? How often? (Responses depend on the age of the child.)
- Does the child wash her hands before snacks and meals?
- Has there been a recent change in hygiene practices?

Nutrition

Nutritional assessment is an important portion of a health assessment because it influences health so strongly (Rolfes, Pinna & Whitney, 2009). Taking a history of a child's food intake can help determine whether there are any foods missing in a typical meal plan or whether any quantities seem inadequate or excessive. Be certain to assess not only the quantity of food eaten but the quality as well; for example, for the infant, cereal should be iron fortified.

Food intake is best obtained by asking a parent to describe a typical day (24-hour recall), listing what the child ate for each meal and between meals as well. With an older child, the 24-hour recall can be a joint parent–child venture. Providing this history can be difficult when the child consumes some meals at home and others at daycare or school. It may be necessary to ask for a weekend history to get a complete picture.

When assessing the adolescent, take a 24-hour recall nutritional history without a parent present, if possible. In front of a parent, adolescents may add nutritional foods to a food intake history or leave out foods they have eaten, such as milkshakes, potato chips or pizza, to avoid a lecture later; on the other hand, they may leave out healthy items or add less desirable ones because they may enjoy the obvious parental disapproval, indicative of their rebellion against adult authority.

After taking a history of a child's food intake, determine whether the child is receiving foods that comply with the recommendations of the food guide pyramid (see Appendix F). If whole food groups are absent or inadequate, a follow-up evaluation is recommended. This is where a food frequency record is undertaken over a 24-hour period to get a true picture of the child's diet. Remember that children do not have to eat food from all groups at every meal, as long as they eat from them every day. If parents think in terms of days rather than meals, it allows them to exert less pressure on a child to eat at each meal.

Be sure to consider the role of food preferences and cultural, lifestyle and financial variations when assessing food intake. The number of meals eaten at home versus outside the home, the form and content of traditional meals cooked at home and the pattern of meals should all be considered. Any religious dietary restrictions should also be obtained. Do not appear critical of a child's diet. If you convey dismay at erratic eating habits, parents or older children (especially adolescents) may begin to fabricate a food history to make it seem more acceptable.

Past health history

For a past health history, ask whether a child has ever had any serious illnesses. Parents do not generally think of childhood diseases such as measles, chickenpox and mumps as serious illnesses; inquire about these separately. Also inquire about the child's immunisation history and whether the child's immunisations are up to date for their age. (See the discussion of immunisation later in this chapter.) Has the child had any accidents (unintentional injuries)? Any surgery? Parents may not think of a tonsillectomy as surgery because there were no stitches; ask about that separately. Has the child been hospitalised for any reason? How many times has a child been seen in an emergency department? These last questions provide information about the degree of adult supervision and possibly clues to abuse (Riley, 2007).

The health of children is affected by their mother's health during pregnancy. For children under 5 years of age a history of the pregnancy is usually obtained.

Pregnancy history

For a pregnancy history, document which pregnancy this was. Were there complications in any past pregnancies, abortions or miscarriages, stillbirths, children born prematurely? A history of the pregnancy of the child being assessed can begin with a question such as, "How were the pregnancies with Maddie and Kristie?" Usually this allows the mother to answer in both physical and emotional areas. In Dave's situation, it is important to recognise that he can still provide this information even though the mother is no longer in a parenting role with Maddie and Kristie. After exploring details ask about specific events that are known to occur with pregnancy that may have had an effect on a fetus, such as:

- Did the mother have any complications such as bleeding, falls, swelling of hands and feet, high blood pressure, unusual weight gain or gestational diabetes?
- Did she take any medication?
- Did she smoke cigarettes, drink alcohol or use recreational drugs?
- Did the pregnancy/ies end early or late?

Because life contingencies such as loss of finances or illness in the family during a pregnancy may affect a parent's ability to form a bond with a child, the emotional experiences of a woman during pregnancy are also important to obtain.

Next, review labour and birth. Questions to ask include:

- How long was labour? Was it what you expected it to be?
- Were there any complications? Was the birth vaginal or caesarean?
- Was anaesthesia used for the birth?

Ask about the health of the child at birth as well. Questions to ask include:

- Did the baby cry right away?
- Did the baby need care in Neonatal Intensive Care?
- Did the baby need special procedures or equipment at birth?
- Was there cyanosis or jaundice?

Ask about the health of the mother and child in the immediate postpartum (postnatal) period. Questions should include:

- Were there any complications, e.g. postpartum haemorrhage, depression?
- Did baby and mother have a skin-to-skin time?
- Was the baby breastfed?

Family health history

Because some diseases are inherited or familial, it is important to know which ones occur in a family. Ask if any family member has heart disease (childhood or adult type), kidney disease, a congenital anomaly, seizures, diabetes (type 1 or 2), allergies or is cognitively challenged. A health history should close with one last open-ended question: "Is there anything more about Maddie and Kristie we should know?" or "Is there anything I didn't mention that you want to ask about?" A parent may have been reluctant to bring up something earlier. Asking this final question gives a parent a final opportunity to do this.

NURSING ASSESSMENT

Nurses working in primary healthcare are often involved in conducting health assessment and screening tests. The type of assessment or test will vary depending on the child's health needs and developmental health risks. The following section outlines examples of assessments that are undertaken at specific points in a child's development. Each assessment aims to collect information that helps identify actual and potential health risks of the age group concerned.

Newborn assessment

All newborns, or neonates, receive a physical examination immediately after birth and again within the first 48 hours of life. At home births and in birthing centres, the newborn assessment is normally carried out by the attending midwife (or GP), and by the midwife, in conjunction with the medical team, in a maternity hospital.

First test: Apgar score

The very first test following birth is called the Apgar score. This occurs in the delivery or birthing room right after the baby's birth. This test is designed to quickly evaluate the baby's physical condition and identify whether there is any immediate need for extra medical or emergency care. Five factors are used to evaluate the baby's condition and each factor is scored on a scale of 0 to 2, with 2 being the best score (see Chapter 18). The scores for these five factors are combined to identify the Apgar score. An initial score of 8 or above is desirable; however, a lower score does not necessarily mean that the baby is unwell or abnormal: it might mean the baby needs, for example, suctioning of the airways or oxygen to improve breathing. The Apgar score is recalculated at 5 minutes after birth and if the baby's score was low at the initial assessment and hasn't improved, the medical team will undertake any medical intervention that may be necessary.

Before giving the baby to the mother, a brief screening examination is conducted to exclude major abnormalities (e.g. spina bifida). The presence of a strong cry and a pink blush over the face and body are good signs that all is well. The sex of the child is also identified; however, this can sometimes be unclear and may require further investigation. At this point the baby is given to the mother for "skin to skin" contact. Being skin to skin with mother protects the newborn from the well-documented negative effects of separation, supports optimal brain development and facilitates bonding. The father is often encouraged to participate as well.

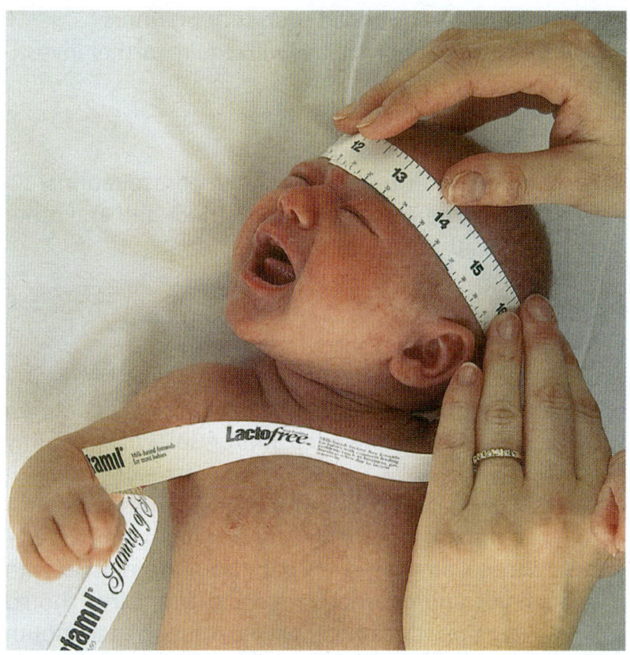

FIGURE 34.1 Measuring head circumference. The measuring tape passes just above the eyebrows and around the prominent posterior aspect of the head.

Newborn examination

It is recommended that a more detailed physical examination is carried out as soon as possible after birth (within 48 hours), preferably before the mother and baby are discharged from the hospital or birthing unit. This examination will form the baseline for all subsequent examinations, and would normally include the following.

General observation

- Overall appearance, including general condition, proportions and maturity
- General tone, sleepiness and rousability
- Evidence of jaundice
- Any birthmarks, rashes or other skin abnormalities
- The baby's cry and how it sounds
- The baby's weight—plotted on the growth chart

Systematic "head to toe" examination

This should be done carefully and in good light to detect abnormalities.

Head

- Shape, presence of fontanelle and whether normal, sunken or bulging
- Head circumference (see Fig. 34.1)—plotted on the growth chart
- Facial appearance and eye position
- Any asymmetry or abnormality of facial shape

Eyes

- Normal shape and appearance
- Presence of red reflex
- Cataracts and signs of infection

Ears

- Shape and size
- Normal level or "low-set"
- Patency of external auditory meatus

Mouth

- Colour of the mucous membrane
- Hard and soft palate
- Suckling reflex—insert a clean, little finger gently inside the baby's mouth

Arms and hands

- Normal shape and moving normally
- Evidence of birth trauma (e.g. traction injury such as Erb's palsy) by checking the neck, shoulders and clavicles
- Number of fingers. Observe their shape; check for any evidence of clinodactyly (incurving of fingers)
- Palmar creases—whether they are multiple or single. A single palmar crease may be normal, but can be a sign of Down syndrome (trisomy 21)

Peripheral pulses

- Rate, rhythm and volume of brachial, radial and femoral pulses
  - A hyperdynamic pulse may suggest patent ductus arteriosus
  - A weak pulse may occur with a congenital cardiac anomaly, that could be impairing cardiac output
  - Radio-femoral delay could indicate aortic coarctation

Heart

- Cardiac position—checked by palpation and feeling for any thrill or heave

- Heart sounds—any added sounds or murmurs
- Any suspected abnormalities will require further investigation

Lungs

- Respiratory pattern—rate and depth of respirations
- Evidence of intercostal recession, stridor and any other sounds (by auscultation)

Abdomen

- Abdominal girth and shape
- Umbilical stump for infection or surrounding hernia
- Palpation for organs, masses or herniae—it is common to be able to feel the liver and/or spleen in healthy newborns
- External genitalia—palpate for testes in boys
- Anus—establish whether meconium has been passed
- Oesophageal atresia—every baby born to a mother with hydramnios and/or who is mucousy after birth should have a large plastic catheter passed through their mouth into the stomach to check for patency of the oesophagus

Back

- The skin over the back and at the spinal curvature/symmetry
- Any evidence of spina bifida occulta or pilonidal sinus hidden by flesh creases or dimples
- Palpation of the spine for any anomalies

Hips

- Congenital dislocation of the hip (congenital hip dysplasia) using a combination of Barlow and Ortolani manoeuvres

Legs and feet

- Watch movements at each joint
- Check for any evidence of talipes equinovarus/varus
- Count toes and check their shape

Central nervous system

- Observe tone, behaviour, movements and posture
- Presence of newborn reflexes

Documentation

The findings of the examination are recorded in the postnatal care plan and the personal child health record. To ensure a safe transition to independent life, further ongoing assessment of the baby should continue. This will include, but is not limited to:

- Assessment of colour, heart rate, respiratory rate, temperature, airway integrity and overall condition
- Tone and activity
- Ability to breastfeed/feed.

A detailed list can be found in the Queensland Department of Health Routine Newborn Assessment guideline at <www.health.qld.gov.au/qcg/documents/g-newexam.pdf>.

Early childhood assessment

From birth to 4/5 years of age it is recommended that all children have routine screening checks to monitor developmental progress. These are normally carried out by specialist nurses working for the Child and Family Health Service (Australia) and the Well Child/Tamariki Ora Service (New Zealand). However, parents can choose to have these examinations done by their general practitioner.

In 2005, the Royal Australian College of General Practitioners (RACGP), in collaboration with the National Aboriginal Community Controlled Health Organisation (NACCHO), developed a national guide to a preventive health assessment for Aboriginal and Torres Strait Islander people (the "National Guide"). The guide has recently been updated and provides primary healthcare providers with practical guidance in the delivery of primary healthcare to Aboriginal and/or Torres Strait Islander people (NACCHO/RACGP, 2012).

Assessing developmental milestones

It would be ideal if children demonstrated all the developmental skills of which they are capable every time they are asked to demonstrate them. Rarely, however, do they accomplish this. Infants may become hungry, sleepy or upset during testing. Older children may become shy. A portion of developmental information on almost all health assessments, therefore, must be elicited by history taking. All previous developmental milestones must be obtained this way.

Developmental history

Many parents keep careful records of their first child's development, a less careful record of their second, a scanty record of their third and so on. The best information, therefore, may rely on the parent's memory. Parents may not be able to recall the exact month during which a skill was first demonstrated so it is often helpful to ask them to try to remember in terms of holidays or seasons. For example, they may not know in which month their infant first used a pincer grasp (grasped cleanly with index finger and thumb) but do recall the way the child pinched the ear of the family dog at a summer picnic. Getting the parents' description of the skills a child has mastered is helpful, however, it is important to assess the child's skills and rate them according to the standard criteria.

On the birth of a new baby, parents are provided with a parent-held personal health record booklet.

- Australia: Each state has its own version of a parent-held personal health record. For example: 'My ACT Personal Health Record' published in 2014 by the Australian Capital Territory, <www.health.act.gov.au/c/health?a=glob&object=1400023710>
- New Zealand: The Ministry of Health has produced a universal document called "Well Child Tamariki Ora My Health Book". This is distributed throughout all District Health Boards, <www.healthed.govt.nz/resource/well-child-tamariki-ora-my-health-book>

These booklets provide parents with a range of information promoting health and wellness, available services, immunisation information and schedules, plus a record of all health assessments from birth to 4 years, therefore providing the parents and health professionals with a complete record of the child's growth and development, health issues and immunisation status.

Health professionals working with Aboriginal and Torres Strait Islander peoples can find specific guidance in the National guide to a preventive health assessment for Aboriginal and Torres Strait Islander people, Chapter 2—Child Health (NACCHO/RACGP, 2012). The National Guide Lifecycle chart provides a summary of the key screening and health assessment areas <www.racgp.org.au/download/documents/AHU/2012lifecyclechart-child.pdf>.

Screening and developmental assessment

Figure 34.2 provides a summary of the routine screening and developmental checks that are typically carried out in Australia and New Zealand for children from birth to 4/5 years of age.

Physical examination techniques

Infant

Infants are usually examined most effectively if a parent holds them during most of the examination. Use an "isn't this fun?" or "this is a game" approach. As a rule, assess heart and respiration rate per minute first; do intrusive procedures, such as ear and oral assessment, last so an infant does not cry and complicate the remainder of the examination. Blood pressure is not taken routinely in younger children. Include assessment of the reflexes until 6 months of age; continue to take the heart rate apically and the temperature per axilla. Measure head circumference and monitor the closure of the fontanelles over the first year.

Towards the end of the first year, children become fearful of strangers. Taking an extra minute to become well acquainted with an infant at the beginning of an examination can help to counteract this problem.

Toddler and preschooler

Both toddlers and preschoolers may be afraid of examination equipment. To alleviate their fears, let them handle items such as stethoscopes, otoscopes and blood pressure cuffs before the examination (see Fig. 34.3). Leave intrusive procedures such as assessment of the genitalia, ears and throat until last. Give generous praise for cooperation (anything short of hysterical screaming or kicking is good cooperation for intrusive procedures in this age group).

Begin to include blood pressure as part of routine assessment at 3 years of age, taking an axillary temperature with a digital thermometer. Before beginning an examination, establish a good rapport with the child's parents, because children this age sense parental trust or suspicion.

School-aged child and adolescent

Some school-aged children and adolescents may still be unaware of what a physical examination includes and whether it will cause discomfort. Offer good explanations so they are not frightened by the unknown. Provide older children with a choice about having a parent with them during the examination. Some may enjoy having a parent with them. Be certain to assess height and weight, as more children are obese than ever before. It is increasingly important to take blood pressure, beginning in early school age (see Fig. 34.4), because as more children are overweight today, more have elevated blood pressure (Chiolero et al., 2007). Obesity in school-aged children and adolescents is also associated with the development of type 2 diabetes mellitus and future cardiovascular disorders. There is also an association between being overweight and suicide in children (Whetstone, Morrissey & Cummings, 2007).

School-aged children and adolescents are particularly modest. Respect this by careful use of gowns. Teach breast examination for girls and testicular self-examination for boys at the end of puberty.

CASE STUDY QUESTION

5. When assessing Maddie's sister Kristie, at what age should you include blood pressure as a routine procedure?

a. 1 year
b. 2 years
c. 3 years
d. 6 years

Adolescent assessment

Adolescence is the period of growth and development that occurs after childhood and before young adulthood (10 to19 years). It characterised by rapid physical growth and is driven by changes in biological processes that begin with puberty. Although the biological determinants of adolescence are relatively universal, the characteristics, commencement and duration vary from individual to individual. Adolescence has seen many changes over the past century. The average onset of puberty is earlier than previously; young adults are marrying later; changes in how we live, e.g. urbanisation, global communication; and changes in sexual attitudes and behaviour, have all contributed to factors that can have a positive, or indeed negative, impact on the health and welfare of this age group.

It is not reasonable to expect an adolescent to discuss sensitive and personal information unless privacy and confidentiality can be assured. Reinforcing that personal information will not be disclosed without their permission is paramount, except where the information reveals that someone might harm them, or if they might harm themselves or someone else. It is reasonable that the nurse give some indication prior to the interview of how

Contact	Health and development assessments	Family/whānau care and support	Health education
Postnatal core visits			
Birth–24 hours (LMC)	Child health and wellbeing, including: brief initial examination at birth, giving Vitamin K (oral or IM) and facilitating access to hepatitis B vaccine and immunoglobulin for infants of hepatitis B surface antigen positive mothers within 12 hours of birth (refer *to Immunisation Handbook 2011*, p 98)	Maternal wellbeing Needs assessment and appropriate referral	
Within 48 hours (LMC)	Child health and wellbeing, including: full clinical examination within 48 hours and facilitating access to BCG vaccine if indicated for infants at risk of tuberculosis (refer to *Immunisation Handbook 2011*, p 259) Newborn baby vision and eye Metabolic screening as soon as possible after 48 hours	Maternal wellbeing Family health and wellbeing Family violence assessment Appropriate information and education about screening Needs assessment and appropriate referral	Breastfeeding and maternal nutrition SUDI prevention Parenting support, including dealing with baby's crying and understanding infant development Shaken baby syndrome prevention
Up to 1 week (LMC)	Child health and wellbeing, including: clinical examination within 7 days (postnatal assessment), and giving 2nd dose of Vitamin K if oral administration chosen by parents	Maternal wellbeing Family health and wellbeing Safe sleep assessment Family violence assessment ABC smoking cessation Needs assessment and appropriate referral	Recognition and management of minor illnesses Safety/injury prevention Maternal and family/whānau support networks
	Hearing screener: Universal newborn hearing screening (generally carried out prior to discharge from maternity facility)		Immunisation
Transition core visits			
2–6 weeks (LMC)	Child health and wellbeing, including: clinical examination at discharge from maternity services, and giving third dose of Vitamin K if oral administration chosen by parents	Maternal wellbeing Family health and wellbeing Family violence assessment ABC smoking cessation Handover care to Well Child provider/GP team Needs assessment and appropriate referral	
6-week check (GP team)	Limited assessment including 6-week immunisations, 6-week vision screen, hip screen using the Ortolani and Barlow tests Address any health issues for mother and baby To provide ongoing medical and primary health care services to the baby and family/whānau Needs assessment and appropriate referral		
4–6 weeks	Comprehensive assessment, including full physical history, at entry into WCTO Provider services	Family health and wellbeing PND screen Family violence assessment ABC smoking cessation Assess breastfeeding status Needs assessment and appropriate referral	Breastfeeding and maternal/infant nutrition Immunisation SUDI prevention Recognition of childhood illness Parenting for child age and stage Safety/injury prevention

FIGURE 34.2 *Well Child/Tamariki Ora National Schedule.* (New Zealand Ministry of Health, 2013; reproduced with the kind permission of the New Zealand Ministry of Health.)

Contact	Health and development assessments	Family/whānau care and support	Health education
Infant and child core visits			
8–10 weeks	Child growth and development	Family health and wellbeing Family violence assessment ABC smoking cessation Needs assessment and appropriate referral	Breastfeeding and infant nutrition SUDI prevention Recognition of childhood illness Parenting for child age and stage Safety/injury prevention
3–4 months	Child growth and development Developmental assessment (PEDS)	Family health and wellbeing PND screen Family violence assessment ABC smoking cessation Assess breastfeeding status Needs assessment and appropriate referral	Breastfeeding and infant nutrition Immunisation SUDI prevention Recognition of childhood illness Parenting for child age and stage Child development Safety/injury prevention
5–7 months	Child growth and development Developmental assessment (PEDS)	Family health and wellbeing Family violence assessment ABC smoking cessation Assess breastfeeding status Needs assessment and appropriate referral	Breastfeeding and infant nutrition Immunisation SUDI prevention Recognition of childhood illness Parenting for child age and stage Child development Oral health Safety/injury prevention
9–12 months	Child growth and development Developmental assessment (PEDS) Oral health (Lift the Lip)	Family health and wellbeing Family violence assessment ABC smoking cessation Needs assessment and appropriate referral	Breastfeeding and nutrition Safety/injury prevention SUDI prevention Recognition of childhood illness Parenting for child age and stage Child development Oral health Early childhood education
15–18 months	Child growth and development Developmental assessment (PEDS) Oral health (Lift the Lip)	Family health and wellbeing Family violence assessment ABC smoking cessation Needs assessment and appropriate referral	Nutrition and activity Immunisation Safety/injury prevention Recognition of childhood illness Parenting for child age and stage Child development Oral health Early childhood education
2–3 years	Child growth and development (plot BMI centiles) Developmental assessment (PEDS) Oral health (Lift the Lip)	Family health and wellbeing Family violence assessment ABC smoking cessation Needs assessment and appropriate referral	Nutrition and activity Safety/injury prevention Recognition of childhood illness Parenting for child age and stage Child development Oral health Early childhood education

FIGURE 34.2 *(Continued) Well Child/Tamariki Ora National Schedule.* (New Zealand Ministry of Health, 2013; reproduced with the kind permission of the New Zealand Ministry of Health.) *(continued)*

Contact	Health and development assessments	Family/whānau care and support	Health education
4 years B4 School Check	Child growth and development (plot BMI centile) Child Health Questionnaire (CHQ) Developmental assessment (PEDS) Behavioural assessment (SDQ) Oral health (Lift the Lip) Vision and hearing	Family health and wellbeing Family violence assessment ABC smoking cessation Needs assessment and appropriate referral	Nutrition and activity Immunisation Safety/injury prevention Recognition of childhood illness Parenting for child age and stage Child development Oral health Preparing for school

FIGURE 34.2 (*Continued*) *Well Child/Tamariki Ora National Schedule.* (New Zealand Ministry of Health, 2013; reproduced with the kind permission of the New Zealand Ministry of Health.)

the information will be stored and who can access it. For example, digital information may be stored on a password protected computer database, where the nurse is the only password holder.

In Australia and New Zealand it is now accepted that children and young people can give consent without parental permission. It is generally accepted that most young people over the age of 16 are capable of giving their own informed consent. However, those younger than 16 year may sometimes be considered to have sufficient maturity to give informed consent. "Children may be able to give consent to medical procedures where they are either over a statutory age (fourteen to sixteen depending on the jurisdiction), or, of sufficient maturity that they are able to comprehend the procedure and give informed consent" (Library of Congress, 2015).

The young person may be happy for their parents to attend the interview. Indeed, in some cultures it is common for family members or friends to attend as support people. It is important that the nurse is aware of who the support people are and their relationship to the client. Problems can arise where the young person does not wish to be interviewed with their parent in attendance and/or does not wish them to have any information about what was said or done. In these situations the nurse must have a strategy in place to defuse any potential disagreement, and, where appropriate, encourage and empower the young person to talk to their parents about important issues.

Specific guidance for health professionals working with Aboriginal and Torres Strait Islander peoples can be found in the national guide to a preventive health assessment for Aboriginal and Torres Strait Islander people (NACCHO/RACGP, 2012). The National Guide Lifecycle Chart provides a summary of the key screening and health assessment areas <www.racgp.org.au/download/documents/AHU/2012lifecyclechart-child.pdf>.

HEEADSSS assessment

The HEEADSSS assessment is a tool that is commonly used to assess adolescent psychological status. Indications for psychosocial screening include but are not limited to:

- drug and alcohol abuse
- mental health concerns
- other problems (e.g. abuse, self-care issues for chronic conditions such as asthma).

HEEADSSS is an acronym for:

- **H**ome
- **E**ducation/employment
- **E**ating
- **A**ctivities

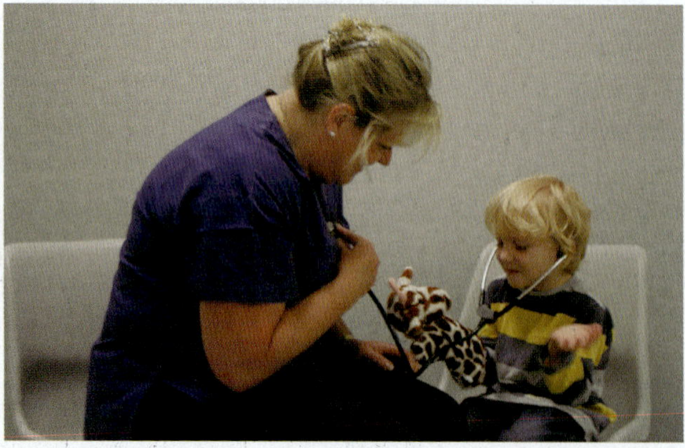

FIGURE 34.3 Puppet or doll play is a great way to prepare a preschooler for physical examination. (© Gavin Crawford.)

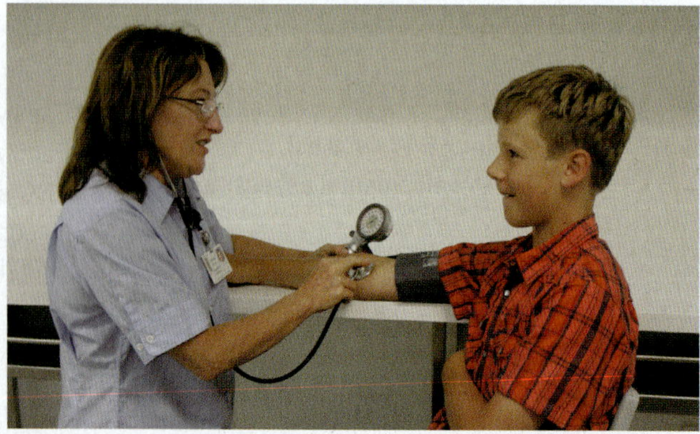

FIGURE 34.4 Measuring blood pressure for a child or an adolescent requires a cuff that is appropriately sized. (© Gavin Crawford.)

TABLE 34.1 Examples of "more" and "less" positive questions

	More positive	Less positive	Reason
Home	Where do you live and who lives there with you?	Tell me about your mother and father?	Parent(s) may have separated, divorced or died. Open-ended questions enable collection of environmental as well as personal history.
Education/employment	What are your favourite subjects at school? What are you good at?	How are you doing at school?	Poor questions can be answered "okay" or "dunno". Open-ended questions ask for information about strengths and weaknesses
Eating	What do you like and not like about your body?	Do you think you are over-weight?	Issues of body image are often complex
Activities	What do you and your friends enjoy doing for fun?	Do you have activities outside of school?	Good questions are open-ended and allow young people to express themselves
Drugs	Have any of your friends experimented with tobacco, alcohol or other drugs?	Do you take drugs?	Asking about friends allows the adolescent to reveal information without implicating themselves
Sexuality	Have you ever been involved in a romantic relationship? How would you describe your feelings towards guys/girls?	Have you ever had sex?	What does the term "had sex" really mean to teenagers? Asking only about heterosexual relationships closes doors at once.
Suicide/depression	Have you ever felt sad or down?	Have you ever tried to kill yourself?	These questions should focus on identifying thoughts or feelings that may lead to suicidal ideation (thoughts or preoccupation)
Safety from injury and violence	Are there any people or situations where you feel unsafe?	Are you being abused by anyone?	Open-ended questions are more likely to uncover issues or concerns

- **D**rugs
- **S**exuality
- **S**uicide/depression
- **S**afety from injury and violence.

Some organisations/agencies will have set questions or example questions, which relate to the subjects which make up the HEEADSSS acronym. The interviewer can create their own questions and the order of questioning. This will result in a more natural conversation, directed by the young person rather than the acronym, with the interviewer asking more specific questions where required. It is important that the interview highlights what is going well in the young person's life. This helps provide a positive tone to the interview and a source of encouragement for the young person. For examples of "more" or "less" positive questions, see Table 34.1.

On conclusion of the HEEADSSS assessment, giving positive feedback on things that are going well provides positive reinforcement and promotes self-esteem. A positive experience helps create trust and will help ensure that future encounters are positive and therapeutic (see Fig. 34.5). However, for young people who engage in significant health risk behaviours it may be necessary to consider the young person's health concerns in terms of the risk and protective factors. Protective factors discourage behaviour that might lead to negative health outcomes (e.g. unprotected sex) or encourage behaviour that might prevent a negative health outcome (e.g. using condoms and contraception).

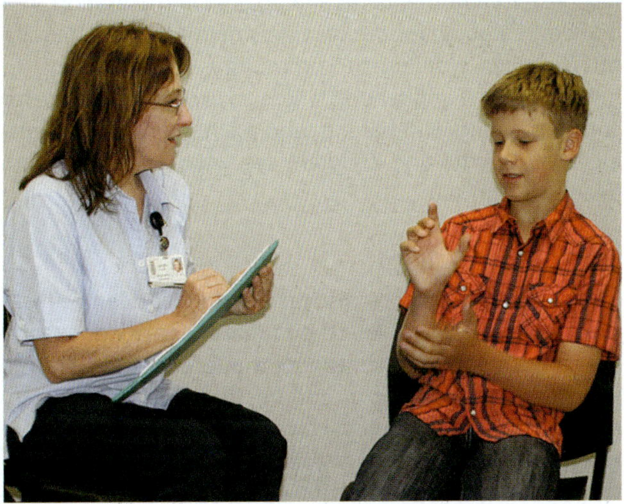

FIGURE 34.5 It is important to establish trust and genuineness when talking to adolescents. (© Gavin Crawford.)

Consequently, a 'risk' factor is the opposite of a protective factor and encourages behaviour that might lead to a negative health outcome or discourage behaviour that might prevent it (World Health Organization, 2004).

Based on the issues identified the nurse and young person, and possibly the parents, should discuss an action plan for potential follow up. The main challenge is that many young people do not always recognise dangerous risk-taking behaviour. The challenge for the nurse is to help them see these behaviours as problems and encourage and empower them to develop better strategies to deal with them.

IMMUNISATION STATUS

One of the most important health assessment and promotion measures for children is to establish that their immunisation status is up-to-date. Routine immunisation schedules call for children to receive vaccines against a number of potentially dangerous infections, including measles, mumps, rubella, diphtheria, tetanus, pertussis, hepatitis B, poliomyelitis, pneumococcal pneumonia, *H. influenzae* meningitis and rotavirus. New influenza vaccines are developed yearly to help ward off influenza viruses. Human papillomavirus vaccination (HPV) is recommended for prepubertal girls (and boys in Australia). Research continues on the development of vaccines to combat other diseases, including HIV infection.

The role of the nurse is to help parents understand that although diseases such as measles and mumps are referred to as common childhood illnesses, they are also potentially serious illnesses, possibly leading to complications such as pneumonia and encephalitis. When children develop these common communicable diseases, they need to be seen by a primary healthcare provider to minimise the risk of possible complications.

Immunisation: myths and realities

The Australian Government has developed a booklet in response to arguments for and against immunisation. The booklet is a guide for the providers of immunisation, quite often nurses working in community health nursing in medical centres and schools, and is an excellent resource for communicating with parents who are hesitant in immunising their infants and children, see <www.immunisation.health.nsw.gov.au>.

Definitions

Most people use the terms "vaccination" and "immunisation" interchangeably but their meanings are not exactly the same. A vaccine is a product that produces immunity from a disease and can be administered by injections, by mouth or by aerosol. A vaccination is the injection of a killed or weakened organism that produces immunity in the body against that organism. Immunisation means receiving a vaccine and then becoming immune to a disease as a result of being vaccinated. Therefore, immunisation is the process by which a person becomes protected from a disease.

Immunisation through vaccination

Vaccines have been successful in providing children with artificially acquired active or passive immunity. Vaccines are prepared in a number of forms. Attenuated vaccines are made from live organisms that have been reduced in virulence to a point where they will not cause active disease but will ensure a good antibody response. Because they are strong and effective solutions, a single dose usually provides a good degree of active immunity.

Because some bacteria, such as diphtheria, cause disease by producing a toxin, the vaccine against such a disease, a toxoid, is actually an extract of the toxin with reduced virulence. The antibodies produced against toxin-producing bacteria are antitoxins. The solution given for passive immunity against diphtheria is an antitoxin.

Gamma globulin is serum obtained from the pooled blood of many people. Because it combines the serum of many people, it probably has antibody protection against measles, rubella, poliomyelitis, varicella and hepatitis B, among many other infectious diseases. When administered, it offers artificially acquired passive immunity (see Box 34.1).

BOX 34.1 ✻ Active versus passive immunity

Immunity, the ability to combat a particular antigen, may be either active or passive:

- *Active immunity*. When a child produces antibodies after the natural invasion of a pathogen (the child has measles, for example), the child is said to have **naturally acquired active immunity**. Active antibodies (or the child's ability to produce antibodies rapidly should the specific antigen [measles] invade again) last a lifetime. When pathogens are artificially injected into the child by immunisation, the child receives **artificially acquired active immunity**. If the specific antigen should enter again, antibodies are produced against the pathogen that are just as lasting as those produced in naturally acquired active immunity.
- *Passive immunity*. IgG antibodies that a woman possesses either through immunisation or through having had a disease are transferred across the placenta to a fetus in utero. Because the fetus does not make these antibodies but merely receives them, this is termed **naturally acquired passive immunity**. Passive immunity lasts only months. Some antibodies transferred across the placenta may have slightly longer lifetimes than this. For example, measles antibodies have been isolated up to age 1 year, which is why measles immunisation is delayed until age 12 to 15 months.

When children are exposed to a disease against which they have no antibodies, antibodies made synthetically or obtained from animal serum may be injected into the child to give rapid immunity **(artificially acquired passive immunity)**. Like naturally acquired passive antibodies, these last only approximately 6 weeks. A child who is susceptible to tetanus, for example, would receive tetanus antibodies after a stab wound.

Available vaccines

Diphtheria, tetanus, pertussis (DTaP) vaccines

Diphtheria, tetanus toxoid and acellular pertussis (whooping cough) vaccines are supplied in a single vial as DTaP and given in one intramuscular injection. It is recommended that children receive a primary series of four immunisations with the vaccine (2, 4, 6 and 12 to 18 months). A booster is then given between 4 and 6 years, or before entry into school. In the past, no further pertussis vaccine was administered after this point. Now, because of whooping cough outbreaks in the teenage or young adult population, a further combined injection of diphtheria, tetanus toxoid and acellular pertussis (Tdap vaccine) is recommended at 11 to 12 years. Teenagers who did not receive the 11 to 12-year booster, or received only a diphtheria/tetanus (Td) injection at that time are encouraged to receive one dose of Tdap 5 years after the last Td/DTaP dose. It is recommended that adults continue with tetanus prophylaxis every 10 years throughout life to keep tetanus immunisation current. There has been a current increase in the incidence of pertussis amongst infants. For this reason, parents and family members are encouraged to have their own immunity levels reassessed.

In the past, a great deal of controversy arose about the safety of the diphtheria-tetanus-pertussis vaccine, most of it directed at the pertussis component. Severe reactions, such as high fever, persistent crying and even seizures, were reported. For this reason, the former DTP vaccine has been modified to DTaP and contains a less reactive pertussis component. Side effects can still include drowsiness, fretfulness, low-grade fever, and redness and pain at the injection site. Some parents, after hearing about reactions to the former vaccine, may refuse immunisation for their children. This is their right, but children who are not immunised against pertussis (unless there is a medical or moral contraindication) may be refused admittance to preschool or beginning school programs. Parents should be informed of this when they refuse to sign consent for immunisation.

Pertussis vaccination is contraindicated in children who have a progressive or unstable neurological disorder or who have had a severe allergic reaction to pertussis in a previous DTaP vaccination. If pertussis immunisation is contraindicated, the Td, or diphtheria-tetanus vaccine, is substituted.

Polio vaccines

Inactivated polio vaccine (IPV) contains all three strains of poliovirus and is the type preferred for routine immunisation. IPV is administered in a primary series of three doses and given along with DTaP at 2, 4 and 6 to 18 months of age. A fourth booster dose is given between the ages of 4 and 6 years, before school entry (AAP, 2009).

Measles, mumps, rubella (MMR) vaccines

Measles, mumps, rubella vaccine is furnished in one injection and routinely administered between 12 and 15 months. A second dose of MMR is generally given between the ages of 4 to 6 years or, if the child did not receive the 4 to 6-year dose, at 11 to 12 years. Until this passive immunity has faded, the injected vaccine will be neutralised by passive antibodies and no immunity will result. For the same reason, children who have recently received immune globulin or other blood products that contain antibodies should not receive MMR vaccination for about 3 months because the passively acquired antibodies could interfere with the child's immune response to the vaccine.

Side effects of the vaccine include transient rash and a fever, which may begin 5 to 12 days after vaccination and last several days. Adverse reactions include joint pain, low-grade fever, rash and lymphadenopathy 5 to 12 days after vaccination. Formerly, there was a concern that the administration of the MMR vaccine was associated with the development of autism in children, as symptoms of autism often begin to be apparent during the second year or close to the time of MMR vaccine administration. Further research has shown there to be no causal relationship between the vaccine and autism, dispelling this fear (Clifton, 2007). Parents may ask about this and refuse to have their child immunised against MMR for this reason.

CASE STUDY QUESTION

6. Dave is not sure if Maddie and Kristie have been immunised for measles varicella. You would inform him that it is usually given at what age?

a. At 12 to 18 months of age
b. At 2 and 4 months of age
c. At 16 years of age
d. It is not recommended for children

Hepatitis B vaccine

The vaccine for hepatitis B virus (HBV) is recommended for all infants soon after birth as hepatitis B is associated with liver cancer later in life. Three doses are required following the birth dose. Those born to hepatitis B surface antigen (HBsAg)-negative mothers should receive the first dose in the newborn period before hospital discharge, a second dose 1 month after the first dose, and a third dose 2 months later. In addition, HBV immunisation is recommended for populations at increased risk of contracting hepatitis B infection, including (but not limited to) healthcare workers with significant exposure to blood, clients receiving haemodialysis, those with haemophilia and others receiving clotting factor concentrates, illicit injectable drug users and sexually active individuals with multiple sexual partners.

Hepatitis A vaccine

Two doses of hepatitis A vaccine are required for Aboriginal and Torres Strait Islander children living in high risk areas. Children who did not receive this as toddlers can be vaccinated against hepatitis A at any time.

Rotavirus vaccine

Rotaviruses are responsible for the majority of severe gastrointestinal disease in infants so immunisation against these viruses is important in preventing outbreaks of diarrhoea in infants, particularly those who attend a daycare setting. The vaccine is given at 2, 4 and 6 months. No doses should be given to children older than 32 weeks.

H. influenzae type b vaccines

H. influenzae type b conjugate vaccine (Hib) protects against *H. influenzae* bacteria, a major cause of meningitis in children. You may need to explain the difference between *H. influenzae* (a bacteria) and influenza virus, so that parents do not think that a "flu shot" protects against this. Several formulations of this vaccine are available, and three of them are currently licensed for use in infancy. Depending on the individual vaccine, they are administered in a two-dose (at age 2 and 4 months) or a three-dose regimen (at 2, 4 and 6 months, with an additional booster at 12 months). Local reactions include tenderness at the injection site. Systemic reactions such as crying and fever may also occur (AAP, 2009).

Varicella vaccine

Varicella (chickenpox) vaccine was a difficult vaccine to develop because of the complex structure of the herpes-zoster virus. It is an important vaccine because once a generation of children has been successfully immunised, it should mark the end of epidemic childhood diseases. Infants may receive varicella vaccine at any visit after their first birthday (usually scheduled at 18 months) and again at 10 to 13 years. Those who did not receive the vaccine as infants and who lack a reliable history of chickenpox should be immunised during adolescence with two doses of vaccine, administered at least 1 month apart.

Pneumococcal pneumonia vaccine

The pneumococcal vaccine is recommended for all children between 2 and 23 months. The vaccine is administered at 2, 4, 6 and 12 months and provides protection for 6 to 10 years (AAP, 2009). It is especially recommended for children (and adults) who would be prone to a pneumococcal infection (those with pulmonary or cardiac disease, those without a spleen and those who are immune-suppressed).

Human papillomavirus vaccine

The human papillomavirus (HPV) is associated with the development of cervical cancer in women. To help prevent HPV, it is recommended that all girls receive three injections of this vaccine beginning at 11 to 12 years of age. The second dose should be administered 2 months after the first and the third dose 6 months after the first dose. Those who did not receive the vaccine in early adolescence can receive it at any time, respecting the proper monthly intervals for administration. Some teenagers who have taken abstinence pledges not to have sexual relations until they are married may say that they do not need the vaccine. Counselling them about the safety of prophylaxis may be necessary.

Meningococcal vaccine

Children receive a meningococcal vaccine between 2 and 10 years of age. As meningitis occurs frequently on university campuses, previously unvaccinated university and high school students (particularly at private schools with dormitory accommodation) should also receive the vaccine.

Influenza vaccine

Influenza is caused by A, B or C retroviruses, which mutate so easily it has been impossible to design a vaccine that is effective for longer than 1 year. All children, infants through to adolescents, particularly those who have chronic pulmonary or cardiovascular disorders or are immune-suppressed, should receive a yearly injection of the vaccine. As the vaccine can be supplied as a nasal spray, receiving the vaccine is painless (AAP, 2009).

Immunisation schedules for Australia and New Zealand can be found in Figures 34.6 and 34.7. Additional guidance for health professionals working with Aboriginal and Torres Strait Islander people can be found in the National guide to a preventive health assessment for Aboriginal and Torres Strait Islander people (NACCHO/RACGP, 2012).

Administration of a vaccine

Vaccines are normally given by a registered nurse who has additional training. For example, in New Zealand, prospective vaccinators must undertake a 2-day vaccinator training course run by the Immunisation Advisory Centre (IMAC).

The immunisation status of ill children admitted to hospital should be assessed to identify those who need their immunisations updated. Children who are seriously ill should not receive immunisation. Infants and preschoolers often have common cold symptoms (the average toddler has 10 to 12 colds a year) that should not deter from receiving their scheduled vaccination. If children were not immunised at health maintenance visits when they have slight cold symptoms, many would never receive their scheduled vaccines. Children who do not receive primary immunisation or are behind in a vaccination schedule can receive a catch-up schedule.

Children who are immune-suppressed, receiving corticosteroids, or receiving chemotherapy or radiation therapy should not receive live virus vaccines. The live-attenuated viruses such as measles, rubella, oral polio (OPV) and mumps must not be given to girls who are pregnant because these vaccines could cross the placenta, causing actual disease in the fetus. Before travelling internationally, parents should consult their local medical practitioner to see what additional vaccines are required for overseas travel.

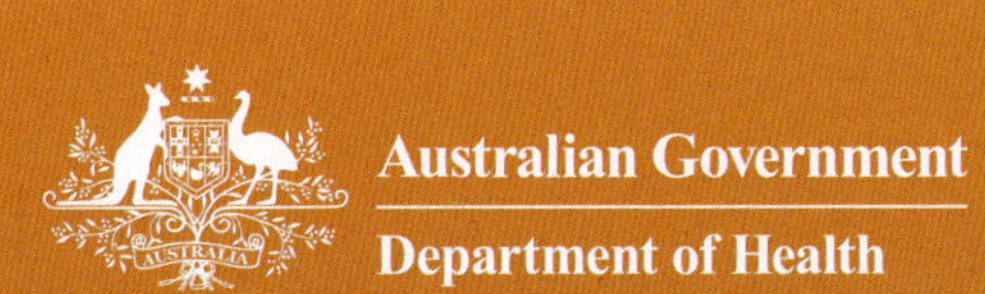

National Immunisation Program Schedule

From 20 April 2015

Age	Vaccine
Child programs	
Birth	• Hepatitis B (hepB) [a]
2 months	• Hepatitis B, diphtheria, tetanus, acellular pertussis (whooping cough), *Haemophilus influenzae* type b, inactivated poliomyelitis (polio) (hepB-DTPa-Hib-IPV) • Pneumococcal conjugate (13vPCV) • Rotavirus
4 months	• Hepatitis B, diphtheria, tetanus, acellular pertussis (whooping cough), *Haemophilus influenzae* type b, inactivated poliomyelitis (polio) (hepB-DTPa-Hib-IPV) • Pneumococcal conjugate (13vPCV) • Rotavirus
6 months	• Hepatitis B, diphtheria, tetanus, acellular pertussis (whooping cough), *Haemophilus influenzae* type b, inactivated poliomyelitis (polio) (hepB-DTPa-Hib-IPV) • Pneumococcal conjugate (13vPCV) • Rotavirus [b]
12 months	• *Haemophilus influenzae* type b and meningococcal C (Hib-MenC) • Measles, mumps and rubella (MMR)
18 months	• Measles, mumps, rubella and varicella (chickenpox) (MMRV)
4 years	• Diphtheria, tetanus, acellular pertussis (whooping cough) and inactivated poliomyelitis (polio) (DTPa-IPV) • Measles, mumps and rubella (MMR) (to be given only if MMRV vaccine was not given at 18 months)
School programs	
10–15 years (contact your State or Territory Health Department for details)	• Varicella (chickenpox) [c] • Human papillomavirus (HPV) [d] • Diphtheria, tetanus and acellular pertussis (whooping cough) (dTpa)
At-risk groups	
Aboriginal and Torres Strait Islanders	
12–18 months (in high risk areas)[e]	• Pneumococcal conjugate (13vPCV)
12–24 months (in high risk areas)[f]	• Hepatitis A
6 months to less than 5 years	• Influenza (flu)
15 years and over	• Influenza (flu) • Pneumococcal polysaccharide (23vPPV) (medically at risk)
50 years and over	• Pneumococcal polysaccharide (23vPPV)
Other at-risk groups	
6 months and over (people with medical conditions placing them at risk of serious complications of influenza)	• Influenza (flu)
12 months (medically at risk)[e]	• Pneumococcal conjugate (13vPCV)
4 years (medically at risk)[e]	• Pneumococcal polysaccharide (23vPPV)
Pregnant women (at any stage of pregnancy)	• Influenza (flu)
65 years and over	• Influenza (flu) • Pneumococcal polysaccharide (23vPPV)

* Please refer to reverse for footnotes

IMMUNISATION

FIGURE 34.6 Recommended national immunisation schedule, Australia. **National Immunisation Programme Schedule from 20 April 2015.** (© 2015 Commonwealth of Australia as represented by the Department of Health.) *(continued)*

Footnotes to the National Immunisation Program (NIP) Schedule

a. Hepatitis B vaccine: should be given to all infants as soon as practicable after birth. The greatest benefit is if given within 24 hours, and must be given within 7 days.

b. Rotavirus vaccine: third dose of vaccine is dependent on vaccine brand used. Contact your State or Territory Health Department for details.

c. Varicella vaccine: contact your State or Territory Health Department for details on the school grade eligible for vaccination.

d. HPV vaccine: is for all adolescents aged between 12 and 13 years. Contact your State or Territory Health Department for details on the school grade eligible for vaccination.

e. Pneumococcal vaccine:
   i. Medically at risk children require a fourth dose of 13vPCV at 12 months of age and a booster dose of 23vPPV at 4 years of age.
   ii. Aboriginal and Torres Strait Islander children require a fourth dose of pneumococcal vaccine (13vPCV) at 12-18 months of age for children living in high risk areas (Queensland, Northern Territory, Western Australia and South Australia). Contact your State or Territory Health Department for details.

f. Hepatitis A vaccine: two doses of Hepatitis A vaccine for Aboriginal and Torres Strait Islander children living in high risk areas (Queensland, Northern Territory, Western Australia and South Australia). Contact your State or Territory Health Department for details.

Further information

Further information and immunisation resources are available from the Immunise Australia Program website at **www.immunise.health.gov.au** or by contacting the infoline on **1800 671 811**.

You should contact your State or Territory Health Department for further information on the program specific to your State or Territory:

State/Territory	Contact Number
Australian Capital Territory	(02) 6205 2300
New South Wales	1300 066 055
Northern Territory	(08) 8922 8044
Queensland	13 HEALTH (13 4325 84)
South Australia	1300 232 272
Tasmania	1800 671 738
Victoria	1300 882 008
Western Australia	(08) 9321 1312

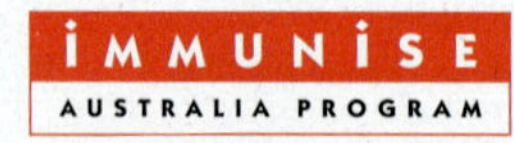

A joint Australian, State and Territory Government initiative

www.immunise.health.gov.au

All information in this publication is correct as at June 2015

11178 June 2015

FIGURE 34.6 *(Continued)* Recommended national immunisation schedule, Australia. **National Immunisation Programme Schedule from 20 April 2015.** (© 2015 Commonwealth of Australia as represented by the Department of Health.)

The National Immunisation Schedule

immunise
our best protection

Age	Disease to protect against	Vaccine
6 Weeks	Rotavirus (start first dose before 15 weeks)	**RotaTeq**® (oral)
	Diphtheria + tetanus + whooping cough (pertussis) + polio + hepatitis B + *Haemophilus influenzae* type b (Hib)	**INFANRIX**® ***hexa***
	Pneumococcal disease	**PREVENAR 13**®
3 Months	Rotavirus	**RotaTeq**® (oral)
	Diphtheria + tetanus + whooping cough + polio + hepatitis B + *Haemophilus influenzae* type b (Hib)	**INFANRIX**® ***hexa***
	Pneumococcal disease	**PREVENAR 13**®
5 Months	Rotavirus	**RotaTeq**® (oral)
	Diphtheria + tetanus + whooping cough + polio + hepatitis B + *Haemophilus influenzae* type b (Hib)	**INFANRIX**® ***hexa***
	Pneumococcal disease	**PREVENAR 13**®
15 Months	Haemophilus influenzae type b (Hib)	**Act-HIB**®
	Measles + mumps + rubella	**M-M-R**® **II**
	Pneumococcal disease	**PREVENAR 13**®
4 Years	Diphtheria + tetanus + whooping cough + polio	**INFANRIX**® **IPV**
	Measles + mumps + rubella	**M-M-R**® **II**
11 Years	Tetanus + diphtheria + whooping cough	**BOOSTRIX**®
12 Years	Human papillomavirus (HPV) *(girls only)*	**GARDASIL**® (3 doses over 6 months)
45 Years	Tetanus + diphtheria	**ADT**® **Booster**
65 Years	Tetanus + diphtheria	**ADT**® **Booster**
	Influenza	Given annually. Supplier varies

MINISTRY OF HEALTH MANATŪ HAUORA hpa health promotion agency New Zealand Government

This resource is available from healthed.govt.nz or the Authorised Provider at your local DHB. Revised July 2014. **Code HE1308**

FIGURE 34.7 Recommended national immunisation schedule, New Zealand. **National Immunisation Schedule from 1 July 2014.** (© New Zealand Ministry of Health. Available at <www.health.govt.nz/system/files/documents/pages/national_immunisation_schedule_july_2014_0.pdf>)

When preparing to administer a vaccination, be sure to follow the manufacturer's recommendations for storage and handling of vaccines, such as whether to avoid exposure to light or whether to refrigerate. Failure to follow these precautions may significantly reduce the potency and effectiveness of vaccines.

Although measles, mumps and rubella vaccines are prepared from chick embryo cultures, egg sensitivities are not likely to occur because egg albumin and yolk components of the egg are absent from the culture. Children with egg allergy should obtain their doctor's permission for immunisation, however, to rule out the possibility of a hypersensitivity Thorogood, C reaction.

What if...

Maddie's father tells you they have moved so often he does not know what immunisation she or her sister have had, but he knows Maddie has never received a full series of anything? What would your recommendation be to their father? What information could you provide to ensure that both girls are fully immunised?

Providing information about immunisation

A major reason why parents do not bring children for routine vaccination relates to a lack of knowledge about what immunisation actually is, or fears about side effects. The vaccinator should fully inform parents, and, when old enough, children, about why immunisation is needed in childhood. When vaccines are given, be certain parents know what is being given and what adverse events to expect. Adverse events following immunisation (AEFI) can be caused by:

- The inherent properties of the vaccine (vaccine reaction)
- An error in the immunisation process
- Injection-related reactions arising from anxiety about or pain of the injection.

The more common vaccine reactions, such as local erythema, irritability and fever, are usually minor and self-limiting. More serious reactions are rare and do not generally lead to long-term problems. Indeed, anaphylaxis, while potentially fatal, is treatable without leaving any long-term effects (Immunisation Advisory Centre, 2012).

Prior to vaccination the following have been shown to reduce pain and distress during vaccination:

- Holding the baby
- Distracting the baby
- Breastfeeding
- Giving sucrose (up to 12 months of age)
- The parent being calm
- Rubbing (or vibration) of the skin near to the injection site
- Using EMLA cream (topical anaesthetic agent).

Following vaccination the baby may be unsettled or sleepy and the injection site may become swollen and red. Cooling the area with a cold flannel helps the swelling and redness. Often a lump can be felt under the skin, which can be present for several days or even weeks.

Paracetamol, or ibuprofen, should only be given if the child is unsettled, in pain, or miserable because of fever. It is important to remind parents to follow the dosage instructions on the bottle/packaging and warn them of the dangers of giving more than the recommended dose. The routine administration of paracetamol before and after immunisation, "just in case" the child feels unwell, is not recommended. Indeed, there is some evidence that paracetamol may reduce the effectiveness of childhood vaccinations.

Key points for review

- Health assessment always causes some degree of apprehension for both parents and children because of concerns some illness will be detected. Giving reassurance of wellness during examinations helps to alleviate this worry.
- A health history is an important part of a health assessment. The purpose is to gather information that will supplement physical or laboratory examinations to provide a more thorough health evaluation.
- The parts of a complete health history are introduction, primary concern, present health, family profile, history of past illnesses, day history, family health history and review of systems.
- Assessment of immunisation status is included as part of health assessment. Childhood immunisations are a major safeguard for children against common illnesses.

CASE STUDY QUESTIONS

7. Maddie's sister, Kristie, is very resistant to being examined. What distraction or other techniques would you use to improve the child's participation in the examination? With reference to child protection guidelines, consider how you would proceed with the assessment.
8. Maddie's father is reluctant to proceed with further immunisation as Maddie experienced a high temperature and hospitalisation after the last vaccine. How would you respond to his concerns?
9. During the assessment you observe bruising on Maddie's upper body. With reference to child protection guidelines, consider how you would proceed with the assessment.

Resources

For an extensive range of additional resources to enhance teaching and learning and to facilitate understanding of this chapter, please see the text's accompanying website located on thePoint at http://thepoint.lww.com.

References

Aboriginal and Torres Strait Islander Cultural Practice Program, Queensland Health. (n.d.). Communicating effectively with Aboriginal and Torres Strait Islander people. Accessed 24 March 2015, <www.health.qld.gov.au/deadly_ears/docs/hp-rescomeffect.pdf>.

Adolescent Health Research Group. (2015,). Youth2000 survey series: National youth health and wellbeing surveys. Accessed 24 March 2015, <www.fmhs.auckland.ac.nz/en/faculty/adolescent-health-research-group/youth2000-national-youth-health-survey-series.html>.

American Academy of Pediatrics (AAP) Committee on Practice and Ambulatory Medicine. (2009). *Recommendations for Preventive Pediatric Health Care.* Washington, DC: Author.

Australian Government Department of Health. (2013). Immunisation myths and realities: Responding to arguments against immunisation (5th ed.). Accessed 24 March 2015, <www.immunise.health.gov.au/internet/immunise/publishing.nsf/Content/uci-myths-guideprov>.

Australian Institute of Health and Welfare. (2011). Young Australians: Their health and wellbeing 2011. Accessed 24 March 2015, <www.aihw.gov.au/publication-detail/?id=10737419261>.

Barnes, M. & Rowe, J. (2013). *Child, Youth and Family Health: Strengthening Communities* (2nd ed.). Sydney: Elsevier Australia.

Bisanz, A. (2007). Chronic constipation. *American Journal of Nursing, 107*(4), 72–78.

Chiolero, A., et al. (2007). Has blood pressure increased in children in response to the obesity epidemic? *Pediatrics, 119*(3), 544–553.

Clifton, J. C. (2007). Mercury exposure and public health. *Pediatric Clinics of North America, 54*(2), 237–269.

Geller, K. H. (2007). Advice of counsel. Quote parents in pediatric patient history. *RN, 70*(8), 23.

Immunisation Advisory Centre. (2012). Adverse events following immunisation (AEFI). Accessed 26 March 2015, <www.immune.org.nz/category/tags/aefi>.

Library of Congress. (2015). Children's rights: Australia. Accessed 26 March 2015, <http://www.loc.gov/law/help/child-rights/australia.php>.

Medical Council of New Zealand. (2008). Best health outcomes for Maori: Practice implications. Accessed 24 March 2015, <www.mcnz.org.nz/assets/News-and-Publications/Statements/Best-health-outcomes-for-Maori.pdf>.

Ministry of Health. (2013). *Well Child/Tamariki Ora Programme Practitioner Handbook: Supporting Families and Whānau to Promote Their Child's Health and Development.* Wellington: Ministry of Health.

NACCHO/RACGP. (2012). National guide to a preventive health assessment for Aboriginal and Torres Strait Islander people. Accessed 25 March 2015, <www.naccho.org.au/download/aboriginal-health/1.National%20guide%20to%20a%20preventive%20health%20assessment%20for%20Aboriginal%20and%20Torres%20Strait%20Islander%20people%20(2).pdf>.

Riley, J. (2007). Do you know how to recognize child abuse? *Nursing Made Incredibly Easy! 5*(2), 54–63.

Rolfes, S. R., Pinna, K. & Whitney, E. N. (2009). *Understanding Normal and Clinical Nutrition.* New York: Wadsworth/Cengage Learning.

Royal Australasian College of Physicians. (2008). National standards for the care of children and adolescents. Accessed 24 March 2015, <www.racp.org.nz/index.cfm?objectid=393E4ADA-CDAA-D1AF-0D543B5DC13C7B46>.

Sleeper, E. J., Ariza, A. J. & Binns, H. J. (2009). Do hospitalized pediatric patients have weight and blood pressure concerns identified? *Journal of Pediatrics, 154*(2), 213–217.

Sundborn, G., Metcalf, P. A., Gentles, D., Scragg, R., Dyall, L., Black, P. & Jackson, R. (2010). Overweight and obesity prevalence among adult Pacific peoples and Europeans in the Diabetes Heart and Health Study (DHAHS) 2002–2003, Auckland New Zealand. *New Zealand Medical Journal, 123*(1311), 30–42.

Whetstone, L. M., Morrissey, S. L. & Cummings, D. M. (2007). Children at risk: The association between perceived weight status and suicidal thoughts and attempts in middle school youth. *Journal of School Health, 77*(2), 59–66.

World Health Organization. (2004). *Risk and Protective Factors Affecting Adolescent Reproductive Health in Developing Countries.* Geneva: WHO.

Suggested readings

My ACT Personal Health Record <www.health.act.gov.au/c/health?a=glob&object=1400023710>.

Queensland Department of Health Routine Newborn Assessment guideline <www.health.qld.gov.au/qcg/documents/g-newexam.pdf>.

Well Child/Tamariki Ora My Health Book <www.healthed.govt.nz/resource/well-child-tamariki-ora-my-health-book>.

Chapter 35

Communication and teaching with children and families

Previous chapters discussed normal growth and development and how children's understanding increases with age. This chapter adds information about techniques for effective communication and health teaching with children. This type of information forms the foundation of successful disease prevention, health promotion and an increase in health literacy.

LEARNING OBJECTIVES

After studying the contents of this chapter, you should be able to:

1. Describe principles of effective communication, teaching and learning as they relate to health teaching with children.
2. Use critical thinking to analyse ways therapeutic communication and health teaching can be further incorporated into the nursing care of children and families to make it more family-centred.
3. Assess children for their ability to communicate and readiness to learn.
4. Plan nursing care based on the use of communication and health teaching priorities.
5. Identify areas of care related to effective communication or health teaching of children that could benefit from additional nursing research or application of evidence-based practice.
6. Integrate knowledge of effective communication and teaching–learning with the nursing process to achieve quality child and family health nursing care.

KEY TERMS

- affective learning
- behaviour therapy
- clarifying
- cognitive learning
- communication
- demonstration
- empathy
- feedback
- focusing
- health literacy
- non-therapeutic communication
- paraphrasing
- perception checking
- positive reinforcement
- psychomotor learning
- reflecting
- teaching plan
- therapeutic communication

CASE STUDY

You meet two patients of very different ages in an outpatient clinic.

- Nathan Jones is a 3-year-old boy with chronic asthma who is scheduled for repair of syndactyly (webbed fingers) next week. One of his favourite activities is colouring. His mother tells you she is concerned Nathan will be hard to entertain after surgery because the large pressure bandage he will have afterwards will prevent him from colouring with that hand. "I don't even want to begin to talk to him about surgery", she tells you.
- James Price is a 15-year-old with asthma. His mother tells you health teaching with James will be ineffective because he never listens to anything adults say.

CASE STUDY QUESTIONS

1. What would be a good strategy for teaching about this type of surgery to a 3-year-old child?
2. Would you try to teach James more about his condition?
3. How would your communications with these children vary because of their age difference?

Health literacy is an individual's ability to read, understand, and use health information in order to make decision and follow advice (Taylor, Nicolle & Maguire, 2013). Both communication and health teaching are independent nursing actions that accompany all nursing care. They are probably the most frequently used interventions for nurses working with childbearing and childrearing families because health promotion is such a priority for this population. Education is a prime method of empowering families to assume responsibility for their own health. It is as important as any other intervention for families experiencing illness or injury, particularly when preparing a child for any sort of healthcare procedure. New areas that require teaching are constantly arising as the healthcare environment continues to become more focused on technology.

Communication is fundamental to social interaction and is one of the first and most important skills that children learn (Cruz et al., 2013). Health teaching may be offered to an individual or to a group of children with similar learning needs. It can be both formal, such as teaching a group of preschoolers about hospitalisation, or informal, such as assuring a parent that a child is getting enough nutrition, even though the child snacks rather than sits down to regular meals. The same principles of effective teaching and learning apply no matter which technique is used or whether it is offered to an individual or to a group.

COMMUNICATION

Communication is the exchange of ideas between two or more persons. It can be verbal, using words, or non-verbal, using actions such as touch or eye contact or even a remote system such as email. It is an important process in the care of children because it can make or break an effective relationship. As a process, communication can be divided into two major categories: non-therapeutic (casual, everyday conversations) and therapeutic (helpful and constructive interchanges).

Non-therapeutic communication

Non-therapeutic communication is identified by its lack of structure or planning—that is, it lacks deliberate purpose other than socialising. Dinner conversation is an example of non-therapeutic communication.

Therapeutic communication

Therapeutic communication is an interaction between two people that is planned (you deliberately intend to determine the true way a child feels), has structure (you use specific wording techniques that will encourage the response you expect to elicit), is helpful and constructive (at the end of the exchange you will know more about the child than you did at the beginning, and the child, ideally, also knows more about a particular problem or concern) (Forchuk, 2010).

In some cases, the interventions you are able to provide to a child and their family may be limited to palliative ones. However, the use of therapeutic verbal and non-verbal communication techniques will allow you to continue to offer comfort and support. This is often the most valued, most appreciated and most helpful aspect of all the care you offer (Svavarsdottir, Tryggvadottir & Sigurdardottir, 2012).

Components of good communication

Communication can be broken down according to essential components: the encoder, the code, the decoder and response or feedback (Arnold, 2011).

The encoder

The encoder (sender) is the person who originates a message. Such a person desires to share a thought or feeling with someone else. The person moulds this thought into a form suitable for transferring to another person (a code). Communication can be ineffective if a person omits cognitive processing or speaks without thinking, chooses the wrong words for the message, or accompanies the spoken words with a facial expression, tone of voice or gesture inappropriate for the message.

The code

The code is the message that is conveyed, as well as the medium or system used to convey it. Although this usually involves a simple spoken system, messages can also be conveyed by such methods as a painting, poem, novel, Morse code, Braille, computer, television, CD, radio, audio or videotape, DVD, camcorder, movie projector, telephone or text messaging. Communication can be ineffective when a person chooses the wrong medium for a message, such as delivering a lecture with many technical words when a drawing with carefully-labelled parts would have made the message much clearer or emailing when confronting a person directly would have been more effective.

The decoder

The decoder (receiver) of the message is the person who not only receives it (hears it, reads it, views it) but interprets or decodes its meaning (cognitive processing). Messages are interpreted in light of the receiver's previous knowledge. They may be misinterpreted if a receiver's store of knowledge is too different from that of the sender. Messages may also be misinterpreted if the receiver misses part of the transmission, such as the wink accompanying the spoken words that would have let the receiver know the sender was joking. Under stress, children tend to narrow their ability to receive information to a small area of concern. When you are dealing with children who are extremely anxious, you may find that although you gave excellent instructions (both sender and message components of communication were adequate), a child did not "hear" you (did not receive or could not interpret the message because of anxiety).

Feedback or response

Feedback is the reply the decoder returns to the sender to acknowledge the message has been received and interpreted. This could be a spoken statement, a nod of the head, a facial grimace, a return email or the sudden slamming of a telephone receiver. With feedback, the roles of sender and receiver become reversed and another communication cycle is begun. Communication can be ineffective if children do not offer feedback (the message was either not received or understood) or offer feedback before the message is fully interpreted (acting before thinking). When you are caring for children with sensory challenges such as vision or hearing problems, you may need to change your usual feedback mechanisms in order to be understood, because a nod of the head or quiet response may not be received.

The development of language

Development of language involves not only physically being able to form and voice words but also comprehension of what they mean and how they are used. One of the first responses an infant makes at birth is to cry. This first cry is important because it signals the infant is breathing well. It also announces to the parents the birth is real and stimulates the beginning of parent–child interaction. By the age of 2 years, children have mastered language well enough to be able to put together two-word sentences (a noun and a verb). By preschool age, they not only have a vocabulary of about 900 words but also can code them into simple jokes or stories (Levine, 2011).

School-age children enlarge their ability to communicate from oral exchanges to use of email or the telephone. They can write poetry and, by the end of the period, demonstrate an adult sense of humour in the jokes they create. Adolescents progress to a new phase in which they originate new words for objects or feelings ("cool" and "whatever" as responses). This form of communication helps them separate their world from adults and keeps their adolescent culture distinct.

Levels of communication

Not every conversation you engage in has the same depth level, nor should it. Throughout a day, a person may use as many as five levels of communication, from clichés to peak communication.

First level: cliché conversation

Cliché conversation is pleasant chatting or comments such as, "Have a nice day" between people who do not intend their relationship to extend beyond a superficial level. It is important when meeting a child for the first time that you introduce yourself not only with your name but also your position and function ("I'm a nursing student who is going to take care of you"). This information leads the family to move the conversation from the cliché level to a more meaningful one.

Second level: fact reporting

Fact reporting is simply stating facts about oneself ("I'm 12; I'm in Year 6"). Fact reporting is necessary for you to understand children, but it does not tell you anything about their feelings or needs. Children can move from this level to a higher level of communication only when they feel they can trust you with more information.

Third level: shared personal ideas and judgements

When children know you well, they are able to share ideas such as, "I always wanted to be an astronaut" and judgements ("This is too hard for me; I need to learn a different way"). This level of communication exposes them to loss of self-esteem if their views are not respected. It is the level that is the beginning of therapeutic interactions.

Fourth level: shared feelings

It is difficult to share feelings until you truly trust another person, because feelings are tenuous, fragile concepts, easily destroyed and crushed by inept or uncaring comments. Listen carefully for an expression of feeling from children such as, "I hate always being sick". These admissions are telling you much more than how a child experiences the world; they represent trust in you and the depth of the relationship the child has established with you.

Fifth level: peak communication

The fifth level of communication is a sense of oneness or being able to know what the other person is experiencing without it actually being voiced. It sometimes occurs spontaneously in high-intensity situations but generally arises out of long-term relationships. For example, you notice that a parent sits soundlessly beside her daughter's bedside for hours at a time. When she leaves, the daughter says, "She makes me feel so much better when she's here". It would be easy to view this mother as non-supportive (she says almost nothing during the time she's there), but by using fifth level communication, she has given her daughter more comfort than other visitors who talk the entire time they visit.

Non-verbal communication

Non-verbal communication involves a variety of factors that are important as accomplishments to effective communication. Non-verbal communication can be especially important in areas such as intensive care units when a child may be unable to speak because of endotracheal tubes and ventilators. Non-verbal communication can be expressed in a variety of ways.

Distance

Although it is affected by cultural and personal variables, the distance at which you position yourself from the person you are talking to can indicate your feelings or the type of conversation you want to have. The space created by this distance can be deemed as intimate, personal, social or public space. People generally consider the space directly surrounding them as *intimate* space, to be crossed only by people who know them well or with whom they are comfortable having close body contact. It is worth noting that people from Middle Eastern cultures may define a wider space as intimate than those from Western cultures (see Box 35.1 for a discussion on respecting cultural diversity).

BOX 35.1 ✻ Respecting cultural diversity

Cultural difference between a teacher and a learner can complicate health teaching and the evaluation of its effectiveness. Even when language is not a barrier, the way children and adolescents show that they are listening or comprehending varies between cultures. For example, making direct eye contact during conversation may be considered to be disrespectful in some Asian countries and among Aboriginal and Torres Strait Islander people. In South Africa and some Middle Eastern countries, the "thumbs up" sign is considered to be an insult. In India, the way people move their head to express "yes" and "no" can be the opposite to the way it is usually done in Australia and New Zealand. A hand raised to indicate "stop" to a child may be interpreted as a "go-ahead" sign by children from some Middle Eastern cultures.

Being aware of these cultural differences is important when planning health teaching for diverse cultural groups so that neither the teaching nor the responses to teaching are misinterpreted.

When you touch a child, it may be perceived as a violation of personal space, so always ask permission to touch ("Is it okay if I change your bandage now?") or with small children, announce what you are going to do ("It's time to change your bandage now"). If children agree to let you enter this space, it means they see you as safe, protective and helpful.

Personal space is the distance people usually stand apart from each other for casual conversation. It is a comfortable hand-shaking distance. When you stand by the side of a bed or sit next to a person at home, you are within this space. It does not invade personal space but allows for private and confidential information to be exchanged. This is the appropriate space in which to conduct health assessment interviews with children and their families.

Social space is, the distance used to conduct business or teach a class. Conversation spoken at this distance is readily heard by others. Therefore, social space should not be used to exchange personal information. If you ask a child, "How are you feeling?" as you pass in a hallway, for example, the child will probably answer, "Fine, thank you", a programmed reply almost everyone is taught in early childhood. In contrast, if you ask that same question from a personal or intimate distance, providing privacy, the answer might be, "I'm scared I'm never going home again".

Although separated widely in terms of distance, most people perceive speaking on the telephone or using email as either social or personal space. The tone of voice or the words used help to differentiate which area they consider it to be. A message such as, "Have I got news for you!" suggests social space. "Can you keep a secret?" brings it into intimate space.

Finally, there is public space. To communicate from this distance, you need to shout; privacy is not respected at all. Waving to a friend in a hallway or across a car park is an example of public space communication.

Genuineness

Genuineness is the quality of projecting sincerity or being yourself. Children will have difficulty trusting you and therefore will be unable to move to an effective therapeutic relationship with you if you change your behaviour from one encounter to the next, such as from very patient to irritable, because they have to spend energy trying to predict your reactions. The best way to convey genuineness is not to try to be what you are not, as the insecurity that comes from pretending can manifest itself as negative feelings such as aggressiveness or a bored attitude.

Warmth

Warmth is an innate quality and some people manifest it more spontaneously than others. Basic ways in which warmth is demonstrated are direct eye contact, use of a gentle tone of voice, listening attentively, approaching a child within a comfortable space and using touch appropriately. Warmth is a quality that you display best when you know another person well. Any action that helps you to know a person better (taking a health history, talking about school or family or how a child feels about the present situation) not only lets you plan care but also allows you to become increasingly comfortable with the child and deepen the warmth of your relationship.

CASE STUDY QUESTION

4. You want to review some health education material with James. In order to maximise his learning and his comfort level, this activity should take place in which type of physical space?

a. Intimate space
b. Social space
c. Public space
d. Personal space

Empathy

Empathy is the ability to put yourself in another person's place in order to understand and be sensitive to their feelings (McMillan & Shannon, 2011). People who are capable of empathy are the best support people because they can anticipate a child's reactions or fears. Feeling empathy may be emotionally draining because, when you assume another person's emotions, you experience them at the same depth as that person. Nurses therefore need to seek both formal and informal support when required.

Gestures

Children vary a great deal in the gestures they use to accompany their spoken words. Although this is culturally influenced, it is also an individual trait. Be careful not to assess emotion only by a child's gestures. Some children wave their arms wildly describing an everyday occurrence; others would use that degree of expression only when in extreme distress. Be aware also that your own gestures are always being read by children. A statement that you approve of something can be contradicted by placing your arms across your chest as you speak because this gesture may convey disapproval.

Body posture and gait

Children who feel good about themselves usually assume an upright body posture and walk rapidly and surely; those who are depressed or insecure tend to slouch and move more slowly and timidly, while those who are threatened tend to either draw back or act aggressively. Children who are in agreement with you usually maintain eye contact with you as you speak to them. Very depressed or insecure children do not do that nor do children who are very angry. Children from some cultures may not meet your gaze because it is not culturally appropriate.

Facial expression is an important accompanying gesture. Clenched teeth, frowns and smiles are easily interpreted by everyone. The degree of pain a child is experiencing may be more evident by facial expression than words.

Touch

Touch is the most intimate and meaningful of non-verbal techniques. When words are inadequate, touch rarely is. Learn to use touch such as patting a child's shoulder or squeezing a hand to accompany reassuring words or in place of words as a strong support signal (I'm here; I understand; it's all right to be afraid). On the other hand, be aware that some children enjoy being touched more than others. Because of individual preferences or cultural variations, some children do not like you to use this non-verbal signal with them. Assess individually for the appropriateness of using touch.

Use of humour

Be careful of the use of humour with children because they are usually at school-age before they appreciate most adult jokes. If they are fatigued or ill, they may be looking for a firm support person to be with them more than someone who is amusing. You can often measure a child's progress by noting the first time after a procedure the child responds to you with a humorous statement. Remember, though, that laughter and joking can also be signs of increasing anxiety. Evaluate the use of humour to be certain a child really finds a situation amusing.

Use of drawings

A useful non-verbal technique to learn how children feel about a frightening experience is to ask them to draw a picture of what happened or a picture of themselves. A child hospitalised for heart surgery, for example, might draw themselves with a large heart. A child's use of colour may be a clue regarding mood (happy children tend to use bright colours; depressed children use black or dark colours). A child with good self-esteem usually fills the full page with a drawing; one with less self-esteem crowds a drawing into a corner.

Techniques to encourage therapeutic communication

Several techniques are effective in deepening communication patterns and relationships. These techniques can be learned if they are not a spontaneous part of your present communication pattern.

Attentive listening

No one likes to talk to someone who does not appear to be listening or responding. Good listening, therefore, like speaking, is not passive but active. Be aware that your posture reveals to a great extent whether you are listening (sitting, not standing, to convey that you are not on the run; leaning forwards, not backwards; stooping to meet a child's level). Nodding, maintaining eye contact and stopping all other activities are strong indicators you are attuned to what is being said. Making it clear that you are concentrating on what another is saying by such a motion as nodding indicates you value what the other person is saying. Children who feel valued are much more likely to confide feelings and concerns than those who sense you consider them unimportant.

Open-ended questions

A pointed or direct question used in discussion asks for a specific response; it implies all you are interested in hearing about is that one fact. An example of a direct question is, "Do you take Panadol when you have a headache?" An open-ended question is not limited to a simple answer but invites a wide variety of responses because it is so comprehensive, such as, "Tell me what you do when you have a headache". A child might answer this question by not only describing the amount of analgesic they take but also offer other important information such as putting a cold towel on their forehead and staying home from school.

Open-ended questions are not effective if the topic is difficult for a child to describe (a preschooler has difficulty responding even yes or no; a paragraph of material would be impossible) or if the child is naturally shy or defensive about the subject. Most communication is a combination of direct and open-ended questions. Listen carefully the next time you ask someone to explain something to see if you make use of mostly direct (information-limiting) questions or open-ended (information-expanding) ones.

Reflecting

Reflecting is another technique, like attentive listening, that is so simple that its importance is easy to discount. Reflecting is restating the last word or phrase a child has said when there is a pause in the communication. A child says, "I'm worried", and then stops. You repeat the last word, "Worried?" The child, assured you are listening and interested, will generally elaborate on the first statement: "I'm worried I won't make the football team this year". Older school-age children may not respond well to reflection; they may interpret it as imitating them, not seeking information.

Clarifying

Clarifying consists of repeating statements others have made so both of you can be certain you understood them. This is particularly helpful if a child has been describing a set of symptoms or series of actions. You would clarify such a statement by saying, "Let me see if I understand this. You said you always get the pain first in your stomach. Then it spreads to your chest". If you are not quoting correctly, the child will interrupt and restate the problem: "No, the chest pain comes first".

Paraphrasing

Paraphrasing is restating what children have said not only to assure them you have heard correctly (as in clarifying) but also to help them explain what they have been trying to say in other words. In clarifying, you repeat a child's exact words; in paraphrasing, you retain the meaning of the words but repeat them in a clearer or more condensed form. The child says, for example, "I don't talk about my problems with my parents". A paraphrasing statement might be, "You're telling me you and your parents haven't discussed how you are feeling. Is that right?" When paraphrasing, ask for confirmation that your interpretation is correct; otherwise, you may find yourself putting words in a child's mouth.

Perception checking

Perception checking documents a feeling or emotion reported to you. This makes it a step deeper than paraphrasing. In paraphrasing, you document a statement or fact; in perception checking, you document a feeling or emotion. The child says, "I'm not at all worried about surgery. I know a lot of kids have the same thing done every day. I mean, what could happen?" You say, "You're telling me you're not worried, but the number of times you've said it makes me wonder if you really are worried. Are you?"

Always ask for validation that your perception is correct so you do not make false assumptions. Perception checking is helpful because, as a rule, children are not ready to deal with emotions until they can admit they are experiencing them. When you bring an emotion out on the table in this way, it allows them to confront it and deal with it for the first time. They may lose their reluctance to admit other worries because you have implied that worrying is acceptable.

> ***What if...***
>
> *Luke has a family history of hyperchlorerolaemia and therefore needs to modify his diet? Who would be the most important person to educate about a low cholesterol diet? Luke? His mother who prepares most of his meals? Or his father who usually does the grocery shopping?*

Focusing

Focusing helps children to centre on a subject you suspect is causing them anxiety because they comment about it indirectly or else completely avoid it. It is done by repeating something they said ("You mentioned you feel tired all the time") or by mentioning the avoided topic ("You haven't said a word about how you feel about this surgery. Is that a problem?"). Once a subject is brought up for discussion, most children respond to it. As long as it can be avoided, however, they do not have to face the problem and begin to solve it.

Supportive statements

Supportive statements let children know you accept their behaviour or at least appreciate they have dealt well with unfortunate circumstances. For example, an adolescent boy says, "My girlfriend dumped me while I've been here in the hospital". Such a statement deserves a supportive reply such as, "That must not feel good". The adolescent will take this response to mean you want to discuss the topic and, encouraged by your empathy, may elaborate on it as it still affects him.

Silence

If you ask a question and a child does not respond immediately, it is natural to ask another question or perhaps change the subject, assuming the child is not interested in the topic. This is a social custom that allows you not to put someone into the awkward position of having to discuss a sensitive topic. Silence, however, is an effective therapeutic technique. If you ask an emotion-laden question ("Are you worried?") and the child does not answer immediately, allow a period of silence to pass. Because you do not hurry to fill in the silence, the child is likely to respond by hurrying an answer (to fill in the silence); when this happens, the answer is usually spontaneous and often open and uninhibited. In other instances, a child may answer the question deliberately and cautiously and, because you have provided a period of time to answer, offer additional information.

Factors that can interfere with effective communication

Because so much of nursing care is influenced by verbal communication, it is important to avoid miscalculations in communication and to recognise common situations in which meanings can easily be distorted.

Age and developmental level

Age and developmental levels are important to communication ability because they influence vocabulary and reading ability so greatly. A 3-year-old child may not have the vocabulary to explain the way their knee feels. Early school-age children have difficulty describing the blurring they experience as they focus on a blackboard with less-than-perfect eyesight, because this is the way they have always seen. The ability to describe inner feelings such as anger, sadness and fear comes only with adolescence.

Intellectual level

Intellectual level, like age, affects vocabulary and ability both to encode and decode messages. It influences the number of languages a child speaks, reading ability and the depth of explanation a child is capable of understanding. Children with cognitive challenges or autism spectrum disorder can have difficulty both transmitting and receiving messages (Johnson et al., 2012).

Physical factors

Physical factors such as speech impairments and hearing or vision challenges interfere with the transmission and reception of messages (Decarlo et al., 2012). When children are distracted by such sensations as fatigue or pain, they also may have a reduced ability to transmit or receive messages correctly.

Technical terminology

Adults have heard common medical words and so usually have little difficulty understanding an explanation of one. Children, in contrast, have not heard many medical words. It may helpful to ask yourself if you would have understood your explanation at the same age.

Showing disapproval

Parents and children do not seek healthcare to be criticised; they do so to learn more about how to stay well or recover from illness. If they are criticised, they may not reveal any further information to you because they do not want you to react in the same way as you did to their preliminary statements.

For example, an adolescent says, "I never drink milk. That's for babies". Knowing milk is an important source of calcium, you respond, "That's not healthy. You should drink at least two glasses a day". This discourages the adolescent from telling you any more about their eating habits. Be aware that non-verbal disapproval (frowning, sighing) can be just as conversation-stopping as spoken disapproval. On the other hand, this does not mean you should show approval of wrong actions. Merely listen to them with no action or comment and make a mental note. At the end of your interaction, introduce the change in behaviour you'd like to see, for example, "Let's plan some ways you can include more calcium with your meals without drinking milk".

Communication situations that require special skills

Some communication situations require special skills in addition to the usual therapeutic communication techniques to promote understanding.

The shy child

As a rule, shy children have much more difficulty talking to new people and establishing peer relationships than other children (Coplan et al., 2013). A reluctance or inability to express their needs to others can lead to these needs being unrecognised and unmet. If they do not give you much verbal feedback, the tendency is to believe they do not have any concerns. That leaves them without support people when they most need them.

Fortunately, in most instances, once children realise they know and can trust you, shyness fades. A therapeutic response, therefore, would be not to leave them alone but to maintain an active relationship despite the lack of feedback. This does not necessarily involve talking to children but may involve checking on them frequently, remaining in the room while a doctor completes an examination or sitting with them for a few minutes while a medication takes effect.

The angry child

All children will experience anger at some point, although boys may express anger more openly than girls (Olino et al., 2013). It can be difficult to work with angry children at times because you may feel yourself becoming angry in response to their behaviour. The natural response at hearing an angry outburst is to imitate it (a child is radiating anger as tight-lipped silence, so you say nothing as well; a child shouts at you and you shout back). This is not therapeutic, however. Make a point of not allowing yourself to be drawn into children's anger, while at the same time acknowledging it is all right to be angry ("I understand that you're angry but please don't shout"). Help them to focus their anger if at all possible so they can better understand it and begin to deal with it.

To encourage focusing, ask children to detail why they are angry. An adolescent who feels angry at the entire healthcare system is highly frustrated because they cannot begin to handle the whole bureaucracy; establishing that what they are really angry about is one nurse's action, for example, builds a base for resolving the problem. If a child uses silence as a method of maintaining anger, suggesting possible reasons for the anger may be helpful ("I know Dr Smith was just talking to you. Are you angry about something they said?" or, "I know you were asking about crutch walking before. Does it have something to do with that?"). Once the subject is out in the open, few children can resist describing the extent of, or reason for, their anger. Be aware, too, that when you ask someone to explain why they are angry, you ask for the emotion and the distress that go with it to be expressed as well. Even if you are the object of the anger, you are committed to listening to the child's views.

Helping children focus anger this way moves them towards a constructive solution. If necessary, censor the way the anger is expressed, not the right to be angry. Keep anger from affecting you by reacting to the explanation, not the tone or force of it. Keep any response on your part a tone gentler and quieter than that used towards you.

The demanding child

Demanding behaviour generally stems from insecurity or fear. For example, afraid that something will happen to them while you are out of the room they constantly find more for you to do to keep you in the room. Give more of yourself, not less, to counteract this response. When you have proven you are dependably there for them, children do not feel so insecure, and the need to be demanding usually fades. Withdrawing may increase the child's insecurity and the demanding behaviour.

The child who is not proficient in English

It is not unusual in any nursing care setting to encounter children who have a different first language from yours;

in other instances, a child's speech may be limited or difficult to understand because of an accent, dialect or speech impairment; some children may speak your language but their use of words is so different from yours that the words have different meanings (Kirk et al., 2012). In some cases, the child may have a parent or another support person who can act as an interpreter. However, it is important not to assume that the child's parents or other support people are proficient in English. Relatives and friends should be used as interpreters with caution because it cannot be guaranteed that they will correctly convey your meaning to the child. It is therefore most appropriate to use a professional interpreter wherever possible.

If a translator is not available or present at the time you need to give instructions, hand gestures or drawings can be used to convey your meaning. The child can be encouraged to draw pictures. You can also ask the interpreter to write out instructions in the child's language for later use (Weldon et al., 2014).

The unconscious child

Hearing is the last sense lost with unconsciousness and the first sense regained with consciousness. As with adults, you need to be aware that an unconscious child may still be able to hear and interpret anything you say (Munjal, Panda & Pathak, 2010). Therefore, never say anything to unconscious children or within their hearing that you would not say if they were fully alert. Continue to use nonverbal communication such as touch to help convey your message.

The hearing-impaired child

It is difficult for hearing-impaired children to enunciate words clearly because they are not aware that the voice sound they are forming is not clear (Williams, 2012). When communicating with hearing-impaired children, check whether they use a hearing aid; if so, be certain it is turned on. Face them when you speak so they can follow your lip movements. Use hand gestures as necessary to convey your message or write out instructions. If you have difficulty understanding what they are trying to say, ask them to write it down if they are old enough. Use common sense about how loud to raise your voice to facilitate communication. As a rule, at the point that privacy is lost, it is time to resort to written words or sign language. Children who use sign language to communicate have a right to have an interpreter present to facilitate communication.

What if...

Nathan, aged 3, refuses to tell you whether he has pain because you are a stranger and he is not allowed to talk to strangers? What would you do?

HEALTH TEACHING IN A CHANGING HEALTHCARE ENVIRONMENT

In the past, when children were admitted to hospitals well in advance of surgery and remained in the hospital after surgery or therapy until they were almost totally well, there was a wide window of time for health teaching. Today, when surgery is often a 1-day experience, the window for teaching has greatly narrowed (Hee et al., 2012). This means nurses must use more creative approaches to achieve the same health education results. Discharge instructions may require both verbal and written approaches (Yang & Chen, 2012).

In addition, children are now exposed to a wide range of sophisticated learning strategies and may find some of the more traditional approaches to health teaching unhelpful. Before beginning, assess each child to find out what the child expects to learn, identify individual learning style and determine what teaching techniques would suit the child best.

The teacher–learner relationship

Effective teaching and learning depend a great deal on the teacher–learner relationship. As a teacher, you can only influence an individual to learn; you cannot force learning. Before teaching can be considered effective, learning has to have occurred in a way in which change in behaviour is measurable. Conversely, before learning occurs, teaching must have occurred in some form. For example, a parent teaching a child about the need to brush teeth daily must not only elicit the child's statement that daily brushing is important but also see that the child is, in fact, brushing their teeth every day. If the topic is abstract, such as helping a child change a concept about a chronic illness, change can still be measured (the child not only talks about the illness but also begins to take actions to prevent complications). Common principles of teaching are summarised in Table 35.1. Principles of effective learning are summarised in Table 35.2.

An equal partnership encourages learning more readily than a relationship in which a teacher maintains ultimate control and authority. A teacher–learner relationship based on mutual sharing empowers and motivates an individual to learn. To foster mutual sharing in the learning process, first negotiate with the learner to establish learning needs and goals. Allow this negotiation to continue throughout the entire learning process as needs and goals change. Next, focus on the whole person by considering the learner's cognitive and developmental abilities, values, beliefs, feelings, experiences and learning style. Finally, the teacher–learner relationship should be interactive. The teacher and learner should both actively participate in the process and modify the teaching plan as they learn from one another.

Types of learning

There are several different types of learning. Learning the mathematical formula necessary to change pounds to

TABLE 35.1 Principles of teaching

Principle	Rationale
Know the subject.	To effectively teach children, you must be able not only to present material but also to answer questions about it. Children's questions can be as probing as an adult's and they can often be more frequent, because children are used to asking questions of a teacher or a parent.
Know the audience.	Children vary a great deal in cognitive development depending on their age group. To teach preschoolers about health, you might choose to teach how to brush teeth using puppets as a teaching aid. The same clever puppet and toothbrushing presentation would most likely be not well received among adolescents.
Know yourself.	Analyse which teaching techniques (lecture, role playing, small group discussion, audiovisual aids) fit your teaching style. Using techniques that are comfortable allows teaching to be most effective.
Assess individual learning styles.	Most children respond well to visual images (seeing a demonstration or drawing) to complement learning. Assessing individual learning styles helps to meet each child's best way of learning.
Define expected outcomes.	Expected outcomes serve as guidelines to help you select from all you know about a subject that part which is most pertinent to an individual child. They should be realistic, measurable and mutually established. Instructions on how to walk using crutches for an early school-age child would include how to carry school books while using crutches; for an adolescent, instruction might include how to board a bus so they can get to and from a part-time job.
Provide an environment conducive to learning.	Children are easily distracted from learning because of so many new experiences in their world. Divide material into segments to keep teaching sessions short; avoid competing factors such as television or mealtime.
Be consistent.	Nothing is more confusing to a person learning something for the first time than to be told two different ways to do it. Choose one method that should work best for a child and then consistently stress that method. After a child has learned the one method, then suggest alternative methods if the child is interested.
Be honest.	Abstract concepts such as "little white lies" cannot be understood by children younger than adolescents.
Recognise that actions teach as much as or sometimes more than verbal statements.	Children watch facial expressions and non-verbal gestures as much as they listen. Be certain that a non-verbal statement is not contradicting a verbal one.
Teach from the simple to the complex.	Fundamentals must be grasped before extensive learning can proceed. Many children have little idea of body anatomy. Often you need to begin with the basics; when these are mastered, you can proceed to teach about a disease condition.
Teach principles.	Teaching children the principle behind why they are doing something gives them reason to do it. It expands learning in that it allows children to modify and change to an alternative method as long as the principle is fulfilled.
Emphasise what the child should do; mention, but do not emphasise what the child should not do.	Teaching from a positive standpoint makes learning more enjoyable. Because healthcare information should last a lifetime, thinking of it in a positive way makes it applicable to lifetime use. However, children need to know both the do's and don'ts regarding health issues.
Include evaluation as a final step.	The only way to determine the effectiveness of teaching is to test or evaluate if learning has occurred. Structure the time and method of evaluation when first establishing a teaching plan.

kilograms, for example, is different from learning how to fill a syringe. Learning to be kind to a brother with a chronic illness is yet another type of education. Before you begin teaching, analyse the type of learning you want to see take place. This helps in setting goals and designing teaching strategies.

Cognitive learning

Cognitive learning involves a change in the individual's level of understanding or knowledge (Baskale & Bahar, 2011). Learning the principle behind why a particular medicine must be injected into a muscle, as opposed to subcutaneous tissue, is cognitive learning. Cognitive learning requires adequate development, intelligence and attention span. It can be gained through exposure to any teaching technique but is usually learned through lecture, reading and audiovisual aids. Techniques for teaching when cognitive learning is the goal must be based on the learner's cognitive ability (Singer, 2013). During the school-age years, learning capability is concrete (children have difficulty picturing body parts functioning unless they actually see them doing this); during the adolescent years,

TABLE 35.2 Principles of learning

Principle	Rationale
Learning occurs best when children are ready to learn.	Interferences with learning may be physical (e.g. pain or hunger) or psychological (e.g. fear or anxiety). The first time children are told that they must inject insulin daily, for example, they may be too anxious to learn about it.
Learning occurs most quickly if children can see how the new information will benefit them.	Sixteen-year-old children learn how to drive a car quickly because they grasp readily that being able to drive will immediately enlarge their world. Children are not ready to learn about insulin injections until they can see an advantage of giving them. Make a habit of including the benefit of learning in the introduction of learning.
Learning occurs best if rewards, not penalties, are offered.	Notice the amount of encouragement that sports coaches engage in (rewarding by praise). Giving positive reinforcement immediately like this makes it more effective than if such reinforcement is delayed. If you must criticise the way a task was done, first compliment children on some aspect they did well and then explain the part that needs improvement. This increases self-esteem and allows children to feel good enough about themselves so that they can accept the criticism. Never be reluctant to praise in public; always criticise in private.
Children learn best by actively participating in learning.	Active participation requires involvement in learning. Ask questions to involve participation; allow children to touch and handle equipment to increase participation.
Learning occurs best in a non-stressful and accepting environment.	No-one wants to take a chance redemonstrating a procedure or asking a question if they believe that actions or opinions will not be respected. People do learn from "top sergeants", but the learning experience has so many unpleasant memories attached to it that they may not retain the learning. Health teaching is too important to be presented in a way that will lead to its being quickly discarded.
Children learn best those things that hold a particular interest for them.	Everyone is more interested in some things than in others. A child with diabetes mellitus who enjoys dancing might be most interested in learning regulation of insulin for exercise; an adolescent anxious to leave for university might be most interested in selecting a diabetic diet from a cafeteria.
Learning ability plateaus.	Children learn to the point of saturation; learning and interest in learning halt at that point and do not continue until the material learned is thoroughly digested and understood. Wait until information is processed, and, at that point, the child will be interested once more.

it becomes possible to learn abstract concepts and children at that point can accept that liver enzymes are released with liver damage even though they never see that occur (Piaget, 1969).

Psychomotor learning

Psychomotor learning requires a change in a person's ability to perform a skill. Learning to hold a syringe, fill the syringe with medicine and inject it into a muscle is an example of psychomotor learning. Acquiring psychomotor skills depends on muscle and neurological coordination. It is mastered best through demonstration and repetition.

Affective learning

Affective learning involves a change in a person's attitude and is the most difficult area in which to bring about change. To teach a child the reason for and the skill of giving a self-injection, for example, may be easy; teaching the child to *like* giving a self-injection may never be possible. The best goal accomplished could be that the child will *value* the procedure because it will prevent them from developing hyperglycaemia. Affective learning is gained best through role modelling, role playing or shared-experience discussion.

Influence of age and stage on ability to learn

Learning ability varies a great deal depending on a child's stage of development and the past experiences the child has had in the specific area of learning.

The infant

Infants learn by exploring the environment with their senses (psychomotor learning). They learn best from a primary carer because that is whom infants most want to please. Few healthcare points are actually taught at this age. Any that are taught must be presented not as a structured activity but as a game or an amusing or attractive activity. For example, an infant could be encouraged to exercise their leg by hanging a ball near their foot.

The toddler

Toddlers are developing a sense of autonomy or learning to be independent (Erikson, 1993). Trying to teach toddlers a new activity such as eating a new food or brushing their teeth may be met with a sharp "No!" as children this age enjoy exerting their new independence. This response does not necessarily mean that the activity is unappealing to a child. Instead, it may be an indication that the child is aware they do not have to do everything they are asked to do.

Toddlers also sometimes resist a change in routine because they need rituals to feel secure. If an activity will allow children to increase a level of independent functioning, they will usually learn it rapidly. Teaching activities such as exercise or deep breathing by having children imitate the action is an effective teaching method because it presents the activity as a game (so there is nothing to be resisted). Parents can be instrumental in maintaining a new skill their child has learned by incorporating it into a daily routine or a ritual.

The preschooler

Preschool children are interested in learning, because developing a sense of initiative is the main developmental task of the period. Provided that instructions are geared to their small vocabularies, they "soak up" new methods of doing things. Because they are so imaginative and uninhibited, they have few reservations about the "right" way to do things. They will experiment with trial-and-error methods. They will both watch eagerly and freely demonstrate a skill. They ask many questions about equipment and procedures. Keep explanations short and words simple; a preschooler's attention span rarely exceeds 5 minutes.

In terms of cognitive development, preschool children "centre" or can learn only one characteristic of an object. This can limit their ability to learn all aspects of care or more than one method of doing something on any one day (Piaget, 1969).

Preschoolers tend to be frightened of intrusive procedures such as rectal temperature taking, bladder catheterisation or nasopharyngeal suction. They typically remove adhesive bandages minutes after application to check on the condition of their skin underneath (that it has not disappeared); they worry that any blood removed may be the last they have. Teaching this type of procedure or explaining to children why it is necessary calls for clear explanations and praise for learning. Use dolls or puppets to help children visualise details whenever possible, because pointing to a place on a puppet's body is not as intrusive as pointing to the child's own body. Parents are often most aware of the technique that will be best to motivate their child. Often, this begins with reading or telling a story about the problem.

The school-aged child

School-aged children enjoy short projects that offer an immediate reward. Therefore, they learn best if a procedure is broken down into different stages and presented as separate short procedures rather than one long one. Games can be an effective way to promote learning.

School-aged children are used to learning things and accept learning a new procedure or new information as just another experience in a busy day. The "staying power" of school-age children is notoriously short; the ability to continue to perform at the level taught tends to decrease sharply if learning is not reinforced. Be certain, therefore, that a backup person in the home knows the healthcare information as well as the child so that person can reinforce it or carry out a procedure if necessary.

Towards the end of the school-age period, children become interested in doing only those things their friends are also doing. Children may interpret as unreasonable, therefore, a request to do something after school (come home and take a medication). Modify a teaching plan as necessary to help children fit what they must learn into a school and social schedule. Otherwise, the teaching may be very short-lived.

As part of moral development, school-age children thrive on rules or the "right way" to do things (Kohlberg, 1984). This means that if two or more people are going to be involved in teaching, they must be consistent in their approach. It is frustrating for school-aged children to be shown two ways or not have a "right way" to do something. Parents who have been supervising their child's school learning through checking homework easily assume a role in supervising health learning. Parents who have not been monitoring learning previously may need support to fulfil this role.

The adolescent

Adolescents struggling for identity like to learn things separately from their parents. As a rule, they can be responsible for their own self-care; if they understand how the new actions they have been taught will directly benefit them, unlike school-age children, they will continue to carry those actions out conscientiously. Adolescents have a strong need to be exactly like their friends; they rarely continue any action that makes them different or conspicuous in front of their peers.

Remember that adolescents are present-oriented; they learn procedures and new information best if they can see how it will immediately benefit them. They also focus best on things they can do rather than on things they cannot do. They learn poorly if the only benefit of new information presented to them is something that will affect them at some future date. Rotating insulin injection sites, for example, prevents "pockmark" formations (*lipoatrophy*) in the skin when the person reaches approximately 30 years of age. Given this information, adolescents tend not to rotate injection sites because the benefit is not relevant to them at the moment. An explanation such as, "Rotating injection sites will ensure insulin absorption and allow you to play football this season" is a better adolescent motivator.

For the first time, adolescents are able to think abstractly or use scientific reasoning. This means they can create hypotheses ("what if" questions) and think through what will be the consequences of an action (Piaget, 1969). This allows them to understand the principle of what they are being taught and reinforces the reason for the learning. Parents may find they are not as effective with teaching their child as they were when the child was younger. They may need to "step aside" and let you introduce the subject until the phase of adolescent rebellion passes.

CASE STUDY QUESTION

5. You want to help James to increase his understanding of his condition. After teaching sessions, which statement from him would best show that his cognitive knowledge has improved?
   a. "I feel so much better now about the care that I need."
   b. "I understand that I have to take two types of medication."
   c. "I've finally learnt to use my inhaler."
   d. "I hate having to take medications but I will do it."

DEVELOPING AND IMPLEMENTING A TEACHING PLAN

A **teaching plan** is a design of the content to be taught and the teaching–learning techniques to be used. The first step in developing a teaching plan consists of assessing a child's current level of knowledge, ability and motivation to learn new knowledge.

Areas of assessment

Important areas for assessment include a child's current level of understanding; cognitive, physical, psychosocial aspects; and how the new knowledge will meld with the child's and family's lifestyle.

Language level

Assessing language development includes assessing both the child's spoken vocabulary (how well the child speaks) and comprehensive vocabulary (how many words the child understands). Most children have a comprehensive vocabulary well above their speaking one or can understand about three times the words they actually use. Assess "family vocabulary" or specific words the family uses. Be aware that if English is not a child's primary language, comprehensive vocabulary may not be greater than spoken vocabulary in English. Additional pictures, drawings or diagrams may be necessary to convey meaning (Weldon et al., 2014).

Child's current knowledge

Assessing how much a child currently knows about the health area in question helps to establish the needs and goals for the teaching plan. Current knowledge is in part developmentally based and in part experience based. Parents can tell you if a young child has had experience with the subject area. Some school-age children have had excellent anatomy and health classes as part of their science curriculum and are well aware of body organs. A helpful method of assessment, which promotes mutual sharing in the learning process, is asking children to list what they know about the health area on one side of a piece of paper and what they want to know more about on the opposite side. To reveal this type of information, young children can be asked to draw pictures of themselves, of someone with their illness or of a good thing to do to keep well.

Child's intellectual capability

In many instances, intellectual capability can be inferred from developmental milestones however, most children regress at least slightly with illness; what one would normally expect from a 10-year-old, therefore, may be impossible for an *ill* 10-year-old. Children with chronic illnesses may not have met developmental milestones because of their lack of experiences, not because they do not have the cognitive ability to learn.

Child's physical/cognitive capabilities

If a procedure that requires a certain level of psychomotor skill, such as medicine injection, will be necessary for care, assess a child's physical ability to perform the procedure. If you omit this step, the procedure will be frustrating because you will be asking a child to perform a skill above their capability. Assess vision and hearing ability and right- or left-hand dominance as well; these are important considerations for determining not only whether a child can accomplish procedures but also how the material will be presented.

Child's psychological or emotional capabilities

To learn best children need some motivation to learn or at least appreciate how their life will be improved through learning this new skill. It may be difficult for young children to grasp how the new skill will make them feel better. Some children are too ill or too exhausted or have too much pain to be ready for learning until these factors can be alleviated. With early hospital discharge, a great deal of health education may have to be delayed until the child has returned home and feels better.

Child's sociocultural values

Different cultures have different values related to good health. If a child from a family that values sports develops an illness that impairs the ability to run, for example, the family might consider the disability overwhelming. If the family believes that being able to write and read well are the keys to succeeding in life, the same leg impairment might be viewed as merely a minor complication. Study each family individually to determine which aspect of health will be most important to emphasise when teaching.

An important aspect of culture is whether children are raised in an environment where they are urged to be active participants in learning or whether they are encouraged to be "watchers". Male/female roles are also culturally determined. How long children are expected to be children (carefree, no responsibility) also varies from culture to culture. In a family where children are expected to be out working and contributing to the family income by the age of 15, a child might have a very different attitude towards learning a self-care activity than the same age child in a family where children are expected to remain non-contributing family members until after university.

Child's attention span

The attention span of children and their capability to comprehend concepts and perform psychomotor skills differ a great deal depending on individuality and age. In general, the younger the child, the shorter the attention span. This means you must use more "attention-getting" teaching to hold attention in younger children. Think about the clever puppet shows or animation children are exposed to today. Teaching that is not accompanied by these same attention-holding techniques needs to be very short to be effective.

Child's lifestyle

Lifestyle refers to the common pattern of a child's life. For example, a child who attends school daily and returns home every day at 4 p.m. has a fairly consistent lifestyle. A busy adolescent who works part-time, participates in several clubs after school and socialises on weekends may have a varied pattern of activity every day.

Knowing family patterns helps to plan the timing of such activities as medication administration or exercise or meal times. If both parents work during the day and do not return home until 6 p.m., medication may have to be administered after this time; exercises may have to be supervised in the evening, not the morning.

Teaching techniques

Teaching techniques vary with the content to be covered, teacher–learner characteristics and the environment for teaching.

Formal versus informal teaching

Both formal and informal teaching formats are used in health education. Careful assessment is necessary to determine which format would be the best technique for a given situation. An example of formal teaching would be conducting an in-service on healthy eating as part of a health education course. An example of informal teaching would be explaining to a child who refuses to eat that they need to at least drink something because their body needs more fluids to get better. Sometimes informal teaching occurs so spontaneously that it is easy to be unaware of it. It may occur, for example, in response to a question such as, "How long will I have to take this medicine?" If you answer, "For 2 weeks," that is just answering a question. If you answer, "For 2 weeks because . . . ," that is teaching. Table 35.3 lists suggestions for incorporating informal teaching into care.

Group versus individual teaching

Although most health teaching is done on an individual basis, teaching groups of children is common in some situations. Individual instruction more directly addresses a child's unique needs; group teaching can meet individual needs while adding depth to learning as children discuss information within

TABLE 35.3 Ways to incorporate informal teaching into care

Activity	Type of teaching
Medication administration	Children as young as early school age should know the type and action and any expected side effects of all medication they are taking. Present medicine not by saying, "Here is your pill" but "Here is your [name of medication], medicine to help your temperature come back to normal. After you take this, you might feel yourself start to sweat. That means it's working."
Vital sign measurement	When taking vital signs such as blood pressure, temperature and pulse, tell children what normal levels are: "Your blood pressure is 100/70. That's normal." If the child is in a high-risk category for hypertension, add some prevention measures to teaching.
Any procedure	Always tell children the purpose and principle of procedures, not "You need to drink a lot of fluid," but "You need to drink a lot of fluid because . . ."
Dressing changes	Dressing changes provide an opportunity to teach the danger of introducing infection into an open wound. The parents or child may not change this dressing, but they will apply bandages to small cuts in the future and so will benefit from teaching.
Mealtime	Provide information about nutrition: "I know you're not hungry enough to eat the entire sandwich, but could you try the meat? Meat is high in protein and that's important for healing."
Hygiene	Emphasise the necessity of good perineal hygiene to decrease the possibility of urinary tract infection.
Physical assessment	Explain aspects of testicular self-examination and describe "normal" findings as both education and reassurance.
Positioning	Teach the hazards of immobility and how change of position and ambulation increase circulation and respiratory function.
Sleep	Teach that sleep is a healing therapy and should not be considered a waste of time.
Bowel elimination	Teach children that elimination patterns vary; occasional variations in their elimination patterns are normal.

the group. For many children, hearing that they are not the only person with their problem is comforting. Hearing another child discuss how to solve a problem may be more meaningful than hearing the same information from an adult. Peer learning in this way, therefore, not only improves knowledge but may also improve children's attitude and motivation to learn (Deibel & Wagner, 2013).

Home versus institutional teaching

Health teaching is just as important in the home as it is in a healthcare, school or community setting. Teaching in the healthcare system usually focuses on immediate acute care concerns. Teaching in the school setting may focus on topics such as basic health promotion and hygiene, reproductive and sex education, and drug prevention. Teaching in the home may focus on medication regimens, dressing changes or measures to prevent complications of a particular illness. It may also involve helping a child and parents adapt a procedure to the home setting, such as accommodating a wheelchair at home. Be sure parents have obtained the supplies they will need to learn and perform the procedure in the home.

> ***What if....***
>
> You organise a discussion group for adolescents on special diets so they can learn more about nutrition in general? James, who needs to follow a low cholesterol diet, says he won't participate in the group because nutrition is "boring". Would you insist that he comes to the meetings or take some extra time to provide him with the information at his bedside?

Determining teaching strategies

Because children's knowledge base, capabilities, learning styles and attention spans vary, teaching strategies are most effective when they are intermixed and when they are selected in response to the individual situation and child to be taught. The more interactive the method, the more appealing it might be to a particular child. Engaging parents and carers is essential to the success of any family-centred teaching program (see Box 35.2).

Lecture

Directly explaining information is the most efficient and time-saving method of offering information to both individual children and groups. This strategy, however, does not allow for much participation and it is effective only in short, well-structured periods. It is rarely effective for children who are not yet school-age.

Demonstration

Demonstration is actually performing a procedure such as a dressing change or administration of eye drops so the child can see clearly how the procedure should be done. Do not demonstrate a procedure unless you have all the necessary

> **BOX 35.2 * Educating parents**
>
> It is important to note that the parents/carers must be included in the development and implementation of any family-centred teaching plan for infants, toddlers, preschool and school-aged children. Parents and carers know their children best and can provide you with valuable information about the child's developmental stage, temperament and preferences. They will also be required to supervise and reinforce any learnt health behaviours on a long-term basis in the home environment. It is good practice to ensure that at least one adult in the household has the necessary information and can perform the required skill. If possible, allowing for cultural practices that may dictate child-care responsibilities within the family, allow the child to choose who this person will be. This person then needs to be provided with as much education as the child.

equipment to do it. If you stop in the middle of a demonstration to say, "Be sure to use a sterile syringe, not what I'm using", the poor technique demonstrated may be the lesson learned, not the good technique. The purpose of demonstration is to show how the procedure actually is done; having to imagine steps is little different to reading about it. School-age children, because of their stage of cognitive development (concrete operations), learn best by demonstration.

Discussion

Discussion is a shared learning experience in which children ask questions about particular concerns and these are answered based on their individual circumstances, or children are asked questions about some problem, such as how they anticipate managing some aspect of care and together the problem is solved. At the beginning of health education, children tend to ask few questions because they do not know enough about an illness or health issue to anticipate concerns. As their knowledge increases, so does their ability to project and modify information to fit their own lifestyle. Remember that children tend to think in the present: a problem that will arise once tomorrow is usually more important to a child than one that can be predicted to arise repeatedly in years to come. Because it recognises and respects their opinions, younger children and adolescents enjoy discussion.

Role modelling

Role modelling is demonstrating a certain attitude or behaviour you want a child to learn. Be certain when health teaching not only to present facts but also to radiate a positive attitude. Showing frustration at getting a bubble out of medicine in a syringe demonstrates, for example, that giving injections is frustrating; showing a bored attitude towards nutrition instructions implies that nutrition information is boring. The child picks up the role modelling cues as readily as the spoken message.

Behaviour therapy

Typically, learning occurs best with **positive reinforcement** (a child tries to understand a new procedure, is praised for the effort and tries even harder). **Behaviour therapy**, also called *behaviour modification,* is a term used for a system aimed at *modifying* behaviour that interferes with healthy functioning. It was originally designed to help people who are cognitively challenged modify socially unacceptable behaviour. Currently it has many uses, such as controlling disruptive classroom behaviour. The basic premise of behaviour modification is that a child is rewarded for healthy behaviour, whereas unhealthy behaviour is ignored or unrewarded. For example, a cognitively challenged child may have a socially unacceptable habit of constantly rocking back and forth. The child is not scolded or criticised for rocking, but the action is ignored. On the other hand, preferred behaviour (sitting for 5 minutes without rocking) is praised. As another example, a child might be ignored for being a picky eater, then praised for the few bites he does eat well. Children respond best to behaviour modification if, in addition to praise, they receive a tangible reward such as a star on a chart or an extra privilege of some sort for good behaviour.

A behaviour modification program should be discussed with the child before it is begun, because no behaviour can be modified, just as no new behaviour can be learned, until a child truly wants a change to occur. It might be necessary to ask older children to sign a learning contract to be certain that both teacher and learner agree on the method to be used. Many older children are able to use self-rewards to reinforce a behaviour modification program such as rewarding themselves by playing a computer game or going to a movie after an afternoon of efficient studying or an hour of doing breathing exercises.

Behaviour modification is a technique that must be used with common sense and concern so that children are not being manipulated more than they are being helped to achieve a healthy lifestyle. It is a legitimate device to use in helping a child with attention deficit/hyperactivity disorder sit still long enough to eat a meal or learn at school. It can be helpful in encouraging children to do as much self-care as possible or discourage disorders such as obsessive compulsive behaviour (May et al., 2012).

Selecting teaching tools

Teaching tools are the mechanical devices used to present content. They vary based on content, teacher–learner characteristics and environment.

Visual aids

"A picture is worth a thousand words" is not an idle quotation but a realistic one. Because small children know little about their bodies or where body organs are located, using visual aids such as drawings or photographs of anatomy can be very helpful (see Fig. 35.1).

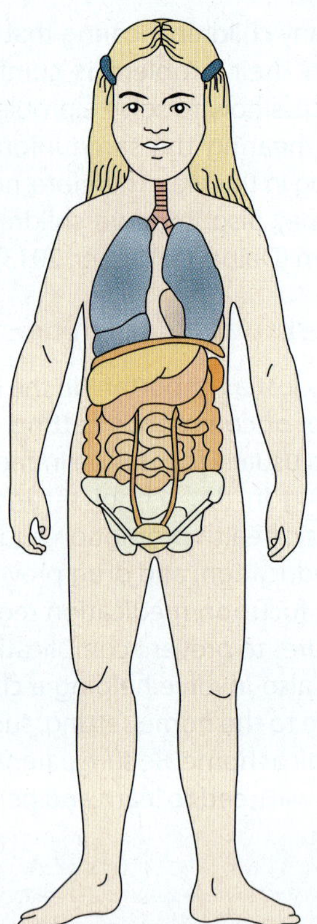

FIGURE 35.1 Anatomical drawings are helpful to illustrate basic health education topics and healthcare procedures.

Pamphlets

Pamphlets are helpful teaching aids with school-age children, adolescents and parents (Pile, 2013). They usually contain brief, easy to read, easily understood information and are often cleverly illustrated with cartoon characters to make them enjoyable. Be certain to read any pamphlet before offering it to a child to make sure the information included in it is accurate. Medical advances are made so quickly that a 1-year-old pamphlet may contain inaccuracies in the light of subsequent knowledge.

Learning games

For memorising certain kinds of information, such as what foods are high or low in potassium or sodium, flashcards are a helpful learning tool. Many children enjoy playing trivia-type board games. Instead of the usual categories of information, make up new cards with questions such as, "Where is insulin produced in your body?" If the child can answer the question correctly, a token is allowed to advance a designated number of spaces on the board. Children learn information quickly in this way because the reward for learning is so immediate. Having parents play the game with their child educates the parents at the same time.

Computers and DVDs

Most children are exposed to computers, tablets and/or smart phones in the home, and these devices are easily accessed in most healthcare facilities. They can be used to show short clips and PowerPoint presentations as part of a health education program. Viewing these can give children a sense of power in that the program seems to be talking directly to them. They can also be used over and over again to refresh children's knowledge of the steps they need to take to remain well (Crawford et al., 2012). It is important to view and assess the material first before showing it. In particular, be certain to check that the vocabulary used is appropriate for an individual child or family. The internet can also be a useful source of information for children and their families. However, they need to be warned that not all the information they find will be reliable.

Puppets and dolls and play

Many children are shy about talking to strangers; this shyness, in addition to their concerns about what will happen to them, may make it difficult for them to discuss or explain what they know about their health, illness or intended surgery. However, they may be able to relate to an uncritical puppet or doll because they see this as a usual part of play. Preschool children are particularly receptive to these techniques (Meghan, 2012) (see Fig. 35.2).

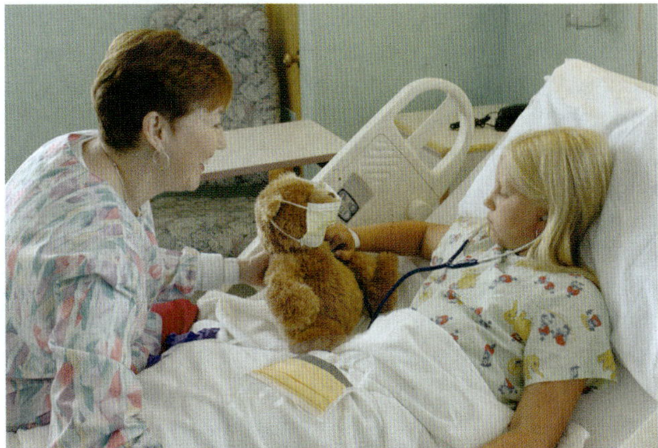

FIGURE 35.2 Teaching with dolls or toys can help to make an intrusive procedure seem less frightening for a preschooler.

Evaluating the effectiveness of teaching

Evaluation or assessing whether teaching has been effective is the final step in the teaching process. Evaluation should occur not only after the teaching plan has been implemented, but also throughout the entire learning process. This continuous evaluation helps both the teacher and the learner to modify the teaching plan to better meet changing needs. Demonstration of a change in behaviour or attitude is the best indication that learning has occurred.

CASE STUDY QUESTION

6. You want to teach James more about his asthma and he has expressed a preference for video clips. In order to ensure that any such materials are safe, age-appropriate and accurate, you should do which of the following?
   a. Preview any potential materials before referring them to James
   b. Encourage James to search YouTube and then report back to you
   c. Tell James that written materials are usually better than video materials
   d. Refer James to his local public or school library and have him liaise with a librarian

HEALTH TEACHING FOR A SURGICAL EXPERIENCE

Teaching to prepare a child for surgery is an example of teaching that requires planning for several stages of learning. The child and the child's parents often feel anxious about surgery because this is always a potentially frightening experience, so teaching must first address this anxiety. Such preparation differs according to the type of surgery being performed, but certain activities apply to all surgery and all children. Psychological preparation of both child and parents is aimed at reducing a child's fears about the procedure and consists primarily of providing health teaching and opportunities for therapeutic play. Physical preparation includes providing for restrictions on food and fluid intake before surgery, preparing the incision site on the child's skin and arranging for transportation of the child to surgery. Because many children's surgical procedures are done on an ambulatory basis, preparation must also include informing parents about the details of the preparation techniques, the surgery, the postoperative period and the steps they must take towards preparation.

Assessing current level of knowledge

On admission to a surgical ward or day surgery unit, discuss with parents the preparation they have made for this experience and what specifically they have told a child about what will happen. It is good to ask whether a child's concerns about the experience seem more or less than the parents had anticipated. Is the child emotionally prepared?

Emotional preparation

Preparing a child emotionally for surgery requires minimising fears common to all children such as fear of separation, fear of mutilation or fear of death. This can be accomplished by telling a child about the procedure and describing any specific equipment and techniques that will be used, such as anaesthetic, eye bandages, nasogastric tubes, sutures or special aftercare. Most children requiring surgery will be administered a general anaesthetic as they are likely to find procedures done under local or regional anaesthetic to be too frightening and will therefore be unable to cooperate adequately during the procedure. Be certain all preparation is appropriate to the child's age. A recent systematic review found that more detailed and formal preoperative education is most effective in children above the age of four (Copanitsanou & Valkeapää, 2014).

It is important to discuss preparations for surgery such as coming for blood tests and not eating the morning of surgery. If the child is to have a general anaesthetic, it is important to emphasise that anaesthetised sleep is "special" sleep. Otherwise, toddlers or preschoolers may be reluctant to fall asleep after surgery for fear people will come and do strange things to them. The surgery procedure should be discussed but minimised. "After you're asleep, the doctor will fix your tummy. You won't feel anything because of the special sleep. When you wake up, you'll be in a room called a recovery room where you'll stay until you are wide awake". Be honest concerning pain: "Your tummy will feel sore afterward, but I'll give you something to make it feel better" is a fair statement.

It is important to alert children that nurses and doctors in the operating theatre wear surgical masks. Assure toddlers and preschoolers that the persons behind the masks are doctors and nurses, some of whom the child has probably already met.

What to expect in the recovery room should also be included in preparation for surgery. In most cases, a parent will be able to be with the child during this period. Explain post-surgery items, such as the use of oxygen, monitors, bedpans, bandages or intravenous equipment (see Fig. 35.3). Furnishing a doll with such equipment is especially helpful in preparing younger children. Older children may benefit from being taken to a surgical ward so that they can see what to expect first hand. After surgery, be certain to evaluate whether a child's preparation was adequate, both to document that the experience caused as little distress to the child as possible and to evaluate your expertise in teaching children.

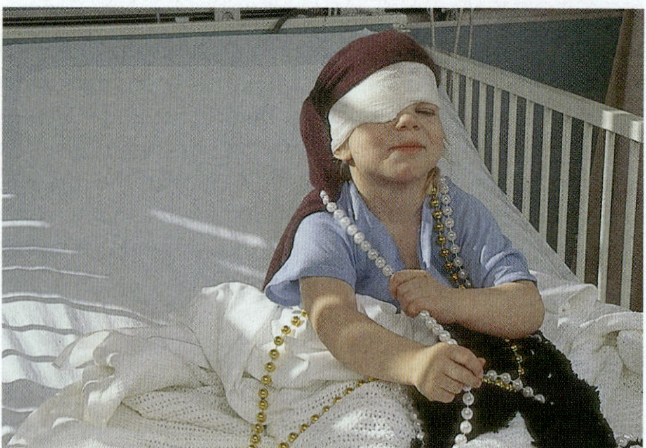

FIGURE 35.3 Pretending to be a pirate helps this young child prepare for having to wear an eye patch after surgery.

CASE STUDY QUESTION

7. You need to teach Nathan, aged 3, how to perform the hand exercises he will need to do post-operatively. When collaborating with the physiotherapist, which technique would be likely to be the most effective?
   a. A pamphlet that you read together
   b. A lecture from a sporting hero
   c. Playing a game of Simon Says
   d. A group discussion on hand pain

Physical preparation

Most children will be placed "Nil by Mouth" (NBM) prior to surgery. The length of time a child will remain NBM depends on the child's age. For example, adolescents and school-aged children may be restricted from taking food or fluids from midnight until the time of surgery the following morning; however, this may be reduced to as little as 4 hours for infants younger than 6 months.

Implementing the plan

Check children's identification bands to ensure they are legible and secure before the child is transported to surgery. If not, replace or secure them before surgery. Immediately before transport, check the mouth for loose teeth (particularly in children aged 6, 7 and 8 years, who are losing their central and lateral incisors). Braces do not need to be removed. Make certain the anaesthetist knows about any loose teeth before an airway for surgery is inserted (a loose tooth could be knocked totally free and aspirated during the procedure).

Preschoolers may enjoy taking a favourite toy or blanket to surgery with them. Ideally, they should be allowed to keep this with them until they are under an anaesthetic. It is standard practice in Australia and New Zealand for a parent to accompany their child into the operating theatre and remain with them until the anaesthetic has been administered. This has been found to reduce some of the fear associated with unfamiliar environment and procedures (Matziou, Chrysostomou & Perdikaris, 2013). Exceptions may include babies under 6 months of age and emergency surgery. Check your local policy and/or with the anaesthetist before telling a parent that they will be able to accompany their child to theatre.

Key points for review

- Communication is the exchange of ideas between two or more persons. It can be verbal or non-verbal.
- Therapeutic communication is a planned interaction, has structure and is constructive. Non-therapeutic communication lacks deliberate purpose other than socialising.
- Successful communication requires an encoder, a code, a decoder and feedback or response.
- Typical methods of non-verbal communication are using distance, gestures, body posture and gait, touch, use of drawings and empathy.
- Techniques that encourage therapeutic communication are attentive listening, open-ended questions, reflecting,

clarifying, paraphrasing, perception checking, focusing, supportive statements and silence.

- Some situations require special communication techniques such as interacting with demanding or shy children, children who are visually or hearing impaired or children from non-English speaking backgrounds.
- There are three types of learning: cognitive, psychomotor and affective. For something to be learned well, all of these areas may need to be involved.
- To individualise a teaching program for a child, assess the child's attention span, cognitive or intellectual capability and lifestyle, and learning style.
- The format and strategies of teaching used with children vary depending on a child's age and developmental level. Various types to consider are formal versus informal, single or group teaching, lecture, discussion and role playing.
- Behaviour modification is a special technique aimed at modifying some form of behaviour that interferes with good health.

CASE STUDY QUESTION

8. Nathan is scheduled for surgery next week and his mother, Linda has stated that she does not want to accompany him to theatre or be with him in recovery because she "won't be able to bear to see him upset or in pain. It will be better for him if I am not there". How would you respond to this and why?

Resources

For an extensive range of additional resources to enhance teaching and learning and to facilitate understanding of this chapter, please see the text's accompanying website located on thePoint at http://thepoint.lww.com.

References

Arnold, E. C. (2011). Theoretical perspectives and contemporary dynamics. In E.C. Arnold & U.K. Boggs (Eds.), *Interpersonal Relationships: Professional Communication Skills for Nurses* (6th ed., pp. 1–21). Philadelphia: Elsevier/Saunders.

Baskale, H. & Bahar, Z. (2011). Outcomes of nutrition knowledge and healthy food choices in 5-to 6- year old children who received a nutrition intervention based on Piaget's theory. *Journal for Specialists in Paediatric Nursing*, *16*(4), 263–279.

Copanitsanou, P. & Valkeapää, K. (2014). Effects of education of paediatric patients undergoing elective surgical procedures on their anxiety: A systematic review. *Journal of Clinical Nursing*, *23*(7/8), 940–954.

Coplan, R. J., Rose-Krasnor, L., Weeks, M., et al. (2013). Alone in a crowd: Social motivations, social withdrawal, and socioemotional functioning in later childhood. *Developmental Psychology*, *49*(5), 861–875.

Crawford, D., Texter, T., Hurt, K., et al. (2012). Traditional nurse instruction versus 2 session nurse instruction plus DVD for teaching ostomy care. *Journal of Wound, Ostomy and Continence Nursing*, *39*(5), 529–537.

Cruz, I., Quittner, A. L., Marker, C., et al. (2013). Identification of effective strategies to promote language in deaf children with cochlear implants. *Child Development*, *84*(2), 543–559.

Decarlo, D. K., McGwin, G. Jr., Bixler, M. L., et al. (2012). Impact of pediatric vision impairment on daily life: Results of focus groups. *Optometry and Vision Science*, *89*(9), 1409–1416.

Deibel, M. D. & Wagner, M. J. (2013). Small group discussion skills. In R. L. Rogers, A. Mattu, M. Winters, et al. (Eds.), *Practical Teaching in Emergency Medicine* (pp. 180–191). Hokoben, NJ: Wiley-Blackwell.

Erikson, E. H. (1993). *Childhood and Society.* New York: W. W. Norton.

Forchuk, C. (2010). Communication and the therapeutic relationship. In W. Austin & M. A. Boyd (Eds.), *Psychiatric Mental Health Nursing for Canadian Practice* (2nd ed.). Philadelphia: Lippincott Williams & Wilkins.

Hee, H. I., Lim, E. H., Tan, Q. C., et al. (2012). Effect of preoperative education on behaviour of children during induction of anaesthesia: A randomised controlled trial of efficacy. *Anasthesia & Intensive Care*, *40*(5), 795–802.

Johnson, N., Lashley, J., Stonek, A. V., et al. (2012). Children with developmental disabilities at a pediatric hospital: Staff education to prevent and manage challenging behaviours. *Journal of Pediatric Nursing*, *27*(6), 742–749.

Kirk, K. I., Prusick, L., French, B., et al. (2012). Assessing spoken word recognition in children who are deaf or hard of hearing: A translational approach. *Journal of the American Academy of Audiology*, *23*(6), 464–475.

Kohlberg, L. (1984). *The Psychology of Moral Development.* New York: Harper & Row.

Levine, D. A. (2011). Growth and development. In K. J. Marcdante, R. M. Kliefman, H. B. Jenson, et al. (Eds.), *Nelson Essentials of Pediatrics* (6th ed., pp 13–44). Philadelphia: Saunders/Elsevier.

McMillan, L. R. & Shannon, D. (2011). Program evaluation of nursing school instruction in measuring students' perceived competence to empathetically communicate with patients. *Nursing Education Perspectives*, *32*(3), 139–143.

Matziou, V., Chrysostomou, A. & Perdikaris, E. V. P. (2013). Parental presence and distraction during painful childhood procedures. *British Journal of Nursing*, *22*(5), 470–475.

May, A. C., Rudy, B. M., Davis, T. E., et al. (2012). Evidence-based behavioural treatment of dog phobia with young children: Two examples. *Behaviour Modification*, *37*(1), 143–160.

Meghan, L. (2012). Children at play: An innovative method for studying and teaching nutritional behaviours. *Pediatric Nursing*, *38*(3), 139–143.

Munjal, S. K., Panda, N. K. & Patchak, A. (2010). Dynamics of hearing status in closed head injury. *Journal of Neurotrauma*, *27*(2), 309–316.

Olino, T, M., Durbin, C. E., Klein, D. N., et al. (2013). Gender differences in young children's temperament traits: Comparisons across observational and parent-report methods. *Journal of Personality*, *8*(12), 119–129.

Piaget, J. (1969). *The Origins of Intelligence in Children.* New York: International Universities Press.

Pile, D. (2013). Does using an asthma prompting form improve asthma care in a pediatric office? *Journal of Pediatric Nursing*, *28*(3), 275–281.

Singer, B. (2013). Perceptions of school nurses in the care of students with disabilities. *Journal of School Nursing*, *29*(5), 329–336.

Svavarsdottir, E. K., Tryggvadottir, G. B. & Sigurdardottir, A. O. (2012). Knowledge translation in family nursing: Does a short-term therapeutic conversation intervention benefit families of children and adolescents in a hospital setting? *Journal of Family Nursing*, *18*(3), 303–327.

Taylor, S. P., Nicolle, C. & Maguire, M. (2013). Cross-cultural communication barriers in health care. *Nursing Standard*, *27*(31), 35–43.

Weldon, J. M., Langan, K., Miedema, F., et al. (2014). Special needs populations: Overcoming barriers for pediatric surgical patients and their family members. *AORN*, *99*(5), 616–629.

Williams, C. (2012). Promoting vocabulary learning in young children who are deaf or hard of hearing: Translating research into practice. *American Annals of the Deaf*, *156*(5), 501–508.

Yang, C. & Chen, C. M. (2012). Effects of post-discharge telephone calls on the rate of emergency department visits in paediatric patients. *Journal of Paediatric and Child Health*, *48*(10), 931–935.

Suggested readings

Brown, A. B. & Elder, J. H. (2014). Communication in autism spectrum disorder: A guide for pediatric nurses. *Pediatric Nursing*, *40*(5), 219–225.

Campos, D. (2011). *Jump Start Health! Practical Ideas to Promote Wellness in Kids of All Ages*. New York: Teachers College Press.

Davis, D. W., Gordon, M. K. & Burns, B. M. (2011). Educational interventions for childhood asthma; a review and integrative model for preschoolers from low-income families. *Paediatric Nursing*, *37*(1), 31–38.

Fisher, M. J. & Broome, M. E. (2011). Parent-provider communication during hospitalisation. *Journal of Pediatric Nursing*, *26*, 58–69.

Kelo, M., Martikainen, M. & Eriksson, E. (2013). Patient education of children and their families: Nurses' experiences. *Pediatric Nursing*, *39*(2), 71–79.

Nabors, L., Bush, A., Buchanon, R., et al. (2011). Preschoolers knowledge about hospital and emergency equipment and care. *Issues in Comprehensive Pediatric Nursing*, *34*, 131–143.

Unit 6

The nursing role in supporting the health of ill children and their families

Chapter 36

Nursing care of a family with an ill child

Previous chapters described the normal growth and development of children and their special needs at each stage of development. This chapter adds information about the additional needs of children when they become ill. Such information builds a base for nursing care and health teaching.

LEARNING OBJECTIVES

After studying the contents of this chapter, you should be able to:

1. Describe illness and illness experiences as they may appear to children.
2. Use critical thinking to analyse ways in which illness care can be made more family-centred, culturally safe and less traumatic for children.
3. Assess the impact of an illness, especially one requiring a hospital stay, on a child.
4. Establish expected outcomes for an ill child.
5. Plan nursing care to reduce the stress of illness, such as helping parents plan for ambulatory care or hospitalisation.
6. Implement measures such as orientation, education and therapeutic play to reduce the stress of illness.
7. Evaluate expected outcomes for achievement and effectiveness of care.
8. Identify areas related to illness in children that could benefit from additional nursing research or application of evidence-based practice.
9. Integrate knowledge about a child's response to illness with the nursing process to achieve quality child and family health nursing care.

KEY TERMS

- kilojoule counting
- play therapy
- primary nursing/case management nursing
- sensory deprivation
- sensory overload
- separation anxiety
- sleep deprivation
- therapeutic play

CASE STUDY

Becky is a 7-year-old who burned her foot in a campfire accident. She is going to be admitted to the hospital for 1-day surgery to have the wound debrided. Becky's parents tell you that Becky "hasn't been herself" since the injury. She has reverted to temper tantrums and sulking, more like a 3-year-old than one of primary school-age. Even though she has been told eating meat is important because it provides protein for healing, she refuses to eat anything but jelly or soup. In the admission ward of the hospital, she picked up a doll and twisted its leg off. "How can we get our old daughter back again?" her mother asks you.

CASE STUDY QUESTIONS

1. Becky is obviously showing some effects of her accident. What type of additional explanation might be helpful to her?
2. What advice would you give her mother to help her better prepare Becky for the upcoming debridement procedure?

Many illnesses that require the attention of healthcare professionals are outside the usual occurrences of childhood, so most children typically have little knowledge about them. Helping a child and family prepare for or adjust to such an experience is a fundamental nursing role. This role goes well beyond just providing information on what to expect throughout an illness. It involves providing emotional support as well.

Gordon, (2012) identified in her research the benefits of preparation for hospitalisation for children and their families and carers and suggested that inclusive models of healthcare and collaboration in healthcare settings are necessary. As well Gordon (2012) argues that transformational approaches to leadership to engage staff and facilitate person-centred ways of working together will improve preparation for childhood hospitalisation. Upon hospitalisation it is most important for the child's voice to be heard. A study by Livesley and Long (2013) found that children's voices were often not heard on the ward and if they were it was seen as a challenge by staff. Quiet, sick and shy children who were alone were most likely to have their needs overlooked. Livesley and Long (2013) maintain that a more inclusive and participatory model of nursing care is needed. Alternatively nurses can help families establish a therapeutic environment for the care of an ill child at home. For individual families, nurses can perform several interventions that promote comfort, safety, security and continued growth and development. Therapeutic play is one of the more powerful tools available to a nurse working towards this objective.

NURSING AN ILL CHILD

Assessment

The ill child requires accurate assessment, observation and monitoring. Children's hospitals in Australia and New Zealand provide guidelines for the care of the ill child. The Royal Children's Hospital Melbourne provides Clinical Guidelines for the observation and continuous monitoring of sick children. These include estimation of haemoglobin-oxygen saturation (SpO2, pulse oximetry), oxygen therapy, respiratory rate, heart/pulse rate, blood pressure (systolic, diastolic and mean), temperature (including measurement method), sedation and pain. In certain clinical circumstances further observations (for example neurological) may be required (Royal Children's Hospital Melbourne, 2012). In NSW the Medical Emergency Team (MET) aims to detect changes in the seriously ill child's condition to allow intervention before a cardiac arrest occurs. This team consists of an intensive care doctor, a senior intensive care nurse and a medical registrar who have advanced resuscitation skills and are on call 24 hours a day seven days a week. Staff refers to criteria relating to changes in the child's airway, breathing, circulation, neurology and any matter that the staff member is worried about that does not fit the criteria. If an emergency response is triggered the MET team will assess the child. Recently New South Wales Health has introduced "Between the Flags" which builds on the MET system concept, in an attempt to identify deteriorating patients before they reach MET calling criteria (NSW Health, 2012).

NSW Health (2011) has produced Clinical Guidelines for the recognition of a sick baby or child in the emergency department. These Guidelines are aimed at providing the highest level of paediatric care and are to be used to guide the health professional in their clinical decision making. A structured, continuous and dynamic assessment of the baby or child must be undertaken. The Standard Paediatric Observation Chart (SPOC) is colour coded and developed by expert clinicians. Sensitive indicators enable the doctor or nurse to identify when the baby or child's condition is deteriorating.

Middleton (2012), in an interview about signs indicating that a child is seriously ill, maintains that the first impressions of the child are really important such as, is the child interacting with their parents and taking notice of their surroundings? He makes the point that a structured assessment of specific symptoms using a system such as the ABCDE method is essential. This refers to airway, breathing, circulation, disability and exposure where a thorough assessment of the child from head to toe is carried out.

Where an emergency does not exist an assessment of the ill child should begin with an interview of the child and parents to identify ways they think the illness will change their lives. This could include a wide range of situations such as increased expenses, changes in schedules to visit or stay with a hospitalised child, the need for one parent to take leave from work to care for an ill child at home, the need to schedule frequent ambulatory visits, consultation to handle body image changes and the need to arrange for childcare for other children. Because these needs change as the course of an illness changes, assessment must be ongoing.

Nursing considerations

Nursing considerations vary greatly depending on the extent of a child's illness, the care needed and the age of a child. Needs to be addressed with families of children seen in ambulatory and in-hospital settings include:

- Health-seeking behaviours related to lack of knowledge regarding illness
- Anxiety related to pending hospital admission
- Risk of social isolation related to hospitalisation
- Fear related to being away from home for the first time
- Activity intolerance related to fatigue from illness
- Potential for injury related to high-tech equipment.

Kearvell and Grant (2010) believe that hospitalisation and ill health can interrupt the natural attachment process between mother and infant. A review of the literature on how nurses can support mother-infant attachment in the neonatal intensive care unit found that kangaroo care, breastfeeding and participation in routine care was found to enhance the mother's role including feelings of closeness, confidence and inclusion. Further it was found that nurses who provided psychosocial care by communicating and engaging with mothers assisted them in developing positive and trusting relationships alleviating the mother's anxiety and improving her confidence interacting with her sick infant.

Planning for the care of an ill child requires consideration of all aspects of the child's and family's life: financial, social and personal. When children become ill, many of their needs, such as those for nutrition, play and family support, change. If a child will need long-term care or hospitalisation, the entire family may find their priorities changing. Unless these changing needs are examined, recognised and met, a child may achieve physical wellness again but not mental or emotional health. A family may be left severely disadvantaged. Identifying additional needs in this way and putting in place necessary services or interventions is an important nursing role. Children's hospitals in Australia and New Zealand provide information and support for hospitalised children and their parents or carers. The Sydney Children's Hospital provides information on their website about preparing the child for hospital and support services for children and families. (Sydney Children's Hospital, 2013). The Wellington Children's Hospital "Just for Kids" website in New Zealand provides information to support hospitalised children and their families or carers who are encouraged to share a story about their experiences in hospital to assist children who will soon be admitted to hospital (Wellington Children's Hospital, 2014). The Royal Children's Hospital Melbourne, has information about preparing your child for hospital and a guide for parents/carers (Royal Children's Hospital Melbourne, 2010). The Association for the Wellbeing of Children in Healthcare provides hospital familiarisation programs designed to prepare preschool children for hospital (Association for the Wellbeing of Children in Healthcare, 2014) Information about the hospitalisation of children can also be accessed at the following website: <www.starship.org.nz/patients-and-families/your-childs-hospital-or-daystay-admission>.

Five differences that may occur with children with all illnesses are: (a) experiencing harm or injury, such as physical discomfort, pain, mutilation and death; (b) being separated from routines, parents, peers and respected adults; (c) facing the unknown (new and strange sights and sounds and happenings); (d) facing uncertain limits (unclear definition of acceptable and expected behaviour); and (e) experiencing a loss of control (loss of competence or loss of the ability to make decisions).

Being aware of these potential problems is important to guard against those that are preventable and to reduce a child's anxiety associated with those that cannot be prevented (such as facing new sights and sounds). Discussing these differences with older children is important so that implementations to reduce their impact can be tailored to each child. Reading to a child, role playing and puppetry are all useful techniques for reducing the number of new experiences and easing the impact on the child. Be certain that the techniques you use are appropriate not only for a child's age and development but also for the child's individual learning style and level of illness. Be certain that children participate in making any decision that is age and developmentally appropriate for them.

Evaluation of expected outcomes for ill children should include specific measures such as whether discomfort was kept to a minimum during the experience. Indicators to evaluate outcomes that are long-term should include whether children were able to return to usual behaviours after the experience. The following are examples that suggest achievement of outcomes regarding a hospital experience:

- Parents state their level of anxiety regarding hospitalisation of their infant is now at a tolerable level
- Parents have effectively changed work schedules to be able to stay with their child in the hospital
- Separation anxiety in a toddler is minimised by parental involvement in their care.

THE MEANING OF ILLNESS TO CHILDREN

The response of children to illness depends on their cognitive ability, past experiences and level of knowledge. From primary school-age, children generally know quite a bit about the workings of their major body parts. As a general guideline, primary school children are usually able to name the function of the heart, lungs and stomach. They may not be able to do that for the bowel, kidneys or bladder. This reflects the difficulty some parents have in discussing these body parts with their children.

Younger children may think the cause of illness is magical (no one knows where it comes from) or that it occurs as a consequence of breaking a rule, such as walking in the rain or eating sweets after school. With this perspective, they may also think that getting well again is possible only if they follow another set of rules, such as staying in bed and taking medicine. By Year 4, children are generally aware of the role that germs play in illness but may mistakenly think that all illness is caused by germs. Because of this, they may see a passive role for themselves in getting well, because illness comes from outside influences. At about Year 8, children are able to voice an understanding that illness can occur from several causes, such as being susceptible to chickenpox because they did not get the vaccine or knowing that by their actions they carelessly caused an accident. Once they understand this, they can take an active role in getting better. These concepts parallel cognitive development (see Chapter 28).

Knowing how children of each age group view illness affects the planning of nursing care, influencing how explanations should be worded. For example, saying this will be like a mosquito bite, could be interpreted by young children as meaning they are actually going to be bitten by a mosquito. Saying a child will receive a dye for a test could be interpreted as meaning the child will "die" during the procedure. Children who think illness comes as punishment for breaking rules can interpret nursing procedures such as giving an injection as punishment. They can be confused about explanations of procedures because some words sound alike or have double meanings ("drawing" as in making a picture versus drawing blood). Because of these distorted perceptions, explanations of procedures do not always relieve children's stress.

Differences in responses of children and adults to illness

Keeping in mind that children are not just small adults is important when evaluating how children react to illness, perceive an illness or react to healthcare. Their body images, as evidenced in their drawings, are different from those of adults. They can have difficulty telling which body parts are indispensable and which are not (this is why it is wise to talk to preschool and primary school children about "fixing" body parts, such as tonsils, rather than "taking them out").

Inability to communicate

Very young children do not have the vocabulary to describe symptoms. Headache is an example of a symptom that children younger than 5 years have a great deal of difficulty describing. Dizziness and nausea can be equally bewildering because children this age do not know the words to express these phenomena.

By the time they reach school age, most children can describe symptoms with accuracy. They may intensify their concerns, however, if they believe someone expects symptoms to be more serious. They may minimise symptoms if they are afraid illness will interfere with an activity.

Evaluating and observing a child's symptoms is as important as listening to their perception of their condition. A crying, whining preschooler who is "just not herself" probably has a symptom she cannot describe. A school-age child who guards her abdomen (keeps abdominal muscles rigid) is in pain just as clearly as a child who verbalises a source of discomfort. This makes keen, astute observations necessary to ascertain the extent of a child's illness at any given time (see Fig. 36.1). Age appropriate pain scale charts are a very useful way to establish a child's level of pain.

Inability to monitor own care and manage fear

Adults who are ill often ask about medications prescribed for them or procedures they are scheduled to undergo. School age and younger children cannot monitor their own care because they may not know which medicine or procedures they are to receive. The infant, for example, fears separation above all else; the toddler and preschooler fear such things as separation, the dark, the unknown, intrusive procedures and mutilation of body parts. The school-age child and adolescent are concerned about the loss of body parts, loss of life and loss of friends. Adults have fears also, but most have learned to cope with them. Children in a strange environment (such as a hospital) require proportionally more support and active intervention to cope with their stress and fears (Gordon, 2012).

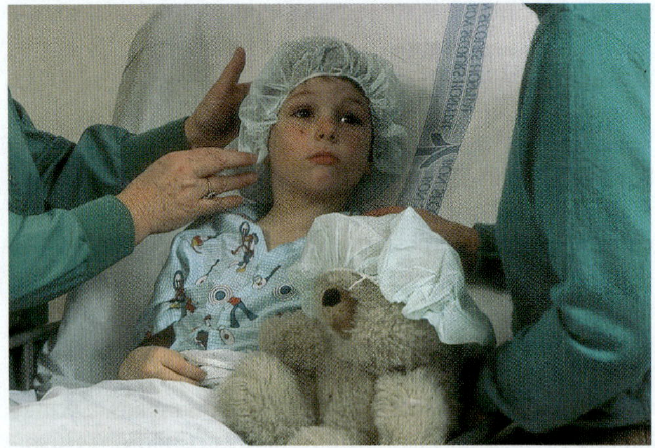

FIGURE 36.1 Illness is potentially traumatic because of the unknown and the pain and discomfort that may be involved. Children need extra attention and reassurance to calm their fears.

Nutritional needs

In addition to psychological differences, there are major physiological differences in the way illness affects children and adults. This is because children have different physiological needs and respond to imbalances in different ways. Children need more nutrients (kilojoules, protein, minerals and vitamins) per kilogram of body weight than adults, for example, because their basic metabolic rate is faster and they must take in not only enough to maintain body tissues but also enough to allow for growth. The infant requires 504 kJ per kilogram of body weight per day; the adult requires only 30 to 35 kJ per kilogram. An ill child who must limit food intake because of nausea or vomiting, therefore, may require hospitalisation, even though this might be unnecessary for an adult under the same circumstances.

Fluid and electrolyte balance

In the adult, extracellular water (that in plasma and outside body cells) represents approximately 23% of total body water; in a newborn, extracellular water is closer to 40%. This means that an infant does not have as much water stored in the cells as an adult does and so is more likely to lose a devastating amount of body water with diarrhoea or vomiting. Because of this, there is no such thing as "only diarrhoea" or "simple diarrhoea" in a child younger than 1 year. The full implications of both vomiting and diarrhoea are discussed in Chapter 45.

Systemic response to illness

Because their bodies are immature, young children tend to respond to disease systemically rather than locally. The child with pneumonia, for example, may be brought to an emergency department not because of a cough (although the child has one) but because of accompanying systemic symptoms such as fever, vomiting and diarrhoea. Nausea and vomiting, in fact, occur so frequently in children with any type of illness that these symptoms do not have the diagnostic value they have in adults. Systemic reactions of these kinds can delay diagnosis and therapy and cause increased fluid and nutrient loss, circumstances that compound an initial illness and can result in hospitalisation.

Age-specific diseases

Because of their growth requirement and their immaturity, children are susceptible to some diseases that do not affect adults. Most adults have achieved immunity to common infectious diseases; children, however, are susceptible to childhood diseases such as measles, mumps and chickenpox. Children younger than 5 years who have a high temperature may respond with generalised seizures (febrile convulsion). Ojha, Shakya and Aryal (2012) report, in research conducted, that almost half of the children who had a febrile seizure were at risk of recurrence at a later date. They suggest that the risk factors for these recurrences are modest rise in body temperature at the onset of febrile seizure, onset of seizure within 12 hours of fever and atypical presentation. When children do not receive adequate iron, those younger than 1 year of age are subject to iron-deficiency anaemia because fetal red blood cells are destroyed after birth and are replaced by mature red blood cells only very slowly.

✔ *Checkpoint question 36.1*

Young children are more at risk of dehydration with vomiting than adults. This is because:

a. They have a smaller stomach and intestines than adults
b. They have proportionally more extracellular water than adults
c. Children metabolise fluid more slowly than most adults
d. They maintain more fluid inside body cells than adults

CARE OF THE ILL CHILD AND FAMILY IN THE HOSPITAL

The parents of children admitted to intensive care or neonatal intensive care units (ICUs and NICUs) can be predicted to experience a high degree of stress during their child's hospitalisation both because of the severity of their child's illness and the high-tech paediatric ICU or NICU setting (Kearvell & Grant, 2010). Based on the theory, that hospitalisation creates a high degree of stress for children, only those children who cannot be managed successfully on an ambulatory basis are now admitted to hospital. This was not always true. For example, in the past, most children with head injuries automatically stayed overnight for observation. Currently, unless a child is unconscious or shows other signs of neurological injury, the child may be sent home to be observed by parents for signs of increased intracranial pressure. This policy requires that time be spent to teach parents skills such as how to take a pulse or evaluate consciousness. Teaching them requires patience because parents under stress can have difficulty comprehending instructions. However, because psychological trauma and excessive healthcare costs are prevented by allowing a child to return home, it is important teaching. Children who are seen in the emergency departments for acute gastritis and vomiting were also once automatically admitted to hospital so they could receive intravenous fluid. Today, they are given an oral hydrating solution or probiotics so they no longer need to be admitted. Evidence-based guidelines developed by the Medical Services Commission (2010) address the oral rehydration of children from 6 months to 17 years. These guidelines emphasise the importance of an accurate clinical assessment of the degree of dehydration and point out that only mild dehydration should be treated at home.

Some paediatric surgery procedures can be done on an inpatient or day-patient basis. This prevents the major problem of separation anxiety, but it does not necessarily reduce parents' or children's anxiety about the procedure. Some parents actually feel less confident and more anxious with ambulatory procedures than they did with in-hospital admissions because they sense their responsibility for preparation and follow-up care will be significantly greater. Cagiran and colleagues (2014) point out that in the preoperative period parents may experience increased anxiety and children may experience fear, anger and guilt. The findings of their study indicated that high levels of maternal anxiety maybe related to increased levels of anxiety in the child undergoing surgery. These researchers emphasise the importance of education and support for the family who has a child undergoing surgery. Although it is true that short hospital stays reduce cost, it is helpful to inform parents that ambulatory or outpatient procedures are as safe as those performed with hospital admissions, and that ambulatory procedures can be helpful in preventing the detrimental effects of separation.

Decreasing separation anxiety

While **separation anxiety** is a normal stage in the growth and development of the child it is clear that separation during hospitalisation has the potential to impact significantly on children. It is difficult to explain the meaning that a primary carer has for a child, but the intensity of the relationship can be demonstrated. As early as 4 months of age, the infant registers disapproval if a primary carer walks away. As early as 5 months of age, an infant registers anxiety when strangers are present or when a person other than the usual carer gives care. Infants fix their eyes on the stranger, become restless, perhaps thrash arms or legs, and begin to cry. This activity peaks at approximately 8 months of age, so it is commonly called "8-month anxiety". It is a developmental milestone that shows an infant is able to distinguish a primary carer from other persons. It also means the child has reached a vulnerable stage in emotional development and will react poorly to separation or to the threat of it (Livesley & Long, 2013).

TABLE 36.1 Stages of separation anxiety

Stage	Manifestations
Protest	The child cries loudly and demandingly rejects any attempts to be comforted by nurse or substitute primary carers.
Despair	The child becomes less active and cries monotonously or wails in a state of mourning; may turn away from parents' approach; often lies on abdomen, facial expression flat; may lose weight and develop insomnia; loses developmental skills; prone to minor ailments such as upper respiratory infections; IQ will measure lower than previous measurement.
Denial	The child is silent, face expressionless; represses feelings for absent carer to protect self; deterioration in developmental milestones is apparent; may respond quickly but superficially to all carers; may have difficulty forming close relationships later in life.

Toddlers and preschoolers can be as affected by separation as infants. In many instances, they express their feelings better, louder and longer than infants. Although many toddlers and preschoolers attend daycare and have had prior experiences with separation, others may have had only limited experiences. Being hospitalised may be the first time they are away from parents in a strange setting or away from home overnight. If this is so, many preschoolers may wonder whether they will ever live with their parents again. Problems of separation are especially intense in younger children because they do not understand time. Statements such as, "Mum will visit again tomorrow" or "Dad will be here by 6 o'clock" are meaningless to children younger than 5 years because they do not know what either "tomorrow" or "6 o'clock" means. Most paediatric units now adopt a model of family-centred care in an attempt to reduce separation anxiety for hospitalised children. Livesley and Long (2013) maintain that while family centred care and parental participation have become standard practice in child health nursing, the delivery of care to hospitalised children in partnership with families still remains a complex and contingent matter impacted by parenting styles, cultural differences and health beliefs and values.

School-aged children and adolescents react better than younger children to the separation imposed by hospitalisation because they have experiences they can use for comparison. They have been to school for whole days; perhaps they have stayed with a grandparent or a friend overnight. They may have been on a school excursion. This can make hospitalisation a time for developing self-esteem and confidence in their ability to be independent. Even in light of this, ill school-age children and adolescents may still feel anxious about being separated from their parents. They appreciate their parents' presence and need reassurance that their parents support and love them. Remember that parents may have an equally difficult time being separated from children. You may need to spend time with them assuring them that their child will receive good care at all times, even if they are absent.

To appreciate why preventing separation is so important, it is helpful to review the research that provided the foundation for this method of care. Spitz (1945) was one of the first researchers who documented the effects of separation on children. He observed children who were separated from their mothers for both short and long periods. From this observation, he was able to document how poorly children responded to separation from their parents. Bowlby conducted additional studies after World War II (Bowlby et al., 1966). Building on Spitz's and Bowlby's work, Robertson (1958) studied the effect of hospitalisation on children and supplied labels for separation effects (see Table 36.1). Although defined over 50 years ago, these findings are still applicable to children today.

Effects of hospitalisation can be severe. Children may develop symptoms of anxiety such as difficulty falling asleep, irritability, outbursts of anger, difficulty concentrating or completing tasks, or stomach aches and headaches. They re-experience the traumatic event through dreams or flashbacks. Nicholas et al. (2014) evaluated the use of videophones as a means of support among families who had limited opportunities to remain with their hospitalised child due to geographical distance. The findings of this study indicated that the use of the videophone decreased feelings of isolation and anxiety and increased feelings of connection between family members.

Reducing the ill effects of separation and hospitalisation to the extent possible should be a high priority for nurses and healthcare providers. Nurses play a major role in this on both direct care and management levels. Unfortunately, despite the best preparation by parents or nurses, not all of these effects of hospitalisation can be prevented.

CASE STUDY QUESTION

3. Suppose Becky shows signs of separation anxiety. The first stage of separation anxiety is marked by:
   a. Loud, demanding crying
   b. Silent, sullen protest
   c. Quiet, introspective thought
   d. Inability to respond verbally

Preparing the ill child and family for hospitalisation

Many childhood illnesses such as febrile convulsions, appendicitis, poisonings and asthma attacks strike suddenly, making advance preparation for hospital admission impossible. However, when hospitalisation for surgery is scheduled, preparation is possible. As a rule, parents eagerly seek guidance from nurses on what and how much to tell their children about an anticipated admission. The preparation parents make for a child obviously varies according to the child's age and individual experience. No matter what the child's age, parents do best when they convey a positive attitude towards the hospitalisation or surgery. Statements such as, "They'll make you behave in the hospital" or "Wait until you have to stay in bed all day" should be avoided.

Children can worry unnecessarily if they are told about their approaching hospitalisation too far in advance. Conversely, few things are more frightening for children than to hear conversation halt as they enter a room or to hear adults spelling out unknown words. As a rule, therefore, children between 2 and 7 years of age should be told about a scheduled ambulatory or inpatient hospitalisation as many days before the procedure as the child's age in years. For example, a 2-year-old should be informed 2 days before hospitalisation; a 4-year-old, 4 days before; and so forth. Children older than 7 years should be told as soon as the parents are aware of it.

On the day of hospital admission, it is important for you to discuss the preparation the child has received to ensure that the child and family accurately understand the child's condition and upcoming procedures. Based on that, you can provide further health teaching and clear up any misunderstandings.

Family carers

Planning for hospitalisation should begin as soon as parents know that hospitalisation will be necessary. Some parents, however, may be so concerned about the reason for hospitalisation that they cannot begin to prepare their child until they are better-prepared themselves. Easing parental anxiety regarding illness and hospitalisation is particularly important because infants and children can keenly sense a parent's stress. No amount or type of preparation for children will be effective if they react to their parents' unspoken tension.

As part of preparation, urge parents to ask questions, contact the hospital or access information online about the hospitalisation so they are as familiar as possible with what will happen. If they are well informed in this way, they will (at least theoretically) have as low an anxiety level as possible. Excellent resources are available for parents and carers. Examples of the type of information available for families can be accessed at the following websites: <www.justforkids.org.nz>, <www.sch.edu.au/general/stay/>, <www.awch.org.au> and <www.starship.org.nz/patients-and-families/your-childs-hospital-or-daystay-admission>.

Infant

Because an infant cannot understand explanations of surgery or treatments, preparation is minimal. Special items such as a favourite toy, blanket or dummy should be packed. These objects provide a special kind of security for which there is no substitute.

A primary carer should plan to spend a great deal of time in the hospital with an infant. For rooming-in, a parent needs to make plans for older children or a spouse ahead of time. If a parent cannot arrange to stay with the infant make the nurse aware so alternative arrangements can be put in place. This can both help decrease parental anxiety and minimise separation anxiety in the infant (Livesley & Long, 2013).

Toddler or preschooler

Three main fears of toddlers or preschoolers are fear of the unknown, fear of abandonment or separation, and fear of pain. Preparation for children of this age, therefore, should clearly aim at alleviating these fears. Bringing a favourite toy or personal item such as a blanket can help.

When making hospital beds or changing paper on examining tables, watch for ragged blankets and threadbare stuffed animals; these can cling to sheets and can be easily discarded. Throw nothing away without first asking a child or parent if it is important. What looks like a useless alphabet block to you may mean security and home to a child. When children are admitted to a hospital in an emergency, parents rarely have time to bring toys. In these instances, suggest a parent give a child a familiar object, such as the parent's scarf or jumper. The child will hold these in the same way as a favourite toy.

Several helpful books about hospitalisation are available for parents to read with children and also learn more about children's healthcare. These can be obtained from local bookstores, libraries or online from organisations such as the Association for the Wellbeing of Children in Healthcare (AWCH) or Child Health in New Zealand, New Zealand Ministry of Health: Manatū Hauora. Because the imagination of preschoolers is at a peak, role playing is an effective means of preparing a child of this age for a new experience. Remind parents it is always better to use the word "fix" rather than "cut" when talking about surgery with young children, because "cut" automatically suggests pain and mutilation.

School-aged child or adolescent

School-aged children enjoy reading, so books about surgery and hospitalisation can be helpful. Be sure both school-age children and adolescents receive factual explanations of what will happen during such an experience. This should include also what will not happen: for example, surgery will require a small abdominal incision, but it will not create a scar that will show when wearing a swimming costume.

Many hospitals organise orientation programs for children's groups or school groups during which hospitalisation is discussed. These programs are beneficial because they lay a foundation for all children about what to expect

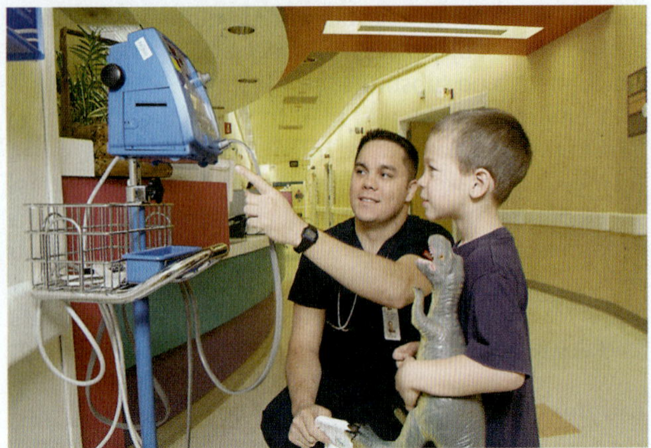

FIGURE 36.2 Children learn what to expect from hospitalisation by becoming familiar with some of the equipment that might be used.

in a hospitalisation; then, if they must be admitted on an emergency basis, they may not be so frightened. Programs are offered by nurses at the hospital or on visits to children's groups or schools (see Fig. 36.2).

At approximately 9 years of age, when children first begin to understand the full meaning of death, parents need to be especially careful to explain that an anaesthetic causes a "special sleep", not that a child is "put to sleep". Animals that are "put to sleep" are not seen again. If hospitalisation is to be more than 1 week long, a parent must think about the means to continue the child's schooling. Advise parents to ask their doctor at what point their child will be able to do homework. Some children's hospitals often have their own teachers from the local education system to carry out this service.

> ***What if...***
>
> Becky's mother brought pots and pans to the hospital as Becky's favourite play items? Would you suggest she bring an actual toy?

Child with a different cultural background

Perhaps the most important aspect to consider when preparing a child from a different culture for hospitalisation is to identify what traditions or practices will be in opposition to healthcare facility practices (Henry & Kurzak, 2013). Make every effort to allow the child to continue to do those things that are culturally important to them. Engage the assistance of an interpreter who can stay at the hospital with the parent if necessary. Low-cost accommodation is available, for example, in facilities such as Ronald McDonald House. The Indigenous Children's Health Report, Health Assessment in Action, can be viewed at the following website: <www.onemda.unimelb.edu.au/docs/ichrreport.pdf>. The Haakuitanga Haakorotanga Maori Parenting Programme can be accessed at <www.net-inc.org.nz/?cID=haakuitanga_haakorotanga_parenting_programme>. Ask enough questions and practise good listening skills to gain information about the particular needs of a child and family. When cultural differences do exist, be prepared to act as a liaison between the family and the healthcare team. If a different language is interfering with communication, a translator may be necessary in this preparation phase. Provide the opportunity for parents to voice their fears and ask questions at the time of hospitalisation or treatment. When families speak a different language or are unfamiliar with hospital routine, allow more time and more opportunities for discussion and communication.

Physically challenged or chronically ill child

Physically challenged or chronically ill children frequently come to ambulatory healthcare settings for care; they often are admitted to the hospital for care, possibly remaining in the hospital for an extended time with continuing care at home. Think about ways in which a new hospitalisation or visit will be like past ones and other ways in which it will be different to determine how best to prepare the child. Help children to maintain contact with their families and school friends during a long hospitalisation by encouraging telephone calls, emails, text messaging, letters and visits.

Admitting an ill child and family

Whether for an ambulatory or inpatient hospital ward admission, children and parents need to be admitted as a single entity to encourage parents to feel they are true partners in care. A child coming to a hospital for an elective admission in some hospitals will attend a pre-admission clinic a couple of days prior to admission to receive information about their hospitalisation. Otherwise the parents and the child will generally arrive at a reception area, where significant facts are obtained, such as name, age, address and private hospital insurance coverage. The child and parents are then brought to the hospital ward. Remember that first impressions count. On arrival at the ward the nurse should:

- Take the time to meet and greet the parents and child and find a comfortable place for the family to wait until someone is available.
- Introduce yourself to children by stooping down so that your face is level with the child's face (see Fig. 36.3). Call the child by name or ask for a nickname. Calling all children "honey" or "pumpkin" can cause children to worry they have been confused with another child.
- Attach an armband giving their name and hospital identification number. Because their hands are not much larger than their wrists and their feet are not much larger than their ankles, neonates (infants younger than 1 month of age) often need two bands in place as an extra safeguard. If a band falls off, secure it back onto the child. Never tape the band to the cot or bedside stand, as this is not adequate protection: if an infant is placed in the

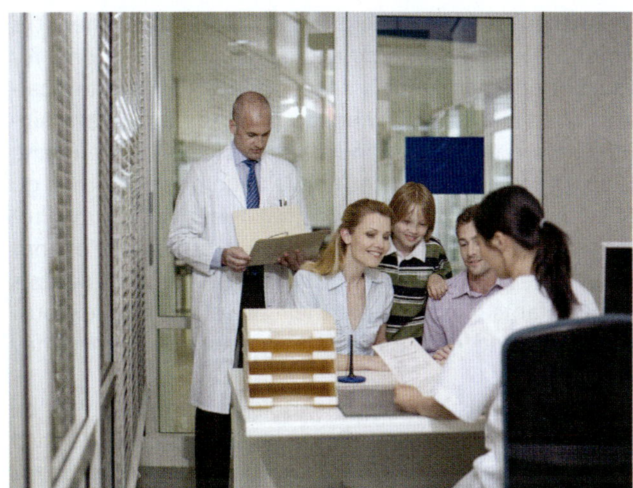

FIGURE 36.3 A child is admitted to a hospital unit. Notice how the nurse engages all the family's members (© F1online digitale Bildagentur GmbH/Alamy).

wrong cot by mistake, the infant could be given a medicine that is lethal before the mistake is realised.

- Provide an orientation for the family to the ward, explaining any routines that need to be followed. Explain if the child can wear their own clothes while in hospital.
- Provide information to the child and family about any special procedures or requirements.
- Ask the parents or carer if they have any questions about the child's condition or care.

Assessment on admission

This involves:

- Assessment of each child's level of preparation for a hospitalisation.
- Awareness of not only what the child describes orally but also what facial expressions or nervous manifestations may be indicating.
- Interviewing parents on hospital admission for a nursing history to obtain the information needed to plan nursing care (Chapter 34 describes a full child interview history). Make a note of any medication or food allergy on the child's plan of care and, if pertinent, post this information by the child's bed because, unlike an adult, a child cannot call these things to the attention of staff when food or medication is offered. If medication has been administered, note when it was last given.
- Taking and recording the child's temperature, pulse, blood pressure and respirations. Information about the Child Early Warning Tool (CEWT) can be viewed at <www.safetyandquality.gov.au/wp-content/uploads/2012/11/The-Children-s-Early-Warning-Tool.pdf>. In addition, in young infants a head circumference measurement is recorded.
- Measuring height and weight to determine overall growth and to allow for determination of surface area, the measurement on which medication dosage is calculated.
- Obtaining information about the child's immunisation status.
- Obtaining a specimen for urinalysis is another routine procedure. Be sure to explain all equipment used and allow the child to touch and handle it as much as possible to help reduce anxiety.
- Inspecting for gross motor ability when weighing a child and measuring height.
- Listening for language ability (although children in strange situations may say nothing).

Promoting a positive hospital stay

Promoting a positive hospital stay is important to the health of both children and their families. Several nursing actions are important to make the difference between a successful and an unsuccessful hospital experience.

Minimising length of hospital stay

Hospitalisation should be limited to the shortest time possible. Be certain that diagnostic procedures are scheduled for a child's, not the hospital's, convenience so that no child stays in a hospital longer than is necessary. Pressure from concerned nurses who insist on having a voice in policies can make a big difference in a department's willingness to cooperate with scheduling.

Providing continuity of care

The best way to ensure that children are exposed to as few substitute care people as possible and to maintain the consistency and quality of care, is to encourage parents to remain with the child during hospitalisation. The Association for the Wellbeing of Children in Healthcare (AWCH) recommends that hospitals provide sleeping accommodation for parents/carers beside their child in the hospital ward. Nursing allocations that work best in achieving continuity of care for the child are those where one nurse gives as much care to the same child as possible (either **primary nursing** or **case management nursing**; see Fig. 36.4). These staffing patterns allow the same nurse to admit the child, take the nursing history, set goals for care in cooperation with the parents and the child and evaluate progress towards achieving goals. It allows children to have one main nurse to call their own. It allows parents to establish meaningful contact with hospital staff and maintains continuity of care, planning and implementation.

A positive hospital stay can be promoted in the following ways.

Promoting open parent visiting

When possible, children younger than 5 years should have their primary carer room-in with them when they are in a hospital (see Fig. 36.5). Children younger than 10 to 12 years continue to enjoy the feeling of security this provides. This practice is essential to reduce the separation anxiety experienced by the child.

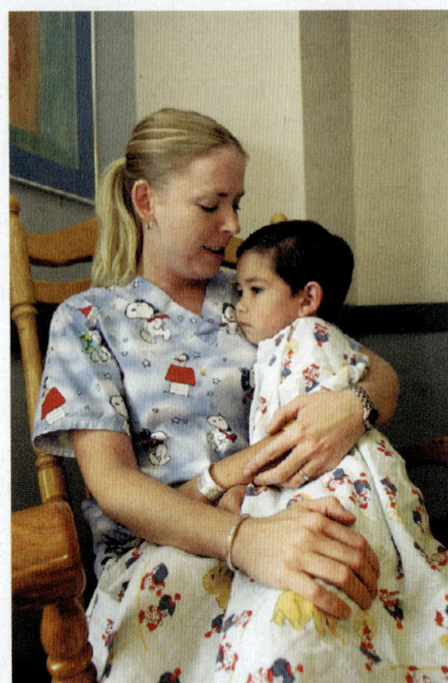

FIGURE 36.4 Hospitalised children should have one nurse who is "theirs" to minimise the effect of separation from parents (primary care nursing).

Not all parents can stay in the hospital continuously. Mothers and fathers who cannot stay may need help in smoothing the transition of their coming or going. For example, when a toddler first sees his parents after being separated, his reaction might be to ignore them (a sign of despair). This is a defence mechanism: "I won't show them I love them until they show me they love me; that way I won't be hurt again". The parents' reaction to being treated this way may be anger. If this makes the parents go and play with a child in the next bed—a "well, be that way then" reaction—the toddler's worst fears are fulfilled: his parents do not love him anymore. However, if you urge the parents to speak to the child for a few minutes or try to interest the child in a toy, a child will generally reach out to be comforted and act relieved the parents are there.

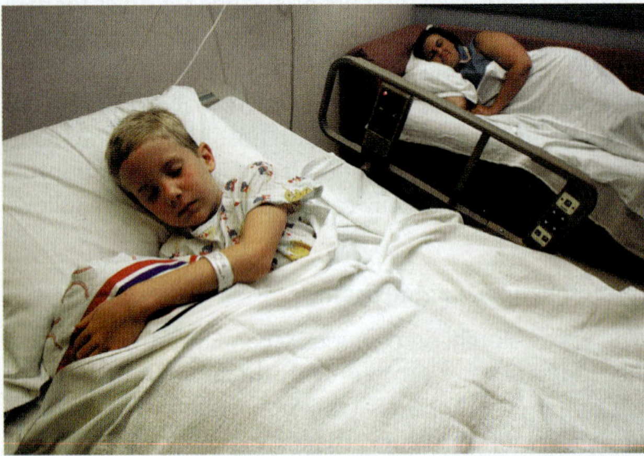

FIGURE 36.5 Rooming-in helps alleviate separation anxiety for both the child and the carer.

Parents often need help in saying goodbye when it is time to leave a child to go and eat a meal or go home for the night (if the parent is not rooming-in). When the parents of an infant are leaving, go into the room a few minutes before they leave and hold or play with the infant. Help a parent to say once, "I have to go now" and then go after explaining to the child that they will return. Prolonged departures only delay the process and do not reduce the amount of crying that may occur. After parents leave, infants may cry until they fall asleep from exhaustion. Hold and rock them, letting them know that they are safe.

When parents leave a preschooler it is best to say "I'll be back" in relation to a specific event, such as after the child has eaten lunch. In the case of a school-age child or adolescent, urge parents to provide definite times when they will return and to leave suggestions for activities a child could do to occupy the time ("Why don't you finish your book?", "Start your homework and I'll check it when I come back").

Providing opportunities for parents to participate in their child's care

Participating in their child's care can make parents feel more in control, thereby reducing anxiety. Therefore, encourage parents to give as much care as possible during a hospital stay, such as bathing or feeding their child, giving oral medicine or being with their child as they wake from anaesthesia. Be certain that parents receive proper instruction on the tasks they will be able to do. Be sure parents who change nappies or feed children know whether the number of nappy changes or the amount of food intake should be recorded; ask them to report when they do these things or write them down on a flow sheet attached to the child's door or cot. Do not have them restrain children for a procedure that will be painful except in cases where it can be helpful for a cooperative parent to firmly cuddle a child lovingly in order to ensure that the child remains still for a procedure to be performed. Assure parents that in the best interests of the child, the parent is the better carer while the nurse is always there if necessary.

Children may be apprehensive about undergoing a procedure without a parent present. There is rarely any reason a parent cannot accompany a child into a treatment room to help with undressing, measuring weight and height, and taking a temperature or accompanying a child to another department for a procedure such as an ultrasound or blood tests. Most importantly, the parent can comfort the child in these strange surroundings.

Although helping with procedures can strengthen the parent–child relationship, remind parents their most important role is being parents. Sitting and rocking or reading to their child and just being there will be their best role to minimise the adverse effects of hospitalisation. When a child is to have surgery, it may be especially difficult for parents to separate from their child. Helping them do this is an important part of preoperative nursing care.

Supporting sibling visits

Children in a family are under considerable stress while a sibling is hospitalised because their world changes so much (Newton et al., 2010) Sibling visits refer to allowing the brothers and sisters of hospitalised children to visit the ill child in the hospital. Allowing this alleviates loneliness on both sides and helps prevent other children at home from imagining the ill child is sicker than is true. It helps the ill child continue to feel part of the family. Siblings who visit need to be free of communicable disease. Nurses may need to help parents divide their time between the ill child and siblings during a visit (short, frequent visits may be better for young children than long ones). Prior to siblings visiting, especially if they are young, ensure that the safety of the room has been maintained in line with hospital policy and best evidence-based practice standards.

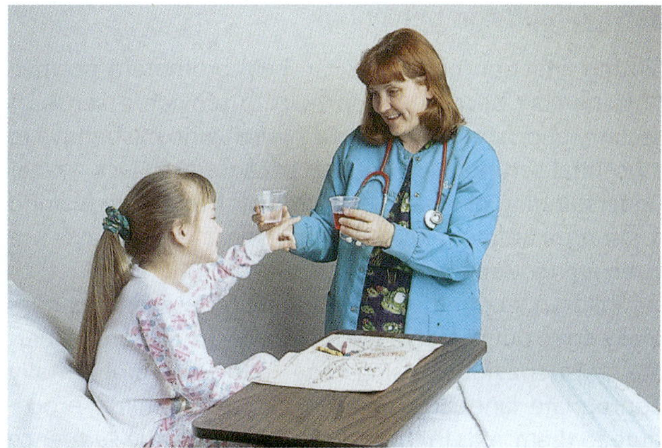

FIGURE 36.6 Include children in procedures whenever possible to offer them a feeling of control. Here a nurse gives a child a choice of fluids to drink with her medication.

Minimising negative effects of procedures

Ill children often undergo numerous diagnostic and therapeutic procedures that have the potential to cause pain, fear and anxiety. Details related to specific procedures are discussed in Chapter 37. General guidelines to make any procedure less painful or frightening are discussed in the following sections.

Reducing or eliminating pain

Some pain and discomfort is unavoidable in association with healthcare. The administration of sucrose sublingually for newborns and young infants up to 12 months of age is an effective short-term analgesic which can be initiated by the nurse. Pain should be reduced or eliminated whenever possible by measures such as advocating for the use of infusion devices (see Chapter 37) to eliminate multiple punctures for intravenous medication or blood sampling. The administration of ample analgesia, including alternative therapy techniques such as distraction or imagery, providing traditional comforts such as a change of clothing or position, reading to a child and planning a special project should be undertaken. Children do not always express discomfort as freely as adults; therefore, closer assessment may be necessary to reveal how they feel. Because pain increases with anxiety, reducing a child's anxiety with good preparation and encouraging a sense of control can also help to eliminate discomfort (see Chapter 39). Dooley et al. (2013) report on the development of an innovative approach to predicting and treating procedural pain in children involving the Liverpool Anticipatory Procedural Pain Score (LAPPS). The introduction of the LAPPS assessment tool and treatment protocol reduced pain and distress during the removal of chest drains.

Maintaining the child's bed as a safe area

To assure children that their bed is an area that is safe, all painful procedures should be done in a treatment room, away from the child's bed. Be sure this rule is not broken, because only one painful experience at the bedside can be enough to significantly increase a child's anxiety. This rule should include finger punctures for blood tests: although done quickly, these can cause as much pain and stress as venepunctures. In addition, dressing changes, although not necessarily painful, can cause worry and so should be done in a treatment room, not at a child's bedside as well. Unfortunately this rule cannot be maintained when the child is in isolation.

Helping children to maintain control

Events are always more frightening if they appear to be beyond our control. Explaining to children what will happen, such as what they will feel or what they will see and helping them to make choices whenever possible limits this type of fear because these actions offer a sense of control (see Fig. 36.6). In almost any procedure, there is some choice a child can make (use a straw to drink or not, decide what size of tape to use on a bandage or walk one way in the hall or the other).

Providing adequate play facilities

Play is the medium through which children learn. To continue development during hospitalisation, children need to be able to play as normally as possible, no matter how long their stay. Children's hospital wards should be equipped with a playroom or play space in which children can feel secure and in which they know they will not be hurt. No medical procedures, not even painless ones, should be performed in this area. Children who are on bed-rest can have their bed wheeled into the playroom or have toys or crafts brought to their bed.

Because hospitalisation is a traumatic experience, children need the opportunity to express their feelings through therapeutic play before painful procedures Ford et al. (2013) argue that clown doctors have a primary role to play in bringing play, fun and laughter in hospitalised children. The uses of play and guidelines for providing therapeutic play are discussed later in this chapter.

Setting limits on behaviour

Setting limits on behaviour can help promote a positive hospital stay because it can help to provide a sense of security and safety for a child. Children who misbehave in a hospital setting usually do so because they lack a clear understanding of what is expected of them or are making a strong statement that their personal needs have not been recognised and met.

Children who refuse to cooperate for procedures generally do so out of fear of the unknown rather than deliberate misbehaviour. Using age and developmentally appropriate language, when explaining a child's procedure to them, aids in their understanding of the sequence of events. This also often improves their cooperation and may lower their anxiety levels, especially if illustrations are available to further support your verbal explanation. If limit setting is necessary, such as with a child who hits or bites other children, confer with the child's parents about the need for limit setting and what measures they would suggest. Gain their cooperation and approval so that what you do is consistent with their care (Pudney & Whitehouse, 2012). Using "time out" periods or removing the child to a non-stimulating area for a short time is an effective measure. Be certain a child understands the rules (if the child bites or hits, sitting alone for a designated period will be necessary).

Discharge planning

Discharge planning is an important link between hospital and home. Many children, particularly those having surgery, are hospitalised for only a few hours; as soon as they are able to take and retain fluid and have voided once, they are discharged. This represents such a short time that preparation for discharge must start even before they are admitted to the hospital (Gordon, 2012). If a child has been admitted on an inpatient basis, preparation for discharge should begin on the day of admission. If some procedures will need to be continued at home, allow parents to perform them in the hospital at least once so that they can become comfortable with the necessary technique and discover any problems while help is still available. Urge parents to think about problems they might have with a procedure at home. There could be real problems that must be worked out before a parent can perform the procedure at home. Do not leave this kind of instruction until the last day, because then there will not be time left to solve such problems (Sydney Children's Hospital, 2013).

Discharge planners can be indispensable in helping ready parents for home care. Teach the parents what they must do on the first day they are at home before they leave the hospital. Be certain they know the person to contact if plans do not work out as anticipated and that they have a definite return appointment for follow-up care.

Many preschool children manifest behavioural problems such as thumb-sucking, bed wetting, temper tantrums and nightmares after returning home from a hospital stay; school-age children may manifest these behaviours to a lesser extent. You can reassure parents these behaviours are part of a child's normal response to hospitalisation. These behaviours do not happen because the child has been "spoiled" by the hospital staff or by the parents during the illness but because the experience was too intense for the child to handle easily, even with all the precautions taken to prevent stress. As children realise they are safely back home and the experience is over, these behaviour reactions become less frequent and eventually disappear.

NURSING RESPONSIBILITIES FOR CARE OF AN ILL CHILD AND FAMILY

Nursing responsibilities will vary, naturally, with the type, extent and seriousness of a child's illness, age, care setting and individual circumstances. Several responsibilities, however, such as promotion of normal growth and development, sleep, stimulation and play apply across all ages and phases of care. Chapter 37 discusses specific responsibilities related to diagnostic tests or interventions. Chapter 39 discusses the important role of promoting comfort in an ill child. It is easy for children to fall behind in growth and development because of an illness unless healthcare providers monitor for this.

Growth and development

Infants

To promote optimal growth and development, try to change an infant's normal routine as little as possible. Sameness provides security to a child and encourages the development of trust. When admitting an infant to a hospital, ask parents what type of bed the child usually sleeps in. A child who is used to sleeping in a bassinet may feel loose and insecure in a large cot.

Also, attempt to change the infant's diet as little as possible. Unless a child is diagnosed with failure to thrive or is obviously underweight, illness is not an ideal period in which to introduce new foods or formula. Unless their physical condition warrants a change, infants who breastfeed should continue to do so for as many feedings as possible. Expressed breast milk can be given by bottle to the child when the mother is not available. Ensure that the child receives comfort and stimulation and play opportunities as their condition improves.

Toddlers or preschoolers

Because illness can limit autonomy and prevent children from learning how to do new things, try to find opportunities to promote both autonomy in toddlers and initiative in preschoolers. Urge parents to encourage children to make choices about their care whenever possible. For example, colouring in a medication schedule is the kind of task that helps to encourage initiative in a preschooler.

As with infants, illness is a poor time to change the eating habits of toddlers and preschoolers. Because children of this age insist on self-feeding, they generally do poorly eating in bed and often do better sitting at low tables. Illness is also a poor time to begin toilet training, even if it is appropriate to the child's age. If the parents have already begun toilet training, continue with as normal a routine as possible.

School-aged children

School-aged children need to continue to work on a sense of industry while ill. This means learning more about how and why things are done. Explain about specific procedures and involve them as much as possible in planning their care to help foster a sense of industry. Encourage school-age children to carry out self-care and, if cared for at home, to contribute to household routines, such as helping with dishes, as much as they are able. This not only takes some burden off carers but also makes a child feel like an intrinsic part of the family.

School-age children and adolescents should continue schooling if they are ill for a long time, provided their condition will allow it. During the times a child will not be attending school, working on projects such as craft, helping plan family menus, writing for brochures about the place the family plans to visit on holidays next year or viewing DVDs on science or nature are activities that not only help pass the time but also encourage learning. School-age children also are developing moral responsibility and may find comfort in spiritual practices.

Adolescents

An adolescent who is struggling to develop a sense of identity may find it tricky coping with constraints associated with their illness. This may involve behaviour that has a temporary detrimental effect on their self-worth. Help adolescents to continue to participate in activities they did before becoming ill, if possible, to help them feel their world is not totally changing. Encourage them to maintain self-care activities and good hygiene practices to help preserve self-esteem.

Illness can be difficult for adolescents because peer relationships are so important to them. For this reason, it is important for them to have visitors from their peer group, just as much as infants need visits from parents. Using a mobile phone to send text messages is an easy way to contact friends and maintain relationships with individuals who are important to them.

Adolescents appreciate being hospitalised in a special adolescent unit or at least in a room free of childish decor. Although adolescents enjoy having parents stay overnight because it is reassuring to know they are concerned, adolescents also enjoy being separated from their parents (assuming everything is going all right) so may not want their parent present all day and night. Often adolescents convey a blasé attitude towards procedures: having x-rays taken is nothing; surgery is a cinch; a cast change is a snap. Listen carefully to make certain adolescents really feel this way and are not trying to convince themselves that a procedure is harmless. It is easy to assume from their attitude that they know more than they do.

Nutrition

Nursing responsibilities related to nutrition for ill children include maintaining optimal nutritional status in the face of illness or treatment that interferes with adequate intake. Correcting nutritional deficiencies or otherwise helping children and families to follow the nutritional care plan devised by the healthcare team and educating a child and family regarding specific nutritional needs as well as overall sound nutritional health needs to be discussed. Specific procedures for promoting nutrition such as measuring fluid intake and output and providing enteral feedings, gastrostomy tube feedings, and total parenteral nutrition are discussed in Chapter 37.

An acute illness in a child, such as pneumonia, is often accompanied by a loss of appetite. Gastrointestinal illnesses often cause nausea and vomiting. As most acute illnesses last only a few days, there is no need for children to eat more than a small amount during this time provided they can drink fluid. Trying to force them to eat only increases nausea and vomiting, which increases the possibility of creating an electrolyte imbalance. When an illness lasts for more than a few days, however, providing adequate nutrition becomes increasingly important because children need nutrients not only to repair ill or diseased tissue but also to maintain normal childhood growth.

Children who are hospitalised often tolerate hospital-prepared food, which can be repetitious and bland, better than adults do. These children, as well as those receiving care at home, require good nutrition at a level which sustains them, ensuring their growth and developmental requirements are adequately met. Aiming for a healthy, age-appropriate, nutritionally-balanced intake will promote healing and aid recovery.

Encouraging fluid intake

The following are some practical guidelines for encouraging fluid intake at any age:

- Offer small, full glasses frequently rather than half-full larger glasses; children are mid-school-age before they can evaluate the amount of fluid in a container rather than the size of the container
- Determine the child's favourite fluid and then offer it
- Try changes of temperature in fluid offered (hot cocoa, then cold juice, then hot soup) for variety—soup can be a nice change of liquid (many commercial types are quick to prepare, but be aware of their high sodium content)
- Iceblocks and jelly count as fluids (see Fig. 36.7)
- Children can drink more of a clear fluid (lemonade, water) than a thicker fluid (milkshakes or cream soups),

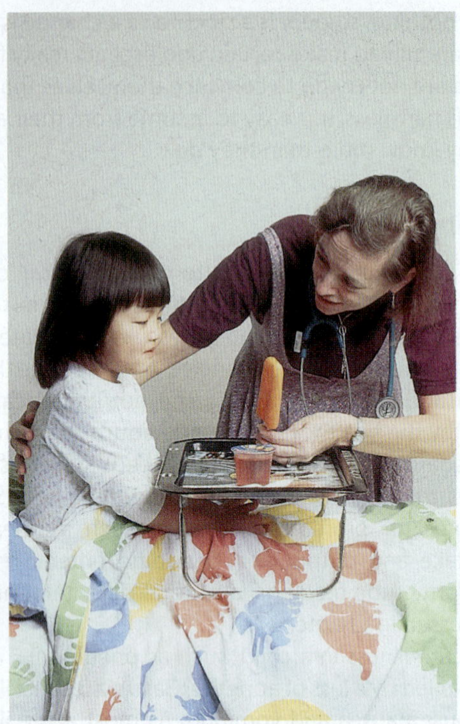

FIGURE 36.7 A nurse offers this young child an ice block, a good source of fluid when children do not feel thirsty or hungry.

because thicker fluids are absorbed from the stomach much more slowly

- Suggest soothing beverages such as water, fruit-flavoured drink or milk for children with mouth lesions; they may be unable to drink fruit juices because the acid content stings their mouths; carbonated beverages may also cause discomfort
- Because ice melts to one half its volume, count a glass of ice chips as only a half-full glass of fluid
- Unless contraindicated, let children drink fluids with a straw; this is a novelty to many who do not normally use these, so encourages intake
- Introduce a game, such as "Simon Says" (Simon says, "Drink")

CASE STUDY QUESTION

4. You want to encourage Becky to drink a lot of water. Which action would do this best?
   a. Scold her for not cooperating to make herself well again
   b. Offer her small glasses of fluid so she can drink these frequently
   c. Offer her large glasses of fluid so she does not have to drink so often
   d. Alert her if she does not drink fluid, she will have to receive an IV

Encouraging food intake

Kilojoule counting, as the name implies, involves counting the number of kilojoules that children ingest each day. To do this, record all the foods that a child eats during each 24-hour period, being certain to include snacks, sweets or chewing gum. A dietician will then analyse the list and determine the overall kilojoule intake. Be sure that everyone caring for the child is aware that kilojoules are being counted so that they also record this information accurately.

Safety

A prime consideration of nursing interventions is to keep children safe during illness care. Promoting safety for children is a responsibility for all healthcare providers. Care of an ill or physically challenged child at home includes assessing the safety of the house and providing family teaching. It also includes making provisions for emergencies. For example, a family may need to install a telephone at bench level or purchase a mobile phone so a child in a wheelchair can call for emergency help.

Safety on a children's ward or clinic is the responsibility of everyone. There are some important steps that can be taken to make a child healthcare environment a safer place:

- Always be sure of the location of all children in your care.
- Ensure that doors or gates are provided near stairways or lifts.
- Ensure that back doors of healthcare facilities have working alarms to prevent children from going out and strangers from coming in.
- Be sure windows are covered by screens or guards so children cannot climb up on windowsills and fall out.
- Check that the side rails of beds and cots are in good repair and raised appropriately.
- Always raise bedside rails after a child has received pre-operative or sedative medication.
- Test a cot rail after it is raised to ensure the lock has caught so the rail will remain raised.
- Push bedside tables or stands away from cots so a child cannot climb over the railing and use the stand as a step down.
- Fasten the seatbelt restraint for infants in highchairs. Never leave an infant in a highchair (at home or in a hospital) without someone close enough to reach the child as infants can easily squirm out of a highchair restraint.
- All unused power points should be fitted with safety plugs.
- Ensure that electrical cords or appliances such as hair dryers are not used in bathrooms, where they could come in contact with water.
- Be careful of the placement of television/call cords or Venetian blind cords so they cannot lead to strangulation.
- Never leave children younger than 5 years alone in a bathtub; they could turn on the hot water and scald themselves or slip under the water and drown.
- Never leave equipment or items that would be harmful to eat, within the reach of children.

- Adhere to all fire precaution measures.
- Closely follow standard infection precautions to prevent the spread of infections.

Promoting fire safety

Fire precautions both in the home and in the hospital are essential for preserving the safety of ill or disabled children. Adults can usually take responsibility for removing themselves from a burning structure, but children depend on care providers. Ensure that there is a plan of action in case of a fire and that everyone in the home, in the clinic or on a hospital unit knows it. To be certain a home is safe, having a smoke detector on each floor is recommended and/or legally required in some states.

Do not use equipment with frayed cords or equipment that is not properly grounded. Plugs should be three-pronged for extra safety; do not overload circuits with additional plugs. Electrical outlets should have safety caps to cover them when they are not in use so toddlers cannot poke objects into them and electrocute themselves.

Adhering to standard infection precautions

In every healthcare setting, closely follow standard infection precautions to protect ill children, family and staff from infections. Because of a compromised immune system, ill children may be more susceptible to repeat or secondary infections than usual, especially drug resistant strains of bacteria such as methicillin-resistant Staphylococcus aureus (MRSA), that can spread easily if everyone is not conscientious about precautions. Proper handwashing technique, disposal of tissues and waste materials and efforts to minimise exposure of other ill children or adults are all effective methods to decrease the risk of infection (Phang, Maznin & Yip, 2012). Tande and colleagues (2010) point out the risk of interfamilial transmission of multidrug resistant bacteria among families of internationally adopted children. For more details on infection control, see Chapter 43.

Sleep

Safe sleeping practices in infants have seen a reduction in the number of sudden unexpected deaths in infants and fatal sleeping accidents. The Safe Sleeping Long Brochure produced by Sids and Kids is endorsed by Paediatrics & Child Health Division, The Royal Australasian College of Physicians and the Australian College of Midwives (Sids and Kids, 2014).

Ill children need adequate rest and sleep so their body tissues can effectively use nutrients for repair and normal growth can continue (Keller & El-Sheikh, 2011). Children may not sleep well when they are ill because of discomfort, pain, administration of medications or intensified symptoms of chronic sleep problems. They may not sleep well in a hospital because it is a strange setting; they may have to undergo so many procedures that they do not rest as much during the day as usual. Children who are recovering from trauma such as injuries from a car accident or burns may be unable to sleep because of nightmares about the accident. These nightmares can cause them to suffer sleep deprivation in the same way as a child who is frequently awakened for procedures during the night. Encourage parents to stay with these children for support and comfort. Remember though, that parents who sleep in hospital rooms do not obtain adequate sleep either. Although their presence is healthy for children, it can lower the parent's ability to handle stress or interpret happenings.

Children who do not receive enough sleep can suffer **sleep deprivation** just as adults do. After approximately 4 days of poor sleep, this can cause them to experience difficulty in concentrating and episodes of disorientation and misperception (Keller & El-Sheikh, 2011). If a child states lack of sleep is a problem, an effective way to document how much sleep the child actually obtains is to ask the child to keep a diary listing start and wake times. Keller & El-Sheikh, (2010) report parental use of logs in a study examining relations between children's sleep and emotional security in the mother-child, father-child and parental marital relationships. Because sleep is so important for ill children, you need to take special steps to ensure that children are able to sleep during an illness. Be certain children are as free from pain and worry as possible. Try to let them maintain as normal a bedtime routine as possible (bath, change to nightclothes, night time story, prayers). Provide an atmosphere conducive to sleep (lights out, quiet surroundings, reassuring support people). Children who are bored with bedrest may catnap constantly during the day and then be wide awake at night. Providing more interesting activities for them during the day can help reduce their naps and increase night-time sleep.

Some children may have chronic sleep problems such as night terrors, nocturnal enuresis, somnambulism (sleepwalking), sleep talking and sleep apnoea. These sleep problems can intensify with illness and increase sleep deprivation in ill children.

Stimulation

Children are in constant interaction with both their internal environment (body) and their external environment (surroundings) by means of their five senses and the central nervous system. This makes them capable of responding to changes in environment and by so doing meet basic needs. Any illness that changes their ability to respond can cause either sensory deprivation or sensory overstimulation.

Sensory deprivation

Sensory deprivation is the condition of being deprived of, or lacking, adequate sensory, social, physical or cognitive stimulation. When this happens, children tend to lose the ability to make decisions and become easily confused and depressed. Some children are more prone to sensory deprivation than others.

Ill children may have sensory deprivation because they are confined to their homes or hospital rooms and their varied activities such as school, sports and clubs are replaced with hours of watching television or playing video games. Hospital regulations for ICUs may limit parental visiting. When parental interaction is limited in this way, children generally receive less-than-normal cognitive stimulation. Such children need cognitive stimulation from warm, reassuring nurses.

Children with hearing or visual deficits are more prone than others to sensory deprivation. Children with forms of sensory nerve loss or those receiving chemotherapy may lose their sense of touch, taste or proprioception (sense of where they are in space). Techniques for interacting with sensory-deprived children are discussed in Chapter 50.

Some children receive medication to lessen awareness of the stimulating factors in their environment. To ensure they do not suffer sensory deprivation, give them definite orientation measures, such as always mentioning the time of day and the day of the week in conversations with them. At the same time, they often must have overly stimulating factors reduced, such as the number of visitors, so that perceptions can be interpreted clearly.

Providing stimulation for children on bedrest

Children on bedrest cannot secure materials for cognitive stimulation by themselves or participate in physical activities, except to a limited degree. When possible, encourage a child with restricted mobility to move out of bed into a wheelchair; this can provide some mobility and transportation to a place of interest, such as near a window or, in a hospital, near the nurses' desk. Watching television, a common activity for children on bedrest, provides little cognitive stimulation after the first 24 hours.

Occasionally, a child must remain in bed to reduce stimulation for reasons such as to rest the heart or to increase kidney function, but generally bedrest is prescribed mainly to inactivate one part of the body, such as a fractured bone. When possible, other stimulation, such as a favourite toy, games, books or simply talking with someone, must be provided for children to help them maintain physical bedrest; otherwise, they become bored and irritable and thrash and turn instead of lying still. If a child is at home on bedrest and the bedroom is away from the main home activities, encourage family members to include the ill child in as many family activities as possible. Orient children to the time of day by making frequent references to it or by providing calendars and clocks.

Providing stimulation for children on transmission-based precautions

Children who are placed on infection control precautions because of the possibility of contagious illness may experience severe sensory deprivation if everyone who enters the room must wear a gown and mask or if the number of visitors must be kept to a minimum. If gloves are part of precautions, a child can experience a significant loss of skin-to-skin contact as well. These precautions are discussed in Chapter 43. Careful planning must be done to ensure that a child who is isolated in this way is not psychologically isolated and that every possible measure is carried out to maintain sensory, social, physical and cognitive stimulation. For example: place the bed so the child can see out of the room; encourage the child to telephone or text message friends; make posters for the walls so they're no longer bare; or encourage interactive play such as electronic games.

Sensory overload

Sensory overload, in contrast to deprivation, occurs when children receive more stimulation than they can tolerate or process. Children with sensory overload react similarly to those with sensory deprivation; feel confused, be unable to make decisions and feel severely fatigued. Sometimes it is difficult to determine the cause of these symptoms (whether they are caused by sensory deprivation or overload) unless assessed carefully.

The lights in ICUs, for example, are never turned out. Although children may find this comforting, it can also result in excessive stimulation. In addition to constant light, there is excessive sound such as the whir of machines, buzzing of ventilators, ringing of alarms or mix of voices in consultation. It is easy for a child to become confused about time and place in such a setting. For children who are cared for at home in a family room where people talk constantly, the television is always on and activity never ceases, sensory overload may also occur. An important nursing role is reducing sensory stimulation attributed to overload. If necessary, provide eye covers or ear plugs to reduce stimulation.

PLAY

Play, often described as "the work of children", is an invaluable component of child healthcare. Providing a space and opportunity for play can help children feel more comfortable and allow for an important release of energy for children who are confined to a room or bed. Play also may be used to help assess children's level of knowledge and feelings about their condition so that more individualised nursing care can be planned. Depending on a child's age, play can also be a useful tool in health teaching (see Chapter 35).

Defining play is not a simple task because play activities vary greatly from child to child and among different age, cultural and socioeconomic groups. A common definition is that play is any voluntary activity engaged in for the purpose of enjoyment. If a child views an activity as enjoyment, therefore, no matter what it is and whether it would be fun or not for an adult, it is play. The manner in which children play, differs as they mature. Types of play and the age groups in which these types are seen most frequently are shown in Box 36.1.

BOX 36.1 ✻ Focus on family teaching

Understanding different play types

Q. Becky's mother tells you, "When Becky was younger, she didn't like toys as much as the boxes they came in. What's normal for children and play?"

A. Children play differently at different ages. Examples of typical play patterns include:

Type of play/age		
Observation/Infant	Child watches particular play intently, although not actively engaged in it	Watching a mobile
Parallel/Toddler	Two children play side by side but seldom attempt to interact with each other	Playing separately with similar push toy
Associative/Preschooler	Children play together in a similar activity; there is little organisation of responsibilities	Engaging in typical backyard play
Cooperative/School-age	Children play within an organised structure or compete for desired goal or outcome	Playing organised games with rules

Assessing child health through play

Children who are acutely ill do not play or play very little, because they do not have the strength, the attention span or the interest in activities required for play. They continue, however, to enjoy being read to and they find comfort in holding a favourite toy even if they do not actively manipulate it. Once children are over the acute phase of an illness, interest in play returns. Whether a child is spontaneously playing, then, is a good index of health. The toys children use at play are a good indication of their growth and development level and emotional state.

The average parent knows a child's play preferences and current favourite game or toy. Asking for this information at a health interview helps to assess a child's developmental level and whether it is age-appropriate. It also helps to assess the quality of parenting (if parents view play as important or are familiar with the child's activities).

Providing play in ambulatory settings

Children in ambulatory departments are under a great deal of stress. They sit in a waiting room and glance fearfully at the door that leads to the examining room. They hear children crying beyond the door and wait in terror for what lies in store for them when it is their turn. Most parents know that when their child is coming to a hospital to be admitted, they should pack the child's favourite toy. They should also be encouraged to bring a toy when a child attends for an ambulatory visit.

Providing play in the hospital

Ideally, all hospital wards in which children are cared for should have a play space big enough for most of the children on the ward to come to. There should be enough space to accommodate children who are not fully ambulatory, such as those with casts or in wheelchairs (see Fig. 36.8). Tables for board games and play materials such as crayons and paints should be available. Children can release a great deal of anger or tension by splashing water, squeezing or pouring sand, or smearing finger paint.

School-aged children can play games such as tossing sand bags for tension relief and competition. Some hospitals offer entertainment areas such as Radio Bed Rock, the Starlight Express Room or the Chinese garden and bird aviary (Children's Hospital, Westmead, Sydney). Adolescents enjoy table tennis and pool tables. A great deal of "play" in older school-age children and adolescents centres on conversation with peers.

For safety reasons, children need to be supervised while they play. Because they do not feel well in a hospital or are shy in these different surroundings, they usually

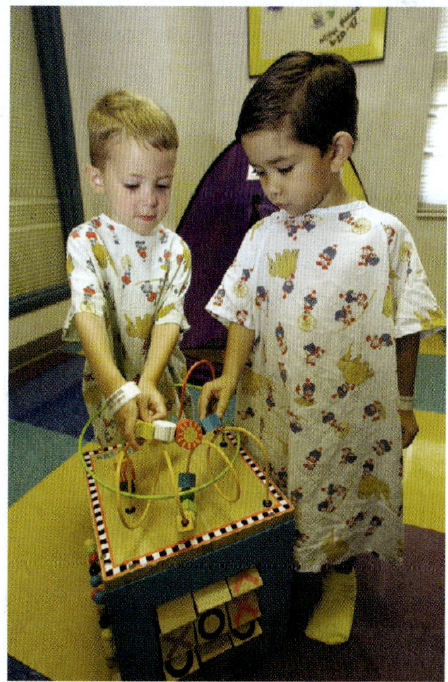

FIGURE 36.8 Children enjoying themselves in a hospital playroom, which is spacious and well-equipped with age-appropriate toys and activities.

enjoy having a concerned adult to watch over them and suggest new activities. Such adults may be volunteers.

Providing play for children on bedrest

Children who are on bedrest, at home or in a hospital, need to have play periods built into their day. The length of time for play and the toys individual children can play with depend on their age and physical and emotional states.

Infants who have toys in their cots, such as mobiles, blocks and rattles must always be supervised when toys are being used and these toys must be removed prior to sleep time. They also need to have time out of cots, sitting on a parent's or a nurse's lap, or sitting in strollers or swings. As soon as they are able, they need some time on the floor (with a sheet under them) to practise crawling or walking. Toddlers need put-in and take-out types of toys, such as blocks, that can be repeatedly dropped into a bottle or that can be stacked to play with in bed. They enjoy listening to tapes of songs and nursery rhymes. Toddlers are in constant motion. They need to be out of bed as much as their physical condition allows, playing with take-apart, put-together or pull-and-push toys. Preschoolers need creative materials such as modelling clay or sand. School-age children need quiet games such as books and crayons or markers by their bedside. While in bed, they enjoy radios, CD players, ipods and mp3 players. Most activities for hospitalised children must be short-term projects because children are called away for treatments or procedures and because when they are ill their attention span is shorter than usual. Short-term projects always appeal to the school-age child because they help this age child achieve a sense of industry. Watching television is a non-participant activity, so it is not the best activity for children. Be certain to screen all toys for safety. They should be washable to prevent spreading disease, with no sharp edges and no small parts that could be swallowed or aspirated.

CASE STUDY QUESTION

5. You worry about Becky aspirating a toy you give her. Which of the following items is most likely to be aspirated?
   a. Pages in a colouring book
   b. Clothing from a doll
   c. Pieces of coloured chalk
   d. Blocks 5 cm square

Therapeutic play

Anything almost automatically becomes less threatening when a person can talk about it. Many children cannot talk about what is happening to them during illness, however, because of fear or because their vocabulary is so limited they cannot describe their feelings. Because play is the language of children, children who have difficulty voicing their thoughts in words can often speak clearly through play.

Play therapy is a psychoanalytical technique used by psychiatrists and play therapists to help children understand their feelings, thoughts and motivations better. In play therapy, the therapist attempts to interpret the child's verbal and non-verbal cues. Interpreting non-verbal cues and helping the child understand them this way requires the skill of a clinical nurse consultant in mental health or others with specialised training. **Therapeutic play** is a play technique that can be used by nurses and doctors to better understand children's feelings and thoughts (Ford et al., 2014). For therapeutic play, only the child's verbal cues are used as responses. Therapeutic play can be divided into three types:

1. Energy release
2. Dramatic play
3. Creative play.

Energy release

Children release energy by pounding, hitting, running, punching or shouting. Furnishing children with materials that allow them to do these things helps them release anxiety as well. For example, toddlers pound pegs with a plastic hammer or pretend to cut wood with a toy saw.

Dramatic play

Dramatic play is acting out an anxiety-producing situation. It is most effective with preschool children because they are at the peak of imagination. During illness, the situations about which children need to express feelings are most often illness related, and therefore the equipment needed for therapeutic play is common healthcare equipment: dolls, doll beds, play stethoscopes, intravenous equipment, syringes, masks and gowns. Puppets of doctors, nurses, mothers, fathers and children help young children express their feelings. Anatomically correct dolls are used to help children describe their feelings about sexual abuse.

Creative play

Some children are too angry to be able to act out their feelings through dramatic play. However, they may be able to draw a picture that expresses their emotions or conveys the extent of their knowledge. To encourage this, give a child a blank piece of paper and crayons or pencils. If a child seems reluctant to draw something spontaneously, suggest a topic: "Why don't you draw a picture of yourself?"

Many ill children draw pictures that reflect punitive images: a boy or girl tied to a bed or shut behind bars, or doctors and nurses frowning at them, obviously unhappy with them. Such children may need assurance that they are not being punished; they need to stay in bed or are being cared for by doctors and nurses to be made well.

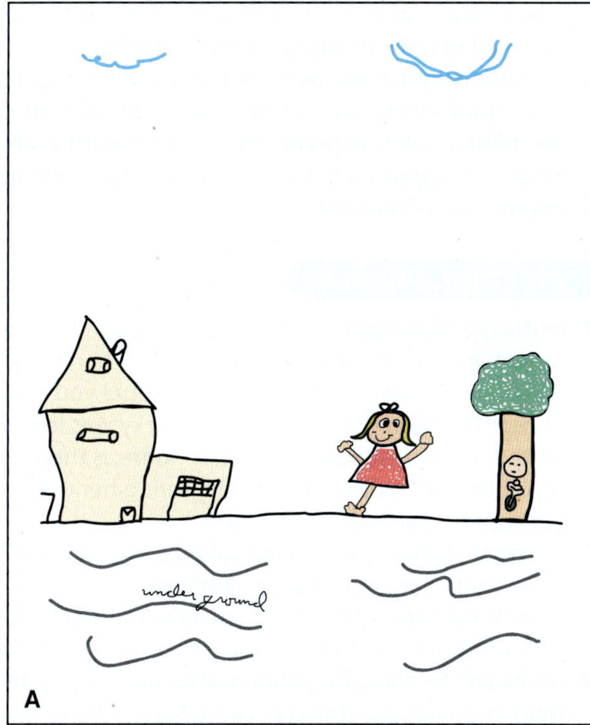

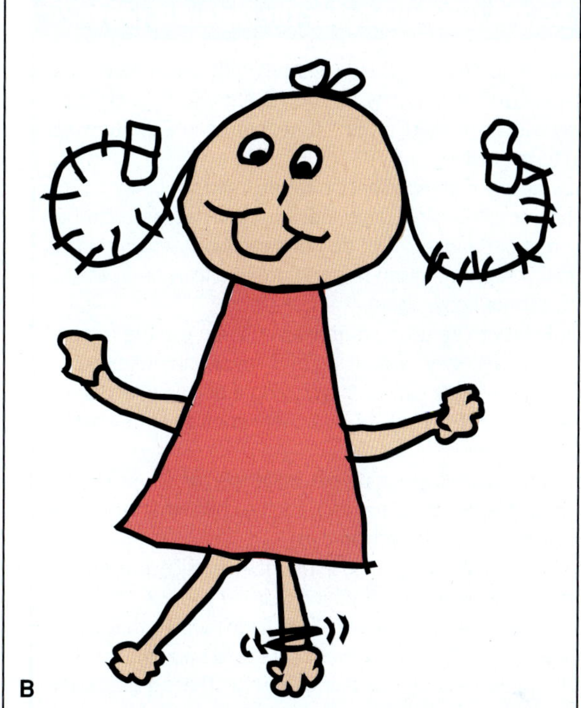

FIGURE 36.9 (**A**) Children who are concerned about body parts may draw pictures with that part missing or exaggerated. Note the missing left leg here. (**B**) After reassurance that her leg will be all right, the girl who did the drawing in (**A**) now draws a girl with two legs.

Other children draw pictures that are symbolic of death: aeroplanes crashing, boats sinking, buildings on fire, children in graveyards. They need reassurance that they will not die (see Figs. 36.9 and 36.10).

> ***What if...***
>
> While you're playing with her, Becky draws a purple person with only three body parts? Would this worry you? Why or why not?

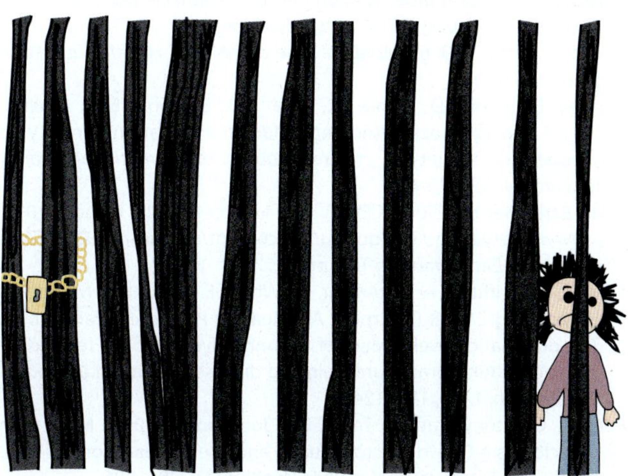

FIGURE 36.10 A picture drawn by a hospitalised child. Note the prison-like appearance of the cot. (Courtesy of Rita Crever.)

Guidelines for conducting therapeutic play

Use commonsense when conducting therapeutic play. Be certain not to interpret a child's black and gloomy drawing as meaning the child is depressed; a black marker may have been the only one available. Many children 4 to 5 years of age draw a person lacking many body parts because that is the best human form they can draw.

Remember, too, that all children occasionally treat dolls badly. A 2-year-old pounding and banging a rag doll may not be expressing anger towards the doll image at all, but may be intent on discovering the feel of a new texture and is unaware for the moment that the object is a doll. A conference with healthcare team members, including a psychologist or a clinical nurse consultant in mental health, may be called for if a child continues to express mutilating behaviour after normal reassurance. See Box 36.2 for some helpful guidelines for therapeutic play.

CASE STUDY QUESTION

6. Becky will have a large bandage on her foot after surgery. Which type of therapeutic play would be best for her?

a. Letting her hold and handle a medicine syringe
b. Giving her a doll and a bandage to change
c. Helping her insert a nasogastric tube into a puppet
d. Teaching her a rhyme about good girls

BOX 36.2 Guidelines for therapeutic play

1. Allow children to choose the articles with which they want to play (something may be too frightening for a child to play with immediately; more time may be needed to work up to the activity).
2. Provide the materials specific to the child's experiences of which you, the nurse, are aware such as a nasogastric tube, syringe or bandages, but do not supply only those things; a child may have misunderstandings and fears of situations you cannot know about.
3. Allow play to be unstructured; let children use the materials however they wish. If a child seems uninterested in materials, initiate play such as giving a doll an injection to see if this reduces the child's anxiety enough to be able to handle items.
4. If a child cannot manipulate materials for some reason such as a large cast or traction, ask the child what would be good for you to do with an item.
5. Reflect only what the child expresses (verbal expression).
6. Do not criticise play; this inhibits further expression.
7. Use a therapeutic response—not "Don't worry, that won't happen", but "Are you worried that could happen?"
8. Ask children to describe paintings, not "That's a good picture of yourself", but "Tell me about your picture".
9. Do not be reluctant to use real equipment such as real catheters and blood lancets. Handling real equipment best helps to reduce stress.
10. Supervise therapeutic play, because some equipment could cause an accident (and therapeutically responding to the child's comments is necessary).

Key points for review

- Illness may be more traumatic for children than for adults because of children's inability to communicate and monitor their own care and because they have different nutrition, fluid and electrolyte needs. The stress of hospitalisation can be so acute that it can result in post-traumatic stress syndrome.
- Separation from parents because of hospitalisation can have permanent psychological effects on children. Methods to reduce this include keeping hospital stays as brief as possible, promoting open parent and sibling visiting and providing primary or case management nursing.
- Currently, many medical procedures can be done on an ambulatory basis. Nurses can advocate for care to be done in such settings while being mindful of other constraints which sometimes prevent procedures from being undertaken on an ambulatory basis.
- The presence of parents during healthcare can help reduce trauma to children. Making parents as welcome as possible in healthcare facilities makes it possible for them to room-in. Include parents in both the planning and the implementation of care. Parents transmit fear to children if their own fear is not reduced.
- Preschoolers may have the most difficult time during hospitalisation because they have so many fears. Preparation and promotion of therapeutic play may be essential to reduce trauma to a tolerable level.
- Because hospitalisations currently are so brief, parents need good discharge instructions to continue to care for children safely at home. Providing clear instructions including suggestions for play or how to avoid sleep deprivation is important.

CASE STUDY QUESTIONS

7. In the hospital playroom, Becky picked up a doll and tore off its leg. Her mother asked you why her daughter is acting this way. What suggestions would you make to her? The burn occurred because Becky was left momentarily unsupervised by a campfire. Is there a possibility her mother may not be acting her usual self because of guilt over the injury?
8. Suppose Becky's parents are called away on a family emergency, so Becky has no family with her for 3 days. What measures would you take to help make hospitalisation and separation less traumatic for her?
9. Becky will be cared for at home after her surgery. Her mother is concerned that because Becky's home-stay will be lengthy, she will be cut off from her friends for a long time. What suggestions could you make to help Becky maintain contact with her friends? Her mother is concerned she will become exhausted because of the need for round-the-clock care. What suggestions could you offer to make care easier?

Resources

For an extensive range of additional resources to enhance teaching and learning and to facilitate understanding of this chapter, please see the text's accompanying website located on thePoint at http://thepoint.lww.com.

References

Association for the Wellbeing of Children in Healthcare (AWCH). (2014), accessed 28 January 2015, <www.awch.org.au>.

Bowlby, J., et al. (1966). *Maternal Care and Mental Health*. New York: Schocken Books.

Cagiran, E., Sergin, D., Deniz, M., Tanatti, B., Emirogly, N. & Alper, I. (2014). Effects of sociodemographic factors and maternal anxiety on preoperative anxiety in children. *Journal of International Medical Research*, *42*(2), 572–580.

Child Early Warning Tool (CEWT). (2011), accessed 28 January 2015, <www.safetyandquality.gov.au/wp-content/uploads/2012/11/The-Children-s-Early-Warning-Tool.pdf>.

Dooley, F., Griffiths, L., McArthur, L., White, E. & Cunlife, M. (2013), Introducing LAPPS (Liverpool Anticipatory Procedural Pain Score). The pragmatic development of an innovative approach to predicting and treating procedural pain and distress in children. *Journal of Child Health*, *17*(2), 114–124.

Ford, K., Courtney-Pratt, H., Tesch, L. & Johnson, C. (2014). More than just clowns—Clown Doctor rounds and their impact for children, families and staff. *Journal of Child Health*, *18*(3), 286–296.

Gordon, B., (2012). An action research study with health care professionals aiming to improve preparation for childhood hospitalisation.

Thesis submitted in total fulfilment of the requirements for the degree of Doctor of Philosophy, University of Technology, Sydney.

Haakorotanga Maori Parenting Programme, accessed 28 January 2015, <www.net-inc.org.nz/?cID=haakuitanga_haakorotanga_parenting_programme>.

Henry, N. & Kurzak, K. (2013). The Australian Collaboration. A Collaboration of National Community Organisations. A Multicultural Australia, accessed 28 January 2015, <www.australiancollaboration.com.au/pdf/FactSheets/Multicultural-Australia-FactSheet.pdf>.

Indigenous Children's Health Report. (2014). Health assessment in action, accessed 28 January 2015, <www.onemda.unimelb.edu.au/docs/ichrreport.pdf>.

Kearvell, H. & Grant, J. (2010). Getting connected: How nurses can support mother/infant attachments in the neonatal intensive care unit. *Australian Journal Advanced Nursing*, *27*(3), 75–82.

Keller, P. & El-Sheikh, M. (2011). Children's emotional security and sleep: Longitudinal relations and direction of effects. *Journal of Child Psychology and Psychiatry*, *52*(1), 64–71.

Livesley, J. & Long, T. (2013). Children's experiences as hospital in-patients: Voice, competence and work. Messages for nursing from a critical ethnographic study. *International Journal of Nursing Studies*, *50*(10), 1292–1303.

Medical Services Commission. (2010). Oral rehydration therapy (ORT) in children, accessed 28 January 2015, <www.bcguidelines.ca/guideline_ort.html>.

Middleton, P. (2012). Signs that a child is seriously ill: Interview with Professor Middleton, Child Health News, accessed 28 January 2015, <www.news-medical.net/news/20120704/Signs-that-a-child-is-seriously-ill-Interview-with-Professor-Middleton.aspx>.

NSW Health. (2011). Children and infants—Recognition of a sick baby or child in the emergency department (2nd ed.). Clinical practice guidelines, accessed 27 January 2015, <www.health.nsw.gov.au/policies/pd/2011/pdf/PD2011_038.pdf>.

NSW Health. (2012). Liverpool Hospital Intensive Care Unit, Medical Emergency Team, accessed 27 January 2015, <www.swslhd.nsw.gov.au/liverpool/ICU/met.html>.

New Zealand Ministry of Health Manatū Hauora. (2011). Child health, accessed 28 January 2015, <www.health.govt.nz/our-work/life-stages/child-health>.

Newton, A., Wolgemuth, A., Gallivant, J. & Wrightson, D. (2010). Providing support to siblings of hospitalised children. *Journal of Paediatrics and Child Health*, *46*(3), 72–75.

Nicholas, D., Fellner, K., Koller, D., Chow, K., & Brister, L. (2014). Evaluation of videophone communication for families of hospitalised children. *Social Work in Health Care*, *50*(3), 215–229.

Ojha, A., Shakya, K.. & Aryal, U. (2012). Recurrence risk of febrile seizures in children. *Journal of Nepal Paediatric Society*, *32*(1), 33–36.

Phang, K., Maznin, N. & Yip, W. (2012). Hand hygiene in the nursery during diaper changing. *International Journal of Evidence-Based Healthcare*, *10*(4), 382–387.

Pudney, W. & Whitehouse, E. (2012). *Little Volcanoes: Helping Young Children and Their Parents to Deal with Anger*. London: Jessica Kinglsey.

Robertson, J. (1958). *Young Children in Hospitals.* London: Tavistock.

Royal Children's Hospital Melbourne. (2012). Clinical guidelines (nursing), observation and continuous monitoring, accessed 27 January 2015, <www.rch.org.au/rchcpg/hospital_clinical_guideline_index/Observation_and_Continuous_Monitoring/#refs>.

Royal Children's Hospital Melbourne. (2010). Preparing your child for hospital and Preparing for hospital—a guide for parents/carers, accessed 28 January 2015, <www.rch.org.au/rch/patients-families.cfm>.

Sids and Kids. (2014). Safe sleeping, accessed 28 January 2015, <www.sidsandkids.org/safe-sleeping/>.

Spitz, R. A. (1945). Hospitalism: An inquiry into the genesis of psychiatric conditions in early childhood. *Psychoanalytic Study of the Child*, *1*(3), 53–59.

Starship Children's Health Service. (2015). Your child's hospital or daystay admission, accessed 28 January 2015, <www.starship.org.nz/patients-and-families/your-childs-hospital-or-daystay-admission/>.

Sydney Children's Hospital. (2013). Child and family health, accessed 28 January 2015, <www.sch.edu.au/departments/child_family_health/>.

Sydney Children's Hospital. (2013). Your stay in hospital, accessed 28 January 2015, <www.sch.edu.au/general/stay/>.

Tande, D., Boisrarne, S., Munck, M., Hery-Arnaud, G., Gouriou, S., Jallot, N., Nordmann, P. & Nass, T. (2010). Intrafamilial transmission of extended-spectrum-β-lactamase-producing *Escherichia coli* and *Salmonella enterica* Babelsberg among the families of internationally adopted children. *Journal of Antimicrobial Chemotherapy*, *65*(5), 859–865.

Wellington Children's Hospital. (2014). Just for kids, accessed 28 January 2015, <www.justforkids.org.nz/>.

Suggested readings

Australian Institute of Health and Welfare. (2012). A picture of Australia's children 2012, accessed 28 January 2015, <www.aihw.gov.au/WorkArea/DownloadAsset.aspx?id=10737423340>.

New Zealand Ministry of Health. (2015). The health of New Zealand children 2011/12, accessed 28 January 2015, <www.health.govt.nz/publication/health-new-zealand-children-2011-12>.

Chapter 37

Nursing care of a family when a child needs diagnostic or therapeutic modalities

Previous chapters described the growth and development of well children. This chapter adds information about how to care for children who are having diagnostic or therapeutic procedures. This is important information because it builds a base for both care and health teaching.

LEARNING OBJECTIVES

After studying the contents of this chapter, you should be able to:

1. Describe common nursing considerations used in the healthcare of children to aid diagnosis and therapy.
2. Use critical thinking to analyse ways in which diagnostic and therapeutic procedures can be modified to be more family-centred.
3. Assess children regarding developmental stage and knowledge level before beginning diagnostic or therapeutic procedures in order to promote positive experiences.
4. Identify common diagnostic or therapeutic procedures used with children.
5. Demonstrate an understanding of expected outcomes for a child who needs a diagnostic or therapeutic procedure.
6. Develop an understanding of nursing considerations to aid in diagnosis or therapy for children, including working within a multidisciplinary team across different modalities.
7. Develop an understanding of differing nursing considerations relevant to diagnostic or therapeutic procedures such as preparing a child for magnetic resonance imaging.
8. Identify areas of own practice in which current research and evidence based medicine can benefit nursing procedures.
9. Integrate knowledge of common diagnostic and therapeutic procedures with nursing process to achieve high quality nursing care for children and families.

KEY TERMS

- aspiration studies
- barium contrast studies
- bronchoscopy
- colonoscopy
- computed tomography (CT)
- electrical impulse studies
- endoscopy
- fever
- gastrostomy tube feedings
- magnetic resonance imaging (MRI)
- mid-stream urine specimen
- nasogastric tube feedings
- ostomy
- positron emission tomography (PET)
- radiopharmaceuticals
- single-photon emission computed tomography (SPECT)
- total parenteral nutrition (TPN)
- ultrasound
- vital signs

CASE STUDY

Hamish Brown is a preschooler who is scheduled to have a magnetic resonance imaging (MRI) study because of a head injury. "How can I agree to this?" his mother asks you. "He's afraid of the dark. How can I allow him to be wheeled into a long dark machine that way?"

CASE STUDY QUESTION

1. How would you explain MRI to Hamish to make the procedure more acceptable to him?

Illness can be particularly stressful if many diagnostic and therapeutic procedures are necessary for diagnosis or care. In today's healthcare climate, there is less time for teaching and preparation than was once available, so good planning and follow-through become essential when these procedures are scheduled (Thalange et al., 2013). The underpinning principle for nurses working with children is to ensure that all care including interventions and procedures maximise the interests of the child and family while minimising the potential harms (Delaney & Conwell, 2012). Everything that nurses do with and for ill children can have a major influence on children's progress towards better health as well as on children's and their families' perception of professional healthcare and the ability to carry out healthful practices in the future.

Many nursing actions offer an opportunity to accomplish several goals. Supporting a child and family during a diagnostic procedure, for instance, can not only aid in efficient consideration but may also help establish a trusting relationship between the family and healthcare providers that will make all future interactions more successful. This chapter describes the most common diagnostic and therapeutic techniques used in the care of ill children, including modifications needed to make these procedures safe and reduce associated stress, depending on the child's age and condition.

CHILDREN REQUIRING DIAGNOSTIC OR THERAPEUTIC PROCEDURES

Assessment

Before performing procedures such as assisting with a diagnostic test or collecting laboratory specimens, first carefully evaluate a child's age and developmental stage, as well as any special needs a child may have. Even the most common and painless procedures create a certain amount of stress for children and parents. During complex diagnostic procedures, this stress level is almost certain to increase even further. Unfamiliar doctors and nurses, high-tech supplies and equipment, and strange surroundings all add up to a frightening experience for most adults; imagine how frightening they can seem to children.

It is important to acknowledge that some procedures can cause pain or discomfort. Assess a child's level of anxiety associated with unfamiliar equipment, circumstances and surroundings as well as the child's knowledge concerning a technique before initiating a therapeutic procedure or beginning health teaching. Respecting a child's past experience with similar procedures can lay a foundation for knowledge and cooperation.

Nursing considerations

Common nursing considerations related to diagnostic and therapeutic procedures are as varied as the procedures themselves. Some examples of specific considerations that nurses are required to address are:

- Fear related to the new and strange surroundings of the procedure room
- Pain related to an invasive procedure
- Diversionary activities related to hospitalisation and lengthy procedures
- Imbalanced nutrition, related to the need for food restriction pre-procedure and post-procedure.

Interventions and procedures can result in higher stress levels than that caused by the primary illness. An important nursing goal is to cause the least degree of anxiety possible while completing interventions. To achieve this goal, plan specific ways to prepare children in advance, such as the best way to explain a procedure to a particular child. Also ensure the child is not overwhelmed by the number of diagnostic or therapeutic procedures performed in any one day. With small children, it may make more sense to stagger ambulatory diagnostic tests over several days to preserve a child's coping ability. Conversely, some older children (and parents) do better if they can complete all necessary tests in 1 day, so they do not have to anticipate more testing over a long period. Use nursing judgement and data from periodic assessments to help primary care providers determine the type of schedule that is in the best interest of each individual child and their family. Helpful websites to recommend for parents to help them prepare children for procedures include:

- Kids Health the Children's Hospital at Westmead Fact sheets <http://kidshealth.schn.health.nsw.gov.au/fact-sheets>
- Sydney Children's Hospital Network <www.schn.health.nsw.gov.au>
- The Royal Children's Hospital Melbourne <www.rch.org.au/kidsinfo>
- Starship Foundation <www.starship.org.nz>.

Whether assisting with a procedure or performing a therapeutic intervention it is necessary to function in several roles at the same time: performing (or assisting with) the procedure; providing active support to the child and parents; and observing and then documenting the child's reactions. Providing support is a major role and there are many ways to do this, such as holding a child's hand or placing a hand on the parent's shoulder. Playing a distracting game with an older child can also be helpful. Important observations to be made include signs of discomfort, changes in vital signs or other signals of distress such as pallor or dizziness. Maintain a flow sheet of observations during a procedure. After a procedure the child's reaction and specimens obtained can then be documented accurately and efficiently in the child's record.

Evaluating expected outcomes related to diagnostic and therapeutic procedures not only helps in determining the effect of the procedure on a child but also aids in future planning, should other procedures be required. Recording that a particular child who did not appear nervous during a procedure later admitted to being "more scared than I've ever been before", for example, can help another nurse provide reassurance to this child, even when the child is masking emotions the next time.

As a final follow-through step, think of therapeutic play techniques to introduce that would be helpful in relieving stress caused by the procedure, debriefing can be very useful. In some hospitals play therapists are available and can assist with pre-procedural education, desensitisation to medical equipment using play, behavioural stress reduction techniques, procedural support and debriefing sessions after procedures.

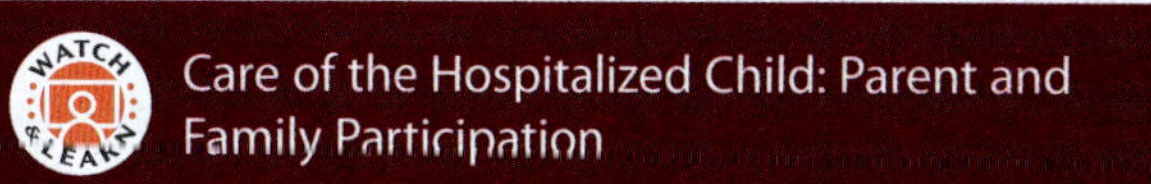

NURSING RESPONSIBILITIES WITH DIAGNOSTIC AND THERAPEUTIC TECHNIQUES

The most efficient way to reduce children's stress from hospitalisation is to reduce the number of hospitalisations necessary. When hospitalisation does become necessary, reducing the stress of the experience by being certain that procedures are carried out in the least stressful way possible is necessary. Responsibilities when assisting with procedures performed on children include:

- Helping obtain informed consent as needed, including the use of healthcare interpreters if necessary.

- Explaining the procedure to the child and the parents to be certain both are well informed; acting out procedures with toys can aid children's understanding
- Scheduling the procedure and obtaining necessary documentation
- Preparing the child physically and psychologically by discussing what will be involved in the procedure and how this will affect the child
- Obtaining necessary equipment for the procedure
- Accompanying a child to a treatment room or hospital department where the procedure will be performed
- Providing support during the procedure
- Ensuring adherence to standardised or specialised infection control precautions
- Assessing a child's response to the procedure
- Providing care to a child and specimens obtained once the procedure is completed
- Coordination or cooperating with other healthcare disciplines.

Obtaining informed consent

Any medical procedure or intervention which carries potential risk must have valid documentation of informed consent, without consent the procedure cannot be performed. For a parent to sign a consent form, they must be knowledgeable about the procedure, the steps involved and the risks of having or not having it performed. If a family is not able to understand the consent form, the procedure or the risks of the procedure it is essential that the nurse advocates on their behalf to ensure they are fully informed. This can involve further discussions with a medical officer and/or use of healthcare interpreters. Important considerations to be aware of include in single-parent families, the custodial parent is the one who is asked to give consent, and adolescents' capability to provide consent. Laws differ in individual states and territories (RANZCOG, 2013).

Explaining procedures

To be able to explain procedures clearly and answer questions about them appropriately, try to observe as many procedures as you can. Asking children after any procedure what sensations they experienced can help children work through possibly frightening situations (often called "debriefing") and also increase your knowledge of common procedures. As a general guide, a child needs a detailed description of the procedure, such as, "I'll clean your finger. You will feel a small pin prick", as well as an explanation of:

- Why the procedure is being performed—for example, "The doctor needs to look at your blood to see why you're so sick".
- Where the procedure will be performed—for instance, the medical imaging department or a treatment room.
- Any unusual sensations to be expected during the procedure, such as, "this is for cleaning your skin and it will feel cold".
- Any pain involved: "The injection will sting, although I'll put some cream on first to dull the feeling".
- Any strange equipment used, such as an x-ray machine.
- The approximate length of time the procedure will take.
- Any special care after the procedure—for example, "You will need to lie quietly for 15 minutes afterwards".

Be certain to use age-appropriate language when explaining procedures. Also be careful not to use words that might be confusing during an explanation, such as "transducer" or "electrode", without defining them. Try to associate the procedure with something with which a child is already familiar and comfortable such as describing an x-ray machine as "a big camera". Try not to use the word "test" in explanations because school-aged children associate the word "test" with a pass/fail situation. This can make them unduly worried after a procedure about whether they have "passed" it. If you are unfamiliar with the steps of the procedure do not guess the answers, as this can generate further stress and anxiety if different to information already given or what actually happens. Reducing parental anxiety by providing clear explanations of the procedure can be very useful in reducing children's anxiety. Encourage parents to stay with a child during procedures whenever appropriate. Parental presence can be extremely helpful in reducing a procedure's perceived threatening aspects (Forsey et al., 2011).

Scheduling

Most diagnostic procedures are scheduled on an ambulatory basis. Try to arrange for a child to have time for meals and some free play time between procedures. If food or fluid must be restricted for procedures, monitor the child's degree of discomfort and physiological needs related to this; advocate as necessary for a time lapse between examinations or improved coordination in scheduling to decrease the time spent without food or fluid. In some circumstances small sips of water or ice are allowed while waiting. This is dependent on the procedure and medical officer's advice.

Preparing a child and family physically and psychologically

Physical preparation varies depending on what procedure is to be performed. In many instances, preparing a child for an examination such as a barium enema involves another procedure such as a saline enema, so physical preparation becomes education for the actual examination. In all instances, explain both the preparative and actual procedures. Appropriate explanations aid in reducing anxiety and fear.

For many procedures, conscious sedation may also be used (Havidich & Cravero, 2012). Conscious sedation refers to a depressed level of consciousness induced by the intravenous administration of a sedative. About 60 minutes before the procedure, children may be given an oral sedative to relieve both apprehension and make them feel sleepy.

Accompanying the child

If a procedure is to be done at a different department from the hospital ward with which a child is comfortable, ideally a nurse, whom the child knows, should accompany the child as well as a parent to the other department and remain with the child for the procedure, or at least until the child has met a primary person who will be responsible for the procedure. Having a parent accompany a child is of additional invaluable help. Older children do well with being accompanied by only a nursing assistant as long as they have been introduced in advance to the new person who will give them care.

Before leaving the child's care unit, have the child void for comfort unless this is contraindicated. Check for any medication or specific assessment procedures, such as a blood pressure recording, that should be given or done before leaving the unit for another department, in case the child is away from the primary unit for an extended time. If a child is an inpatient, check also that the identification band is securely in place and readily visible despite any intravenous equipment. If there will be a considerable wait in another department, ask the child if they would like to bring along an activity such as a game or book. Hallways can be cool. Provide adequate blankets for comfort, especially for infants. Always ensure side rails are locked for safety.

Providing support

Children do well with diagnostic and evaluative procedures as long as they have adequate support from a concerned provider or parent. Try to provide this both verbally (explain what is going to happen; assure the child everything is going well) and non-verbally (a hand on the arm or a nearby presence).

Modifying procedures according to a child's age and developmental stage

A child's age and potential understanding of procedures must be considered when planning the number and order of tests and the way they are performed. For children with developmental delay additional preparation time, education, play therapy and debriefing may be necessary, to ensure understanding and reduce anxiety.

The infant

The number of painful or uncomfortable procedures done on infants should be kept to an absolute minimum to avoid interfering with an infant's developing sense of trust. Parents should be allowed to accompany their infant to hospital departments and remain during procedures to offer support. Some parents may ask to hold their child during a procedure that causes pain, but do not ask parents to restrain the child during such a procedure. Their role should be a supportive and comforting one, not a policing one. Sucrose is a common technique used to settle infants during a painful or distressing procedure, but should be used with caution.

Infants become dehydrated quickly so the time for procedures must be limited. You may need to advocate for time for breastfeeding before and after procedures for both an infant's and mother's comfort. If a procedure continues longer than 3 to 4 hours, provide the mother a room in which to use a breast pump, if needed.

The toddler and preschooler

Toddlers and preschoolers resist any diagnostic testing that involves any degree of discomfort or pain or that is unfamiliar to them. Give children of this age short explanations of what to expect close to the time of the procedure, so that little time can be spent worrying about it. Try to associate any new equipment with things which they are already familiar.

The school-aged child and adolescent

School-aged children are interested in the theory and reason for procedures. Often they can be persuaded to cooperate for a procedure by being promised a look at their x-rays. Be careful to ensure that viewing the results is actually possible before promising this to children; otherwise, it can be difficult to obtain any further cooperation. Adolescents may project an air of maturity or sophistication beyond their years to remain in control of themselves in the face of frightening procedures. Do not be misled into thinking a child this age would not appreciate an explanation or a comforting hand on a shoulder during a procedure.

Promoting safety during procedures

Safety is an important component of all patient care. Children's immaturity, which makes them unable to form mature judgements, leaves them vulnerable to harm unless their carers give special consideration to promoting safety during procedures.

As a basic safety measure, before giving any food or performing any procedure, read the name on a child's identification armband. If an armband must be removed because it interferes with an intravenous infusion site, cut it away but immediately anchor it to another extremity with adhesive tape. Ask the admissions department to provide a new armband as soon as possible. Do not leave the old one off while waiting for a replacement band; this leaves the child susceptible to the danger of mistaken identity during the waiting period.

Because of their natural curiosity, children tend to fuss with equipment to see what will happen if they turn a knob or spin a dial. This means they need close monitoring while procedures are performed to ensure they do not touch any buttons or in other ways accidentally harm

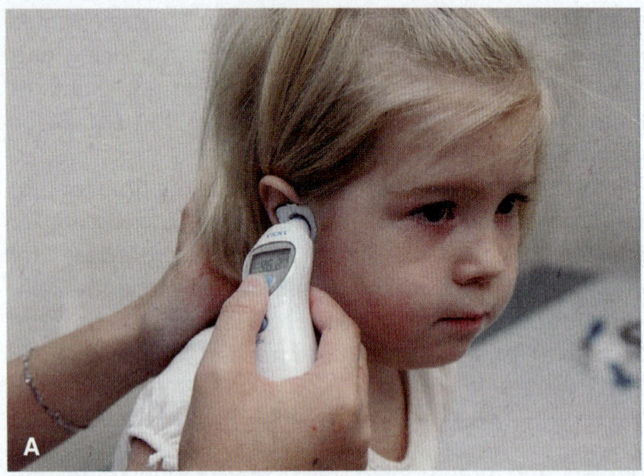

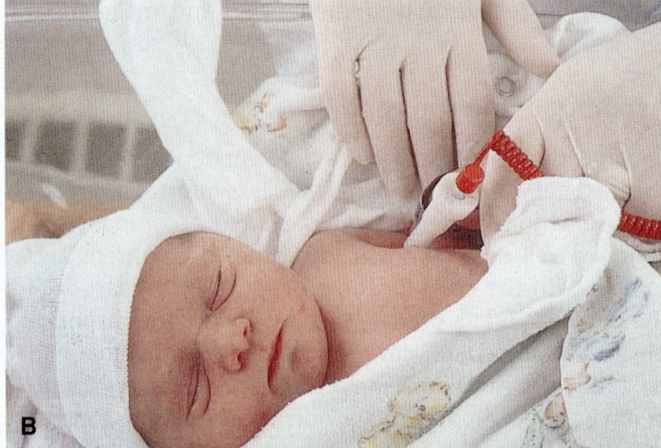

FIGURE 37.1 Taking temperature. (**A**) Tympanic membrane temperature. (**B**) Axillary temperature.

themselves. After a procedure, be sure to remove all equipment from a room.

Providing care after procedures

After a procedure, assess how well a child reacted to the procedure by both observation and history. Allowing children to explain what happened helps them retrace the procedure in their mind so they can conquer their fear of it. Fill in gaps in information as necessary to improve a child's perception of the procedure. Providing therapeutic play is another measure to reduce anxiety.

Children can be discharged as soon as 30 minutes after conscious sedation if they are awake and oriented; the airway is patent and respiratory status is stable (no retraction, stridor or wheezing); oxygen saturation is 95% or greater in room air; blood pressure, heart rate and respiratory rates are appropriate for age; and the child is reasonably free of pain.

MEASURING VITAL SIGNS

Vital signs for children consist of temperature, pulse, respiratory rate, blood pressure and pain assessment. All of these vital signs need to be recorded both conscientiously and with knowledge of the child's underlying condition so they can be analysed meaningfully. Be especially alert that assessing any of these measures is not enough; if they are abnormal or if a child has pain, a measure to relieve the problem needs to be initiated. Appendix C shows the average pulse rates, respiration rates and blood pressures for children of different ages, as these differ according to the size and age of the child.

Temperature

Normal temperature values in children are the same as in adults: axillary (36.5°C); oral or tympanic (37.0°C); and rectal (37.6°C). Electronic thermometers that assess axillary temperature are ideal for assessment in children. Axillary measurement of temperature is recommended for routine clinical use, but staff should be aware that axillary temperatures are up to 1°C lower than rectal temperatures (see Fig. 37.1). Rectal and oral temperatures are not recommended because of safety concerns and problems with acceptability. There is also a lack of data for oral temperatures. Tympanic temperatures are not recommended as they are unreliable (NSW Health, 2010).

Rectal temperatures are the 'gold standard' for measuring central body temperature [Level IV]. There are safety concerns, however, (particularly in the very young) with its routine use as well as issues concerning lack of acceptability (NSW Health, 2010). Newborns should not have their temperature taken rectally because of the danger of damaging their rectal mucosa with a thermometer; it should be taken by the axillary route instead. Because preschoolers generally fear intrusive procedures, consider taking axillary recordings in children until 4 or 5 years of age.

For an axillary recording, place the tip of an electronic thermometer in the axilla and hold the child's arm down to the side to keep the thermometer firmly in place until it registers. For the rare occasions when a rectal temperature must be taken, insert a thermometer only to the length of the bulb (1 cm) in infants and not over 2 cm in older children and hold it in place for 5 minutes.

Pulse rate

As children grow older, the heart rate slows and the range of normal values narrows. If possible, measure a child's pulse rate at rest. An apical pulse (listening at the heart apex through a stethoscope) is taken in children younger than 1 year because their radial (wrist) pulse is too faint to be palpated accurately. In an infant, the point of maximum intensity, or the point on the chest wall where the heartbeat can be heard most distinctly, is just above and outside the left nipple (just lateral to the midclavicular line at the third or fourth intercostal space). This point gradually becomes more medial and slightly lower up to 7 years of age. By 7 years, it is at the fourth or fifth interspace at the midclavicular line.

Respiratory rate

Respirations should be measured while an infant is calm because the respiratory rate increases with crying. Take the respiratory rate while a child is sitting on a parent's lap or lying quietly in a cot before lowering the side rail if possible. Infants tend to breathe with their abdominal muscles; therefore, it is as accurate to take respirations by counting movements of the abdomen as it is to count chest movements.

Blood pressure

Blood pressure is included in the routine physical assessment of all children. Offer a good explanation of the procedure, especially to young children, because wrapping their arm and applying pressure can be frightening if they are not prepared for it. Blood pressure is difficult to measure in infants because of mechanical problems. The cuff used should be no more than two-thirds and not less than one-half the length of their upper arm; a wider cuff (larger bladder size) gives a lower reading and a narrower cuff gives a higher reading. Doppler ultrasound blood pressure recording is especially effective with infants. This technique bounces high-frequency sound waves off body parts; the rate and pitch at which they return depends on the density of the body part that is struck. If a Doppler lead is placed over an artery, either the movement of the blood (pulse wave) or its tension (blood pressure) can be registered on a digital readout or monitor print. Doppler examinations can be adapted to broadcast the sound of the pulse waves for auscultatory assessment.

Electronic blood pressure recording is most helpful when a continuous assessment is necessary, but it can be used for a single recording. Watching the digital readout numbers is interesting for preschoolers. Electronic pressure readings are typically 5 mmHg higher for diastolic and 10 mmHg higher for systolic blood pressure compared with auscultatory techniques (Brayden, Daley & Brown, 2008). Direct measurement (intra-arterial monitoring by an indwelling catheter into the radial or femoral artery) is used with children who are critically ill.

Lower extremity blood pressure can be obtained by wrapping the cuff over the thigh and palpating or auscultating the popliteal pulse (posterior knee). In infants younger than 1 year, the thigh and arm blood pressure should be equal. In children older than 1 year, the systolic pressure in the thigh tends to be 10 to 40 mmHg higher, while diastolic pressure remains the same. If the thigh blood pressure reading is lower than that in the arm, suspect that coarctation of the aorta or an interference with circulation to the lower extremities may be causing this.

When assessing blood pressure, be certain to pay attention to the pulse pressure—the difference between systolic and diastolic readings. Both unusually wide (more than 50 mmHg) or narrow (less than 10 mmHg) ranges may suggest congenital heart disease. An abnormally narrow pulse pressure, for instance, is a sign of aortic stenosis. An abnormally low diastolic pressure (causing a wide pulse pressure) occurs with patent ductus arteriosus.

REDUCING ELEVATED TEMPERATURE IN CHILDREN

Fever is such a common symptom in children that reducing temperature or giving a parent instructions on how to reduce a child's temperature at home is a common intervention with children. Because the temperature-regulating mechanism in children is immature, fever tends to be more marked in children than in adults and may even be out of proportion to the seriousness or extent of their disease. An increased temperature occurs because a child's temperature-regulating point (set point) has been elevated. The child's temperature cannot be reduced until the set point returns (or is returned) to normal. Currently recommended antipyretics such as paracetamol and ibuprofen are the drugs most often prescribed to reduce fever in children (NSW Health, 2010).

Parents often do not give an adequate dose of an antipyretic such as paracetamol because they are afraid their child will have a bad reaction to it. This results in the high fever continuing. Paracetamol is given every 4 hours, up to 4 doses a day, until their child's temperature is reduced (NSW Health, 2010). Teach parents that fever is actually a body protection measure and unless it is exceptionally high (more than 41.1°C) it does no specific harm. In fact, there is some evidence that fever may be of value in helping to combat infection, because it aids in destroying microorganisms (Edwards et al., 2007). For this reason, parents can be cautioned that low grade fever itself is not harmful and does not need treatment. Over treatment of fever with regular high doses of an antipyretic or severe overdose can result in liver or kidney toxicity (McKenna & Mirkov, 2014). In hospital settings an antipyretic is generally ordered for any child whose oral or tympanic temperature is more than 38.4°C or whose rectal temperature is more than 39.0°C. It is important to caution parents not to give acetylsalicylic acid (aspirin) to children with fever because aspirin is associated with Reye's syndrome, a severe neurological disorder.

Parents should dress children with fever in lightweight clothing, such as summer pyjamas or with an infant remove all clothing but the nappy. Tepid sponging and other physical methods of reducing temperature are not recommended and may be counterproductive. Although sponging children to lower their temperature may be effective in a small group of children, it is no longer recommended for children as a whole, because it can lead to extreme chilling and shock to an immature nervous system and has little advantage over the use of oral antipyretics (Meremikwu & Oyo-Ita, 2009). Unwrapping an overdressed child is appropriate. In fever above 38.4°C antipyretic administration is advisable (NSW Health, 2010). Many parents dress febrile children warmly in flannel nightgowns to keep them from "getting a chill". This actually increases the child's temperature and does not prevent the shaking, trembling reaction that comes with high fever.

COMMON DIAGNOSTIC PROCEDURES

Diagnostic and therapeutic procedures used with children vary depending on a child's condition and age but are similar to those used with adults. Blood, urine and stool studies are commonly ordered.

Electrical impulse studies

Electrical impulse studies are those that include electrical conduction. Children need special preparation for studies such as electrocardiograms (ECGs) (see Fig. 37.2) or electroencephalograms (EEGs) because they have been warned not to play with electric wires and so may worry about being burned or electrocuted. They can be reassured that the electricity passes from their body to the machine, not the other way around. Except for electromyelograms (study of the conduction paths of the spinal cord), children can be assured that these tests are painless. Electrodes are attached to the body by paste, which is easily removable. If possible, give the child a portion of the test strip afterward as a souvenir.

Radiological studies

A variety of radiological studies are used to inspect internal body tissues. These range from simple x-rays to the more complicated computed tomography (CT) scan or dye contrast study. Radiological studies expose children to ionising radiation which could increase the risk of certain cancers as children's bodies are more susceptible to mutagenic changes than adults. Because of this, each procedure should be considered carefully in order to reduce unnecessary exposure to ionising radiation (Tompane et al., 2013).

Flat-plate (plain) x-rays

X-rays are used to diagnose fractures, illnesses or check the placement of apparatus such as gastrointestinal feeding tubes. As a rule, children accept x-rays well because an x-ray machine can be compared with a camera, an instrument with which they are familiar. If it is necessary for you to remain in the room to restrain a child, a lead apron must be worn. Such protection is also necessary for portable x-rays taken at a child's or infant's bedside.

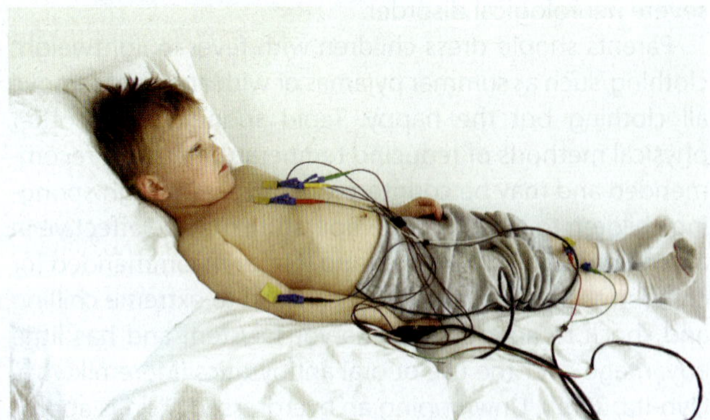

FIGURE 37.2 Administering an electrocardiogram (ECG). Children can be assured this is a painless procedure. (© Fotosearch.com.)

Dye contrast studies

To visualise a body cavity, radiopaque dyes may be swallowed or injected into the cavity and then examined by a series of x-ray's. **Barium contrast studies**, for example, are used to observe the outline of the gastrointestinal tract. Barium may be swallowed to outline the upper gastrointestinal tract or instilled by enema to outline the lower portion. Caution a child that barium, even if flavoured, does not taste terribly nice. In studies such as an intravenous pyelogram (IVP), dye is injected intravenously; as it circulates to the kidneys and bladder, x-ray's are taken. Iodine is incorporated in most radiopaque contrasts, be sure to check whether a child is allergic to iodine or seafood before the procedure. When the dye is injected, the child may feel a hot flush, or the sensation of passing urine. This sensation can be embarrassing and frightening if the child is unprepared.

Computed tomography

Computed tomography (CT) is a radiological procedure in which many views of an organ or body part are obtained to represent what the organ would look like if it were cut into thin slices (see Fig. 37.3A). As with any x-ray, dense structures appear white and less dense structures appear grey to black on the films. Because a CT scan involves so many films, it is a lengthy procedure. The scanning table will move in and out of the centre of the machine several times. In order to clearly visualise the desired area, oral and/or intravenous contrast are sometimes necessary. Children must lie still during the long procedure to avoid creating shadows on the film. This can be difficult as the machinery is complex, large, noisy and potentially frightening.

Magnetic resonance imaging

Magnetic resonance imaging (MRI) combines a magnetic field, radiofrequency and computer technology to produce diagnostic images to aid in the imaging of soft tissue (Fig. 37.3B). Disorders such as the cause of renal or brain pathology can be easily identified without the need for ionising radiation (Akpinar, Koroglu & Ptak, 2007). The child lies on a moving table that is pushed into the core of the machine—the magnet. When the magnetic field surrounding the child is turned on, it causes tissue atoms to line up in a parallel fashion. As radio waves are turned on and off, the atoms change position. This change is sensed and converted into a visual display on a computer screen. MRI scans are made up of several magnetic sequences

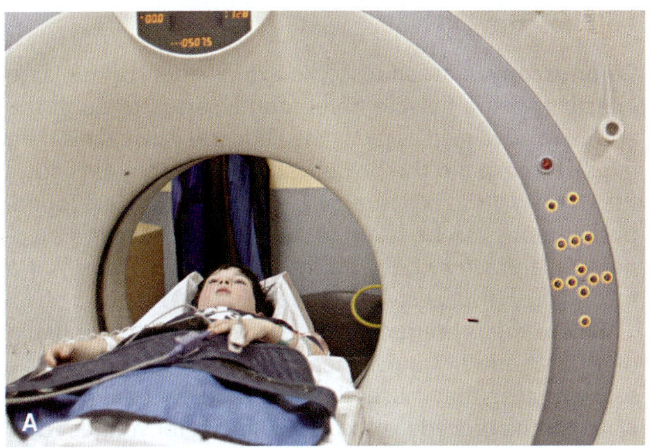

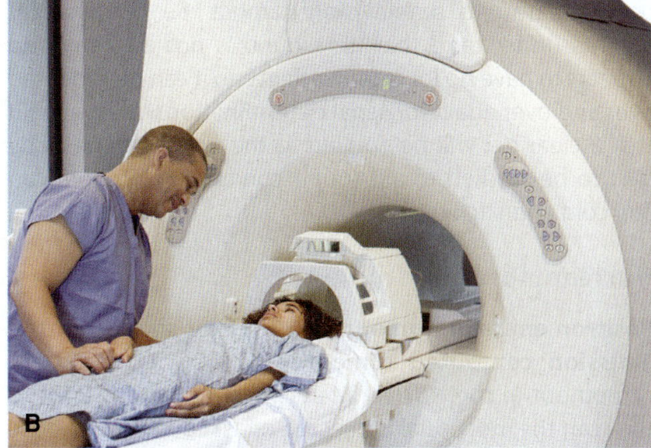

FIGURE 37.3 Some procedures are potentially frightening because of the size of the machinery used. (**A**) A computed tomography (CT) scanner. (From Michelle Del Guercio/Photo Researchers, Inc.) (**B**) A magnetic resonance imaging (MRI) scanner. (© Fotosearch.com.)

between 2–10 minutes long. They are very noisy and can be frightening for some. Any movement during a sequence blurs the image meaning the sequence will need to be repeated. Some MRI units can offer music via headphones, a mirror to see parents standing inside or outside the room and sometimes a DVD for children to watch. Local options can be checked prior to the scan. Infants less than 2 months, can often be scanned using a feed and wrap technique with a bean bag device, which prevents movement.

Sedation for CT and MRI procedures

The use of sedation and general anaesthesia in paediatric radiology is common for several reasons: it avoids memories of painful processes attached to procedures, reduces anxiety during procedures and improves image quality as children are kept still. In children 3 years and above trialling procedures without sedation can often be successful and in those unable to keep still, conscious sedation can be used via oral, IV or inhalation techniques (see Box 37.1). General anaesthetic (GA) is the preferential choice for infants and preschoolers or children with developmental delays or neurological impairment. GA is a safer and more controlled technique often allowing for several procedures to be completed in one anaesthetic episode (Arlachov & Ganatra, 2012).

BOX 37.1 ✻ Focus on evidence-based practice

Methods to reduce procedural distress in children

A recent study discusses a systemic review of non-invasive interventions to reduce procedural distress in children undergoing MRI scans. The study reviewed three randomised controlled trials, the highest level of evidence available. The review found statistical improvements in children aged 3–10 years when offered mock MRI scans to trial before the actual procedure date, audiovisual distraction during the scan and cognitive behavioural therapy such as guided meditation. The children in both the younger and the older age brackets had noticeably less improvement, but some children were still able to avoid sedation or anaesthetic.

Based on these findings, what could you suggest to help children preparing for diagnostic imaging procedures? Could music or videos help? Could children be given breathing exercises or imagery to help them through the procedure?

Source: Munn, Z. & Jordan, Z. (2013). Interventions to reduce anxiety, distress and the need for sedation in pediatric patients undergoing magnetic resonance imaging: A systemic review. *Journal of Radiology Nursing, 32*(2), 87–96.

Ultrasound

Ultrasound is a painless procedure in which images of internal tissue and organs, such as the appendix, are produced by the use of sound waves (Dingemann & Ure, 2012; see Fig. 37.4). Because it is non-invasive, children accept ultrasound easily and may even enjoy watching the oscilloscope screen during the procedure. The transducer that is used on the body surface to pick up internal images can

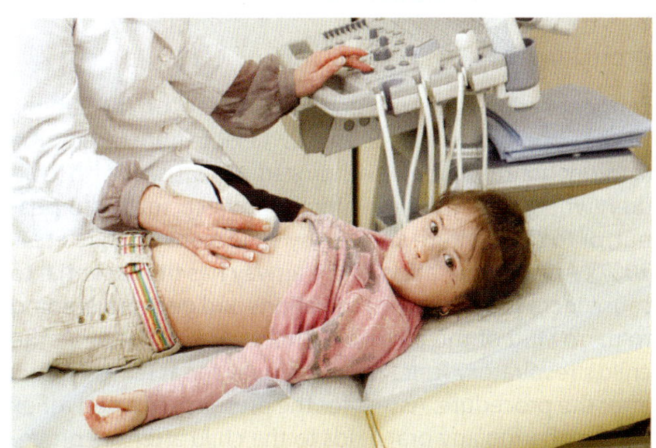

FIGURE 37.4 Children should receive good preparation for ultrasound to help with their understanding of the procedure. (© iStockphoto/Thinkstock.)

be compared to a television camera. Be certain that parents understand that ultrasound is not an x-ray and appears to have no long-term effects, so it can be repeated over and over again for serial determinations. Alert a child that a clear gel will be applied to the skin over the body part to be studied to aid sound conduction. The gel can feel cold and sticky.

Nuclear medicine studies

Positron emission tomography (PET) or **single-photon emission computed tomography (SPECT)** scans are carried out in the Nuclear Medicine department. Prior to the scan the individual is injected or asked to drink a dose of radioactive-combined substances also known as **radiopharmaceuticals**. These flow to designated body organs. When a scintillation machine (a form of Geiger counter) is passed over the organ where the radiopharmaceutical has collected, the pattern of the collected material outlines the organ; some tissues absorb more of the radioactive isotope than others and appear brighter in the images. The pattern can be produced as a screen image or a photograph.

Direct visualisation procedures

Direct visualisation procedures involve the observation of an internal body cavity by way of a thin tube inserted through a body surface opening. Types of direct visualisation include endoscopy, bronchoscopy and colonoscopy.

Endoscopy

Endoscopy involves an endoscope passed through the mouth to examine the gastrointestinal tract. It has become a common method of examination for gastrointestinal disorders in children. When first developed, endoscopes were straight, stiff metal instruments, so their use was limited. Currently, endoscopes are fibre optic (using a flexible, easily manoeuvred, brightly-lit tube), so these examinations have become more common and certainly not as uncomfortable as before.

Bronchoscopy

Bronchoscopy is the direct visualisation of the larynx, trachea and bronchi through a lit, flexible fibre optic tube (a bronchofibrescope). The procedure is used with children who have aspirated a foreign object, such as a peanut, or to take culture and biopsy specimens (Righini et al., 2007). Any manipulation of the airway has the potential to cause increased bronchial secretions and oedema, leading to narrowing of the airway. Therefore, closely observe the child's respiratory function and airway for at least 4 hours after the procedure. Assess for the presence of a gag reflex before offering any oral fluids to the child after the procedure and observe them carefully, the first time they drink after the procedure, to be certain their gag reflex is intact and they do not choke.

Colonoscopy

Colonoscopy is an endoscopic examination of the large intestine with a flexible fibrescope inserted through the anus and advanced as far as the ileocecal valve. Air is then infused to expand the bowel walls. The technique allows the colon walls to be visualised; if abnormalities are found, photographs can be taken for analysis. It is used to diagnose inflammatory bowel disease or obtain biopsies if a malignancy is suspected (Thakkar et al., 2012).

Before the procedure, children are given a clear liquid diet for about 24 hours. Then they are given an isotonic saline laxative that causes fluid diarrhoea so their bowel is clean for the procedure. It can be difficult for younger children to drink as much of the laxative solution as is needed to completely clear their bowel.

Aspiration studies

Aspiration studies (removal of body fluids by such techniques as lumbar puncture or bone marrow aspiration) are always anxiety-causing procedures; just looking at the size of the needle that will be used is frightening. Children may need a sedative so that they can lie quietly. Support and restrain them by talking and using touch as appropriate. Assess for bleeding at the puncture site after the procedure and apply pressure as needed to halt bleeding completely.

COLLECTING SPECIMENS FOR ANALYSIS

The collection of body fluids, secretions and excretions is a collaborative nursing function essential to the complete assessment of a child. Elements of these fluids can be measured by a variety of means and compared with baseline standards of health. Findings may be used to help diagnose an illness, evaluate the progress of a condition or evaluate a child's response to therapy. As with all procedures, use of standard infection precautions is essential when obtaining, transporting, discarding or storing specimens.

Obtaining blood specimens

Never underestimate how frightening obtaining a blood specimen can be to a child. For many children, their experience with losing blood has involved a nosebleed or a cut knee, which they remember as causing discomfort or pain. They have also had injections for immunisations, so they know that injections sting. Putting the two experiences together makes having blood withdrawn an extremely frightening procedure.

Venepuncture

Even for very small infants, the usual sites for venepuncture (entrance into a vein) are the same as for adults: the superficial veins of the dorsal surface of the hand or the antecubital fossa. Apply topical anaesthetic (such as EMLA) cream 30 minutes before venepuncture, if possible, to reduce pain. Use distraction techniques such as "I spy" or blowing bubbles for preschoolers, and videos or computer programs for school-aged children and adolescents (Hanrahan et al., 2012). Children need a simple explanation of what will be done: "I need to take some blood from your hand. First, I'll put some cream on your skin. Then in a little while, when I come back to get the blood you won't feel the needle as much because of the cream". Let the child know you understand how difficult it is to agree to the procedure.

Capillary puncture

Capillary blood heel or fingertip punctures are often obtained for glucose and haematocrit determinations. For fingertip punctures, be certain to use the side of the finger, not the centre, to reduce discomfort afterwards; for heel punctures, use the lateral aspect of the heel to avoid striking the medial plantar artery or the periosteum of the bone. Apply topical anaesthetic cream (EMLA) before the procedure to reduce discomfort, if possible. Comfort the child afterwards, because puncture techniques can be as painful as venepuncture. In infants, studies have shown that administration of oral sucrose can reduce pain associated with venepuncture and capillary puncture procedures but must be used with caution as hyperglycaemia can occur with too frequent use (Shah & Ohlsson, 2009).

Obtaining urine specimens

Depending on the type of test required, urine may be collected with a usual voiding, after the external meatus has been cleaned (a clean-catch specimen) by catheterisation or by suprapubic aspiration. A procedure may require a single specimen or collection of all voidings in a 24-hour period.

Routine urinalysis

Routine urinalysis requires only a single voiding specimen. The specimen will then be analysed for appearance, glucose, specific gravity (see Fig. 37.5B) and microscopic analysis. Specimens must be collected in clean containers to prevent contamination.

The infant or toddler

A child who has not been toilet-trained cannot be expected to urinate on command, so it is necessary to attach a collecting device to a girl's perineum or a boy's penis and scrotum to collect the next voiding (see Fig. 37.5A). Be certain to wash and dry the site where the collecting device will be attached to ensure good adherence and avoid contaminents. Offer the child something to drink. Most infants void shortly after a feeding, so if the collector is applied just before a regular feeding, voiding will probably result soon afterwards. Remove the collector as soon as the infant voids and transfer the specimen to a specimen cup by cutting a bottom corner of the bag.

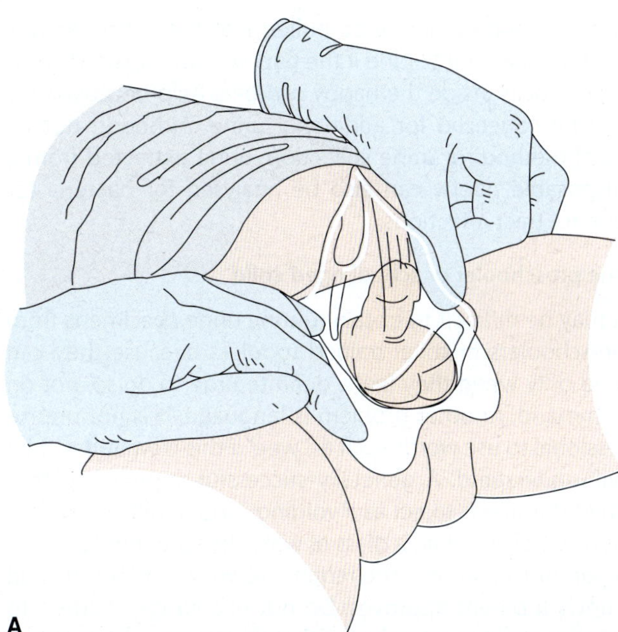

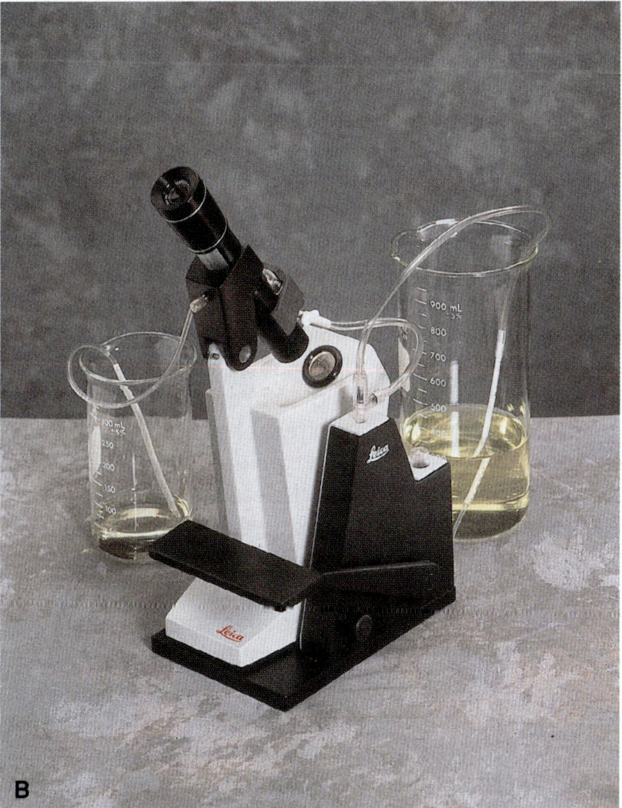

FIGURE 37.5 (**A**) Urine collector for infants. The trick to making the collector adhere is to be certain the child's skin is dry. (**B**) Testing specific gravity of urine with a refractometer. The advantage of this is that only one drop of urine is required.

Urine may be aspirated from nappies for tests such as specific gravity, dipstick protein, pH or glucose. Even with cloth nappies, this does not pull enough lint into the specimen to change its specific gravity. With disposable nappies, urine tends to be pulled into the nappy, so it is best available for testing if the nappy is torn apart. Placing cotton balls inside the nappy can be a help because they can be squeezed for additional urine. Although not an ideal method for urine collection, urine extracted from a disposable nappy can also be analysed for bacteria for urinary tract infections.

The preschooler or school-aged child

It may be difficult to obtain routine urine specimens from preschoolers or toilet-trained toddlers because they can void only when they feel a definite urge to do so, not on command. Another problem is language. It is not unprofessional to use words such as "wee" if this is what the child will understand. A generally successful approach with a child this age is to act as if voiding is not a difficult procedure. Offer the child a glass of water or other fluid and ask a parent to reinforce the request to void so that the child knows a parent approves. Do not encourage children to drink more than one glass of fluid to induce voiding, however, or else their urine production may be so diluted that the specific gravity, protein and glucose levels can be inaccurate. A school-aged child is usually able to void when asked, although the child may find it more difficult than the adult.

The adolescent

Adolescents are usually knowledgeable and cooperative about providing urine specimens. As with adults, give them a clean specimen container and tell them what is needed. Unless they have voided recently, they are usually able to void on command. Remember, however, that adolescents are concerned and self-conscious about body functions and therefore are often reluctant to carry a urine specimen through a crowded waiting room to the desk area. They may be too self-conscious to void if they know someone is nearby—just outside a curtain, for example. Send them to a nearby bathroom with a closed door or leave the area to give them privacy.

Adolescent girls may be embarrassed to mention they are menstruating. Be sure to question an adolescent girl about this so the presence of any red blood cells in a urine specimen can be explained. To avoid having a urine specimen contaminated by menstrual blood (which changes the specific gravity, protein and red blood cell analysis), ask the girl who is menstruating to wash her perineum well and rinse and dry it to remove menstrual blood. Next, supply a sterile cotton ball for her to insert gently into her vagina just before voiding (and remove again following voiding). Mark the specimen "possibly contaminated by menstrual blood" even though it does not appear discoloured, because red blood cells may be present microscopically.

Twenty-four–hour urine specimens

Although urinalysis of a single urine specimen will indicate the presence of substances such as protein or glucose, a 24-hour urine specimen may be necessary to determine how much of a substance is excreted during a day (quantitative analysis). To begin a 24-hour urine collection, ask a child to void (with an infant, attach a collecting bag and wait for the child to void). This specimen (the discard specimen) is then thrown away so that a specific time for the ensuing collection is known. If the urine collection was started early in the morning and this first specimen was counted as part of the collection, the urine collected during the next 24 hours would include urine that had been forming all night, resulting in an approximately 32-hour collection period that would distort the analysis.

Record the start of the collection period as the time of the discarded urine. Save all urine voided for the next 24 hours and place it in one collection bottle. Have the child void (or watch for an infant to void) at the end of the 24-hour period and add the final specimen to the collection bottle. Record the time of the collection as being from the time of the discarded urine to the final specimen added to the collection.

A mid-stream urine specimen

A **mid-stream urine specimen** is ordered when a urine culture for bacteria is desired. The objective of the specimen is to obtain urine that is uncontaminated by external organisms that would increase the organism count of the urine. Specimens used for protein or blood analysis may be ordered as mid-stream specimens because this careful cleaning also reduces the possibility that vaginal or foreskin secretions, which contain protein or blood, would be added to the specimen. This type of specimen requires that the urinary meatus and the surrounding structures be cleaned before voiding.

The technique for obtaining a mid-stream urine specimen from an older child is the same as that for an adult. Some modifications are necessary for the young child or infant, as it is not always possible to obtain a mid-stream urine specimen from young children. To collect a specimen from a young child, ask the child to void into a sterile emesis basin or sterile container attached to a toilet or potty seat after you have washed the perineum or penis. Then dip a sterile container into the urine stream to obtain the specimen.

Suprapubic aspiration

Suprapubic aspiration is the withdrawal of urine by insertion of a sterile needle into the bladder through the anterior wall of the abdomen. The technique is used to obtain urine for culture in infants who cannot void on command, congenital abnormality prevents urethral catheterisation or to avoid contamination that may occur from urethral catheterisation. The bladder is the most anterior of abdominal organs and, when distended with urine, is easily accessible just under the abdominal wall. Pain relief should be considered for this procedure, as the needle can induce bladder spasm leading to sharp discomfort (Hockenberry & Wilson, 2013). The steps for suprapubic aspiration are:

1. The anterior abdominal wall is cleaned with an antiseptic.
2. The urinary meatus is blocked by gloved finger pressure, confining urine in the bladder.
3. A needle is inserted just above the pubis into the bladder.
4. Urine is aspirated through the needle into a sterile syringe and the syringe and needle are withdrawn.

Catheterisation

Bladder catheterisation is when a thin catheter passes readily through the meatus of even an infant. Before beginning catheterisation, be certain to observe the perineum of girls to locate the urinary meatus; it is not as readily observable in infants and young children as it is in adult women. Cleanse the perineum or penis well before inserting the tube to reduce the risk of infection.

Catheterisation is an invasive procedure, so children must be prepared in advance. Caution children that the catheter will sting for an instant as it is inserted and they will have to lie still until the urine specimen is obtained. They need both support to submit to the procedure and praise afterwards for their cooperation. Preschool boys may need assurance that the procedure has no long-term consequences to reduce their fear of castration.

Obtaining stool specimens

Stool specimens are frequently obtained to be analysed for blood or ova and parasites. Obtain stool specimens from children who are toilet-trained by asking them to use a potty seat or by placing a collector cap device on a toilet. For effective communication, be certain you know the word the child uses for stool. Transfer the specimen to a collection cup with tongue blades. To obtain a specimen from a child who is not toilet-trained, scrape the stool from a nappy using tongue blades and place it in a stool collection cup. Some stool specimens need a preservative added to the container. If it is important to keep urine from contaminating the stool specimen, place a separate urine collector bag on an infant.

Be certain stool specimens are sent to the laboratory promptly so they do not dry and have to be collected a second time, because they can be difficult to obtain for at least 24 more hours. If the stool specimen is for ova and parasites, see that it arrives in the laboratory in less than 1 hour. Do not refrigerate ova and parasite specimens because refrigeration destroys the organisms to be analysed.

CASE STUDY QUESTION

2. Hamish will have a 24-hour urine specimen collected. You would time this from:

   a. The time of the discard specimen
   b. The first urine voided in the morning
   c. A set time, such as 8 a.m.
   d. The first voiding after the discard urine

MEASURING FLUID INTAKE AND OUTPUT

Fluid is an essential element of nutrition because of the water supplied and because it can also be a source of kilojoules and vitamins. To document fluid balance, some children may have fluid intake and output measured and recorded. This is especially true for children with vomiting, diarrhoea, burns, haemorrhage, dehydration, cardiac and kidney disease, draining wounds, gastrointestinal suction, oedema and diuretic or intravenous therapy.

Fluid intake

Estimating the intake of infants who are formula-fed is simply a matter of estimating the kind and amount of fluids that were swallowed. Intake in breastfed infants is merely recorded as "breastfed". If it is necessary to estimate the amount more closely than this, an infant can be weighed in the same clothing and nappy before and after a feeding. The difference in weight (in grams) is the number of millilitres of breast milk ingested. This measurement is not very accurate, however, because if the child voided or had a bowel movement, weight is affected by these losses.

With preschool children, be certain to record fluids ingested during snacks as well as meals, because children this age usually have many during the day. At approximately 10 years of age, children can be depended on to record their own intake as long as they have a list of how many millilitres are contained in each glass or cup they use (an average cup is 150 mL; a glass, 180 mL). Remind them that soup and flavoured frozen ice-blocks are liquids and should be counted.

Fluid output

Nappies can be readily used as a method of measuring urine output. Weigh a nappy before it is placed on an infant and record this weight conspicuously (mark it on the front of the plastic covering with a ballpoint pen). Reweigh the nappy after it is wet and subtract the difference to determine the amount of urine present. This difference will be in grams. Because 1 g = 1 mL, the amount can be recorded in millilitres. In infants who have liquid stools, it is difficult to separate stool from urine because these blend together in a nappy. Separate urine from stool by applying a urine collector; check it frequently for filling. Girls often void along with bowel movements when they use a toilet, which means that a urine specimen is easily lost. To separate urine from bowel movements, teach older children to void first before trying to move their bowels.

SUPPLEMENTAL FEEDING

Enteral feedings

Enteral feedings, also called **nasogastric tube feedings**, are a common means of supplying adequate nutrition to an infant who is unable to suck or tires too easily when sucking, or to an older child who cannot eat. Enteral feedings have the advantage over parenteral nutrition because they preserve the stomach mucosa and also decrease the risk of intravenous infection.

Whether enteral catheters should be passed through the nares or the mouth is controversial. Orogastric insertion allows for easier breathing because the nose is not blocked. Because newborns are nose breathers, it seems reasonable that passing a catheter through the mouth in this size infant will lead to less distress than passing it through the nose. Orogastric insertion can also decrease the possibility of striking the vagal nerve and causing bradycardia. If the tube is to be left in place, however, it may be passed through a nostril. For the older child, insertion through a nostril is more comfortable.

Children with long-term neurological disabilities may have enteral tubes left in place for continuous feedings administered by an enteral feeding pump. Give mouth care at least twice a day to children who are receiving nasogastric tube feedings; otherwise, their mouths become dry and ulcers can form.

Gastrostomy tube feedings

Children may have gastrostomy tubes inserted for feeding (see Fig. 37.6). **Gastrostomy tube feedings** may be necessary for children who cannot swallow or have an oesophageal stricture (Ramelli et al., 2007). With the use of regional anaesthesia, the tube is inserted through a puncture wound in the abdominal wall into the stomach. The tube used in children is usually an indwelling urinary catheter (Foley catheter) rather than a true gastrostomy tube. This is because a Foley catheter can be removed easily and changed, should it become plugged. In addition, the balloon used to secure the tube is small enough so it does not obscure and fill the small stomach space.

Infants who are fed by gastrostomy tube miss the pleasure of sucking. Offer a dummy to suck on during the procedure unless contraindicated. Talk or sing to the child as if the feeding were being given orally. The biggest problem with gastrostomy tubes is that they may not fit snugly, so formula or gastric secretions can leak around the tube onto the abdominal skin. Gastric secretions are irritating because of their high hydrochloric acid content. Often commercially available skin protectants can be placed around the tube to protect the skin.

A major complication associated with the use of a gastrostomy tube is that it can move into the duodenum through the pyloric sphincter and cause obstruction. Observe and report any vomiting, abdominal distension, or brown or green tube drainage (duodenal secretions that would suggest the tube has moved). Testing residual aspiration fluid to see that it is acid is a guarantee that the tube is in the stomach (stomach secretions are acid; duodenal secretions are alkaline). Putting a mark on the tube with an indelible pen just above the nipple lets you check that the tube is remaining securely in place.

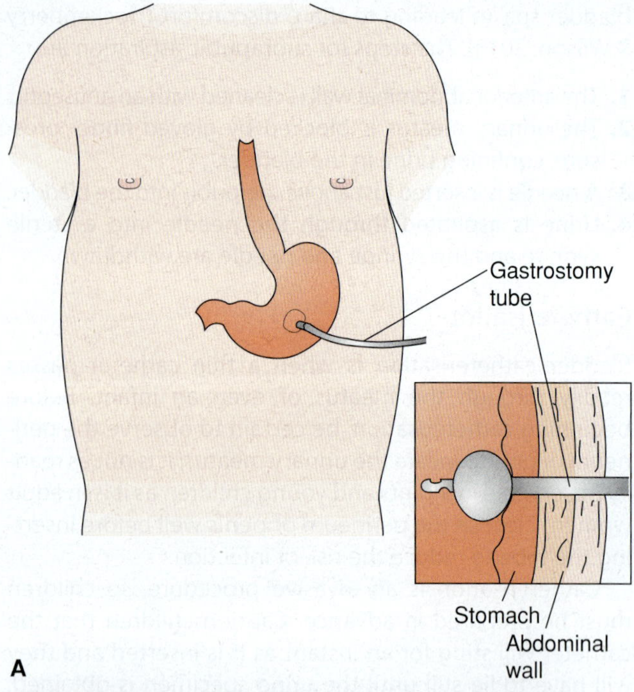

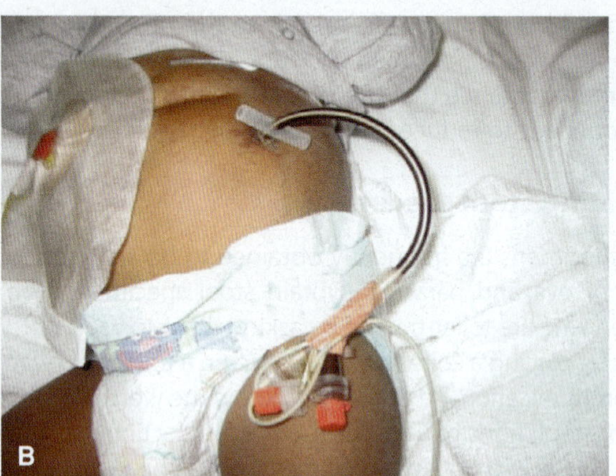

FIGURE 37.6 Children who are ill often need supplemental feeding by nasogastric or gastrostomy tube feedings. (**A**) Internal placement of a gastrostomy tube. (**B**) An infant with a gastrostomy tube in place. (Ricci, S. S., Kyle, T. & Carman, S. (2012). *Maternity and Pediatric Nursing*. Philadelphia: Lippincott Williams & Wilkins.)

Tubes are replaced approximately every 6 weeks. Most children receiving gastrostomy feedings will have the tube in place for an extended time. Teach the child's parents how to feed the child by this method, how to remove and to replace a tube, and the danger signs to watch for such as vomiting, abdominal discomfort or skin excoriation. Help parents to view this as an alternative way of feeding rather than a totally different one. Be certain they are comfortable with the procedure before the child is discharged from the hospital, so they can effectively feed the child by this method. Reinforce with them the understanding that it does not hurt their child to have the tube replaced or to have pressure put against the tube, so that they need not worry about holding their child snugly. Many children on long-term gastrostomy feedings have gastrostomy buttons implanted for easier stomach access. For feeding, a catheter is inserted through the device; the catheter is removed following the feeding. With a gastrostomy button in place, only a small access device is visible, not a large bulky tube.

What if...

A parent whose child has a gastrostomy tube in place tells you she's going to take the child to a restaurant so the child learns about "eating out"? Would you agree with her that this is a good idea?

Total parenteral nutrition

Total parenteral nutrition (TPN) has become one of the most important therapies for children who are unable to tolerate enteral feeding such as those with gastrointestinal disease/malformation, liver failure or prematurity resulting in an inability to absorb necessary nutrients for life. Parenteral nutrition bypasses the gut and the first pass through the liver in those unable to absorb nutrients due to existing bowel or liver disease (Jeejeebhoy, 2012). TPN differs from traditional intravenous therapy in that it contains not only sugars and electrolytes but also protein, carbohydrates, amino acids, trace minerals and fats that are essential for the maintenance and growth of body tissues. With TPN, all of a child's nutritional needs can be met by a concentrated hypertonic solution of intravenous therapy administered over long periods, usually 15–20 hours via a central venous catheter (CVC) or peripherally inserted central catheter (PICC).

The most common sites for PICC or CVC lines are the right external jugular vein into the superior vena cava or directly into the subclavian vein under strict aseptic conditions. The catheter is secured at the site of insertion with sutures and covered with a sterile dressing to help reduce bacterial contamination. A major vein of this type is chosen to avoid inflammation reactions and resulting venous thrombosis from the high-kilojoule and high-osmotic fluid that will be infused (Ainsworth, Clerihew & McGuire, 2009).

Infection is a major danger of TPN because the solution is a perfect medium for the growth of bacteria or *Candida* organisms. In order to reduce the risk of infection the dressing over the insertion site and the intravenous tubing are changed every 1 to 2 days using aseptic technique. Infection can quickly lead to sepsis or thrombosis. At each dressing change the insertion site should be inspected for indications of infection such as redness, tenderness or discharge (Marra, 2007). Unless a double lumen catheter is in place the CVC or PICC line should not be used to obtain blood samples or administer medications, as these processes have the potential to introduce contaminants. Tubing and bottle changes should be attended using either aseptic or non-touch technique, to reduce the risk of contamination (King Edward Memorial Hospital, 2014). Some healthcare facilities require nurses to wear sterile gloves, aprons and masks to avoid airborne and direct contamination; local guidelines must be adhered to in all instances.

TPN solution is prepared in a pharmacy under sterile conditions according to individualised prescription based on the person's electrolyte balance. A Millipore filter, which removes small particles in the solution that might cause an embolus to form, is inserted into the tubing prior to connection to the individual. In order to maintain the infusion rate as per the prescribed hourly volume of administration a constant infusion pump should always be used. Infusions that have fallen behind schedule must not be increased as this can lead to serious cardiovascular fluid overload or fat embolus because of the concentrated nature of the solution. Those receiving TPN should have close monitoring of vital signs, blood sugars, biochemistry, fluid balances and weight (King Edward Memorial Hospital, 2014).

ASSISTANCE WITH ELIMINATION

Two aspects of intestinal elimination that require special care are administration of enemas and stoma care.

Administering enemas

Enemas are rarely used with children unless they are therapy for Hirschsprung's disorder or a part of preparation for surgery or an x-ray study. If an enema is necessary, offer a careful explanation of what the child can expect. As the sizes of children's bowels vary greatly, the usual amounts of enema solutions used are titrated as follows:

- Infant: Less than 250 mL (exact amount should be stipulated by doctor's prescription)
- Preschooler: 250–350 mL
- School-aged child: 300–500 mL
- Adolescent: 500 mL.

Providing ostomy care

An **ostomy** is an opening of the bowel on the surface of the abdomen (see Fig. 37.7). Ostomies in newborns are created to relieve bowel obstruction caused by conditions such as ileal atresia, necrotising enterocolitis and imperforate anus. In older children they are constructed for conditions such as inflammatory bowel syndrome and Hirschsprung's disorder (Sharma & Gupta, 2012). If an ostomy is created in the ileum (an ileostomy), the stoma is located on the right side of the abdomen and drains liquid stool, which is extremely irritating to the skin because of the digestive enzymes it contains. If an ostomy is created in the sigmoid portion of the bowel (colostomy), the stoma is on the left lower abdomen and passes normally-formed stool.

An ileostomy requires the use of a collecting ostomy appliance to contain acid stool and prevent excoriation of the abdominal skin. Older children also may use an appliance with a colostomy. For an infant colostomy, parents may choose (with support and advice) whether to use an appliance.

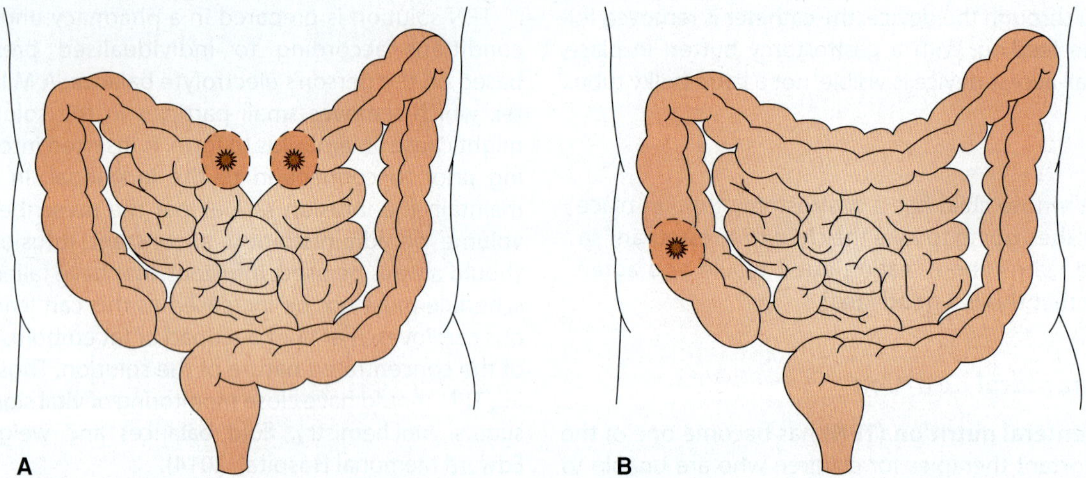

FIGURE 37.7 Different sites for ostomies. (**A**) A double-barrel colostomy. (**B**) A single-barrel colostomy.

Two basic problems commonly arise when using an ostomy appliance with an infant: it may be difficult to locate one small enough to contain liquid drainage without leaking and the skin under the appliance may become extremely irritated. Clear plastic colostomy bags without a ring can often be cut more easily to fit the size of the stoma and the contour and size of an infant's abdomen than a ring type. A commercial skin sealant is helpful to harden the skin surrounding the stoma. Apply it according to the brand directions and fan to dry. Apply the chosen stoma collection appliance. Check the appliance or bag for collecting stool at least every 4 hours. To protect the underlying skin, do not remove a self-adhering bag if it is full, but drain collected stool from the bottom of the appliance into a basin or paper cup for disposal. Change the bag no more frequently than the point at which leakage occurs (perhaps as long as 1 week) to reduce skin irritation. To remove a bag that was placed with a sealant, be certain to use the designated solvent to prevent pulling or harming underlying skin. Wash the solvent away with soap and water or it will become an irritant itself. Because most infants enjoy tub bathing, a long, soaking bath is an excellent way to loosen an appliance.

Stress to parents that the stoma has no nerves, so a parent can feel free to wash it without hurting the child and that compression against the stoma will not cause a child pain. These explanations can help the parents feel comfortable placing an infant on the abdomen or holding the infant closely against their body for comfort.

WOUND CARE

Children frequently have a dressing or bandage in place to cover a surgical incision or sutured laceration. Such dressings differ from adult dressings in terms of material, size and methods used to secure them. Keeping a dressing dry to avoid introducing infection to the wound in infants and toddlers who are not toilet-trained can be a major problem. In many instances after surgery, collodion (a clear substance similar to nail polish) or other commercially available "wound glues" are used to cover the incision. Wound glue not only takes the place of stitches but also serves as a dressing to keep the incision line from coming into contact with urine or faeces. Since these materials are clear, they allow good visualisation of the healing surface as well. Assure parents that such a covering is adequate and actually preferable if the incision is in the groin, such as a hernia repair. They are also preferable if an incision or laceration is on the face, as they heal with less scarring than if sutures were used.

Occlusive dressings (hydrogel sheets, hydrocolloids or polyurethane films) are specially designed to provide a healing surface over a wound. These need to be applied and removed according to each product's directions. The skin of infants and young children is usually too sensitive for adhesive tape to be used to secure dressings. Use non-adhesive tape instead or secure a dressing with a non-adhering bandage (Kling) or roller gauze. Young children, as a rule, find bandages comforting and accept them as a "badge of courage", displaying them proudly. Apply adhesive bandages (Band-Aids) generously after venepuncture or finger punctures for this reason. Teach parents and children how to continue wound dressings when they return home.

CASE STUDY QUESTION

3. Hamish's younger brother receives total parenteral nutrition. Why does dehydration tend to occur with this?

a. The glucose solution leads to diuresis
b. Infection occurs easily and causes fever
c. Only 100 mL of fluid can be infused daily
d. Children tend to develop diarrhoea

Key points for review

- Preparing children for procedures reduces anxiety. Prepare a child and parents by trying to relate a procedure to something with which a child is already familiar, such as comparing an x-ray machine to a camera.
- Include parents in both the planning and implementation of care, as parents can reinfect children with fear if their own fear is uncontrolled.
- Minimise the number of painful procedures; for instance, combine blood sampling procedures, if possible.
- Perform treatments without chilling or exposure; modesty should be respected at all times, as even small children are aware of social norms.
- Allow a child to voice anger or fear of a procedure. Provide therapeutic play before and after a procedure to help reduce these reactions.
- Children enjoy adults who are secure in their actions. Practice, as necessary, the steps of a procedure before you begin so you can demonstrate confidence and skill.
- Once you have announced that a procedure needs to be done, proceed to do it; waiting for something to happen is often as stressful as actually having it done.
- Involve children in procedures; praise children for cooperation or bravery even if none was visibly obvious.
- Following the use of conscious sedation, observe children carefully until they are fully awake. Check for the return of the child's gag reflex before offering any fluids to minimise the risk of aspiration.
- Help make feeding by a route such as a gastrostomy tube as close to normal as possible by talking to the child to simulate mealtime conversation and socialisation.

CASE STUDY QUESTIONS

4. Hamish is also scheduled for a CT scan with dye injected. His mother asks you to assure her that her son will not have a reaction to the dye. How will you answer her?
5. Hamish's new brother had bowel surgery at birth and now has a temporary colostomy. His grandmother cares for him two mornings a week while his mother attends work. The grandmother tells you that she cannot imagine how she can care for an infant with a colostomy. What could you do to try to make her feel more comfortable with the baby's care? Will his care really be much different from that for other newborns?
6. What would be a possible research topic to explore pertinent to preparing children for medical interventions that would be applicable to Hamish's family and also advance evidence-based practice?

Resources

For an extensive range of additional resources to enhance teaching and learning and to facilitate understanding of this chapter, please see the text's accompanying website located on thePoint at http://thepoint.lww.com.

References

Ainsworth, S. B., Clerihew, L. & McGuire, W. (2009). Percutaneous central venous catheters versus peripheral cannulae for delivery of parenteral nutrition in neonates. *Cochrane Database of Systematic Reviews, 2009*(1), (CD004219).

Akpinar, E., Koroglu, M. & Ptak, T. (2007). Diffusion tensor MR imaging in pediatric head trauma. *Journal of Computer Assisted Tomography, 31*(5), 657–661.

Arlachov, Y. & Ganatra, R. H. (2012). Sedation/anaesthesia in paediatric radiology. *The British Journal of Radiology, 85*(1019), e1018–e1031.

Brayden, R. M., Daley, M. F. & Brown, J. M. (2008). Ambulatory and community pediatrics. In W. W. Hay, et al. (Eds). *Current Pediatric Consideration and Treatment* (18th ed.). Columbus, OH: McGraw-Hill.

Delany, C. & Conwell, M. (2012). Ethics and teamwork for pediatric medical imaging procedures: Insights from educational play therapy. *Pediatric Radiology, 42*(2), 139–146.

Dingemann, J. & Ure, B. 2012). Imaging and the use of scores for the diagnosis of appendicitis in children. *European Journal of Pediatric Surgery, 22*(3), 195–200.

Edwards, H., Walsh, A., Courtney, M., Monaghan, S., Wilson, J. & Young, J. (2007). Improving paediatric nurses' knowledge and attitudes in childhood fever management. *Journal of Advanced Nursing, 57*(3), 257–269.

Forsey, M., Salmon, P., Eden, T., et al. (2011). Comparing doctors' and nurses' accounts of how they provide emotional care for parents of children with acute lymphoblastic leukaemia. *Psychooncology, 22*(2), 260–267.

Hanrahan, K., McCarthy, A. M., Kleiber, C., et al. (2012). Building a computer program to support children, parents, and distraction during healthcare procedures. *Computers, Informatics, Nursing, 30*(10), 554–561.

Havidich, J. E. & Cravero, J. P. (2012).The current status of procedural sedation for pediatric patients in out-of-operating room locations. *Current Opinion in Anaesthesiology, 25*(4), 453–460.

Hockenberry, M. J. & Wilson, D. (2013). *Wong's Essentials of Pediatric Nursing* (9th ed.). Elsevier Mosby: St Louis, Missouri.

Jeejeebhoy, K. N. (2012). Parenteral nutrition in the intensive care unit. *Nutrition Reviews, 70*(11), 623–630.

King Edward Memorial Hospital. (2014). Total parenteral nutrition, accessed 13 February 2015, <www.kemh.health.wa.gov.au/development/manuals/O&G_guidelines/sectiona/4/a4.11.pdf>.

Marra, A. R. (2007). Epidemiology of bloodstream infections in patients receiving long-term total parenteral nutrition. *Journal of Clinical Gastroenterology, 41*(1), 19–28.

McKenna, L. & Mirkov, S. (2014). *McKenna's Drug Handbook for Nursing & Midwifery* (7th ed.). Sydney: Lippincott Williams & Wilkins.

Meremikwu, M. & Oyo-Ita, A. (2009). Physical methods for treating fever in children. *Cochrane Database of Systematic Reviews, 2009*(1), (CD004264).

Munn, Z. & Jordan, Z. (2013). Interventions to reduce anxiety, distress and the need for sedation in pediatric patients undergoing magnetic resonance imaging: A systemic review. *Journal of Radiology Nursing 32*(2), 87–96.

New South Wales Health. (2010). Policy directive [PD2010_063]. Children and infants with fever—acute management, accessed 13 February 2015, <www.health.nsw.gov.au/policies/pd/2010/pdf/PD2010_063.pdf>.

Ramelli, G. P., Alaysius, A., King, C., Davis, T. & Muntoni, F. (2007). Gastrostomy placement in paediatric patients with neuromuscular disorders: Indications and outcome. *Developmental Medicine & Child Neurology, 49*(5), 367–371.

Righini, C. A., Morel, N., Karkas, A., Reyt, E., Ferretti, K., Pin, I. & Schmerber, S. (2007). What is the diagnostic value of flexible bronchoscopy in the initial investigation of children with suspected foreign body aspiration? *International Journal of Pediatric Otorhinolaryngology, 71*(9), 1383–1390.

Royal Australian & New Zealand College of Obstetricians and Gynaecologists (RANCOG). (2013) Statement: Consent and provision of information to patients in Australia and New Zealand regarding proposed treatment, accessed 13 February 2015, <www.ranzcog.edu.au/search.html?searchword=Consent&searchphrase=all&areas[0]=docman&areas[1]=656>.

Shah, V. & Ohlsson, A. (2009). Venipuncture versus heel lance for blood sampling in term neonates. *Cochrane Database of Systematic Reviews, 2009*(1), (CD001452).

Sharma, S. & Gupta, D. K. (2012). Hirschsprung's disease presenting beyond infancy: Surgical options and postoperative outcome. *Pediatric Surgery International, 28*(1), 5–8.

Thakkar, K., Alsarraj, A., Fong, E., et al. (2012). Prevalence of colorectal polyps in pediatric colonoscopy. *Digestive Diseases & Sciences, 57*(4), 1050–1055.

Thalange, N., Beach, R., Booth, D., & Jackson, L. (2013). *Essentials of Paediatrics Pocket Edition* (2nd ed.). UK: Elsevier Saunders.

Tompane, T., Bush, R., Dansky, T. & Huang, J. S. (2013). Diagnostic imaging studies performed in children over a nine-year period. *Pediatrics, 131*(1), e45–e52.

Suggested readings

Carter, A. J., Greer, M. L. C., Gray, S. E. & Ware, R. S. (2010). Mock MRI: Reducing the need for anaesthesia in children. *Pediatric Radiology, 40*, 1368–1374.

Mikkelsen, G. & Frederiksen, K. (2011). Family-centred care of children in hospital—A concept analysis. *Journal of Advanced Nursing, 67*(5), 1152–1162.

Rogers, J. & Saunders, C. (2008). Urine collection in infants and children. *Nursing Times, 104*(5), 40–42.

Scott, J. T., Harmsen, M., Prictor, M. J., Sowden, A. J. & Watt, L. (2009). Interventions for improving communication with children and adolescents about their cancer. *Cochrane Database of Systematic Reviews, 2009*(1), (CD002969).

Wennstrom, B., Hallberg, L. R. & Bergh, I. (2008). Use of perioperative dialogues with children undergoing day surgery. *Journal of Advanced Nursing, 62*(1), 96–106.

Chapter 38

Nursing care of a family when a child needs medication administration or intravenous therapy

Previous chapters described the difficulty children may have adjusting to illness and also diagnostic and therapeutic procedures that are frequently used with children. This chapter adds information about techniques for administering medication and intravenous (IV) therapy to children. Because therapy for almost all illnesses today involves some form of medicine or IV administration, and safe medication administration is one of the most important parts of a child health nurse's role, this information is pertinent to the care of almost all children.

LEARNING OBJECTIVES

After studying the contents of this chapter, you should be able to:

1. Describe common methods of medication and intravenous therapy used in the healthcare of children.
2. Use critical thinking to analyse ways that medication or intravenous therapy can be modified to be more family-centred.
3. Consider the developmental stage and knowledge level of children and adolescents before beginning medication or intravenous therapy.
4. Identify expected outcomes for children receiving medication or intravenous therapy.
5. Plan nursing interventions to aid in making medication and intravenous therapy optimally effective.
6. Implement nursing interventions concerned with medication and intravenous therapy and children.
7. Evaluate expected outcomes for achievement and effectiveness of care.
8. Identify areas related to medication or intravenous therapy with children that could benefit from additional nursing research or application of evidence-based practice.
9. Integrate knowledge of medication and intravenous therapy with nursing care to achieve quality child and family health nursing care.

KEY TERMS

- absorption
- distribution
- excretion
- intermittent infusion
- metabolism
- pharmacokinetics

CASE STUDY

Ava, an 8-year-old with Down syndrome, is brought to the emergency department by her parents because she has pain in her ankle. She is diagnosed with osteomyelitis. When you give her a paracetamol tablet for pain, she spits it out. She does the same with a second tablet. Her mother tells you Ava can't swallow pills. Her father tells you "You'll have to give her medication intravenously."

CASE STUDY QUESTIONS

1. What technique would you use to help Ava learn to swallow pills?
2. How would you gain her cooperation?

Most adults understand that taking medication is important to relieve the symptoms they are experiencing. Children do not necessarily have this same level of understanding. They may resist taking medication unless its importance is thoroughly explained to them and the medication is given to them by a method that best meets their preference. Most children are unable to swallow tablets or capsules until they are 6 or 7 years of age. Most children fear intrusive procedures and will therefore resist medications given by a rectal, nasal, intramuscular (IM) or intravenous (IV) route. Due to the fact that children range in size it is imperative that accurate doses of medication and IV therapy are given. This is achieved by calculating the dosage based on the child's weight. Children may also have difficulty reporting any adverse effects of medication as accurately as adults. This can make it difficult to determine if side effects or adverse effects are occurring. Each of these factors makes medication administration for children one of the most challenging interventions in nursing (Walsh et al., 2013). Cooperation is needed to be successful with medicating a child. In most situations the parent/guardian is the best person to utilise. Parents and guardians have knowledge of the child's individual traits. They understand how to best pacify the child to relieve anxieties and to then encourage compliance with taking medication. Even with parents, this can be a difficult process and the nurse will need to appraise the situation in view of the most appropriate way for the child to obtain the medical care required for health improvement.

Medication Safety is one of the 10 National Safety and Quality Health Service (NSQHS) Standards. The standard on Medication Safety "describes the systems and strategies to ensure clinicians safely prescribe, dispense and administer appropriate medicines to informed patients" (see *National Safety and Quality Health Service Standards*, available from <www.safetyandquality.gov.au/wp-content/uploads/2011/09/NSQHS-Standards-Sept-2012.pdf>).

THE CHILD NEEDING MEDICATION/ INTRAVENOUS THERAPY

Assessment

Medication administration to children begins by assessing their height and weight so a correct dose of medication or amount of IV fluid can be calculated. It is also important to establish the child's chronological age and cognitive level. This will reveal if a child is able to swallow oral medication or use self-medication methods such as patient-controlled analgesia. It also aids planning the level of explanation required. Include an assessment of the child's past experience with taking medication to help predict what a present response to medication administration might be. Finally, inquire about the family's cultural beliefs and attitudes towards medications, including use of over-the-counter and complementary medications (see Box 38.1).

Following medication administration, careful observation must continue to determine if the medication is having its desired effect and if any unwanted or adverse effects are occurring (Dickinson et al., 2012).

Nursing considerations

Nursing considerations related to medication administration vary widely. Some examples are:

- Disturbed sleep pattern related to q4h (every 4 hours) timing of medication administration
- Deficient knowledge related to action and side effects of a medication
- Fear related to parenteral medications
- Discomfort related to injections or side effects of medication.

BOX 38.1 * Nursing care planning to respect cultural diversity

Assessing children's attitudes about the worth or wisdom of medicine is important because attitudes are not consistent across cultures. Some families, for example, would rather depend on a herb or home remedy rather than a prescribed medicine. Because of this, a family may accept a prescription but then not fill it or administer the medicine. A herbal remedy they use may duplicate or counteract a prescribed medicine's effect. Socioeconomic factors effect medicine administration as well because medicine is expensive and difficult to afford for many families who do not have health insurance.

As part of health histories, always ask if a child commonly takes any type of herbal or home remedy or if the child has been given anything specific for the present illness. Because medicine is expensive, when discussing a prescription with parents, ask them if they think they will have any difficulty with obtaining or giving it, as well as assessing for the medicine's effect, or returning for a follow-up appointment to evaluate the medicine's effect. Such inquiries allow parents to say they have questions about the medicine or are uncertain whether they should give it because of a cultural belief.

Planning for medication administration for children involves the same safety rules as those for adults. Extra consideration is necessary at each step, however, because determining the right form and route of administration is important. All paediatric medication preparations and calculations must be checked by a second nurse or medical officer to ensure accuracy. However, it is important to ensure that hospital/clinical facility policy is reviewed, as in some institutions oral medications do not require double checking before administration

In addition to administering medications and IV therapy to children, the nurse is also responsible for teaching parents and children how to continue to take the medication when at home or at school. The reason for giving the medication, the administration schedule and the route of administration should be clearly explained in order to ensure that the child continues to take the medication correctly for the desired period of time.

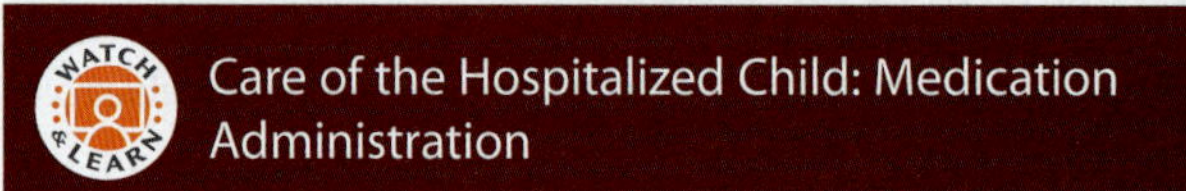

MEDICATION ADMINISTRATION

Medications in children are given by a variety of routes: orally, intranasally, transdermally, topically, rectally, via injection (subcutaneous, IM, IV, intraosseous, or epidural) or by inhalation. Epidural administration is described in Chapter 16. Inhalation techniques are discussed in Chapter 40.

Pharmacokinetics in children

To administer medications safely, it is important to have a good understanding of **pharmacokinetics** (the way medications are absorbed, distributed throughout the body, metabolised, inactivated and excreted). The four basic processes of absorption, distribution, metabolism and excretion determine the intensity and duration of a medication's action. The immaturity of body systems in children (and especially in newborns) plays a major role in medication action throughout each of these processes (Johnson & Rostami-Hodjegan, 2010).

Absorption

Medication **absorption** (transfer of the medication from its point of entry in the body into the bloodstream) is influenced by the route of administration as well as by the concentration and acidity of the medication. Some routes of administration are not appropriate for children. For example, infants are likely to remove transdermal patches and are unable to swallow tablets. The small muscle size of young children limits sites available for IM injection. Gastrointestinal absorption is reduced in newborns, while vomiting and diarrhoea can also interfere with absorption.

Distribution

Distribution refers to the movement of the medication through the circulation to a specific site of action. Many medications are distributed bound to serum albumin (manufactured by the liver). This binding action limits the amount of free medication in the circulation, thereby providing protection against toxic levels. Newborns with immature liver function may not have enough serum albumin to transport medications readily. In addition, newborns have sluggish peripheral circulation, so distribution in children this young may not be effective. Any child with cardiovascular disease may also have limited distribution of medications because of poor circulation.

Metabolism

Metabolism involves the conversion of the medication into an active form (biotransformation) or an inactive form (inactivation). A child's basic metabolic rate is faster than that of an adult. This means that certain medications are metabolised more rapidly in children. As a result, the medication must be administered more frequently in order to maintain therapeutic levels. Some medications are metabolised directly by liver enzymes which are not fully developed in newborns. These medications will therefore reach toxic levels rapidly in this group of patients. Older children with liver disease also have a decreased ability to inactivate or transform medications.

Excretion

The **excretion** (elimination of raw medication or medication metabolites) of medications is potentially limited until about 12 months of age, when kidney function becomes mature. If a child has kidney disease, excretion potential is limited at any age. Some medications are excreted in bile. In the newborn with sluggish bile formation, excretion of these medications is questionable. Monitoring intake and output is important in children receiving medications to be certain that urine excretion or an outlet for medication metabolites is adequate.

Adverse medication effects in children

Children respond to medications in much the same way as adults, but they may experience unique or exaggerated side effects because of immature liver function or rapid metabolism during periods of rapid growth. The newborn may suffer adverse effects from medications taken by the mother prenatally or from medications taken by a breastfeeding mother.

Safe storage of medications

All medications should always be stored in a safe place, a fact which should be stressed to parents for implementation at home. In most homes, this is in a locked cabinet or drawer above the height their child can reach.

Safe administration of medications

Administering medications safely to children requires that you first determine that you are giving the right medication to the right child, in the right dosage and by the right route, at the right time.

Right medication

Most medication errors are made in situations where the number of medications being given is high and speed in administration is crucial. Intensive care units and emergency departments, therefore, are the areas highest at risk for medication errors, often because of interruptions during the medication administration process (Kalisch & Aebersold, 2010; Pham et al., 2011). A prescriber should only write a prescription using a generic name.

Right child

Children cannot be depended on to give their correct names. A preschooler is likely to answer the question, "Are you Jack Jones?" with "Yes." To prevent these types of errors, never ask children their names for identification. Instead, read their identification arm bands and compare them with the medication sheet or medical record. Parents or guardians are an integral component in communicating with children in all settings and they can be asked to confirm the child's identity.

CASE STUDY QUESTION

3. You are going to give paracetamol to Ava in the emergency department. She has no ID band in place as yet. What would be the best way to identify her?
   a. Ask her to tell you her name
   b. Tell her you need to know her name
   c. Ask a parent to confirm her identify for you
   d. Ask to see her school bus pass

Right dosage

Before administering any medication to a child, confirm that the dose ordered is correct for the child's weight or body surface area (see Fig. 38.1). The MIMS and other medication dosage guidelines approved by the local health service can be used to help identify the correct medication dose.

However, there are always exceptions to a rule. For example, a child with a compound fracture may receive more than the usual dose of antibiotics because the risk of infection is so high. Therefore, an ordered dose that does not conform to the standard dose may still be correct. If there is any doubt concerning the dose of a medication, the order should be rechecked with the prescriber and pharmacist before it is administered.

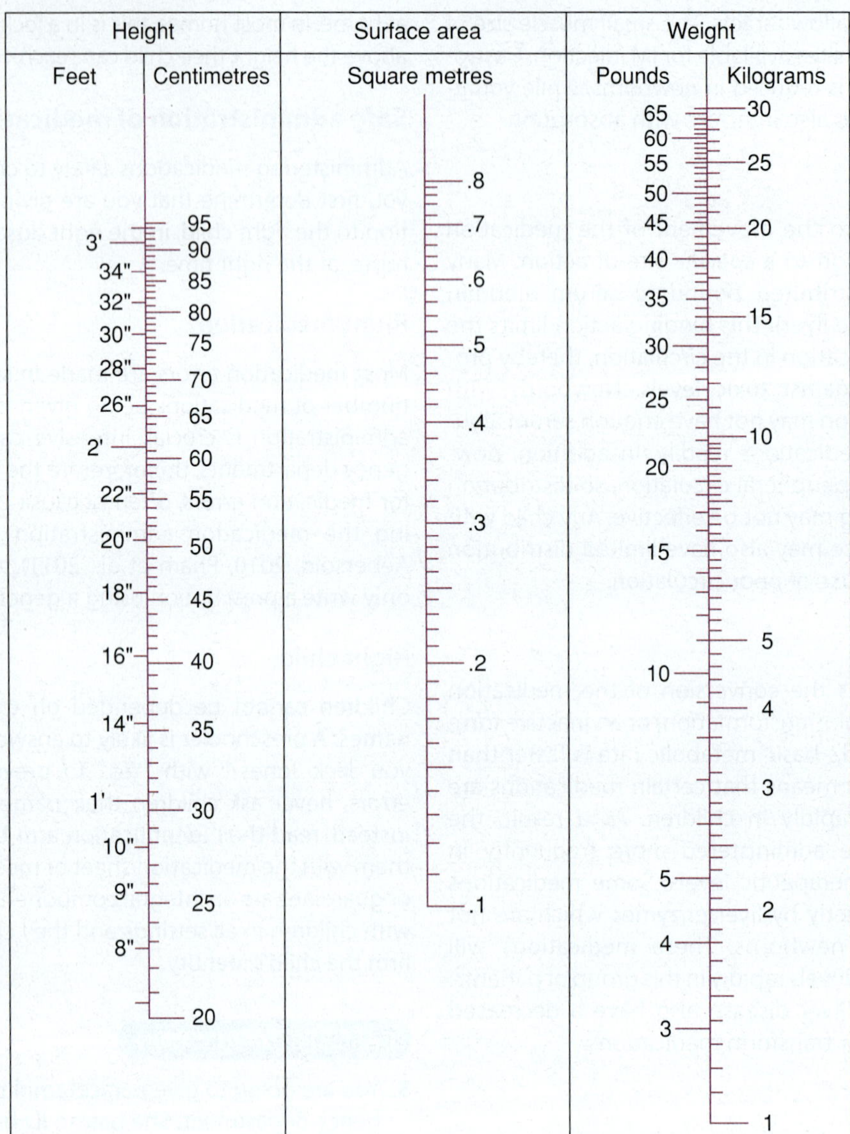

FIGURE 38.1 A nomogram to estimate body surface area. To use such a chart, draw a line from the child's height to the child's weight. The point at which it crosses the middle line is the child's surface area.

Right route and time

Possible routes of administration for medications in children are discussed below. Each of these methods requires special techniques, as most children do not enjoy taking medication and need strong support during administration.

Oral administration

Children younger than 9 years often have difficulty swallowing tablets. For children younger than 3 years, it is virtually impossible. Most oral medication for young children, therefore, is supplied in liquid, chewable or dissolvable form (El-Alfy et al., 2010).

In infants, oral medication can be given with a dropper or a unit dose syringe. To prevent aspiration, medications are never given if the child is lying completely flat or crying. The infant should be held in the nurse's lap or preferably the lap of a parent or guardian with the head elevated. The syringe or dropper is then inserted into the side of the infant's mouth. It is important to allow the fluid to flow slowly so that the child has time to swallow (see Fig. 38.2). Many hospitals within Australia and New Zealand now have colour coded syringes for oral medications. This practice has been introduced to avoid errors in administrating oral medications through intravenous routes.

If a child has difficulty swallowing tablets, they can be crushed (not enteric-coated tablets) and added to a teaspoonful of yoghurt or custard. Some children are old enough to swallow tablets but have never done it before. Whole tablets can also be added to a spoonful of ice cream as children will tend to swallow ice cream without chewing. This should be done in front of the child. The intent is not to hide the medication but to help the child learn how to swallow tablets (see Box 38.2).

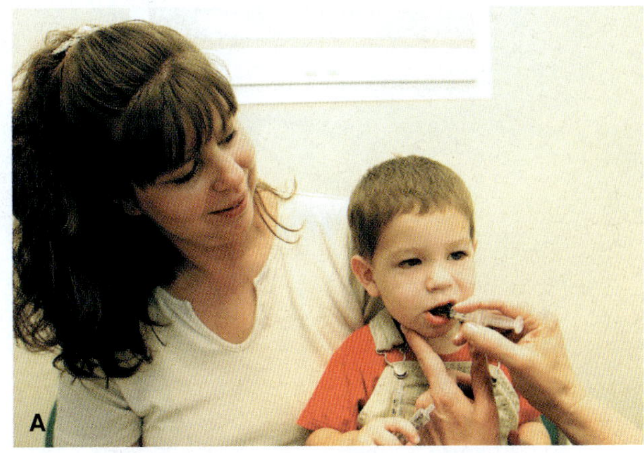

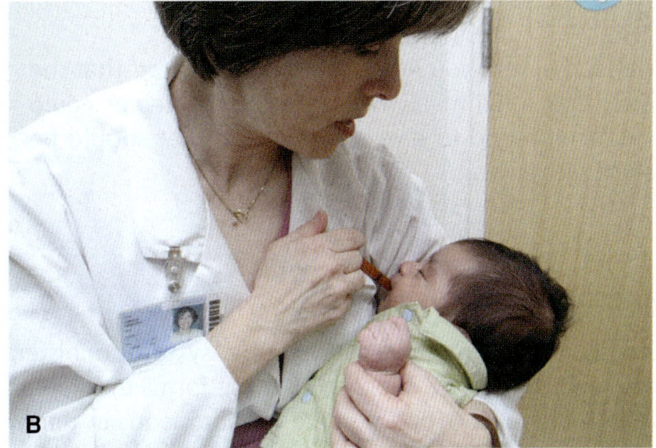

FIGURE 38.2 To administer oral medicine with a syringe, place the medicine at the side of the child's mouth (**A**). Note that infants should be positioned at least at a 45° angle (**B**).

CASE STUDY QUESTION

4. Although Ava is 8 years old, she doesn't know how to swallow pills. If you needed to delegate the administration of an oral medication to a licensed practical nurse, what instruction would you provide to your colleague?

a. "Draw a picture of a child swallowing medicine and talk about it"
b. "Tell the child that all medicine tastes sweet so she'll take it readily"
c. Give the child a small ice chip to use to practise swallowing"
d. "Tip the child's head forwards to avoid the possibility of choking"

BOX 38.2 * Focus on family teaching

Guidelines for administering oral medication

Q. Ava's mother tells you, "All my children fight me anytime they need to be given medication. How can I get them to take medication without a battle?"

A. Use the following guidelines to help make this task a bit easier:

- Do not say, "*Can* you drink this for me?" If an adult seems unsure whether children can do a task, children can develop grave doubts themselves.
- Do not say, "*Will* you drink this for me?" This leaves a child the opportunity to say no and creates the awkward position of having to admit that the child really does not have a choice in the matter; the child *must* take the medication.
- Do not state, "It's time for you to drink your medicine now." Give the child a secondary choice that allows a sense of control: "It is time to drink your medicine now; do you want milk or water to swallow after it?" is a suitable choice, assuming both milk and water are compatible with the medication.
- Never refer to medication as lollies. If they think it is lollies, children may help themselves to fatal amounts of medication when everyone's back is turned.
- Do not bribe children to take medication. Bribing may work for one dose, but when a second dose is due, the child will ask for a bigger bribe; for a third dose, an even bigger one. At some point (generally reached quickly), it is impossible to supply such large bribes and therefore it is impossible to enforce the rules.
- Do not threaten. Statements such as, "Take this quickly or I'll ask the doctor to make it into a needle" cannot be followed through. The child calls the bluff (many medicines do not come in a form that can be injected intramuscularly) and once more the child is in control. A statement such as, "Take this or I'll call your doctor" is unfair (the doctor has been made the villain) and ultimately undermines your authority (it is obvious that you must not have much power, or you would not need help).
- Do not lie about the taste of medication. Children expect honesty from adults. If in doubt about the taste, taste it (with the obvious exception of drugs such as digitoxin). Most children's medications are artificially flavoured with raspberry, orange or cherry syrup, so they do not taste bad.
- If a medicine tastes bitter, mix it with a spoonful of strained yoghurt or a teaspoonful of flavoured syrup. Do not mix medication with a full jar of baby food, because the child will then have to eat the entire jar of food to get all of the medication. As a rule, encourage children to take medication straight, then follow it with a pleasant-tasting drink to take away any bitter taste.
- If medication is supplied in tablet form, crush or dissolve it in water and mix it with syrup or yoghurt for a better taste if appropriate. Be certain before removing the particles from a capsule that the medication will work properly when not in capsule form: some are encapsulated to keep them from dissolving in the stomach and to bring them into the intestine, where they have their therapeutic effect. The same precaution must be followed when giving enteric-coated tablets.
- Never leave medication by a child's bed for the child to take "in a minute" or "after your shower." The child may become involved with another activity "in a minute" and will not take it, or a smaller child could find the medication appealing and swallow it.

What if...

Ava's father tells you Ava is such a "picky eater" that she rarely eats a full meal? What possible strategies could you recommend to give a medication that should be taken with a meal?

Intranasal administration

Because nasal drops and sprays are easy to administer, more medications are supplied in these forms every year (Wolfe & Braude, 2010). These are advantageous in that a nasal spray is easy for a parent to administer. Medications are well absorbed across the nasal mucosa creating an effective means of medication administration including some life-sustaining medications. Dropping medication into the nose can be very uncomfortable, so you will need to ensure an age-appropriate explanation is given.

The child should be lying on their back. A school-aged child could extend the head over the side of the bed so that it is lower than the trunk. Preschoolers may be too frightened by this position and do better with a pillow under their shoulders so that their head extends over the pillow and rests downward. An infant may need to be restrained in a mummy restraint for nose drop administration.

Instil the appropriate number of drops into one nostril. Turn the child's head to the side—to the left after the left nostril, to the right after the right nostril—so that the medication stays in the nose longer. If the child is a preschooler or older, ask him or her to further "sniff" the medication. Have the child remain in the head-flat position for at least 1 minute to let the medication come in contact with the mucous membrane of the nose.

Children over about age 6 can use nasal sprays competently after they have been introduced to the technique. Acknowledge it may be uncomfortable and cause tickling or a sneezing sensation. Have the child sit or stand upright, hold the spray bottle upright with the tip just inside one side of the nose and gently squeeze the spray bottle. In most instances, a child should then tip the head to the side (the right side for the right nostril, the left side for the left nostril) or sniff, depending on the bottle instructions, for best absorption. Spray bottles should be individually prescribed for children.

Ophthalmic administration

Eye medications, in particular antibiotics to treat eye infections, are administered by being dropped into the conjunctival sac of the eye (Wong & Nischal, 2010). This type of administration, like nose drops, is often frightening for children. As a result, infants and preschoolers may need to be restrained in a mummy restraint for eye drop administration and the following procedure can be implemented.

- Avoid direct contact of container on eyelid as this will cross-contaminate.

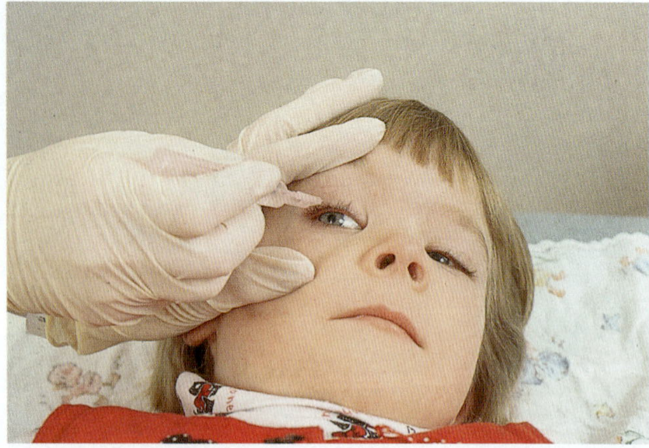

FIGURE 38.3 Administering eye drops.

- Eye medication should be individually prescribed and not used by other children.
- Explain the procedure at an age-appropriate level.
- Place the child on their back, open the eye of infants or preschoolers by gently but firmly pressing on the lower lid with the thumb and on the upper lid with the index finger.
- A school-age child or adolescent will open their eyes cooperatively, but you may need to rest a hand on the eyelid to keep the eye open long enough for the medication to be administered (see Fig. 38.3).
- Instil the correct number of drops into the conjunctiva of the lower lid.
- Allow the eyelid to close. Avoid placing the drops directly on the cornea, because that can be painful.
- Make sure the child has blinked two or three times before sitting up.
- To instil an ophthalmic ointment, apply a fine line of ointment along the inside rim of the conjunctival sac, working from the inner to the outer eye canthus.

Otic administration

Otic administration refers to administering medication, primarily drops, into the ear canal. Like other forms of medication administration, this can be frightening for children. When explaining the procedure tell the child that ear drops can feel funny, like tickling the ear. Ear drops must always be used at room temperature or warmed slightly. Cold fluid, such as medication taken from a refrigerator, may cause pain and severe vertigo as it touches the tympanic membrane.

The following procedure can then be implemented.

- Place the child on their back, in a mummy restraint if necessary. Turn the head to one side.
- If the child is younger than 2 years, straighten the external ear canal by pulling the pinna down and back.
- If the child is older than 2 years, pull the pinna of the ear up and back (see Fig. 38.4).
- Instil the specified number of drops into the ear canal.

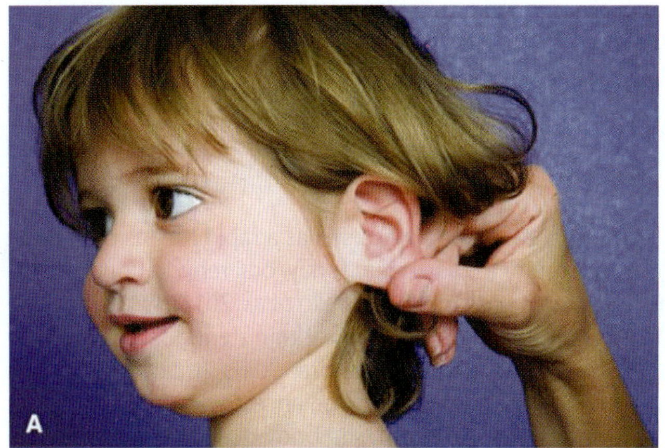

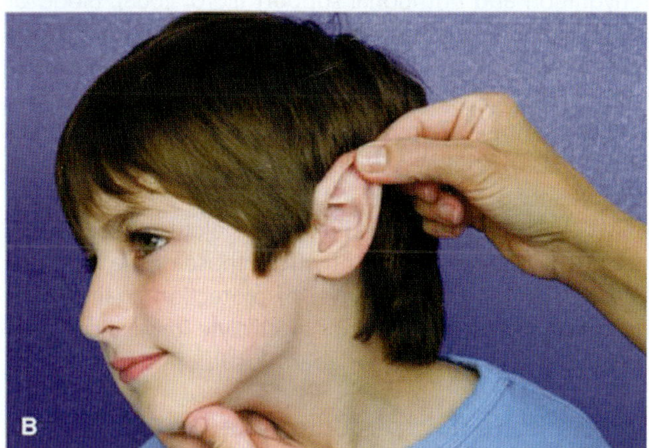

FIGURE 38.4 Administering ear drops. For the child over 2 years old, the pinna of the ear is pulled up and back. (Kyle, T. & Carman, S. (2012). *Essentials of Pediatric Nursing*. Philadelphia: Lippincott Williams & Wilkins.)

- Hold the child's head in the sideways position for at least 1 minute to ensure that the medication fills the entire ear canal.

✓ Checkpoint question 38.1

Suppose Zoe, 9 years old, needs to have ear drops administered. If you consult the unit's policies and procedures, you should expect what directive?

a. Have the child self-administer the drops to give the child a sense of control.
b. Refrigerate the drug for at least 30 minutes so it numbs the ear canal.
c. Pull the pinna of the child's ear down to straighten the canal.
d. Keep the child's head turned to the side to help retain the drops.

Rectal administration

A good route for administering medication to children who are having a seizure or who are unconscious is by rectal insertion, because this not only allows a drug to be absorbed across the mucous membrane of the intestine but also avoids the danger of aspiration (de Haan et al., 2010). Rectal administration may also be used to give medications to uncooperative young children or those who are vomiting. Most children, however, rate this as the least desirable method of receiving medication so it is not a common route of administration.

Some medications are given by rectal suppository; a few are given by retention enema. Because the child cannot see what is happening with rectal administration, they can be frightened by this procedure. Show the child the medication so that they can be certain it is not an injection. Remember that invasive procedures are particularly threatening to the preschooler.

The following procedures should be implemented:

- Many suppositories are supplied already lubricated. If not, add a drop of water-based lubricant such as K-Y jelly to the tip.
- Use a glove and insert the suppository gently but quickly beyond the rectal sphincter (approximately 2.5 cm or as far as the first knuckle of the little finger for infants and approximately 5 cm or as far as the first knuckle of the index finger for older children).
- Carefully withdraw your finger and press the child's buttocks together for a count of approximately 10, or until the child's urge to evacuate the suppository passes.
- If the medication is to be administered by a retention enema to a young child, use the usual enema technique, but with as small an amount of fluid as possible so the child can retain it.
- Press the child's buttocks together for approximately 15 seconds after administering the enema or a child will expel the solution almost immediately.
- Using a distraction technique, such as asking the child to count backward or saying the alphabet backward, can also help a defecation reflex to pass.

Transdermal/topical administration

Children who have a skin irritation or need medications to relieve itching or dryness may have topical creams or lotions prescribed. Most children accept this type of application well because the medication brings almost immediate relief. Children as young as toddlers can help apply this type of medication with supervision. Be certain they wash their hands afterwards.

Several children's medications are available by transdermal patch, because absorption of medications through the skin can be yet another effective and pain-free route of administration. Be certain that the child's skin is dry and intact at the site where the patch will be applied. For optimal absorption, apply patches over the trunk or a major muscle, not on distal extremities. Assess the skin under the patch every time a patch is changed to be certain the site is not becoming irritated. Change the site every time a new patch is applied to decrease the possibility of irritation to the skin.

Young children tend to remove transdermal patches the same as they do Band-Aids because of normal curiosity about what is underneath. Putting clothes on the young child immediately, so the patch is out of sight, is helpful. Be certain patches applied to children wearing nappies are not placed where a leak could wet the patch and irritate the skin or dilute the medication.

Intramuscular and subcutaneous administration

IM injections are rarely prescribed for children because many children do not have sufficient muscle mass for easy deposition of medication and they are often painful. For IM injections in infants, the mandatory site for administration is the vastus lateralis muscle of the anterior thigh (see Figs 38.5 and 38.6). Using the gluteal muscle in children younger than 1 year is extremely hazardous as this muscle does not develop until a child walks. This means that the sciatic nerve occupies a larger portion of the area and could be permanently damaged. In older children, as in adults, the deltoid muscle or a ventrogluteal site should be used (see Fig. 38.6).

Always give a short explanation of what you are about to do. Be honest about the pain involved; try to describe it accurately so that the child knows it has limits (a small amount of pain for a short time) with an explanation such as, "I have some medication for you. I'm going to put it into your leg. It will sting for a second just like a pinprick. Then it will be over." To reduce pain further, ask for a prescription for an analgesic cream to be applied an hour before the injection (see Chapter 39).

Statements such as "Don't cry" are not therapeutic. When children feel pain, they should be allowed to cry. As a way of giving children a better sense of control, you can tell them to say "ouch" or yell or scream when the needle is inserted. Most children appreciate being given approval to vent their feelings in this way. It may be necessary to ask for help in restraining a child when giving an injection to ensure safe administration. Allow a parent or guardian to hold and comfort a young child after all painful procedures.

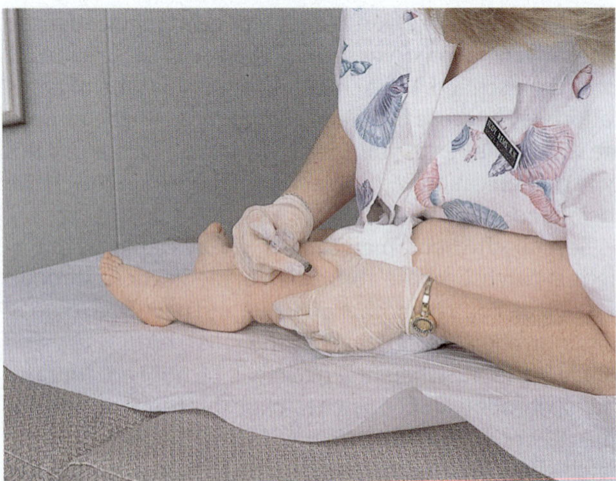

FIGURE 38.5 Technique for administering an intramuscular injection to an infant. Note the way the nurse uses her body to restrain and stabilise the infant.

INTRAVENOUS THERAPY

Historically IV therapy was used as a rapid means of hydrating children with diarrhoea. Today, oral rehydration therapy is preferred if possible (Passariello et al., 2011). IV therapy is a fast and effective means of administering fluid when a patient is unable to tolerate oral fluids. It can be used to maintain fluid and electrolyte balance, to produce therapeutic levels of medications in the body quickly and to provide rehydration and nutritional support (Ford, 2008). Blood or blood product replacement is another common therapy (see Chapter 44). IV fluid may be infused into a peripheral vein, a central venous access device or a peripherally-inserted central venous catheter. The amount, type and rate of IV fluids for children are prescribed carefully to prevent fluid overload. It is important to understand the principles of IV therapy, including the fluid and kilojoule needs of children (which differ significantly from those of the adult) so you can act as a second level of protection against over hydration, under hydration or electrolyte imbalances such as hyponatremia (Hanna & Saberi, 2010).

Determining fluid and kilojoule needs of the child

The fluid and kilojoule needs of children differ significantly to those of an adult. IV fluid administered to children and infants must be isotonic (exerts the same osmotic pressure as their bloodstream) to prevent the destruction of red blood cells or the development of water intoxication. The use of isotonic fluid prevents fluid shifting from the bloodstream into interstitial tissue (as would happen if the IV fluid were hypotonic) or fluid shifting from interstitial tissue into the bloodstream (as would happen if the IV fluid were hypertonic). Maintenance fluids are given to children in order to provide enough water and electrolytes to produce a normal urine output when the child is unable to maintain their oral fluid intake (see Table 38.1). Hypotonic fluids are no longer recommended for children due to the high risk of hyponatraemia. It is now widely accepted that isotonic fluids such as normal saline or Hartmann's solution are the most appropriate for children (Moritz & Ayus, 2011).

TABLE 38.1 A method to calculate fluid requirements

Body weight	Fluid requirement per 24 hours
Up to 10 kg	100 mL/kg
11–20 kg	1000 mL + 50 mL/kg for each additional kg over 10 kg
More than 20 kg	1500 mL + 20 mL/kg for each additional kg over 20 kg

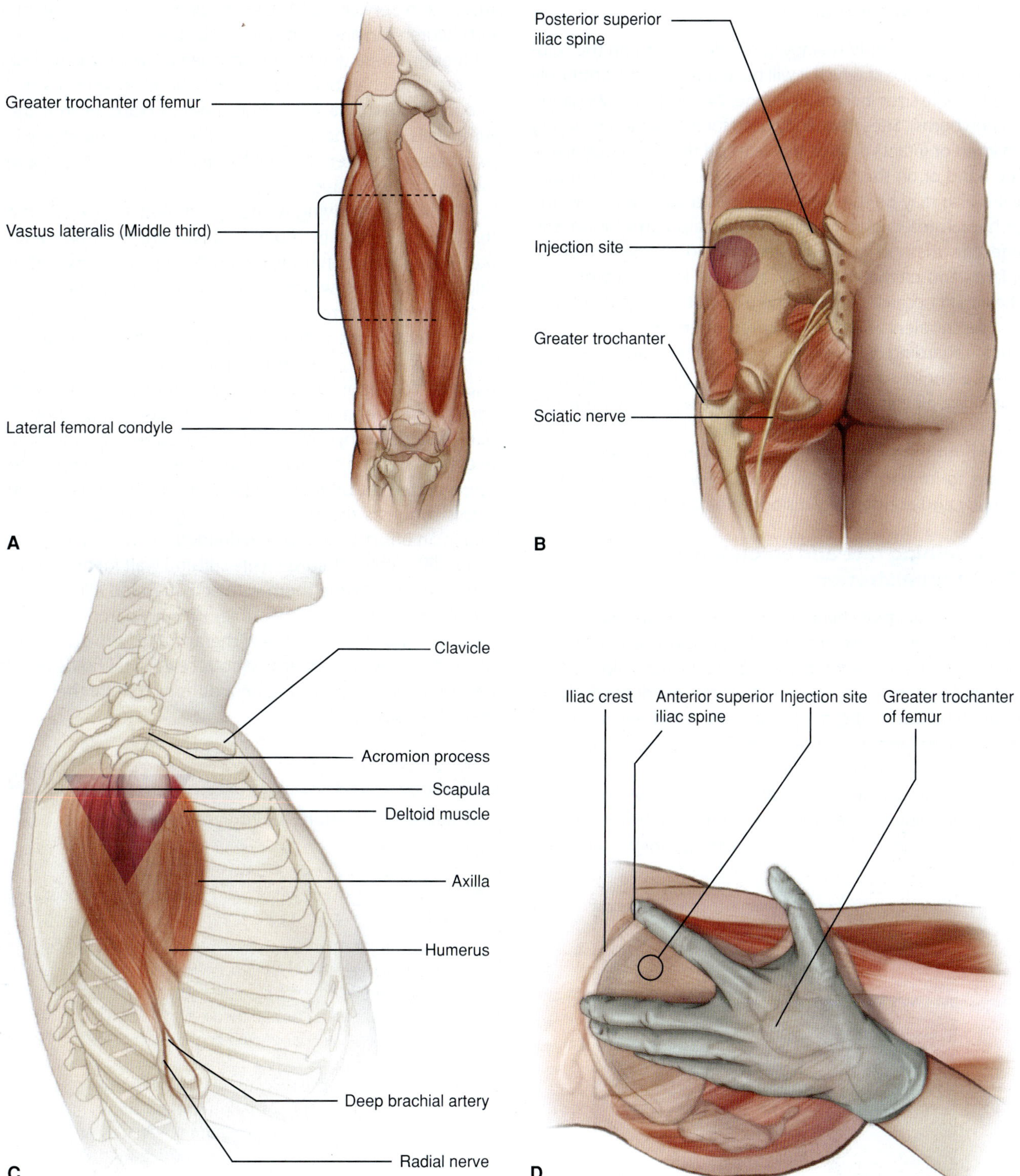

FIGURE 38.6 Locating intramuscular injection sites. (**A**) Vastus lateralis: identify the greater trochanter and the lateral femoral condyle; inject in the middle third and anterior lateral aspect. (**B**) Dorsogluteal: place your hand on the iliac crest and locate the posterosuperior iliac spine; inject in the outer quadrant formed when an imaginary line is drawn between the trochanter and the iliac spine. (**C**) Deltoid: locate the lateral side of the humerus, one to two finger widths below the acromion process; inject into the upper third of the muscle. (**D**) Ventrogluteal: place the palm of your left hand on the right greater trochanter so your index finger points towards the anterosuperior iliac spine and spread your middle finger to form a V; inject in the middle of the V. (Kyle, T. & Carman, S. (2012). *Essentials of Pediatric Nursing*. Philadelphia: Lippincott Williams & Wilkins.)

Obtaining venous access

The needle size for IV therapy varies depending on the solution and the rate at which it will be administered. Commonly used needle sizes include 22 gauge, 24 gauge and 25 gauge (in newborns). Sites frequently used for IV insertion in young children or infants include the veins on the dorsal surface of the hand or on the flexor surface of the wrist. Leg and foot veins also may be used. Another site is a scalp vein over the temporal area. Explain to parents that scalp vein infusion is an effective method of administering fluid or medication to infants and ultimately might cause the least discomfort to their child because cannulas there do not infiltrate readily.

Preschoolers and older children often express a preference regarding where they want an infusion inserted. Offer a choice, if possible, or suggest the non-dominant hand. For all children (including adolescents), IV infusions are usually secured in place with at least a small arm board. Although children may be careful without an arm board to immobilise the area it is easy to move unintentionally and accidentally dislodge the cannula.

Determining rate and amount of fluid administration

Due to the fact that children's hearts and circulatory systems are smaller than those of adults, IV fluid must be infused at a slower rate. If administered at an adult rate, the child's cardiovascular system could quickly become overloaded. Automatic rate-flow infusion pumps are used when giving medications and they are mandatory for small children because they regulate the flow accurately (see Fig. 38.7). In addition, the use of pressure alarms can be set on most IV pumps to minimise trauma to the internal lumen of the vein and reduce the incidence of infiltration (Sydney South West Area Health Service, 2010). Overloading of IV fluid in infants and children can also be prevented by use of fluid chambers or burettes. These devices are attached between the IV flask and the drip chamber and can only be filled with a small amount of fluid at a time. With these in place, even if the pump fails, only the amount of fluid in the burette will be allowed to enter the child's circulation, not the entire contents of the IV flask.

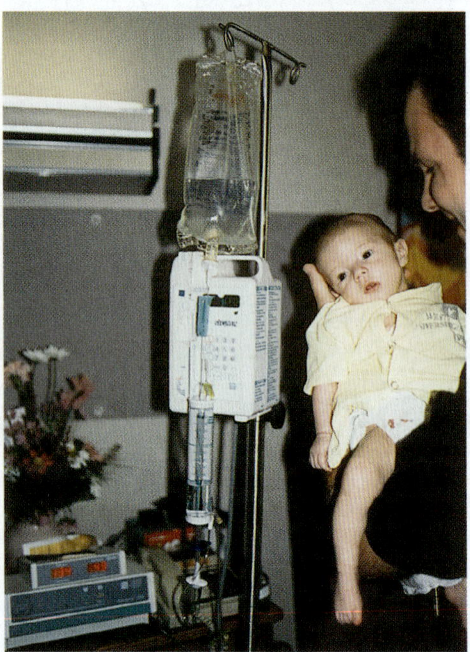

FIGURE 38.7 An infusion pump and calibrated infusion chamber are safety features used with children's intravenous infusions.

All children receiving IV therapy should be placed on a fluid balance chart in order to guard against fluid overload. At least once an hour, record the type and amount of fluid, the rate of flow (including the number of drops per minute and pressure values if available) and, for a cross-check, the amount of fluid remaining in the bag. In addition, the cannula site and surrounding area should be assessed for signs of infiltration or inflammation. Vital signs should be monitored closely for signs of fluid overload such as tachycardia and hypertension. In addition, assess the specific gravity of urine at least every 4 hours to detect extremely dilute urine (specific gravity under 1.003) as this suggests the child is excreting a large quantity of fluid in an effort to reduce overloaded circulating volume.

It is difficult for children to lie still and wait for an IV infusion to finish. Provide them with activities and allow them out of bed as much as possible. Be sure parents understand the importance of the IV therapy and help guard the infusion site as well. Infants who receive total fluids by IV infusion may enjoy sucking on a dummy to fulfil their oral needs (see Box 38.3).

BOX 38.3 ✻ Focus on family teaching

General considerations for intravenous therapy

Q. Ava's mother asks you a lot of questions about intravenous therapy, such as "Why can't Ava just drink fluid?"

A. Parents and children often want to know more about IV therapy. Some of the typical questions parents ask are:

- Will the insertion hurt? (Yes, but only as the needle is inserted; after that the infusion will be pain-free.)
- How long will the infusion be necessary? (The duration differs depending on the medication and fluid prescription and can vary depending on the effect of the medication or fluid.)
- Isn't there another way to administer the same medication? (Usually, no. IV administration allows medication to reach the bloodstream immediately and so is the method of choice when immediate effect is important; also, some medications can only be given intravenously.)
- What can the child do during the infusion? (Any activity that will not interfere with the infusion. If a child will have medication administration daily, help the child plan a special activity such as to play a board game, listen to special music, or watch a favourite TV program, an activity reserved for only that time. This changes the IV infusion from a dreaded activity to a "can't wait for" activity.)
- Will it hurt when the needle is removed? (No, although taking off the tape that holds the needle in place may cause some discomfort.)

CASE STUDY QUESTION

5. Ava has her IV site changed to her dominant hand. She has stated that she is "bored and kind of sad." What would be the best activity for her while her medication infuses?
   a. Listening to a story you read
   b. Playing kick ball in the hallway
   c. Playing Simon Says with her parents
   d. Building a tower in the play area with another child

Intravenous medication administration

IV medications are administered to children in several ways including added directly to an IV cannula or line as a bolus, or administered as an **intermittent infusion** via a burette, or as a piggyback. Analgesics may be administered to children over the age of five by patient controlled analgesia (PCA) machines. The child must be able to understand the concept of PCA and be physically able to press the button to be suitable for this mode of analgesia.

Using central venous access catheters and devices

The insertion of a central venous access catheter is indicated in children who have poor peripheral access, require long-term venous access and/or medications or IV fluids that cannot be given peripherally, such as TPN and chemotherapy. These catheters are inserted into the superior vena cava just above the right atrium and may be tunnelled or non-tunnelled (see Fig. 38.8A). Tunnelled central venous catheters are inserted by a surgeon or radiologist and have separate entry and exit sites. Examples of these catheters include Broviac, Hickman and Groshong catheters. There is less risk of infections with tunnelled devices and they are therefore recommended when treatment is expected to last for more than 14 days. Non-tunnelled central venous catheters are inserted directly into the blood vessel and advanced to the desired point (see Fig. 38.8C). Due to the higher risk of infection, they are only recommended if treatment is expected to last less than 14 days (Royal Children's Hospital Melbourne, 2009). Central venous access devices may be single lumen or multi-lumen. Due to the fact that infection risk increases with the number of lumens, single lumen devices should be used wherever possible (Royal Children's Hospital Melbourne, 2009).

Care of central venous catheters will depend on individual hospital policy and includes weekly dressing changes with a transparent semi-permeable dressing, using strict aseptic technique (see Fig. 38.8B). The dressing should cover the insertion site and hub, to reduce infection as well as secure and stabilise the catheter. A designated securement device dressing, such as Grip Lok, may also be applied (in lieu of suturing) when the catheter is inserted and should be changed as per local policy. Regular saline flushes may be used to ensure patency for lumens not accessed and/or the use of positive pressure displacement capless valves (ACI NSW Agency for Clinical Innovation, 2014; NSW Health, 2011).

Vascular access ports

Vascular access ports (infusion ports that can be implanted) are small plastic devices that are implanted under the skin, usually on the anterior chest just under the clavicle, dependent on the child's age, size and proposed timeframe use. They are used for long-term fluid or medication administration via bolus or continuous administration (see Fig. 38.8D). A small catheter threads from the port internally into a central vein. Common brands include Port-A-Cath and Infus-A-Port. After skin cleansing, blood samples can be removed or medication can be injected by a puncture through the chest skin into the port. Although this device requires a skin puncture, it may be well-accepted by children because it is not as visible as a central venous catheter, no dressing is required (expect when the port is accessed) and it allows a full range of activities, such as showering and swimming. Special port access needles are only to be used as a regular needle tends to "core" or remove a small circle of the membrane over the port and destroy the integrity of the device. Use EMLA cream to decrease discomfort as necessary. Some older children may be considered competent to access their own port for home therapy. It is important to involve them in their care. However, local policy will dictate inpatient port access guidelines and at all times nurses must adhere to strict aseptic techniques when accessing the port or attached lines. As with central lines, air emboli, bleeding from a disconnected line and infection are major concerns with VAPs.

Peripherally inserted central catheters

Children also may have peripherally inserted central catheters (PICC lines) for IV therapy (Levy et al., 2010). These are advantageous, particularly for in-home care, because they can remain in place for up to 4 months without being changed. These catheters are inserted into a peripheral vein (usually in the non-dominant arm) and advanced until the tip rests in the superior vena cava. Care of a PICC line is similar to central lines. However PICCs must be assessed closely for mechanical complications such as migration, particularly in young children which is accentuated by excessive movement of the related limb. Peripheral insertion decreases infection risks. However, the smaller catheter size results in decreased intra-luminal flow rates which restricts infusion flow rates as per manufacture guidelines. The dressing over the insertion site is changed periodically according to agency policy. It is common to have post insertion mechanical irritation, seen as a red mark tracking up the vein from the insertion site, but it should resolve within 48 hours. Assessment of the PICC should include insertion site, migration of line (check correct length at securement device as well as any signs of internal migration such as headache or pulmonary dysfunction), dressing and line integrity, ensuring there is no pulling on the catheter. Measurement of the mid-upper limb circumference is compared to initial value and reported if a significant

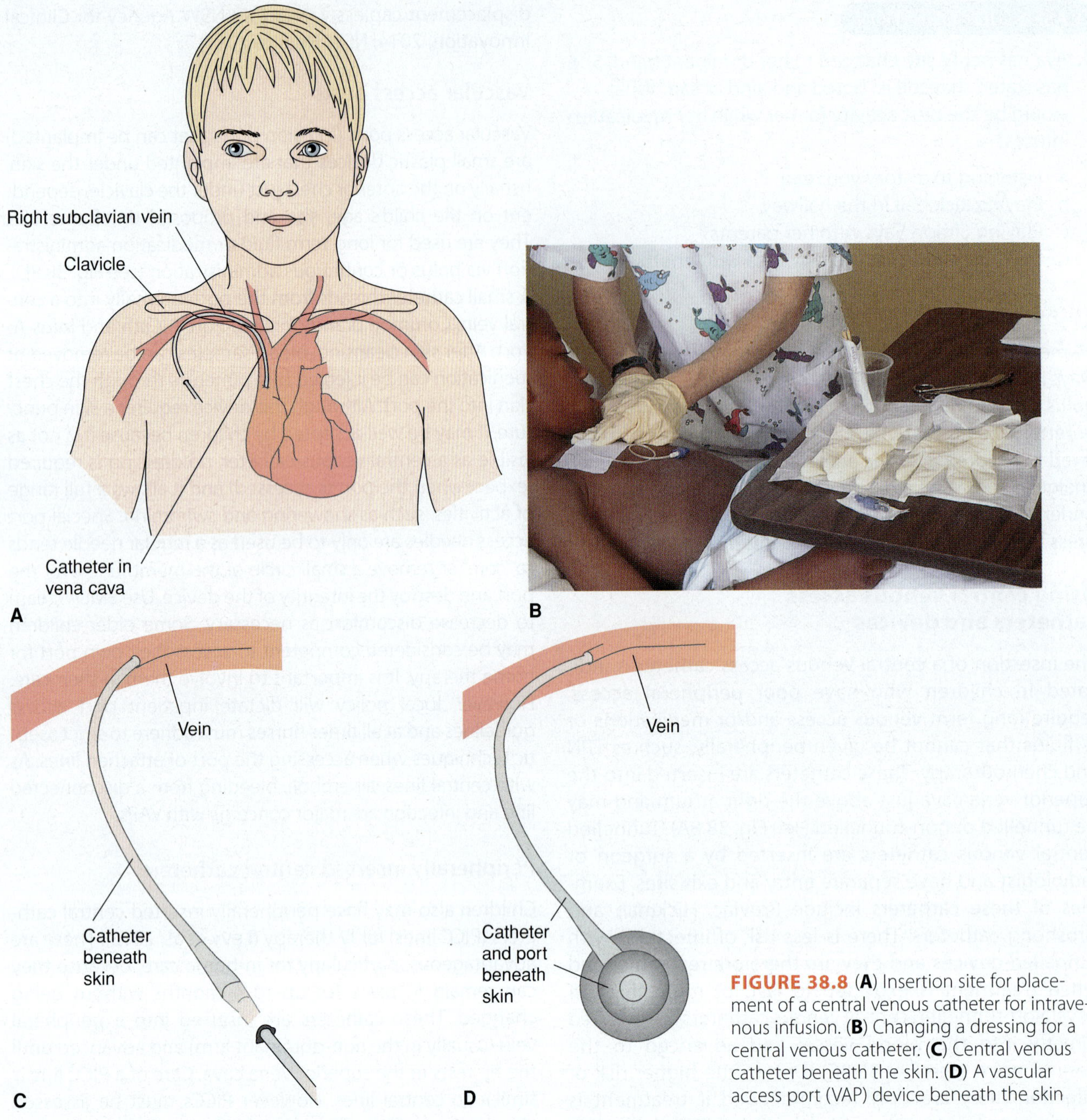

FIGURE 38.8 (**A**) Insertion site for placement of a central venous catheter for intravenous infusion. (**B**) Changing a dressing for a central venous catheter. (**C**) Central venous catheter beneath the skin. (**D**) A vascular access port (VAP) device beneath the skin

increase occurs, as this may reflect potential venous thrombosis. Remember that when caring for children with central venous access systems in place, all the various types have the potential to result in haemorrhage, infection, air embolism and thrombosis. Be certain to use strict aseptic techniques when changing the dressings over them to prevent infections because this is a major area of emphasis (O'Grady et al., 2011).

Administering an intraosseous infusion

Intraosseous infusion is the infusion of fluid into the bone marrow cavity of a long bone, usually the distal or proximal tibia, the distal femur, or the iliac crest (Nagler & Krauss, 2011). Bone marrow communicates directly with the circulatory system so fluid reaches the bloodstream as quickly as if it were administered intravenously. Intraosseous infusion is used in an emergency when usual IV access is poor, or with such extensive burns that the usual sites for IV infusion are not available. Intraosseous infusion is a temporary measure until a usual route of administration can be obtained because of the danger of osteomyelitis. It must be initiated with a sterile technique and, if continued for an extended time, the infusion point is rotated about every 2 to 3 days to minimise the risk of infection.

Key points for review

- The effectiveness of medications varies depending on the pharmacokinetics (absorption, distribution, metabolism and excretion) of the medication.
- The principles of safe medication administration for adults also apply to children: right medication, right child, right dose, right route, right time and right patient instructions.
- The correct medication dose in children is usually calculated according to the child's body surface area.
- It is important to teach parents safe actions for giving medication at home so children continue to receive accurate doses after hospital discharge.
- In children, the majority of medications are given orally or intravenously to avoid the pain of IM injection. Subcutaneous pumps infuse medication such as insulin.
- IV therapy may be administered peripherally or via a central venous access site.

CASE STUDY QUESTIONS

6. Ava's mother tells you that she does not believe in introducing any "foreign" substance into her child's body, so she does not intend to give her the antibiotic for her infected foot. Would there be a way to change her mind? How would you counsel her?

Resources

For an extensive range of additional resources to enhance teaching and learning and to facilitate understanding of this chapter, please see the text's accompanying website located on thePoint at http://thepoint.lww.com.

References

ACI NSW Agency for Clinical Innovation (2014). IC Manual. Central venous access device post insertion management. Accessed 13 April 2015, <www.aci.health.nsw.gov.au/__data/assets/pdf_file/0010/239626/ACI14_CVAD-2-2.pdf>.

de Haan, G., van der Geest, P., Doelman, G., et al. (2010). A comparison of midazolam nasal spray and diazepam rectal solution for the residential treatment of seizure exacerbations. *Epilepsia, 51*(3), 478–482.

Dickinson, C. J., Wagner, D. S., Shaw, B. E., et al. (2012). A systematic approach to improving medication safety in a pediatric intensive care unit. *Critical Care Nursing Quarterly, 35*(1), 15–26.

El-Alfy, M., Sari, T. T., Lee, C. L., et al. (2010). The safety, tolerability, and efficacy of a liquid formulation of deferiprone in young children with transfusion iron overload. *Journal of Pediatric Hematology/Oncology, 32*(8), 601–605.

Ford, D. M. (2008). Fluid, electrolyte and acid-base disorders and therapy. In W. W. Hay, et al. (Eds). *Current Pediatric Diagnosis and Treatment* (18th ed.). Columbus, OH: McGraw-Hill.

Hanna, M. & Saberi, M. S. (2010). Incidence of hyponatremia in children with gastroenteritis treated with hypotonic intravenous fluids. *Pediatric Nephrology, 25*(8), 1471–1475.

Johnson, T. N. & Rostami-Hodjegan, A. R. (2010). Resurgence in the use of physiologically based pharmakinetic models in pediatric clinical pharmacology. *Pediatric Anesthesia, 21*(3), 291–301.

Kalisch, B. J. & Aebersold, M. (2010). Interruptions and multitasking in nursing care. *Joint Commission Journal on Quality and Patient Safety, 36*(3), 126–132.

Levy, I., Bendet, M., Samra, Z., et al. (2010). Infectious complications of peripherally inserted central venous catheters in children. *Pediatric Infectious Disease Journal, 29*(5), 426–429.

Moritz, M. L. & Ayus, J. C. (2011). Prevention of hospital acquired hyponatremia: Do we have the answers? *Pediatrics, 128*(5), 980–983.

Nagler, J. & Krauss, B. (2011). Intraosseous catheter placement in children. *New England Journal of Medicine, 364*(8), e14.

NSW Health. (2011) Central venous access device insertion and post insertion care, accessed 30 March 2015, <www.health.nsw.gov.au/policies/pd/2011/PD2011_060.html>.

O'Grady, N. P., Alexander, M., Burns, L., et al. (2011). Guidelines for the prevention of intravascular catheter-related infections. *Clinical Infectious Diseases, 52*(9), e162–e193.

Passariello, A., Terrin, G., de Marco, G., et al. (2011). Efficacy of a new hypotonic oral rehydration solution containing zinc and prebiotics in the treatment of childhood acute diarrhea: A randomized controlled trial. *Journal of Pediatrics, 158*(2), 288–292.

Pham, J. C., Story, J. L., Hicks, R. W., et al. (2011). National study on the frequency, types, causes, and consequences of voluntarily reported emergency department medication errors. *The Journal of Emergency Medicine, 40*(5), 485–492.

Royal Children's Hospital Melbourne. (2009). Clinical practice guidelines: Intravenous fluids. Accessed 30 March 2015, <www.rch.org.au/clinicalguide/cpg.cfm?doc_id=5203>.

Sydney South West Area Health Service. (2010). Cannula: Insertion & management of peripheral intravenous cannulae in paediatric patients, accessed 30 March 2015, <www.sswahs.nsw.gov.au/pdf/policy/SSW_PD2010_015.pdf>.

Walsh, K. E., Mazor, K. M., Roblin, D., et al. (2013). Multisite parent centered risk assessment to reduce pediatric oral chemotherapy errors. *Journal of Oncology Practice, 9*(1), e1–e7.

Wolfe, T. R. & Braude, D. A. (2010). Intranasal medication delivery for children: A brief update. *Pediatrics, 126*(3), 532–537.

Wong, I.B.Y. & Nischal, K. K. (2010). Managing a child with an external ocular disease. *Journal of American Association for Pediatric Ophthalmology and Strabismus, 14*(1), 68–77.

Suggested readings

Adhikan, A., Tocher, J., Smith, P., Corcoran, J. & MacAuthur, J. (2014). A multidisciplinary approach to medication safety and the implication for nursing education and practice. *Nurse Education Today, 34*(2), 185–190.

Australian Commission on Safety and Quality in Healthcare <www.safetyandquality.gov.au/our-work/medication-safety>.

Clinical Excellence Commission <www.cec.health.nsw.gov.au/programs/medication-safety>.

de Maria, C., Lussier, M. & Bajcar, J. (2011). What do children know about medications? A review of the literature to guide clinical practice. *Canadian Family Physician, 57*(3), 291–295.

Hamrin, V., McCarthy, E. M., & Tyson, V. (2010). Pediatric psychotropic medication initiation and adherence: A literature review based on social exchange theory. *Journal of Child and Adolescent Psychiatric Nursing, 23*(3), 151–172.

Health Quality and Safety Commission New Zealand <www.hqsc.govt.nz/our-programmes/medication-safety>.

Jones, J. H. & Treiber, L. (2010). When the 5 rights go wrong: Medication errors from the nursing perspective. *Journal of Nursing Care Quality, 25*(3), 240–247.

Landier, W. (2011). Age span challenges: Adherence in pediatric oncology. *Seminars in Oncology Nursing, 27*(2), 142–153.

Medsafe New Zealand Medicines and Medical Devices Safety Authority <www.medsafe.govt.nz>.

Chapter 39

Pain management in children

Previous chapters described the growth and development of children and general care of ill children. This chapter adds information about the care of children when they need pain management. Such information builds a base for care and health teaching in a crucial area.

LEARNING OBJECTIVES

After studying the contents of this chapter, you should be able to:

1. Describe the major methods and techniques of pain management for children.
2. Use critical thinking to analyse ways nursing care for a child in pain could be more family-centred.
3. Assess a child regarding whether pain management is needed or adequate.
4. Formulate nursing considerations for a child in pain.
5. Identify expected outcomes for a child in pain.
6. Plan nursing care for a child in pain.
7. Implement nursing care related to a child in pain.
8. Evaluate outcomes for achievement and effectiveness of care of a child in pain.
9. Identify areas related to care of children in pain that could benefit from additional nursing research or application of evidence-based practice.
10. Integrate knowledge of pain in children with nursing considerations to achieve quality child and family health nursing care.

KEY TERMS

- distraction
- epidural analgesia
- guided imagery
- pain
- patient-controlled analgesia (PCA)
- transcutaneous electrical nerve stimulation (TENS)

CASE STUDY

Amy Johnson is a 3-year-old girl who was admitted to your hospital unit and has just returned from a bone marrow aspiration to rule out the possibility of leukaemia. Amy received intravenous morphine sulphate during the procedure. Her mother, Jackie, asks if Amy could have some more. "I know she's not having pain yet", her mother tells you, "but I want her to have something before the pain comes back".

CASE STUDY QUESTIONS

1. Is Jackie's assessment of Amy's pain accurate or should you ask Amy about her pain?
2. Would anticipating pain in this way be the best intervention for Amy?

Pain is a difficult concept to define because it is experienced uniquely. It is important to remember that it is subjective (experienced by the person), not objective (able to be determined by observation). McCaffery's classic description of pain (Pasero & McCaffery, 2004) is the one most useful with children: "The sensation of pain is whatever the person experiencing it says it is and it exists whenever the person says it does."

For children, pain is not only a hurting sensation, it can also be a confusing one because a child often does not anticipate the pain, does not have words to explain how it feels and cannot always understand its cause. In addition, preschoolers and younger children lack an understanding of time, which makes it difficult to explain when the pain will go away. Children may feel frustrated or angry because no one can prevent their hurt or give them relief. As children may have difficulty describing pain in a manner adults can understand, it is difficult to assess the extent of their discomfort. As pain is an individualised sensation, it may be experienced and expressed differently by different children. In some families pain may be expressed very openly and freely. In others, children are expected to be stoic. This means that children experiencing procedures that are less intrusive but who feel maximum anxiety from them may describe the degree of pain felt as more intense than they otherwise might have because of the accompanying anxiety (Vervoort et al., 2010). Helping children describe the type and extent of pain they are feeling and performing active interventions to relieve pain are important nursing roles. Assessing for pain should be considered the "fifth vital sign" (Harrison et al., 2013).

CHILDREN AND PAIN

Assessment

Children experience pain differently depending on the type and cause of the pain, their temperament, their previous experience with pain and their expectation of relief. Infants and young children cannot verbalise what they are feeling so have the most trouble communicating how they feel.

Preschoolers can indicate where they feel pain and can learn to express the degree of pain through a system such as comparing it to drawings of faces. Older children and adolescents can be asked to rate their pain on a scale of 1 to 10. Be aware that children may be reluctant to admit pain because they are trying to be brave. Some may be reluctant to say they have pain because they are afraid they will receive a "needle" to relieve it, causing more pain. As a rule, including assessment of pain level along with vital sign measurement is one way to ensure that pain is regularly assessed. However, this is only the first step in pain management. If children have pain, they need intervention as a second step to relieve it. Let children know that admitting to having pain is necessary for them to obtain adequate relief.

Parents might be unclear about their role in pain management, assuming nurses and doctors are the experts and so will automatically treat their child's pain. Conversely, nurses might assume that parents will speak up if their child is in pain. How pain will be assessed, the parents' role and what is available for pain relief should be discussed clearly and openly. Ensure that pain is reassessed to ascertain that interventions such as administration of an analgesic, distraction or improved positioning were effective.

Nursing considerations

Nursing considerations for children with pain focus not only on the pain but also on the stress, fear or anxiety that pain produces. These include:

- Pain related to invasive procedures
- Fear and anxiety related to anticipation of pain
- Disturbed sleep patterns related to pain.

The mark of efficient pain control is to anticipate when pain will occur and plan interventions to prevent it, rather than let it occur and then relieve it. Three common reasons why nurses may not provide adequate pain relief to children are a belief that infants and young children do not experience pain, a fear that children will become addicted to analgesic medications and a fear of causing respiratory depression. Infants and young children do experience pain, but there is no confirmation that children receiving opioids short term will become addicted to them or that opioids cause greater respiratory depression in children than in adults (Fanning et al., 2012).

Implementation of pain relief includes choosing the specific method of pain relief best for each child. All persons involved in a child's care need to be aware of the signs and symptoms an individual child uses to express pain and specific ways that will help the child manage pain. If children are reluctant to admit they have pain because of the fear of receiving an injection, advocate for an oral form of analgesia or an intermittent intravenous (IV) infusion device or patient-controlled analgesia (PCA) as appropriate options.

Evaluation of expected outcomes is a key aspect of managing pain because no one pain relief measure is effective for everyone. After a child is given an analgesic, look for non-verbal clues, assess vital signs and listen to the child's statements about pain to determine whether a medication was effective. It may become clear that the pain management technique chosen needs to be modified or increased. A new technique may need to be added to the regimen so a child receives maximum pain relief.

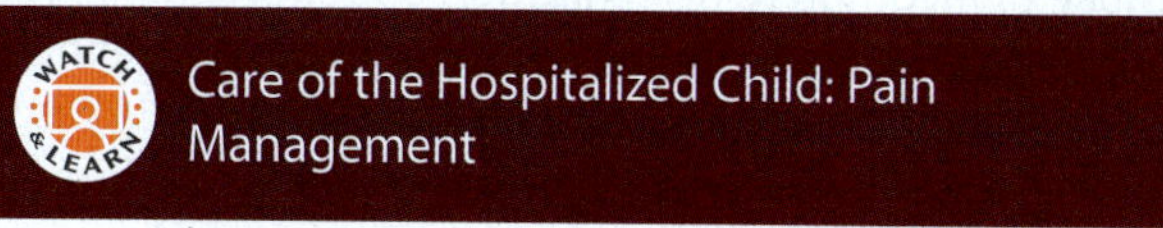

ASSESSING THE TYPE AND DEGREE OF PAIN

Pain assessment is difficult with children, not only because children have difficulty describing pain, but also because some children will suffer with pain rather than report it, unaware that someone could make it go away. Other children may distract themselves by methods such as concentrating on play. Some children may sleep, not from comfort but from the exhaustion caused by pain. Cultural differences also influence how pain is expressed (see Box 39.1). All of these things can make using only subjective measures to assess pain, such as observation, misleading.

Pain assessment in children is also difficult because techniques vary widely from assessment of a non-verbal infant to an older adolescent. Keep in mind a child's developmental level as well as chronological age when assessing pain.

BOX 39.1 Assessment * Assessing a child with pain

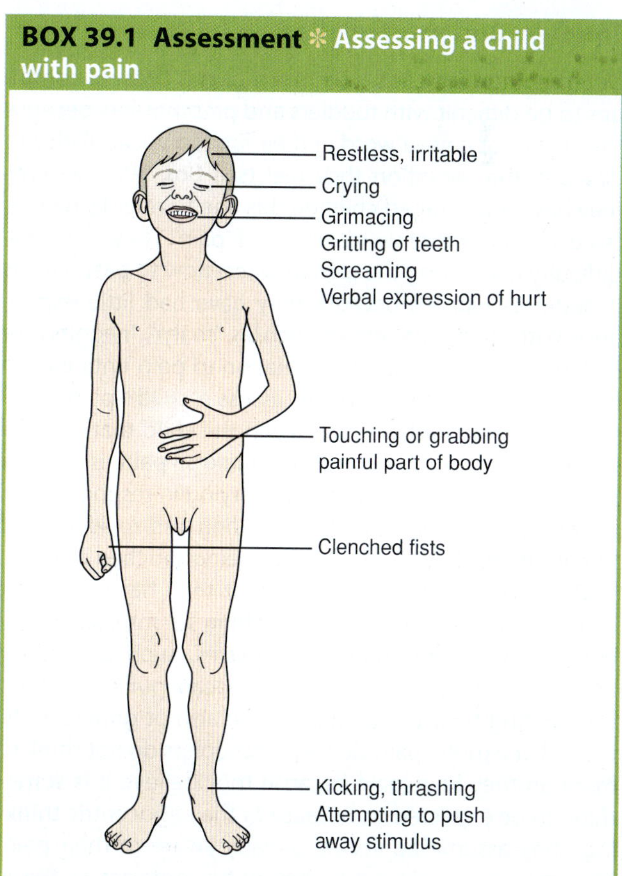

Infants

It was previously believed that infants do not feel pain because of incomplete myelinisation of peripheral nerves. This is no longer believed to be true, because myelinisation is not necessary for pain perception.

A second argument against needing to provide pain relief to infants was that they have no memory. However, physiological changes occur with pain even in premature infants, so despite a lack of memory, it is clear pain is experienced. In all ages, pain has been shown to have the potential for serious physical harm. Any procedure or condition that causes pain in an adult will also cause pain in a child.

As infants are preverbal, observing for cues such as diffuse body movement; tears; a high-pitched, sharp, harsh cry; stiff posture; lack of play; and fisting are all cues to reveal discomfort (Schiavenato, Butler-O'Hare & Scovanner, 2011). Even newborns instinctively guard a body part by holding an extremity still or tensing the abdomen. Perhaps the chief mark of pain in infants is that when pain is present, they cannot be comforted completely. Preterm neonates may have a particularly difficult time organising a distress response to alert a healthcare provider to the presence of pain. When working with infants of this age, be sensitive to situations that could cause pain and reduce them to the maximum extent possible. Be alert for subtle alterations in facial expression, such as eyes squeezed shut or a quivering chin that might signify pain.

BOX 39.2 * Focus on communication

Amy has just returned from surgery. You want to assess her level of pain.

Less effective communication

Nurse: Amy? How are you feeling?

Jackie Johnson: I don't think she hurts yet.

Nurse: I'm going to show you some faces, Amy. Just point to the one that looks the way you feel. If you point to a sad one, I'll get you a needle to take away your pain.

Amy: (Points to the first face—the "no pain" face.)

Nurse: No pain? Good. That's probably because your anaesthetic is still working.

More effective communication

Nurse: Amy? How are you feeling?

Jackie Johnson: I don't think she hurts yet.

Nurse: Amy, remember the faces we looked at this morning before surgery? I want you to use them to tell me how you feel. This one means "no hurt". This one means "the most hurt you could have". Point to the one that shows how much hurt you have.

Amy: (Points to the middle face—the "hurts even more" face.)

It is important when using pain rating scales to introduce them to children before surgery or before they have pain from procedures, so that both the pain and the rating tool are not new to the child. It is also important to give the correct instructions for standardised assessment tools, or the results will not be accurate. Mentioning a "needle for pain" can cause children not to report pain because they imagine the injection will cause even more pain, rather than relieve it.

Toddlers and preschoolers

Determining when and how much pain is present continues to be difficult with toddlers and preschoolers because they may not have a word in their limited vocabularies to describe the sensation they feel (see Box 39.2). Parents may have encouraged children this age to refer to pain as "sore" or some other word instead of "pain". They may have difficulty comparing the pain they feel now to past pain (is it better or worse?) because they have had little experience with past pain. Words such as "sharp", "nagging" or "aching" have no meaning in relation to pain until a child has experienced each type. To assess a child's pain accurately, use the child's term or teach the child that "pain" is the same as "sore". For some toddlers, pain is such a strange sensation that, aside from crying in response to it, they may react aggressively (pounding and rocking) as if to fight it off. They also may avoid being touched or held.

Preschool children can state that they have pain but continue to have difficulty describing its intensity. They begin to use comforting mechanisms, such as gritting teeth, pressing a hand against a forehead, pulling on their ear, holding their throat, rubbing an arm or grimacing to control or express pain. Some preschoolers do not think to mention they have pain because they believe it is something to be expected or, because of their egocentric thinking, they assume adults are already aware of their pain. They may think pain is punishment for some act, so this is what they deserve. It is sometimes difficult to comfort children this age during painful procedures because they do not yet have a perception of time. Soothing statements such as, "It's only for a minute" are not comforting to the preschooler who does not know how long that is.

For all young children who cannot fully verbalise their pain state, carefully examine their behaviour. In addition, young children may regress or become very withdrawn when in pain. Ask yourself, "What would this child normally be doing (for example, playing, eating, sleeping)?" Deviations from usual behaviour may, in the absence of any other verbal description, be signs a child is in pain. Input from parents on how their child usually behaves can be valuable in evaluation. In a non-verbal child, a trial dose of analgesia may be used. You can then evaluate behaviour changes after the dose is given. Children who resume their usual behaviour after analgesia were probably in pain before the analgesia took effect.

School-aged children and adolescents

Children who think concretely (pre-adolescents) can have difficulty envisioning that a word like "sharp" applies both to knives and to the feeling in their abdomen. As a result, they continue to have difficulty describing pain. They may

TABLE 39.1 Common fallacies about pain in children

Fallacy	Fact
Nurses can accurately estimate children's pain from physical appearance or activity	Nurses commonly underestimate children's pain when they do not rely on children's self-reports
Young children, particularly newborns, do not feel pain	Newborns and children do feel pain
A child who resumes usual activity or sleeps cannot be in pain	Some children distract themselves with play or music while in pain. They may sleep from exhaustion from the pain
Because of the possible adverse effects, opioid analgesics are too dangerous for young children	Opioids can be used safely with children, including low-birth-weight infants
Experiencing pain will not harm an infant or young child	Newborns with pain can become cyanotic and bradycardic; no-one knows the psychological stress of pain at this age
If children deny they are feeling pain, you should believe them	Children may deny pain to avoid a procedure, such as an injection, which they view as more painful. They may be afraid, fearing that they are being punished, or believe others know how they feel.

also assume that you, as an authority figure, already know they have pain.

Some children of school age will regress with pain such as baby-talk or lying in a fetal position. Children this age can understand that if pain will last only an instant, such as with an injection, it can be controlled through non-pharmacological activities such as distraction techniques.

Children may be at school before they can understand how to use a numerical pain rating scale or that the scale intensifies from left to right. Doing some pre-assessment work with them, such as giving them 10 different-sized triangles and asking them to arrange them from smallest to largest, is a good way to evaluate if they understand incremental measurements. The child who can arrange triangles in this way understands the concept of least to most. Once children have grasped this concept, they can describe pain intensity in a very measurable way. A scale of 1 to 5 can be used in younger children if 1 to 10 seems overwhelming. Yet another technique is to turn the scale vertically so it measures bottom (little pain) to top (a lot of pain).

Adolescents commonly use adult mechanisms for controlling pain. Some are even more stoic in the face of pain than adults, trying to avoid stereotypes of "cry-baby" or "wimp". This tendency makes assessment for body motions that could indicate pain, such as clenched hands, clenched teeth, rapid breathing and guarding of body parts, not as helpful as it may be in adults.

PAIN ASSESSMENT

Common fallacies about pain in children are shown in Table 39.1. The techniques to assess pain must vary depending on the age of the child and the type and extent of pain. Although monitoring for changes in vital signs might give some indication that a child is under stress, these are not the most dependable indicators of pain. Pain is a subjective finding, so once children can speak, asking them to tell you about their pain (self-reporting on a pain rating scale) is the most accurate method of assessment (Downey & Zun, 2012; see Box 39.3).

A variety of pain rating scales have been devised for use with children. None has been proven to be consistently better than the others, mainly because both children and the type of pain they can be experiencing vary so much. As a rule, pick a well-documented effective scale and use that consistently for a child, rather than asking a child to adapt to different assessment techniques. Be sure to follow the specific instructions for that scale.

The FLACC Pain Assessment Tool

The FLACC (Face, Legs, Activity, Cry and Consolability) Pain Assessment Tool is a scale by which healthcare providers can rate a young child's pain when a child cannot give input, such as during circumcision (Merkel, Voepel-Lewis & Malviya, 2002). It incorporates five types of behaviours

BOX 39.3 ✻ Pain experience questions

Questions for the child

Tell me what pain is.
Tell me about the hurt you have had before.
What do you do when you hurt?
Do you tell others when you hurt?
What do you want others to do for you when you hurt?
What do you not want others to do for you when you hurt?
What helps the most to take away your hurt?
Is there anything special that you would like me to know about you when you hurt? (If yes, have child describe).

Questions for the parents

Describe any pain your child has had before.
How does your child usually react to pain?
Does your child tell you or others when pain is experienced?
How do you know when your child is in pain?
What do you do for your child when your child is hurting?
What does your child do to help relieve pain?
Which of these actions work best to decrease or take away your child's pain?
Is there anything special that you would like me to know about your child and pain? (If yes, have parents describe) (Hester & Barcus, 1986).

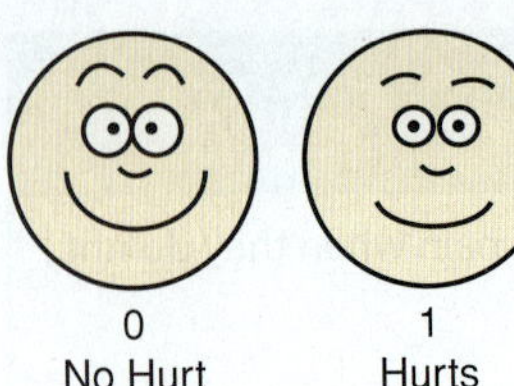
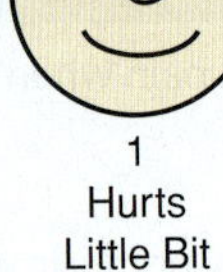
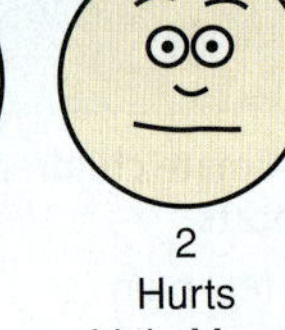

FIGURE 39.1 The Wong-Baker FACES pain rating scale. (Copyright 1983, Wong Baker FACES Foundation, www.WongBakerFACES.org. Used with permission. Originally published in Whaley & Wong's Nursing Care of Infants and Children. © Elsevier Inc.)

that can be used to rate pain: facial expression, leg movement, activity, cry and consolability. Because a child does not provide active input, older children may prefer a pain rating system in which they actively participate.

CRIES neonatal postoperative pain measurement scale

The CRIES inventory is a 10-point scale on which five physiological and behavioural variables frequently associated with neonatal pain can be assessed and rated (Krechel & Bildner, 1995):

- Amount and type of crying
- Need for oxygen administration
- Increased vital signs
- Facial expression
- Sleeplessness.

Each area is scored from 0 to 2 and then a total score is obtained (see Table 39.2). On the scale, infants with a score of 4 or more are most likely to be in pain and need interventions to reduce discomfort. The scale cannot be used with infants who are intubated or paralysed for ventilatory assistance because they would have no score for cry, and because their faces are obscured, it is difficult to rate them for facial expression.

The COMFORT behaviour scale

The COMFORT behaviour scale is a pain-rating scale devised by nurses to rate pain in very young infants (Boerlage et al., 2012; van Dijk et al., 2005). On the first part of the scale, six different categories (alertness, calmness/agitation, crying, physical movement, muscle tone and facial expression) are rated from 1 to 5. Six is the lowest score (no pain) and 30 is the highest (a great deal of pain). In addition to rating physical parameters, the infant is then observed for 2 minutes and the evaluation of the baby's pain is documented on an analogue (1-to-10) visual scale.

Wong-Baker FACES pain rating scale

The FACES pain-rating scale consists of six cartoon-like faces ranging from smiling to tearful (see Fig. 39.1). Explain to the child that each face from left to right corresponds to a person who has no hurt up to a lot of hurt (Wong & Baker, 1996). Use the words under each face to describe the amount of pain the face represents. Next, ask the child to choose the face that best describes the child's pain and record the number under the face the child chooses. Children as young as 3 years can effectively use this scale (Pagé et al., 2012).

Numerical or visual analogue scale

A numerical or visual analogue scale (see Fig. 39.2) uses a line with end points marked "0 no pain" on the left and "10 worst pain" on the right. Explain to children that the left end of the line (the 0) means a person feels no pain. At the other end is a 10, which means a person feels the worst pain possible. The numbers 1 to 9 in the middle are for "a little pain" to "a lot of pain". Ask children to choose a number that best describes their pain. As soon as they can count and have a concept of numbers, children can use a numerical scale. Be certain to show school-age children the scale; do not just say "score your pain from 0 to 10". Until children reach late

TABLE 39.2 CRIES neonatal postoperative pain measurement scale

	Infant's score		
Assessment	**0**	**1**	**2**
Crying	No	High-pitched	Inconsolable
Oxygen required for saturation above 95%	No	≤30%	>30%
Increased vital signs	Heart rate and blood pressure within 10% of preoperative value	Heart rate or blood pressure 11–20% higher than preoperative value	Heart rate or blood pressure 21% or more above preoperative value
Expression	None	Grimace	Grimace/grunt
Sleepless	No	Waking at frequent intervals	Constantly awake
Total infant score			

Source: Krechel, S. W. & Bildner, J. (1995). CRIES: A new neonatal postoperative pain management score. *Pediatric Anesthesia*, *5*(1), 53.

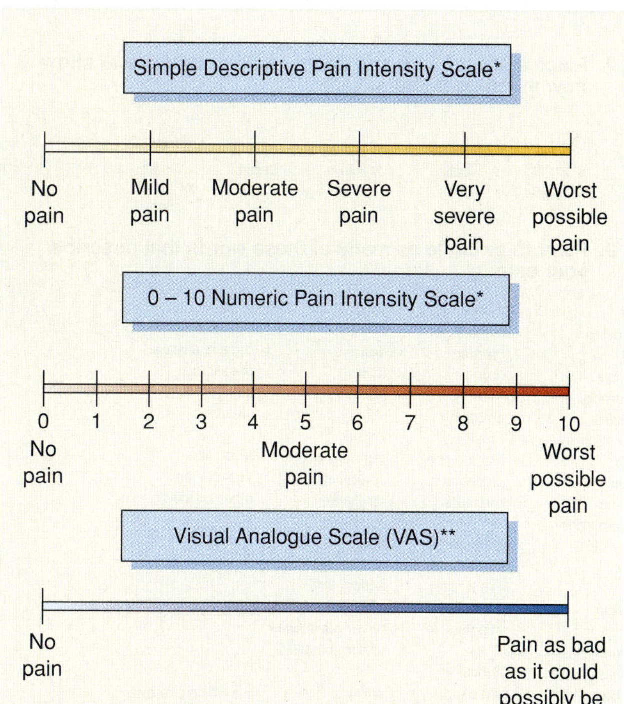

* If used as a graphic rating scale, a 10-cm baseline is recommended.
** A 10-cm baseline is recommended for VAS scales.

FIGURE 39.2 Numerical and visual analogue scales.

adolescence, they use concrete thought processes so need the help of seeing the line to rate their pain accurately.

Adolescent Paediatric Pain Tool

The Adolescent Paediatric Pain Tool (APPT) combines a visual activity and a numerical scale (Savedra et al., 1992). On one half of the form (see Fig. 39.3) is an outline figure showing the anterior and posterior view of a child. To use the tool, tell a child to colour in the figure drawing where pain is felt. In addition, on the right side of the form, tell the child to rate present pain in reference to "no pain", "little pain", "medium pain", "large pain" and "worst possible pain". For a third activity, tell children to point to or circle as many words as possible on the form that describe their pain (words such as horrible, pounding, cutting and stinging). The scale is suggested for use in children from 8 to 17 years. As many children below this level need so much help reading and interpreting the multitude of words that pain, it makes the form impractical below this age.

This is a useful tool for involving parents to talk with their child about pain. Reading the words together helps children examine the type, location and level of pain they are experiencing. It also helps parents to better understand what their child is experiencing.

Logs and diaries

Having children keep logs or diaries in which they note when pain occurs and then rate the pain each time it occurs is useful for assessing children with chronic but intermittent pain. Examining such a diary can not only reveal when pain occurs but also provide direction for pain management. For example, if the diary shows the child always awakens with pain in the morning, the child may need a longer-acting analgesic to take at bedtime.

PAIN MANAGEMENT

Pain management techniques vary greatly depending on the age of a child and the degree and type of pain a child is experiencing. Some healthcare agencies employ nurses specially trained in pain management to serve on an interdisciplinary team of healthcare providers, including doctors, anaesthetists, patient advocates and wound therapy nurses, to plan individual pain management programs for children (see Box 39.4).

BOX 39.4 ✻ Focus on evidence-based practice

Pain assessment

Pain assessment is recognised universally as one of the most common symptoms when caring for children. Assessing pain is also recognised as an essential nursing skill that, if implemented expertly, can avoid adverse effects.

A cross-sectional study of 82 paediatric nurses from all paediatric departments of a tertiary hospital in Israel examined in-hospital pain assessment methods nurses report using and assessed challenges, difficulties and barriers nurses report to assessing pain in hospitalised children. A self-report questionnaire was developed to examine how nurses assess children's in-hospital pain and barriers to in-hospital pain assessment. Nearly all nurses (90%) reported having enough knowledge to assess children's pain in the hospital, relying on child's self-report (86%) and being familiar with commonly used validated pain scales (90%). However, a majority (75%) reported not using pain scales recently and only half (58%) reported using an alternative method involving the child. Most nurses (86%) reported relying on their own overall impression of the child's pain and only a third (34%) reported involving the parents in their pain assessments. Nurses included comments stressing the importance of pain assessments and their frustration with the current validated measures available.

This study adds to a growing body of literature demonstrating a gap between recommended paediatric pain assessment guidelines and reported practice, with nurses showing a resistance to relying on single-item or unidimensional measures to assess and evaluate the rich and complex pain experience. A multidimensional approach involving child self-report, parent report and nurses' own overall impression based on clinical assessment skills of pain is discussed.

Based on these findings, would you try to change the attitude of healthcare providers towards pain management?

Source: Yaffa Zisk-Rony, R., Lev, J. & Havit, H. (2014). Nurses' report of in-hospital pediatric pain assessment: Examining challenges and perspectives. *Pain Management Nursing, 16*(2), 112–120.

CODE ____________

DATE ____________

Adolescent and Paediatric Pain Tool (APPT)

1. INSTRUCTIONS

Colour in the areas on these drawings to show where you have pain. Make the marks as big or as small as the place where the pain is.

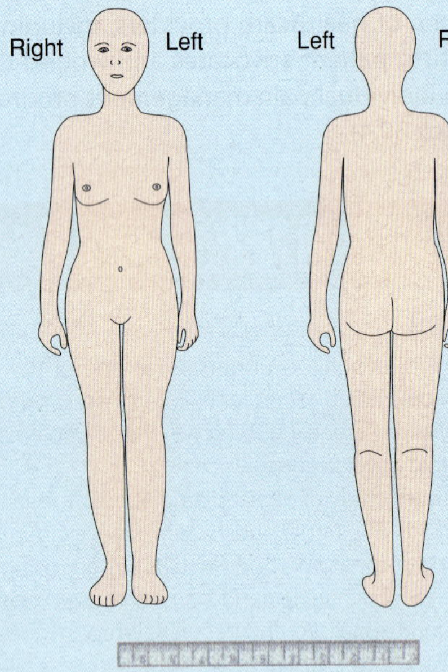

Right Left Left Right

2. Place a straight, up and down mark on this line to show how much pain you have.

No pain — Little pain — Medium pain — Large pain — Worst possible pain

3. Point to or circle as many of these words that describe your pain

1
annoying
bad
horrible
miserable
terrible
uncomfortable

2
aching
hurting
like an ache
like a hurt
sore

3
beating
hitting
pounding
punching
throbbing

4
biting
cutting
like a pin
like a sharp knife
pin like
sharp
stabbing

5
blistering
burning
hot

6
cramping
crushing
like a pinch
pinching
pressure

7
itching
like a scratch
like a sting
scratching
stinging

8
shocking
shooting
splitting

9
numb
stiff
swollen
tight

10
awful
deadly
dying
killing

11
crying
frightening
screaming
terrifying

12
dizzy
sickening
suffocating

13
never goes away
uncontrollable

14
always
comes and goes
comes on all of a sudden
constant
continuous
forever

15
off and on
once in a while
sneaks up
sometimes
steady

If you like you may add other words:

____

____

____

For office use only

BSA: ______
IS: ______

#S (2-9) ____/37= ____ %
#A (10-12) ____/11= ____ %
#E (1,13) ____/8= ____ %
#T (14,15) ____/11= ____ %

Total ____/67= ____ %

FIGURE 39.3 Adolescent Paediatric Pain Tool (APPT). (From Savedra, M. C., Tesler, M. D., Holzemer, W. L., et al., [1992]. *Adolescent Pediatric Pain Tool: User's Manual.* San Francisco, CA: University of California/San Francisco.)

Children with chronic pain or pain not relieved with standard approaches may benefit from a referral to a pain management specialist or team. Relief of frequent pain episodes or prolonged pain may require intense, consistent assessment and intervention, which is difficult to achieve in an acute care setting or during infrequent medical visits. Whatever assessment tools or methods of pain relief are used, staff should become familiar and comfortable with their use. It is important that pain be assessed in an organised and consistent manner so relief and interventions do not vary based on the healthcare provider.

In the past, children were frequently not prescribed potent analgesics because of the fear that the opioids commonly used, such as morphine, would decrease their respiratory rate to an unsafe level. Children who had adequate analgesia prescribed may not have received it because a nurse was overly concerned about causing respiratory distress. Today, it is recognised that if the dosage of an opioid such as morphine is based on the child's size, there is no more danger of respiratory depression in children than in adults. Therefore, after checking that the correct dosage has been prescribed, opioids can be given with confidence to decrease pain without untoward effects. To give nurses more leeway in pain management, it is helpful if a range is given for a dose, rather than a set number so the dose can be adjusted based on the degree of pain (Pasero, Manworren & McCaffery, 2007).

Healthcare professionals such as laboratory technicians, doctors and x-ray or endoscopy assistants are often called on to perform procedures that could cause a child pain. Assist these individuals to schedule procedures at times when a child can be administered optimal pain relief and help them institute non-pharmacological measures of pain management such as distraction (Riddell et al., 2012).

NON-PHARMACOLOGICAL PAIN MANAGEMENT

Non-pharmacological pain relief measures can be used independently or as complements to pharmacological

BOX 39.5 * Focus on family teaching

Pain management with children

Q. Mrs Johnson asks you, "How can I be sure I can keep my daughter free from pain after she returns home from the hospital?"

A. Here are some ways to offer pain relief in addition to just giving medicine:

- Let your child know it is important to you to try to take the pain away and you will work with her to relieve it. Use a positive approach: "This medicine will take away your pain" not "Take this and let's hope it works".
- Administer pain medication before pain becomes intense to help prevent pain rather than just relieve it. If your child is in hospital, inform the staff if a particular approach works or does not work.
- Never just give an analgesic. Make your child comfortable in ways such as straightening the sheets or offering a backrub.
- Ask your child about measures she thinks will be helpful, such as an additional pillow, the television turned on, a favourite toy nearby.
- Help your child talk about and describe the pain she is experiencing. This can help make it more concrete and not as psychologically frightening.
- Relieve anxiety about other phases of life, if possible. Relaxation reduces muscle strain and tension that add to pain.
- Offer emotional support to your child. Pain never seems as bad when a support person is present. Reassuring your child that she is loved and that you will be there for her can be very comforting.
- Try not to use such statements as, "Be a big girl" or "Stop crying" when a child is in pain from a procedure such as an injection. Say instead, "It's all right to cry. I know it hurts" to avoid shaming a child who cannot stop crying.

pain relief (see Box 39.5). They fit under the umbrella of complementary and alternative therapies.

Distraction

Distraction techniques aim at shifting a child's focus from pain to another activity or interest (see Fig. 39.4). Blowing soap bubbles, for example, could be used during an injection to accomplish this. If oral glucose is offered to infants during painful procedures, the pain they experience appears to be significantly less (Kassab et al., 2011). It is hypothesised that drinking glucose not only serves as a distraction technique but also activates endorphins and produces a central analgesic effect (Harrison, Beggs & Stevens, 2012). When helping parents teach a distraction technique such as blowing soap bubbles to their child, be certain they do not interpret "distraction" as just talking to the child or suggesting a video game to divert attention. Although these are distractions, simple distraction can help the child focus more on the play activity, rather than the clinical procedure.

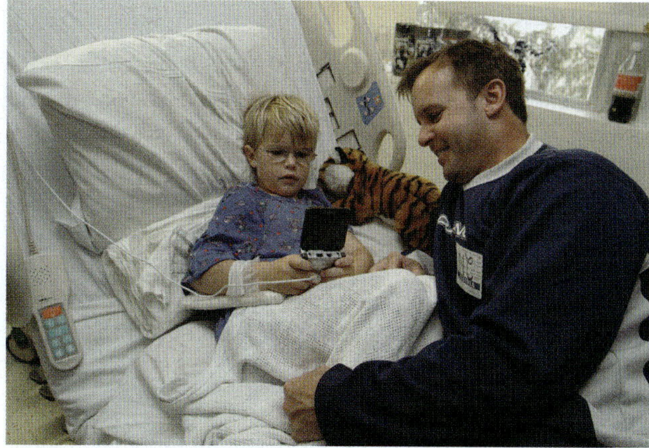

FIGURE 39.4 Distraction with electronic games and parental presence may help reduce pain perception. (Bowden, V. & Greenberg, C. S. (2013). *Bowden: Children and Their Families*. Philadelphia: Lippincott Williams & Wilkins.)

Guided imagery

Guided imagery is a distraction technique to help a child place another meaning (a non-painful one) on a painful procedure (Kline et al., 2010). Children are often more adept at imagery than adults because their imagination is less inhibited. Success with this technique requires practice, so it has limited application in an acute care setting. This technique works well with quick, simple procedures such as venepunctures or chronic pain. A venepuncture, for example, could be viewed as a silver rocket probing the moon to transport specimens back to Earth. Be certain a child thinks of a specific image. Help them elaborate on the image to make it more concrete each time it is used so their mind stays on the image (What colour is the rocket ship? Are there stripes on the sides? What does the pilot look like?).

Aromatherapy and essential oils

Aromatherapy is based on the principle that the sense of smell plays a significant role in overall health. When an essential oil is inhaled, its molecules are transported via the olfactory system to the limbic system in the brain. The brain responds to particular aromas with emotional responses. When applied externally, the oils are absorbed by the skin and then carried throughout the body. Essential oils may be able to penetrate cell walls and transport nutrients or oxygen to the inside of cells. Jasmine and lavender are oils thought to be responsible for relieving pain (Miller, Jacob & Hockenberry, 2011).

Music therapy

Music therapy is the use of music for calming or improving wellbeing and can be effective even for premature infants. It can help to relieve pain both because it can be relaxing and is a distraction (Nguyen et al., 2010). Children may "blast" music, not because they enjoy hearing it that loud, but because they are feeling great pain and need that level of distraction to feel free of pain.

Acupuncture

Acupuncture involves the insertion of needles into critical positions (meridian lines) in the body to achieve pain relief (Chiou & Nurko, 2010). Although acupuncture is almost painless, children can be very afraid of it at first because of the sight of the needles. This level of stress can make it an unattractive option for pain management for children. Children who consent to either technique, however, particularly those with chronic pain, report that the overall process is pleasant and the method offers relief from stress (Das, Nayak & Margaret, 2011).

Herbal therapies

Parents may believe that specific herbs are helpful in relieving pain for their child. Some examples include chamomile tea (inflammation reduction), garlic (anti-inflammatory, anticancer), ginger (nausea or vomiting reduction), goldenrod (urinary tract inflammation reduction) or peppermint (abdominal pain relief) (Hunt & Ernst, 2011). Always ask when taking health histories if a child is being given any herbs, both to be informed about common herbs and to be certain that what the child is receiving will complement, not interfere with, the effects of any pain medication.

Therapeutic touch

Therapeutic touch is the use of touch to provide comfort and relieve pain (Hall, 2012). It is based on the concept that the body contains energy fields. When these are plentiful, they lead to health, but when they are in lesser supply, ill health results. Proponents believe it is possible to redirect energy fields to increase the release of endorphins. Therapeutic touch may also be effective as it serves as a form of distraction.

Transcutaneous electrical nerve stimulation (TENS)

Transcutaneous electrical nerve stimulation (TENS) involves applying small electrodes to the dermatomes that supply the body portion where pain is experienced (Ali et al., 2010). When children sense pain, they push a button on a control box, which then delivers a small electrical current to the skin. The principle underlying this technique is the same as rubbing an injured part: the current interferes with the transmission of the pain impulse across small nerve fibres.

Some children (and parents) dislike TENS therapy because they are nervous about the electrical current. Assure them the current is a very mild one and will not harm their child. TENS is not recommended if the child is incontinent or has a wound that is likely to cause the electrodes to get wet.

Heat or cold application

Cold reduces pain by constricting capillaries and therefore reducing vessel permeability and oedema and pressure at an injured site. After the first 24 hours of an injury, applying heat may be more helpful because this dilates capillaries, increases blood flow to the area and again helps reduce oedema.

CASE STUDY QUESTION

3. You teach Amy imaging to help reduce pain. Why does a technique such as imagery work well for children?
   a. Children's pain is not as acute as is adults' pain
   b. Intravenous pain relief is not effective in children
   c. Children's imaginations are at their peak
   d. Children's muscles are less tense than adults' muscles

PHARMACOLOGICAL PAIN RELIEF

Pharmacological pain relief refers to the administration of a variety of analgesic medications. Many children need analgesic agents in addition to non-pharmacological techniques for pain relief, especially for acute pain. Medications can be applied topically, inhaled or given orally, intravenously, or by epidural injection. Intramuscular injections should be avoided because some children fear injections. Be certain children understand it is acceptable to ask for medication for pain; they may not know they can unless this is stressed by healthcare providers.

Topical anaesthetic cream

To reduce the pain of procedures such as venepuncture, lumbar puncture and bone marrow aspiration, a local anaesthetic cream that contains 4% lignocaine can be used (Jorge, Feres & Teles, 2011; Poonai et al., 2012). The cream is applied to the skin and the site is then covered with an occlusive dressing (see Fig. 39.5). To be most effective, it must be applied at least 1 hour before an expected procedure

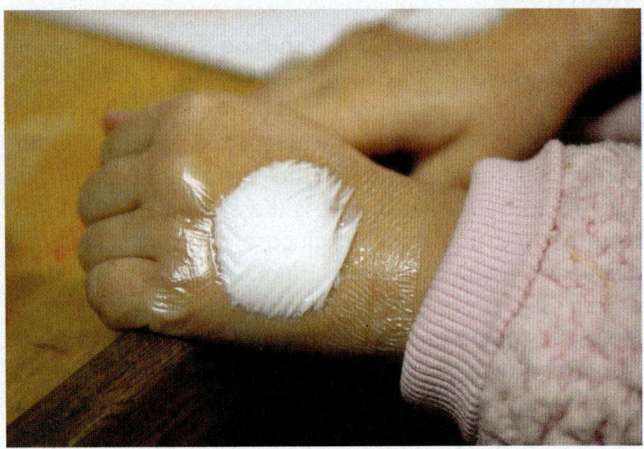

FIGURE 39.5 The local anaesthetic cream can be applied to a child's hand and held in place with a transparent dressing at home prior to surgery. (© Sheldon Levis/Alamy.)

BOX 39.6 ✻ Focus on pharmacology

EMLA cream

Classification: EMLA (an eutectic mixture of local anaesthetics) is a topical analgesic cream containing lignocaine and prilocaine.

Action: Acts to anaesthetise skin before potentially painful procedures (McKenna & Mirkov, 2014).

Pregnancy risk category: B

Dosage: Dollop of cream to intended skin site for at least 1 hour before procedure (2–3 hours before deeper procedures such as lumbar puncture or bone marrow aspiration)

Possible adverse effects: Hypersensitivity

Nursing implications

- Explain to the child that the cream will help prevent pain during a procedure.
- Apply a dollop of cream to the intended site and cover with a transparent occlusive dressing at least 1 hour before the procedure. Do not spread cream or rub it in.
- If the cream is to be applied at home, instruct the parents how to apply the cream and the occlusive dressing. Suggest that the parents use plastic wrap for the occlusive dressing.
- Instruct the child not to touch the dressing while it is in place. If necessary, cover the occlusive dressing with an opaque material to prevent the child from touching or playing with the dressing.
- Just before the procedure, remove the dressing and then wipe the skin to remove the cream.
- Observe the skin. Look for reddened or blanched skin, which indicates that the medication has penetrated the skin.
- Do not use the medication for a child with a known history of sensitivity or allergy to local anaesthetics such as lignocaine.
- The medication is not approved for use in infants younger than 1 month.

(see Box 39.6). Parents can apply anaesthetic cream at home before bringing a child to hospital for a procedure such as bone marrow aspiration. Caution them not to allow their child to remove the dressing and eat the cream (it could anaesthetise the gag reflex). It also is potentially dangerous if rubbed into the eyes.

What if…

Amy is scheduled to have blood taken at 10 a.m. so you apply an anaesthetic cream at 9 a.m.? However, the blood collector arrives early. Would you ask the blood collector to wait or explain to Amy the cream is not going to work?

Oral analgesia

Oral analgesia is advantageous because it is cost-effective and relatively easy to administer. Many analgesics can be prepared as elixirs or suppositories for children unable to swallow pills. Analgesia can be adequately achieved if dosing is correct.

Over-the-counter analgesics, such as paracetamol (Panadol), are flavoured to make them more palatable. Reinforce with parents the need for proper storage (locked away or out of the child's reach). Toxicity from too-frequent or overly large doses of paracetamol can lead to severe liver damage in children (McKenna & Mirkov, 2014).

Non-steroidal anti-inflammatory drugs (NSAIDs) are excellent for reducing the pain that accompanies inflammation in injuries such as sprained ankles or rheumatic conditions. However, long-term administration of any NSAID can lead to severe gastric irritation and may be associated with adverse cardiac effects, so they should not be used longer than prescribed. Help parents, who are giving any analgesia around the clock for several days, to make out a medication sheet to hang on their refrigerator door. This reminds them when the next dose is due and alerts them not to give the doses too close together.

For managing severe or acute pain, such as postoperative pain or the pain of a sickle-cell crisis, opioids (such as morphine and codeine), are the drugs of choice. Preparations often include paracetamol due to its opioid-sparing effects.

Intravenous (IV) administration

Intravenous (IV) administration is the most rapid-acting and preferred route in emergency situations in the child with acute pain and in a child requiring frequent doses of analgesia but in whom the gastrointestinal tract cannot be used. Common opioids given by this route include morphine and fentanyl. Fentanyl has a shorter duration of action than morphine. Side effects of pruritus and vasodilation are less, making it an ideal drug to use for short, painful procedures such as debriding a wound.

These analgesics can be given by bolus injection or by continuous infusion. If doses will be given periodically by an IV line, advocate for the use of an intermittent infusion device to avoid repeated venepunctures with each dose or the need for a confining IV line to be in place.

If a child's pain is frequent or constant, continuous IV administration may be necessary to reduce the level of pain. As the child becomes able to take medications by mouth, oral forms of analgesics are then administered. When switching from IV to oral medications it is important to use equianalgesic doses. As-needed (Pro Re Nata) dosing should be avoided because it leads to inconsistent administration.

All opioids have the potential to decrease respiratory rate, although this is reduced with accurate dosing. Other side effects include nausea, pruritus, vasodilation, cough suppression and constipation. If toxicity with opioids should occur, naloxone (Narcan) can be administered to counteract the effects.

CASE STUDY QUESTION

4. Amy was given analgesia intravenously. Why is the intramuscular route infrequently used to administer analgesia to children?
   a. The average child has a fear of injections
   b. Intramuscular doses must be larger in children than in adults
   c. Intramuscular medications must be administered cold or chilled
   d. Intramuscular solutions are readily confused with IV solutions

Patient-controlled analgesia

Patient-controlled analgesia (PCA) is a form of IV administration that allows a child to self-administer boluses of medication, usually opioids, with a medication pump (see also Chapter 24). Children as young as 5 or 6 years may be able to assess when they need a bolus of medicine and press the button on the pump to deliver the new dose through an established IV line. Morphine is a common analgesic used for PCA administration (Anghelescu et al., 2012). The pump is set with a lock-out time so that after each dose the pump will not release further medication even if the button is pushed again; so that children cannot over medicate themselves. If pain is constant, a background infusion should be used so that pain relief continues even while the child sleeps. The pump can still be programmed for bolus dosing to cover episodes of increased pain.

Intranasal administration

Intranasal administration is becoming a preferred way to dispense medicine for children. Midazolam (Hypnovel) is a short-acting adjuvant sedative that can be administered intranasally by nasal drops or nasal spray before surgery or procedures such as nuclear medicine scanning (McKenna & Mirkov, 2014). Because it has a very short duration of action, it may require repeat administration. As midazolam has no analgesic action, additional analgesia, such as morphine, should also be used if the procedure will be painful.

Local anaesthesia injection

Local anaesthetics stop pain transmission by blocking nerve conduction of the impulse at the site of pain. Children receive local anaesthetic injections, such as lignocaine, before procedures such as bone marrow aspiration and peritoneal dialysis. The use of an anaesthetic cream before the injection relieves the needle-stick pain and allows the anaesthetic to numb the deeper tissues to prevent pain (Crowley et al., 2011).

Epidural analgesia

Epidural analgesia, injection of an analgesic agent into the epidural space, can be used to provide analgesia to the lower body for 12 to 24 hours. An opioid, often combined with a long-acting anaesthetic, is instilled continuously or administered intermittently. Children who have orthopaedic or chest surgery, for example, may have an epidural catheter inserted in the operating room and continue to receive analgesia by this method to relieve post-surgical pain (Wu & Raja, 2011). This is a very effective route of analgesia in the postoperative child in the first few days.

ONGOING PAIN RELIEF

Be certain children who begin a pain management program in a healthcare setting are provided with support and follow-up pain management to the extent necessary when they return home. Early discharge and the increased use of outpatient services necessitate adequate pain management in the home setting.

Either oral or IV analgesia may be needed, so be certain parents have instructions on dosing, administration, frequency, expected outcomes and expected level of relief. Provide them with the name and telephone number of a healthcare professional whom they can call if they have questions about pain management (Johnston et al., 2011).

CASE STUDY QUESTION

5. Amy is scheduled for conscious sedation to have her repeat bone marrow aspiration. Which would be the best explanation to prepare her for this?
   a. "You'll be given a special medicine to put you to sleep for surgery."
   b. "I'll give you some medicine, but you'll still be awake and feel pain."
   c. "Conscious sedation is an analgesic, not anaesthetic, method of pain relief."
   d. "I'll give you medicine so you're very sleepy but can still talk to me."

Key points for review

- Children and infants are often under-medicated for pain because of common misconceptions of healthcare personnel.
- Inviting parents and the child, if preschool age or older, to participate in assessment and pain management is an important aspect of pain therapy.
- Pain in children is best assessed by means of a standardised self-report tool such as the Wong-Baker FACES tool or numerical analogue scale. Without self-report forms, both nurses and parents may underestimate children's pain.
- Children will benefit from a combination of non-pharmacological and pharmacological methods of pain management.
- Few analgesics are administered intramuscularly to children. Instead, IV administration is the method of

choice for the child with acute pain. Patient-controlled analgesia, commonly used to administer morphine, can be used effectively with children.

CASE STUDY QUESTIONS

6. Amy was given IV morphine in surgery 1 hour ago for a bone marrow aspiration. Her mother asks you now if Amy can have some more, not because her pain has returned, but because the mother wants it given before any pain comes back. Is this mother's assessment or Amy's assessment of her pain likely to be most accurate? Would anticipating pain in this way be the best intervention for Amy?
7. Amy is prescribed an intravascular antibiotic twice daily. She always screams the second she sees the syringe even though the addition of the medicine to her IV line should cause minimal pain. What type of pain management should be used? How should the child's anxiety be addressed?
8. A fellow nurse tells you that she does not use self-report tools with children; she feels they take the place of her nursing judgment. You like to use rating scales. How would you justify your view? What are the pros and cons of pain assessment tools?
9. What would be a possible research topic that would be applicable to Amy's family and would also advance evidence-based practice?

Resources

For an extensive range of additional resources to enhance teaching and learning and to facilitate understanding of this chapter, please see the text's accompanying website located on thePoint at http://thepoint.lww.com.

References

Ali, S., Drendel, A. L., Kircher, J., et al. (2010). Pain management of musculoskeletal injuries in children: Current state and future directions. *Pediatric Emergency Care, 26*(7), 518–524.

Anghelescu, D. L., Faughnan, L. G., Oakes, L. L., et al. (2012). Parent controlled PCA for pain management in pediatric oncology: Is it safe? *Journal of Pediatric Hematology/Oncology, 34*(6), 416–420.

Boerlage, A. A., Ista, E., de Jong, M., et al. (2012). The COMFORT behavior scale: Is a shorter observation period feasible? *Pediatric Critical Care Medicine, 13*(2), e124–e125.

Chiou, E. & Nurko, S. (2010). Management of functional abdominal pain and irritable bowel syndrome in children and adolescents. *Expert Review of Gastroenterology & Hepatology, 4*(3), 293–304.

Crowley, M. A., Storer, A., Heaton, K., et al. (2011). Emergency nursing resource: Needle-related procedural pain in pediatric patients in the emergency department. *Journal of Emergency Nursing, 37*(3), 246–251.

Das, R., Nayak, B. S. & Margaret, B. (2011). Acupressure and physical stress among high school students. *Holistic Nursing Practice, 25*(2), 97–104.

Downey, L. V. & Zun, L. S. (2012). The impact of watching cartoons for distraction during painful procedures in the emergency department. *Pediatric Emergency Care, 28*(10), 1033–1035.

Fanning, J. J., Stucke, A. G., Christensen, M. A., et al. (2012). Perioperative opiate requirements in children with previous opiate infusion. *Paediatric Anaesthesia, 22*(3), 203–208.

Hall, R. W. (2012). Anesthesia and analgesia in the NICU. *Clinical Perinatology, 39*(1), 239–254.

Harrison, D., Beggs, S. & Stevens, B. (2012). Sucrose for procedural pain management in infants. *Pediatrics, 130*(5), 918–925.

Harrison, D., Elia, S., Royle, J., et al. (2013). Pain management strategies used during early childhood immunisation in Victoria. *Journal of Paediatric Child Health, 49*(4), 313–318.

Hester, N. O. & Barcus, C. S. (1986). Assessment and management of pain in children. *Pediatrics: Nursing Update, 1*(14), 2–6.

Hunt, K. & Ernst, E. (2011). The evidence-base for complementary medicine in children: A critical overview of systematic reviews. *Archives of Disease in Childhood, 96*(8), 769–776.

Johnston, C., Barrington, K. J., Taddio, A., et al. (2011). Pain in Canadian NICUs: Have we improved over the past 12 years? *Clinical Journal of Pain, 27*(3), 225–232.

Jorge, L. L., Feres, C. C. & Teles, V.E.P. (2011). Topical preparations for pain relief: Efficacy and patient adherence. *Journal of Pain Research, 20*(4), 11–24.

Kassab, M., Sheehy, A., King, M., et al. (2011). A double-blind randomized controlled trial of 25% oral glucose for pain relief in 2-month old infants undergoing immunization. *International Journal of Nursing Studies, 49*(3), 249–256.

Kline, W. H., Turnbull, A., LaBruna, V. E., et al. (2010). Enhancing pain management in the PICU by teaching guided mental imagery: A quality improvement project. *Journal of Pediatric Psychology, 35*(1), 25–31.

Krechel, S. W. & Bildner, J. (1995). CRIES: A new neonatal postoperative pain measurement score. *Paediatric Anesthesia, 5*(1), 53–57.

McKenna, L. & Mirkov, S. (2014). *McKenna's Drug Handbook for Nursing & Midwifery* (7th ed.). Sydney: Lippincott Williams & Wilkins.

Merkel, S., Voepel-Lewis, T. & Malviya, S. (2002). Pain assessment in infants and young children: The FLACC scale. *American Journal of Nursing, 102*(10), 55–58.

Miller, E., Jacob, E. & Hockenberry, M. J. (2011). Nausea, pain, fatigue, and multiple symptoms in hospitalized children with cancer. *Oncology Nursing Forum, 38*(5), e382–e393.

Nguyen, T. N., Nilsson, S., Hellstrom, A., et al. (2010). Music therapy to reduce pain and anxiety in children with cancer undergoing lumbar puncture: A randomized clinical trial. *Journal of Pediatric Oncology Nursing, 27*(3), 146–155.

Pagé, M. G., Katz, J., Stinson, J., et al. (2012). Validation of the numerical rating scale for pain intensity and unpleasantness in pediatric acute postoperative pain: Sensitivity to change over time. *Journal of Pain, 13*(4), 359–369.

Pasero, C., Manworren, R. C. B. & McCaffery, M. (2007). Pain control: IV opioid range orders for acute pain management. *American Journal of Nursing, 107*(2), 52–60.

Pasero, C. & McCaffery, M. (2004). Comfort-function goals: A way to establish accountability for pain relief. *American Journal of Nursing, 104*(9), 77–81.

Poonai, N., Alawi, K., Rieder, M., et al. (2012). A comparison of amethocaine and liposomal lidocaine cream as a pain reliever before venipuncture in children: A randomized control trial. *Pediatric Emergency Care, 28*(2), 104–108.

Riddell, P., Racine, N. M., Turcotte, K., et al. (2012). Non-pharmacological management of infant and young child procedural pain. *Evidence-Based Child Health: A Cochrane Review Journal, 7*(6), 1905–2121.

Savedra, M. C., Tesler, M. D., Holzemer, W. L., et al. (1992). *Adolescent Pediatric Pain Tool: User's Manual.* San Francisco, CA: University of California/San Francisco.

Schiavenato, M., Butler-O'Hare, M. & Scovanner, P. (2011). Exploring the association between pain intensity and facial display in term newborns. *Pain Research and Management, 16*(1), 10–12.

van Dijk, M., Peters, J. W., van Deventer, P., et al. (2005). The COMFORT Behavior Scale: A tool for assessing pain and sedation in infants. *American Journal of Nursing, 105*(1), 33–36.

Vervoort, T., Eccleston, C., Goubert, L., et al. (2010). Children's catastrophic thinking about their pain predicts pain and disability 6 months later. *European Journal of Pain, 14*(1), 90–96.

Wong, D. & Baker, C. (1996). *Reference Manual for the Wong-Baker FACES Pain Rating Scale.* Duarte, CA: CHNMC.

Wu, C. L. & Raja, S. N. (2011). Treatment of acute postoperative pain. *Lancet, 377*(9784), 2215–2225.

Yaffa Zisk-Rony, R., Lev, J. & Havit, H. (2014). Nurses' report of in-hospital pediatric pain assessment: Examining challenges and perspectives. *Pain Management Nursing, 16*(2), 112–120.

Suggested readings

Carter, B. & Ford, K. (2013). Researching children's health experiences: The place for participatory, child-centred, arts-based approaches. *Research in Nursing and Health, 36*(1), 95–107.

He, H., Lee, T., Jaha, R., et al. (2011). The use of non-pharmacological methods for children's postoperative pain relief: Singapore nurses' perspective. *Journal for Specialists in Pediatric Nursing, 16*(1), 27–38.

Landier, W. & Tse, A. M. (2010). Use of complementary and alternative medical interventions for the management of procedure-related pain, anxiety, and distress in pediatric oncology: An integrative review. *Journal of Pediatric Nursing, 25*(6), 566–579.

Selimen, D. & Andsoy, I. I. (2011). The importance of a holistic approach during the perioperative period. *Association of Operating Room Nurses Journal, 93*(4), 482–490.

Starship Children's Health. (2015). Starship clinical guidelines, accessed 22 April 2015, <www.starship.org.nz/for-health-professionals/starship-clinical-guidelines>.

The Royal Children's Hospital Melbourne. (2011). Procedural pain management, accessed 22 April 2015, <www.rch.org.au/rchcpg/hospital_clinical_guideline_index/Procedural_Pain_Management/>.

The Sydney Children's Hospital Network. (2014). Pain research unit at Sydney Children's Hospital, Randwick, accessed 22 April 2015, <www.schn.health.nsw.gov.au/parents-and-carers/our-services/pain-medicine/sch-0>.

Unit 7

The nursing role in restoring and maintaining the health of children and families with physiological disorders

Chapter 40

Nursing care of a family when a child has a respiratory disorder

LEARNING OBJECTIVES

After mastering the contents of this chapter, you should be able to:

1. Describe common respiratory disorders in children.
2. Use critical thinking to analyse ways nursing care for a child with a respiratory disorder could be more family-centred.
3. Undertake a nursing assessment on a child with a respiratory disorder.
4. Identify nursing considerations related to respiratory disorders in children.
5. Identify expected outcomes that address the priority needs of a child with a respiratory disorder.
6. Plan nursing care for a child with a respiratory disorder.
7. Implement nursing care for a child with a respiratory disorder such as administering oxygen.
8. Evaluate expected outcomes for achievement and effectiveness of care.
9. Identify areas related to care of children with respiratory disorders that could benefit from additional nursing research or application of evidence-based practice.
10. Integrate knowledge of respiratory disorders in children with nursing process to achieve quality child and family health nursing care.

KEY TERMS

- adventitious sounds
- anoxia
- aspiration
- atelectasis
- crackles
- cyanosis
- hypoxia
- paroxysmal coughing
- pneumothorax
- retractions
- steatorrhoea
- stridor
- tachypnoea
- tracheostomy
- tracheotomy
- wheezing

CASE STUDY

Michael is a 4-year-old who is brought to the emergency department by paramedics after responding to an emergency call from his grandmother at his home. He has a sharp, barking cough, is crying loudly and is obviously short of breath. "He can't breathe!" his grandmother shouts at you. "I gave him some chocolate. Is he allergic to that?" his grandmother asks. Michael is diagnosed as having laryngotracheobronchitis (croup) and admitted to the paediatric ward.

CASE STUDY QUESTIONS

1. What emergency care does Michael need?
2. What about Michael's action would lead you to believe his airway is not yet completely obstructed?

Respiratory disorders are among the most common causes of illness and hospitalisation in children. Overall, respiratory dysfunction in children tends to be more serious than in adults because the lumens of a child's respiratory tract are smaller and therefore more likely to become obstructed.

Respiratory disorders range from minor illnesses to life-threatening lower respiratory tract diseases. Because the level of acuity can change quickly, respiratory disorders are often difficult for parents to evaluate. Both a child and parents need a great deal of nursing support when disease interferes with the function of breathing because even very young children can panic when breathing becomes laboured. Early diagnosis and treatment are essential in preventing a minor problem from turning into a more serious one (Southern et al., 2009).

CARING FOR A CHILD WITH A RESPIRATORY DISORDER

Assessment

Respiratory illness can begin as early as moments after birth if a newborn has difficulty initiating a first breath or establishing regular respirations. Rating a newborn using an Apgar score can help to quickly identify a newborn who may be experiencing respiratory difficulty at this early stage.

As a nurse you are often the first healthcare provider to talk to a parent about a child's respiratory illness. It is important to establish both the onset and duration of the problem so that its seriousness can be rapidly determined. A child admitted to hospital with a respiratory disorder is usually in an acute stage of the illness. Nursing assessment that a child is developing tachypnoea or retractions may be the first indication of a child's worsening condition.

Nursing considerations

Nursing considerations established for children with respiratory disorders focus both on the alteration in mechanisms of breathing and on the emotional distress such problems can create. "Ineffective airway clearance" is a common diagnostic category used in this area. The problem may be related to any one of a variety of factors, such as ineffective cough, fatigue, weakness, viscous secretions, pain, aspiration (inhalation of a foreign object into the airway), or lack of knowledge about the importance of coughing.

The terms "impaired gas exchange" and "ineffective breathing pattern" may also be used, although because a nurse does not generally prescribe definitive treatment for these problems (except when caused by hyperventilation), it may be more appropriate for nursing considerations to focus on the effects of impaired gas exchange or ineffective breathing on daily activities and psychosocial health. Examples of nursing considerations are:

- Activity intolerance related to insufficient oxygenation
- Fatigue related to impaired gas exchange
- Fear related to inability to breathe without effort
- Impaired social interaction related to difficulty in keeping up with physical activities of peers
- Deficient knowledge related to need for continued treatment.

If a child is experiencing an acute respiratory problem, the expected outcomes and plan of care will focus on supporting the child and family through prescribed therapy and keeping parents informed about their child's health status and response to treatment. Helping parents to plan programs of exercise and teaching chest physiotherapy as well as the actions of prescribed medications are some of the related nursing activities.

Collaborative nursing interventions in the care of a child with respiratory dysfunction include suctioning to remove respiratory secretions, administering oxygen and providing humidification and expectorant therapy to help maintain clear airways. Some of the most important nursing interventions in this area are independent nursing functions: placing a child in an upright position to help the child cough more effectively; providing an interesting game to teach a child the importance of strengthening chest muscles; supporting a child and family through the anxiety created when a child is not breathing normally; and teaching parents of a child with chronic respiratory dysfunction the basics of percussion or chest physiotherapy techniques. All of these interventions require sound nursing judgement and skill to carry out or teach effectively.

An acute respiratory illness can be extremely frightening for parents as well as the child. After the child has recovered, talk with the parents to determine whether they have come to terms with their fear and can treat the child as a well child again. Otherwise, over protection of a child by the parents may result in a well but dependent child. This pattern is one that nursing evaluation can help to prevent.

Expected outcomes for a child with chronic respiratory disease will change as a child grows and develops. No matter what the specific concerns are, however, evaluation should always include examination of how well a child individually and the family as a whole have adapted to managing the limitations imposed by the disorder while maintaining a lifestyle that fosters growth and development for all family members.

RESPIRATORY TRACT DIFFERENCES IN CHILDREN

The respiratory tract grows and changes until the child is about 12 years of age. During the first 5 years, the child's airway increases in length but not in diameter. Infants and young children have larger tongues in proportion to their mouths, shorter necks, narrower airways and the structures are closer together. This leads to the possibility of respiratory obstruction, especially if there is oedema, swelling or increased mucus in the airways. The ability to breathe through the mouth when the nose is blocked is not automatic but develops as the child's neurological development increases. The tonsillar tissue is enlarged in the early school-aged child, but the pharynx, which contains the tonsils, is still small, so the possibility of obstruction of the upper airway is more likely.

Embryological development of the respiratory tract is discussed in Chapter 9. Because the respiratory tract continues to mature during childhood, children have several important differences in respiratory anatomy and physiology than adults. The ethmoidal and maxillary sinuses are present at birth; the frontal sinuses (the sinuses most frequently involved in sinus infection) and the sphenoidal sinuses do not develop until 6 to 8 years of age. Due to rapid growth of lymphoid tissue, tonsillar tissue is normally enlarged in early school-aged children.

Respiratory mucus functions as a cleaning agent by moving invading organisms or other particles out of the lungs. However, newborns produce little respiratory mucus, which makes them more susceptible to respiratory infection than older children. Excessive production of mucus in children up to 2 years of age can actually lead to obstruction because the bronchial lumens are so small in children of this age.

After 2 years of age, the right bronchus is noticeably shorter, wider and more vertical than the left. This is the reason that inhaled foreign bodies most often lodge in the right bronchus. Infants' chest muscles are not fully developed so they use their abdominal muscles to assist in inhalation. The change to thoracic breathing begins at 2 to 3 years of age and is complete at 7 years. Because accessory muscles are used more in children than in adults, weakness of these muscles from disease may more easily result in respiratory failure in children than in adults (Hatfield, 2013).

In infants, the walls of the airways have less cartilage than in older children and adults and so are not as strong and more likely to collapse after expiration. An advantage of immature development is that a lessened amount of smooth muscle in the airway means an infant does not develop bronchospasm as readily as an older child or adult. Therefore, **wheezing** (the sound of air being pushed through constricted bronchioles) may not be a prominent finding in infants even when the lumen of the airway is severely compromised and hence an important point to consider in the assessment of young children.

BOX 40.1 Assessment ❋ Assessing a child for signs and symptoms of respiratory dysfunction

History

Chief concern: Cough, rapid respirations, noisy breathing, rhinitis, reddened sore throat, lethargy, cyanosis, difficulty sucking, fever.

Past medical history: Poor weight gain, difficulty with respirations at birth, prematurity.

Family history: History of family member with asthma; other family members with respiratory infection.

Physical examination

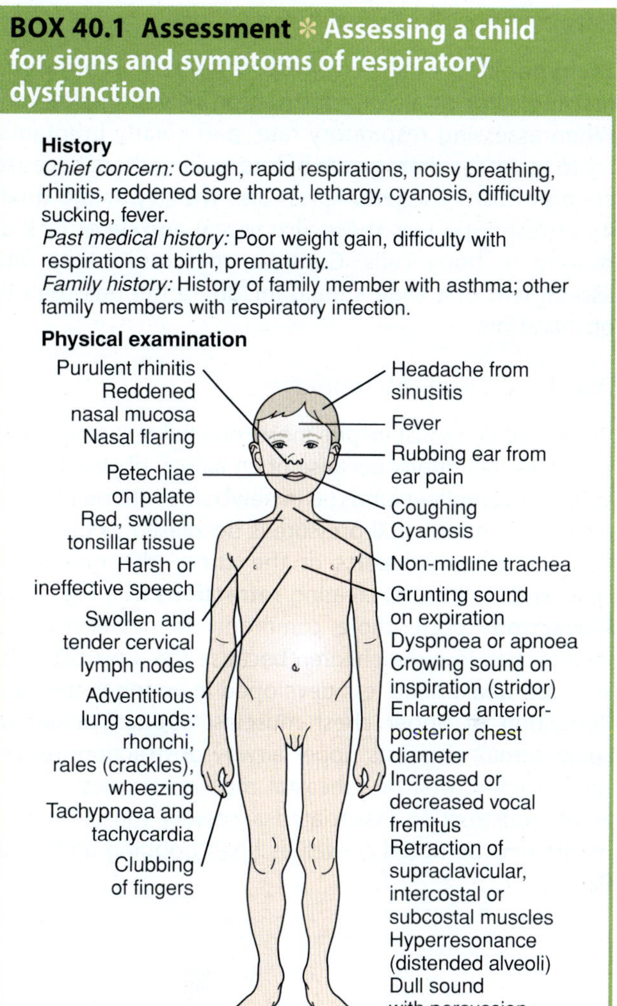

ASSESSING RESPIRATORY ILLNESS IN CHILDREN

Assessment of respiratory illness in children includes an interview, physical examination and laboratory testing. If the child is in acute distress, the interview and health history may cover only the most important details: when the child first became ill and what symptoms are present. All emergency presentations will follow paediatric emergency assessment protocols based on the primary ABCD format and as per local protocols/ pathways. It is important, however, to get as accurate a picture as soon as possible, because the problem could be the result of a variety of circumstances. Non-acute presentations are to be assessed against local MET call and/or rapid response criteria, age related as appropriate.

Physical assessment

Physical assessment of a child with a respiratory disorder includes observation of symptoms such as cough, cyanosis or pallor, as well as evaluation of respirations and breath sounds (Carter & Marshall, 2014). In addition assessment of the associated signs or symptoms of other organ or body systems involvement is needed to look for systemic effects of hypoxia and other respiratory implications (see Box 40.1).

Cough

A cough reflex is initiated by stimulation of the nerves of the respiratory tract mucosa by the presence of irritants or inflammation. The sound of coughing is caused by rapid expiratory air movement past the glottis. Coughing is a useful procedure to clear excess mucus or foreign bodies from the respiratory tract. It only becomes harmful and needs suppression when there is no mucus or debris to be expelled and the amount of coughing becomes exhausting. This might occur with respiratory tract inflammation. **Paroxysmal coughing** refers to a series of expiratory coughs after a deep inspiration. Commonly, this occurs in children with pertussis (whooping cough) or those who have aspirated a foreign body or a liquid they attempted to drink. Because young children often vomit after a series of coughs, they may be suspected initially of having a gastric disturbance even though their main illness is respiratory.

Rate and depth of respiration

Tachypnoea (an increased respiratory rate) is often the first indicator of airway obstruction in young children. When assessing respiratory rate, particularly in infants, try to count respiratory rate before waking them because crying distorts the rate. Assess also the depth and quality of respiration, as these also reveal **anoxia** or lack of oxygen in body cells. Consider that respiratory rate assessment in a child should include a full one minute observation.

Recessions and retractions

When children must inspire more forcefully than normally to inflate their lungs because of an airway obstruction or stiff, non-compliant lungs (as in newborns with pulmonary dysplasia), intrapleural pressure is decreased to the point that the non-rigid parts of the chest (the intercostal spaces) draw inward, creating **retractions** (see Fig. 40.1). **Retractions** occur more commonly in newborns and infants than in older children because the intercostal tissues are weaker and less developed in younger children. Retraction of upper chest muscles (supraclavicular or suprasternal) suggests upper airway obstruction; retraction of intercostal or subcostal muscles suggests lower airway obstruction. Associated accessory muscle movements may be noted as well as head bobbing and nasal flaring.

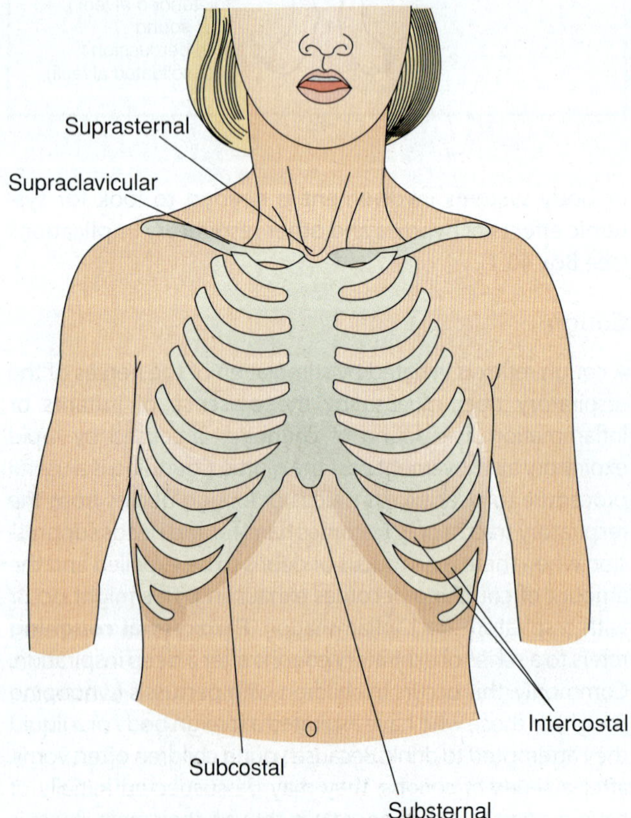

FIGURE 40.1 Sites of respiratory retraction.

Restlessness

When children or infants have decreased oxygen in body cells **(hypoxia)**, they become anxious and restless. Be careful not to interpret the excessive movements of infants with respiratory distress as a sign that they are improving; anxious, restless stirring may be their only way of signalling that their respiratory obstruction is becoming acute; it may be one of the first signs of airway obstruction.

Cyanosis

Cyanosis (a blue tinge to the skin) indicates hypoxia. If children have a low red blood cell count, cyanosis may not be apparent because there are not enough red blood cells to give the arterial blood its blue tinge. The degree of cyanosis present, therefore, is not always an accurate indication of the degree of airway difficulty. When children have accompanying peripheral vasoconstriction caused by shock, cyanosis of the extremities may or may not also be apparent. Be aware of variations based on skin colour pigmentation.

As the Po_2 drops and cyanosis results, children increase their respiratory effort in an attempt to supply more oxygen to their tissues. When they do this, the difference in pressure between the intralumen of a not yet fully developed trachea and the surrounding tissue becomes so great that the trachea may collapse, compounding the obstruction problem.

Adventitious sounds

Adventitious sounds (extra or abnormal breathing sounds) are caused by pathological conditions and can be heard on lung assessment in children with respiratory disorders. Accessory sounds of respiration result from the vibrations produced as air is forced past obstructions such as mucus. If the obstruction is in the nose or pharynx, the noise produced is a snoring sound (*rhonchi*). If the obstruction is at the base of the tongue or in the larynx, you will hear a harsh, strident sound on inspiration. This is laryngeal ***stridor***. If an obstruction is in the lower trachea or bronchioles, it is most noticeable on expiration. An expiratory whistle sound (*wheezing*) occurs. If alveoli become fluid-filled, fine crackling sounds **(crackles)** are heard. Diminished or absent breath sounds occur when the alveoli are so fluid-filled that little or no air can enter them. The absence of sound may indicate a silent chest which is a life-threatening condition resulting from limited or no air movement.

Chronic respiratory disease changes

Children with chronic respiratory conditions may have varying degrees of anatomical changes to their chest wall reflective of extended hyperinflation of lungs resulting in an elongated anteroposterior diameter of the chest, sometimes termed a "pigeon breast." In addition clubbing of the digits may occur in conditions which result from chronic alterations in gaseous exchange.

Laboratory tests

Several laboratory tests can be used to confirm or rule out the presence and severity of a respiratory disorder. These include analysis of arterial blood gases, nasopharyngeal culture and sputum analysis. The nurse must identify and implement the appropriate level of comfort and support as part of these invasive procedures.

Blood gas analysis

Blood gas analysis is an invasive method for determining the effectiveness of ventilation and acid-base status. Blood gas analysis therefore provides important information about oxygenation of the blood, as values may indicate not only whether the arterial partial pressure of oxygen (Po_2) is adequate but also whether the oxygen saturation of haemoglobin is adequate. The oxygen saturation level will fall if adequate oxygen cannot reach the bloodstream because of respiratory distress or if the haemoglobin is defective and cannot carry a full complement of oxygen (as with sickle cell anaemia or thalassaemia major). If a child has a severe anaemia, the saturation level may be adequate (95–100%), but body cells may still not be receiving enough oxygen because of the limited number of red blood cells carrying oxygen. To analyse blood gases, arterial blood rather than venous blood must be used. In the young infant, the temporal artery may be used as a site for blood gases; in newborns, an umbilical artery catheter can be used. In older children, the radial artery is the site of choice because of the collateral circulation present at the wrist. (If clotting should occur in the radial artery, the hand would still be well nourished by collateral circulation). An Allen test must be performed by an experienced practitioner to assess the effectiveness of collateral circulation in the hand. This involves briefly obstructing both radial and ulnar arteries and then releasing the ulnar vessel to see the effectiveness of collateral supply.

For an arterial blood gas (ABG) assessment, a specimen is withdrawn into a heparinised syringe (to prevent clotting). After any arterial puncture, always firmly compress the site. Otherwise, blood from the punctured vessel can seep into subcutaneous tissue, possibly causing a large haematoma and obscuring the site for further assessment. If frequent specimen collections are required, an arterial catheter, inserted either peripherally or centrally, may be used. Doing so allows frequent specimen collections without the trauma of additional punctures. Be sure to apply dressings over the area where an arterial catheter exits the skin to help prevent a young child from fussing or playing with the site.

Indicate oxygen therapy in situ as well as collection site on the specimen. While being transported to the laboratory, ABG specimens should be kept on ice to ensure accurate results (CO_2 levels decline in room air).

Pulse oximetry

Pulse oximetry is a non-invasive technique for measuring oxygen saturation. The pulse oximeter may be attached to the foot, finger or forehead of a child to detect the saturation of oxygen on haemoglobin within the underlying vascular bed (see Fig. 40.2). Advantages of pulse oximetry are that it is non-invasive and can provide continuous monitoring of oxygen saturation and pulse (see Box 40.2). A disadvantage is excess light in a room can distort the reading and the sensor may need to be covered with a blanket for readings to be accurate. Ensure the probe is repositioned regularly to an alternate site to minimise skin irritation or pressure points. Haemoglobin saturation will be obscured in carbon monoxide poisoning and therefore the saturation level will be an inaccurate reflection of oxygenation status.

Transcutaneous oxygen monitoring

Transcutaneous monitoring is another means of continuous, non-invasive measurement of oxygen saturation. Electrodes

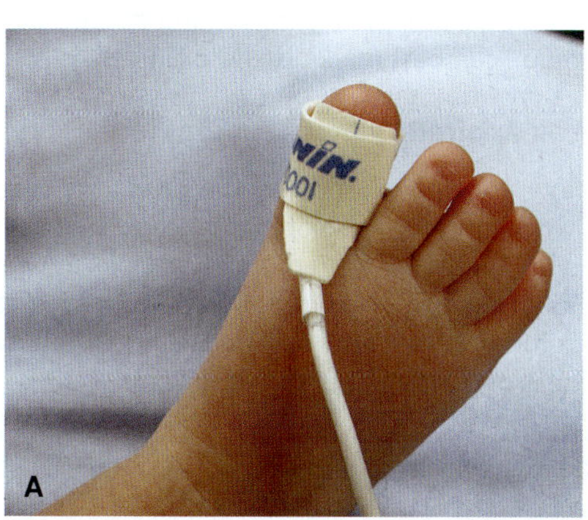

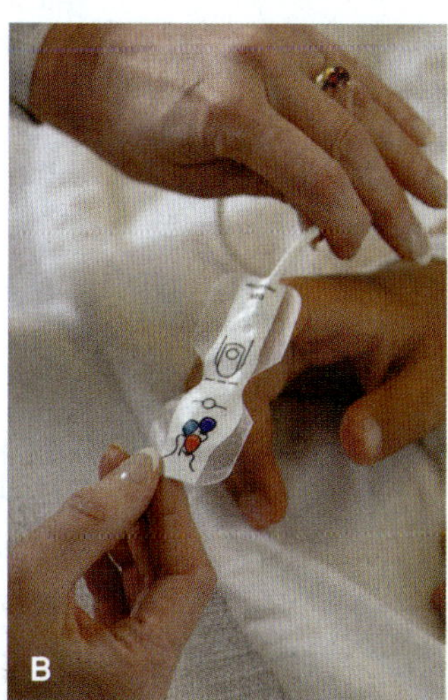

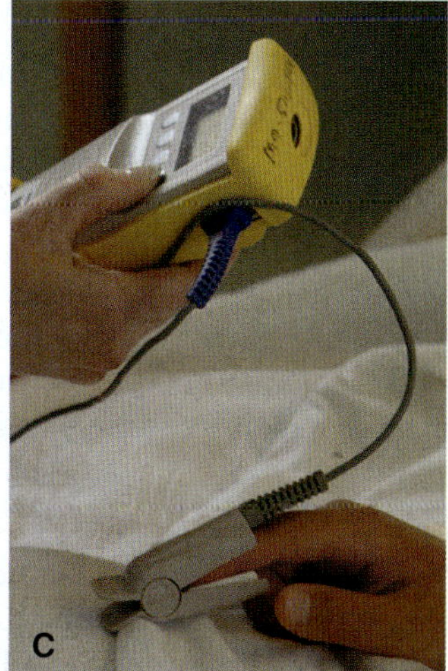

FIGURE 40.2 Types of pulse oximetry probes include (**A**) infant continuous; (**B**) finger continuous; and (**C**) finger intermittent. (From Ricci, S., Kyle, T. & Carman, S. (2012). *Maternity and Pediatric Nursing.* (2nd ed.). Philadelphia: Lippincott Williams & Wilkins.)

BOX 40.2 * Frequency of infant observations and related documentation

Oxygen flow rate, inspired oxygen concentration and/or oxygen saturation of the infant should be monitored and recorded to prevent hyperoxia and hypoxia, regardless of the delivery system.

- Minimum of hourly for ventilated or CPAP
- Less frequent for stable infants with nasal prongs, headbox or incubator
- Each time there is a change in the oxygen delivery system and/or change in the gas mixture given to an infant it is recommended two staff members check and record the changes
- Recommended two staff members check and record the changes and status of the baby at every bedside shift handover.

The following observations are to be carried out and documented on all infants receiving supplemental oxygen as a minimum at every bedside shift handover by TWO staff members

- Range of oxygen levels that the infants readings are to be kept between
- Method of supplemental oxygen administration as per flow meter
- Percentage of supplemental oxygen administered via headbox or incubator (measured by an analyser positioned near the infant's airway)
- Range of oxygen level in the baby by oxygen saturation monitor or transcutaneous oxygen monitor readings since the previous recording
- Physical assessment of the infant and documentation of respiratory/cardiac status
- Tolerance of the infant to supplemental oxygen administration during handling and post feeds.

Summary from NSW Health (2006). *Newborn Infants—Safe Oxygen Administration. Policy Directive.* PD2006_103. <www.health.nsw.gov.au/policies>.

heated to 44°C are attached to an infant's chest. The heat causes vasodilation underneath the skin and brings the peripheral arterial blood to the surface to be read for oxygen content. This is converted to mmHg on a monitor readout. The oxygen saturation level read by this method correlates with intra-arterial Po_2, the same as with pulse oximetry. Transcutaneous monitoring has a disadvantage compared with pulse oximetry because the probe position needs to be changed every 3 to 4 hours to prevent a burn to the skin and sensor recalibration is necessary with each position change.

Nasopharyngeal culture

When done efficiently, nasopharyngeal cultures cause little discomfort and allow identification of microorganisms present. The procedure involves touching a moistened swab to the mucous membrane of the nose or throat in a swift process applying only light pressure. The site of specimen collection will only reflect organisms in that location, hence the nose and throat reflect the upper respiratory tract (e.g. RSV) and will not identify potential lower respiratory tract organisms.

Respiratory syncytial virus nasal washings

Nasal washings are obtained to diagnose an infection caused by the respiratory syncytial virus (RSV). For this, a child is placed in the supine position, and 1 to 2 mL of sterile normal saline is dropped with a sterile needleless syringe into one nostril. The nose is then aspirated using a small, sterile bulb syringe or designated RSV suction catheter reservoir. The secretions removed are placed in a sterile container to be sent to the laboratory for analysis. Nasal washings are more uncomfortable for children than nasal swabbing because of the saline that is instilled.

Sputum analysis

Because they cannot raise sputum with a cough, sputum collection is rarely feasible in children younger than school age. Older children, however, are able to cough and raise sputum. Ask them to breathe in and out several times, cough deeply and spit mucus they have raised from coughing, as opposed to just the back of the throat, into a sterile specimen jar using a non-touch technique.

Diagnostic procedures

As well as cultures, several other common diagnostic procedures are used to identify respiratory disorders in children. A child may require specialised investigations such as bronchoscopy, bronchography, to visualise internal lumens of the airways, and pulmonary function tests to ascertain lung volumes and compliance related problems.

Chest x-ray films

Chest x-ray films will show areas of infiltration or consolidation in the lungs; if a foreign body is opaque, an x-ray study will show its location. Chest x-ray films are more difficult to obtain in infants as they cannot take a breath and hold it when instructed. Computed tomography (CT) scans may be ordered for children with chronic lung disease because this technique can best mark disease progress.

PEFR: Peak expiratory flow reading

A "peak flow" reading is used in some paediatric cases for children who have the developmental capacity to understand and complete the test accurately. A peak flow measures the volume of forced expired air and gives an indication of lung volume. A pre and post measure can show the effectiveness of treatment, e.g. a nebuliser.

HEALTH PROMOTION

Advocating and educating appropriate infection control measures to children and their parents such as hand-washing, properly disposing of tissues and covering their mouth while coughing are pivotal health promotion strategies to minimise cross-contamination of contact and airborne organisms. Furthermore routine immunisation and following relevant public health guidelines for flu vaccines helps reduce incidence of preventable respiratory conditions. Children with chronic respiratory illnesses should also receive the pneumococcal vaccine. Reducing respiratory irritation by removing secondary smoke can help prevent upper respiratory infections, lower the incidence of asthma attacks, as well as otitis media (middle ear infection).

THERAPEUTIC TECHNIQUES USED IN THE TREATMENT OF RESPIRATORY ILLNESS IN CHILDREN

The primary goal of nursing interventions in the care of children with respiratory disorders is to maintain or re-establish the airway to help ensure that adequate oxygen reaches the blood. Often this includes interventions aimed at liquefying and removing mucus secretions so they do not clog the bronchial pathways. Such clogging prevents adequate oxygenation and contributes to the development of bronchial and alveolar infections.

Expectorant therapy

Any irritation of the respiratory tract causes the production of large amounts of mucus. The amount produced can become so great that the natural mechanisms for clearing it (coughing and upward cilia action) are no longer adequate. If a child is breathing rapidly because of respiratory distress, the frequent passage of air over the mucus tends to dry it and make it more viscid, compounding the removal. Several measures may be used to liquefy dried mucus and help raise it.

Liquefying agents

Expectorants such as guaifenesin (Robitussin), given orally, are designed to liquefy mucus in the trachea and bronchi. Instilling saline nose drops or using saline nasal sprays can be effective in moistening and loosening dried mucus in the nose (McKenna & Mirkov, 2014).

Humidification

Humidification is the provision of moisture to the airway. Common methods of delivering moisture include vaporisers and nebulisers. It is not always standard practice and therefore may be implemented on a medical order or as deemed appropriate.

Nebulisers

Nebulisers are mechanical devices that provide a stream of moistened air directly into the respiratory tract. Most are hand-held masks that fit over the nose and mouth and are attached to an electrical pump as a power source (see Fig. 40.3). Ultrasonic nebulisation delivers such minuscule droplets into the respiratory tract that even the smallest bronchioles can be moistened. Nebulisers also serve as an important means for the delivery of respiratory tract medications (Facts and Comparisons, 2014). Medications such as antibiotics or bronchodilators can be combined with the nebulised mist and delivered directly into the lungs.

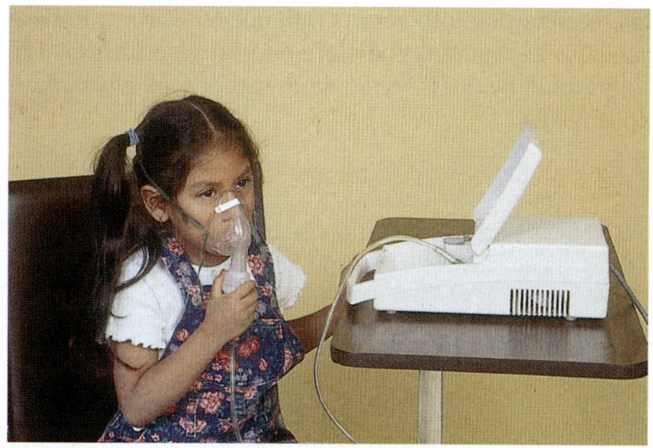

FIGURE 40.3 Child using a nebuliser.

Many children find nebuliser treatments uncomfortable because the feeling of the mist in their upper respiratory tract can be frightening or irritating. Assure them that aerosol administration is the most effective route for moisture and medication to reach and cause an effect in the respiratory tract. During aerosol medication administration, watch carefully for signs of both local tracheal or bronchial effect (spasm or oedema) that might result from airway irritation as well as systemic symptoms that might result from absorption of a medication by the membrane (such as tachycardia).

Coughing

As a rule, encourage coughing rather than suppressing it, because coughing is an effective method of raising mucus, if it is a productive cough. Helpful techniques to initiate coughing include changing a child's position and suggesting mild exercise or deep breathing.

Chest physiotherapy

Three techniques are involved with chest physiotherapy to loosen mucus for expectoration: postural drainage, percussion and vibration. Each technique can be used alone, but they are usually more effective at moving mucus towards the main stem bronchus when performed together.

An infant may be positioned on your lap, whereas a slant board or other surface is needed for postural drainage with an older child. Not all positions are tolerated well. Be ready to modify the positions used depending on the child's condition and tolerance. It is common practice for chest physiotherapy regimens to be initiated and overseen by physiotherapists with nurses assisting in these activities as required. Therefore refer to a person's clinical notes for individualised requirements or seek physiotherapist review.

> ***What if...***
>
> Michael needs to cough to raise bronchial mucus? What if he refuses to? How can you get him to cough?

Therapy to improve oxygenation

Oxygen administration

Oxygen administration elevates the arterial oxygen saturation level by supplying more oxygen to red blood cells through the respiratory tract. Oxygen may be delivered to infants by flooding an incubator or by using a plastic hood, mask or cannula. Plastic oxygen hoods are tight-fitting enclosures that can keep oxygen concentration at nearly 100% (see Fig. 40.4). Always check that a hood fits snugly over the infant's head, making sure it does not rub against the infant's neck, chin or shoulders. Be sure the gas does not blow directly into the infant's face.

Although a nasal catheter or nasal prongs can be used for infants, there is risk of airway obstruction as they are nasal breathers and therefore nasal prongs are usually reserved for older children. Most children do not like nasal prongs because they are intrusive. Assess their nostrils carefully when using these as the pressure of prongs can cause areas of necrosis, particularly on the nasal septum. Nasal prongs have a maximum flow rate of 2 L/min in children, higher flows require alternate device.

General guidelines for oxygen administration in children are simple flow mask 6–10 L/min and non-rebreather face mask greater than 10 L/min (NSW Health, 2012).

A correct fitting oxygen mask receiving the correct oxygen flow rate will provide the stated oxygen concentration as per manufacturer's guidelines. However, masks are also often not well tolerated by children and if necessary, let them hold a mask rather than strapping it in place.

In some incidences humidification and warming may be combined with oxygen therapy. In any child, administering oxygen concentrations of 70% to 80% for an extended period may lead to a thickening of the lung alveoli and a loss of lung pliancy (oxygen toxicity or bronchopulmonary dysplasia). For these reasons, oxygen should not be given in high concentrations for long periods unless adequate facilities for blood gas analysis are available (Marino, 2007).

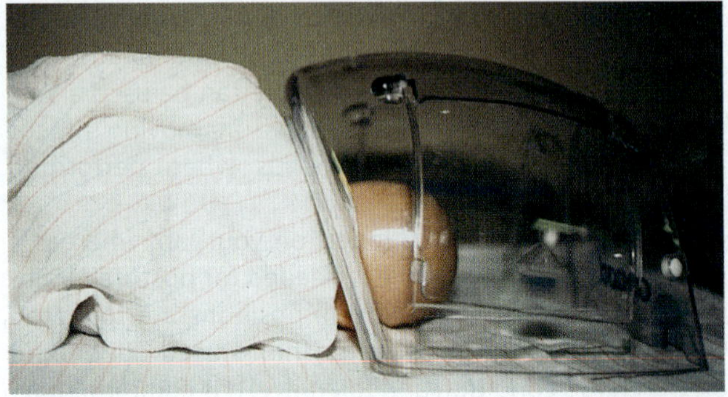

FIGURE 40.4 Oxygen hood for an infant.

Also ensure safety and infection control guidelines are adhered to during oxygen administration. It is recommended that when there is a change in oxygen delivery regimens for neonates that two staff check and record these changes. In addition the two staff members should also check and record changes and status at the bedside shift handover. Oxygen therapy is considered a drug and requires a medical prescription for its use.

Pharmacological therapy

Children notice difficulty with exchange of air when their airways become obstructed because of unusual mucus production, bronchoconstriction or inflammation. Several medications may be used to reverse these processes. Nasal sprays such as normal saline can be administered to moisten and loosen nasal secretions. Antihistamines given by this route can reduce mucus production and thereby open the airway. Decongestants cause vasoconstriction, leading to shrinkage of the mucous membranes, which expands breathing space. Expectorants help to raise mucus but most of these agents also cause drowsiness, so their doses must be regulated, especially in adolescents who may be driving. Bronchodilators are used to open the lower airway. Antibiotics may be given intravenously, intramuscularly, orally or inhaled through nebulisation to reduce infection and limit purulent mucus and inflammation. Corticosteroids taken either orally or by inhalation enlarge the airway by reducing further inflammation (Vallerand & Sanoski, 2014). Caution parents not to give cough and cold medications to children under 2 years of age unless specifically prescribed by their healthcare provider.

Metered-dose inhalers

A metered-dose inhaler (MDI) is a hand-held device that provides a route for medication administration directly to the respiratory tract. The child inhales while pressing a trigger on the apparatus. Some devices include a spacer attached to the apparatus, a plastic extension tube or chamber that helps better coordinate inhalation with the medication delivery. For successful use, children need to follow five general rules: shake the canister; exhale deeply; activate the inhaler as they begin to inhale; take a long slow inhalation; and then hold their breath for 5–10 seconds. They should take only one puff at a time, with a 1-minute wait between puffs (McKenna & Mirkov, 2014). MDIs require that children trigger the inhaler at the same time as they breathe in (see Fig. 40.5A). Because it is difficult for children younger than approximately 12 years of age to do this, placing a spacer tube between the inhaler and the mouthpiece better coordinates inhaling and trigger release

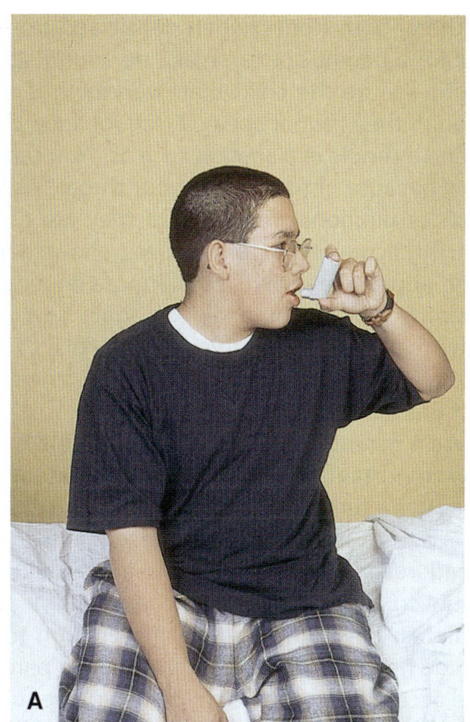

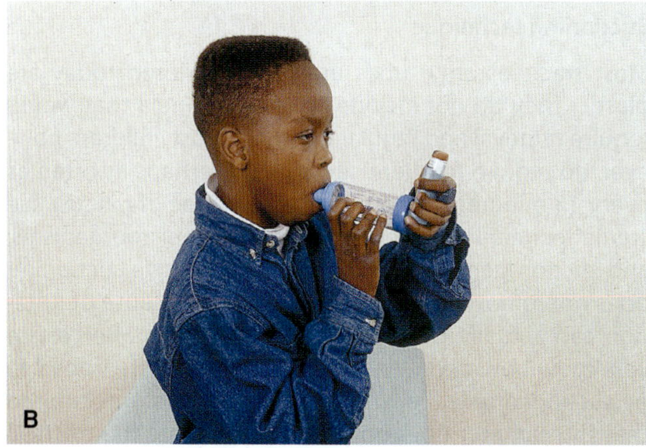

FIGURE 40.5 (**A**) Many children use a metered-dose inhaler to administer a bronchodilator to themselves. Be certain children respect such medicine as medicine so they use sensible precautions. (**B**) Younger children need a "spacer" with inhalers so they do not need to correlate administration with inhalation.

(see Fig. 40.5B). Refer to the specific manufacturer's guidelines for further details. Important education points are to ensure the child breathes normally and takes two breaths per puffer dose then repeats if a second dose and/or subsequent doses are required. Clean the spacer and ensure it is for the exclusive use of one child.

Inhalation and breathing techniques

Physiotherapy regimens may include actions and devices to increase exhalation to improve alveoli expansion and oxygenation. Incentive spirometers are devices that encourage children to inhale deeply to aerate the lungs fully or move mucus. Children need instruction on how to use this type of device because their first impression is that they should blow out against the mouthpiece rather than inhale. Breathing techniques can also include blowing through straws or blowing up balloons as well as pursed lip breathing which all aim to better inflate alveoli or more effectively empty alveoli.

Emergency airway management

Few medical emergencies are as frightening to a child or parents as an acute obstruction of a child's upper airway requiring an endotracheal intubation or tracheotomy. The child suddenly becomes limp and breathless, with colour changing quickly to systemic cyanosis. Assistance in an emergency intubation will involve procedural assistance with either an oral or nasal intubation process followed by the connection to the required ventilator. In addition the nurses will provide support to the child who will commonly be given sedation as well as support to the carers witnessing or being made aware of the event.

Endotracheal intubation

Endotracheal intubation (nasal or oral intubation) is the preferred means of bypassing upper airway obstruction and allowing free entry of air to the trachea. There is little difference in efficiency between oral and nasal methods (Spence & Barr, 2000). However, since intubation tubes cause oedema and local irritation, they cannot be left in place as a permanent solution. As with tracheostomies, children cannot speak while intubated. Age-appropriate communication strategies may include a pencil and paper, pictures, or simple drawings or photos (a drink, a straw, a blanket, the television turned on, a toilet) to make needs known. In young children endotracheal tubes are held in place by being taped to the face (see Fig. 40.6). Make sure tubes are carefully secured because children can easily dislodge them. As much as possible, limit the number of tape changes to protect the skin on the child's cheeks.

A capnometer is a device that measures the amount of CO_2 in inhaled or exhaled breaths. It is attached to the distal end of the endotracheal tube and measures the percentage of CO_2 in expired air, so the arterial CO_2 (Pco_2) can be estimated. Used in this way, a capnometer can reduce the number of arterial punctures needed for ABG analysis.

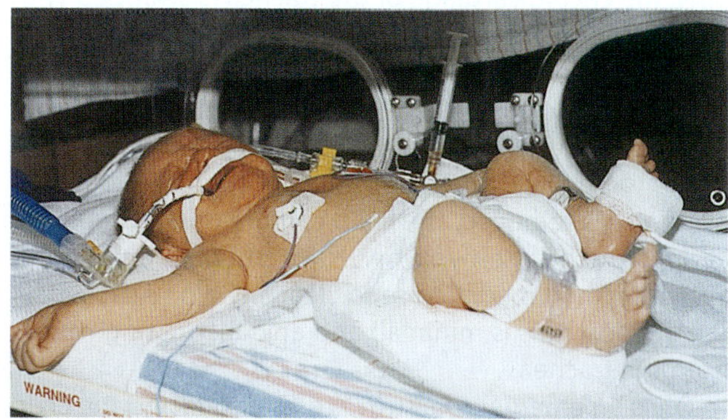

FIGURE 40.6 An infant with an endotracheal tube receiving assisted ventilation.

Assisted ventilation

When it is not possible to improve oxygen saturation to sufficient levels by the methods described above, assisted ventilation may be necessary (Abadesso et al., 2012). Positive-pressure machines deliver moistened or nebulised air or oxygen to the lungs under enough pressure and with appropriate timing to produce artificial, periodic inflation of alveoli. They rely on the elastic recoil of the lungs to empty the alveoli.

There are several types of assisted ventilation ranging from full ventilation support, which takes complete control of breathing for the child, to less invasive forms. Before full ventilation is used less invasive forms are generally implemented. The more common and less invasive form of assisted ventilation is called NIV (non-invasive ventilation). One common form of NIV is CPAP (continuous positive airway pressure). CPAP provides a sustained level of positive pressure set by the operator to provide end expiratory support to hold the alveoli open. The CPAP machine also works to sense the child starting to take a breath and provides the delivery of air at the preset pressure to sufficiently inflate the child's lungs to the end point pressure.

NIV including CPAP are advanced skills in most facilities and will require further accreditation. All assisted ventilation situations will require a high dependency acuity rating. Therefore, have the required observation monitoring in situ and do not leave the child unattended.

Children who need respiratory assistance are understandably frightened. Muscle relaxants and sedation may be administered intravenously to a point of abolishing spontaneous respiratory action to overcome resistance and allow mechanical ventilation to be accomplished at lower pressures because without normal respiratory action, there is no normal muscle resistance to overcome. Clearly, children who receive pancuronium have no spontaneous respiratory function and need critical observation and frequent ABG analysis because they depend totally on carers at that point.

Tracheotomy

Tracheotomy is used when airway obstruction does not allow for oral or nasal intubation methods. For tracheotomy, the cricoid cartilage of the trachea is swabbed with an antiseptic; if readily available, a local anaesthetic may be injected into the cartilage ring. (This is not necessary in the unconscious child.) An incision is made just under the ring of cartilage and a tracheostomy tube with its obturator in place is inserted into the opening. When the obturator is removed, the child can breathe through the hollow tracheostomy tube. Have suction equipment available for immediate use to clear any blood caused by the incision (this is minimal) and any obstructing mucus from the trachea.

Once an emergency airway is established and the child begins to breathe normally and, if unconscious, regain consciousness, they often thrash and push at people around them, both from oxygen deficit and from fright. They call for a parent but can make no sound, adding to their fright. Assure the child that everything is all right, even though they cannot speak. A school-aged child can understand a simple explanation such as, "You can't speak right now because of the tube in your throat." As soon as the child's respirations are even and they are no longer experiencing acute respiratory distress, show them how, (in an age-appropriate child), by placing a finger over the tracheostomy tube opening, air will again flow past the larynx and they can speak. If this causes a child to become short of breath, supply a paper and pencil or whiteboard for communication.

Be certain parents understand why the tube is in place and how important it is that it remains patent. Assure them that it is a temporary measure to give oxygen (provided this is true). If they were not present in the room for the procedure, encourage them to visit the child as soon as possible to assure themselves their child is again all right. Children have difficulty relaxing enough to accept this strange new way of breathing until their parents can relax and accept it also. Some children hyperventilate, not because of respiratory difficulty, but because of this fear.

Suctioning technique

Most tracheostomy tubes used with children today are plastic. They do not include an inner cannula that would require removal and regular cleaning. Most children, however, do require frequent suctioning (perhaps as often as every 15 minutes) to keep their airway free of mucus. Use sterile technique to prevent introducing microorganisms, and suction gently, yet thoroughly. Ineffective suctioning does not remove obstructive mucus and because of irritation can actually cause more mucus to form. Be certain you know how deeply to suction. Some children need to be suctioned only the length of the tracheostomy tube so that the catheter does not touch and irritate the tracheal mucosa. Others need to be deeply suctioned to reduce the possibility that mucus will become so copious or so thickened that it obstructs the trachea below the tube.

Because suctioning removes air as well as secretions from the trachea, children may become oxygen-deprived during the procedure. Although not evidence-based, pre-oxygenating them by "bagging" or administering oxygen for approximately 5 minutes before the procedure may help reduce this problem (Pritchard, Flenady & Woodgate, 2009). Occasionally, a child may have such thick mucus that it is necessary to insert a drop or two of normal saline into the tracheostomy tube before suctioning. This should not be routine, however, as fluid running into the trachea produces a frightening, suffocating feeling.

Check frequently on children with tracheostomies to assess for possible respiratory difficulty. Tracheostomy tubes are held in place by cloth straps that fasten at the back of the child's neck. Change straps when they become soiled or loose, and check them frequently (at least once every 8 hours) to be certain they remain tied. Assess that the ties fit snugly but allow for one finger to be inserted underneath so they do not rub and cause pain. For preschoolers or younger children, it is a good idea to cover the tracheostomy opening with a gauze square tied to the child's neck like a bib while they eat, and ensure no small objects are accessible which may be inserted and obstruct the airway.

Lung transplantation

Lung transplantation is a possibility for some children with a chronic respiratory illness such as cystic fibrosis (Visner & Goldfarb, 2007). The transplant may involve a single lung, or it can be done in conjunction with heart transplantation if chronic respiratory disease has caused ventricular hypertrophy of the heart.

As with any organ transplantation, children need continued immunosuppression therapy following a lung transplant to decrease cell-mediated immunity. Children may need to have chest physiotherapy or use a portable spirometry device daily to help mobilise secretions resulting from loss of nerve innervation or a reaction to accumulating mucus in the transplanted lung.

DISORDERS OF THE UPPER RESPIRATORY TRACT

The upper respiratory tract warms, humidifies and filters the air that enters the body. As such, the structures of the upper respiratory tract constantly come into contact with a barrage of foreign organisms, including pathogens that can lead to airway irritation and illness. Congenital malformations of respiratory structures also cause some upper respiratory tract disorders.

Choanal atresia

Choanal atresia is congenital obstruction of the posterior nares by an obstructing membrane or bony growth, preventing a newborn from drawing air through the nose and down into the nasopharynx (Eladl, 2010). It may be either unilateral or bilateral.

Newborns up to approximately 3 months of age are naturally nose-breathers. Infants with choanal atresia, therefore, develop signs of respiratory distress at birth or immediately after they become quiet for the first time and attempt to breathe through their nose. Passing a soft gauge 8 or 10 French catheter through the posterior nares to the stomach is a part of birthing room procedure in many healthcare facilities. If such a catheter will not pass bilaterally, the diagnosis of choanal atresia is confirmed immediately at birth.

The treatment for choanal atresia is either local piercing of the obstructing membrane or surgical removal of the bony growth. Some infants may need an oral airway inserted so they can continue to breathe through their mouths. Following surgery, most children have no further difficulty or symptoms.

Acute nasopharyngitis (common cold)

The common cold is the most frequent infectious disease in children, which is caused by one or several viruses (Friedman et al., 2014). Symptoms begin with nasal congestion, a watery rhinitis and a low-grade fever. The mucous membrane of the nose becomes oedematous and inflamed, constricting airway space and causing difficulty breathing. Posterior rhinitis, plus local irritation, leads to pharyngitis (sore throat). Upper airway secretions that drain into the trachea lead to a cough. Cervical lymph nodes may be swollen and palpable. The process lasts about a week and then symptoms fade. In some children, a thick, purulent nasal discharge occurs because bacteria such as streptococci invade the irritated nasal mucous membrane and cause a secondary infection.

Infants can be critically ill yet not develop a fever because their temperature-regulating system is still immature. With the common cold, they often develop a fever elevated out of proportion to the symptoms, possibly as high as 38.8° to 40°C. Infants also may develop secondary symptoms, such as vomiting and diarrhoea, as a general response. Because they cannot suck and breathe through their mouth at the same time, they refuse feedings. This can lead to dehydration. Older children rarely develop as high a fever, rarely above 38.8°C. Because older children can breathe through their mouth, nasal congestion does not seem as acute.

There is no specific treatment for a common cold as they are caused by a virus, antibiotics are not effective unless a secondary bacterial invasion has occurred. Fever symptoms can be reduced by antipyretics. If infants have difficulty nursing because of nasal congestion, saline nose drops or nasal spray may be prescribed to liquefy nasal secretions and help them drain. Removing nasal mucus via a bulb syringe before feedings also allows infants to breathe more freely and be able to suck more efficiently. Caution parents that if they use a bulb syringe, they must compress the bulb first, then insert it into the child's nostril. If they insert the bulb syringe first, then depress the bulb, they will actually push secretions further back into the nose, causing increased obstruction.

Pharyngitis

Pharyngitis is infection and inflammation of the throat. It may be either bacterial or viral in origin. It may occur as a result of a chronic allergy in which there is constant post-nasal discharge that results in secondary irritation.

Viral pharyngitis

The causative agent of pharyngitis is usually an adenovirus (Martin, 2010). The symptoms are generally mild: a sore throat, fever and general malaise. On physical assessment, regional lymph nodes may be noticeably enlarged. Erythema will be present in the back of the pharynx and the palatine arch. Laboratory studies will indicate an increased white blood cell count.

If the inflammation is mild, children rarely need more than an oral analgesic or ibuprofen for comfort. Gargling may be indicated in an age-appropriate child. Due to sore throats children often prefer liquids to solid food. Infants, especially, must be observed closely until the inflammation and tenderness diminish to be certain that they take in sufficient fluid to prevent dehydration.

Streptococcal pharyngitis

Group A beta-haemolytic streptococcus is the organism most frequently involved in bacterial pharyngitis in children. All streptococcal infections must be taken seriously because they can lead to cardiac and kidney damage from the accompanying autoimmune process (Altamimi et al., 2012).

Streptococcal infections are generally more severe than viral infections. The fact that symptoms are mild, however, does not rule out streptococcal infection. With a streptococcal pharyngitis, the back of the throat and palatine tonsils are usually markedly erythematous (bright red); the tonsils are enlarged and may have white exudates. Petechiae may be present on the palate. A child typically appears ill with a high fever (as high as 40°C), an extremely sore throat, difficulty swallowing and overall lethargy. The child often has a headache. Swollen abdominal lymph nodes may cause abdominal pain. A throat culture confirms the presence of the *Streptococcus* bacteria.

Treatment consists of a full course of oral antibiotics as prescribed following culture sensitivity, or broad-spectrum macrolides if resistant organisms are known to be in the community. Advice should be given regarding need for rest, relief of throat pain and maintaining hydration, which are the same actions as for a common cold.

CASE STUDY QUESTION

3. Suppose Michael is diagnosed as having streptococcal pharyngitis. The chief danger of such an infection is:

a. Lymph nodes will swell and obstruct the airway
b. Infection may spread and cause a tooth abscess
c. A small number of children develop kidney disease
d. Four out of five children will develop lung abscesses.

Retropharyngeal abscess

In infants, the lymph nodes that drain the nasopharynx are located just behind the posterior pharynx wall. These nodes may become infected following acute nasopharyngitis or pharyngitis. Since these nodes disappear by preschool age, the problem is usually limited to young infants (Lin & Lee, 2011). Swallowing may be impaired requiring suctioning the upper airway. Caution must be taken so as not to rupture the abscess and surgical intervention may be required if obstruction is severe.

Tonsillitis

Tonsillitis refers to infection and inflammation of the palatine tonsils. *Adenitis* refers to infection and inflammation of the adenoid (pharyngeal) tonsils. Infection of the palatine tonsils presents with all of the symptoms of a severe pharyngitis. Children may drool because their throat is too sore for them to swallow saliva and complain of pain. High fever, lethargy, as well as bright red enlarged tonsillar tissue may be evident. Pus can be detected on or expelled from the tonsillar crypts (Lin & Lee, 2011). In addition to fever, lethargy, pharyngeal pain and oedema, the symptoms of adenoidal tissue infection also include a nasal quality of speech, mouth breathing, difficulty hearing and perhaps halitosis or sleep apnoea. Mouth breathing, change in speech and apnoea result from the postpharyngeal obstruction by the enlarged tissue. The difficulty with hearing occurs because of eustachian tube obstruction. Long-term obstruction this way can further cause serious and acute otitis media.

Tonsillitis occurs most commonly in school-aged children. The responsible organism is identified by a throat culture. In children younger than 3 years of age, the cause is often viral. Therapy may include antipyretics, analgesia and antibiotics as prescribed.

Tonsillectomy

Tonsillectomy is removal of the palatine tonsils. *Adenoidectomy* is removal of the pharyngeal tonsils. Tonsillectomy is now only recommended after an ear, nose, throat (ENT) review following recurrent episodes of tonsillitis. It is the surgeon's preference as to whether surgery is undertaken during or after an active episode.

Tonsillectomies are done as day surgery or 1-day surgery followed by generic guidelines for home rest for a week or so. Preadmission preparation includes completion of a complete history and physical examination and laboratory tests, including bleeding and clotting times, complete blood count and urinalysis. An important aspect of immediate assessment on the day of surgery is to observe for loose teeth; if present, they could be dislodged during surgery and aspirated. If loose teeth are present, mark this on the front of the child's chart and pre-op checklist and report it to the theatre admission nurse and anaesthetist.

The most dangerous periods for a child after a tonsillectomy are the first 24 hours, when the clots covering the denuded surgical area are forming, and days 5 to 7, when the clots begin to lyse or dissolve. If new granulation tissue is not yet present when the clots dissolve, haemorrhage from the denuded surface can occur.

CASE STUDY QUESTION

4. Suppose Michael's 4-year-old roommate spits up dark-red blood following her tonsillectomy. Your best action in relation to this would be:

a. Suction the back of her throat
b. Encourage her to cough vigorously
c. Make an MET call
d. Continue to observe her for bleeding.

Epistaxis

Epistaxis (nosebleed) is extremely common in children and usually occurs from trauma, such as picking at the nose, from falling or from being hit on the nose (Robertson, King & Tomkinson, 2010). In homes that lack humidification, the hot, dry environment causes children's mucous membranes to dry, feel uncomfortable and be susceptible to cracking and bleeding. In all children, epistaxis tends to occur during respiratory illnesses. It also may occur after strenuous exercise, and it is associated with several systemic diseases, such as rheumatic fever, scarlet fever, measles or varicella infection (chickenpox). It can occur with nasal polyps, sinusitis or allergic rhinitis. Some families have a predisposition towards nosebleeds. Nosebleeds are always frightening because of the visible bleeding and a choking sensation if blood should run down the back of the nasopharynx. The fear is generally out of proportion to the seriousness of the bleeding.

Keep children with nosebleeds in an upright position with their head tilted slightly forwards to minimise the amount of blood pressure in nasal vessels and to keep blood moving forwards, not back into the nasopharynx. Apply pressure to the sides of the nose with your fingers. Make every effort to calm the child and to help stop crying, because crying increases pressure in the blood vessels of the head and prolongs bleeding. A nasal pack may be necessary to provide continued pressure. Every child has an occasional nosebleed. Chronic nasal bleeding, however, should be investigated to rule out a systemic disease or blood disorder.

Sinusitis

Sinusitis is infection and inflammation of the sinus cavities. It is rare in children younger than 6 years of age because the frontal sinuses do not develop fully until the age of 6. Children develop a fever, a purulent nasal discharge, headache and tenderness over the affected sinus. A nose and throat culture will identify the infectious organism.

Treatment for acute sinusitis consists of an antipyretic for fever, an analgesic for pain, and an antibiotic for the specific organism, supplied as nose drops or a nasal spray, which shrinks the oedematous mucous membranes and allows infected material to drain from the sinuses and relieve pain. To avoid a rebound effect, this type of nasal spray should be used for only 3 days at a time; otherwise, it actually causes more nasal congestion. Warm compresses to the sinus area may also encourage drainage and relieve pain. Some children need analgesia for pain.

Sinusitis may cause serious complications if the infection spreads from the sinuses to the facial bone (osteomyelitis) or the middle ear (otitis media).

Laryngitis

Laryngitis is inflammation of the larynx. It results in brassy, hoarse voice sounds or inability to make audible noise. It may occur as a complication of pharyngitis or from excessive use of the voice, as in shouting or loud cheering. Sips of fluid (either warm or cold, whichever feels best), offer relief from the annoying tickling sensation often present. The most effective measure, however, is for the child to rest the voice for at least 24 hours, until inflammation subsides. For infants with laryngitis, attempt to meet their needs before they cry. Simply caution older children not to speak. Provide them with a paper and pencil for communication.

Congenital laryngomalacia/tracheomalacia

Congenital laryngomalacia means that an infant's laryngeal structure is weaker than normal and collapses more than usual on inspiration (Adil, Rager & Carr, 2012). This produces laryngeal **stridor** (a high-pitched crowing sound on inspiration) present from birth, possibly intensified when the infant is in a supine position or when sucking. Most children with congenital laryngomalacia need no routine therapy other than to have parents feed them slowly, providing rest periods as needed. The condition improves as infants mature and cartilage in the larynx becomes stronger at about 1 year of age.

Tracheomalacia is the weakening of the tracheal walls and may require surgical Intervention.

Croup (laryngotracheobronchitis)

Croup (inflammation of the larynx, trachea and major bronchi) is one of the most frightening diseases of early childhood for both parents and children. In children between 6 months and 3 years of age, the cause of croup is usually a viral infection such as parainfluenza virus. In previous years, the most common cause was *H. influenzae*. However, since immunisation against this organism is now included in the routine immunisation schedule, the incidence of croup from this virus has declined by 90% (Federico et al., 2011).

With croup, children typically have only a mild upper respiratory tract infection at bedtime. Temperature is normal or only mildly elevated. During the night, they develop a barking cough (croupy cough), inspiratory stridor and marked retractions. They wake in extreme respiratory distress. The larynx, trachea and major bronchi are all inflamed. These severe symptoms typically last several hours and then, except for a rattling cough, subside by morning. Symptoms may recur the following night. Cyanosis is rarely present, but the danger of glottal obstruction from the laryngeal inflammation and hypoxaemia is very real. Pulse oximetry and transcutaneous Sao_2 monitors are helpful measures to document whether hypoxaemia is occurring.

One emergency method of relieving croup symptoms at home is for a parent to run the shower or hot water tap in a bathroom until the room fills with steam, then keep the child in this warm, moist environment. If this does not relieve symptoms, parents should bring the child to

TABLE 40.1 Clinical assessment: Stridor/respiratory distress

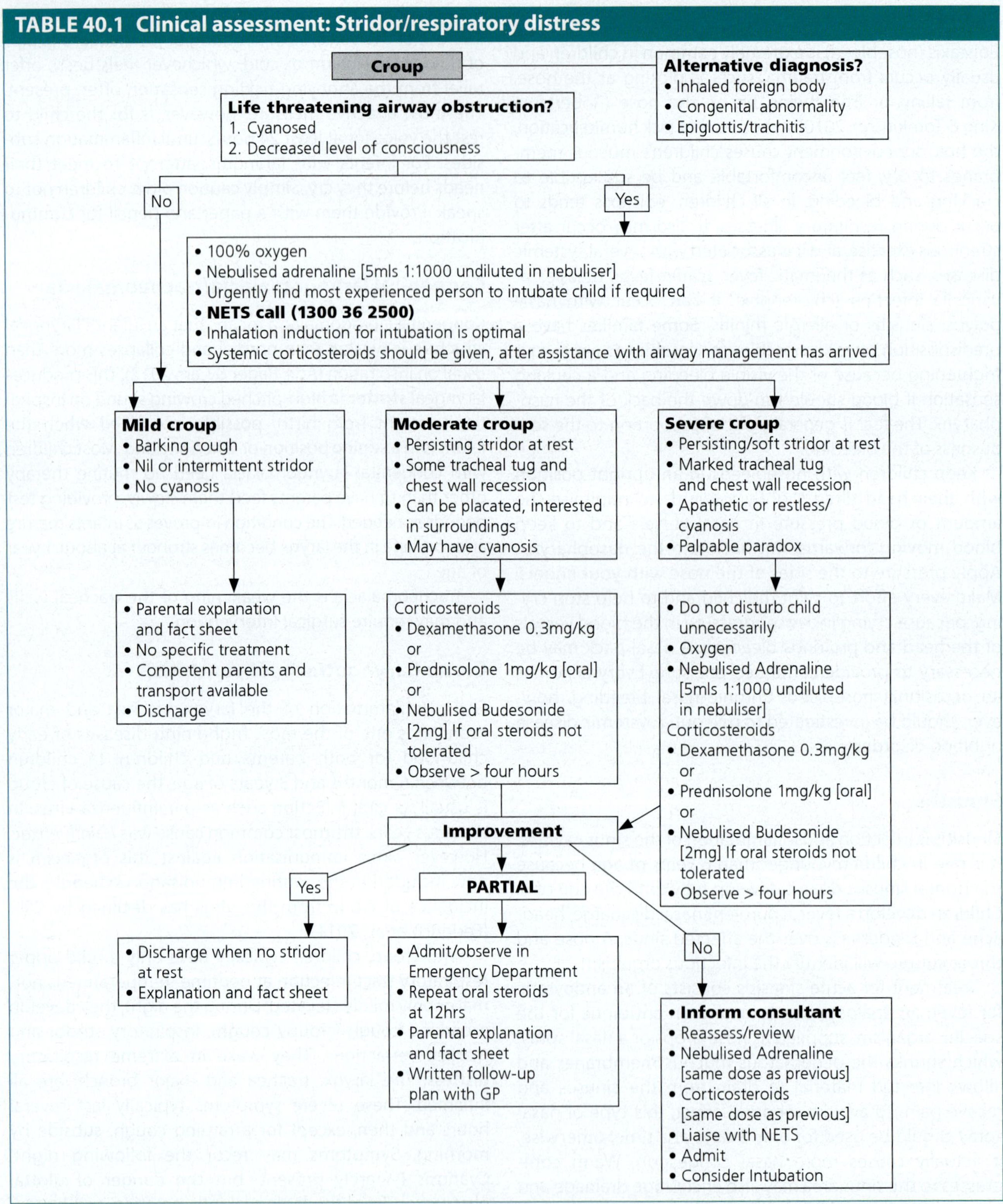

Source: NSW Health. (2010). Infants and children: Acute management of croup. Policy directive: PD2010_053. <www.health.nsw.gov.au/policies/pages/default.aspx>. Reproduced by permission, NSW Ministry of Health ©2015.

an emergency department for further evaluation and care. When a child is seen at an emergency room, cool moist air with a corticosteroid such as dexamethasone, given by nebuliser, reduces inflammation and produces effective bronchodilation to open the airway. Humidification is a common part of the acute treatment plan. Dependent on volume of oedema medical management may include adrenaline as per local policy. Intravenous therapy may be prescribed to keep the child well hydrated. Maintain accurate intake and output records and test urine specific gravity to ensure that hydration is adequate (see Table 40.1).

What if...

Michael, who had loud stridor when he was admitted, suddenly has no stridor present? Would you be relieved (his condition must be improving) or worried (his airway may be so blocked that not enough air is entering to make the sound of stridor)? How should you respond?

Epiglottitis

Epiglottitis is inflammation of the epiglottis and may be either bacterial or viral in origin. It occurs most frequently in children from 2 to about 8 years of age (Smith, 2011; see Table 40.2).

Although it is rare, inflammation of the epiglottis is potentially a medical emergency because the swollen epiglottis cannot rise and allow the airway to open. Complete airway obstruction may be present or occur if the airway is stimulated. Always be aware that the action of visualising the airway may be a precursor to stimulating the airway to obstruct. Care must be taken to keep the child calm and ensure appropriate medical staff are available if respiratory distress occurs.

Symptoms begin as those of a mild upper respiratory tract infection. After 1 or 2 days, as inflammation spreads to the epiglottis, the child suddenly develops severe inspiratory stridor, a high fever, hoarseness and a very sore throat. Children may have such difficulty swallowing that they drool saliva. They may protrude their tongue to increase free movement in the pharynx.

If a child's gag reflex is stimulated with a tongue blade (by a medical practitioner), the swollen and inflamed epiglottis is observed to rise in the back of the throat as a cherry-red structure. It can be so oedematous, however, that the gagging procedure causes complete obstruction of the glottis and shuts off the ability of the child to inhale. Therefore, in children with symptoms of epiglottitis (dysphagia, inspiratory stridor, cough, fever and hoarseness), never attempt to visualise the epiglottis directly with a tongue blade or obtain a throat culture unless a means of providing an artificial airway, such as tracheostomy or endotracheal intubation, is readily available. This is especially important for the nurse who functions in an expanded role and performs physical assessments and routinely elicits gag reflexes.

Children need moist air to reduce the epiglottal inflammation. If cyanosis is present, they need oxygen. An antibiotic may not be prescribed until a throat culture indicates a specific bacteria. Because they cannot swallow, children need intravenous fluid therapy to maintain hydration. They may need a prophylactic tracheostomy or endotracheal intubation to prevent total airway obstruction, although it is often difficult to intubate children with epiglottitis because the tube cannot be passed beyond the oedematous epiglottis. After antibiotic therapy begins, the epiglottal inflammation recedes rapidly. Antibiotic administration will continue for a full 7 to 10 days. Siblings of the ill child may be prescribed prophylactic antibiotic therapy to prevent them from developing the same symptoms.

Aspiration

Aspiration (inhalation of a foreign object into the airway) occurs most frequently in infants and toddlers. When a child aspirates a foreign object such as a coin or a peanut, the immediate reaction is choking and hard, forceful coughing. Usually, this dislodges the object. However, if the airway becomes so obstructed that coughing is impossible (no sound with cough) or if there are signs of increased respiratory difficulty accompanied by stridor, some intervention is essential. A series of subdiaphragmatic abdominal thrusts are recommended for children, the same as for

TABLE 40.2 Comparison of laryngotracheobronchitis (croup) and epiglottitis

Assessment	Laryngotracheobronchitis	Epiglottitis
Causative organism	Usually viral	Usually pneumococci or streptococci
Usual age of child	6 months–3 years	3–6 years
Seasonal occurrence	Late autumn and winter	None
Onset pattern	Preceded by upper respiratory infection; cough becomes worse at night	Preceded by upper respiratory infection; suddenly very ill
Presence of fever	Low grade	Elevated to about 39.4°C
Appearance	Retractions and stridor; prolonged inspiratory phase of respirations; not very ill-appearing	Drooling; very ill-appearing; neck hyperextended to breathe. (Do not attempt to view enlarged epiglottis or immediate airway obstruction can occur.)
Cough	Sharp, barking	Muffled cough
Radiography findings	Lateral neck x-ray showing subglottal narrowing	Lateral neck x-ray showing enlarged epiglottis
Possible complications	Asphyxia because of subglottic obstruction	Asphyxia because of supraglottic obstruction

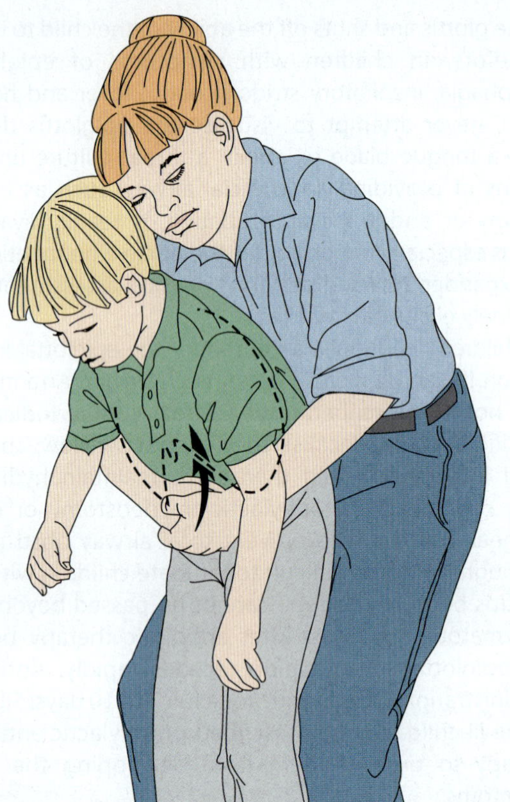

FIGURE 40.7 Subdiaphragmatic abdominal thrust on a school-aged child.

adults. This recommendation does not extend to infants, however, because of the great risk of rupturing the liver (American Heart Association, 2011).

To perform this manoeuvre, stand behind the child and place a fist just under the child's diaphragm (a point immediately below the anterior rib cage). Embrace the child, grip your fist with your other hand, and pull back and up with a rapid thrust (see Fig. 40.7). The pressure created by this action of pushing up on the diaphragm forces the aspirated material out of the trachea.

If a child is lying on their back at the time of the aspiration, stand at the head of the bed or table, place your hands in the same position as described above, and exert the same inward and upward thrust. A subdiaphragmatic abdominal manoeuvre may cause a child to vomit as well as expel an aspirated object. Turn the child's head to the side to prevent aspiration of vomitus.

For infants, use back thrusts to dislodge an aspirated object. Turn the infant prone over your arm and administer up to five quick back blows forcefully between the infant's shoulder blades, using the heel of the hand. If the object is not expelled, turn the infant while carefully supporting the head and neck and hold the infant in a supine position draped over your thigh. Be sure to keep the infant's head lower than their chest (see Fig. 40.8). This is generally enough to dislodge the foreign object. However, if this does not occur, rescue breathing may then be attempted.

Bronchial obstruction

The right main bronchus is straighter and has a larger lumen than the left bronchus in children older than 2 years of age. For this reason, an aspirated foreign object that is not large enough to obstruct the trachea may lodge in the right bronchus, obstructing a portion or all of the right lung. The alveoli distal to the obstruction will collapse as the air remaining in them becomes absorbed **(atelectasis)**, or hyperinflation and pneumothorax may occur if the foreign body serves as a ball valve, allowing air to enter but not leave the alveoli.

After aspirating a small foreign body, the child generally coughs violently and may become dyspnoeic. If the article is not expelled, haemoptysis, fever, purulent sputum and leucocytosis will generally result as infection develops. Localised wheezing (a high whistling sound on expiration made by air passing through the narrowed lumen) may occur. Because this is localised, it is different from the generalised wheezing of a child with asthma.

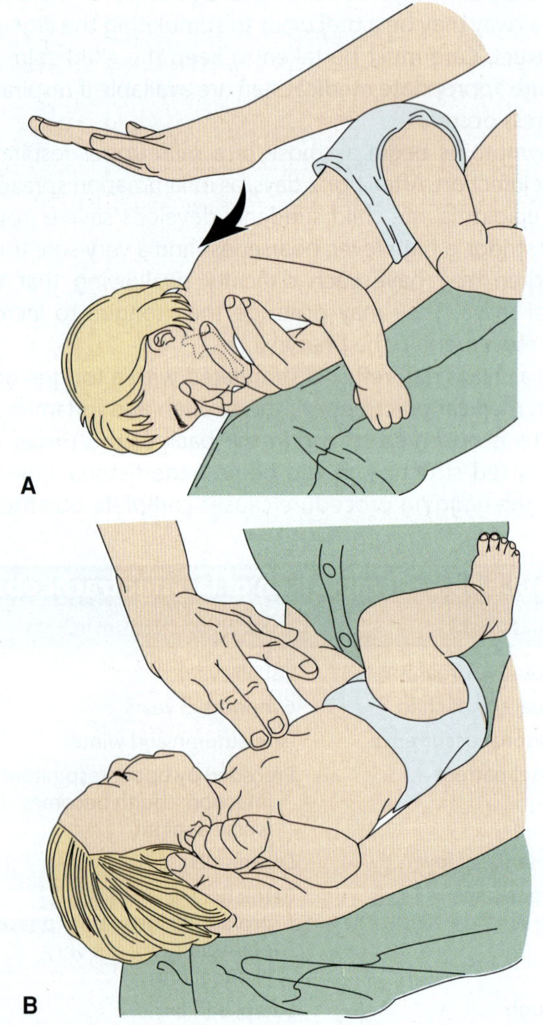

FIGURE 40.8 Back blows (**A**) and chest thrusts (**B**) to relieve complete foreign body airway obstruction in an infant. (From American Heart Association. (2008). *Resuscitation in the Newborn*. Dallas, TX: Author.)

A chest x-ray will reveal the presence of a radiopaque object. Objects such as plastic and nuts cannot be visualised well on x-ray film so an x-ray study may be inconclusive. Children who are seen in emergency departments after aspirating a foreign body are in distress from pain and are choking and coughing. Throughout, be vigilant in observing the child for coughing up the foreign body or developing increasing respiratory distress.

A bronchoscopy may be necessary to remove the foreign body (Bhat et al., 2010). Children are often given conscious sedation for a bronchoscopy. After bronchoscopy, assess the child closely for signs of bronchial oedema and airway obstruction that occurs from mucus accumulation because of the bronchus manipulation. Obtain frequent vital signs (increasing pulse and respiratory rates suggest increased oedema and obstruction).

DISORDERS OF THE LOWER RESPIRATORY TRACT

The structures of the lower respiratory tract are subject to infection by the same pathogens that attack the upper respiratory tract. Inflammation and infection of the lungs or bronchi is particularly troublesome: it occurs in various forms and is caused by several organisms. Other illnesses that occur in the lower respiratory tract, such as bronchiectasis, can lead to secondary pneumonia infections and chronic illness.

Influenza

Influenza involves inflammation and infection of the major airways. It is marked by a cough, fever, fatigue, aching pains, a sore throat and often accompanying gastrointestinal symptoms such as vomiting or diarrhoea. The disease spreads readily through close or confined contact with infected people who are contagious on the day before symptoms appear and for about the next 5 days.

Children usually need an antipyretic to control fever. Other regimens may include antiviral medications as well as influenza vaccines. Because the influenza virus mutates yearly, the influenza vaccine is specific for only that year and must be readministered yearly (Zimmerman, 2014).

Bronchitis

Bronchitis, or inflammation of the major bronchi and trachea, is one of the more common illnesses affecting preschool and school-aged children. It is characterised by fever and cough, usually in conjunction with nasal congestion. Children usually have a mild upper respiratory tract infection for 1 or 2 days; they then develop a fever and a dry, hacking cough, which is hoarse and mildly productive in older children. The cough is serious enough to wake a child from sleep. These symptoms may last for a week, with full recovery sometimes taking as long as 2 weeks.

On auscultation, rhonchi and coarse crackles can be heard. A chest x-ray will reveal diffuse alveolar hyperinflation and some markings at the hilus of the lung. Therapy is aimed at relieving respiratory symptoms, reducing fever and maintaining adequate hydration. An antibiotic is prescribed for bacterial infections. If mucus is viscid, an expectorant may be necessary to help the child raise sputum. It is important that children with bronchitis cough to raise accumulating sputum. Cough syrups to suppress coughing, therefore, are rarely indicated.

Bronchiolitis

Bronchiolitis is inflammation of the fine bronchioles and small bronchi. It is the most common lower respiratory illness in children younger than 2 years, peaking in incidence at 6 months of age. The infection occurs most often in the winter and spring. Many children who develop asthma later in life have numerous instances of bronchiolitis during their first year of life. Viruses, such as adenovirus, parainfluenza virus and RSV, in particular, appear to be the pathogens most responsible for the infection (Black & Brennan, 2011).

Typically, infants have 1 or 2 days of an upper respiratory tract infection, then suddenly begin to demonstrate nasal flaring, intercostal and subcostal retractions on inspiration, and an increased respiratory rate. They may have a mild fever, leucocytosis, and an increased erythrocyte sedimentation rate, indicating the amount of bronchial inflammation present. Both accumulating mucus and inflammation block the small bronchioles, so air can no longer enter or leave alveoli freely. Most infants develop alveolar hyperinflation because air enters more easily than it leaves inflamed, narrowed bronchioles. This increases the expiratory phase of respiration and can create wheezing. After initial hyperinflation, areas of atelectasis in alveoli may occur as the air that cannot be expired is absorbed. Tachycardia and cyanosis develop from hypoxia. Infants soon become exhausted from rapid respirations. A chest x-ray may show pulmonary infiltrates caused by a secondary infection or collapse of alveoli (atelectasis). Pulse oximetry shows low oxygen saturation. A throat culture will identify the offending organism.

For children with less severe symptoms, antipyretics, adequate hydration and maintaining a watchful eye for progression to more serious illness is all that is necessary. Hospitalisation is warranted for children in severe distress such as when an infant is tachypnoeic, has marked retractions, seems listless or has a history of poor fluid intake.

Antibiotics are not commonly used in the treatment of bronchiolitis because bacteria are rarely a causative factor (Spurling et al., 2011). Children with chronic pulmonary disease may receive anti-RSV immunoglobulin if RSV (respiratory syncytial virus) was identified as the causative agent. If symptoms are severe, children need humidified oxygen to counteract hypoxaemia and adequate hydration to keep respiratory membranes moist. Nebulised bronchodilators, adrenaline and anti-inflammatory medications such as nebulised budesonide (a glucocorticoid steroid) may be used, although there is little evidence they make a major difference in reducing symptoms. Some children need ventilatory assistance to achieve adequate ventilation. All infants with bronchiolitis need to be carefully observed because if RSV is the cause, apnoea may occur. In some infants, extracorporeal membrane oxygenation (the same as that used for heart surgery) is necessary to maintain adequate oxygenation (Babl et al., 2008). Feeding is often a problem because infants tire easily and therefore cannot finish a feed. Intravenous fluids may be given for the first 1 or 2 days of illness to eliminate the need for oral feeding.

Respiratory syncytial virus bronchiolitis

RSV is the most common cause of bronchiolitis in young children. Symptoms begin as a mild upper respiratory infection that quickly extends to include the bronchioles. The infant becomes lethargic and possibly cyanotic. Dehydration occurs as the child becomes too fatigued to suck. Respiratory distress with nasal flaring, retractions, grunting, rales, rhonchi and expiratory wheezing noted on auscultation occur. All infants with an RSV infection must be monitored closely because the virus tends to cause apnoea or periodic halting of respirations. The diagnosis is confirmed by throat or nasal culture.

Therapy is supportive (supplemental oxygen and hydration therapy), although life-threatening apnoea may require ventilatory support with mechanical ventilation. Ribavirin, an antiviral agent, is effective against RSV, but is controversial as the medication is teratogenic and could be harmful to pregnant carers (Ventre & Randolph, 2007). Because RSV infection spreads readily from one child to the next, infants should be isolated for care. Nursing care should be organised so nurses do not care for infants other than those infected with RSV.

The disease peaks in severity between 48 to 72 hours. Recurrent apnoeic episodes are rare, so home monitoring for apnoeic episodes is usually not necessary. Two products are available for the prevention of RSV infection: RSV immune globulin intravenous (RSV-IGIV), made from RSV antibody-positive donor serum, and Palivizumab, a humanised monoclonal antibody produced by recombinant DNA technology. These may be given prophylactically to premature infants during the winter months (Federico et al., 2011).

Asthma

Asthma primarily affects the lower airways and involves three separate processes: bronchospasm, inflammation of bronchial mucosa and increased bronchial secretions (mucus). All three processes act to reduce the size of the airway lumen, leading to acute respiratory distress. Children's smaller airway lumens predispose them to higher levels of mucus plugging which may present as altered breath sounds within a lobe and is a precursor to hypoxia. The diagnosis of asthma is based on the assessment of cough, breathlessness and wheeze. This is further supported by a clinical response to medications, particularly bronchodilators.

Assessment

History

Assessment should include a thorough history of the development of a child's symptoms—for example, what the child was doing at the time of the attack, and what actions were taken by the parents or child to decrease or stop the symptoms. A thorough family history will be completed including respiratory and inflammatory conditions as well as common triggers such as smoking exposure. When an acute attack has passed, ask the parent or child to describe the home environment, including pets, the child's bedroom, outdoor play space, classroom environment, and type of heating, flooring and furnishing coverings in the house, to see whether more environmental control could reduce future occurrences.

Physical assessment

A physical assessment includes examining for the specific symptoms of asthma. Listen for air entry and compare across all zones. Ascertain if wheeze is audible with or without a stethoscope as well as lung zones affected. Audible wheezing in only one lobe suggests that only one bronchus is plugged, which may suggest a mucus plug (or foreign body). Cyanosis may be present. The eosinophil count is commonly elevated.

Bronchospasm leads to CO_2 trapping and retention; therefore, arterial oxygen saturation monitored by a pulse oximeter will begin to decrease because of the child's inability to fully aerate and oxygenate the lungs. The child becomes frightened because of an acute feeling of suffocation. A peak flow meter (if applicable) shows decreased ability to exhale.

Also observe for retractions (the chest wall is drawn inward with breaths) because children have to use intercostal accessory muscles to achieve full breaths. As constriction increases, wheezing may decrease because so little air can leave the alveoli. Hypoxaemia and possibly cyanosis will become severe. When blood gases show an increased P_{CO_2} level and the sound of wheezing suddenly stops, respiratory failure is imminent.

During attacks, children with asthma are generally more comfortable in a sitting, tripod or standing position. An age-specific assessment of mental state will assist in determining effects of hypoxia. The carers will need to be included, as appropriate, to advise on any alterations they have noted.

Peak expiratory flow rate monitoring

Adolescent children with asthma often use a home peak flow meter daily to measure gross changes in peak expiratory flow over time and help in planning an appropriate therapeutic regimen. Children with asthma should be able to tell you their usual reading and personal best score. This is all predetermined on their asthma action plan designed with their local doctor. It is considered that a symptom-based action plan can be superior to a peak flow plan providing earlier identification of deterioration as peak flow measure is a subjective effort dependent reading (NSW Health, 2012).

Therapeutic management

Therapy for children with asthma involves planning for the three goals of all allergic disorders: avoidance of the allergen by environmental control; skin testing and hyposensitisation to identified allergens; and relief of symptoms by pharmacological agents (McMullen et al., 2007). Cough suppressants are contraindicated with asthma because, as a rule, as long as children can continue to cough up mucus, they are not in serious danger. When they stop coughing up mucus, thick plugs form that then may lead to pneumonia, atelectasis and further acidosis.

A child with mild but persistent asthma is usually prescribed an inhaled anti-inflammatory corticosteroid daily. Children who have moderate persistent symptoms are usually prescribed a long-acting bronchodilator at bedtime in addition to the inhaled anti-inflammatory daily corticosteroid. Children who have severe persistent asthma symptoms take a high dose of both an oral corticosteroid and an inhaled corticosteroid daily as well as a long-acting bronchodilator at bedtime. In addition, children may be prescribed a short-acting beta$_2$-agonist bronchodilator, to use if an attack should begin. Another group of medications used in the treatment of asthma are leukotriene receptor antagonists (Blakey & Wardlaw, 2012). These medications are used for prophylaxis and chronic treatment of asthma in children over 6 years of age. They are not effective in an acute attack.

Dehydration occurs rapidly in children during an asthma attack because they have decreased oral intake (children stop drinking because they are coughing, or coughing makes them vomit and parents stop offering fluid) as well as increased insensible loss that occurs from tachypnoea. Dehydration may contribute to increased mucus plugging and further airway obstruction. Encourage children to continue to drink fluids (ask about favourite beverages and offer small sips of them). Avoid milk or milk products because they cause thick mucus and difficulty swallowing. In an emergency setting, an intravenous line is established to supply continuous fluid therapy and also provide a route for emergency medication administration.

Status asthmaticus

Under ordinary circumstances, an asthma attack responds readily to the aerosol administration of a bronchodilator. When children fail to respond and an attack continues, they are in *status asthmaticus*. This is an extreme emergency because, if the attack cannot be relieved, a child may die of heart failure caused by the combination of exhaustion, atelectasis and respiratory acidosis from bronchial plugging. A child with status asthmaticus is in acute respiratory distress. Elevated heart and respiratory rates are seen as well as low oxygen saturation. In contrast to the loud wheezing initially heard in an asthma attack, children with status asthmaticus may have so little air able to pass in or out of their lungs that breath sounds are limited.

Continuous nebulisation with an inhaled beta$_2$-agonist and intravenous corticosteroids may be necessary to reduce symptoms. Oxygen is given to maintain the Po_2 above 90 mmHg. To prevent drying of pulmonary secretions, oxygen may be given with humidification. If oxygen concentrations greater than 40% are needed, a Venturi mask that allows for greater accuracy of oxygen delivery and decreases rebreathing may be used. In severe cases adrenaline may be indicated as per local policy.

During the acute stage of status asthmaticus, children need increased fluid to combat dehydration and keep airway secretions moist. Drinking tends to increase coughing, so an intravenous infusion is usually ordered. If a child can drink, do not offer cold fluids because these tend to aggravate bronchospasm. Monitor intake and output and measure the specific gravity of urine to reflect hydration status. An increasing Pco_2 is a danger sign because it indicates the degree of hypoventilation. In severe attacks, endotracheal intubation and mechanical ventilation may be necessary to maintain effective respirations (Lim et al., 2012; see Table 40.3).

Bronchiectasis

Bronchiectasis is chronic dilation and plugging of the bronchi. It may follow pneumonia, aspiration of a foreign body, pertussis or asthma. Children develop a chronic cough with mucopurulent sputum (Federico et al., 2011). Young infants may have accompanying wheezing or stridor. If a large area of lung is involved, children may have cyanosis. As the disease becomes chronic, children develop symptoms of chronic lung disease, such as clubbing of the fingers and easy fatigability. Their physical growth may become restricted. Their chest may become enlarged from overinflation of alveoli caused by the air trapped behind inflamed bronchi. Inhaled mucolytic agents or bronchodilators and chest physiotherapy may be necessary to raise the tenacious sputum. An antibiotic will be necessary if infection is present.

Pneumonia

Pneumonia (infection and inflammation of alveoli) may be of bacterial origin (pneumococcal, streptococcal, staphylococcal or chlamydial) or viral in origin, such as RSV. Aspiration of lipid or hydrocarbon substances also causes pneumonia. The disease is commonly divided into two types: hospital acquired (pneumococcal or streptococcal

TABLE 40.3 Infants and children: Acute management of asthma

Initial severity assessment

Treat in the highest category in which any symptom occurs

Symptoms	Mild Likely to go home	Moderate Possibly be admitted	Severe and life threatening will be admitted or transferred
Oximetry in air	>94%	90-94%	<90%
Heart rate	Close to normal range for age	Mild-Moderate Tachycardia for age	Marked Tachycardia - beware relative Bradycardia for age
(age appropriate) **Ability to talk in:**	Sentences or Long vigorous Cry	Phrases or Shortened Cry	Words / Weak Cry or Unable to Speak / Cry
Accessory muscle use	None	Mild to Moderate	Moderate to Severe
Altered consciousness	Alert Age Appropriate	Easily Engaged Age Appropriate	Be concerned if Agitated or Drowsy or Confused
Cyanosis in air	None	None	Any Cyanosis is very concerning
			Get consultant help then Call NETS 1300 36 2500
Treatment			
Oxygen	No	To maintain SaO2 >94%	To maintain SaO2 >94% Consider High flow Oxygen
Salbutamol 100 micrograms metered dose inhaler (MDI) & spacer	<6 years **6 x** puffs stat ≥6 years **12 x** puffs stat **review frequently and repeat when required**	<6 years **6 x** puffs ≥6 years **12 x** puffs **Give 20 minutely x 3 then repeat as required**	**Severe – see page 10** <6 years **6 x** puffs ≥6 years **12 x** puffs **Give 20 minutely x 3** with Ipratropium **Reassess**
			OR
Salbutamol nebulised	Not recommended	Not recommended	**Life threatening** - Continuous nebulised Salbutamol **(5mg/mL undiluted)** with Ipratropium (3 doses as below) until improvement **Reassess**
Ipratropium (atrovent) 20 micrograms (3 doses always together with Salbutamol)	No	Consider **20 minutely x 3** <6 years - 4 puffs MDI ≥6 years - 8 puffs MDI	**Yes - 20 minutely x 3** <6 years - 4 puffs MDI or 250mcg Neb Ipratropium ≥6 years - 8 puffs MDI or 500mcg Neb Ipratropium
No or Poor response to Treatment	Check diagnosis and treat as per Moderate	Check diagnosis and treat as per Severe and Life Threatening	**Immediate Senior Review -Consult PICU (via NETS if outside a children's hospital)**
If contemplating giving any of IV salbutamol, IV aminophylline or IV magnesium sulphate	Not applicable	Not applicable	If no or poor response to Nebulised Salbutamol, contact **senior help or PICU via (NETS 1300 36 2500) for discussion regarding retrieval**
Systemic corticosteroids	Consider Oral Prednisone 1-2mg/kg depending on history and response to treatment	Oral Prednisone 1-2mg/kg	Hydrocortisone IV 4mg/kg or Methylprednisone IV 1mg/kg
Investigations	Nil (routine) required	Nil routine required Consider Chest X-ray if focal signs	Consider Blood Gases, Chest X-ray and UEC
Observation & review	Observations (HR, RR and O2 Sats) pre and post treatment – minimum hourly for 3 hours. MO review prior to discharge	Continuous observations (HR, RR and O2 Sats). Observations pre and post treatment –initially Q 30min then MO review within 1 hour	Continuous cardiorespiratory monitoring (HR, RR and O2 Sats) Regular medical review
Disposition	Home if Salbutamol requirement >3hourly See 'Discharge Criteria'	Observe for 3 hours after last dose. If not suitable for discharge then – Admit or Transfer. Otherwise home.	Admit to Level 4 facility or above if improving or retrieve to Paediatric ICU (call NETS)

Source: NSW Health. (2012). Infants and children: Acute management of asthma. Policy directive: PD2012_056. <www.health.nsw.gov.au/policies/pages/default.aspx>. Reproduced by permission, NSW Ministry of Health © 2015.

pneumonia) and community acquired (chlamydia, viral pneumonias). It is the most common pulmonary cause of death in infants younger than 48 hours of age. It occurs most often in late winter and early spring. Newborns, who are born more than 24 hours after rupture of the amniotic membranes and those who aspirated amniotic fluid or meconium during birth are particularly prone to developing pneumonia in their first few days of life (Raab, 2013). When it is known that the fetal membranes have been ruptured for more than 24 hours before birth, prophylactic broad-spectrum antibiotics may be given to prevent pneumonia.

Pneumococcal pneumonia

The onset of pneumococcal pneumonia is generally abrupt and follows an upper respiratory tract infection. In infants, pneumonia tends to remain bronchopneumonia with poor consolidation (infiltration of exudate into the alveoli). In older children, pneumonia may localise in a single lobe and consolidation may occur. With this, children may have blood-tinged sputum as exudative serum and red blood cells invade the alveoli. After 24 to 48 hours, the alveoli are no longer filled with red blood cells and serum but fibrin, leucocytes and pneumococci. At this point, the child's cough no longer raises blood-tinged sputum but thick purulent material.

Children develop a high fever, nasal flaring, retractions, chest pain, chills and dyspnoea. Some children report the pain as being abdominal. Febrile convulsions may occur in severe cases. Children with pneumococcal pneumonia appear acutely ill. Tachypnoea and tachycardia develop. Crackles may be present as a result of the fluid in the alveoli. Dullness on percussion over a lobe indicates that total consolidation has occurred. Chest x-rays will usually show this type of lung consolidation in older children but only patchy diffusion in young children. Laboratory studies will indicate leucocytosis.

Therapy for pneumococcal pneumonia is antibiotics (Federico et al., 2011). Children need rest to prevent exhaustion. Plan nursing care carefully to conserve the child's strength. At the same time, turn and reposition a child frequently to avoid pooling of secretions. Intravenous therapy may be necessary to supply fluid, especially in infants, because infants tire so readily with sucking they may not be able to achieve a good oral intake. They may need an antipyretic to reduce fever.

Humidified oxygen may be necessary to alleviate laboured breathing and prevent hypoxaemia. Assess oxygen saturation levels frequently via pulse oximetry. Chest physiotherapy encourages the movement of mucus and prevents obstruction. Older children may need to be encouraged to cough so that secretions do not pool and become further infected. Following pneumonia, children usually have a period of at least a week when they tire easily and need frequent, small feedings. Parents need to be cautioned that this degree of fatigue is an expected outcome and not a complication in itself. Children with chronic illness, those who have had a splenectomy or those who are immunocompromised should receive a pneumococcal vaccine to prevent pneumococcal pneumonia.

Viral pneumonia

Viral pneumonia is generally caused by the viruses of upper respiratory tract infection. Symptoms begin as an upper respiratory tract infection. After a day or two, additional symptoms such as a low-grade fever, non-productive cough and tachypnoea begin. There may be diminished breath sounds and fine crackles on chest auscultation. Chest x-rays will show diffuse infiltrated areas.

Because this is a viral infection, antibiotic therapy is usually not effective. The child needs rest and, possibly, an antipyretic for the fever. Intravenous fluid may be necessary if a child becomes exhausted or is dehydrated and refusing fluids. After recovery from the acute phase of illness, a child will have a week or two of lethargy or lack of energy, the same as occurs with bacterial pneumonia.

Atelectasis

Atelectasis is the collapse of lung alveoli. It may occur in children as a primary or secondary condition. It must be considered as a possibility in all children with respiratory distress.

Primary atelectasis

Primary atelectasis occurs in newborns who do not breathe with enough respiratory strength at birth to inflate lung tissue or whose alveoli are so immature or so lacking in surfactant that alveoli cannot expand. When atelectasis occurs, the newborn's respirations become irregular, with nasal flaring and apnoea. After a few minutes, a respiratory grunt and cyanosis may occur. The sound of a respiratory grunt is caused by the newborn's glottis closing on expiration. At first this is a helpful action because it increases pressure in the respiratory tract, keeps alveoli from collapsing and allows for better alveoli exchange surfaces. This action is also tiring, however, and as the infant tires, hypoxaemia will increase and the infant will become hypotonic and flaccid. The Apgar score will invariably be low. As infants cry or are administered oxygen, more alveoli become aerated and cyanosis may decrease. The cause of the atelectasis must be established, however, so that therapy directed to the specific cause can be initiated.

Secondary atelectasis

Secondary atelectasis occurs in children when they have a respiratory tract obstruction that prevents air from entering a portion of the alveoli. As the residual air in the alveoli is absorbed, the alveoli collapse. The causes of obstruction in children include mucus plugs that may occur with chronic respiratory disease or aspiration of foreign objects. In some children, atelectasis occurs because of pressure on lung tissue from outside forces, such as compression from a diaphragmatic hernia, scoliosis or enlarged thoracic lymph nodes.

The signs of secondary atelectasis depend on the degree of collapse. Asymmetry of the chest may be noticed. Breath sounds on the affected side are decreased. If the process is extensive, tachypnoea and cyanosis will be present. A chest x-ray will show the collapsed alveoli (a "whiteout"). Children with atelectasis are prone to secondary infection because mucus, which provides a good medium for bacteria, becomes stagnant without air exchange.

Atelectasis caused by inspiration of a foreign object will not be relieved until the object is removed by bronchoscopy. Atelectasis caused by a mucus plug will resolve when the plug resolves, is moved or expectorated. Children may need oxygen and assisted ventilation to maintain adequate respiratory function until this time (Carter & Marshall, 2014). A semi-Fowler's position generally allows for the best lung expansion because it lowers abdominal contents and increases chest space. Raise the humidity of the child's environment to prevent further bronchial plugging; suction and chest physiotherapy may be necessary to keep the respiratory tract clear and free of mucus. Observe closely for increased respirations or cyanosis, as these indicate failing oxygenation.

Pneumothorax

Pneumothorax is the presence of atmospheric air in the pleural space; its presence causes the alveoli to collapse (atelectasis). Pneumothorax in children usually occurs when air seeps from ruptured alveoli and collects in the pleural cavity. It can also occur when external puncture wounds allow air to enter the chest (Janssen & Cardillo, 2011). The infant develops tachypnoea, grunting respirations, flaring of the nares and cyanosis. Auscultation reveals absent or decreased breath sounds on the affected side. Percussion may not be revealing, despite the hollow air space; as so much air is present, this may be hyperresonant. A more revealing sign may be the shift of the apical pulse (mediastinal shift) away from the site of the pneumothorax and the resulting atelectasis. A chest film will show the darkened area of the air-filled pleural space.

A child with a pneumothorax needs oxygen therapy to relieve respiratory distress. A thoracotomy catheter or needle may be placed in the pleural space (by the doctor) and atmospheric air aspirated or low-pressure suction with water-seal drainage applied to remove accumulated air. In most children with pneumothorax, symptoms are relieved within 24 hours after suction is begun.

If the air in the pleural space is from a puncture wound such as a stab wound, cover the chest wound immediately with an impervious material, such as gauze, to prevent further air from entering and help decrease the possibility of atelectasis. In an emergency, an impervious object can be your gloved hand.

Pneumothorax is always a potentially serious respiratory problem. The extent of the symptoms and the outcome will depend on the cause of entry of air into the pleural space and whether it can be removed.

Bronchopulmonary dysplasia

Bronchopulmonary dysplasia is chronic pulmonary involvement that occurs in 10–40% of infants who are treated for acute respiratory distress in the first days of life (Hayes et al., 2010). The condition most often occurs in infants who received mechanical ventilation for respiratory distress syndrome at birth. The condition is thought to occur from a combination of surfactant deficiency (decreased from lung trauma), barotrauma (lung damage from ventilator pressure), oxygen toxicity (from high levels needed to counteract the original respiratory distress) and continuing inflammation. It occurs most often in infants born weighing less than 1000 g.

Tuberculosis

Tuberculosis is a highly contagious pulmonary disease. The mode of transmission is inhalation of infected droplets. The incubation period is 2 to 10 weeks (Starke, 2007). Children generally contract this disease from someone in the immediate family. When any member of a family contracts tuberculosis, all family members must be tested (a Mantoux skin test) to screen for the disease. In some children, the contact is not known, and the disease is first detected when symptoms appear. Children who are homeless or severely impoverished or who have chronic illness or malnutrition tend to be more susceptible than others because of their overall susceptibility to infection. It also occurs at a higher incidence in internationally adopted children (Raviglione et al., 2012).

When *tuberculosis* invades a child's lung, there is primary inflammation. The child develops a slight cough. As the disease progresses, anorexia, weight loss, night sweats and a low-grade fever occur. If a child is in poor health or does not have adequate calcium intake for the body to confine the infection, tuberculosis may spread to other lung areas or to other parts of the body (miliary tuberculosis). Common body sites that may be affected are bones and joints, lymph nodes, kidneys and the subarachnoid space (tuberculous meningitis).

A positive Mantoux reaction (the formation of 5–15 mm of reddened induration) indicates the child has been exposed to tuberculosis or has developed antibodies to the foreign products of the tuberculosis organism. Children with positive reactions need follow-up with a chest x-ray to ascertain whether a current infection exists. Skin testing should not be done on children who are known to have had tuberculosis. Such a child will have such an intense reaction that the skin at the site of the test may slough and necrose.

In the early course of tuberculosis, because the initial focus of the tuberculosis is so small, it may not be evident on a chest x-ray. As local inflammation occurs, however, cloudiness in the inflamed area will be noticeable on the film, as will calcification.

To confirm a diagnosis of active disease, sputum may be analysed. Children who have primary tuberculosis are not infectious because they have a minimal pulmonary lesion and little or no cough. They need not be isolated. As soon as medication therapy has been started, they can return to regular activities, including school. Treatment regimens will vary and be case specific dependent on the severity and length of illness of the individual child.

Cystic fibrosis

Children with cystic fibrosis (CF) have a generalised dysfunction of the exocrine glands (Brashers, 2012). Mucous secretions of the body, particularly in the pancreas and the lungs, are so tenacious that they have difficulty flowing through gland ducts. There is also a marked electrolyte change in the secretions of the sweat glands (chloride concentration of sweat is two to five times above normal). The cause of the disorder is an abnormality of the long arm of chromosome 7. This results in the inability to transport small molecules across cell membranes; this leads to dehydration of epithelial cells in the airway and pancreas, and dried secretions.

Boys with CF may not be able to reproduce because they have persistent plugging and blocking of the vas deferens from tenacious seminal fluid. Girls may have such thick cervical secretions that sperm penetration is limited. Artificial insemination or in vitro fertilisation can be accomplished if they desire to become pregnant.

Pancreas involvement

The pancreas normally produces enzymes lipase, trypsin and amylase, that flow into the duodenum to digest fat, protein and carbohydrate. With CF, these enzyme secretions become so thickened they plug the ducts; eventually, there is such back-pressure the pancreas is no longer capable of producing the enzymes. Without pancreatic enzymes in the duodenum, children cannot digest fat, protein and some sugars. The child's stools become large, bulky and greasy **(steatorrhoea)**. The intestinal flora increases because of the undigested food; this, when combined with the fat in the stool, gives the stool an extremely foul odour, often compared to that of a cat's stool. Meconium in a newborn is normally thick and tenacious. In approximately 10% of children with CF, it may be so thick, because pancreatic enzymes are lacking, that it obstructs the intestine (meconium ileus). The newborn develops abdominal distension with no passage of stool.

Lung involvement

Thickened mucus pools in bronchioles. Pockets of infection then begin in these secretions. Bronchiectasis and pneumonia result. Respiratory acidosis occurs and atelectasis is common. The child's fingers become clubbed because of the inadequate peripheral tissue perfusion. The anterior-posterior diameter of the chest becomes enlarged.

Sweat gland involvement

Although the sweat glands themselves do not appear to be changed in structure, the electrolyte composition of perspiration is changed.

Assessment

Children who are not diagnosed at birth may be seen in a healthcare setting at about 1 month of age because of a feeding problem. Using only about 50% of their intake because of their poor digestive function, they are always hungry. This causes them to eat so ravenously they tend to swallow air. This leads to colic or abdominal distension and vomiting. The appearance of typical CF stools (large and greasy) is an important finding because children with simple colic do not show these changes in stool consistency.

Respiratory infections develop at 4–6 months of age. Even at this early stage of the disease, wheezing and rhonchi may be heard on chest auscultation. By the time a child with CF is a preschooler, a cough is a prominent finding. On percussion, the chest is hyperresonant, reflecting the emphysema present. Rales and rhonchi are heard. Clubbing of the fingers may already be apparent. It is rare for a child to go undiagnosed beyond this time because the symptoms of the illness have become so persistent and evident.

Sweat testing

Sweat testing may occur at the doctor's request and assesses the sodium chloride content on the skin.

Duodenal analysis

Analysis of duodenal secretions for detection of pancreatic enzymes reveals the extent of the pancreatic involvement. This is done by passing a nasogastric tube into the duodenum and then aspirating secretions for analysis.

Stool analysis

Stool may be collected and analysed for fat content and lack of trypsin, although description of the large greasy appearance may be all that is necessary.

Pulmonary testing

A chest x-ray generally confirms the extent of the pulmonary involvement (pockets of emphysema and perhaps the beginning of pneumonia infiltration are present). Pulmonary function tests may be done to determine if atelectasis and emphysema are present.

Nursing considerations

Imbalanced nutrition

The child's height and weight follow percentile growth curves; the quantity of stool decreases; signs and symptoms of vitamin deficiency are absent. Children with CF are placed on a high-kilojoule, high-protein and moderate-fat diet. Water-soluble forms of vitamins A, D and E are supplemented. Generally, infants with CF cannot be totally breastfed because there is not enough protein in breast milk for them (they need large amounts because they cannot make use of all the protein they ingest). Breastfeeding with supplementary formula is required. Because children with CF have a ravenous appetite, they eat well. Before each meal or snack, they need to take a synthetic pancreatic enzyme, pancreatic lipase (Cotazym or Pancrease), to replace the enzyme they cannot produce.

Ineffective airway clearance

The child's temperature is below 38.0°C and decreased work of breathing is evident. Unfortunately, the pulmonary effects of CF progress despite supplementation with pancreatic enzyme; infection from plugged airways is always a possibility. Therefore, it is important to try to keep bronchial secretions as moist and freely flowing as possible so they can drain from the bronchial tree. This is done by frequent nebulisation or aerosol therapy followed by chest physiotherapy.

Be certain to observe children with CF frequently because their condition can change rapidly. If a portion of a lung becomes obstructed by a plug of mucus, a child can quickly experience respiratory difficulty. The right side of the heart tends to enlarge in children with chronic respiratory disease because the congestion in the lungs increases pressure in the pulmonary artery and the right ventricle. After a period of stress or exercise, children may begin to show signs of cardiac failure because their already enlarged heart cannot compensate any further.

Humidified oxygen. Oxygen is supplied to children by mask or nasal prongs and mist delivery may be applicable to decrease droplet size.

Aerosol therapy. Aerosol therapy, by means of a nebuliser, to provide antibiotics or bronchodilators may be given three or four times a day. A mucolytic, such as acetylcysteine (Mucomyst), can be added to the mist to aid in diluting and liquefying secretions. Children's coughs will become loose and productive after using aerosol therapy. Never give cough syrups to suppress a cough because getting secretions out is essential for air exchange and to prevent infection. Likewise, question an order for codeine as an analgesic because codeine suppresses the cough reflex.

Chest physiotherapy. Because the bronchial secretions with CF are so tenacious, and to aid drainage of secretions, children need chest physiotherapy frequently, approximately three or four times a day.

Activity

Children with CF need to maintain their usual activities as much as possible within their exercise tolerance levels.

Respiratory hygiene

The sputum that a child coughs up may have a disagreeable taste or odour. Offer frequent mouth care, tooth-brushing and a good-tasting mouthwash to make the child's mouth feel fresh.

Risk of compromised family coping related to chronic illness in a child

Adequate rest and comfort. Any child who has compromised lung function has a degree of dyspnoea that leads to exhaustion. Plan a rest period before meals so that a child is not too tired to eat. Also plan for a long rest period before chest physiotherapy so that a child will be able to tolerate it better. Achieving a balance between allowing periods of rest and yet not doing all procedures at once, is not an easy task.

Continuing care. It is particularly important that children with CF receive the pertussis and measles vaccines because these two infections cause severe respiratory complications. Children also should receive influenza, meningococcal and pneumococcal vaccines. As children with CF reach adolescence, they are candidates for lung transplants. Some of these are done as lower lobe transplants from a living donor. People who donate a single lobe in this manner report that they feel little loss of lung capacity afterward. A lung transplant is advantageous for children with CF because the new lung does not possess the defective gene that caused mucus to be so thick. Lifespan can greatly improve.

Key points for review

- Respiratory tract disorders tend to occur more frequently in children than adults because the lumens of children's bronchi are narrow and obstruction and infection can occur more easily.
- Acute nasopharyngitis (common cold) is the most common infectious disease in children. There is no specific therapy for a common cold other than comfort measures.
- Tonsillitis is infection and inflammation of the tonsils. Adenitis is infection and inflammation of the adenoid tonsils. Children with recurring infections may have their tonsils surgically removed.
- Laryngotracheobronchitis (croup) is inflammation of the larynx, trachea and major bronchi. Epiglottitis is inflammation of the epiglottis. Both of these conditions can cause severe impairment of the airway.
- Bronchitis is inflammation of the major bronchi and trachea. Bronchiolitis is inflammation of the fine bronchioles. Both conditions are caused by bacterial or viral invasion.
- Respiratory syncytial virus infection is an infection that accounts for the majority of lower respiratory infections in young children. Infants with RSV infections must be observed closely because they are prone to apnoea.
- Pneumonia may occur from a variety of organisms (except for viral pneumonia, children need specific antibiotics, depending on the organism present). Infants with respiratory illness need extremely close observation because they cannot describe oxygen deprivation.
- Tuberculosis is a lung infection, with some strains becoming very resistant to the usual therapy.
- Cystic fibrosis is a disease in which there is generalised dysfunction of the exocrine glands. This results in malabsorption and tenacious pulmonary secretions, leading to infection and pneumonia. Lung transplantation can be used to replace the diseased lung tissue and increase the child's life span.

CASE STUDY QUESTIONS

5. Michael's grandmother brought him to the emergency room because his respirations were rapid and he had a sharp, barking cough. He is diagnosed as having laryngotracheobronchitis (croup). He was crying loudly. What about Michael's actions would lead you to believe his airway is not yet extremely constricted? Would you encourage him to lie down and rest? What emergency care does Michael need?
6. One of Michael's observation unit roommates has a permanent tracheostomy tube in place from pulmonary dysplasia as an infant. Her parents are going to enrol her in kindergarten starting next month. What precautions would you want to review with her parents to keep this experience safe?
7. When the 4-year-old in the ambulatory bed next to Michael returns from tonsillectomy surgery, what observations would be most important to make? Why is the seventh day after tonsillectomy surgery a particularly important day for close observation?

Resources

For an extensive range of additional resources to enhance teaching and learning and to facilitate understanding of this chapter, please see the text's accompanying website located on thePoint at http://thepoint.lww.com.

References

Abadesso, C., Nunes, P., Silvestre, C., Matias, E., Loureiro, H. & Almeida, H. (2012). Non-invasive ventilation in acute respiratory failure in children. *Pediatric Reports*, *4*(2), e16.

Adil, E., Rager, T. & Carr, M. (2012). Location of airway obstruction in term and preterm infants with laryngomalacia. *American Journal of Otolaryngology*, *33*(4), 437–440.

Altamimi, S., Khalil, A., Khalaiwi, K. A., Milner, R. A, Pusic, M. V. & Al Othman, M. A. (2012). Short-term late generation antibiotics versus longer term penicillin for acute streptococcal pharyngitis in children. *Cochrane Database of Systematic Reviews*, (8), (CD004872).

American Heart Association. (2011). *Pediatric Advanced Life Support Provider (PALS) Manual*. Dallas, TX: Author.

Babl, F., Sheriff, N., Neutze, J., Borland, M. & Oakley, E. (2008). Bronchiolitis management in pediatric emergency departments in Australia and New Zealand: A PREDICT study. *Pediatric Emergency Care*, *24*(10), 656–658.

Bhat, K. V., Hegde, J. S., Nagalotimath, U. S. & Patil, G. C. (2010). Evaluation of computed tomography virtual bronchoscopy in paediatric tracheobronchial foreign body aspiration. *Journal of Laryngology and Otology*, *124*(8), 875–879.

Black, A. & Brennan, R. A. (2011). Breathing easy: Implementing a bronchiolitis protocol. *Pediatric Nursing*, *37*(3), 129–135.

Blakey, J. D. & Wardlaw, A. J. (2012). What is severe asthma? *Clinical & Experimental Allergy*, *42*(5), 617–624.

Brashers, V. L. (2012). Alterations in pulmonary function. In S. E. Huether & K. L. McCance (Eds). *Understanding Pathophysiology*. St Louis: Elsevier/Mosby.

Carter, E. R. & Marshall, S. G. (2014). The respiratory system. In K. J. Marcdante & R. M. Kliegman. *Nelson Essentials of* Pediatrics. (7th ed.). Philadelphia: Saunders/Elsevier.

Eladl, H. M. (2010). Transnasal endoscopic repair of bilateral congenital choanal atresia: Controversies. *Journal of Laryngology and Otology*, *124*(4), 387–392.

Facts and Comparisons. (2014). *Drug Facts and Comparisons 2014*. St Louis: Wolters Kluwer Health.

Federico, M. J., Kerby, G. S., Deterding, R. R., Baker, C. D., Balasubramaniam, V., Zemanick, E. T., Sagel, S. D., Cavanaugh, K. L. & Accurso, F. J. (2011). Respiratory tract and mediastinum. In W. W. Hay et al. (Eds), *Current Diagnosis & Treatment: Pediatrics* (21st ed.). New York: McGraw-Hill/Lange.

Friedman, N. R., Scholes, M. A. & Yoon, P. J. (2014). Ear, nose and throat. In W. W. Hay et al. (Eds). *Current Diagnosis & Treatment: Pediatrics* (22nd ed.). New York: McGraw-Hill/Lange.

Hatfield, N. T. (2013). *Introductory Maternity and Pediatric Nursing* (3rd ed.). Philadelphia: Lippincott Williams & Wilkins.

Hayes, D., Feola, D. J., Murphy, B. S. et al. (2010). Pathogenesis of bronchopulmonary dysplasia. *Respiration*, *79*(5), 425–436.

Janssen, J. & Cardillo, G. (2011). Primary spontaneous pneumothorax: Towards outpatient treatment and abandoning chest tube drainage. *Respiration*, *82*(2), 201–203.

Lim, W. J., Mohammed-Akram, R., Carson, K. V., Mysore, S., Labiszewski, N. A., Wedzicha, J. A., Rowe, B. H. & Smith, B. J. (2012). Non-invasive positive pressure ventilation for treatment of respiratory failure due to severe acute exacerbations of asthma. *Cochrane Database of Systematic Reviews*, (12), (CD004360).

Lin, Y. Y. & Lee, J. C. (2011). Bilateral peritonsillar abscesses complicating acute tonsillitis. *Canadian Medical Association*, *183*(11), 1276–1279.

McKenna, L. & Mirkov, S. (Eds). (2014). *Australia New Zealand Nursing & Midwifery Drug Handbook* (7th ed.). Sydney: Lippincott Williams & Wilkins.

McMullen, A., Yoos, H. L., Anson, E., Kitzmann, H. & Halterman, J. S. (2007). Asthma care of children in clinical practice: Do parents report receiving appropriate education? *Pediatric Nursing*, *33*(1), 37–44.

Marino, P. L. (2007). *The ICU Book*. Philadelphia: Lippincott Williams & Wilkins.

Martin, J. M. (2010). Pharyngitis and streptococcal throat infections. *Pediatric Annals*, *39*(1), 22–27.

NSW Health. (2012). *Infants and Children: Acute Management of Asthma*. Policy directive PD2012_056, accessed 18 February 2015, <www.health.nsw.gov.au/policies/pages/default.aspx>.

Pritchard, M., Flenady, V. & Woodgate, P. (2009). Preoxygenation for tracheal suctioning in intubated, ventilated newborn infants. *Cochrane Database of Systematic Reviews*, (1), (CD000427).

Raab, E. L. (2013). Neonatal resuscitation. In A. H. DeCherney, L. Nathan, L. Laufer & A. S. Roman (Eds). *Current diagnosis & treatment: Obstetrics and Gynecology* (11th ed.). Columbus, OH: McGraw-Hill.

Raviglione, M., Marais, B., Floyd, K., Lönnroth, K., Getahun, H., Migliori, G. B., Harries, A. D., Nunn, P., Lienhardt, C., Graham, S., Chakaya, J., Weyer, K., Cole, S., Kaufmann, S. H., Zumla, A. (2012). Scaling up interventions to achieve global tuberculosis control: Progress and new developments. *Lancet*, *379*(9829), 1902–1913.

Ricci, S., Kyle, T. & Carman, S. (2012). *Maternity and Pediatric Nursing*. (2nd ed.). Philadelphia: Lippincott Williams & Wilkins.

Robertson, A., King, R. & Tomkinson, A. (2010). Frequency and management of epistaxis in schools. *Journal of Laryngology and Otolaryngology*, *124*(3), 302–305.

Smith, S. (2011). Infectious diseases. In K. J. Marcdante & R. M. Kliegman (Eds). *Nelson Essentials of Pediatrics* (7th ed.). Philadelphia: Saunders/Elsevier.

Southern, K. W., Mérelle, M. M., Dankert-Roelse, J. E. & Nagelkerke, A. D. (2009). Newborn screening for cystic fibrosis. *Cochrane Database of Systematic Reviews*, (1), (CD001402).

Spence, K. & Barr, P. (2000). Nasal versus oral intubation for mechanical ventilation of newborn infants. *Cochrane Database of Systematic Reviews*, (2), (CD000948).

Spurling, G.K.P., Doust, J., Del Mar, C. B. & Eriksson, L. (2011). Antibiotics for bronchiolitis in children. *Cochrane Database of Systematic Reviews, (1)*, (CD005189).

Starke, J. R. (2007). New concepts in childhood tuberculosis. *Current Opinion in Pediatrics*, *19*(3), 306–313.

Vallerand, A. H. & Sanoski, C. A. (2014). *Davis's Drug Guide for Nurses*. (14th ed.). Philadelphia: F. A. Davis.

Ventre, K. & Randolph, A. G. (2007). Ribavirin for respiratory syncytial virus infection of the lower respiratory tract in infants and young children. *Cochrane Database of Systematic Reviews*, (1), (CD000181).

Visner, G. A. & Goldfarb, S. B. (2007). Posttransplant monitoring of pediatric lung transplant recipients. *Current Opinion in Pediatrics*, *19*(3), 321–326.

Zimmerman, R. K. (2014). Influenza. In F. J. Domino (Ed). *The 5-Minute Clinical Consult Standard 2015*. Philadelphia: Lippincott Williams & Wilkins.

Suggested readings

Advanced Paediatric Life Support (Heimlich manoeuvre): <www.apls.org.au>.

Asthma Foundation Victoria: <www.asthma.org.au>.

Asthma Foundation: <www.asthmafoundation.org.nz>.

Asthma New Zealand: The Lung Association: <www.asthma-nz.org.nz>.

Centers for Disease Control and Prevention. (2015). Influenza vaccine 2014–2015: What you need to know. Accessed 14 February 2015, <www.cdc.gov/vaccines/hcp/vis/vis-statements/flu.pdf>.

Cystic Fibrosis Federation Australia: <www.cysticfibrosis.org.au>.

Kelsall-Knight, L. (2012). Clinical assessment and management of a child with bronchiolitis. *Nursing Children & Young People*, *24*(8), 29–34.

National Asthma Council Australia: <www.nationalasthma.org.au>.

Peacock, J. & Stanik-Hutt, J. (2013). Translating best care practices to improve nursing documentation regarding pediatric patients dependent on home mechanical ventilation and tracheostomy tube support: A quality improvement initiative. *Home Healthcare Nurse*, *31*(1), 10–17.

Royal Children's Hospital Melbourne:

- assessment of severity of respiratory conditions: <www.rch.org.au/clinicalguide/guideline_index/Assessment_of_Severity_of_Respiratory_Conditions>.
- asthma fact sheet: <www.rch.org.au/kidsinfo/fact_sheets/Asthma>
- inhaled medications for asthma and rhinitis: <www.rch.org.au/genmed/clinical_resources/Inhaled_medications_for_asthma_and_rhinitis>.
- using a puffer with spacer and mask: <www.rch.org.au/genmed/clinical_resources/Asthma_-_using_a_puffer_with_spacer_and_mask>.

Upton, C. & Thalange, N. (2013). Respiration. In N. Thalange, R. Reach, D. Booth & L. Jackson (Eds), *Essentials of Paediatrics* (2nd ed.). Philadelphia: Elsevier/Saunders.

Watson, P. (2012). Inhaler spacer devices to treat asthma in children. *Nursing Times*, *108*(46), 18–20.

Chapter 41

Nursing care of a family when a child has a cardiovascular disorder

Previous chapters described the growth and development of well children. This chapter adds information about the child who is ill with a cardiovascular disorder and the stress that such a serious diagnosis places on families. Such information builds a base for care and health teaching for children with these disorders.

LEARNING OBJECTIVES

After mastering the contents of this chapter, you should be able to:

1. Describe the common cardiovascular disorders of childhood.
2. Use critical thinking to analyse ways that nursing care of children with cardiovascular disorders could be more family-centred.
3. Discuss the assessment of a child with a cardiovascular dysfunction.
4. Demonstrate an understanding of nursing considerations for a child with a cardiovascular disorder.
5. Identify appropriate outcomes based on the priority needs of a child with a cardiovascular disorder.
6. Demonstrate an understanding of planning care for a child with a cardiovascular disorder.
7. Discuss the implementation of nursing care for a child with a cardiovascular disorder such as teaching about the importance of taking prescribed medication.
8. Demonstrate an understanding of health outcomes for achievement and effectiveness of care.
9. Identify areas related to the care of children with cardiovascular disorders that could benefit from additional nursing research or application of evidence-based practice.
10. Integrate knowledge of cardiovascular disorders with nursing process to achieve quality child and family health nursing care.

KEY TERMS

- cardiac catheterisation
- cardiopulmonary arrest
- congestive heart failure (CHF)
- cyanosis
- innocent heart murmur
- left-to-right shunt
- organic heart murmur
- right-to-left shunt
- vasculitis

CASE STUDY

Megan is a newborn who was born with tetralogy of Fallot. By 1 hour of age, she had developed rapid respirations, tachycardia and cyanosis. An echocardiogram revealed the typical four structural defects of the syndrome. Megan's parents will be taking her home for a month to await cardiac surgery. They tell you their doctor instructed them to "watch her carefully" during that time. "What does that mean?" they ask you. Will they be able to take her outside in a stroller? Should she sleep in their bedroom? Exactly what should they watch for?

CASE STUDY QUESTION

1. What advice would you give Megan's parents?

The cardiovascular system, the body system on which all other systems depend, consists of the heart, which acts as a pump; the blood, which provides the fluid and cells for transport of oxygen and nutrients; and the blood vessels, which provide the means and routes for transport throughout the body. The regular pumping of the heart propels oxygen and needed nutrients through the bloodstream to cells and allows waste products to be removed from cells and transported to the lungs or kidneys for excretion. The cardiovascular system also transports regulatory materials such as hormones, enzymes and antibodies to the body systems. It can adapt to changing body needs by adjusting the rate and force of heart pumping, modifying the size of the blood vessels and altering the volume and composition of the blood (Bashore & Granger, 2011).

Most cardiovascular disorders in children occur as a result of a congenital anomaly; either the heart developed inadequately in utero or the heart cannot adapt to extrauterine life for some reason. Open-heart surgery is often the only treatment that will correct the primary congenital problem. Children also may experience acquired cardiovascular disorders, such cardiomyopathy. All these disorders can lead to inadequate heart function.

Cardiovascular disorders are frightening for both children and parents, as even small children realise the importance of their hearts in sustaining life and they recognise the seriousness of any illness that undermines the heart's activity. For the families of children with a cardiovascular disorder, understanding the functioning of the heart and circulation is an important first step towards coping with the illness.

CARE OF A CHILD WITH A CARDIOVASCULAR DISORDER

Assessment

Assessment of a child with a cardiovascular disorder includes both careful history taking and physical examination, because many of the signs and symptoms of heart disease in children are subtle. A variety of diagnostic studies such as echocardiography, electrocardiography (ECG) or cardiac catheterisation may be used to confirm the diagnosis and prepare a child for surgery. Teaching about these tests and providing psychological support to children and their families are two major responsibilities of nurses.

Remember that hypertension, hypercholesterolaemia and congenital heart disorders occur at higher incidences in some families than others because these disorders tend to be familial. Nurses have a responsibility to educate adolescents about the importance of maintaining a sensible weight and sodium intake and reducing saturated fat and cholesterol intake, in an attempt to minimise these familial disorders. Be knowledgeable about cultural preferences in foods when planning preventive healthcare.

Nursing considerations

Nursing considerations associated with heart disease in children usually speak to the effect of poor circulation on body tissues or the effect a serious disorder can have on the child or parents. Planning nursing care is essential to help parents and children understand heart anatomy. A sound knowledge base will help them understand the need for diagnostic testing. Additional teaching is necessary to prepare parents and children for procedures or surgery and recovery at home. Teaching parents to conscientiously administer cardiac medications is another area where planning plays an important role. This includes establishing appropriate outcomes to help a child and parents adjust to a serious diagnosis, now and in the future, such as coping with their present fears and caring for the child at home. Parents may wish to contact Heartkids Australia <www.heartkids.org.au/index.php> or Heart kids NZ at <www.heartnz.org.nz> for educational materials and family support groups in their area.

Nursing interventions in the care of children with a cardiovascular disorder include teaching, providing an opportunity for children and their families to express fears about a child's illness and treatment plan, providing physiological and psychological support such as comfort measures after surgery, and caring for a child in cardiac failure. An equally important role is teaching prevention of heart disease. Measures such as promoting non-smoking and exercise, maintaining appropriate weight and eating a low-fat diet are also important.

It is important for families to receive adequate immediate support during procedures and treatment. If long-term care is necessary, evaluating the family's ability to think of their child not in terms of illness but in terms of wellness is also key. Provide opportunities for parents to express their concerns about their child at follow-up visits to help address any misconceptions about their child's future.

ASSESSMENT OF HEART DISORDERS IN CHILDREN

The assessment of heart disease in children begins with a thorough history and a physical assessment. More specific diagnostic studies, such as ECG or echocardiography, are ordered as indicated. Because all children with heart disorders have an increased risk of poor tissue perfusion, which may affect growth and development, developmental testing also is incorporated into the assessment.

History

Some congenital heart disorders, such as atrial septal defects, may have a polygenic inheritance pattern. Because the heart arises from the same embryonic origin as the kidney, heart disorders often occur in conjunction with renal disease. Heart disorders also occur as an anomaly in chromosomal disorders such as Down syndrome (Marian, Brugada & Roberts, 2011).

As a result of technological advances in antenatal healthcare, such as prenatal ultrasound, which can show poor heart action or an enlarged heart, heart disease may be recognised as early as fetal life. However, even with these advances, heart disease may not be detected before birth. In the newborn period, due to the newborn heart rate being so rapid, extra sounds of abnormal circulation may not be heard thus heart disease still may not be detected. Because of relatively high pulmonary resistance, defects of the septum may not be readily apparent until about 2 weeks after birth. Infants with heart disease generally have tachycardia and tachypnoea. The infant who is breathing rapidly has to stop sucking on a bottle or breast frequently to breathe. The infant who is easily fatigued because of ineffective heart action has to stop sucking to rest before finishing feeding. Heart disease may be first discovered, therefore, when an infant is brought to a primary care setting at 1 or 2 weeks of age because the child is so fatigued they are unable to suck long enough to obtain adequate kilojoules or fluid.

A history should include a thorough pregnancy history to try to determine whether an intrauterine insult could have led to poor fetal formation. Cardiac anomalies can occur as a result of intrauterine infections such as toxoplasmosis, cytomegalovirus or rubella. Also ask whether the mother took any medication during pregnancy, whether nutrition was adequate, or whether she was exposed to any radiation, because these may also contribute to congenital heart disorders.

A mark of older children with heart disease is that they become easily fatigued. When obtaining the history, ask how much activity it takes before a child becomes tired: an hour of strenuous play? A short walk? Be sure parents are not confusing sedentary activities (the child who prefers to sit and read) with activities that are the result of fatigue, such as coming home from school and falling asleep day after day.

Ask about a child's usual position when resting. Some infants with congenital heart disease prefer a knee–chest position, whereas older children often voluntarily squat. These positions are unusual in children but trap blood in the lower extremities because of the sharp bend at the knee and hip, allowing the child to oxygenate the blood remaining in the upper body more fully and easily. Also ask about frequency of infections, because children with heart disease have a higher incidence of lower respiratory tract infections than do other children, probably due to less than usual pulmonary circulation. Children with **left-to-right shunts** tend to perspire excessively because of sympathetic nerve stimulation. Ask if there is an indication of this. Urine is produced only when cardiac function is adequate to perfuse the kidneys. Ask if an infant is wetting nappies or if an older child is voiding normally to discover this. Oedema from retained fluid is a late sign of heart disease in children. If it does occur, periorbital oedema generally occurs first. **Cyanosis** (a blue tinge to the skin) may occur if a shunt allows deoxygenated blood to enter the arterial system. Such infants generally fail to thrive and are below usual height and weight on a standard growth chart. Children with coarctation of the aorta, discussed below, who have high blood pressure in the head and upper extremities, have a history of nosebleeds and headaches. Because of corresponding low blood pressure in the lower extremities, such children may have pain in the legs on running (reported as "growing pains").

BOX 41.1 Assessment ✻ Assessing a child with cardiovascular disorder

History

Chief concern: Fatigue, cyanosis, frequent upper respiratory infections, feeding difficulty, poor weight gain, growth failure.
Past medical history: Infection during pregnancy, difficulty with resuscitation at birth.
Family history: Other members with heart disorders.

Physical examination

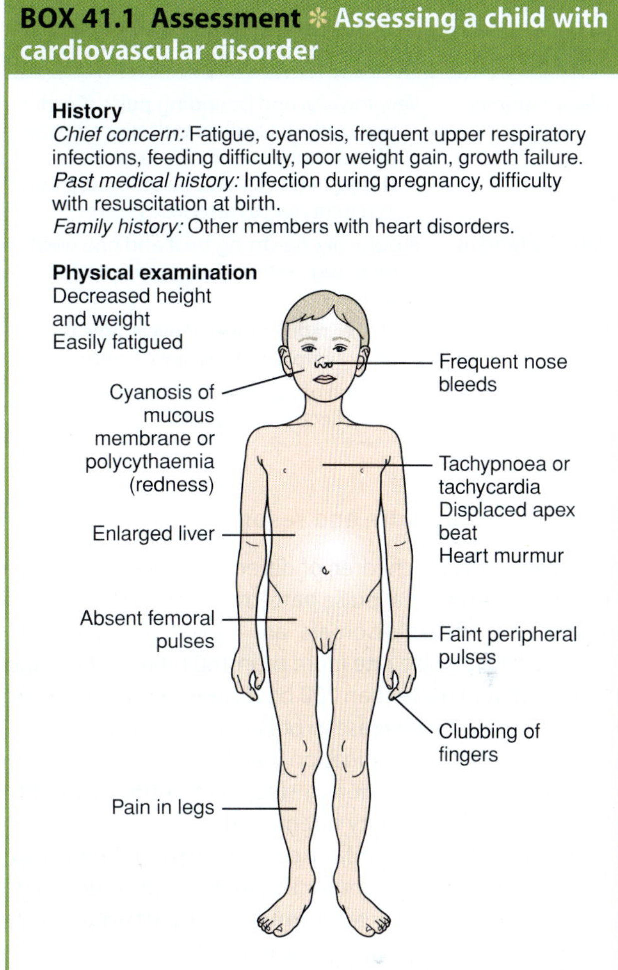

Physical assessment

Physical assessment of a child with a suspected heart disorder begins with measuring height and weight and comparing these findings against standard growth charts. A thorough physical examination should then be done, with particular emphasis on certain body parts or systems (see Box 41.1).

Because a major part of the physical assessment will include inspection, palpation and auscultation of the chest for heart function, it is best if a child is relaxed and not crying. Provide age-appropriate toys to distract the child. A bottle of formula or breast milk (or asking the mother to breastfeed) can help comfort an infant. Play with both children and infants if possible before an examination so they are acquainted and not afraid of you.

General appearance

Inspect toes and fingers (particularly the thumbs) for clubbing and colour. Assess capillary refill time by applying slight pressure on a fingernail and quickly releasing. The nail bed will blanch white and then quickly return to pink in a child with good circulation and oxygenation. In a child with poor tissue perfusion, the pink colour returns slowly (more than 5 seconds).

The mucous membranes of the mouth are the most likely place for cyanosis to be visible, so always assess the buccal membrane and lips for a blue colour. Any time haemoglobin is reduced below 4 to 6 g per 100 mL, cyanosis may not be evident because the severe anaemia masks it. Cyanosis persisting for over 20 minutes after birth (except for acrocyanosis—persistent cyanosis of the extremities) suggests serious cardiopulmonary dysfunction. If the cyanosis increases with crying, cardiac dysfunction is suggested, as this implies the infant cannot meet the increased circulatory demands of extrauterine life. If the cyanosis decreases with crying, pulmonary dysfunction is suggested because crying deepens respirations and aerates more lung tissue.

A ruddy complexion may be present in some children with heart disease because the body overproduces red blood cells (polycythaemia) in an attempt to better oxygenate body cells. Also observe for lethargy and rapid respirations, symptoms that the heart is an ineffective pump.

Inspection of the chest may reveal a prominence of the left side and obvious heart movement (the apex beat or point of maximum impulse). If a chest is extremely flat, loud innocent murmurs, accentuated heart sounds and palpable cardiac activity may be very noticeable because of the proximity of the heart to the chest wall.

TABLE 41.1 Abnormal pulse patterns

Pulse pattern	Description
Water hammer	Very forceful and bounding pulse (Corrigan's pulse); capillary pulsations possibly apparent even in the fingernails; suggestive of cardiac insufficiency, as in patent ductus arteriosus
Pulsus alternans	A pulse of one strong beat and one weak beat; suggestive of myocardial weakness
Dicrotic	A double radial pulse for every apical beat; symptomatic of aortic stenosis
Thready	Weak and usually rapid pulse; suggestive of ineffective heart action

Pulse, blood pressure and respiration

Normal findings for children of different ages are shown in Appendix C. Abnormal pulse patterns that tend to occur in children with heart disorders are shown in Table 41.1. Tachycardia is a pulse rate more than 160 beats per minute in an infant and more than 100 beats per minute at 3 years of age or older. An increase in pulse rate over these standards needs further investigation. Tachycardia is particularly significant if it persists during sleep, when the possibility of excitement and activity is removed.

Murmurs of no significance are termed functional, insignificant or innocent murmurs. In discussing such murmurs with parents, the term **innocent heart murmur** is best to use because it most clearly describes that the sound heard is not important or is nothing to worry about. Such murmurs probably reflect a normal variation of vibration in the heart or pulmonary artery.

Although innocent murmurs are of no consequence, parents need to be told when their child has one because this finding will undoubtedly be discovered again at a future health assessment. Activities need not be restricted when a child has an innocent murmur and the child requires no more frequent health appraisals than other children. Innocent murmurs do not turn into serious murmurs so parents should not view them as a prelude to heart disease. Innocent murmurs may become more pronounced during febrile illness, anxiety or pregnancy. This is why they may be audible for the first time at a hospital admission or at a sick-child visit. At future health assessments, parents may need to be reassured again that a murmur is innocent.

If a murmur occurs as the result of heart disease or a congenital defect, it is an organic heart murmur. To help differentiate innocent from organic murmurs, describe any murmur that you hear according to:

- Its position in the cardiac cycle, that is, early systolic, midsystolic, late diastolic, etc.
- Duration (how long the sound lasts)
- Quality (blowing, rasping, rumbling)
- Pitch (high- or low-sounding noise)
- Intensity (loudness)

TABLE 41.2 Comparison of innocent and organic murmurs

Characteristic	Innocent	Organic
Timing	Systolic	Systolic or diastolic
Duration	Short	Longer
Quality	Soft, musical	Harsh, blowing
Intensity	Soft	Loud
Position in which heard	Usually supine position	Heard in all positions
Affected by exercise	Yes	No

- Location (where it is heard best or the point of maximum intensity)
- Presence of a thrill (a palpable purring sensation)
- The response of the murmur to exercise or change of position (see Table 41.2).

Diagnostic tests

The diagnostic studies performed on a child with suspected heart disease vary with the specific lesion suspected.

Electrocardiogram

An *electrocardiogram* (ECG) is a written record of the electrical voltages generated by the contracting heart. It provides information about heart rate, rhythm, state of the myocardium, presence or absence of hypertrophy (thickening of the heart walls), ischaemia or necrosis due to inadequate cardiac circulation and abnormalities of conduction. It also can provide information about the presence or effect of various drugs and electrolyte imbalances.

On an ECG waveform tracing, an upward pattern indicates a positive voltage, whereas a downward pattern indicates a negative voltage. The heartbeat is initiated by the sinoatrial (SA) node in the right atrial wall near the entrance of the superior vena cava. From the SA node, the electrical impulse spreads over the atria, reaching the atrioventricular (AV) node in the lower right atrium. From there, it spreads through the AV bundle (bundle of His) and the Purkinje fibres to the walls and septum of the ventricles. At the point that the ventricles have filled, the electrical flow has reached a peak, causing the ventricles to contract.

A normal ECG consists of an atrial wave (the P wave, denoting atrial contraction), a brief hesitation before the AV node is activated, then the prominent peak as the ventricles contract (the QRS spike), another brief hesitation and then a large slow wave caused by ventricular recovery (the T wave) with often an incompletely understood additional slow wave (the U wave). A longer-than-normal P wave suggests that the atria are hypertrophied and it is taking longer than usual for the electrical conduction to spread over the atria. A lengthened P-R interval suggests that there is difficulty in coordination between the SA and

AV nodes (first-degree heart block). A heightened R wave indicates that ventricular hypertrophy is present. An R wave that is decreased in height means that the ventricles cannot contract fully, as happens if they are surrounded by fluid (pericarditis). Elongation of the T wave occurs in hyperkalaemia; depression of the T wave is associated with anoxia; depression of the ST segment is associated with abnormal calcium levels.

CASE STUDY QUESTION

2. Megan has a heart murmur from tetralogy of Fallot, a congenital heart disorder. This type of murmur is termed:

a. Innocent
b. Functional
c. Organic
d. Symmetrical

Radiography

X-ray examination can furnish an accurate picture of the heart size and the contour and size of the heart chambers. It can reveal fluid collecting in the lungs or pulmonary artery from cardiac failure. It also can be used to confirm the placement of pacemaker leads. In a posteroanterior view (in children over 1 year of age), if the cardiac width is more than half the chest width, it indicates that the heart is unusually enlarged. In infants, because of the more horizontal position of the heart, this ratio must be increased to more than half.

In addition to a chest x-ray, an upper gastrointestinal (UGI) series may be done. This is because the oesophagus is located so close to cardiac chambers that when it is visualised with barium, it can help define cardiovascular structures. Even with this technique, interpretation of atrial or ventricular hypertrophy in infants and children by radiography is difficult. X-ray findings are therefore usually complemented by ECG, a more sensitive and accurate measure of ventricular enlargement (see Fig. 41.1).

Fluoroscopy, a form of x-ray, provides a permanent motion-picture record of the size and configuration of the heart and great vessels, lungs, thoracic cage and diaphragm. Because prolonged observation is necessary to record this information, special precautions must be taken to protect a child and healthcare personnel from radiation during an assessment.

In *radioangiocardiography*, a radioactive substance such as Technetium is injected intravenously into the bloodstream. As the substance circulates through the heart, it may be traced and recorded. The procedure involves a low dose of radiation and may be used to demonstrate, in particular, septal shunts.

Generalised angiography, or instillation of dye followed by x-rays, has little value in demonstrating paediatric heart defects. *Selective angiocardiography*, however, performed as part of a cardiac catheterisation, allows identification of specific heart abnormalities if followed by serial x-ray films. After a contrast medium has been introduced into a specific heart chamber, closed-circuit video equipment records fluoroscopy pictures. Although an excellent diagnostic technique, angiocardiography is not without hazard: deaths have been reported from sensitivity to the dye used, cardiac arrhythmias and pulmonary oedema.

Echocardiography

Echocardiography, or ultrasound cardiography, has become the primary diagnostic test for heart disease (Bharucha & Mertens, 2013). High-frequency sound waves, directed towards the heart, are used to locate and study the movement and dimensions of cardiac structures, such as the size of chambers, thickness of walls, relationship of major vessels to chambers, and the thickness, motion and pressure gradients of valves. This technique is referred to as: M-mode, a single beam that reveals chamber contractility; two-dimensional, a technique used to reveal chamber and vessel size; and Doppler technique, which reveals the velocity of blood flow. Remind parents that echocardiography does not use x-rays so it can be repeated at

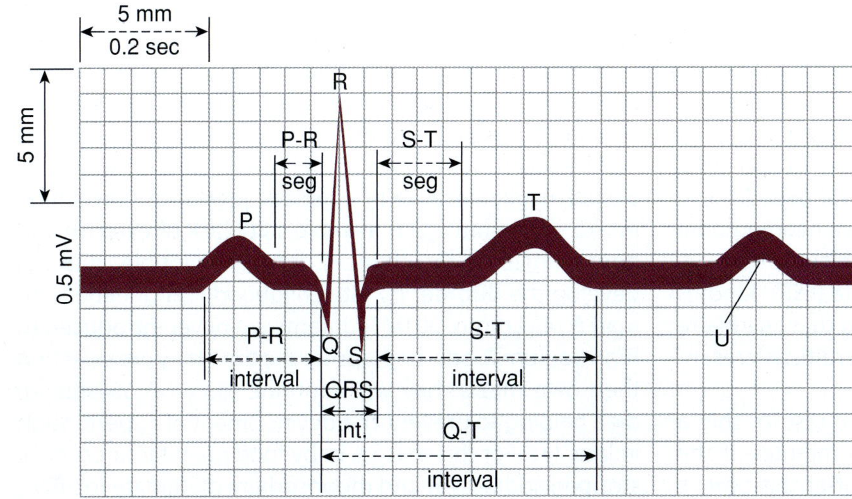

FIGURE 41.1 A normal ECG configuration.

frequent intervals without exposing children to the possible risk of radiation. It may be done using a transoesophageal probe to better reveal heart chambers (Lim & Matherne, 2007). Fetal echocardiography can reveal heart anomalies as early as 18 weeks into a pregnancy. This can alert staff to be prepared with immediate resuscitation or other needed equipment at the baby's birth (Brown & Fulton, 2011).

Phonocardiography and magnetic resonance imaging

A *phonocardiogram* is a diagram of heart sounds translated into electrical energy by a microphone placed on the child's chest and then recorded as a diagrammatic representation of heart sounds. The technique can measure the timing of heart sounds that occur too quickly or at too high or too low a sound frequency for the human ear to detect by direct auscultation. Magnetic resonance imaging (MRI) may also be used to evaluate heart structure or size or blood flow (Meziani, Debbal & Atbi, 2012).

Exercise testing

Exercise tests using treadmill walking to demonstrate that the pulmonary circulation can increase to meet the increased respiratory demands of exercise may be performed with children, although these tests are not used as extensively with children as they are with adults. With children who have heart defects that obstruct the flow of blood to the lungs (such as pulmonary stenosis), accommodation to exercise is not possible and such a test can cause extreme exertional dyspnoea. Such tests are difficult to perform successfully with young children because they require the child's cooperation.

Laboratory tests

Children with heart disease usually undergo a number of blood tests to support the diagnosis of heart disease or to rule out anaemia or clotting disorders. Haematocrit or haemoglobin studies are usually obtained to assess the rate of erythrocyte production, which may increase in an attempt to produce more oxygen-carrying red blood cells. If the increase in the number of red blood cells is extreme (polycythaemia), there will be a corresponding increase in blood volume and possibly an increase in blood viscosity. Newborns are normally slightly polycythaemic. In a newborn, polycythaemia is defined as a haemoglobin level over 25 g per 100 mL or a haematocrit level over 70%. In an older child, polycythaemia is defined as a haemoglobin level over 16 g per 100 mL or a haematocrit level over 55%. An elevated erythrocyte sedimentation rate (ESR) denotes inflammation and is useful in documenting that an inflammatory process, such as occurs with myocarditis, is present (Modi & Beaudoin, 2014).

Blood gas levels also are determined. To test for this, a child is given 100% oxygen for about 15 minutes. If the child still has a Po_2 less than 150 mmHg after this time, a shunt directing deoxygenated blood into oxygenated blood can be suspected. Oxygen saturation levels are also assessed; children with a deoxygenated to oxygenated shunt will have a lower-than-normal oxygen saturation level in arterial blood. Normally, arterial blood oxygen saturation is 95% to 100%; oxygen saturation is usually less than 92% when venous arterial shunts are present.

HEALTH PROMOTION

Cardiac disease prevention in adults has received extensive attention in health literature. Because the risk factors that lead to adult heart disease (such as obesity, high cholesterol serum levels and lack of consistent exercise) involve health habits that begin in childhood, prevention of cardiac disease has shifted from an adult to a child focus. Early interventions to reduce risk factors in early life should have a major impact on reducing the incidence of heart disease in the next generation.

Congenital heart disease

The cause of congenital heart disease often cannot be documented, although it is associated with familial patterns of inheritance and possibly triggers such as infection during pregnancy. All women of childbearing age should be immunised against rubella (German measles) and varicella (chickenpox) because these viruses are known to cause heart damage in a fetus if the mother contracts them during pregnancy. Because some types of congenital heart disorders have a familial incidence, parents who have a family member born with a heart defect need to alert their primary care provider so that other children can be carefully screened prenatally and at birth for a similar disorder.

Acquired heart disease

Acquired heart diseases in children that have identified risk factors include rheumatic fever, hypertension and hyperlipidaemia. Rheumatic fever is an autoimmune response that follows a group A beta-haemolytic streptococcal infection. Ensuring that all parents know that children with streptococcal infections from otitis media, streptococcal pharyngitis and impetigo should receive adequate antibiotic therapy is essential for disease prevention (Mayosi & Carapetis, 2011).

Although hypertension (elevated blood pressure) occurs mainly because of a genetic predisposition, a high intake of sodium (such as table salt), lack of exercise and obesity increase the chances that a susceptible child will develop the disorder by late childhood (Sondheimer, Yetman & Miyamoto, 2014). If infants are never introduced to high-sodium foods, perhaps by the time they are selecting their own meals they will continue to eat a low-sodium diet, helping to prevent the development of hypertension in later life. For this reason, baby food manufacturers have stopped adding salt and monosodium glutamate to infant food. Urging school-age children and adolescents to reduce their intake of canned soups, cheese, lunch meats and hot dogs, all foods with high sodium content, can reduce salt intake in these age groups. School nurses can play an important role in this effort by monitoring the foods served daily in school canteens and advocating for more nutritious menus.

The use of vegetable oils in place of saturated fat should begin when children start on solid food. Children from high-risk families (a family member has had an early myocardial infarction or hyperlipidaemia) should be regularly screened for elevated cholesterol and triglyceride levels beginning at about 3 years of age.

NURSING CARE OF THE CHILD WITH A CARDIAC DISORDER

Most parents have many questions about how to care for a child with heart disease. Encourage them to learn as much as possible about their child's disorder. Encourage them to handle and feed their newborn in the hospital so they can feel secure in caring for the infant at home. Be certain parents recognise that not all children with heart disease have the same disease or need the same degree of restriction.

Information for parents

Parents generally ask whether it is safe to let a baby with heart disease cry. If the infant has a cardiac disorder such as tetralogy of Fallot in which hypercyanotic episodes tend to develop, the baby should not be allowed to cry for long periods of time (no baby should). However, crying for a few minutes while a parent warms formula or fully awakens at night will, as a rule, not harm the baby.

Another common question is, *"Does our child need special nutrition?"* As with all newborns, breastfeeding is the preferred method of feeding and the average infant with heart disease can be successful at this. Salt is rarely restricted during early life because infants need sodium to regulate water balance. Because anaemia stresses the heart, infants are generally given an iron supplement, either with formula or separately, to prevent iron deficiency anaemia during the first year. They may be prescribed supplemental vitamins with formula or when breastfeeding is stopped. Because some infants with congenital heart disease tire readily, frequent small feeds during the day may be necessary. If a child is an extremely poor eater, a high-kilojoule formula or enteral or gastrostomy feeds may be necessary to supply enough kilojoules for growth.

"How much activity can we allow the baby?" This answer depends on the type and extent of the heart disorder. As a rule, infants or young children naturally limit their own activity. Parents may need guidance, however, in setting sensible limits. Encourage parents to observe their infant carefully to recognise the first signs of respiratory distress and the point at which a child's activity is beginning to exceed tolerance. Caution parents to observe a child carefully and thoughtfully as new activities are introduced and new interests are gained, so that the child's activity is limited to what the heart can accommodate.

"What do we do if our child becomes ill?" Although children with congenital heart disorders are usually seen by a cardiologist for health supervision, it is important that they are also seen by healthcare personnel for routine care and to receive normal childhood immunisations and health guidance. As a rule, infants with heart disorders need prompt treatment for minor illnesses. The fever that accompanies a cold, for instance, can increase the metabolic rate of a child who has a severe congenital heart disorder beyond the point at which their heart can compensate. Children with congenital heart disorders or rheumatic fever need prophylactic antibiotic therapy before they have oral surgery (tooth extractions or tonsils removed). This is because the streptococcal organisms generally present in the mouth can lead to infectious endocarditis if the organisms enter the bloodstream during surgery (Sykes & Farrington, 2007). It is a good rule for parents of children with structural heart defects to ask that their children be given prophylactic antibiotics before they visit the dentist at all, because they cannot always anticipate what procedures the dentist will do at any one visit. Oral penicillin is the preferred prophylactic antibiotic; erythromycin can be used for a child sensitive to penicillin. Some parents need reassurance that their child will not become immune to penicillin if it is taken this way over long periods. Children with congenital heart disorders should receive routine immunisations and influenza vaccines and should be considered for pneumonia vaccine.

The child having cardiac catheterisation

Cardiac catheterisation, a procedure in which a small radiopaque catheter is passed through a major vein in the arm, leg or neck into the heart to secure blood samples or inject dye, helps to evaluate cardiac function (Sondheimer, Yetman & Miyamoto, 2014; see Fig. 41.2). Diagnostic

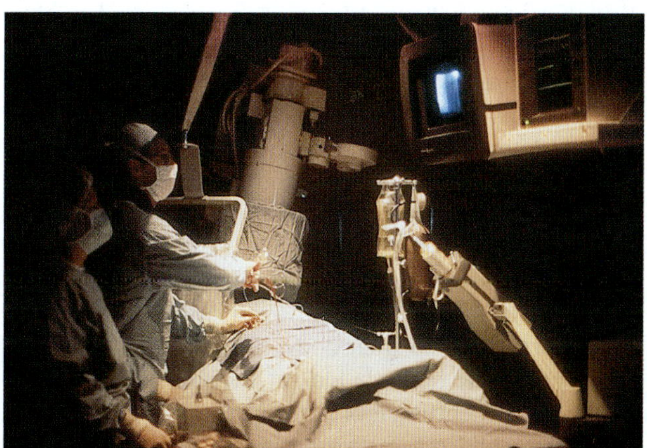

FIGURE 41.2 A child undergoing a cardiac catheterisation. (© Hough/Custom Medical Stock Photograph.)

cardiac catheterisation is used to help diagnose specific heart disorders in anticipation of surgery. Interventional cardiac catheterisation is used to correct an abnormality, such as dilating a narrowed valve by the use of a balloon catheter or other device. With both types, the pressure of blood flow in all heart chambers and total cardiac output can be evaluated. Blood specimens can be obtained to determine oxygen saturation levels or a contrast dye can be injected for angiography. Electrodes can be introduced to record electrical activity and diagnose arrhythmias.

In the cardiac catheterisation room, ECG and pulse oximetry leads are attached. The site for catheter insertion is locally anaesthetised and a catheter is threaded through a large-bore needle into a blood vessel. The specific vessel used differs according to the technique being planned. In neonates, an umbilical artery can be catheterised. For right-side heart catheterisation, a right femoral vein or a vein in the antecubital fossa is usually used. Left-side heart catheterisation can be performed using either a venous or an arterial approach. If done by the arterial route, a catheter is inserted into either the femoral or brachial artery. If a venous route is used, the catheter is inserted into the right femoral vein. Under fluoroscopy, the catheter is advanced to the right atrium and then through the foramen ovale. Once the catheter is in a selected heart chamber, radiopaque dye can be injected to outline the heart configuration.

Cardiac catheterisation has a mortality rate of under 0.1% when done as an elective procedure and approximately 2–5% when performed in a severely distressed child (Kern & King, 2011). Arrhythmias may occur while the catheter is being passed through the heart chambers or when contrast dye is being injected. Other complications include bleeding from the insertion site (secondary to heparin introduced into the catheter to reduce the possibility of clot formation) and thrombophlebitis (from platelet aggregation due to irritation by the catheter, a foreign body).

Because most cardiac catheterisations are done with children under sedation, children may need more information about what is going to happen during this procedure than they will need for cardiac surgery, when they will be fully anaesthetised. Provide explanations about the procedure for the child with the parents present, if possible. This allows parents to help reinforce the information. After this explanation, provide parents with a more detailed explanation of the procedure and allow time to ask any questions they do not want to ask in the child's presence.

Do not underestimate what children know about their heart's purpose and function; even preschoolers know their heart is vital to their body. Reassure them that the doctors are only taking a look at their heart during this procedure, not cutting it or removing any part of it.

When a child returns from the procedure, assess the pressure dressing over the catheter insertion site to be certain the dressing is snug and intact and no bleeding is present. Instruct the child not to bend the hip (if the femoral site was used) or the elbow (if the brachial site was used) to keep the pressure dressing secure and to prevent haematoma formation. This is particularly important when an artery was used for catheterisation. Palpate pulses and assess colour, temperature and circulation (blanch the toe or fingernail and watch to see that it turns pink again readily) distal to the insertion site to ensure that blood flow in the extremity is unobstructed. If there is bleeding at the insertion site, apply firm, continuous pressure and notify the doctor who performed the procedure immediately.

Keep the child flat in bed for 2–3 hours until they are completely awake from sedation. This helps to prevent not only oozing at the insertion site but also postural hypotension, which may occur when a child rises suddenly after lying flat while under sedation for such a long period. In the immediate post-catheterisation period, a child's blood pressure may be 10–15% lower than the pre-catheterisation level because of the hypotensive effect of the radiopaque dye.

Assess pulse, blood pressure and respiration at frequent intervals (about every 15 minutes) for the first several hours to help detect if this has occurred. Monitor the pulse for a full minute to aid in recognising abnormalities. Be alert for signs of arrhythmias. Small children cannot describe the odd feeling that accompanies an arrhythmia. Older children might describe it as their heart "fluttering" or "skipping beats".

Assess temperature immediately after the procedure to determine a baseline. Some children have a transient elevation in temperature already due to physiological dehydration as a result of having been nil by mouth (NBM) or as a reaction to the dye. Others have slightly subnormal temperature readings from lying in a cool procedure room for a lengthy period. The adverse effects of cardiac catheterisation may be episodes of apnoea, sternal retractions or dyspnoea. If oxygen was administered during the catheterisation procedure, it may be continued for a period of time after the procedure to reduce the stress of respiration. Like arrhythmias, dyspnoea, bradycardia and blood pressure anomalies may be transient, but all should be reported so they can be evaluated.

Nursing considerations

Risk of infection related to presence of cardiac catheterisation

If the dressing for a cardiac catheterisation is over the femoral artery or vein, keep it clean of stool and urine. Waterproofing the dressing with plastic may be necessary. Also check the insertion site for signs of infection, because any opening in the skin is a portal of entry for bacteria. Alert parents to observe the catheter insertion site daily for redness. Most parents are advised to monitor their child's temperature daily for about 3 days and to omit baths and strenuous exercise for their child for 2 to 3 days to aid healing.

CASE STUDY QUESTION

3. Megan is scheduled for a cardiac catheterisation. Why might a child develop cardiac arrhythmias after this procedure?
    a. The dye inserted can create inflamed heart chambers
    b. The many x-rays taken lead to a weakened heart muscle
    c. The catheter can irritate nerves in the heart septum
    d. Latex allergy can cause symptoms of unusual heart rate

The child scheduled for cardiac surgery

There are many different types of congenital heart disorders and many different procedures are available to correct them. Open-heart or intra-catheter surgery, however, remains the chief cure for congenital heart disease (Brown & Fulton, 2011). Open-heart surgery is made possible by the use of cardiopulmonary bypass or extracorporeal membrane oxygenation (ECMO). With this, the venous return to the heart is diverted from the right atrium or inferior and superior vena cava to a heart–lung machine, where it is artificially oxygenated. It is returned to the body's arterial system by way of the aorta, bypassing the heart. The heart, practically bloodless, now can be opened and operated on. Blood returns to the coronary and pulmonary capillary beds under pressure from the aorta so that even though blood bypasses the heart, it still receives an adequate blood supply for self-maintenance during the bypass procedure (Fynn-Thompson & Almond, 2007). Very ill infants may be maintained on ECMO using the same technique after surgery.

During surgery, hypothermia (reducing the child's body temperature to 20°–26°C) is used to reduce the child's metabolic needs and slow the heart rate. If extreme hypothermia is used (15°–20°C), usually in an infant, the body temperature drops so low that the heart stops beating and the surgeon can work in a quiet and bloodless field. Measuring temperature to be certain the infant is rewarmed is a major responsibility afterward.

Preoperative care

Before surgery, obtain vital signs (blood pressure, temperature, pulse and respiration) to establish baselines. Count pulse and respiratory rates for a full minute for accuracy. Some children may need baseline pulse determinations done at several pulse points or blood pressures taken in both upper and lower extremities. Before obtaining a blood pressure, have a child rest for about 15 minutes and take the recording with the child lying down so it closely mimics what the child's position will be following surgery. Also record height and weight—these parameters are necessary for the estimation of blood volume for the heart-lung machine and for medication dosages. Weighing is also helpful in estimating blood loss or oedema after surgery. The immediate surgical preparation of children varies from one institution to another but usually includes preparing the skin incision site.

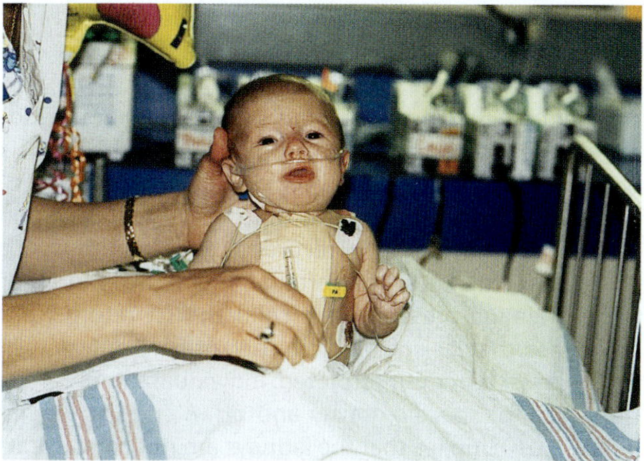

FIGURE 41.3 Because children after cardiac surgery typically have a myriad of wires and tubes attached to monitors, pumps and equipment, parents need to be prepared for how their child will look. As the child's condition improves, use of the equipment is discontinued. Here, an infant is 2 days post-cardiac surgery. Note his level of alertness and the use of only a few monitoring devices and equipment. (© Caroline Brown, RNC, MS, DEd.)

Bringing a child to the hospital for cardiac surgery is a large responsibility for parents. They want their child to be made well, but they are also aware there is a definite risk from this surgery. They may have been protecting and guarding their child for months or years, and they feel no less protective the morning of surgery. Prepare them for the amount of equipment that will surround their child after surgery, such as cardiac monitors, oxygen and IV equipment, chest tubes and a ventilator (see Fig. 41.3).

Preparing a child for surgery and postoperative care

It is best if a child is prepared for surgery with the parents present. Children can be very frightened because many children having cardiac surgery have had previous cardiac catheterisations. Talking to them about their previous hospitalisation experiences is helpful. After surgery, a child will need to cough and deep-breathe and use incentive spirometry to help the lungs expand. Introduce these exercises preoperatively to let a child know what will be expected. Familiarise children with chest tubes. In addition, introduce them to the form of oxygen therapy they will receive after surgery (mask, cannula or ventilator) to avoid surprises. Orienting children to oxygen equipment is discussed in Chapter 40.

Taking accurate vital signs, as often as every 15 minutes, is essential in the immediate postoperative period following cardiac surgery. Continuous cardiac monitoring and assisted ventilation with endotracheal intubation also are usually necessary. Blood pressure will probably be monitored directly by means of an intra-arterial catheter or indirectly with an automated blood pressure recording device. Haemodynamic monitoring by way of a pulmonary artery or central venous catheter will reveal information about chamber pressures and oxygen saturation.

Adequate voiding after surgery indicates that the kidneys are receiving an adequate blood flow or the heart is working effectively. An indwelling urinary (Foley) catheter is usually inserted at the time of surgery so urine output can be carefully recorded postoperatively (it should be 1 mL/kg/hr). Be certain to mark the amount of urine drainage present when children first return from surgery so that lack of, or diminished urinary output, will not be missed or misinterpreted. Individual samples may be tested for specific gravity and pH. A specific gravity below 1.010 implies that the kidneys are not concentrating urine well, perhaps because of the stress of surgery. The pH should remain slightly acidic; however, extreme acidity may indicate respiratory acidosis from poor pulmonary perfusion.

Carefully record all IV fluid administered to the child after surgery. Fluid overload can pose a severe threat to the heart during the immediate postoperative period. Use an infusion control device to regulate the amount and rate of infusion.

Laboratory tests such as arterial blood gases (Po_2 and Pco_2), haemoglobin, haematocrit, clotting time and electrolytes (particularly sodium and potassium) should be monitored closely to assess cardiac and pulmonary function postoperatively. Oxygen saturation levels may be monitored by pulse oximetry or transcutaneous oxygen monitoring. A drug such as dopamine may be administered to improve cardiac output.

Central venous pressure (CVP) monitoring

CVP may be recorded by inserting a catheter into a brachial, jugular or subclavian vein and ultimately into the right atrium. CVP is an excellent way to evaluate a child's fluid volume status. CVP will rise with heart failure, indicating that the heart cannot handle the blood arriving at the atria (see Fig. 41.4).

Pulmonary artery pressure monitoring

To assess pressure in the left side of the heart parallel to CVP measurement, a multilumen pulmonary artery catheter, such as a Swan-Ganz catheter, can be threaded through the venous circulation through the right side of the heart and into the pulmonary artery. The pressure, registered there as a waveform on a cardiac monitor, reflects both the resistance of the lungs to the passage of blood (pulmonary artery resistance) and the ability of the left side of the heart to handle the circulating fluid volume.

Measures to prevent pooling of secretions in lungs

Suction as necessary while a child is receiving ventilatory assistance to prevent pooling of secretions in the respiratory tract. As soon as the endotracheal tube and ventilator are removed, encourage the child to cough and deep-breathe or use an incentive spirometer at hourly intervals to help mobilise secretions. Although children may have practised such procedures preoperatively, they may have difficulty carrying them out now because, unless continuous epidural anaesthesia is used for pain relief, coughing or deep-breathing can be very painful. To minimise pain, administer the prescribed analgesia or alert the child to use the patient-controlled analgesia (PCA) pump 10 to 15 minutes before it is time to deep-breathe. For optimal effectiveness, demonstrating coughing again, sometimes deep-breathing with the child, may be necessary. Chest physiotherapy with percussion and vibration may be prescribed to keep lung secretions mobile. Be certain parents

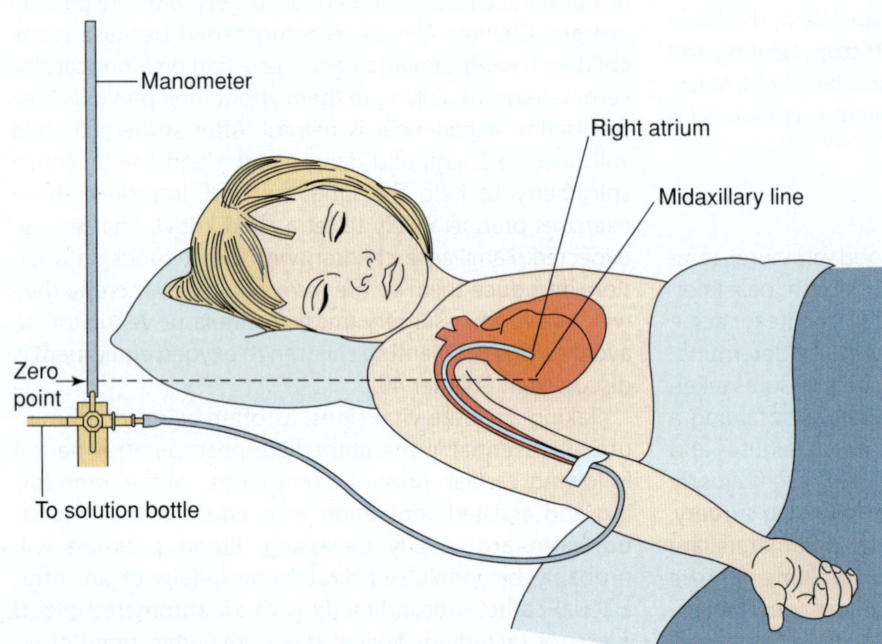

FIGURE 41.4 A CVP catheter may be inserted after cardiac surgery to monitor fluid volume. The zero point on the scale is at the level of the right atrium.

understand that games such as blowing cotton balls or blowing up a balloon are not really games but important exercises to help achieve lung expansion. Otherwise, they may interpret these exercises as too tiring for the child and discourage them.

Most children have two thoracotomy chest tubes inserted following surgery. The upper tube drains air to aid lung re-expansion and the lower one drains fluid to encourage lung expansion and decrease the possibility of infection. These tubes are connected to a water-seal drainage apparatus.

Underwater-seal drainage apparatus consists of three chambers: one to collect drainage, one to furnish a water seal and one that can be attached to suction. A thoracotomy tube connects to the first drainage compartment. Because of the water seal, atmospheric air cannot enter the tube and flow back into the pleural space. Note how much drainage is occurring and if the level of fluid fluctuates (proof that the apparatus is airtight). On the third or fourth postoperative day, the fluctuation will cease, indicating that the lungs are fully expanded. Then it is time for the tubes to be removed.

Maintain children with chest tubes in place in a semi-Fowler's position because thoracotomy tubes drain best in this position; often there is less dyspnoea as well, because the chest is elevated and the abdominal contents do not press on the lungs. Always keep thoracotomy chest tube drainage systems below the level of the child's chest so that fluid does not flow back into the pleural space. Check that tube connections are secure and not cracked or broken. Otherwise, air can enter the chest cavity and collapse the lungs (pneumothorax).

Mark the fluid level in the collecting chamber immediately after surgery. Continue to mark the level of fluid in the drainage chamber every hour so the hourly amount of drainage can be evaluated (approximately 5 mL/kg/hr is typical). Also note the colour and the presence of any clots in the drainage. Drainage fluid may be blood-tinged but should not contain fresh blood. If it does, this suggests active bleeding.

A chest x-ray taken on the third or fourth postoperative day will confirm that full lung expansion has returned. The tubes are then removed by a doctor or nurse practitioner while an impervious dressing is simultaneously applied to the puncture wound. Do not change any dressings over former thoracotomy tube sites, because lifting them to change them could allow air to enter.

Children tend to develop hypervolaemia after cardiac surgery because of increased production of aldosterone by the adrenal glands and an increase in antidiuretic hormone secretion by the pituitary gland in response to stress. Also, if cardiopulmonary bypass was used, some fluid may have been shifted from the intravascular system to the interstitial spaces during surgery. After surgery, this fluid returns by osmosis to the vessels, causing hypervolaemia. On the other hand, an individual child may have experienced excessive bleeding because of the heparin used during surgery and may subsequently develop hypovolaemia.

Monitor central venous or pulmonary artery pressure to evaluate a child's haemodynamic status. Monitor IV fluid administration carefully to prevent fluid overload. Typically, oral fluid intake is withheld for at least the first 24 hours after surgery. Once bowel sounds have returned, oral fluids can be introduced gradually.

Most children recover quickly from heart surgery. Passive range-of-motion exercises may be prescribed the day of surgery. By 24 hours, children are out of bed and ambulating. Encourage parents to do whatever they want to do for their child's care during this period. It may be difficult for them to accept the fact the surgery is over and their child is now a well child (or will be at the end of the recovery period; see Box 41.2). Offering the child sips of water or helping the child with bathing (under supervision) helps parents see that their child is returning to usual activities and doing well.

BOX 41.2 * Focus on evidence-based practice

Parents' quality of life when their child has cardiac surgery

When caring for children undergoing cardiac surgery, always consider the parent's quality of life. In one study, researchers assessed both parents (mother (n = 135) and father (n = 97)) of 138 children after discharge following cardiac surgery. The results showed that in both parents, several domains of health-related quality of life were decreased at their child's hospital discharge, with mothers showing lower health-related quality of life than fathers. Mental domains were more affected than physical domains. At 6 months, parental health-related quality of life was within or above population norms. At discharge, symptoms of post-traumatic stress and at 6 months a high impact of the child's disease on family life were associated with low mental health-related quality of life in both parents. In mothers, lower socioeconomic status and foreign nationality were also associated with a higher risk for low mental health-related quality of life at discharge.

Based on the above study, what support mechanisms would you suggest to parents following child cardiac surgery?

Source: Landolt, M., Buechel, E. & Latal, B. (2011). Predictors of parental quality of life after child open-heart surgery: A 6 month prospective study. *Journal of Pediatrics, 158*(1), 93.

CASE STUDY QUESTION

4. Megan will be scheduled for open-heart surgery. What type of fluid imbalance is likely to occur after cardiac surgery?

a. Hypervolaemia from aldosterone production
b. Hypercalcaemia from calcium release from bones
c. Hypernatraemia from excess sodium retention
d. Hypokalaemia from excess urine diuresis

CONGENITAL HEART DISORDERS

About 8% of term newborns are born with a congenital cardiovascular abnormality (Brown & Fulton, 2011). This rate is even higher in preterm infants. Overall, these disorders affect equal numbers of male and female infants, but specific defects show a tendency towards sex differences. Patent ductus arteriosus and atrial septal defect, for example, are found more commonly in girls. Conditions such as valvular aortic stenosis, coarctation of the aorta, tetralogy of Fallot and transposition of the great vessels occur more often in boys.

The usual cause of congenital heart disorders is failure of a heart structure to progress beyond an early stage of embryonic development. Maternal rubella is an example of an infection known to lead to disorders such as patent ductus arteriosus, pulmonary or aortic stenosis, atrial or ventricular septal defects, or pulmonary stenosis. Atrial and ventricular septal defects can also be familial. If a parent has an aortic stenosis, atrial septal defect, ventricular septal defect or pulmonic stenosis, the incidence of this occurring also in the child is about 10–15% (Brown & Fulton, 2011).

Disorders with increased pulmonary blood flow

Congenital heart disorders associated with increased pulmonary blood flow involve blood flow from the left side of the heart, which is under greater pressure, to the right side of the heart, which is under less pressure, through some abnormal opening or connection between the two systems or the great arteries. Disorders of this type include ventricular septal defect (VSD), atrial septal defect (ASD), artioventricular canal defect (AVC) and patent ductus arteriosus (PDA).

Ventricular septal defect (VSD)

VSD, the most common type of congenital cardiac disorder seen, accounts for about 30% of all instances of congenital heart disease or about 2 in every 1000 live births (Brown & Fulton, 2011; see Fig. 41.5). With this defect, an opening is present in the septum between the two ventricles. Because pressure in the left ventricle is greater than that in the right ventricle, blood shunts from left to right across the septum (an acyanotic disorder). This impairs the effort of the heart because blood that should go into the aorta and out to the body is shunted back into the pulmonary circulation, resulting in right ventricular hypertrophy and increased pressure in the pulmonary artery.

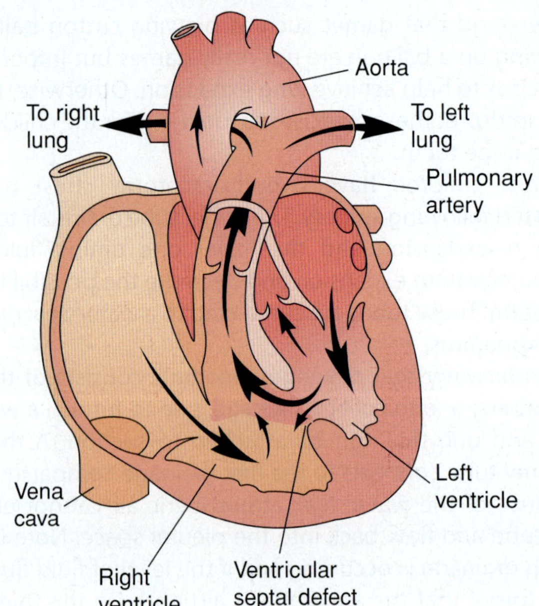

FIGURE 41.5 A ventricular septal defect (VSD).

Atrial septal defect (ASD)

An ASD is an abnormal communication between the two atria, allowing blood to shift from the left to the right atrium (an acyanotic defect; see Fig. 41.6). It is more common in girls than boys (Brown & Fulton, 2011). Blood flow is from left to right (oxygenated to deoxygenated) because of the stronger contraction of the left side of the heart. This causes an increase in the volume in the right side of the heart and generally results in ventricular hypertrophy and increased pulmonary artery blood flow, the same as with a VSD. There are two types of ASD: ostium primum (ASD1), where the opening is at the lower end of the septum and ostium secundum (ASD2), where the opening is near the centre of the septum. ASD2 defects may be asymptomatic and not discovered until infection from recirculating blood occurs.

Atrioventricular canal defect (AVC)

AVC, also called an endocardial cushion defect, results from incomplete fusion of the endocardial cushion, which is the septum of the heart at the junction of the atria and

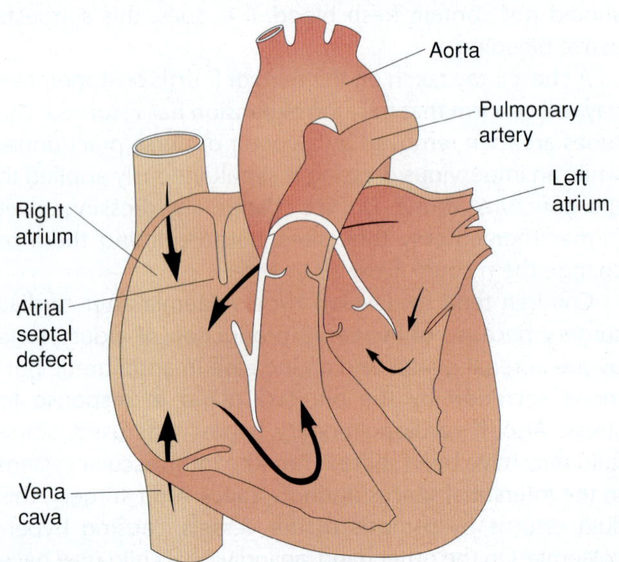

FIGURE 41.6 Atrial septal defect (ASD).

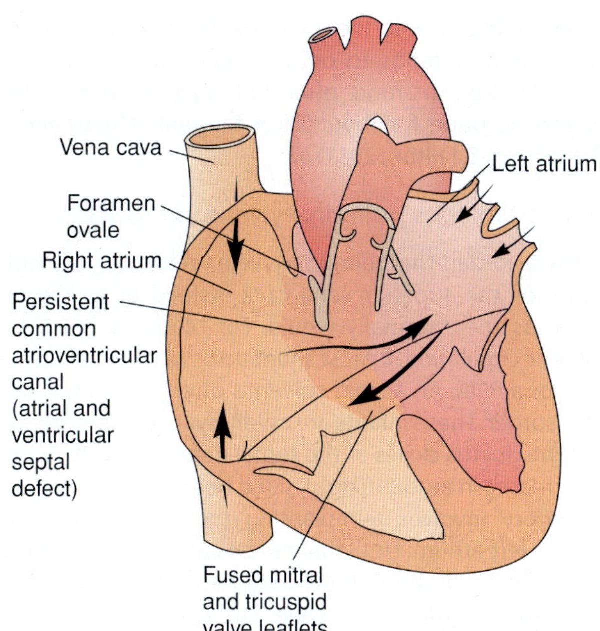

FIGURE 41.7 Atrioventricular canal defect (AVC).

the ventricles (see Fig. 41.7). Usually there is a low ASD continuous with a high VSD and distortion of the mitral and tricuspid valves (Keller, Hoying & Markwald, 2011). Although blood flow is generally left to right, blood may flow between all four heart chambers with this defect. Although rare in the general population, as many as 50% of children with trisomy 21 (Down syndrome) who have heart disease have this type of congenital cardiac defect (Marian, Brugada & Roberts, 2011). The defect leads to the same symptoms as other ASDs (right ventricular hypertrophy, increased pulmonary blood flow and fixed S2 splitting). An ECG often will reveal first-degree heart block as impulse conduction is halted before the AV node. Echocardiography will confirm the diagnosis. Pulmonary artery banding may be done as a palliative treatment in selected infants. This increases pressure in the pulmonary artery and right side of the heart, reducing the amount of shunting. Surgery, however, is always necessary for a final repair because these defects are too large to close spontaneously.

Patent ductus arteriosus

The ductus arteriosus is an accessory fetal structure that connects the pulmonary artery to the aorta (see Fig. 41.8). If it fails to close at birth (closure begins with the first breath and is usually complete between 7 and 14 days of age, although full closure may not occur until 3 months of age), blood will shunt from the aorta (oxygenated blood) to the pulmonary artery (deoxygenated blood) because of the increased pressure in the aorta (Thilo & Rosenberg, 2014). The shunted blood returns to the left atrium of the heart, passes to the left ventricle, out to the aorta and shunts back to the pulmonary artery. This causes increased pressure in the pulmonary circulation from the extra

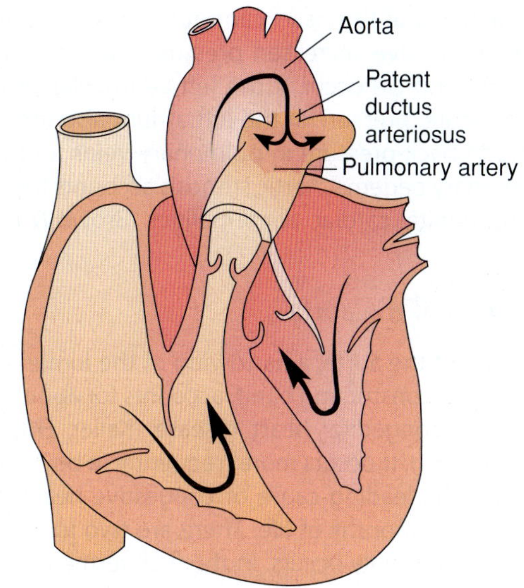

FIGURE 41.8 Patent ductus arteriosus.

shunted blood; this leads to right ventricle hypertrophy and ineffective heart action.

CASE STUDY QUESTION

5. Megan has a simple ventricular septal defect. With this condition, in which direction would blood shunt?
   a. From the left to the right ventricle
   b. From the right ventricle to the aorta
   c. From the right to the left ventricle
   d. From the left ventricle to the left atria

Disorders with obstruction to blood flow

A number of congenital anomalies cause the blood flow leaving the heart to be obstructed because a vessel or a valve is narrower than usual. Pressure from blood flow increases prior to the narrowing and decreases after the narrowing. These are problematic defects in that they prohibit enough blood from reaching its intended site, the lungs or the rest of the body; they threaten to overwhelm the heart because of back-pressure. Obstructive defects of this category include pulmonary stenosis, aortic stenosis and coarctation of the aorta.

Pulmonary stenosis

Pulmonary stenosis is narrowing of the pulmonary valve or the pulmonary artery just distal to the valve. It accounts for about 10% of congenital heart anomalies (Brown & Fulton, 2011). Inability of the right ventricle to evacuate blood by way of the pulmonary artery because of the obstruction leads to right ventricular hypertrophy.

Aortic stenosis

Stenosis, or stricture, of the aortic valve prevents blood from passing freely from the left ventricle of the heart into the aorta. Because the heart cannot force blood through the strictured valve, increased pressure and hypertrophy of the left ventricle occur. If the left ventricular pressure becomes acute, pressure in the left atrium also increases, resulting in back-pressure in pulmonary veins and possibly pulmonary oedema. Aortic stenosis accounts for about 7% of congenital cardiac abnormalities (Brown & Fulton, 2011).

Coarctation of the aorta

Coarctation of the aorta, a narrowing of the lumen of the aorta due to a constricting band, accounts for about 6% of instances of congenital heart disease (Keller, Hoying & Markwald, 2011). It occurs more frequently in boys than in girls and is the leading cause of congestive heart failure in the first few months of life. There are two locations in which this commonly occurs. In the first, termed "preductal", the constriction occurs between the subclavian artery and the ductus arteriosus. In the second, termed "postductal", the constriction is distal to the ductus arteriosus.

Because it is difficult for blood to pass through the narrowed lumen of the aorta, blood pressure increases proximal to the coarctation and decreases distal to it. This results in increased blood pressure in the heart and upper portions of the body as pressure in the subclavian artery increases. Elevated upper-body blood pressure produces headache and vertigo. Because a child under 3 years of age has difficulty describing these sensations, exceptional irritability may be the main clue that these symptoms are present. Epistaxis (nosebleed) and cerebrovascular accident, an event not generally associated with children, can occur from this dangerously elevated blood pressure.

Disorders with mixed blood flow

Mixed disorders are cardiac anomalies that involve mixing of blood from the pulmonary and systemic circulation in the heart chambers. This mixing results in a relative deoxygenation of systemic blood flow, although cyanosis is not always visible. Mixed defects include transposition of the great arteries, total anomalous pulmonary venous return, truncus arteriosus and hypoplastic left heart syndrome.

Transposition of the great arteries

In transposition of the great arteries, the aorta arises from the right ventricle instead of the left and the pulmonary artery arises from the left ventricle instead of the right. Blood enters the heart from the vena cava to the right atrium, then flows to the right ventricle and goes out into the aorta to the body completely deoxygenated; it returns again by the vena cava. A secondary source of blood enters the heart from the pulmonary veins, goes to the left atrium, left ventricle and out the pulmonary artery to the lungs to be oxygenated and returns to the left atrium, a second closed circulatory system. This severe defect is incompatible with life. In most instances, atrial and ventricular septal defects occur in connection with this transposition, making the entire heart one mixed circulatory system. It tends to occur in large newborns (4 to 4.5 kg) and occurs more often in boys than in girls. This disorder accounts for about 5% of congenital heart anomalies (Brown & Fulton, 2011).

Total anomalous pulmonary venous return

In this disorder, the pulmonary veins return to the right atrium or the superior vena cava instead of to the left atrium as they normally would. For blood to reach the systemic circulation, it must shunt across a patent foramen ovale or a PDA. An absent spleen is often associated with the disorder. These infants are mildly cyanotic and tire easily. If the ductus closes or the septal defect is small, cyanosis increases in amount; right-sided heart failure develops.

Surgery involves reimplanting the pulmonary veins into the left atrium. Until this can be carried out, a balloon atrial septal pull-through procedure may be necessary to enlarge a small foramen ovale. The child may be maintained on a continuous IV infusion containing PGE_1 to help keep the ductus arteriosus open (Brown & Fulton, 2011).

Truncus arteriosus

In truncus arteriosus, a rare defect (approximately 1% of initial cardiac lesions), one major artery or "trunk" arises from the left and right ventricles in place of separate aorta and pulmonary artery vessels. There is usually an accompanying VSD. The child is cyanotic and may have a typical VSD murmur. Repair involves restructuring the common trunk to create separate vessels. Some children need a second surgical procedure by school age as the graft inserted to separate the aorta and pulmonary artery is outgrown.

Hypoplastic left heart syndrome

In hypoplastic left heart syndrome, a rare disorder accounting for only 1% to 3% of congenital heart disease, the left ventricle is non-functional. There may be accompanying mitral or aortic valve atresia. The non-functioning left ventricle lacks adequate strength to pump blood into the systemic circulation. This causes the right ventricle to hypertrophy as it tries to maintain the entire heart action (Naguib et al., 2013). The disorder may be detected by ultrasound prenatally (Rasiah et al., 2008). At birth, mild to moderate cyanosis develops as deoxygenated blood is shunted across the foramen ovale because of the greater pressure on the right. Echocardiography effectively diagnoses this condition. Prostaglandin therapy to maintain a PDA will be initiated to increase blood supply to the aorta. Inhaled nitrogen combined with oxygen may be prescribed to decrease Po_2; this increases pulmonary resistance and allows the right heart to shift more blood into the left heart and aorta. Surgery has limited success in this syndrome, although a great deal of research is being done in this area and a two- or three-stage procedure (restructuring of the heart; a Norwood procedure) is possible.

Heart transplantation is the ultimate answer for prolonging the child's life, but the number of donor hearts available for newborns is limited (Tjang et al., 2007).

Disorders with decreased pulmonary blood flow

As the category implies, disorders with decreased pulmonary blood flow involve some type of obstruction to blood flow in the pulmonary artery. Because of the obstruction, pressure increases in the right side of the heart. If an ASD or VSD also is present, deoxygenated blood shunts from right to left. This results in deoxygenated blood invading the systemic circulation. Common disorders include tricuspid atresia and tetralogy of Fallot.

Tricuspid atresia

Tricuspid atresia is an extremely serious disorder because the tricuspid valve is completely closed, allowing no blood to flow from the right atrium to the right ventricle. Instead, blood crosses through the patent foramen ovale into the left atrium, bypassing the lungs and the step of oxygenation. It reaches the lungs for oxygenation by being shunted back through a PDA. As long as the foramen ovale and ductus arteriosus remain open, the child can obtain adequate oxygenation. At the point they close, however, the infant will develop extreme cyanosis, tachycardia and dyspnoea. An IV infusion of PGE_1 is begun to ensure that the ductus remains open. Surgery consists of the construction of a vena cava-to-pulmonary artery shunt, which deflects more blood to the lungs, or a Fontan procedure (sometimes termed a Glenn Shunt baffle), which restructures the right side of the heart.

Tetralogy of Fallot

Tetralogy of Fallot, one of the first types of congenital heart disease described, occurs in about 10% of children with congenital cardiac disease (Haley, 2014). It is called a tetralogy because four anomalies are present: pulmonary stenosis, VSD (usually large), dextroposition (overriding) of the aorta and hypertrophy of the right ventricle. Because of the pulmonary stenosis, pressure builds up in the right side of the heart. Blood then shunts from this area of increased pressure into the left ventricle and the overriding aorta. The extra effort involved to force blood through the stenosed pulmonary artery causes the fourth deformity, hypertrophy of the right ventricle. A number of children with this disorder show a deletion abnormality of chromosome 22 (22q11.2) or the disorder can result from a documented chromosome disorder.

ACQUIRED HEART DISEASE

The most commonly acquired heart disease in children is congestive heart failure (CHF) or a condition where the heart is overwhelmed and unable to effectively pump blood forwards (see Box 41.3).

BOX 41.3 Assessment ✻ Assessing a child with heart failure

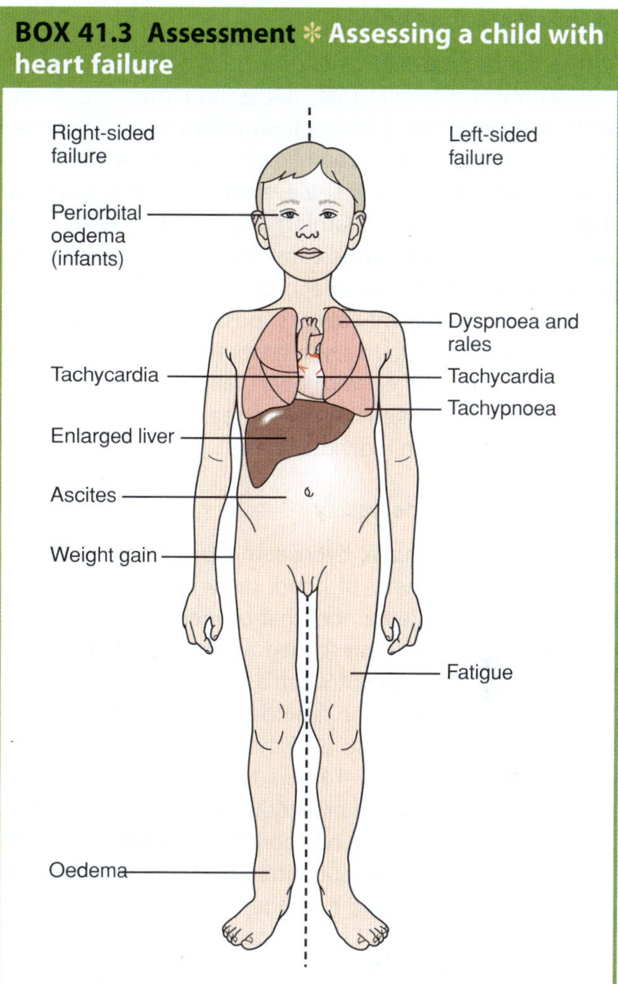

Congestive heart failure

Congestive heart failure (CHF) usually occurs as a result of a congenital heart disorder or a disease such as rheumatic fever, Kawasaki disease or infectious endocarditis. This occurs when the myocardium of the heart cannot pump and circulate enough blood to supply oxygen and nutrients to body cells (Fenton & Burch, 2007). Blood pools in the heart (excessive preload) or in the pulmonary or venous systems. This may result from a congenital disorder that lessens the effectiveness of the heart's pumping action or it may occur after cardiac surgery or rheumatic fever, when the myocardium is weakened. Severe anaemia, hypocalcaemia and myocarditis may contribute to the heart's inability to function effectively. CHF is most apt to occur in children under 1 year of age (Brown & Fulton, 2011).

Nursing considerations

Be certain that outcomes established for the care of a child with congestive heart disease are realistic in light of the child's condition as well as individualised for each child. Interventions focus on helping support heart function and helping parents deal with this crisis until the child's heart is again strong enough to maintain strong heart action.

Provide for rest periods

Rest, a major aspect of care for a child with heart failure, reduces the metabolic rate, decreasing myocardial and body oxygen demand. Most children with heart failure feel more comfortable in a semi-Fowler's position than in a supine position. This chest-elevated position lowers the abdominal contents, enlarging the thoracic cavity and allowing for easier, more comfortable lung expansion. Babies are most comfortable in an infant seat, which supports them in a semi-Fowler's position. Sedation with morphine may be necessary to encourage bedrest in some children. Most children with heart failure, however, automatically limit their activity, so the need for sedation must be considered on an individual basis.

Provide oxygen as necessary

If a child has dyspnoea, hypoxaemia or cyanosis, supplemental oxygen by way of hood, mask or nasal prongs is usually necessary. Remember that oxygen is considered to be a drug so must be prescribed according to amount or oxygen parameters except when associated with resuscitation and oxygen saturation should be monitored with pulse oximetry. Assess the nostrils of the child receiving oxygen with nasal prongs every 4 hours to prevent pressure and subsequent irritation and breakdown of the interior nostrils (this is a major problem in newborns). For a child with heart failure, it is a strain to be submitted to strange, frightening equipment. Orient a child to oxygen equipment before it is brought to the bedside. Children generally experience such relief from dyspnoea when they are receiving oxygen that their apprehension quickly disappears.

Administer drugs as prescribed to improve heart action

Digoxin, a cardiac glycoside made from digitalis, acts directly on the heart to increase the contractility of the myocardium (and the force of contraction). It also slows the ventricular response in atrial arrhythmias. Digoxin is a potent drug, so doses must be prepared with extreme accuracy. For safest administration, digoxin should be prescribed with the dose designated in both milligrams and millilitres. When this is done, the milligram dose can be checked against the millilitre dose to be certain the decimal point of the milligram dose has not been inadvertently misplaced (0.03 mg, not 0.3 mg, for example). Digoxin may also be ordered in micrograms or μg (0.02 mg = 20 μg). Digoxin preparations are typically administered IV first in a large dose (the digitalising dose). Six to 8 hours later, a quarter of the initial dose is given; another quarter is given again in 6–8 more hours. An ECG and serum digoxin level are generally obtained before the second or third dose of digoxin to assess the adequacy of the dose. Following this, maintenance doses are given once daily. For children under 10 years of age, the dosage could be divided into two doses given at 12-hour intervals.

Before administering a dose of digoxin, to be certain that the child's heart rate is not abnormally low, always obtain a child's apical pulse. As a rule, the pulse rate should be above 100 beats per minute in infants and above 70 beats per minute in older children. When effective, digoxin improves the strength of the heart's contraction. Diuresis begins and relieves any oedema present. Changes in the ECG (a lengthening of the P-R interval or a depression of the S-T segment) confirm that digitalisation has taken place.

The "window" between effective digitalisation and digoxin toxicity is very narrow. Monitor serum digoxin levels closely as prescribed. Symptoms of toxicity include anorexia, nausea and vomiting, dizziness, diarrhoea, headache and arrhythmia.

Many children are discharged on long-term medications and it is important that parents and carers are educated on the incremental requirements and precautions required to ensure safe administration. They must be aware of the drug's correct dose and frequency of administration. Help them choose a specific time for administration to which they can adhere faithfully. Diuretics may be administered to decrease pulmonary oedema, which will reduce afterload. This choice appears to be more effective than restricting salt and fluid in young children. Daily weights are a good way to gauge the diuretic's effectiveness. Be certain children are weighed at the same time, with the same scale, in the same clothing (or nude) every day so measurements are as accurate as possible and any weight loss can be noted easily. As large quantities of fluid can be lost through diuretics, so can potassium, which could lead to hypokalaemia (low serum potassium levels). For these reasons, monitor urine output and serum electrolyte levels, including the potassium.

Maintaining proper nutrition may be a problem for children with heart failure because they tire easily. Eating six to eight small meals daily is often less tiring than eating three large meals. Smaller meals also prevent the child's stomach from pressing upward on the diaphragm and compromising an enlarged heart. Sucking is hard work, so infants may need to drink smaller amounts frequently to maintain adequate fluid intake or receive a higher-kilojoule formula to allow for adequate kilojoules without added fluid volume.

By school age, children with heart failure are usually aware of the seriousness of their condition. They learn this from the frequent procedures and visits to cardiologists and from the exhaustion they feel because their heart is not working well.

Persistent pulmonary hypertension

Persistent pulmonary hypertension (PPH) results when the pulmonary vascular resistance present at birth because of unopened alveoli fails to fall to normal. The disorder occurs most often in full-term infants who have experienced perinatal asphyxia from conditions such as post-term birth (Lange & Hillis, 2013). PPH occurs because hypoxia and acidosis from respiratory difficulty cause vasoconstriction of the pulmonary artery. The infant develops tachypnoea. Pulse oximetry shows a low Po_2 from inability of blood to perfuse the lungs because of the pulmonary artery constriction. The resulting hypoxia and acidosis cause even greater vasoconstriction of the pulmonary artery. An echocardiogram slows a **right-to-left shunt** across the patent ductus or foramen ovale.

PPH is a serious threat to newborns, both because of the original insult from respiratory distress that produced the syndrome and the prolonged therapy course. Because of this, a newborn may be left with neurological challenge from severe hypoxia and inadequate brain cell oxygen perfusion.

Rheumatic fever

Rheumatic fever is an autoimmune disease that occurs as a reaction to a group A beta-haemolytic streptococcal infection (Bashore & Granger, 2011). Inflammation from the immune response leads to fibrin deposits on the endocardium and valves, in particular the mitral valve, as well as in the major body joints. The disease often follows an attack of pharyngitis, tonsillitis, scarlet fever, "strep throat" or impetigo, because the organism common to these infections is a group A beta-haemolytic streptococcus. In 95% of children with acute rheumatic fever, an elevation of one or more antistreptococcal antibodies, an indication of a recent streptococcal infection, can be documented (Ivory & Folzenlogen, 2009). It occurs most often in children 6 to 15 years of age, with a peak incidence at 8 years. It is seen most often in poor, crowded, urban areas. Because children do not develop immunity to streptococcal infections, streptococcal infections recur; rheumatic fever also recurs.

The symptoms of the original streptococcal infection subside in a few days with or without antimicrobial therapy. Children appear well again. After 1 to 3 weeks, however, if the child was not treated with an appropriate antibiotic for the original infection, the onset of rheumatic fever symptoms can begin. Because nurses are the primary people who advise parents when to seek healthcare and how to adhere to medicine administration, nurses have contributed greatly to the decline of this disorder.

Kawasaki disease

Kawasaki disease (mucocutaneous lymph node syndrome) is a febrile, multisystem disorder that occurs almost exclusively in children before the age of puberty. It has replaced rheumatic fever as the most likely cause of acquired heart disease in children. The peak incidence is in boys under 4 years of age. The incidence is higher in late winter and spring. **Vasculitis** (inflammation of blood vessels) is the principal (and life-threatening) finding because it can lead to formation of aneurysm and myocardial infarction (Rowley & Shulman, 2007).

The cause of Kawasaki disease is unknown, but it apparently develops in genetically predisposed individuals after exposure to an as-yet-unidentified infectious agent. After the infection (perhaps an upper respiratory infection), altered immune function occurs. An increase in antibody production creates circulating immune (antibody–antigen) complexes that bind to the vascular endothelium and cause inflammation. The inflammation of blood vessels leads to aneurysms, platelet accumulation and the formation of thrombi or obstruction in the heart and blood vessels.

Endocarditis

Endocarditis is inflammation and infection of the endocardium or valves of the heart (Vorasettakarnkij, 2014). It may occur in a child without heart disease but more commonly occurs as a complication of congenital heart disease such as tetralogy of Fallot, VSD or coarctation of the aorta. The infection is generally caused by streptococci of the viridans type, although staphylococcal or fungal organisms may be at fault. The streptococcal infection tends to invade the body during oral surgery, such as with dental extractions. It also can enter from a urinary tract infection or a skin infection, such as impetigo. As the disease progresses, vegetation composed of bacteria, fibrin and blood appears on the endocardium of the valves and heart chambers. This tends to occur more commonly on the left side of the heart, although if a heart defect is present the erosion begins at the site of the defect. Over a period of time, the invading process destroys the endocardial lining of the heart, underlying muscle and valves (Sondheimer, Yetman & Miyamoto, 2014).

Arrhythmias

Children have fewer cardiac arrhythmias than adults, but the number of these is increasing as more and more children survive cardiac surgery for congenital heart disease but are left with a cardiac arrhythmia due to septal trauma (Prystowsky & Fogel, 2011). Better means of monitoring cardiac rhythm patterns through the use of Holter monitors has also made detection of cardiac arrhythmia easier. Remember that most children show a normal sinus arrhythmia or a slowing of the heart rate during inspiration (increased lung size slows lung perfusion, putting enough back-pressure on the heart to slow the heartbeat), with the normal rate resuming on expiration.

Ventricular tachycardia and atrial fibrillation are syndromes that occur because of multiple or abnormal initiation of the heartbeat and can occur following surgery for congenital heart disease. These can cause episodes of syncope, palpitations and exercise intolerance. If bradycardia occurs, it can be treated with a drug such as atropine to counteract vagal stimulation; digoxin is commonly used for decreasing and strengthening the heart rate if needed. A few children may require pacemakers implanted to maintain a steady heart rhythm.

Hypertension

Although primary hypertension may occur in children, hypertension in children usually occurs as a secondary manifestation of another disease such as a kidney disorder.

As obesity in children is increasing, the incidence of hypertension in children is also increasing. It is difficult to define hypertension in children because normal blood pressure varies with the age of the child. A systolic pressure reading above the 95th percentile for a given age may be used as a practical criterion (American Academy of Pediatrics [AAP], 2009).

Beginning at 3 years of age, blood pressure should be included as a part of routine health assessment. Normal blood pressure and the technique of blood pressure recording in children are discussed in Chapter 34. To ensure accuracy, be sure a child is relaxed, after at least 1 or 2 minutes of rest, before taking blood pressure. When children are discovered on routine physical assessment to have hypertension, the reading should be repeated at a successive visit to confirm that the abnormal reading was not a reaction to the stress of the examination or some other emotional event of that day. Only when the blood pressure is still elevated on a third occasion is hypertension diagnosed.

Dyslipidaemia

Dyslipidaemia (increased lipids in blood serum) can involve cholesterol or triglycerides. Risk factors include: familial hypercholesterolaemia, a dominantly inherited disease occurring in 5% to 25% of children; obesity; a sedentary lifestyle; and a high-fat diet (Pignone & McPhee, 2011). For this reason, all children of parents with premature coronary artery disease (disease before the age of 55) or a family history of hypercholesterolaemia (parents with blood cholesterol levels above 200 mg/dL or low-density lipoprotein [LDL] levels above 130 mg/dL) should be screened for total serum cholesterol, because there is an association between high total cholesterol and LDL and the incidence of coronary artery disease. This is particularly important if the child smokes, is obese or has a sedentary lifestyle.

Cardiomyopathy

The term "cardiomyopathy" refers to a structural or functional abnormality of the ventricular myocardium that occurs following an infection such as adenovirus, cytomegalovirus or HIV/AIDS infection and results in severe dilation of the left or both ventricles (Colam et al., 2007). This impairs systolic function and leads to heart failure. Idiopathic dilated cardiomyopathy (IDC) is a rare form that presents before 2 years of age, usually after a viral respiratory or gastrointestinal illness. Hypertrophic cardiomyopathy (HCM) is a relatively common autosomal dominant disease that occurs at an incidence of about 1 in 500 young adults (Marian, Brugada & Roberts, 2011).

In the older child, symptoms appear gradually. Physical examination reveals an ill-appearing child with severe respiratory distress. Peripheral pulses are weak and blood pressure is decreased. Pulsus alternans (beat-to-beat variation) is a common finding. The liver is enlarged from backflow pressure. A chest x-ray, echocardiogram and ECG all reveal the enlarged heart.

Therapy is directed at controlling the heart failure by bedrest, fluid restriction and pharmacological agents to decrease the cardiac load, improve myocardial contractility and decrease afterload. Immune globulin may help reverse the process. If a child fails to respond to medical therapy, the prognosis is poor unless the child is eligible for cardiac transplantation.

CARDIOPULMONARY ARREST

Children with heart disease are at high risk of cardiopulmonary arrest, although this may occur in any child for reasons such as airway obstruction, trauma, anaphylactic reaction, central nervous system depression, drowning or electrocution. Management of cardiopulmonary arrest may vary according to the cause of the arrest and the age of the person, but the basic considerations are the same (see Fig. 41.9).

Many healthcare facilities and public buildings provide automated external defibrillators (AEDs) for use in cardiac resuscitation. To familiarise yourself with the Australian Resuscitation Council & New Zealand Resuscitation Council standards, you can read more about CPR on the following websites <http://resus.org.au/guidelines> and <www.nzrc.org.nz/guidelines>. There are *Clinical Standards for Resuscitation* available at <http://resus.org.au/download/general/clinical-standards-for-resuscitation-amended.pdf>.

Respiratory failure is the most frequent cause of cardiac arrest because anoxia in the heart muscle quickly leads to cardiac arrest. When cardiac arrest occurs, no audible heart sounds or pulses can be obtained. No blood pressure can be recorded (do not waste time trying to obtain one). If a cardiac monitor was attached before the arrest, it will show no ECG complex. This is a helpful assessment if available, but again do not waste time attaching monitor leads if they are not already in place. The outcome for the child in arrest will depend to a great extent on the speed with which resuscitation is begun, so it is better to err on the side of unnecessary resuscitation rather than delayed resuscitation.

Secondary measures

IV access for drug administration must be accomplished as a next step. If it is not possible after several attempts to locate an accessible vein, an intraosseous catheter can be inserted. Drugs administered through an intraosseous route reach the circulation as rapidly as IV administration because of the rich blood supply in bone. Drugs such as adrenaline and atropine also may be given by an endotracheal tube. An endotracheal dose is calculated by multiplying the IV dose by 2 or 3. The drug is then diluted with normal saline, administered by a catheter inserted deeply into the tube, and followed by an additional 1 or 2 mL of normal saline and several positive-pressure breaths to move the drug into the lungs.

Common drugs helpful in resuscitation procedures that should be available on a paediatric emergency resuscitation cart include:

- *Atropine:* Reduces bronchial secretions, keeping the airway clear during resuscitation attempts. It also reduces vagus nerve effects, relieving bradycardia
- *Calcium chloride:* Increases heart contractility. A contraindication to its use is the presence of digitalis toxicity
- *Adrenaline:* Strengthens or initiates cardiac contractions; increases heart rate and blood pressure; bronchodilates
- *Adenosine:* Relieves arrhythmias
- *Lignocaine:* Counteracts ventricular arrhythmias
- *Amiodarone (Cordarone):* An antidysrhythmic
- *Dopamine:* Increases cardiac output. It acts on alpha-receptors to cause vasoconstriction
- *Dobutamine:* Acts as a direct-acting beta-agonist that increases contractility and heart rate.

Psychological support

A **cardiopulmonary arrest** is an acute emergency and everyone who arrives at the scene should know what course of action to take. Even after heart action has been initiated, ventricular fibrillation may occur, requiring defibrillation. As soon as children begin to respond to resuscitation, be aware that they begin to hear. Children may be frightened by the number of people and all the equipment surrounding them, such as cardiac monitor leads, IV tubing and possibly an endotracheal tube. A child may have vivid memories of frightening body sensations just before going into cardiac arrest. A child may regain consciousness, therefore, struggling and fighting. Assure the child that everyone is there to help. It is extremely frightening for parents to see their child suddenly cease breathing. Although it is comforting to see emergency personnel arrive promptly and efficiently, parents will be frightened to realise their child is ill enough to need such skilled personnel. Assist, inform and comfort parents, therefore, as well as the child.

Provide specific information on the child's condition as soon as it is available and update the parents often. Allow them to see their child as soon as possible after the resuscitation attempt is complete so they can assure themselves their child is breathing and has heart function once again. Be certain they know that follow-up procedures such as ECG monitoring or blood-gas measurements are being scheduled to prevent another emergency. In contrast, offer support to help them begin grieving if the child does not survive.

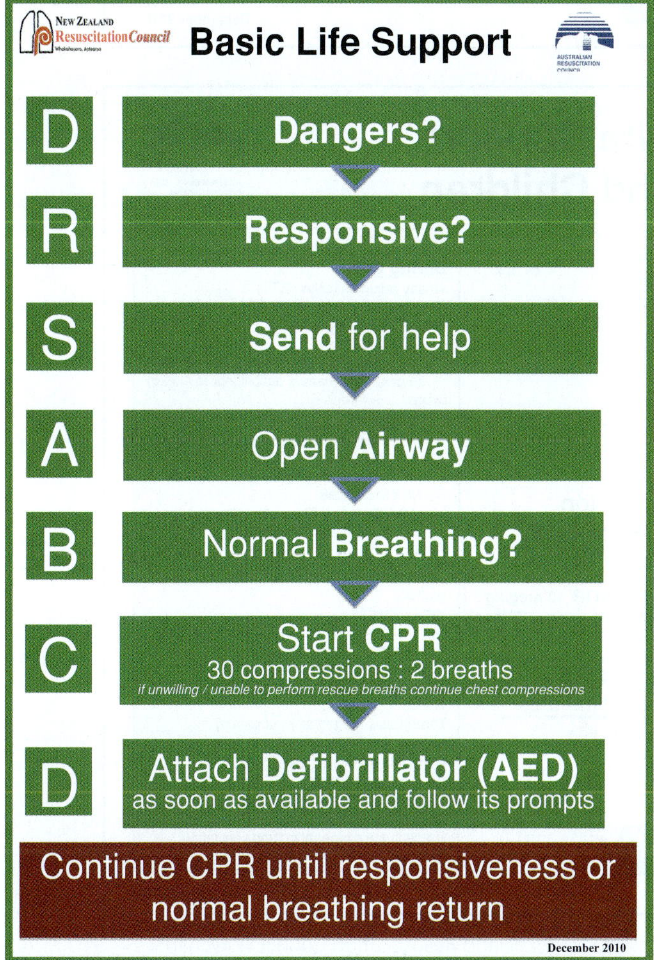

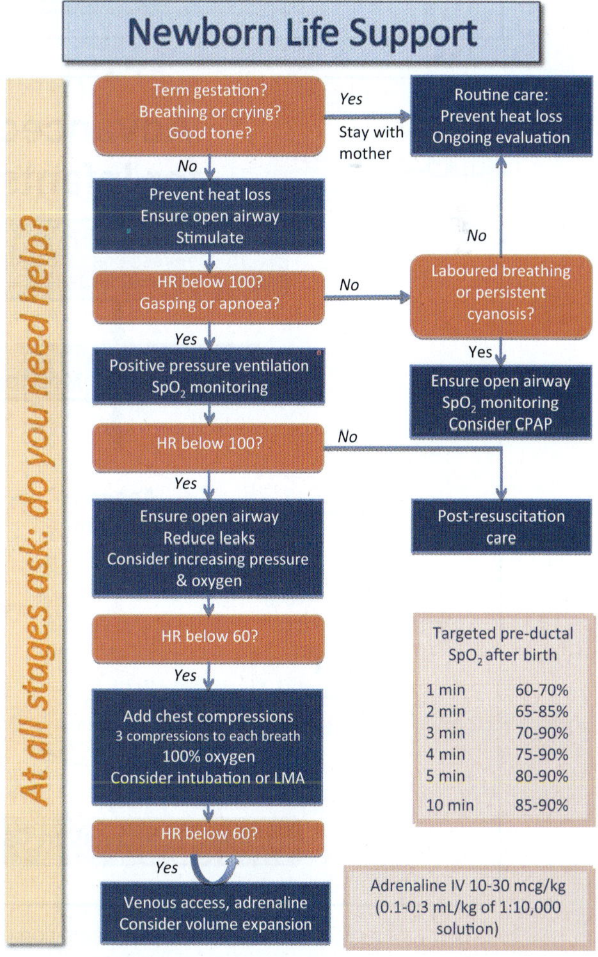

FIGURE 41.9 Australian Resuscitation Council and New Zealand Resuscitation Council flowcharts. (Reproduced by kind permission of the Australian Resuscitation Council and the New Zealand Resuscitation Council.) (*continued*)

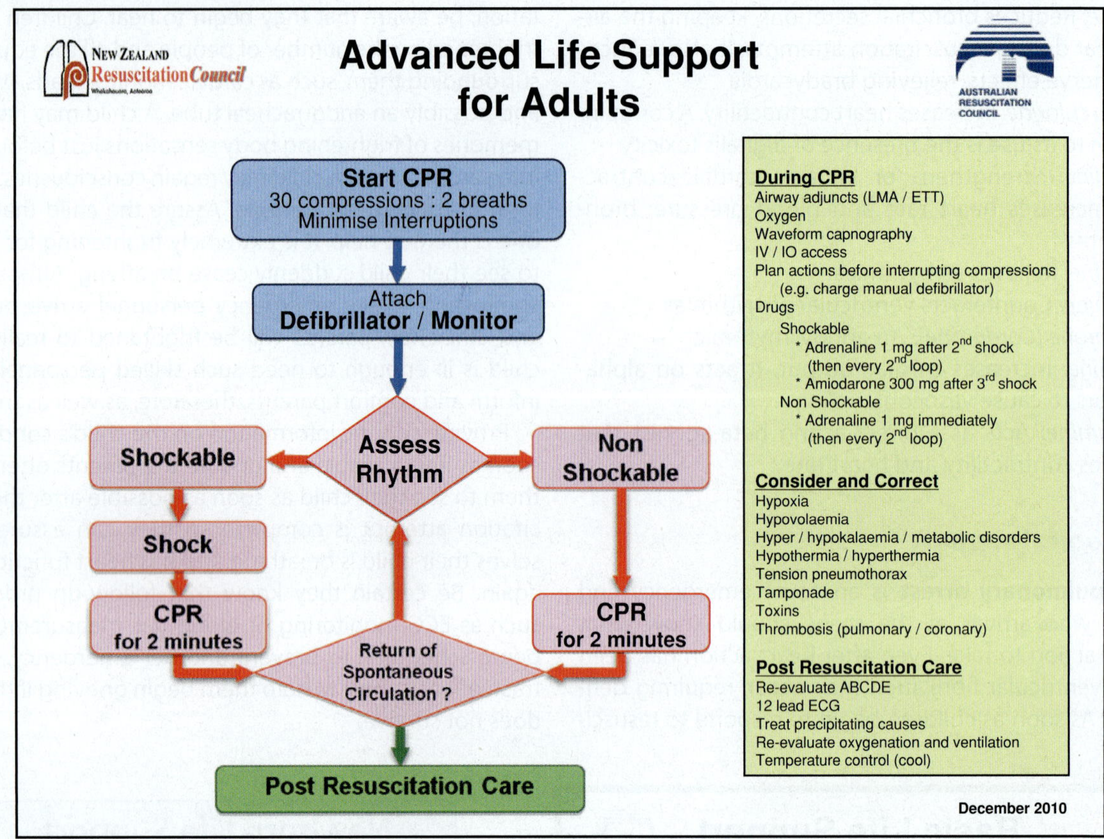

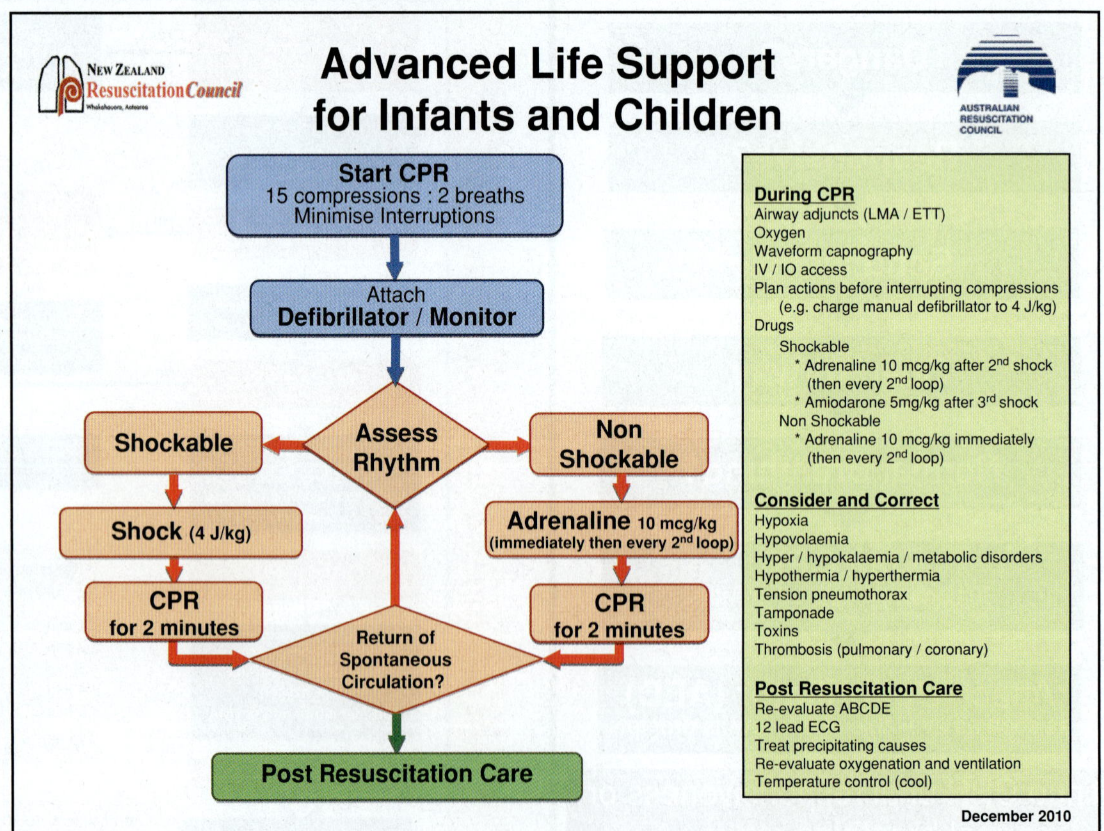

FIGURE 41.9 *(Continued)* Australian Resuscitation Council and New Zealand Resuscitation Council flowcharts. (Reproduced by kind permission of the Australian Resuscitation Council and the New Zealand Resuscitation Council.)

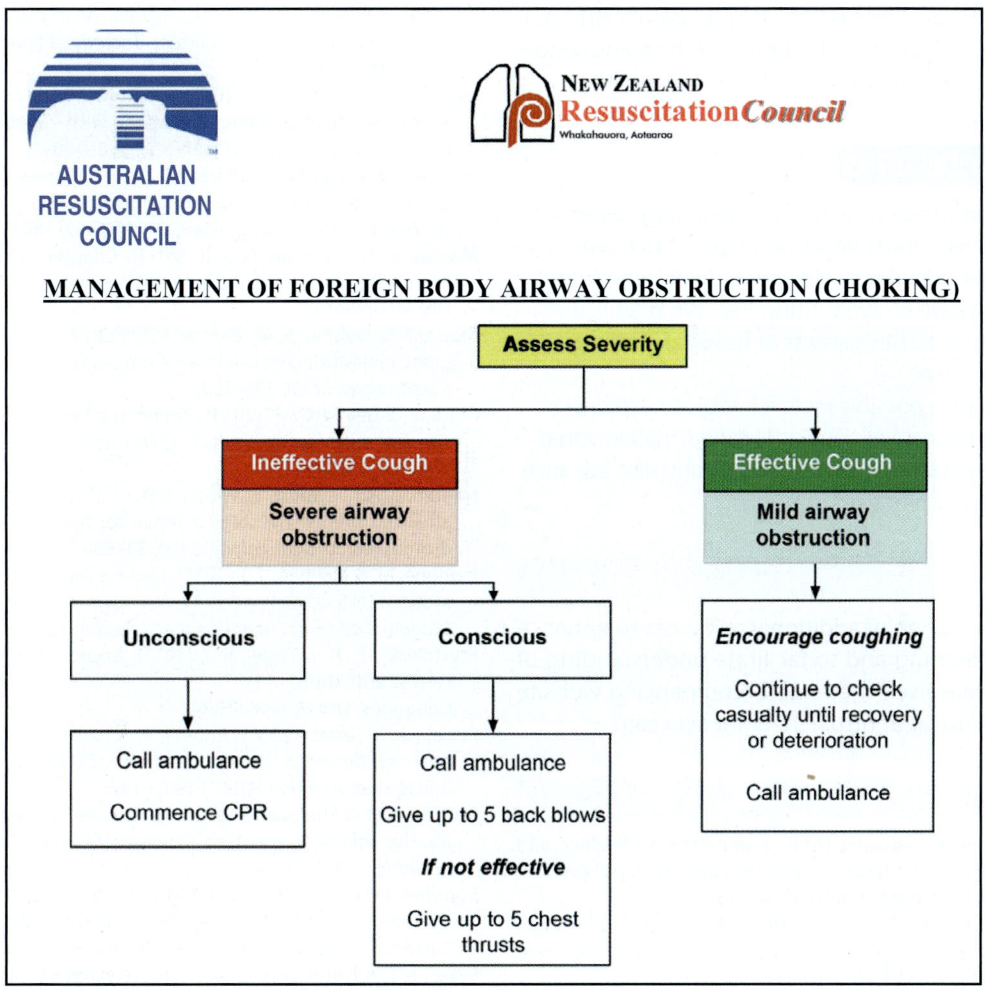

FIGURE 41.9 *(Continued)* Australian Resuscitation Council and New Zealand Resuscitation Council flowcharts. (Reproduced by kind permission of the Australian Resuscitation Council and the New Zealand Resuscitation Council.)

CASE STUDY QUESTION

6. You need to teach CPR to Megan's parents before hospital discharge. What is the ratio of ventilation to compressions used for resuscitating an infant (one person rescue)?

a. 2:30
b. 1:10
c. 2:15
d. 3:15

Key points for review

- Cardiovascular disorders in children may be either structural, such as congenital heart disease, or acquired, such as Kawasaki disease, rheumatic fever or cardiomyopathy. Assessment of children with heart disease includes history and physical examination. Echocardiogram, magnetic resonance imaging and cardiac catheterisation are procedures used frequently for diagnosis.
- Children with cardiac disease may fall behind in development because they do not have the energy to play usual childhood games. Help parents to think of games that are intellectually or developmentally stimulating without being physically exhausting.
- Limiting saturated fat intake and following a consistent exercise program are important strategies for children to prevent heart disease in later life.
- The families of children undergoing cardiac surgery need a great deal of support from healthcare personnel so they can cope well enough with this major event to provide effective support to their child.
- Congenital heart disorders are classified as those associated with increased pulmonary blood flow, decreased pulmonary blood flow, obstruction to blood flow and mixed blood flow.
- Common signs of heart failure seen in children include tachycardia, tachypnoea, enlarged liver, dyspnoea and cyanosis. Signs tend to be subtle in infants and may be manifested chiefly by difficulty in feeding from exhaustion and dyspnoea.
- Infectious endocarditis is an infection of the endocardium of the heart. It may be a complication of congenital heart disease.
- Hypertension in children usually occurs as a result of a secondary disorder. A diet that is moderate in cholesterol content along with regular exercise and maintenance of weight proportional to height can help prevent this condition.

- Children with heart disease are at high risk of cardiopulmonary arrest. Nurses and parents need to know how to perform CPR to be prepared for this emergency.

CASE STUDY QUESTIONS

7. Megan is admitted to the hospital with beginning heart failure. Her most important need is to have sustained periods of rest. How would you schedule your nursing care to avoid tiring her? What advice would you give to her parents at hospital discharge about home care?
8. What would be a possible research topic to explore pertinent to the care of paediatric cardiac patients that would be applicable to Megan's family and also advance evidence-based practice?

Resources

For an extensive range of additional resources to enhance teaching and learning and to facilitate understanding of this chapter, please see the text's accompanying website located on thePoint at http://thepoint.lww.com.

References

American Academy of Pediatrics (AAP), Committee on Practice and Ambulatory Medicine. (2009). *Recommendations for Preventive Pediatric Health Care*. Washington, DC: Author.

Bashore, T. M. & Granger, C. B. (2011). Heart disease. In S. J. McPhee & M. A. Papadakis (Eds). *Current Medical Diagnosis and Treatment* (52nd ed.). Columbus, OH: McGraw-Hill.

Bharucha, T. & Mertens, L. (2013). Recent advances in pediatric echocardiography. *Expert Review of Cardiovascular Therapy, 11*(1), 31–47.

Brown, D. W. & Fulton, D. R. (2011). Chapter 83: Congenital Heart Disease in Children and Adolescents. In V. Fuster et al. (Eds). *Hurst's the Heart* (13th ed.). Columbus, OH: McGraw-Hill.

Colam, S. D., et al. (2007). Epidemiology and cause-specific outcome of hypertrophic cardiomyopathy in children: Findings from the pediatric cardiomyopathy registry. *Circulation, 115*(6), 773–781.

Fenton, M. & Burch, M. (2007). Understanding chronic heart failure. *Archives of Disease in Childhood, 92*(9), 812–816.

Fynn-Thompson, F. & Almond, C. (2007). Pediatric ventricular assist devices. *Cardiology, 28*(2), 149–155.

Haley, J. (2014). Ventricular septal defect. In F. J. Domino (Ed). *The 5-Minute Clinical Consult*. Philadelphia: Lippincott Williams & Wilkins.

Ivory, D. & Folzenlogen, D. (2009). Post streptococcal syndromes, a rheumatologist perspective. *The Internet Journal of Rheumatology, 6*(2), accessed at <https://ispub.com/IJRH/6/2/12159>.

Keller, B. B., Hoying, J. & Markwald, R. R. (2011). Chapter 9: Molecular development of the heart and vasculature. In V. Fuster et al. (Eds). *Hurst's the Heart* (13th ed.). Columbus, OH: McGraw-Hill.

Kern, M. J. & King, S. B. (2011). Chapter 19: Cardiac catheterisation, cardiac angiography, and coronary blood flow and pressure measurements. In V. Fuster et al. (Eds). *Hurst's the Heart* (13th ed.). Columbus, OH: McGraw-Hill.

Landolt, M., Buechel, E. & Latal, B. (2011). Predictors of parental quality of life after child open-heart surgery: A 6 month prospective study. *Journal of Pediatrics, 158*(1), 93.

Lange, R. A. & Hillis, L. D. (2013). Congenital heart disease. In E. T. Bope & R. D. Kellerman, *Conn's Current Therapy*. Philadelphia: Elsevier/Saunders.

Lim, D. S. & Matherne, G. P. (2007). Percutaneous device closure of atrial septal defect in a premature infant with rapid improvement in pulmonary status. *Pediatrics, 119*(2), 398–400.

Marian, A. J., Brugada, R. & Roberts R. (2011). Chapter 82: Cardiovascular diseases due to genetic abnormalities. In V. Fuster et al. (Eds). *Hurst's the Heart* (13th ed.). Columbus, OH: McGraw-Hill.

Mayosi, B. M. & Carapetis, J. R. (2011). Chapter 75: Acute rheumatic fever. In V. Fuster et al. (Eds). *Hurst's the heart* (13th ed.). Columbus, OH: McGraw-Hill.

Meziani, F., Debbal, S. M. & Atbi, A. (2012). Analysis of phonocardiogramsignals using wavelet transform. *Journal of Medical Engineering &Technology, 36*(6), 283–302.

Modi, P. & Beaudoin, F. (2014). Rheumatic fever. In F. J. Domino (Ed). *The 5-Minute Clinical Consult.* (22nd ed.). Philadelphia: Lippincott Williams & Wilkins.

Naguib, A. N., Dewhirst, E., Winch, P. D., et al. (2013). Pain management after comprehensive stage 2 repair for hypoplastic left heart syndrome. *Pediatric Cardiology, 34*(1), 52–58.

Pignone, M. & McPhee, S. J. (2011). Disease prevention and health promotion. In S. J. McPhee & M. A. Papadakis (Eds). *Current Medical Diagnosis and Treatment* (52nd ed.). Columbus, OH: McGraw-Hill.

Prystowsky, E. N. & Fogel, R. I. (2011). Approach to the patient with cardiac arrhythmias. In V. Fuster et al. (Eds*). Hurst's the Heart* (13th ed.). Columbus, OH: McGraw-Hill

Rasiah, S. V., et al. (2008). Antenatal perspective of hypoplastic left heart syndrome: 5 years on. *Archives of Disease in Childhood Fetal and Neonatal Edition, 93*(3), F192–F197.

Rowley, A. H. & Shulman, S. T. (2007). New developments in the search for the etiologic agent of Kawasaki disease. *Current Opinion in Pediatrics, 19*(1), 71–74.

Sondheimer, H. M., Yetman, A. T. & Miyamoto, S. D. (2014). Cardiovascular diseases. In W. W. Hay, et al. (Eds.). *Current Pediatric Diagnosis and Treatment* (22nd ed.). Columbus, OH: McGraw-Hill.

Sykes, R. B. & Farrington, E. (2007). Prophylaxis for bacterial endocarditis prior to dental procedures in children. *Journal of Pediatric Health Care, 21*(4), 256–260.

Thilo, E. H. & Rosenberg, A. A. (2014). The newborn infant. In W. W. Hay, et al. (Eds.). *Current Pediatric Diagnosis and Treatment* (22nd ed.). Columbus, OH: McGraw-Hill.

Tjang, Y. S., et al. (2007). Heart transplantation in children: Clinical outcomes in a single center. *Annals of Thoracic Surgery, 84*(5), 1640–1644.

Vorasettakarnkij, Y. (2014). Mitral regurgitation. In F. J. Domino (Ed). *The 5-Minute Clinical Consult* (23rd ed.). Philadelphia: Lippincott Williams & Wilkins.

Suggested readings

Cho, A. K., & Siberry, G. K. (2012). Chest pain in child with persistent fever. *Contemporary Pediatrics, 29*(4), 28–31.

Conway, J., & Dipchand, A. I. (2010). Heart transplantation in children. *Pediatric Clinics of North America, 57*(2), 353–373.

Gerding, R. (2011). Kawasaki syndrome: A review. *Journal of Pediatric Health, 25*(6), 379–387.

Knirsch, W., & Nadal, D. (2011). Infective endocarditis in congenital heart disease. *European Journal of Pediatrics, 170*(9), 1111–1127.

Lemson, J., Nusmeier, A. & vander Hoeven, J. G. (2012). Advanced hemodynamic monitoring in critically ill children. *Pediatrics, 128*(3), 560–571.

Pate, M. F. D. & Alexander, E. (2012). Pharmacotherapy for pediatric acute and critical care. *American Association of Critical-Care Nurses, 23*(4), 396–397.

Chapter 42

Nursing care of a family when a child has an immune disorder

Previous chapters described normal growth and development of children. This chapter adds information about the dramatic changes, both physical and psychosocial, that can occur when a child is born with or develops a disorder of the immune system.

LEARNING OBJECTIVES

After mastering the contents of this chapter, you should be able to:

1. Discuss the immune process as it relates to childhood illnesses.
2. Use critical thinking to analyse ways that nursing care for a child with an immune disorder can be more family-centred.
3. Demonstrate an understanding of the assessment of a child with a disorder of the immune system.
4. Develop a knowledge base of nursing considerations for a child with a disorder of the immune system.
5. Demonstrate an understanding of health outcomes for a child with a disorder of the immune system.
6. Demonstrate an understanding of nursing care planning pertinent to a child with an immune system disorder and their family.
7. Display an understanding of preventive nursing care for a child with an immune disorder such as teaching about environmental control.
8. Identify areas related to care of a child with an immune disorder that could benefit from additional nursing research or application of evidence-based practice.
9. Integrate knowledge of immune disorders and the nursing process to achieve quality child and family health nursing care.

KEY TERMS

- allergen
- anaphylactic shock
- antigen
- environmental control
- hypersensitivity
- hyposensitisation
- immunity
- lymphocytes
- tolerance

CASE STUDY

Jack Goodwell is a 6-year-old boy you meet in an ambulatory setting. He had atopic dermatitis (infantile eczema) as an infant. Today, his eyes look reddened and are watering; his nose is draining a clear discharge. His mother tells you he is constantly listless and other children make fun of him because of his appearance. His grades are "terrible" because the minute he gets to school, his symptoms begin. Jack is diagnosed as having atopic rhinitis (hay fever). "Thank heavens", his mother exclaims. "I thought when I heard he had an immune system disease he had AIDS. What a relief to know it's only an allergy."

CASE STUDY QUESTIONS

1. In the light of the effect this condition is having on Jack's life, is this "only" an allergy?
2. What additional information would you want his mother to know about his condition?
3. Knowing his problem is worse at school, what environmental control measures would you want to suggest for Jack?

The immune system consists of a complex network of cells interacting to protect the body against invasion by foreign substances. The study of the immune system has grown immensely over the past several years and almost every day brings new findings. More diseases are being attributed at least in part to malfunctioning of the immune system, all of which makes an understanding of how the immune system works in health and disease essential for safe and effective nursing care.

Disorders of the immune system include deficiencies of immune substances and function that affect the body's ability to ward off infection (immunodeficiency disorders); abnormal and excessive immune response to foreign substances (**hypersensitivity** disorders or allergies); and abnormal and excessive immune response to self (autoimmune disorders). Immune disorders are a focus of much research and study because they potentially hold the key to understanding why major illnesses such as HIV/AIDS and possibly even cancer occur. Immunodeficiencies and examples of allergic disorders are described in this chapter. Autoimmune disorders, which include a wide range of illnesses, often affect a particular body system. These are addressed in the chapters that discuss the affected system (rheumatoid arthritis, which affects the joints, for example, is discussed in Chapter 51).

THE CHILD WITH IMMUNODEFICIENCY

Assessment

The immune system provides protection for the body from invading organisms or **antigens**. A deficiency of *immunocompetent* cells (cells capable of resisting these types of foreign invaders) or alteration in their function can limit this protection. Assessment focuses on analysis of blood components, particularly the white blood cells, to determine exactly what components are altered, missing or not functioning properly. When the immune system reacts excessively or inappropriately to the invasion of certain antigens, a thorough history and analysis of presenting symptoms is usually the best way to identify the problem and develop appropriate interventions.

Nursing considerations

Nursing considerations for children experiencing allergic responses focus on their particular allergic symptoms. Some examples of these are:

- Low self-esteem related to effects of contact dermatitis
- Ineffective breathing pattern related to bronchospasm of anaphylaxis
- Anxiety related to continued allergic response
- Powerlessness related to difficulty determining cause of allergy
- Risk of delayed growth and development related to chronicity of HIV/AIDS.

Relief of immediate symptoms is the first priority. This is followed by planning for long-term care and prevention of future attacks. Researching organisations that can supply information for parents or children is key. Information and support organisations that can be helpful are:

- Kids Health the Children's Hospital at Westmead: Allergy fact sheets <http://kidshealth.chw.edu.au/fact-sheets>
- The Royal Children's Hospital Melbourne: Kids health info. Fact sheets <www.rch.org.au/kidsinfo>
- Royal Prince Alfred Hospital Allergy Unit <www.sswahs.nsw.gov.au/rpa/allergy>
- Food Standards Australia New Zealand: Food allergies and intolerances <www.foodstandards.gov.au/consumer/foodallergies>
- Australasian Society of Clinical Immunology and Allergy (ASCIA) <www.allergy.org.au>
- Allergy & Anaphylaxis Australia <www.allergyfacts.org.au>
- Allergy & Anaphylaxis Australia: Schooling and Childcare <www.allergyfacts.org.au/how-to-manage/schooling-childcare>
- Allergy New Zealand: Managing allergies and anaphylaxis in schools and preschools <www.allergy.org.nz/shop/schools+and+pre-schools.html>.

THE IMMUNE SYSTEM AND IMMUNE RESPONSE

The immune system functions to protect the body from invasion by foreign substances via several mechanisms. The first line of defence is the physical barriers created by the skin cilia and mucous membranes. Phagocytosis, or the destruction of the invader cells, begins if the pathogen successfully penetrates the initial physical barriers. Finally, macrophages (mature white blood cells) engulf, ingest and neutralise the pathogen. At the same time the inflammatory response creates vascular and cellular changes that assist with the removal of the inactivated pathogen.

The immune response refers to the actions carried out by the human body to combat the effects of an invading organism or substance. An antigen is any foreign substance capable of simulating an immune response. If an antigen is one that can be readily destroyed by the immune response and **immunity** (the ability to destroy like antigens) results, the antigen is classified as a simple immunogen. Conversely if the mediating substances cause tissue damage and allergic symptoms the antigen is termed an **allergen**.

Immune system organs and cells

The organs of the immune system consist of the lymph nodes, bone marrow, thymus, spleen and tonsils. Bone marrow produces two types of **lymphocytes**: *B-lymphocytes* and *T-lymphocytes*. After leaving the bone marrow, lymphocytes travel throughout the lymphoid system and are stored in the lymph nodes and spleen. Both B- and T-lymphocytes are able to recognise invading organisms and attack specific antigens (see Fig. 42.1).

B-lymphocytes originate in the bone marrow (hence their name) and develop into *plasma cells* and *memory cells* when exposed to antigens. Plasma cells excrete large quantities of immunoglobulins (Ig) or antibodies which bind to, and destroy, specific antigens. This process is referred to as humoral immunity, Memory cells are responsible for retaining the formula or ability to produce specific immunoglobulins.

T-lymphocytes account for 70–80% of blood lymphocytes and are responsible for cell-mediated immunity. These cells are produced by the bone marrow and mature under the influence of the thymus gland (hence their name). T-lymphocytes leave the thymus to enter specific body regions (thymus-dependant zones), mainly the lymph nodes and spleen; there they react specifically to viruses, fungi and parasites, but have an effect on all antigens.

T cells can be divided into three subtypes. The first type, cytotoxic (killer) T cells, are T-lymphocytes that have the ability to bind to the surface of antigens, directly destroy the cell membrane, and, therefore the cell. A second type, helper T cells (CD4 cells), serve the purpose of stimulating B-lymphocytes to divide and mature into immunoglobulins. The third type, suppressor T cells, are cells that reduce the production of immunoglobulin against a specific antigen and prevent their overproduction.

Types of immunity

As discussed in the previous section, the action of B- and T-lymphocytes leads to two different types of immunity: humoral and cell mediated. There is a third type of immune

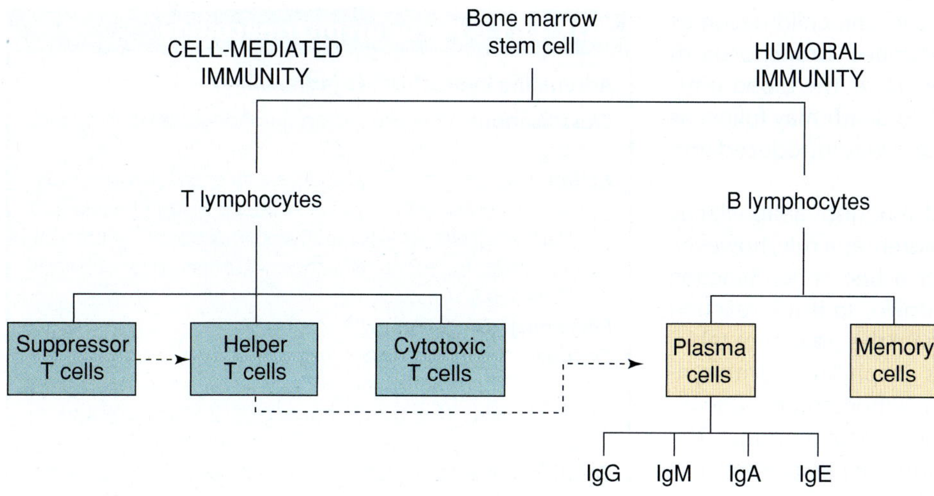

FIGURE 42.1 Lymphocyte production. From the bone marrow stem cell, T- and B-lymphocytes are formed. T-lymphocyte action leads to cell-mediated immunity. B-lymphocyte action results in humoral immunity. Ig, immunoglobulin.

response referred to as autoimmunity. Autoimmunity is the result of the immune system being unable to distinguish self from non-self, causing the immune system to carry out immune responses against normal cells and tissue rather than invading antigens. Autoimmune responses may be limited to one organ or may be generalised.

IMMUNODEFICIENCY DISORDERS

When any one portion of the immune system is not functioning adequately, an immunodeficiency results. The immunodeficiency disorder may be primary (congenital) or acquired (secondary to viral invasion or exposure to a toxic substance). A part, or the entire system, may fail in its goal of protecting the body from invading organisms.

Primary (congenital) immunodeficiency

Children with primary congenital immunodeficiencies are born without an essential immune substance or function or with inadequate amounts of immune substances. Usually these deficiencies become apparent relatively early in life. However, it may take a few months for B-lymphocyte deficiencies to produce symptoms, because a newborn is born with enough maternal IgG (which crossed the placenta during pregnancy) to supply protection for approximately the first 6 months of life.

Secondary (acquired) immunodeficiency

Secondary immunodeficiency, or loss of immune system response, can occur from factors such as severe systemic infection, cancer, renal disease, radiation therapy, severe stress, malnutrition, immunosuppressive therapy and ageing. There can be complete or partial loss of both B- and T-lymphocyte responses.

Stress appears to alter the immune response by stimulating the release of corticosteroids from the adrenal gland. This suppresses the inflammatory response by inhibiting macrophage action. Immunosuppressive medications, such as prednisone, can also suppress the inflammatory response. Radiation or chemotherapy can act to limit or destroy rapidly growing cells. Because both T and B lymphocytes are rapidly growing and dividing cells, they are killed by these medications or radiation. Extreme infection is yet another cause for a decreased immune response because the body's continued ability to combat infection becomes exhausted.

Malnutrition can decrease immunity because rapidly growing cells need protein for synthesis; renal disease with protein loss will also deplete the amount of protein available for new lymphocyte production.

ALLERGIES

Allergic diseases occur as a result of an abnormal antigen–antibody response. Allergic symptoms can be chronic and minor, such as those that occur with seasonal rhinitis, or acute and severe, as in an anaphylactic reaction. They can disrupt a child's life and development and the life of the family. When the cause of an allergic response is difficult to pinpoint, the child and parents often become frustrated. Even when the child has a known allergy, symptoms can vary from minor to acute without warning, ultimately disrupting family functioning.

Anaphylactic shock

Anaphylactic shock is an immediate, life-threatening, type I hypersensitivity reaction that occurs after exposure to an allergen in a previously sensitised child. Within minutes of antigen invasion (being stung by an insect or receiving an injection of a medication to which a child has been sensitised), symptoms begin (Boguniewicz, 2008).

Initially, a child may become nauseated, with vomiting and diarrhoea, because of the sudden increase in gastrointestinal secretions produced by the stimulation of histamine. This is followed by urticaria and angio-oedema.

Bronchospasm can become so severe the child becomes dyspnoeic and hypoxaemic. Continued bronchospasm leads to hypoxia. As blood vessels dilate, the blood pressure and pulse rate fall. Seizures and death may follow as soon as 10 minutes after the allergen was introduced into the child's body.

It is sometimes difficult to distinguish anaphylactic shock from fainting (syncope). Children, as a rule, however, do not faint after an injection or a bee sting. Syncope rarely occurs if a person is lying down, so if the reaction occurred while the child was lying on the treatment table, it is most likely that the reaction is anaphylactic. With syncope, although the child falls and is momentarily unconscious, the pulse and blood pressure remain normal. The child appears pale and may have intense perspiration, but can be roused readily after breathing amyl nitrite (smelling salts). The child with an anaphylactic reaction cannot be roused in this way.

Preventing and recognising anaphylaxis is as important as knowing how to respond when it occurs. Before giving medications that are known to have a high incidence of anaphylactic reactions such as penicillin, aspirin or antitoxin serums, be certain to ask parents if their child has ever had a reaction to the medication before. If in doubt, withhold the medication until its safety can be confirmed. Check the child's medication chart/medical notes to be certain that no prior reactions are noted. People who have hypersensitivity reactions to any injectable substance should wear a bracelet or necklace identifying the medication to which they are allergic. Some children object to this safety measure because they do not want to look conspicuous. Generally, children who have hypersensitivity reactions to insect stings are advised to undergo hyposensitisation therapy, because they cannot totally avoid insects.

Adrenaline is the medication of choice to treat anaphylaxis (James, 2013; Box 42.1). If anaphylaxis follows an injection or an insect sting, give the adrenaline in the opposite arm. Place a tourniquet on the extremity of the allergenic injection or sting, proximal to the injection site, to prevent further absorption of the allergen. Release the tourniquet every 15 minutes for a few seconds to avoid totally compromising blood flow.

Parents and children need practice to inject EpiPens correctly or they can accidentally puncture their thumb. If that happens, the vasoconstriction action of the adrenaline could potentially lead to tissue necrosis (Baris et al., 2011). Evaluation of the child after an anaphylactic reaction involves not only a physical examination but also education to help the child avoid such a serious reaction from occurring again. This involves education about the substance that caused the reaction and related substances that could have the same effect.

The Australasian Society of Clinical Immunology and Allergy (ASCIA) provides information and educational resources on its website <www.allergy.org.au/health-professionals/anaphylaxis-resources> for health professionals. The site includes directions for the following procedures:

- Action plans: allergic reactions
- How to give Epipen
- Action plan: anaphylaxis
- First aid for anaphylaxis.

BOX 42.1 * Focus on pharmacology

Adrenaline hydrochloride (adrenaline)

Classification: Adrenaline is an autonomic nervous system drug

Action: Acts on both alpha- and beta-receptor sites of sympathetic receptor cells to cause increased blood pressure and heart rate. It also relaxes the smooth muscles of the bronchi. It is used to counteract the symptoms of anaphylaxis (McKenna & Mirkov, 2014)

Pregnancy risk category: A

Dosage: For hypersensitivity reactions and anaphylaxis in children: 0.01 mg/kg (10 mcg) of a 1:1000 solution subcutaneously every 20 min to 4 hours p.r.n. (McKenna & Mirkov, 2014)

Possible adverse effects: Anxiety, restlessness, headache, nausea, arrhythmias, hypertension, palpitations, pallor

Nursing implications

- Be sure to calculate the drug dosage and check the solution strength carefully; solution is available in different concentrations and adrenaline is a very potent drug
- Obtain blood pressure, pulse and respirations and auscultate breath sounds before and immediately after administration. Assess the child for signs indicating resolution of anaphylaxis
- Rotate injection sites to prevent necrosis
- Have a rapidly acting alpha-adrenergic blocking agent or vasodilator readily available in case of hypertensive reaction; have a beta-adrenergic blocking agent readily available in case of arrhythmias
- Protect the drug from light and heat. Use only solutions that are clear and colourless.

✔ Checkpoint question 42.1

Any child can have an anaphylactic reaction to a food or medication. What is the medication of choice you would want to have available to treat anaphylactic reactions?

a. Prednisone
b. Adrenaline
c. Penicillin
d. Ibuprofen

Urticaria and angio-oedema

Urticaria, or hives, refers to flat wheals surrounded by erythema arising from the chorion layer of skin; they are intensely pruritic (often described as a burning sensation). Elevations may occur so close together they tend to coalesce (blend together). Urticaria occurs from a type I or immediate hypersensitivity reaction created by the release of histamine from an antibody-antigen reaction, similar to but of lesser intensity, than anaphylaxis. In chronic urticaria, no causative allergen may be found. There is dilation of capillaries and venules with increased permeability.

Angio-oedema is oedema of the skin and subcutaneous tissue. This occurs most frequently on the eyelids, hands, feet, genitalia and lips—areas where skin is loosely bound by subcutaneous tissue. Angio-oedema can be distinguished from other oedemas because it is not dependent, is generally asymmetrically distributed and usually occurs with urticaria. There are different classifications of angio-oedema based on their cause, these include: hereditary (type I, II and III), acquired, IgE mediated ("allergic"), medication induced and idiopathic (Busse, 2011). With severe angio-oedema, the larynx may be involved. This is serious because laryngeal oedema may lead to airway obstruction and subsequently asphyxiation and death.

The allergens that most frequently cause urticaria and angio-oedema include medications, foods and insect stings. Exposure to hot or cold can also cause these reactions. The cause of the reaction should be identified so it can be avoided in the future. Although hot and cold exposure is a rare cause, children with this form must be identified, because if they swim in cold water, the sudden release of histamine could cause dizziness so severe that they could drown. Therapy for urticaria or angio-oedema is subcutaneous adrenaline or an oral antihistamine.

Serum sickness

Serum sickness is a type III hypersensitivity response to a foreign serum antigen or medication (Ko & Chung, 2013). Examples of foreign sera given to children include tetanus antitoxin, diphtheria antitoxin and rabies antiserum. These are obtained from horse serum. Children may also experience a serum sickness reaction to medication such as penicillin, but this is rare.

Symptoms of serum sickness begin 7 to 12 days after the serum injection. If the child has received the same type of foreign serum previously, symptoms may occur as early as 1 to 5 days. Children experience itching, oedema and erythema at the injection site and generalised urticaria (hives) with or without angio-oedema (generalised oedema). Erythematous maculopapular rashes, erythema multiforme (a generalised macular eruption with dark red papules) or purpura (haemorrhage into the skin) may result.

Common symptoms include fever and arthralgia (joint pain). Swollen lymph nodes may be present, especially of the regional nodes near the site of the injection. The child may have weight gain, nausea, vomiting and abdominal pain. In more extreme instances, the child's nervous system may be involved and optic neuritis, stupor and coma may occur. If oedema is severe, laryngeal oedema will become the paramount symptom that needs treatment.

Serum sickness lasts days to weeks. In its usual form (symptoms of urticaria, oedema, arthralgia or pruritus), the treatment is symptomatic as the condition will improve by itself with time. However, an antihistamine such as diphenhydramine (promethazine hydrochloride, Phenergan) or adrenaline may be helpful in relieving symptoms. A non-steroidal anti-inflammatory medication (NSAID) such as ibuprofen or a corticosteroid may be necessary to relieve the fever and joint pain.

Like anaphylactic reactions, serum sickness reactions are a frightening experience for a child and their parents. Parents need an explanation of why the reaction occurred (their child has a low threshold of sensitisation to this particular substance) and reassurance that it was not anyone's fault and that it did not occur from administration of the wrong compound (assuming that proper precautions to ascertain sensitivity to the solution were taken before the incident). Because serum sickness mimics so many other disorders, parents need to be aware that it is not a condition such as arthritis (the arthralgia may make them think it is) and that their child will not have long-term effects from it.

The child should not receive the foreign serum or medication that was responsible for this primary occurrence of serum sickness again. If administered again the manifestation of the reaction may be anaphylaxis. Children should wear a bracelet or necklace stating the solutions to which they are hypersensitive. Children should have their immunisations (and records) kept current so health professionals are aware of their immunisation history.

Assessment of allergies in children

History

Taking a health history of a child with an allergy can be time-consuming because many factors must be considered. A family history is important because there are familial tendencies with allergic diseases. Obtaining the exact symptoms of the allergy is important to help identify the allergen: rhinitis, for example, is probably because of an airborne antigen; urticaria (swelling and itching) is often caused by ingested antigens; and contact dermatitis (often a rash) must be from something that contacts the skin in that area. The time of the year that the allergy occurs may also give a clue to its cause. If the child's allergy exists all year, the antigen must be one that is present all year (house dust mites, pet dander or a common food).

Children with allergic rhinitis (hay fever) develop common symptoms such as a horizontal crease across the nose (called a Dennie's line) from their habit of constantly wiping away nasal secretions. They also may develop dark patches under their eyes from back-pressure from nasal congestion.

Many symptoms of allergy are vague, described as "colds all winter", "itching" or "runny nose". Listen carefully: even though no one symptom is acute, together such symptoms can interfere with a child's comfort, school experience and long-term health. Having the parents and the child keep a chart of when symptoms are worse and better, often helps identify a specific allergen. Children with allergic rhinitis (hay fever), for example, have more symptoms on a windy day and fewer after a rainstorm (the rain washes pollen out of the air). Children are often poor reporters of when they have symptoms because they cannot remember clearly whether they had the same rhinitis and watery eye symptoms last summer as they do this summer. A record that details when symptoms start—for example, on arising or only after the child reaches school—can also help identify an allergen.

Skin testing

Skin testing is conducted to detect the presence of IgE in the skin or to isolate an antigen (allergen) to which the IgE is responding or to which a child is sensitive. When an allergen is introduced into the child's skin and the child is sensitive to that allergen, a wheal or flare response appears at the site of the test (Fig. 42.2). This is because of the release of histamine, which leads to local vasodilation. Because this reaction appears quickly, the test should be read in 20 minutes. Systemic or aerosol administration of an antihistamine will inhibit the flare response, so the child should not receive these medications for 8 hours before skin testing. Corticosteroid therapy does not affect immediate skin reactivity and so may be continued during skin testing.

Skin testing may be done by applying a patch or using a scratch or an intracutaneous injection technique. Patch testing has become the method of choice because it is painless and more efficient. For the child with rare allergies not typically provided for, commercial patches, scratch or intracutaneous testing may still be necessary. Scratch testing is done by placing a drop of allergen solution on the skin, then scratching through the drop of liquid with a sterile needle. A relatively concentrated extract of allergen must be used for scratch testing because little allergen enters the child's skin.

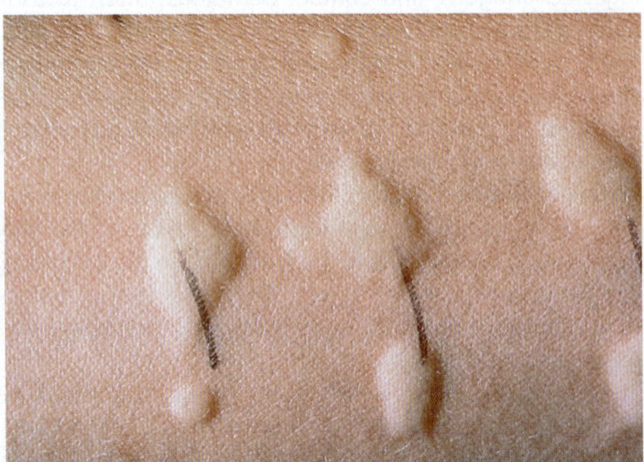

FIGURE 42.2 Allergy skin testing. Note the positive reactions. (© SPL/Custom Medical Stock Photograph.)

Intracutaneous injections are done by injecting a small amount of a solution of allergen below the epidermis of the skin. This is usually done on the forearm so that if a sensitivity reaction does occur, a tourniquet can be applied proximal to the test site to prevent further absorption of the antigen. If the categories to be tested are extensive, the back can be used. Solutions used for intracutaneous injections are more dilute than those used for scratch testing (1:500 dilution compared with 1:5 for scratch testing). This means that the allergen extracts are not interchangeable from a group prepared for scratch testing to a group prepared for intracutaneous injections (or vice versa).

After all forms of skin testing, if the child is allergic to the test solution, a wheal and erythema (redness) will occur at the test site. The size of the reaction is measured and graded from 11 to 41, or as slight, moderate or marked. No matter what the symptoms of a child's allergy, there are three goals for therapy: reduce the child's exposure to the allergen; hyposensitise the child to produce a state of increased clinical tolerance (a state of not responding) to the allergen; and modify the child's response to the allergen with a pharmacological agent.

Reducing the child's exposure to the allergen is possible when the offending allergen is a medication, food or irritant. Reducing exposure is much more difficult when the child is found to be allergic to allergens such as moulds, dust, feathers or other substances found almost everywhere.

ATOPIC DISORDERS

Individuals with atopy are prone to all allergic responses. Three disorders occur most frequently: hay fever (allergic rhinitis), eczema (atopic dermatitis) and asthma (discussed in Chapter 40). Although these diseases show a familial tendency, different family members may have different symptoms. In one family, for example, the father may have allergic rhinitis, one child may have asthma and another may have atopic dermatitis.

The gene responsible for an immune response is located near the human leucocyte antigen that is responsible for graft rejection. In certain children, a tendency for sensitivity to antigens or abnormality of this gene is inherited. These children have a higher-than-normal production of IgE antibody that makes them more responsive to allergens than other people. However, there is also a strong environmental component to these diseases. Children whose parents smoke have a greater incidence of atopic disorders compared with children of parents who do not smoke (Nieto et al., 2014).

Allergic rhinitis

Allergic rhinitis affects approximately 1 in 5 people in Australia and New Zealand. The condition affects both adults and children (ASCIA, 2012). Common symptoms of allergic rhinitis include sneezing, nasal engorgement and

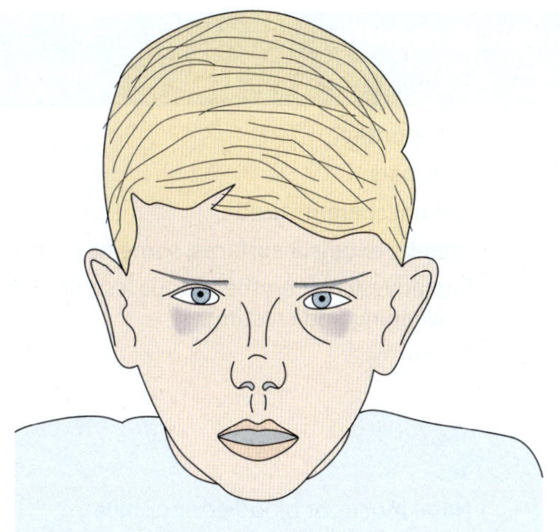

FIGURE 42.3 Back-pressure to the blood circulation around the eye orbit from allergic rhinitis may lead to dark areas under the eyes (allergic shiners). The frequent rubbing of the nose in an upward direction can lead to a peculiar horizontal crease (Dennie's line).

a profuse watery nasal discharge. The mucous membrane of the nose is generally paler than normal and may be oedematous, adding to nasal congestion. The eyes tend to water and the conjunctivae may be pruritic, often with a distinctive pebbly appearance. Children constantly rub their noses in an upward motion, termed an allergic salute. Over a long period, rubbing the nose in this way leads to a horizontal crease across the tip of the nose, called an allergic crease, known as Dennie's line. Because of congestion in the nose, there tends to be back-pressure to the blood circulation around the eye orbit, which leads to blackened areas under the eyes, termed allergic shiners (see Fig. 42.3). Children older than 6 years (when frontal sinuses develop) may report a full frontal headache. This becomes more marked with adolescence. Some children feel exhausted and lethargic and cannot function well at school. Recurrent otitis media may occur because of the swollen pharyngeal tissue (eustachian tubes are blocked to the middle ear). A smear of the nasal discharge will reveal an increased eosinophil count (more than 10% of the white cell count). RAST analysis may reveal the offending allergens.

The allergens that cause allergic rhinitis are generally pollens or moulds rather than foods or medicines. Children with allergic rhinitis are often brought to a healthcare setting during peak pollen months because parents think they have a "summer cold". However, with an upper respiratory infection, the mucous membrane of the nose is more likely to be reddened than pale and the secretions draining from the nose are likely to be thick white or yellow rather than the thin, watery secretions of allergic rhinitis. Children with an upper respiratory infection often have a fever; children with allergic rhinitis do not. With an upper respiratory infection, a sore throat and cervical adenopathy may be present, but these are rare with allergic rhinitis.

Perennial allergic rhinitis

Allergic rhinitis becomes perennial (year-round) when the allergen is one that is capable of affecting the child year-round, such as house dust mites or pet hair. Although the child's symptoms may not result in the obvious distress associated with seasonal allergic rhinitis, the child still requires adequate treatment and attention. Because the agent that causes perennial allergic rhinitis is often house dust, environmental control plays a big role in the control of the disorder. Serous otitis media may be a long-term consequence of perennial allergic rhinitis (see Chapter 50).

Atopic dermatitis (infantile eczema)

Atopic dermatitis is primarily a disease of infants, beginning as early as the second month of life and possibly lasting until the child is from 2 to 3 years old (see Fig. 42.4). It may be related to food allergy because it tends to occur more often in formula-fed infants than in breastfed infants and is more common if infants are fed solid food before 6 months. Sweating, heat, tight clothing and contact irritants, such as soap, increase the pruritus. Symptoms may be more annoying in winter (when additional irritating clothing is present) with marked improvement in the summer.

With infantile atopic dermatitis, capillary permeability increases, causing a loss of serous fluid out into the tissues. Children develop papular and vesicular skin eruptions with surrounding erythema. The vesicles rupture and exude yellow, sticky secretions that form crusts on the skin as they dry. Because the lesions are extremely pruritic, the child scratches and further irritates the lesions, causing linear excoriations. Secondary infections of open lesions may then occur. As the infected lesions heal, the skin becomes depigmented and lichenified (shiny), and dry, flaky scales form. If secondary infection occurs, local lymph nodes will be swollen. The child may have a low-grade fever. An increased eosinophil count reveals that the condition is allergy-based.

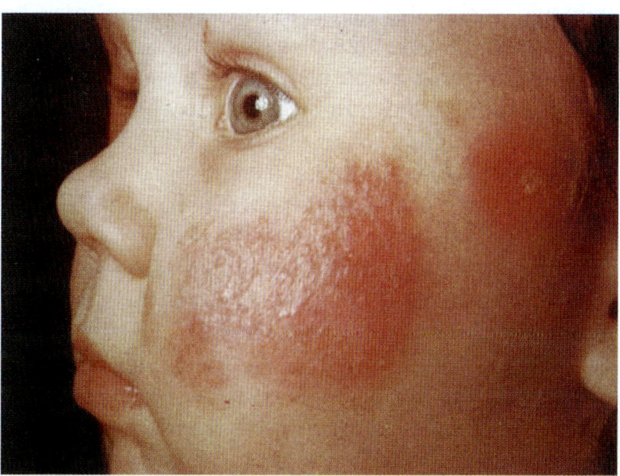

FIGURE 42.4 Infant with atopic dermatitis. (From Sauer, G. C. & Hall, J. C. (1996). *Manual of Skin Diseases* [7th ed.]. Philadelphia: Lippincott-Raven Publishers.)

TABLE 42.1 Comparison of seborrhoeic dermatitis and atopic dermatitis

Finding	Seborrhoeic dermatitis	Atopic dermatitis
Age at onset	0–6 months	2–6 months
Length of disease	Rarely 1 year	2–3 years
Mood of child	Happy; parents happy	Irritable; parents tired
Location of lesions	Scalp, behind ears, near umbilicus	Cheeks, extensor surfaces, some flexor surfaces
Types of lesions	Salmon-coloured erythematous lesions with greasy scales	Papulovesicular erythematous lesions with weeping and crusting
Itching	No	Severe
Depigmentation	No	Yes
Lichenification	No	Yes
White dermographism	No	Yes
Eosinophilia	No nasal mucus or blood eosinophilia	Nasal mucus or blood eosinophilia
IgE serum levels	Low	High

The common sites for lesions include the scalp and forehead, cheeks, neck, behind the ears and the extensor surfaces of the extremities. The palms of the hands and the soles of the feet are uninvolved. Because the lesions are uncomfortable, children with infantile atopic dermatitis may be overly fussy and irritable. Children with this condition may not eat well because of the generalised discomfort.

Although infantile atopic dermatitis is generally diagnosed while taking the family history (considering other allergic individuals in the family) and noticing the characteristic lesions and their patterns, it is sometimes difficult to distinguish from seborrhoeic dermatitis (cradle cap; see Chapter 29). Seborrhoeic dermatitis is a benign condition of infants, requiring little treatment other than frequent shampooing of the hair and soaking the lesions in mineral oil and combing them away. A child with infantile atopic dermatitis, on the other hand, will not respond to these measures but must be referred for additional treatment (see Table 42.1). Skin testing is ineffective because the allergen causing infantile atopic dermatitis is often a food allergen. However, it may also be caused by pollens, dust or mould spores. For this reason, skin testing may be attempted to isolate a causative allergen.

The treatment of atopic dermatitis is aimed at reducing allergen exposure. The most likely foods to which infants are allergic are milk, eggs, wheat, chocolate, fish, tomatoes and peanuts. The use of elimination diets to identify food allergens is discussed later in this chapter. A second major consideration in treatment is aimed at reducing pruritus so children do not irritate lesions and cause secondary infections by scratching. Hydrating the skin by bathing or applying wet dressings (wet with tap water or Burow's solution) for 15–20 minutes, followed by application of a hydrating emollient such as petroleum jelly (Vaseline) or even vegetable oil, is helpful. Do not allow infants to become chilled if a large portion of the body is to be covered with wet dressings. A stockinette dressing, with holes cut out for the eyes, nose and mouth, pulled over the head will hold wet dressings in place on the face and neck. To prevent corneal irritation, be careful that such dressings do not come in contact with the eyes.

Some infants need an antihistamine to reduce itching. Topical steroids such as 1% hydrocortisone cream do a great deal to relieve the discomfort and appearance of lesions by reducing the inflammation and pruritus. If the lesions are dry, a corticosteroid ointment is most effective; if moist, a lotion may be most effective. Applying the cream or lotion and then covering the area with an occlusive dressing such as plastic wrap overnight may assist the healing process. If the lesions are secondarily infected, hydrocortisone mixed with an antibiotic and a suitable base is prescribed. Caution parents not to discontinue application of cortisone cream abruptly. Although absorption with topical application is limited, some does occur. This reduces adrenal gland functioning. If the cream is discontinued abruptly, the infant's adrenal response (ability to produce adrenaline) in an emergency might be limited. Also caution the parents not to overuse the cortisone cream. More is not better and may increase the risk of systemic absorption.

Nursing considerations

Parents of children with infantile atopic dermatitis need a great deal of support through the course of the disease because infants can be irritable from the constant pruritus. Parents need a listening ear so they can vent these concerns and maintain their self-esteem as parents. Support groups also can help meet this need.

When lesions begin to heal, a skin emollient and moisturiser, such as Eucerin, or baths with a substance to lubricate the skin, such as Alpha-Keri, are prescribed to prevent excessive skin dryness. The infant should soak in the bath with the lubricant for approximately 15 minutes, then be patted, not rubbed, dry so the lesions are not aggravated. Caution parents not to use soap, because it can be drying.

Suggest that parents trim their infant's fingernails short or cover hands with cotton socks to prevent scratching. Exposure to the herpes virus can cause a generalised reaction. Caution parents to screen babysitters or alert childcare personnel with active herpes lesions not to care for their infants while atopic dermatitis is active.

In most infants, the lesions of infantile atopic dermatitis clear by the time a child is 3 years old. Unless secondary infection with scarring results, the skin surface will not be marked. Many of these children go on to develop other allergies, however, as they grow older. In the preschool years, the child's parents may report that the child has "one cold after another" (allergic rhinitis). By early school years, the child may show signs of asthma.

Atopic dermatitis in the older child

Atopic dermatitis in the older child may occur at any age, but frequently it occurs at puberty or late adolescence (Horii et al., 2007). Atopic dermatitis that occurs at these later ages is prominent on the flexor surface of the extremities and on the dorsal surfaces of the wrists and ankles. It often occurs in the eyebrows; if the child scratches the lesions, the child may be left with scant eyebrows. Depigmentation or hyperpigmentation is usually present and lichenification is marked. The fingernails often have a glossy sheen from the buffing action of constant rubbing and scratching. In some children, an itch-scratch cycle in response to stress may lead to an exacerbation of symptoms. For example, children begin to feel pressured at school or upset because they are left out of the neighbourhood group of children. Children rub their skin, a nervous, comforting mannerism and the rubbing or scratching leads to irritation of lesions. Then the lesions itch and the child scratches vigorously because of discomfort. The more a child scratches, the worse the lesions become; the more lesions there are, the more the child scratches and so on.

HIV INFECTION AND AIDS

AIDS is the end stage of acquired immunodeficiency caused by infection with the RNA human immunodeficiency retrovirus HIV (McFarland, 2008). The virus has at least two divisions, HIV-1 and HIV-2, with a variety of further subtypes. The virus acts by attacking the lymphoreticular system, in particular CD4-bearing helper T lymphocytes. The virus enters, substitutes its own RNA and DNA for the cell's DNA and replicates in these lymphocytes, destroying them in the process.

There is no defence against the virus, so it remains in the body for life. Infection results in loss of CD4 lymphocytes and the ability to initiate an effective B-lymphocyte response. A CD4 cell count in the laboratory determines how many cells are still present and functioning. Because B-lymphocyte or humoral immune function, which initiates the production of antibodies, is affected, antibody formation will be decreased (hypogammaglobulinaemia). When monocytes and macrophages become affected as well, the person with HIV infection cannot resist normal infection. When this CD4 count falls below 500 cells/mm^3 or the viral load rises above 5000 copies/mL, it is difficult for infected individuals to resist opportunistic infections such as fungal infections. The final result is that both the immune response and the ability to screen and remove malignant cells from the body are lost.

HIV infection is spread by exposure to blood and other body secretions through sexual contact, sharing of contaminated needles for injection, transfusion of contaminated blood or blood products, and perinatally from mother to fetus or newborn and through breastfeeding. A few children have acquired the infection because of sexual abuse. Healthcare providers must maintain vigilance to guard against incidents such as needle punctures, as these injuries are a source of blood transfer.

Although it is decreasing in incidence, mother-to-child transmission of HIV during pregnancy, labour, delivery or breastfeeding is still the most common reason for childhood HIV infection. In the absence of intervention transmission rates vary from 15% to 45%. This rate can be reduced to below 5% with effective interventions (WHO, 2014).

In the past, many children with haemophilia, because they received so many blood product transfusions, received HIV-contaminated blood and were infected. This source of transmission now almost never occurs. The increasing rate of sexual activity and the rapidly rising incidence of sexually-transmitted infections among adolescents make this group, next to newborn infants who received the virus from their mother, the most vulnerable to growing rates of HIV infection (McFarland, 2008). HIV is not transmitted by animals or through usual casual contact, such as shaking hands or kissing.

An estimated 25,708 people were living with diagnosed HIV infection in Australia at the end of 2012. A total of 1253 cases of HIV infection was newly diagnosed in Australia in 2012, a 10% increase from the number recorded in 2011. The annual number of new HIV diagnoses has gradually increased over the past 13 years, from 724 diagnoses in 1999 (The Kirby Institute, 2013).

HIV has a long incubation period of about 10 years in adults. The disorder appears to progress more rapidly in children and infants who receive the virus through placental transmission if they do not receive treatment. These individuals are usually HIV positive by 6 months and develop clinical signs by 1 to 3 years of age. Children who receive the virus from another source usually convert to HIV positivity by 2 to 6 weeks or at least by 6 months after exposure. During this preconversion time, a child may display preliminary symptoms such as poor resistance to infection, fever, swollen lymph nodes, respiratory tract infections and thrush. All infants born to infected mothers test positive for antibodies to the virus at birth because of passive antibody transmission. This persists for about 18 months. The disease is diagnosed, therefore, by recovery of the HIV antigen in children under this age and antibodies to the virus in children over this age.

CASE STUDY QUESTION

4. When Jack's mother learned he had an immunological disease, she was concerned that he had developed acquired immunodeficiency syndrome (HIV infection or AIDS). What is the transmission method by which most children acquire HIV infection?

   a. Blood transfusion
   b. Shared bath towels
   c. Placental transfer
   d. Sneezing and coughing

Nursing considerations

Children with HIV infection and their families must maintain strict personal hygiene by measures such as frequent hand-washing and avoiding close contact between the child and anyone who has a respiratory infection to try to prevent the child from contracting dangerous opportunistic infections. It is important to assess the oral cavity of children with AIDS for herpes and thrush lesions (Gennaro, Naidoo & Berthold, 2008). When infections do occur, antiviral and antifungal treatments should be prompt and aggressive.

Combating the infection requires specific antiretroviral medications to prevent progressive deterioration of the immune system and to provide prophylactic measures against opportunistic infections. Three classes of medication are the mainstay of therapy: nucleoside reverse transcriptase inhibitors (NRTIs), non-nucleoside reverse transcriptase inhibitors (NNRTIs) and protease inhibitors. NRTIs are designed to block production of viral DNA, limiting the ability of the virus to infect cells; zidovudine is an example (see Box 42.2). NNRTIs also inhibit the DNA synthesis of viruses but act at different sites on the viral enzyme; nevirapine and efavirenz are examples. Protease inhibitors stop the ability of the virus to produce protease, limiting metastasis; amprenavir, nelfinavir, atazanavir and ritonavir are examples of protease inhibitors used in children (Chadwick et al., 2008).

The diagnosis of HIV infection in an infant or child can prove devastating for a family. When the infection is transmitted maternally, this diagnosis may be the first indication of the existence of HIV infection in the mother; as such, this signals tremendous stress for the whole family. When it occurs in an adolescent, parents may blame themselves for not supervising the child's activities more closely or not providing better safe sex information. In any instance, the family's coping skills are certain to be compromised. Siblings may feel left out of the family circle because of the many healthcare appointments needed for the ill child. They may also fear contracting the infection themselves. One of the first nursing priorities in the care of such a family should be to help the family re-establish their previous level of functioning so they can turn their attention to their child's emotional and physical care needs and to their own needs as well.

BOX 42.2 ✻ Focus on pharmacology

Zidovudine (ZDV)

Classification: Zidovudine is an anti-infective drug

Action: Zidovudine inhibits the replication of some retroviruses, including HIV (McKenna & Mirkov, 2014)

Pregnancy risk category: B3

Dosage: 2 mg/kg every 6 hours to infants born to HIV-positive mothers, starting within 12 hours of birth to 6 weeks of age. 180 mg/m^2 (720 mg/m^2/dose) orally or intravenously every 6 hours to children ages 3 months to 12 years (dosage not to exceed 200 mg every 6 hours)

Possible adverse effects: Nausea, loss of appetite, change in taste, paraesthesia, headache, fever, agranulocytopoenia and rash

Nursing implications

- When administering the drug intravenously, infuse the drug over 60 minutes to avoid too rapid an infusion
- Administer the drug around the clock for maximum effectiveness
- Monitor blood studies frequently for changes
- Advise child to eat frequent small meals to counteract change in taste and loss of appetite
- If the child experiences paraesthesias, institute safety precautions and instruct the child and parents in measures to prevent injury related to loss of feeling
- Caution child and parents that ZDV does not reduce the risk of HIV transmission, except placentally. Reinforce the importance of hygiene and infection control measures

Physical care requirements for the child with HIV infection may be extensive, depending on the child's symptoms and disease progression. No matter what the child's physical needs, however, love and emotional support are essential to the child's well-being and psychological health. Parents or carers need extensive support, education and anticipatory guidance from nurses and other members of the healthcare team.

MEDICATION AND FOOD ALLERGIES

Medication allergies

One of the hazards of giving any medication is the risk that a child may experience a reaction to it or exhibit allergic symptoms. Because reactions to medications differ, it is important to be familiar with the symptoms of an allergic reaction, a toxic reaction or a known side effect of a medication.

A toxic reaction is one that occurs when a child has received too much of a medication. Side effects of medications are those that are known to occur in addition to a therapeutic effect. When an allergic effect occurs, unpredictable symptoms occur. The medication itself may not be an allergen, but when the medication combines with body protein, it becomes an allergen. This is why allergic responses occur not with the initial administration of a medication but only after the protein interaction (hapten formation or sensitivity) has occurred. When medications are applied to skin or mucous membrane, the chance of a medication allergy is highest. With the exception of acetylsalicylic acid (aspirin), allergy occurs rarely to orally-administered medications. Children with atopic diseases appear to be most prone to allergic medication reactions, although anyone can have such a reaction.

Reactions to medications differ, however, skin manifestations seen frequently include urticaria, angio-oedema, allergic contact dermatitis, pruritus and purpura. Respiratory symptoms include wheezing or rhinitis. Thrombocytopenia and haemolytic anaemia may also develop. Anaphylactic shock and serum sickness may occur. Children with a known medication allergy should wear a medical identification bracelet stating the medication to which they are sensitive.

Medications that are frequently involved in allergic reactions include parenteral penicillin and vaccines. In most instances, discontinuing the medication or never again administering the vaccine is the only therapy needed. If urticaria or serum sickness occurs, an antihistamine (such as diphenhydramine hydrochloride [promethazine hydrochloride, Phenergan]) is needed to relieve the symptoms. If anaphylaxis results, the treatment would be the same as for any anaphylaxis.

Food allergies

Food allergies manifest themselves differently from one child to another, but urticaria, angio-oedema, pruritus, stomach pain, colic, cramps, diarrhoea, respiratory symptoms and atopic dermatitis are common symptoms (Roberts, 2007). A symptom such as urticaria begins to manifest itself only minutes after an offending food is eaten. Other symptoms may be delayed, making the offending food difficult to recognise. Whole protein is probably the cause of immediate reactions; delayed reactions are likely the result of sensitivity to some protein breakdown product.

Skin testing is unreliable with food allergies because it is done with whole protein extracts. Delayed reactions, therefore, will not be detected in this way. The most common foods that cause immediate allergy symptoms include egg whites, fish and other seafood, berries and nuts. Delayed food reactions are commonly caused by cereals (wheat and corn), milk, chocolate, pork, legumes, white potatoes, beef, food additives and colourings, and oranges. If children are allergic to milk, they are probably allergic to milk products as well. Children who are allergic to eggs often cannot eat any foods that contain egg, such as puddings or baked goods. Some vaccines are still manufactured using eggs in the production process. The process to reduce the amount of egg protein available is continually improving, however, the actual amount may vary by manufacturer, year of production, batch and country of origin. For this reason it is important that health practitioners are made aware of a child's egg allergy prior to vaccination (ASCIA, 2010).

Young children cannot describe why they do not enjoy eating because they do not know the word for "headache", "stomach ache" or "itchiness", but they tend to avoid foods that affect them. This gives them a reputation of being "fussy eaters". This is not diagnostic of food allergies, however, because children may refuse to eat foods as a form of toddler rebellion or may be reported as fussy eaters because parents are expecting them to eat more than their small size requires.

Encouraging a child or parents to keep a food diary or a record of everything a child eats each day often is the best way to detect offending foods. They should note the presence of symptoms, if any. An elimination diet is another method that can be used to detect food allergens. For this, parents feed the child only foods that rarely cause allergy, such as rice, lamb, carrots, peas and sweet potatoes, for about 7 days. Then they add, one by one, at 2- to 3-day intervals, foods that are suspected of causing allergy. The treatment of food allergy is to permanently eliminate offending foods from the child's diet. This is relatively easy to do if there are only a few offending foods, but it becomes difficult when the foods are great in number or, like milk, wheat and eggs, are found in many products. Parents must become careful shoppers, reading labels carefully to be certain the foods they are buying do not contain products to which their child is sensitive. Help school-age children learn to choose foods they can eat safely at the school canteen or at school camps.

Milk hypersensitivity

The true incidence of milk hypersensitivity is probably not as high as the number of diagnoses made. Allergy to milk is typified by failure to gain weight, diarrhoea, vomiting and abdominal pain. Because these symptoms may also occur in a gastroenteritis infection, an infant may be misdiagnosed with an infection. Some infants with colic (characterised by abdominal pain, no change in stools and no failure to gain weight) or those with lactase deficiency (they cannot ingest the lactose in milk) may also be incorrectly diagnosed as having a milk allergy. If milk allergy is suspected, children are given a casein hydrolysate or soybean formula (Sondheimer, 2008). When this is done, symptoms are usually dramatically relieved.

Peanut hypersensitivity

A growing number of children are identified yearly as being so allergic to peanuts that even smelling peanut butter in a canteen or another child's lunch can provoke acute wheezing or anaphylaxis (Banerjee et al., 2007). School staff need to be very aware of this danger and may need to advocate for "peanut-free" school grounds. Desensitisation to peanuts can minimise children's responses.

BOX 42.3 * Focus on evidence-based practice

Food allergies

Food allergies are an important concern for nurses working in child-care and preschool settings because at such sites children often eat meals and snacks and so a child may eat an allergenic food and experience a possibly fatal reaction. To examine the circumstances of why allergic reactions occur in young children, researchers collected data on 512 infants aged 3 to 15 months who had documented allergies to milk or egg. The incidence of reactions in the study group was less than one reaction per child per year. Reactions occurred mostly because of unintentional exposure to milk or egg through label-reading errors and cross-contact. In 50% of reactions, the offending food was provided by a person other than a parent. Of the reactions, 29% were severe enough that the child was treated with adrenalin. Factors resulting in undertreatment included a lack of recognition of the severity of symptoms, adrenalin being unavailable and fears about adrenalin administration.

How would the results of this study help you in your teaching?

Source: Fleischer, D. M., Perry, T. T., Atkins, D., et al. (2012). Allergic reactions to foods in preschool-aged children in a prospective observational food allergy study. *Pediatrics, 130* (1), e25–e32.

Food allergy and food intolerance

Food allergies are an immune response to a particular food type entering the body. This should not be confused with a food intolerance, which relates to an inability to correctly digest food (NSW Food Authority, 2014). Food allergies are generally associated with common immune system symptoms including itchiness, swelling and even anaphylaxis in extreme cases (see Box 42.3). An intolerance to food results in a physical response that does not involve the immune system. Symptoms of food intolerance are unpleasant (headache, drowsiness, irritability etc.) but they are usually not life-threatening and are dose dependant.

STINGING INSECT HYPERSENSITIVITY

Allergic reactions to stinging insect bites are common. Children tend to suffer from less severe reactions to insect stings than adults. Children tend to commonly suffer from large local reactions and skin symptoms. For those who have experienced initial systemic reactions the risk of subsequent anaphylaxis is estimated to be around 20% (Tan & Campbell, 2013).

The history of stinging insect bites and the associated reactions is important in identifying a child who may have developed a hypersensitivity. The first time a child is stung, the total reaction is probably only local oedema at the site. The second time, generalised urticaria, pruritus and oedema may develop. The third time, symptoms may progress to wheezing and dyspnoea. The next time, the reaction could be so severe that shock and death result. The progression of symptoms may be slower than this (involving 10 to 12 stings) if the stings occur far apart. If the stings are received close together (1 or 2 days apart, or even 3 weeks apart), the progression to fatal symptoms may occur as early as the second or third exposure.

The time interval between the fatal sting and death is extremely short, approximately 10 minutes. For this reason, these children must be identified and given medication to combat shock immediately (there is no time to transport them for emergency care). The best way to protect children with allergies to stinging insects is to begin hyposensitisation against insect stings after the first reaction. An extract of wasp or bee venom accomplishes this.

The child who has not been hyposensitised must be treated immediately after the sting. This can be done by subcutaneous injection of adrenaline, which will give rapid relief (EpiPens are available for self-injection). If a child is stung during recess or an outside exercise period, it is the school nurse's responsibility to give the injection. In schools where there is no full-time nurse, another person must be designated and taught how to give the injection. If the child has antihistamine medication in addition to adrenaline, this should also be taken. Ice applied to the site minimises the amount of venom absorbed. The child should then be transported to the nearest hospital in case additional adrenaline is needed (the initial injection will be effective for only approximately 20 minutes).

CASE STUDY QUESTION

5. Jack is atopic or prone to allergies. In the hospital he has no toys. What material would you avoid if you wanted to make a toy for him?

a. A paper deck of cards
b. A cloth beanbag
c. A latex glove balloon
d. A tongue-blade puppet

CONTACT DERMATITIS

Contact dermatitis is an example of a delayed or type IV hypersensitivity response; it is a reaction to skin contact with an allergen (a substance irritating to the child only with prior sensitisation). The first reaction is generally erythema, followed by intensely pruritic papules and then vesicles. The allergen causing the irritation is often suggested by the part of the child's body that is affected. For example, dermatitis from a nappy-washing compound appears in the nappy area. Allergy to cosmetics appears on the face. Oozing at the site of pierced ears suggests an allergy to the nickel used in earring posts. Poison ivy appears on the hands and arms where the child brushed against the plant. Many children, especially those who have had many surgical procedures, such as children with spina bifida, as well as healthcare providers, are developing reactions to latex gloves (Cremer et al., 2007). Footwear, because of the chemicals used to tan leather, is also a frequent offender.

> ***What if…***
>
> Jack, who is allergic to leather, develops an erythematous, pruritic area on his right buttock? What would be a likely object causing the irritation?

MANAGEMENT OF IMMUNE DISORDERS

Environmental control

Environmental control, means removal of as many common allergens as possible from a child's environment (see Table 42.2). Some parents carry out instructions to reduce potential allergens in their house without difficulty but for others the process seems too involved to undertake. Help parents understand that environmental control can make a great deal of difference to their child's symptoms. If environmental control is effective with a child, this is preferable to hyposensitisation, which involves numerous visits to the doctor and several injections.

Hyposensitisation

Hyposensitisation, or immunotherapy, is carried out when the child's allergy symptoms cannot be controlled by avoidance of an allergen or conventional medication therapy. Because it is expensive and may not be successful, it is usually considered only after environmental control has been tried.

Hyposensitisation works by increasing the plasma concentration of IgG antibodies. IgG acts to prevent or block IgE antibodies from coming in contact with the allergen. After specific allergens have been recognised with skin testing, small amounts of the allergy extract (dilute enough to be clinically subreactive) are injected into the child subcutaneously at 3 to 5 day intervals. The dose of antigen is increased in strength, each time, until a peak concentration is reached. The peak dose corresponds to the greatest strength that does not give clinical symptoms after injection. Following this, the child's allergy symptoms should be greatly reduced or absent. The child then needs periodic injections every 3 to 4 weeks to maintain hyposensitisation to the allergen. If a child is going to have an anaphylactic reaction to an injected allergen, it generally

TABLE 42.2 Common measures for environmental control of allergens

Area of concern	Measures	Rationale
Child's bedroom	Encase mattress and pillow in sturdy plastic.	Reduces dust and dust mites
	Cover the zipper of plastic pillow and mattress case with adhesive tape.	Keeps dust confined
	Use blankets or quilts made of or stuffed with smooth, synthetic material; avoid wool.	Minimises dust; wool is a good dust collector or may be an allergen itself
	Take down any ornamental items, such as a bed canopy.	Prevents dust collection
	Remove stuffed chairs and replace with wooden ones.	Removes dust collectors
	Remove venetian blinds and curtains that need to be dry-cleaned; replace with easily laundered types.	Removes dust collectors
	Remove stuffed toys unless filled with synthetic material.	Removes dust collectors and possible sources of allergens
	Remove aquariums and plants.	Removes mould spores
	Clean wardrobe so it contains only currently used items.	Eliminates dust collectors
	Remove any fur or woollen items from child's wardrobe.	Removes possible allergens
Living room	Remove all carpets. If a rug is necessary, replace an animal hair pad with a foam rubber one.	Avoids containers for dust collection
	Provide a wooden chair for sitting.	Provides space free from allergens
	Vacuum frequently.	Minimises dust collection
	Use linoleum or plastic laminate surface on carpet if child sits on the floor.	Provides space free from allergens
	Discourage child from lying on rug.	Reduces exposure to allergens
Bathroom	Use non-scented toilet paper, soaps, cleaners.	Minimises exposure to potential irritants
School room	Have child sit away from blackboard, caged animals or fish tanks.	Minimises exposure to chalk, mould spores, and animal dander, which are allergens
	Keep locker free of collectibles.	Reduces dust collection
General	Purchase a dehumidifier; add compounds to paint to decrease mould spores.	Reduces mould spores
	Use HEPA filters on furnaces, vacuums.	Filters air of possible allergens
	Do not keep a pet.	Reduces exposure to animal dander
	Dust daily with a moist cloth.	Controls dust better than dry dusting

occurs within 30 minutes after the injection. Therefore, always have children wait in the healthcare setting for 30 minutes after the injection before going home.

Immunotherapy is generally continued for 2 to 3 years because the longer it is used, the longer the period of relief from symptoms after it is stopped. A newer technique of immunotherapy is the sublingual administration of chosen allergen solutions. SLIT (sublingual immunotherapy) is administered for an equal length of time as injection therapy, but SLIT has the advantage of being painless while producing equal results.

Caring for children with immune disorders and their families

The indeterminate and irregular nature of many physical manifestations of immunodeficiency disorders can pose social and psychological challenges to nursing care. The physical restrictions faced by children with immune conditions may also be socially restrictive, especially in a school setting. The often reduced ability to participate in social or cultural activities that are "normal" for the affected individual may lead to stigmatisation for both the child and their families.

Extra consideration needs to be given to the physical context of the child's family and social situation when developing prevention strategies and education for both the child and those providing direct support. Focusing on the medical treatment of an immunodeficiency without considering context may significantly reduce the compliance and resultant patient outcomes. For example, Jack Goodwell's mother reports that Jack's symptoms begin immediately after he arrives at school. It is not realistic to suggest that Jack avoid the area as it is necessary for him to attend. It is important that Jack's care plan evaluates his current school environment and routine in order to establish a realistic prevention strategy.

A major nursing consideration in the care of children with immune disorders is child and family education. The family of a child with an immunodeficiency may need help in identifying ways to keep the child from contracting life-threatening infections while at the same time providing enough stimulation and social contact to promote normal growth and development. A similar teaching goal must be established for a child with a chronic allergic disorder. Parents need to learn ways to help their child avoid triggers or situations that provoke allergy, but they must not keep the child so isolated or fearful that the child misses out on important experiences.

In Jack's case the next question to ask is what are the realistic management outcomes in relation to his home situation? This seems like a lot to think about. Put simply you are applying your knowledge of the physical aspects of the disease and causative agents to the actual context in which it is it is occurring, to achieve maximum benefits for the individual child and their family. As discussed throughout this chapter immunological disease varies greatly in both physiology and context of disease. This inevitably results in there being no "one size fits all" solution for patient management.

Health outcomes with immune disorders must be ongoing because new triggers for allergies can arise at any time. As the field of immunology is continually evolving, theories about immune diseases and associated treatments may change from visit to visit. Be certain parents are kept abreast of developments in the field, especially those that will affect their ability to provide an environment that is safest for their child.

Health promotion

It is estimated that as many as 40% of children living in Australia and New Zealand will have an allergic disorder some time in their life, with 20% having current symptoms (ASCIA, 2010). Preventing allergies, therefore, could have a major impact on the health of children. Early prevention can begin with encouraging women to breastfeed so that infants are not exposed to cow milk protein. Delaying the introduction of solid food until 6 months of age, once thought to reduce the development of allergies, may not be as beneficial as once thought (Tham, Rajakulendran & Shek, 2014). Delaying solid food because infants' gastrointestinal tracts are not ready for digestion, however, is still a valid reason to delay early feeding.

Environmental control to reduce the number of allergens in a home can drastically reduce allergy symptoms. This should begin when parents choose furniture for a child's room, such as eliminating woollen blankets, choosing toys carefully and keeping the room free of dust. Teach parents to use a minimum of washing compounds so that children are exposed to as few chemical products as possible. Avoiding spray products such as perfumes and air fresheners and discontinuing cigarette smoking also help (see Box 42.4). These are sensible rules for parents to follow beforehand, rather than waiting for a child to develop

BOX 42.4 ✻ Focus on family teaching

Avoiding secondary smoke

Q. Jack's mother says to you, "Neither my husband nor I smoke, but some of our relatives and friends do. How can we keep our child from being exposed to secondary smoke?"

A. Use the following guidelines to help avoid secondary smoke:

- Declare your home a smoke-free zone
- If family members smoke, ask them to smoke outside
- If at a restaurant, ask to sit in a no-smoking area or visit only smoke-free restaurants
- If staying at a hotel, ask for a non-smoking room
- Do not be reluctant to ask people around your child at a social gathering to stop smoking
- As smoke adheres to people's clothing, suggest that a person who smokes not hold a young baby
- Encourage your friends or family members who smoke to take quit-smoking courses (for their own benefit as well as yours).

allergic rhinitis or atopic dermatitis and then having to put more extreme measures into effect.

Latex is a common substance which causes allergy in children. Avoiding the use of latex gloves for healthcare procedures can help reduce the incidence of this (Rapp, 2008). Environmental pollutants such as exhaust from motor vehicles or ash from forest fires are other triggers for atopic diseases.

Because some families are more prone to allergies than others, some communities have a higher incidence of children with allergies than others. As a result, these communities may have more services and specialists to treat these children, a situation that develops a "community culture" of allergy acceptance and treatment. Children typically may leave school early for immunotherapy. School canteens commonly offer allergy-free foods. In other communities where fewer children have allergies, a child with an allergy is viewed as unique or not typical and so may need additional support.

Allergies are a type of disorder that typically cause chronic, rather than acute, symptoms. For this reason, children who develop allergies often need to be encouraged to be vigilant in taking their medicine. For the same reason, once parents begin a child on an immunotherapy program, they may need to be encouraged to continue it. It helps if children and their parents understand how allergic reactions lead to symptoms and how important it is for them to play a role in their own therapy.

Although it is probably impossible to keep children with atopic allergies free of reactions and manifestations of allergies, parents who know of familial allergy patterns can take some preventive steps in this direction. If parents are going to prepare allergy-free foods, be sure they consider the child's likes and dislikes and think about the child's weekly intake, to ensure the child receives all essential nutrients. If a child eats at school or has a meal prepared every day at a childcare centre, remind parents to make sure the centre, babysitter or school is aware of the child's allergies. If a child's allergies involve pollen sensitivities, planning holidays at a time when the pollen count is lowest may make the holiday more pleasant for the family. If desensitisation against a specific pollen is necessary, assist parents in planning to start desensitisation so it will be effective by the time the pollen count of the offending allergen rises.

Health promotion is also important to prevent HIV/AIDS. Teaching young people safer sex practices is an important part of this. All healthcare providers can help prevent the spread of HIV/AIDS by using standard infection precautions. The parents of children with immune deficiencies may need to be reminded periodically to take measures to keep their children free of disease, such as keeping immunisations updated and seeking help immediately for infections.

Key points for review

- An antigen is a foreign substance capable of stimulating an immune response. The immune system protects the body from invasion by foreign substances.
- Humoral immunity refers to immunity created by antibody production. B-lymphocytes are involved in this type of reaction. Cell-mediated immunity refers to T-lymphocyte involvement.
- Immunodeficiency disorders can be primary, such as B-lymphocyte and T-lymphocyte deficiencies, or secondary, such as acquired immunodeficiency syndrome (AIDS). HIV/AIDS is spread by the retrovirus HIV through blood and body secretions. Conscientious use of standard infection precautions is essential to prevent transmission.
- Allergic disorders occur as a result of an abnormal antigen-antibody response. As many as 40% of children in Australia and New Zealand have some form of allergy, 20% with current symptoms.
- Immune disorders, as a category, are long-term disorders, and children must participate in their own care to remain well, such as avoiding allergens and conscientiously taking an antihistamine to remain well. Involving children from the start helps them play an active role in their own care.
- Anaphylactic shock is an acute type I hypersensitivity reaction characterised by extreme vasodilation and bronchoconstriction. If action is not taken immediately, the reaction can be fatal. Subcutaneous adrenaline is the medication of choice to reduce symptoms.
- Atopic disorders include allergic rhinitis (hay fever), atopic dermatitis and asthma.
- Environmental control refers to ways to reduce the number of allergens to which children are exposed.
- Promoting breastfeeding may be a prime intervention to help prevent food allergies in allergy-prone families.

CASE STUDY QUESTIONS

6. Jack is diagnosed as having allergic rhinitis. His symptoms begin when he arrives at school. Knowing this problem is worse at school, what environmental control measures would you suggest for Jack?
7. When Jack had atopic dermatitis (infantile eczema) as an infant, almost his entire face was covered with weeping, crusting lesions. His forehead was lined with scratch marks. His mother was exhausted because Jack never slept because of the constant itching. What suggestions could you have made to his mother to make him more comfortable? What would you have suggested she do for herself?
8. Jack's mother was concerned he might have AIDS. What would you want to explain to Jack's mother about how the HIV virus is spread?
9. What would be a possible research topic to explore pertinent to these allergies that would be applicable to Jack's family and also advance evidence-based practice?

Resources

For an extensive range of additional resources to enhance teaching and learning and to facilitate understanding of this chapter, please see the text's accompanying website located on thePoint at http://thepoint.lww.com.

References

Australasian Society of Clinical Immunology and Allergy (ASCIA). (2012). Is it allergic rhinitis (hay fever)? Accessed 24 February 2015, <www.allergy.org.au/patients/allergic-rhinitis-hay-fever-and-sinusitis/allergic-rhinitis-or-hay-fever>.

Australasian Society of Clinical Immunology and Allergy (ASCIA). (2010). Guidelines for medical practitioners. Influenza vaccination of the egg-allergic individual. Accessed 24 February 2015, <www.allergy.org.au/images/stories/pospapers/ascia_guidelines_influenza_vaccination_egg_allergic_individual_2010.pdf>.

Australasian Society of Clinical Immunology and Allergy (ASCIA). (2010). Allergy prevention in children, accessed 24 February 2015, <www.allergy.org.au/images/stories/aer/infobulletins/2010pdf/AER_Allergy_Prevention_in_Children.pdf>.

Banerjee, D. K., et al. (2007). Peanut-free guidelines reduce school lunch peanut contents. *Archives of Disease in Childhood, 92*(11), 980–982.

Baris, S., Saricoban, H. & Ozdemir, C. (2011). Papaverine chloride as a topical vasodilator in accidental injection of adrenaline into a digital finger, *Allergy-European Journal of allergy and clinical immunology, 66*(11), 1495–1496.

Boguniewicz, M. (2008). Allergic disorders. In W. W. Hay et al. (Eds). *Current Pediatric Diagnosis and Treatment* (18th ed.). Columbus, OH: McGraw-Hill.

Busse, P. J. (2011). Angioedema: Differential diagnosis and treatment. *Allergy and Asthma Proceedings, 32*(5) S3–11.

Chadwick, E. G., et al. (2008). Pharmacokinetics, safety and efficacy of lopinavir/ritonavir in infants less than 6 months of age: 24 week results. *AIDS, 22*(2), 249–255.

Cremer, R., et al. (2007). Natural rubber latex sensitisation and allergy in patients with spina bifida, urogenital disorders and oesophageal atresia compared with a normal paediatric population. *European Journal of Pediatric Surgery, 17*(3), 194–198.

Gennaro, S., Naidoo, S. & Berthold, P. (2008). Oral health & HIV/AIDS. *American Journal of Maternal Child Nursing, 33*(1), 50–57.

Horii, K. A., et al. (2007). Atopic dermatitis in children in the United States, 1997–2004: Visit trends, patient and provider characteristics, and prescribing patterns. *Pediatrics, 120*(3), e527–e534.

James, B. (2013). Anaphylaxis: Diagnosis and treatment, *Nursing Standard, 27*(41), 49–56.

Ko, J. & Chung, W. (2013). Serum sickness. *Lancet, 381*(9862), e1.

McFarland, E. J. (2008). Human immunodeficiency virus infection. In Hay, W. W., et al. (Eds). *Current Pediatric Diagnosis and Treatment* (18th ed.). Columbus, OH: McGraw-Hill.

McKenna, L. & Mirkov, S. (2014). *McKenna's Drug Handbook for Nursing and Midwifery* (7th ed.). Sydney: Lippincott Williams & Wilkins.

Morgenstern, V., et al. (2008). Atopic diseases, allergic sensitization, and exposure to traffic-related air pollution in children. *American Journal of Respiratory and Critical Care Medicine, 177*(12), 1331–1337.

NSW Food Authority. (2014). Allergy and intolerance, Accessed 24 February 2015, <www.foodauthority.nsw.gov.au/consumers/problems-with-food/allergy-and-intolerance>.

Nieto, A. et al. (2014). Allergy and asthma prevention 2014. *Paediatric Allergy and Immunology, 25*(6), 516–533.

Rapp, S. M. (2008). Hospitals adopt latex-safe practices for patient, health care worker safety. *Orthopedics Today, 28*(5), 83.

Roberts, G. (2007). Anaphylaxis to foods. *Pediatric Allergy and Immunology, 18*(6), 543–548.

Sondheimer, J. M. (2008). Gastrointestinal tract. In W. W. Hay et al. (Eds). *Current Pediatric Diagnosis and Treatment* (18th ed.). Columbus, OH: McGraw-Hill.

Tan, J. W. & Campbell, D. E. (2013). Insect allergy in children. *Journal of Paediatrics and Child Health, 49*(9), e381–e387.

Tham, E. H., Rajakulendran, M. & Shek, L. P. (2014). Prevention of food allergy in the real life. *Asian Pacific Journal of Allergy and Immunology, 32*(1), 16–24.

The Kirby Institute, (2013). HIV, viral hepatitis and sexually transmissible infections in Australia. Annual surveillance report 2013. Accessed 24 February 2015, <https://kirby.unsw.edu.au/sites/default/files/hiv/resources/2013AnnualSurvReport.pdf>.

World Health Organization (2014). Mother-to-child transmission of HIV, accessed 24 February 2015, <www.who.int/hiv/topics/mtct/en>.

Suggested readings

Beyer, K., Eckermann, O., Hompes, S., et al. (2012). Anaphylaxis in an emergency setting—Elicitors, therapy and incidence of severe allergic reactions. *Allergy, 67*(11), 1451–1456.

Boyle, R. J., Elremeli, M., Hockenhull, J., et al. (2012). Venom immunotherapy for preventing allergic reactions to insect stings. *Cochrane Database of Systematic Reviews*, (10), CD008838.

Kramer, M. S., & Kakuma, R. (2012). Maternal dietary antigen avoidance during pregnancy or lactation, or both, for preventing or treating atopic disease in the child. *Cochrane Database of Systemic Reviews*, (9), CD000133.

Mullins, R. J., Clark, S. & Camargo, C. A. (2010). Socio-economic status, geographic remoteness and childhood food allergy and anaphylaxis in Australia. *Clinical and Experimental Allergy, 10*(10), 1523–1532.

Rebouças, C., Souza Paiva, S. D., Costa, E., et al. (2012). Proxemic communication between HIV-infected mother-child pairs. *British Journal of Nursing, 21*(18), 1098–1101.

Sanagavarapu, P. (2012). Don't forget to pack my EpiPen® please: What issues does food allergy present for children's starting school? *Australian Journal of Early Childhood, 37*(2), 56.

Chapter 43

Nursing care of a family when a child has an infectious disorder

Previous chapters described the growth and development of well children. This chapter adds information about the dramatic changes, both physical and psychosocial, that can occur when children contract an infectious disorder. This is important information to protect child health because many of these disorders spread easily to other children.

LEARNING OBJECTIVES

After mastering the contents of this chapter, you should be able to:

1. Describe the causes and manifestations of common infectious disorders of childhood.
2. Use critical thinking to analyse how the nature of the infectious disease effects the child and family at home.
3. Assess a child with an infectious disorder.
4. Discuss nursing considerations for a child with an infectious disorder.
5. Identify nursing care specific to the child with an infectious disorder, such as helping alleviate the pruritus of a rash.
6. Identify areas of nursing care related to children with infectious diseases that could benefit from additional nursing research or application of evidence-based practice.
7. Integrate knowledge of infectious diseases and nursing process to achieve quality child and family health nursing care.

KEY TERMS

- catarrhal stage
- chain of infection
- convalescent period
- enanthem
- exanthem
- incubation period
- Koplik's spots
- portal of entry
- prodromal period
- mode of transmission

CASE STUDY

Sam Ireland, a 10-year-old boy, was admitted to hospital for appendicitis. The morning after surgery, his throat was painful and his arms were covered by a very itchy, red, macular rash. Sam was diagnosed as having scarlet fever.

CASE STUDY QUESTIONS

1. What advice would you give Sam's mother?
2. Is it likely that Sam contracted this new disease while he was in hospital or before he was admitted?
3. What is a measure you would recommend to help reduce the itching?

Despite the number of preventive measures available, infectious diseases remain a leading cause of morbidity in children. Nurses play a key role in educating parents and the public about common childhood infectious disorders and appropriate preventive measures. They must be able to identify the symptoms of common infectious diseases of childhood, as they are often the first to see evidence of infection. For example, a school nurse needs to be able to effectively screen children for potentially communicable infections such as impetigo or tinea capitis (ringworm). In healthcare settings, nurses often perform triage, identifying children who must be seen immediately, those who can wait to be seen and those who should not stay in a waiting room with other children because they may have an infectious disorder. For example, occasionally children admitted to an inpatient unit develop diarrhoea soon after admission. It is vital that a nurse quickly recognises that this could be contagious so other children in the hospital, especially those who are immunosuppressed, and staff can be protected (Chambers, 2009).

A CHILD WITH AN INFECTIOUS DISORDER

Assessment

Many infectious diseases begin subtly. Parents report general symptoms such as, "he doesn't act like himself" or "she's so listless". In many syndromes, children are infectious during this period. Following the prodomal period, an **exanthem** (rash) can develop. Rashes can be difficult to identify, so it is important to obtain a full description and history of the rash.

Nursing considerations

Common nursing considerations directly related to the infectious process are:

- Pain
- Impaired skin integrity
- Risk of infection
- Altered body temperature
- Fluid volume deficit.

When planning care of children with infectious disorders, include steps that help parents deal with the current infection and also prevent another infection. This is particularly important if the child has siblings at home. Education should include information about necessary infection-control precautions and immunisations. Parents often ask about communicability to their other children and to the infected child's playmates or schoolmates, so these issues need to be addressed. Planning care for a child who requires restrictions to prevent disease transmission requires thoughtful consideration as it may involve extended periods of social isolation while avoiding contact with peers and other family members. Guidelines relating to isolation times for children with infectious diseases can be found in the Australian Government document *Staying healthy: Preventing infectious diseases in early childhood education and care services* available at <www.nhmrc.gov.au/guidelines/publications/ch55>.

The Australian Government releases annual reports on notifiable disease status titled the Annual Report of the National Notifiable Diseases Surveillance System. You can learn more about communicable diseases or disease groups in Australia at <www.health.gov.au/internet/main/Publishing.nsf/Content/cda-pubs-annlrpt-nndssar.htm>.

Nursing responsibilities when caring for a child with an infectious disorder depend on the setting in which the child is seen. Often, a child will not be brought into a hospital. Counselling parents about techniques to relieve the irritation of rashes and other symptoms of infectious illness can be given over the telephone, however, it is important to ensure a correct diagnosis is made. Administering prescribed medications and being alert for potential adverse effects are other major nursing responsibilities.

THE INFECTIOUS PROCESS

A *pathogen* is any organism that causes disease. Pathogens can be classified into five types of microorganisms: viruses, bacteria, rickettsiae, helminths and fungi.

Stages of infectious disease

Infectious diseases follow certain stages during which the communicability (ability to be spread to others) or severity of the illness can be predicted (see Fig. 43.1).

- The **incubation period** is the time between the invasion of an organism and the onset of symptoms of infection. During this time, microorganisms grow and multiply. The incubation period varies depending on the pathogen. A common interval is 7–10 days, but it can be longer. The incubation period for tetanus, for example, is 2–21 days.
- A **prodromal period** is a time between the beginning of non-specific symptoms and disease-specific ones. Non-specific symptoms include lethargy, low-grade fever, fatigue and malaise. Children are infectious (capable of spreading the microorganisms to others) during this time, but because their symptoms are so vague they do not generally take any precautions against spreading disease. Therefore, during a prodromal period, infectious diseases spread readily through communities to any susceptible individuals. Prodromal stages are generally short, ranging from hours to a few days.
- *Illness* is the stage during which specific symptoms are evident. Most illnesses have local symptoms related to the body organ affected and also systemic symptoms that affect the entire body, such as fever, increased white blood cell count or headache. Many childhood infections have an accompanying rash on the skin **(exanthem)** or mucous membrane (**enanthem;** see Box 43.1).

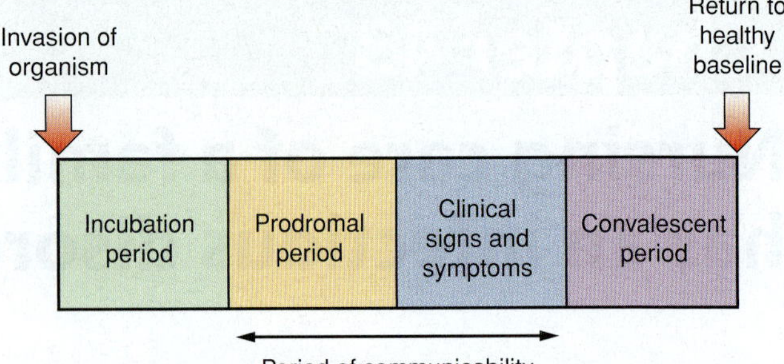

FIGURE 43.1 The time frame for infectious diseases. The period of communicability is the time during which the disease can be transmitted to other people.

BOX 43.1 Assessment ✻ Assessing a child with common signs and symptoms of infectious disorders

History

Chief concern: Does child have a fever, general malaise, vomiting or diarrhoea? Was child recently exposed to someone with an infection?

Past medical history: Are child's immunisations current?

Physical examination

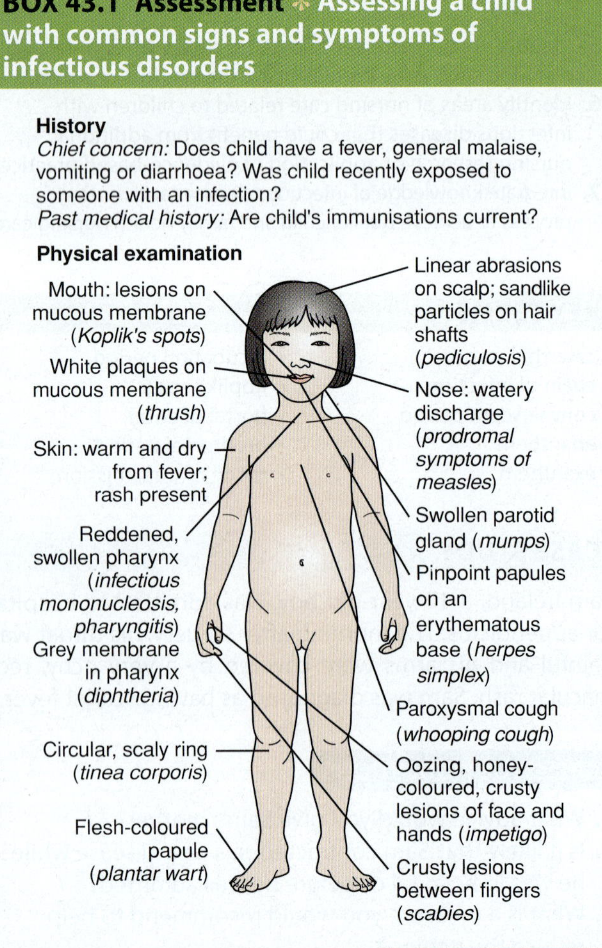

TABLE 43.1 Methods by which infections spread

Portal of exit	Means of transmission	Portal of entry	Prevention measures
Blood	Arthropod vectors Blood sampling Transfusion	Injection into the bloodstream	Decreasing exposure to vectors Careful handing of blood sampling equipment Prescreening of blood for organisms such as HRV or hepatitis B
Respiratory secretions	Airborne droplets Fomites	Respiratory tract	Wearing a mask Droplet and airborne precautions Hand washing
Faeces	Water, food Fomites Vectors such as flies	Gastrointestinal tract	Hand washing before eating, after using bathroom or after handling nappies
Exudate from lesions	Direct contact Contact with soiled dressings	Skin, mucous membranes	Contact precautions Self-screening for sexual contacts Gloves

- The **convalescent period** is the interval between when symptoms first begin to fade and the child returns to full wellness. Because fatigue is often an accompanying symptom of infection, the convalescent period, or the time until full energy is restored, is often longer than anticipated.

Chain of infection

The **chain of infection** is the method by which organisms are spread and enter a new individual to cause disease. Breaking the chain at one of its susceptible points is the most efficient way to prevent infection from spreading (Smith, 2011). The chain of infection consists of the reservoir, portal of exit, mode of transmission, portal of entry and a susceptible host.

The reservoir is the container or place in which an organism grows and reproduces. This could be another person with the disease, a contaminated object, or an animal or insect. The portal of exit is the route by which an organism leaves the infected child's body to be spread to others. A **portal of entry** refers to the opening through which a pathogen enters a child's body such as by inhalation, ingestion, or breaks in skin from bites, abrasions or burns. Understanding the portal of entry of a pathogen assists in breaking the chain of infection at this point, through education. For example, teaching children to wash their hands after sneezing or coughing or teaching parents to wash a cut or abrasion before bandaging them. Finally, for infection to occur there must be a susceptible host (see Table 43.1).

Certain characteristics make some individuals more prone to infection than others. Age, gender, virulence of the pathogen and body defences (physical, chemical and immune responses) all effect the susceptibility of a child to a specific infectious disease. Immunisation plays a large role in decreasing the susceptibility of children to many infectious diseases.

Consider the elements of the chain of infection when reading the information relating to specific infectious conditions later in this chapter. Refer back to this section and identify the reservoir, portal of exit, mode of transmission, portal of entry and susceptible host for each condition. Applying this knowledge to specific conditions allows for effective patient management and education. This knowledge also assists in determining the appropriate precautions to be adopted, both in the healthcare setting and at home, to avoid the spread of further infection and protect susceptible individuals including healthcare workers.

Mode of transmission

The **mode of transmission** refers to whether the infection is spread by contact (direct or indirect), droplet or airborne modes. Contact, involves transmission by touch or via contact with blood or body substances. Direct transmission occurs when a pathogen is transferred from one person to another, for example, direct exposure to blood from one child to another with an open cut in the skin. Indirect transmission relates to the transmission of a pathogen through a contaminated object or person, for example a child's toy or drinking vessel. Droplet transmission, generally occurs when an infected person coughs, sneezes or talks. Respiratory droplets transmit infections when they land on a susceptible mucosal surface. Airborne pathogens are spread in a similar manner to droplet pathogens. The difference being these aerosols can be dispersed over long distances and the infective agents may remain infective for a period of time.

Understanding the route of transmission is important as it directly relates to the type of infection control precautions that need to be implemented to avoid the spread of disease. Modes of transmission include contaminated food and water, medications, and medical devices and equipment (National Health and Medical Research Council, 2010).

HEALTH PROMOTION

Preventing infectious diseases is important because these disorders are responsible for a high percentage of hospital admissions in children. Prevention begins with being certain all children are generally in good health. Adequate nutrition is important to provide protein and vitamins to support immune system function.

The incidence of childhood disease from vaccine preventable diseases (VPDs) is low in both Australia and New Zealand due to strong immunisation programs (New Zealand Ministry of Health, 2014c; Australian Government Department of Health, 2013). In Australia today there is an average vaccination coverage of 90% for children at 12 months, 24 months and 60 months of age. These rates have improved dramatically over the last 30 years, which has been reflected in the decreased rates of VPDs reported. While we do enjoy excellent immunisation rates, it should be noted that some VPDs require even higher rates of community immunity to avoid outbreaks. For example, for measles, the required rate is 95%. The result of not having the required coverage rate was highlighted in a measles outbreak in Sydney in 2012 when 170 cases of the disease were identified.

The reduction in VPDs due to a successful immunisation program in both Australia and New Zealand and resultant lack of exposure to the related diseases has, in some instances, lead to a complacency in relation to immunisation. This situation has been exacerbated by concerns held by some parents relating to the potential adverse side effects of immunisation. It is important that parents are aware of the need for their children to be immunised and of the detailed guidelines that are in place in relation to immunising high risk children. Nurses need to ensure that immunisations are offered to children at well-child and illness healthcare visits. Further reading regarding immunisation guidelines for Australia and New Zealand can be found at <www.health.gov.au/internet/immunise/publishing.nsf/Content/Handbook10-home> and <www.health.govt.nz/publication/immunisation-handbook-2014>. It is important that parents also understand that although diseases such as chickenpox (varicella) and mumps (infectious parotitis) are referred to as "common" childhood illnesses, they have the potential to be serious illnesses, leading to complications such as pneumonia and encephalitis. When children develop these common communicable diseases, parents need to seek medical assistance as soon as possible, to minimise the risk of complications.

The responsibility of parents and children to help prevent the spread of communicable diseases differs from country to country and varies among cultures. In Australia and New Zealand both federal and state governments have taken an active role in preventing the spread of infectious disease by requiring children to have immunisations against the most common illnesses. Parents are expected to obtain immunisations for children by school-age. Schools and school nurses take an active role in promoting these recommendations. Community health nurses are also instrumental in administering immunisation and counselling families on how to prevent the spread of disease in their home. Nurses can also make certain that parents are aware of the latest studies available on the safety of vaccines so they do not associate common vaccines with the development of autism, for example.

Developing countries have a great deal of difficulty maintaining this same level of disease prevention as Australia and New Zealand. Remember when caring for children newly-arrived from another country that the child may not have the same level of immunisation usually seen here. This opens an important area of health teaching, as the parents may not be aware of the importance or availability of immunisation, or the community services available to supply them.

Healthcare-associated infections

Nosocomial or healthcare-associated infections (HAI) are infections that are contracted while in a hospital or other healthcare setting. They represent a major threat to hospitalised children. Children younger than 2 years, or children with a nutritional deficit, those who are immunosuppressed, those who have indwelling vascular lines or catheters, those receiving multiple antibiotic therapy or those who remain in the hospital for longer than 72 hours are at highest risk of contracting such an infection. Nurses provide a line of defence against such infections by always implementing standard precautions, including frequent and thorough hand-washing (Harding, Almquist & Hashemi, 2011). Nurses and other healthcare providers must also take precautions to protect themselves from acquiring communicable diseases, including HIV and hepatitis, by adhering to standard infection precautions.

CARING FOR THE CHILD WITH AN INFECTIOUS DISEASE

As almost all childhood infectious diseases include a fever or rash, nursing care must address identification and relief of these symptoms.

Pruritis

Providing comfort for the pruritus of skin lesions is important for many childhood infections. No matter what agent is causing the disease, a rash tends to be extremely itchy and uncomfortable. Fortunately, several simple remedies are available for reducing both pain and inflammation associated with this condition. An antihistamine is extremely helpful in reducing symptoms. A topical treatment such as Calamine lotion is a non-prescription lotion that is cooling and soothing and often helps to relieve itching. Colloidal baths, such as baking soda or oatmeal (approximately 1 cup to 8 cm of bath water), are soothing for some children. Caution parents to use only lukewarm water, not hot, because heat usually increases the sensation of itching. Bathing serves two purposes, it can not only be soothing but also distracting. A child, especially a preschooler, may splash for 15–20 minutes in a bath without noticing the discomfort of a rash.

Social isolation

A child who is restricted from others because of infection control precautions can begin to feel lonely and depressed unless stimulation and social needs are met. Children easily associate isolation and restriction with being punished. In a hospital setting, make as few trips as possible in and out of the room to limit the possibility of pathogen spread; on the other hand, do not make care visits seem hurried. If there is a procedure scheduled at 9.00 a.m. and another at 9.30 a.m., stay in the room rather than leave to return again, if possible. Use the time to read a story to the child, play a card game or talk about how strange and lonely it feels to be separated from other people.

When a child is hospitalised and requires transmission-based infection control precautions, parents must follow these precautions, just as all hospital personnel do, when they visit. Making them feel comfortable with these procedures is a nursing responsibility. If a child has an infectious condition and is being cared for in the home it is important to consider what (if any) restrictions need to apply to other family members and visitors. Similarly consideration needs to be given to whether the child needs to be excluded from attending a childcare facility or school for a period of time depending on the nature of their condition.

VIRAL INFECTIONS

Viruses are the smallest infectious agents known; so small they cannot be seen through an ordinary microscope. Although a body cell may not be outwardly altered by a virus invasion, it could fail to function or die because of lysis of internal components or rupture. Symptoms usually do not become apparent until many cells have been interrupted in this way, so the incubation period of viral infections can be long. Some viruses are capable of invading only specific cells. The Epstein-Barr virus, for example, invades only *viral exanthems*.

The majority of childhood exanthems (rashes) are caused by viruses and each of these diseases has specific symptoms, characteristic lesions and a specific distribution or pattern to the rash that allows it to be identified (see Appendix G).

Exanthem subitum (roseola infantum)

- Causative agent: Human herpes virus 6 (HHV-6)
- Incubation period: Approximately 10 days
- Period of communicability: During febrile period
- Mode of transmission: Unknown
- Immunity: Contracting the disease offers lasting natural immunity; no artificial immunity is available

Roseola is a disease with symptoms that appear to be more severe than is warranted. It generally occurs in children between 6 months and 3 years, mainly in spring and autumn, although it can occur any time of the year. The first symptom is a high fever (40.0° to 40.6°C). Infants may be irritable and anorexic but rarely appear as ill as this high a fever suggests. They usually remain playful and alert. The pharynx may be slightly inflamed. The occipital, cervical and postauricular lymph nodes may be enlarged. The white blood count is usually decreased, with the proportion of lymphocytes increased.

After 3 or 4 days, the fever falls abruptly and a distinctive rash appears. The lesions are discrete, rose-pink macules approximately 2–3 mm in size. They fade on pressure and occur most prominently on the trunk. The rash resembles that of rubella or measles, but it is darker and children have no accompanying coryza (upper respiratory symptoms), conjunctivitis or cough. Because it occurs mainly on the child's trunk, parents may report it as a heat rash. The rash lasts 1–2 days. The diagnosis of roseola is based on the physical signs and symptoms. The hallmark of roseola is the appearance of a rash immediately after the sharp decline in fever (Dyer, 2007).

Treatment focuses on measures to reduce the discomfort of the rash and fever. The fever will respond to medication but after 4 hours it is apt to rise again to the high level. The most frequent complication of roseola is a febrile seizure with the onset of the disease because the temperature rises so rapidly.

Rubella (German measles)

- Causative agent: Rubella virus
- Incubation period: 14–21 days
- Period of communicability: 7 days before, to approximately 5 days after, the rash appears
- Mode of transmission: Direct and indirect contact with droplets
- Immunity: Contracting the disease offers lasting natural immunity; a high rubella titer reveals infection has occurred

Rubella is a disease rarely seen today in developed countries. When it does occur, it affects older school-age and adolescent children. It occurs most commonly during spring. The symptoms begin with a 1- to 5-day prodromal period, during which children or adolescents have a low-grade fever, headache, malaise, anorexia, mild conjunctivitis, possibly a sore throat, a mild cough and swollen lymph nodes such as those in the suboccipital, postauricular and cervical chains (Weinberg & Levin, 2014).

After 1–5 days of prodromal signs, a discrete pink-red maculopapular rash begins on the face, then spreads downwards to the trunk and extremities. On the third day, the rash disappears. There is generally no desquamation (peeling); if present, it is primarily fine flaking of the skin. Fever with rubella is not marked, although arthritis (joint pain) with effusion into the joints occurs in some children on the second or third day, lasting as long as 5–10 days.

If rubella occurs during pregnancy, it can cause extensive congenital malformation in the fetus (see Chapter 12). Because of this, it can never be considered a simple disease. It is important that girls be immunised against it before they reach child-bearing age (Thilo & Rosenberg, 2008). This said, it is equally important to ensure boys are also immunised to avoid transmission to females who do not seroconvert following immunisation.

Measles (rubeola)

- Causative agent: Morbillivirus
- Incubation period: 10–12 days
- Period of communicability: Fifth day of incubation period until the first few days of rash
- Mode of transmission: Direct or indirect contact with droplets
- Immunity: Contracting the disease offers lasting natural immunity

Measles is a viral condition with potentially series physical complications. Measles is sometimes called brown or black, regular or 7-day measles, to differentiate it from rubella (German or 3-day measles). Like rubella, because of high vaccination rates, it is rarely seen today except for periodic outbreaks that occur in newly under-immunised immigrant populations or an under-immunised young adult population (Muller et al., 2007). The incidence of the disease is highest in winter and spring. Complications associated with measles include ear infections, diarrhoea and pneumonia potentially requiring hospitalisation in severe cases. Approximately 1 in 1000 people with measles will develop encephalitis (New South Wales Health, 2014).

This disease has a 10 to 11-day prodromal period, during which lymphoid tissue, particularly postauricular, cervical and occipital lymph nodes, become enlarged. Children develop a high fever (39.5° to 40.0°C) and malaise. By the second day of the prodromal period, coryza (rhinitis and a sore throat), conjunctivitis with photophobia (sensitivity to light) and a cough develop. **Koplik's spots** (small, irregular, bright-red spots with a blue-white centre point) appear on the buccal membrane. Unfortunately, the coryza of measles is indistinguishable from that of a common cold (nasal congestion, a mucopurulent discharge and a deep brassy, bronchial cough) when it begins. As a result, many children with measles are diagnosed as having a simple upper respiratory infection at this point.

Koplik's spots distinguish the disease because none of the other exanthems has this finding. They appear first on the buccal membrane opposite the molars and then extend to cover the entire buccal surface (see Fig. 43.2). The raised base of the spots may coalesce so that the blue-white centres stand out as grains of salt on the erythematous membrane. It should be noted that Koplik's spots only appear briefly and are often missed by the time a child is brought to a medical facility for assessment.

By the fourth day of fever, the rash appears. A deep-red maculopapular eruption begins at the hairline of the forehead, behind the ears and at the back of the neck, and then spreads to the face, the neck, upper extremities, trunk and finally the lower extremities (see Fig. 43.3). After several days, the rash typically turns from red to brown. While the rash is red, it fades on pressure; when it is brown, it does not fade. This differentiates it from the rash of scarlet fever, which always fades on pressure. After 5–6 days, the rash completely fades. There is a fine desquamation after this. However, the skin of the hands and feet does not desquamate, a feature again differentiating it from scarlet fever.

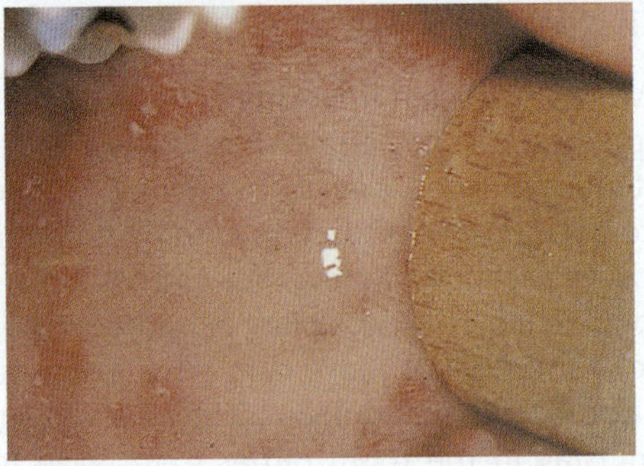

FIGURE 43.2 Koplik's spots on the oral mucous membrane. (SPL/Custom Medical Stock Photograph.)

Children with measles appear very ill because their cough is loud and frequent, the coryza is acute, the fever is high and the rash is pruritic. Fortunately, on the third or fourth day of rash, when the temperature begins to fall, the other symptoms clear quickly and children feel better. Fever that lasts beyond the third or fourth day of rash or coughing that continues, generally suggests that a complication of measles, such as pneumonia, has occurred.

Children with measles need comfort measures for the rash and an antipyretic for the fever. Because children with

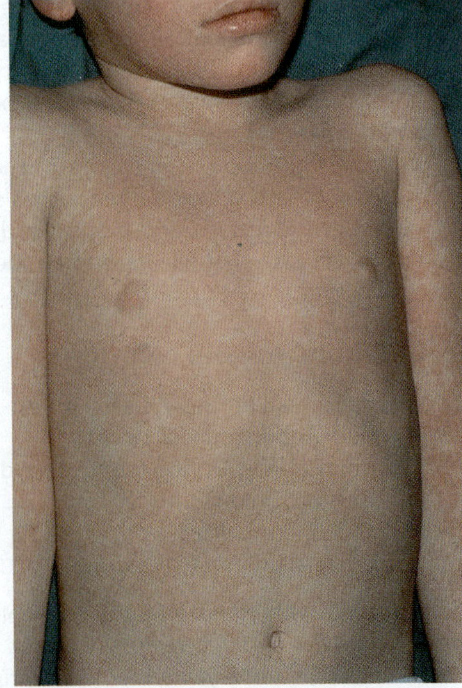

FIGURE 43.3 The typical rash of measles on a child's upper body. (© NMSB/Custom Medical Stock Photograph.)

measles have photophobia, it is painful for them to look at bright lights, so it may be painful for them to watch television. They are often more comfortable with the blinds or curtains drawn or wearing dark glasses, so these measures should be instituted. Children need to be seen by a healthcare provider because the complications of measles include otitis media (middle ear infection), pneumonia, airway obstruction and acute encephalitis (Weinberg & Levin, 2008). If a child is hospitalised, follow airborne precautions for the duration of the illness in addition to standard infection precautions.

Chickenpox (varicella)

- Causative agent: Varicella-zoster virus
- Incubation period: 10–21 days
- Period of communicability: 1 day before the rash to 5–6 days after its appearance, when all the vesicles have crusted
- Mode of transmission: Highly contagious; spread by direct or indirect contact of saliva or vesicles
- Immunity: Contracting the disease offers some natural immunity to chickenpox; because the same virus causes herpes zoster, it may be reactivated at a later time as herpes zoster (shingles). Varicella-zoster vaccination is available to children in both Australia and New Zealand.

Chickenpox is another common childhood infection that is decreasing in incidence due to high immunisation rates. Individuals who have not been vaccinated, such as older children and young adults are at a higher risk of infection. The disease is marked by a low-grade fever, malaise and, in 24 hours, the appearance of a rash. The lesion begins as a macula, then progresses rapidly within 6 to 8 hours to a papule, then a vesicle that first becomes umbilicated and then forms a crust. Each lesion is approximately 2–3 mm in diameter and is surrounded by an erythematous area. When the first crop of lesions appears, the child's temperature may rise markedly to 40.0° or 40.6°C.

Most of the chickenpox lesions are found on the trunk, although the face, scalp, palate and neck also may be involved. They appear in approximately three separate series or crops, with each new lesion moving through progressive stages (see Fig. 43.4). At one time, all four stages of lesions (macule, papule, vesicle and crust) are present.

If the scabs from crusting are allowed to fall off naturally and lesions do not become secondarily infected, no scarring results. Scabs removed prematurely may leave a white, round, slightly indented scar at the site. For this reason, it is important that children do not scratch and remove scabs. However, because the rash of chickenpox is extremely pruritic, preventing scratching becomes a difficult problem for parents. A prescribed antihistamine usually helps to reduce the itchiness to a bearable level and an antipyretic will counteract the high fever. The development of Reye's syndrome has been associated with aspirin use during varicella and influenza virus illnesses (see Chapter 49), so caution parents to avoid aspirin and to use acetaminophen or ibuprofen to control fever instead.

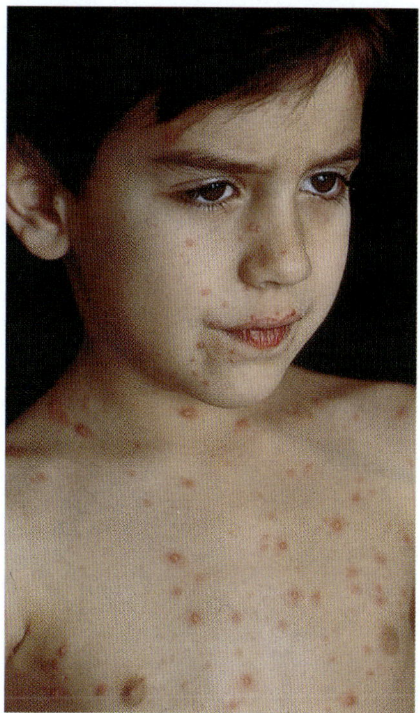

FIGURE 43.4 An older school-aged boy with varicella. (© Martin/Custom Medical Stock Photograph.)

If the child is hospitalised, follow airborne and contact precautions until all lesions are crusted, in addition to standard infection precautions. Children may return to school as soon as all the lesions are crusted (the crusts are not infectious). Complications include secondary infections of the lesions, pneumonia and encephalitis.

Herpes zoster

Herpes zoster is caused by a reactivation of latent varicella-zoster virus, the same virus that causes chickenpox. The first time the virus invades, children have symptoms of chickenpox. With a second invasion, herpes zoster symptoms appear. Herpes zoster tends to occur in older children or young adults, although it can occur at any age.

The first manifestations are pruritus and cutaneous vesicular lesions on erythematous bases that follow the distributions of the lumbar and thoracic nerves (usually on the trunk, face or upper back) and cause deep nagging pain (see Fig. 43.5). In the majority of cases the prodromal phase for this disease is 48–72 hours before the appearance of lesions (Australian Government Department of Health, 2013). Treatment for herpes zoster includes measures to reduce pruritus and analgesia for pain.

Viral infections of the integumentary system

Viral infections of the skin include the herpes infections and warts (verrucae).

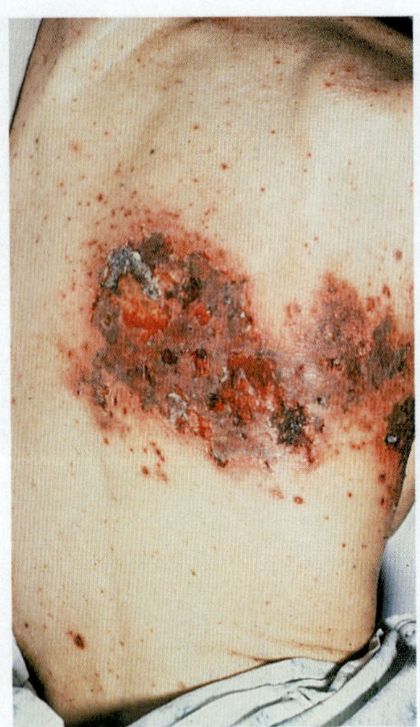

FIGURE 43.5 Herpes zoster on a child's back. (© Dr. P. Marazzi/SPL/Science Source/Photo Researchers.)

Herpes virus infections

Herpes viruses are responsible for several infections in children.

- Causative agent: Herpes simplex virus type 1 or type 2
- Incubation period: 2–12 days
- Period of communicability: Greatest early in the course of the infection
- Mode of transmission: Direct contact
- Immunity: Immunity to a primary herpes response is gained after one incident. There is no immunity to recurrent herpes infections because the virus lies dormant in the body until it is activated by stress, sun exposure, fever, other illness or menstruation

HSV type 1

Initial infection with HSV type 1 usually occurs in early childhood (Department of Health, Victoria, 2015). Herpes simplex infection, popularly known as a cold sore or fever blister, represents the recurrent form of a type 1 herpes virus invasion that has remained dormant in the ganglia of the trigeminal or fifth cranial nerve. Herpes simplex typically appears as clusters of painful, grouped vesicles surrounded by an erythematous base on the lips or skin surrounding the mouth. After 2 or 3 days, vesicles crust, then gradually dry. Keeping lesions dry helps them to fade sooner, but keeping them lubricated with an ointment reduces pain. Topical or oral acyclovir reduces pain and increases healing. Children feel conspicuous about the appearance of herpes simplex lesions. They may need counselling to assure them that the lesions are not as obvious to others as they seem to them (Berger, 2009).

HSV type 2

HSV type 2 is the primary cause of genital warts (however this can also be caused by HSV type 1). This disease is sexually transmitted and generally occurs in adults.

Warts (verrucae)

Warts, one of the most common dermatological diseases in children, are caused by the papillomavirus. The virus has an incubation period of 1 to 6 months. The mode of transmission is unknown, but it is probably by direct contact (Androphy & Lowy, 2008).

Warts are flesh-coloured, dirty-appearing papules. They generally occur on the dorsal surface of the hands, although they may occur anywhere. Plantar warts appear on the soles of the feet and are painful when children walk. They may be differentiated from calluses in that they obliterate skin lines as they grow, whereas calluses do not.

Warts on the hands or the face are generally removed if they are cosmetically unattractive to children. Plantar warts may have to be removed because of the discomfort they cause. Parents can use over-the-counter wart-removing preparations to dissolve them. Application of 40% salicylic acid may be prescribed to remove plantar warts. Carbon dioxide snow, liquid nitrogen, electrodesiccation and curettage are also effective for removal, but these methods are painful and rarely necessary.

Children need reassurance that people do not catch warts from frogs or toads and even if left without any treatment, warts will eventually fade by themselves after about 24 months. Anogenital warts need special consideration as they can be a mark of sexual abuse (Ornstein & Hatchette, 2012).

Other viral infections

Mumps (epidemic parotitis)

- Causative agent: Mumps virus
- Incubation period: 14–21 days
- Period of communicability: Shortly before and after onset of parotitis
- Mode of transmission: Direct or indirect contact
- Immunity: Contracting the disease gives lasting natural immunity

Mumps is now a rare disease in Australia and New Zealand due to successful immunisation programs. It is most likely to be seen in adolescents who have not been immunised. If the disease occurs, it begins with fever, headache, anorexia and malaise. Within 24 hours, an "earache" occurs. When the child points to the site of the pain, however, they point to the jawline just in front of the ear lobe. Chewing movements aggravate the pain. By the next day, the parotid gland (located just in front of the earlobe) is swollen and tender. As the parotid gland swells, it displaces the ear upwards and backwards. Boys also may develop testicular pain and swelling (orchitis).

It is often difficult to differentiate mumps from submaxillary adenitis (swelling of lymph nodes). The best method of differentiation is to place a hand along the child's jaw line. If the major amount of swelling is above the hand, it is probably mumps. If the largest amount of swelling is below the hand line, it is probably adenitis.

Because chewing movements are so painful, children may need soft or liquid foods until the major portion of the swelling recedes (about 6 days). It is also more difficult for them to swallow sour foods than sweet ones. They may need an analgesic for pain and an antipyretic for fever. If a child is hospitalised, follow droplet precautions in addition to standard infection precautions. Children should not return to school or childcare for 9 days or until the swelling goes down (whichever is sooner) (National Health and Medical Research Council, 2010).

Mumps is a potentially serious illness because several serious complications can occur. If mumps orchitis develops, it is generally unilateral. A single testis swells rapidly and is painful and tender. When the fever declines, testicular swelling also decreases, although the tenderness may exist for weeks. Atrophy of the testis may result, leading to a low sperm count.

The complication of meningoencephalitis occurs in a few children. Severe permanent hearing impairment is a rare complication that may occur because of neuritis of the auditory nerve.

✔ Checkpoint question 43.1

Which is the best description of mumps (infectious parotitis)?

a. Cervical lymph nodes become swollen
b. Swelling behind the child's ear occurs
c. Swelling above the jaw line occurs
d. The adenoid tonsils are red and swollen

Infectious mononucleosis

- Causative agent: Epstein-Barr virus
- Incubation period: Unknown; probably 2–8 weeks
- Period of communicability: Unknown; probably only during acute illness
- Mode of transmission: Direct and indirect contact
- Immunity: One episode apparently gives lasting immunity—no vaccination is available

Infectious mononucleosis is also known as glandular fever or, because it was first discovered as a disease that is transferred readily from one person to another by kissing, the *kissing disease*. It occurs most commonly in adolescents and young adults, although it may occur in any age child.

The beginning symptoms include chills, fever, headache, anorexia and malaise. Children develop enlarged lymph nodes and a severe sore throat. The fever is generally high (39.5°C) and lasts approximately 6 days. The cervical lymph nodes, most markedly affected, feel firm and tender. The tonsils feel painful and are enlarged and erythematous. A thick, white membrane may cover the tonsils and often petechiae appear on the palate. If the mesenteric lymph nodes enlarge, children may experience abdominal pain that simulates appendicitis. The spleen enlarges, placing the child at risk for spontaneous rupture. A maculopapular eruption similar to the rash of rubella, pneumonitis and central nervous system involvement such as encephalitis, meningitis or polyneuritis may occur.

Children with infectious mononucleosis need bed rest during the acute stage of the illness (7 to 10 days) because, with the splenomegaly, there is a danger of spleen rupture with any trauma to that area. If a child is hospitalised, follow standard infection precautions. Be careful in helping children with this disease turn in bed so that no pressure is placed over the splenic area. If palpating the spleen, do so gently to avoid inadvertent rupture.

Teach children and parents the importance of maintaining a good fluid intake despite the sore throat. Cool, non-acidic fluids are often tolerated best.

Neurological complications such as meningitis or encephalitis may occur. Children may notice weakness and general fatigue for up to 6 weeks after the illness. Caution them to avoid contact sports as long as their spleen is enlarged. Because infectious mononucleosis occurs primarily in young adults, it may interrupt school or career plans. Help these young adults to voice their frustration with this illness. Offer support to help them through this unexpected interruption in their life.

✔ Checkpoint question 43.2

For a child with infectious mononucleosis, why must abdominal palpation be performed gently?

a. Regional lymph nodes are painful
b. The enlarged spleen can rupture
c. Red cells pocket just under the skin
d. Petechiae form easily from bruising

BACTERIAL INFECTIONS

Streptococcal diseases

Streptococci, gram-positive organisms, are found normally in the respiratory, alimentary and female genital tracts. Most severe diseases in children result from infection with *Streptococcus pyogenes* (beta-haemolytic streptococci, group A). Beta-haemolytic, group B streptococcal infection can be contracted from vaginal secretions at birth (see Chapter 26) and so tends to occur in newborns. Streptococcal pharyngeal infection is discussed in Chapter 40 with other throat infections.

Scarlet fever

- Causative agent: Beta-haemolytic streptococci, group A
- Incubation period: 2–5 days

- Period of communicability: Greatest during acute phase of respiratory illness; 1–7 days
- Mode of transmission: Direct contact and large droplets
- Immunity: One episode of disease gives lasting immunity to scarlet fever toxin—no vaccination is available

Scarlet fever occurs most commonly in the 6- to 12-year-old age group, although it may be seen in preschoolers. The incidence is highest in temperate climates and the disease occurs usually in late winter or early spring.

The symptoms of scarlet fever begin abruptly and are those of a streptococcal pharyngitis: fever, sore throat, perhaps headache, chills and malaise. As the beta-haemolytic, group A *Streptococcus* grows in the child's body, it produces several toxins; erythrogenic toxin is the one responsible for the rash of scarlet fever. The rash appears 12–48 hours after the onset of the pharyngeal symptoms. The fever is high (39.5° to 40.0°C) on the first day of throat symptoms and again on the day the rash appears and then gradually returns to normal. The pulse rate may be increased out of proportion to the fever.

The rash of scarlet fever is both enanthematous and exanthematous (on both mucous membrane and skin). The tonsils are inflamed and enlarged and usually covered with white exudate. The uvula and pharynx are beefy red. The palate is usually covered with erythematous punctiform (pinpoint) lesions and perhaps scattered petechiae. The tongue, during the first 2 days of the illness, is white and appears furry. By day 3, papillae enlarge and protrude through the white coat, giving the tongue a "white strawberry" appearance. By day 4 or 5, the white coat disappears and the prominent papillae of the tongue give it a "red strawberry" appearance. A "strawberry tongue" is distinctive for scarlet fever and helps to differentiate the disease from other rashes. A throat culture reveals streptococci.

The skin rash is typically red, pinpoint lesions that blanch on pressure and feel rough like sandpaper. Lesions are densest on the trunk and in skin folds. Few lesions appear on the face. The area around the mouth tends to be abnormally pale (circumoral pallor). There are areas of hyperpigmentation in skin folds at the joints (Pastia's sign). The rash persists for approximately 1 week. It desquamates, with large areas of skin peeling off in fine flakes.

Children with scarlet fever usually appear ill. They need a soft or liquid diet for a few days until their throat soreness has diminished. They may need an analgesic and antipyretic for pain and fever. The rash of scarlet fever tends to be pruritic, so comfort measures are necessary. Because the underlying cause of the illness is a streptococcal infection, a course of penicillin is prescribed (Travers & Mousdicas, 2008). Caution parents to give the full amount prescribed for the full course to prevent the complications of beta-haemolytic, group A streptococcal infections (acute glomerulonephritis or rheumatic fever). If a child is hospitalised, follow droplet precautions until 24 hours after therapy is started, in addition to standard infection precautions.

Impetigo

- Causative agent: Beta-haemolytic streptococcus, group A (non-bullous); *Staphylococcus aureus* (bullous)
- Incubation period: 2–5 days
- Period of communicability: From outbreak of lesions until lesions are healed
- Mode of transmission: Direct contact with lesions
- Immunity: None

Impetigo (school sores) is spread by direct contact with sores or mucus from the nose or throat of an infected person. The lesions carry a large number of bacteria resulting in this condition being very contagious if left untreated (Department of Health Goverment of Western Australia, 2014). It is not uncommon to see several children in a family with identical lesions. Parents may be upset at being told their child has impetigo because at one time the lesions (dirty and crusty-appearing) were associated with low socioeconomic status and poor hygiene.

Impetigo is a superficial infection of the skin. It begins as a single papulovesicular lesion surrounded by localised erythema. As more vesicles appear, they become purulent, ooze and form honey-coloured crusts (see Fig. 43.6). They are found most commonly on the face and extremities. They are often seen as secondary infections of insect bites or in children who have body piercings. If there are several lesions, children may have local swollen lymph nodes.

Treatment is oral administration of antibiotics. The lesions heal most quickly if a parent or the child washes the crusts daily with soap and water.

Although rare, complications of rheumatic fever or acute glomerulonephritis may occur after impetigo, as they may after other streptococcal infections. If a child develops impetigo while in hospital, follow contact precautions until 24 hours after initiation of therapy.

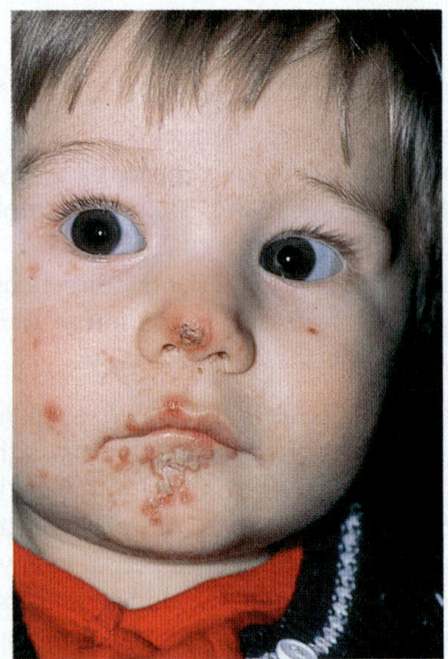

FIGURE 43.6 Impetigo in a toddler. Note the honey-coloured crust appearance of some of the lesions. (© Dr. P. Marazzi/SPL/Science Source/Photo Researchers.)

Staphylococcal infections

Staphylococcal organisms are gram-positive. Colonies of staphylococci are normally found on the skin, so they are generally the organisms involved in skin infections (pyodermas). Because the organisms grow rapidly in cream foods that are not well-refrigerated, such as potato salad or cream pies, they are often the organisms involved in summer food poisoning episodes. Because food poisoning produces gastrointestinal symptoms, these infections are discussed in Chapter 45.

Furunculosis (boils)

A furuncle is a staphylococcal infection of a hair follicle. A yellow pustule forms at the site. There is localised redness, pain and oedema of the surrounding skin. Moist heat, for 20 minutes, applied to the lesion can help relieve pain. Urge children not to rupture these lesions but rather, to allow them to run their self-limiting course so the infection is not spread to surrounding tissue and does not become a cellulitis.

Cellulitis

Cellulitis is a staphylococcal inflammation of the deeper layers of skin. It occurs generally on the extremities or face, or surrounding wounds. The skin feels warm and is oedematous and reddened. Cellulitis is treated with a systemic antibiotic. Warm soaks relieve pain and inflammation.

Methicillin-resistant staphylococcus aureus

Methicillin-resistant *staphylococcus aureus* (MRSA) is a strain of staphylococcus that causes skin infections and has become resistant to common broad-spectrum antibiotics. When an infection occurs in a healthcare setting, it is referred to as healthcare–associated MRSA or HA-MRSA. If it occurs in a community setting, it is CA-MRSA. Children with weakened immune systems are at most risk of contracting the infection.

An infection usually begins as a boil. It can spread to become a painful abscess or invade deeper body structures such as joints and heart valves. Children who are identified as having MRSA are isolated to help prevent spread of the bacteria to others. Vancomycin is the medication of choice for treatment of hospital-based lesions because the bacteria are still susceptible to its design. Trimethoprim-sulfamethoxazole is commonly used with community infections. Use strict standard infection precaution measures when caring for a child with an MRSA infection. Teach children that the best way to prevent staphylococcal infections of the skin is good handwashing and reporting skin wounds to a healthcare provider before an open wound can become infected (Pallin et al., 2008).

Other bacterial infections

Whooping cough (pertussis)

- Causative agent: *Bordetella pertussis*
- Incubation period: 7–20 days
- Mode of transmission: Direct or indirect contact
- Period of communicability: Greatest in catarrhal (respiratory illness) stage
- Immunity: Contracting the disease offers lasting natural immunity
- Active artificial immunity: Pertussis vaccine given as part of DTaP vaccine
- Passive artificial immunity: Pertussis immune serum globulin

Pertussis is a serious disease of childhood. Like diphtheria, pertussis rates have decreased significantly as a result of increased immunisation rates. This said, there is still a portion of the population who are not vaccinated against this disease and outbreaks occur every 3–4 years. These outbreaks result in large numbers of persons becoming ill in unvaccinated populations (Australian Government Department of Health, 2013). Those most susceptible are children who have not been immunised.

Pertussis manifests itself in three stages: catarrhal, paroxysmal and convalescent. The **catarrhal stage** begins with upper respiratory symptoms such as coryza, sneezing, lacrimation, cough and a low-grade fever. Children are irritable and listless. In some children, a mild cough is the only symptom during this stage, which lasts from 1 to 2 weeks (Knox, 2008).

The paroxysmal stage lasts 4–6 weeks. During this time, the cough changes from mild to paroxysmal involving 5–10 short, rapid coughs, followed by a rapid inspiration, which causes the "whoop" or high-pitched crowing sound associated with whooping cough. Children are in obvious distress while coughing. They may become cyanotic or red-faced and their nose may drain thick, tenacious mucus. They often vomit after a paroxysm of coughing and they are exhausted afterwards from the effort. Attacks of coughing tend to be more severe at night.

During the convalescent stage, there is a gradual cessation of the coughing and vomiting. The cough may be present for some time, but as single, not paroxysmal coughs. During the next year, if children develop an upper respiratory infection, they may again have a return of the paroxysmal coughing with vomiting.

Pertussis is diagnosed by its striking symptoms, although in children younger than 6 months of age, the "whoop" of the cough may be absent, making it more difficult to diagnose. The *B. pertussis* bacillus may be cultured from nasopharyngeal secretions during the catarrhal and paroxysmal stages. The white cell count, particularly the lymphocyte count, increases with whooping cough. This count may be as high as 20,000 to 30,000/mm^3 at the end of the catarrhal stage (normal is 5000–10,000/mm^3).

Children with pertussis should be restricted to bed rest until the paroxysms of coughing subside. They need to be secluded from environmental factors that initiate coughing episodes such as cigarette smoke, dust and strenuous activity. Nutrition may be a problem if the child is constantly coughing and vomiting. As a rule, frequent small meals are vomited less than larger meals. Infants with pertussis may be admitted to a healthcare facility for observation because they may have such tenacious secretions with coughing episodes that they need airway suction.

Complications of pertussis include pneumonia, atelectasis or emphysema from plugged bronchioles. Seizures from asphyxia as a result of severe paroxysms of coughing may occur. Epistaxis, subconjunctival and subarachnoid bleeding from the force of coughing, may also occur. If sufficient fluid intake cannot be maintained, alkalosis and dehydration from persistent vomiting may occur.

Little passive immunity is transferred to the newborn, meaning children in their early months are particularly susceptible to this disease. As a result pertussis vaccine is one of the first immunisations scheduled. Infants who have not yet been immunised or are immunocompromised and are exposed may be given pertussis immune serum globulin to protect them from contracting the disease (Wood et al., 2008). Pertussis is highly infectious for an undiagnosed child, with the condition spreading to 90% of susceptible household contacts (Australian Government Department of Health, 2013).

Tetanus (lockjaw)

- Causative agent: *Clostridium tetani*
- Incubation period: 3 days to 3 weeks
- Period of communicability: None
- Mode of transmission: Direct or indirect contamination of a closed wound
- Immunity: Development of the disease gives lasting natural immunity
- Active artificial immunity: Tetanus toxoid (given in combination with diphtheria toxoid and acellular pertussis (DPTa) vaccine for children)
- Passive artificial immunity: Tetanus immune globulin

Tetanus, a potentially fatal disease if untreated, is caused by an anaerobic, spore-forming bacillus. The bacillus, found in soil and the excretions of animals, enters the body through a wound. If the wound is deep, such as a puncture wound, where the distal end of the wound is shut off from an oxygen source, the tetanus bacilli begin to reproduce. The organism may also enter through a burn site, which crusts, creating an anaerobic environment. As the bacilli grow, they produce exotoxins, that cause the disease symptoms by affecting the motor nuclei of the central nervous system (Ogle & Anderson, 2008).

The entrance site of the bacillus does not appear infected (no pus or reddened area is present unless a secondary infection also exists). After the incubation period, the exotoxins have developed to such an extent, however, that they are capable of disrupting the nervous system. The first symptoms that are noticeable are stiffness of the neck and jaw (lockjaw). Within 24–48 hours, muscular rigidity of the trunk and extremities develops. The back becomes arched (opisthotonos), the abdominal muscles are stiff and board like, and the face assumes an unusual appearance, with wrinkling of the forehead and distortion of the corners of the mouth (a "sardonic grin" sign). Any stimulation, such as a sudden noise, a bright light or a touch, causes painful, paroxysmal spasms. The sensorium is clear throughout the course of the disease, so the child is aware of the pain associated with muscle spasms. As these spasms begin to include laryngospasm, respiratory obstruction and a collection of secretions in the respiratory tract, death by asphyxiation may occur. Fever is an ominous sign accompanying tetanus. Children who survive the disease rarely have more than a low-grade fever.

A child needs to be cared for in a quiet, stimulation-free room. If the wound has necrotic tissue, it may be débrided to ensure that no secondary infections arise. Tetanus immune globulin (human) is administered to supply passive antitoxins to combat the growing organisms. Antibiotics are administered to reduce the number of growing forms of the bacillus. Sedation and a muscle relaxant may be necessary to reduce the severity and pain of the muscle spasms.

Tetanus is a serious disease, but it can be prevented through active immunisation and suitable booster immunisation. Children routinely receive tetanus immunisation as part of routine DTaP. If a child's immunisation record cannot be obtained or if it has been more than 10 years since the child received a booster injection or an initial injection for tetanus, a child will probably be treated with a booster injection and tetanus immune globulin.

OTHER INFECTIOUS PATHOGENS

Chlamydial infections

Chlamydiae are gram-negative non-motile organisms. Chlamydial pneumonia or vaginitis may occur in children (see Chapters 40 and 47). In Australia 81% of cases occur in the 14–24 year age group with the highest overall rates recorded in remote areas (The Kirby Institute, 2013). Psittacosis is a chlamydial infection caused by the bacteria *Chlamidia psittaci* and is usually transmitted to humans from birds. Infection is commonly transmitted by inhaling the bacteria from dried bird droppings or handling infected birds (New South Wales Health, 2012a).

Parasitic infections

Parasites are organisms that live on and obtain their food supply from other organisms. Frequently seen parasites in children include head lice and scabies. Parents are often embarrassed when they learn that their child has lice. Reassure them that this infestation can happen to any child. Parents can help to prevent their children getting head lice by frequently checking their child's hair for cleanliness and the presence of lice. This is particularly important once the child reaches an age where they are attending school or a care facility. Other preventive measures include: frequently brushing hair, tying back long hair, avoid sharing any item that comes into contact with the head (brushes, hats etc.) and regular checking of children (e.g. weekly) for the presence of lice. If head lice are detected, all family members should be treated at the same time (New Zealand Ministry of Health, 2014b).

Helminthic infections

Helminths are pathogenic or parasitic worms. They may be roundworms (nematodes), flukes (trematodes) or tapeworms (cestodes). Most helminths begin life when the eggs or larvae are eliminated in the faeces or urine of humans. They are then transmitted to the oral cavity by contaminated foods or hands. Because children tend to be careless about washing their hands before eating or tend to suck their thumbs, they are prone to these infections (Wilson & Caumes, 2008).

Roundworms

Ascariasis is an infection caused by the roundworm parasite. The parasite lives in the intestinal tract and its eggs are excreted in the faeces. Children typically ingest the eggs when they eat food with hands that are improperly washed. Larvae, which hatch from the ingested eggs, penetrate the intestinal wall and enter the circulation. From there, they may migrate to any body tissue. If left untreated, ascariasis can migrate to the lungs or liver, which may result in vital organ damage. Children have a loss of appetite and in some cases nausea and vomiting. Intestinal obstruction may occur from a mass of roundworms in the intestinal tract. Ascariasis can be prevented by the sanitary disposal of faeces to prevent contamination of the soil.

Hookworms

Hookworm eggs, like roundworm eggs, are found in human faeces. They enter children's bodies through the skin and then migrate to the intestinal tract, where they attach themselves onto the intestinal villi. They suck blood from the intestinal wall to sustain themselves. If a great number of hookworms are present, severe anaemia may result. Treatment is with anthelmintics to destroy the worms. Children may also need therapy for the anaemia.

Pinworms

Pinworms are small, white, threadlike worms that live in the caecum. At night, the female pinworm migrates down the intestinal tract and out the anus to deposit eggs on the skin in the anal and perianal region. The movement of the worms causes the anal area to itch, and the child awakens at night crying and scratching. Some of the eggs are then carried from the child's fingernails to the mouth. They hatch in the child's intestinal tract and the cycle is repeated (Weinberg & Levin, 2008).

The worms are large enough to be seen if children's buttocks are separated when they are sleeping. Pressing a piece of cellophane tape against the anus and then looking at it under a microscope will generally reveal pinworm eggs.

Treatment is with a single dose of mebendazole (Vermox). All family members are treated for pinworm infestation because the worms are easily transmitted from person to person. Underclothing, bedding, towels and nightclothes should be washed before reuse. Teach children to avoid nail-biting and to wash their hands before food preparation or eating, to avoid transfer of pinworm eggs to the gastrointestinal tract.

Strongyliodes

Strongyliodes is an infection caused by the *Strongyloides stercoralis* worm. Transmission of the disease relates to poor sanitation as the larva lives in soil which has been contaminated by faeces of an infected person. Transmission to a susceptible host occurs when the larvae burrows through the skin, following contact with contaminated soil. The larvae then establishes itself in the gut or lungs and forms adult worms. Strongyliode infection in Australia is most commonly seen in remote Aboriginal communities, WWII veterans and immigrants from South East Asia, Africa and South American tropical and subtropical regions (Northern Territory Government Centre for Disease Control, 2014).

Other helminthic infections

Rat lung disease (*angiostrongylus catonesis*) is a parasite that lives in rodents and can infect snails and slugs that come into contact with the faeces of infected animals. People can be infected if they ingest infected snails or slugs. Children are at risk as they sometimes ingest infected snails or slugs and adults and children may be exposed to infected animals when eating raw produce (New South Wales Health, 2012b).

Protozoan infections

Protozoa are unicellular organisms. They absorb fluid through the cell membrane and can move from place to place by pseudopod, flagella or cilia action. They are most pathogenic in the gastrointestinal, genitourinary and circulatory systems. Some protozoa reproduce by simple binary fission; other forms have complex life cycles. Protozoa have the ability to form cysts or surround themselves with a membrane; this makes them resistant to destruction.

Giardiasis

Giardia lamblia is a protozoan infection. Transmission occurs when the child ingests the cysts of the organism on unclean hands. In the intestine, the cysts develop into the mature form of the organism, causing symptoms such as diarrhoea, weight loss, abdominal cramps and nausea. Diagnosis is made by history and recognition of the mature form of the organism in the stool or on duodenal aspiration. Treatment includes rehydration and antibiotic therapy. Giardia is a notifiable disease in New Zealand. Adults need to check with their medical practitioner prior to returning to work or children returning to school or a care facility (New Zealand Ministry of Health, 2014a).

Fungal infections

Fungi are larger than bacteria; some are unicellular (yeasts), but generally they are multicellular (moulds). Fungal infections are most often divided into groups according to the body tissue they infect. Deep mycoses invade internal organs. Transmission is by the inhalation of spores. Subcutaneous mycoses invade skin, subcutaneous tissue and bone. Infections usually occur from introduction of the fungi into a wound. Superficial mycoses invade only the hair, skin or nails.

Superficial fungal infections

Tinea (ringworm) is a superficial fungal infection caused by one of several types of fungus. Tinea can occur anywhere in the body, however, it typically affects the scalp, body, feet and nails. This condition is transmitted via direct contact with an infected person or animal. A child may also be exposed to tinea in the environment (e.g. warm moist areas such as change room showers). The appearance of tinea infection varies depending on where it is occurring. Skin lesions usually appear red, dry and scaly with the central area of the lesion clearing to form a ring-like appearance (Queensland Government, 2014).

Tinea cruris

Tinea cruris (crotch itch) occurs on the inner aspects of the thighs and scrotum. A red itchy rash appears in the moist skin folds. As the rash spreads, the centre clears to produce the characteristic ring appearance (The Royal Children's Hospital Melbourne, 2010).

Tinea pedis

Tinea pedis (athlete's foot) produces skin lesions between the toes and on the plantar surface of the foot. Pruritic, pinpoint vesicles and fissuring, especially between the toes, may occur.

Tinea capitis

Tinea capitis (ringworm) is a fungal infection that begins as an infection of a single hair follicle but spreads rapidly in a circular pattern to produce a lesion, usually approximately 2–3 cm in diameter. The hairs involved in the lesion generally break off. The circle becomes filled with dirty-appearing scales. Some strains of tinea capitis may be detected because they glow green under a Wood's light. Newer strains of the organism do not do this, however, so the test is losing its accuracy.

Treatment is with griseofulvin, given orally. Adolescents should be cautioned not to use alcohol while taking this medication; this may cause tachycardia. Safety during pregnancy is not established. Children need to avoid strong sunlight during therapy because photosensitivity may occur.

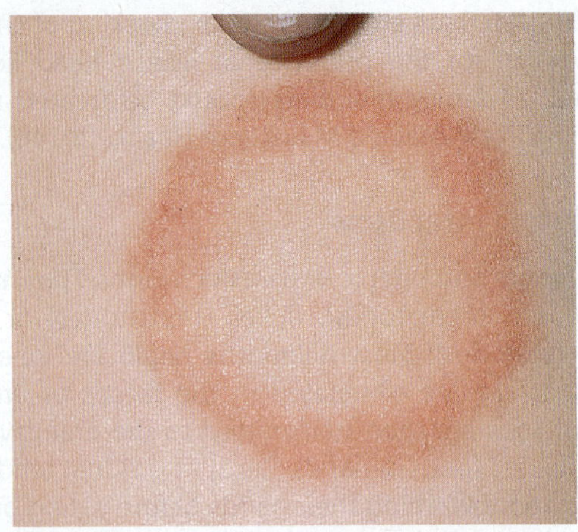

FIGURE 43.7 Ringworm (tinea corporis). The fungus spreads rapidly, producing a circular, ring-like lesion. (© SPL/Science Source/Photo Researchers.)

Tinea capitis is not as contagious as was once assumed. Children need not be kept home from school, although they should be cautioned not to exchange towels or combs or other potential fomites. The course of the disease may be long; it may be 3 months before all lesions have faded (Ali, Graham & Forgie, 2007).

Tinea corporis

Tinea corporis is a fungal infection of the epidermal layer of the skin. It presents as a scaly ring of inflammation, with a clear area in the centre, anywhere on the body (see Fig. 43.7).

Candidiasis

Candida albicans is the fungus responsible for candidal (monilial) infections. Candidal organisms grow in the vagina of many adult women and adolescents (candidal vaginitis) (see Chapter 47). Newborns born vaginally may develop an infection of the mucous membrane of the mouth (thrush or oral candidal infection). Thrush, is characterised by white plaques on an erythematous base on the buccal membrane and the surface of the tongue. It resembles a milk curd left from a recent milk feeding. Thrush plaques do not scrape away, however, whereas milk curds do. The mouth is painful and the child does not eat well due to the inflammation and local pain.

Candida albicans can also cause a severe, bright red, sharply circumscribed nappy-area rash (see Fig. 43.8). Satellite lesions are usually also present. The rash is marked by its intense colour and that it does not improve with the usual nappy rash measures.

Nystatin is an example of an antifungal medication (McKenna & Mirkov, 2014). For oral thrush, it is generally administered by mouth, approximately four times a day. It should be dropped into the mouth after feeding so it will remain in contact with the lesions rather than being washed away immediately. For nappy rash, a nystatin ointment is prescribed.

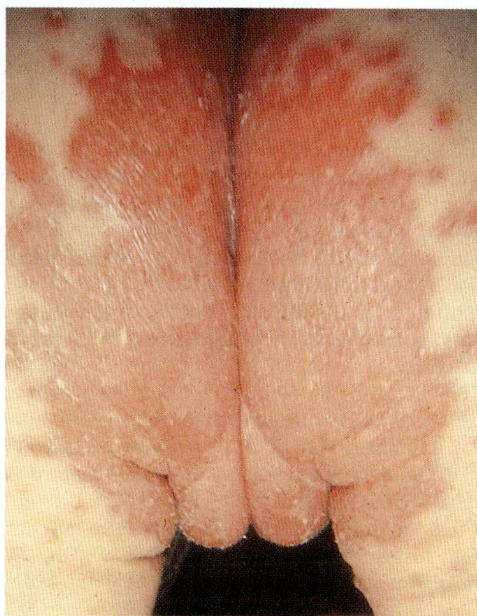

FIGURE 43.8 Monilial nappy rash. Note the intense red colour of the rash. (© Custom Medical Stock Photograph.)

Candidiasis can become a generalised infection, especially in a newborn. It can spread easily through a neonatal unit (Mohan, Eddama & Weisman, 2009). There is a tendency to think of thrush as a common, almost expected disease of infants. This said, the condition needs to be treated to prevent it from becoming more serious or systemic or epidemic.

CASE STUDY QUESTION

4. Sam had a pinworm infection last year. A typical symptom of this infection to assess for would be:

   a. Nausea and vomiting
   b. Anal itching on awakening
   c. Loose, bloody stools
   d. Mild jaundice and itching

Key points for review

- The incubation period of an infectious disease is the time between the invasion of an organism and the onset of symptoms. The prodromal period is the time between the beginning of non-specific symptoms and specific symptoms. Children are infectious during the prodromal period. Illness is the stage during which specific symptoms are evident. The convalescent period is the interval between the time symptoms begin to fade and the time the child returns to full wellness.
- Understanding the elements of the chain of infection and the different modes of transmission for diseases is imperative for preventing the spread of disease and providing appropriate education to children and their family.
- Common viral infections of childhood include rubella (German measles), measles (rubeola), chickenpox (varicella), herpes zoster, mumps (epidemic parotitis), infectious mononucleosis and verrucae (warts).
- Streptococcal diseases include scarlet fever and impetigo. Staphylococcal infections include furunculosis (boils). Outbreaks of whooping cough (pertussis) still occur.
- Parasitic infections are pediculosis capitis (head lice), pediculosis pubis and scabies. Helminthic infections are roundworms, hookworms and pinworms. Fungal infections are tinea capitis and tinea corporis (ringworm).
- Teaching parents and children about the manner by which an infectious condition is spread, associated infection control measures and the need for keeping immunisation up-to-date is essential to reduce the risk of infectious disorders in children.

CASE STUDY QUESTIONS

5. Sam was diagnosed as having scarlet fever the morning after surgery for appendicitis. Is it likely that Sam contracted this infection while he was hospitalised or is it more likely that the contact occurred before hospitalisation? What is the typical pattern of scarlet fever lesions? What would you recommend to his parents to help reduce the itchiness of the rash?
6. Suppose Sam's mother tells you she doesn't intend to have her newborn immunised because she feels the risk of developing a complication from vaccine administration is higher than letting her child contract simple childhood illnesses. How would you counsel her?
7. What would be a possible research topic to explore pertinent to these goals that would be applicable to the Ireland family and also advance evidence-based practice?

Resources

For an extensive range of additional resources to enhance teaching and learning and to facilitate understanding of this chapter, please see the text's accompanying website located on thePoint at http://thepoint.lww.com.

References

Ali, S., Graham, T. A. & Forgie, S. E. (2007). The assessment and management of tinea capitis in children. *Pediatric Emergency Care, 23*(9), 662–665.

Androphy, E. J. & Lowy, D. R. (2008). Warts. In K. Wolff et al. (Eds). *Fitzpatrick's Dermatology in General Medicine* (7th ed.). Columbus, OH: McGraw-Hill.

Australian Government Department of Health. (2013). National immunisation strategy for Australia 2013–2018, accessed 2 March 2015, <www.immunise.health.gov.au/internet/immunise/publishing.nsf/Content/immunisation-strategy-2013-18-cnt>.

Australian Government Department of Health. (2013). *The Australian Immunisation Handbook* (10th ed.), accessed 3 March 2015, <www.health.gov.au/internet/immunise/publishing.nsf/Content/Handbook10-home>.

Berger, T. G. (2009). Dermatology. In S. J. McPhee & M. A. Papadakis (Eds). *Current Medical Diagnosis and Treatment.* Columbus, OH: McGraw-Hill.

Chambers, H. F. (2009). Infectious diseases: Bacterial and chlamydial. In S. J. McPhee & M. A. Papadakis (Eds). *Current Medical Diagnosis and Treatment*. Columbus, OH: McGraw-Hill.

Department of Health Government of Western Australia. (2014). Impetigo fact sheet, accessed 3 March 2015, <www.public.health.wa.gov.au/2/1661/2/impetigo.pm>.

Department of Health, Victoria. (2015). Herpes simplex infections, accessed 3 March 2015, <http://ideas.health.vic.gov.au/bluebook/herpes.asp>.

Dyer, J. A. (2007). Childhood viral exanthems. *Pediatric Annals, 36*(1), 21–29.

Harding, A., Almquist, L. & Hashemi, S. (2011). The use and need for standard precautions and transmission-based precautions in the emergency department. *Journal of Emergency Nursing, 37*(4), 744–749.

Knox, M. A. (2008). Common infections in children. In J. E. South-Paul, S. C. Matheny & E. L. Lewis (Eds). *Current Diagnosis and Treatment in Family Medicine* (2nd ed.). Columbus, OH: McGraw-Hill.

McKenna, L. & Mirkov, S. (2014). *McKenna's Drug Handbook for Nursing & Midwifery* (7th ed.). Sydney: Lippincott Williams & Wilkins.

Mohan, P., Eddama, O. & Weisman, L. E. (2009). Patient isolation measures for infants with Candida colonization or infection for preventing or reducing transmission of Candida in neonatal units. *Cochrane Database of Systematic Reviews, 2009*(1), (CD006068).

Muller, C. P., et al. (2007). Reducing global disease burden of measles and rubella. *Vaccine, 25*(1), 1–9.

National Health and Medical Research Council, (2010). Australian guidelines for the prevention and control of infection in healthcare, accessed 2 March 2015, <www.nhmrc.gov.au/guidelines/publications/cd33>.

New South Wales Health. (2014) Measles fact sheet, accessed 2 March 2015, <www.health.nsw.gov.au/Infectious/factsheets/Factsheets/measles.pdf>.

New South Wales Health. (2012a). Psittacosis fact sheet, accessed 3 March 2015, <www.health.nsw.gov.au/Infectious/factsheets/Pages/Psittacosis.aspx>.

New South Wales Health. (2012b). Rat lung worm (angiostrongylus catonensis), accessed 3 March 2015, <http://www.health.nsw.gov.au/Infectious/factsheets/Pages/Rat-Lung-Worm.aspx>.

New Zealand Ministry of Health. (2014a). Giardia, accessed 3 March 2015, <www.health.govt.nz/your-health/conditions-and-treatments/diseases-and-illnesses/food-and-water-borne-diseases/giardia>.

New Zealand Ministry of Health. (2014b). Head lice, accessed 3 March 2015, <www.health.govt.nz/your-health/conditions-and-treatments/diseases-and-illnesses/head-lice>.

New Zealand Ministry of Health. (2014c). *Immunisation Handbook 2014*, accessed 3 March 2015, <www.health.govt.nz/publication/immunisation-handbook-2014>.

Northern Territory Government Centre for Disease Control. (2014). Strongyloidiasis factsheet, accessed 3 March 2015, <www.health.nt.gov.au/library/scripts/objectifyMedia.aspx?file=pdf/57/42.pdf&siteID=1&str_title=Strongyloidiasis June 2014.pdf>.

Ogle, J. W. & Anderson, M. S. (2008). Infections: Bacterial and spirochetal. In W. W. Hay et al. (Eds). *Current Pediatric Diagnosis and Treatment* (18th ed.). Columbus, OH: McGraw-Hill.

Ornstein, A. & Hatchette, T. (2012). Human papillomavirus and anogenital warts in children. *Canadian Medical Association Journal, 184*(3), 321.

Pallin, D. J., et al. (2008). Increased US emergency department visits for skin and soft tissue infections, and changes in antibiotic choices, during the emergence of community-associated methicillin-resistant *staphylococcus aureus. Annals of Emergency Medicine, 51*(3), 291–298.

Queensland Government. (2014). Tinea (ringworm), accessed 3 March 2015 <http://conditions.health.qld.gov.au/HealthConditions/2/Infections-Parasites/39/Fungal-Infections/639/Tinea-Ringworm>.

Smith, S. (2011). Infectious diseases. In K. J. Marcdante, R. M. Kliegman, H. B. Jenson, et al. (Eds), *Nelson Essentials of Paediatrics* (6th ed.), p. 355–462. Philadelphia: Saunders/Elsevier.

The Kirby Institute. (2013). *HIV, viral hepatitis and sexually transmissible infections in Australia, Annual Surveillance Report 2013*. Sydney: University of New South Wales.

The Royal Children's Hospital Melbourne. (2010). Ringworm, accessed 3 March 2015, <www.rch.org.au/kidsinfo/fact_sheets/Ringworm>.

Thilo, E. H. & Rosenberg, A. A. (2008). The newborn infant. In W. W. Hay et al. (Eds). *Current Pediatric Diagnosis and Treatment* (18th ed.). Columbus, OH: McGraw-Hill.

Travers, J. B. & Mousdicas, N. (2008). Gram-positive infections associated with toxin production. In K. Wolff et al. (Eds). *Fitzpatrick's Dermatology in General Medicine* (7th ed.). Columbus, OH: McGraw-Hill.

Weinberg, A. & Levin, M. J. (2008). Infections: Parasitic and mycotic. In W. W. Hay et al. (Eds). *Current Pediatric Diagnosis and Treatment* (18th ed.). Columbus, OH: McGraw-Hill.

Wilson, M. E. & Caumes, E. (2008). Helminthic infections. In K. Wolff et al. (Eds). *Fitzpatrick's Dermatology in General Medicine* (7th ed.). Columbus, OH: McGraw-Hill.

Wood, N., et al. (2008). Pertussis in infants: Preventing deaths and hospitalisations in the very young. *Journal of Paediatrics and Child Health, 44(*4), 161–165.

Yorita, K. L., et al. (2008). Infectious disease hospitalizations among infants in the United States. *Pediatrics, 121*(2), 244–252.

Suggested readings

Campbell, D. (2010). Teen with a genital lesion. *Pediatric Nursing, 36*(5), 273–274.

Government of Western Australia Department of Health. (2014). A-Z of diseases, accessed 3 March 2015, <www.public.health.wa.gov.au/1/10/2/az_diseases.pm>.

Leung, V., Harper, S., Slavin, M. et al. (2014). Are they protected? Immunity to vaccine preventable diseases in healthcare workers at an Australian hospital. *Australian and New Zealand Journal of Public Health, 38*(1), 83–86.

National Health and Medical Research Council. (2013). Staying healthy: Preventing infectious diseases in early childhood education and care services, (5th ed.), accessed 3 March 2015, <www.nhmrc.gov.au/guidelines/publications/ch55>.

Popovich, D. & McAlhany, A. (2007). Accurately diagnosing commonly misdiagnosed circular rashes. *Pediatric Nursing, 33*(4), 315–320.

Rollins, J. A. (2010). Back to school? The "no nit" policy. *Pediatric Nursing, 36*(5), 236–237.

Shapiro, R. (2012). Prevention of vector transmitted diseases with clove oil insect repellent. *Journal of Pediatric Nursing, 27*(4), 346–349.

Chapter 44

Nursing care of a family when a child has a haematological disorder

Previous chapters described the growth and development of well children. This chapter adds information about the dramatic changes both physical and psychosocial that occur when children have a haematological disorder.

LEARNING OBJECTIVES

After studying the contents of this chapter, you should be able to:

1. Describe the major haematological disorders of childhood.
2. Use critical thinking to analyse ways that nursing care for a child with a haematological disorder could be more family-centred.
3. Develop an understanding of assessing a child with a haematological disorder.
4. Identify nursing considerations for a child with a haematological disorder.
5. Discuss expected nursing outcomes for a child with a haematological disorder.
6. Discuss nursing care for a child with a haematological disorder.
7. Discuss expected outcomes for achievement and effectiveness of care.
8. Identify areas related to care of children with haematological disorders that could benefit from additional nursing research or application of evidence-based practice.

KEY TERMS

- allogeneic transplantation
- anaemia
- autologous transplantation
- blood dyscrasias
- blood transfusion
- bone marrow
- haematological
- haemophilia
- haemosiderosis
- hypodermoclysis
- leucopenia
- pancytopenia
- petechiae
- purpura
- stem cells
- synergeneic transplantation
- thrombocytopenia

CASE STUDY

Lena is a 4-year-old girl diagnosed with thalassaemia major. She has a prominent mandible and wide-spaced upper front teeth from overgrowth of bone marrow centres. Her skin is bronze from the number of transfusions (64) she has received in her short lifetime. Joey, a 7-year-old with sickle-cell anaemia, is seen at the same clinic. His growth is only in the 5th percentile. He has had two vaso-occlusive crises in the past year. "Why did this happen?" Lena's mother asks you. "Why were our two families so unlucky? What could we do to help our children have better lives?"

CASE STUDY QUESTION

1. What additional health teaching does Lena's mother need to help her better understand these haematological diseases?

The blood and blood-forming tissues that make up the **haematological** system play a vital role in body metabolism: transporting oxygen and nutrients to body cells; removing carbon dioxide from cells; and initiating blood coagulation when vessels are injured. As a result, any alteration in the substance or function of blood or its components can have immediate and life-threatening effects on the functioning of all body systems. For instance an alteration in the process of coagulation can result in death from acute and uncontrollable blood loss. Inadequate red cell formation results in decreased oxygenation in tissues (Linker, 2009).

Blood dyscrasias occur when components of the blood are formed incorrectly or either increase or decrease in amount beyond normal ranges. Most blood dyscrasias in children originate in the **bone marrow** where blood cells are formed.

Blood dyscrasias do not occur at equal rates in all countries, because many of these disorders are inherited. Sickle-cell anaemia, for example, occurs mainly in African Americans; thalassaemia occurs in children from Mediterranean countries. Iron-deficiency anaemia, an example of a non-inherited disorder, tends to occur in children from lower socioeconomic areas of many countries because iron-rich foods are often expensive. Treatment for blood disorders can be culturally influenced as well. For example, families who are Jehovah's Witnesses may refuse blood transfusions on religious grounds.

ANATOMY AND PHYSIOLOGY OF THE HAEMATOPOIETIC SYSTEM

Blood components originate in the bone marrow, circulate through blood vessels and ultimately are destroyed by the spleen.

Blood formation and components

The total volume of blood present in the human body is roughly proportional to body weight: 85 mL/kg at birth, 75 mL/kg at 6 months old and 70 mL/kg after the first year. Although blood plasma is important in diseases that cause vomiting and diarrhoea, plasma is not a major site of haematological disease. The formed elements—the erythrocytes (red blood cells [RBCs]), leucocytes (white blood cells [WBCs]) and thrombocytes (platelets)—are the portions most effected by haematological disorders in children.

Erythrocytes

Erythrocytes function chiefly to transport oxygen and carry carbon dioxide away from body cells. They are formed in the bone marrow under the stimulation of erythropoietin, a hormone formed by the kidneys that is produced whenever a child has tissue hypoxia.

Haemoglobin

The component of RBCs that allows them to carry out the transport of oxygen is haemoglobin, composed of globin, a protein, and haem, an iron-containing pigment. It is the haem portion that combines with oxygen for transport.

Bilirubin

After a RBC reaches its life span of approximately 120 days, it disintegrates and its protein component is preserved by the reticuloendothelial cells of the liver and spleen for further use. Iron is reused by the bone marrow to construct new RBCs. As the haem portion is degraded, it is converted into protoporphyrin; protoporphyrin is then further broken down into direct bilirubin. Indirect bilirubin is fat soluble and so cannot be excreted by the kidneys. It is therefore converted by the liver enzyme, glucuronyl transferase, into direct bilirubin which is water soluble and excreted in bile.

In the newborn, liver function is generally so immature that the conversion from indirect to direct bilirubin is difficult, allowing a portion of bilirubin to remain in the indirect form. When the level of indirect bilirubin in the blood rises to more than 7 mg/100 mL, it permeates outside the circulatory system, and the infant begins to show signs of yellowing or jaundice from the colour of the bilirubin. At any point in life, if excessive destruction of RBCs occurs from other than usual causes, a child will show signs of jaundice.

Leucocytes

Leucocytes are nucleated cells and are few in number compared with red blood cells (there is approximately 1 WBC to every 500 RBCs). Their primary function is the defence against antigen invasion; their life span ranges from approximately 6 hours to unknown intervals. With the exception of neutropenia (a reduced number of WBCs), leucocytes are not a major haematological concern.

Thrombocytes

Thrombocytes are round, non-nucleated bodies formed by the bone marrow; their function is capillary haemostasis and primary coagulation.

HAEMATOLOGICAL DISORDERS IN CHILDREN

Assessment

Many of the symptoms of **haematological** disorders begin insidiously with symptoms such as pallor, lethargy and bruising. These are such minor symptoms that parents may not bring their child to a healthcare facility for some time. They are surprised to learn when they do that such subtle symptoms can signify the presence of a serious illness.

Many haematological disorders are inherited. When a child is diagnosed with such a disorder, parents may feel guilty or blame themselves or their partner for their child's disease. It may be difficult for parents to support a child during an illness when they need intensive support themselves, due to feelings of guilt. Be certain both parents and children receive the support and comfort that they need.

Asking at routine checkups about a child's dietary intake often reveals iron-deficiency anaemia. Many infants with this problem have been drinking too much milk and not eating enough iron-containing foods. This makes them iron-deficient, but aside from paleness and irritability, they appear plump and "healthy". Their parents do not suspect their baby's appearance masks a nutritional deficiency.

Nursing considerations

Nursing considerations for children who have haematological disorders are:

- Knowledge deficiency related to the cause of a child's illness
- Imbalanced nutrition related to parental lack of knowledge of need for iron-rich foods
- Anxiety related to frequent blood-sampling procedures
- Pain related to tissue ischaemia
- Developing family coping mechanisms related to long-term care needs of a child with a chronic haematological disorder.

When helping parents plan outcomes be sure that the health related goals are realistic for both the child and family. For example, it may not be possible to reduce the number of blood-sampling procedures, however, a child can be helped to deal with the pain and anxiety the procedures produce with the use of distraction techniques.

Children with haematological disorders are often prescribed long-term medication such as a corticosteroid. When a child appears very ill parents are usually very conscientious about giving such medicine. When a child has a disorder with few symptoms, however, like a blood dyscrasia, it is easy for parents to forget to give the medication. In addition, a child may refuse to take the medication for a long time because of taste or because it may upset the stomach. Planning includes helping parents devise ways to disguise the taste or remember to give the medication over the long term.

Nutritional planning is another area that needs consideration. Parents of children with iron-deficiency anaemia, for example, may need to modify meal plans not only for the child but also for the entire family; this is not necessarily easy to do because iron-rich foods are expensive. If children are "fussy eaters", parents may need a great deal of support to insist that children eat foods containing iron rather than giving them what they want to eat. If a child will be restricted in activity for long periods because the immune system is compromised as a part of the illness, planning must include ways to keep the child engaged with friends to promote development. Parents may need help investigating possible resources for education and support to do this. The Women's and Children's Hospital South Australia provides an overview of childhood blood disorders at <www.wch.sa.gov.au/services/az/divisions/paedm/clinhaem/files/blood_disorders/index.html>.

Nursing children with haematological disorders includes helping to obtain specimens for testing and assisting with blood or haematopoietic stem cell transfusions. Remember that a finger puncture for blood is often as painful as a venepuncture (and more painful afterwards because the fingertip is irritated every time the child attempts to use it). Suggesting that blood be drawn by means of an intermittent device may reduce the number of times a child is subjected to venepuncture. Applying an anaesthetic cream before finger punctures or venepunctures also helps to reduce pain and improve cooperation with these procedures.

ASSESSMENT OF AND THERAPEUTIC TECHNIQUES FOR HAEMATOLOGICAL DISORDERS

Assessment of children with haematological disorders begins with a history to identify inherited disorders. For specific diagnosis, children generally require several diagnostic procedures such as blood cell or bone marrow analysis.

Blood transfusion

Transfusions of blood or its products are used in the treatment of many disorders, including the anaemias and primary immunodeficiency disorders (see Chapter 42). A variety of forms of blood are available including: whole blood, packed RBCs (red blood cells), washed RBCs (as much "foreign" matter is removed as possible to reduce the possibility of blood reaction), plasma, plasma factors, platelets, WBCs (white blood cells) and albumin. No matter what the blood product, it is important that it has been carefully matched with the child's blood type. Blood must be infused accompanied with a solution as nearly isotonic as possible (normal saline). If blood is given with a hypertonic solution, fluid will be drawn out of the RBCs, causing them to shrink; if infused with a hypotonic solution, fluid will be drawn into the cells and they will burst. In both instances, they will be destroyed.

Packed RBCs is the most common form of transfusion used with children as they minimise the risk of fluid overload. The volume and rate at which blood products are to be transfused is prescribed by a medical officer. Rates will vary between facilities and will be dependent on the clinical scenario. Guidelines for the delivery of blood products are provided by the Australian and New Zealand Society of Blood Transfusion Ltd and can be accessed at <www.anzsbt.org.au/publications/documents/ANZSBT_Guidelines_Administration_Blood_Products_2ndEd_Dec_2011_Hyperlinks.pdf>. Guidance relating to specific volumes and flow rates for paediatric patients can be found in current policy from Australian and New Zealand Children's Hospitals including The Children's Hospital at Westmead <www.chw.edu.au/about/policies/pdf/2007-8092.pdf> and The Royal Children's Hospital Melbourne <www.rch.org.au/clinicalguide/guideline_index/Blood_product_transfusion/>.

Even if given slowly, a **blood transfusion** is always a strain on a child's circulation beyond that of a regular intravenous infusion because the circulatory system must accommodate a thick, difficult-to-mobilise fluid.

Before any transfusion, ensure that a signed consent form is obtained to respect sociocultural or religious beliefs. Also obtain vital signs to establish a baseline. Monitor vital signs about every 15 minutes during the first hour and approximately every half hour for the remainder of the transfusion. A standard rate of infusion is slowly for the first 15 minutes; then increase the rate to 10 mL/kg/hr if no reaction occurs. This will vary between facility and individual patient scenario. Common symptoms of blood transfusion reactions are shown in Table 44.1.

Bone marrow aspiration and biopsy

Bone marrow aspiration provides samples of **bone marrow** so that the type and quantity of cells can be determined (Beattie, 2007). In children, the aspiration sites used are the iliac crests or spines rather than the sternum which is commonly used in adults because these sites have larger marrow compartments during childhood. Performing the test at these sites is usually less frightening for children. In neonates, the anterior tibia can be used (see Fig. 44.1).

For a bone marrow aspiration, a child lies prone on a treatment table. Use of a hard table rather than a bed is advantageous because pressure is needed to insert the needle

TABLE 44.1 Common symptoms of blood transfusion reactions

Symptoms	Cause	Time of occurrence	Nursing interventions
Headache, chills, back pain, dyspnoea, hypotension, haemoglobinuria (blood in urine)	Anaphylactic reaction to incompatible blood; agglutination of red blood cells occurs; kidney tubules may become blocked, resulting in kidney failure	Immediately after start of transfusion	Discontinue transfusion. Maintain normal saline infusion for accessible intravenous line. Administer oxygen as necessary. Anticipate doctor order for diuretic to increase renal tubule flow and reduce tubule plugging and/or heparin to reduce intravascular coagulation.
Pruritus, urticaria (hives), wheezing	Allergy to protein components of transfusion	Within first hour after start of transfusion	Discontinue transfusion temporarily. Give oxygen as needed. Anticipate doctor order for antihistamine to reduce symptoms.
Increased temperature	Possible contaminant in transfused blood	Approximately 1 hour after start of transfusion	Discontinue transfusion. Obtain blood culture to rule out bacterial invasion as ordered.
Increased pulse, dyspnoea	Circulatory overload	During course of transfusion	Discontinue transfusion. Give oxygen as needed. Provide supportive care for pulmonary oedema and congestive heart failure. Anticipate doctor order for diuretic to increase excretion of fluid.
Muscle cramping, twitching of extremities, convulsion	Acid-citrate-dextrose anticoagulant in transfusion is combining with serum calcium and causing hypocalcaemia	During course of transfusion	Discontinue transfusion. Anticipate doctor order for calcium gluconate intravenously to restore calcium level.
Fever, jaundice, lethargy, tenderness over liver	Hepatitis from contaminated transfusion	Weeks or months after transfusion	Obtain transfusion history of any child with hepatitis symptoms. Refer for care of hepatitis.
Bronze-coloured skin	Haemosiderosis or deposition of iron from transfusion in skin	After repeated transfusions	Support self-esteem with altered body image. Administer iron-chelating agent (deferoxamine) as ordered to help reduce level of accumulating iron.

through the surface of the bone into the marrow compartment. Conscious sedation may be used to help reduce the child's fear. Topical anaesthesia helps to reduce pain.

The area of the aspiration is cleaned with an antiseptic solution and draped. The overlying skin is infiltrated with a local anaesthetic. After a few minutes, a large-bore needle and stylus is introduced through the overlying tissue into the bone. This involves considerable pressure. When the marrow cavity is reached, the stylus is removed, a syringe is attached to the needle and bone marrow is aspirated (appears as thick blood in the syringe). The syringe is then removed and marrow is expelled onto a slide and allowed to dry. After being sprayed with a preservative it is taken to the laboratory for analysis. The aspiration needle is removed and pressure is applied to the puncture site to prevent bleeding. After another few minutes a pressure dressing is applied.

A child feels pain from the local anaesthetic injection and hard pressure while the needle is inserted. Some patients report a sharp pain when the marrow is actually aspirated. If conscious sedation is used monitor vital signs until the child is fully awake. Monitor pulse and blood pressure and observe the dressing every 15 minutes for the first hour after the procedure to be certain that no bleeding is occurring. Keep the child fairly quiet for the first hour by playing a quiet game or other activity. If the procedure was done as an ambulatory procedure, instruct parents to take the child's temperature 12 and 24 hours after the procedure to detect infection.

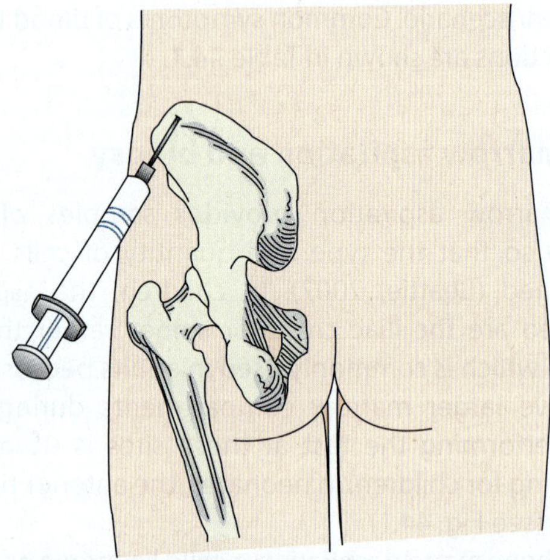

FIGURE 44.1 A common site used for bone marrow aspiration in children is the iliac crest. In neonates, the anterior tibia may be used.

Haematopoietic stem cell transplantation

Stem cell transplantation is the intravenous infusion of haematopoietic **stem cells** from bone marrow obtained by marrow aspiration or from peripheral or umbilical cord blood drawn from a donor. The purpose of this procedure is to re-establish marrow function in a child with defective or non-functioning bone marrow. Donors are compatible when their human leucocyte antigen (HLA) system matches that of the recipient.

Haematopoietic stem cell transplantation has become a relatively common procedure for children with blood disorders such as acquired aplastic anaemia, sickle-cell anaemia, thalassaemia and leukaemia, and some forms of immune dysfunction diseases. Although a stressful procedure to undertake stem cell transplantation remains the optimal curative therapy (Cutler & Ballen, 2012). There is no guarantee that the graft will be accepted by the recipient or that improvement will occur. However with good tissue compatibility in the absence of infection, this can be effective in most children.

Haematopoietic stem cells can be recovered from circulating peripheral blood after the stimulation of stem cell production by a cytokine or stem cell colony-stimulating factor. Stem cell transplants are most successful when recipients have not already received multiple blood transfusions that have sensitised them to blood products. Success also depends on the HLA compatibility of donated stem cells to the child's blood. An identical twin is the ideal donor; a parent or sibling may be next best, although compatibility is not guaranteed. Siblings have about a 25% chance of being HLA compatible.

Stem cell transplants are allogeneic, synergeneic or autologous. **Allogeneic transplantation** involves the transfer of stem cells from an immune-compatible (histocompatible) donor, usually a sibling. **Synergeneic transplantation** involves a donor and recipient who are genetically identical (identical twins). **Autologous transplantation** involves use of the child's own stem cells. The source of most autologous transfusions is cord blood that was banked at the child's birth (Tse, Bunting & Laughlin, 2008). If this is not available stem cells are aspirated from the bone marrow or obtained from circulating blood, treated to remove abnormal cells and then reinfused.

Parents who are found to be incompatible donors may feel guilty and frustrated they cannot do more for their child. If the most compatible person for transplant is a young sibling, the ethical issues faced by parents and healthcare providers and associated implications for care (including socioeconomic status of the family) must be addressed (Bendorf & Keridge, 2011). This assessment will assist in providing the best clinical and psychological outcome for all parties involved.

Be certain children are well prepared for all procedures. Allow them to make as many choices as they can about their care to help them preserve a sense of control over their treatment. Children who receive a transplant need periods of therapeutic play incorporated into their care so they can begin to express their anger and frustration at the number of intravenous therapies or follow-up bone marrow aspirations they require. Measures to help children cope with pain, such as imagery, can help a child accept one more painful procedure. Encourage parents to spend time with their child during long periods of hospitalisation for additional support.

Provisions for completing schoolwork need to be made as soon as a child has a return of RBCs in the peripheral blood (approximately 3 weeks). On the day of discharge, parents may be surprised that the child's blood replacement is not complete and that they will need to continue infection control measures and restrictions at home. Help them to locate a support group in their community if possible. Be certain they feel free to call the transplant centre after discharge if they have any problems. Once the danger of infection has passed and the restrictions can be discontinued some parents may still be reluctant to allow their child outside, fearing that the child may still be susceptible to infection. Frequent follow-up for the next year is not only necessary to ensure that a child is free of infection but also to assess whether the parents allow their child to pursue age-appropriate activities.

If children are prepared adequately for these painful or restrictive procedures and supported throughout, they should have no long-term consequences. Not all haematopoietic stem cell transplants are successful, however, and some children will die of the original disease that necessitated the transplant. There is also a risk that some children will develop an infection despite all precautions and die of sepsis in the weeks immediately after the transplant.

Graft-versus-host disease

Graft-versus-host disease (GVHD) refers to a condition where lymphocytes of the donor identify the cells of the recipient as being different and try to reject the tissues of the recipient. The targeted tissues generally include the skin, the gut and the liver, causing rash, diarrhoea and jaundice (yellow skin). This condition may be acute or chronic (Royal Children's Hospital Melbourne, 2015). The symptoms range from mild to severe and include a rash and general malaise beginning 7 to 14 days after the transplant. Latent virus infections may become active. Severe symptoms include high fever and diarrhoea and liver and spleen enlargement as cells are destroyed.

Because there is no known cure for GVHD, prevention is essential. Careful tissue typing, Intravenous administration of an immunosuppressant such as methotrexate, a corticosteroid or cyclosporine before transplant and irradiation of blood products (which helps to inactivate mature T lymphocytes) before stem cell infusion can all help reduce the incidence of this complication. Medications such as methotrexate and cyclosporine kill all rapidly growing cells including WBCs and T lymphocytes. Administration of these medications after transplantation cannot be continued because they would also slow the growth of the host's new stem cells. Depletion of mature T lymphocytes from donor bone marrow before it is infused into the child offers good results, as does the administration of corticosteroids or anti-thymocyte globulin (ATG), an immune serum, to children after the transplant (Grosskreutz et al., 2007).

Splenectomy

One of the purposes of the spleen is to remove damaged or aged blood cells. This poses a problem with diseases such as sickle-cell anaemia and the thalassaemias because the spleen recognises the typical cells of these diseases as damaged and destroys them. This causes children with these disorders to have a continuous **anaemia** with haemoglobin levels as low as 5 to 9 g/mL. In a high number of cases removal of the spleen (splenectomy) will not cure the basic defect of the blood cells but will limit the degree of anaemia. Splenectomy formerly required a large abdominal incision but today it can be performed by laparoscopy (Wood et al., 2011).

A second function of the spleen is to strain the plasma for invading microorganisms so that phagocytes and lymphocytes can destroy them. This causes children who have had their spleen removed to be very susceptible to pneumococcal infections because this bacteria is no longer removed systematically from the body (Rosado et al., 2013). After surgery antibiotic therapy is given prophylactically for a year or two to guard against infection. The child should receive pneumococcal and meningococcal vaccines as well as routine immunisations, including influenza vaccine. Teach parents about signs of infection (cough, fever, general malaise) and encourage them to report these signs immediately.

HEALTH PROMOTION

Haematological disorders cover a wide range of diseases and produce multiple symptoms in children. Many disorders such as sickle-cell anaemia and haemophilia are inherited. Health promotion and disease prevention therefore begin with ensuring that families have access to genetic counselling so they can be aware of the incidence of a disorder in their family and the potential for the disease to develop in their child.

The most frequently occurring anaemia in children, iron-deficiency anaemia, is preventable. This condition could be virtually eliminated if all infants were breastfed and those infants who are formula-fed were fed iron-fortified formula for the full first year, then iron-fortified types of cereals. The disorder occurs again with a high incidence in adolescents because adolescent diets tend to be low in meat and green vegetables, the chief dietary sources of iron. Adolescents who begin vegetarian diets become especially prone to developing the disorder. Counselling parents of young children to maintain well child healthcare visits and urging adolescents to ingest iron-rich foods could have a major impact on decreasing the incidence of the disorder.

Aplastic anaemia, or the inability to form blood elements, can be acquired if a child is exposed to a toxic medication or chemical. Educating parents about the importance of keeping poisons out of the reach of children could help decrease the incidence of this disorder.

Nurses can also help make the therapy for these disorders much less painful and distressing than it was in the past. All haematological disorders require obtaining blood specimens for diagnosis and continued testing for follow-up. Many therapies include blood product transfusion. The use of EMLA cream or topical anaesthetic agent can greatly reduce the pain of venepuncture. Helping a child to use a distraction technique such as imagery can reduce apprehension or fear associated with the procedures or treatments (see Box 44.1).

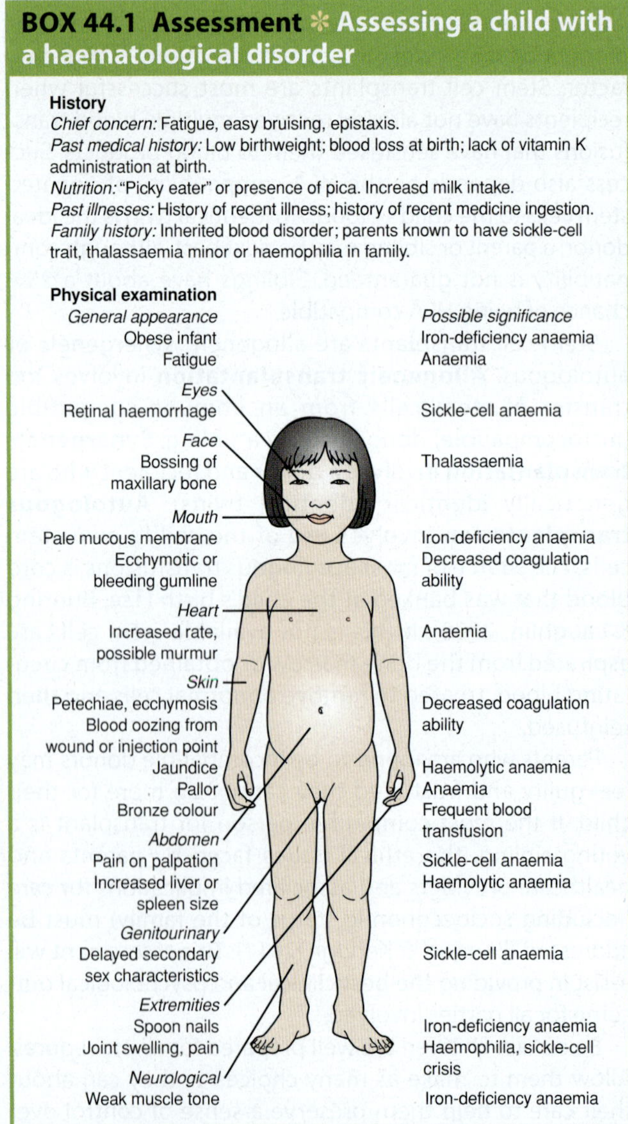

DISORDERS OF THE RED BLOOD CELLS

Most RBC disorders fall into the category of the anaemias, or a reduction in the number or function of erythrocytes. Polycythaemia, or an increase in the number of RBCs, can also occur and may be as dangerous to a child as a reduction in RBC production.

Anaemia occurs when the rate of RBC production falls below that of cell destruction, or when there is a loss of RBCs, causing their number and the haemoglobin level to fall below the normal value for a child's age. Anaemias are classified according to the changes seen in RBC numbers or configuration, or according to the source of the problem. Although any reduction in the amount of circulating haemoglobin lessens the oxygen-carrying capacity, clinical symptoms are not apparent until the haemoglobin level reaches 7 to 8 g/100 mL.

Normochromic, normocytic anaemias

Normochromic, normocytic anaemias are marked by impaired production of erythrocytes by the bone marrow, or by abnormal or uncompensated loss of circulating RBCs as with acute haemorrhage. The RBCs are normal in both colour and size, but there are simply too few of them.

Acute blood-loss anaemia

Blood loss sufficient to cause anaemia might occur from: trauma such as a motor vehicle accident with internal bleeding; from acute nephritis in which blood is lost in the urine; or in the newborn from disorders such as placenta praevia, premature separation of the placenta, maternal-fetal or twin-to-twin transfusion, or trauma to the cord or placenta, as might occur with caesarean birth. It can also occur from intestinal parasites such as tapeworm (Barnett et al., 2007).

The causative condition is a medical emergency. Children are in shock from acute blood loss and appear pale. As the heart attempts to push the reduced amount of blood through the body more rapidly, tachycardia will occur. Loss of RBCs needed for oxygen transport causes body cells to register an oxygen deficit and children begin to breathe rapidly. Newborns may have gasping respirations, sternal retractions and cyanosis. They will not respond to oxygen therapy because they lack RBCs to transport and use the oxygen. Such infants become listless and inactive.

This type of acute blood-loss anaemia is generally transitory because the sudden reduction in available oxygen stimulates the release of erythropoietin from the kidney and a regeneration response in the bone marrow. The reticulocyte count becomes elevated which is evidence the bone marrow is trying to increase production of erythrocytes to meet the sudden shortage.

Treatment involves control of bleeding by addressing its underlying cause. The child or infant should be placed in a supine position to provide as much circulation as possible to brain cells. Keep the child warm with blankets; place an infant in an incubator or under a radiant heat warmer. Blood transfusion may be necessary to provide an immediate increase in the number of erythrocytes. Until blood is available for transfusion, a blood expander such as plasma or intravenous fluid such as normal saline or Hartmann's may be given to expand blood volume and improve blood pressure.

Anaemia of acute infection

Acute infection or inflammation, especially in infants, may lead to increased destruction or decreased production of erythrocytes. Common conditions include osteomyelitis, ulcerative colitis and kidney infection. Management involves treatment of the underlying condition. When this is reversed, the blood values should return to normal.

Anaemia of renal disease

Either acute or chronic renal disease can cause loss of function in kidney cells and result in a decrease in erythropoietin production. This decreases the stimulation for RBC production in the bone marrow and a resultant normocytic, normochromic anaemia occurs. Administration of recombinant human erythropoietin can increase RBC production and correct the anaemia, however, the renal disease must still be addressed (Lum, 2012).

Anaemia of neoplastic disease

Malignant growths such as leukaemia or lymphosarcoma (common neoplasms of childhood) result in normochromic, normocytic anaemias because invasion of bone marrow by proliferating neoplastic cells impairs RBC production. There may be accompanying blood loss if platelet formation has also decreased. The treatment of such anaemia involves measures designed to achieve remission of the neoplastic process and transfusion to increase the erythrocyte count.

Hypersplenism

Under normal conditions, blood is filtered rapidly through the spleen. If the spleen is enlarged and functioning abnormally, blood cells pass through more slowly, resulting in cells being destroyed in the process. This increased destruction of RBCs can cause anaemia and may lead to **pancytopenia** (deficiency of all cell elements of blood). Virtually any underlying splenic condition can cause this syndrome.

Therapeutic management consists of treating the underlying splenic disorder, including possible splenectomy. Although the spleen's role in the body's defence mechanisms against infection is not well documented, the organ is important in early infancy. Its function decreases as a child grows older and it may serve no immune function at all in adulthood. There is evidence to suggest removal of the spleen's filtering function may be associated with an increased susceptibility to meningitis or pneumonia due to pneumococci (Di Sabatino, Carsetti & Corazza, 2011). For this reason, a splenectomy may be delayed until after 2 years of age, when the risk of meningitis decreases. Such children should receive immunisation against influenza, pneumococci and *H. influenzae* in addition to prophylactic penicillin for 2 years after the splenectomy.

Aplastic anaemias

Aplastic anaemias result from depression of haematopoietic activity in the bone marrow. The formation and development of WBCs, platelets and RBCs can all be affected.

Congenital aplastic anaemia (Fanconi syndrome) is inherited as an autosomal recessive trait. A child is born with several congenital anomalies such as skeletal and renal abnormalities, hypogenitalism and short stature. Between 4 and 12 years of age a child begins to manifest symptoms of **pancytopenia** or reduction of all blood cell components (Linker, 2009).

Acquired aplastic anaemia is a decrease in bone marrow production that can occur if a child is exposed excessively to radiation, medications or chemicals known to cause bone marrow damage. Medications that may cause this include chloramphenicol, sulfonamides, arsenic (contained in rat poison, sometimes eaten by children), benzene or quinine. Exposure to insecticides also may cause severe bone marrow dysfunction. Chemotherapeutic medications temporarily reduce bone marrow production. A serious infection such as meningococcal pneumonia might cause autoimmunological suppression of the bone marrow.

When symptoms begin, a child appears pale, fatigues easily and has anorexia. These symptoms reflect the lower RBC count (anaemia) and result in tissue hypoxia. Because of reduced platelet formation **(thrombocytopenia)**, the child bruises easily or has **petechiae** (pinpoint, macular, purplish-red spots caused by intradermal or submucous haemorrhage). A child may have excessive nosebleeds or gastrointestinal bleeding. As a result of a decrease in WBCs **(leucopenia)**, a child may contract an increased number of infections and respond poorly to antibiotic therapy. Observe closely for signs of cardiac decompensation such as tachycardia, tachypnoea, shortness of breath or cyanosis from the long-term increased workload on the heart. Ask about any exposure to medications or chemicals or recent infection. Bone marrow samples will show a reduced number of blood elements; blood-forming spaces become infiltrated by fatty tissue.

Infection related to dramatic decrease in number of WBCs

Exposure to other children must be limited as long as WBC production is inadequate to prevent infection. Remind parents of the signs and symptoms of infection and advise them to come for treatment promptly if their child shows any of these signs. In the absence of granulocytes antibiotic therapy may be ineffective and severe septicaemia can result. WBCs (granulocytes) may be transfused to counteract a severe infection. Parents should monitor their child to ensure the child's temperature remains below 38.0°C (axillary) and symptoms of infection such as cough, vomiting or diarrhoea are absent.

Disturbed body image related to changed appearance

Children who receive corticosteroids such as prednisone to suppress the immune response almost always experience some of the medication's side effects such as cushingoid appearance, hirsutism, hypertension and marked weight gain. Long-term therapy with testosterone can result in masculinising effects, such as growth of facial and body hair, the development of acne and deepening of the voice. Be sure both children and their parents know that these effects are related to the medication and that they will remain for an extended period but will fade when the medication is withdrawn.

Adolescents may have an especially difficult time accepting weight gain and increased acne. They need a chance to express their feelings about their changed appearance. Reinforce and emphasise positive attributes. Signs a child is coping with the alteration in body image include the child viewing themselves as a worthwhile person and the child appearing not to be excessively shy or reluctant to interact with peers.

Injury related to ineffective blood clotting mechanisms

Inadequate platelet formation interferes with blood coagulation placing a child at risk of bleeding. Parents and clinicians need to monitor susceptible children to ensure the child exhibits no ecchymotic skin areas, gingival bleeding or epistaxis, and stools are negative for occult blood.

Hypoplastic anaemias

Hypoplastic anaemias also result from depression of haematopoietic activity in bone marrow; they can be either congenital or acquired. Unlike aplastic anaemias, in which WBCs, RBCs and platelets are affected, in hypoplastic anaemias only RBCs are affected.

Congenital hypoplastic anaemia (Blackfan-Diamond syndrome) is a rare disorder that shows symptoms as early as the first 6 to 8 months of life. It affects both sexes and is caused by an inherent defect in RBC formation. No changes in the leucocytes or platelets occur. An acquired form is caused by infection with parvovirus, the infectious agent of fifth disease (Blümel et al., 2010).

The onset of hypoplastic anaemia is insidious and at first it may be difficult to differentiate it from iron-deficiency anaemia. In iron-deficiency anaemia, blood cells appear hypochromic and microcytic; in hypoplastic anaemia, they are normochromic and normocytic but few in number.

With acquired hypoplastic anaemia, the reduction of RBCs is transient, so no therapy is necessary. Children with the congenital form show increased erythropoiesis with corticosteroid therapy. Long-term transfusions of packed RBCs are needed to raise erythrocyte levels. As a result of the necessary number of transfusions, **haemosiderosis** (deposition of iron in body tissue) can occur. Therefore, an iron chelation program such as subcutaneous infusion **(hypodermoclysis)** of deferrioxamine (Desferal) may be started concurrently with transfusions.

CASE STUDY QUESTION

2. Lena has received iron chelation therapy in the past. Iron chelation therapy is:

a. A procedure to remove excess iron from the child's body
b. A procedure to help iron move effectively into haemoglobin
c. A therapy to increase the iron level in bone and muscle cells
d. A therapy to convert iron into calcium to increase heart action

Hypochromic anaemias

When haemoglobin synthesis is inadequate, the erythrocytes appear pale (hypochromia). Hypochromia is generally accompanied by a reduction in the diameter of cells (RBCs are also microcytic).

Iron-deficiency anaemia

Although the incidence of iron-deficiency anaemia is decreasing in the developed world due to improved infant nutrition, it is still the most common anaemia of infancy and childhood. It also is the only nutrient deficiency that is prevalent in industrialised countries (World Health Organization, 2015). Most iron in the body is incorporated in haemoglobin but an additional amount is stored in the bone marrow to be available for haemoglobin production. Inadequate dietary iron prevents proper haemoglobin formation. With iron-deficiency anaemia, RBCs are both small in size (hypocytic) and pale (hypochromic) due to the altered haemoglobin.

Children are at high risk of iron-deficiency anaemia because, compared to adults, they need more daily iron in proportion to their body weight to maintain an adequate iron level. Specific guidelines for the daily iron intake for children in Australia and New Zealand can be found in the nutrient reference values of Australia and New Zealand available at <www.nhmrc.gov.au/guidelines-publications/n35-n36-n37>. Iron-deficiency anaemia occurs most often between the ages 9 months and 3 years; its frequency rises again in adolescence when iron requirements increase for girls who are menstruating. It is also found in overweight teenagers if they ingest most of their kilojoules from high-carbohydrate, not iron-rich, foods (Brotanek et al., 2007).

Causes in infants

There are several causes of iron-deficiency anaemia in infants. When an infant's diet lacks sufficient iron the child usually has enough in reserve to last for the first 6 months of life. After that, if the infant's diet continues to be iron deficient there will be difficulty forming adequate RBCs. Infants of low birth weight have fewer iron stores than those born at term because iron stores are laid down near the end of gestation. Because low-birth-weight infants also grow rapidly and their need for RBCs expands accordingly, they tend to develop iron-deficiency anaemia before 5 to 6 months. As a preventive measure they may be given an iron supplement beginning around 2 months of age.

Women with iron deficiency during pregnancy tend to give birth to iron-deficient babies because the babies do not receive iron stores.

Iron-deficiency anaemia can be prevented in formula-fed infants by giving them iron-fortified formula. If an infant is breastfed, iron-fortified cereal should be introduced when solid foods are introduced in the first year. Fortunately, these cost no more than non-fortified foods. Occasionally, an infant becomes constipated while ingesting iron-rich formula, but this is the exception rather than the rule.

Causes in older children

In children older than 2 years, chronic blood loss is the most frequent cause of iron-deficiency anaemia. This is caused by gastrointestinal tract lesions such as polyps, ulcerative colitis, Crohn's disease, protein-induced enteropathies, parasitic infestation or frequent epistaxis.

Adolescent girls can become iron deficient because of frequent attempts to diet and over consumption of snack foods low in iron. Without sufficient iron, their body cannot compensate for the iron lost with menstrual flow.

Children with iron-deficiency anaemia appear pale. Because the pallor develops slowly parents may not realise how extensive it is. They may describe their child as "fair-skinned" even though the child's pallor is so extreme the skin is transparent. In dark-skinned infants, pale mucous membranes may be the most significant finding.

Infants may show poor muscle tone and reduced activity. They are generally irritable from fatigue. Their heart may be enlarged and there may be a soft systolic precordial murmur as the heart increases its action, attempting to supply body cells with more oxygen. The spleen may be slightly enlarged. Fingernails become typically spoon-shaped or depressed in contour (see Box 44.2).

Therapy for iron-deficiency anaemia focuses on treatment of the underlying cause. Sources of gastrointestinal bleeding must be ruled out. The diet must be rich in iron and should contain extra vitamin C, as this enhances iron absorption. Once other underlying causes have been ruled out and/or addressed, oral iron supplements may be prescribed. The patient and their family should be advised of the possible side effects of these medications (gastrointestinal, including abdominal pain, constipation and black stools, diarrhoea, dyspepsia and nausea). Encourage parents to report any of these symptoms if they occur (Hussain, 2014; see Box 44.3).

BOX 44.2 Assessment ✻ Assessing a child with iron-deficiency anaemia

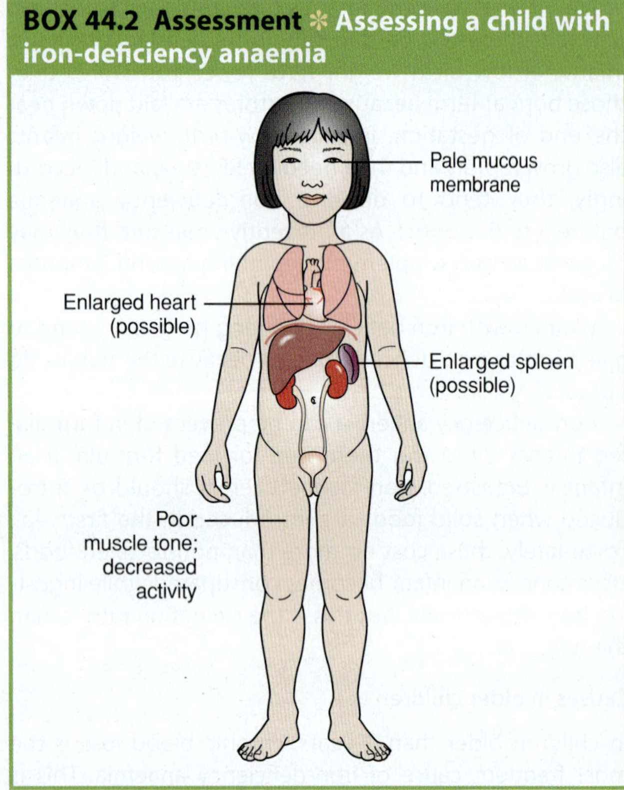

Imbalanced nutrition

When planning care for an infant with iron-deficiency anaemia, it is helpful to minimise the child's activities to prevent fatigue, particularly at mealtime, as a fatigued child is more reluctant to eat any food, let alone eat iron-rich foods.

Counsel parents on measures to improve their infant's nutrition such as adding iron-rich foods while decreasing formula or breast milk intake. If the child is not fond of meat, suggest parents substitute cheese, eggs, green vegetables or fortified cereal. Because iron-rich foods are often expensive, remind parents that these items are important and that they should not substitute less expensive, high-carbohydrate foods. Before iron therapy is started, help parents create reminder sheets so they can manage to give the supplement over a long period of time. Alert parents to possible side effects, such as stomach irritation, constipation, and that liquid iron preparations can stain teeth if not taken through a straw. Iron is absorbed best with an accompanying acid medium so ascorbic acid may also be prescribed (or the parent be advised to give the iron medication with orange juice) to increase absorption. To avoid constipation, the child may need additional fibre like that supplied by green leafy vegetables. If oral iron is not tolerated or if there is a doubt the child will take it, an iron-dextran injection (Imferon) can be given intramuscularly. Imferon stains the skin and is extremely irritating unless it is given by deep Z-track intramuscular injection.

Of all age groups, adolescents tend to do the least well with taking medicine consistently. Help them plan a daily time for taking their iron supplement with a medication reminder chart. At first they may reject this as childish, but assure them that everyone needs these charts. Review with them the iron-rich foods they will need to eat daily. An iron supplement is effective only if taken with iron-rich foods.

BOX 44.3 ✻ Focus on pharmacology

Ferrous sulfate

Classification: Ferrous sulfate is an iron salt.

Action: Supplies iron for red cell production. It elevates the serum iron concentration and then is converted to haemoglobin or trapped in the reticuloendothelial cells for storage and eventual conversion to a usable form of iron (McKenna & Mirkov, 2014).

Pregnancy risk category: A

Dosage: For iron-deficiency: Children over 12 years 15–30 mL PO daily. Children 7–12 years 5–20 mL PO daily. Children 2–6 years up to 5 mL PO daily. Children under 2 years—administer only under medical advice (McKenna & Mirkov, 2014).

Possible adverse effects: Gastrointestinal upset, anorexia, nausea, vomiting, constipation, dark stools, stained teeth (liquid preparations).

Nursing implications

- Instruct parents to administer the drug on an empty stomach with water to enhance absorption. If this causes gastrointestinal irritation, administer it after meals. Avoid giving it with milk, eggs, coffee or tea.
- If the liquid preparation is ordered, advise parents to mix it with water or juice to mask the taste and prevent staining of teeth. Encourage the parents to have the child drink the medication through a straw to avoid staining of the teeth.
- Keep in mind that iron is absorbed best in the presence of vitamin C. Suggest parents give the iron with a citrus juice such as orange juice to help absorption. Some children may be prescribed vitamin C to take concurrently to increase absorption.
- Inform child and parents that iron may turn stools black.
- Encourage parents to include high-fibre foods in the child's diet to minimise the risk of constipation.
- Reinforce the need for thorough brushing of teeth to prevent staining.
- Remind parents about the need for follow-up blood tests to evaluate the effectiveness of the drug.

Pernicious anaemia (vitamin B_{12} deficiency)

Vitamin B_{12} is necessary for maturation of RBCs. Pernicious anaemia results from deficiency or inability to use this vitamin (Waterbury, 2007). In children, the cause is more often lack of ingestion of vitamin B_{12}. The vitamin is found primarily in foods of animal origin, including both cow's milk and breast milk. Adolescents may be deficient in vitamin B_{12} if they are ingesting a long-term, poorly formulated vegetarian diet.

For absorption of vitamin B_{12} from the intestine, an intrinsic factor must be present in the gastric mucosa. In adults, lack of the intrinsic factor is the most frequent cause of the disorder. If a child has an intrinsic factor deficiency, symptoms can occur as early as the first 2 years of life (once the intrauterine stores of vitamin B_{12} have been exhausted). The child appears pale, anorexic and irritable, with chronic diarrhoea. The tongue appears smooth and beefy red due to papillary atrophy. In children, neuropathological findings such as ataxia, hyporeflexia, paraesthesia and a positive Babinski reflex are less noticeable than in adults.

Sickle-cell anaemia

Sickle-cell anaemia is the presence of abnormally shaped (elongated) RBCs. It is an autosomal recessive inherited disorder on the beta chain of haemoglobin; the amino acid valine takes the place of the normally appearing glutamic acid. The erythrocytes become characteristically elongated and crescent-shaped (sickled) when they are submitted to low oxygen tension (less than 60–70%), a low blood pH (acidosis), or increased blood viscosity such as occurs with dehydration or hypoxia. When RBCs sickle, they cannot move freely through vessels. Stasis and further sickling occurs (a *sickle-cell crisis*). Blood flow halts and tissue distal to the blockage becomes ischaemic, resulting in acute pain and cell destruction (Linker, 2009).

Both parents of the child with the disease will have either normal adult haemoglobin S or be carriers (heterozygous) of the *sickle-cell trait* (have haemoglobin AS). In people with the trait, approximately 25% to 50% of haemoglobin produced is abnormal. They produce enough normal haemoglobin to compensate for the haemoglobin that is sickled and therefore show no symptoms. A child with the disease (homozygous) produces no normal haemoglobin and so shows characteristic symptoms of sickle-cell anaemia see (see Box 44.4). A very few children have combinations of haemoglobin S and haemoglobin C or E, leading to mild anaemia (Creary, Williamson & Kulkarni, 2007; see Box 44.5).

BOX 44.4 Assessment ✻ Assessing a child with sickle-cell crisis

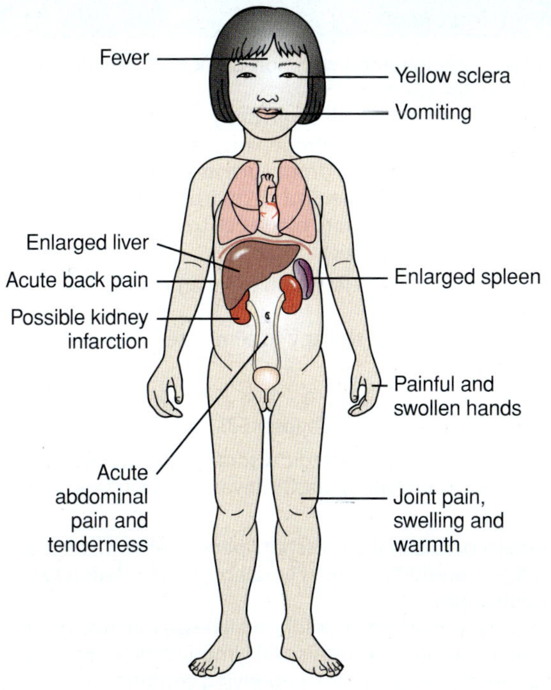

Fever
Yellow sclera
Vomiting
Enlarged liver
Acute back pain
Possible kidney infarction
Enlarged spleen
Painful and swollen hands
Acute abdominal pain and tenderness
Joint pain, swelling and warmth

BOX 44.5 ✻ Focus on communication

Joey Harrow, who has sickle-cell disease, is seen in the emergency department with a new vaso-occlusive crisis. His right knee is discoloured by a large brush burn. He's crying from pain.

Less effective communication

Nurse: Hello, Mr Harrow. I need to ask some questions to see if anything triggered this new crisis.

Mr Harrow: He better not have been doing something he's not allowed to do.

Nurse: His knee looks like he fell. Were you running, Joey? So you got dehydrated?

Mr Harrow: He better not say he was doing that!

Nurse: Joey, how did you hurt your knee?

Joey: I don't know.

Nurse: Okay. Let's get you better and not worry about what started this.

More effective communication

Nurse: Hello, Mr Harrow. I need to ask some questions to see if anything triggered this new crisis.

Mr Harrow: He better not have been doing something he's not allowed to do.

Nurse: His knee looks like he fell. Were you running, Joey? So you got dehydrated?

Mr Harrow: He better not say he was doing that!

Nurse: Mr Harrow, I need to get an accurate history of what happened. I'd like Joey to tell us how he thinks the accident happened. Then later on, we can talk about what are good rules for him to be following.

Children with blood disorders have to follow a great many rules to avoid clotting or bleeding episodes, such as not playing contact sports or playing too hard in the sun. Because these forbidden activities are appealing, children occasionally break the rules. In an emergency room, it is important that children and parents both recognise that the priority at the moment is obtaining an accurate history. Until they realise this, they may be so concerned with the broken rule that they are unable to move beyond that to secure adequate therapy.

Thalassaemias

The thalassaemias are autosomal recessive anaemias associated with abnormalities of the beta chain of adult haemoglobin (HgbA). The highest rates of thalassaemias occur in Asia, the Mediterranean basin and the Middle East (World Health Organization, 2011).

Thalassaemia minor (heterozygous beta-thalassaemia)

Children with thalassaemia minor, a mild form of this anaemia, produce both defective beta haemoglobin and normal haemoglobin. Because there is some normal production, the RBC count is normal, but the haemoglobin concentration is decreased 2–3 g/100 mL below normal levels. The blood cells are moderately hypochromic and microcytic because of the poor haemoglobin formation.

Children may have no symptoms other than pallor. They require no treatment and life expectancy is normal. They should not receive a routine iron supplement because their inability to incorporate it well into haemoglobin may cause them to accumulate too much iron. The condition represents the heterozygous form of the disorder or can be compared with children having the sickle-cell trait.

Thalassaemia major (homozygous beta-thalassaemia)

Thalassaemia major is also called Cooley's anaemia or Mediterranean anaemia. Because thalassaemia is a beta chain haemoglobin defect, symptoms do not become apparent until a child's fetal haemoglobin has largely been replaced by adult haemoglobin during the second half of the first year of life. Unable to produce normal beta haemoglobin, the child shows symptoms of anaemia: pallor, irritability and anorexia (Muncie, 2008; see Table 44.2).

RBCs are hypochromic (pale) and microcytic (small). Fragmented poikilocytes and basophilic stippling (unevenness of haemoglobin concentration) are present. The haemoglobin level is less than 5 g/100 mL. The serum iron level is high because iron is not being incorporated into haemoglobin; iron saturation is 100%.

TABLE 44.2 Effects of thalassaemia major

Body organ or system	Effect of abnormal cell production
Bone marrow	Overstimulation of bone marrow leads to increased facial-mandibular growth
Skin	Bronze-coloured from haemosiderosis and jaundice
Spleen	Splenomegaly
Liver and gallbladder	Cirrhosis and cholelithiasis
Pancreas	Destruction of islet cells and diabetes mellitus
Heart	Failure from circulatory overload

DISORDERS OF THE WHITE BLOOD CELLS

Most disorders characterised by a decrease or increase in the number of WBCs or specific WBC components occur in response to another disease (often infection or an allergic reaction) in the body. Laboratory values of WBCs, therefore, provide one of the first objective indicators of infectious disease, often aiding in specific diagnoses. These diseases are discussed in Chapter 43. Leukaemia, overproduction of WBCs, is discussed with other malignant conditions in Chapter 53. Table 44.3 outlines disorders associated with white blood cells.

TABLE 44.3 Disorders of white blood cells

Disorder	Description	Causes/Treatment
Neutropenia	Reduced number of white blood cells	Transient phenomenon with non-pyrogenic infections such as viral disease Response to therapy with some drugs, such as 6-mercaptopurine or nitrogen mustard Possible side effect from drugs such as phenytoin sodium (Dilantin), chloramphenicol or chlorpromazine Treatments: Possibly white blood cell transfusion; prophylactic antibiotics
Neutrophilia	Increased number of circulating white blood cells, primarily neutrophils (total number of cells increases and the proportion of mature neutrophils changes, with an increase in immature cells)	Usually in response to infection or inflammation (see Chapter 43) Treatment: antibiotic therapy to eliminate infectious organisms
Leukaemia	Uncontrolled proliferation of white blood cells	Neoplastic disorder (see Chapter 53)
Eosinophilia	Increased number of eosinophils	Associated with many allergic disorders, such as atopic dermatitis, and with parasitic invasion (see Chapters 42 and 43)
Lymphocytosis	Increased number of lymphocytes	Normally occurs in the preschool period, when there is a marked predominance of lymphocytes in relation to neutrophils Abnormally elevated in childhood illnesses such as pertussis, infectious mononucleosis and lymphocytic leukaemia Treatment: Therapy for the underlying condition

DISORDERS OF BLOOD COAGULATION

Effective blood coagulation depends on a complex series of four events, including a combination of blood and tissue factors released from the plasma (the intrinsic pathway) and from injured tissue (the extrinsic pathway) (Schwartz, Rote & McCance, 2012).

When a vessel is injured, vasoconstriction occurs in the area proximal to the injury, thus narrowing the vessel lumen and reducing the amount of blood that can flow to the injured area. Platelets begin to adhere to the damaged vessel site and to one another, forming a platelet plug and initiating the first stage of clotting. In the second stage, factors from either the intrinsic or the extrinsic system combine with platelet phospholipids to form complete thromboplastin. In the third stage, thromboplastin converts prothrombin (factor II) to thrombin if ionised calcium is present. The production of prothrombin and factors VII, IX, and X all depend on the presence of vitamin K. This stage will be incomplete, therefore, if levels of any of factors VIII through XII, vitamin K or calcium are deficient. In the fourth stage, thrombin converts fibrinogen (factor I) to fibrin. Fibrin strands form a mesh incorporating RBCs, WBCs and platelets to form a permanent protective seal at the site of injury. Factor XIII (fibrin stabilising factor) then acts to make the fibrin clot insoluble and permanent.

Platelets are necessary for blood coagulation, so disorders that limit the number of platelets limit the effectiveness of this process. A normal platelet level is 150,000/mm^3. Thrombocytopenia (decreased platelet count) is defined as a platelet count of less than 40,000/mm^3. Thrombocytopenia often leads to purpura, or blood seeping from vessels into the skin. In one rare disorder, children are born with thrombocytopenia and are also missing the radius bone in the forearm (TAR [thrombocytopenia/absent radius] syndrome).

Purpuras

Purpura refers to a haemorrhagic rash or small haemorrhages in the superficial layer of skin. Two main types of purpura occur in children: idiopathic thrombocytopenia purpura and Henoch-Schönlein syndrome.

Idiopathic thrombocytopenic purpura

Idiopathic thrombocytopenic purpura (ITP) is the result of a decrease in the number of circulating platelets in the presence of adequate megakaryocytes (precursors to platelets). The disease is characterised by isolated thrombocytopenia without a clinically apparent cause (Kayal, Jayachandran & Khushboo Singh, 2014).

In most instances, ITP occurs approximately 2 weeks after a viral infection such as rubella, rubeola, varicella or an upper respiratory tract infection. Congenital ITP may occur in the newborn of a woman who has had ITP during pregnancy. An antiplatelet factor crosses the placenta and causes platelet destruction in the newborn in the same way that Rh incompatibility or haemolytic disease of the newborn develops (see Chapter 26). However in ITP, the platelets, not the RBCs, are sensitised.

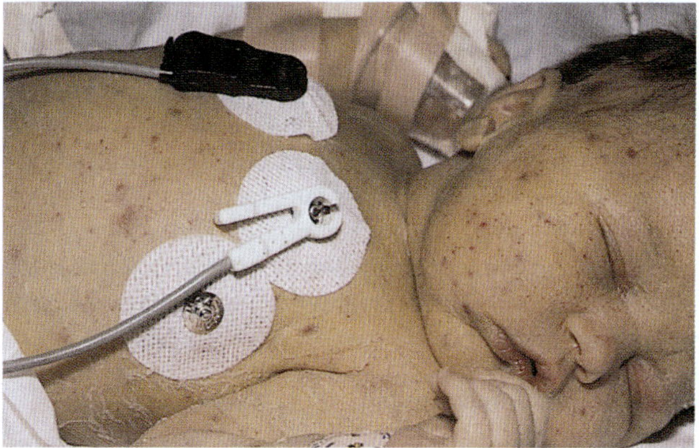

FIGURE 44.2 An infant with ITP. Notice the tiny petechiae and larger ecchymotic areas. (From Zitelli, B. J. & Davis, H. W. [1997]. *Atlas of Pediatric Physical Diagnosis* [3rd ed.]. St Louis: Mosby.)

Manifestations often begin abruptly, first evidenced as miniature petechiae or as large areas of asymmetric ecchymosis most prominent over the legs, although they may occur anywhere on the body (see Fig. 44.2). Epistaxis or bleeding into joints may be present.

Laboratory studies reveal marked thrombocytopenia. The platelet count may be as low as 20,000/mm^3. Bone marrow examination reveals a normal number of megakaryocytes.

Oral prednisone to reduce the immune response and intravenous immunoglobulin (IVIG) or, in Rh-positive children, anti-D immunoglobulin which is believed to coat RBCs that are positive for D antigen, are strategies used to treat ITP (Bredlau, Semple & Segel, 2011). Platelet transfusion will temporarily increase the platelet count. However, because the life span of platelets is relatively short, a platelet transfusion has only limited effect. Children with central nervous system bleeding may require a splenectomy, although this is rarely necessary.

If the child experiences joint pain from bleeding, paracetamol, rather than salicylates or ibuprofen is prescribed for pain. Both salicylates and ibuprofen increase the chance of bleeding as they prevent the aggregation of platelets at wound sites.

In most children, ITP runs a limited, 1- to 3-month course. A few children develop chronic ITP. A course of immunosuppressive medications may be attempted if the chronic state persists. All children need to be vaccinated against the viral diseases of childhood so that diseases such as rubella, rubeola and varicella are eradicated and can no longer lead to this defective coagulation process.

Health-seeking behaviours related to injury-prevention measures

Education for parents and carers needs to include: parents ability to state precautions necessary to reduce the possibility of bleeding, repeat correct dose and timing of medication therapy, ensure the child's skin is free of ecchymotic areas and monitor results for when the childs platelet count rises to normal values.

The chief danger to the child from ITP is intracranial haemorrhage. Although this is rare, be alert for signs such as persistent headache, nuchal rigidity and lethargy. The psychological stress of living with a perplexing illness must also be considered when planning nursing care for both the patient and family.

Compromised family coping

Parents need to fully understand the nature of their child's illness and identify ways they can continue to carry out daily activities. Because symptoms such as the easy bruising of ITP mimics the beginning ones of leukaemia, parents may be extremely frightened when symptoms first occur. You can assure them after the diagnosis is made that this bruising is not leukaemia. If the ITP follows a long course (2 or 3 months), reassure them that this process will not later become leukaemia. A child may have so many bruises that the parents are initially suspected of child abuse. This can cause them to become very defensive and angry at healthcare personnel. Allow them time to express their anger and regain confidence in their healthcare team.

It is always bewildering for parents to be told that no-one knows exactly what is causing their child's illness. To feel comfortable that healthcare personnel can manage their child's care without knowing the exact cause, they need careful explanations of all procedures.

Henoch-Schönlein syndrome

Henoch-Schönlein purpura (also called anaphylactoid purpura) is caused by increased vessel permeability (see Fig. 44.3). Although no definite allergic correlation can be identified, it is generally considered to be a hypersensitivity reaction to an invading allergen. It occurs most frequently in children between 2 and 8 years of age, and more frequently in boys than girls (Hellmann & Imboden, 2009). Usually, there is a history of a mild infection before the outbreak of symptoms. The syndrome presents (because of the purpura) as a possible platelet disorder until a differential diagnosis is made.

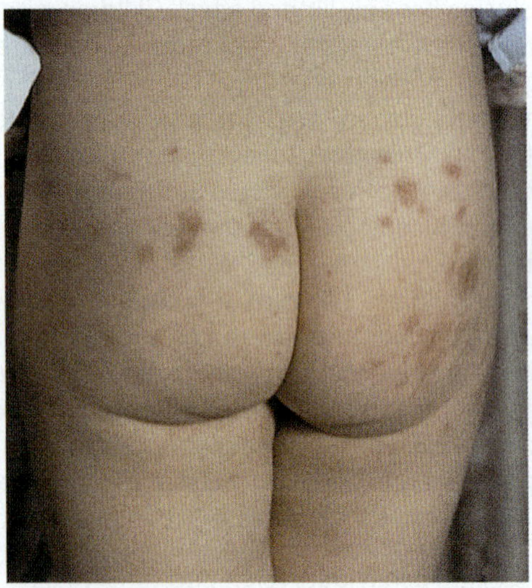

FIGURE 44.3 The distinctive purpural rash of Henoch-Schönlein syndrome appearing on the buttocks of a young child. (From Zitelli, B. J. & Davis, H. W. [1997]. *Atlas of Pediatric Physical Diagnosis* [3rd ed.]. St Louis: Mosby.)

Disseminated intravascular coagulation

Disseminated intravascular coagulation (DIC) is an acquired disorder of blood clotting that results from excessive trauma or some similar underlying stimulus (Bowman, 2007). Normal blood clotting is a balance between the haemostatic (clotting) system and the fibrinolytic (dissolving) system of the bloodstream. After a blood vessel injury, local vasoconstriction rapidly prevents additional blood loss at the site. With the tear in the vessel wall, the underlying collagen is exposed. This causes platelets to swell and become adherent and irregular in shape. They release adenosine diphosphate, which attracts additional platelets and binds them together (platelet aggregation). This phenomenon results in a platelet plug to seal the vessel. The plug is strengthened by fibrin threads that form as a result of an intrinsic and extrinsic coagulation process into a firm, fixed structure. To prevent too much clotting from occurring, plasmin or fibrinolysin, a proteolytic enzyme formed from plasminogen, digests fibrin threads and causes lysis of the clot along with consumption of blood clotting factors. As plasmin, fibrinogen and fibrin are lysed, fibrin degradation products are formed. These products prevent the laying down of further fibrin and platelet aggregation.

With DIC, an imbalance occurs between clotting activity and fibrinolysis. Extreme clotting due to endothelial damage begins at one point in the circulatory system, depleting the availability of clotting factors such as platelets and fibrin from the general circulation. A secondary initiation of fibrinolysis begins as well. A paradox exists: the child has both increased coagulation and a bleeding defect at the same time. Many of the complications of pregnancy (abruptio placentae or death of a fetus) initiate DIC, so this is a common complication seen accompanying bleeding during pregnancy (see Chapter 21). DIC also tends to occur in children with acute infections or trauma.

A child begins to have uncontrolled bleeding from puncture sites from injections or intravenous therapy. Ecchymoses and petechiae form on the skin. The toes and fingers may appear pale, cyanotic or mottled and feel cold because small blood vessels are so filled with coagulated blood that circulation to the extremities is impaired. If coagulation is acute, neurological or renal symptoms may occur from occlusion of vessels supplying the brain and kidneys. Observe all children with a serious illness carefully for signs of increased bleeding such as petechiae or oozing from blood-sampling sites to help identify that this is happening.

With DIC, laboratory tests usually reveal:

- Thrombocytopenia (level depends on the rate at which bone marrow can replace platelets)
- Large platelets on blood smear, possibly fragmented (from passing through meshes of collecting fibrin)
- Prolonged prothrombin and partial thromboplastin times
- Markedly low serum fibrinogen levels (less than 100 mg/100 mL)
- Elevated fibrin split products.

To halt the process of DIC the underlying insult that began the phenomenon must be halted. Intravenous heparin administration helps to interfere with the marked coagulation. Although blood transfusion may be necessary to correct blood loss, it may be delayed until after heparin has been administered so that the new blood factors are not also consumed by the coagulation process. Fresh-frozen plasma, platelets or fibrinogen may be administered.

With adequate therapy, the results of blood coagulation studies will return to normal. If renal or brain cells were damaged from occluded capillaries, permanent injury to these areas can result.

✔ Checkpoint question 44.1

Disseminated intravascular coagulation can occur in any child with a critical illness. The medication of choice you would expect to administer for this condition is:

a. Erythropoietin, to stimulate new red cells
b. Methotrexate, to decrease red cell number
c. Heparin, to halt abnormal coagulation
d. Prednisone, to decrease the immune reaction

Haemophilias

Haemophilia is an inherited disorder of blood coagulation. There are numerous haemophilia types, each involving deficiency of a different blood coagulation factor.

Haemophilia A (factor VIII deficiency)

The classic form of haemophilia is caused by deficiency of the coagulation component factor VIII, the antihaemophilic factor. It is transmitted as a sex-linked recessive trait. The female carrier may have slightly lowered but sufficient levels of the factor VIII component so that she does not manifest a bleeding disorder. Males with the disease also have varying levels of factor VIII and their bleeding tendency varies accordingly, from mild to severe (Ambruso, Hays & Goldenberg, 2008).

Factor VIII is an intrinsic factor of coagulation, so the intrinsic system for manufacturing thromboplastin is incomplete. The child's coagulation ability is not absent because the extrinsic or tissue system remains intact. Because of this system, the child's blood will eventually coagulate after an injury.

Haemophilia often is recognised first in the infant who bleeds excessively after circumcision. If the disease has not shown itself for several generations in a family, the parents may be unaware of its existence. For this reason, all infants need careful and thoughtful observation after circumcision.

Because infants do not receive many injuries, children's bleeding tendencies may not become apparent until they become active (crawling, climbing or walking).

Suddenly the lower extremities (where the child bumps into things) become heavily bruised. There is soft tissue bleeding and painful haemorrhage into the joints, which become swollen and warm. The child holds the injured joint stiffly. Repeated bleeding into a joint causes damage to the synovial membrane (haemarthrosis), possibly resulting in severe loss of joint mobility.

Severe bleeding may also occur into the gastrointestinal tract, peritoneal cavity or central nervous system. Interestingly, nosebleeds are common but are not as severe as with the platelet deficiency syndromes. The child must be identified as having haemophilia before surgery is performed for any reason; otherwise, fatal bleeding could occur.

With haemophilia, the platelet count and prothrombin time are normal. The whole blood clotting time is markedly prolonged or normal, depending on the level of factor VIII present. A thromboplastin generation test is abnormal. Partial thromboplastin time (PTT) is the test that best reveals the low levels of factor VIII.

With even minor abrasions, bleeding must be controlled by the administration of factor VIII. This may be supplied by fresh whole blood or by fresh or frozen plasma, but it is best supplied by a concentrate of factor VIII. Powdered forms of factor VIII that can be stored at home and reconstituted as needed are available. In some children, administration of desmopressin (DDAVP), which stimulates the release of factor VIII, may be helpful. Prophylactic administration, although expensive, may best reduce bleeding episodes.

In a few children, antibodies (termed inhibitors) to factor VIII develop, rendering the factor ineffective. If this happens, epsilon-aminocaproic acid, a fibrinolytic enzyme that helps to stabilise clot formation and promote wound healing, can be self-administered every 6 hours if needed. Children with inhibitors to factor VIII can also be given a factor IX concentrate. This concentrate enters the coagulation cascade after factor VIII and halts bleeding.

Strategies for protecting child from injury

Parents need information about how to prevent bleeding episodes and also how to respond when one occurs (see Box 44.6). Prevention of injury is the most important intervention with these children. Help parents to set appropriate limits. An active infant may need to have cot sides padded; all toys need to be inspected for sharp edges or parts.

Parents (and the older child) can be taught to administer a replacement factor intravenously to prevent bleeding

BOX 44.6 ✻ Techniques for reducing bleeding with thrombocytopenia

Some techniques for reducing bleeding due to inadequate platelet formation include:

- Limit the number of blood-drawing procedures; combine samples whenever possible.
- Use a blood pressure cuff instead of a tourniquet to reduce the number of petechiae.
- Apply pressure to any puncture site for a full 5 minutes before applying a bandage.
- Minimise use of adhesive tape to the skin (pulling for removal may tear the skin and cause petechiae).
- Pad side and cot rails to prevent bruising.
- Protect intravenous sites to avoid numerous reinsertions.
- Administer medication orally or by intravenous infusion when appropriate to minimise the number of injection sites.
- Assess that the child is offered foods that can be chewed without irritation (avoid toast crusts, for example).
- Urge the child to use a soft toothbrush.
- Check toys for sharp corners, which may cause scratches. Urge the child to be careful with paper, because paper cuts can bleed out of proportion to their size.
- Assess the need for routine blood pressure determinations. Tight cuffs could lead to petechiae.
- Distract the child from rough play; suggest stimulating but quiet activities to minimise risk of injury.
- Keep a record of blood drawn; do not draw extra amounts "just in case" so children do not become more anaemic.

immediately after an injury. Although the child needs to be assessed by a healthcare provider, this action, combined with immobilisation of the injured extremity and an ice pack applied locally, almost always eliminates the need for hospital admission. Pressure should be applied to a laceration to halt bleeding directly. "Butterfly bandages" are used in place of suturing for lacerations whenever possible, because sutures make additional puncture sites that could bleed.

Joint pain

The child with haemophiliac bleeding experiences discomfort because of the bleeding into joints and may be frightened because their parents are also scared by the confronting presentation. Immobilisation of the affected joint helps to decrease bleeding and also helps provide relief. Be certain that immobilised joints are in good alignment. As soon as the acute bleeding episode has halted (after approximately 48 hours), perform passive range of motion as ordered to maintain function. Paracetamol (Panadol) is the recommended first line drug for pain management. Other types of analgesia such as ibuprofen should only be prescribed following an analysis of the possible side effects of these medications for a patient with this condition (Holstein et al., 2012). As soon as effective levels of factor VIII have been provided, the pain in the bleeding joint is generally relieved, despite the continued heat or swelling.

Fears regarding child's prognosis and long-term nature of illness

Parents of children with haemophilia are frightened during a time of acute bleeding, not just because of what is currently happening but also because they may have seen other family members or even a previous child die of the disease. Be certain to give them a chance to talk about how the bleeding began ("I should have noticed that toy had a sharp edge" "He fell from his bike. I should have watched him more closely"). It is extremely important for parents to allow the child to lead a normal life. Remind them that it is impossible to prevent all injuries. Assist them with measures that offer them a sense of control over the situation. As children reach school age, they must learn to monitor their own activities to prevent bleeding episodes.

von Willebrand's disease

Von Willebrand's disease, an inherited autosomal dominant disorder affecting both sexes, is often referred to as angiohaemophilia. Along with a factor VIII defect, there is also an inability of the platelets to aggregate. In addition, the blood vessels cannot constrict to aid in coagulation. Bleeding time is prolonged, with most haemorrhages occurring from mucous membrane sites.

Epistaxis is a major problem, because all children tend to rub or pick at their nose as a nervous mechanism. In girls, menstrual flow is unusually heavy and may cause embarrassment from stained clothing. Childbirth is obviously a risk for women with von Willebrand's disease with pregnant patients requiring close monitoring (Hitch, 2014)). Bleeding is controlled with factor VIII replenishment as with haemophilia, or by administration of DDAVP, which stimulates factor VIII release.

Christmas disease (haemophilia B, factor IX deficiency)

Christmas disease, caused by factor IX deficiency, is transmitted as a sex-linked recessive trait. Only approximately 15% of people with haemophilia have this form. Treatment is with a concentrate of factor IX, available for home administration (Linker, 2009).

Haemophilia C (factor XI deficiency)

Haemophilia C or plasma thromboplastin antecedent deficiency, caused by factor XI deficiency, is transmitted as an autosomal recessive trait occurring in both sexes. The symptoms are generally mild compared with those in children with factor VIII or factor IX deficiencies. Bleeding episodes are treated with administration of DDAVP or transfusion of fresh blood or plasma (Ambruso, Hays & Goldenberg, 2008).

✔ *Checkpoint question* 44.2

Justin is a 5-year-old boy with haemophilia who wants to join a preschool soccer program. How would you counsel his family regarding this plan?

Key points for review

- Haematopoietic stem cell transplantation is the main therapy for numerous blood dyscrasias. Transplantation can be allogeneic (from a histocompatible donor), autologous (using the child's own marrow or umbilical cord blood) or synergeneic (the donor and recipient are identical twins).
- Splenectomy, another possible treatment, may increase a child's susceptibility to pneumococcal infections. Assess whether a child has received pneumococcal vaccine after a splenectomy.
- Disorders of the RBCs that commonly occur in children include acute blood-loss anaemia and anaemia of acute infection. Aplastic and hypoplastic anaemias occur from depression of haematopoietic activity in bone marrow. These anaemias can be congenital or acquired.
- A major hypochromic anaemia that develops in children is iron-deficiency anaemia. Children invariably fatigue easily because they cannot oxygenate body cells well. Their care must include measures to keep them from tiring; oxygen administration may be necessary.
- Macrocytic anaemias occur from folic acid deficiency and pernicious anaemia (vitamin B_{12} deficiency).
- Disorders of WBCs that occur include neutropenia (reduced number of WBCs) and neutrophilia (increased number). Neutropenia makes children susceptible to infection.
- Disorders of blood coagulation include the purpuras (idiopathic thrombocytopenic purpura and Henoch-Schönlein syndrome), disseminated intravascular coagulation and the haemophilias.
- Children with blood coagulation disorders must carefully guard against injury. This includes monitoring types of toys and activities. It may include padding a cot or side rail.
- Disorders of the blood tend to be long-term illnesses. Education of the parents and child is important to promote adaptation to the condition and enhance long-term medication therapy.

CASE STUDY QUESTIONS

3. Lena has a prominent mandible and wide-spaced upper front teeth from overgrowth of bone marrow centres. Her skin is bronze from the number of transfusions (64) she has received in her short lifetime. "Why is my daughter starting to look different?" Lena's mother asks you. What additional health teaching does Lena's mother need to help her better understand her daughter's disease? How would you explain why skin colour changes have happened to her daughter?
4. Joey's growth is only in the fifth percentile and he has had two vaso-occlusive crises in the past year. Every summer for the past 2 years, while he has been home from school on holidays, he has had an acute episode of his illness. What assessments would you want to make of his family before this summer? What precautions would you want to discuss with them?

Resources

For an extensive range of additional resources to enhance teaching and learning and to facilitate understanding of this chapter, please see the text's accompanying website located on thePoint at http://thepoint.lww.com.

References

Ambruso, D. R., Hays, T. & Goldenberg, N. (2008). Hematologic disorders. In W. W. Hay et al. (Eds). *Current Pediatric Diagnosis and Treatment* (18th ed.). Columbus, OH: McGraw-Hill.

Australian and New Zealand Society of Blood Transfusion Ltd & Royal College of Nursing Australia. (2011). Guidelines for the administration of blood products (2nd ed.), accessed 3 February 2015, <www.anzsbt.org.au/publications/documents/ANZSBT_Guidelines_Administration_Blood_Products_2ndEd_Dec_2011_Hyperlinks.pdf>.

Barnett, K., et al. (2007). Tapeworm infestation: A cause of iron deficiency anemia shown by capsule endoscopy. *Gastrointestinal Endoscopy, 66*(3), 625–627.

Beattie, S. (2007). Hands-on help: Bone marrow aspiration and biopsy. *RN, 70*(2), 41–43.

Bendorf, A. & Keridge, I. (2011). Ethical issues in bone marrow transplantation in children, *Journal of Paediatrics and Child Health, 47*(9), 614–619.

Blümel, J., et al., (2010). Parvovirus B19—Revised, *Transfusion Medicine and Hemotherapy, 37*(6), 339–350.

Bowman, S. H. (2007). Disseminated intravascular coagulation. In J. Schaider et al. (Eds). *Rosen & Barkin's 5-Minute Emergency Medicine Consult*. Philadelphia: Lippincott Williams & Wilkins.

Bredlau, A. L., Semple, J. & Segel, G. (2011). Management of immune thrombocytopenic purpura in children, *Paediatric Drugs, 13*(4), 213.

Brotanek, J. M., et al. (2007). Iron deficiency in early childhood in the United States: Risk factors and racial/ethnic disparities. *Pediatrics, 120*(3), 568–575.

Children's Hospital Westmead. (2014). Transfusion of blood and blood components—policy and procedure, accessed 3 February 2015, <www.chw.edu.au/about/policies/pdf/2007-8092.pdf>.

Creary, M., Williamson, D. & Kulkarni, R. (2007). Sickle-cell disease: Current activities, public health implications and future directions. *Journal of Women's Health, 16*(5), 575–582.

Cutler, C. & Ballen, K. (2012). Improving outcomes in umbilical cord blood transplantation: State of the art, *Blood Reviews, 26*(6), 241–246.

Di Sabatino, A., Carsetti, R. & Corazza, G. R. (2011). Post-splenectomy and hyposplenic states. *Lancet, 378*(9785), 86–97.

Grosskreutz, C., et al. (2007). Graft versus host disease after stem cell allotransplantation with low-dose total body irradiation, fludarabine, and antithymocyte globulin. *Transplantation, 84*(5), 598–604.

Hellmann, D. B. & Imboden, J. B. (2009). Musculoskeletal disorders. In S. J. McPhee & M. A. Papadakis (Eds). *Current Medical Diagnosis and Treatment*. Columbus, OH: McGraw-Hill.

Hitch, D. (2014). von Willebrand disease 101, *American Nurse Today*, 9(6), accessed 3 February 2015, <www.americannursetoday.com/von-willebrand-disease-101/>.

Holstein, K., et al., (2012). Pain management in patients with haemophilia: A European survey, *Haemophilia, 18*(5), 743– 752.

Hussain, N. (2014). Iron-deficiency anaemia, *Innovait, 7*(7), 398–403.

Kayal, L., Jayachandran, S. & Khushboo Singh. (2014). Idiopathic thrombocytopenic purpura, *Contemporary Clinical Dentistry, 5*(3), 410.

Linker, C. A. (2009). Hematology. In S. J. McPhee & M. A. Papadakis (Eds). *Current Medical Diagnosis and Treatment*. Columbus, OH: McGraw-Hill.

Lum, G. M. (2012). Kidney and urinary tract. In W. W. Hay et al. (Eds.), *Current Pediatric Diagnosis and Treatment* (20th ed.). Columbus, OH: McGraw-Hill.

McKenna, L. & Mirkov, S. (2014*). McKenna's Drug Handbook for Nursing and Midwifery* (7th ed.). Sydney: Lippincott Williams & Wilkins.

Muncie, H. L. (2008). Thalassemia. In F. J. Domino (Ed). *The 5-Minute Clinical Consult*. Philadelphia: Lippincott Williams & Wilkins.

National Health and Medical Research Council (Australia). (2014). Nutrient reference values for Australia and New Zealand including recommended daily intakes, accessed 3 February 2015, <www.nhmrc.gov.au/guidelines-publications/n35-n36-n37>.

Rosado, M. et al. (2013). Preserved antibody levels and loss of memory B cells against pneumococcus and tetanus after splenectomy: Tailoring better vaccination strategies, *European Journal of Immunology*, *43*(10), 2659–2670.

Royal Children's Hospital Melbourne. (2015). Blood product transfusion, accessed 3 February 2015, <www.rch.org.au/clinicalguide/guideline_index/Blood_product_transfusion/>.

Royal Children's Hospital Melbourne. (2015). Bone marrow transplants, accessed 2 February 2015, <www.rch.org.au/ccc/treatments/Bone_marrow_transplants/>.

Schwartz, A., Rote, N. S. & McCance, K. L. (2012). Alterations of hematologic function. In S. E. Huether & K. L. McCance (Eds), *Understanding Pathophysiology* (5th ed.), pp. 500–534. New York: Elsevier.

Tse, W., Bunting, K. D. & Laughlin, M. J. (2008). New insights into cord blood stem cell transplantation. *Current Opinion in Hematology*, *15*(4), 279–284.

Waterbury, L. (2007). Anemia. In N. H. Fiebach et al. (Eds). *Principles of Ambulatory Medicine* (7th ed.). Philadelphia: Lippincott Williams & Wilkins.

Women's and Children's Hospital South Australia. (2014). Childhood blood disorders—information for your family, accessed 3 February 2015, <www.wch.sa.gov.au/services/az/divisions/paedm/clinhaem/files/blood_disorders/index.html>.

Wood, J., et al. (2011). Contemporary pediatric splenectomy: Continuing controversies, *Pediatric Surgery International*, *27*(11), 1165–1171.

World Health Organization. (2011). Sickle-cell disease and other haemoglobin disorders. Fact sheet number 308, January 2011, accessed 3 February 2015, <www.who.int/mediacentre/factsheets/fs308/en/>.

World Health Organization. (2015). Micronutrient deficiencies, Iron deficiency anaemia, accessed 3 February 2015, <www.who.int/nutrition/topics/ida/en/>.

Suggested readings

Anionwu, E., Leary, A., & Johnson, K. (2012). Protecting specialist roles in haemoglobin disorders. *Nursing Times*, *108*(26), 18.

Cassis, F., et. al., (2014). Haemophilia experiences, results and opportunities (HERO) study: Influence of haemophilia on interpersonal relationships as reported by adults with haemophilia and parents of children with haemophilia, *Haemophilia*, *20*(4), e287–e295.

Rodgers, C., et al. (2008). Growth patterns and gastrointestinal symptoms in pediatric patients after hematopoietic stem cell transplantation. *Oncology Nursing Forum*, *35*(3), 443–448.

Schaider, J. et al. (Eds). (2014). *Rosen & Barkin's 5-Minute Emergency Medicine Consult*. Philadelphia: Lippincott Williams & Wilkins.

Thalassaemia International Federation. (2015). Epidemology, accessed 3 February 2015, <www.thalassaemia.org.cy/about-haemoglobin-disorders/alpha-thalassaemia/epidemiology.shtml>.

Chapter 45

Nursing care of a family when a child has a gastrointestinal disorder

Previous chapters described growth and development of well children and the nursing care for children with disorders of other systems. This chapter describes dramatic changes, both physical and psychosocial, that can occur when children develop gastrointestinal disorders.

LEARNING OBJECTIVES

After studying the contents of this chapter, you should be able to:

1. Describe common gastrointestinal disorders seen in children.
2. Analyse nursing care of a child with a gastrointestinal disorder.
3. Discuss the assessment of a child with a gastrointestinal disorder.
4. Develop an understanding of expected outcomes for a child with a gastrointestinal disorder.
5. Demonstrate knowledge of nursing care for a child with a gastrointestinal disorder.
6. Discuss nursing care for a child with a gastrointestinal disorder.
7. Display an understanding of expected outcomes for effective care.
8. Identify areas of care related to gastrointestinal disorders and children that could benefit from additional nursing research or application of evidence-based practice.

KEY TERMS

- coeliac disease
- dehydration
- gastro-oesophageal reflux
- hiatal hernia
- intussusception
- irritable bowel syndrome
- kwashiorkor
- liver transplantation
- Meckel's diverticulum
- volvulus

CASE STUDY

Jacob Abraham is a 2-year-old boy diagnosed with coeliac disease who you see at a birthday party. His abdomen is protuberant, yet his arms and legs seem thin and wasted. He refuses to eat a piece of birthday cake even though his mother sits beside him insisting on it. "See the problem I have with him?" she asks you. "He eats nothing. When he does, he gets diarrhoea."

CASE STUDY QUESTIONS

1. Does Jacob's mother understand her son's disease?
2. Is she choosing wise food selections for him?

The gastrointestinal (GI) system involves a long body tract and numerous organs (see Fig. 45.1). A multitude of possible disorders can occur, including both congenital disorders and acquired illnesses. The GI system is responsible for taking in and processing nutrients for all parts of the body. Any problem can quickly affect other body systems and, if not adequately treated, can affect overall health, growth and development.

Health education is extremely important for children and their families with GI disorders as it can be difficult to appreciate the seriousness of GI illness. Often parents are surprised to find that what they thought was a simple illness has caused serious electrolyte imbalances and possibly a life-threatening state for their child. Some GI disorders require both parents and child to learn new nutritional patterns.

THE CHILD WITH A GASTROINTESTINAL DISORDER

Assessment

Children with GI disorders quickly become dehydrated, especially if vomiting or diarrhoea is a symptom. Complete assessment is needed. This means they need to be assessed for signs of fluid loss, such as poor skin turgor, dry mucous membranes or lack of tears. Urine output needs to be considered, including the number of wet nappies in an infant. Compare the child's current weight with past weight measurements, if available.

Ask parents to describe what they mean by diarrhoea as some parents mistakenly confuse normal newborn or infant stools with diarrhoea. As a rule, all children with diarrhoea, especially small children, need to be seen by a healthcare provider because fluid and electrolyte changes occur rapidly in children.

Nursing considerations

Nursing considerations relevant to children with GI disorders invariably centre on imbalanced nutrition. Most GI diseases alter the kind and amount of nutrients ingested or absorbed into the body in some way. Feeding is one of the primary ways mothers bond with their newborns, so bonding can be seriously threatened when a newborn develops a GI disorder, especially when hospitalisation is required. The process of eating and the types of food eaten are also integral components of family life and

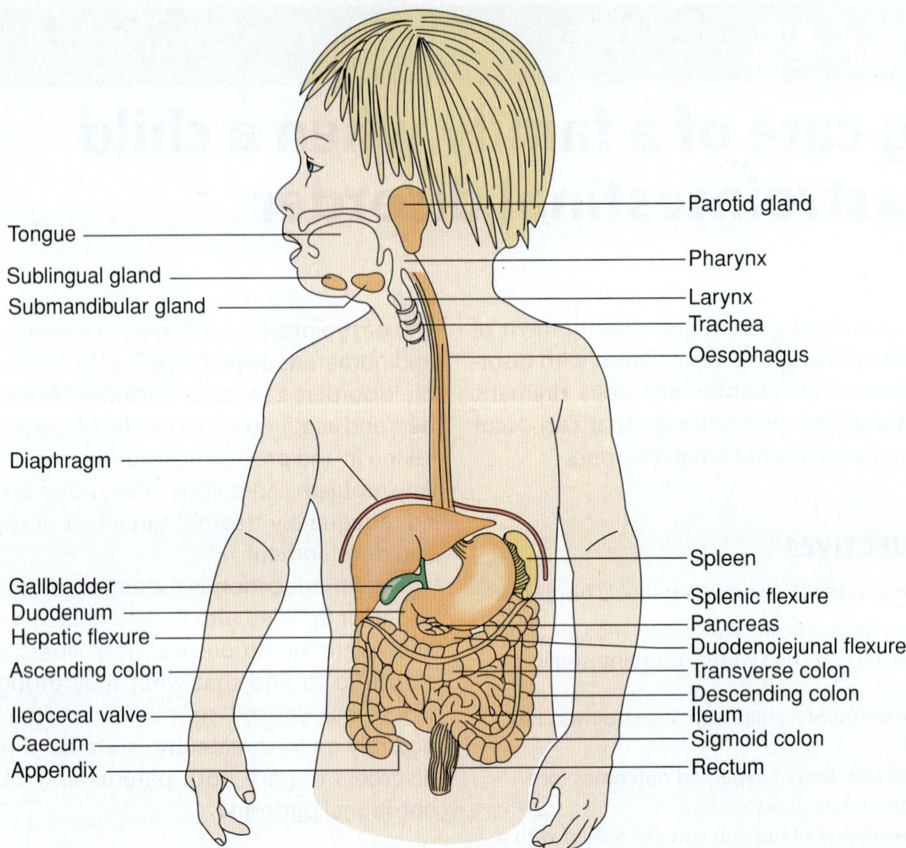

FIGURE 45.1 The gastrointestinal tract.

culture, so any disruption caused by illness can place a strain on the entire family.

Examples of nursing considerations are:

- Interference with establishing parent–infant bond
- Family processes related to chronic illness in child
- Deficient fluid volume related to chronic diarrhoea
- Imbalanced nutrition, related to malabsorption of necessary nutrients
- Low self-esteem related to feelings of being different resulting from special dietary restrictions.

Parents need to be educated with regard to specialised dietary requirements for a child with a GI illness. When a special diet is requested a referral to a dietician is important. If feeding by nasogastric or gastrostomy tube, parents need to be comfortable with the equipment and the technique before they are expected to do it at home. If the parents are not able to replace the feeding tube, if needed, a plan for care should be in place for the child.

Anticipate the need for additional support for the family and child with a chronic GI disorder. Organisations that may be helpful for referral include:

- NSW Health <www.health.nsw.gov.au>
- Coeliac Australia <www.coeliac.org.au>
- Coeliac New Zealand <www.coeliac.org.nz>
- Crohn's and Colitis Australia <www.crohnsandcolitis.com.au>
- Crohn's and Colitis New Zealand <http://crohnsandcolitis.org.nz>.

Parents need appropriate support to adapt their life to alternative methods of feeding and caring for a child with a GI disorder. Recording children's height and weight is a primary method to evaluate nutritional outcomes. Even if a diet is limited in a special way, if it is adequate, children should gain weight and maintain growth.

Children will ultimately be responsible for their own nutrition; expected outcomes should include making certain that children gradually learn more about their specific nutritional measures so they can become responsible for their own intake. Often, only when they are at this stage can their parents feel secure. Children who require special nutritional plans need to be evaluated for self-esteem at periodic health visits. This is done to provide support to maintain self-esteem and may enable problems or issues to be recognised and discussed.

Diagnostic and therapeutic techniques

Several typical procedures are used in the diagnosis and treatment of GI disorders. Common diagnostic procedures include fibre-optic endoscopy, colonoscopy and barium enema. Therapy may include alternative methods of feeding such as enteral (nasogastric or gastrostomy tube feeding) or nutrition sources such as total parenteral nutrition and intravenous (IV) therapy to rest the GI tract. A colostomy or ileostomy may be created to further rest the GI tract. As these are used for other disorders as well, these procedures, their meaning, their impact on children and nursing responsibilities are discussed in Chapters 37 and 38.

HEALTH PROMOTION

Health promotion relating to GI disorders focuses on a wide area. Some disorders, such as appendicitis, cannot be prevented because they occur for unpredictable reasons. **Coeliac disease** (sensitivity or abnormal immunological response to protein) involves genetic aspects that cannot be changed. Crohn's disease and ulcerative colitis are associated with an autoimmune response. Other conditions, such as vomiting and diarrhoea, can be viral and due to poor hygiene or food preparation. A vaccine to prevent rotavirus infections is recommended for infants (Soares-Weiser et al., 2009). Hepatitis A can be prevented by good hand-washing and immunisations are available for hepatitis A and B. Vitamin and protein deficiency disorders can be prevented by educating about good food choices.

Since any interference with nutrition pervades many aspects of children's lives, families often need help with planning care. Planning for necessary adaptations to their lifestyle will minimise the impact of the disease on family functioning. For the family with a child who has a feeding problem such as gastrostomy feeding or total parenteral nutrition, this can be difficult. Families should try to have meals together to help with unity. Urge such families to bring the child to the table for a social time even if the child cannot eat with the family. Educating parents about normal nutrition and how to distinguish things such as vomiting from illness or severe diarrhoea from a simple GI upset helps parents bring their children for care at the earliest possible time. Early intervention prevents the child from becoming dehydrated and seriously ill.

FLUID, ELECTROLYTE AND ACID–BASE IMBALANCES

The GI system plays a major role in maintaining fluid, electrolyte and acid–base balance. It is the main route by which substances are taken into the body and can be a major source of loss if vomiting or diarrhoea occurs (Smith, 2011).

Fluid balance

Retaining fluid is of greater importance in the body chemistry of infants than adults because fluid constitutes a greater proportion of the infant's total weight. In adults, body water accounts for approximately 60% of total weight. In infants, it accounts for as much as 75% to 80% of total weight; in children, it averages approximately 65% to 70%.

Fluid is normally obtained by the body through oral ingestion of fluid and by the water formed in the metabolic breakdown of food. Primarily, fluid is lost from the body in urine and faeces. Minor losses, *insensible losses*, occur from evaporation from skin and lungs and from saliva. Infants do not concentrate urine as well as adults because their kidneys are immature. As a result, they have a proportionally greater loss of fluid in their urine. In infants, the relatively greater surface area to body mass also causes a greater insensible loss. Fluid intake is altered when a child is nauseated and unable to ingest fluid or is vomiting and losing fluid ingested. When diarrhoea occurs or when a child becomes diaphoretic because of fever, the fluid output can be markedly increased. **Dehydration** occurs when there is an excessive loss of body water (Porth, 2011).

Seven kg infants have an ECF (extracellular fluid) volume of only 1750 mL. They ingest approximately 700 mL daily and excrete approximately 700 mL daily. Therefore, they exchange approximately 40% of their volume daily. As a result of this increased exchange rate, infants' fluid balance may be more critically affected when they are ill. Adults, when they do not eat for a day because of a GI upset and whose kidneys continue to excrete at the normal rate, will have 14% less fluid in the extracellular space by the end of the day. Infants who do not eat for a day (providing kidney function remains constant) will be 40% short of ECF by the end of the day. This is obviously a more important loss of fluid than the same loss would be in an adult; therefore, dehydration is always a more serious problem in infants than in older children and adults. Requirements of fluid for infants and children are shown in Table 45.1.

Fluid imbalances

Under most circumstances, water and salt are lost in proportion to each other (*isotonic dehydration*). Occasionally, water is lost out of proportion to salt or water depletion and so *hypertonic dehydration* occurs. Occasionally, electrolytes are lost out of proportion to water (*hypotonic dehydration*). Each of these abnormal states produces specific symptoms.

Isotonic dehydration

When a child's body loses more water than it absorbs (as with diarrhoea) or absorbs less fluid than it excretes (as with nausea and vomiting), the first result will be a decrease in the volume of blood plasma. The body compensates for this

TABLE 45.1 A method to calculate fluid requirement

Body weight	Fluid requirement per 24 hours
Up to 10 kg	100 mL/kg
11–20 kg	1000 mL + 50 mL/kg for each additional kg over 10 kg
More than 20 kg	1500 mL + 20 mL/kg for each additional kg over 20 kg

TABLE 45.2 Signs and symptoms of dehydration

	Isotonic	Hypotonic	Hypertonic
Thirst	Mild	Moderate	Extreme
Skin turgor	Poor	Very poor	Moderate
Skin consistency	Dry	Clammy	Moderate
Skin temperature	Cool	Cool	Warm
Urine output	Decreased	Decreased	Decreased
Activity	Irritable	Lethargic	Very lethargic
Serum sodium level	Normal	Reduced	Increased

rapidly by shifting interstitial fluid into the blood vessels. However, this replacement phenomenon can proceed only until the interstitial fluid reserve is depleted—a danger point for a child because it is difficult for the body to replace interstitial fluid from the intracellular fluid (the fluids in these two compartments have different electrolyte contents). If an infant continues to lose fluid after this point, the volume of the plasma will continue to fall rapidly, resulting ultimately in cardiovascular collapse. Typical signs and symptoms of isotonic dehydration are summarised in Table 45.2.

Hypertonic dehydration

Water is lost in a greater proportion than electrolytes when fluid intake decreases, as might occur in a child with: nausea and fever (increased fluid loss through perspiration); profuse diarrhoea; or renal disease associated with polyuria such as nephrosis with diuresis. In these instances, fluid loss is out of proportion to the loss of electrolytes and increases electrolyte concentration in the blood. Fluid shifts from the interstitial and intracellular spaces into the bloodstream (from areas of less osmotic pressure to areas of greater pressure). Dehydration occurs in the interstitial and intracellular compartments. The red blood cell count and haematocrit will be elevated because the blood is more concentrated than usual. Levels of electrolytes such as sodium, chloride and bicarbonate are also likely to be increased. Additional signs and symptoms are summarised in Table 45.2.

Hypotonic dehydration

With hypotonic dehydration, there is a disproportionately high loss of electrolytes relative to fluid lost. The plasma concentration of sodium and chloride will be low. This could result from excessive loss of electrolytes by vomiting or from low intake of salt associated with extreme losses through diuresis. It also occurs when there is extreme loss of electrolytes in diseases such as adrenocortical insufficiency or diabetic acidosis. When low levels of electrolytes occur, the osmotic pressure in extracellular spaces decreases. The kidneys begin to excrete more fluid to decrease ECF volume and bring the proportion of electrolytes and fluid back into line. This may lead to a secondary extracellular dehydration.

Overhydration

Overhydration may be as serious as dehydration. It generally occurs in children who are receiving IV fluid. The excess fluid in these instances is usually extracellular. The condition is serious because the ECF overload can lead to cardiovascular overload and cardiac failure.

When large quantities of salt-poor fluid (hypotonic solutions) such as tap-water are ingested, the body transfers water from the extracellular space into the intracellular space to restore normal osmotic relationships. This transfer results in intracellular oedema manifested by headache, nausea, vomiting, dimness and blurring of vision, cramps, muscle twitching and seizures.

Acid–base imbalance

The GI system often is involved with two severe acid–base imbalances: metabolic acidosis and metabolic alkalosis. These imbalances occur with severe diarrhoea or vomiting.

Metabolic acidosis

Metabolic acidosis may result from diarrhoea. When diarrhoea occurs, a great deal of sodium is lost with stool.

Metabolic alkalosis

With vomiting, a great deal of hydrochloric acid is lost. When alkalosis occurs from vomiting, a secondary electrolyte problem often occurs. Low K^1 levels (hypokalaemia) invariably accompany metabolic alkalosis.

CASE STUDY QUESTION

3. Jacob has frequent bouts of vomiting. What secondary electrolyte problem often occurs when metabolic alkalosis results from vomiting?
   a. Acidosis
   b. Hyponatraemia
   c. Hypokalaemia
   d. Hyperchlorosis

COMMON GASTROINTESTINAL SYMPTOMS OF ILLNESS IN CHILDREN

Vomiting and diarrhoea in children commonly occur as symptoms of disease of the GI tract as well as symptoms of disease in other body systems. Pneumonia or otitis media, for example, may present first with vomiting or diarrhoea. The danger is that either can lead to a disturbance in hydration, electrolyte or acid-base balance. In many infants, these secondary disturbances can be more threatening to the child than the primary disease.

Vomiting

Many children with vomiting are suffering from a mild gastroenteritis (infection) caused by a viral or bacterial organism.

Some children develop persistent or cyclic vomiting (Fitzpatrick et al., 2007). Vomiting is always potentially serious because a metabolic alkalosis and dehydration may result.

It is important that vomiting be described correctly because different conditions are marked by different forms of vomiting and a correct description can aid greatly in diagnosis. The treatment for vomiting is to withhold food from the stomach; if there is nothing in the stomach, vomiting cannot occur. Most parents treat vomiting in the opposite way. Every time a child vomits, they attempt to feed the child again. This prolongs the vomiting and intensifies the potential for electrolyte imbalance.

Nursing considerations

Deficient fluid volume related to vomiting

Skin turgor remains good; specific gravity of urine is 1.003 to 1.030; urine output is more than 1 mL/kg/hr; episodes of vomiting decrease in frequency and amount.

To decrease vomiting, withhold food and fluid for a time, depending on the age of the child. On average, a period of 3 to 6 hours is usually sufficient. In the older child, after this period of fasting, offer a few ice chips, then water or oral rehydration solution (ORS) in small amounts. Suitable volumes should be offered; 0.5 mL/kg every 5 minutes.

Children may become hungry and/or thirsty and want whole glasses of fluid, but keeping the quantity to small sips prevents vomiting. Children can take an age-appropriate diet as soon as vomiting settles. For the infant, introduce fluid after a fasting period of approximately 3 hours in the same slow manner.

A commercial ORS such as Gastrolyte or Hydralyte may be given as fluid during this time to help the infant maintain electrolyte balance. Infants who are breastfed should receive small frequent breastfeeds to ensure normal urine output. If vomiting is prolonged, infants may need IV therapy to restore hydration (Leung & Robson, 2007).

Teach parents the importance of following these routines of gradually increasing fluid at intervals.

TABLE 45.3 Differentiation between infant normal stool and diarrhoeal stool

Characteristic	Infant normal stool	Diarrhoeal stool
Frequency	1–3 daily	Unlimited number
Colour	Yellow	Green
Effort of expulsion	Some pushing effort	Effortless; may be explosive
pH	More than 7.0 (alkaline)	Less than 7.0 (acidic)
Odour	Odourless	Sweet or foul smelling
Occult blood	Negative	Positive; blood may be overt
Reducing substances	Negative	Positive

Diarrhoea

Diarrhoea caused by a virus is the major cause of infant gastroenteritis in developing countries. The most common viral pathogens that invade the GI tract include rotaviruses and adenoviruses (Rabin, 2011). The most common bacterial pathogens include *Campylobacter jejuni, Salmonella, Clostridium difficile and Escherichia coli (Porth, 2011).* Both viral and bacterial infections are easily spread in common nappy-changing areas in day-care centres or public areas (Rimon & Freedman, 2010). Diarrhoea that is acute is usually associated with infection; chronic diarrhoea is more likely to be related to a malabsorption or inflammatory cause.

Mild diarrhoea

Normal and diarrhoeal stool characteristics are compared in Table 45.3. If diarrhoea is mild, fever of 38.5° to 39.0°C may be present. Children usually are anorectic and irritable and appear unwell. The episodes of diarrhoea consist of 2 to 10 loose, watery bowel movements per day.

The mucous membrane of the mouth appears dry and the skin feels warm although skin turgor will not yet be decreased. The pulse will be rapid and out of proportion to the low-grade fever. Urine output is usually normal.

At this stage, diarrhoea is not yet serious and children can be cared for at home. As with vomiting, treatment for diarrhoea must involve resting the GI tract, but this is necessary for only a short time. At the end of approximately 1 hour, parents can begin to offer an ORS such as Gastrolyte or Hydralyte in small amounts on a regimen similar to that for vomiting (Smith, 2011). For breastfed infants, breastfeeding should continue. Children also need measures to reduce the elevated temperature. Zinc and probiotics (dietary supplements containing potentially beneficial bacteria or yeasts) to change the bacterial flora of the intestine may be administered (McFarland, 2010), when the normal diet of the child has been reintroduced.

Caution parents to contact their healthcare provider rather than use over-the-counter medications such as antimotility or anti-diarrhoeal to halt diarrhoea because, as a rule, these are too strong for young children (McKenna & Mirkov, 2014). Also caution parents to wash their hands after changing nappies to prevent the spread of infection to themselves and to notify their healthcare provider if fever, pain or diarrhoea worsens.

Severe diarrhoea

Severe diarrhoea may result from progressive mild diarrhoea or it may begin in a severe form. Infants with severe diarrhoea are obviously ill. Rectal temperature is often as high as 39.5° to 40.0°C. Both pulse and respirations are weak and rapid. The skin is pale and cool. Infants may appear apprehensive, listless and lethargic. They have obvious signs of dehydration such as a depressed fontanelle, sunken eyes and poor skin turgor. The episodes of diarrhoea usually consist of a bowel movement every few minutes. The stool is liquid green, perhaps mixed with mucus and blood, and it may be passed with explosive force. Urine output will be scanty and concentrated.

It is difficult to measure the amount of fluid a child has lost, but an estimate can be made from the loss in body weight, if known. Mild dehydration occurs with a loss of 2.5–5% of body weight. In contrast, severe diarrhoea quickly causes a 5–5% loss. Any infant who has lost 10% or more of body weight requires immediate treatment.

Treatment focuses on regulating electrolyte and fluid balance by oral or IV rehydration therapy, initiating rest for the GI tract and discovering the organism responsible for the diarrhoea.

All children with severe diarrhoea or diarrhoea that persists longer than 24 hours should have a stool culture taken so definite antibiotic therapy can be prescribed. Stool cultures may be taken from the rectum or from stool in a nappy or a bedpan. Blood pathology needs to be done, including FBC, EUC and BGL. If a child can drink, the most effective way to replace fluid is by offering oral rehydration therapy. For a child who will not drink, administer an IV solution such as 0.9% normal saline +2.5% glucose or 0.45% normal saline +2.5% glucose. The solution will provide replacement of fluid, sodium and kilojoules. Although infants usually have a potassium depletion, potassium cannot be given until it is established that they are not in renal failure. Giving potassium IV when the body has no outlet for excessive potassium can lead to excessively high potassium levels and heart block. Before this initial IV fluid is changed to a potassium solution, therefore, be certain that the infant or child has voided—proof that the kidneys are functioning. Do not give electrolyte replacement until review of pathology.

Fluid must be given to replace the deficit that has occurred, for maintenance therapy and to replace the continuing loss until the diarrhoea improves. If infants have lost less than 5% of total body weight, their fluid deficit is approximately 50 mL/kg of body weight. If infants have lost 10% of body weight, they need approximately 100 mL/kg of body weight to replace their fluid deficit. If the weight loss suggests a 12–15% loss of body fluid, they require 125 mL/kg of body weight to replace the fluid lost.

Nursing considerations

Deficient fluid volume related to loss of fluid through diarrhoea

Skin turgor remains good; specific gravity of urine is 1.003 to 1.030; urine output is more than 1 mL/kg/hr; bowel movements are formed and fewer than four per day. Stool tests negative for reducing substances and blood pH is more than 7.

During the time infants are nil by mouth (NBM), maintain oral hygiene. Offer them a dummy to suck if this seems to comfort them. (They want to suck because they are very thirsty and, if they have intestinal cramping with the diarrhoea, they interpret this as hunger.)

As the infant's condition improves, oral intake can be increased, changing to a soft then a regular diet. If the child with severe diarrhoea also has a fever, measures to reduce the fever will be necessary. Do not obtain rectal temperatures to assess fever, because stimulating the anal sphincter could initiate more diarrhoea. Assess perianal skin for irritation from liquid stools and keep the skin clean and dry.

Much of the nursing care of children with diarrhoea focuses on careful recording of fluid intake and output. As children may have dehydration when first seen, oral rehydration or IV therapy are important.

In children who are not toilet-trained, apply a disposable urine collection bag to help separate urine from faeces. This makes it obvious that the child is voiding, confirming kidney function.

Separating urine from stools also helps to judge the appearance of stools or their water content. For each stool passed, record its colour, consistency, odour, size and the presence of any blood or mucus. Weigh soiled nappies to reveal the number of grams of stool in the nappy. Testing the stool for acidity and for reducing substances (sugars) indicates how quickly the stool has passed through the irritated tract. (Diarrhoeal stools are green from lack of time for bile to be modified in the intestine.) As diarrhoea improves and stool remains in the intestine for a longer period, the stool deepens in colour and the acid and sugar contents fade. Testing stools for occult blood shows the extent of bowel irritation that is occurring from the acid stool. As the diarrhoea improves and the irritation to the bowel lessens, the finding of occult blood disappears.

Impaired skin integrity related to presence of diarrhoeal stool on skin

Because diarrhoeal stool is extremely irritating to the skin, change nappies immediately after infants pass any stool. Wash the skin of the nappy area well after each stool and use an ointment if required to protect it from further irritation.

> ***What if...***
>
> Jacob's mother tells you her doctor has told her to "force fluids" for Jacob whenever he has diarrhoea? She asks how much she should force the child to drink. How would you answer her?

Bacterial infectious diseases that cause diarrhoea and vomiting

Several common microorganisms are responsible for diarrhoea in children.

Salmonella

- Causative agent: One of the *Salmonella* bacteria
- Incubation period: 6–72 hours for intraluminal type; 7–14 days for extraluminal type

- Period of communicability: As long as organisms are being excreted (may be as long as 3 months)
- Mode of transmission: Ingestion of contaminated food, especially chicken and raw eggs

Salmonella is the most common type of food poisoning and a major cause of diarrhoea in children. The diagnosis of the infection can be made from stool culture. Children develop diarrhoea, abdominal pain, vomiting, high temperature and headache. They are listless and drowsy. The diarrhoea is severe and may contain blood and mucus (Chambers, 2009). *Salmonella* infection may remain in the bowel as an intraluminal disease. When it does, it is treated, like severe diarrhoea, with fluid and electrolyte replacement. Antibiotics are rarely prescribed as they may actually prolong the length of the infection (Sirinavin & Garner, 2009). If the infection becomes systemic (extraluminal disease), it is treated with the addition of an antibiotic such as ampicillin or a third-generation cephalosporin (Ogle & Anderson, 2008).

Complications such as meningitis, bronchitis and osteomyelitis may occur. Because the source of *Salmonella* generally is infected food (contaminated chicken and eggs are common sources), caution parents to carefully wash utensils used to prepare raw chicken (such as cutting boards) and to cook eggs thoroughly.

Listeriosis

- Causative agent: *Listeria monocytogenes*
- Incubation period: Variable, ranging from 1 day to more than 3 weeks
- Mode of transmission: Ingestion of unpasteurised milk or cheeses or vegetables grown in contaminated soil

Listeriosis is a serious infection caused by eating food contaminated with the gram-positive bacterium *Listeria monocytogenes*. The cause of the infection may be difficult to locate as the incubation period can last for almost a month. After this time, however, a child develops fever, muscle aches, nausea and diarrhoea. If infection spreads to the nervous system, symptoms such as headache, stiff neck, confusion, loss of balance or convulsions can occur. The infection is particularly important to avoid during pregnancy as infections can lead to miscarriage or stillbirth, prematurity or infection of the newborn. The bacteria is found in soil and water. The most frequent source, however, is unpasteurised milk or foods made from unpasteurised milk such as soft cheese.

Shigellosis (dysentery)

- Causative agent: Organisms of the genus *Shigella*
- Incubation period: 1–7 days
- Period of communicability: Approximately 1–4 weeks
- Mode of transmission: Contaminated food, water or milk products

Shigella organisms, like the *Salmonella* group, cause extremely severe diarrhoea that contains blood and mucus. The child needs intense fluid and electrolyte replacement. *Shigella* infection can be prevented by safe food-handling and drinking only from safe water sources (Ogle & Anderson, 2008).

Staphylococcal food poisoning

- Causative agent: Staphylococcal enterotoxin produced by some strains of *Staphylococcus aureus*
- Incubation period: 1–7 hours
- Period of communicability: Carriers may contaminate food as long as they harbour the organism
- Mode of transmission: Ingestion of contaminated food

With staphylococcal food poisoning, a child has severe vomiting and diarrhoea, abdominal cramping, excessive salivation and nausea within 2 to 6 hours of eating (Ogle & Anderson, 2008). It is often difficult to culture the causative organism from the contaminated food because although the staphylococci may have been destroyed by cooking, the enterotoxin that actually causes the disorder will not have been destroyed. The child needs intensive supportive therapy with fluid and electrolyte replacement with possible use of antibiotics. Food poisoning from this source can be prevented by proper refrigeration of food.

CASE STUDY QUESTION

4. Jacob's mother tells you she often makes milkshakes with raw eggs. What infectious organism is easily spread this way?

a. Pneumococcus
b. Salmonella
c. Streptococcus A
d. *H. pylori*

COMMON DISORDERS OF THE STOMACH AND DUODENUM

Disorders of the upper GI tract in children tend to involve inadequate valve function or infection.

Gastro-oesophageal reflux

Gastrointestinal reflux or the regurgitation of stomach secretions into the oesophagus through the gastro-oesophageal (cardiac) valve occurs mainly in infants and adolescents.

Gastro-oesophageal reflux in infants

Gastro-oesophageal reflux in infants occurs from a neuromuscular disturbance in which the gastro-oesophageal (cardiac) sphincter and the lower portion of the oesophagus spasm and allow easy regurgitation of gastric contents into the oesophagus. It usually starts within 1 week after birth and may be associated with a hiatal hernia. Children with cerebral palsy or other neurological involvement are at particular risk. The regurgitation occurs almost immediately after feeding or when the infant is laid down after feeding. If the amount of the reflux is large or constant, an infant does not retain sufficient kilojoules and will fail to thrive. In addition, aspiration pneumonia or oesophageal stricture from the constant reflux of hydrochloric acid into the oesophagus can occur (Sundaram et al., 2011).

Assessment

The diagnosis is suggested by the history. Vomiting appears effortless and is not projectile; it begins much earlier in life than the vomiting associated with pyloric stenosis. The child may be irritable and may experience periods of apnoea. Fibre optic endoscopy or oesophagography (barium swallow) will further show the involved sphincter and the reflux of stomach contents into the oesophagus, especially if the infant's head is tilted downwards.

Therapeutic management

The traditional treatment of GI reflux is to feed infants a formula thickened with rice cereal while holding them in an upright position and then keeping them upright in an infant chair for 1 hour after feeding so gravity can help prevent reflux (Craig et al., 2009). An H_2 receptor antagonist such as ranitidine or a proton pump inhibitor such as omeprazole may be prescribed daily to reduce the possibility of the stomach acid contents irritating the oesophagus.

Gastro-oesophageal reflux is usually a self-limiting condition. As the oesophageal sphincter matures and the child begins to eat solid food and is maintained in a more upright position, the problem disappears. If not, botulinum toxin may be injected into the lower oesophageal sphincter to temporarily relieve symptoms of obstruction. If medical therapy this way is ineffective, a laparoscopic or surgical myotomy procedure (narrowing of the oesophageal sphincter) may be performed.

When infants are first fed after surgery, they may display signs of abdominal discomfort and distension because food can no longer reflux into the oesophagus as readily as it could before surgery. As their stomach adjusts to this, symptoms fade.

Nutritional issues related to oesophageal reflux

Teach parents the importance of monitoring intake, output (urination) and weight. Also reinforce the need to keep the infant upright, such as in an infant seat, after feeding. Be certain parents understand how much cereal to mix with formula or breast milk.

Gastrointestinal reflux in adolescents—gastro-oesophageal reflux disease (GORD)

Irritation to the oesophagus occurs when stomach contents, including hydrochloric acid, reflux through the lower oesophageal sphincter and irritate the oesophageal lining. Reflux occurs because of an incompetent sphincter especially when the adolescent lies supine or when intra-abdominal pressure is increased by a full stomach, lifting or bending, or tight clothing. It is potentially dangerous because it can lead to erosion of the oesophagus with perforation or stricture of the oesophagus. It may be associated with the development of oesophageal cancer in later life (Wang & Souza, 2011).

The typical symptom is heartburn that occurs 30–60 minutes after a meal. Diagnosis is based on history (typical symptoms of heartburn) and, if symptoms are severe, endoscopy to reveal the irritated oesophagus (oesophagitis). The goal of treatment is to provide symptomatic relief and to heal any oesophagitis.

Adolescents should avoid lying down until 3 hours after a meal and should sleep at night with their upper body elevated on a foam wedge. They should avoid acidic foods such as tomato products, citrus fruits or spicy foods. Avoiding foods that delay gastric emptying such as fatty foods, chocolate or alcohol and eating smaller portions may also be helpful. Antacids relieve pain immediately by decreasing the concentration of the stomach acid and are sold over the counter. H_2-receptor antagonists such as famotidine or ranitidine are also available over the counter and can be taken before meals to prevent heartburn symptoms. Proton pump inhibitors such as omeprazole or rabeprazole medications that halt the release of stomach acids, are prescription medications that offer the best long-term relief. Adolescents generally take these for 6 to 8 months until oesophageal healing is complete.

Pyloric stenosis

The pyloric sphincter is the opening between the lower portion of the stomach and the beginning portion of the intestine, the duodenum. If hypertrophy or hyperplasia of the muscle surrounding the sphincter occurs, it is difficult for the stomach to empty, a condition called *pyloric stenosis* (see Fig. 45.2). With this condition, at 4 to 6 weeks of age, infants begin to vomit almost immediately after each feeding. The vomiting grows increasingly forceful until it is projectile. The exact cause is unknown.

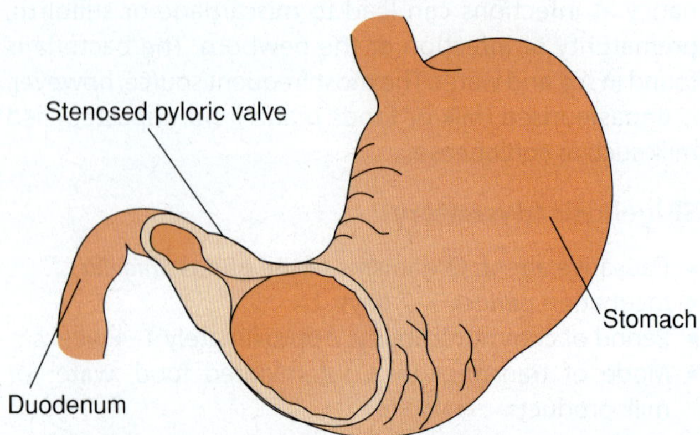

FIGURE 45.2 Pyloric stenosis. Fluid is unable to pass easily through the stenosed and hypertrophied pyloric valve.

Vomitus usually smells sour because it has reached the stomach and has been in contact with stomach enzymes. There is never bile in the vomiting of pyloric stenosis because the feeding does not reach the duodenum to become mixed with bile. Infants are usually hungry immediately after vomiting because they are not nauseated. Although it is difficult to assess whether nausea is present in infants, signs such as a disinterest in eating, excessive drooling or chewing on the tongue may suggest this.

The diagnosis of pyloric stenosis is made primarily from the history. Whenever parents say that their baby is vomiting or spitting up, be certain to get a full description:

- Duration? *Begins at 6 weeks of age*
- Intensity? *Projectile vomiting*
- Frequency? *Immediately after eating*
- Description of the vomitus? *Sour but contains no bile*
- Is the infant ill in any other way? *No.*

Many infants have signs of dehydration from the vomiting when they are first seen. Lack of tears (many infants younger than age 6 weeks do not tear), dry mucous membrane of the mouth, sunken fontanelles, fever, decreased urine output, poor skin turgor and weight loss are common signs. A definitive diagnosis is made by watching the infant drink. Before the child drinks, attempt to palpate the right upper quadrant of the abdomen for a pyloric mass. If one is present, it feels round and firm, approximately the size of an olive. As the infant drinks, observe for gastric peristaltic waves passing from left to right across the abdomen. The olive-size lump becomes more prominent. The infant vomits with projectile emesis. If the diagnosis is still in doubt, an ultrasound will show the hypertrophied sphincter (Oldham & Aiken, 2007). Endoscopy also may be used for diagnosis by directly visualising the hypertrophied sphincter.

Treatment is surgical or laparoscopic correction (a pyloromyotomy), performed before electrolyte imbalance from the vomiting or hypoglycaemia from the lack of food occurs. For surgical correction, the muscle of the pylorus is split down to the mucosa, allowing for a larger lumen. Although the procedure sounds simple, it is technically difficult to perform and there is a high risk for infection afterwards because the abdominal incision is near the nappy area. The prognosis for infants with pyloric stenosis is excellent if the condition is discovered before an electrolyte imbalance occurs.

Nursing considerations

Deficient fluid volume related to inability to retain food

Skin turgor remains good; specific gravity of urine is 1.003 to 1.030; vomiting episodes have ceased; weight is within acceptable age-appropriate parameters.

Preoperative care. Preoperative management consists of fluid and electrolyte replacement based on laboratory determinations. A baseline weight is essential for establishing the extent of dehydration.

Postoperative care. The postoperative feeding regimen differs from one surgeon to another but usually involves frequent feeding of small amounts of fluid. Approximately 4–6 hours after surgery, infants are started on a small amount of an oral rehydrating solution by bottle. If no vomiting occurs, the amount is increased. By 24–48 hours, infants are taking their full formula diet or being fully breastfed. They are usually discharged from hospital at the end of 48 hours.

Postoperatively, it is important that infants be given no more than the amount of fluid ordered at a time so the surgical repair site is not overwhelmed. Infants need to ingest these small amounts because a small quantity of fluid passing through the sphincter in the immediate postoperative days helps to keep adhesions of the sphincter from forming. Infants should be burped well after feeding so there is no pressure from air in the stomach. Lay them on their side after feeding so that if vomiting does occur, there is little chance of aspiration. Laying them on their right side may aid the flow of fluid through the pyloric valve by gravity. Continue to monitor daily weights to confirm that the child is receiving adequate intake. Usually no vomiting occurs postoperatively, but if it does occur, report it immediately. Some infants have short-term diarrhoea (dumping syndrome) after surgery because of rapid functioning of the pyloric sphincter, but this tends to resolve without additional therapy.

As with any surgical intervention, pain assessment and monitoring in regards to analgesic requirements needs to be appropriate for the individual child's needs and within facilities' policies.

Infection at site of surgical incision because of proximity to nappy area

Infant's temperature is below (37.0°C) axillary; incision is clean, dry and intact, without erythema or drainage. The surgical incision for pyloric stenosis may be covered with a dry dressing, to help keep urine and faeces from touching it. Change nappies frequently. If the incision should be exposed to faeces, clean wound as appropriate.

Hiatal hernia

Hiatal hernia is the intermittent protrusion of the stomach up through the oesophageal opening in the diaphragm. When this occurs, the volume of the stomach is suddenly restricted, leading to periodic vomiting similar to that of gastro-oesophageal reflux. With a hiatal hernia, however, pain usually accompanies the vomiting.

Hiatal hernia is diagnosed by history and an ultrasound or barium swallow. Keeping a baby in an upright position helps prevent the condition from recurring. Medication to reduce acid secretions may also be helpful. If the condition has not corrected itself by the time the infant is 6 months old, even with maintaining an upright position most of the day, laparoscopic surgery may be performed to reduce the stomach's ability to protrude through the diaphragm.

Peptic ulcer disease

A *peptic ulcer* is a shallow excavation formed in the mucosal wall of the stomach, the pylorus or the duodenum. In infants, ulcers tend to be gastric; in adolescents, they are usually duodenal.

The small ulceration of the gastric or duodenal lining leads to pain, blood in the stool and vomiting (with blood). If left uncorrected, peptic ulcer disease can lead to bowel or stomach perforation with acute haemorrhage or pyloric obstruction (Hua et al., 2007). A chronic ulcer condition may lead to anaemia from the constant, gradual blood loss.

Assessment

An ulcer occurring in a neonate usually presents with haematemesis (blood in vomitus) or melaena (blood in the stool). Such ulcers are usually superficial and heal rapidly.

If an ulcer occurs in a toddler, the first symptoms are usually anorexia or vomiting. Bleeding follows in several weeks. If an ulcer begins when children are of preschool or early school-age, pain may be the presenting symptom.

In older, school-aged children and adolescents, symptoms are generally a gnawing or aching pain in the epigastric area before meals that is relieved by eating. Vomiting (because of spasm and oedema of the pylorus) occurs in a small number of children. On abdominal palpation, epigastric tenderness is noted.

Endoscopy is the most reliable diagnostic test to confirm the diagnosis of peptic ulcer disease; it allows for visual inspection and cultures for *H. pylori*. Children with this condition must have blood tests done periodically to be monitored for blood-loss anaemia.

Nursing considerations

Pain related to ulceration in intestinal tract

Children with peptic ulcer disease should be able to eat a normal diet, avoiding heavily spiced food if such food causes discomfort. Be certain that the outcomes planned are realistic. It may not be possible to relieve symptoms of peptic ulcer immediately. Children can be helped to understand why the pain occurs and what they can do to help relieve it.

CASE STUDY QUESTION

5. Jacob's older sister had pyloric stenosis as an infant. Vomiting with pyloric stenosis typically occurs:
   a. Immediately after feeding
   b. An hour after feeding
   c. On arising in the morning
   d. When the infant cries

HEPATIC DISORDERS

Hepatic disorders include both acquired disorders, such as hepatitis or cirrhosis, and congenital disorders, such as obstruction or atresia of the biliary duct.

Liver function

The liver assists in the catabolism of fatty acids and protein and serves as a temporary storage space for both fat and protein. The liver, by means of the enzyme glucuronosyltransferase, converts indirect (or unconjugated) bilirubin into direct (or conjugated) bilirubin so it can be excreted in bile and eliminated from the body. This is an important function in the newborn and jaundice can result if the level of glucuronosyltransferase is low because of immaturity.

The liver manufactures bile, a secretion necessary for the digestion of fat; fibrinogen and prothrombin, substances essential for blood clotting; heparin, a substance necessary to keep blood from clotting in intact vessels; and blood proteins. It produces large amounts of body heat. It destroys red blood cells and detoxifies many harmful absorbed substances, such as drugs.

Hepatitis

Hepatitis (inflammation and infection of the liver) is caused by invasion by hepatitis A, B, C, D or E virus (Tan & Lok, 2007).

Hepatitis A

- Causative agent: *A picornavirus*, hepatitis A virus (HAV)
- Incubation period: 25 days on average
- Period of communicability: Highest during 2 weeks preceding onset of symptoms
- Mode of transmission: In children, ingestion of faecally contaminated water or shellfish; day-care centre spread from contaminated changing tables
- Immunity: Natural; one episode induces immunity for the specific type of virus
- Active artificial immunity: Vaccine–immunisation as per current guidelines
- Passive artificial immunity: Immune globulin

Hepatitis B

- Causative agent: *A hepadnavirus*; hepatitis B virus (HBV)
- Incubation period: 120 days on average
- Period of communicability: Later part of incubation period and during the acute stage
- Mode of transmission: Transfusion of contaminated blood and plasma or semen
- Immunity: Natural; one episode induces immunity for the specific type of virus
- Active artificial immunity: Vaccine–immunisation as per current guidelines
- Passive artificial immunity: Specific hepatitis B immune serum globulin

Hepatitis C, D and E

Hepatitis A and B are the viruses that are most frequently diagnosed as hepatitis. Hepatitis C, D and E viruses also exist. Hepatitis C (HCV) is a single-strand RNA virus. Transmission, as with HBV, is primarily by blood or blood products, IV drug use or sexual contact. The virus produces mild symptoms of disease, but there is a high incidence of chronic infection.

Hepatitis D (HDV) or the delta form is similar to HBV in transmission, although it apparently requires a coexisting HBV infection to be activated. Disease symptoms are mild, but there is a high incidence of fulminant hepatitis after the initial infection.

The E form of hepatitis is enterically transmitted similarly to hepatitis A. Disease symptoms from the E virus are usually mild.

Assessment

No matter which virus is involved, hepatitis is a generalised body infection with specific intense liver effects. Type A occurs in children of all ages. Hepatitis B tends to occur in newborns from placental-fetal transfer and in adolescents after intimate contact or the use of contaminated syringes.

Clinically, it is impossible to differentiate the type of hepatitis from the signs that are present. All hepatitis viruses cause liver cell destruction, leading to increased serum aspartate amino transaminase (AST), alanine aminotransaminase (ALT) and alkaline phosphatase levels. The type of virus causing the disease can be determined by the recognition of a specific antibody against the virus (anti-HAV IgM, anti-HBV IgM). Symptoms with hepatitis A are generally mild. Children notice headache, fever and anorexia. Jaundice occurs as liver function slows. This lasts for approximately a week and then symptoms fade with full recovery.

Symptoms of hepatitis B are more marked. Children report generalised aching, right upper quadrant pain and headache. They may have a low-grade fever. They feel ill and can be irritable from pruritus (itching). After 3 to 7 days of such symptoms, the colour of the urine becomes darker (brown) because of the excretion of bilirubin. In another 2 days, the sclerae of the eyes become jaundiced; soon a child has generalised jaundice. With the generalised jaundice, there is little excretion of bilirubin into the stool, so the stools become white or grey. This icteric (jaundiced) phase lasts from a few days to 2 weeks. Some children have an anicteric form of infection, in which they develop the beginning symptoms but then never develop the jaundice. They are as infectious, however, as children with overt jaundice. Laboratory studies will show elevations of the liver enzymes: AST and ALT. Levels of bilirubin are increased in the urine. Bile pigments in the stool are decreased. Serum bilirubin levels are increased.

Therapeutic management

Strict hand-washing and infection control precautions are mandatory when caring for children with hepatitis. Faeces must be disposed of carefully because the type A virus can be cultured from faeces. Standard precautions should be used at all times.

The treatment for hepatitis A is increased rest and maintenance of a good kilojoule intake. Children are generally hungrier at breakfast than later in the day, so encourage them to eat a healthy breakfast. Children can be cared for at home. They should not return to school or a day-care centre until 2 weeks after the onset of symptoms.

An antiviral agent may be effective in reducing viral replication with hepatitis B. Interferon may also be prescribed. Of those with type B, 90% will recover completely, but 10% will develop chronic hepatitis and become hepatitis carriers. As hepatitis B is a sexually-transmitted infection, preadolescent children with the infection need to be screened for the possibility of sexual abuse (Lewin, 2007).

Pruritus

Pruritus from jaundice results in extreme discomfort for some children (Cies & Giamalis, 2007). Being certain that a child is not overheated and not perspiring reduces the itching. A cool bath is often comforting. Skin moisturisers or an antihistamine may be prescribed. Cholestyramine is a bile acid sequestrant which binds bile in the GI tract to prevent its reabsorption and so helps prevent pruritus.

Chronic hepatitis

Hepatitis is considered chronic when it persists for longer than 6 months. This is most often the result of hepatitis B, D or C infection. Abnormal liver enzyme levels and a liver biopsy establish the diagnosis and can also predict the severity. With chronic hepatitis, fatty infiltration and bile duct damage can occur. The disease may progress to cirrhosis and eventually liver failure. Therapy is supportive to compensate for decreased liver function (Friedman, 2009).

Fulminant hepatic failure

Fulminant hepatic failure is present when acute, massive necrosis or sudden, severe impairment of liver function occurs, leading to hepatic encephalopathy. Hepatic encephalopathy is the result of ammonia intoxication caused by the inability of the liver to detoxify the ammonia being constantly produced by the intestine in the process of digestion (Cochran & Losek, 2007).

Children may show such symptoms as confusion, drowsiness or disorientation. Treatment involves reducing protein intake and administering lactulose to prevent absorption of ammonia in the colon or administering nonabsorbable antibiotics such as neomycin to decrease the production of ammonia by the intestinal bacteria. Liver transplantation may be necessary. As adults have excess liver tissue, a donor liver may be provided by a living donor. Otherwise, many children cannot survive the long wait for a donor organ.

Obstruction of the bile ducts

Obstruction of the bile ducts in children generally occurs from congenital atresia, stenosis or absence of the duct. It also can occur from the plugging of biliary secretions, though this is rare. When the bile duct is obstructed, bile that is unable to enter the intestinal tract accumulates in the liver. Bile pigments (direct bilirubin) enter the bloodstream and jaundice occurs, increasing in intensity daily.

Although bile duct obstruction is a congenital disorder, the chief sign (jaundice) does not develop until approximately 2 weeks of age. This delay differentiates it clinically from physiological jaundice, which occurs in almost all newborns on the third day of life or the jaundice of Rh or ABO isoimmunisation, which typically occurs during the first 24 hours of life. Physiological jaundice and isoimmunisation jaundice occur from a rise in indirect bilirubin, whereas the jaundice of bile duct obstruction is a result of a rise in direct bilirubin. The infant's stools appear light in colour from lack of bile pigments. The pressure on the liver from the obstruction becomes so acute with time that cell destruction or cirrhosis occurs. Ultimately, without liver transplantation, death from liver failure will result (Kaido et al., 2012).

Pathology and a liver biopsy under local anaesthesia may be obtained to rule out hepatitis. If atresia of the bile duct is the problem, a surgical option (kasai procedure) is the treatment. However, surgical correction is impossible in all infants with atresia because the atresia tends to occur too far back in the liver to be in an operable area. Liver transplantation is needed for children with extensive involvement or in whom a kasai procedure is not successful.

Cirrhosis

Cirrhosis is fibrotic scarring of the liver. Cirrhosis means "yellow" or the typical colour of hepatic scar tissue. It occurs rarely in children, although it may be seen as a result of congenital biliary atresia or as a complication of chronic illnesses such as protracted hepatitis, sickle-cell anaemia or cystic fibrosis.

Oesophageal varices

Oesophageal varices (distended veins) is a frequent complication of liver disorders such as cirrhosis (Hussey, Kelleher & Ling, 2010). Varices may bleed if children cough vigorously or strain to pass stool.

Rupture of oesophageal varices is an emergency because children can lose a large quantity of blood quickly from the engorged vessels. Vasopressin or nitroglycerine may be given IV to lessen hypertension and reduce the haemorrhage. Injection of a sclerosing agent into veins may be attempted to decrease their size. A Sengstaken-Blakemore tube or Linton-Nachlas catheter may be passed into the stomach. Children must be monitored for future bleeding episodes. Frequent vital sign measurements and testing of stool and any vomitus for the presence of blood will indicate new oesophageal bleeding.

LIVER TRANSPLANTATION

Liver transplantation is the surgical replacement of a malfunctioning liver by a donor liver. Donor livers are not readily available, so the waiting time for surgery may be months. Finding an acceptable, child-sized liver may be especially difficult, so adult livers can be reduced in size for transplantation. A lobe of a liver from a living donor is frequently used. Often, the child is extremely ill with ascites, GI bleeding, extreme pruritus, hepatic encephalopathy or renal dysfunction before the surgery can be performed. This makes nursing care after liver transplantation in a child complex.

Despite the severity of illness and the length of surgery, however, children tend to recover quickly after liver transplantation (Mouzaki & Ng, 2010). Both children and parents must have thorough preoperative preparation. Counselling and support groups are also often beneficial.

Preoperative management

Preoperative management consists of keeping the child in the best physical condition possible. For many children, this includes dialysis and severe nutritional restrictions.

Postoperative management

Nursing care after liver transplantation surgery focuses on preventing complications that may arise from the surgery and the continued immunosuppression. Children may need assisted ventilation for approximately 24 hours postoperatively to prevent pulmonary complications such as atelectasis and pneumonia because the large abdominal incision makes coughing and deep breathing difficult. In addition, ascites often places pressure against the diaphragm, interfering with lung expansion. After discontinuation of mechanical ventilation and extubation, chest physiotherapy may be started to mobilise lung secretions.

Pain assessment and analgesia is a priority. Assess all vital signs, capillary refill, peripheral pulses and skin colour frequently to ensure adequate cardiovascular function. Assess neurological status hourly using a modified Glasgow Coma Scale.

Typically, children have a nasogastric tube inserted during surgery. Assess the gastric pH by aspirating stomach contents every 4 hours; based on this assessment, administer antacids or H_2 receptor antagonists as prescribed to help prevent stress ulcer. If preoperative oesophageal varices are present, assess nasogastric drainage carefully for frank or occult blood.

A T-tube inserted into the bile duct for drainage allows the amount of bile being produced by the new liver to be monitored. If vomiting occurs and is persistent, total parenteral nutrition may be used for 3 or 4 days to rest the intestinal tract before fluid is reintroduced (The Royal Children's Hospital Melbourne, 2013).

Hypoglycaemia is a danger postoperatively because glucose levels are regulated by the liver and the transplanted organ may not yet function efficiently. Assess blood glucose levels hourly by fingertip sample.

Continuous cardiac monitoring is usually necessary to detect arrhythmias that may be indicative of hyperkalaemia (hyperkalaemia causes elevation of T waves or ventricular fibrillation) or hypokalaemia.

Many children develop hypertension within 72 hours after surgery. This occurs because of alterations in the renin–angiotensin system because of the not yet fully functioning transplanted liver or as a side effect of immunosuppressant medications, which are continued postoperatively to guard against transplant rejection. IV therapy with hypotensive agents such as hydralazine may be needed to reduce hypertension. Hypotension will occur if the transplanted liver becomes dysfunctional or if there is bleeding caused by poor blood coagulation. To help detect bleeding, observe and measure abdominal girth, the incision line and drainage from any catheters or tubes. Document any findings.

Take axillary or tympanic, not rectal, temperatures, because many children with liver damage have haemorrhoids that could rupture from the trauma of a thermometer insertion.

Nursing considerations

Administration of immunosuppressive medication

Temperature remains within normal range; no presence of exudate or inflammation around abdominal incision. Immunosuppressive agents must be continued postoperatively to prevent graft rejection. Because children are prone to infection while receiving immunosuppressive therapy, be sure to use strict aseptic technique, standard infection precautions and careful hand-washing.

After successful liver transplantation, a child should be able to function normally, attending school and enjoying age-appropriate activities. Ensure that parents have a plan of care, education with regard to graft rejection symptoms and follow-up appointments, prior to discharge.

CASE STUDY QUESTION

6. Jacob's family likes to eat shellfish. What form of hepatitis is most apt to be contracted by eating contaminated shellfish?

a. Hepatitis B
b. Hepatitis A
c. Hepatitis E
d. Hepatitis C

INTESTINAL DISORDERS

Because the intestines form a long body system, several either congenital or acquired disorders can occur.

Intussusception

Intussusception, the invagination of one portion of the intestine into another, usually occurs in the second half of the first year of life (Kaiser, Applegate & Ladd, 2007).

In infants younger than 1 year, intussusception generally occurs for idiopathic reasons. In infants older than 1 year, a "lead point" on the intestine likely cues the invagination. This may include Meckel's diverticulum, a polyp, hypertrophy of *Peyer's patches* (lymphatic tissue of the bowel that increases in size with viral diseases) or bowel tumours.

Children with this disorder suddenly draw up their legs and cry as if they are in severe pain; they may vomit. After the peristaltic wave that caused the discomfort passes, they are symptom-free and play happily. In approximately 15 minutes, another episode occurs. Vomitus will begin to contain bile because the obstruction is below the point in the intestine where bile empties into the duodenum. After approximately 12 hours, blood appears in the stool and possibly in vomitus, described as a "currant jelly" appearance. The abdomen becomes distended as the bowel above the intussusception distends.

If necrosis occurs, children generally have an elevated temperature, abdominal guarding and tenderness may be evident, an increased white blood cell count and often, a rapid pulse.

Diagnosis is suggested by the history. When a parent is describing a child who is crying, be certain to ask enough questions to recognise the possibility of intussusception:

- The duration of the pain? *It lasts a short time, with intervals of no crying in between.*
- The intensity? *Severe*
- The frequency? *Approximately every 15 to 20 minutes*
- The description? *The child pulls up legs with crying*
- Other Symptoms? Yes. *Vomits; refuses food; states stomach feels "full".*

The presence of the intussusception is confirmed by ultrasound or a CT scan (Applegate, 2008).

The condition is a surgical emergency. Reduction of the intussusception must be done promptly by either instillation of a water-soluble solution, barium enema or air (pneumatic insufflation) into the bowel or surgery to reduce the invagination before necrosis of the effected portion of the bowel occurs. If there is no lead point, just the pressure of these non-surgical techniques may reduce the intussusception. After this type of reduction, children are observed for 24 hours as some children will have a recurrence.

Nursing considerations

Risk of deficient fluid volume related to bowel obstruction diarrhoea

Infants are kept on NBM before surgery or non-surgical reduction. Because they have abdominal pain, they may find comfort in sucking a dummy. Because they have been

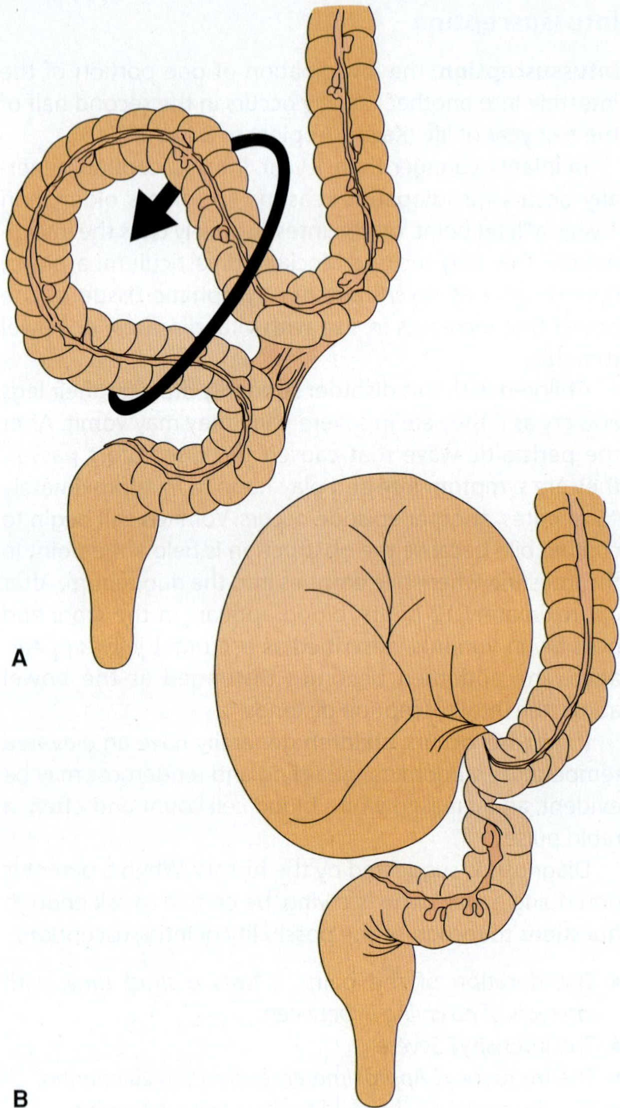

FIGURE 45.3 Volvulus of the sigmoid colon. (**A**) The unattached loop of bowel twists. (**B**) The bowel lumen is obstructed, leading to inability of stool to pass and compression of the blood supply to the looped bowel segment.

vomiting, IV fluid therapy may be started to re-establish their electrolyte balance and to supply adequate fluid to hydrate them.

Following a non-surgical reduction, infants are kept NBM for a few hours and then introduced gradually to regular feedings. Infants who have surgery will return with a nasogastric tube and an IV infusion in place.

Volvulus

A **volvulus** is a twisting of the intestine (see Fig. 45.3). The twist leads to obstruction of the passage of faeces and compromise of the blood supply to the loop of intestine involved. Usually, the symptoms are those of intestinal obstruction and occur during the first 6 months of life. Symptoms may include intense crying and pain, pulling up the legs, abdominal distension and vomiting. The diagnosis is made based on the history and an abdominal examination, which reveals an abdominal mass. Surgery is used to relieve the volvulus and reattach the bowel so it is no longer so free moving. This must be done promptly before necrosis of the intestine occurs from a lack of blood supply to the involved loop of bowel. Preoperative and postoperative care will be the same as for infants with intussusception.

Necrotising enterocolitis

With *necrotising enterocolitis* (NEC) the bowel develops necrotic patches that interfere with digestion and possibly lead to paralytic ileus, perforation and peritonitis (Huether, 2012). The necrosis appears to result from ischaemia or poor perfusion of blood vessels in sections of the bowel. The entire bowel may be involved or it may be localised. The incidence of NEC is highest in immature infants, those who have suffered anoxia or shock and those fed by enteral feeding.

Signs of NEC usually appear in the first week of life. The infant's abdomen becomes distended and tense. The stomach does not fully empty by the next feeding time because of poor intestinal action; if the stomach contents are aspirated before a feeding, a return of undigested milk of more than 2 mL will be obtained. Stool may be positive for occult blood. Periods of apnoea may begin or increase in number. Signs of blood loss because of intestinal bleeding, such as lowered blood pressure and inability to stabilise temperature, may also be present.

Abdominal x-ray films show a characteristic picture of air invading the intestinal wall; if perforation has occurred, there will be air in the abdominal cavity.

As soon as the condition is recognised, the infant is maintained on IV or total parenteral nutrition solutions to rest the GI tract with the additional supplement of enteral probiotics (Al Faleh & Bassler, 2009). An antibiotic may be given to limit secondary infection.

If the area of necrosis appears to be localised, surgery to remove that portion of the bowel may be successful. If a large portion of the bowel is removed, the infant may be prone to "short-bowel" syndrome or may have a problem with digestion of nutrients in the future. If the bowel perforates, peritoneal drainage or a laparotomy will be necessary to help remove faecal secretions from the abdomen. An infant may need a temporary colostomy performed to allow for bowel function.

Appendicitis

Appendicitis (inflammation of the appendix) is the most common cause of abdominal surgery in children. It occurs most frequently in school-age children and adolescents, although it can occur in preschoolers and even in newborns (Ladd et al., 2012). If the condition is not discovered early enough, the necrotic area will rupture and faecal material will spill into the abdomen, causing peritonitis.

Most parents assume that appendicitis begins with sharp pain, so they may dismiss a child's early symptoms for some time as simple gastroenteritis. Pain is a late symptom. Diagnosis is made on a cluster of symptoms: anorexia, pain or tenderness in the right lower quadrant, nausea or vomiting, elevation of temperature and leucocytosis (Ebell, 2008). The history typically begins with anorexia for 12–24 hours. Children do not eat and do not act like their usual selves. Nausea and vomiting may then occur. The abdominal pain, when it does start, is at first diffuse. Gradually, it becomes localised to the right lower quadrant. The point of sharpest pain is often one-third of the way between the anterior superior iliac crest and the umbilicus (*McBurney's point*). If the child's appendix is displaced from this usual position, the pain will not be at this typical point, so pain at any other point does not rule out appendicitis. Temperature is a late symptom.

Until the pain becomes localised, appendicitis is difficult to distinguish from acute gastroenteritis. Often, it is difficult to palpate children's abdomens because they guard their abdomen or make abdominal muscles stiff and hard by tensing them. Although this interferes with abdominal examination, it is in itself an important sign that children have abdominal pain.

Rebound tenderness is a phenomenon in which a child feels relatively mild pain when the area over the appendix is palpated, but, once an examiner's hand is withdrawn, the child experiences acute pain caused by the shifting of the abdominal contents. This is diagnostic for appendicitis, but it should be done with children only when necessary because it does cause acute pain. On auscultation, bowel sounds will be reduced: only one or two are heard in the same length of time that 30 are normally heard. Absence of bowel sounds on auscultation suggests peritonitis or an appendix that has already ruptured.

An ultrasound reveals the swollen appendix. It can also be confirmed by a CT scan. Because ultrasound can successfully reveal appendicitis, however, analgesia to make the child comfortable can be given (Bromberg & Goldman, 2007).

Therapy for appendicitis is surgical removal of the appendix by laparoscopy before it ruptures (Sauerland, Lefering & Neugebauer, 2009).

Nursing considerations

Pain related to inflamed appendix

Child states that level of pain is tolerable. Diagnosis may be confirmed by ultrasound, in all cases analgesia should be provided when required.

Deficient fluid volume related to NBM status

Child's skin fold returns to place quickly when turgor is assessed; pulse and blood pressure are within normal age limits; weight is maintained. Preoperatively, obtain a urine sample for urinalysis and blood for a complete blood count. IV fluid therapy may be initiated to hydrate a child who has been vomiting a great deal. Postoperatively, children will be maintained on IV fluids until they can take adequate oral feedings. With unruptured appendicitis, the postoperative course is uneventful; children are up a few hours after surgery and are discharged within several days.

Ruptured appendix

If a child's appendix has already ruptured when the child is seen in the emergency department, the potential for peritonitis increases greatly. Children generally appear severely ill. Position the child in a semi-Fowler's position, if possible, so that infected drainage from the caecum drains downwards into the pelvis rather than upwards towards the lungs. The child needs an IV fluid line inserted for hydration. Antibiotics will be begun preoperatively or as soon as the ruptured appendix is confirmed (Hung, Lin & Chen, 2012).

Intraoperatively, a drain may be placed in the wound bed. The drain should be observed and the output documented. The drain insertion site should also be assessed and dressings changed as required. IV fluid and antibiotic therapy are continued until full bowel function is restored.

Also assess for signs of peritonitis. Assess the child's vital signs, including temperature, and observe the wound area for signs of infection. Although the postoperative course is slower (approximately 3 weeks) after a ruptured appendix, the prognosis is still good.

Meckel's diverticulum

In embryonic life, the intestine is attached to the umbilicus by the omphalomesenteric (vitelline) duct. This duct becomes a vestigial ligament as infants reach term. In 2% or 3% of all infants, a small pouch of this duct remains, located off the ileum, approximately 45 cm from the ileum–colon junction: a **Meckel's diverticulum** (Kloss, Bronton & Sullivan, 2010). In this structure, there may be some misplaced gastric mucosa, which secretes gastric acids that flow into the intestine and irritate the bowel wall. This can lead to ulceration and bleeding. Infants will have painless, tarry (black) stools or grossly bloody stools. On occasion, the diverticulum may serve as the lead point causing an intussusception. In some instances, a fibrous band extending from the diverticulum pouch to the umbilicus acts as a constricting band, causing bowel obstruction.

The history of the child suggests the diagnosis. Because the pouch is small, it does not fill, and therefore it may not be evident on x-ray or ultrasound. Treatment is laparoscopy exploration and removal of the vestigial structure.

Coeliac disease

The basic problem in **coeliac disease** is a sensitivity or abnormal immunological response to protein, particularly the gluten factor of protein found in grains—wheat, rye, oats and barley. When children with the disorder ingest gluten, changes occur in their intestinal mucosa or villi that prevent the absorption of foods, especially fat, across the intestinal villi into the bloodstream. As a result, children develop *steatorrhoea* (bulky, foul-smelling, fatty stools); deficiency of fat-soluble vitamins A, D, K and E (the vitamins are not absorbed because the fat is not absorbed); malnutrition; and a distended abdomen from the fat, bulky stools. Because vitamin D is one of the fat-soluble vitamins, rickets or loss of calcium from bones may occur. Hypoprothrombinaemia may occur from loss of vitamin K. In addition, children may have hypochromic anaemia (iron-deficiency anaemia) and hypoalbuminaemia from poor protein absorption (Holmes, 2010).

Children with the syndrome tend to be anorectic and irritable. They gradually fall behind other children their age in height and weight. They appear skinny, with spindly extremities and wasted buttocks. The face, however, in contrast to children with true starvation, may be plump and well-rounded.

The diagnosis is based on the history; clinical symptoms such as bulky stools, malnutrition, distended abdomen and anaemia which become noticeable between 6 and 18 months of age; serum analysis of antibodies against gluten (IgA antigliadin antibodies); and a biopsy of the intestinal mucosa (done by endoscopy), which establishes the typical changes in intestinal villi. In addition, the child's response to gluten is observed by placing the child on a gluten-free diet. In most instances, the response to this diet is dramatic: the child begins to gain weight, steatorrhoea improves and the irritability fades.

Treatment is to continue the gluten-free diet for life, because there is some suggestion that these children are more prone to GI carcinoma later in life if they do not continue the diet into adulthood. In addition to this, children need to have water-soluble forms of vitamins A and D administered. Both iron and folate may be necessary as well to correct any anaemia present.

Nursing considerations

Imbalanced nutrition, related to malabsorption of food

Child's weight is maintained on a percentile curve on a growth chart; skin turgor is good; steatorrhoea is minimal; parents verbalise appropriate gluten-free food choices.

Parents need to record the consistency, appearance, size and number of stools that the child passes. The disappearance of steatorrhoea is a good indicator that the child's ability to absorb nutrients is improving.

Parents need a great deal of nutritional counselling when their child is first placed on a gluten-free diet so that they can recognise foods that contain gluten (wheat, rye, oats and barley products). Because children are anorectic when they are first introduced to the new diet, getting them to eat it may be a problem. Remember that toddlers often eat small servings better than larger ones. As children reach school age, preparing a gluten-free diet becomes more and more difficult. A referral to a dietician is very important to help educate both parents and children to make appropriate food choices.

Coeliac crisis

When children with coeliac disease develop any type of infection, a crisis of extreme symptoms may occur. Both vomiting and diarrhoea become acute. Children can quickly experience electrolyte and fluid imbalances and need intensive therapy to correct them. Gradually, after such an episode, they are placed back on a gluten-free diet.

DISORDERS OF THE LOWER BOWEL

In children, disorders of the lower bowel mainly create problems with evacuation.

Constipation

Constipation or difficulty passing hardened stools may occur in children of any age (Greenwald, 2010). Constipation is distressing to children because passing hardened stool is painful and may cause anal fissures. A child then represses the next urge to defecate because of pain. The rectum gradually becomes distended and adjusts to the ever-present bulk of stool. The urge to defecate becomes less frequent. When the child does pass stool, it is larger and firmer than before and causes even more anal pain. This vicious cycle continues until the child becomes severely constipated. Children may have episodes of diarrhoea or *encopresis* (involuntary release of stool) when their rectum can hold no more. They may experience abdominal pain from forceful intestinal contractions.

Some children begin holding stool for psychological reasons. Once the process begins, however, the hardened stool, the anal fissures and the pain on defecation soon occur, and what began for an emotional reason becomes a physical ailment. This is important to understand, because with these children, therapy involves both counselling to correct the initial problem and treatment of the physical symptoms (McQuaid, 2009).

When taking a history, be certain to have parents describe what they mean by constipation. Some children normally pass stool every 2 to 3 days. As long as the stool is not hard and there is no discomfort associated with passing stool, this is not constipation. Examine the circumstances that may have led to constipation e.g. diet (fibre, fresh fruit and vegetables) and stressors.

Children with constipation should be examined carefully to see if they have anal fissures. If these are present, sexual abuse must be ruled out. Constipation must be differentiated from aganglionic disease of the intestine. In constipation, on rectal examination, hard stool is found in the rectum; in aganglionic disease of the intestine, no stool is normally present.

Treatment of chronic constipation is aimed at softening stool so it will pass painlessly. Children also need help to form good bowel habits so that stools are passed before they become large and hardened (Reading, 2007).

Nursing considerations

Constipation related to pain from anal fissure and hardened stool

Child has a soft bowel movement without pain every other day. For initial therapy, an enema may be administered to loosen hard stool. The use of a stool softener, ingestion of a high-fibre, high-fluid diet and being urged to evacuate their bowels at the same time every day to form a habit helps reduce constipation.

Inguinal hernia

Inguinal hernia is a protrusion of a section of the bowel into the inguinal ring. It occurs usually in boys because, as the testes descend from the abdominal cavity into the scrotum late in fetal life, a fold of parietal peritoneum also descends, forming a tube from the abdomen to the scrotum (García-Hernández et al., 2012). In most infants, this tube closes completely. If it fails to close, intestinal descent into it (hernia) may occur at any time when there is an increase in intra-abdominal pressure. In girls, the round ligament extends from the uterus into the inguinal canal to its attachment on the abdominal wall. In girls, an inguinal hernia may occur because of a weakness of the muscle surrounding the round ligament.

A hernia appears as a lump in the left or right groin. In some instances, the hernia is apparent only on crying (when abdominal pressure increases) and not when children are less active. Inguinal hernias are painless. Pain at the site implies that the bowel has become incarcerated in the sac, an emergency that requires immediate action to prevent bowel obstruction and ischaemia.

The diagnosis is established by history and physical appearance. When taking a history of a well child, be certain to ask parents whether they have ever noticed any lumps in the child's groin area. The hernia may not be noticeable at the time of a healthcare visit, so, unless asked specifically, parents may not mention it. If present, the herniated intestine can be palpated in the inguinal ring on physical examination.

Treatment of an inguinal hernia is by laparoscopic surgery. To prevent the complication of bowel strangulation, infants with an inguinal hernia may have surgery before 1 year of age. If surgery is proposed as a prophylactic measure, setting outcomes may be difficult for parents as they weigh the value of surgical repair against the risks of anaesthesia and surgery.

During surgery, the bowel is returned to the abdominal cavity and retained there by sealing the inguinal ring. Pneumoperitoneum (instillation of carbon dioxide into the perineal cavity) during surgery may be performed to reveal the presence of an enlarged inguinal ring on the opposite side. If this is present, both sides may be repaired and the child will return from surgery with dressings on both groins.

Postoperatively, keep the suture line dry and free of urine or faeces to prevent infection by performing frequent nappy changes and care. Most incisions in this area are closed by a tissue adhesive, which is waterproof and seals the incision from urine and faeces. Assess circulation in the leg on the side of the surgical repair to be certain that oedema of the groin is not compressing blood vessels and obstructing blood flow to the leg.

Gastroschisis

Gastroschisis is a birth defect in which an infant's intestines are outside the body due to a hole in the abdominal wall (Lee, 2015). It is considered a type of hernia. The child's intestines usually protrude through the hole. The condition looks similar to an omphalocele, which is a birth defect in which the infant's intestine or other abdominal organs protrude through a hole in the umbilical area, however, they are covered with a membrane. Surgical intervention is used to correct the defect. Other treatments may include intravenous nutrients and antibiotics to prevent infection.

Hirschsprung's disease (aganglionic megacolon)

Hirschsprung's disease or *aganglionic megacolon* is absence of ganglionic innervation to the muscle of a section of the bowel—in most instances, the lower portion of the sigmoid colon just above the anus (Pakarinen et al., 2013; see Fig. 45.4). The absence of nerve cells means there are no peristaltic waves in this section to move faecal material through the segment of intestine. This results in chronic constipation or ribbon-like stools (stools passing through such a small, narrow segment look like ribbons).

Occasionally, infants are born with such an extensive section of bowel involved that even meconium cannot pass. This is suggested if infants fail to pass meconium by 24 hours of age and have increasing abdominal distension (Hartman et al., 2007).

Because newborn stools are normally soft, however, symptoms of aganglionic megacolon generally do not become apparent until 6 to 12 months of age. By the time children are seen by a healthcare provider, they generally have a history of constipation or intermittent constipation and diarrhoea. A careful history helps to document the illness:

- The duration of the constipation? *It may have been a problem from birth*
- What do parents mean by constipation? *Children do not have a bowel movement more than once a week*
- Consistency of the stool? *Ribbon-like or watery*
- Is the child ill in any other way? *Children with aganglionic disease of the intestine tend to be thin and undernourished, sometimes deceptively so because their abdomen is large and distended.*

If a gloved finger is inserted into the rectum of a child with true constipation, the examining finger will touch hard, caked stool. With aganglionic colon disease, the rectum is

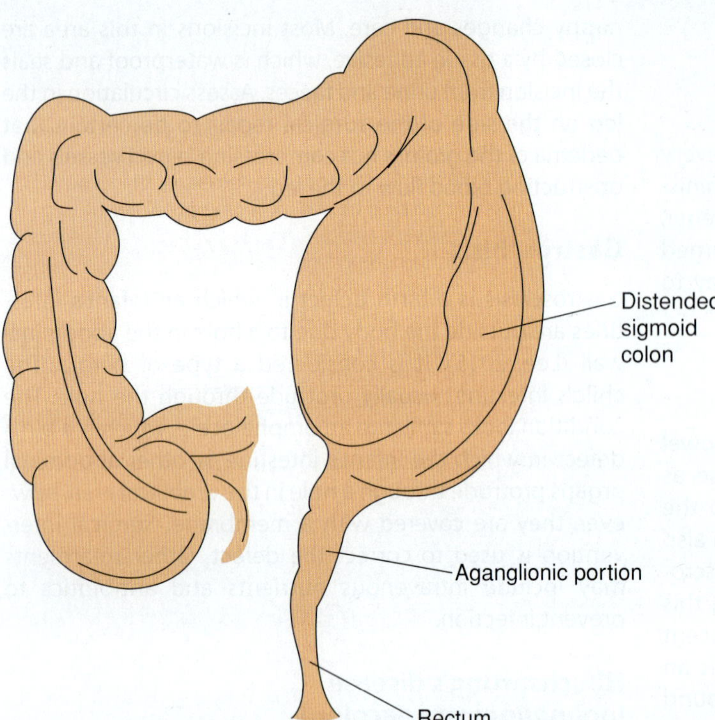

FIGURE 45.4 Aganglionic megacolon (Hirschsprung's disease). The distal portion of the bowel lacks nerve innervation. Because there is no peristalsis in this narrowed segment, the bowel proximal to it distends markedly.

empty because faecal material cannot pass into the rectum through the obstructed portion.

Repair of aganglionic megacolon involves dissection and removal of the affected section, with anastomosis of the intestine. Because this is a technically difficult operation to perform in a small abdomen, the condition is generally treated in the newborn by two-stage surgery: first a temporary colostomy is established, followed by bowel repair at 12 to 18 months of age. After the final surgery, children should have a functioning, normal bowel. In the few instances in which the anus is deprived of nerve endings, a permanent colostomy will be established.

Nursing considerations

Constipation related to reduced bowel function

Child has a daily bowel movement through either a colostomy or by enema. Before surgery, the child may be prescribed daily enemas to achieve bowel movements. Teach parents how to prepare and administer enemas at home. Caring for a child with a colostomy is discussed in Chapter 37.

Imbalanced nutrition, related to reduced bowel function

Child ingests a low-residue diet; weight follows a percentile curve on a growth chart. Preoperatively, older children may be in poor health from poor food intake over a long period. If this is so, they may be returned home on a minimal-residue diet, stool softeners, vitamin supplements and perhaps daily enemas until their condition improves. Parenteral nutrition can offer another source of nutrition. It is a sterile intravenous solution of protein, dextrose and fat in combination with electrolytes, vitamins, trace elements and water. It is used to treat children who are unable to be fed by the oral or enteral route. If a child is to be cared for at home, help the parents learn about a low-residue diet. Fried foods and highly seasoned foods are omitted to eliminate chemical irritants in the intestinal tract.

When children are beginning a special diet, it may be advisable to have parents refrain from introducing new feeding methods, such as a cup or spoon, unless children are at that developmental point where they will quickly adapt to the new procedure and are, in fact, so eager to feed themselves that they will actually eat better this way.

Postoperatively, observe the infant for abdominal distension. Assess bowel sounds and observe also for passage of flatus and stools. As soon as peristalsis has returned (approximately 24 hours after surgery), the child will be offered small, frequent feeding of clear fluids. The child is then introduced gradually to full fluids, a soft diet, a low-residue diet and finally a normal diet for age.

Compromised family coping related to chronic illness in child

Parents state they are able to cope with the level of stress present from their child's condition. Most parents feel tremendous relief after the second-stage surgery is complete. Caution parents that the child may still remain a "fussy eater" for a few months, because feeding problems that begin for physical reasons can continue for emotional or psychological reasons.

Inflammatory bowel disease: Ulcerative colitis and Crohn's disease

Two conditions are categorised as inflammatory bowel disease: *ulcerative colitis* and *Crohn's disease* (Danese &

TABLE 45.4 Comparison of Crohn's disease and ulcerative colitis

Comparison factor	Crohn's disease	Ulcerative colitis
Part of bowel affected	Ileum	Colon and rectum
Nature of lesions	Intermittent	Continuous
Diarrhoea	Moderate	Severe and bloody
Anorexia	Severe	Mild
Weight loss	Severe	Mild
Growth retardation	Marked	Mild
Anal and perianal lesions	Common	Rare
Association with carcinoma	Rare	Common

Fiocchi, 2011). Both involve the development of ulcers of the mucosa or submucosa layers of the colon and rectum. They both occur most frequently in young adults and adolescents (see Table 45.4).

The cause of these disorders is obscure, but they probably represent an alteration in immune system response or are autoimmune processes. Psychological factors have not been supported as a primary contributory factor to inflammatory bowel disease, but psychological problems often occur secondary to the disease, possibly intensifying symptoms. Smoking and frequent use of antibiotics or aspirin are correlated with the occurrence of Crohn's disease (Ananthakrishnan, 2013).

Crohn's disease is an inflammation of segments of the intestine; it may affect any part of the GI tract but most commonly involves the terminal ileum. Inflamed segments are separated by normal bowel tissue. The wall of the colon becomes thickened and the surface is inflamed, leading to a "cobblestone" appearance of mucosa.

In ulcerative colitis, typically the colon and rectum are involved, with the distal colon and rectum most severely affected, and inflammation involves continuous segments.

As inflammation becomes acute with these disorders, children develop abdominal pain from contractions of the irritated portions. These areas do not absorb nutrients or fluid well, so diarrhoea and malnutrition develop. To reduce abdominal pain (which is most acute after eating, when the bowel becomes active), children begin to skip meals. They may be malnourished and have a vitamin or iron deficiency at the time the condition is diagnosed.

Several complications may occur. Haemorrhage from bowel perforation during the active disease is possible. Perforation can lead to peritonitis or the formation of fistulas between bowel loops. Rectal fistula is often present. A relapse is apt to occur 6 to 12 months after therapy. With ulcerative colitis, there is an association between the disease and bowel carcinoma if the disease persists over 10 years (McQuaid, 2009).

In both conditions, diarrhoea and steatorrhoea develop from the irritation and the unabsorbed fluid. If inflamed portions ulcerate, there will be blood in the stool. Weight loss occurs; growth failure occurs in prepubertal children. A recurring fever may be present.

Diagnosis is established by colonoscopy and barium enema. On colonoscopy, the shallow ulcerations along the bowel can be seen; the mucosa is friable (easily irritated) and bleeds easily from inflammation. A biopsy may be performed for definite diagnosis. Observe children carefully after a bowel biopsy to detect rectal bleeding from an internal bleeding point, including full vital signs and assess for occult blood.

The child's bowel heals best if it is allowed to rest for a time. Enteral or total parenteral nutrition is usually provided for nutrition during the resting period (Wiskin, Wootton & Beattie, 2007).

When food is reintroduced after the resting period, a high-protein, high-carbohydrate, high-vitamin diet is prescribed to replace nutrients. Children may eat cautiously at first to avoid reintroducing diarrhoea so assess intake and output. A combination of an anti-inflammatory medication, an immunosuppressive agent or monoclonal antibodies generally bring about a great improvement in symptoms. If medical therapy is ineffective, bowel resection to remove a portion of the bowel (colectomy) may be necessary. Bowel surgery is a serious step; because it reduces the possibility of the child developing intestinal cancer in association with ulcerative colitis, it may be necessary in children whose disease is running a long-term, debilitating course that does not improve (Ba'ath et al., 2007). Children who recover from inflammatory bowel disease should have a colonoscopy yearly for the rest of their lives.

Nursing considerations

Imbalanced nutrition related to poor absorption because of disease process

Child's weight follows a percentile growth curve; child states that alternative feeding method is tolerable. Nutrition is a priority concern for children with both Crohn's disease and ulcerative colitis because malnutrition can occur from the combination of poor intestinal absorption and chronic diarrhoea. Unless active steps are taken to supplement nutrition, children with inflammatory bowel disease can be left both short in stature and light in weight. Anorexia with protein, vitamin, fat and mineral deficiencies all may occur.

Ineffective coping related to chronic illness

Child expresses feelings and understanding of the disease and therapy. Caution children about the possible side effects, such as excessive weight gain, a round facial appearance and facial acne, that may occur if corticosteroid therapy is used so they are not surprised by this. Assess blood pressure, intake and output, weight and sleep patterns for any child taking steroids. Caution children that sulfasalazine turns urine an orange-yellow so they do not mistake this colour change as bleeding.

The disorder follows a chronic course and can involve embarrassing episodes of diarrhoea or acute abdominal pain. Counselling and support groups are often invaluable to help with coping.

Irritable bowel syndrome (chronic non-specific diarrhoea)

Irritable bowel syndrome involves intermittent episodes of loose and normal stools or recurrent abdominal pain. It is most often seen in infants 6 to 36 months of age. Most children outgrow the symptoms by 3 years of age. The cause is unknown, but it is associated with low fat intake (without fat slowing absorption, stool passes rapidly through the bowel). Excessive fluid intake also may play a role.

The symptoms are usually vague. The episodes of diarrhoea may occur several times a week or as frequently as twice a day. There seems to be no relationship to meals.

Children are encouraged to eat a regular diet. Psyllium bulk agents will almost always reduce the frequency of symptoms. Probiotics or foods supplemented with lactic acid-producing bacteria may improve symptoms (Walter & Isolauri, 2007).

Chronic recurrent abdominal pain

Some children develop episodes of recurring abdominal pain. Although such episodes can occur for reasons such as lactose intolerance or muscle strain from sports activities, in most instances the cause is unknown (Collins & Lin, 2010). Children who experience this are commonly 6 or 7 years of age or in prepuberty (11–12 years of age). The pain is not accompanied by a change in bowel habits. There is no association with meals. Episodes of pain can last for only a few minutes or for hours. The intensity of the pain is mild or "annoying" rather than severe. It is generally poorly localised, although children may point to the umbilicus as the primary site. On physical examination there is no abdominal tenderness, distension, guarding or muscle spasm.

Symptoms of stress such as sleep disturbances, fears or eating problems may be present. Although the cause of the pain cannot be identified, the pain is real. For some children, just having the opportunity to talk to an understanding person about the problem is all that is necessary to stop the attacks. Other families need counselling regarding the underlying problem. The family may need to be referred to a family service agency for counselling.

DISORDERS CAUSED BY FOOD, VITAMIN AND MINERAL DEFICIENCIES

There are many underfed and malnourished children in every part of the world. Although extreme diseases of food or vitamin deprivation are rare in western countries, they do exist. The average child does not develop a deficient intake of essential nutrients because, even if the child is occasionally a fussy eater, over the space of a week, a child does ingest foods containing the necessary nutrients. Carefully assess any child who has an interference in nutrition such as a GI illness or a child who is receiving enteric feedings or total parenteral nutrition to make sure that nutrient deficiencies do not exist. Assess abused or neglected children closely for nutritional deficiencies, because they may not have been given adequate food.

Kwashiorkor

Kwashiorkor, a disease caused by protein deficiency, occurs most frequently in children of ages 1 to 3 years, because this age group requires a high protein intake. It is a disease found almost exclusively in developing countries (Boyd, Andea & Hughey, 2012). Growth failure is a major symptom. Because oedema is also a symptom, children may not appear light in weight or show severe wasting of muscles until the oedema is relieved.

Oedema results from hypoproteinaemia, which causes a shift of body fluid from the intravascular compartments to the interstitial space, causing ascites. The oedema tends to be dependent, so it is first noted in the lower extremities. Children also have diarrhoea, iron-deficiency anaemia and enlarged livers. Without treatment, kwashiorkor is fatal. For therapy, a diet rich in protein is essential.

Nutritional marasmus

Nutritional marasmus is caused by a deficiency of all food groups, basically a form of starvation. They have many of the same symptoms as children with kwashiorkor, including growth failure, muscle wasting, irritability, iron-deficiency anaemia and diarrhoea. Whereas children with kwashiorkor are anorectic, children with nutritional marasmus are invariably hungry (starving) and will suck at any object offered to them, such as a finger or their clothing. Treatment is a diet rich in all nutrients.

Vitamin and mineral deficiencies

Both vitamin and mineral deficiencies occur at a low rate in children because so many foods are enriched or fortified. Common foods such as milk and bread are enriched with vitamins and minerals. For vitamin deficiency disorders see Table 45.5.

Iodine deficiency

Because iodine is not supplemented in food except as iodised salt, a diet deficient in iodine may lead to either hypothyroidism or goitre of the thyroid gland. Supplemental iodine or synthetic thyroxine is needed to correct the deficiency. Children must also be maintained on a diet adequate in iodine, found most abundantly in seafood (Rolfes, Pinna & Whitney, 2009).

TABLE 45.5 Vitamin deficiency disorders

Vitamin	Cause of deficiency	Signs and symptoms
Vitamin A	Lack of yellow vegetables in diet	Tender tongue; cracks at corners of mouth; night blindness **Xerophthalmia** (dry and lusterless conjunctivae) **Keratomalacia** (necrosis of the cornea with perforation, loss of ocular fluid and blindness)
Vitamin B_1	Most common in children who eat polished rice as dietary staple, because B_1 is contained in hull of rice	**Beriberi** (tingling and numbness of extremities; heart palpitations; exhaustion) Diarrhoea and vomiting Aphonia (cry without sound) Anaesthesia of feet
Niacin	Common in children who eat corn as dietary staple, because corn is low in niacin	**Pellagra** (dermatitis; resembles a sunburn) Diarrhoea Mental confusion (dementia)
Vitamin C	Lack of fresh fruits in diet	**Scurvy** (muscle tenderness; petechiae)
Vitamin D	Lack of sunlight	Poor muscle tone; delayed tooth formation **Rickets** (poor bone formation) Craniotabes (softening of the skull) Swelling at joints, particularly of wrists and cartilage of ribs Bowed legs Tetany (muscle spasms)

✔ *Checkpoint question 45.1*

Kwashiorkor is a disorder common in developing countries. This disorder occurs because of lack of which nutrient?

a. Water-soluble vitamins
b. Fats and triglycerides
c. Quality protein
d. Vitamin K

Key points for review

- Some gastrointestinal disorders lead to long-term therapies such as colostomy or gastrostomy feeding. Because these disorders interfere with common body functions such as eating and elimination, they are difficult for children to accept without the support of concerned healthcare providers.
- Children lose proportionately more fluid with vomiting and diarrhoea than adults, so they need rapid assessment and interventions to avoid dehydration.
- Fluid, electrolyte and acid–base imbalances tend to occur rapidly with vomiting and diarrhoea. Vomiting leads to alkalosis. Diarrhoea leads to acidosis.
- Gastrointestinal disorders almost always interfere with nutrition to some degree. This is a greater problem in children than adults because children need to ingest adequate nutrients and fluid daily for growth as well as body maintenance.
- Gastro-oesophageal reflux is a neuromuscular disturbance in which the cardiac sphincter is lax, allowing for easy regurgitation of gastric contents into the oesophagus. It is treated by feeding a thickened formula and keeping an infant upright after feeding.
- Pyloric stenosis is hypertrophy of the valve between the stomach and duodenum. It impedes the passage of feedings, leading to vomiting.
- Peptic ulcer disease may occur in children of all ages. The disorder causes a shallow excavation to form in the mucosal wall of the stomach. It is treated, like adult ulcers, with antibiotics and agents to suppress gastric acidity.
- Forms of hepatitis seen in children include hepatitis A and C (usually caused by eating contaminated shellfish) and hepatitis B, D and E (caused by contaminated blood or placental transfer).
- Congenital obstruction of the bile ducts occurs from failure of the bile duct to recanalise in utero. This can lead to fibrotic scarring of the liver (cirrhosis). Most of these children need a liver transplant to restore liver function.
- Intussusception is the invagination of one portion of the intestine into another. Volvulus is twisting of the intestine. Both may lead to bowel obstruction.
- Necrotising enterocolitis is the development of necrotic patches on the intestine. It occurs almost exclusively in immature infants.
- Appendicitis is inflammation of the appendix. It is always an emergency and is the most common reason for abdominal surgery in children. Laparoscopy is done to remove the appendix, ideally before it ruptures.
- Coeliac disease (gluten-induced enteropathy) is a change in the ability of the intestinal villi to absorb. It is a dominantly inherited illness.
- Both inguinal and hiatal hernia can occur in children. These are surgically corrected when recognised.
- Hirschsprung's disease (aganglionic megacolon) is absence of ganglionic innervation in a section of the lower bowel.

- Inflammatory bowel disease can occur as either ulcerative colitis or Crohn's disease. Therapy is long-term. If medical therapy is unsuccessful, portions of the bowel may be surgically removed. Ulcerative colitis is associated with the development of colon cancer later in life.
- Kwashiorkor (protein deficiency), nutritional marasmus (starvation), vitamins A and D (rickets), B_1 (beriberi) and C (scurvy) deficiencies, or iodine deficiencies occur in children when they are not provided with or cannot absorb adequate nutrients. Although more common in developing countries, they can occur in a child in any community.

CASE STUDY QUESTIONS

7. Jacob was diagnosed with coeliac disease. When you met him, his mother was insisting that he eat a piece of birthday cake. What health education does his mother need to help her choose a better diet for her son? What would have been a better food, probably available at a birthday party, that he could have eaten?
8. Suppose Jacob is seen in a hospital emergency department with severe diarrhoea. What emergency interventions does he need to prevent an electrolyte or fluid imbalance? What measures could you take to reduce his fear of the strange hospital environment?
9. Jacob's older sister, who has Crohn's disease, is being cared for at home with total parenteral nutrition. How can you help her keep pace with her friends at school? How can you help her maintain a sense of high self-esteem in the light of her many hospitalisations and home care?

Resources

For an extensive range of additional resources to enhance teaching and learning and to facilitate understanding of this chapter, please see the text's accompanying website located on thePoint at http://thepoint.lww.com.

References

Al Faleh, K. & Bassler, D. (2009). Probiotics for prevention of necrotizing enterocolitis in preterm infants. *Cochrane Database of Systematic Reviews,* (1), (CD005496).

Ananthakrishnan, A. N. (2013). Environmental triggers for inflammatory bowel disease. *Current Gastroenterology Reports*, *15*(1), 302.

Applegate, K. E. (2008). Intussusception in children: Imaging choices. *Seminars in Roentgenology, 43*(1), 15–21.

Ba'ath, M. E., et al. (2007). Surgical management of inflammatory bowel disease. *Archives of Disease in Childhood, 92*(4), 312–316.

Boyd, K. P., Andea, A. & Hughey, L. C. (2012). Acute inpatient presentation of kwashiorkor: Not just a diagnosis of the developing world. *Pediatric Dermatology*, *30*(6), e240–e241.

Bromberg, R. & Goldman, R. D. (2007). Pediatric pearls: Current practice. Does analgesia mask diagnosis of appendicitis among children? *Canadian Family Physician, 53*(1), 39–41.

Chambers, H. F. (2009). Infectious diseases: Bacterial and chlamydial. In S. J. McPhee & M. A. Papadakis (Eds). *Current Medical Diagnosis and Treatment.* Columbus, OH: McGraw-Hill.

Cies, J. J. & Giamalis, J. N. (2007). Treatment of cholestatic pruritus in children. *American Journal of Health-System Pharmacy, 64*(11), 1157–1161.

Cochran, J. B. & Losek, J. D. (2007). Acute liver failure in children. *Pediatric Emergency Care, 23*(2), 129–135.

Collins, B. & Lin, H. (2010). Chronic abdominal pain in children is associated with high prevalence of abnormal microbial fermentation. *Digestive Diseases and Sciences*, *55*(1), 124–130.

Craig, W. R., et al. (2009). Metoclopramide, thickened feedings, and positioning for gastro-oesophageal reflux in children under two years. *Cochrane Database of Systematic Reviews,* (1), (CD003502).

Danese, S. & Fiocchi, C. (2011). Medical progress: Ulcerative colitis. *The New England Journal of Medicine*, *365*(18), 1713–1725.

Ebell, M. H. (2008). Diagnosis of appendicitis: Part II. Laboratory and imaging tests. *American Family Physician, 77*(8), 1153–1155.

Fitzpatrick, E., et al. (2007). Outcomes for children with cyclical vomiting syndrome. *Archives of Disease in Childhood, 92*(11), 1001–1004.

Friedman, L. S. (2009). Hepatology. In S. J. McPhee & M. A. Papadakis (Eds). *Current Medical Diagnosis and Treatment.* Columbus, OH: McGraw-Hill.

García-Hernández, C., Carvajal-Figueroa, L., Suarez-Gutiérrez, R., et al. (2012). Laparoscopic approach for inguinal hernia in children: Resection without suture. *Journal of Pediatric Surgery*, *47*(11), 2093–2095.

Greenwald, B. (2010). Clinical practice guidelines for pediatric constipation. *Journal of the Academy of Nurse Practitioners*, *22*(7), 332–338.

Hartman, E. E., et al. (2007). Explaining change in quality of life of children and adolescents with anorectal malformations or Hirschsprung disease. *Pediatrics, 119*(2), e374–e383.

Holmes, S. (2010). Coeliac disease: Symptoms, complications and patient support. *Nursing Standard*, *24*(35), 50–56.

Hua, M. C., et al. (2007). Perforated peptic ulcer in children: A 20-year experience. *Journal of Pediatric Gastroenterology and Nutrition*, *45*(1), 71–74.

Huether, S. E. (2012). Alterations of digestive function in children. In S. E. Huether & K. L. McCance (Eds.), *Understanding Pathophysiology* (5th ed.), Philadelphia: Elsevier Mosby.

Hung, M. H., Lin, L. H. & Chen, D. F. (2012). Clinical manifestations in children with ruptured appendicitis. *Pediatric Emergency Care*, *28*(5), 433–435.

Hussey, S., Kelleher, K. T. & Ling, S. C. (2010). Emergency management of major upper gastrointestinal hemorrhage in children. *Clinical Pediatric Emergency Medicine*, *11*(3), 207–216.

Kaido, T., Mori, A., Ogura, Y., et al. (2012). Pre- and perioperative factors affecting infection after living donor liver transplantation. *Nutrition*, *28*(11–12), 1104–1108.

Kaiser, A. D., Applegate, K. E. & Ladd, A. P. (2007). Current success in the treatment of intussusception in children. *Surgery, 142*(4), 469–475.

Kloss, B. T., Bronton, C. E. & Sullivan, A. M. (2010). Perforated Meckel diverticulum. *Internal Journal of Emergency Medicine*, *3*(4), 455–457.

Ladd, M. R., Neff, L. P., Becher, R. D., et al. (2012). Computerized tomography in the workup of pediatric appendicitis: Why are children scanned? *America Surgeon*, *78*(6), 716–721.

Lee, K. G. (2015). Medline plus: Gastroschisis, accessed 23 February 2015, <www.nlm.nih.gov/medlineplus/ency/article/000992.htm>.

Leung, A. K. & Robson, W. L. (2007). Acute gastroenteritis in children: Role of anti-emetic medication for gastroenteritis-related vomiting. *Paediatric Drugs*, *9*(3), 175–184.

Lewin, L. C. (2007). Sexually transmitted infections in preadolescent children. *Journal of Pediatric Health Care*, *21*(3), 153–161.

McFarland, L. V. (2010). Probiotics and diarrhea. *Annals of Nutrition and Metabolism*, *57*(Suppl. 1), 10–11.

McKenna, L. & Mirkov, S. (2014). *McKenna's Drug Handbook for Nursing and Midwifery* (7th ed.). Sydney: Lippincott Williams & Wilkins.

McQuaid, K. R. (2009). Gastroenterology. In S. J. McPhee & M. A. Papadakis (Eds). *Current Medical Diagnosis and Treatment.* Columbus, OH: McGraw-Hill.

Mouzaki, M. & Ng, V. L. (2010). Acute liver failure in children. *Clinical Pediatric Emergency Medicine, 11*(3), 198–206.

Ogle, J. W. & Anderson, M. S. (2008). Infections: Bacterial and spirochetal. In W. W. Hay et al. (Eds). *Current Pediatric Diagnosis and Treatment* (18th ed.). Columbus, OH: McGraw-Hill.

Oldham, K. T. & Aiken, J. J. (2007). Congenital pyloric stenosis and duodenal obstruction. In J. E. Fischer (Ed). *Mastery of Surgery.* Philadelphia: Lippincott Williams & Wilkins.

Pakarinen, M. P., Kurvinen, A., Koivusalo, A. I., et al. (2013). Surgical treatment and outcomes of severe pediatric intestinal motility disorders requiring parenteral nutrition. *Journal of Pediatric Surgery, 48*(2), 333–338.

Porth, C. M. (2011). Gastrointestinal & hepatobiliary function. In C. M. Porth (Ed.), *Essentials of Pathophysiology* (3rd ed.). Philadelphia: Lippincott Williams & Wilkins.

Rabin, R. F. (2011). Gastroenterology. In M. M. Tschudy & K. M. Arcara (Eds), *The Harriet Lane Handbook* (19th ed.), pp. 293–308. Philadelphia: Elsevier Mosby.

Reading, R. (2007). Clinical review: chronic constipation in children. *Child: Care, Health and Development, 33*(3), 350–351.

Rimon, A. & Freedman, S. B. (2010). Recent advances in the treatment of gastroenteritis. *Clinical Pediatric Emergency Medicine, 11*(3), 163–170.

Rolfes, S. R., Pinna, K. & Whitney, E. N. (2009). *Understanding Normal and Clinical Nutrition.* New York: Wadsworth/Cengage Learning.

Sauerland, S., Lefering, R. & Neugebauer, E.A.M. (2009). Laparoscopic versus open surgery for suspected appendicitis. *Cochrane Database of Systematic Reviews,* (1), (CD001546).

Sirinavin, S. & Garner, P. (2009). Antibiotics for treating salmonella gut infections. *Cochrane Database of Systematic Reviews,* (1), (CD001167).

Smith, S. (2011). Infectious diseases. In K. J. Marcdante, R. M. Kliegman, H. B. Jenson, et al. (Eds.), *Nelson Essentials of Pediatrics* (6th ed.). Philadelphia: Saunders/Elsevier.

Soares-Weiser, K., et al. (2009). Rotavirus vaccine for preventing diarrhoea. *Cochrane Database of Systematic Reviews,* (1), (CD002848).

Sundaram, S., Hoffenberg, E., Kramer, R., et al. (2011). Gastrointestinal tract. In W. W. Hay et al. (Eds.), *Current Diagnosis & Treatment Pediatrics* (21st ed.). New York: McGraw-Hill/Lange.

Tan, J. & Lok, A.S.F. (2007). Update on viral hepatitis. *Current Opinion in Gastroenterology, 23*(3), 263–267.

The Royal Children's Hospital Melbourne. (2013). Clinical guidelines (nursing): Parenteral nutrition PN, accessed 23 February 2015, <www.rch.org.au/rchcpg/hospital_clinical_guideline_index/Parenteral_Nutrition_PN>.

Walter, A. & Isolauri, E. (2007). Understanding the use of probiotics in pediatric populations. *Contemporary Pediatrics, 24*(5), 1–6.

Wang, D. H. & Souza, R. F. (2011). Biology of Barrett's esophagus and esophageal adenocarcinoma. *Gastrointestional Endoscopy Clinics of North America, 21*(1), 25–38.

Wiskin, A. E., Wootton, S. A. & Beattie, R. M. (2007). Nutrition issues in pediatric Crohn's disease. *Nutrition in Clinical Practice, 22*(2), 214–222.

Suggested readings

Aworanti, O. M., et al. (2012). Comparative review of functional outcomes post surgery for Hirschsprung's disease utilizing the paediatric incontinence and constipation scoring system. *Pediatric Surgery International, 28*(11), 1071–1078.

El-Radhi, A. S. (2015). Management of abdominal pain in children. *British Journal of Nursing, 24*(1), 44–47.

Halber, K. L. (2011). Nissen vs. Toupet fundoplication in the treatment of gastroesophageal reflux disease. *Pediatric Nursing, 37*(4), 171–174.

Rollins, H., Arnold-Jellis, J., & Taylor, A. (2012). How accurate are X-rays to check NG tube positioning? *Nursing Times, 108*(42), 14–16.

van Tilburg, M.A.L. & Murphy, T. B. (2015). Quality of life paradox in gastrointestinal disorders. *Journal of Pediatrics, 166*(1), 11–14.

Chapter 46

Nursing care of a family when a child has a renal or urinary tract disorder

LEARNING OBJECTIVES

After studying the contents of this chapter, you should be able to:

1. Describe common renal and urinary disorders that occur in children.
2. Describe methods for making nursing care of the child with a renal or urinary disorder more family-centred.
3. Assess a child for a renal or urinary tract disorder.
4. Formulate nursing considerations related to renal or urinary disorders in children.
5. Establish expected outcomes for a child with a renal or urinary disorder.
6. Plan nursing care related to urinary or renal disorders in children.
7. Discuss nursing care for a child with a renal or urinary disorder such as preparing a child for peritoneal dialysis.
8. Evaluate expected outcomes for achievement and effectiveness of care.
9. Integrate knowledge of renal and urinary tract disorders with the nursing process to achieve quality child and family health nursing care.

KEY TERMS

- Alport's syndrome
- azotaemia
- dialysis
- enuresis
- epispadias
- exstrophy of the bladder
- glomerular filtration rate
- glomerulonephritis
- hydronephrosis
- hypospadias
- nephrosis
- patent urachus
- polycystic kidney
- postural proteinuria
- prune belly syndrome
- vesicoureteral reflux

CASE STUDY

Emily Smith is a 4-year-old girl admitted to the hospital with nephrotic syndrome. She has marked ascites and oedema. "I kept asking everyone why she was gaining so much weight when she doesn't eat anything", her grandmother tells you. "My daughter said this happened because she drank part of a beer I left on the coffee table. Do you think that's what caused it? What if she needs a kidney transplant? Will I be allowed to give a kidney to her?"

CASE STUDY QUESTIONS

1. How would you answer Emily's grandmother?
2. What information does she need to better understand her grandchild's condition?

Normally, the urinary system maintains the proper balance of fluid (water) and electrolytes in the blood. When disease occurs, such as with structural abnormalities or kidney malfunction, children may be left with excessive amounts of fluid in the body or with an imbalance of electrolytes essential to their body's functioning. Disorders involving the kidneys and urinary tract often are long term. Urinary tract disorders can ultimately (if not originally) affect the kidneys, resulting in kidney dysfunction, with potentially fatal consequences ((Martini, Nath & Bartholomew, 2015).

Unfortunately, because symptoms may be vague, or because a child or parents do not realise the seriousness of urinary disease or are embarrassed by discussing it (either for cultural, religious or personal reasons), children may not be evaluated at the first sign of illness. Health education to increase the awareness of the symptoms of urinary tract and kidney disorders is an important area of family health teaching.

CARE OF A CHILD WITH A RENAL OR URINARY TRACT DISORDER

Assessment

Because the symptoms of many urinary tract and renal disorders are subtle such as mild abdominal pain, slowly increasing oedema, or low-grade fever, parents may not bring their child for evaluation early in the disease. A hallmark of kidney or bladder infection is pain. If children have had bladder surgery, they also may experience pain on urination or pain from bladder spasms. Be sure to assess the degree of any pain, including its location and intensity, before administering an analgesic or antispasmodic. Urine specimens also provide valuable assessment information.

Nursing considerations

Nursing considerations used with children with urinary tract or renal disorders are related to the symptoms these disorders cause. Some examples are:

- Pain related to bladder irritation from urinary tract infection
- Excess fluid volume related to decreased kidney function and fluid accumulation
- Fear related to as yet unknown outcome of kidney transplant
- Imbalanced nutrition related to effects of dietary restrictions

- Social isolation related to immunosuppressant therapy
- Risk of injury related to body's inability to excrete waste products properly.

Because the entire family becomes involved in long-term renal disease, other appropriate nursing diagnoses might include:

- Interrupted family processes related to the effects and stresses of child's chronic illness
- Compromised family coping related to the chronic nature of child's illness.

Be certain that outcomes established for care are relevant to a child's age, condition and cultural background and beliefs. Renal disease may become chronic, expected outcomes may need to be modified frequently to meet changing needs. Nursing care considerations must also include cultural awareness and culturally appropriate care—families from different cultural groups and backgrounds may not always respond to "European" standards of care. Carers should also consider a possible language barrier. For example, there are many different Indigenous dialects and many Indigenous Australians and Māoris have English as a second or third language.

Planning for a child with a urinary tract or renal disorder often involves helping parents remember to give medicine. A child with nephrotic syndrome or a renal transplant, for example, may take three or four different types of medicine every day at home. Ensure parents have a sound understanding of action and regimen needs. Ensure parents and the child are educated regarding the importance of their medications. School-aged children may need altered regimens outside school hours. If a child has severe renal impairment, parents may be asked to make decisions regarding kidney removal and transplantation. Helping parents to schedule times for haemodialysis or peritoneal dialysis or to supervise cyclic/automated peritoneal dialysis (CPD/APD), to care for their other children and to provide a life apart from their child requires nursing planning.

Many children with kidney disease take a corticosteroid for immunosuppression and so develop a typical cushingoid (typically "moon" faced) appearance. They may have oedema or ascites, which makes them appear obese. A child may be teased or criticised by others because of this "different" appearance. If kidney damage is extensive and the child's kidneys fail or a transplant is rejected, nursing care needs to be refocused on helping the family to face the possibility of the child's terminal illness

Children with urinary or renal disease often need follow-up care after their acute illness. Because they are followed by a specialty renal group or clinic, parents may assume that routine health maintenance care is being given as well. Check to see that children are receiving routine childhood immunisations (remember that children taking steroid or other immunosuppressive therapy should not receive live virus immunisations) and that parents have their questions about day-to-day childrearing concerns answered.

Nursing care should also include the family's ability to attend follow-up appointments. Where families live in rural and isolated areas, distance and socioeconomic issues may hinder/increase non-compliance with follow-up.

ANATOMY AND PHYSIOLOGY OF THE KIDNEYS

Embryonic development of the urinary tract is discussed in Chapter 9. Figure 46.1 identifies the structures of the tract while the function of the kidney is summarised in Table 46.1.

Urine production

The amount of urine excreted in a 24-hour period depends on fluid intake, kidney health and age. Approximate urine output from different age groups is shown in Table 46.2. A significant decrease in urine production is *oliguria;* absence of urine production is *anuria.*

When renal disease occurs and glomerular or tubular function becomes impaired, non-protein nitrogenous substances such as creatinine, urea, ammonia and purine bodies are retained in the blood rather than being excreted.

TABLE 46.1 Functions of the nephron

Site	Activity
Glomerulus	Secretion of water and all solutes except protein from blood
Proximal convoluted tubule	Reabsorption of 80% of glomerular filtrated water, all of glucose, amino acids, vitamins and proteins; most of sodium, chloride, and ascorbic acid; secretion of creatinine
Descending and ascending loop of Henle	Reabsorption of additional water; fluid becomes neutral in reaction; specific gravity 1.010; additional reabsorption of sodium and chloride
Distal convoluted tubule	Reabsorption of water, sodium, chloride, phosphate and sulfate as needed; secretion of potassium, H^+ ions, and ammonia (secretion of $NH4^+$ and H^+ ions conserves base because H^+ ions are substituted for sodium ions; sodium is reabsorbed as sodium bicarbonate)

TABLE 46.2 Child's average urine output in 24 hours

Age	Amount of urine (mL)
6 months–2 years	540–600
2–5 years	500–780
5–8 years	600–1200
8–14 years	1000–1500
Over 14 years	1500

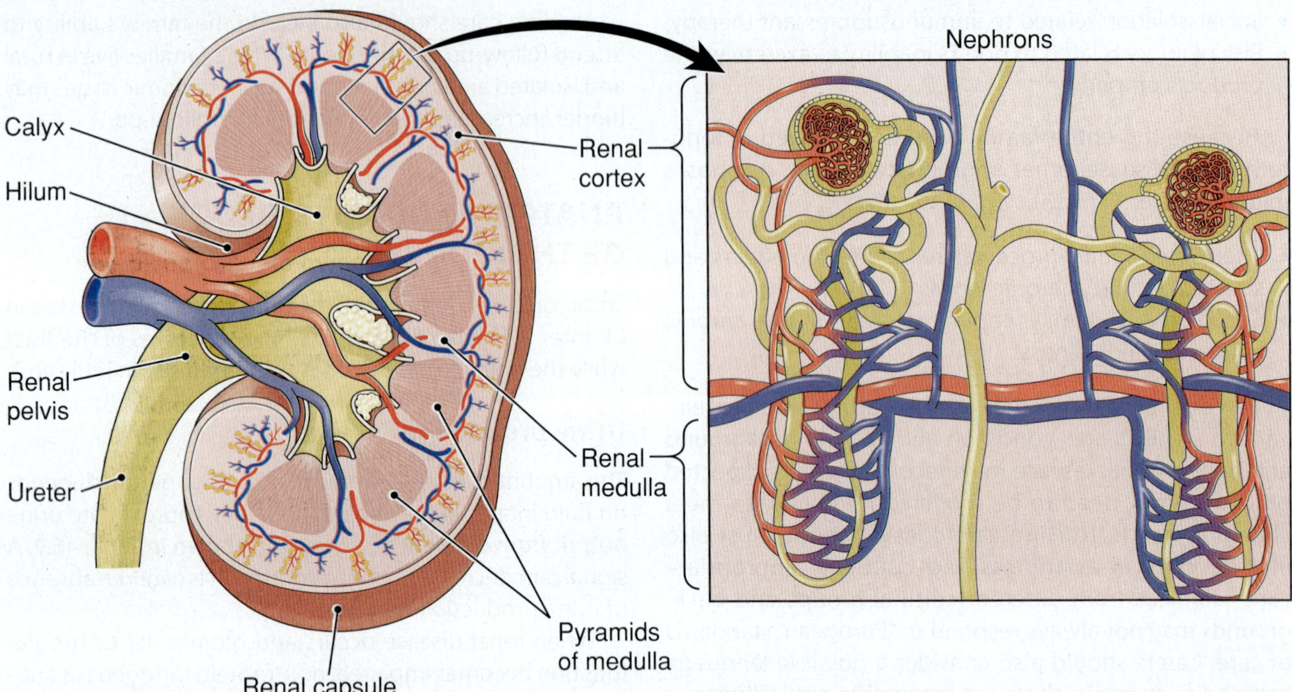

FIGURE 46.1 Longitudinal section through the kidney. Its internal structure is shown (left), along with an enlarged diagram of nephrons (right). Each kidney contains more than 1 million nephrons (Cohen, B. J. & Taylor, J. J. (2009). *Memmler's the Human Body in Health and Disease* (11th ed.). Baltimore: Wolters Kluwer Health.)

Urea is formed from the breakdown of amino acids by the liver. The amount of urea in urine is an indirect indication of kidney and liver function.

ASSESSMENT OF RENAL AND URINARY TRACT DYSFUNCTION

Assessment of urinary or renal tract disorders is based on the history, physical examination and laboratory/diagnostic tests (see Box 46.1).

Laboratory/diagnostic tests

Urinalysis

One of the most revealing tests of kidney function is also one of the simplest: urinalysis. For best results, specimens collected should be fresh because urine that stands at room temperature for any length of time changes composition. A chemical reagent strip can be used to detect glucose, protein and occult blood, and to measure pH. Normal constituents of urine are shown in Table 46.3.

Creatinine clearance rate

The **glomerular filtration rate** is the rate at which substances are filtered from the blood to the urine. It is measured by the amount of creatinine (the breakdown product of creatine from muscle contraction) excreted in 24 hours as determined by a 24-hour urine sample. A venous blood sample is taken during the 24-hour period and compared with the urine findings (if urine creatinine is decreased,

BOX 46.1 Assessment ✻ Assessing a child for renal and urinary tract dysfunction

History

Chief concern: Child reports burning or cries on urination; bloody or "dark" urine, frequency of urination; abdominal pain, flank pain, enuresis. Parents report increase in size of abdomen, periorbital oedema, poor appetite, frequent thirst, weight gain, strong odour to urine; nappy rash in infants. A school-aged child may be described as a behaviour problem because he or she frequently asks to use the bathroom.

Family history: History of renal disease, such as polycystic kidney, enuresis; hypertension.

Pregnancy history: Exposure to nephrotoxic drugs (antibiotics) during pregnancy. Oligohydramnios at birth.

Past illness history: Child recently had a throat or skin infection.

Physical assessment

General appearance
Fatigue, paleness
Growth restriction
Low-grade temperature

Mouth
Pale mucous membrane, caries

Cardiovascular
Hypertension

Respiratory
Rapid respirations

Back
Pain over kidney area

Genitals
Reddened urethra
Nappy area rash in infants
Round urethra in males
Constant dripping of urine
A stronger than usual arc of urine in males
Displaced urethral opening

Skin
Poor skin turgor
White crystals on skin
Oedema

Head
Swelling around eyes
Odd facies; beaklike nose, small chin, prominent epicanthal folds, low-set ears

Chest
Gynaecomastia

Abdomen
Tenderness over bladder area
Abdominal mass
Slack abdominal muscles
Protuberant abdomen

Extremities
Bowed legs

Neurological
Confusion, muscle twitching

TABLE 46.3 Characteristics of urine

Assessment	Normal finding	Description/implications
Colour	Pale yellow	Colour is influenced by urine concentration and ingredients; if fresh blood is present, urine may be red; if old blood, it may be brown or black.
Appearance	Clear	Bacteria, excessive crystals, or cells cause cloudiness; if protein content is high, it foams like beer when it is poured.
pH	4.6–8.0	Urine becomes alkaline (pH more than 7) with urinary tract infection or severe alkalosis; urine left at room temperature also becomes alkaline.
Specific gravity	1.003–1.030	Specific gravity is elevated in dehydration as kidneys try to conserve fluid and decreased in overhydration as they try to rid the body of fluid.
Protein	0	Due to inflammation, protein molecules pass into urine; in adolescent girls, protein in urine may occur as a result of pregnancy; some children have orthostatic proteinuria, slight to mild proteinuria occurring only when they are standing.
Ketones	0	Ketones are released after breakdown of body protein, because of starvation.
Glucose	0	Glucose in urine occurs most frequently as a symptom of diabetes mellitus; in adolescent girls, glucosuria may occur with pregnancy.
Red blood cells	Less than 1 per high-power field Negative on dipstick	Blood may be present in urine as a result of such diseases as glomerulonephritis, urinary tract infection, or trauma; may also suggest systemic diseases such as leukaemia or blood dyscrasias.
White blood cells	Less than 5 per high-power field	White blood cells are round, small configurations on a microscopic slide; they are present with bacteriuria.
Casts	0	Casts (protein configurations) are found most often in concentrated urine specimens; with cast formation, there is invariably proteinuria; casts comprise red blood cells, white blood cells or desquamated renal epithelium; as an epithelial cast moves along the nephron, the cells begin to disintegrate, leaving a coarse granular cast; some disintegrate still further to become fine granular casts. The last stage of the process is a configuration in the shape of the tubule, termed a waxy cast (translucent and may be shiny and reflect light). The stage of the cast is important in indicating the flow of urine through the kidney. Hyaline casts are formations of protein appearing dull and reflecting light poorly; fatty casts are casts caused by the degeneration of tubular epithelial cells and are found in children with nephrosis. Red blood cells, white blood cells and fatty casts are evidence of disease; other casts suggest urine stasis and probably proteinuria.
Crystals	Possibly present or not	Crystal formation is possibly an indication of urine pH; uric acid, cystine and calcium oxalate crystals are examples of crystals found in acid urine; phosphate crystals tend to be present in alkaline urine. Infection (particularly Proteus infection) is the most usual cause of alkaline urine. Sulfur crystals may be present if the child is receiving a sulfa drug (such as sulfamethoxazole).

this will be increased). A normal creatinine clearance rate is 100 mL/min. A normal urine creatinine level is 0.7 to 1.5 mg/100 umoL; creatinine in blood serum rarely exceeds 1 mg/umoL (Huether & McCance, 2013).

Radioisotope scanning

The administration of radioisotopes is a second way to assess glomeruli filtration ability. Radioactively tagged substances are given intravenously (IV); the rate at which these substances can be observed flowing through the kidney and excreted in urine is then determined. The level of radioisotopes used in these studies is small and easily excreted in urine afterwards. Children do not remain radioactive, so parents should not be afraid to stay near them or to hold them after such a study.

Urine culture

A urinary tract infection (UTI), the presence of bacteria in urine, is diagnosed by a urine culture. Bladder catheterisation can introduce bacteria into the bladder and also is painful and intrusive. Most urine specimens in children are obtained by a clean-catch procedure or sterile suprapubic aspiration.

Blood studies

A blood urea nitrogen (BUN) test measures the level of urea in blood and is used to assess glomerular function. However, this level may not increase until approximately 50% of glomeruli are destroyed, because the remaining glomeruli can increase in size and function to accommodate urine production. A normal value is 5 to 20 mg/100 umoL.

Ultrasonography and magnetic resonance imaging

An *ultrasound* or *magnetic resonance imaging* (MRI) scan can detect differing sizes of kidneys or ureters and can differentiate between solid or cystic kidney masses. They do not involve x-rays and so may be repeated at frequent intervals for follow-up without danger of radiation exposure (Nelson et al., 2012). Sedation may need to be considered to enable the child to lay still for the length of the MRI scan.

Computed tomography

Computed tomography (CT) scans of the kidneys are used to show the size and density of kidney structures and adequacy of urine flow. Conscious sedation may be needed to assist the child to lie still and decrease confinement anxiety caused by the enclosure of the CT machine. A contrast medium may be injected before the procedure to better outline urine flow. If this medium is iodine-based, be certain to ask about allergy to iodine before the study. A support person is not allowed to remain in the room during the procedure. Thoroughly prepare children so they can comfortably remain still for the procedure.

X-ray studies

An x-ray film can provide information about the size and contour of the kidneys. This x-ray may be referred to as a *KUB* (*k*idney, *u*reters and *b*ladder). A small kidney shown this way is generally a hypoplastic or an underdeveloped organ. A large kidney may indicate hydronephrosis or a polycystic kidney.

Intravenous pyelogram

An *intravenous pyelogram* (IVP) is an x-ray study of the upper urinary tract. However MRI and CT are now more conclusive tests. For an IVP, a radio-opaque dye is injected into a peripheral vein, circulates through the bloodstream, and is almost immediately identified as a foreign substance by the kidney and filtered out into the urine by the glomeruli. X-ray films taken at frequent intervals show the outline of collecting systems in the kidney and of the ureters as the radio-opaque dye passes through them.

In preparing children for an IVP, tell them that they will receive an injection and will need to lie still during the procedure. This may be difficult for young children due to the hard cold surface and intimidating x-ray camera overhead. Caution children that they may experience flushing of the face, warmth and a salty taste in their mouth after the injection of medicine. The dye used is iodine-based, ask the parents if the child has a known allergy to iodine. This is rarely known in children because they may have had no previous studies of this kind. Adequate hydration is required after this procedure as the radio-opaque dye is nephrotoxic.

Voiding cystourethrogram

A *voiding cystourethrogram* (VCUG), a study of the lower urinary tract, reveals the structure of the urethra and bladder and the presence of reflux into the ureters) (Bogaert & Slabbaert, 2012). After bladder catheterisation, a radio-opaque dye is injected into the bladder and the catheter is then removed. The child is asked to void into a bedpan while serial x-ray films are taken. Although the catheterisation is unpleasant and the first void may be slightly painful children may find the need to void while being x-rayed the most stressful aspect of the procedure.

A VCUG should not be done if a child has an active UTI as there is a danger that the radio-opaque material injected into the bladder could spread, carrying bacteria from the infection into the ureters and kidneys. Report any symptoms of UTI such as frequency, pain on voiding or low back pain to the radiographer. A clean-catch urine specimen for culture may be ordered before the VCUG to rule out infection.

Cystoscopy

Cystoscopy, examination of the bladder and ureter openings by direct examination with a cystoscope introduced through the urethra, is done to diagnose possible reflux or stenosis. Radio-opaque dye may be introduced into the bladder at the time of cystoscopy so the bladder can be visualised on radiography (cystography). The procedure is painful and requires a child to lie still, so it is usually done under conscious sedation. After the procedure, the first voiding may be painful. Once allowed, urge children to drink plenty of fluids so they urinate frequently to flush out any pathogens introduced at the time of the procedure.

Renal biopsy

Renal biopsy involves passing a thin biopsy needle into the kidney through the skin over the kidney. The procedure is used to diagnose the condition and extent of renal disease to thereby predict disease outcome or progress or reveal the beginning of rejection of a transplanted kidney (Tse et al., 2013). Sedation with or without intubation may be required for the child as it is necessary to lie still while the biopsy specimen is taken. A support person for the child may be required prior, during or after the procedure depending on the situation.

Post biopsy, a sterile gauze square is applied over the biopsy site for 5–10 minutes to assist clot formation. A pressure dressing is then applied and remains intact for 24 hours. Parental education is required regarding the amount of tissue removed (lumen needle length), which is not reflective of dressing size.

The child is instructed to remain flat for 4 hours after the procedure. For the following 2 hours they are then encouraged to progress slowly from lying to sitting to standing and mobilising. During this time vitals and the biopsy site are monitored, generally every 15 minutes for at least the first hour then hourly until discharge. Urine output is monitored for signs of haematuria from the time of admission and parental instruction is given to continue this for a minimum of 24 hours after discharge. Fluid intake is encouraged to sustain filtration within the tubules. If there is an absence of complications discharge is generally 6 hours after the procedure. The child is instructed to refrain from any activities that require exertion for a period of 7 days. A haematocrit may be ordered 24 hours after the procedure to ensure that no bleeding is continuing.

STRUCTURAL ABNORMALITIES OF THE URINARY TRACT

Because the urinary tract is a system of hollow tubes, congenital disorders can arise from faulty recanalisation in intrauterine life.

Patent urachus

When the bladder first forms in utero, it is joined to the umbilicus by a narrow tube, the *urachus*. When this fails to close properly during embryological development, a fistula is left between the bladder and umbilicus **(patent urachus)**. This occurs more commonly in males than in females. Nurses are frequently the ones to discover this condition as they notice clear fluid draining from the base of the umbilical cord while changing a newborn's nappy. If you test the fluid with Nitrazine paper for pH, its acid content will identify it as urine. An ultrasound will confirm the patent connection. A few patent urachus abnormalities heal spontaneously, but most require surgical correction to prevent pathogens from entering the fistula site and causing persistent bladder infection. This is done in the immediate neonatal period using only a small subumbilical incision (Tsai & Yeh, 2011).

Exstrophy of the bladder

Exstrophy of the bladder is a midline closure defect that occurs during the embryonic period of gestation (first 8 weeks). As a result, the bladder lies open and exposed on the abdomen. It occurs more frequently in males than females at a ratio of 2:1 (Mahan, 2011).

Hypospadias

Hypospadias is a urethral defect in which the urethral opening is not at the end of the penis but on the ventral (lower) aspect of the penis. The meatus may be near the glans, midway back or at the base of the penis. This anomaly occurs in approximately 1 in 300 male neonates. It tends to be familial or may occur from a multifactorial genetic focus. **Epispadias** is a similar defect in which the opening is on the dorsal surface of the penis; this is corrected the same way.

Children with hypospadias should not be circumcised as the surgeon may wish to use a portion of the foreskin for the repair. In the newborn, a *meatotomy*—a surgical procedure in which the urethra is extended to a normal position—may be performed to establish better urinary function. If the repair will be extensive, surgery may be delayed until the child is 3 to 4 years of age.

INFECTIONS OF THE URINARY SYSTEM AND RELATED DISORDERS

As the urinary system drains to the outside of the body, infection can easily spread to the bladder or kidneys.

Urinary tract infection

UTI occurs more often in females than in males at a rate of about 8–2% (Lum, 2014). Pathogens appear to enter the urinary tract most often as an ascending infection from the perineum. UTIs are a common consequence of nosocomial or healthcare-acquired infections in children with urinary catheters.

UTIs tend to occur more often in girls than in boys because the urethra is shorter in girls and it is located close to the vagina (allowing the spread of vulvovaginitis) and close to the anus, from which *E. coli* spreads. Changing nappies frequently can help reduce the risk of infection in infants. Teach girls to wipe themselves from front to back to avoid contaminating the urethra. Products such as bubble bath, feminine hygiene sprays and spas possibly increase the incidence of UTI in girls so use of these should be discouraged or minimised (Gaylord & Peterson-Smith, 2012). Infection also often occurs after sexual intercourse. Teach both adolescent males and females to void after sexual intercourse.

UTIs need vigorous treatment in childhood so they do not spread to involve the kidneys (pyelonephritis). Girls who have more than three UTIs or boys with their first UTI should be referred to an urologist to determine whether they have a congenital anomaly such as urethral stenosis or bladder–ureter reflux that causes recurrent urinary stasis. A secondary problem is more likely in boys with a UTI.

Although it may be possible to diagnose a UTI precisely as urethritis, cystitis, ureteritis or pyelonephritis, the signs and symptoms in young children often are not clear-cut. When the exact location or extent of the infection is unknown, it is referred to simply as a UTI. The typical symptoms that occur in older children or in adults—pain on urination, frequency, burning and haematuria—may not be present. If the infection is confined to the bladder (cystitis), the child may have a low-grade fever, mild abdominal pain and enuresis (bedwetting). If the infection is a pyelonephritis, the symptoms generally are more acute, with high fever, abdominal or flank pain, vomiting and malaise. Any child with a fever and no demonstrable cause on physical examination should be evaluated for UTI (Jadresic, 2014).

Urine for culture can be collected by a clean-catch technique, suprapubic aspiration or catheterisation, so that bacteria from the vulva or foreskin do not contaminate the sample and give a false reading. Suprapubic aspiration is generally limited to infants because the sight of the syringe is so frightening for older children and the procedure can introduce infection. The use of catheterisation, also frightening and a potential source of infection, is limited in children of all ages.

The medical treatment for UTI is oral antibiotics specific to the causative organism that is cultured (Paintsil, 2013). In addition to the antibiotics, oral fluid intake is encouraged to "flush" the infection out of the urinary tract. Cranberry juice is often recommended as being highly effective in acidifying urine and making it more resistant to bacterial growth. However in actual practice, there is little proof of its effectiveness. A mild analgesic may help reduce pain enough to allow voiding.

A repeat clean-catch urine sample is usually obtained after 72 hours to assess the effectiveness of the antibiotic treatment. After antibiotic therapy is stopped, it is helpful if parents obtain another clean-catch urine specimen to be tested to prove that bacteria are not still present. After recurrent UTIs, children may be prescribed a prophylactic antibiotic for 6 months.

"Honeymoon" cystitis

Honeymoon cystitis refers to lower UTI in women after they initiate a first sexual relationship. Such infections occur in connection with the local irritation and inflammation caused by initial coitus. Antibiotic therapy may be effective and voiding after coitus may help to flush pathogenic organisms from the urethra and prevent such infections. Educate about UTI prevention, sexually-transmitted infections and reproductive planning if indicated. Recurrent UTIs in a school-aged or preschool girl may suggest sexual abuse.

Vesicoureteral reflux

Normally, urine flows from the ureters into the bladder, with almost no flow re-entering the ureters from the bladder. **Vesicoureteral reflux (VUR)** refers to retrograde flow of urine from the bladder into the ureters (Tullus, 2015). This reflux occurs because the valve that guards the entrance from the bladder to the ureter is defective (either from birth or scarring from repeated UTIs), bladder pressure that is stronger than usual, or ureters that are implanted at abnormal sites or angles. This backflow of urine happens at micturition (voiding) when the bladder contracts (see Fig. 46.2).

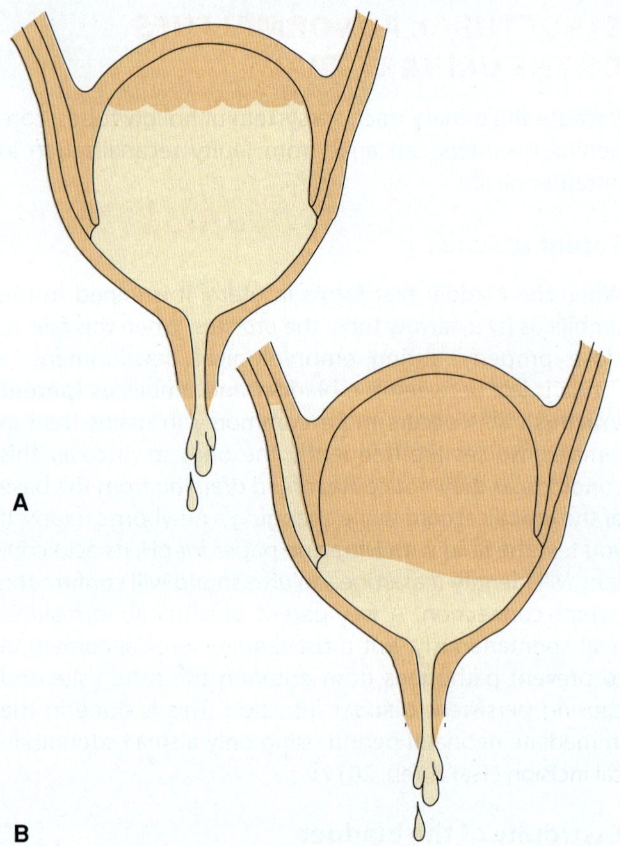

FIGURE 46.2 Vesicoureteral reflux. (**A**) Normal voiding pattern. (**B**) Reflux into ureters with voiding.

Reflux leads to bladder infection because urine is retained in the ureters after voiding and stasis of any fluid is subject to infection. It also appears that the capacity for normal bladder tissue to lyse bacteria becomes reduced due to the large residual urine volume that is always present. In addition, reflux is a potentially serious condition because it can lead to back-pressure on the kidneys, possibly leading to nephron destruction and subsequently hydronephrosis or dilation of the renal pelvis. As it is prone to appear in families, it is most likely a heterogeneous gene disorder (Hunziker & Puri, 2012).

A child with reflux usually has a history of repeated UTIs. In younger/smaller children recurrent otitis media or failure to thrive may delay (or mask) a diagnosis of VUR (Bogaert & Slabbaert, 2012). A voiding cystourethrogram, CT scan, cystoscopy, or cystography with contrast will show the ureteral reflux. Based on diagnostic studies, reflux is graded from I to V by degree of reflux, with V being the most serious.

The majority of instances of vesicoureteral reflux resolve with maturity without a need for surgery. However, the condition must be rigorously treated to decrease the possibility of glomerular scarring from infection or back-pressure. Teaching double voiding (having the child void, then a few minutes later attempting to void again) may help to empty the bladder and prevent recurrent infection from urinary stasis. Long-term maintenance with antibiotics may be as effective as surgery in reducing renal scarring from recurrent UTI in lower grades of reflux; however, in recent studies, the prophylatic use of antibiotics has come under some scrutiny as to advantages of their usage (Bogaert & Slabbaert, 2012).

If continuous antibiotic therapy does not prevent recurrent UTIs, reflux can be corrected by cystoscopy. Laparoscopic surgery may be needed to correct the placement of ureters at a more oblique angle, creating the usual valve effect.

After surgery, a suprapubic catheter remains in place to keep the bladder empty and prevent pressure against the surgical area. Two ureteral catheters (stents) also exit at the suprapubic tube site into sterile collection bags. Sterile gauze dressings and antibiotic cream are placed around the tube insertion sites.

Preoperative education includes the explanation of the number and types of tubes inserted, principles of closed drainage systems and the need to keep these below the height of the bladder to prevent backflow. Encourage gentle postoperative ambulation as ordered.

Check catheter drainage tubes every hour for the first 24 hours and then at least every 4 hours. Record the colour and the amount of drainage (urine). Initially, drainage will be bloody, but will clear in 1 or 2 days. Assess drainage for clots (should not be over pinpoint in size). The stents should drain an equal amount, to ensure that kidney production is equal on both sides. Urine will drain primarily from the stents for approximately the first 3 days after surgery; thereafter, drainage will flow around the stents and will be mainly from the suprapubic tube.

Incisional pain and painful bladder spasms may occur for the first 3 days, so antispasmodics may be prescribed to reduce bladder spasm. Also, not touching or not moving the suprapubic tube helps to reduce spasms by limiting bladder irritation. The suprapubic tube is removed between 4 to 7 days after surgery. Remind the child and parents to avoid immersion in water until the suprapubic tube site has closed completely.

Hydronephrosis

Hydronephrosis is enlargement of the pelvis of the kidney with urine as a result of back-pressure in the ureter. The back-pressure is generally caused by obstruction, either of the ureter or of the point where the ureter joins the bladder, as with vesicoureteral reflux. Although this may occur at any age, it occurs most often in the first 6 months of life.

Children with hydronephrosis are usually asymptomatic. They may have repeated UTIs from urinary stasis. Elevated blood pressure caused by increasing tubular pressure may be detected on a routine health assessment. With severe back-pressure, the infant experiences flank or abdominal pain. Abdominal palpation may reveal an abdominal mass (the dilated kidney pelvis). An IVP or ultrasound will show the enlarged pelvis and the point of obstruction.

Hydronephrosis is a serious disorder because if the pressure in the pelvis becomes too acute, back-pressure on the kidney will interfere with tubular function or destroy the nephrons. The treatment is surgical correction of the obstruction before glomerular or tubular destruction occurs.

DISORDERS AFFECTING NORMAL URINARY ELIMINATION

Interference with urine elimination can arise from innocent conditions such as enuresis or extremely serious disorders such as kidney agenesis.

Enuresis

Enuresis is involuntary passage of urine past the age when a child should be expected to have attained bladder control (Fleming, 2012), which is usually age 2–3 years for daytime control and age 4 years for night-time control. Enuresis occurs at approximately 5–7 years of age. Enuresis occurring at night is termed nocturnal enuresis (NE) and during the day it is known as daytime incontinence (Harari, 2013). It is also known as primary if bladder training was never achieved, and acquired or secondary if control was established but has now been lost. Box 46.2 discusses the impact of enuresis on families. Treatment for NE may include a decrease in oral intake prior to bed-time, a bedwetting alarm or medication—predominantly desmopressin acetate (Harari, 2013; see Box 46.3).

BOX 46.2 ✻ Focus on evidence-based practice

Bedwetting (nocturnal enuresis)

The purpose of this study was to assess the effect of nocturnal enuresis on the quality of life of the mother. For the study, 60 women who reported that their child had nocturnal enuresis and 90 women whose child had no urinary symptoms were included. The women undertook a Short-Form Health Survey (SF-36) Questionnaire, Spielberg's State-Trait Anxiety Inventory (STAI) and the Beck Depression Inventory (BDI). All SF-36 subscales except social functioning were significantly lower in the mothers of children with nocturnal enuresis; and the trait-anxiety score (the subcomponent of the STAI) and the mean BDI score were both higher in the mothers of children with nocturnal enuresis. This study shows that the quality of life of the mother is negatively affected by having a child with nocturnal enuresis.

Suppose a parent tells you that her child has nocturnal enuresis but she knows it is only a stage of growth so she is not worried. Based on the above study, would you ask any further questions?

Source: Meydan, E. A., Civilibal, M. et al. (2012). The quality of life of mothers of children with monosymptomatic enuresis nocturna. *International Urology and Nephrology, 44*(3), 655–659.

BOX 46.3 ✻ Focus on pharmacology

Desmopressin acetate (DDAVP)

Classification: A synthetic form of human antidiuretic hormone

Action: Promotes reabsorption of water in the renal tubule or decreases bladder filling; drug of choice for enuresis (McKenna & Mirkov, 2014)

Pregnancy risk category: B2

Dosage: In children 6 years of age and older, 20 mg (0.2 mL) intranasally at bedtime, possibly increasing the dose up to 40 mg if necessary; or 0.2 mg orally at bedtime, titrated up to 0.6 mg to obtain the desired response

Possible adverse effects: Transient headache, nausea, flushing, mild abdominal cramps, fluid retention

Nursing implications

- Instruct parents and child that child should restrict fluid after dinnertime in addition to taking medication.
- If given intranasally, advise parents to refrigerate the solution.
- Teach parents and child the proper method for intranasal administration.
- Caution child and parents that nasal administration is less effective if the child develops a cold with draining rhinitis.

Postural (orthostatic) proteinuria

A few children will spill albumin into the urine when they stand upright for an extended period (**postural proteinuria**, also called postural albuminuria). The amount of spilling decreases when they rest in a supine position. Children with this condition have no apparent damage to glomeruli; the phenomenon is apparently attributable to the effect of gravity on glomerular function.

To determine whether postural proteinuria exists, urine is collected after the child has been recumbent during the night (a first-voided specimen) and then again after the child has been up and active for several hours. Make certain when collecting these urine specimens to record the child's activity accurately. If the child stood in a cot crying for a parent or was held in a nurse's lap for most of the night, the urine may show protein in the morning specimen because it is not truly a "resting specimen". Likewise, for the specimen to be collected after the child has been active, make certain that the child is up and active, not lying in a supine position for most of the time. Play a game if necessary, such as "follow the leader", so the child is active.

Postural proteinuria needs no therapy. However, be sure to document the condition because some of these children develop some form of kidney disorder later in life.

Kidney agenesis

Agenesis means lack of growth (literally, lack of a beginning) or that no organ formed in utero. Absence of kidneys in a newborn is suggested when the volume of amniotic fluid on ultrasound or at birth is less than normal (oligohydramnios). This occurs because urine normally adds to the volume of amniotic fluid in utero. The infant with kidney agenesis often has *Potter's syndrome* or accompanying misshapen, low-set ears and hypoplastic (stiff, inflexible) lungs from the lack of amniotic fluid in utero. Without kidneys, the fetus cannot void urine. Bilateral absence of kidneys is obviously incompatible with life unless a renal transplant can be accomplished, but the associated condition of non-functioning lungs makes a successful transplant highly unlikely.

Polycystic kidney

Polycystic kidney means that large, fluid-filled cysts have formed in place of normal kidney tissue. The most frequent type of polycystic kidney seen in children is inherited as an autosomal recessive trait. A more rare form is inherited as an autosomal dominant trait (Mahan, 2011). With either type, there is abnormal development of the collecting tubules. The kidneys are large and feel soft and spongy. If the disorder is bilateral, an infant will not pass urine. The mother will have had oligohydramnios during pregnancy. Children often have a typical appearance (*hypertelorism*—wide-spaced eyes, epicanthal folds, flattened nose; or *micrognathia*—small jaw) consistent with Potter's syndrome.

If the condition is unilateral, urine production will be decreased (oliguria), not absent. Because kidneys are difficult to locate in newborns, a unilateral polycystic kidney may be missed until later in life, when, with increased kidney growth, an abdominal mass can be palpated. The cystic growth offers such resistance to blood circulation that systemic hypertension often results by school age.

In many children, the liver is filled with identical cysts. This is most evident later in life when increased difficulty with portal circulation occurs (blood cannot perfuse the cystic liver structures either).

The treatment for polycystic formation is surgical removal of a kidney if only one is cystic. If both kidneys are cystic, treatment is renal transplant. This kidney disease is inherited, so parents, and children at adolescence, need genetic counselling to inform them that future children may also have this problem.

Renal hypoplasia

Hypoplasia means reduced growth. Hypoplastic kidneys contain fewer lobes than normal kidneys and are small and underdeveloped. The child with hypoplastic kidneys, in addition to having poor kidney function, may develop hypertension from stenosis of the renal arteries. If hypoplasia is bilateral, the child may need a kidney transplant in later life to maintain kidney function and prevent extreme hypertension.

Prune belly syndrome

Prune belly syndrome is severe urinary tract dilation that develops as early as intrauterine life from an unknown cause. Occurring mainly in boys, the severe dilation causes back-pressure and destruction of kidneys. The infant is born with oligohydramnios and pulmonary dysplasia because of the lack of amniotic fluid in utero (Hassett et al., 2012).

The condition is marked by the presence of three symptoms: deficiency of usual abdominal muscle tone, bilateral undescended testes, and the dilated faulty development of the bladder and upper urinary tract. The infant's abdomen appears wrinkled (like a prune) because of the poorly-developed abdominal muscles. Without surgical remodelling, the infant will develop repeated UTIs, leading to end-stage renal disease. Teach parents to protect their child's abdomen from trauma associated with lap belts or baby walkers because their child lacks abdominal support. Some children with the syndrome will require a renal transplant, due to end stage renal failure, most commonly as the result of chronic pyelonephritis, repeated UTI's (from incomplete bladder drainage) and obstructive nephropathy (Hassett et al., 2012).

Acute poststreptococcal glomerulonephritis

Glomerulonephritis, inflammation of the glomeruli of the kidney, may occur as a separate entity but usually occurs as an immune complex disease after infection with nephritogenic streptococci (most commonly subtypes of group A beta-haemolytic streptococci). Tissue damage occurs from a complement fixation reaction in the glomeruli.

Intravascular coagulation occurs in the minute renal vessels. Ischaemic damage leads to scarring and decreased glomerular function. This results in a reduction in the glomerular filtration rate, leading to an accumulation of sodium and water in the bloodstream. Inflammation of the glomeruli increases permeability, allowing protein molecules to escape into the filtrate.

Acute glomerulonephritis is most common between the ages of 5 and 10 years. It is more prevalent in boys than girls and occurs more often in winter and spring. The child typically has a history of a recent respiratory infection (within 7 to 14 days) or impetigo (within 3 weeks). In Indigenous children the most common skin infection is from scabies (Northern Territory Government, Department of Health and Families, 2010).

All children who have had a "strep" throat, tonsillitis, otitis media, or impetigo caused by streptococcal infection, ideally, should have a urinalysis 2 weeks after the infection to ensure that glomerulonephritis is not occurring.

Acute glomerulonephritis is characterised by a sudden onset of haematuria and proteinuria. The protein content both of individual urine specimens and of total 24-hour urine volume is measured.

The haematuria associated with acute glomerulonephritis is usually so extensive that the child's urine appears tea-coloured, reddish-brown or smoky. After these initial urine changes, the child develops oliguria. Specific gravity of urine is elevated. Hypertension from hypervolaemia occurs. The child may have abdominal pain, a low-grade fever, oedema, anorexia, vomiting or headache. There may be cardiac involvement related to fluid excess. Such children show signs of orthopnoea, cardiac enlargement, enlarged liver, pulmonary oedema and a galloping heart rhythm. Heart failure may occur from circulatory overload.

Blood analysis will show a lowered blood protein level (hypoalbuminaemia) caused by the massive proteinuria. Low serum complement will be present and, as the blood volume expands, a mild anaemia will also occur. As in all inflammatory diseases, the erythrocyte sedimentation rate will increase. Because the glomeruli cannot filter properly, concentrations of urea, non-protein nitrogen (BUN) and creatinine in blood will increase. If blood pressure reaches 160/100 mmHg as part of the acute process, encephalopathy may occur, with symptoms of headache, irritability, seizures, vomiting, coma or lethargy, and perhaps transitory paralysis. This extreme elevation in blood pressure is probably related to the expanded circulatory volume. The cerebral symptoms are caused by *cerebral ischaemia* (vasoconstriction of cerebral vessels to reduce cranial pressure).

The course of acute glomerulonephritis is 1 to 2 weeks. During this time, there is little therapy specific for the disorder. Antibiotics usually are ineffective and diuretics are of little value because obstructed glomeruli bases cannot be made to function. If heart failure occurs, specific measures such as placing the child in a semi-Fowler's position, digitalisation and oxygen administration may be necessary. If diastolic blood pressure rises to more than 90 mmHg, antihypertensive therapy with a calcium channel blocker may be necessary. Phosphate binders to reduce phosphate absorption in the GI tract, or a potassium-removing resin agent may be necessary in children who have rising phosphate and potassium levels.

Bedrest is unnecessary, although children should be encouraged to participate in quiet play activities. Normal activity may resume in 1 or 2 weeks, but competitive activity should be limited until kidney function has returned to normal.

Diet is controversial. Although limiting protein intake reduces the amount of protein lost in urine, many children who are losing large quantities of protein need high-protein diets to supplement this loss. Salt restriction may be needed to reduce severe oedema. Most do well on a normal diet. Daily weighing and calculating intake and output are important assessments to review the disease.

In most children, acute glomerulonephritis runs a limited, benign course. After most symptoms fade, proteinuria and impaired urea and creatinine clearance may remain for up to 2 months. Advise parents that the results of a urine protein test may remain abnormal for up to a year. A few children will not completely recover from acute glomerulonephritis but will develop chronic nephritis. These children appear to suffer destruction from the initial inflammation that results in chronic renal insufficiency.

IGA glomerulonephritis

Acute glomerulonephritis may occur when there is no evidence of a prior infection. In these children, immunoglobin A is elevated. The gross haematuria resolves within a few days and is not apt to produce serious sequelae. Because of the benign course of the illness, no therapy is indicated except for careful observation for more serious signs such as severe proteinuria, hypertension or renal insufficiency. If these symptoms occur, corticosteroids will halt the disease process.

✔ *Checkpoint question 46.1*

What is typically the first symptom of acute glomerulonephritis?

a. Low blood pressure from excessive aldosterone
b. "Old blood" in urine from kidney bleeding
c. Dependent oedema from protein accumulation
d. Pain on urination from urethra inflammation

Chronic glomerulonephritis

Although chronic glomerulonephritis occasionally follows acute glomerulonephritis or nephrotic syndrome, it also occurs as a primary disease. Proteinuria is found at a routine check-up plus hypertension and the presence of red cell or white cell casts and occult blood in urine. The specific gravity of the child's urine is below normal (below 1.003). Blood studies may indicate an increased BUN or creatinine level. A renal biopsy will show permanent destruction of glomeruli membranes.

Chronic glomerulonephritis may result in either diffuse or local nephron damage. The remaining functioning nephrons increase their glomerular filtration rate to compensate for those that are damaged. At some point in this chronic disease destruction process, however, compensatory mechanisms fail, and renal insufficiency or failure will result. **Alport's syndrome**, which also includes hearing loss and ocular changes, is a progressive chronic glomerulonephritis inherited as an X-linked or autosomal recessive disorder (Kruegel, Rubel & Gross, 2013).

During the illness, if the child has acute symptoms of oedema, haematuria, hypertension or oliguria, bedrest may be necessary. If children have only a chronic manifestation, such as proteinuria, and if they feel well, they can maintain normal activity, including attending school. Children should not engage in competitive activities such as contact sports, however, because of the risk of kidney injury.

Therapy is non-specific and directed at symptom relief rather than the disease process itself, because the cause of the disease is unknown. Therapy with antihypertensive medications or with diuretics to increase urine output may be necessary. Corticosteroid therapy may reduce or halt the progress of the disorder by reducing inflammation. Children have difficulty accepting long-term corticosteroid therapy because of the side effects, in particular a typical "moon face" and extra body hair (Cushing's syndrome). Children receiving corticosteroids are at an increased risk of infection because of the immunosuppressive activity of these medications. They need to be shielded from other children and healthcare personnel with infection. Parents need to learn to take their child's temperature and recognise and report the earliest signs of infection.

Generally, the prognosis for children with chronic glomerulonephritis is poor. Although the illness may run a long-term course, eventually it leads to renal insufficiency and renal failure. Children may be maintained for long periods by peritoneal dialysis or haemodialysis. Kidney transplant is a possibility.

Nephrotic syndrome (nephrosis)

Nephrosis, altered glomerular permeability due to fusion of the glomeruli membrane surfaces, causes abnormal loss of protein in urine. Immunological mechanisms are involved in instigating the process. The highest incidence is at 3 years of age and it occurs more often in boys than in girls (Mahan, 2011).

Nephrosis can be classified according to the amount of membrane destruction. Minimal change nephrotic syndrome (MCNS) is the type most often seen in children (80%). As the name implies, with this type, little scarring of glomeruli occurs. Children with this degree of scarring respond well to therapy. Other types are focal glomerulosclerosis (FGS) and membranoproliferative glomerulonephritis (MPGN). Both of these types involve scarring of glomeruli and both have a poorer response to therapy (Hahn et al., 2015).

The four characteristic symptoms of nephrotic syndrome are proteinuria, oedema, hypoalbuminaemia (low serum albumin level) and hyperlipidaemia (increased blood lipid level). Proteinuria occurs because increased glomerular permeability leads to protein loss in the urine and subsequently hypoalbuminaemia. With a low level of protein in the bloodstream, osmotic pressure causes fluid to shift from the bloodstream into interstitial tissue, causing oedema. As the blood volume decreases, the kidneys begin to conserve sodium and water, adding to the potential for oedema. The hyperlipidaemia occurs because the liver increases production of lipoproteins to try to compensate for protein loss. Lipids are too large to be lost in urine, so they rise to high levels in the blood serum. Some children have such high lipid levels that, when blood is drawn and placed into a test tube, a circle of white fat forms on the top of it. Figure 46.3 illustrates the process that leads to these common symptoms.

Symptoms usually begin insidiously. Children develop oedema around the eyes (periorbital oedema). Clothing may no longer fit a child around the waist, because oedematous fluid is beginning to collect in the abdominal cavity (ascites). As oedema progresses, the child's skin becomes pale, stretched and taut. In boys, scrotal oedema becomes extremely marked. Ascites may become so extensive that the resultant pressure on the stomach leads to anorexia or vomiting. Children may have diarrhoea caused by intestinal oedema and poor absorption by the oedematous membrane. Because of poor nutrition, growth may stop. The child may become malnourished and yet appear deceptively obese because of the extensive oedema. When the ascites become even more extensive, children may have difficulty breathing as the abdominal fluid presses

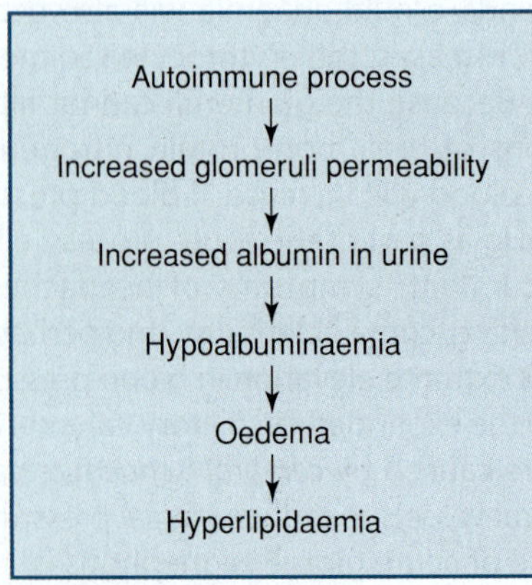

FIGURE 46.3 The process that results in the signs and symptoms of nephrotic syndrome.

TABLE 46.4 Comparison of features of acute glomerulonephritis and nephrotic syndrome

Factor	Acute glomerulonephritis	Nephrotic syndrome
Cause	Immune reaction to group A beta-haemolytic streptococcal infection	Idiopathic; possibly a hypersensitivity reaction
Onset	Abrupt	Insidious
Haematuria	Profuse	Rare
Oedema	Mild	Extreme
Hypertension	Marked	Mild
Hyperlipidaemia	Rare or mild	Marked
Peak age frequency	5–10 years	2–3 years
Interventions	Limited activity; antihypertensives as needed; symptomatic therapy for congestive heart failure	Corticosteroid administration; cyclophosphamide administration; possibly a diuretic and potassium supplement
Diet	Normal for age	High-protein, low-sodium diet
Prevention	Prevention or thorough treatment of group A beta-haemolytic streptococcal infections	None known

against the diaphragm, decreasing lung expansion. Parents report that children are irritable and fussy, probably from the feeling of abdominal fullness and generalised oedema. An increased risk of clotting can occur from the decreased intravascular fluid volume.

Laboratory studies will reveal marked proteinuria. The protein loss with nephrotic syndrome is almost entirely albumin, differentiating it from the proteinuria of glomerulonephritis. Some children with nephrotic syndrome exhibit haematuria at the onset, but it is minimal in contrast to that seen with acute glomerulonephritis. The erythrocyte sedimentation rate (demonstrating the inflammation of the glomeruli membrane) is elevated. Features of acute glomerulonephritis and nephrotic syndrome are compared in Table 46.4. A renal biopsy will show whether there is scarring of the glomerular membrane and document the type of nephrotic syndrome present.

Therapy aims to reduce the proteinuria and subsequently the oedema with a course of corticosteroids, keeping the child free of infection while the immune system is suppressed. An initial dose of prednisone is given until diuresis without protein loss is accomplished; the dosage is then reduced for maintenance and continued for as long as 1–2 months.

Instruct parents to test the first urine specimen of the day for protein with a chemical reagent strip and keep an accurate chart showing the pattern of protein loss. Approximately once a week, they are usually asked to collect a 24-hour urine specimen so total protein loss can be measured.

After the initial 4 weeks, prednisone is generally given every other day rather than every day. Prednisone has the potential to halt growth and to suppress adrenal gland secretion. However, growth is apparently not delayed when the medication is given on alternate days and there is less alteration of adrenal steroid production (McKenna & Mirkov, 2014). Prednisone tastes bitter, so parents may welcome suggestions regarding how to disguise the taste, such as mixing it with jam.

Be certain that both the parents and the child are aware that prednisone causes a cushingoid appearance or a "moon face", extra fat at the base of the neck and increased body hair. Advise parents prednisone cannot be stopped abruptly as it will lead to adrenal insufficiency. Diuretics are not commonly used to reduce the oedema because they tend to decrease blood volume, which is already decreased. This could lead to acute renal failure. Children who respond poorly to prednisone alone, however, may need diuretic therapy with a medication such as furosemide (Lasix). When children are taking furosemide for extended periods, there is always a danger that too much potassium will be excreted, causing hypokalaemia. Children on long-term diuretic therapy need frequent blood studies to determine that electrolyte levels, especially potassium, are adequate. Supplemental potassium may be needed and the children should eat foods high in potassium. IV albumin may be administered to temporarily correct hypoalbuminaemia. As the serum albumin level rises, fluid shifts from subcutaneous spaces into the bloodstream. Children are then administered a rapid-acting diuretic to remove the extra fluid. It is important that the diuretic be administered after the albumin infusion or the child could develop a fluid overload and subsequently heart failure.

Some children are prednisone resistant or do not respond to corticosteroid therapy and may require stronger medications—that is, a cytoxic agent or stronger immunosuppressive medications (Banaszak & Banaszak, 2012). It is important to ensure adequate fluid intake with these medications to prevent bladder irritation and bleeding.

The prognosis for children with nephrotic syndrome varies. Almost all children with MCNS respond initially to steroid therapy. Although they may have a relapse, they will then remain free of the disease. Those with FGS and MPGN will have relapses at frequent or infrequent intervals.

Children who have frequent relapses have a relatively poorer chance of ever being free of the disorder. Many develop renal failure later. A kidney transplant may be necessary to sustain life. All children and families need emotional support while the disease runs a long-term course.

Systemic lupus erythematosus

SLE is an autoimmune disease in which autoantibodies and antigens cause deposits of complement in the kidney glomerulus. Some children with SLE develop symptoms of acute or chronic glomerulonephritis, the ultimate cause of death in many adults with SLE (Lateef & Petri, 2012). Therapy with corticosteroids or cytotoxic agents may be effective. If a kidney transplant is required, the same damage rarely occurs in the transplanted kidney.

Haemolytic-uraemic syndrome

With haemolytic-uraemic syndrome, the lining of glomerular arterioles becomes inflamed, swollen and occluded with particles of platelets and fibrin. The child's red blood cells and platelets are damaged as they flow through the partially-occluded blood vessels. As the damaged cells reach the spleen, they are destroyed by the spleen and removed from circulation. This leads to haemolytic anaemia.

Ninety percent of children who develop this syndrome have recently experienced an *E. coli* GI infection. The most likely source of the *E. coli* is undercooked beef as it is found in the intestine of beef cattle. It occurs more frequently in infants who have their initial *E. coli* infection treated with an antibiotic than those who are not treated (Geerdes-Fenge et al., 2013).

Children may have transient diarrhoea increasing to severe fluid loss and bowel-wall necrosis, fever, plus possible stupor and hallucinations. Oliguria accompanied by proteinuria, haematuria and urinary casts in urine follows. The oliguria will lead to increased serum creatinine, BUN and extensive oedema. Children appear pale from anaemia; easy bruising or petechiae may be present from *thrombocytopenia*. Thrombocytopenia is present because platelets are damaged by the irregular blood vessels.

Children need supportive therapy to maintain kidney and heart function. The extreme oliguria can be treated with peritoneal dialysis; anaemia can be corrected by careful transfusion of packed red cells.

Despite the extent of the illness, most infants with haemolytic-uraemic syndrome recover completely. Some children, however, die of the acute illness or continue to have chronic renal involvement.

Acute renal failure

Renal failure occurs in either an acute or chronic form. The acute form most often occurs because of a sudden body insult, such as severe dehydration. The chronic form results from extensive kidney disease, such as haemolytic-uraemic syndrome or glomerulonephritis (Lum, 2014).

Other causes of acute renal failure include prolonged anaesthesia, haemorrhage, shock, severe diarrhoea or sudden traumatic injury. It also can occur in children who are placed on cardiopulmonary bypass while undergoing heart surgery, who receive common antibiotics (aminoglycosides, penicillin, cephalosporins and sulfonamides), who swallow a poison such as arsenic (found in rat poison) or who are exposed to industrial wastes such as mercury. All of these conditions can lead to renal ischaemia, which ultimately results in acute renal failure.

One of the first symptoms noted with acute renal failure is *oliguria,* a urine output of less than 1 mL/kg of the child's body weight/hour. An indwelling urinary catheter may be inserted to exclude the possibility that urinary retention in the bladder rather than kidney dysfunction is causing the severe oliguria.

Azotaemia (accumulation of nitrogen waste in the bloodstream) will occur because of the oliguria. *Uraemia* (extra accumulation of nitrogen wastes in the blood, with additional toxic symptoms such as cerebral irritation) also may occur. The BUN rises progressively as renal insufficiency continues and the breakdown products of protein cannot be excreted. A BUN level greater than 80 to 100 mg/100 umoL is toxic and needs correction. Urine creatinine is another measure that can be used as an indicator of function, because it is normally excreted at a uniform rate. A rate of less than 10 mg/100 umoL indicates severe renal failure. As the kidneys become unable to dilute or concentrate urine, the specific gravity of urine often becomes "fixed" at 1.010.

Hyperkalaemia (elevated potassium level) may occur if potassium cannot be excreted. Hyperkalaemia is manifested by a weak, irregular pulse, abdominal cramps, lowered blood pressure and muscle weakness. As total output decreases, phosphorus levels will rise in the bloodstream. A high serum phosphorus level leads to a low calcium serum level. Severe hypocalcaemia can lead to muscle twitching and seizures (*tetany*); chronic hypocalcaemia can lead to withdrawal of calcium from bones (*osteodystrophy*).

An IVP or radioactive uptake scan may be ordered to substantiate the lack of kidney function. If the child is dehydrated, IV fluid is needed to replace plasma volume. Administer such fluid slowly enough to avoid heart failure. The fluid should not contain potassium until it is established that kidney function is adequate; build-up of potassium may otherwise cause heart block. Potassium correction will need to be undertaken and is dependent on serum levels.

A diuretic such as furosemide (Lasix) may be ordered in an attempt to increase urine production. Diet should be low in protein, potassium and sodium, and high in carbohydrate to supply enough kilojoules for metabolism. Fluid restriction may be indicated. Daily weighing plus strict accumulative fluid balance including input and output measures are indicated. If children are so ill that they cannot eat, total parenteral nutrition may be necessary. During recovery a degree of diuresis occurs as the extra fluid accumulated by the body is cleared. The increase in urine may necessitate additional fluid intake to prevent hypovolaemia.

Chronic renal failure

Chronic renal failure results from developmental abnormalities, when acute failure becomes long-term, or when chronic kidney disease has caused extensive nephron destruction (Braun et al., 2012). The nephrons that are not destroyed by long-term disease appear to function normally; they simply are inadequate in number to sustain kidney function. Glomeruli can adjust so that kidney functions continue normally until 50% of nephrons are destroyed. After this point, kidney function diminishes until the child develops end-stage kidney disease, where the kidneys cannot maintain normal function.

With loss of nephron function, kidneys cannot concentrate urine. This results in polyuria, possibly manifested as enuresis. The few functioning nephrons present cannot reabsorb enough sodium to maintain a functioning level of body fluid, so dehydration occurs. As additional nephrons are lost, oliguria and anuria occur. Inability to excrete H^1 ions leads to acidosis. Hypocalcaemia and hyperphosphataemia occur from the kidney's inability to excrete phosphate. Osteodystrophy occurs as calcium is withdrawn from the bones to compensate. Kidneys are responsible for synthesising vitamin D to its active form. With poor kidney function, vitamin D cannot be used. Without this, calcium cannot be absorbed from the GI tract and deposited in bones. Bones become so calcium-depleted that growth halts and the bones lose strength (renal rickets).

Erythropoietin, formed by the kidneys, stimulates red cell production. With decreased erythropoietin production, anaemia develops. Pruritus may be present from skin irritation due to excretion of nitrogenous wastes in sweat from high levels of BUN and serum creatinine. These changes are summarised in Figure 46.4.

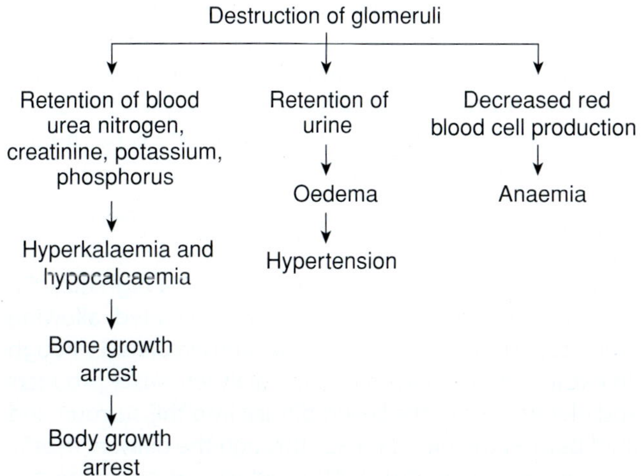

FIGURE 46.4 Pathology of chronic renal failure.

Children with chronic renal failure are generally placed on a low-protein, low-phosphorus, low-potassium diet to prevent rapid urea and phosphate build-up. Children may take aluminium hydroxide gel with meals to bind phosphorus in the intestines and prevent absorption. Milk usually is not given because it is high in sodium, potassium and phosphate—electrolytes children may have difficulty clearing. Meat is restricted and even beans are high enough in protein to be eliminated from the diet. Letting children have some choice about what foods they eat each day helps to promote adjustment to this restricted diet.

Total daily fluid intake may need to be restricted, although the restriction should be as minimal as possible or it can present an area of tremendous conflict between the child and parents. Many children need sodium intake restricted and others need a normal sodium intake. Other children may actually need additional salt because of poor tubular re-absorption. Low-sodium formulas are recommended for children with heart failure who need a low-sodium intake. Use them cautiously in children with renal insufficiency, because their high potassium content can lead to toxic potassium blood levels. Diuretics may be ordered to help children regulate sodium and fluid levels and prevent oedema.

As renal failure becomes prolonged, a child may need supplemental calcium to prevent muscle cramping, rickets, tetany or seizures. A daily antihypertensive medication may be prescribed for increasing hypertension from fluid excess. A blood transfusion may be needed to correct anaemia, but it must be given cautiously so volume overload does not occur. Recombinant human erythropoietin may be prescribed to stimulate red blood cell formation. Effective excretion of urea can be accomplished by dialysis or by replacing the non-functioning kidneys with a kidney transplant. Growth hormone may increase height in some children who have fallen behind in stature (Vimalachandra et al., 2009).

THERAPEUTIC MEASURES FOR THE MANAGEMENT OF RENAL DISEASE

As kidney function is necessary for life, if it deteriorates, some method to replace function must be instituted or a decision for conservative management made.

Peritoneal dialysis

Dialysis is the separation and removal of solutes from body fluid by diffusion through a semipermeable membrane. *Peritoneal dialysis* (PD) uses the membrane of the peritoneal cavity to do this (see Fig. 46.5). Haemodialysis uses an outside synthetic membrane to do this.

In children and adolescents requiring renal replacement therapy (RRT), PD is the preferred dialysis modality. It has improved preservation of residual renal function and is technically easier in small children (Bordador et al., 2010).

Peritoneal dialysis may be used as a temporary measure for children who experience sudden renal

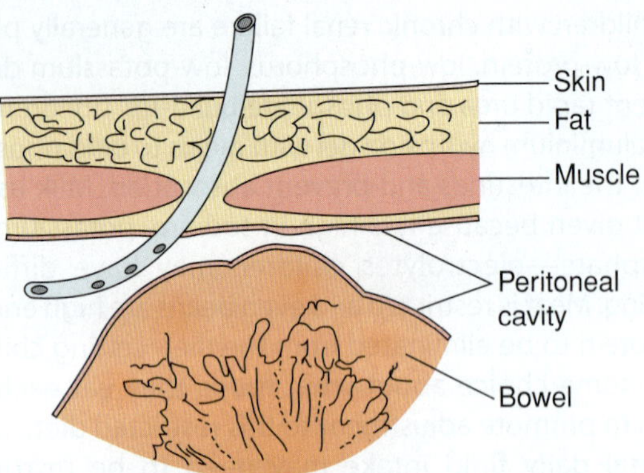

FIGURE 46.5 Insertion site for peritoneal dialysis catheter.

failure caused by trauma or shock. It is used for fairly long periods for children with end-stage kidney disease at home to allow them to live until a kidney transplant can be arranged (Issa et al., 2012). Commencement of treatment is individualised for each person but generally when the serum creatinine level reaches 10 mg/100 umoL. Other indications are congestive heart failure, BUN of more than 100 mg/100 umoL, hyperkalaemia (potassium level of more than 6 mEq/L) and ureamic encephalopathy (confusion or coma).

Method for performing peritoneal dialysis

Generally a double-cuffed curled peritoneal catheter is inserted into the peritoneal cavity via the abdomen using a sharp tunnelling device under general anaesthetic. The exit site of the catheter is determined prior to surgery in consultation with the child, surgeon and experienced paediatric nephrology nurse. After the insertion, intraoperatively, the catheter is flushed to determine patency and then capped off.

The postoperative dressing remains intact for 1 week. It is evaluated then redressed and again remains intact for a further week. For the following 6-week postoperative period the exit site is dressed daily (if wet, change immediately) and observed for signs of healing and infection. The dressing of choice is either non-occlusive or sterile gauze enabling the absorption of any exudate (see Fig. 46.6).

The catheter is rested to allow for tissue granulation post-insertion for a period of 2 weeks. If dialysis is required to start immediately due to the medical condition of the child then small volumes 10 mL/kg/cycle are used with the child nursed in a supine position during the cycle to prevent catheter leakage. The catheter remains taped to the abdomen at all times when not in use to prevent trauma to the exit site.

The child is able to mobilise 24 hours after the procedure and should be instructed to avoid any physical exertion, showering or swimming for a period of 6 weeks. After this time swimming in public pools or spas is discouraged, however, if unavoidable, an occlusive dressing over the catheter and exit site should be used. A fresh dressing should be applied immediately afterwards.

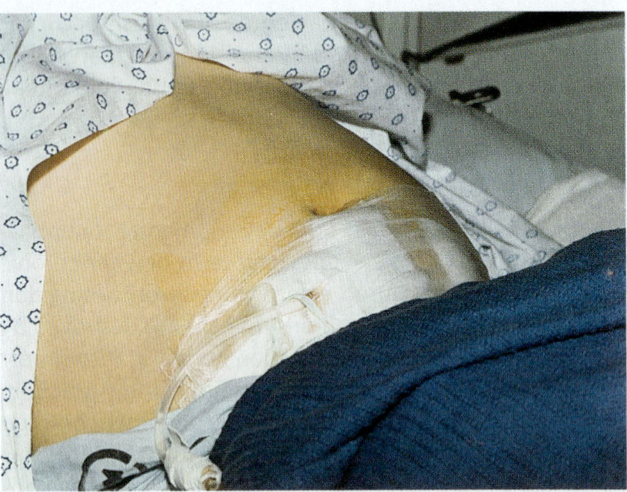

FIGURE 46.6 Peritoneal catheter inserted into a child's abdomen. A secure dressing surrounds the insertion site to prevent infection. (Courtesy of Karen M. Polise, MSN, RN, Division of Nephrology, The Children's Hospital of Philadelphia.)

Cycling peritoneal dialysis or automated peritoneal dialysis

CPD/APD allows a child to go to school or participate in other activities while receiving dialysis. With CPD/APD, a permanent dialysis catheter is inserted into the abdomen. A nephrologist determines the PD prescription initially which is reviewed monthly in renal clinics. This also involves review by a renal dietician. The dietary requirements of the child are monitored closely to ensure growth parameters are met. Monitoring weekly by a nephrology nurse and daily by the parents, dependent on individual patient parameters, is also necessary. Infection is a risk due to the nature of the treatment. Signs and symptoms require immediate intervention. Possible complications of CPD/APD are summarised in Table 46.5.

CPD/APD is a continuous process. Fluid, electrolytes and waste products are maintained at more constant levels than with intermittent dialysis. CPD/APD allows normal activities of daily living for the child and family during the day. Each night a bag of dialysis fluid is attached to an automated PD machine and the child's catheter. A prescribed dialysis solution is cycled overnight according to the programmed parameters. The cycle continues for the period of sleep. Once awake the bag is disconnected and the catheter capped off (as per guidelines from the renal team).

Haemodialysis

Haemodialysis removes body wastes using a high flux dialyser. For haemodialysis, an access is created allowing blood to be removed from the child and circulated through an extra-corporeal circuit and the dialyser. Waste products and electrolytes in the blood diffuse into the surrounding fluid bath as the blood passes through the dialyser (Hothi, Stronach & Harvey, 2013). After diffusion is complete, the blood is returned to the child's circulation (see Fig. 46.7).

TABLE 46.5 Possible complications of CPD/APD

Assessment	Problem	Interventions
Redness or pain or swelling at tube insertion site	Infection	Take culture at site; administer antibiotics as prescribed; continue site care as ordered; notify doctor.
Abdominal pain, increased temperature, nausea and vomiting, cloudy return in drainage solution	Peritonitis	Notify doctor; administer antibiotics as prescribed; auscultate for bowel sounds.
Cramps as fluid is infused	Irritation of peritoneal cavity	Infuse solutions more slowly; warm temperature of solution to body temperature.
Difficulty with infusion or drainage of fluid	Kinked or clotted tubing; malpositioned catheter	Assess tubing for kinking; change position of child; ask child to cough to increase abdominal pressure; add prescribed amount of heparin to dialysate bag (prevents clotting).
Weight increase; moist cough, shortness of breath	Fluid overload	Decrease sodium and fluid oral intake; assess blood pressure and weight; use 4.25% exchange solution until weight is again decreased.
Weight loss, hypotension, poor skin turgor, tachycardia	Fluid loss	Increase fluid and sodium intake; assess blood pressure and weight; do not use 4.25% solution.
Blood-tinged dialysis return	Ruptured blood vessel	Assess pulse and blood pressure; observe for further bleeding in drainage; flush catheter with prescribed amount of heparin to keep clots from forming.

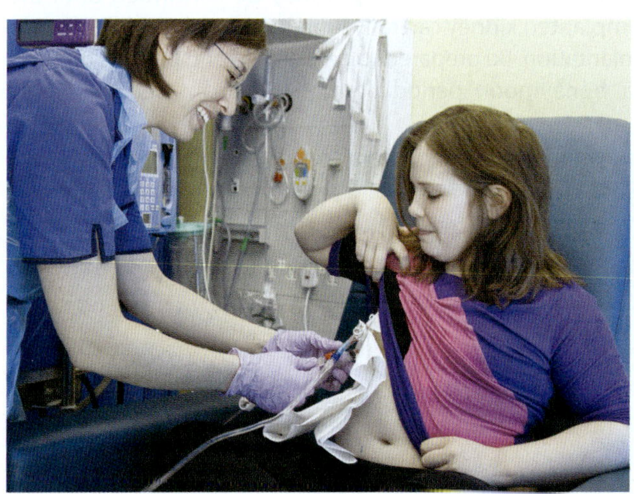

FIGURE 46.7 A nurse preparing a 10-year-old girl for a haemodialysis session. A subclavian catheter from the child is connected to the haemodialysis equipment (in the background). Blood flows from the child through the catheter to the haemodialysis equipment and is then returned to the child's venous circulation. (© Life in View/Science Source.)

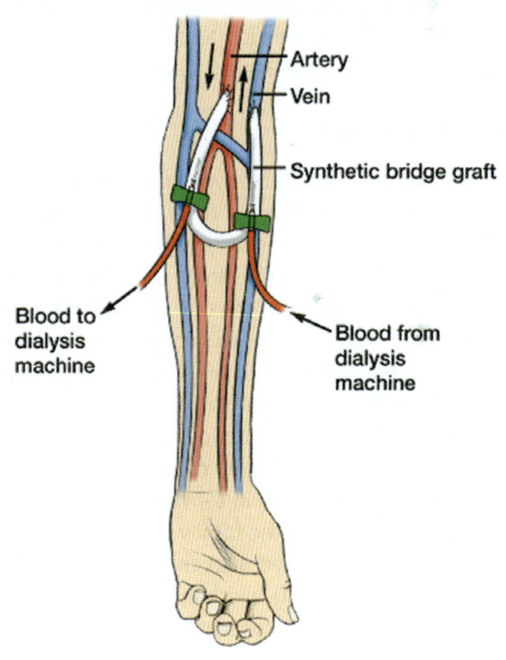

FIGURE 46.8 Arteriovenous graft. (Lippincott's Nursing Advisor.)

Children who have renal failure or whose kidneys have been removed while they await a kidney transplant can be maintained almost indefinitely on haemodialysis. A haemodialysis prescription determined by the nephrologist is generally three times a week for approximately 3 hours. A renal dietician is closely involved as there are both fluid and dietary restrictions with this form of RRT.

There are three forms of access. The first is a central venous tunnelled catheter. This is inserted into the internal jugular, as there is a lower risk of stenosis of the vessel. The next two are an arteriovenous fistula (uses existing native artery and vein) and an arteriovenous graft (attachment of PTFE graft to existing artery and vein; see Fig. 46.8). Surgical anastamosis of a vein and artery either create a vessel large enough or give graft access, to allow insertion of large bore needles to remove and return blood during treatment (see Fig. 46.9).

KIDNEY TRANSPLANTATION

The ultimate possibility for prolonging the life of children with end-stage renal disease (ESRD) is kidney transplantation. With complete renal failure, children who have extensive hypertension may have their damaged kidneys

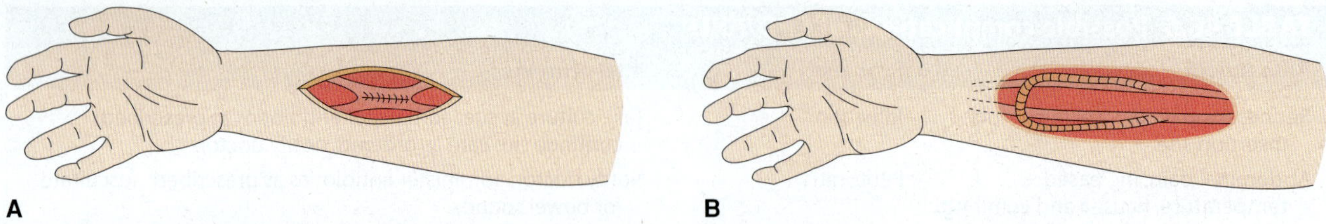

FIGURE 46.9 (**A**) An internal arteriovenous fistula. (**B**) An internal arteriovenous graft.

removed and may be placed on haemodialysis or CPD/APD to await kidney transplant. Kidney removal this way is an important step for parents and the child. Although parents realise that their child's kidneys are no longer functioning, this step removes hope of a miracle to make them function once more. Parents may ask whether it is possible to leave one of the child's kidneys, because only one kidney will be transplanted (not recommended as the hypertension would continue). Parents need a thorough explanation of why hypertension is destructive, as it could lead to cerebrovascular accident or coronary artery disease.

Indigenous Australians have higher rates of renal disease and low transplantation rates among people on RRT. Indigenous children in particular suffer higher rates of renal disease and infant mortality (Grace et al., 2013).

Preoperative care

Kidney transplant is most effective (the kidney is less likely to be rejected) if the kidney is taken from a living twin, parent or sibling (Butani, Troppmann & Perez, 2012). Rejection is higher if a kidney comes from a cadaver or recently deceased child. Most people consider that children should be of legal age to give consent to supply a kidney for transplant, so few children have a sibling who is eligible to donate a kidney. Tissue studies done to determine the best donor (matched for human leucocyte antigens [HLA]) may show that the person in a family most willing to donate a kidney is not the best person in terms of tissue compatibility, increasing stress within the family dynamics. Adult-sized kidneys may be transplanted into children, although if the child weighs less than 10 kg, a kidney this large may lead to hypertension, excessive diuresis and abdominal complications because of the lack of space. Transplanted kidneys are placed in the abdomen, not the usual kidney space.

In some Indigenous families, close family members may not be deemed suitable donors, as there is an increased prevalence of morbidity and some health related issues, for example smoking (Grace et al., 2013).

Before surgery, those children on haemodialysis (scheduled for living donor transplant) should have their dialysis the day before surgery. Those on peritoneal dialysis are dialysed the night before scheduled surgery (CHW, 2014). If the donated kidney will be from a relative, there is adequate time for thorough preoperative preparation. If the donor kidney is from a cadaver, the announcement of surgery will be sudden and time for preoperative instruction and procedures may be limited.

Debate over pretransplant blood transfusions, as a treatment for anaemia, continues. Recent studies suggest that transfusions should be avoided as first line treatment, as they can lead to high sensitisation (Scornik et al., 2013).

Postoperative care

After renal transplant, children are cared for in an environment that is as sterile as possible. They are placed on immunosuppressive therapy to reduce the possibility of kidney rejection. Antilymphocyte globulin and antithymocyte globulin may be added to aid immunosuppression.

Although some transplanted kidneys begin to function immediately, haemodialysis may be continued until the implanted kidney can fully function after the insult of transplantation. Be prepared to help a child and parents through a "honeymoon" period after the transplant (see Box 46.4).

BOX 46.4 ✻ Focus on communication

Emily's grandmother tells you Emily has "changed completely" since she became ill.

Less effective communication

Nurse: Mrs Smith, in what way has Emily changed?
Mrs Smith: She used to whine all the time and constantly ask for things. Now she entertains herself. It's like heaven.
Nurse: That sounds wonderful. Let's review her medicine routine to be sure that's going well.
Mrs Smith: That's another thing she does perfectly: never fusses a bit about anything she has to take.

More effective communication

Nurse: Mrs Smith, in what way has Emily changed?
Mrs Smith: She used to whine all the time and constantly ask for things. Now she entertains herself. It's like heaven.
Nurse: Do you think she's acting a little too perfect?
Mrs Smith: Well, it does seem a bit strange for her.
Nurse: Do you think she could be worrying that if she misbehaves, her medicine won't work?
Mrs Smith: I never thought of that. I would feel better if she started to act like her old self.

What the grandmother above is describing is a "honeymoon" period that children may pass through after being told their kidneys are important for life. Parents often need help seeing this for what it is so they can begin to reassure children that behaving perfectly will not influence the outcome of their illness and that, because they loved them as they were, they will continue to love them regardless.

Postoperative complications can include hypertension, hyperkalaemia (K >5.5 mmol/L), fever and rising creatinine levels (CHW, 2014). Each complication requires immediate action and treatment.

Children with end-stage renal disease usually fail to grow despite treatment. Although growth is improved after kidney transplant, they will probably never reach full height. Part of this growth restriction is related to the need for corticosteroid maintenance therapy to continue immunosuppression.

Transplant rejection

Acute transplant rejection, if it occurs, usually develops within the first 3 months after transplant. Children begin to develop fever, proteinuria, oliguria, weight gain, hypertension and tenderness over the kidney. Serum creatinine and BUN levels will rise. Increasing the dose of immunosuppressants may be effective in relieving this type of rejection.

Rejection may also be *chronic,* in which the transplanted kidney gradually loses function after the first 6 months. This type of rejection is difficult to halt, although it may be such a slow, steady process that it is 2 or 3 years before the kidney fails. If a kidney is rejected, it is removed and a child is returned to a program of haemodialysis. Malignant disease is more common in transplant recipients than in the normal population, probably because of the long-term immunosuppression (Ponticelli & Graziani, 2012). The original disease for which the child underwent transplant may recur in the transplanted kidney. This is most apt to occur in glomerulonephritis.

Key points for review

- Many urinary tract disorders, such as polycystic kidneys, urethral obstruction and bladder exstrophy, are evident on a fetal ultrasound. Early identification allows therapy to begin in utero or immediately after birth.
- Many urinary tract disorders, such as polycystic kidneys or chronic renal failure, are long-term conditions requiring years of therapy. Be certain that parents are well-informed about their child's condition so they can continue to participate in planning their child's care.
- Congenital structural abnormalities of the urinary tract include patent urachus, exstrophy of the bladder, hypospadias and epispadias. Surgical correction is required for all of these.
- Urinary tract infection tends to occur more often in girls than boys. "Honeymoon cystitis" refers to a urinary tract infection occurring with first-time sexual intercourse.
- Vesicoureteral reflux is the backflow of urine into ureters with voiding. It occurs because the valve that guards the entrance to the ureters is lax or misplaced. Surgical correction may be necessary to prevent repeated urinary tract infections.
- Kidney dysfunction can occur for structural reasons such as kidney agenesis, polycystic kidney and renal hypoplasia.
- Acute poststreptococcal glomerulonephritis is inflammation of the glomeruli after a streptococcal infection. It is characterised by an acute episode of haematuria and proteinuria.
- Nephrotic syndrome is an immunological process that results in altered glomerular permeability.
- Diminished kidney function leads to both fluid and electrolyte imbalances. Creative techniques are necessary to encourage children to continue to ingest a restricted-protein diet.
- Renal failure can be acute or chronic. Peritoneal dialysis or haemodialysis may be used to remove body wastes until kidney function can be restored.
- Kidney transplant may be an option for some children with kidney disorders. This is extensive surgery and requires the child to remain on immunosuppressive therapy to counteract transplant rejection.

CASE STUDY QUESTIONS

3. Emily's grandmother asked you whether a sip of beer could have caused Emily's kidney disease. What would you tell her is the cause of nephrosis? What discharge instructions can you anticipate you will need to review with Emily's grandmother?
4. Emily's grandmother is afraid Emily will need a kidney transplant. Emily tells you she hopes she has been good enough to deserve being chosen for a transplant. What would you want to teach this family about the transplant selection process?
5. Suppose Emily receives continuous ambulatory peritoneal dialysis and wants to go to her church camp in the holidays. Her grandmother asks you whether this would be a good experience for her. What factors would you want to know about the camp? About Emily? About her procedure?

Resources

For an extensive range of additional resources to enhance teaching and learning and to facilitate understanding of this chapter, please see the text's accompanying website located on thePoint at http://thepoint.lww.com.

References

Banaszak, B. & Banaszak, P. (2012). The increasing incidence of initial steroid resistance in childhood nephrotic syndrome. *Pediatric Nephrology, 27*(6), 927–932.

Bogaert, G. A. & Slabbaert, K. (2012). Vesicoureteral Reflux. *European Urology Supplements, 11*, 16–24.

Bordador, E. B, Johnson, D. W., Henning, P., Kennedy, S. E., McDonald, S. P., Burke, J. R. & McTaggart, S. J. (2010). On behalf of the Australian and New Zealand dialysis and transplant registry. *Pediatric Nephrology, 25*, 1739–1745.

Braun, L., Sood, V., Hogue, S., et al. (2012). High burden and unmet patient needs in chronic kidney disease. *International Journal of Nephrology Renovascular Disease, 5*, 151–163.

Butani, L., Troppmann, C. & Perez, R. V. (2012). Outcomes of children receiving en bloc renal transplants from small pediatric donors. *Pediatric Transplantation*, *17*(1), 55–58.

Children's Hospital at Westmead (CHW). (2014) Kidney transplantation—CHW—Procedure. Procedure No; O/C/08;8137-01;01, accessed 4 March 2015, <www.schn.health.nsw.gov.au/_policies/pdf/2008-8137.pdf>.

Fleming, E. (2012). Supporting children with nocturnal enuresis. *Nursing Times*, *108*(41), 22–25.

Gaylord, N. M. & Peterson-Smith, A. M. (2012). Genitourinary disorders. In C. E. Burns, A. M. Dunn, M. A. Brady, et al. (Eds), *Pediatric Primary Care* (5th ed.). Philadelphia: Elsevier/Saunders.

Geerdes-Fenge, H. F., Lobermann, M., Nurnberg, M., Fritzsche, C., Koball, S., Henschel, J., Hohn, R., Schober, H. C., Mitzner, S., Podbielski, A. & Reisinger, E. C. (2013). Ciprofloxacin reduces the risk of hemolytic uremic syndrome in patients with Escherichia coli 0104: H4-associated diarrhea, *Infection*, *41*(3), 669.

Gomella, L. G. & Haist, S. A. (2007). *Clinician's Pocket Reference* (11th ed.). Columbus, OH: McGraw-Hill.

Grace, B. S., Kennedy, S. E., Clayton, P. A. & McDonald, S. P. (2013). Racial disparities in paediatric kidney transplantation. *Pediatric Nephrology*, *29*, 125–132.

Hahn, D., Hodson, E. M., Willis, N. S. & Craig, J. C. (2015). Corticosteroid therapy for nephrotic syndrome in children. *Cochrane Database of Systematic Review*, (3), (CD001533).

Harari, M. D. (2013). Nocturnal enuresis. *Journal of Paediatrics and Child Health*, *49*(4), 264–271.

Hassett, S., Smith, G. H. & Holland, A. J. (2012). Prune belly syndrome. *Pediatric Surgery International*, *28*(3), 219–228.

Hothi, D. K., Stronach, L. & Harvey, E. (2013). Home haemodialysis. *Pediatric Nephrology*, *28*(5), 721–730.

Huether, S. E. & McCance, K. L. (2013). *Understanding Pathophysiology* (5th ed.), New York: Elsevier Publishing.

Hunziker, M. & Puri, P. (2012). Familial vesicoureteral reflux and reflux related morbidity in relatives of index patients with high grade vesicoureteral reflux. *Journal of Urology*, *188*(4, Suppl.), 1463–1466.

Issa, N., Lankireddy, S. & Kukla, A. (2012). Should peritoneal dialysis be the preferred therapy pre-kidney transplantation? *Advances in Peritoneal Dialysis*, *28*(1), 89–93.

Jadresic, L. (2014). Symposium: Nephrology. *Paediatrics and Child Health*, *24*(7), 289–292.

Kruegel, J., Rubel, D. & Gross, O. (2013). Alport syndrome. Insights from basic and clinical research. *Nature Reviews: Nephrology*, *9*(3), 170–178.

Lateef, A. & Petri, M. (2012). Unmet medical needs in systemic lupus erythematosus. *Arthritis Research Therapy*, *14*(Suppl. 4), S4.

Lu, D. F., et al. (2007). A descriptive study of individuals with membranoproliferative glomerulonephritis. *Nephrology Nursing Journal: Journal of the American Nephrology Nurses' Association*, *34*(3), 295–302.

Lum, G. M. (2014). Kidney and urinary tract. In W. Hay, M. Levin, R. Deterding, et al. (Eds), *Current Diagnosis & Treatment Paediatrics* (22nd ed.). New York: McGraw-Hill/Lange.

Mahan, J. D. (2011). Nephrology and urology. In K. J. Marcdante, R. M. Kliegman, H. B. Jenson, et al. (Eds), *Nelson Essentials of Paediatrics* (6th ed.). Philadelphia: Saunders/Elsevier.

Martini, F. H., Nath, J. L. & Bartholomew, E. F. (2015). *Fundamentals of Anatomy & Physiology* (10th ed.), Pearson Education: San Francisco.

McKenna, L. & Mirkov, S. (2014). *McKenna's Drug Handbook for Nursing and Midwifery* (7th ed.). Sydney: Lippincott Williams & Wilkins.

Meydan, E. A., Civilibal, M. et al. (2012). The quality of life of mothers of children with monosymptomatic enuresis nocturna. *International Urology and Nephrology*, *44*(3), 655–659.

Nelson, C. P., Chow, J. S., Rosoklija, I., et al. (2012). Patient and family impact of pediatric genitourinary diagnostic imaging tests. *Journal of Urology*, *188*(4, Suppl.), 1601–1607.

Northern Territory Government, Department of Health and Families (2010). Acute post-streptococcal glomerulonephritis, accessed 4 March 2015, <www.health.nt.gov.au/library/scripts/objectifyMedia.aspx?file=pdf/10/84.pdf>.

Paintsil, E. (2013). Update on recent guidelines for the management of urinary tract infections in children: The shifting paradigm. *Current Opinion in Pediatrics*, *25*(1), 88–94.

Ponticelli, C. & Graziani, G. (2012). Education and counseling of renal transplant recipients. *Journal of Nephrology*, *25*(6), 879–889.

Scornik, J. C., et al. (2013). An update on the impact of pre-transplant transfusions and allosensitization on time to renal transplant and on allograft survival. *BMC Nephrology*, *14*, 217.

Tsai, M. S. & Yeh, M. L. (2011). Images in clinical medicine. Patent urachus. *New England Journal of Medicine*, *365*(14), 1328.

Tse, Y., Yadav, P., Herrema, I., et al. (2013). Performing renal biopsies in children under general anesthesia in the lateral position. *Pediatric Nephrology*, *28*(4), 671–673.

Tullus, K. (2015). Vesicoureteric reflux in children. *Lancet*, *385*(9965), 371–379.

Vimalachandra, D., et al. (2009). Growth hormone for children with chronic kidney disease. *Cochrane Database of Systematic Reviews*, (1), (CD003264).

Suggested readings

ANZDATA-Australian and New Zealand dialysis and transplantation registry <www.anzdata.org.au>.

Auron, A., et al. (2007). Prevention of peritonitis in children receiving peritoneal dialysis. *Pediatric Nephrology*, *22*(4), 578–585.

Bethel, J. (2012). Acute pyelonephritis: Risk factors, diagnosis and treatment. *Nursing Standard*, *27*(5), 51–56.

Kidney Health Australia: Home dialysis <www.kidney.org.au/ForPatients/Treatmentoptions/HomeDialysis/tabid/811/Default.aspx>.

Marks, S. D. (2007). How have the past 5 years of research changed clinical practice in paediatric nephrology? *Archives of Disease in Childhood*, *92*(4), 357–361.

Murphy, F. (2007). The role of the nurse post-renal transplantation. *British Journal of Nursing*, *16*(11), 667–675.

The Royal Children's Hospital Melbourne: 126 Guidelines for Paediatric Haemodialysis <www.rch.org.au/nephrology/protocols/126_Guidelines_For_Paediatric_Haemodialysis/>.

The Sydney Children's Hospital Network <www.schn.health.nsw.gov.au>

Watkins, J. (2007). Urinary tract infections in children. *Practice Nursing*, *18*(10), 516.

Zioni, N. (2007). Improving the nutritional condition of infants and young children undergoing hemodialysis. *EDTNA/ERCA Journal of The European Dialysis and Transplant Nurses Association/European Renal Care Association*, *33*(1), 11–16.

Chapter 47

Nursing care of a family when a child has a reproductive disorder

Previous chapters described the growth and development of well children and illnesses. This chapter adds information about the dramatic changes, both physical and psychosocial, that occur when children develop reproductive disorders. Such information forms the basis for care and health teaching in this area.

LEARNING OBJECTIVES

After studying the contents of this chapter, you should be able to:

1. Describe common reproductive disorders in children.
2. Analyse ways that nursing care for a child with a reproductive disorder can be more family-centred.
3. Discuss the assessment of a child with a reproductive disorder.
4. Demonstrate an understanding of expected outcomes for a child with a reproductive disorder.
5. Demonstrate an understanding of nursing care related to reproductive disorders in children.
6. Discuss nursing care for a child with a reproductive disorder.
7. Discuss expected outcomes for achievement and effectiveness of care.
8. Identify areas related to the care of children with reproductive disorders that could benefit from additional nursing research or application of evidence-based practice.
9. Integrate knowledge of reproductive disorders in children with the nursing process to achieve quality child and family health nursing care.

KEY TERMS

- amenorrhoea
- dysmenorrhoea
- endometriosis
- gynaecomastia
- hermaphrodite
- hydrocoele
- menorrhagia
- metrorrhagia
- mittelschmerz
- orchiectomy
- pelvic inflammatory disease (PID)
- premenstrual dysphoric disorder (PDD)
- pseudohermaphrodite
- sexually-transmitted infections (STIs)
- toxic shock syndrome (TSS)
- varicocoele
- vulvovaginitis

CASE STUDY

Alicia is a 15-year-old girl you meet in a paediatric clinic. She has been diagnosed with gonorrhoea because of a purulent vaginal discharge and burning on urination. When you ask her if she is sexually active, she says no; she thinks she contracted the infection from sharing a towel in a changing room. As she leaves the clinic, you hear her tell the receptionist, "I'm glad I got this early in life. Now I won't have to worry about getting it again."

CASE STUDY QUESTION

1. What kind of health education does Alicia need?

Reproductive disorders in children range from mild infections to serious anatomical malformations. All of these disorders require prompt and careful treatment so that children can reach adulthood in good reproductive health, with unaltered fertility, and a positive sense of sexuality. Reproductive infections may suggest child abuse, so children with these also need careful assessment to rule out this possibility (see Chapter 55).

CARE OF A CHILD WITH A REPRODUCTIVE DISORDER

Assessment

Assessment of reproductive health begins with the first physical examination at birth and continues at health assessments throughout childhood and adolescence. As this is a sensitive area for many people to discuss, parents may not be as comfortable inquiring about or describing disorders of the reproductive tract as they are about other disorders. Unless they have clear, thorough explanations of the disease process and prescribed therapy, their reluctance to pursue the subject may leave them confused or misinformed. Even young children can sense that illness affecting the genitalia or their reproductive tract is viewed by some adults as different from other diseases, so may not ask as many questions as they do about other diseases.

Assessment of a child's knowledge about the reproductive system and ways that illness can affect reproductive and sexual functioning forms the foundation for developing appropriate outcomes. Educating the child about reproductive health may be one of the first areas to plan.

Nursing considerations

Working with children with reproductive disorders should always include education about reproductive functioning and measures for maintaining reproductive and sexual health, and preventing illness. Health education regarding the importance of testicular self-examination for adolescent males should be stressed at healthcare visits. Guidelines for teaching about menstrual health and safer sex (covered in Chapter 5) are also important.

Essential nursing interventions also include supporting parents and children through difficult decisions and frightening procedures, as well as providing close observation and empathetic counselling after surgery. For example, surgery for undescended testes is a procedure that can be traumatic for a child, especially if it is performed during a developmental stage in which a boy views such surgery as castrating (a psychological reason in addition to a physical reason why it is done early in life). As all children with any reproductive disorder reach puberty, they need honest explanations about any effect such a condition will have on interpersonal relationships, sexual functioning or childbearing.

The responses of children to reproductive dysfunction vary both with the severity of the illness and the specific age and fears of the child. It is safe to assume that children who have experienced such an illness are at risk of a loss of self-esteem or confusion about their body image. If a child contracts a sexually transmitted infection (STI), evaluation should also address the child's knowledge about avoiding STIs in the future and willingness to seek help should an infection recur.

BOX 47.1 Assessment ✻ Assessing a child with a reproductive disorder

Gynaecomastia in males
Breast lumps in females
Early breast growth in females (precocious puberty)
Accessory nipples
Undescended testes in males
Vulvar or vaginal discharge or pruritus in females
No breast or genital changes (delayed puberty)
Abdominal pain
Early pubic hair growth (precocious puberty)
Abnormal genitalia
Lesion on genitalia

ASSESSING REPRODUCTIVE DISORDERS IN CHILDREN

Reproductive disorders in children may be congenital or acquired so assessment for these must be ongoing throughout childhood (Fitzgerald, 2014; see Box 47.1). As with other parts of a health interview, questions regarding reproductive health and illness are generally addressed to the parents until the child is able to answer history questions reliably and independently. Once a girl has reached adolescence, a gynaecological history should be included in the health assessment. To preserve their privacy, adolescents of both genders may prefer not to be accompanied by a parent during a physical examination for reproductive dysfunction (see Box 47.2).

Some adolescents visit healthcare facilities by themselves. They may be worried that they have contracted an STI. They may suspect that they have become pregnant or want to receive some form of contraception. Before they can admit their chief concern they may "test" a healthcare provider by eliciting a reaction to a minor problem. Be aware that an adolescent who consults a healthcare provider with a seemingly minor concern may be misinterpreting symptoms and may actually be worried that a minor symptom is serious; on the other hand, the adolescent may also be seeking help for another problem. Asking the adolescent "Is there anything else that worries you? Is there any other way I can help you today?" may help you elicit the adolescent's primary concern (see Box 47.3).

For the adolescent girl, pelvic examination becomes part of routine healthcare around the age of 18 to 20 years if the teenager is not sexually active and is not having problems. Because the first pelvic examination can be stressful for some teens, spend time with the girl before the procedure to teach her about what is being assessed. A three-dimensional model of internal organs and some representative instruments may be more useful when describing the examination than a verbal description of anatomy. Remaining beside an adolescent as a support person helps to reduce the stress the teenager may be experiencing. To protect her self-esteem, be sure a girl meets the person who will examine her beforehand. Different cultures have different attitudes towards reproductive disorders and may be more comfortable if the examiner is a woman (Lewis & Foley, 2014).

HEALTH PROMOTION

A thorough physical examination of a newborn seeks early identification and intervention of congenital reproductive disorders. All children need education about sexually-healthy decisions and caring for their bodies. Adolescents may state they are not interested in this information because they are certain that they are choosing abstinence. It is still

BOX 47.2 ✻ Taking a gynaecological history

When assessing an adolescent for a gynaecological health history, be especially conscious of an adolescent's sense of modesty and need for privacy. To ensure privacy, conduct the interview without the parent or carer present.

Menstrual history

- At what age did you begin menstruating?
- How often do your menstrual periods occur and how long do they usually last?
- What is the amount of menstrual flow? (Document by number of pads or tampons used).
- Do you experience discomfort? (Document if discomfort occurs on first day, all days and so forth, and action taken to relieve it).
- Do any sisters or your mother have discomfort or pain during their menstrual periods (dysmenorrhoea or endometriosis)?
- Do you experience any symptoms of irritability, moodiness, headache or diarrhoea (premenstrual dysphoric disorder) 1 or 2 days before menses?
- What were the dates of your last two menstrual periods? How long did they last (duration)? Was the flow light or heavy?

Reproductive tract history

- Have you had any vaginal discharge? (Document amount and whether pad is necessary—include duration, frequency, description, associated symptoms, action taken).
- Is there vaginal itching (pruritus)?
- Is there any vaginal odour?
- Have you had reproductive tract surgery? Have you ever been pregnant? Have you ever had an abortion or miscarriage?

Sexual history

- Have you had a sexually transmitted infection such as herpes, gonorrhoea or syphilis?
- Are you currently sexually active? What is the gender of your partner?
- Do you experience any discomfort during sexual activity (dyspareunia) or any spotting afterward (postcoital spotting)?
- Do you have any concerns such as being worried about frequency, position or partner's satisfaction with coitus? Do you experience orgasm?

Contraception history

- Do you use any type of birth control? If so, what contraceptive do you use? (Document length of time used, satisfaction, any problems.)
- Have you used any other type in the past?

Breast health

- Have you ever noticed any abnormality such as a lump, discharge or pain in your breasts?
- Have you ever had breast surgery?
- Have you breastfed a child?
- Do you have a yearly breast examination by a healthcare provider?

BOX 47.3 ✻ Focus on communication

Alicia, age 15 years, is seen at your paediatric clinic. She has mild upper respiratory tract symptoms.

Less effective communication

Nurse: Alicia? Doctor Jensen doesn't believe you need anything for your cold. Just drink a little extra fluid and take it easy for a couple days.

Alicia: Don't I need a prescription? Some penicillin or something?

Nurse: No. Colds are caused by viruses. Penicillin isn't necessary.

Alicia: I want to be sure I get over this. I'd really like an antibiotic of some kind.

Nurse: One really isn't necessary.

Alicia: I have a bad cough. I don't think I mentioned that.

Nurse: Doctor Jensen listened to your chest. You don't have anything serious there.

Alicia: My stomach doesn't feel very good either. Can't I have something?

Nurse: Sorry. Goodbye now.

More effective communication

Nurse: Alicia? Doctor Jensen doesn't believe you need anything for your cold. Just drink a little extra fluid and take it easy for a couple days.

Alicia: Don't I need a prescription? Some penicillin or something?

Nurse: No. Colds are caused by viruses. Penicillin isn't necessary.

Alicia: I want to be sure I get over this. I'd really like an antibiotic of some kind.

Nurse: One really isn't necessary.

Alicia: I have a bad cough. I don't think I mentioned that.

Nurse: Doctor Jensen listened to your chest. You don't have anything serious there.

Alicia: My stomach doesn't feel very good either. Can't I have something?

Nurse: It seems that you have more symptoms than you mentioned. Are you worried about something other than cold symptoms?

Alicia: Well, I have this rash and . . .

Nurse: And . . . ? Go on . . .

Alicia: And I'm scared I might have a sexually transmitted infection.

Adolescents can have difficulty discussing reproductive tract symptoms. If they have too much difficulty, they can try to obtain an antibiotic by describing respiratory or abdominal symptoms. Being alert to this possibility helps you to recognise a "growing" history of this type.

important to provide the education about making sexually-healthy decisions and reward positive choices.

Caring for Aboriginal and Torres Strait Islander peoples irrespective of age requires carers to be mindful of cultural needs. Reproductive health issues are generally referred to as "men's business" or "women's business" by Indigenous people (Lewis & Foley, 2014); however, discussions may be enhanced if carers are of the same gender and age-appropriate pictures, diagrams and models are used. Similar considerations should be exercised when caring for New Zealand Māori as the population on average have poorer health outcomes (Lewis & Foley, 2014).

DISORDERS CAUSED BY ALTERED REPRODUCTIVE DEVELOPMENT

Genetic sex or *biological gender* (sex chromosomes XX or XY) is determined at conception. However, development of the reproductive system, including external genitalia, occurs over two distinct periods. Reproductive organs and genitalia begin to differentiate in utero by the eighth week followed by growth and refinement occurring over the next few months. This period constitutes the first phase of reproductive development. The second phase occurs with specific endocrine changes that are triggered during puberty with maturation of primary and secondary sexual characteristics.

Ambiguous genitalia

When the genitalia cannot be identified on observation due to incomplete or abnormally formed genitalia it is known as ambiguous genitalia (Gollu et al., 2007). Under normal circumstances XX and XY chromosomes determine female and male gender, respectively; however, under certain circumstances it is possible for structures usually considered "male" or "female" to develop in individuals of either chromosomal gender. For example, hypospadias where the urethral opening is on the underside of the penis (see Chapter 46) or cryptorchidism (undescended testes) may first appear as female genitalia.

For a chromosomal female (XX) fetus exposure to androgen in utero may cause clitoral enlargement and fusion of the labia so that it looks like a male penis and perineum. Likewise, if there is a very forward displacement of the urethra towards the clitoris, the newborn will appear to be a boy on initial inspection, or a chromosomal male (XY) may become "feminised", with a lack of fusion of the labioscrotal folds and an incompletely formed penis.

If testosterone was produced in utero but development of the müllerian duct (female) was not suppressed, a child may be intersexed (formerly termed hermaphrodite), with both ovaries and testes and either male or female external genitalia. Pseudointersexed individuals or pseudohermaphrodites have some external features of both sexes although only either ovaries or testes (or neither) are present.

Precocious puberty

Development of breasts or pubic hair before 8 years of age or menses before 9 years of age may be "early" maturation, but is known as precocious sexual development (Cesario & Hughes, 2007). Development is mostly limited to breast tissue or pubic hair growth but can proceed to complete secondary sex characteristics, spermatogenesis or menstrual function. Precocious puberty occurs more often in girls than in boys (Carel & Leger, 2008).

This condition is caused by the early production of gonadotropins by the pituitary gland; gonadotropins stimulate the ovaries or testes to produce sex hormones. Because of this, children suffering precocious puberty should be investigated for oestrogen-secreting pituitary cysts, tumours of the ovary or testosterone-secreting cysts of the testes. In rare instances, it occurs because of an oestrogen-secreting or testosterone-secreting adrenal tumour.

In the absence of a sinister cause of precocious puberty, age-appropriate social groups, family support and adherence to cultural beliefs help to avert any deleterious outcomes (Hoffnung et al., 2010).

Delayed puberty

Delayed puberty is the failure of secondary (pubertal) sex characteristics to occur by 14 years of age in girls and 15 years of age in boys with familial tendency for late maturation. It is necessary for the child to have a thorough physical examination to disclose whether some secondary sex characteristics are present or whether endocrine stimulation is beginning.

In the absence of abnormal pathology if girls have not begun to menstruate by 17 years of age menstrual cycles can be initiated by administering oestrogen. However with reassurance and education they are usually willing to wait for menarche to occur on its own. Similarly, boys who are distressed by their lack of development may receive testosterone supplements to stimulate pubic hair and genital growth.

✔ Checkpoint question 47.1

Suppose a school-aged girl develops precocious puberty. What advice would you give her parents?

a. Excess oestrogen causes children to be intersexed or hermaphrodites
b. Although her sexual appearance is advanced, the girl cannot conceive
c. Treat the child appropriately for her chronological, not appearance age
d. Do not allow the girl to eat processed meats which contain hormones

REPRODUCTIVE DISORDERS IN MALES

Common reproductive disorders in males include structural alterations in the penis or testes such as phimosis and cryptorchidism, inflammation such as balanoposthitis, and in adolescents, testicular cancer.

Balanitis (balanoposthitis)

Balanoposthitis is inflammation of the glans and prepuce of the penis. The prepuce and glans become red and swollen, a purulent discharge may be present, crusting at the meatal opening which can interfere with voiding and acidic urine touching the denuded surface of the glans causes pain (Hsieh, Chang & Chang, 2007).

Although balanoposthitis is painful, a boy may tolerate the discomfort for several days because he is too embarrassed to discuss the problem. He may think it was caused by masturbation (which can contribute to the irritation) or by sexual activity and may be reluctant to seek help for fear of being criticised. He can be reassured that the problem is local and will have no long-term effect. Any discharge should be cultured to rule out an STI such as gonorrhoea.

Phimosis and paraphimosis

Phimosis is the inability to retract the foreskin from the glans of the penis (see Fig. 47.1A). This is normal with newborns as with age the adhesions dissolve and the foreskin becomes retractable; if it does not, the infant has phimosis. It can interfere with voiding. Balanoposthitis may develop because the foreskin cannot be retracted for cleaning. Circumcision of newborns is no longer routinely advised but it is an option to relieve phimosis (Johnson et al., 2007). Paraphimosis is the inability to replace the prepuce over the glans once it has been retracted (see Fig. 47.1B). This is an emergency situation to address before circulation to the glans is impaired (Yigiter, Arda & Hicsonmez, 2008).

Cryptorchidism

Cryptorchidism is failure of one or both of the testes to descend from the abdominal cavity into the scrotum (Kollin et al., 2007; see Fig. 47.1C). Normally, the testes descend into the scrotal sac during months 7 to 9 of intrauterine life or during the first 6 months after birth. Fibrous bands at the inguinal ring or inadequate length of spermatic vessels may prevent descent. About 17% of premature infants and 3% to 4% of full-term infants are born with undescended testes.

Hydrocoele

Testis descends into the scrotum in utero preceded by a fold of tissue known as *processus vaginalis.* Occasionally fluid collects in this fold (see Fig. 47.1D). If this occurs, the **hydrocoele** (the fluid) can be seen on prenatal ultrasound. At birth the collection of fluid makes the scrotum of the newborn appear enlarged (Bouhadiba, Godbole & Marven, 2007). *Transillumination* through the scrotal sac illuminates the water which shines or glows. Uncomplicated hydrocoele gradually reabsorbs without treatment and parents can be reassured the scrotal enlargement is not caused by an abnormal testis, tumour or hernia.

Formation of a hydrocoele later in life can be due to an *inguinal hernia* (abdominal contents extruding into the scrotum through the inguinal ring, with accompanying fluid). If this happens, the hernia must be repaired for the hydrocoele to be reabsorbed (see Chapter 45). Injection of

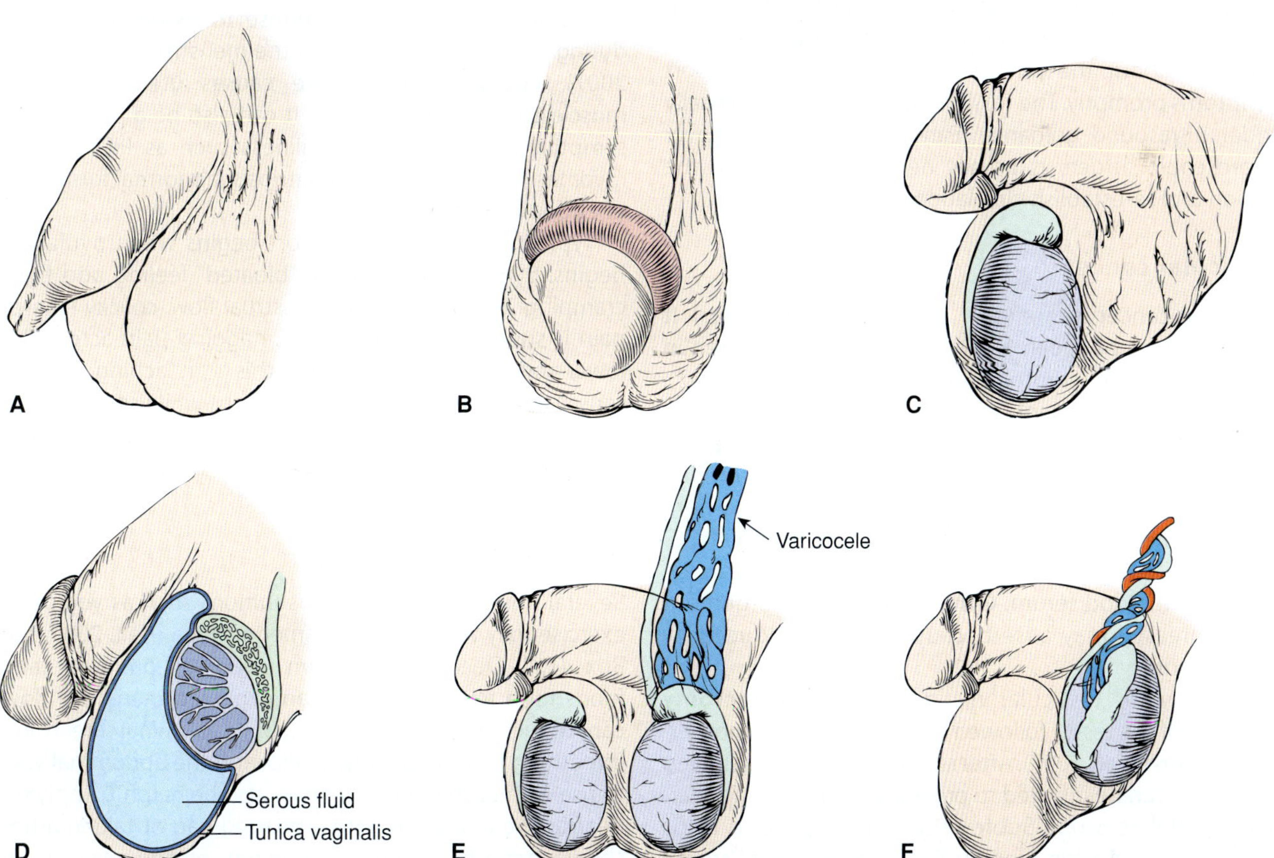

FIGURE 47.1 Common reproductive disorders in males: (**A**) phimosis; (**B**) paraphimosis; (**C**) cryptorchidism; (**D**) hydrocoele; (**E**) varicocoele; (**F**) testicular torsion.

a medication to decrease fluid production (*sclerotherapy*) may also be effective.

Varicocoele

A **varicocoele** is abnormal dilation of the veins of the spermatic cord (see Fig. 47.1E). It is important to identify varicocoeles in adolescents because the increased heat and congestion in the testicles could be a cause of subfertility (Zampieri et al., 2007). No treatment is necessary unless fertility becomes a concern, at which time the varicocoele can be surgically removed. The adolescent may report some local tenderness and oedema for a few days after surgery which is eased with the application of ice during the first few postoperative hours.

Testicular torsion

Testicular torsion (twisting of the spermatic cord) is a surgical emergency (see Fig. 47.1F). Although it can be present in newborns it occurs most frequently during early adolescence (Brown-Guttovz, 2007). Less than normal testicular support apparently allows the spermatic cord to twist. Testicular torsion usually results from a sports activity. The boy experiences severe scrotal pain, and perhaps nausea and vomiting, from the severity of the pain. The testis feels tender to palpation and oedema begins to develop. If the condition is not recognised promptly (within 4 hours), irreversible changes in the testis can occur from lack of circulation to the organ. Boys need to be educated about the phenomenon so that they report symptoms promptly. The torsion can be reduced manually under ultrasound guidance (Park et al., 2007) however laparoscopic surgery is usually necessary to reduce the torsion and re-establish circulation.

Testicular cancer

Testicular cancer is rare (only 1% of all malignancies). It usually occurs between 15 and 35 years of age, often in association with cryptorchidism (Walsh et al., 2007). Symptoms include painless testicular enlargement and a feeling of heaviness in the scrotum. The disease metastasises rapidly leading to abdominal and back pain due to retroperitoneal node extension, weight loss and general weakness. Human chorionic gonadotropin (hCG) and alpha-fetoprotein (AFP), tumour markers, can be detected in blood serum. **Gynaecomastia** (enlargement of the breasts) may arise because of hCG produced by the tumour.

Therapy for testicular malignancy is **orchiectomy** (removal of the testis) followed by radiation or chemotherapy (Einhorn et al., 2007). After surgical removal, a gel-filled prosthesis can be inserted to provide a symmetric appearance to the scrotum. Subfertility in the opposite testis results after radiation therapy. For some patients, "sperm banking" or preserving frozen sperm before the procedure, may be presented as an option for future family planning.

REPRODUCTIVE DISORDERS IN FEMALES

The most frequent reproductive disorders in females involve vaginal or menstrual irregularities. Other disorders are caused by structural alterations of the reproductive organs such as imperforate hymen, pelvic inflammatory disease (PID) or infections caused by STIs.

Menstrual disorders

Because menstruation is an ongoing process throughout half of a woman's life, it affects her self-image significantly. An irregularity such as painful cycles can exert a major influence on daily activities. Menstrual disorders fall into two categories: (a) menstruation that is painful or uncomfortable; and (b) infrequent or too-frequent cycles.

Mittelschmerz

Mittelschmerz is a sharp crampy pain that occurs when a small amount of follicular fluid or blood spills into the abdominal cavity during prostaglandin release and ovulation. It is typically felt on one side of the abdomen (near an ovary) and may be accompanied by scant vaginal spotting.

Dysmenorrhoea

Dysmenorrhoea is painful menstruation caused by the prostaglandin release in response to tissue destruction during the ischaemic phase of the menstrual cycle (Harel, 2007). Prostaglandin release causes uterine smooth muscle contraction and pain. It can also be a preliminary symptom of an underlying illness such as PID, uterine myomas (tumours) or endometriosis (abnormal formation of endometrial tissue).

Typical menstrual discomfort begins when ovulation begins. Symptoms include a "bloated" feeling and light cramping 24 hours before menstrual flow, colicky (sharp) pain is superimposed on a dull, nagging pain across the lower abdomen. Accompanying this is an "aching, pulling" sensation of the vulva and inner thighs while some experience mild diarrhoea, abdominal cramping, breast tenderness, abdominal distension, nausea and vomiting, headache and facial flushing.

Pain related to dysmenorrhoea

Several non-pharmacological solutions such as yoga and exercise may help relieve dysmenorrhoea (Hall, 2009; see Box 47.4). Decreasing sodium intake by omitting salty foods for a few days before an expected menstrual flow can reducing bloating and pain. Abdominal breathing (breathing in and out slowly, allowing the abdominal wall to rise with each inhalation) may also be helpful. Applying heat to the abdomen with a heating pad or taking a hot shower or bath may relax muscle tension and relieve pain. Acupressure, although short lived, might also be of help (Jun et al., 2007). Caution young girls not to apply heat to

BOX 47.4 * Focus on evidence-based practice

The pain of dysmenorrhoea

Non-pharmacological interventions are being used with increasing frequency to help reduce the pain of dysmenorrhoea. To discover if yoga exercises could achieve this, a researcher recruited 92 female students aged 18 to 22 years. Half of them were assigned to an experimental group where they were taught and asked to perform yoga poses during the second half of their next cycle; the other half were assigned to a control group. Results of the study showed a significant difference in both the intensity of pain and its duration between the experimental group and the control group during their next menstrual period.

Based on the above, would you recommend yoga if a woman asks you what she can do to reduce the pain of dysmenorrhoea?

Source: Rakhshaee, Z. (2011). Effect of three yoga poses (cobra, cat and fish poses) in women with primary dysmenorrhea: A randomized clinical trial. *Journal of Pediatric & Adolescent Gynecology, 24*(4), 192–196.

their abdomen for abdominal pain until their menstrual flow begins; if the pain results from an inflamed appendix, heat can cause rupture of the appendix and life-threatening peritonitis. Resting may help to relieve vulvar pain; abdominal massage (effleurage or light massage) may feel soothing. Adolescents who remain sexually active during their menses may discover that orgasm helps relieve pelvic engorgement and cramping.

Menorrhagia

Menorrhagia is an abnormally heavy menstrual flow, usually defined as greater than 80 mL per menses. It may occur in girls close to puberty and in women nearing menopause because of anovulatory cycles. Without ovulation and subsequent progesterone secretion, oestrogen secretion continues and causes extreme proliferation of endometrium. Menorrhagia signifies the presence of many conditions such as endometriosis, anaemia, blood clotting dyscrasia, myoma (fibroid) tumour, PID or a coincidental indication of early pregnancy loss. It can occur from breakthrough bleeding from an oral contraceptive (Grover, 2007). There is often an unusual amount of flow in girls using intrauterine devices (IUDs). With oral contraceptives, the flow is often light; for this reason, it may seem alarmingly heavy once the pill is discontinued, when in reality this is just a return to the adolescent's normal flow.

Metrorrhagia

Metrorrhagia is bleeding between menstrual periods (Gray & Emans, 2007). It can occur in teenagers taking oral contraceptives during the first 3 or 4 months of use or from infection which causes vaginal irritation. Spotting may also represent a temporarily low level of progesterone production and endometrial sloughing (dysfunctional uterine bleeding or a luteal phase defect), although this condition most often occurs near the end of the reproductive years.

If metrorrhagia occurs for more than one menstrual cycle in a teenager who is not taking oral contraceptives, she should be referred to her primary care provider for examination, because abnormal vaginal bleeding can be an early sign of uterine carcinoma or ovarian cysts.

Endometriosis

Endometriosis is the abnormal growth of extrauterine endometrial cells, often in the cul-de-sac of the peritoneal cavity or on the uterine ligaments or ovaries. This abnormal tissue results from excessive endometrial production and a reflux of blood and tissue through the fallopian tubes during a menstrual flow. Unfortunately for Australian adolescent girls suffering endometriosis the median time to diagnosis is 12.1 years compared to 3.1 years for older females (Parker, 2009).

The condition tends to occur most often in white primiparous women, but there is also a familial tendency. Daughters of women with endometriosis may develop symptoms of dysmenorrhoea early in life. They may want to consider having children before overgrowth of the endometrium becomes so extensive that it interferes with conception. Statistically about 20% of women with a diagnosis of endometriosis experience infertility (ECCA, 2008).

The excessive production of endometrial tissue may be related to a deficient immunological response. In many women, it appears to be related to excess oestrogen production or a failed luteal menstrual phase. Many women with endometriosis do not ovulate or ovulate irregularly. Therefore, endometriosis is discovered at a higher than usual rate among women undergoing subfertility testing (Vercellini et al., 2007).

In these women, oestrogen secretion continues through the cycle rather than becoming secondary to progesterone late in the cycle, as happens with normal ovulation. The resulting proliferation of tissue forces the blood back into the fallopian tubes.

Endometriosis causes dysmenorrhoea when the abnormal tissue responds to oestrogen and progesterone stimulation by swelling and then sloughing its layers in the same manner as the uterine lining. This causes inflammation of surrounding tissue in the abdominal cavity and an even greater release of prostaglandins. Abnormal tissue in the pelvic cul-de-sac can cause *dyspareunia* (painful coitus) because it puts pressure on the posterior vagina. Subfertility may result if the fallopian tubes become immobilised and blocked by tissue implants or adhesions, preventing peristaltic motion and transport of ova (see Chapter 8).

Amenorrhoea

Amenorrhoea, or absence of a menstrual flow, strongly suggests pregnancy but is by no means definitive, because it can also result from tension, anxiety, fatigue, chronic illness, extreme dieting or strenuous exercise. Amenorrhoea as a sign of pregnancy is discussed in Chapter 10. Competitive swimmers, long-distance runners (80 to 120 km weekly) and ballet dancers notice that intensive training causes their periods to become scant and irregular. This appears to be associated with their low ratio of body fat to body muscle, which leads to excessive secretion of prolactin. An elevation in prolactin causes a decrease in GnRH from the hypothalamus, followed by declines in follicle-stimulating hormone (FSH), follicular development and oestrogen secretion. Menstrual cycles usually return to normal within 3 months of discontinuation of strenuous training and conditioning.

Adolescents who wish to maintain a normal cycle while training for a sports event may take bromocriptine (Parlodel), which can reduce high prolactin levels by acting on the hypothalamus and initiating menstruation each month. Many adolescents, however, view the absence of menstrual periods as a benefit during sports training. If a menstrual flow is delayed and pregnancy is suspected, bromocriptine should be discontinued, because it is potentially teratogenic.

Amenorrhoea also occurs among females who diet excessively, partially as a natural defence mechanism to limit ovulation and as a means of conserving body fluid. Adolescents with *anorexia nervosa* or *bulimia* (eating disorders described in Chapter 54) often develop amenorrhoea after approximately 3 months of excessive dieting or binging and dieting; as in athletes, this is caused by an increase in prolactin.

Premenstrual dysphoric disorder

Premenstrual dysphoric disorder (PDD) is a condition that occurs in the luteal phase of the menstrual cycle and is relieved by the onset of menses. It has both behavioural and physiological symptoms. Because of the variety of possible symptoms, as many as 30% of women experience some degree of PDD; at least 3% experience a cluster of symptoms that include anxiety, fatigue, abdominal bloating, headache, appetite disturbance, irritability and depression. For about 3% of women, these symptoms are so extreme that they are incapacitating (Stotland, 2007).

The cause of PDD is unproved but, contrary to previous beliefs, it must be due to more than a drop in progesterone just before menses. A syndrome similar to PDD can occur in women after tubal ligation; a decrease in the blood supply to the ovary apparently results in decreased luteal function. In some women, a vitamin B–complex deficiency may lead to oestrogen excess, causing an abnormal ratio of oestrogen to progesterone; other related causes may be poor renal clearance leading to water retention, or hypoglycaemia leading to a surge of adrenaline and low calcium levels and interference with serotonin synthesis.

Symptoms of PDD vary from cycle to cycle and throughout life. Therapy is aimed at correcting specific symptoms (Yonkers, O'Brien & Eriksson, 2008). Adolescents who think they have PDD should keep a diary of when symptoms occur. If they are aware of recurring patterns that indicate PDD, they will be better able to recognise the cause. They should be certain their diet is high in vitamins and calcium, and low in salt.

Female genital mutilation (FGM)

Female genital mutilation (FGM) describes all practices that purposefully alter or injure the female genital organs through partial or total removal of the external genitalia without a medical need (WHO February 2014). Because such procedures are performed on young girls between infancy and 15 years of age, severe bleeding is an initial complication but longer term these girls and women endure problems with urination, cyst development, infections, infertility, childbirth complications and increased risk of death in the newborn (WHO, 2014). WHO estimates that 125 million girls and women across Africa and the Middle East have endured female genital mutilation. It is now considered a violation of the human rights of girls and women and is strongly campaigned against around the world.

Although not a custom practised in Australia or New Zealand, adolescents or women who have had such procedures performed on them in another country may be seen in gynaecological settings. They may have difficulty with childbirth because of vulvar scarring and contraction.

Imperforate hymen

An imperforate hymen occurs as a result of abnormal hymen development in the embryo. A thin membranous ring of tissue partly obstructs the vaginal opening blocking outflow thus it is commonly detected with the girls first period (Dane et al., 2007). Palpation of the abdomen reveals pain and a lower abdominal mass. On vaginal examination an intact bulging hymen is evident. Imperforate hymen can be rectified with surgery once detected.

Careful explanation of this condition will help the girl understand that it will not interfere with sexual relations or future childbearing. Because most girls of early menstrual age have scant knowledge of anatomy, pictures of the reproductive tract help to explain that this is a local and minor problem.

Toxic shock syndrome

Toxic shock syndrome (TSS) is an infection that usually is caused by toxin-producing strains of *Staphylococcus aureus* organisms. Although organisms can enter the body by other means, they typically enter through vaginal walls that have been damaged by the insertion of tampons at the time of a menstrual period (Kansal et al., 2007), TSS can also occur in males (South Australian Health, 2015). The symptoms of TSS are described in Box 47.5. Some women have mild diarrhoea as a normal accompaniment to

BOX 47.5 ✻ Symptoms of toxic shock syndrome

- Sudden onset of high fever
- Vomiting
- Diarrhoea
- Dizziness from low blood pressure
- Muscle aches
- Confusion and collapse
- Sunburn-like rash followed by skin peeling on palms and soles 1–2 weeks after illness

(South Australian Health, 2015)

BOX 47.6 ✻ Focus on family teaching

Preventing toxic shock syndrome

Q. Alicia says to you, "I've heard so much about a disease called toxic shock syndrome. What is it and how can I make sure that I don't get it?"

A. Although toxic shock syndrome can occur for other reasons, it most often occurs during a menstrual flow when tampons are used. The following are measures to help prevent the syndrome:

- Use only tampons made of natural materials such as cotton, not synthetics such as cellulose or polyester and avoid high-absorbency tampons.
- Change tampons at least every 4 hours during use.
- Alternate use of tampons with use of sanitary pads.
- Avoid handling the portion of the tampon that will be inserted vaginally.
- Do not use tampons near the end of a menstrual flow, when excessive vaginal dryness can result from scant flow.
- Do not insert more than one tampon at a time, to avoid abrasions and to keep the vaginal walls from becoming too dry.
- Avoid deodorant tampons, deodorant sanitary pads and feminine hygiene sprays; these products can irritate the vulvar–vaginal lining.
- If fever, vomiting or diarrhoea occurs during a menstrual period, discontinue tampon use and immediately consult a healthcare provider, because these are symptoms of TSS.
- Anyone who has had one episode of TSS is well advised not to use tampons again, or at least not until two vaginal cultures for *Staphylococcus aureus*, the bacteria usually responsible for TSS, are negative.

dysmenorrhoea, but any female who develops fever with diarrhoea and vomiting during a menstrual period should suspect TSS. Once occurring at epidemic proportions because of superabsorbent tampons, it now can be prevented by simple steps (see Box 47.6).

Vulvovaginitis

In **vulvovaginitis**, inflammation of the vulva or vagina is accompanied by pain, odour, pruritus and a vaginal discharge (Hansen et al., 2007). Vaginal bleeding may be present. This condition may occur in a girl of any age, but it tends to be more frequent as girls reach puberty. The change to adult pH and the presence of vaginal secretions make the vagina more receptive to infections (see Table 47.1).

Preschool and school-aged children

Vaginal discharge may occur before menarche, but bleeding is rarely seen at this age. If bleeding is present, its cause must be determined. Cystitis can cause urethral bleeding; scratching due to rectal pruritus can lead to rectal bleeding. The cause of true vaginal bleeding in this early age group is usually either irritation caused by an inserted foreign object in the vagina, infestation of pinworms or *vaginitis* (vaginal inflammation or infection). Sexual abuse must be investigated as a cause of any bleeding, tenderness or infection (see Chapter 55). Precocious puberty must also be ruled out.

Treatment for pinworm is discussed in Chapter 43. If there is a foreign body in the vagina, vaginal examination is necessary to locate the object and then to confirm that it has been fully removed. This may be difficult for girls to accept, because vaginal manipulation and stretching can be painful. Use of a small speculum helps reduce the pain. A local antibiotic ointment or warm bath may be ordered to reduce accompanying infection and inflammation afterwards. Sometimes, daily bubble baths cause vulvar irritation. This can be quickly remedied by discontinuing the bubble baths; irritation from such compounds can lead not only to local discomfort but to urinary tract infection as well (Schilling McCann et al., 2007).

A few preschool or school-aged children develop a vaginitis due to *Streptococcus* or *E. coli* introduced from the anus by improper perineal care after voiding or bowel movements. A tight hymen then traps the micro-organisms in the vagina and leads to infection. The girl needs to be reminded to wipe from front to back after voiding or bowel movements.

Adolescents

As a girl enters puberty, she may notice a slight vaginal discharge caused by increased vaginal secretions. She can be reassured that this is normal. To keep from developing vulvar irritation, caution girls to wear cotton underpants rather than nylon (so that moisture is absorbed better) and to dry the vulva thoroughly after bathing or swimming.

Some girls develop vulvar irritation after using personal hygiene sprays or douches. These products are unnecessary so should be discontinued. Good hygiene can be achieved by daily washing and frequent changing of tampons or sanitary pads during menstruation. This will prevent chafing or stasis of menstrual blood and help prevent irritation and excessive odour.

Box 47.7 discusses common measures to relieve vulvovaginal discomfort.

TABLE 47.1 Common vulvovaginal infections

Causative agent	Symptoms	Common therapy
Candida	Vulvar reddening and pruritus; thick, white, cream cheese-like vaginal discharge	Nystatin or miconazole (Monistat) suppositories or fluconazole (Diflucan) orally; bathing with dilute sodium bicarbonate solution may relieve pruritus
Trichomonas	Thin, irritating, frothy, grey-green discharge; strong, putrid odour; itching	Metronidazole (Flagyl) orally; douching with weak vinegar solution to reduce pruritus
Herpes virus type II	Painful pinpoint vesicles on an erythematous base with a watery vaginal discharge possible; voiding may be irritating and painful	Bathing with dilute sodium bicarbonate solution, applying lubricating jelly to lesions or an oral analgesic such as aspirin may be necessary for pain relief; topically applied acyclovir (Zovirax) helps heal lesions
Gardnerella	Oedema and reddening of vulva, milky grey discharge, fishlike odour	Metronidazole (Flagyl) or clindamycin
Chlamydia trachomatis	Watery, grey-white vaginal discharge, vulvar itching	Tetracycline or doxycycline; erythromycin during pregnancy
Neisseria gonorrhoeae	Possibly symptomless; may have profuse yellow-green vaginal discharge	Ceftriaxone and doxycycline; oral amoxicillin
Enterobius vermicularis (pinworm)	Rectal pruritus, especially on rising in the morning	Oral administration of an anthelmintic, such as mebendazole (Vermox)
Treponema pallidum (syphilis)	Painless ulcer on vulva or vagina	Benzathine penicillin, administered intramuscularly
Streptococcus	Vaginitis, vulvar itching; oedema and reddening of vulva	Antibiotic (e.g., amoxicillin)
Foreign body	Vaginal discharge; odour	Removal of foreign body during pelvic examination

BOX 47.7 * Focus on family teaching

Tips for relieving the pain of vulvitis

Q. Alicia says to you, "I have a vaginal discharge. The itching is awful. Is there anything I can do to relieve it?"

A. Here are some tips that might help:

- Wash the area twice a day with mild, non-perfumed soap and water, and pat dry. This removes secretions and decreases irritation. Wash and dry from front to back, to prevent spreading rectal contamination forwards.
- Take sitz baths or apply warm, moist compresses three times a day to soothe the area and keep it free of irritating drainage.
- After drying the cleansed area, apply cornflour for comfort and to absorb residual moisture.
- Avoid bubble baths and feminine hygiene sprays, because the ingredients may cause additional local irritation or contribute to urinary tract infections.
- Take acetaminophen (Tylenol) every 4 hours. Acetaminophen is an analgesic that relieves pain and reduces itching, a mild pain sensation.
- Avoid scratching, which may increase abrasions and introduce a secondary infection. Instead, apply a cold compress to relieve the itching sensation.
- Wear cotton underwear, which allows air to circulate and moisture to evaporate, rather than nylon or silk, which prevents air circulation and retains moisture.
- Sleep without underwear.
- Use an anaesthetic spray or hydrocortisone cream only as prescribed.
- Carefully follow instructions from your healthcare provider about caring for a vaginal infection; only after the infection subsides will the vulvitis clear.

Pelvic inflammatory disease

Pelvic inflammatory disease (PID) is infection of the pelvic organs: the uterus, fallopian tubes, ovaries, and their supporting structures. The infection can extend to cause pelvic peritonitis. Although sexual transmission accounts for approximately 75% of all instances of PID (gonorrhoeal and chlamydial organisms are frequently responsible), infections from other causes such as *E. coli* or *Streptococcus* are beginning to occur more frequently and may be as severe. Adolescents and young adults have a higher incidence of PID than other age groups (Soper, 2007).

PID begins with a cervical infection that spreads by surface invasion along the uterine endometrium and then out to the fallopian tubes and ovaries. It is most likely to occur at the end of a menstrual period, because menstrual blood provides an excellent growth medium for bacteria and there is loss of the normal barrier of cervical mucus during this time.

With acute PID an adolescent notices severe pain in the lower abdomen. She may have an accompanying heavy, purulent discharge. As the infection progresses, she will develop a fever. Leucocytosis and an elevated erythrocyte sedimentation rate will be present on laboratory testing. During a pelvic examination, any manipulation of the cervix causes severe pain. It may be difficult to palpate the ovaries because of tenderness and abdominal guarding. As peritoneal tissue becomes inflamed and oedematous, a purulent exudate forms. If the process is untreated, it enters a chronic phase and fibrotic scarring with stricture of the fallopian tubes results. If the PID enters a chronic phase the abdominal pain lessens but dyspareunia and dysmenorrhoea may be extreme. If the ovaries are affected intermenstrual spotting may occur. Diagnosis can be aided by ultrasound or laparoscopy. Although treatment can be prolonged it is important for the healthcare provider to reiterate the significance of an uninterrupted treatment schedule to increase the likelihood of success (ASHM, 2014).

SEXUALLY TRANSMITTED INFECTIONS

Sexually transmitted infections (STIs) are diseases that are spread through sexual contact with an infected partner. In Australia, 75% of STIs diagnoses occur in the 15- to 29-year-old group (Latreille, Collyer & Temple-Smith, 2014). A similar trend is seen in New Zealand (Institute of Environmental Science & Research, 2012). In Australia, Aboriginal and Torres Strait Islander populations have been identified as priority groups for action due to consistent STI rates and the potential for wider transmission (The Kirby Institute 2014). Unlike Australia, STIs are not notifiable diseases in New Zealand making it more difficult to estimate STI rates and surveillance (Institute of Environmental Science & Research, 2012).

Generally STIs range in severity from easily treated infections, such as trichomoniasis, to human immunodeficiency virus (HIV) infection, which, despite advances in therapy, is still life-threatening. If these diseases are discovered in young children, the possibility of sexual abuse has to be considered (Reading & Rannan-Eliya, 2007). STIs may be spread among women having sex with women or men having sex with men (Evans et al., 2007). Male circumcision does not appear to reduce the spread.

Abstinence or condom use provides the best protection against STIs. Additional measures are voiding immediately after coitus, washing the genitals well with soap and water, and choosing sexual partners who are at low risk of infection (avoiding persons who are intravenous drug users or those with multiple sexual partners). Educating adolescents about safer sex practices, including the need for condom use and the importance of health screening for these disorders, is an important nursing responsibility. STIs are becoming more difficult to treat because the causative organisms are becoming more and more resistant to antibiotics. Always reinforce the fact that little immunity develops from STIs, so such diseases can be contracted repeatedly. In most instances, an infected partner should also be treated or the disease can recur from cross-infection. Treatment of most STIs begins with determining the causative organism so that the appropriate antimicrobial or antifungal agent can be prescribed. Above all, it is imperative that the young population are aware that a vast proportion of STI's are asymptomatic thus the need to engage in screening programs for early detection and intervention and to prevent the spread of infection (ASHM, 2014).

Opportunities to discuss sexual health issues with young people may occur unexpectedly therefore it is essential that the healthcare provider has the knowledge and skills to assist. Health promotion includes offering accurate information on the diagnosed infection, prevention and treatment, offering both printed and electronic sources of information (ASHM, 2014).

Pregnancy and sexually transmitted infections

Several STIs such as syphilis are known to be teratogenic. All of them are suspected of being a causative factor of preterm birth.

Candidiasis

Candidiasis is a vaginal infection spread by the fungus *Candida,* an organism that thrives on glycogen. Candidiasis is so common that as many as 90% of women will have it at some time in their life. As many as 40% of sexually active females have asymptomatic candidal vaginal infections; this rate rises even higher during pregnancy, when high oestrogen levels lead to glycogen levels that produce a favourable environment for fungal growth. Because oral contraceptives produce a pseudopregnancy state, women using oral contraceptives also have frequent vaginal candidal infections. When a woman is being treated with an antibiotic (which destroys normal vaginal flora and lets fungal organisms grow more readily), she is also particularly susceptible to this infection. Incidence is also strongly associated with immune suppression and diabetes mellitus because hyperglycaemia provides a glucose-rich environment for candidal growth (Tanner & Alexander, 2007).

Because of the scant mucus production in the period before menses, symptoms may be most acute at this time. An adolescent will notice vulvar and vaginal reddening, burning and itching, and even bleeding from hairline fissures. The vagina sometimes shows white "patches" on the walls. The patches are adherent and cannot be scraped away without bleeding. A thick, cream cheese-like discharge can usually be observed at the vaginal introitus. There may be pain on coitus or on tampon insertion. Candidal infections may also be present at other body sites, such as the oral cavity or a moist area such as the umbilicus. In immunosuppressed individuals, it can become systemic (Blyth, Palasanthiran & O'Brien, 2007).

Candidal infections are confirmed through microscopic examination: typical fungal hyphae indicate the presence of *Candida* organisms or alternatively use of an at-home test kit.

Pregnancy and candidiasis

Candidiasis occurs more frequently than usual during pregnancy because of the increased oestrogen level present which causes the vaginal pH to be less acidic. It occurs frequently in pregnant women with gestational diabetes and in women with HIV infection. Women with repeated infections should have their urine tested for glucose to determine whether gestational diabetes is present.

Both miconazole (Monistat) for 7 days or a single dose of oral fluconazole (Diflucan) are approved for use during

BOX 47.8 ✻ Focus on pharmacology

Fluconazole (Diflucan)

Classification: Antifungal agent
Action: Increases fungal cell wall permeability, thereby exerting fungicidal or fungostatic action (McKenna & Mirkov, 2014)
Pregnancy risk category: C
Dosage: 150 mg orally as a single dose
Possible adverse effects: Nausea, vomiting; diarrhoea, abdominal pain, headache

Nursing implications

- Instruct the adolescent that this drug is given as a one-time single dose.
- Teach the adolescent about safer sex measures and hygiene practices to help prevent reinfection after therapy.
- Urge the adolescent to watch for signs and symptoms of possible reinfection and report them to the primary care provider.

pregnancy (see Box 47.8). Treating the infection during pregnancy is important not only because the profuse vaginal discharge and pruritus can be uncomfortable but if the infection is still present in the vagina at the time of childbirth, it may cause a candidal infection, or thrush, in the newborn (see Chapter 43). Caution pregnant women to call their primary healthcare provider before using an over-the-counter product and to alert them of her vaginal infection. Antifungal use during the first trimester of pregnancy is possibly associated with hypoplastic heart disease in newborns (Carter et al., 2008).

What if...

Alicia tells you she feels safe from contracting an STI because she knows she is up-to-date with her immunisations? How would you counsel her?

Trichomoniasis

Trichomonas vaginalis is a single-cell protozoan that is spread by coitus. It is most prevalent in the Indigenous populations of Australia and in travellers from countries where prevalence is high (ASHM, 2014). The incubation period is from 4 to 20 days.

With a trichomonal infection, females notice vaginal irritation and a frothy white or greyish-green vaginal discharge. The frothiness of the discharge is an important typical finding. The upper vagina is reddened and may have pinpoint petechiae. Extreme vulvar itching is present. By contrast males with the same infection rarely report any symptoms.

The infection is diagnosed by microscopic examination of a sample of the vaginal discharge after it is combined with lactated Ringer's or normal saline solution. Trichomonads typically appear as rounded, mobile structures. Be aware that *Trichomonas* infections cause such inflammatory changes in the cervix or vagina that a pap smear taken during this time may be misinterpreted as showing abnormal tissue.

Pregnancy and trichomoniasis

Trichomoniasis infections are associated with preterm labour, premature rupture of membranes and post-caesarean infection (Hay & Czeizel, 2007). The medication of choice is single-dose oral metronidazole. Metronidazole was once thought to be teratogenic but is now considered to be safe in either early or late pregnancy (McKenna & Mirkov, 2014).

Bacterial vaginosis

Bacterial vaginosis is the invasion of an organism such as *Gardnerella vaginalis*. This organism thrives in the vagina, a body area with a reduced oxygen level. When the infection is present vaginal discharge appears milk-white to grey and has a fish-like odour. Pruritus can be intense. Microscopic examination of the discharge in normal saline solution shows gram-negative rods adhering to vaginal epithelial cells termed *clue cells* (Burke & Rogers, 2007).

The treatment is oral or vaginal metronidazole for 7 days; the woman's sexual partners should also be treated to prevent recurrence of the infection.

Pregnancy and bacterial vaginosis

The treatment during pregnancy is oral metronidazole or clindamycin for 7 days. Untreated *G. vaginalis* infections are associated with amniotic fluid infections and, perhaps, preterm labour as well as premature rupture of the membranes (Soper, 2007).

Chlamydia trachomatis infection

Chlamydia trachomatis infections are on the increase in Australia, with numbers rising steadily over the last decade. Currently, it is the most prevalent STI (The Kirby Institute, 2014). This rise is attributed to improved testing techniques and greater sexual freedom among the 15–39 age group (ASHM, 2014). In New Zealand, *Chlamydia* is more prevalent in 15- to 19-year-old females and 20- to 24-year-old males (Institute of Environmental Science & Research, 2012). Symptoms include a heavy, greyish-white discharge and vulvar itching, however some women may be asymptomatic. The incubation period is 1 to 5 weeks. Diagnosis is made by culture of the organism. Therapy is oral doxycycline or tetracycline for 7 days or azithromycin in a single dose. Because it has become so common, most public health departments require that cases now be reported. Long-term effects of chlamydial infections are PID, possibly leading to subfertility. Because there is a strong association between gonorrhoea and *Chlamydia*, if a chlamydial infection is documented, all women should be tested for gonorrhoea as well (Cook et al., 2007).

Pregnancy and *Chlamydia*

Screening for *Chlamydia* via a urine culture is usually done during a woman's first prenatal visit. If a woman has multiple sexual partners, screening may be repeated again in the third trimester. Doxycycline (Vibramycin), the therapy for non-pregnant women, is contraindicated during pregnancy because of possible fetal long-bone deformities; azithromycin (Zithromax) or amoxicillin (Amoxil) is used instead (Tanner & Alexander, 2007). A woman's partner also should be treated to prevent re-infection.

Chlamydial infections must be treated during pregnancy because they are associated with premature rupture of the membranes, preterm labour and endometritis in the postnatal period. An infant who is born while a chlamydial infection is present can suffer conjunctivitis or pneumonia after birth (Hahn & Giunta, 2007) (see Chapter 40).

Human papillomavirus

The human papillomavirus (HPV) causes fibrous tissue overgrowth (sometimes called genital warts) on the external vulva, vagina or cervix (condyloma acuminatum). At first, lesions appear as discrete papillary structures; they then spread, enlarge and coalesce to form large, cauliflower-like lesions (see Fig. 47.2). The infection may be present in as many as 10–30% of women and is most common in women who have multiple sexual partners (Howley & Lowy, 2007). Therapy for such lesions is aimed at dissolving the lesions and also ending any secondary infection present. Small growths may be removed by applying podophyllotoxin (Wartec). Large lesions may be removed by laser therapy, cryocautery or knife excision. With cryocautery, oedema at the site is evident immediately; lesions become gangrenous and sloughing occurs in 7 days. Healing will be complete in 4–6 weeks with only slight depigmentation at the site. Salt baths and a lignocaine cream may be soothing during the healing period. Children (both male and female) with HPV infections should be further investigated for sexual abuse (Reading & Rannan-Eliya, 2007). HPV infections are serious because they are associated with the development of cervical cancer later in life (Soper, 2007). Women who have had one episode of infection should be conscientious about having yearly pap smears for the rest of their lives. The vaccine, Gardasil, is recommended to be routinely administered to early teenage girls in three doses. A second dose is given 2 months after the first dose and the third dose is 6 months after the first dose. Immunising young teenage girls against HPV infection should reduce not only the incidence of HPV infections in the future but the rate of cervical cancer as well (Deglin & Vallerand, 2009).

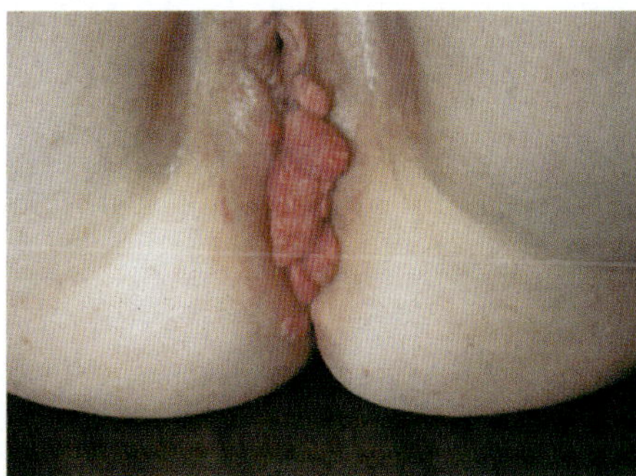

FIGURE 47.2 Genital warts. (Courtesy Reed & Carnrick Pharmaceuticals. From Lewis, P. & Foley, D. (2014). *Health Assessment in Nursing* (2nd ed.). Sydney: Lippincott Williams & Wilkins.)

Pregnancy and human papillomavirus infection

HPV lesions tend to increase in size during pregnancy because of the high vascular flow in the pelvic area. They may become secondarily ulcerated and infected; when this occurs, a foul vulvar odour may develop.

Podophyllotoxin (Wartec) is contraindicated during pregnancy because of possible toxic effects on the fetus. Women who do not find the lesions bothersome may choose to leave them in place during pregnancy and have them removed during the postnatal period.

The presence of vulvar lesions appears to have no effect on the fetus during pregnancy, but if they are present at the time of birth and so large that they obstruct the birth canal, a caesarean birth may be scheduled.

Herpes genitalis (herpes simplex type 2)

Genital herpes is caused by *herpes virus hominis* type 2 (also called herpes simplex virus type 2 or HSV-2). This is one of four similar herpes viruses: cytomegalovirus, Epstein-Barr, varicella-zoster and herpes types 1 and 2. Genital herpes occurs in epidemic proportions in the developed world and its incidence appears to be growing yearly (Wendel & Zenilman, 2007). Unlike most other STIs, although the virus can be contained, there is no known cure. The disease involves a lifelong process. Although it is not a precursor to cervical cancer, women with cervical cancer tend to have more antibodies against herpes genitalis than others or probably have been exposed to the virus more than others. The virus is spread by skin-to-skin contact, entering through a break in the skin or mucus membrane. In the newborn, the virus can be systemic or even fatal.

Herpes is diagnosed by culture of the lesion secretion from its location on the vulva, vagina, cervix or penis, or by isolation of HSV antibodies in serum. The incubation period is 3 to 14 days. On first contact, extensive primary lesions originate as a group of pinpoint vesicles on an erythematous base. Within a few days, the vesicles ulcerate and become moist, painful, draining, open lesions (see Fig. 47.3). An adolescent may have accompanying flu-like symptoms with increased temperature; vaginal lesions may cause a profuse discharge. Pain is intense on contact with clothing or acidic urine.

After the primary stage that lasts approximately 1 week, lesions heal but the virus lingers in a latent form, affecting the sensory nerve ganglia. The condition will flare up and become an active infection during illness, just prior to

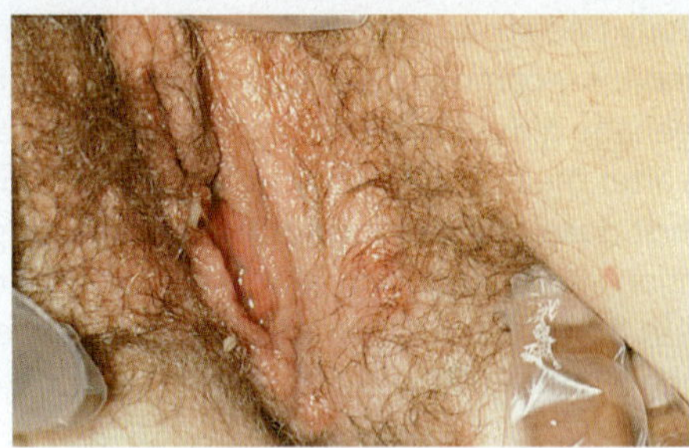

FIGURE 47.3 Small, painful, redbased, ulcer-like lesions of herpes simplex virus, type 2. (© 1992. Science Photo Library/CMSP. From From Lewis, P. & Foley, D. (2014). *Health Assessment in Nursing* (2nd ed.). Sydney: Lippincott Williams & Wilkins.)

menstruation, fever, overexposure to sunlight or stress. A secondary response usually produces only local lesions rather than systemic symptoms.

Pregnancy and herpes simplex virus type 2 infection

If a woman contracts a herpes type 2 infection during pregnancy, herpes can be transmitted across the placenta to cause congenital infection in the newborn. If a woman has primary or secondary active lesions in the vagina or on the vulva at the time of birth, herpes infection can be transmitted to the newborn at birth. When infection in the newborn occurs, congenital herpes, a severe systemic infection that is often fatal, can result. To help avoid transmission, women with active lesions are scheduled for caesarean birth. If no lesions are present a vaginal birth is preferable (Tanner & Alexander, 2007).

Diagnosis of the disorder is made by the appearance of the lesions and on the results of a pap smear and an enzyme-linked immunosorbent assay (ELISA). The medication of choice for the treatment of herpes infection is the same as for non-pregnant women (acyclovir [Zovirax] or valacyclovir [Valtrex]) (McKenna & Mirkov, 2014). Women can reduce the pain of the lesions by taking salt baths or applying warm, moist tea bags to the area.

Hepatitis B and hepatitis C

Both hepatitis B and hepatitis C can be spread by semen as well as blood and therefore are considered STIs. These are discussed in Chapter 45, with other forms of hepatitis. Because hepatitis B can be spread by sexual intercourse, adolescents who did not receive immunisation as an infant need immunisation updated.

Gonorrhoea

Gonorrhoea is transmitted by *Neisseria gonorrhoeae,* a gram-positive diplococcus. Symptoms begin after a 2- to 7-day incubation period. In males, they include *urethritis* (pain on urination and frequency of urination) and a urethral discharge. Without treatment, the infection may spread to the testes, scarring the tubules and causing permanent sterility. Untreated, the infection is easily spread among sexual partners. It often occurs concurrently with chlamydial infection (Wendel & Zenilman, 2007).

Although symptoms of gonorrhoea in females are not as visible, there may be a slight yellowish vaginal discharge. Bartholin's glands may become inflamed and painful (see Fig. 47.4). If left untreated, the infection may spread to pelvic organs, most notably the fallopian tubes (PID). Tubal scarring can result in permanent sterility. In both males and females, untreated gonorrhoea can lead to arthritis or heart disease from systemic involvement.

A urine culture for the gonococcal bacillus, in addition to vaginal and urethral cultures, should be obtained from all children with vulvovaginitis or a urethral discharge. In males a first voiding may reveal gonococci if a midstream urine specimen is inconclusive.

Of recent concern is the rise of drug-resistant gonorrhoea strains as has been the case in Auckland (Institute of Environmental Science & Research, 2012). Although the number of gonorrhoea cases in Australia is increasing this is not yet a problem (ACYS, 2014).

Pregnancy and gonorrhoea

Gonorrhoea is associated with spontaneous miscarriage, preterm birth and endometritis in the postnatal period. Pregnant women cannot be administered doxycycline because it has the potential to be teratogenic. Instead, they are prescribed amoxicillin or azithromycin. It is important that gonorrhoea be identified and treated during pregnancy because if the infection is present at the time of birth, it can cause a severe eye infection that can lead to blindness in the newborn (ophthalmia neonatorum; see Chapter 26) (Heidary & Kazlas, 2008).

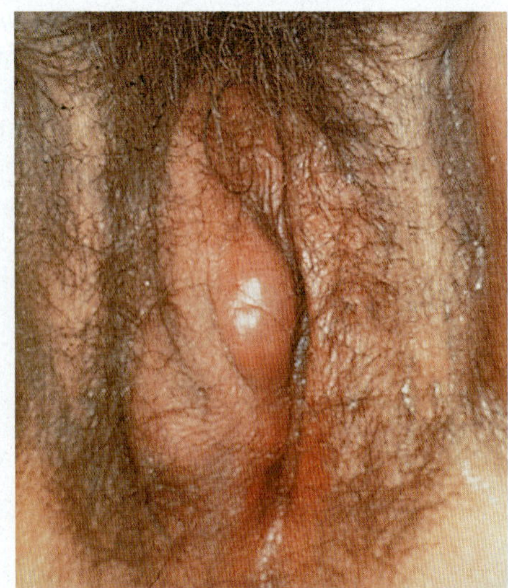

FIGURE 47.4 Abscess of a Bartholin's gland, a painful condition and common sign of *Neisseria gonorrhoeae* infection. (© 1992, National Medical Slide Bureau, CMSP. From From Lewis, P. & Foley, D. (2014). *Health Assessment in Nursing* (2nd ed.). Sydney: Lippincott Williams & Wilkins)

Syphilis

Syphilis is a systemic disease caused by the spirochete *Treponema pallidum* transmitted by sexual contact with a person who has an active lesion (Tanner & Alexander, 2007). Like gonorrhoea and Chlamydia, it must be reported to public health departments. Although the Institute of Environmental Science & Research Surveillance report (2012) shows a significant drop in infection rates in New Zealand surveillance centres, a significant proportion of these infections occur in male subjects.

After an incubation period of 10 to 90 days, a typical lesion appears, usually on the genitalia (penis or labia) or on the mouth, lips or rectal area from oral–genital or genital–anal contact. The lesion (termed a *chancre*) is a deep ulcer and is usually painless despite its size (see Fig. 47.5). Swollen lymph nodes may be present but these are unlikely to be noticed by the affected person. A lesion in the vagina may not be detected. Without treatment a chancre lasts approximately 6 weeks and then fades.

Approximately 2–4 weeks after the chancre disappears, a generalised, macular, copper-coloured rash appears. Unlike many other rashes, it affects the soles and the palms. A serologic test for syphilis yields a positive result at this time. There may be secondary symptoms of generalised illness such as low-grade fever. With or without treatment this stage of syphilis also fades. The next stage is a latency period that may last from only a few years to several decades. The only indication of the disease is the serologic test, which continues to yield a positive result. The final stage of syphilis is a destructive neurological disease that involves major body organs such as the heart and the nervous system. Typical symptoms are: blindness; paralysis; severe, crippling neurological deformities; mental confusion; slurred speech; and lack of coordination. This third stage must be identified before the disease becomes fatal.

Syphilis is diagnosed by recognition of the various symptoms of the three stages and by serologic serum tests, usually the Venereal Disease Research Laboratory test (VDRL), the automated reagin test (ART), the rapid plasma reagin test (RPR) or the fluorescent treponemal antibody–absorption test (FTA-ABS).

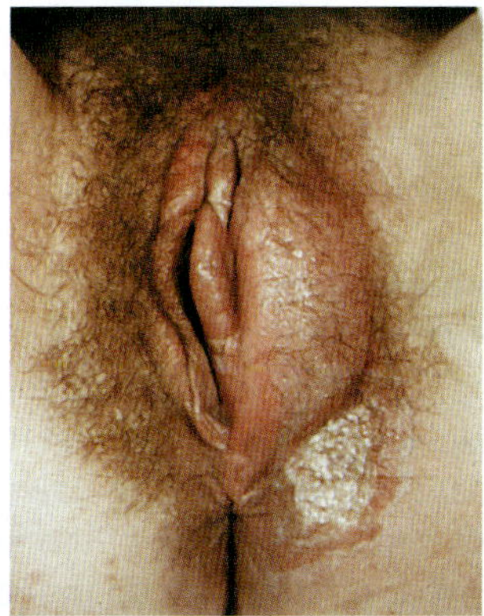

FIGURE 47.5 Chancre typical of syphilis. (Courtesy of Upjohn Co. From Lewis, P. & Foley, D. (2014). *Health Assessment in Nursing* (2nd ed.). Sydney: Lippincott Williams & Wilkins.)

Pregnancy and syphilis

Early in pregnancy (before week 18), the placenta appears to provide some protection against syphilis. After this time, however, the spirochete crosses the placenta freely and may be responsible for spontaneous miscarriage, preterm labour, stillbirth or congenital anomalies in the newborn (see Chapter 12). All pregnant women are screened for syphilis at a first prenatal visit with a VDRL, ART or FTA-ABS antibody reaction test. Those who have multiple sexual partners are tested again at about week 36 of pregnancy. In some institutions, women are screened again at the beginning of labour and newborns are screened for congenital syphilis by a cord blood sample. One injection of benzathine penicillin G is the medication of choice for the treatment of syphilis during pregnancy, the same as for those who are not pregnant.

If a woman does contract syphilis during pregnancy and it is untreated, a congenital form of the disease can occur in the newborn as the spirochete crosses the placenta readily in the last four months of pregnancy. Severely infected infants will be stillborn; others, less infected, are born with congenital anomalies. Moist lesions of the infant (the cord and nasal secretions) are generally infectious.

When the child's permanent teeth erupt at 5 or 6 years of age, they may be pegged or notched (Hutchinson's teeth). This is most noticeable in the upper central incisors. All teeth tend to be of poor quality and decay easily. If the disease remains untreated, interstitial keratitis, an inflammatory reaction of the cornea that can result in scarring and blindness, may develop when the child is school age. As the disease progresses further, it may become tertiary or lead to severe neurological symptoms.

Infants born to a woman with a positive VDRL are given a course of penicillin at birth. FTA-ABS is a sensitive, specific test for IgM antibodies against syphilis and may be helpful for diagnosis in the newborn.

Group B streptococcal infection

Although streptococcus B infection is a less publicised disease than STIs such as herpes type 2 or gonorrhoea, it may actually occur at a higher incidence than those diseases. It produces few symptoms. For a pregnant adolescent, consequences can be urinary tract infection (UTI), intra-amniotic infection, perhaps preterm birth and postnatal endometritis.

Pregnant women are screened for streptococcus B at 35 to 38 weeks of pregnancy. This screening is important, because approximately 40–70% of newborns whose mothers have an active infection at the time of birth will become infected from placental transfer or from direct contact with the organisms. Infected newborns may develop severe pneumonia, sepsis, respiratory distress syndrome or meningitis (Heath & Schuchat, 2007).

A broad-spectrum penicillin such as ampicillin is the treatment of choice. Women who experience rupture of membranes at less than 37 weeks of pregnancy and so have not yet been screened may be treated with intravenous ampicillin to reduce the risk of spreading the infection to the newborn.

Human immunodeficiency virus (HIV)

HIV is carried by semen as well as other body fluids, so infection with this virus is considered an STI. Invasion of the virus is discussed with other immune disorders in Chapter 42.

Anxiety related to having contracted a reportable STI

People who seek treatment for an STI need to believe that they can trust healthcare personnel and reveal information without fear of criticism. In notifiable STI cases the adolescent should be assured of absolute confidentiality in naming sexual contacts so they themselves are not put at risk. All contact partners can be notified that they have been exposed to a particular STI and should be advised to seek screening. This vital information helps prevent further spread of the disease.

Reassure people that the treatment is not prolonged and is as simple as taking medication. This is an insidious disease, and, even though no symptoms are apparent, it can have disastrous long-term effects if left untreated.

✔ *Checkpoint question 47.2*

Candidal vaginal infections can occur as an opportunistic infection when adolescents are prescribed antibiotics. What are the typical symptoms of a candidal vaginal infection?

a. Yellow pinpoint vaginal lesions
b. Puritic reddened vaginal walls
c. White, cream cheese-like vaginal discharge
d. Vaginal atrophy with final scarring

Key points for review

- Children who are born with a reproductive tract disorder frequently adjust well when young. They may need counselling at puberty or when they become aware of the impact of their disorder on sexual functioning or their ability to reproduce.
- The cause of ambiguous genitalia is unknown but may be related to the level of testosterone produced in utero. The true gender of children is established by a karyotype of chromosomes.
- The development of breast or pubic hair before 8 years of age or menses before 9 years of age is considered precocious sexual development. Children may be treated with a synthetic analogue of gonadotropin-releasing hormones to reduce development. Without effective support, such children are at high risk of disturbed body image.
- Delayed puberty is the failure to develop secondary sex characteristics by the age of 17 years. Girls may be administered oestrogen to promote development; boys may be administered testosterone.
- Balanoposthitis (inflammation of the glans and prepuce of the penis) and phimosis (constricted foreskin) occur in boys. Phimosis can be treated with circumcision.
- Cryptorchidism is a failure of one or both testes to descend during intrauterine life. The condition is surgically corrected to prevent subfertility and to detect testicular cancer later in life.
- Testicular cancer is rare but tends to occur in young men. Boys need to be taught testicular self-examination for early detection.
- Dysmenorrhoea, or painful menstruation, occurs frequently in adolescent girls. Therapy is the use of a prostaglandin inhibitor such as ibuprofen.
- Untreated endometriosis (the abnormal growth of extrauterine endometrial tissue) can lead to subfertility later in life. Therapy is the administration of a synthetic androgen or gonadotropin-releasing hormone receptor inhibitor or surgery to reduce the size of the abnormal tissue.
- Vulvovaginitis (inflammation of the vulva and vagina) and pelvic inflammatory disease are infections that can occur in adolescents. Therapy to prevent fallopian tube scarring and subfertility later in life is essential. Girls need to be taught, in addition, ways to avoid toxic shock syndrome (TSS).
- Sexually transmitted infections (STIs) such as candidiasis, trichomoniasis, *C. trachomatis* infection, genital warts, herpes genitalis, gonorrhoea and syphilis are increasing in incidence in the adolescent population. An important education area for adolescents is the need to follow safer sex practices.
- STIs such as candidiasis, trichomoniasis, *Chlamydia*, syphilis, herpes type 2, gonorrhoea, papilloma and HIV may occur during pregnancy. These illnesses need to be treated promptly. Women need to use safer sex practices to help prevent these diseases.
- When teaching about STIs, it is important to stress that they do not confer immunity and therefore can be contracted more than once. If an STI occurs in a young child, the potential for child abuse should be investigated.

CASE STUDY QUESTIONS

2. Alicia says she is glad she contracted the disease early in life, because now she will never get it again. She also states that she is not sexually active. What health teaching does Alicia need to be better informed about her disease? What other follow-up is needed?
3. Alicia has almost no breast development and also has not menstruated yet. She asks you if it is time to worry. How would you counsel her?

4. Ryan, the boy whom Alicia dates, was born with undescended testes. He had surgery for this condition when he was 2 years old. He is concerned now that he is at high risk of testicular cancer. How would you counsel him?

Resources

For an extensive range of additional resources to enhance teaching and learning and to facilitate understanding of this chapter, please see the text's accompanying website located on thePoint at http://thepoint.lww.com.

References

Australian Clearinghouse for Youth Studies (ACYS). (2014). Face the facts briefing: Young Australians and sexual health. Australian Government Department of Education, accessed 25 February 2015 <www.acys.info/facts>.

Australian Society of HIV Medicine (ASHM) (2014). *HIV, Viral Hepatitis and STI's: A Guide for Primary Health Care*, accessed 25 February 2015 <www.ashm.org.au/images/Publications/Monographs/Multi_Mono_2014/4th_Edition_2014.pdf>.

Blyth, C. C., Palasanthiran, P. & O'Brien, T. A. (2007). Antifungal therapy in children with invasive fungal infections: A systematic review. *Pediatrics, 119*(4), 772–784.

Bouhadiba, N., Godbole, P. & Marven, S. (2007). Laparoscopic excision of abdominoscrotal hydrocele. *Journal of Laparoendoscopic and Advanced Surgical Techniques, 17*(5), 701–703.

Brown-Guttovz, H. (2007). Testicular torsion. *Nursing 2007, 37*(10), 72.

Burke, A. E. & Rogers, L. C. (2007). Nonmalignant vulvovaginal disorders, pelvic inflammatory disease, and chronic pelvic pain. In N. H. Fiebach, et al. (Eds). *Principles of Ambulatory Medicine* (7th ed.). Philadelphia: Lippincott Williams & Wilkins.

Carel, J. C. & Leger, J. (2008). Clinical practice. Precocious puberty. *New England Journal of Medicine, 358*(22), 2366–2377.

Carter, T. C., et al. (2008). Antifungal drugs and the risk of selected birth defects. *American Journal of Obstetrics and Gynecology, 198*(2), 191–197.

Cesario, S. K. & Hughes, L. A. (2007). Precocious puberty: a comprehensive review of literature. *JOGNN: Journal of Obstetric, Gynecologic, and Neonatal Nursing, 36*(3), 263–274.

Cook, R. L., et al. (2007). Home screening for sexually transmitted diseases in high-risk young women: Randomized controlled trial. *Sexually Transmitted Infections, 83*(4), 286–291.

Dane, C., et al. (2007). Imperforate hymen—a rare cause of abdominal pain. Two cases and review of the literature. *Journal of Pediatric and Adolescent Gynecology, 20*(4), 245–247.

Deglin, J. H. & Vallerand, A. H. (2009). *Davis's Drug Guide for Nurses* (11th ed.). Philadelphia: F. A. Davis Company.

Dickson, N. P., et al. (2008). Circumcision and risk of sexually transmitted infections in a birth cohort. *Journal of Pediatrics, 152*(3), 383–387.

Einhorn, L. H., et al. (2007). High-dose chemotherapy and stem-cell rescue for metastatic germ-cell tumors. *New England Journal of Medicine, 357*(4), 340–348.

Endometriosis Care Centre of Australia (ECCA). (2008). About endometriosis, accessed 25 February 2015 <www.ecca.com.au/about-endometriosis>.

Evans, A. L., et al. (2007). Prevalence of bacterial vaginosis in lesbians and heterosexual women in a community setting. *Sexually Transmitted Infections, 83*(6), 470–475.

Fitzgerald, P. A. (2014). Endocrine disorders. In S. J. McPhee & M. A. Papadakis (Eds). *Current Medical Diagnosis and Treatment*. Columbus, OH: McGraw-Hill.

Gollu, G., et al. (2007). Ambiguous genitalia: an overview of 17 years' experience. *Journal of Pediatric Surgery, 42*(5), 840–844.

Gray, S. H. & Emans, S. J. (2007). Abnormal vaginal bleeding in adolescents. *Pediatrics in Review, 28*(5), 175–182.

Grover, S. (2007). Bleeding disorders and heavy menses in adolescents. *Current Opinion in Obstetrics and Gynecology, 19*(5), 415–419.

Hahn, B. & Giunta, Y. P. (2007). Images in emergency medicine. *Chlamydia* conjunctivitis. *Annals of Emergency Medicine, 49*(6), 823–831.

Hall, J. E. (2009). Menstrual disorders and pelvic pain. In A. S. Fauci (Ed). *Harrison's Principles of Internal Medicine* (17th ed.). Columbus, OH: McGraw-Hill.

Hansen, M. T., et al. (2007). *Streptococcus pyogenes* pharyngeal colonization resulting in recurrent, prepubertal vulvovaginitis. *Journal of Pediatric and Adolescent Gynecology, 20*(5), 315–317.

Harel, Z. (2007). Dysmenorrhea in adolescents and young adults: Etiology and management. *Journal of Pediatric and Adolescent Gynecology, 19*(6), 363–371.

Hay, P. & Czeizel, A. E. (2007). Asymptomatic trichomonas and candida colonization and pregnancy outcome. *Best Practice and Research in Clinical Obstetrics and Gynaecology, 21*(3), 403–409.

Heath, P. T. & Schuchat, A. (2007). Perinatal group B streptococcal disease. *Best Practice and Research in Clinical Obstetrics and Gynaecology, 21*(3), 411–424.

Heidary, G. & Kazlas, M. (2008). Pediatric ophthalmology. In D. Pavan-Langston (Ed). *Manual of Ocular Diagnosis and Therapy*. Philadelphia: Lippincott Williams & Wilkins.

Hoffnung, M. et al. (2010) *Lifespan Development* (1st Australasian ed.). Brisbane: John Wiley & Sons.

Howley, P. M. & Lowy, D. R. (2007). Papillomaviruses. In D. M. Knipe & P. M. Howley (Eds). *Fields Virology*. Philadelphia: Lippincott Williams & Wilkins.

Hsieh, T. F., Chang, C. H. & Chang, S. S. (2007). Foreskin development before adolescence in 2149 schoolboys. *International Journal of Urology, 13*(7), 968–970.

Institute of Environmental Science & Research, (2012). Sexually transmitted infections in New Zealand: Annual surveillance report 2011, accessed 25 February 2015 <https://surv.esr.cri.nz/PDF_surveillance/STISurvRpt/2011/2011AnnualSTIRpt.pdf>.

Johnson, T. R., et al. (2007). Why and how a Department of Obstetrics and Gynecology stopped doing routine newborn male circumcision. *Obstetrics and Gynecology, 109*(3), 750–752.

Jun, E. M., et al. (2007). Effects of acupressure on dysmenorrhea and skin temperature changes in college students: A non-randomized controlled trial. *International Journal of Nursing Studies, 44*(6), 973–981.

Kansal, R., et al. (2007). Structural and functional properties of antibodies to the superantigen TSST-1 and their relationship to menstrual toxic shock syndrome. *Journal of Clinical Immunology, 27*(3), 327–338.

The Kirby Institute for infection and immunity in society, (2014) *HIV, viral hepatitis and sexually transmissible infections in Australia: Annual surveillance report 2014*. Sydney: The Kirby Institute, The University of New South Wales, accessed 25 February 2015 <http://kirby.unsw.edu.au/sites/default/files/hiv/resources/ASR2014.pdf>.

Kollin, C., et al. (2007). Surgical treatment of unilaterally undescended testes: Testicular growth after randomization to orchiopexy at age 9 months or 3 years. *Journal of Urology, 178*(4.2), 1589–1593.

Latreille, S., Collyer, A. & Temple-Smith, M. (2014) Finding a segue into sex: Young men's views on discussing sexual health with a GP. *Australian Family Physician*, *43*(4), 217–222.

Lewis, P. & Foley, D. (2014). *Health Assessment in Nursing* (2nd ed.). Sydney: Lippincott Williams & Wilkins.

McKenna, L. & Mirkov, S. (2014). *McKenna's Drug Handbook for Nursing and Midwifery* (7th ed.). Sydney: Lippincott Williams & Wilkins.

Park, S. J., et al. (2007). Manual reduction of torsion of an intrascrotal appendage under ultrasonographic monitoring. *Journal of Ultrasound in Medicine, 26*(3), 293–299.

Parker, M.A. (2009) The menstrual disorder of teenager (MDOT) study: Determining typical menstrual patterns and menstrual disturbances in large population-based study of Australian teenagers. *BJOG: An International Journal of Obstetrics & Gynaecology, 117*, 185–192.

Rakhshaee, Z. (2011). Effect of three yoga poses (cobra, cat and fish poses) in women with primary dysmenorrhea: A randomized clinical trial. *Journal of Pediatric & Adolescent Gynecology, 24*(4), 192–196

Reading, R. & Rannan-Eliya, Y. (2007). Evidence for sexual transmission of genital herpes in children. *Archives of Disease in Childhood, 92*(7), 608–613.

Schilling McCann, J. A., et al. (Eds). (2007). *Professional Guide to Signs and Symptoms*. Philadelphia: Lippincott Williams & Wilkins.

Soper, D. E. (2007). Genitourinary infections and sexually transmitted diseases. In J. S. Berek (Ed). *Berek & Novak's Obstetrics and Gynecology*. Philadelphia: Lippincott Williams & Wilkins.

South Australian Health (2015). Toxic shock syndrome, accessed 25 February 2015, <www.sahealth.sa.gov.au/wps/wcm/connect/Public+Content/SA+Health+Internet/Health+topics/Health+conditions+prevention+and+treatment/Infectious+diseases/Toxic+shock+syndrome/Toxic+shock+syndrome+TSS+-+including+symptoms+treatment+and+prevention>.

Stotland, N. L. (2007). Common psychiatric problems. In J. S. Berek (Ed). *Berek & Novak's Obstetrics and Gynecology*. Philadelphia: Lippincott Williams & Wilkins.

Tanner, E. & Alexander, C. J. (2007). Infections of the genital tract. In K. B. Fortner, et al. (Eds). *The Johns Hopkins Manual of Gynecology and Obstetrics*. Philadelphia: Lippincott Williams & Wilkins.

Vercellini, P., et al. (2007). Association between endometriosis stage, lesion type, patient characteristics and severity of pelvic pain symptoms: A multivariate analysis of over 1000 patients. *Human Reproduction, 22*(1), 266–271.

Walsh, T. J., et al. (2007). Prepubertal orchiopexy for cryptorchidism may be associated with lower risk of testicular cancer. *Journal of Urology, 178*(4.1), 1440–1446.

Wendel, K. A. & Zenilman, J. M. (2007). Sexually transmitted diseases. In N. H. Fiebach, et al. (Eds). *Principles of Ambulatory Medicine* (7th ed.). Philadelphia: Lippincott Williams & Wilkins.

World Health Organization (WHO) (2014). Female genital mutilation, accessed 25 February 2015, <www.who.int/mediacentre/factsheets/fs241/en>.

Yigiter, M., Arda, I. S. & Hicsonmez, A. (2008). An unusual cause of paraphimosis: Hemangioma of the glans penis. *Journal of Pediatric Surgery, 43*(2), e31–e33.

Yonkers, K. A., O'Brien, P. M. & Eriksson, E. (2008). Premenstrual syndrome. *Lancet, 371*(9619), 1200–1210.

Zampieri, N., et al. (2007). Varicocele and adolescents: semen quality after 2 different laparoscopic procedures. *Journal of Andrology, 28*(5), 727–733.

Suggested readings

Auckland Sexual Health Service <www.ashs.org.nz>.

Australian Government STI <www.sti.health.gov.au/internet/sti/publishing.nsf>.

Australian Government. The Department of Health. National Women's Health Policy <www.health.gov.au/womenshealthpolicy>.

Australian Institute for Health and Welfare. Child health development and wellbeing <www.aihw.gov.au/child-health-development-and-wellbeing>.

Leung-Chen, P. (2008). Syphilis makes another comeback: Nurses can help in containing transmission, above all through education. *American Journal of Nursing, 108*(2), 28–31.

Massey, M. T. & Winterburn, S. A. (2008). Managing minor illness—vaginal discharge. *Journal of Community Nursing, 22*(1), 20–21.

Public Health Surveillance: information for public health action <https://surv.esr.cri.nz/surveillance/annual_sti.php>.

Roberts, S. C., Hodgkiss, C., DiBenedetto, A., et al. (2012). Managing dysmenorrhea in young women. *Nurse Practitioner, 37*(7), 47–52.

Sass, A. E. & Kaplan, D. W. (2014). Adolescence. In W. W. Hay, et al. (Eds). *Current Pediatric Diagnosis and Treatment* (22nd ed.). Columbus, OH: McGraw-Hill.

Sexual Reproductive Health in New Zealand <www.health.govt.nz/our-work/preventative-health-wellness/sexual-and-reproductive-health>.

Sexually Transmitted Infections Summary of Guidelines, 2013 <www.nzshs.org/guidelines/STI_Summary_of_Guidelines_2013.pdf>.

STI Handbook, New Zealand <www.bpac.org.nz/resources/handbook/sti/sti.asp>.

The Australians Longitudinal Study on Women's Health <www.alswh.org.au>.

Varty, A. (2008). Establishing best practice for premenstrual syndrome. *Nursing Times, 104*(20), 23–24.

Watkins, J. (2008). Genital herpes simplex. *Practice Nursing, 19*(6), 296–297.

Women's & Children's Health Network, Parenting and Child Health <www.cyh.com/HealthTopics/HealthTopicCategories.aspx?p=122>.

World Health Organization; Child development <www.who.int/topics/child_development/en>.

Chapter 48

Nursing care of a family when a child has an endocrine or a metabolic disorder

This chapter provides information about the changes, both physical and psychosocial, that occur when children develop an endocrine or metabolic disorder.

LEARNING OBJECTIVES

After studying the contents of this chapter, you should be able to:

1. Briefly describe the structure and function of the endocrine glands and why metabolic illnesses occur.
2. Analyse ways that care of a child with altered endocrine or metabolic function can be made more family-centred.
3. Assess a child with a disorder of endocrine or metabolic function.
4. Discuss the nursing care for a child with endocrine or metabolic dysfunction.
5. Evaluate expected outcomes for achievement and effectiveness of care.
6. Identify areas of care related to endocrine or metabolic disorders and children that could benefit from additional nursing research or application of evidence-based practice.

KEY TERMS

- exophthalmos
- hormones
- hyperglycaemia
- hypoglycaemia
- ketoacidosis
- latent tetany
- manifest tetany
- polydipsia
- polyuria

CASE STUDY

Jack West is a 16-year-old boy with type 1 diabetes whom you meet in the emergency department, where he was taken after he became comatose while running. His diabetes was diagnosed when he was 7 years old. His records indicate that his disease has generally been under good control over the past years, but in the last 6 months he has "forgotten" to take his insulin at least once a week. When you ask him about this, he tells you that triathlon training every morning and a new girlfriend have occupied his time and interrupted what used to be a strict schedule of home-cooked meals and a rigid routine.

CASE STUDY QUESTIONS

1. Is Jack's history unusual for an adolescent?
2. What health teaching do you think will most help him re-establish control?

The endocrine system is composed of a small group of ductless glands that work together with the neurological system to regulate and coordinate all body systems (see Fig. 48.1). The glands produce chemicals called **hormones**, which are secreted into surrounding tissue and picked up by the bloodstream, where they act individually and in concert to affect various organ systems. (The word *hormone* is from the Greek *hormaein,* which means "to set in motion".) Each gland of the endocrine system acts on a specific target (or designated) organ or has specific duties that are necessary for regulating body processes (Thalange & Beach, 2013).

Dysfunction of the glands or action of the hormones results in a variety of disorders, most of which have long-term implications. Parents and children, as soon as they are old enough, need to understand the causes and symptoms of these diseases and to participate in their long-term plan of care.

CARE OF A CHILD WITH AN ENDOCRINE OR METABOLIC DISORDER

Assessment

Endocrine and metabolic disorders as a group commonly cause changes in normal growth or activity patterns. This is usually detected when a child's height and weight are assessed and compared with standards for the child's age at a health visit. An acute loss in weight is often the first symptom of type 1 diabetes mellitus in children. Thyroid deficiencies or type 2 diabetes mellitus may be revealed by a child being overweight. As more children become obese, more children develop type 2 diabetes. Pituitary difficulties may be revealed by short or unusually tall stature.

To obtain information on activity, take an accurate history by asking a parent or child to describe all of the child's actions on a typical day. This type of information yields clues that are helpful in distinguishing between a normally "quiet" child and one who is experiencing inactivity and chronic fatigue as a result of decreased endocrine function. For example, the quiet child lies down after school and reads; the ill child lies down and sleeps. Taking a day history also helps to differentiate between a child who is merely active and one who is overly active because of hyperthyroidism. For example, the healthy child appears to "go constantly" but can sit through a favourite television

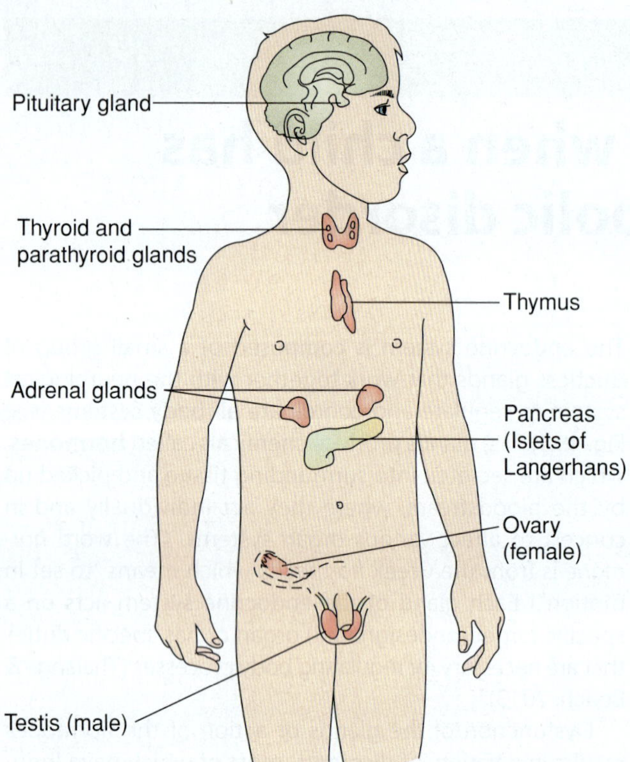

FIGURE 48.1 Location of the endocrine glands.

program or a meal. The child with increased thyroid hormone production may be unable to sit quietly at all.

Also assess dietary and elimination habits. Extreme thirst or appetite may occur with an endocrine disorder such as diabetes insipidus or type 1 diabetes mellitus. Frequent voiding in children most often reflects a urinary tract infection, but it may be evidence of excessive urine excretion **(polyuria)**, possibly from pituitary dysfunction or diabetes mellitus.

On physical examination, observe a child's general appearance, noting any excessive tiredness, scaly or dry skin, drooping eyelids, protrusion of the eyeballs **(exophthalmos)** or poor muscle tone, all indications of endocrine disorders.

Nursing considerations

Although most endocrine and metabolic disorders have long-term implications, parents and children may initially find it easier to work with outcomes that are short term—particularly if they are having difficulty accepting the diagnosis and the long-term nature of the disorder. Because symptoms are usually not acute, children and/or parents may forget to take medication. Helping parents create reminder charts is an effective measure to increase adherence.

Evaluate the school as well as the home situation for any child with a chronic illness. Information may need to be provided to the child's school about their health problem (with the parents' permission) so that appropriate care can be maintained. Selected organisations for referral include:

- Diabetes Australia <www.diabetesaustralia.com.au>
- Diabetes New Zealand <www.diabetes.org.nz>
- Kids and Teens with Diabetes <www.diabeteskidsandteens.com.au>
- Congenital Adrenal Hyperplasia Support Group Australia Inc. <www.cah.org.au>
- Association for Children with a Disability <www.acd.org.au>
- Australian Pituitary Foundation Ltd <www.pituitary.asn.au>.

Interventions for children with endocrine or metabolic disorders must always be carried out with long-term aspects of care in mind. Bribing children to take medicine, for example, is never good practice. It quickly becomes ineffective with children who must continue to take a medication for the rest of their lives. Simple explanations for younger children, becoming more detailed as the child grows older and can better understand their disorder, should be carried out.

Children with disorders of endocrine or metabolic function need to be evaluated periodically throughout childhood, because growth and changing activities necessitate changes in medication dosages or schedules. These check-ups provide good opportunities for health teaching to equip children to meet new situations that arise as they mature. For example, body appearance becomes increasingly important as children enter adolescence. Because of this, seemingly well-adjusted school-age children may develop extreme difficulty continuing to accept their illness as they get older. Adherence to a medication program may become erratic. Only by periodic re-evaluation

BOX 48.1 Assessment ✻ Assessing a child with an endocrine disorder

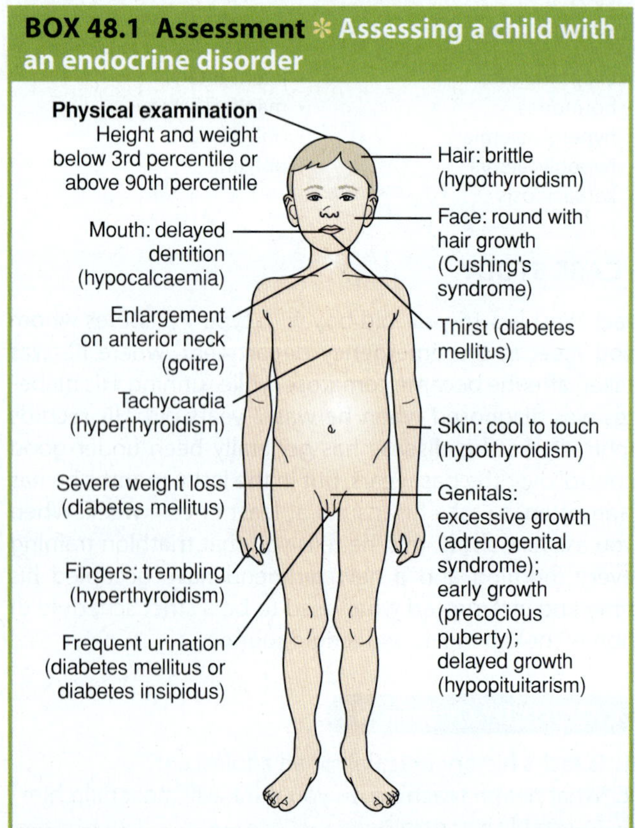

can these problems be identified so that healthcare plans can be modified and adapted to the child's needs, enabling the child and family to continue coping with a long-term illness.

HEALTH PROMOTION

Many endocrine and metabolic disorders are inherited so education and genetic counselling are important preventive measures (see Box 48.1). Type 2 diabetes mellitus is strongly associated with obesity so is at an epidemic incidence as obesity in school-aged children is also at epidemic proportions.

PITUITARY GLAND DISORDERS

Pituitary gland disorders are caused by pituitary dysfunction which can result from a tumour growing in the pituitary or hypothalamus, interference with circulation to the gland, trauma, inflammation, structural abnormalities, erratic or non-functional feedback mechanisms, and, possibly, autoimmune responses (see Table 48.1). This can

TABLE 48.1 Common pituitary hormones and their purposes

Pituitary hormone	Source and target organs	Actions and effects
Antidiuretic hormone (ADH)	Secreted by the neurohypophysis *Target organ:* Kidney	• ADH helps regulate fluid volume and urine output. It decreases urinary output by increasing water resorption. This action increases extracellular fluid volume, resulting in a vasoconstrictor effect (increased blood pressure). When the plasma concentration increases or overall circulating vascular volume decreases, more ADH is released. • If blood pools in the body periphery, decreasing core body volume, ADH is released. • Postural changes (from a lying to a standing position) and exposure to high temperatures (blood shifts to peripheral structures to begin the cooling process) stimulate ADH release. • Trauma, pain and anxiety increase ADH release. • When ADH levels fall, little or no water is reabsorbed, and urinary output increases. • Alcohol consumption inhibits ADH secretion; as a result, urine output increases.
Corticotropin (ACTH)	Secreted by the adenohypophysis *Target organ:* Adrenal glands	• ACTH stimulates the adrenal gland to produce glucocorticoid and mineralocorticoid hormones. Increased production of adrenal gland secretions decreases ACTH production and vice versa. • If a child receives synthetic ACTH or a corticosteroid, natural ACTH production is temporarily depressed. If these synthetic hormones are given for a long time, then stopped abruptly, the decreased amount of natural ACTH may not be enough to stimulate adrenal gland activity. The child will experience symptoms of adrenal insufficiency. • When discontinuing ACTH and high doses of long-term corticosteroids, dosage must be reduced gradually to protect adrenal function. The medication should never be stopped abruptly.
Somatotropin (growth hormone [GH])	Secreted by the adenohypophysis *Target organ:* None; acts on all body cells	• GH increases bone and cartilage growth and increases gastrointestinal absorption of calcium. If GH production is inhibited, undergrowth will occur; if GH production is excessive, overgrowth will occur. • GH decreases catabolism of protein in cells by freeing fatty acids for energy, which, in turn, frees glucose for glycogen storage (GH is both protein and glucose sparing). • GH production increases when hypoglycaemia occurs and during sleep. • GH is released from the adenohypophysis based on a release factor from both the hypothalamus and the liver. • The amount of GH secretion is influenced by exercise, sleep, nutrition and thyroid and adrenal function.
Thyrotropin (TSH)	Secreted by the adenohypophysis *Target organ:* Thyroid gland	• TSH stimulates the thyroid gland to produce thyroid hormones (thyroxine and triiodothyronine). • Too little TSH leads to atrophy and inactivity of the thyroid gland; too much TSH causes hypertrophy (increase in size) and hyperplasia (increase in the number of cells) of the gland. • A feedback message of increased thyroid secretion lowers TSH production; decreased thyroid production increases TSH production.

result in partial or total hypopituitarism which results in conditions such as growth hormone deficiency, diabetes insipidus and congenital adrenal hyperplasia. Partial or total hyperpituitarism results in conditions such as Cushing's syndrome.

Growth hormone deficiency

If production of human growth hormone (GH or somatotropin) is deficient, children cannot grow to full size (Dahlgren, 2011). As a result, children remain in proportion but well below the average on a standard growth chart. In most children with hypopituitarism, the cause of the defect is unknown. It may have a genetic origin (Hernandez, Lee & Camacho-Hubner, 2007).

If a child with hypopituitarism is not treated, predicting exactly what height the child will reach is difficult because height varies with each individual. Without treatment, however, most children will not reach more than 1 to 1.2 m in height.

Assessment includes growth history, family history, as well as history of chronic illnesses and nutrition. A pituitary tumour must be ruled out as the cause of decreased GH production. Sudden halted growth suggests a tumour; gradual failure suggests an idiopathic involvement. Signs of increased intracranial pressure also suggest a pituitary tumour. The history of a child with GH deficiency typically reveals a well child except for the abnormal lack of growth. A physical assessment, including neurological testing, is necessary to detect a lesion or tumour. Blood studies for hypothyroidism, hypoadrenalism, hypoaldosteronism and growth factor binding proteins are performed as well as radiographical studies of epiphyseal closure of long bones and bone age. A head computed tomography (CT) scan or magnetic resonance imaging (MRI) will be performed to detect a possible pituitary tumour.

GH deficiency is treated by the administration of subcutaneous (SC) recombinant human growth hormone (rhGH) two or three times a week (see Box 48.2). GH is usually given at bedtime, the time of day at which GH normally peaks. Because these children have delayed epiphyseal closure, if treatment is started early, they will be able to reach a targeted height. Some may need suppression of luteinising hormone-releasing hormone (LHRH) or gonadotropin-releasing hormone (GnRH) to delay epiphyseal closure. Other children may need supplements of gonadotropin or other pituitary hormones if these are deficient as well (Zeitler et al., 2014). Children who do not respond to growth hormone stimulation may be offered a course of synthetic recombinant insulin-like growth factor I (Ali & Wyatt, 2011).

✓ *Checkpoint question 48.1*

A 12-year-old girl with GH deficiency is only 90 cm tall and has been told she probably will not grow taller than 135 cm. Her parents tell you they find her "cute" so they do not want her to receive GH. How would you approach this family? To what extent should the child be able to contribute to this decision?

Diabetes insipidus

Diabetes insipidus is a disease in which there is a decreased release of antidiuretic hormone (ADH) by the pituitary gland (Chamarthi et al., 2010). This causes less reabsorption of fluid in the kidney tubules. Urine becomes extremely diluted and a great deal of fluid is lost from the body. Diabetes insipidus may reflect an X-linked dominant trait or it may be transmitted by an autosomal recessive gene. It may result from a lesion, tumour or injury to the posterior pituitary; or it may have an unknown cause. In a rare type of diabetes insipidus, pituitary function is adequate, but the kidneys' nephrons are not sensitive to ADH (a kidney-related aetiology).

The child with diabetes insipidus experiences **polydipsia** (excessive thirst that is relieved only by drinking water) as well as **polyuria** (excessive urine excretion). The specific gravity of the urine is low (1.001 to 1.005); normal values are more often 1.010 to 1.020. Urine output may reach 4 to 10 L in a 24-hour period (normal range, 1 to 2 L, depending on age).

BOX 48.2 ✻ Focus on pharmacology

Somatropin (nutropin, humatrope)

Classification: Somatropin is a recombinant human growth hormone (rhGH).

Action: Used for the long-term treatment of children who have growth failure from inadequate production of pituitary hormone, renal failure or Turner's syndrome; may be used to promote healing in severe burns (McKenna & Mirkov, 2014)

Pregnancy risk category: C

Dosage: Somatropin dosage is individualised. The drug is administered by injection.

Possible adverse effects: Injection site pain, glucose intolerance, hypothyroidism, bone problems (particularly the hip), blood abnormalities, rare intracranial hypertension in first 8 weeks of therapy

Nursing implications

- Advise parents that x-rays of the wrist or hip are performed before therapy begins. Thereafter, parents should be alert for limping or knee or hip pain, which should be reported to their primary care provider. Slipped capital epiphysis is associated with rhGH supplementation.
- Reinforce the need for periodic thyroid function tests and fundoscopical examination (to detect rare intracranial hypertension).
- Tell parents that rhGH may interact with glucocorticoid therapy such as prednisone, causing a decrease in the effectiveness of the rhGH. Urge parents to inform all healthcare practitioners that the child is receiving rhGH.
- Keep in mind that administration of rhGH is associated with a possible increased risk of leukaemia.

Signs and symptoms of diabetes insipidus usually appear gradually. Parents may notice the polyuria first as bedwetting in a toilet-trained child. Weight loss occurs because of the large loss of fluid. If the condition remains untreated, the child will lose such a quantity of water that dehydration and death can result.

Surgery is the treatment of choice of diabetes insipidus if a tumour is present. If the cause is idiopathic, the condition can be controlled by the administration of desmopressin (DDAVP), an arginine vasopressin. In an emergency, this drug can be given intravenously (IV). In older children, treatment consists of desmopressin intranasally or orally, in addition to thiazide diuretics and a low-sodium diet. For infants and small children, the intranasal route is unreliable, therefore desmopressin is given subcutaneously. The preferred treatment regimen in infants and small children is a thiazide diuretic combined with low-solute (low sodium and low protein) diet, with or without SC desmopressin (Chamarthi et al., 2010; Blanco et al, 2006).

Carers need to be taught to monitor their child's urine output, in particular for infants and small children. Education should also be given on identifying hyponatraemia and hypernatraemia, in addition to the management of diabetes insipidus during periods of intercurrent illness that affect fluid intake or fluid loss.

Syndrome of inappropriate antidiuretic hormone

Syndrome of inappropriate antidiuretic hormone (SIADH) is the overproduction of antidiuretic hormone by the posterior pituitary gland. This results in a decrease in urine production and water intoxication. As sodium levels fall in proportion to water, the child develops hyponatraemia or a lowered sodium plasma level. It can be caused by central nervous system infections such as bacterial meningitis (see Chapter 49), long-term positive pressure ventilation or pituitary compression such as could occur from oedema.

Mild symptoms of hyponatraemia are weight gain, concentrated urine (increased specific gravity), nausea and vomiting. As the hyponatraemia grows more severe, coma or seizures occur from brain oedema.

Therapy consists of treating the underlying cause in addition to restriction of fluid and supplementation of sodium by IV fluid if needed. Demeclocycline may be prescribed. Demeclocycline is a tetracycline antibiotic which has the side effect of blocking the action of ADH in renal tubules and reducing resorption of water, however it is contraindicated in young children (Frederick & Danzl, 2008; Ranadive, 2011).

THYROID GLAND

The thyroid gland is responsible for controlling the rate of metabolism in the body through production of the hormones thyroxine (T_4) and triiodothyronine (T_3) by its follicular cells. A third hormone, thyrocalcitonin, is produced by the interstitial cells of the gland. Thyrocalcitonin is released if a high serum calcium level occurs. This hormone inhibits bone resorption, thereby slowing the rate of release of calcium from bone to plasma and resulting in a lowered serum calcium level. It reflects the reverse action of parathyroid hormone, which elevates serum calcium levels.

THYROID GLAND DISORDERS

Congenital hypothyroidism

Thyroid hypofunction causes reduced production of both T_4 and T_3. Congenital hypofunction (reduced or absent function) occurs as a result of an absent or non-functioning thyroid gland in a newborn. The disorder occurs in 1 in every 4000 live births and about twice as often in girls as in boys (Jameson & Weetman, 2012). The cause of the disorder is usually unknown, although if a woman has hyperthyroidism during pregnancy this can cause the fetal thyroid to not fully develop as it does not need to function (Kempers et al., 2007). The symptoms of congenital hypothyroidism become apparent during the first 3 months of life in a formula-fed infant and at about 6 months in a breastfed infant. Because congenital hypothyroidism causes progressive physical and cognitive challenges, early diagnosis is crucial.

A screening test for hypothyroidism is mandatory at birth (using the same few drops of blood obtained for a Guthrie or phenylketonuria [PKU] test) (Korada et al., 2008).

The treatment for hypothyroidism is oral administration of synthetic thyroid hormone, sodium levothyroxine. The child needs to continue taking medication indefinitely to supplement that which the thyroid does not make. Supplemental vitamin D may also be given to prevent the development of rickets when, with the administration of thyroid hormone, rapid bone growth begins (Delvecchio et al., 2007).

Acquired hypothyroidism (Hashimoto's thyroiditis)

Hashimoto's disease is the most common form of acquired hypothyroidism in childhood; the age at onset is often 10 to 11 years. It occurs more often in girls than in boys. The decrease in thyroid secretion is caused by the development of an autoimmune phenomenon that interferes with thyroid production. Excretion of thyroid-stimulating hormone (TSH) from the pituitary increases when thyroid hormone production decreases, in an attempt to cause the thyroid to be more effective (Fitzgerald, 2014). In response to TSH, hypertrophy of the thyroid gland (goitre) occurs and body growth is impaired by lack of thyroxine.

Treatment for acquired hypothyroidism is the administration of synthetic thyroid hormone (sodium levothyroxine), the same as for congenital hypothyroidism. With adequate dosage, the obesity diminishes and growth begins again. It is important that the disease be recognised as early as possible so there is time to stimulate growth before the epiphyseal lines close at puberty.

If acquired hypothyroidism exists in a woman during pregnancy, her infant can be born cognitively challenged. Therefore, it is important that girls with this syndrome be identified before they reach childbearing age.

Hyperthyroidism (Graves' disease)

Hyperthyroidism is oversecretion of thyroid hormones by the thyroid gland. In children, it usually occurs at the time of puberty or during adolescence and is more common in girls than in boys (Lee & Masharani, 2012). Over activity of the thyroid gland can occur due to a pituitary tumour. More frequently, hyperthyroidism in children is caused by an autoimmune reaction that results in overproduction of immunoglobulin G (IgG), which stimulates the thyroid gland to overproduce thyroxine. An exophthalmos-producing pituitary substance causes the prominent-appearing eyes that accompany hyperthyroidism in some children.

Therapy consists first of a course of a beta-adrenergic blocking agent, such as propranolol, to decrease the antibody response (Glaser & Styne, 2008). After this, the child is placed on an antithyroid medication, such as methimazole (Tapazole), to suppress the formation of thyroxine. Propylthiouracil (PTU) can also be used, however it has more frequent and severe side effects, including severe hepatotoxicity (LaFranchi, 2014).

Radioiodine ablative therapy with ^{131}I to reduce the size of the thyroid gland (Rivkees & Dinauer, 2007) or surgical removal of part or almost all of the thyroid gland, can also be completed safely (Lee, Grumbach & Clark, 2007). After both radioiodine ablative therapy and thyroidectomy, supplemental thyroid hormone therapy may be needed. It is important that adolescent girls be carefully regulated before they consider childbearing as high hyperthyroidism during pregnancy can lead to hypothyroidism in a fetus (Kempers et al., 2007).

THE ADRENAL GLAND

The two adrenal glands are located retroperitoneally, just above each kidney (because of their location, they are also referred to as suprarenal glands). The adrenal glands are made up of two distinct parts, which differ not only in tissue origin but also in function. The *adrenal medulla* is a small core surrounded by the *adrenal cortex*. Although each of these parts have different functions and release different hormones, together they protect the body against acute and chronic forms of stress.

ADRENAL GLAND DISORDERS

Disorders of the adrenal glands include those related to hypofunction, which can lead to acute or chronic insufficiency, and those related to hyperfunction (overactivity), which most often leads to overproduction of androgen or cortisol.

Acute adrenocortical insufficiency

Insufficiency (hypofunction) of the adrenal gland may be either acute or chronic. In many adrenal syndromes, only one hormone is involved, and the symptoms are directly related only to that hormone. In acute adrenocortical insufficiency, the function of the entire cortical adrenal gland suddenly becomes insufficient. Usually this occurs in association with severe overwhelming infection, typically involving haemorrhagic destruction of the adrenal glands. It can also occur when corticosteroid therapy that has been maintained at high levels for long periods is stopped abruptly.

The symptoms of acute adrenocortical insufficiency are acute and sudden. Blood pressure drops to extremely low levels and the child appears ashen grey and may be pulseless. Temperature becomes elevated; dehydration and hypoglycaemia are marked. Sodium and chloride blood levels are very low but serum potassium is elevated, because there is usually an inverse relationship between sodium and potassium values. The child is prostrate and seizures may occur. Without treatment, death can occur abruptly (Thalange & Beach, 2013).

Treatment involves the immediate replacement of cortisol with IV hydrocortisone sodium succinate; administration of deoxycorticosterone acetate (DOCA), the synthetic equivalent of aldosterone; and IV rehydration with 0.9% saline to restore blood pressure and sodium. Intravenous 5% glucose is given to replace blood glucose levels. A vasoconstrictor may be necessary to further elevate the blood pressure.

Congenital adrenal hyperplasia

Congenital adrenal hyperplasia (CAH) is a syndrome that is inherited as an autosomal recessive trait. The primary defect is an inability of the adrenal glands to synthesise cortisol from its precursors. Because the adrenal gland is unable to produce cortisol, the level of adrenocorticotropic hormone (ACTH) increases, stimulating the adrenal glands to improve function. Although the adrenals enlarge (hyperplasia), they still cannot produce cortisol; instead, they overproduce androgen.

There are two main forms of CAH, classical salt wasting and simple virilising. In classical salt wasting CAH there is a complete blockage of cortisol formation, leading to aldosterone deficiency. This results in severe salt wasting and Addisonian crisis. This most commonly occurs in the neonatal period; however it can occur at any time whenever there is a deficiency in cortisol and aldosterone (Claahsen-van der Grinten et al., 2011). In simple virilising CAH there is impaired cortisol synthesis with near normal aldosterone production. For both forms of CAH, girls usually present with ambiguous genitalia ranging from nearly complete male appearance to clitoromegaly. Girls with simple virilising CAH usually present before 8 years of age. Boys with simple virilising CAH may present with normal genitalia with hyperpigmentation and develop pubic and axilliary hair before 9 years of age. Newborn screening should detect the majority of children with CAH (Witchel & Azziz, 2011).

Treatment of CAH is based on clinical goals of normal growth, skeletal maturation, puberty onset and weight status. Both male and female infants are given a corticosteroid agent, such as oral hydrocortisone, to replace what they cannot produce naturally. Stimulation by ACTH decreases, production of androgen returns to normal limits and no further masculinisation occurs. Corticosteroid therapy needs to continue for life. The child needs periodic analysis of serum cortisol levels and growth measurements to estimate the effectiveness of the therapy.

Children with salt wasting CAH also require replacement of mineralocorticoid, such as with fludrocortisone, to prevent salt loss. Infants also require salt supplementation until they are 6–8 months of age (Claahsen-van der Grinten et al., 2011).

Parents of females with congenital adrenogenital hyperplasia may need a great deal of support during the first few days of their child's life if they feel that their child is imperfect in an embarrassing, hard-to-explain way. When they are told the results of the chromosome analysis, parents may react with grief for the loss of the son they thought had been born to them.

Parents and children, as they grow older, need to understand the importance of continuing to take the oral medication prescribed. Cortisol is necessary for glucose and protein metabolism, however, the body needs adequate levels to allow it to react to physical and emotional stress. Children may need to have a routine dose increased when they are undergoing periods of stress, such as surgery or infection.

✔ *Checkpoint question 48.2*

A newborn is diagnosed as having the salt-losing form of congenital adrenal hyperplasia. What would be the most important measure to teach her parents before she is discharged from the hospital? How may having a child with this disorder change this family's life?

Cushing's syndrome

Cushing's syndrome is caused by overproduction of the adrenal hormone cortisol; this usually results from increased ACTH production due to a pituitary tumour. It may also occur from a malignant or benign tumour of the adrenal cortex. The peak age of occurrence is 6 or 7 years, but the syndrome can occur in infancy (Batista et al., 2007). Overproduction of cortisol results in increased glucose production; this causes fat to accumulate on the cheeks, chin and trunk, causing a moon-faced, stocky appearance. Cortisol is catabolic, so protein wasting occurs leading to muscle wasting and osteoporosis. Cortisol also suppresses humoral immunity, leaving children susceptible to infection. Additionally, it causes vasoconstriction, so extreme hypertension may occur.

Treatment of Cushing's syndrome is by surgical removal of the causative tumour. The prognosis depends on whether the tumour is benign or malignant; carcinoma of this type tends to metastasise rapidly. If a major part of the adrenal gland is surgically removed, the child will need replacement cortisol therapy for life.

If a major portion of the pituitary gland is removed because the problem was overproduction of ACTH, replacement of all pituitary hormones may be necessary. After adrenal surgery, observe the child carefully for signs of shock: without adrenaline from the adrenal gland, the body's ability to maintain blood pressure is severely compromised, and severe hypotension can result.

CASE STUDY QUESTION

3. Jack has his adrenal gland function assessed. What is the effect on a child when sufficient aldosterone cannot be produced?

a. Substantially fewer red blood cells are produced
b. There is an overall decreased urine output
c. An excessive amount of sodium is lost in urine
d. The child's growth rate increases abnormally

THE PANCREAS

The pancreas is a unique organ in that it has both endocrine (ductless) and exocrine (with duct) types of tissue. The *islets of Langerhans* form the endocrine portion; these cells are scattered in-between the exocrine cells like small islets—hence, their name. The islet cells represent only about 1% of the total weight of the pancreas. Alpha islet cells secrete glucagon; beta islet cells secrete insulin.

Insulin is essential for carbohydrate metabolism and is important in the metabolism of fats and protein. When serum glucose that passes through the pancreas exceeds 5.5 mmol/L, beta cells immediately increase insulin production. When blood serum levels are lowered, production decreases. Both the ability to secrete additional insulin and the action to decrease production are immediate responses.

Other hormones that stimulate insulin production include gastrin, glucagon, cortisol, GH, progesterone and oestrogen. In contrast, increasing levels of adrenaline or noradrenaline inhibit the secretion of insulin to preserve glucose.

Type 1 diabetes mellitus

Type 1 diabetes is a disorder that involves an absolute or relative deficiency of insulin in contrast to type 2 where insulin production is only reduced (see Table 48.2). Type 1 diabetes (formerly referred to as juvenile diabetes or insulin-dependent diabetes), which occurs almost exclusively in childhood, affects as many as 1 in 1500 children before

TABLE 48.2 Comparison of type 1 and type 2 diabetes

Assessment	Type 1	Type 2
Age at onset	5–7 years or at puberty	40–65 years (may occur in adolescents as maturity-onset diabetes of youth [MODY])
Type of onset	Abrupt	Gradual
Weight changes	Marked weight loss often initial sign	Associated with obesity
Other symptoms	Polydipsia Polyuria (often begins as bedwetting) Fatigue (marks fall at school) Blurred vision (marks fall at school) Glycosuria Polyphagia (excessive eating) Pruritus Mood changes (may cause behavioural problems at school)	Polydipsia Polyuria Fatigue Blurred vision Glycosuria Pruritus Mood changes
Therapy	Hypoglycaemic agents never effective; insulin required Diet recommended as 55% carbohydrates, 15% protein and 30% fat; no dietary foods used Commonsense foot care for growing children	Diet, oral hypoglycaemic agents or insulin Nutrition concentrating on no excess weight gain and balanced intake of carbohydrates, protein and fat Meticulous skin and foot care necessary
Period of remission	Period of remission for 1–12 months ("honey-moon period") generally after initial diagnosis	Not demonstrable

5 years of age and this increases to 1 in 350 by the age of 16 (Masharani, 2014). Children with this type of diabetes must take insulin to replace what their pancreas cannot produce.

Assessment

Laboratory studies

In some children, diabetes is detected at a routine health screening. For others, although the disease has been progressing internally for some time, outward symptoms have such an abrupt onset that the child is very acidotic and hyperglycaemic by the time it is detected. Laboratory studies usually show a random plasma glucose level greater than 11 mmol/L (normal range, 3.6 to 6.1 mmol/L fasting, 3.6 to 7 mmol/L not fasting) and significant glycosuria.

Two diagnostic tests, the fasting blood glucose test and the random blood glucose test, are used to diagnose diabetes. A diagnosis of diabetes is confirmed based on finding one of the following three criteria on two separate occasions:

- Symptoms of diabetes with a random blood glucose level greater than 11 mmol/L
- Fasting blood glucose level greater than 7 mmol/L
- Two-hour plasma glucose level greater than 11 mmol/L during an oral glucose tolerance test (GTT).

Other diagnostic tests

If diabetes is detected, the diagnostic workup also usually includes: analysis of blood samples for pH; partial pressure of carbon dioxide (P_{CO_2}), sodium and potassium levels; a white blood cell count; and glycosylated haemoglobin (HbA_{1c}) evaluation.

Therapy for children with type 1 diabetes involves five measures: insulin administration; regulation of nutrition and exercise; stress management; and blood glucose and urine ketone monitoring (Clar, Waugh & Thomas, 2009).

Therapeutic management

Initial regulation of insulin

When children are first diagnosed with diabetes, they are usually hyperglycaemic and perhaps ketoacidotic. To correct the metabolic imbalance, they are given insulin administered IV at a dose of 0.1 to 0.2 units per kg of body weight per hour. This initial IV infusion of insulin is followed by dose reductions once the blood glucose level is lower than 11 mmol/L. Ideally, the blood glucose level should reduce by 1–2 mmol/L each hour. Within 12 hours, the acidosis should be mostly resolved and the serum glucose level at near the normal range.

After 24 hours, as the child's serum glucose returns to normal, oral feedings replace the IV route. Further management in the days after this first crucial 24-hour period is based on the serum glucose measurement. A child may remain on regular insulin alone (given three or four times a day) for the first 1 or 2 days. Typically, intermediate-acting insulin is then prescribed as soon as oral fluids are taken, usually on the second day of therapy.

Insulin administration

Types of insulin vary as to their time of onset, peak action and duration of action. There are five main types of insulin; very short acting; short acting; intermediate acting; long acting; and premixed.

Injection technique. When insulins are mixed in one syringe, the regular or short-acting insulin should be drawn into the syringe first. Then, if mixing accidentally occurs in the bottle, the time of effectiveness of the

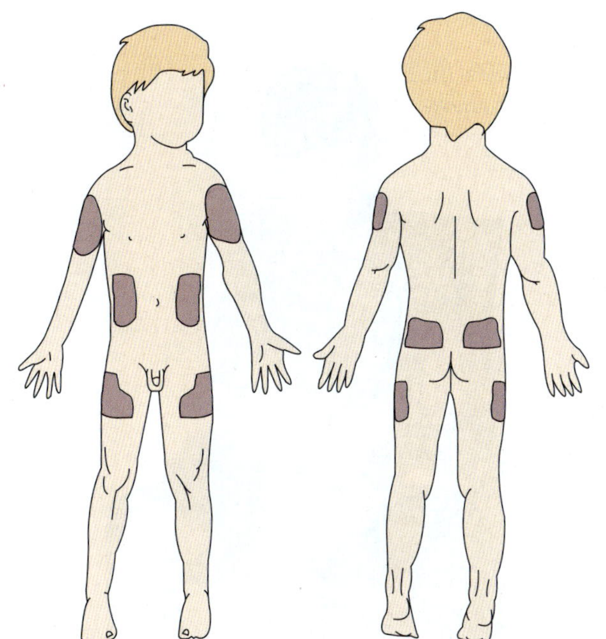

FIGURE 48.2 According to the American Diabetes Association, insulin injection sites in children and adults are the upper outer portions of the arms; the thighs—10 cm below the hip and 10 cm above the knee (adjusted proportionally for children); and the abdominal area just above and just below the waist. The navel and a circular area just around it are excluded as injection sites. In some children, the abdominal area may not be an appropriate injection site.

short-acting insulin (which needs to be kept short-acting for emergency treatment) will not be lengthened by the addition of the intermediate-acting insulin.

Insulin is always injected subcutaneously except in emergencies, when short-acting insulin may be given intravenously. Subcutaneous tissue injection sites include those of the upper outer arms and the outer aspects of the thighs (see Fig. 48.2). The abdominal subcutaneous tissue injection sites may be preferred for injection, because many children have a greater amount of subcutaneous tissue there.

Work out a plan of rotation with children so that everyone who will be working with the child and giving injections knows what injection site should be used next. In the hospital, record the injection site in the child's chart or nursing plan of care, so that each nurse can check it before an injection and not repeat an injection site. If the same injection site is used repeatedly, a great deal of subcutaneous atrophy (lipodystrophy) can occur at the site, causing deep, obvious pockmarks. This, however, is less of a problem now that synthetic human insulin is available.

Insulin should be given at room temperature. This diminishes subcutaneous atrophy and ensures peak effectiveness. Parents may keep additional bottles in the refrigerator to increase the insulin's shelf life.

Insulin pens. Insulin pens are an alternative to syringes and needles. Each 'pen' is specific to a brand of insulin, which may prevent mixing. This means that two injections may need to be given or a syringe and needle will need to be used.

Insulin pumps. An insulin pump is a computerised device approximately the size of an iPod. It delivers insulin at a constant background rate, with boluses for meals and corrections. The pump regulates serum glucose levels better than periodic injections (Buchko et al., 2012). It has the potential to decrease future complications (Marschilok, 2007).

Inhalation insulin. In the future, insulin may be administered by way of inhalation, because it is absorbed well across mucus membranes. This method releases the child from the chore of daily injections. However, if the child develops a cold or allergies that cause oedema of the nasal membrane, drug absorption is reduced. Absorption can also be influenced by whether the child is upright or lying down at the time of administration (McKenna & Mirkov, 2014).

Nutrition

Children with type 1 diabetes need to consume a diet appropriate for their age in the proportion of 55% carbohydrate, 15% protein and 30% fat. The meal pattern should include three spaced meals high in fibre plus a snack in the mid-morning, mid-afternoon and evening (Rolfes, Pinna & Whitney, 2009).

Urine testing

Urine testing has the disadvantage of not being as accurate as blood serum testing to detect glucose levels; it is now used only to test for ketonuria if the child's blood glucose level is above 11 mmol/L. A dipstick technique is used. Acetone appearing in the urine is a sign that fat is being used for energy; a situation which occurs with infection or if not enough food has been ingested.

Self blood glucose monitoring (SBGM)

Children as young as early school-age can learn the techniques of finger puncture and reading a computerised monitor. Using a spring-loaded puncture device and a glucometer simplifies the procedure.

Stress adjustment

Whenever children with diabetes undergo a stressful situation, either emotionally or physically, they may need increased insulin to maintain glucose homeostasis. When children are seen at healthcare facilities for periodic check-ups, ask them whether they are having any difficulty with blood testing or insulin injection and how things are at home and school.

Try to interview children separately from their parents, so they can feel free to talk about anything that may be happening or going wrong. There must be cooperation between primary healthcare personnel and school healthcare personnel so that conflicts about the child's regimen do not cause problems or tensions at school. Parents may have to meet with schoolteachers to help them view the child as well, not ill, so that they will allow participation in all activities, including sports. Sometimes children are embarrassed to have to do blood glucose testing at school, especially in the school toilet. It may be easier for them if they can go to the school's office for privacy when testing.

Complications

If temperature rises and infection occurs, counter-regulatory hormones increase, causing insulin resistance and increasing the need for more insulin. If a child with diabetes is scheduled for surgery, careful regulation on the day of surgery and in the immediate postoperative period is essential, especially if oral fluids will be restricted.

Many long-term body changes that occur because of chronic hyperglycaemia are not a major part of disease management in childhood because their onset does not begin until late adolescence or adulthood. These changes include arteriosclerosis (hardening of artery walls), which can lead to general poor circulation and kidney disease, and thickening of retinal capillaries and cataract formation, which ultimately can result in blindness. Some children may notice blurred vision when their disease is not under control, but this should not be confused with the final retinopathy that may result with older age. The blurred vision is caused by a temporary change in depth of the eye globe related to hyperglycaemia.

Pancreas transplantation

For children who develop severe kidney disease or retinopathy, pancreas transplantation may be considered. In contrast to other organ transplantation procedures, the original pancreas is not removed entirely. The portion that supplies digestive enzymes is still functioning and is left in place. During surgery, a new pancreas is grafted to the iliac artery and vein, to allow insulin from the new organ to enter the systemic circulation. For this reason, pancreatic replacement is more accurately called grafting. The digestive enzymes of the new pancreas can be diverted into the intestine or bladder, or the pancreatic ducts can be sclerosed so that the digestive enzymes do not leave the transplanted organ.

Pancreatic transplantation is a last-resort solution for children, because the outcome is guarded (about 50% of transplanted organs are rejected) and the outcome—continuous immunosuppressive medication for life—may not be regarded as a major improvement over the original illness, which would require continuous daily insulin for life (Chase & Eisenbarth, 2014).

Nursing considerations

Self-administration of insulin

From about 8 years of age, children can be taught to administer their own insulin (see Fig. 48.3). Many children younger than this do not have the dexterity to handle a syringe or an understanding of the importance of sterile technique and proper dosage. They may skip injections if they are tired or busy.

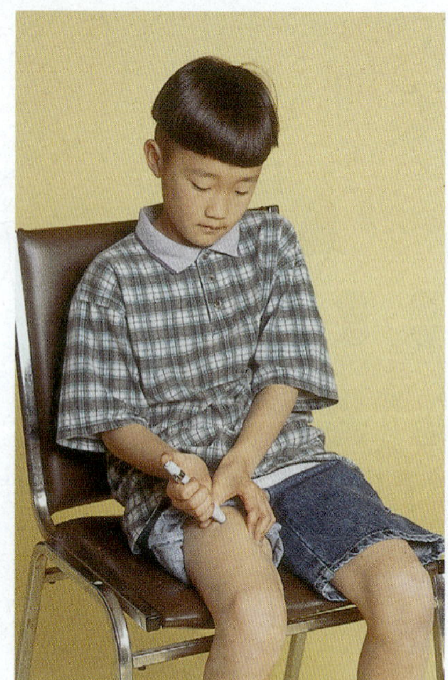

FIGURE 48.3 A school-aged child practises insulin administration. (© Lesha Photography.)

Even if children are taught to give their own insulin from the beginning, at least one adult in the family should be taught to give it as well. There will be days when the child refuses to administer their own insulin or is not feeling well and needs to have or appreciates having someone to do it for them. Parents may have difficulty giving their child a painful injection; teaching them to view it as a helping action helps to alleviate their distress.

Exercise

Exercise is an important component of care, because it uses up carbohydrates and helps reduce hyperglycaemia. No type of exercise is restricted for children with diabetes.

Hygiene

Skin care, particularly foot care, is extremely important for adults with diabetes, because arteriosclerosis causes loss of circulation to the feet, and decreased circulation leads to poor healing ability. This is not as important a concern with children, but they (and all children) should be taught to cut their toenails straight across, to prevent ingrown toenails, and to tend to cuts and scrapes promptly so that healing can begin right away. Properly fitting shoes are essential. Girls may need to be reminded of good perineal care to prevent vaginal infections.

> ***What if...***
>
> Jack wants to try out for football in his school team, but the coach thinks diabetic children should be excluded from sports? What information can you give the parents about diabetes that they could share with the coach?

Disease and the principles of care

Teaching is one of the main interventions necessary for children newly diagnosed with diabetes. Review general principles of care, including the fact that insulin injections, supervised intake of food and exercise all decrease the blood glucose level, while increased intake of food increases it. Infection and emotional upset also increase insulin requirements. If this process is not explained, parents may attempt to keep the child relatively quiet, unaware that exercise is actually helpful.

Teach that an episode of hypoglycaemia is an extremely serious condition and must be prevented, if possible. If early signs are not recognised and treated, hypoglycaemia can lead to coma and seizures. Severe glucose depletion can lead to permanent brain damage with mental and motor impairment, because brain cells need glucose for metabolism.

Be certain that parents have opportunities to practise supervised insulin injection and blood glucose testing so that they can become familiar with these procedures and any accompanying problems. Urge the parents or the child to begin keeping a log of blood glucose test results in a permanent notebook so that these numbers can be evaluated for any unusual patterns at periodic checkups.

Serving as an active support person for the parents is also necessary. Often parents are so concerned with learning the techniques of insulin administration and blood glucose testing that they do not think about other problems of everyday living that will arise later. Make sure the parents can identify support people and others to contact if they have problems or questions.

Nutrition program

At one time, children with diabetes were placed on rigidly specified diets in which each food item had to be weighed. Then followed a period when children were allowed free diets and any resulting glycosuria was managed by increasing their insulin doses. Today, it is generally accepted that conscientious diet modification, within lifestyle and cultural preferences, is necessary, because chronic hyperglycaemia can lead to vascular disease in later years.

Hypoglycaemic management

Symptoms of hypoglycaemia occur when the blood glucose level falls below 3 mmol/L. Parents and children, as soon as they are old enough to understand, need to be aware of the reasons for hypoglycaemia and what measures they must take to counteract it if it occurs.

Hypoglycaemia can result from the administration of too much insulin, excessive exercise (because exercise uses up glucose) or failure to eat enough food. Typically beginning symptoms include nervousness, weakness, dizziness, sweating or tremors. In many children, the first signs of hypoglycaemia are behavioural problems: temper tantrums, stubbornness, silliness, irritability or simply "not acting their usual self".

When the signs of hypoglycaemia are recognised, a child needs an immediate source of carbohydrate. Fifteen grams of a fast-acting carbohydrate such as that contained in a half-glass of orange juice or regular soft drink is recommended. It is easy for children to always carry glucose tablets or sweets such as Lifesavers with them and have them available for these times. If there is no improvement in symptoms and the blood glucose level has not risen by 1 mmol/L after 15 minutes, more carbohydrate (perhaps juice) should be given.

If the child is comatose when first discovered or is too upset or uncooperative to take oral sugar, glucagon hydrochloride may be injected. This converts the glycogen that is stored in the liver to glucose. The drug is not effective if the child's supply of glycogen is depleted.

If parents cannot give their child an injection and oral sugar cannot be given, honey or glucose gel can be rubbed onto the gums or inside the cheek. As soon as children come out of the coma or are cooperative, they should take a source of complex carbohydrate, such as crackers or toast, to prevent further hypoglycaemia.

Signs of ketoacidosis

It is often difficult to distinguish between **hypoglycaemia** (occurring from too much insulin) and **hyperglycaemia** (occurring from too little insulin for the level of glucose present in the bloodstream) (see Table 48.3). Hyperglycaemia leads to **ketoacidosis**, with symptoms of vomiting and abdominal pain and the same kind of behavioural changes exhibited with hypoglycaemia.

If ketoacidosis is severe, respirations become deep and rapid (Kussmaul breathing) as the body attempts to "blow off" carbon dioxide and lessen the acidotic state. The breath smells sweet, because of the presence of ketone bodies, and the pulse rate may be rapid. Urine output is copious. Children may have signs of dehydration, including dry mucus membranes and skin, sunken eyeballs and no tears. This may be the picture when children with diabetes are first diagnosed. It is often seen in children with diabetes who develop gastroenteritis and hence eat poorly for several meals. Because the child is not eating well, parents may omit giving insulin. In fact, because of an increased metabolic rate due to fever, the child may need more insulin and glucose than usual during these times.

Type 2 diabetes mellitus

Type 2 diabetes (formerly known as non-insulin-dependent diabetes), which is characterised by diminished insulin secretion and not caused by autoimmune factors, is a separate disease from type 1 diabetes (Sherr & Weinzimer, 2012). Usually individuals with type 2 diabetes do not need daily insulin because their disease can be managed with diet alone or with diet and an oral hypoglycaemic agent. Once thought only to occur in older adults, type 2 diabetes is now seen in overweight adolescents, termed maturity-onset diabetes of youth (MODY) (Franks, 2007).

TABLE 48.3 Comparison of hypoglycaemia and hyperglycaemia

Comparison factor	Hypoglycaemia	Hyperglycaemia
Cause	Excessive insulin injection Excessive exercise Limited food intake	Inadequate insulin injection Excessive food intake Stress from infection, surgery, etc.
Symptoms	Hunger Lethargy Sensorium changes Pallor Sweating Seizures Coma	Glycosuria and ketonuria Polyuria, polydipsia Kussmaul respirations Flushing Sweet (acetone) breath Decreased CO_2 combining power Dehydration Lowered sodium, potassium, bicarbonate, chloride and phosphate levels Vomiting, abdominal pain Coma
Danger	Brain cells need glucose for function and survival	Fatty acids are used and acidosis develops
Major nursing interventions	Administration of source of glucose by oral or IV route Education to prevent recurrences	Re-establishment of electrolyte balance and hydration Education to prevent recurrences

Between 8% and 45% of newly diagnosed children with diabetes have type 2. At the time of diagnosis, it may not be possible for the classification to be correctly determined, because symptoms and findings are so similar. Type 2 diabetes usually occurs in children who have a strong family history of diabetes and who are overweight at diagnosis. Because the pancreatic islet cells are not devoid of function, the pancreas continues to secrete at least minimal amounts of insulin. Symptoms often become apparent at puberty because increasing sex hormones naturally increase insulin resistance and require more insulin production. Children will have sugar in their urine but few ketones in urine. They have lessened amounts of thirst and increased urination. About 90% of children with type 2 diabetes have dark shiny patches on the skin (*acanthosis nigricans*), which are most often found between the fingers and between the toes and on the back of the neck ("dirty neck") and in axillary creases. Development of polycystic ovary syndrome (see Chapter 8) is strongly associated with the disorder.

Therapy consists of nutrition and exercise regulation, the same as for type 1 diabetes, combined with an oral antiglycaemic agent such as a biguanide (Metformin), which decreases the amount of glucose produced by the liver and may increase insulin sensitivity in both the liver and muscle cells. If this therapy is not effective, a sulfonylurea (Glibenclamide or Gliclazide), which stimulates the beta cells in the pancreas to produce more insulin, can be added to the child's regimen.

THE PARATHYROID GLANDS

The four parathyroid glands, located posterior and adjacent to the thyroid gland, function to regulate serum levels of calcium in the body; they control the rate of bone metabolism by secretion of parathyroid hormone. This hormone is not under the control of the pituitary gland but is controlled by a negative feedback from the circulating serum levels of calcium. If blood calcium levels fall, parathyroid hormone secretion increases; if blood calcium levels increase, hormone production decreases. Vitamin D is necessary for absorption of calcium from the gastrointestinal tract into the bloodstream, so it also influences parathyroid hormone secretion. Calcitonin (thyrocalcitonin), secreted by the thyroid gland, opposes the action of parathyroid hormone, decreasing blood calcium levels.

Hypocalcaemia

Hypocalcaemia is a lowered blood calcium level. Phosphate and calcium levels are maintained in an inverse proportion to each other in the bloodstream, therefore, if phosphate levels rise, calcium levels decrease; if calcium levels rise, phosphate levels decrease. Hypocalcaemia, therefore, may be caused by changes in either calcium or phosphate metabolism.

Latent tetany

The chief sign of hypocalcaemia is neuromuscular irritability, often referred to as **latent tetany**. This occurs if the blood calcium level is less than 1.9 mmol/L. Newborns with latent tetany are jittery when they are handled or they cry for extended periods.

Four methods can be used to produce the clinical manifestations of tetany for diagnosis of hypocalcaemia (shown in Table 48.4). These are all useful tests to determine or suggest whether a newborn's jitteriness is a result of hypocalcaemia, a central nervous system problem or some other cause.

TABLE 48.4 Tests for detection of hypocalcaemia

Sign	Description
Chvostek's	When skin anterior to external ear (just over sixth cranial nerve) is tapped, facial muscles surrounding eye, nose and mouth contract unilaterally.
Trousseau's	When upper arm is constricted by tourniquet for 2–3 min and area becomes blanched, carpal spasm is elicited (hand abducts, wrist flexes, thumb is positioned across cupped palm).
Peroneal	When fibular side of leg over peroneal nerve is tapped, foot abducts and dorsiflexes.
Erb's	This test is dramatic to see demonstrated, although it requires a mild galvanic current so is not used routinely. A person with tetany has greater muscular irritability than a person with a normal calcium level; therefore, when a mild current is applied over the peroneal nerve just below the head of the fibula, the foot on that side will abduct and dorsiflex.

Manifest tetany

If the blood calcium level falls well below 1.75 mmol/L, **manifest tetany** may result, commonly observed as muscular twitching and carpopedal spasms. Generalised seizures may occur. There may be spasm of the larynx, with the infant emitting a high-pitched, crowing sound on inspiration because of the constricted airway. If the spasm is prolonged, respirations may cease.

Therapeutic management

Treatment is aimed at increasing the calcium level in the blood above the point of latent tetany. Calcium may be administered orally as 10% calcium chloride if the infant can and will suck, or intravenously as a 10% solution of calcium gluconate. Newborns who are having generalised seizures may require anticonvulsant therapy in addition to the calcium gluconate to halt the seizures. Emergency equipment for intubation to relieve laryngospasm should be available.

After immediate therapy to increase the low blood calcium levels, infants are given oral calcium therapy until their calcium level stabilises at greater than 1.9 mmol/L. Because vitamin D is necessary for absorption of calcium and phosphorus from the gastrointestinal tract, the infant also may be given a vitamin D supplement.

METABOLIC DISORDERS

In addition to endocrine disorders, a group of hereditary biochemical disorders also affect metabolism. These are caused largely by some specific defect in the body biochemistry that disrupts one step of the metabolic process. The term *inborn errors of metabolism* is used to refer to these disorders. Most of them are caused by a lack of, or deficiency in, a particular enzyme, which seriously impairs the ability of the body to metabolise properly the components of food for energy.

Inborn errors of metabolism affect the metabolism of amino acids and proteins, carbohydrates, and lipids. Many of these disorders are evident at or soon after birth and can cause severe symptoms rapidly. Early detection and treatment are essential to prevent irreversible cognitive challenge and early death. Gene therapy is expected to be available in the future to reverse symptoms of these disorders.

Phenylketonuria

Phenylketonuria (PKU) is a disease of metabolism that is inherited as an autosomal recessive trait. Absence of the liver enzyme phenylalanine hydroxylase prevents conversion of phenylalanine, an essential amino acid, into tyrosine (a precursor of adrenaline, thyroxine and melanin). As a result, excessive phenylalanine builds up in the bloodstream and tissues, causing permanent damage to brain tissue and leaving children severely cognitively challenged. PKU affects 1 in 10,000 to 14,000 Australians.

Early identification of the disorder is essential to prevent the child from becoming severely cognitively challenged. Infants are screened at birth on routine newborn screening. The screening is done by pricking the infant's heel with a blood lancet and letting a few drops of blood fall onto a specially prepared filter paper. The filter paper is then analysed by mass spectrometry.

Infants in whom this disease is detected during the first few days of life are placed on a formula that is extremely low in phenylalanine. Beginning the diet early allows normal cognitive development. The diet is carefully monitored by a dietician. Providing nutrition for a child with PKU is a difficult task. There is no natural protein with both a low phenylalanine concentration and normal levels of other essential amino acids. A diet that simply restricted protein would result in restriction of all essential amino acids and would be incompatible with life. Foods highest in phenylalanine are those that are rich in protein, such as meats, eggs and milk. Foods low in phenylalanine include orange juice, bananas, potatoes, lettuce, spinach and peas. Children need their blood and urine monitored frequently for phenylalanine levels. Haemoglobin levels should also be closely monitored to ensure that the child is not becoming anaemic, because iron is found primarily in protein-rich foods, which the child must avoid.

When to discontinue the diet is controversial because of reports of progressive neurological deterioration in children who no longer follow a restricted diet. Generally, current advice is for children to follow the diet indefinitely although discontinuing the diet in adolescence may lead to only subtle differences (Channon et al., 2007). A woman who has PKU must anticipate when she wants to have children as an adult; she must maintain a low-phenylalanine diet for about 3 months before conception and remain on the diet during pregnancy. Otherwise, her fetus will be exposed to high levels of phenylalanine during pregnancy and will be born cognitively challenged.

Maple syrup urine disease

Maple syrup urine disease is a rare disorder, inherited as an autosomal recessive trait, in which there is a defect in metabolism of the amino acids leucine, isoleucine and valine that leads to cerebral degeneration similar to that observed in children with PKU.

Like PKU, infants are screened at birth for the disorder. Infants who have the disorder appear well at birth but quickly begin to show signs of feeding difficulty, loss of the Moro reflex and irregular respirations. The symptoms progress rapidly to *opisthotonos,* generalised muscular rigidity and seizures. If the condition remains untreated, an infant may die of the disease as early as 2 to 4 weeks of age.

Although the disorder is rare, it is mentioned here because it is relatively easy to detect. By the first or second day of life, the urine of the child develops the characteristic odour of maple syrup; hence the name of the disease. If the disease is diagnosed during the first day or two of life and the child is placed on a well-controlled diet that is high in thiamine and low in the amino acids leucine, isoleucine and valine, the cerebral degeneration can be prevented, just as it can be prevented in PKU. Such a diet is extremely difficult to maintain, however, because of its low protein content. Parents need intensive nutritional counselling.

Galactosaemia

Galactosaemia is a disorder of carbohydrate metabolism that is characterised by abnormal amounts of galactose in the blood (*galactosaemia*) and in the urine (*galactosuria*). It occurs in about 1 in every 60,000 births, most often as an inborn error of metabolism, transmitted as an autosomal recessive trait. The child is deficient in the liver enzyme galactose 1-phosphate uridyltransferase (Listernick, 2012).

Lactose (the sugar found in milk) normally is broken down into galactose and glucose; galactose is then further broken down into additional glucose. Without the galactose 1-phosphate uridyltransferase enzyme, this second step, the conversion of galactose into glucose, cannot take place, and galactose builds up in the bloodstream and spills into the urine. When it reaches toxic levels in the bloodstream, it destroys body cells.

Symptoms appear as soon as the child begins formula feeding or breastfeeding and include lethargy, hypotonia and perhaps diarrhoea and vomiting. Next, the liver enlarges as cirrhosis develops. Jaundice is often present and persistent; bilateral cataracts develop. The symptoms begin abruptly and worsen rapidly. If the condition remains untreated, a child may die by 3 days of age.

The treatment of galactosaemia consists of placing the infant on a diet that is free of galactose or on a formula made with milk substitutes such as casein hydrolysates (Bosch, 2007).

Glycogen storage disease

Glycogen storage disease refers to a group of genetically transmitted disorders that involve altered production and use of glycogen in the body. Twelve of the 13 described types are inherited as autosomal recessive traits; the other is a sex-linked disorder (Krishnani & Chen, 2012).

Glycogen is normally stored in the liver to provide a reserve supply of glucose. When the body needs glucose for energy, this glycogen is transformed back to glucose. In children with glycogen storage disease, glycogen is deposited normally, but an enzyme deficiency prevents retransformation of the glycogen back to glucose. As a result, children's livers rapidly increase in size from the stored glycogen. Children with this disorder are susceptible to periods of hypoglycaemia, because their only source of ready glucose is oral intake.

A common sign of the disease is liver enlargement, because the liver must store such a large supply of glycogen. Consequently, the abdomen protrudes. Over a long period, the child's growth is stunted because there is not enough glucose for any function but immediate energy. If hypoglycaemic episodes have been severe, brain damage may result. Many children have a tendency towards epistaxis or haemorrhage and are at risk when having surgery performed because of impaired clotting ability due to decreased platelet adhesiveness.

Children with glycogen storage disease need to be maintained on a high-carbohydrate diet with snacks between meals to prevent hypoglycaemia. In addition, a continuous glucose nasogastric or gastrostomy feeding during the night may be necessary to prevent hypoglycaemia while sleeping. Therapy with an antihypoglycaemic that inhibits insulin release, may help regulate the glucose level to provide additional growth. Liver transplantation may be a possibility, but it will not cure the basic enzyme deficiency (Iyer et al., 2007).

Key points for review

- Endocrine disorders are almost all long-term disorders. Helping parents and children remember to take medicine on a long-term basis is an important nursing responsibility.
- Children with endocrine or metabolic disorders often develop height or weight discrepancies. Help children continue to feel high self-esteem by concentrating on the things they are able to do despite a growth lag.
- Growth hormone (GH) deficiency, a pituitary disorder, results in short stature. Therapy for children consists of the injection of synthetic GH. Children can experience

situational low self-esteem if they do not receive adequate emotional support from significant others.

- Other pituitary disorders include diabetes insipidus. With diabetes insipidus, there is decreased release of antidiuretic hormone. Urine becomes dilute and large amounts are excreted. Therapy is administration of desmopressin, an arginine vasopressin. Children with this are at high risk of fluid volume deficit.
- SIADH is an overproduction of antidiuretic hormone, resulting in decreased urine output and water retention. Treatment is with sodium supplementation and fluid restriction or with Demeclocycline.
- Congenital hypothyroidism occurs as a result of an absent or non-functioning thyroid gland. The condition is discovered by a blood test at birth. The therapy is oral administration of synthetic thyroid hormone.
- Acquired hypothyroidism (Hashimoto's disease) is an autoimmune phenomenon that interferes with thyroid gland function. Therapy is administration of a synthetic thyroid hormone.
- Hyperthyroidism or Graves' 'disease may be due to a tumour or an autoimmune reaction. Therapy consists of treating the underlying cause, in addition to methimazole.
- Acute adrenocortical insufficiency can occur in children from causes such as an overwhelming infection in which there is haemorrhagic destruction of the adrenal gland. A more common disease in children is congenital adrenogenital hyperplasia. Girls are born masculinised; either sex may be unable to retain sodium, which results in rapid fluid loss. Therapy is administration of hydrocortisone and aldosterone if sodium loss is also present.
- Cushing's syndrome is caused by overproduction of cortisol by the adrenal gland. This usually results from a tumour in the gland. Children appear abnormally obese. Therapy is by surgical removal of the tumour.
- The most frequently occurring pancreatic disorder is type 1 diabetes mellitus. This may be an autoimmune process in which there has been destruction of insulin-producing islet cells. Therapy is a combination of administration of insulin, diet and exercise. Type 2 diabetes is now also occurring in children. Therapy is diet, exercise and an oral antiglycaemic agent.
- Hypocalcaemia, a parathyroid gland disorder, results in a lowered blood calcium level causing tetany to develop. Therapy is the administration of calcium.
- Various disorders of metabolism that interfere with carbohydrate, amino acid or fat metabolism occur in children. Representatives of these include phenylketonuria, maple syrup disease, galactosaemia and glycogen storage disease.

CASE STUDY QUESTION

4. In the last 6 months, Jack has "forgotten" to take his insulin at least once a week. Is Jack's history unusual for an adolescent? What health teaching do you think will most help him re-establish control?

Resources

For an extensive range of additional resources to enhance teaching and learning and to facilitate understanding of this chapter, please see the text's accompanying website located on thePoint at http://thepoint.lww.com.

References

Ali, O. & Wyatt, D. (2011). Therapy of growth disorders. Current Opinion in Endocrinology, *Diabetes & Obesity*. *18*(1), 3–8.

Batista, D. L., et al. (2007). Diagnostic tests for children who are referred for the investigation of Cushing syndrome. *Pediatrics*, *120*(3), e575–586.

Blanco, E. J., Lane, A. H., Aijaz, N., Blumberg, D. & Wilson, T. A. (2006). Use of subcutaneous DDAVP in infants with central diabetes insipidus. *Journal of Pediatric Endocrinology*. *19*(7), 919–925.

Bosch, A. M. (2007). Classical galactosaemia revisited. *Journal of Inherited Metabolic Disease*, *29*(4), 516–525.

Buchko, B., Artz, B., Dayhoff, S., et al. (2012). Improving care of patients with insulin pumps during hospitalization: Translating the evidence. *Journal of Nursing Care Quality*, *27*(4), 333–340.

Chamarthi, B., Morris, C. A., Kaiser, U. B., et al. (2010). Clinical problem-solving: Stalking the diagnosis. *The New England Journal of Medicine*, *362*(9), 834–839.

Channon, S., Goodman, G., Zlotowitz, S., Mockler, C. & Lee, P. J. (2007). Effects of dietary management of phenylketonuria on long-term cognitive outcome. *Archives of Disease in Childhood*, *92*(3), 213–218.

Chase, P. & Eisenbarth, G. S. (2014). *Diabetes mellitus*. In W. W. Hay, et al. (Eds). *Current Pediatric Diagnosis and Treatment* (22nd ed.). Columbus, OH: McGraw-Hill.

Claahsen-van der Grinten, H. L., et al. (2011). Congenital adrenal hyperplasia—Pharmacological interventions from the prenatal phase to adulthood. *Pharmacology & Therapeutics*, *132*, 1–14.

Clar, C., Waugh, N. & Thomas, S. (2009). Routine hospital admission versus out-patient or home care in children at diagnosis of type 1 diabetes mellitus. *Cochrane Database of Systematic Reviews*, (1), (CD004099).

Dahlgren, J. (2011). Metabolic benefits of growth hormone therapy in idiopathic short stature. *Hormone Research in Paediatrics*, *76*(Suppl. 3), 56–58.

Delvecchio. M., et al. (2007). Longitudinal assessment of levo-thyroxine therapy for congenital hypothyroidism. *Hormone Research*, *68*(3), 105–112.

Fitzgerald, P. A. (2014). Endocrine disorders. In S. J. McPhee & M. A. Papadakis (Eds). *Current Medical Diagnosis and Treatment*. Columbus, OH: McGraw-Hill.

Franks, P. W., et al. (2007). Childhood predictors of young-onset type 2 diabetes. *Diabetes*, *56*(12), 2964–2972.

Frederick, S. & Danzl, D. F. (2008). Metabolic and endocrine emergencies. In C. K. Stone & R. L. Humphries (Eds). *Current Diagnosis & Treatment: Emergency Medicine* (6th ed.). Columbus, OH: McGraw-Hill.

Glaser, N. S. & Styne, D. M. (2008). Predicting the likelihood of remission in children with Graves' disease: a prospective, multicenter study. *Pediatrics*, *121*(3), e481–488.

Hernandez, L. M., Lee, P. D. & Camacho-Hubner, C. (2007). Isolated growth hormone deficiency. *Pituitary*, *10*(4), 351–357.

Iyer, S. G., et al. (2007). Long-term results of living donor liver transplantation for glycogen storage disorders in children. *Liver Transplantation*, *13*(6), 848–852.

Jameson, J. L. & Weetman, A. P. (2012). Disorders of the thyroid gland. In A. S. Fauci, et al. (Eds). *Harrison's Principles of Internal Medicine* (18th ed.). Columbus, OH: McGraw-Hill.

Kempers, M. J., et al. (2007). Loss of integrity of thyroid morphology and function in children born to mothers with inadequately treated Graves' disease. *Journal of Clinical Endocrinology & Metabolism*, *92*(8), 2984–2991.

Korada, M., et al. (2008). The implementation of revised guidelines and the performance of a screening programme for congenital hypothyroidism. *Journal of Medical Screening*, *15*(1), 5–8.

Krishnani, P. S. & Chen, Y. T. (2012). Glycogen storage diseases and other inherited disorders of carbohydrate metabolism. In A. S. Fauci, et al (Eds). *Harrison's Principles of Internal Medicine* (18th ed.). Columbus, OH: McGraw-Hill.

LaFranchi, S. (2014). Evaluation and management of neonatal Graves' disease. In T. W. Post (Ed), *UpToDate*, Waltham: MA.

Lee, G. A. & Masharani, U. (2012). Disorders of the thyroid gland. In A. K. Lalwani (Eds). *Current Diagnosis and Treatment in Otolaryngology* (3rd ed.). Columbus, OH: McGraw-Hill.

Lee, J. A., Grumbach, M. M. & Clark, O. H. (2007). The optimal treatment for pediatric Graves' disease is surgery. *Journal of Clinical Endocrinology & Metabolism*, *92*(3), 801–803.

Listernick, R. (2012). A 2 month old with hyperbilirubinemia. *Pediatric Annals*, *41*(3), 94–97.

McKenna, L. & Mirkov, S. (2014). *McKenna's Drug Handbook for Nursing and Midwifery* (7th ed.). Sydney: Lippincott Williams & Wilkins.

Marschilok, C. (2007). Update on insulin pump therapy. *School Nurse News*, *24*(1), 12–13.

Masharani, U. (2014). Diabetes mellitus and hypoglycaemia. In S. J. McPhee & M. A. Papadakis (Eds). *Current Medical Diagnosis and Treatment*. Columbus, OH: McGraw-Hill.

Masharani, U. & German, M. S. (2007). Pancreatic hormones and diabetes mellitus. In D. G. Gardner & D. Shoback (Eds). *Greenspan's Basic and Clinical Endocrinology* (8th ed.). Columbus, OH: McGraw-Hill.

Menon, K. & Lawson, M. (2007). Identification of adrenal insufficiency in pediatric critical illness. *Pediatric Critical Care Medicine*, *8*(3), 276–278.

Potts, J. T. (2008). Diseases of the parathyroid gland and other hyper- and hypocalcemic disorders. In A. S. Fauci (Ed). *Harrison's Principles of Internal Medicine* (17th ed.). New York: McGraw-Hill.

Powers, A. C. (2008). Diabetes mellitus. In A. S. Fauci et al. (Eds). *Harrison's Internal Medicine* (17th ed.). Columbus, OH: McGraw-Hill.

Ranadive, S. A. (2011). Pediatric disorders of water balance. *Pediatric Clinics of North America*, *58*(5), 1271–1280.

Rivkees, S. A. & Dinauer, C. (2007). An optimal treatment for pediatric Graves' disease is radioiodine. *Journal of Clinical Endocrinology & Metabolism*, *92*(3), 797–800.

Rolfes, S. R., Pinna, K. & Whitney, E. N. (2009). *Understanding Normal and Clinical Nutrition*. New York: Wadsworth/Cengage Learning.

Sherr, J. & Weinzimer, S. (2012). Diabetes types 1 and 2 in the pediatric population. *Pediatric Annals*, *41*(2), 1–7.

Thalange, N. & Beach, R. (2013). Endocrinology & metabolism. In N. Thalange, R. Beach, D. Booth, et al. (Eds.), *Essentials of Paediatrics* (2nd ed.). Philadelphia: Elsevier/Saunders

Witchel, S. F. & Azziz, R. (2011). Mini review. Congenital adrenal hyperplasia. *Pediatric and Adolescent Gynaecology*. *24*, 116–126.

Zeitler, P. S., et al. (Eds). (2014). Endocrine disorders. In W. W. Hay, et al. (Eds). *Current Pediatric Diagnosis and Treatment* (22nd ed.). Columbus, OH: McGraw-Hill.

Suggested readings

Association for Children with a Disability <www.acd.org.au>.

Australian Pituitary Foundation Ltd <www.pituitary.asn.au>.

Congenital Adrenal Hyperplasia Support Group Australia Inc. <www.cah.org.au>.

Crawford, A., & Harris, H. (2012). SIADH: Fluid out of balance. *Nursing*, *42*(9), 50–58.

Diabetes Australia <www.diabetesaustralia.com.au>.

Diabetes New Zealand <www.diabetes.org.nz>.

Fisher, M. S., & Broome, M. E. (2011). Parent-provider communication during hospitalization. *Journal of Pediatric Nursing*, *26*(1), 58–69.

John, C., & Day, M. (2012). Central neurogenic diabetes insipidus, syndrome of inappropriate secretion of antidiuretic hormone and cerebral salt-wasting syndrome in traumatic brain injury. *Critical Care Nurse*, *32*(2), 1–9.

Kids and Teens with Diabetes <www.diabeteskidsandteens.com.au>.

Sarver, P. A. S., Senczakowicz, E. A., & Slovensky, B. M. (2010). Development of simulation scenarios for an adolescent patient with diabetic ketoacidosis. *Journal of Nursing Education*, *49*(10), 578–586.

Sudia-Robinson, T. (2011). Ethical implications of newborn screening, life-limiting conditions, and palliative care. *American Journal of Maternal Child Nursing*, *36*(3), 188–196.

Tourigny, J., Clendinnenq, D., Chartrand, J., et al. (2011). Evaluation of a virtual tour for children undergoing same-day surgery and their parents. *Pediatric Nursing*, *37*(4), 177–183.

Whittemore, R., Jaser, S. S., Jeon, S., et al. (2012). An internet coping skills training program for youth with type 1 diabetes: Six-month outcomes. *Nursing Research*, *61*(6), 395–404.

Winsett, R. P., Stender, S. R., Gower, G., et al. (2010). Adolescent self-efficacy and resilience in participants attending a diabetes camp. *Pediatric Nursing*, *36*(6), 293–296.

Chapter 49

Nursing care of a family when a child has a neurological disorder

Previous chapters described normal growth and development in children and nursing care of children with disorders of other systems. This chapter adds information about the dramatic changes, both physical and psychosocial, that occur when a child is born or develops a neurological disorder. Such information builds a base for care and health teaching for children with these disorders.

LEARNING OBJECTIVES

After studying the contents of this chapter, you should be able to:

1. Describe common neurological disorders in children.
2. Analyse ways in which care of a child with a neurological disorder can be optimally family-centred.
3. Assess a child with a neurological disorder.
4. Establish expected outcomes for a child with a neurological disorder.
5. Plan nursing care for a child with a neurological disorder.
6. Implement nursing care, such as monitoring medicine effectiveness, for a child with a neurological disorder.
7. Evaluate expected outcomes for achievement and effectiveness of care.
8. Identify areas related to care of children with neurological disorders that could benefit from additional nursing research or application of evidence-based practice.
9. Integrate knowledge of neurological disorders and the nursing process to achieve quality child and family health nursing care.

KEY TERMS

- astereognosis
- automatisms
- autonomic dysreflexia
- choreoathetosis
- choreoid
- decerebrate posturing
- decorticate posturing
- diplegia
- dyskinetic
- graphesthesia
- hemiplegia
- infantile spasms
- kinaesthesia
- paraplegia
- pulse pressure
- quadriplegia
- status epilepticus
- stereognosis

CASE STUDY

Harrison is a 4-year-old boy who is brought to an emergency department by his mother. Harrison's mother reported that he had been unwell for 24 hours with a fever and that within the last hour, Harrison appeared to fit. His doctor suspects he may have had a seizure caused by meningitis. His mother is visibly upset. She says, "Does this mean he'll always have seizures? How can he ever be independent? How will I cope?"

CASE STUDY QUESTION

1. What education does this parent need about recurrent seizures?

Parents of children with neurological disorders require a calm and caring approach. Seizures are terrifying events for parents as they fear for the immediate and long-term future of their child. Nurses are in a position to empower parents to cope better with stress by keeping them informed and involved in their child's care. Explaining the Modified Glasgow Coma Scale for Infants and Children aids in the parents' understanding of a reliable way of identifying a child's level of consciousness. (For further information, see Chapter 52.) Questions regarding long-term implications can then be better addressed at each stage of the treatment. Parents or carers should be provided with hope, as their quick action will ensure children receive immediate medical care.

Neurological disorders encompass a wide array of problems resulting from congenital disorders, acquired dysfunction, infection or trauma. Many of these disorders can cause severe illness. Others can result in life-threatening complications. In the future, stem cell research may offer a cure for neurological disorders, but in the present, because neural tissue does not regenerate like other body tissue, any nervous system degeneration is permanent. Whenever possible, prevention must be the highest priority for keeping the nervous system healthy. If degeneration has already occurred, nursing care focuses on helping the child and family develop strategies for dealing with the associated loss of mental or physical functioning, making the child comfortable and providing an environment conducive to the child's development and self-esteem.

CARE OF A CHILD WITH A NEUROLOGICAL SYSTEM DISORDER

Assessment

Neurological disorders often manifest themselves with vague symptoms. Parents may report that their child seems to be "walking strangely" or is "just not herself". A thorough history and neurological examination provide the best sources of information regarding the cause of the child's problem. As with all patients, the nurse–patient relationship begins with the introduction, when nurses explain their roles and the purpose of the interview (Lewis & Foley, 2014).

The neurological examination covers six areas of neurological functioning, including mental or cognitive processes as well as motor and sensory functioning. If more information is needed, numerous diagnostic laboratory tests may be ordered. The parents and child need considerable support throughout the assessment process. Although the neurological examination can be made "fun" for a child, other procedures such as a computed tomography (CT) scan or lumbar puncture can be frightening. Additionally, the anxiety of not knowing what is wrong and fearing the worst can make the waiting period for test results especially difficult for the child's parents.

At this point, it is important to ensure that any cultural issues are identified. Australia and New Zealand are multicultural societies and health is not always viewed the same in each cultural group. Reponses by parents to neurological disorders will differ and fear, due to misconceptions, can impede the assessment process. Other cultural considerations in the interview process are the language used, cultural taboos such as touch and making eye contact (Lewis & Foley, 2014).

Nursing considerations

Children who have permanent limitations may not be able to achieve in some areas. When neurological disorders are first diagnosed, parents may be able to focus only on the short term, such as whether the child will survive meningitis or whether the child has stopped convulsing. Later, they may need help to look at the long-term picture: Will they need assistance to care for the child at home? What type of education setting will be best for their child? What type of exercise program will be required?

Long-term care needs can be a source of stress, physically, emotionally, socially and financially. Numerous organisations are available for assistance and support such as:

- Australia and New Zealand Child Neurology Society (ANZCNS) <www.anzcns.org.au>
- Brain Injury Australia <www.braininjuryaustralia.org.au>
- Cerebral Palsy Australia <www.cpaustralia.com.au>
- Epilepsy Action Australia <www.epilepsy.org.au>
- Neurological Foundation of New Zealand <www.neurological.org.nz/resources/other-neurological-organisations>
- Royal Children's Hospital epilepsy fact sheet <www.rch.org.au/kidsinfo/fact_sheets/Epilepsy_an_overview>
- The Epilepsy Foundation <www.epinet.org.au>.

Nursing interventions for a child with a neurological problem must address both short- and long-term needs. For instance, while feeding an infant with increased intracranial pressure (ICP), demonstrate a caring attitude by showing parents how to gently handle the infant. For parents of a child with seizures, explain that turning him gently to his side will prevent him from choking. This can help them feel less anxious about future seizures. The child, too, will feel more in control of his illness if he believes that both he and his parents will be able to handle any acute symptoms. Providing nursing care that meets everyone's needs takes a great deal of sensitivity and planning.

ASSESSING THE CHILD WITH A NEUROLOGICAL DISORDER

Neurological symptoms, such as headache, an unsteady gait or lethargy, are often insidious. Both a thorough history and a neurological examination are needed to reveal the cause and extent of such symptoms (see Box 49.1).

Health history

The child's history may first reveal symptoms of a neurological disorder. Because many neurological problems result from fetal injury, it is important to obtain the mother's pregnancy history as well. At primary care visits, ask parents about their child's developmental milestones and ability to perform age-appropriate tasks successfully. A Denver Developmental Screening Test (see Appendix C)

BOX 49.1 Assessment ✻ Assessing a child for signs and symptoms of a neurological disorder

History

Chief concern: Seizure, loss of consciousness, delay in developmental tasks, headache, clumsiness at motor tasks.

Past medical history: Infection during pregnancy; difficult birth; difficulty with initiating respirations at birth; head injury from fall or accident.

Family medical history: History of seizures or headaches in other family members.

Physical examination

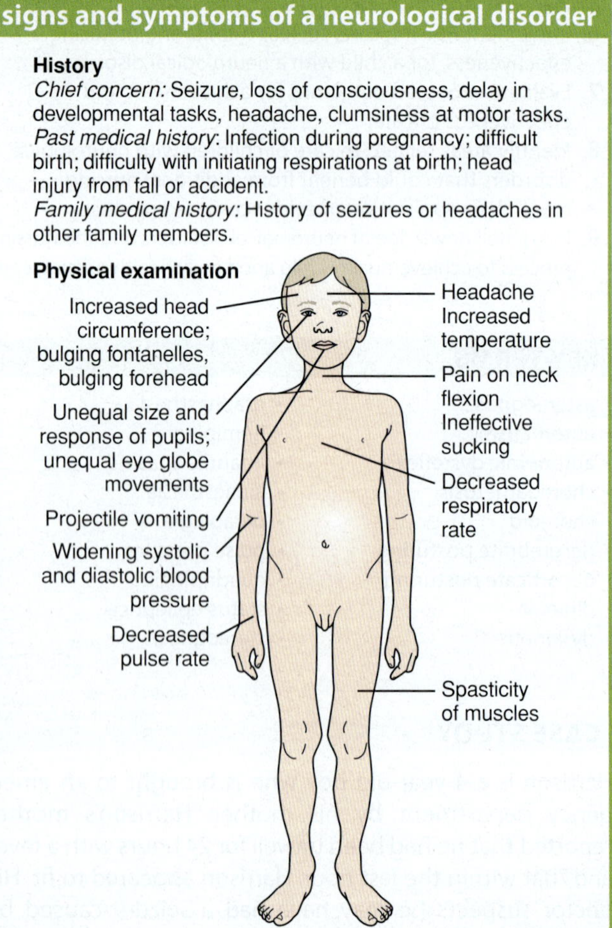

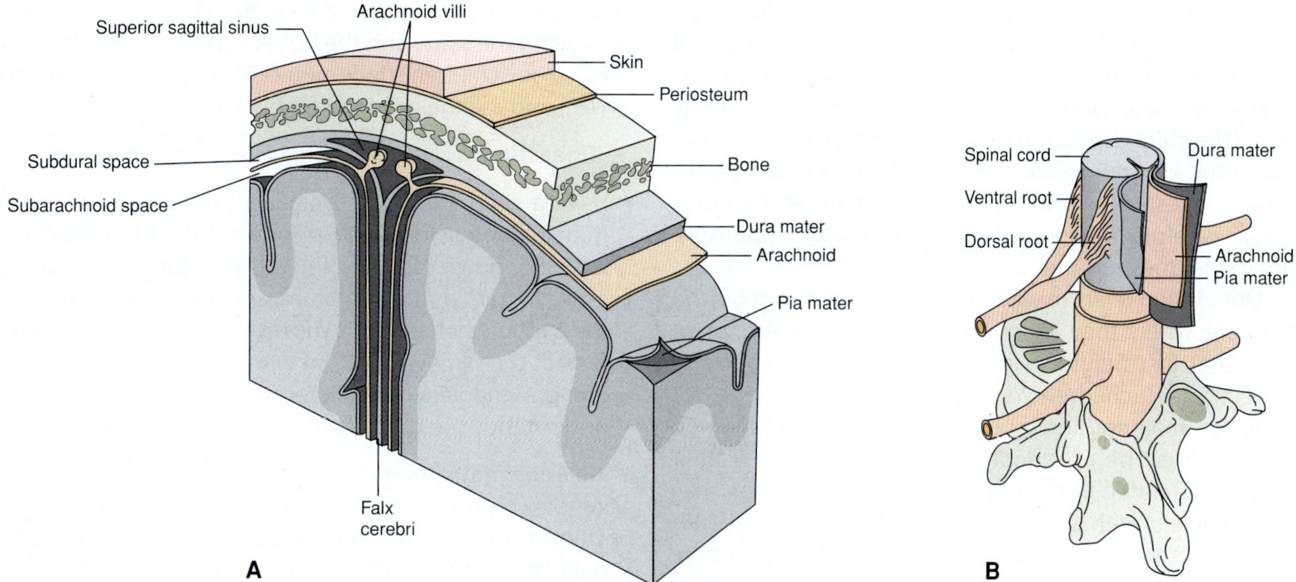

FIGURE 49.1 Meninges of the (**A**) brain and (**B**) spinal cord.

can indicate whether a parent's concern about a preschool child is well founded. The ability to perform well in school is important documentation for an older child. Lewis and Foley (2014) suggest that asking the child or parent to clearly describe health changes enables a comparison with current health status.

Neurological examination

A complete neurological examination takes at least 20 minutes. It requires patience and skill to keep a child's attention while observing for possible indications of neurological disease. For a full examination, six areas are assessed: cerebral, cranial nerve, cerebellar, motor, sensory and reflex function (see Fig. 49.1 and Table 49.1).

Cerebral function

Both general and specific cerebral functions are evaluated. General cerebral function is indicated by level of consciousness, orientation, intelligence, performance, mood and general behaviour (Rust, 2011).

TABLE 49.1 Normal properties of cerebrospinal fluid

Parameter	Normal finding	Abnormal finding: Possible significance
Opening pressure	60–160 cm H_2O	Lowered pressure usually indicates that there is subarachnoid obstruction in the spinal column above the puncture site. Elevated pressure suggests intracranial compression, haemorrhage or infection. Pressure increases if a child coughs or pressure is applied to the external jugular vein (Valsalva manoeuvre).
Appearance	Clear and colourless	If cloudy, indicates possible infection with an increased number of white blood cells (WBCs). If reddened, colour is probably red blood cells (RBCs).
Cell count	0–8/mm^3	Granulocytes suggest CSF infection. Lymphocytes suggest meningeal irritation and inflammation. A few RBCs and WBCs are normally present in the newborn CSF due to the trauma of birth.
Protein	15–45 mg/100 mL	Elevated count (>45/100 mL) occurs if RBCs are present. If both protein content and RBC count are elevated, meningitis or subarachnoid haemorrhage is suggested. If protein content alone is elevated, it suggests a degenerative process such as multiple sclerosis.
Glucose	60%–80% of serum glucose level	Decreased glucose level suggests that a glycolytic process is occurring. Bacterial meningitis causes a marked decrease in CSF glucose; invasion of fungi, yeast, tuberculosis or protozoans into the CSF results in some decrease in glucose level. Viral infections do not cause a decrease in CSF glucose and may occasionally cause a slight increase.
Albumin/globulin (A/G)	8:1	Increased level suggests infection or A/G ratio neurological disorder.

When evaluating a child's cerebral function, conversation with the child is essential. Talking to the child will identify the child's level of consciousness. During this period the nurse will look for signs of drowsiness, lethargy and if the child is oriented to surroundings. It is also essential in the evaluation process that the child is allowed to answer questions without prompting and that the nurse listens carefully to assess whether the answer is appropriate to the question.

Orientation refers to whether children are aware of who they are, where they are and what day it is (person, place and time). Be careful to take into account a child's age and development; children younger than 4 years of age, for example, may not know both their first and last names. Children may be of school age before they know their address. Children younger than 7 or 8 years of age may have difficulty with the days of the week, confusing "yesterday" with "today" or "tomorrow". Intellectual performance (IQ) can be determined by the child's score on a standard intelligence test. Estimates of intellectual function can be made by asking the child questions on common topics.

Immediate recall is the ability to retain a concept for a short time. Ask the child to repeat numbers after you.

- A child who is 4 years old can usually repeat three digits.
- A child older than 6 years can repeat five digits.

Recent memory covers a slightly longer period. Show the preschool child an object such as a key and ask him to remember it because later you will ask him to tell you what it was. After about 5 minutes, ask whether he remembers what object you showed him. Ask older children what they ate for breakfast to test recent memory.

Remote memory is long-term recall.

- Ask preschoolers what they ate for breakfast that morning (to them, that was a long time ago).
- Ask older children the name of their teacher.

Specific cerebral function can be measured by assessing language, sensory interpretation and motor integration. When assessing language, listen to the child's ability to articulate. Remember that many preschoolers substitute "w" for "r", saying "west time" instead of "rest time".

Stereognosis refers to the ability to recognise an object by touch and tests sensory interpretation.

- Ask the child to close her eyes; then place a familiar object, such as a key, a coin or a bottle cap, in her hand and ask her to identify it. This is a skill even preschoolers are able to do successfully.

Graphesthesia is the ability to recognise a shape that has been traced on the skin.

- Ask a pre-schooler to close his eyes; trace first a circle and then a square, on the back of his hand and ask him whether the shapes are the same or different. Be sure that the child understands the concept of "different" by first showing him objects such as two keys and a bottle cap and documenting that he is able to identify the keys as being the same and the bottle cap as being different. For older children, trace numbers (8, 3, 0 and 1 work well) and ask the child to identify each one.

Kinaesthesia is the ability to distinguish movement.

- Have a child close her eyes and extend her hands in front of her. Raise one of her fingers and ask her whether it is up or down. Hold the finger by its sides so that your other fingers do not brush against the child's palm or the back of her hand (this will reveal the finger position). Repeat the same movement with a toe on each foot.
- For preschoolers, first determine whether the child understands the concept of up and down.

Measure motor integration by asking a child to perform a complex motor skill such as folding a piece of paper and putting it into an envelope. A child of 4 years or older should be able to do this neatly. Children do best when these tests are presented as a game. Be certain to convey that there are no right or wrong answers. A child who believes that he has failed these tests may not respond well to further testing.

Cranial nerve function

Testing for cranial nerve function consists of assessing each pair of cranial nerves separately. Cranial nerves and methods of cranial nerve testing are described in Table 49.2. Methods to test pupil constriction and ability to follow into fields of gaze are described in Chapter 34.

Cerebellar function

Tests for cerebellar function are tests for normal balance and coordination. The following points identify activities and exercises the child is asked to undertake during this assessment.

- Observe the child walking. Does he do so naturally and freely? (Most children walk at least a little self-consciously when they know they are being observed.)
- Ask the child to stand on one foot. A child as young as 4 years should be able to do this for as long as 5 seconds.
- Ask the child to attempt a tandem walk (walk in a straight line, one foot directly in front of the other, heel touching toe). A child older than 4 years of age should be able to do this for about four consecutive steps.
- Ask the child to touch his nose with his finger, then reach and touch your finger with the same hand (held about 50 cm in front of him). Tell him to repeat this action and move your finger to a new position each time. The average child rarely reaches past your finger or stops before touching it.
- Ask the child to pat one knee with the palm of her hand, then quickly turn the hand over and pat the knee with the back of her hand; repeat over and over. He should be able to do this rapid, coordinated motion without much difficulty. Always ask him to do the motion one

TABLE 49.2 Cranial nerve function

Cranial nerve	Function	Assessment
I (olfactory)	Sense of smell	Assess child's ability to recognise common odours such as peanut butter or an orange while eyes are closed.
II (optic)	Vision	Assess vision fields and visual acuity; examine retinas.
III (oculomotor)	Motor control and sensation for eye muscles and upper eyelid	Assess pupillary size, equality, reaction to light and ability to follow an object in all directions. Note any nystagmus (an abnormal jerking motion).
IV (trochlear)	Movement of major eye globe muscles	As for nerve III.
V (trigeminal)	Mastication muscles and some facial sensations	Assess ability to discern light touch to test sensory component; assess symmetry and strength of bite to test motor component.
VI (abducens)	Movement and muscle sense of eye globe	As for nerves III and IV.
VII (facial)	Impulses for facial muscles, salivation, and taste	Assess motor strength by asking child to close eyes while you attempt to open them. Note symmetry of facial expression (such as smile) and movement (such as wrinkling forehead). Assess taste by asking child to identify salt or sugar.
VIII (acoustic)	Equilibrium and hearing	Assess hearing by the response to a whispered word or a Weber or Rinne test. Equilibrium is not tested routinely.
IX (glossopharyngeal)	Motor impulses to heart; sensation from pharynx, thorax, and abdominal organs	Assess gag reflex by pressing on back of tongue with tongue blade. Note midline uvula (tested together with nerve X).
X (vagus)	Swallowing and gag reflexes	Assess ability to swallow; elicit gag reflex by pressing a tongue blade on posterior tongue.
XI (accessory)	Impulses to striated muscles of pharynx and shoulders	Ask child to turn head to the side; try to turn it to center. Ask the child to elevate shoulders while you press down on them.
XII (hypoglossal)	Motor impulses to tongue and skeletal muscles; sensation from skin and viscera	Ask child to protrude tongue. Assess for tremors. Ask child to press on side of cheek with tongue; assess tongue strength.

hand at a time. Preschoolers will mirror the movement of the actively moving hand by moving the inactive hand as well. Older children should not demonstrate this (or should show only a small amount of movement).

- Ask the child to touch each finger on one hand with the thumb of that hand in rapid succession.
- Ask him to run the heel of one foot down the front of his other leg while he is lying supine (he should be able to do this without "running off" the leg).
- While he is still lying on the examining table, ask him to close his eyes and draw a circle or figure 8 in the air with his foot.

Tests of cerebellar function are all fun for children to do, as long as they know that there are no passes or failures. Show approval for effort even if they are having difficulty with a task, so that they have confidence to try another one.

Motor function

Muscle size, strength and tone are part of motor function assessment.

- Compare the size of the extremities on each side. If in doubt about symmetry, measure the circumference of the calves and thighs or upper and lower arms for comparison.
- Palpate muscles for tone. Move the extremities through passive range of motion; evaluate for symmetry, spasticity and flaccidity bilaterally.
- Ask the child to extend her arms in front of her and resist your action as you push down or up on her hands or push them out to the side. Do the same with the lower extremities.

Sensory function

If children's sensory systems are intact, they should be able to distinguish light touch, pain, vibration, hot and cold.

- Have a child close his eyes and then ask him to point to the spot where you touch him with an object. Light touch is tested by using a wisp of cotton; deep pressure by pressure of your finger; pain by a safety pin; temperature by test tubes filled with hot or cold water. Warn the child that on testing with a pin, he will feel a momentary prick. Otherwise, he may be unwilling to close his eyes again for further testing.
- Vibration is tested by touching the child's bony prominences (iliac crest, elbows, knees) with a vibrating tuning fork.

Reflex testing

Deep tendon reflex testing, which is part of a primary physical assessment (see Chapter 34), is also a basic part of a neurological assessment. In newborns, reflex testing is especially important, because the infant cannot perform tasks on command to demonstrate the full range of neurological function (see Chapter 18).

CASE STUDY QUESTION

2. Harrison is scheduled for a full neurological examination. What would be the best explanation to prepare him for this?
    a. "You'll need to answer questions carefully so you can pass this test."
    b. "I'll be asking you to move in different ways, almost like a game."
    c. "I need to find out how healthy or unhealthy your brain seems to be."
    d. "Seizures can be caused by a brain tumour, so that needs to be ruled out."

Diagnostic testing

A variety of diagnostic tests may be ordered to provide more information should any abnormalities be detected in the health history, physical examination or neurological examination. Many of these tests are invasive, so it is best to try to schedule the least invasive procedures first, before the painful or more frightening procedures are done, to help promote the child's cooperation. Ensuring that the child and family are well prepared for these procedures is an important nursing responsibility. When explaining tests, take into account not only the child's chronological age, but also the child's level of cognitive functioning, otherwise, explanations may not be well understood. Be sure to provide an explanation that includes a description of all of the sensory experiences the child might undergo—that is, not only what will be done but also how the child might feel, or what the child might see or hear or even smell or taste (if appropriate).

Lumbar puncture

Lumbar puncture involves the introduction of a needle into the subarachnoid space (under the arachnoid membrane) at the level of L4 or L5 to withdraw cerebrospinal fluid (CSF) for analysis. The procedure is used most frequently to diagnose haemorrhage or infection in the central nervous system (CNS) or to diagnose an obstruction of CSF flow. Lumbar puncture is contraindicated if the skin over the needle insertion site is infected (to avoid introducing pathogens into the CSF) or if there is a suspected elevation of CSF pressure. In the latter instance, if fluid is removed, the higher pressure in the intracranial space could cause the brainstem to be drawn down into the spinal cord space, compressing the medulla and compromising the action of the cardiac and respiratory centres. EMLA can be applied to the puncture site 1 hour before the procedure to reduce pain. Alternatively, the child may receive conscious sedation for the procedure (see Chapter 39).

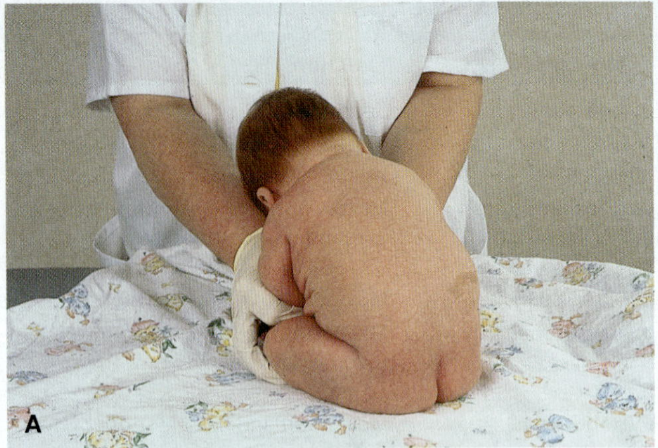

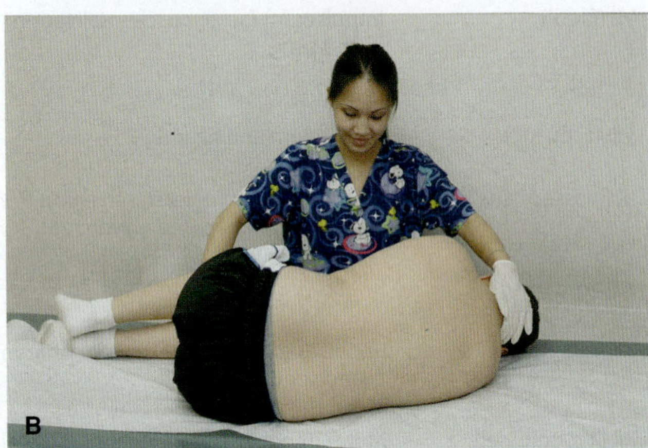

FIGURE 49.2 (**A**) Positioning an infant for a lumbar puncture. (**B**) Positioning an older child for a lumbar puncture. (© Barbara Proud.)

For a lumbar puncture, a newborn is seated upright with the head bent forwards (see Fig. 49.2A). The older infant or child is placed on one side on the examining table. The head is flexed forwards, the knees are flexed on the abdomen and the back is arched as much as possible. This position opens the space between the lumbar vertebrae, facilitating needle insertion (see Fig. 49.2B). Children younger than school-age need to be held in this position, because they may be so frightened by someone working on their back, unseen, that they are unable to hold this arched position; they may try to turn over or turn their head to see what is happening. It helps a school-age child or adolescent if you stand by the table facing him and gently rest your hand on the back of the head, keeping it bent forwards. This helps to maintain a good position without the impression of being restrained.

Children need good preparation for a lumbar puncture.

- Be certain that they know that the healthcare provider performing the procedure will wash their back with a solution that feels cold and inject a local anaesthetic that might sting like a bee sting (if an analgesic cream was not applied before the procedure).

- Caution children that they probably will feel pressure but not pain as the lumbar puncture needle is inserted.
- Remind them to remain absolutely still throughout the procedure. You might describe the position as "rolling into a ball" or "folding up like an astronaut in a small spaceship".
- Occasionally during a lumbar puncture, the needle will press against a dorsal nerve root and the child will experience a shooting pain down one leg. If this happens, reassure the child that this feeling passes quickly and does not indicate an injury.

When the insertion stylette is removed and CSF drips from the end of the needle, the procedure has been successful. An initial pressure reading is made, which varies with the child's age. To confirm that the subarachnoid space in the cord is patent with that in the skull, the examiner may ask a child who is older than 3 years of age to cough, or the examiner may ask you to press on the child's external jugular vein during the procedure. Either of these measures will cause an increase of CSF pressure if fluid is flowing freely through the subarachnoid space. Typically, three tubes of CSF, containing 2 to 3 mL each, are collected, a closing pressure reading is taken and the needle is withdrawn. Samples are usually sent for culture, sensitivity, glucose level and presence of red blood cells. Other evaluations are determining whether there is an alteration in the albumin/globulin ratio in the CSF and measuring the gamma-globulin level. An increased level of gamma-globulin is suggestive of multiple sclerosis or meningitis. The first sample obtained may contain blood or skin pathogens from the puncture, so it should not be the sample sent for determination of red blood cell content or culture. Throughout the procedure, sterile technique must be strictly observed to ensure that an uncontaminated sample of fluid is sent for culture and to avoid the introduction of pathogens into the CSF.

Post lumbar puncture headache

Lumbar puncture involves at least momentary pain, so children need to be comforted afterwards. A child may develop a headache after a lumbar puncture as a result of the reduction in CSF volume or invasion of a small air pocket during the puncture, although this is rare because of the small needle used. Encouraging the child to lie flat for about 30 minutes and to drink a glass of fluid can help prevent cerebral irritation caused by air rising in the subarachnoid space and helps increase the amount of CSF. Some children have a headache despite these precautions and may need an analgesic for pain relief (Bezov, Ashina & Lipton, 2010). Although post lumbar puncture headache is seen less frequently in young children than in adults, assessing for it is important to reduce the risk of pain for the child.

If a child had minimally increased CSF pressure at the time of the puncture, closely observe the child after the procedure to prevent respiratory and cardiac difficulty from medulla pressure. An increase in blood pressure or a decrease in pulse and respiration are important signs of increased intracranial compression. Other important signs include a change in consciousness, pupillary changes and a decrease in motor ability.

Ventricular tap

In infants, CSF may be obtained by a subdural tap into a ventricle through the coronal suture or anterior fontanelle. A small space on the scalp over the insertion site is shaved or clipped and the area is prepared with an antiseptic. The infant's head must be held firmly in a supine position to prevent movement during the procedure, which could cause the needle to strike and lacerate meningeal tissue.

Fluid must be removed from this site slowly, rather than suddenly, to prevent a sudden shift in pressure that could cause intracranial haemorrhage. After the procedure, a pressure dressing is applied to the site and the infant is placed in a semi-Fowler's position to prevent prolonged drainage from the puncture site. After the procedure, comfort the infant or allow the parents to do so; this both reduces the stress of a painful procedure and prevents the infant from crying excessively, an action that could increase ICP.

Cerebral angiography

Cerebral angiography is an x-ray study of cerebral blood vessels that involves the injection of a contrast material into an extracranial artery. Serial x-rays are then taken as the dye flows through the blood vessels of the cerebrum. The injection site chosen is often a femoral artery, although a carotid artery may be used. The study shows any vessel defects or space-occupying lesions that are occluding cranial blood vessels.

Myelography

Myelography is the x-ray study of the spinal cord that involves the introduction of a contrast material into the CSF by lumbar puncture. It is used to show the presence of space-occupying lesions of the spinal cord. After the procedure, keep the head of the child's bed elevated to prevent contrast medium from reaching the meninges surrounding the brain.

Computed tomography (CT) and magnetic resonance imaging (MRI)

CT involves the use of radiography to reveal densities at multiple levels or layers of brain tissue. It is helpful in confirming the presence of a brain tumour or other encroaching lesions. Single-photon emission computed tomography (SPECT) is a similar procedure used mainly for blood flow evaluation. MRI uses magnetic fields to show differences in tissue composition, revealing normal versus abnormal brain tissue. Both CT and MRI are discussed in greater detail in Chapter 37.

Nuclear medicine studies

Brain scan

For a brain scan, a radioactive material is injected intravenously (IV), and, after a fixed time during which the injected material is deposited in cerebral tissue, radioactivity levels over the skull are measured. If the blood–brain barrier is not functioning, the radioactive material will accumulate in specific areas, suggesting possible tumour, subdural hematoma, abscess or encephalitis.

Positron emission tomography

The diagnostic technique of positron emission tomography (PET) involves imaging after injection of positron-emitting radiopharmaceuticals into the brain. These radioactive substances accumulate at diseased areas of the brain or spinal cord. PET is extremely accurate in identifying seizure foci.

Echoencephalography

Echoencephalography involves the projection of ultrasound (high-frequency sound waves above the audible range) towards the child's head or spinal cord (an ultrasound). Ultrasound may be used to outline the ventricles of the brain. Because this technique of scanning is non-invasive, produces no discomfort and has no known complications, it may be repeated frequently to monitor changes in the size of ventricles or an invading lesion.

Electroencephalography

The electroencephalogram (EEG) reflects the electrical patterns of the brain summarising the physical and chemical interactions within the brain at the time of the test (Rapin, 2011). Normally, a tracing indicates four types of waves: delta (1 to 3 waves per second); theta (4 to 7 waves per second); alpha (8 to 12 waves per second); and beta (13 to 20 waves per second).

To reduce extraneous movements of the eyes, head or muscles that would affect the tracing, the child must be cooperative and quiet during the procedure. Traditionally, parents are asked to keep their child up later than usual the night before so that the child will be sleepy. Good preparation and encouragement are also important to help a child relax. Caution children that the room will probably be darkened to help them rest. Compare the electrode wires attached to their scalp with adhesive paste to those attached to astronauts in space. Reassure them that these electrodes are not painful. Be careful not to use the word electrical. Children as young as 3 years of age know that electrical wires are ordinarily dangerous and can hurt them. They cannot relax if they are worried that they may be shocked or even electrocuted by the procedure.

Children who are unable to lie still and cooperate even after careful explanation may need conscious sedation, although sedation alters the electrical pattern of the cortex and should be avoided if possible (Britton & Kosa, 2010). Sedation may be required for children undergoing neurological examinations. The type of sedation is dependent on the medical officer, the hospital protocol and the age and condition of the child. Parents should be given specific instructions about the preparation for the EEG prior to coming for testing as they may need to omit an anticonvulsant medication on the morning of testing.

Although EEGs can show important information about brain activity, they are not helpful in all circumstances. For example, approximately 15% of children who are well demonstrate some abnormality on an EEG. Most brain tumours in paediatric clients are in the posterior fossa, but the activity of this region does not show up well on an EEG. This limitation means that an EEG may appear normal even if a brain tumour is present, unless the tumour is pressing on more distal brain portions. On inspection of the symmetry of hemispheres, local lesions may be suggested. Where there is a lesion, there will be slower waves, a higher voltage pattern and an overall more irregular pattern. A subdural lesion (perhaps from a haematoma) can interfere with transmission of the electrical impulses, lowering the voltage pattern.

Visual stimulation, such as having a child look at a whirling disk, may be used in connection with the EEG, because various types of electrical discharges increase with rapid eye movements. In a child who is sensitive to this type of stimulation, the testing may produce a seizure. If this occurs, the child may be very disturbed and disoriented after the procedure. Describe what has happened, letting him know that the seizure is over to help him relax.

HEALTH PROMOTION

Health promotion for nervous system health begins antenatally with measures to ensure optimal fetal growth and development and prevention of problems associated with anoxia. It continues throughout childhood with routine health maintenance visits, screening for possible neurological or developmental problems and timely immunisations to prevent sequelae of typical childhood infections such as measles or chickenpox. Nurses play a key role in providing education to parents about the importance of obtaining immunisations and completing medication therapy to ensure complete resolution of an infection.

Parents also need anticipatory guidance about safety measures to prevent injury, specifically, head and spinal cord injury. Remind parents that children should wear helmets when riding or using anything that can move faster than the child can run such as scooters, roller skates/blades, ice skates, horses, skis, skateboards or snowboards, bicycles or motorcycles (Riesch et al., 2012). For a child with seizures, parents need instructions to prevent injury during a seizure (see later discussion) and to administer anticonvulsants conscientiously. For a child with a long-term neurological disorder, rehabilitation and early intervention play a major role in reducing the risk of complications and in promoting the child's and family's optimal level of functioning.

INCREASED INTRACRANIAL PRESSURE

Increased intracranial pressure (ICP) is not a single disorder but a sign that may occur with many neurological disorders. When caring for a child with a potential neurological disorder, it is an important sign to detect. Increased ICP may occur with an increase in the CSF volume, blood entering the CSF, cerebral oedema or space-occupying lesions such as tumours. Examples of causes of increased ICP include:

- Birth trauma or hydrocephalus
- Head trauma from an accident
- Infection
- Brain tumour
- Guillain-Barré syndrome.

The rate at which symptoms develop depends on the cause and the ability of the child's skull to expand to accommodate the increased pressure. Children with open fontanelles can withstand more pressure without brain damage than can older children, whose suture lines and fontanelles have already closed.

Assessment of neurological function may involve only a few quick procedures, such as obtaining vital signs, evaluating pupil response and determining level of consciousness and motor and sensory function, or it may include more elaborate electronic monitoring. Common signs and symptoms of increased ICP are shown in Table 49.3.

With increased ICP, symptoms are often subtle at first. The child may report a headache, irritability or restlessness. Headache is difficult to detect in an infant but most infants with headaches become increasingly fussy or difficult to comfort. Growing pressure on the brainstem, which controls respiration and cardiac activity, causes pulse and respirations to slow. Compression of cranial vessels leads to a compensatory increase in blood pressure (or **pulse pressure**, the gap between the systolic and diastolic blood pressures). Pressure on the hypothalamus, the temperature-regulating centre of the body, causes an increase in temperature. These changes may occur gradually, so a single measurement may not show the extent of the change. Always compare the new information with all recordings taken in the last 24 hours.

Ocular changes may indicate that pressure is increasing posterior to the eye globe. One obvious abnormality is a dilated pupil, which suggests compression of cranial nerve II. Test pupil reactivity by shining a light into each eye. To elicit the most dramatic and sudden response, bring the light to the child's eye from the side or down from the forehead, to make it appear suddenly rather than gradually. Repeat this with the other eye. Each pupil should constrict and the constriction should be equal bilaterally. Consensual constriction should also be present. As you shine the light on the right pupil, the left pupil also should constrict and vice versa.

If a child is alert and able to cooperate, have her follow the light through the six cardinal positions of gaze and test convergence (ability to follow the light as it approaches closer and closer to the nose). Note any tendency towards strabismus, nystagmus (constant eye movement), "sunset eyes" (white sclera showing over the top of the cornea), or inability to follow the light into any quadrant. Be specific about what you document. "Inability to follow light" is not as informative as "inability to follow light into left superior field; vertical nystagmus noted as child follows light into other fields".

If a child lies supine and you turn his head gently but rapidly to the right, the eyes will normally turn towards the left and vice versa ("doll's eye" reflex). If a child has increased ICP, this phenomenon will be absent (this test is useful in assessing a comatose child who is unable to cooperate by following a light). An older child may be able to report symptoms such as diplopia. On funduscopic examination, papilloedema may be detected.

Assess the child's level of consciousness. If the child is alert but unable to comprehend surroundings, time or place, this may be the first indication of increased ICP. As pressure increases, a pseudo-awake state may occur, in which the child is awake but unable to follow light or locate a noise. Finally, the child becomes comatose, unable to be roused by any stimuli. Levels of coma are rated by the Glasgow Coma Scale. This is discussed in Chapter 52 in connection with assessment for head injury.

Children, like adults, generally become disoriented about time first, then place, then self. It is useful, therefore,

TABLE 49.3 Signs and symptoms of increased intracranial pressure

Sign or symptom	Indication of increased intracranial pressure
Increased head circumference	An increase >2 cm per month in first 3 months of life, >1 cm per month in the second 3 months, and >0.5 cm per month for the next 6 months
Fontanelle changes	Anterior fontanelle tense and bulging; closing late
Vomiting	Occurring in the absence of nausea, on awakening in morning or after nap; possibly projectile
Eye changes	Diplopia (double vision) from pressure on abducens nerves; white of sclera evident over pupil (setting sun sign); limited visual fields, papilloedema
Vital sign changes	Elevated temperature and blood pressure; decreased pulse and respiration rates
Pain	Headache, often present on awakening and standing; increasing with straining at stool (Valsalva maneuver) or holding breath
Mentation	Irritability, altered consciousness such as sleepiness

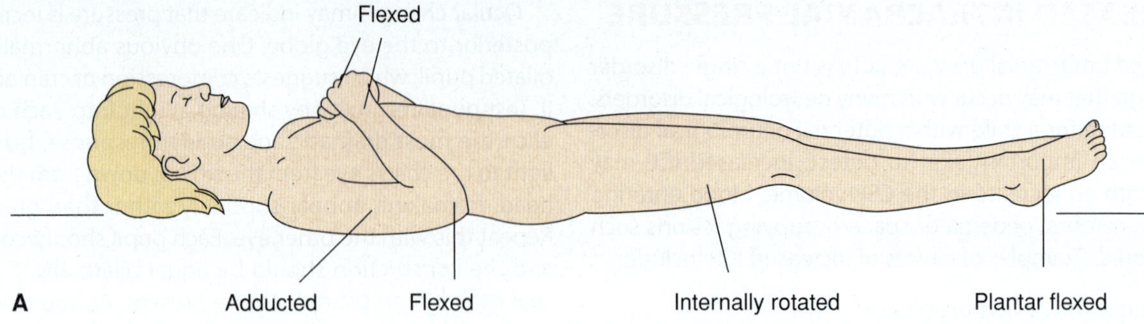

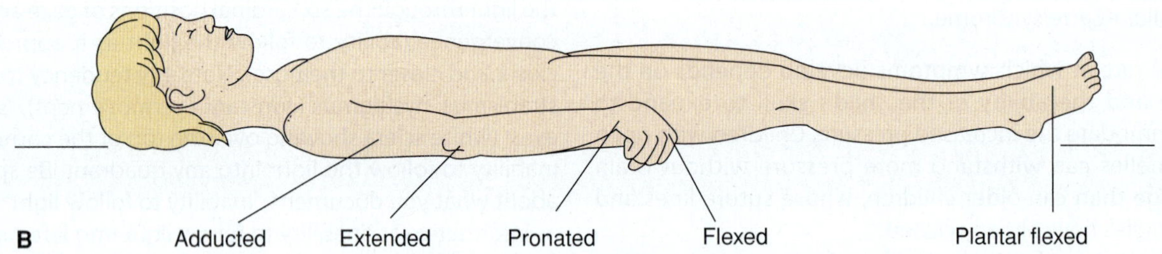

FIGURE 49.3 (**A**) Decorticate posturing. (**B**) Decerebrate posturing.

to assess that the child is alert enough to answer these questions. Explain that you will be asking these seemingly simple questions periodically to make sure the child can answer them accurately each time. Be aware that many children, even when healthy, are groggy when they first wake up; until fully awake they may not be able to say who or where they are on first awakening. Make sure children are fully awake before attempting to determine level of consciousness.

Be certain also that you ask questions appropriate to a child's age. Even if they give the wrong answer, it does not matter. Your concern is that they understood your request. Also remind parents that you are asking these questions to assess their child level of consciousness, not to quiz for right answers or to be intrusive. Remind them not to answer for the child. A good way to test an infant's level of consciousness is to determine whether the child responds to sounds such as a music box or voices, or reaches for an attractive object.

Motor ability can be assessed by asking a child to perform a simple motor task, such as squeezing your hand, pushing against your hand with both feet or performing rapid, alternating hand movements, such as turning a hand over and back several times. Evaluate cranial nerves grossly by having the child make a face, close the eyes tightly or smile. With all these assessments, be sure to evaluate whether the responses are equal and symmetrical bilaterally.

Test deep tendon reflexes, because these decrease in intensity with decreased level of consciousness. Carefully observe a child's resting posture. When motor control grows weaker because of loss of cell function, characteristic posturing (primitive reflexes) occurs. Cerebral loss is shown mainly by **decorticate posturing**. The child's arms are adducted and flexed on the chest with wrists flexed, hands fisted. The lower extremities are extended and internally rotated, and the feet are plantar flexed (see Fig. 49.3A). **Decerebrate posturing**, which occurs when the midbrain is not functional, is characterised by rigid extension and adduction of arms and pronation of the wrists with the fingers flexed. The legs are extended and the feet are plantar flexed (see Fig. 49.3B).

Observe the child carefully for any seizure activity. However, keep in mind that this is a late sign of increased ICP.

Intracranial pressure monitoring

To monitor intracranial pressure intraventricular catheters are threaded into the lateral ventricle, filled with normal saline, and then connected to an external pressure monitor (Bailey et al., 2012). As pressure in the ventricle fluctuates, it is registered through the filled catheter on an oscilloscope screen and a written printout. This method is advantageous over simple scanning because it also enables CSF drainage and administration of medication through the catheter.

ICP normally ranges from 1 to 10 mmHg. A level greater than 15 mmHg is considered abnormal. As blood pressure rises and falls with the influx of blood through vessels, so does ICP. On a monitor, it appears as A waves (plateau waves), which are transient paroxysmal elevations that last for 5 to 20 minutes with an amplitude of 50 to 100 mmHg. If brain ischaemia is present, these waves increase before other signs, such as a change in blood pressure or pulse rate, become apparent. B waves are short-duration waves (1/2 to 2 minutes) with low amplitude (up to 50 mmHg).

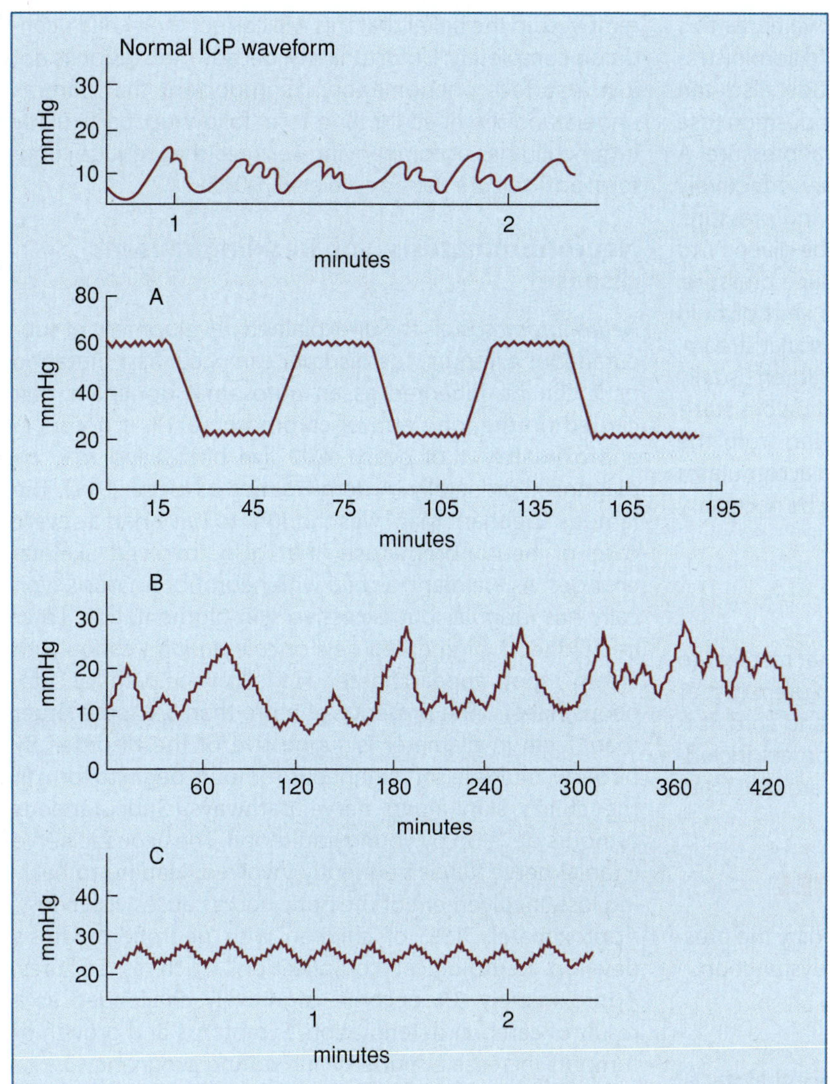

FIGURE 49.4 Normal ICP waveform and generalised shapes of the three types of intracranial pressure waves: A waves or plateau waves, B waves and C waves.

C waves are small, rhythmic waves at a frequency of approximately 6 waves per minute. They are related to deviations in the arterial blood pressure (see Fig. 49.4). Because A waves appear to reflect brain ischaemia, they can be used to signal when a child needs more oxygen.

ICP monitoring also can be used to estimate cerebral perfusion pressure (CPP) or cerebral blood flow.

Parents may have difficulty accepting procedures such as the insertion of intraventricular catheters or screws. Explaining the brain's anatomy will help them see that the catheter or screw does not puncture or tear brain tissue. Be sure to explain that this type of monitoring is advantageous, not only because it enables early detection should problems arise but helps to reduce the risk of further injury or complications.

If ICP increases, the cause of the problem must be identified and remedied as quickly as possible to prevent brain injury (see Box 49.2). In addition to local injury, severe pressure elevation can compress the brainstem and lead to cardiac and respiratory failure. Actions such as coughing, vomiting and sneezing increase the ICP and should be kept to a minimum, if possible. When burping infants after

BOX 49.2 ✻ Calculating cerebral perfusion pressure

Cerebral perfusion pressure (CPP) is calculated by subtracting the mean intracranial pressure (ICP) from the mean arterial pressure (MAP):

$$\text{MAP} - \text{ICP} = \text{CPP}$$

Mean arterial pressure is determined by subtracting the diastolic blood pressure (DBP) reading from the systolic blood pressure (SBP) reading, dividing the result by 3, then adding that sum to 80:

$$\text{MAP} = (\text{SBP} - \text{DBP})/3 + 80$$

Follow this example: A child has a blood pressure of 100/70 and an ICP of 10 mmHg.

Using the formulas above, first calculate the MAP:

$$(100 - 70)/3 + 80 = 90 \text{ mmHg}$$

Next calculate the CPP:

$$90 - 10 = 80 \text{ mmHg}$$

Therefore, a child with a blood pressure of 100/70 and an ICP of 10 has a CPP of 80 mmHg.

feeding, do not put pressure on the jugular veins, as this can increase the ICP. Monitor the rate of IV fluid administration in such children, because overhydration also can increase ICP. Placing a child in a semi-Fowler's position (use an infant seat for babies) can reduce cerebral pressure. A corticosteroid such as dexamethasone may effectively reduce cerebral oedema and its accompanying pressure. An osmotic diuretic, such as mannitol, may be given IV to remove fluid from interstitial tissue and reduce pressure. Because mannitol is hypertonic, it causes a shift of fluid from extravascular compartments into the vascular stream, where it can be eliminated by the kidneys. Children usually have an indwelling urinary catheter inserted before starting this therapy, to ensure bladder emptying from the drug-induced rapid diuresis. If excessive fluid accumulates in the brain's ventricles, a ventricular tap may be necessary for immediate reduction of pressure.

NEURAL TUBE DISORDERS

The neural tube is the embryonic structure that matures to form the CNS. Because this structure forms in utero first as a flat plate, then moulds to form the brain and cord, it is susceptible to malformation. Neural tube disorders, including spina bifida, are present at birth and so are discussed in Chapter 27.

NEUROCUTANEOUS SYNDROMES

Neurocutaneous syndromes are characterised by the presence of skin or pigment disorders with CNS dysfunction.

Sturge-Weber syndrome

A child with Sturge-Weber syndrome (encephalofacial angiomatosis) has a congenital port-wine birthmark on the skin of the upper part of the face that extends inward to the meninges and choroid plexus. The skin manifestation follows the distribution of the first division of the fifth cranial nerve (trigeminal nerve). Because the defect is usually unilateral, the port-wine stain ends abruptly at the midline. In many children, only the ophthalmic branch of the nerve is involved and the lesion is confined to the upper aspect of the face.

Because of involvement of the meningeal blood vessels, blood flow is sluggish and anoxia may develop in some portions of the cerebral cortex. The child may have symptoms of hemiparesis (numbness) on the side opposite the lesion from destruction of motor neurons. The child may experience intractable seizures, be cognitively challenged or develop blindness from glaucoma. A CT scan or an MRI of the skull usually shows calcification in the involved cerebral cortex. Such calcification follows a diagnostic "railroad track" or double-groove pattern. An EEG shows areas of decreased voltage.

When this syndrome is first diagnosed, parents may hope that the defect does not extend beyond the skin lesion. They may ask to have the skin lesion surgically removed, in the belief that this will correct their child's condition completely. Unfortunately, because the lesion is not just a surface phenomenon, it's important that parents understand the need for long-term follow-up, particularly if the child has accompanying seizures that require long-term anti-seizure therapy (Lo et al., 2012).

Neurofibromatosis (von Recklinghausen's disease)

Neurofibromatosis is the unexplained development of subcutaneous tumours. The disorder can occur as a mutation or it can be inherited as an autosomal dominant trait carried on the long arm of chromosome 17. It occurs in approximately 1 of every 4000 live births and may be diagnosed prenatally (Ardern-Holmes & North, 2011). The famous "Elephant Man" was thought to have had a severe case of neurofibromatosis that also involved skeletal changes. As an infant, a child with neurofibromatosis typically has irregular but excessive skin pigmentation. Later in childhood, pigmented nevi or *café-au-lait* ("coffee with cream") spots appear that tend to follow the paths of cutaneous nerves. The presence of more than six spots larger than 1 cm in diameter is suggestive of the disorder. By puberty, multiple soft cutaneous tumours begin to form in the child's skin along nerve pathways. Subcutaneous tumours develop by young adulthood. The acoustic nerve (cranial nerve VIII) is frequently involved, leading to hearing loss. Involvement of the optic nerve causes vision loss. Approximately 15% of children with neurofibromatosis develop neurological complications such as seizures. Approximately 8% become cognitively challenged as a result of cerebral deterioration. Symptoms and growth of tumours increase at puberty and during pregnancy.

Little therapy is available to halt the tumour growth. Mast cell blockers have some effect. If lesions are causing acoustic or optic degeneration, surgical removal of the tumours may be attempted. Be certain that the parents and child have a source of emotional support through the disease's slow but invariably fatal course.

CEREBRAL PALSY

Cerebral palsy (CP) is a group of non-progressive disorders of upper motor neuron impairment that result in motor dysfunction. Affected children also may have speech or ocular difficulties, seizures, cognitive challenges or hyperactivity. Muscle spasticity can lead to orthopaedic or gait difficulties (Crosbie et al., 2012).

The exact cause of CP is unknown, but the disorder is associated with low birth weight, premature birth or birth injury (Gilbert et al., 2010). It apparently is caused by brain anoxia leading to cell destruction of the motor tracts. If intrauterine anoxia occurs for some reason such as faulty placental implantation, placenta praevia or abruptio placentae, this type of brain cell dysfunction may result. Nutritional deficiencies, medications and maternal infections such as cytomegalovirus or toxoplasmosis, as well as direct birth injury, may also contribute to the cause.

CP occurs in approximately 1 of every 400 births in Australia, most frequently in very-low-birth-weight infants and those who are small for gestational age (Cerebral Palsy Australia, 2015). It is increasing in incidence because of the number of very-low-birth-weight infants who survive today. It occurs more frequently in infants born from occipito-posterior rather than anterior birth positions. In these instances, anoxia and resulting brain damage are more likely to occur with birth. In all instances, however, the damage may already have occurred in utero and may be the reason the infant is born abnormally early or presents in an unusual position. Head injury from child abuse, shaken baby syndrome, trauma or severe dehydration in the newborn, with resulting venous thrombosis, also may lead to CP symptoms.

Infections such as meningitis or encephalitis in the newborn are yet another cause of CP. In the past, kernicterus resulting from neonatal hyperbilirubinaemia was considered a cause of the athetoid type of CP (slow, writhing, involuntary movements). This type is rarely seen today because of improved management of hyperbilirubinaemia.

Children with all forms of CP may have sensory alterations such as strabismus, refractive disorders, visual perception problems, visual field defects and speech disorders such as abnormal rhythm or articulation. They may show an attention deficit disorder or autism. Deafness caused by kernicterus occurs in connection with athetoid CP. Cognitive challenge and recurrent seizures also frequently accompany all types of the disorder.

Types of cerebral palsy

CP has been classified in various ways. Traditionally, it is divided into two main categories based on the type of neuromuscular involvement: a pyramidal or spastic type (approximately 40% of affected children) and an extrapyramidal type, which is further subdivided into ataxic (approximately 10%), dyskinetic or athetoid (approximately 30%) and mixed (10%) (Moster et al., 2010).

Spastic type

Spasticity is excessive tone in the voluntary muscles that results in loss of upper motor neurons. A child with spastic CP has hypertonic muscles, abnormal clonus, exaggeration of deep tendon reflexes, abnormal reflexes such as a positive Babinski reflex, and continuation of neonatal reflexes, such as the tonic neck reflex, well past the age at which these usually disappear. If infants with CP are held in a ventral suspension position, they arch their backs and extend their arms and legs abnormally. They fail to demonstrate a parachute reflex if lowered suddenly, failing to hold out their arms as if to break their fall. Children tend to assume a "scissors gait" because tight adductor thigh muscles cause their legs to cross when held upright. This involvement may be so severe that it leads to a subluxated hip. Tightening of the heel cord usually is so severe that children walk on their toes, unable to stretch their heel to touch the ground.

Spastic involvement may affect both extremities on one side **(hemiplegia)**, all four extremities **(quadriplegia)** or primarily the lower extremities (**diplegia** or **paraplegia**). Children with hemiplegia usually have greater involvement in the arm than the leg. This may be demonstrated by asking the child to extend the arms and pronate them. When the child is asked to supinate the arm, the elbow flexes on the involved side. The involved arm may be shorter and may have a smaller muscle circumference than the other arm. Most children with hemiplegia have difficulty identifying objects placed in their involved hand when their eyes are closed **(astereognosis)**.

A child with quadriplegia invariably has impaired speech (pseudobulbar palsy) but may or may not be cognitively challenged. Swallowing saliva may be so difficult that the child drools and has difficulty swallowing food. Upper extremity involvement may be limited to an abnormal, awkward hand movement. If there is no involvement of the arms at all, this is a true spastic paraplegia and a spinal cord anomaly rather than a cerebral anomaly is suggested.

Dyskinetic or athetoid type

The athetoid type of CP involves abnormal involuntary movement. *Athetoid* means "wormlike". Early in life, the child is limp and flaccid. Later, in place of voluntary movement, children make slow, writhing motions. This may involve all four extremities, plus the face, neck and tongue. Because of poor tongue and swallowing movements, the child drools and speech is difficult to understand. With emotional stress, the involuntary movements may become irregular and jerking **(choreoid)** with disordered muscle tone **(dyskinetic)**.

Ataxic type

Children with ataxic involvement have an awkward, wide-based gait. On neurological examination, they are unable to perform the finger-to-nose test or to perform rapid, repetitive movements (tests of cerebellar function) or fine coordinated motions.

Mixed type

Some children show symptoms of both spasticity and athetoid movements. Ataxic and athetoid movements also may be present together. This combination results in a severe degree of physical impairment.

Nursing considerations

Children with CP need promotion of any function that is not already impaired, to prevent further loss of function. Major areas to be addressed include self-care, communication, ambulation, education, safety, nutrition, parental support and establishment of self-esteem.

Parents who are reacting to the news that their child has multiple physical disabilities often find it difficult to make long-term plans. Therefore, focus expected outcomes on short-term concerns to assist with family functioning.

Spasticity of muscles

Learning to be ambulatory is an important part of self-care because it helps determine how independent the child can become. This is difficult for the child to achieve because of lack of muscle group coordination. Surgery to lengthen heel tendons may be needed. Assisted ambulation devices such as wheeled walkers may be necessary (see Fig. 49.5). Medication to reduce spasticity has little effect, although baclofen (Lioresal) may be prescribed for some children to improve motor function. Cerebellar pacemakers may reduce spasticity in some children. Administration of botulism toxin (Botox) has been successful in some children to relieve spasticity and aid in walking (Placzek, Siebold & Funk, 2010).

Preventing contractures is important to maintain motor function. Formerly, children were fitted with extensive braces. The weight of these braces, however, often impeded muscle movement and actually prevented children from learning to walk. Partial lighter-weight leg braces may be prescribed to encourage children to bring their heels down and to keep heel cords from tightening. If leg braces are prescribed, parents may need some encouragement and support to insist that their children wear them. Passive and active muscle exercises also are important to prevent contractures. Teach parents passive exercises and games to play with their child that encourage active exercise. At healthcare visits, remind parents that these exercises are an important part of their child's therapy and must be done consistently each day.

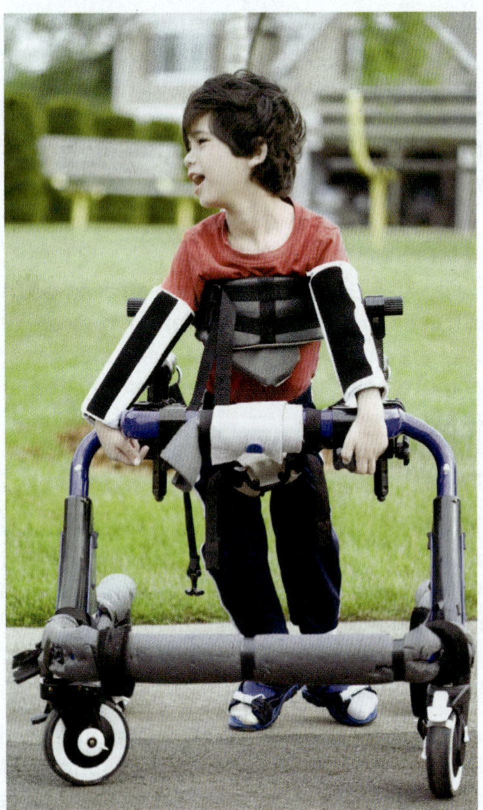

FIGURE 49.5 Wheeled walkers give a child added stability for walking and keep heel cords from shortening. (© fotosearch.com.)

Impaired mobility

Children need to learn self-care measures such as dressing, tooth brushing, bathing and toileting, so they can not only gain self-esteem by accomplishing these tasks but achieve optimal independence. Modifications such as straps attached to their toothbrush or feeding utensils may be necessary so they can hold them more securely. Advise parents to always supervise children during bathing. Lack of coordination could cause them to slip underwater and drown. Toileting is often difficult because the child does not have the muscle group coordination necessary to achieve successful bowel evacuation. A high-fibre diet helps prevent constipation and aids bowel evacuation. Voiding may be equally difficult because the child may lack sufficient voluntary muscle control.

Growth and development

Children with CP may be unable to pursue stimulating activities and surroundings because they are not fully mobile. Choose toys and activities that are appropriate to the child's intellectual, developmental and motor levels, not the child's chronological age. Some children need more stimulating activities than others because they have difficulty concentrating on one activity for any length of time.

A preschool program is important to provide exposure to the outside world. If at all possible, school-aged children with CP should be mainstreamed so that they can be among other children. By law, children who are physically or cognitively challenged must be provided with an education in the least restrictive setting possible. If they are both cognitively and physically challenged, however, the combined mental and motor deficits may severely limit their abilities, making school placement difficult. You may need to advocate that a child be placed in a school setting that is consistent with the child's intellectual ability.

Nutrition

Providing adequate nutrition to children with CP can be difficult. As infants, they often suck poorly because uncoordinated movements of the tongue, lips and jaw, and tongue thrusting cause them to push food out of their mouth (a retained primitive reflex). Lip and tongue control may be poor, with weak or uncoordinated jaw muscles. Older children may have difficulty holding and controlling a spoon to bring food to their mouth. Spasticity causes children to hyperextend the head when leaning forwards to take a bite. Parents may need guidance in finding a feeding pattern that works for their child. Manually controlling the jaw may help control the head, correct neck and trunk hyperextension, and stabilise the jaw to assist with feeding. If a child cannot chew or swallow well, a liquid or soft diet may be necessary. Some children can handle solids and finger foods but may take longer to eat than the average child. They may need protection for their clothing and the floor.

Communication

It is important that a child can verbally make needs known to strangers and family members. Most children with CP benefit from speech therapy, which helps them learn to speak slowly and to coordinate their lips and tongue to form speech sounds. Be patient with children and allow them to form words deliberately. If they try to hurry to please you, their speech will be much less clear and communication will be impaired. For the child who cannot speak clearly, provide an alternative form of communication, such as flash cards or a picture board. Touch-screen computer programs are often used in school settings to aid communication.

Parental education

Help parents to understand that the cause of CP is unknown and that it is a non-progressive disease. The brain damage that occurred during pregnancy or at birth will not recur, although the child's condition may seem to grow more apparent with age. Motor deficits of the upper extremities, for example, may not be strikingly evident until the child attempts fine motor tasks at school. Without follow-up care, contractures from spasticity may result, further reducing existing motor function.

Caution parents also that CP is a single name for a wide variety of diseases of varying consequence. Although another child may have such severe CP that he has no useful function in his extremities, their own child may not be affected to the same extent. Conversely, although they know someone with CP who is able to hold a full-time job, their child may not be able to do as well. Each child's potential must be evaluated individually.

Long-term care

Because CP is not always diagnosed early in infancy, parents may not learn that their child has a chronic disease until 2 to 4 years later. Help them to encourage their child to reach their full potential within the limits of their disorder. Evaluations at healthcare visits should note not only whether the child is achieving goals but also whether the child and family members find satisfaction and acceptance in the child's achievements. Parents may grieve because their child is not able to accomplish all of the major things they had wished for during pregnancy and they may feel defeated by the day-to-day strain of caring for their child's multiple special needs. Care of a child with a chronic illness is discussed further in Chapter 56.

✔ Checkpoint question 49.1

What information would you want parents to know about their child with cerebral palsy?

a. Symptoms of cerebral palsy usually fade by puberty.
b. All children with cerebral palsy are cognitively challenged.
c. Cerebral palsy may be associated with a vaccine reaction.
d. Symptoms may seem to grow worse as fine motor skill is needed.

INFECTION

Nervous system tissue is as susceptible to infection as any other body tissue. Common major infections include meningitis, encephalitis, Guillain-Barré syndrome, Reye's syndrome and botulism.

Bacterial meningitis

Meningitis is an infection of the cerebral meninges. It occurs most often in children younger than 24 months of age. Although the disease can occur at any time during the year, its peak incidence appears to be in the winter. In Australia, it is caused most frequently by *Streptococcus pneumoniae* or group B *Streptococcus*. In children younger than 2 months of age, group B *Streptococcus* and *Escherichia coli* are common causes of meningitis. In children with myelomeningocele who develop meningitis, *Pseudomonas* infection is common. Children who have had a splenectomy are particularly susceptible to pneumococcal meningitis unless they have received a pneumococcal vaccine. *Haemophilus influenzae*, once a major cause of meningitis, is now rarely seen because of routine immunisation against this organism (Greenberg-Kushnir et al., 2012).

Pathological organisms usually are spread to the meninges from upper respiratory tract infections, by lymphatic drainage possibly through the mastoid or sinuses, or by direct introduction through a lumbar puncture or skull fracture. Once organisms enter the meningeal space, they multiply rapidly and spread throughout the CSF. Organisms invade brain tissue through meningeal folds that extend down into the brain itself. The inflammatory response that occurs may lead to a thick, fibrinous exudate that blocks CSF flow. Brain abscess or invasion of the infection into cranial nerves can result in blindness, deafness or facial paralysis. Pus that accumulates in the narrow aqueduct of Sylvius can cause obstruction leading to hydrocephalus. Brain tissue oedema can put pressure on the pituitary gland, causing increased production of antidiuretic hormone, resulting in the syndrome of inappropriate antidiuretic hormone secretion (SIADH). This causes increased oedema because the body cannot excrete adequate urine.

The symptoms of meningitis occur either insidiously or suddenly. Children usually have had 2 or 3 days of upper respiratory tract infection. They become increasingly

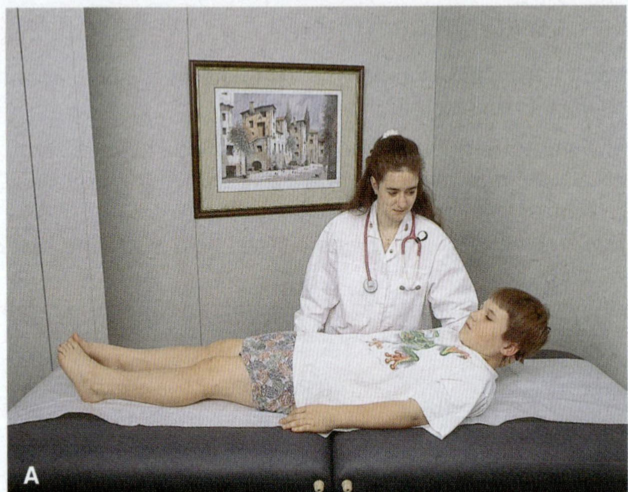

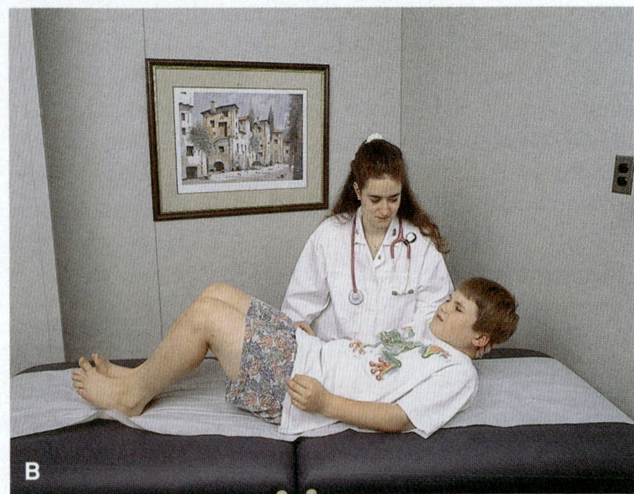

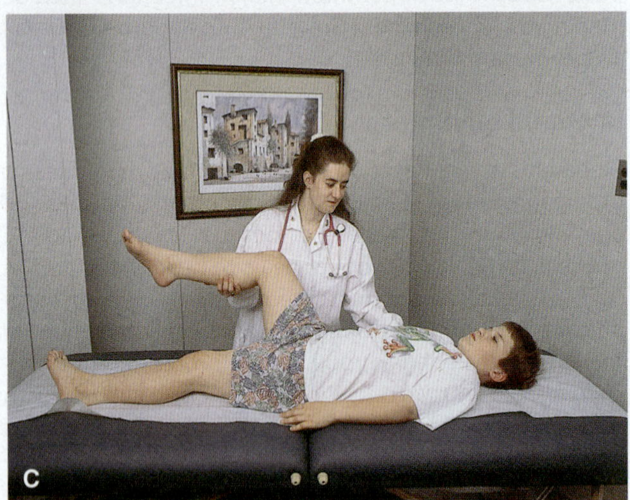

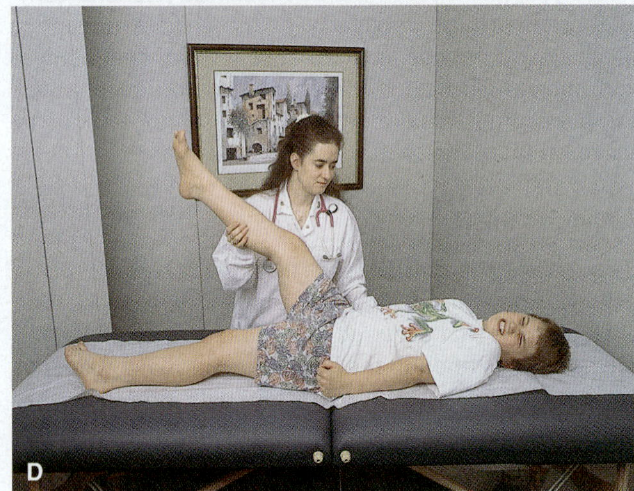

FIGURE 49.6 (**A**) Brudzinski's sign. The nurse flexes the child's neck forwards. (**B**) Positive response. Bilateral hip, knee and ankle flexion indicates meningeal irritation. (**C**) Kernig's sign. The nurse flexes the child's hip and knee, forming a 90° angle. (**D**) Positive response. As the leg is extended, pain, resistance and spasm are noted, indicating meningeal irritation. (Photographs by John Gallagher.)

irritable because of headaches. They have sharp pain on bending their head forwards. They may have seizures. In some children, seizure or shock is the first noticeable sign of illness. As the disease progresses, signs of meningeal irritability occur, as evidenced by positive Brudzinski's sign and Kernig's sign (see Fig. 49.6). Children's backs may become arched and their necks hyperextended (opisthotonos). Cranial nerve paralysis, most typically of the third and sixth nerves, may occur, so that the child is not able to follow a light through full visual fields. If the fontanelles are open, they are bulging and tense; if they are closed, papilloedema may develop. If the meningitis is caused by H. influenzae, the child may develop septic arthritis. If it is caused by *N. meningitidis*, a papular or purple petechial skin rash may occur (Pace & Pollard, 2012).

In the newborn, symptoms such as poor sucking, weak cry or lethargy are often vague. After this generalised beginning, sudden cardiovascular shock, seizures, nuchal rigidity or apnoea may occur. Because the infant has open fontanelles, nuchal rigidity appears late and is not as useful a sign for diagnosis as in the older child.

Meningitis is diagnosed by history and analysis of CSF obtained by lumbar puncture. A child with a febrile seizure should be assumed to have meningitis until CSF findings prove otherwise. CSF results indicative of meningitis include increased white blood cell and protein levels and a lowered glucose level (because bacteria have fed on the glucose). In a healthy child, the glucose level in the CSF is 60% of that of the serum glucose. Because meningitis often spreads and causes septicaemia, a blood culture also is done.

Antibiotic therapy as indicated by sensitivity studies is the primary treatment measure. Usually antibiotics are given IV for rapid effect, but intrathecal injections (directly into the CSF) may be necessary to reduce the infection because the blood–brain barrier may prevent an antibiotic from passing freely into the CSF. If the organism is identified as *H. influenzae*, ampicillin usually is the medication of choice. In other instances, a third-generation cephalosporin, such as cefotaxime (Claforan) or ceftriaxone (Rocephin), may be used for 8–10 days. In some children, it takes a month before the CSF cell count returns to normal. A corticosteroid such as dexamethasone or the osmotic diuretic, mannitol, may be administered to reduce ICP and help prevent hearing loss.

In addition to standard precautions, children with meningitis are placed on respiratory precautions for 24 hours after the start of antibiotic therapy to prevent transmission of the infection. Antibiotics also may be prescribed prophylactically for the immediate family members of the ill child or for others who have been in close contact with the child.

Meningitis is always a serious disorder, because it can run a rapid, fulminating and possibly fatal course. However, if symptoms are recognised early and treatment is effective, a child will recover with no sequelae. Neurological sequelae, such as learning problems, seizures, hearing and cognitive challenges, and inability to concentrate urine from poor antidiuretic hormone secretion, must be assessed after the infection because these can be long-term consequences.

Group B streptococcal infection

A major cause of meningitis in newborns is group B *Streptococcus*. The organism is contracted either in utero or from secretions in the birth canal. It can spread to other newborns if good hand washing technique is not used. Colonisation can result in either early-onset or late-onset illness. With the early-onset form, symptoms of pneumonia become apparent in the first few hours of life. The late-onset type leads to meningitis instead of pneumonia.

At approximately 2 weeks of age, the infant gradually becomes lethargic and develops a fever and upper respiratory tract symptoms. The fontanelles bulge from increased ICP. The disease is extremely serious as mortality from the infection is approximately 25%; surviving infants may develop neurological consequences such as hydrocephalus or seizures (Libster et al., 2012). Treatment is with antibiotics, such as ampicillin and cephalosporins, which are effective against group B streptococcal infections. It can be difficult for parents to understand how their infant suddenly became so ill. They may need considerable support in caring for the infant if the infant is left neurologically challenged.

CASE STUDY QUESTION

3. Harrison is diagnosed as having bacterial meningitis. How long should he be placed on respiratory precautions for this condition after beginning an antibiotic?

   a. 4 hours
   b. 24 hours
   c. 10 days
   d. 30 days

Encephalitis

Encephalitis is an inflammation of brain tissue and, possibly, the meninges as well (Kneen et al., 2012). It can arise from protozoan, bacterial, fungal or viral invasion. Enteroviruses are the most frequent cause, followed by arboviruses such as the togavirus. Several encephalitis viruses, such as those that cause St Louis encephalitis, West Nile encephalitis and Eastern equine encephalitis, are borne by mosquitoes and are seen most often during the summer months. In endemic areas, mosquito repellents are strongly suggested. Encephalitis also can result from direct invasion of the CSF during lumbar puncture. It may occur as a complication of common childhood diseases, such as measles, mumps or chickenpox. Therefore, it is crucial that children receive immunisation against these diseases.

Symptoms of encephalitis begin gradually or suddenly. Symptoms include headache, high temperature, and if meninges are also involved, signs of meningeal irritation, such as nuchal rigidity (positive Brudzinski's sign and Kernig's sign). Symptoms of ataxia, muscle weakness or paralysis, diplopia, confusion or irritability also may occur. A child becomes increasingly lethargic and eventually comatose.

Treatment for a child with encephalitis is primarily supportive. An antipyretic is given to control fever. Take and record vital signs frequently because brainstem involvement can affect cardiac or respiratory rates. An antiviral agent, such as acyclovir (Zovirax), is usually prescribed. Anticonvulsants, such as carbamazepine (Tegretol), phenobarbitone or phenytoin (Dilantin), may be prescribed for seizures. A steroid such as dexamethasone or an osmotic diuretic such as mannitol may be prescribed to decrease brain oedema and ICP.

Encephalitis is always a serious diagnosis because, although a child may recover from the initial attack without further symptoms, there may be residual neurological damage, such as seizures or learning disabilities. Parents may find it hard to believe that their child is so seriously ill at first because in the beginning of the illness, their child only seemed tired and had a slight headache. They can find it even harder to accept a diagnosis of permanent impairment, such as a learning disability. Follow-up care after hospitalisation is important for the child's rehabilitation and to help parents deal with their grief, shock and possible anger.

Reye's syndrome

Reye's syndrome is acute encephalopathy with accompanying fatty infiltration of the liver, heart, lungs, pancreas and skeletal muscle. It occurs in children from 1 to 18 years of age regardless of gender (Stone, 2011). The cause is unknown, but it usually occurs after a viral infection such as varicella (chickenpox) or influenza that was treated with a salicylate such as acetylsalicylic acid (aspirin). Anticipatory guidance to parents and children about avoiding the use of aspirin during viral infections has led to almost total prevention of this syndrome (Bennett et al., 2012).

After seeming to recover from an initial viral illness, children become ill again 1 to 3 weeks later, with lethargy, vomiting, agitation, anorexia, confusion and combativeness. Symptoms in adolescents may be so extreme that they mimic those of drug intoxication. As fatty droplets invade the liver, enzyme abnormalities, hypothrombinaemia, hypoglycaemia and elevated blood ammonia levels occur. Although CSF findings except for a slightly elevated opening pressure remain normal, cerebral symptoms progress from confusion to stupor to deep coma, with seizures and respiratory arrest resulting from pressure on the brainstem.

Left untreated, Reye's syndrome is rapidly fatal. If it is diagnosed early and promptly treated, however, the child usually recovers quickly and without any residual neurological effects. Reye's syndrome is not infectious. It is categorised by stages of involvement from 1 to 5, depending on the degree of the child's lethargy or coma. In stages 1 and 2, the child responds to stimuli but may exhibit lethargy or delirium and possibly combativeness. In stages 3 through 5, a child is unresponsive to stimuli with a progressively deepening coma. Frequent neurological assessments are necessary to evaluate the child's status and possible progression to a more serious stage of involvement. Therapy is directed towards supporting respiratory function, controlling hypoglycaemia and reducing brain oedema.

Guillain-Barré syndrome

Guillain-Barré syndrome (inflammatory polyradiculoneuropathy) is a perplexing syndrome that occurs in about 1 in every 100,000 children. Both motor and sensory portions of peripheral nerves are affected. Boys develop it more often than girls (Yuki & Hartung, 2012). With successful widespread polio eradication efforts, Guillain-Barré syndrome is now the most common cause of acute and subacute flaccid paralysis in childhood (Rosen, 2012). The cause of the condition is unknown, but it is suspected that the reaction is immune mediated, occurring after upper respiratory tract or gastrointestinal illnesses or immunisations. Inflammation of the nerve fibres apparently causes temporary demyelinisation of the nerve sheaths.

Children experience peripheral neuritis several days after the primary infection. Tendon reflexes begin to decrease and then become absent. Muscle paralysis and paraesthesia (loss of sensation) begin first in the legs and then spread to involve the arms, trunk and head. The symmetrical nature of the disorder helps to differentiate it from other types of paraplegia. Cranial nerve involvement leads to facial weakness and difficulty in swallowing. As the respiratory muscles become involved, spontaneous respirations are no longer possible. This can lead to respiratory involvement severe enough to warrant mechanical ventilation.

Treatment of Guillain-Barré syndrome is supportive until the process runs its course; paralysis peaks at 3 weeks and is followed by gradual recovery. A course of prednisone to halt the autoimmune response may be tried, but its use is controversial. Plasmapheresis or transfusion of immune serum globulin may shorten the course of the illness.

Care of a child with Guillain-Barré syndrome includes preventing all of the effects of extreme immobility while guarding respiratory function. Cardiac and respiratory function must be closely monitored. An indwelling urinary catheter is usually inserted to monitor urine output. Enteral or total parenteral nutrition may be used to support protein and carbohydrate needs. If the child has discomfort from neuritis, adequate analgesia should be administered.

To prevent muscle contractures and effects of immobility, the child needs passive range-of-motion exercises every 4 hours. Turning and repositioning every 2 hours also is important to protect skin integrity. Providing adequate stimulation for the long weeks when the child is unable to perform any care independently is also important. Fortunately, most children recover completely, without any residual effects of the syndrome, although they may continue to have minor problems such as residual weakness.

INFLAMMATORY DISORDERS

Carpal tunnel syndrome and facial palsy are two inflammatory disorders found frequently in adolescents.

Carpal tunnel syndrome

Carpal tunnel syndrome is nerve compression of the median nerve that passes through the carpal tunnel at the wrist (Luckhaupt et al., 2013). Compression of the nerve causes numbness and sharp pain and burning in the thumb and the second, third and fourth fingers of the hand. Pain usually occurs at night and is enough to keep a child awake. It occurs more frequently in children who have a rheumatoid process such as arthritis. The usual therapy is application of a splint to the wrist, which holds the wrist in a neutral (neither flexed nor extended) position. An oral anti-inflammatory medication and perhaps a corticosteroid injection into the inflamed wrist both help to relieve pain. If these therapies are not successful, the stricture at the carpal canal can be relieved surgically. Although carpal tunnel syndrome is still rare in children, it is increasing in incidence as more and more teenagers spend hours in repetitive motion while they play electronic games, do word processing or send text messages.

Facial palsy (Bell's palsy)

Facial palsy is facial paralysis of the seventh (facial) cranial nerve, the nerve that innervates the muscles of facial expression. The syndrome occurs abruptly, usually after a herpes or Lyme disease infection. It may occur as a result of cold air from skiing or from riding in a convertible. Therapy consists of prednisone to reduce inflammation and acyclovir if the syndrome is herpes related. If the child is unable to close the eye on the affected side, eye drops 3 or 4 times daily will be needed. Although recovery is slow, usually not until 4 months, most children recover without any permanent disability (McNamara et al., 2013).

PAROXYSMAL DISORDERS

A paroxysmal disorder is one that occurs suddenly and recurrently. Seizures, headaches and breath-holding spells are the most frequent types seen in childhood.

Recurrent seizures

A seizure is an involuntary contraction of muscle caused by abnormal electrical brain discharges. Approximately 5% of children will have at least one seizure by the time they reach adulthood (Baldin et al., 2012). These episodes are always frightening to parents and other children because of the intensity. Although seizures can be idiopathic (without cause), they also can be attributed to infection, trauma or tumour growth. Familiar or polygenic inheritance may be responsible. Fifty percent of seizures are unexplained. Because they are not so much a disease as a symptom of an underlying disorder, all seizures need to be investigated carefully. The degree of understanding about the cause of disorders such as recurrent seizures varies in different cultures. Because the cause of recurrent seizures is often idiopathic, they have, in the past, been attributed to an invasion by evil spirits. Many people today still fear that recurrent seizures will lead to cognitive impairment. Being aware of these common misconceptions can help you appreciate parents' anxiety about the diagnosis of recurrent seizures. This anxiety can accentuate the need for parent education and careful planning to maintain self-esteem in the child (see Box 49.3).

The term *epilepsy* comes from a Greek word meaning "to take hold of". The preferred term now is recurrent seizures, because epilepsy carries the stigma of cognitive challenge, behavioural disorders, institutionalisation or inexplicable strangeness.

The types and causes of seizures vary with age. They are classified into two major categories: partial seizures and generalised seizures (see Box 49.4). With partial seizures, only one area of the brain is involved; with generalised seizures, the disturbance involves the entire brain and loss of consciousness usually occurs. It is important that seizures be differentiated by their degree of severity and type, so that appropriate management and medication can be instituted.

BOX 49.3 ✻ Focus on evidence-based practice

SEISMIC: Sydney Epilepsy Incidence Study To Measure Illness Consequences

Epilepsy Action Australia and The George Institute for International Health are undertaking a major epidemiological research project to measure the impact and incidence of epilepsy. Epilepsy is one of the most common serious neurological disorders in Australia and around the world. An estimated 140,000 people in Australia have epilepsy, which, given the early age of onset in many and the lifelong nature of the condition in most, makes epilepsy a major cause (~1%) of days lost due to ill-health globally.

This large-scale, inter-disciplinary project is the first population-based study of the incidence and outcome of epilepsy to be conducted in Australia. Although many of the consequences of the diagnosis on some elements of psychosocial functioning in adults and children are reasonably well characterised, potentially modifiable determinants are far less understood. Clinical factors such as seizure severity and frequency play some role in determining these consequences; however, the interaction and effects of vulnerability (e.g. psychological disorder) and resilience (e.g. mastery and family support) are only now receiving research and policy attention. The study has a two-stage consent process: participants will be enrolled over 24 months and they or their carer/proxy/guardian will be interviewed at three time points following the diagnosis of their epilepsy: within 28 days (baseline), 4 and 12 months (Epilepsy Action Australia Fact Sheet 2012). The study aims to identify modifiable factors that enhance resilience and reduce vulnerability to the socioeconomic impact of epilepsy.

How might the results of this study help you to educate the parents of children with epilepsy?

More information about this research can be found at Epilepsy Action Australia <www.epilepsy.org.au/research/seismic>.

BOX 49.4 ✻ Classification of seizures

Partial (focal) seizures

- Simple partial seizures (no altered level of consciousness)
- Simple partial seizures with motor signs (includes aversive, Rolandic and Jacksonian march)
- Simple partial seizures with sensory signs
- Complex partial (psychomotor) seizures (some impairment or alteration in level of consciousness)

Generalised seizures

- Tonic–clonic seizures (formerly grand mal)
- Tonic
- Clonic
- Absence seizures (formerly petit mal)
- Atonic seizures (formerly "drop attacks")
- Myoclonic seizures
- Infantile spasms

Seizures in the newborn period

Seizure activity in the newborn period may be difficult to recognise because it may consist only of: twitching of the head, arms or eyes; slight cyanosis; and perhaps respiratory difficulty or apnoea. Afterward, the infant may appear limp and flaccid. Whereas older children often have seizures of unknown cause, 75% of seizures in neonates have a known cause. Some of these possible causes are:

- Trauma and anoxia (head trauma involved with the birth process, tight maternal cervix, use of forceps or placenta praevia)
- Metabolic disorders, such as hypoglycaemia; infants of diabetic mothers; hypocalcaemia; and lack of pyridoxine (vitamin B_6)

- Neonatal infection (CNS infection or prolonged rupture of membranes before birth)
- Kernicterus.

High doses of anticonvulsant medication may be needed to control seizures in newborns because they metabolise more rapidly than older infants. For healthcare guidelines on acute management of newborns with recurrent seizures, including medication used in acute seizures, see the relevant NSW Department of Health policy <www.health.nsw.gov.au/policies/pd/2013/pdf/PD2013_049.pdf>.

Seizures in the infant and toddler periods

Seizures commonly seen in this age group are **infantile spasms**, a form of generalised seizure ("salaam" or "jack-knife"), or infantile myoclonic seizures. These are characterised by very rapid movements of the trunk with sudden strong contractions of most of the body, including flexion and adduction of the limbs. The infant suddenly slumps forwards from a sitting position or falls from a standing position. These episodes may occur singly or in clusters as frequently as 100 times a day.

In approximately 50% of children affected, there is an identifiable cause such as trauma, a metabolic disease such as phenylketonuria, or a viral invasion such as herpes or cytomegalovirus. In other children, the cause is unknown, but the spasms apparently result from a failure of normal organised electrical activity in the brain. Approximately 90% of infants with this type of involvement will be developmentally delayed as intellectual development appears to halt and even regress after the pattern of seizures begins. Most children with infantile spasms show high-amplitude slow waves and spikes, a chaotic discharge called *hypsarrhythmia*, on an EEG tracing.

The response to treatment with anticonvulsant therapy is poor. Parenteral adrenocorticotropic hormone (ACTH) and pyridoxine (vitamin B6) therapy is commonly used. High-dose sodium valproate (Epilim) or a newer anticonvulsant agent such as topiramate (Topamax) may be used in children who do not respond to usual therapy. The infantile seizure phenomenon seems to "burn itself out" by 2 years of age. The associated cognitive or developmental delay remains, however, so children need good follow-up planning and care.

Seizures caused by poisoning or medications

The possibility of poisoning must be considered in any child who has a first seizure. Although poisoning is most likely to occur between 6 months and 3 years of age, it must be considered again in adolescence, when medications may be intentionally self-administered. Seizures also can be a late symptom of encephalopathy caused by lead poisoning (see Chapter 52).

Seizures in children older than 3 years of age

Febrile seizures

Seizures associated with high fever of 38.9°C to 40.0°C are the most common type seen in preschool children (5 months to 5 years), although these can occur as early as 3 months or as late as 7 years of age. Febrile seizures may occur after immunisation because of an accompanying fever. Seizures show an active tonic–clonic pattern, which lasts for 15–20 seconds. The EEG tracing usually is normal. There is often a history of other family members having had similar seizures.

Febrile seizures usually occur due to a sudden spike of temperature. The seizure only lasts 1–2 minutes or less. Such seizures must be taken seriously, however, and investigated for a possible cause, because meningitis often manifests initially with high fever and a seizure (Middleton, 2011).

Prevention of febrile seizures

Because these seizures arise with high fever, they are largely preventable. If paracetamol is given to keep a developing fever below 38.4°C, seizures rarely occur. They happen most often when a child develops a fever at night, when a parent is not aware of it, or when a parent is reluctant to give acetaminophen in large enough doses to be therapeutic. Although this type of seizure can be prevented by phenobarbitone, prophylactic use during an upper respiratory tract infection is not recommended, because phenobarbitone takes 2 or 3 days to reach therapeutic blood levels. By this time, the seizures would already have occurred. In addition, phenobarbitone is associated with sleepiness, which possibly reduces cognitive function in children. If a second febrile seizure occurs, diazepam (Valium) or Midazolam may be prescribed for the parents to administer the next time the child has a high fever.

What if...

Harrison's mother is worried that Harrison will have another febrile convulsion if he develops a cold in the future? She asks if it will be safe to send Harrison to day care. How would you respond to this parent?

Complex partial (psychomotor) seizures

More than half the children who develop recurrent seizures during school age have an idiopathic type. Nevertheless, medication can control idiopathic seizures in almost all affected children. Other seizures in this age group occur because of organic causes, usually from focal or diffuse brain injury that has left residual damage. The injury may have been caused by laceration of brain tissue in a motor vehicle accident or fall, haemorrhage due to a blood dyscrasia, infection (meningitis or encephalitis), anoxia, or toxic conditions such as lead poisoning. The possibility that a growing brain tumour is causing brain irritation must also be considered.

This type of seizure may begin with a sudden change in posture, such as an arm dropping suddenly to the side. Other motor, sensory and behavioural signs may include

automatisms (complex purposeless movements, such as lip smacking or fumbling hand movements). The child then slumps to the ground, unconscious. Circumoral pallor may develop due to a halt in respirations. The child usually regains consciousness in less than 5 minutes. He or she may feel slightly drowsy afterwards but does not have an actual postictal stage as in tonic–clonic seizures.

Common medications used to treat this type of seizure include carbamazepine, sodium valproate, phenytoin and phenobarbitone. Carbamazepine can lead to neutropenia, so white blood cell counts need to be monitored during therapy. If these medications are not effective, surgery to remove the epileptogenic focus or the implantation of a vagus nerve stimulator can significantly reduce seizure frequency.

Partial (focal) seizures

Partial seizures originate from a specific brain area. A typical partial seizure with motor signs begins in the fingers and spreads to the wrist, arm and face in a clonic contraction. If the movement remains localised, there will be no loss of consciousness. If the spread is extensive, the seizure becomes generalised and then is impossible to differentiate from a tonic–clonic seizure. Therefore, it is important to observe children carefully when a seizure begins to distinguish this type. A partial seizure with sensory signs may include numbness, tingling, paraesthesia or pain originating in one area and spreading to other parts of the body. These types of seizures may be caused by a rapidly growing brain tumour. Documenting the spread can help localise the spot in the brain that first initiated the abnormal electrical discharge.

Absence seizures

Absence seizures, formerly known as petit mal seizures, are classified as generalised seizures (Tatum, Ho & Benbadis, 2010). They usually consist of a staring spell that lasts for a few seconds. A child might be reciting in class when she pauses and stares for 1 to 5 seconds before continuing the recitation; she is unaware that time has passed. Rhythmic blinking and twitching of the mouth or an extremity may accompany the staring. Absence seizures can occur up to 100 times per day. An EEG usually shows a typical 3-Hz wave and slow-wave discharge (Mariani, Rossi & Vojani, 2011). Such seizures tend to occur more frequently in girls than in boys. The usual age of occurrence is 6 to 7 years.

Children with absence episodes may be accused of daydreaming at school and may be referred to the school nurse for behavioural problems. These children usually have normal intelligence; however, if they have frequent episodes, they may be doing poorly at school because they are missing instructional content.

If seizures are fully controlled by medication, children can participate in normal school activities and ride a bicycle or scooter. If seizures cannot be controlled fully, parents need to anticipate potentially hazardous situations during the child's day, such as crossing a busy street on the way to school or learning to drive. This is crucial for adolescents who are eager to get a driver's licence.

Approximately one-third to one-half of all children with absence seizures "outgrow" them by adulthood. This does not mean that treatment is not necessary during childhood, however, in order to keep the child safe and maintain self-esteem. Absence seizures usually occur independently of tonic–clonic seizures, although it is possible for a child to manifest both types. Some children's seizure pattern changes from absence involvement to tonic–clonic involvement as they approach adulthood.

Tonic–clonic seizures

Typical tonic–clonic seizures (formerly termed grand mal seizures) are generalised seizures consisting of four stages. There may be a prodromal period of hours or days; an aura, or warning, immediately before the seizure; the tonic–clonic stage; and, finally, a postictal stage. Not all four stages occur with every seizure.

The prodromal period may consist of drowsiness, dizziness, malaise, lack of coordination or tension. Parents may observe simply that their child is acting differently. As a child reaches school age, the child may be able to predict from these vague preliminary feelings when a seizure is about to occur.

The aura, or second phase, may reflect the portion of the brain in which the seizure originates. Smelling unpleasant odours (often reported as faeces) denotes activity in the medial portion of the temporal lobe. Seeing flashing lights suggests the occipital area; repeated hallucinations arise from the temporal lobe; numbness of an extremity relates to the opposite parietal lobe; and a "Cheshire-cat grin" relates to the frontal lobe. Young children, unable to describe or understand an aura, may scream in fright or run to their parent with its onset. Noting exactly what symptoms the child experiences during this time helps to localise the involved brain portion.

The third phase is the tonic stage. All muscles of the body contract and the child falls to the ground. Extremities stiffen and the face distorts. Although this phase lasts only about 20 seconds, the respiratory muscles are contracted, so the child may experience hypoxia and turn cyanotic. Contraction of the throat prevents swallowing, so saliva collects in the mouth. The child may bite the tongue when the jaws contract. As the chest muscles contract initially, air is pushed through the glottis, producing a guttural cry.

The seizure then enters a clonic stage in which muscles of the body rapidly contract and relax, producing quick, jerky motions. The child may blow bubbles or foamy saliva and, if the tongue was bitten when the jaw shut with a spasm, saliva will be bloody. A child will be incontinent of stool and urine. This phase usually lasts 20 to 30 seconds.

After the tonic–clonic period, the child falls into a sound sleep, called the postictal period. He will sleep soundly for 1 to 4 hours and will rouse only to painful stimuli during this time. When he awakens, he often experiences a severe headache. He has no memory of the seizure.

Seizures may occur only at night. The child wakes in the morning with a bitten tongue, blood on the pillow or a bed wet with urine. In a child with persistent bedwetting, the possibility of nocturnal seizures must be considered.

Therapy includes the daily administration of an anticonvulsant such as sodium valproate (Epilim) and carbamazepine (Tegretol). Phenobarbitone has the advantage of being an inexpensive anticonvulsant and so may be prescribed as well, however, drowsiness and sleepiness from this may interfere with a child's ability to perform in school. Phenobarbitone dosages should be tapered, never stopped suddenly, because the body becomes dependent on it. Rapid withdrawal may precipitate a seizure.

Children with tonic–clonic seizures also may be given phenytoin sodium (Dilantin) for control. One non-toxic side effect of phenytoin is painless hypertrophy of the gums. Unless the gum hypertrophy is extensive, it is not sufficient reason to discontinue. Medications are usually continued until the child has been seizure free for 2 to 3 years.

Some children are prescribed a ketogenic diet. This diet is high in fat and low in protein and carbohydrate. It causes the child to have a high level of ketones, which is believed to decrease myoclonic or tonic–clonic seizure activity. Because the diet is monotonous for children and difficult for parents to prepare, however, it may be hard for children to continue this for a long time (Kossoff et al., 2010).

Status epilepticus

Status epilepticus refers to a seizure that lasts continuously for longer than 30 minutes or a series of seizures from which the child does not return to the previous level of consciousness (Dobrin, 2015; Singh, et al., 2010). This is an emergency situation requiring immediate treatment, otherwise exhaustion, respiratory failure, permanent brain injury or death may occur. Oxygen may be necessary to relieve cyanosis. An IV benzodiazepine such as diazepam (Valium) or Midazolam (IV or bucccal) halts seizures dramatically. This may be followed by IV phenobarbitone or phenytoin (Dilantin). Diazepam must be administered with extreme caution because the medication is incompatible with many others and any accidental infiltration into subcutaneous tissue causes extensive tissue sloughing. Parents may administer diazepam by enema at home.

Assessment of the child with seizures

A thorough pregnancy history must be obtained for any child with seizures. Events that occurred immediately before the seizure and an accurate description of the seizure itself also should be recorded. Investigate the child's overall behaviour in the last few weeks. Is the child an A student who has been getting Ds lately? Has the parent noticed bedwetting? These might be signs of absence or nocturnal seizures that have occurred but gone unnoticed.

A complete physical and neurological examination and blood tests are necessary to rule out metabolic or infectious processes. Prepare a child for a lumbar puncture to rule out meningitis or bleeding into the CSF. A CT scan, MRI, skull x-ray or EEG may be obtained if indicated. During the EEG, the child may be stimulated with rhythm patterns or flashing lights or asked to hyperventilate to see whether a seizure can be provoked.

Nursing considerations

Protecting the child

Protecting a child from being hurt during a tonic–clonic seizure is crucial. Restraining the child's thrashing extremities is not advisable because it is difficult for an adult to do and could result in injury to the parent or child because of the amount of force needed to keep the child still. In early school-aged children, it is particularly important to avoid inserting a tongue blade between the teeth because these children often have loose anterior teeth that are on the verge of falling out. Such teeth could be loosened and aspirated.

Remaining calm is important; be aware that people are frightened by the sight of a child having a seizure because the action is so forceful and violent. It is reassuring for them to see someone calm and in control of the situation and to know that there is no reason to be afraid. If the child passes rapidly from one seizure into another (status epilepticus), be prepared to provide supplemental oxygen and administer anticonvulsant therapy as needed.

Long-term considerations

As soon as the diagnosis of a seizure disorder is made, parents and children need to be told that it is likely to signify a long-term disorder as, although seizures can be controlled with medication, these do not cure the underlying cause. If children neglect their medication, seizures are apt to recur. Most children are given tablets rather than liquid medication, because the latter tends to settle at the bottom of the bottle, resulting in over-diluted or over-concentrated doses that can allow seizures to break through. Parents need instruction to plan on always having an adequate supply of medications, especially for a trip away from home or for activities like school camp. Abrupt discontinuation of seizure medications (particularly phenobarbitone) may result in severe seizures.

The child needs to be monitored frequently during childhood to be certain that the medication dosage is adequate. Children need periodic blood sampling to ascertain whether therapeutic blood levels of the medication are being maintained. Provide parents with as much information as possible about the cause of their child's seizures. This helps them feel that they are dealing with a known disease, not an inexplicable and unpredictable illness. If the cause of the seizures is unknown, parents can be reassured that the treatment is known. Many new anticonvulsant medications are available today and are being introduced into therapy.

Therapeutic management

General guidelines for safe administration of anticonvulsants include:

- Cautioning children to be careful around motor vehicles and electrical equipment because many anticonvulsants cause drowsiness
- Advising the child and parents to observe for easy bruising because several anticonvulsants may suppress bone marrow function
- Cautioning the adolescent to avoid alcohol while taking anticonvulsants because alcohol can potentiate the CNS effects of some anticonvulsants
- Using caution when administering anticonvulsants to children with liver disease; because many of these medications are metabolised by the liver, they may not be fully effective in such children
- Cautioning the child and parents not to discontinue anticonvulsant therapy abruptly because this may lead to uncontrolled seizures
- Reminding parents about the need for follow-up blood tests to evaluate the medication level.

Maintaining a therapeutic blood level enhances the medication's effectiveness and minimises the risk of toxicity. Assure parents that occasional seizures in children are not harmful. Unless status epilepticus occurs and the child becomes anoxic, the chance that their child will be injured during a seizure is remote. Knowing this helps parents not to worry about the child becoming cognitively challenged or other misconceptions about seizures. Although some children who have seizures are cognitively challenged, this and the seizures were caused by the same event; the seizures did not cause the impairment. At every healthcare visit, be certain that parents have time to ask questions about their child's care and to express any concerns they have. There are so many myths about seizures that every parent is likely to believe some of these stories unless counselled otherwise.

In many children, seizures increase at puberty. This may be the result of glandular changes or sudden growth and the need for an increased medicine dosage. It may result in part from adolescent rebellion against following prescribed medication routines. Respect the adolescent's feelings and need for independence, but assist the adolescent with channelling feelings to a more positive area.

CASE STUDY QUESTION

4. Harrison had a generalised, or tonic–clonic, seizure. What is the usual description of this type of seizure?
   a. A momentary halt of about 10 seconds in respirations
   b. Stiffening of the extremities, then shaking of the body
   c. Extreme pain and twitching of one of the extremities
   d. Rapid blinking, then foaming of the mouth

Breath holding

Breath holding is a phenomenon that occurs in young children when they are stressed or angry. The child breathes in and, because of anger or stress, does not breathe out again or else breathes out and then does not inhale again. As brain cells become anoxic, the child becomes cyanotic and slumps to the floor, momentarily unconscious. With loss of consciousness, the child begins breathing again. The child's colour returns to normal and they awaken. Breath holding is frightening but represents the immaturity of the child's neurological control. This differs from a temper tantrum, in which a child deliberately attempts to hold their breath and pass out (see Chapter 30). The child needs no therapy except reassurance that the episode is over.

Headache

Headache in children younger than school age is rare, although children may report "headache" in imitation of their parents. Headache may occur with a fever because of increased ICP caused by increased cerebral blood flow. As children reach school age, headaches may occur as a result of conditions as simple as eyestrain and sinusitis or as serious as a brain tumour. Headache pain results from meningeal or vascular irritation. The brain itself is insensitive to pain, so a cerebral tumour can be present for a long time before meningeal irritation occurs and pain symptoms become apparent. With a brain tumour, pain becomes evident on changing body position, so a young child who reports a headache after getting up should be carefully evaluated. Pain from a brain tumour is also usually occipital, so asking the child to indicate where it hurts helps determine whether a tumour could be the cause.

Migraine headache

Migraine headache refers to a specific type of headache that may or may not begin with an aura or visual disturbance such as diplopia or a zigzag pattern across the visual field. The pain that follows is usually unilateral and extremely intense, with throbbing that is moderate to severe. The headache is aggravated by routine physical activity and menstrual periods, and may be compounded by nausea and vomiting and intolerance to bright lights and noise (Cleves-Bayon, 2014).

The cause of migraine headache in any age group is not well-understood. It probably results from abnormal constriction of intracranial arteries that temporarily reduces cerebral blood supply. This is followed by compensating over-distension of cranial blood vessels. The aura accompanying such headaches is the result of the temporary ischaemia, whereas the headache is the result of the over-distension. Some children who have migraine headaches have an abnormal EEG. Most children with migraine headaches have a positive family history. This syndrome may be inherited as a dominant trait.

ATAXIC DISORDERS

Ataxia is failure of muscular coordination or irregularity of muscle action. Ataxic disorders are often manifested by an awkward gait or lack of coordination. Causes of ataxia differ, but degeneration of cerebellar or vestibular function is always involved.

Ataxia-telangiectasia

Ataxia-telangiectasia, transmitted as an autosomal recessive trait attributable to a defect of chromosome 11, is a primary immunodeficiency disorder that results in progressive cerebellar degeneration. This is a multisystem disease with neurological and immunological aspects. In addition, endocrine abnormalities may occur and there is an increased risk of cancer, particularly brain tumour. Telangiectasia (red vascular markings) appear on the conjunctiva and skin at the flexor creases (Buckley, 2008). Both immunological and neurological symptoms of this disorder vary in severity and onset. Serum immunoglobulin A (IgA) and immunoglobulin E (IgE) levels may be low and there is often evidence of reduced T-cell function. Children develop frequent infections (primarily sinopulmonary) because of the immunological deficits. Tonsillar tissue in the pharynx is scant.

Neurological symptoms caused by the degeneration process can usually be detected in early infancy when developmental milestones are not met. Children develop an awkward gait when they begin to walk. **Choreoathetosis** (rapid, purposeless movements), nystagmus, an intention tremor or scoliosis may develop. Children may be unable to move their eyes on demand or follow movement through visual fields. Eye changes (conjunctival telangiectasia) develop by 5 years of age. There is no effective treatment. Children with this disorder often die in late adolescence of infection, respiratory failure or a malignant brain tumour.

SPINAL CORD INJURY

Because of the resilience of their vertebrae, children have fewer spinal cord injuries than adults. However, the incidence among adolescents is increasing because more adolescents are involved in motor vehicle accidents, particularly motorcycle accidents, than previously (Martin-Herz, Zatzick & McMahon, 2012). Another frequent cause of spinal cord injury is diving into too-shallow water. Any child with multiple traumatic injuries should be assessed for spinal cord damage. Spinal cord injury without radiographic abnormality (SCIWRA syndrome) may occur. Stabilising the neck is the best protection against further injury in these children (Hazinski, 2012).

Recovery phases

Spinal injuries result when the spinal cord becomes compressed or severed by the vertebrae; further cord damage can be caused by haemorrhage, oedema or inflammation at the injury site as the blood supply becomes impeded. Table 49.4 summarises functional ability after spinal cord injury. The first questions commonly asked after the injury are: "How much damage is there?" and "Will our child be able to walk again?" Predictions of useful body function

TABLE 49.4 Functional ability after spinal cord injury

Injury site	Highest key functions still present	Effects and possible interventions
C1–3	Head and neck muscles intact	Respiratory paralysis from loss of phrenic nerve innervation; will need ventilatory assistance No voluntary motion below chin; possibly able to learn to use mouth to control pen for writing and mouthstick to reach objects
C4	Diaphragm intact	Loss of motor function of upper and lower extremities and trunk; able to learn to use abdominal muscles to breathe independently
C5	Shoulder control; biceps, deltoid function	Able to feed self and operate wheelchair if fitted with self-care aids
C6	Forearm pronation; wrist extension	Use of upper extremities for self-care. Can transfer to wheelchair and so have increased independence
C7	Triceps function	Able to transfer to wheelchair readily; increasing independence
C8	Thumb and finger function	Able to do fine motor tasks; increases self-care ability
T1–7	Intercostal muscles (able to breathe with chest, not abdominal, muscles)	Full use of upper extremities but is still dependent on wheelchair Possibly able to drive car with hand controls Possibly able to have high leg braces fitted for standing
T10–12	Abdominal muscles	Use of long leg braces and four-point crutch to ambulate
L2–4	Hip flexion Leg extension	Use of long or short leg braces to ambulate
L5–S1	Gluteus maximus muscle function	Walking without aids
S4	Bladder and anal sphincter control	Controlling bladder and bowel function Penile erection and ejaculation possible

cannot be made at the time of the accident, however, as three phases of recovery must first take place.

First recovery phase

Immediately after the injury, the child experiences spinal shock syndrome or loss of autonomic nervous system function (loss of anterior nerve fibres travelling through the anterior horn of the spinal canal). This leads to loss of motor function, sensation and reflex activity, as well as flaccid paralysis in body areas below the level of the injury. If a cervical injury is present, there is loss of respiratory function because of flaccidity of the diaphragm. In high thoracic lesions, use of accessory muscles of the chest is lost, so the child has difficulty maintaining effective respirations. The child has no ability to sweat or shiver to change body temperature below the level of the lesion because of loss of autonomic nerve control; therefore, hypothermia or hyperthermia becomes a threat. Blood vessels below the level of the injury are no longer able to constrict, so blood tends to pool in the lower body, leading to hypotension, especially if the upper body is elevated. Loss of bladder control occurs (when flaccid, the bladder over distends and continually empties). The bowel becomes equally distended and bowel sounds are absent. This phase of spinal cord injury lasts from 1 to 6 weeks. As a rule, the shorter the phase of spinal shock, the better the final outcome.

Second recovery phase

During the second phase of recovery, the flaccid paralysis of the shock phase is replaced by spastic paralysis. Normally, motor impulses begin in the brain cortex and are transmitted to the medulla, where they cross to the opposite side of the cord; they then travel down the descending motor tracts of the spinal cord. They synapse in the anterior horn of the spinal cord and travel by way of the spinal and peripheral nerves to the designated muscle group, which they set in motion. The nerve pathways of the brain and the descending tracts are termed *upper motor neurons*. Those in the anterior horn cells and the spinal and peripheral nerves are termed *lower motor neurons*. Whether a motor neuron has upper or lower function, therefore, does not depend on its height in the spinal tract but rather on its position in relation to an anterior horn: between the brain and the anterior horn, it is an upper motor neuron; between the anterior horn and the point of innervation, it is a lower motor neuron.

Spasticity in the second phase is caused by the loss of upper level control or transmission of meaningful innervation to the lower muscles. Lacking upper motor neuron function because of a severed cord, the lower motor neurons or reflex arcs cause the muscles to contract and remain that way. Parents and children are quick to interpret the sudden spastic movement of a lower extremity as meaningful activity. This is particularly easy to believe with an infant who cannot tell you that he has no control over his leg movement. Differences between upper and lower neuron damage are listed in Table 49.5. If the injury is very low in the spinal tract, affecting mostly lower motor neurons, the muscles will remain flaccid because the lower motor neurons cannot send impulses for contraction.

During this phase, if the child's bladder is allowed to fill, the resultant sensory stimulation relayed to the damaged cord will initiate a powerful sympathetic reflex reaction **(autonomic dysreflexia)** and the child will show signs of hypertension, tachycardia, flushed face and severe occipital headache. This is an emergency situation; if the severe hypertension is not relieved, cerebral vascular accident can result (Pellatt, 2010). Assess that the child's urinary catheter is not obstructed, so urine can flow freely and reduce the sensory stimulation.

Third recovery phase

The third phase of recovery from spinal cord injury is the final outcome, or permanent limitation of motor and sensory function. If the compression of the spinal cord is caused by oedema that is then relieved, no permanent motor and sensory disability will occur.

> ***What if...***
>
> You are caring for a child with a spinal cord injury and he suddenly develops hypertension, tachycardia, diaphoresis and headache? What would you initially assess for? How would you intervene?

TABLE 49.5 Characteristics of upper and lower motor nerve lesions after spinal shock phase

Finding	Upper motor lesion	Lower motor lesion
Spasticity	Present	Absent (flaccidity present)
Clonus	Present, increased	Absent
Tendon reflexes	Increased	Absent
Babinski reflexes	Present	Absent
Reflexes below level of lesion	Present	Absent
Reflex at level of lesion	Absent	Absent
Atrophy of muscles	Absent or present only to slight degree	Present (muscle fasciculations may be present)

Assessment of spinal cord injury

Cervical and thoracolumbar areas of the spine are the ones most likely to sustain injury. Spinal cord injury should be suspected whenever a child has sustained a forceful trauma of any kind. The signs of spinal cord injury vary according to the level of the injury.

Do not move a child with suspected spinal cord injury until the back and head can be supported in a straight line to prevent further injury to the spinal column from twisting or bending. In the emergency department, do not attempt to move the child from a stretcher to an examining table until spinal x-ray films have been obtained. This reduces any unnecessary movement. When moving the child onto the x-ray table, use a gentle log-rolling technique to avoid additional injury. If resuscitation is necessary, maintain the head in a neutral position; do not hyperextend it. To keep the neck immobilised, do not remove a child's sports helmet or neck brace.

The child will need a thorough neurological assessment to determine the level of injury. Help maintain spinal immobilisation during such procedures.

Nursing considerations

During the first phase of recovery, a child's major problems are those resulting from almost complete immobility: pressure ulcers on bony prominences; loss of appetite and subsequent poor nutrition from depression or being in the supine position; urinary calculi caused by excessive calcium loss from bones; atrophy of flaccid muscle groups; and urinary retention and bladder infection.

Impaired physical mobility related to effects of spinal cord injury

To relieve oedema at the injury site and prevent further injury, IV corticosteroids will be administered. Children may be placed in cervical traction with Crutchfield tongs and a traction belt (see Fig. 49.7) or with halo traction (see Chapter 51). Having tongs inserted into the skull is a very frightening procedure for children. They worry that the tongs will burrow into their skull and strike their brain.

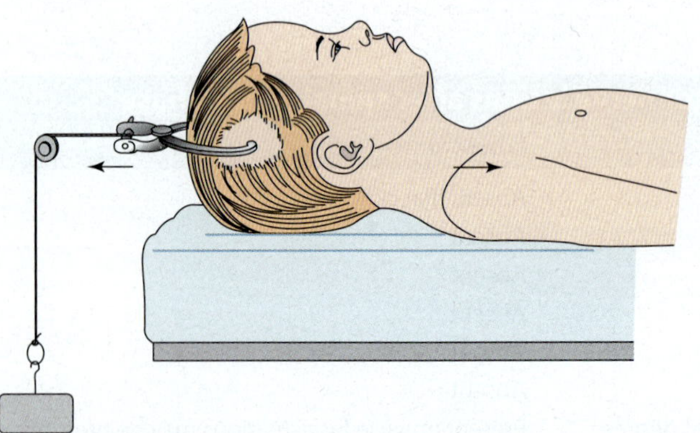

FIGURE 49.7 Crutchfield tongs used to create spinal traction.

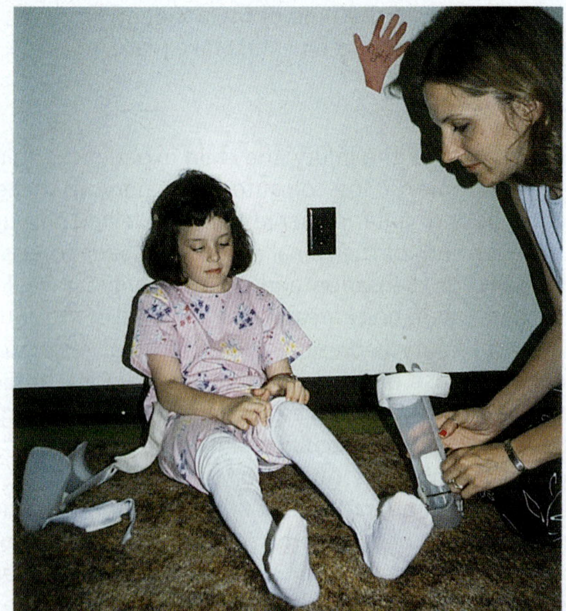

FIGURE 49.8 Specialised splints are used for a child with a low spinal cord injury to prevent contractures and foot drop. Here the physiotherapist prepares to apply the splint to the child's leg. (Photograph courtesy of Sue Moses.)

Children need someone they know and trust to help them lie still during the procedure.

To promote circulation and prevent loss of calcium that results from inactivity, full range-of-motion exercises must be done approximately three times per day. These are time-consuming but important in maintaining joint function.

During the second phase of recovery, when spasticity of muscle groups occurs, preventing contractures becomes an important nursing responsibility. Specialised splints, boots or even high-top sneakers may be used to prevent footdrop (see Fig. 49.8). If children have upper extremity mobility but will be left with lower extremity paralysis, exercises to strengthen the upper extremity muscle groups are needed. Strengthening the arms helps children to be able to lift themselves from bed to a wheelchair or raise themselves with a trapeze over the bed when changing positions. Holding legs and arms at the joints while moving them helps reduce muscle spasms.

One major problem of ambulation after spinal cord injury is helping a child's body readjust to a vertical position after being maintained in the supine position for so long. When the child's head is raised, blood tends to pool in dilated blood vessels below the level of the lesion. This pooling of blood results in pseudohypovolaemia and hypotension, and the child may faint. Gradually increasing the angle of the bed helps the child become acclimatised to the upright position without experiencing vascular pooling.

Learning to self-care

As soon as possible, children should be introduced to self-help methods for activities of daily living. Most parents need to be encouraged to allow a child to become as self-sufficient as possible and not to take over complete care. The child may well outlive them and will someday need to be able to function as independently as possible.

With autonomic nervous system dysfunction, a child is unable to sweat and becomes hyperthermic if covered too warmly; if not covered warmly enough, the capillaries dilate and the child loses considerable heat into the environment. If the room temperature cools at night, be careful to dress the child appropriately for sleeping.

Specific measures for bowel evacuation may be necessary, depending on the level of the injury. A bowel program incorporating the use of stool softeners, suppositories and bowel retraining may be required. The child and parents need support and instructions in accomplishing this task and gaining independence.

When the child reaches sexual maturity, limitations in this area may become apparent. If a male has had an upper motor neuron injury, he will not be able to achieve spontaneous erection or ejaculation. However, with manual stimulation of the penis (stimulation of lower motor neuron function), he may be able to achieve an erection and engage in coitus. Ejaculation and fertility remain limited. At the time of injury, lack of lower extremity motor control may seem to be the greatest loss. In adolescence, loss of normal sexual function may become even more disturbing. With most spinal cord injuries, a female is not able to experience orgasm but is able to conceive and bear children.

The limitations caused by a spinal cord injury become especially evident to the child (and the parents) when choosing a vocation and selecting an appropriate school program (children cannot be denied normal education by law, even with a severe physical disability). Counselling and rehabilitation are crucial aspects to achieve an optimal level of functioning and independence.

Ventilation assistance

If the cervical level of the cord is involved, a child will need ventilatory assistance. The child may be intubated at first, but orotracheal or nasotracheal intubation is only a temporary measure to maintain a patent airway. A tracheostomy may be done for long-term airway management and to prevent sloughing of pharyngeal tissue from the pressure of the intubation tube. If this is required, parents need instruction about caring for the tracheostomy and working with a mechanical ventilator. A phrenic nerve pacemaker may be used to stimulate the diaphragm to contract and initiate respirations. If the child has a thoracic level injury (which is rare because the rib cage gives extra strength to thoracic vertebrae), the child will be able to breathe independently but will have reduced vital capacity. Periodic positive-pressure breathing treatments may be necessary to encourage increased lung filling. Be careful when positioning a child not to compromise chest movement with equipment or other restricting objects. Other respiratory care measures, such as suctioning and chest physiotherapy, are also important.

Skin integrity

A child's skin should remain clean, dry and intact without signs of erythema or ulceration. To prevent skin breakdown, a child should be turned about every 2 hours (always be sure to log-roll or maintain immobilisation with a striker frame or a continuously moving, automatically controlled bed). The use of an alternating-pressure mattress may be helpful. With loss of sensation in body parts, the child is unable to report skin irritation from a wrinkled sheet or wet clothing. If the child is incontinent, the bedding must be changed immediately to prevent skin breakdown. Once children begin to be ambulatory, their legs and buttocks should be checked regularly to prevent pressure ulcers caused by sitting in a wheelchair or using leg braces.

Urinary elimination

To prevent urinary retention during the first phase of recovery, a Foley catheter is inserted, or the bladder can be emptied by periodic suprapubic aspiration or intermittent catheterisation. Second-stage spasticity causes periodic reflex emptying. This rarely empties the bladder completely, however, so the same problems of stasis and infection continue. To live independently, the child will need to learn self-catheterisation to empty the bladder.

Anticipatory grieving

The second recovery phase is the time for parents and children to begin thinking about what this degree of disability will mean to them and to face its full extent. Children and parents typically react to the initial diagnosis with grief. They may still be in denial or shock when the second phase begins. With no sudden miracle cure in sight, they may begin to move through stages of anger, bargaining, depression and then acceptance (the accident happened; we must go on from this point). They need assistance and support to work through these feelings. Both the parents and the child may need counselling to reach acceptance (see Fig. 49.9). Incorporation of a rehabilitation program can

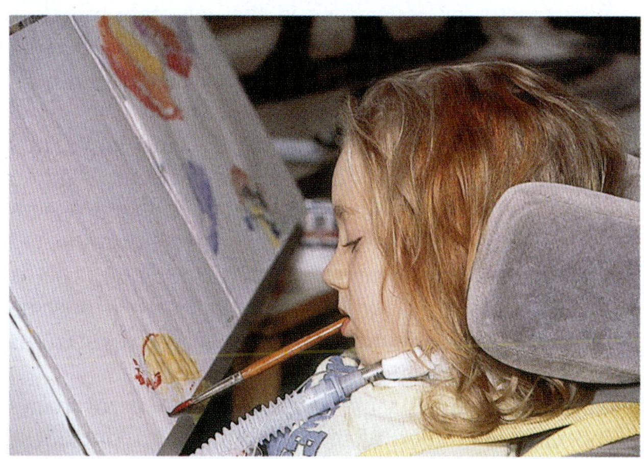

FIGURE 49.9 A 6-year-old girl with a cervical spine injury adapts to her disability by using her mouth to hold a paintbrush and participate in age-appropriate activities. (© Elisa Peterson/Stock Boston)

help in maximising the child's potential despite the limitations imposed by the injury.

✔ Checkpoint question 49.2

Spinal cord injuries usually occur from accidental injuries. Which is the most common type of injury seen in adolescents that leads to spinal cord injury?

a. Cervical fracture from a diving accident
b. Sacral fracture from a bicycle accident
c. Thoracic fracture from a bullet injury
d. Thoracic/sacral injury from lifting weights

✔ Checkpoint question 49.3

A spinal cord injury can cause severe disability in adolescents. If you were designing a program to teach measures to prevent spinal cord injury, what topics would you include in your presentation?

Key points for review

- Nerve cells are unique in that they do not regenerate if damaged. This makes neurological disease a long-term condition. Parents and children alike need support from healthcare providers to cope with problems that continue to occur over a long period.
- Increased intracranial pressure arises from an increase in the volume of cerebrospinal fluid or from blood accumulation, cerebral oedema or space-occupying lesions. Neurological changes, such as increased temperature and blood pressure and decreased pulse and respirations, that occur with increased intracranial pressure are subtle. Always compare assessments with previous levels to detect that a consistent, although minor, change is occurring.
- Cerebral palsy is a non-progressive disorder of upper motor neurons. The exact cause is usually unknown, but the condition is associated with anoxia occurring before, during or shortly after birth. Four major types are identified: spastic (excessive tone in the voluntary muscles), dyskinetic or athetoid (abnormal involuntary movement), atonic (decreased muscle tone) and mixed (symptoms of both spasticity and athetoid movements).
- Meningitis is infection of the cerebral meninges. It is caused most frequently by bacterial invasion. Children need follow-up afterwards to monitor for hearing acuity and impaired secretion of antidiuretic hormone.
- Encephalitis is inflammation of brain tissue. This is always a serious diagnosis because the child may be left with residual neurological damage, such as seizures or learning disabilities.
- Reye's syndrome is acute encephalitis with accompanying fatty infiltration of the liver, heart and lungs; it is associated with the administration of acetylsalicylic acid (aspirin) to children with a viral infection. Its incidence is declining.
- Guillain-Barré syndrome is inflammation of motor and sensory nerves. The reaction may be immune mediated, occurring after an upper respiratory tract illness. Temporary demyelinisation of the nerve sheath causes loss of function.
- Recurrent seizures are involuntary contractions of muscle caused by abnormal electrical brain discharges. Common types seen in children include febrile seizures, infantile spasms, partial (focal) seizures, absence seizures and tonic–clonic seizures. Therapy is by administration of anticonvulsant medication.
- Spinal cord injury is occurring at increased rates in children involved in sports and motor vehicle accidents. Children pass through a first, second and third recovery phase after the injury.

CASE STUDY QUESTIONS

5. Harrison is the 4-year-old boy you met at the beginning of the chapter, who was diagnosed with bacterial meningitis after a febrile seizure. His mother is concerned about long-term problems because of the seizure. Would you encourage her to concentrate on this or on more short-term concerns?
6. Harrison is diagnosed with bacterial meningitis. He has severe neck pain when he is moved. His mother asks you not to worry so much about measuring intake and output, so her son can rest. How would you answer her? Suppose you call the child's name and he does not answer you? Why is this a particular cause of concern in a child with meningitis?

Resources

For an extensive range of additional resources to enhance teaching and learning and to facilitate understanding of this chapter, please see the text's accompanying website located on thePoint at http://thepoint.lww.com.

References

Ardern-Holmes, S. L. & North, K. N. (2011). Therapeutics for childhood neurofibromatosis type 1 and type 2. *Current Treatment Options in Neurology*, *13*(6), 529–543.

Bailey, B. M., Liesemer, K., Statler, K. D., et al. (2012). Monitoring and prediction of intracranial hypertension in pediatric traumatic brain injury: Clinical factors and initial head computed tomography. *Journal of Trauma & Acute Care Surgery*, *72*(1), 263–270.

Baldin, E., Ludvigsson, P., Mixa, O., et al. (2012). Prevalence of recurrent symptoms and their association with epilepsy and febrile seizures in school-aged children: A community-based survey in Iceland. *Epilepsy & Behavior*, *23*(3), 315–319.

Bennett, C. L., Starko, K. M., Thomsen, H. S., et al. (2012). Linking drugs to obscure illnesses: Lessons from pure red cell aplasia, nephrogenic systemic fibrosis, and Reye's syndrome. A report from the Southern Network on Adverse Reactions (SONAR). *Journal of General Internal Medicine*, *27*(2), 1697–1703.

Bezov, D., Ashina, S. & Lipton, R. (2010). Post-dural puncture headache: Part II—Prevention, management, and prognosis. *Headache: The Journal of Head and Face Pain*, *50*(9), 1482–1498.

Britton, J. W. & Kosa, S. C. (2010). The clinical value of chloral hydrate in the routine electroencephalogram. *Epilepsy Research*, *88*(2–3), 215–220.

Buckley, R. H. (2008). Primary immunodeficiency diseases. In W. E. Paul (Ed). *Fundamental Immunology* (6th ed.). Philadelphia: Lippincott Williams & Wilkins.

Cerebral Palsy Australia, (2015). The facts. Accessed 20 April 2015, <https://cpaustralia.com.au/learning-center/the-facts/>.

Cleves-Bayon, C., et al. (2014). Headache in children and adolescents. In S. J. Tepper & D. E. Tepper (Eds), *The Cleveland Clinic Manual of Headache Therapy* (2nd ed.). New York: Springer.

Crosbie, J., Alhusaini, A. A., Dean, C. M., et al. (2012). Plantar flexor muscle and spatiotemporal gait characteristics of children with hemiplegic cerebral palsy: An observational study. *Developmental Neurorehabilitation, 15(*2), 114–118.

Dobrin, S. (2015). Seizures and epilepsy in adolescents and adults. In E. T. Bope & R. D. Kellerman (Eds), *Conn's Current Therapy 2015*. Philadelphia: Elsevier/Saunders.

Gilbert, W. M., Jacoby, B. N., Xing, G., et al. (2010). Adverse obstetric are associated with significant risk of cerebral palsy. *American Journal of Obstetrics and Gynecology, 203*(4), 328.e1–328.e5.

Greenberg-Kushnir, N., Haskin, O., Yarden-Bilavsky, H., et al. (2012). Haemophilus influenzae type b meningitis in the short period after vaccination: A reminder of the phenomenon of apparent vaccine failure. *Case Reports in Infectious Diseases*, 2012, 950107.

Hazinski, M. F. (2012). Neurologic disorders. In M. F. Hazinski (Ed), *Nursing Care of the Critically Ill Child* (3rd ed.). St Louis: Elsevier Health Sciences.

Kneen, R., Michael, B. D., Menson, E., et al. (2012). The management of suspected viral encephalitis in children. *The Journal of Infection, 64*(5), 449–477.

Kossoff, E. H., Bosarge, J. L., Miranda, M. J., et al. (2010). Will seizure control improve by switching from the modified Atkins diet to the traditional ketogenic diet? *Epilepsia, 51*(12), 2496–2499.

Lewis, P. & Foley, D. (2014). *Health Assessment in Nursing* (2nd ed.). Sydney: Lippincott William & Wilkins.

Libster, R., Edwards, K. M., Levent, F., et al. (2012). Long-term outcomes of group B streptococcal meningitis. *Pediatrics, 130*(1), e8–e15.

Lo, W., Marchuk, D. A., Ball, K. L., et al. (2012). Updates and future horizons on the understanding, diagnosis and treatment of Sturge-Weber syndrome brain involvement. *Developmental Medicine & Child Neurology, 54*(3), 214–223.

Luckhaupt, S. E., Dalhamer, J. M., Ward, B. W., et al. (2013). Prevalence and work-relatedness of carpal tunnel syndrome in the working population. *American Journal of Industrial Medicine, 56*(6), 615–624.

Mariani, E., Rossi, L. N. & Vojani, S. (2011). Interictal paroxysmal EEG abnormalities in childhood absence seizures. *Seizures, 20*(4), 299–304.

Martin-Herz, S. P., Zatzick, D. F. & McMahon, R. J. (2012). Health related quality of life in children and adolescents following traumatic injury: A review. *Clinical Child and Family Psychology Review, 15*(3), 192–214.

McGrath-Morrow, S. A., Gower, W. A., Rothblum-Oviatt, C., et al. (2010). Evaluation and management of pulmonary disease in ataxiatelangiectasia. *Pediatric Pulmonology, 45*(9), 847–859.

McNamara, R., Doyle, J., McKay, M., et al. (2013). Medium term outcome in Bell's palsy in children. *Emergency Medicine Journal, 30*(6), 444–446.

Middleton, D. B. (2011). Seizures. In J. E. South-Paul, S. C. Matheny & E. L. Lewis (Eds). *Current Diagnosis and Treatment in Family Medicine* (3rd ed.). Columbus, OH: McGraw-Hill.

Moster, D., Wilcox, A. J., Voilset, S. E., et al. (2010). Cerebral palsy among term and postterm births. *JAMA: Journal of the American Medical Association, 304*(9), 976–982.

Pace, D. & Pollard, A. J. (2012). Meningococcal disease: Clinical presentation and sequelae. *Vaccine, 30*(2), B3–B9.

Pellatt, G. C. (2010). Spinal surgery for acute traumatic spinal cord injury: Implications for nursing. *British Journal of Neuroscience Nursing, 6*(6), 271–275.

Placzek, R., Siebold, D. & Funk, J. F. (2010). Development of treatment concepts for the use of botulinum toxin A in children with cerebral palsy. *Toxins, 2*(9), 2258–2271.

Rapin, I. (2011). Child neurologists as evaluators of developmental disorders. *Seminars in Pediatric Neurology, 18*(2), 104–109.

Riesch, S. K., Kedrowski, K., Brown, R. L., et al. (2012). Health-risk behaviors among a sample of US pre-adolescents: Types, frequency, and predictive factors. *International Journal of Nursing Studies, 50*(8), 1067–1079.

Rosen, B. A. (2012). Guillain-Barré syndrome. *Pediatrics in Review, 33*(4), 164–171.

Rust, R. (2011). What the child neurologist should know at the conclusion of training: History taking, examination, and formulation (and a few other generalizations). *Seminars in Pediatric Neurology, 18*(2), 59–65.

Singh, R. K., Stephens, S., Berl, M. M., et al. (2010). Prospective study of new-onset seizures presenting as status epilepticus in childhood. *Neurology, 74*(8), 636–642.

Stone, C. K. (2011). Neurologic emergencies. In C. K. Stone & R. L. Humphries (Eds). *Current Diagnosis and Treatment: Emergency Medicine* (7th ed.). Columbus, OH: McGraw-Hill.

Tatum, W. O., Ho, S. & Benbadis, S. R. (2010). Polyspike ictal onset absence seizures. *Journal of Clinical Neurophysiology, 27*(2), 93–99.

Yuki, N. & Hartung, H. (2012). Guillain-Barré syndrome. *New England Journal of Medicine, 366*(24), 2294–2304.

Suggested readings

Boldt, C., Velstra, I., Brach, M., et al. (2013). Nurses' intervention goal categories for persons with spinal cord injury based on the International Classification of Functioning, Disability, and Health. *Journal of Advanced Nursing, 69*(5), 1109–1124.

Chiocca, E. M. (2011). *Advanced Pediatric Assessment*. Philadelphia: Lippincott Williams & Wilkins.

Duffy, L. V. (2009). The nurse's role in treatment decisions for the child with neurological impairment. *Journal of Neuroscience Nursing, 41*(5), 270–276.

Hancock, E., Osborne, J. P. & Edwards, S. W. (2013). Treatment of infantile spasms. *Cochrane Database of Systematic Reviews, 2013*(6), (CD001770).

NSW Department of Health. (2009). Infants and children: Acute management of seizures (2nd ed.), Clinical Practice Guidelines. Accessed 9 March 2015, <www.health.nsw.gov.au/policies/pd/2009/pdf/pd2009_065.pdf>.

Reilly, C., Atkinson, P., Das, K. B., et al. (2014). Neurobehavioral comorbidities in children with active epilepsy: A population-based study. *Pediatrics, 133*(6), e1586–1593.

Chapter 50

Nursing care of a family when a child has a vision or hearing disorder

Previous chapters discussed the growth and development of well children. This chapter adds information about the changes, physical and psychosocial, that occur when a child develops a disorder of the eyes (vision) or ears (hearing). This is important information because it builds a base for care and health teaching.

LEARNING OBJECTIVES

After mastering the contents of this chapter, you should be able to:

1. Describe the structure and function of the eyes and ears and disorders of these organs as they affect children.
2. Use critical thinking to analyse ways that nursing care of children with a disorder of vision or hearing could be more family-centred.
3. Assess a child who has a disorder of vision or hearing.
4. Implement nursing care to meet the specific needs of a child who has a disorder of the eyes or ears, such as educating parents about the symptoms of otitis media.
5. Identify areas related to care of children with vision or hearing disorders that could benefit from additional nursing research or application of evidence-based practice.

KEY TERMS

- accommodation
- amblyopia
- astigmatism
- diplopia
- enucleation
- fovea centralis
- goniotomy
- hyperopia
- light refraction
- myopia
- nystagmus
- orthoptics
- photophobia
- ptosis
- stereopsis
- strabismus
- tympanocentesis

CASE STUDY

Amy Smith, a 4-year-old child, presents with her mother to the doctors' surgery. Her mother states, "She's always had a lot of problems. She had strabismus as a baby. Now, I think she has another ear infection. It started out as a head cold but now she's pulling at her ear. Why does she get so many of these?"

CASE STUDY QUESTIONS

1. How would you answer Ms Smith?
2. What information does she need to know about ear infections?

Any interference with vision or hearing poses a threat to normal growth and development, because so much of what and how a child learns about the world is achieved through these sensory organs. Infants first learn how to interact with others by watching their parents' faces. They learn to speak by listening to words spoken to them. They continue to depend on sensory input for stimulation and to protect their safety throughout life (Sininger, Grimes & Christensen, 2010).

Eye and ear disorders may be transitory. However, they always have the potential for becoming long-term illnesses if they permanently affect vision and hearing. Subsequently, this will impact on a child's education, employment and long-term health. This is an area, therefore, in which health promotion, illness prevention and health rehabilitation are all important aspects of nursing care.

HEALTH PROMOTION

Identification of significant hearing loss is achieved through universal hearing screening of all newborns. In Australia, approximately one to two in every 1000 babies has significant hearing loss. Initiatives such as the NSW Statewide Infant Screening–Hearing (SWISH) Program aim to identify those babies and introduce them to appropriate services as soon as possible after birth (NSW Department of Health, 2012b). The goals of universal neonatal hearing screening within Australia are to identify and assist their families to reduce the impacts of the child's hearing impairment. Each territory and state conducts universal hearing screening (Australian Institute of Health and Welfare, 2013).

Avoidable blindness has been raised as a significant issue by the World Health Organization (WHO). In July 2004, a National Health Plan for Australia for eye health promotion was proposed. This was also to ensure the system was proactive rather than reactive. $13.8 million was allocated over 4 years in the 2006–2007 Federal Budget for a National Health Initiative (NEHI) to promote eye health. Reviews were conducted, with the resultant outcome being that there was a lack of evidence that preventative screening would be of much assistance, with further research required. This was to be reviewed in 2008 (National Children's Vision Screening Project). Most current screening is reliant on the vigilance of parents with many checks having poor uptake rates.

TABLE 50.1 Assessment parameters for vision and hearing screening

Age	Vision assessment parameters	Hearing assessment parameters
Infant	Ability to follow objects Corneal reflex Ability to turn to light stimuli	Startle reflex (at birth) Ability to track sounds (3–6 months) Ability to recognise sounds (6–8 months) Ability to locate sounds (8–12 months)
Toddler	Corneal light reflex Cover test Smooth ocular movements Hand–eye coordination	Ability to react to soft sounds (whispers) Ability to track source of sounds Ability to form a noun–verb sentence by 2 years Ability to follow simple directions Awareness of pitch and tone
Preschooler	Corneal light reflex Cover test Snellen E chart (or modification)	Pure tone audiometry (starting at age 4 years) Understandable language with increasing vocabulary
School-age	Visual acuity testing every 1–2 years	Pure tone audiometry at ages 6, 8 and 11 years
Adolescent	Visual acuity testing every 1–2 years	Pure tone audiometry at ages 14 and 18 years

In 2009 it was determined that the vision check during the neonatal period was important with a review recommended around age 4 (National Children's Vision Screening Project, 2009). As a result, in Australia, the healthy kids check is aimed at those 4 years old and those potentially commencing school, where a detailed checklist to improve children's health ranging from dental checks, vision, hearing and social interaction is applied (Australian Government Department of Health, 2014). Several preventative children's services also are available for Aboriginal and Torres Straight Islanders as these groups statistically have much higher incidences of hearing and vision issues (Western Australian Government, 2012; Australian Government Department of Social Services, 2012).

From preschool through to adolescence, children should continue to be screened routinely for vision and hearing problems, so that these problems can be detected and management commenced as early in life as possible (Hopkins et al., 2013; see Table 50.1). If a child has a vision or hearing impairment, safety measures take on even greater importance. It is important to educate parents about measures to adapt the child's environment to meet safety needs while promoting growth and development and independence as much as possible. For example, supplementing verbal explanations with tactile and visual aids and allowing the child to use drawings, writing or gestures to respond and communicate can be useful. Encourage the use of specialised devices, such as a talking picture board or e-mail, if the child is hearing challenged with limited speech. Provide ample time for interaction and incorporate the use of therapeutic play. Children with vision or hearing disorders need to attend regular classrooms at school, if possible, so that they can have contact with seeing and hearing children to promote normal growth and development. In addition to safety measures, parents may need advice about measures to prevent eye and ear infections, so that they do not lead to long-term problems. Mild vitamin A deficiency, for example, leads to loss of night vision and severe vitamin A deficiency, that could occur from an adolescent eating disorder, can lead to blindness (keratomalacia) (Lai, Ng & Srinivasan, 2014).

VISION

Vision occurs because light rays reflect from an object through the corneas, aqueous humours, lenses and vitreous humours to the retinas (see Fig. 50.1). If any of these structures have defects, light rays may not be able to reach the retinas or focus there correctly, resulting in a vision disturbance. The retinas are studded with *rods*, which are instrumental for night vision and movement in the visual field, and *cones*, which register daylight and colour vision. Rods and cones join in a major network to register at the optic nerve. The **fovea centralis** (the centre of the macula)

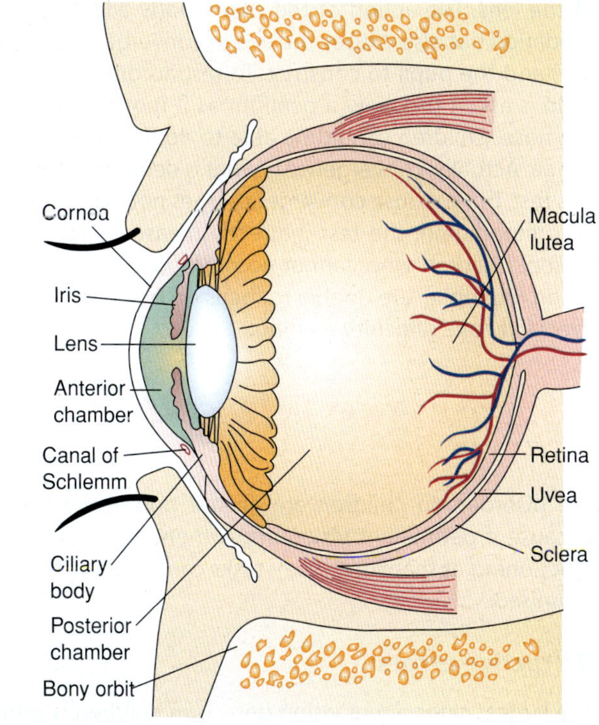

FIGURE 50.1 Anatomy of the eye.

is an area of closely packed cones on the retinas where colour is best perceived.

Each eye globe must develop good central and peripheral vision. However, in addition, *fusion* must occur—that is, both eyes together must interpret a visual image as one image, fusing visual perception into a single image. This is called *single binocular vision.* Infants with poor eye alignment cannot establish single binocular vision but have **diplopia** or double vision.

Stereopsis

Stereopsis is depth perception or the ability to locate an object in space relative to other objects. The right eye sees more of the right side of an object, whereas the left eye sees more of the left side. This makes the object appear to be three-dimensional. Children with vision loss in one eye do not develop stereopsis and, consequently, tend to reach farther than or closer than the actual distance to an object when attempting to grasp it. They have difficulty learning to ride a bicycle and have great difficulty driving a car safely. Children without stereopsis do not realise that their sight is different from that of other people. The *Stereo-Fly* or random dot test, a simple test for depth perception, is a specially constructed picture of a large fly made of coloured dots. When asked to touch the fly's wings, a child with good depth perception touches them accurately. A child with poor depth perception touches a spot 5 or 8 cm above the pattern.

Accommodation

Accommodation is the adjustment the eye makes when focusing on a close image. To focus on a close object, the ciliary bodies of the eye contract, changing the curvature of the lens. The action of the ciliary body allows accommodation but also causes the eye to converge (look medially) and the pupil to constrict. To test accommodation, a child is asked to follow a penlight as it moves in towards the nose. Children should be able to do this by 6 months of age. Actually, convergence is what is demonstrated with this test, but because convergence does not occur without accommodation, the test indirectly measures accommodation. Children who cannot accommodate have double vision (diplopia), are unable to focus on objects near their eyes and have difficulty reading.

DISORDERS THAT INTERFERE WITH VISION

Eye disorders in children are always potentially serious because if permanent vision impairment occurs, a child's functioning at many everyday tasks can be severely compromised.

Refractive errors

The largest category of vision defects in children is refractive errors (Hopkins et al., 2013). **Light refraction** refers to the manner in which light is bent as it passes through a lens. Normally, this bending causes a ray of light to fall directly on the retina. Because the depth of the eye globe in infants and children increases with age, the light rays do not always focus onto the retina accurately as the child grows older, but rather, focuses at a point behind the retina. This results in **hyperopia** (farsightedness), in which vision is blurry at a close range and clear at a far range. The normal hyperopia of a preschooler needs no correction. At about 5 years of age, as a result of developmental changes, hyperopia begins to diminish. Some children, however, remain hyperopic. Focusing on close objects requires such strong accommodation that these children often have headaches or dizziness after completing schoolwork. A finding of hyperopia in a school-age child is cause for referral so that the child can get a prescription for glasses with a convex lens.

Approximately 10% of school-aged children have eye changes that result in **myopia** (nearsightedness), meaning that the light rays focus at a point in front of the retina (Morgan, Ohno-Matsui & Saw, 2012). These children can read a book or a computer screen immediately in front of them but are unable to read the blackboard clearly in a classroom. They have difficulty reading signs across the street or playing sport such as tennis or softball. Once myopia begins, it often progresses into the teenage years, when it plateaus and remains for life. Children with myopia need corrective (concave) lenses to enable them to see at a distance.

Myopia tends to be familial. If both parents are myopic, their children should be screened yearly during the early school years. Children with myopia try to focus on objects by squinting and rubbing their eyes, which changes the shape of the eye globe. Any child who reports difficulty seeing or who shows mannerisms suggestive of refraction errors—rubbing the eyes, tearing, red-rimmed eyes, blinking, squinting or pressing on the eyes—should be screened for visual difficulty (see Fig. 50.2).

In the past, the only correction for refractive errors of vision was by eyeglasses or contact lenses. Today, adolescents can have laser surgery (LASIK) to permanently change the contour of the cornea and correct refractive vision errors.

Although wearing glasses is more acceptable today, children may still experience teasing. It is important to encourage them to persist with wearing glasses, however, as in most instances, glasses improve vision to such an extent that after trying them, children will continue to wear them. However, throughout their development, they may need continued encouragement to keep wearing glasses until they are old enough for contact lenses or surgical correction.

If parents are going to purchase eyeglasses, it is important they choose frames fitted with plastic or safety glass (shatterproof) lenses, so that if the lenses accidentally break, the child's eyes will not be injured. It is possible for contact lenses to be fitted for even young infants. Children

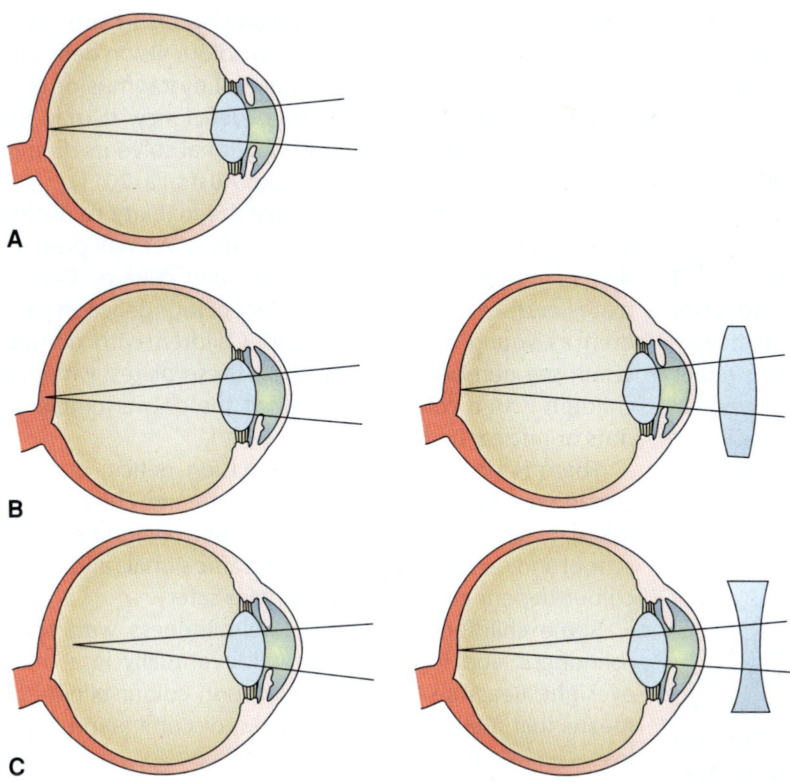

FIGURE 50.2 Corrective lenses for refractive errors of vision. (A) Normal vision. (B) Convex lens for hyperopia (farsightedness). (C) Concave lens for myopia (nearsightedness).

as young as 5 years of age are capable of putting them in and taking them out if taught properly. Contact lenses are a big responsibility, however; they require conscientious cleaning or changing to prevent eye irritation or infection. Children are usually about 12 years of age before they can be relied on to take appropriate care of contact lenses totally independently.

Laser in situ keratomileusis (LASIK)

Laser in situ keratomileusis (LASIK) is laser surgery for correction of myopia (O'Keefe & Kirwan, 2010). It involves making an incision under the cornea to change the contour of the eye globe so that light rays fall more accurately on the retina. Postoperatively, children frequently have disturbed tear function for one or more months and need to be managed with artificial tears or ointments to prevent surface damage. Because having the procedure carried out before the child's eye globe has reached its adult size would require that the surgery be repeated with maturity, the youngest age at which LASIK therapy is appropriate is controversial. The technique is a major method of correcting refractive vision errors in adults and in the future is expected to also be applicable to children.

Astigmatism

Astigmatism is congenital or acquired unevenness of the curvature of the cornea (Huang et al., 2014). This causes light rays coming to the retina to not be all refracted in the same way; the result is an uneven quality of vision. When children with astigmatism look at the letter T, for example, they may see the crossbar but not the letter stem. If they focus on the stem, they cannot see the crossbar. On any given page of print, therefore, they may see only half the letters. For this reason, they can have difficulty reading or following written instructions. They may report headache and vertigo after doing close work. Their vision may appear deceptively normal on vision screening tests because they are able to see all of the numbers on a chart by tilting their head. These children need to be referred to an ophthalmologist, however, on the basis of their other problems such as vertigo, headaches and difficulty with reading. Corrective lenses for close work relieve the symptoms and restore functional vision. Contact lenses may be even more helpful, because they actually smooth out the curvature of the cornea.

Nystagmus

Nystagmus is rapid, irregular eye movement, either vertically or horizontally. It is not a disease in itself but rather a symptom of an underlying disease condition. It is seen in children with vision-impairing lesions such as congenital cataracts. It also occurs as a neurological sign if there is a lesion of the cerebellum or brainstem. Children with nystagmus must be referred to a specialist so that the underlying cause of the symptom can be determined.

Amblyopia

Amblyopia is "lazy eye" or subnormal vision in one eye; the child may be using only one eye for vision while "resting" the other eye. If this process continues for too long, central vision fails to develop (or the central vision that had developed fades), and the child becomes functionally blind in one eye. This can occur in children who have a refractive error in one eye that is significantly different from that of the other eye or in children with astigmatism. Because one eye focuses more readily than the other, they come to depend on only the easily focused eye (West & Williams, 2011).

Amblyopia can also develop from strabismus (crossed eyes). With strabismus, one eye looks straight ahead while the other eye "wanders". Children who have an eye that wanders are constantly looking at two separate images rather than one fused image. To make sense out of what they see, they suppress one visual image; this leads to suppression of central vision in that eye, or amblyopia. The same phenomenon occurs if the vision in one eye is obscured by a lid that does not open fully (ptosis).

Assessment

All preschool children should be screened for amblyopia. A child with amblyopia has 20/50 vision (normal for preschool age) in one eye and the other eye shows lessened vision (perhaps 20/100). In Australia, the StEPS Program (Statewide Eyesight Preschooler Screening) was initiated in order to identify, as early as possible, visual problems in preschool children. The aims of the program are to:

- Address parental concerns regarding a child's vision
- Identify children who may be at risk due to their family history
- Conduct a visual inspection of the eye
- Test visual acuity
- Facilitate referral to an eye health professional when necessary (NSW Department of Health, 2012a).

Therapeutic management

Amblyopia is correctable if treated during the preschool period. Although there are reports of success with older children and adolescents, the prognosis for correction is considerably diminished after 6 years of age. It may not be possible 7 to less than 13 years of age (Holmes et al., 2011). For treatment, the good eye is covered by a patch held firmly in place. This forces the child to use the poor eye, thus developing vision in that eye. Usually, children have some difficulty initially adjusting to a patch; being unable to see well from the unpatched eye, they may develop headaches or dizziness and notice poor depth perception. Only constant attempts to see with the weaker eye, however, will improve binocular vision. The patch is removed for 1 hour each day to prevent amblyopia from developing in the non-amblyopic eye.

Colour vision deficit (colour blindness)

Colour vision deficit is the inability to perceive colour correctly. It occurs because one of the sets of cones of the retina that perceive red, green or blue is absent. It is inherited as a sex-linked disorder and occurs in about 8% of boys. There is a high incidence of colour vision deficit in children with haemophilia, congenital nystagmus or glucose-6-phosphate dehydrogenase deficiency. It may be associated with exposure to occupational solvents during pregnancy (Government of Western Australia, 2011).

The vision problem may involve the inability to distinguish red from green or blue from yellow. A small proportion of children are unable to see any colours. Colour plates or discs can be used to detect colour deficit in children as young as preschool age. Children with normal vision see numbers or patterns on these plates, whereas children with a colour vision deficit see only a jumble of dots or unclear images.

There is no therapy for colour vision deficit, but the condition should be detected early so the child is not asked to complete colour identification assignments in school and can be educated about traffic signals and other colour-dependent signs necessary for safety.

Some children associate colour blindness with total "blindness" and fear that they will eventually lose their eyesight. Reassure them that, although colour blindness means that they have a loss of colour discrimination, their loss is limited to that one area.

✔ *Checkpoint question 50.1*

What if Katie, who is 6 years old, develops amblyopia? Which statement by her mother would assure you that her learning needs are being met?

a. "I place the patch over her weak eye to enhance the vision in her stronger eye."
b. "I place the patch over her good eye to allow the weaker eye to strengthen."
c. "I alternate the patch between eyes every other day so both eyes strengthen."
d. "I can take off the patch while Katie eats to make it easier for her."

STRUCTURAL PROBLEMS OF THE EYE

Structural problems of the eye tend to be congenital or present at birth.

Coloboma

A *coloboma* is the congenital incomplete closure of the facial cleft. The incomplete closure may involve only the lower eyelid (there is a notch in the lid); the iris, giving it the shape of a keyhole, rather than a circle; or it may involve the ciliary body, the lens, the choroid, the retina and the optic nerve (see Fig. 50.3). Children with any degree of coloboma should be referred to an ophthalmologist for further investigation to determine the extent of the condition. Children with retina and optic nerve coloboma will have some vision impairment in the affected eye.

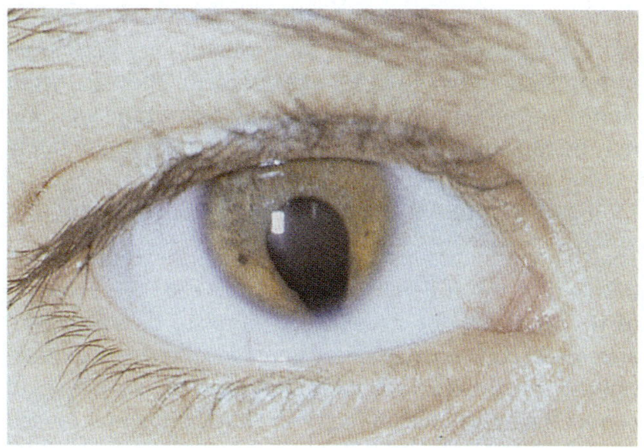

FIGURE 50.3 Coloboma involving the iris, showing a "keyhole" appearance. (From Tasman, W. & Jaeger, E. A. [1996], *Willis Eye Hospital Atlas of Clinical Ophthalmology*. Philadelphia: Lippincott-Raven Publishers.)

Hypertelorism

Hypertelorism is a congenital condition involving abnormally wide-spaced eyes. Children with wide epicanthal folds by the inner canthus may appear to have wide-spaced eyes, but, when the distance between the pupils is measured and compared with standards for the child's age, the true condition is revealed. Detecting true hypertelorism in children is important because this condition is associated with chromosomal abnormalities, most notably Waardenburg's syndrome, which also involves congenital hearing impairment. Children with this syndrome also have a white forelock of hair, different-coloured irises and eyebrows that tend to grow together in the centre line. These signs may not be noticeable in newborns. Therefore, wide-spaced eyes, because of a broad-bridged nose, are the chief clue in a newborn that the child can hear no sound and will need close follow-up to determine whether cochlear implants or hearing aids can provide ability to hear.

Ptosis

Ptosis is the inability to raise the upper eyelid normally so the eyelid always remains slightly closed. The condition may be congenital (frequently hereditary and bilateral) or acquired (usually unilateral). It may be a result of injury to the third cranial nerve (neurogenic) or to the lid or levator muscle. Usually, with injury to the third cranial nerve, paralysis of one or more of the other muscles supplied by that nerve is also present. In addition, children may exhibit:

- A dilated pupil
- Inability to rotate the eye globe upwards, medially or downwards
- Weakness of accommodation (looking at near objects).

Myasthenia gravis, which produces generalised muscle weakness, must always be ruled out as a cause of bilateral ptosis. Children with ptosis tend to wrinkle their forehead and raise their eyebrows more than usual in an attempt to lift the eyelid further. Also, they may cock their heads back to see under the lowered lid.

After careful investigation of the cause has been completed, ptosis is corrected surgically. The correction is usually important to the child from a cosmetic standpoint. More importantly, if the lid obstructs vision, early surgery is necessary to prevent the development of amblyopia (from lack of use of the eye). Be sure that parents understand the importance of surgical correction. Otherwise, they may insist on delaying a corrective procedure "until the child is older". When the child is older, although the ptosis can be corrected, the amblyopia cannot.

Strabismus

The movement of each eye globe is controlled by extraocular muscles. **Strabismus** is unequally aligned eyes (cross-eyes) caused by unbalanced muscle control (see Fig. 50.4). In Australia, approximately 5% of children have strabismus (Lions Eye Institute, 2013). Approximately 30% of children with strabismus have a history of a similar strabismus in the family. If there is a family history of strabismus, the child needs to be observed and examined yearly for this problem (O'Dowd, 2013).

Normally, with good eye alignment, the resting position of the eyes is straight, largely as a result of neuromuscular influences the child cannot control. In strabismus, the resting position of one eye may be *divergent* (turned out) or *convergent* (turned in). One pupil may be higher than the other (vertical strabismus). The strabismus may be monocular, in which the same eye deviates constantly, or it may be an alternating strabismus, in which one eye and then the other deviates.

Both the resting position of eyes and the amount of turning necessary to read small print depend on the eyes' ability to fuse and see only one image. This ability is minimal in infancy but becomes stronger with practice. In adulthood, it is automatic. If children cannot fuse vision effectively early in life because of strabismus, they may be unable to achieve fusion later on or be unable to maintain good eye position.

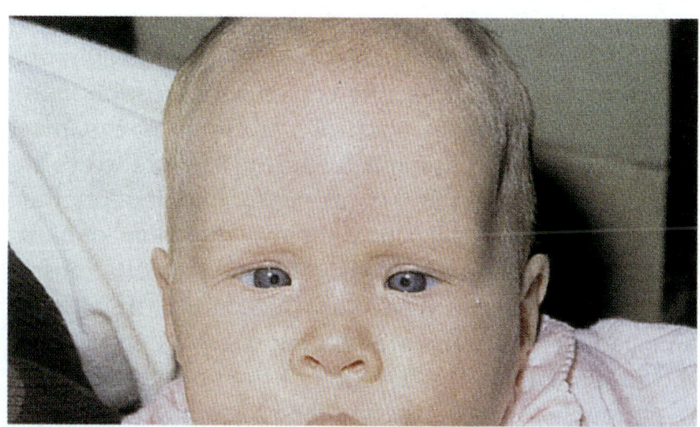

FIGURE 50.4 Strabismus (esotropia) in an infant.

Assessment

Infants' eyes may cross occasionally until 6 weeks of age. If infants demonstrate strabismus past this age, they should be referred for diagnosis and treatment. Infants who demonstrate a constant strabismus before 6 weeks of age need referral immediately.

Definite deviations are obvious. These can be *exotropia* (eye turning out), *esotropia* (eye turning in) or *hypertropia* (eye turning up). If the deviation is not so obvious and occurs only when the child is tired or ill and therefore, less able to maintain fixation, the terms used are *exophoria, esophoria* and *hyperphoria*. If the parents report that the deviation occurs only when the child is tired or sick, attempt to assess the strabismus at such a time, because then the deviation will be most striking.

Strabismus may be best detected when children examine a nearby object. It takes muscular effort to look medially (turn an eye in towards the nose). When children read small print, they turn both eyes medially, or *converge*, to focus at the short distance. If they are farsighted in one eye, they will have to turn the affected eye in more than the other, causing strabismus. If one eye is nearsighted, they will not need to turn that eye in as far as the other one; this results in divergence of the nearsighted eye. Although these children have good eye alignment at rest, they "cross their eyes" when attempting to focus at a reading distance.

Some children have a latent strabismus, but, because they are able to maintain fusion, the strabismus is not overt. They maintain this fusion however, at the expense of eyestrain. They may experience headaches; tired, irritated eyes; and perhaps even nausea and vomiting.

Children who have flat, broad-bridged noses, a narrow interpupillary distance and an epicanthal fold or oval-shaped palpebral fissures may appear to have strabismus when they truly do not (pseudostrabismus). These children have less white sclera visible in the inner margin of the eye than normal, so the eye appears to be turned in (*pseudoesotropia*). A cover test reveals the true condition. If pseudostrabismus is present, the covered eye will not move after being uncovered. It only appears to be turned medially because of the obscured sclera at the inner canthus. Hirshberg's test is another method of detecting true strabismus.

Once strabismus is detected, it is important to attempt to discern whether it is concomitant (measures the same in all directions of gaze) or non-concomitant (greater in one direction than in another; often called *paralytic strabismus*).

Concomitant (non-paralytic) strabismus is the most usual type found in children. All the muscles of the eye are capable of function but they are not functioning together. The deviation is equally apparent in all directions of gaze.

Paralytic strabismus is caused by paralysis of a muscle or nerve, perhaps from an injury, such as a birth injury or an invading lesion. The eyes appear straight except when they are moved in the direction of the paralysed muscle; then double vision occurs and the crossed eye is evident. Such children often close one eye or tilt their head to decrease the double vision. They may tilt their head so much they appear to have a torticollis, or "wry neck"—an orthopaedic rather than an eye problem. They are often clumsy because of the diplopia. They cannot see well and may be too young to describe what is happening to them.

Therapeutic management

The therapy for strabismus depends on the cause of the problem. If the fusion mechanism is weak, eye exercises **(orthoptics)** may be necessary. If eyes are diverging with attempted convergence because of farsightedness or nearsightedness, the child will more than likely require glasses to correct the basic visual defect. If the misalignment is caused by unequal muscle strength, eye-muscle surgery may be necessary to correct the problem (Lions Eye Institute, 2013).

Because strabismus causes the eyes to be viewing two different fields of vision, diplopia occurs. To prevent this, the child suppresses the vision in one eye or looks with one eye (amblyopia). Even if diplopia is not present, the lack of fusion leads to the same consequence. For this reason, eye correction for strabismus must be done early in life, before 6 years of age. Some children whose eyes are crossing because of an accommodation problem caused by hyperopia in one eye, outgrow the condition, as the normal hyperopia of the preschooler lessens. This does not always occur, however. Even if the child's eyes appear to be straighter later, an amblyopia may be present that could have been prevented by earlier treatment.

Nursing care for the child having eye surgery is discussed later in this chapter. After strabismus surgery, eye patches are not required. Postoperatively, antibiotic ointment is applied to the eye for 2 or 3 days. The child may experience some pain on eye movement for the first day. Follow-up visits after surgery are necessary to determine the success of the surgery.

INFECTION OR INFLAMMATION OF THE EYE

Many different types of eye infection or inflammatory conditions can occur in children. Newborns are susceptible to eye infection contracted from vaginal secretions (Women and Newborn Health Service, 2013). Regardless of the condition, parents need specific instructions about instilling eye drops or applying ointment, preventing the transmission of infection, applying compresses and completing systemic antibiotic therapy. Having eye medication applied can be frightening for older children, because they worry that the healthcare provider's or parent's hand might slip and damage their eye. If they have pain, they may be especially reluctant to let anyone touch their eye.

TRAUMATIC INJURY TO THE EYE

The primary cause of vision disorders in children today is ocular trauma, caused by missiles such as dirt or sand, balls, pieces of broken plastic toys, or flying glass in car accidents that strike or even enter the eye globe. Fights with other children, cigarette burns, sports injuries and fingernail scratches are also causes (American Association for Pediatric Ophthalmology and Strabismus, 2011; Armstrong et al., 2012).

Assessment

Children who have eye injuries are usually in acute pain immediately after the accident. Their eyes tear and are sensitive to light, and they blink rapidly. Vision may be blurred or lost in the affected eye. Because of the pain and the fear of not being able to see clearly, most children are very reluctant to let anyone examine or touch their injured eye. A few drops of a topical anaesthetic instilled into the eye may be necessary to relieve the pain and allow the eye to be opened for examination. Even after the anaesthetic is applied, the child needs a thorough explanation of what is happening. Following application of an anaesthetic, a child may not be able to open the eye readily for inspection, because the acute pain of the injury can cause the eyelid to close by reflex spasm. Eyelid oedema also may form quickly, interfering with the eye's ability to open (Pan & Oliver, 2011).

A foreign body, such as a speck of dirt or a fragment of glass, often clings to the inside of the upper lid and can be readily removed by touching it with a moistened, sterile, cotton-tipped applicator while the lid is everted. Keep an eyelid everted no longer than is necessary, because the eye globe tends to become dry when it is exposed. Magnetic resonance imaging (MRI) is an excellent method for documenting internal eye damage after an injury.

Foreign bodies

Foreign bodies such as sand or dirt that are loose on the conjunctiva can be removed by irrigation with a sterile normal saline solution or by gentle wiping with a well-moistened, sterile, cotton-tipped applicator after the eyelid is everted. After the removal, if the conjunctiva is touched with a strip of filter paper impregnated with fluorescein stain, any corneal ulceration or abrasion from the foreign body will stain green and be readily apparent. If the foreign body is easily removed and no corneal ulceration or injury is present, no further treatment is necessary. The child will blink a few times after the upper lid is returned to its place, but, in a matter of minutes, the child will report feeling "fine" again. If the fluorescein stain shows any corneal ulceration, the child should be referred to an ophthalmologist for follow-up care.

If a foreign body adheres to the cornea, it needs to be removed by an ophthalmologist. If the foreign body is metallic and has been in contact with the cornea for a period of hours, a rust ring can form around the particle. This rust ring must also be removed or it will continue to act as a foreign body. After corneal injury, corneal tissue regenerates. To allow for this, the eye is washed with an antibiotic solution and then closed and patched. The patch must be secure enough to keep the eyelid closed yet not put undue pressure on the eye. The child should be educated that the patch must be left in place to prevent the delicate regenerating corneal epithelium from being rubbed off until it is well healed and secure once more.

If a foreign object is relatively large, such as a lollipop stick or piece of broken glass, the fact that it has punctured the eye globe is usually apparent on first inspection (The Royal Children's Hospital Melbourne, 2015). In these instances, the child needs to be examined by an ophthalmologist. Surgery may be necessary to explore the depth of the puncture and save the child's sight in that eye. Iron or copper fragments must be removed to prevent rust formation and continued irritation.

An extremely serious complication called *sympathetic iritis* or inflammation of the opposite eye, may result if the ciliary body was involved in a penetrating injury. As a result, blindness in the non-injured eye may occur. This complication can be prevented by administration of a corticosteroid and antibiotics to reduce inflammation. If this is unsuccessful, removal **(enucleation)** of the injured eye may be necessary. Fortunately, immediate treatment with corticosteroids and antibiotics has significantly reduced the incidence of this complication.

Contusion injuries

Many eye injuries happen not from a sharp object striking the eye but from blunt trauma such as being hit in the eye by a fist, a soccer ball or a motor vehicle dashboard. With this type of injury, the eyelid and the surrounding tissue, including the intraorbital tissue, haemorrhages and becomes oedematous.

The simplest form of contusion injury is a "black eye". When this occurs, the eye globe should be inspected and vision assessed. The child should be asked if they are having any difficulty seeing and extraocular eye movements evaluated for adequate function. Children should be able to look up and down, left and right, upward obliquely and downward obliquely—the six cardinal positions of gaze (Kadappu, Silveira & Martin, 2013).

If there is no apparent eye injury, ocular movement is good and vision is normal (for that child), the only treatment necessary is an ice pack applied to the eye to minimise swelling (20 minutes on, 20 minutes off, and repeat). Reabsorption of haemorrhage in the tissue surrounding the eye will take place over the next 1 to 3 weeks. Often, tissue haemorrhage extends across the nose and surrounds the other eye the day after the injury. Parents and child should be educated that this is not a worsening of the condition but mainly evidence of the severity of the initial blow.

Limited eye movement or reports of diplopia (double vision) are strong evidence that a "blowout" fracture of the floor of the orbit (the maxillary bone) has occurred. This fracture line is trapping intraorbital tissue and preventing the eye globe from moving freely. These children should be referred to an ophthalmologist. Surgery is needed to free the entrapped tissue, prevent interference with vascular flow and restore normal eye movements.

After a blunt contusion to the eye globe, several serious findings in addition to limited motion may be present. These include disturbances of the pupil, such as a dilated, fixed or cloudy pupil; cloudy lens or cornea; loss of vision in the eye; and visible blood in the anterior chamber (hyphaema). These conditions may indicate dislocation of the lens or retinal detachment requiring immediate evaluation by an ophthalmologist.

Eyelid injuries

Eyelid injuries may accompany eye globe injuries or they may be the only finding present after a foreign body has struck the eye. Although such injuries appear to be trivial, the child should still be referred to an ophthalmologist for care. A deep laceration of the eyelid can cause a permanent ptosis. A laceration to the inner canthal area can disrupt the lacrimal drainage system (dacryostenosis).

INNER EYE CONDITIONS

Inner eye conditions are those that affect the lens, the retina or the aqueous humour.

Congenital glaucoma

Glaucoma is increased intraocular pressure (IOP) in the eye globe caused by inadequate or blocked drainage of the aqueous humour (Allingham, et al, 2012). Normally, aqueous humour, produced by the ciliary body, flows from the posterior chamber through the pupil to the anterior chamber and is excreted through the canal of Schlemm at the lateral angle into the venous circulation. In congenital glaucoma, a developmental anomaly in the angle of the anterior chamber prevents proper drainage into the canal (see Fig. 50.5). Later in life, glaucoma occurs when the canal becomes blocked. The increased fluid content that accumulates causes the globe of the eye to increase in size. After it has increased in size to the extent that it can, the pressure in the eye globe continues to rise, compressing and ultimately destroying the optic nerve.

Assessment

Although congenital glaucoma is a rare disease, all infants should be assessed for it because the disease accounts for vision disorders in 5–13% of children in schools for the visually challenged. In most infants the condition is bilateral and is caused by inheritance of a recessive gene. Symptoms begin to be noticeable shortly after birth; readily noticeable symptoms are apparent at 1 year of age. The condition occurs more often in girls than in boys (Strouthidis & Papadopoulos, 2013). Glaucoma can occur after eye trauma in older children if there is scarring at the canal of Schlemm.

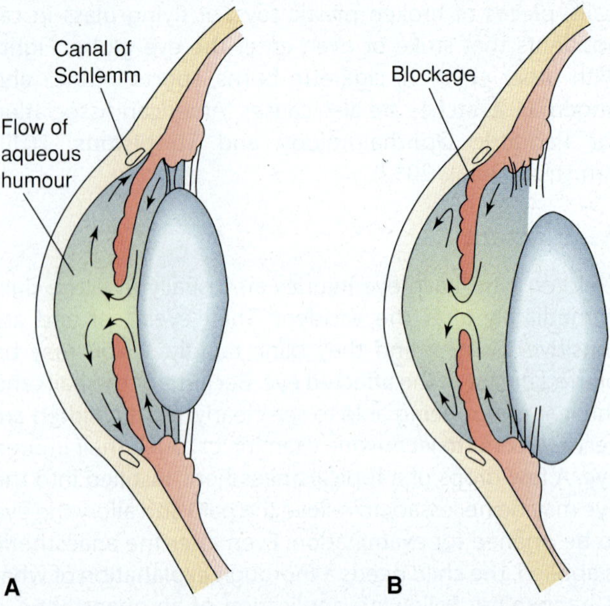

FIGURE 50.5 (**A**) Circulation of aqueous humour. (**B**) Blockage of canal of Schlemm in congenital glaucoma.

The cornea, which appears enlarged, may be oedematous and hazy. In addition, there may be tearing, pain and **photophobia** (sensitivity to light), all difficult to identify in a newborn. The eye globe may feel tense to finger palpation.

Eye pressure is measured by means of a *tonometer,* a pressure-sensitive device that is placed against the anterior eye globe and measures eye pressure by a beam of light directed towards the eye. Tension greater than the normal range of 12 to 20 mmHg is suggestive of glaucoma.

Therapeutic management

Immediate surgery—a **goniotomy** or trabeculotomy, in which a new opening to the canal of Schlemm is constructed—should be scheduled for the infant (Wiese, Heiligenhaus & Heinz, 2014). A medication such as carbonic anhydrase inhibitor that suppresses the formation of aqueous humour, may be used temporarily to reduce eye pressure before surgery can be scheduled. Newer surgical techniques include laser therapy (Song et al., 2013).

Before surgery, the infant should not receive any medication that dilates the pupil, because this will further occlude the canal of Schlemm. After surgery, rough play activities should be restricted for 1 week.

Cataracts

A *cataract* is marked opacity of the lens. This may be present at birth or it may become apparent in early childhood. Some children have cataracts as a dominantly inherited condition. They also can be caused by galactosaemia or inability to metabolise the lactose in milk (Ryan et al., 2013). A few children develop cataracts as a result of steroid use or radiation exposure. It can be caused by trauma to the eye if the lens is injured. If the opacity occurs on the anterior surface of the lens, the cause is thought to be birth injury or possibly contact between the lens and the cornea during intrauterine life. If the opacity is located at the edge of the lens, it may be a result of nutritional deficiency during intrauterine life, such as rickets or hypocalcaemia. Infants who contract rubella prenatally may develop opacity throughout the lens (McLean et al., 2012).

Assessment

In the pupil of a child with a cataract, the pupil opening appears to be white (leucocoria). The red reflex elicited by shining a light into the pupil appears white. Older children may report blurred vision because of cataract formation. In the infant, this can be detected by lack of response to a smile or inability to reach and grasp a nearby object. The infant may also demonstrate nystagmus, being unable to focus the eye on objects. A few other conditions, such as retinoblastoma, retinopathy of prematurity or an abscess of the posterior chamber, simulate this appearance. In congenital glaucoma, the lens may be opaque because of oedema. This can be differentiated from simple cataract by the accompanying enlargement of the eye and pupil opening.

Therapeutic management

Treatment of childhood cataract is surgical removal of the cloudy lens, followed by insertion of an internal intraocular lens. If the total lens is involved, this may be done as early as 3 months of age. If this is not done before 6 months of age, amblyopia may result.

With modern surgical techniques, the incision is so small that eye patching is not necessary. Infants may be given a sedative to help them rest for 24 hours. Fluids should be introduced cautiously after eye surgery so nausea and vomiting do not occur, as vomiting increases increased intraocular pressure (IOP), which could injure the suture line. Infants can be expected to have some discomfort but, in general, they should not have acute pain after surgery. If they are unusually restless or crying and seem to be in pain, notify the doctor immediately. Although this could be unrelated to the surgery, it may be a sign of increased IOP from haemorrhage or from occlusion of the canal of Schlemm, causing a developing glaucoma.

As a rule, children will be given a mydriatic agent to dilate the pupil and steroids to prevent postoperative development of pupillary adhesions. If the eye that had the cataract is now amblyopic, patching of the normal eye (as with usual amblyopia correction) may be necessary to restore vision.

Parents of children with congenital cataracts need support to carry out the procedures necessary and to give the long-term medication and corrective measures required. Outcome evaluation should include children's current vision status and also how they view themselves in light of this early vision problem.

✔ *Checkpoint question 50.2*

Ed is 5 years old and is to have corrective eye surgery for strabismus. Why would the prevention of vomiting from anaesthetic be a high priority?

a. Vomitus could be splashed into the eye.
b. Loss of sodium threatens the integrity of the new lens.
c. Vomiting increases IOP.
d. Loss of fluid causes the globe diameter to shrink.

THE CHILD UNDERGOING EYE SURGERY

Surgery for cataracts or glaucoma in childhood is usually performed during the infant period. Preparation for surgery, therefore, primarily consists of helping a baby to adjust to a strange environment and encouraging parents to spend as much time with the infant as possible. This is particularly important if the eyes will be patched after surgery. Surgery for strabismus is often done during the preschool period. The operation can be explained to the preschooler through the use of puppets or dolls. As with all surgical procedures, talk about the child's affected parts (in this case, the eyes) being "fixed" or "made better", never "cut".

When you meet children before surgery, be certain to speak with them enough so they will be able to recognise your voice afterwards. Practise having the child identify a parent's voice by covering the eyes and then guessing whether it is you or the parent who is speaking.

STRUCTURE AND FUNCTION OF THE EARS

Ear anatomy is shown in Figure 50.6. Most diseases of the ear in children involve the external and middle portions.

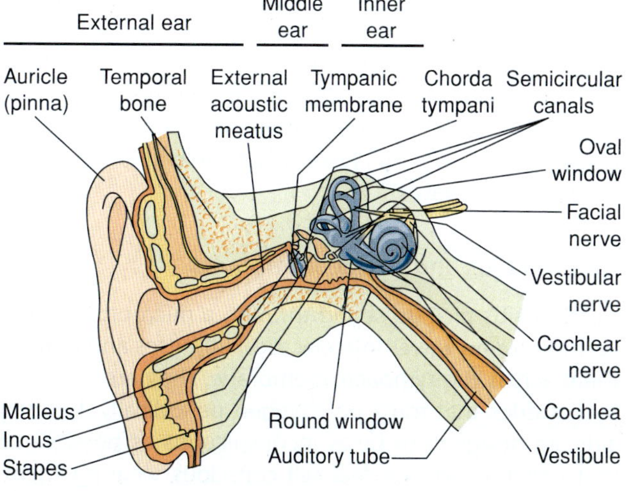

FIGURE 50.6 Structures of the ear.

Physiology of hearing loss

Hearing loss is termed a *conduction loss* if there is interference with sound reaching the inner ear (difficulty with the external canal, the tympanic membrane or the ossicles). It is termed *nerve* or *sensorineural loss* if the inner ear or the eighth cranial nerve is affected. Conduction loss can occur if the external canal is obstructed with cerumen (wax) or a foreign object, if the tympanic membrane is damaged or immobile, or if the middle ear is filled with fluid, as occurs in *serous otitis media.* Sensorineural loss results from diseases that affect the transmission of sound sensation to the cerebral cortex or from a pathological condition of the cochlea. In children, this condition is usually congenital, although it can occur after drug therapy or an infection such as meningitis. It can also occur from exposure to loud sound (Henderson, Testa & Hartnick, 2011).

Because the diseases that lead to inherited hearing challenge tend to be autosomal dominant, there is a strong chance that they will occur in future siblings of the hearing-challenged child.

Hearing impairment

Hearing impairment occurs in many different degrees and is rated by level of severity. In Australia, for every 10,000 births between 9 and 12 children will be born with a moderate or greater hearing loss in both ears and a further 23 children per 10,000 will acquire a hearing impairment that requires hearing aids by the age of 17, either through accident, illness or other causes (Australian Hearing, 2011). Treacher Collins syndrome, otosclerosis, osteogenesis imperfecta and Waardenburg's syndrome, all transmitted by autosomal dominant inheritance, are examples of disorders that result in congenital deafness. Prenatal rubella infection accounts for another large percentage. Causes of slight hearing impairment include serous otitis media, trauma from such things as inflating airbags and untreated acute otitis media with rupture of the tympanic membrane.

Children with congenital hearing impairment should be enrolled in special programs for hearing-challenged children as soon as the hearing loss is discovered (Australian Hearing, 2013). This early exposure is necessary so that the child can learn effective speech. For children who have conductive losses, an improvement in hearing usually can be achieved by use of a hearing aid (which intensifies the level of sound waves).

Hearing aids and cochlear implants

Hearing aids pick up sound through a microphone, convert the sound waves into electrical impulses and amplify them across the tympanic membrane. They are powered by batteries that must be changed periodically. Hearing aids are designed to be as inconspicuous as possible so that children will not feel self-conscious wearing them. The receiver of the hearing aid may be incorporated into eyeglasses, moulded into a plastic form that fits behind or in the ear, or housed in a small box that children wear on a cord around their neck or carry in a blouse or shirt pocket.

Cochlear implants are mechanical devices consisting of a microphone, a speech processor, a transmitter/receiver and an arrangement of electrodes that send impulses from the receiver to the auditory nerve. The auditory nerve then transmits the impulses to the brain where they are interpreted as words or common noises. Cochlear implants have the potential to replace a non-functioning inner ear and create the ability to receive and interpret sounds in an ear that has sustained nerve damage (Cochlear Australia/New Zealand, 2015). The implant consists of an external portion that sits behind the ear and a second portion that is surgically implanted under the skin. After implantation, hearing is often reported as "muffled" but adequate. Months of training are necessary to help a child interpret these distorted impulses correctly.

Speech therapy

If children who are hearing challenged are to interact as fully as possible with the world around them, they need an intensive program of speech therapy. Some therapists believe that learning sign language early is helpful because it allows children to express their needs early. Others believe that by learning sign language, children decrease their need to learn to articulate speech sounds or to lip read and, for this reason, learning sign language should not be encouraged. It is true that, for real independence and to perform in regular school classes, children need to communicate by means other than sign language. For children with a profound impairment, however, learning speech sounds may be a long-term process, making sign language necessary for contact with the world around them until they can learn to speak.

DISORDERS OF THE EAR

Ear disorders are always serious in children, because hearing is such an important function for the growing child.

External otitis

External otitis (otitis externa) is inflammation of the external ear canal. Although external ear inflammation rarely threatens hearing or causes permanent damage, it does cause discomfort in the form of itching and sometimes extreme pain.

Assessment

The history of children with external otitis usually reveals that they have recently been swimming, which is why this condition is popularly called *swimmer's ear.* It can also occur if a young child pushes a foreign object, such as a peanut, into the ear canal. Unlike middle ear infection (otitis media), there is no history of a recent respiratory infection. Children first notice itching of the canal, then pain. When the external ear is touched, the pain becomes acute. The moisture in the canal left from swimming has caused inflammation; a secondary infection then occurs in the closed space. *Pseudomonas* and *Candida* are agents frequently involved in these infections. Otoscopic examination may indicate only the sharply localised, tender swelling of a furuncle, or the entire canal may be swollen shut and tender to the touch. If a fungal infection is present, the entire canal may appear brown or black. If the inflammation is from a foreign body, such as a peanut or the tip of a cotton applicator, white or grey debris may surround the object; the skin under the object will be moist, red and eroded.

In otitis externa, the tympanic membrane must be visualised to ensure that there is no extension of the external otitis into the middle ear (Koch, 2012). In some instances, the eardrum is so inflamed from the external infectious process that it is difficult to tell whether the middle ear is free of disease. Before the tympanic membrane can be visualised, it is often necessary to remove superficial debris from the canal. A Weber test should show that hearing is equal in both ears. A tuning fork vibration that sounds louder in the affected ear suggests that otitis media (middle ear infection) is present.

Therapeutic management

The treatment of otitis externa differs according to the organism causing the infection. If the canal is so swollen that ear drops cannot flow back into the canal, use of an ear wick allows for effective delivery of medication into a swollen and narrow auditory canal.

Most doctors prescribe a combination of drugs to manage otitis externa. For example, hydrocortisone reduces inflammation and antibiotic or antifungal preparations reduce the infection. Some ear drops have an additional alcohol base, which serves to dry the external canal further. If ear pain is present, an analgesic may be necessary to control discomfort. Children must keep the ear canal dry, avoiding swimming and hair washing during this time. If they shower, they should first insert ear plugs into the external meatus, to keep out moisture.

Impacted cerumen

Cerumen (earwax) serves the important function of cleansing the external ear canal as it gradually moves outward, bringing with it shed epithelial cells and any foreign objects. Wax accumulation rarely is extensive enough to interfere with hearing. Cerumen serves a protective function, however, so should not be removed routinely. Caution parents not to clean the child's ears with cotton-tipped applicators as a regular practice, because they may scratch the ear canal, causing an invasion site for a secondary infection. This practice may also push accumulated cerumen farther into the ear canal, causing a true plugging of wax.

Commercial softeners are available if cerumen accumulates to such an extent that hearing is affected.

Acute otitis media

Inflammation of the middle ear (otitis media) is the most prevalent disease of childhood after respiratory tract infections (The Royal Children's Hospital Melbourne, 2015). In Australia, the incidence of otitis media is significantly higher among Indigenous children for whom it represents a serious health and educational issue (Australian Hearing, 2011). There is also a higher incidence of otitis media in formula-fed infants than those who are breastfed. This is due to the fact that formula-fed infants are held in a more slanted position while feeding and this allows milk to enter the eustachian tube. Otitis media is also associated with constant dummy use and is higher in homes in which a parent smokes cigarettes (Jones et al., 2012; Kong & Coates, 2009).

Otitis media is an extremely serious disease of childhood, because permanent damage can occur to middle ear structures leading to hearing impairment.

Assessment

Acute otitis media usually occurs after a respiratory tract infection. Children have a "cold", rhinitis, and perhaps, a low-grade fever for several days. Suddenly, they develop a high temperature and a sharp, constant pain in one or both ears. Older children can verbalise reports of pain. Infants become extremely irritable and frequently pull or tug at the affected ear in an attempt to gain relief from pain. The external canal is usually free of wax because the warmth of the inflammation and fever melts the wax and moves it more readily out of the canal. In contrast to an external ear canal infection, the discomfort does not increase on manipulation of the auricle. It is important that the mastoid process behind the ear does not feel tender to touch. If it does, the infection probably has spread out of the middle ear into the mastoid cells, a very serious complication.

Therapeutic management

Most middle ear infections are caused by *Streptococcus pneumoniae, Haemophilus influenzae* (especially in children younger than 5 years) or *Streptococcus pyogenes*. Doctors will generally prescribe an antibiotic as well as an analgesic and antipyretic. Some healthcare providers may prescribe decongestant nose drops to open the eustachian tubes and allow air to be admitted to the middle ear. Although not proved, this may be helpful in preventing the infection from becoming a serious or long-term otitis media. Nasal decongestant drops are usually given for only 3 days. If they are given longer, a rebound effect may occur, causing oedema and a subsequent increase in mucous membrane inflammation.

During the course of otitis media, most children have a conductive hearing loss; this may last up to 6 months after an acute infection. It is important to educate parents about this, so they will not think the infection is growing worse, if they first notice the impairment after they arrive home. They also need to know about the possible hearing loss, so that if the child is routinely screened for hearing in school during the next 6 months, they can account for the loss. If a child still has a conductive hearing loss after 6 months (or has other symptoms), the child should be examined again to see whether a new infection or serous otitis media is present.

Otitis media with effusion

Otitis media with effusion is a result of chronic otitis media. Normally, the middle ear is an air-filled cavity with air being supplied to it by the eustachian tube. The tube opens with swallowing, yawning or chewing. If this source of air to the middle ear is shut off, the epithelial cells of the middle ear change in function, becoming secretory cells. The middle ear fills with these secretions. Over time the fluid becomes so thick and tenacious that it is described as "gluelike". Some children notice a feeling of fullness or the sound of popping or ringing in their ears. There may be a drop in hearing of 20 to 40 decibels because of the fluid content. Because the loss is gradual, parents and children may not be aware of it, until it is noticed on a routine hearing screening. Involvement is usually bilateral. The condition occurs most frequently in children 3 to 10 years of age (Williamson, 2011).

Assessment

With otitis media with effusion, a child experiences muffled hearing and a feeling of pressure in the ear. Examination of the ears may show a level of fluid behind the tympanic membrane. However, a fluid line will be visible only if there is also a quantity of air in the middle ear to contrast with it. As the collected fluid becomes thick, it tends to retract the eardrum. This makes the malleus more prominent and perhaps displaced to a horizontal angle as the membrane is retracted around it; the light reflex from the otoscope light becomes distorted. If a pneumatic otoscope is used, gentle introduction of air against the eardrum produces no movement of the tympanic membrane (as there would be normally).

Therapeutic management

Therapy for otitis media with effusion may be long term. If the condition appears to be intensified by inflammation from an allergy, measures to control the allergy must be initiated. These may include avoidance of the allergen, hyposensitisation or pharmacological alteration of the allergic response. Treatment of children with allergies is discussed in Chapter 42.

Definitive medical treatment is aimed at supplying air to the middle ear. For mild involvement, the daily administration of an antihistamine or a nasal decongestant to shrink the mucous membrane of the eustachian tube may be enough to achieve an air supply. In a few children, the eustachian tube is blocked by enlarged adenoids, and

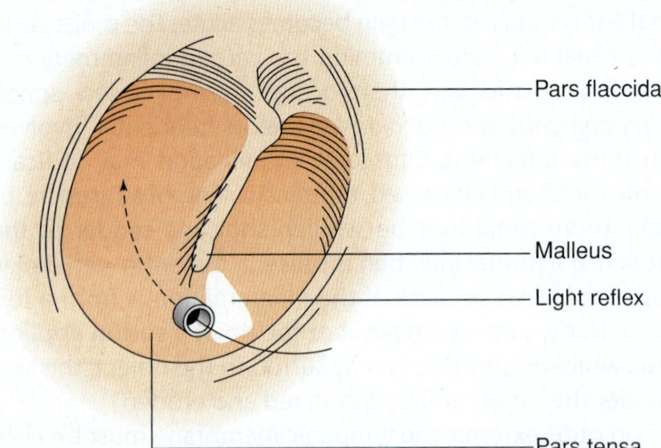

FIGURE 50.7 A myringotomy tube provides air to the middle ear to prevent otitis media with effusion.

their removal is indicated. Fluid from the middle ear can be removed by **tympanocentesis** (a needle inserted through the tympanic membrane); this usually returns, however, unless some intervention to introduce air to the middle ear (tubal myringotomy) is undertaken.

Tubal myringotomy

A source of air can be supplied to the middle ear by the insertion of small plastic (Teflon) tubes (grommets) inserted through the tympanic membrane (tympanostomy). The insertion of such tubes is done after a myringotomy at a point in the tympanic membrane that is not instrumental for hearing, so they do not interfere with hearing (see Fig. 50.7). Tubes tend to be extruded after 6 to 12 months. For many children, this period is long enough to halt the secretory process of the middle ear. In others, tubes must be reinserted to continue the aeration.

When myringotomy tubes are in place, water should not be allowed to enter the child's ears. Most doctors prefer children to bathe rather than shower, but showering may be allowed if ear plugs are used. Hair washing should be done with ear plugs in place. Similarly, swimming is either contraindicated or allowed only with ear plugs in place.

Cholesteatoma

Cholesteatoma is a lesion of the pars flaccida or upper portion of the tympanic membrane. A retraction cyst forms and there is necrosis of the pars flaccida with foul-smelling drainage from the ear. If the retraction cyst is not discovered and surgically removed at this point, it grows gradually deeper and deeper, until it eventually invades the mastoid cells. It can progress to mastoiditis, meningitis and possibly facial nerve paralysis if it is not surgically removed (Diom et al., 2013).

Any child with foul-smelling drainage from the ear should be referred to a doctor for further investigation to rule out this problem.

CASE STUDY QUESTION

3. Amy is diagnosed as having otitis media. When interpreting the documentation in Amy's electronic health record, you should be cognisant that this diagnosis differs from otitis externa in what way?

a. Otitis media occurs from swimming; otitis externa typically follows a common cold.
b. Otitis media involves the middle ear; otitis externa involves the outer canal.
c. Otitis media involves the eardrum; otitis externa involves the cochlear nerve.
d. Otitis media does not cause pain; otitis externa produces throbbing pain.

THE HOSPITALISED CHILD WITH HEARING IMPAIRMENT

A hearing loss greater than 49 decibels is sufficient enough to interfere with hearing normal conversation and developing language. Like visually challenged children, children with hearing loss may be hospitalised for other health problems. It can be difficult for parents to prepare children who cannot hear for hospitalisation. Words such as *surgery, tonsils, hurts, operating room* and *recovery room* are new to them. Showing the child a book with good pictures demonstrating what is going to happen is helpful. Allowing children time to play with dolls or puppets can help them understand hospital routine. Because children who are hearing challenged may not be as well prepared for hospitalisation as those without a hearing impairment, efforts should be made, on admission, to ensure that they receive such instruction.

Always allow hearing-challenged children to see you before you touch them as they will not find this nearly as intrusive as being touched without warning. If children are sleeping when you approach them, use a light touch to waken them gently. Some children turn off their hearing aid or remove it while they sleep. You may need to turn it on before you call them to wake them or they may need to replace the hearing aid as soon as they awaken. Children as young as 2 years of age are effective lip readers as long as you are facing them. Position yourself at eye level, so the child can view your face. In a group, help the child follow conversation by directing him to the person who is speaking. Assigning consistent staff members is also useful.

It is important not to underestimate the intelligence level of hearing-challenged children. Due to the fact they do not speak clearly, incorrect assumptions can be made regarding their cognitive status. As a result, they may not be given information that the average hearing child receives, such as explanations of how things work. In a hospital ward, hearing-challenged children, locked in a silent world, are unable to express how they feel about procedures. They need help from healthcare personnel who understand this and take more than the usual amount of time to offer them explanations and support.

Ask parents of children who are hearing challenged to draw pictures or demonstrate the sign language symbols their children use for important words such as *pain, drink* and *toilet*. Encourage children to use or draw pictures of what they want if they are still too young to write words and you cannot understand what they are saying.

Hearing-challenged children have the right to be provided with a sign language interpreter during care. Advocate for this, especially if the parents will not be present during care.

As the entire family is affected through illness and subsequent hospital and clinic appointments, especially chronic conditions, it is important for nurses to review the implications the medical issue may have upon siblings. The child diagnosed may receive more attention and more gifts; for some children the attention given to the "ill" child may evoke jealousy or resentment. They may feel lonely or worried. Encouraging the spending of time with the family rather than gifts is important and also having special time for the well sibling. Involving social workers and also engaging and acknowledging the entire family and friends is important to ensure the health issue dealt with does not become worse due to other inter-personal family issues.

In conducting the family assessment it may be advisable to incorporate the Australian Family Strengths Nursing Assessment Guide to review the strengths, weaknesses and support required for that particular family (Smith, 2008).

✔ *Checkpoint question* 50.3

The parents of a child displaying hearing issues do not wish their child to have treatment as they feel it will "sort itself out". What are your obligations?

Key points for review

- Refractive errors of vision such as myopia and hyperopia are the most common eye disorders in children. Amblyopia (lazy eye) is subnormal vision in one eye. Children with these disorders need correction at the time the disorder is recognised to prevent further vision distortion.
- Coloboma is congenital incomplete closure of the pupil or lower eyelid. Ptosis is the inability to open the upper eyelid normally. Ptosis needs correction to avoid development of amblyopia. Strabismus is unequally aligned eyes. Like ptosis, it can lead to amblyopia if not corrected.
- Eye injuries such as penetration by a foreign body need follow-up after treatment to be certain that vision remains adequate.
- Children who are either vision or hearing challenged need special preparation and orientation for hospital.
- Otitis media (middle ear infection) is a common childhood illness. Some children who have otitis media with effusion have myringotomy tubes inserted to relieve pressure and supply air access to the middle ear.

Critical thinking exercises

1. List the key factors you need to be aware of when assessing a child's eyesight or hearing.
2. Describe to whom you might refer parents of a child with hearing or visual issues.
3. What might be the outcome for a child who does not obtain assistance in regards to hearing or visual issues?

Resources

For an extensive range of additional resources to enhance teaching and learning and to facilitate understanding of this chapter, please see the text's accompanying website located on thePoint at http://thepoint.lww.com.

References

Allingham, R. R., Damji, K. F., Freedman, S. F., Moroi, S. E., Rhee, D. J. & Shields, M. B. (2012). *Shields Textbook of Glaucoma*. Philadelphia: Lippincott Williams & Wilkins.

American Association for Pediatric Ophthalmology and Strabismus. (2011). Pediatric occular trauma. Accessed 4 March 2015, <www.aapos.org/terms/conditions/135>.

Armstrong, G. W., Kim, J. G., Linakis, J. G., Mello, M. J. & Greenberg, P.B. (2012). Pediatric eye injuries presenting to United States emergency departments 2001–2007. *Graefe's Archive for Clinical and Experimental Opthamology*. *251*(3), 629–636.

Australian Government Department of Health, (2014). Healthy kids check fact sheet. Accessed 4 March 2015, <www.health.gov.au/internet/main/publishing.nsf/Content/health_Kids_Check_factsheet>.

Australian Government Department of Social Services. (2012). Remote hearing and vision services for children. Accessed 4 March 2015, <www.dss.gov.au/our-responsibilities/disability-and-carers/program-services/for-people-with-disability/remote-hearing-and-vision-services-for-children>.

Australian Hearing. (2011). *Australian Hearing Annual Report 2011*. Accessed 30 March 2015, <www.hearing.com.au/wp-content/uploads/2013/09/Australian-Hearing-Annual-Report-2011.pdf>.

Australian Hearing. (2013). Who is eligible for Australian Hearing Services? Accessed 4 March 2015, <www.hearing.com.au/eligible-australian-hearing-services>.

Australian Institute of Health and Welfare. (2013). National performance indicators for neonatal hearing screening in Australia. Accessed 4 March 2015, <www.aihw.gov.au/WorkArea/DownloadAsset.aspx?id=60129545175>.

Cochlear Australia/New Zealand. (2015). Cochlear implants & cochlear implant technology. Accessed 4 March 2015, <www.cochlear.com/wps/wcm/connect/au/home/understand/hearing-and-hl/hl-treatments/cochlear-implant>.

Council of Australian Governments. (2009). Protecting children is everyone's business. National framework for protecting Australia's children 2009–2020. Accessed 4 March 2015, <www.communities.qld.gov.au/resources/childsafety/child-protection/national-framework.pdf>.

Diom, E. S., Cisse, Z., Tall, A., Ndiaye, M., Pegbessou, E., Ndiaye, I. C., et al. (2013). Management of acquired cholesteatoma in children: A 15 year review in ENT service of CHNU de FANN Dakar. *International Journal of Pediatric Otorhinolaryngology*, *77*(12), 1998–2003.

Donahue, S. P. (2007). Paediatric strabismus. *New England Journal of Medicine, 356*(10), 1040–1047.

Government of Western Australia. (2011). Colour blindness. Accessed 4 March 2015, <www.health.wa.gov.au/docreg/Education/Population%5CChild_Health%5CIllnesses_and_Health_Problems%5CHP8856_colour_blindness.pdf>.

Henderson, E., Testa, M. A. & Hartnick, C. (2011). Prevalence of noise-induced hearing-threshold shifts and hearing loss among US youths. *Pediatrics*, *127*(1), e39–e46.

Holmes, J. M., Lazar, E. L., Melia, B., et al. (2011). Effect of age on response to amblyopia treatment in children. *Arch Ophthalmol*, *129*(11), 1451–1457.

Hopkins, S., Sampson, G., Hendicott, P. L. & Wood, J. M. (2013). Review of guidelines for children's vision screenings. *Clinical and Experimental Optometry*, *96*(5), 443–449.

Huang, J., Maguire, M. G., Ciner, E., Kulp, M. T., Cyert, L. A., Quinn, G. E., et al. (2014). Risk factors for astigmatism in the vision in preschoolers study. *Optometry & Vision Science*, *91*(5), 514–521.

Jones, L. L., Hassanien, A., Cook., D. G., Britton, J. & Leonardi-Bee, J. (2012). Parental smoking and the risk of middle ear disease in children: A systematic review and meta-analysis. *Archives of Pediatrir and Adolescent Medicine*. *166*(1), 18–27.

Kadappu, S., Silveira, S. & Martin, F. (2013). Aetiology and outcome of open and closed globe eye injuries in children. *Clinical & Experimental Ophthalmology*, *41*(5), 427–434.

Koch, K. (2012). Managing otitis externa: Review. *SA Pharmaceutical Journal*, *79*(8), 17–22.

Kong, K. & Coates, L. C. (2009). Natural history, definitions, risk factors and burden of otitis media. *Medical Journal of Australia*, *191*(9), 39.

Lai, K. L., Ng, J. Y. & Srinivasan, S. (2014). Xerophthalmia and keratomalacia secondary to diet-induced vitamin A deficiency in Scottish adults. *Canadian Journal of Ophthalmology/Journal Canadien d'Ophtalmologie*, *49*(1), 109–112.

Lions Eye Institute. (2013). Strabismus. Accessed 4 March 2015, <www.lei.org.au/services/eye-conditions/strabismus>.

McLean, H., Redd, S., Abernathy, E., Icenogle, J. & Wallace, G. (2012). Congenital rubella syndrome. *Centers for Disease Control and Prevention, Manual for the Surveillance of Vaccine-Preventable Diseases* (5th ed.), Atlanta, GA: Centers for Disease Control and Prevention.

Morgan, I. G., Ohno-Matsui, K. & Saw, S-M. (2012). Myopia. *The Lancet*, *379*(9827), 1739–1748.

National Children's Vision Screening Project. (2009). Final Report. Accessed 4 March 2015, <www.rch.org.au/uploadedFiles/Main/Content/ccch/Vision_Screening_Final_Report_May_2009.pdf>.

NSW Department of Health. (2012a). Statewide eyesight preschooler screening (StEPS) program. Accessed on 4 March 2015, <www.health.nsw.gov.au/policies/pd/2012/PD2012_001.html>.

NSW Department of Health. (2012b). Statewide infant screening - hearing (SWISH) program. Accessed 17 June 2015, <www0.health.nsw.gov.au/policies/gl/2010/GL2010_002.html>.

O'Dowd, C. (2013). Evaluating squints in children. *Australian Family Physician*, *42*(12), 872–874.

O'Keefe, M. & Kirwan, C. (2010). Laser epithelial keratomileusis in 2010–a review. *Clinical & Experimental Ophthalmology*, *38*(2), 183–191.

Pan, C. K. & Oliver, S.C.N. (2011). Evaluation of poor vision. *Berman's Pediatric Decision Making*, 380.

Ryan, E. L., Lynch, M. E., Taddeo, E., Gleason, T. J., Epstein, M. P. & Fridovich-Keil, J. L. (2013). Cryptic residual GALT activity is a potential modifier of scholastic outcome in school age children with classic galactosemia. *Journal of Inherited Metabolic Disease, 36*(6), 1049–1061.

Sininger, Y. S., Grimes, A. & Christensen, E. (2010). Auditory development in early amplified children: Factors influencing auditory-based communication outcomes in children with hearing loss. *Ear and Hearing*, *31*(2), 166.

Smith, L. M. (2008). Conducting a family strengths assessment using the AFS nursing assessment guide. Accessed 4 March 2015, <http://eprints.utas.edu.au/9486/1/How_to_conduct_family_assessment_using_the__AFS_nursing_assessment.pdf>.

Song, J., Song, A., Palmares, T. & Song, M. (2013). Selective laser trabeculoplasty success in pediatric patients with glaucoma: Two case reports. *Journal of Medical Case Reports*, *7*(1), 198.

Strouthidis, N. G. & Papadopoulos, M. (2013). Clinical evaluation of glaucoma in children. *Current Ophthalmology Reports*, *1*(2), 106–112.

Tasman, W. & Jaeger, E. A. (1996). *Willis Eye Hospital Atlas of Clinical Ophthalmology*. Philadelphia: Lippincott-Raven Publishers.

The Royal Children's Hospital Melbourne, (2015). Acute eye injuries in children. Accessed 4 March 2015, <www.rch.org.au/clinicalguide/guideline_index/Acute_eye_injuries_in_children>.

The Royal Children's Hospital Melbourne, (2015). Acute otitis media. Accessed 4 March 2015, <www.rch.org.au/clinicalguide/guideline_index/Acute_Otitis_Media>.

West, S. & Williams, C. (2011). Amblyopia. *Clinical Evidence, 2011*(0709).

Western Australian Government. (2012). Enhanced Aboriginal child health schedule rationale Document 2012. Child and adolescent community health statewide policy. Accessed 4 March 2015, <www.pmh.health.wa.gov.au/general/CACH/docs/manual/3%20Birth%20to%20School%20Entry/3.2/3.2.4_Enhanced_Aboriginal_Child_Health_Schedule_Rationale.pdf>.

Wiese, K., Heiligenhaus, A. & Heinz, C. (2014). Trabeculectomy in uveitis associated with juvenile idiopathic arthritis: Long-term results in pediatric secondary glaucoma. *Ophthalmologe, 111*(4), 330–338.

Williamson, I. (2011). Otitis media with effusion in children. *Clinical Evidence (online)*, 2011:0502.

Women and Newborn Health Service King Edward Memorial Hospital. (2013). Eye infections in the newborn. Accessed 4 March 2015, <http://kemh.health.wa.gov.au/development/manuals/O&G_guidelines/sectionb/10/b10.5.1.1.pdf>.

World Health Organization. (2010). Action plan for the prevention of avoidable blindness and visual impairment 2009–2013. Accessed 4 March 2015, <www.who.int/blindness/ACTION_PLAN_WHA62-1-English.pdf?ua=1>.

Suggested readings

Australian Hearing <www.hearing.com.au>.

Australian Research Alliance for Children & Youth (ARACY) <www.aracy.org.au>.

Jacoby, P., Carville, K. S., Hall, G., Riley, T. V., Bowman, J., Leach, A. J. & Kalgoorlie Otitis Media Research Project Team. (2011). Crowding and other strong predictors of upper respiratory tract carriage of otitis media-related bacteria in Australian Aboriginal and non-Aboriginal children. *The Pediatric Infectious Disease Journal, 30*(6), 480–485.

Johnson, N. L., Lashley, J., Stonek, A. V., et al. (2012). Children with developmental disabilities at a pediatric hospital: Staff education to prevent and manage challenging behaviors. *Journal of Pediatric Nursing, 27*(6), 742–749.

Lieu, J. E., Tye-Murray, N., Karzon, R. K. & Piccirillo, J. F. (2010). Unilateral hearing loss is associated with worse speech-language scores in children. *Pediatrics, 125*(6), e1348–e1355.

Vision Australia <www.visionaustralia.org>.

Chapter 51

Nursing care of a family when a child has a musculoskeletal disorder

Previous chapters described the growth and development of well children and the nursing care of children with a disorder of other body systems. This chapter adds information about the dramatic changes, both physical and psychosocial, that can occur when a child develops a musculoskeletal disorder.

LEARNING OBJECTIVES

After mastering the contents of this chapter, you should be able to:

1. Describe common musculoskeletal disorders in children.
2. Use critical thinking to analyse ways that care of a child with a musculoskeletal disorder can be more family-centred.
3. Assess a child with a musculoskeletal disorder.
4. Establish expected outcomes for a child with a musculoskeletal disorder.
5. Plan nursing care for a child with a musculoskeletal disorder.
6. Implement nursing care, such as supplying age-appropriate diversional activities, for a child with a musculoskeletal disorder.
7. Evaluate expected outcomes for achievement and effectiveness of care.
8. Identify areas related to care of a child with a musculoskeletal disorder that could benefit from additional nursing research or application of evidence-based practice.
9. Integrate knowledge of musculoskeletal disorders with nursing process to achieve quality child and family nursing care.

KEY TERMS

- apposition
- arthroscopy
- cartilage
- compartment syndrome
- diaphysis
- distraction
- epiphyseal plate
- epiphysis
- fracture
- malleoli
- metaphysis
- myopathy
- periosteum
- remodelling
- resorption
- sequestrum
- sprain
- strain
- traction

CASE STUDY

Will, a 13-year-old boy with scoliosis, is brought to a clinic today because he has pain in his left lower leg. He has a fever, and his leg is warm to the touch and oedematous. His mother tells you he had an infected mosquito bite in that area 2 weeks ago. After further evaluation, Will is diagnosed with osteomyelitis. His mother asks, "How could he get an infection all the way into his bone from such a simple thing? I thought he was just having growing pains".

CASE STUDY QUESTIONS

1. What does Will's mother need to know about bone infections?
2. How would you explain to her what has happened?

The skeletal system, composed of more than 200 bones connected by the joints and tendons, provides a structural casing or protective armour for the internal organs of the body. Skeletal muscles, which are attached to the bones by connective tissue, tendons and ligaments, allow for voluntary movement, including gross motor activity, such as running, and fine motor activity, such as writing. Together, the skeletal and muscular systems support the body and make coordinated movement possible.

Because their bones and muscles are still growing, children suffer from disorders of the musculoskeletal system more frequently than do adults. On the other hand, because bones are still growing, **fractures** (breaks in the continuity or structure of bone) heal much quicker in children than in adults. Injuries that might be simple in an adult become serious in a child; if a growth plate is injured bone growth is halted. Because many musculoskeletal system disorders lead to problems with locomotion and associated limitations of activity, they can threaten a child's ability to develop optimally in other ways. Children gain much of their knowledge by interacting with people and exploring their environment so any self-limiting problem of movement can become a serious impairment. Nurses, along with other allied health staff such as occupational therapists and physiotherapists, play a key role in teaching parents ways to expose their children to the same sorts of stimuli that might be experienced if a child were able to move around independently. Much of this can be achieved by early intervention programs.

CARE OF A CHILD WITH A MUSCULOSKELETAL DISORDER

Assessment

Unlike many other diseases in children, disorders of the skeletal system usually manifest with specific, localised symptoms resulting in parents bringing children to healthcare facilities early in the course of an illness. On the other hand, disorders of the muscles or joints such as juvenile rheumatoid arthritis (JA) may manifest insidiously; when the disorder is diagnosed, parents may feel guilty for not having sought healthcare earlier.

The way that parents and children react to the diagnosis of a musculoskeletal disorder can be culturally influenced. Because an adolescent culture is often one that respects athletics, beauty and conformity, it can be a very difficult time for an adolescent to maintain positive body image and self-esteem when a musculoskeletal disorder is present.

One condition whose seriousness parents may underestimate is a childhood limp. A limp is never normal and it may be the first manifestation of a serious hip or knee problem. When weighing or measuring children at healthcare visits, take the opportunity to assess gait (whether a child walks naturally or stiffly, on tiptoes or on the whole foot; whether the feet are in good alignment; whether the back is held straight). Such assessments may detect that a child brought to a healthcare centre because of an upper respiratory condition, for example, has another, perhaps more important, musculoskeletal problem requiring evaluation. Because scoliosis is a common spinal deformity requiring early detection, school nurses have direct responsibility for instituting scoliosis screening programs in their schools. Skeletal injuries can also be a sign of abuse so careful history taking is necessary to rule out this possibility.

Nursing considerations

The nursing considerations most frequently identified for children with musculoskeletal disorders include those associated with pain, lack of mobility and resultant need for diversional activities. Children, especially adolescents, who require any form of mobility aid in skeletal support or locomotion, may encounter problems with self-esteem. Examples of some typical nursing diagnoses are:

- Pain related to chronic inflammation of joints
- Impaired physical mobility related to limb immobilisation, for example, cast on leg
- Deficient diversional activity related to need for imposed activity restriction for several weeks
- Situational low self-esteem related to continuous use of visible aid such as a body brace.

Many musculoskeletal problems in children require long-term care. Despite current therapies, some disorders may leave a child with a permanent disability. Before a child is discharged from an ambulatory or inpatient setting, help the parents to plan how they will care for the child at home. The often lengthy time periods associated with the treatment of musculoskeletal conditions frequently results in the physical and psychological impact of treatment evolving as time progresses. For example, initially a cast on an arm seems exciting to a school-age child: it is something to show off, an injury to describe or an excuse not to write at school. After a few days, the cast may become more frustrating than enjoyable. Take the time to review what wearing the cast will mean to the child in everyday situations. For example, the cast may not fit through school uniform shirts with tight cuffs. Planning transportation may be a problem if the child has a large cast and is not able to fit in a car seat. If the child must stay home from school, plans for tutoring need to be made. If both parents work outside their home, childcare may be necessary.

Depending on the child's and family's circumstances, the answers to these problems differ. However, taking the time to sit down with the parents and asking them whether these concerns will pose problems initiates problem solving. Doing so helps parents prepare solutions with a concerned person rather than by themselves at home.

Referrals to appropriate organisations may be helpful. Examples of organisations that can be used for referral include Arthritis Australia <www.arthritisaustralia.com.au>, Muscular Dystrophy Australia <www.mda. org.au> and Osteogenesis Imperfecta Society of Australia <www.oiaustralia.org.au>.

Many nursing interventions for children with musculoskeletal disorders involve care of a child in a cast or in **traction** (treatment involving pulling on a body part in one direction against a counterpull exerted in the opposite direction) or teaching about common concerns, such as posture or children's shoes. Parents and children who are kept well informed in these matters are much more likely to be able to cope with changing circumstances.

Children with musculoskeletal disorders invariably need follow-up care after discharge from an ambulatory visit or inpatient care because bone healing can be a slow process. Both parents and children may need support at re-evaluation visits when learning that a cast or brace must stay on longer or that they must continue exercises. Praise for their management thus far is an effective intervention for helping parents realise that they can cope with the situation in the future.

During re-evaluation visits, spend time assessing children's body image and self-esteem. Do children view themselves as basically well persons who, by the way, have a right leg shorter than the left leg, or as deformed persons who are inferior to others? Success of treatment is incomplete if a child's self-concept is diminished. Some examples indicating achievement of outcomes are:

- Child states he feels no pain or numbness in extremity after application of a cast
- Child demonstrates allowable weight-bearing activities with casted lower extremity
- Parents accurately state child's care needs both in and out of the hospital
- Child states positive aspects of self, participates in activities, establishes friendships with peers.

THE MUSCULOSKELETAL SYSTEM

Bones and bone growth

Bones are generally classified by their shape as long, short, flat or irregular. Long bones are the bones of the extremities, including the fingers and toes, in which most childhood bone disorders are found. The short bones are those found in the ankle and wrist. Flat bones are found in the skull, ribs, scapula and clavicle. Irregular bones are found in the vertebrae, the pelvis and the facial bones of the skull.

Long bones are composed of a long central shaft (the **diaphysis**), a rounded end portion (the **epiphysis**) and a thin area between them (the **metaphysis**; see Fig. 51.1). Increase in the length of long bones occurs at the cartilage segment (the **epiphyseal plate**), between the epiphysis and the metaphysis. As **cartilage** (connective tissue) cells grow away from the shaft, they are replaced by bone, thereby increasing bone length. Injury to this area in a growing child is always potentially serious because it may halt growth, stimulate abnormal growth or cause irregular or erratic growth. The central shafts of long bones are covered by an outer sensitive layer of **periosteum**. Bone width increases by growth at the inner surface of the periosteum. Injury to the periosteum, such as may occur with osteomyelitis, can also threaten bone growth (Hellmann & Imboden, 2009).

Although it is easy to think of bones as rigid, solid structures, they are, in fact, living tissue, to which nutrients must be supplied for growth. Calcium, one of the main components of bone, is an important element for bone formation, **remodelling** (replacement of old by new bone tissue) and **resorption** (bone breakdown). These processes are influenced by parathyroid hormone, calcitonin, vitamin D, other minerals, nutrients and enzymes. "Bone age" can be determined by an x-ray of the wrist that shows the ossification level of the bones.

The inner core of long bones is filled with yellow and red marrow and is responsible for the formation of platelets, red blood cells, white blood cells and adipose (fat) cells. Red marrow is primarily involved in blood component production, whereas yellow marrow is chiefly involved in adipose cell formation. The blood supply to bones is abundant, so that the marrow can actively supply enough blood components for the body. As with other tissues, if the blood supply is cut off, bone cells die.

The bones of children tend to be more resilient than those of adults. This means that accidents that might result in severe breaks to adult bones are apt to result in lesser breaks or only torsional twists in children. Because bones heal more quickly in children than in adults, children usually are incapacitated for a shorter time after an injury.

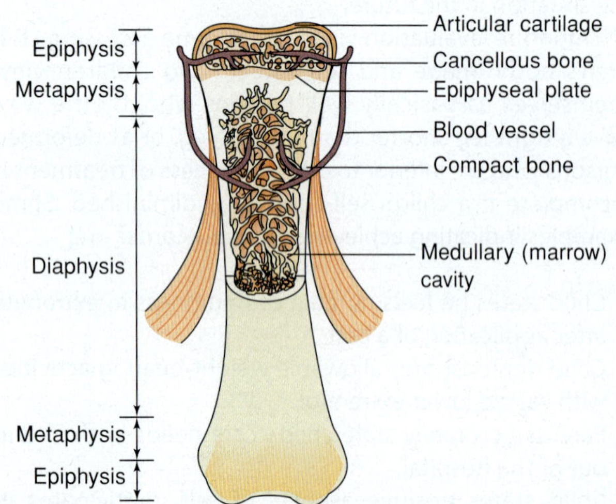

FIGURE 51.1 Structure of a bone.

Muscle

The skeletal muscular system is composed of one type of muscle, called striated muscle, which is the predominant muscle in the body (differentiated from smooth muscle, which is responsible for, among other things, gastrointestinal peristalsis). Activation of skeletal muscle occurs with innervation from a motor nerve and is under voluntary control. **Myopathy**, or disease of the muscular system, can be inherited (as in muscular dystrophy) or acquired (as in myasthenia gravis).

ASSESSMENT OF MUSCULOSKELETAL FUNCTION

In addition to a history and physical examination, it is usually necessary to conduct diagnostic tests to detect musculoskeletal dysfunction in children. These may include x-ray and bone scans, bone and muscle biopsies, electromyography and arthroscopy. Ultrasound and magnetic resonance imaging (MRI) studies are used to reveal soft tissue disease.

Radiography

Because bones are opaque, they outline well on radiography. Information can be provided about a specific bone, groups of bones or a joint. X-rays can also provide information about soft tissue structure, swelling or calcification around bones. However, other tests are indicated to confirm problems with cartilage, tendons and ligaments.

Bone scan

A bone scan is a study of the uptake by bone of intravenously (IV) injected radioactive substances (Brenner et al., 2012). The distribution and concentration of the substance are evaluated to determine the exact problem. For example, areas of increased metabolic activity cause the substance to concentrate in that area. A bone scan provides information on very early stages of bone disease and healing, often before they are visible on x-rays.

Electromyography

Electromyography studies the electrical activity of skeletal muscle and nerve conduction. It can determine the location and cause of disorders such as myasthenia gravis, muscular dystrophy, and lower motor neuron and peripheral nerve disorders.

For the test, needle electrodes are inserted into muscle masses; the electrical activity of the muscle at rest and in motion is detected by audio-amplification and recorded on an oscilloscope screen. Normally, resting muscle is quiet. If defects such as fasciculations are present, abnormal noises or oscilloscope spikes will be observed.

Although the needle electrodes are small, the test may be frightening for children because they are pricked by needles. They need support from someone they know during the procedure. Before and after the procedure, provide opportunities for therapeutic play so a child can express anxiety and feelings.

Muscle or bone biopsy

A muscle or bone biopsy involves removal of a tissue sample for examination of its microscopic structure. It can provide evidence of infection, malignant bone growth, inflammation or atrophy of the area. Either type may be done during surgery or as an ambulatory procedure.

Muscle biopsy is usually done using conscious sedation and a local anaesthetic. If local anaesthesia is used, caution children that they will feel the initial prick of an anaesthetising needle; as the actual biopsy needle enters the muscle mass, they will feel additional momentary pressure. They can be assured that the amount of tissue taken from them is no larger than the inner bore of the biopsy needle, comparable to the size of the lead in a pencil.

Arthroscopy

Arthroscopy involves direct visualisation of a joint with a fibre-optic instrument. It is usually done under local anaesthesia in an ambulatory care setting. Arthroscopy allows a joint, most commonly the knee, but also the hip, shoulder, elbow or wrist, to be examined without a large incision. It is most often used to diagnose athletic injuries and to differentiate between acute and chronic joint disorders.

HEALTH PROMOTION

Health promotion focuses on thorough assessment at all health maintenance visits. A child's ability to achieve developmental milestones, specifically gross and fine motor abilities, provides important information about the child's musculoskeletal function. The ability of a child to be fully mobile directly influences the child's exploration of the environment and exposure to stimuli. If mobility is impaired, it can significantly interfere with growth and development. Screening for musculoskeletal disorders, such as for scoliosis in the prepubescent child and adolescent, is an extremely important health promotion measure.

Safety is paramount for any child to prevent injury. Anticipatory guidance for parents is essential to minimise the risk of injury, specifically to the extremities, in all aspects of daily life. As a child grows and becomes active in sports, parental and child education about the importance of using protective equipment such as helmets for bike riding or protective gear for football, becomes important.

Nutrition education is important to ensure adequate calcium intake for bone growth and healing. However, if a child requires prolonged periods of inactivity (bed rest), calcium intake should be moderated to reduce the risk of renal calculi formation, resulting from immobilisation. The teenage years are an important time for both males and females to build calcium stores to protect against osteoporosis later in life (Kontulainen et al., 2013).

THERAPEUTIC MANAGEMENT OF MUSCULOSKELETAL DISORDERS IN CHILDREN

Various interventions may be used as therapy for children with musculoskeletal disorders, including casts, crutches, traction, distraction and open reduction.

Casting

Casts may be used to treat a variety of musculoskeletal system disorders, from simple fractures in the extremities to correction of congenital structural bone disorders.

Cast application

Casts are created from either plaster of Paris or fibreglass. Fibreglass is an attractive material to use for children's casts because it is: light in weight; comes in attractive colours; and, when a special waterproof liner is used, can be immersed in water. Unfortunately, it is more expensive and may not be practical for casts that need frequent changing, such as those used to correct talipes disorders, a common congenital disorder that requires serial casting.

Children need an explanation of what to expect with casting. To maintain alignment of body parts, a doctor gently exerts a pull on the body part being treated during the cast application. If a large body cast is being applied, children may be positioned on a special cast table with traction apparatus at the chin and pelvis to initiate tension. These are stark, steel tables and may resemble torture racks children have seen in horror movies. Allow a support person to accompany children to a cast room to hold their hand or talk to them during the application. Most children (and adults) are unaware that casts are formed from strips or rolls of material impregnated with the casting material. The normal curiosity of children as they watch a cast grow and mould to their body part

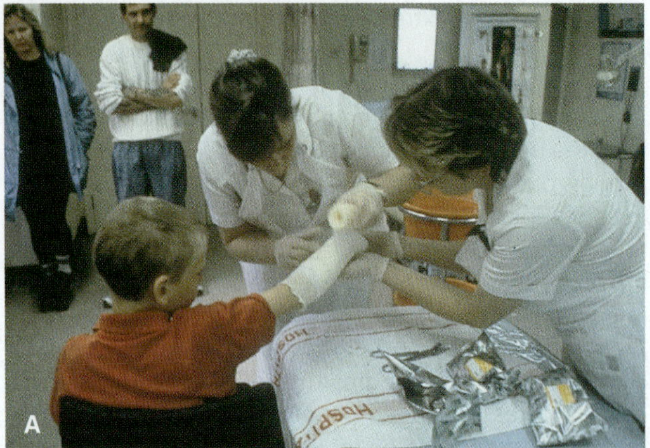

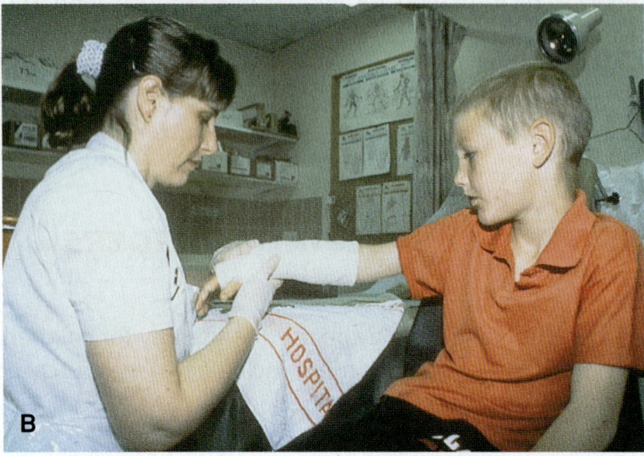

FIGURE 51.2 Cast application. (**A**) A cast is applied to a young boy's arm over a stockinette already in place. (**B**) Casts do not cover the fingers so these can be assessed for colour and warmth. (© Shout Pictures/Custom Medical Stock Photographs.)

makes casting a pleasant procedure. Some children look forward to having a cast applied, regarding it as a badge of courage or a conversation piece.

Before a cast is applied, a tube of stockinette is stretched over the area and soft cotton padding is placed over bony prominences. This stockinette is pulled up and over the raw edges of the cast as it is applied to create a smooth, padded surface (see Fig. 51.2). If a plaster cast is to be applied, caution children that, at first, the wet strips of plaster of Paris feel cool. Almost immediately, the strips begin to generate heat as evaporation begins, and body parts feel warm. If the cast is a full-body cast, children may become uncomfortably warm, with perspiration possibly running from their forehead. Assure them that this feeling of warmth is transient.

A plaster cast takes 10 to 72 hours to dry, depending on its size. Fibreglass casts usually dry within 5 to 30 minutes. A window may be placed in a cast if an infection is suspected, so that the area can be observed. A window also may be used with an open fracture, to permit observation and care of the wound site. If the child has a body or hip spica cast, windowing may prevent uncomfortable abdominal distension.

Compartment syndrome is a phenomenon that occurs when a cast or tight constrictive dressing puts pressure on an enclosed space such as the forearm. This pressure results in severely decreased blood flow that potentially threatens damage to, and necrosis of, surrounding soft tissue or nerves. Assess fingers or toes carefully for warmth, pain and function after application of a cast to be certain a compartment syndrome is not developing. If signs of compartment syndrome are present, the cast needs to be released immediately to prevent permanent nerve and tissue damage. A fasciotomy (surgically opening the compartment) may be necessary to further prevent nerve damage (Najarian, 2013).

Risk of ineffective peripheral tissue perfusion related to pressure from cast

If a cast has been applied to an extremity, keep it elevated to prevent oedema forming in the area. Check circulation frequently, a standard routine is every 15 minutes during the first hour, hourly for the next 4 hours, and then every 4 hours through the first day. Assess for colour, warmth, presence of pulses, and sensations of numbness or tingling. Signs of impaired neurovascular function include pallor (including blueness or distal portion of extremity feeling cool to touch), lack of pulse, pain in the part that has been cast, paraesthesia (numbness or tingling, as if it were "asleep") and paralysis. Children younger than 6 or 7 years of age have difficulty describing paraesthesia; however, they may whine or cry with the discomfort of the sensation. Oedema that does not improve with elevation is also an important sign. Any of these symptoms requires immediate attention as neurovascular impairment can lead to nerve ischaemia and destruction, possibly resulting in permanent paralysis of an extremity.

Cast care and risk of damage to cast

Preventing the flow of urine under the edges of a cast can be a problem with full body or high leg casts. If a cast surrounds the genital area of a nontoilet-trained child, cover the edges of the cast with plastic or a waterproof material. Keeping children in a semi-Fowler's position by using pillows or raising the head of the bed helps to direct urine and faeces downwards away from the cast. Because a cast is heavy, infants tend to slip down in bed a great deal, so they need frequent repositioning to remain in a raised position.

Make certain that children who are being fed or feeding themselves have a bib or cover over the top edge of their cast so that crumbs and fluid do not spill inside. Toys should be chosen carefully for the same reason. A piece of food inside a cast will mould and macerate the skin; a small part of a toy dropped inside a cast can cause irritation and a pressure ulcer. Casts can be cleaned with a damp cloth if food or fluid is spilled on the outer surface.

Parental health-seeking behaviours related to care of child with cast at home

If a child has an upper-extremity cast, be sure the parents understand how to position the extremity properly, such as with a sling. If the cast is on a lower extremity, instruct the child and parents on the amount of weight-bearing allowed to the affected extremity and the use of crutches, if prescribed.

Handling a child in a large cast is a major task for parents. For many, it seems so overwhelming that they do not see how they will be able to care for the child at home. Assure them that the child is quite comfortable in the cast, despite its awkward, constricting appearance. Demonstrate effective methods of moving the child when providing instruction. Be sure to caution carers that, if an abduction bar is used with a cast, it must never be used as a handle for lifting the cast. Such use can break the bar from the cast or weaken its support.

A body cast is heavy, so caution parents to use good body mechanics (lift with the thighs instead of the back) when turning or positioning the child. Parents may also appreciate suggestions on ways to help move the child from room to room, such as using a toy wagon with a flat board on top or using a skateboard for the child to propel themselves forwards. It is important to point out the importance of physical contact for children. Children in large body casts need their head and arms stroked (or any areas of the body that are not covered by the cast). Demonstrate how even a child in a large hip spica cast can be held, cuddled and supported for feeding.

Many children report a sensation of itching inside a cast at about the end of the first week. If the area is immediately under the edge of the cast, the itching is probably the result of dry skin caused by the drying effect of the cast. Reaching a hand under the edge of the cast and massaging the area usually relieves the itching. Applying hand lotion may relieve the dryness. If the area is unreachable, blowing cool air through the cast with a fan or a hair dryer set on cool air may relieve the uncomfortable feeling. Caution the child and parents not to use implements such as a coat hanger or knitting needle to scratch the area. These can injure the skin, causing infection under the cast.

Transporting the child in a car, particularly fitting a bulky cast into an infant car seat, can be a major problem. Before a child is discharged from the healthcare facility, give parents a telephone number to call if they have any questions about cast care or their child's condition (see also Box 51.1).

BOX 51.1 * Focus on family teaching

Cast care at home

Q. Will's sister has a fibreglass cast on her arm. Her parents ask you, "How do we care for this?"

A. Here are some helpful tips to care for your child's cast at home:

- Keep the body part that has been cast elevated on a pillow for the first day to decrease swelling.
- Observe the hands and fingers (the body part distal to the cast) for swelling or blueness, and ask your child to move the part about every 4 hours for the first 24 hours. If she is unable to move distal parts or if swelling, blueness or pain is present, telephone your healthcare provider. These signs could mean the cast is pressing on a nerve or constricting a blood vessel.
- Monitor strenuous activities, such as rough-housing, while the cast is in place, but urge usual activities so your child remains active.
- Ask your child to think through how wearing a cast will change her day, such as making it difficult to eat lunch at school or carry books to classes, and brainstorm how to solve these problems.
- Be certain your child knows not to put anything inside the cast. If itching occurs inside the cast, blowing some cool air into it from a hair dryer can be comforting.
- Be sure that your child keeps the cast dry (cover it with a plastic bag to shower); no swimming is allowed. Remind her that autographs are not allowed because fibreglass is a porous material.
- Be certain to keep your return appointment for follow-up care. Because children grow so quickly, they can outgrow a cast rapidly. Outgrowing the cast could put pressure on nerves and lead to permanent disability.

Cast removal

Most casts remain in place for 4 to 8 weeks and are then removed, using an electric cast cutter with a rapidly vibrating, circular disc (see Fig. 51.3). Cast cutters are frightening because the disc makes a very loud noise as it cuts through the cast material and also generates heat. To the child, the disc appears capable of cutting through not only the plaster but an arm or leg as well. The person removing the cast usually demonstrates that the disc does not cut skin by touching a thumb to the edge of it. Not all children are totally convinced by the demonstration, however, and may require additional support while the disc moves from one end of a cast to the other, such as saying, "It's all right to cry; I know this looks scary" or by holding your hands over the child's ears to lessen the noise.

The skin of the child's extremity looks macerated and dirty after a cast is removed; this usually improves once the area is washed. If an arm has been casted in flexion, the elbow may feel stiff and even sore as the child is asked to extend it for the first time. Children often use extremities with caution after a cast has been removed. Advise parents to allow children to begin using extremities again at their own pace. As children naturally play and reach for objects, they gradually forget to favour the arm or leg, and full function then returns. Once healing has taken place, the extremity is often as strong as it was before the fracture. The child does not need to continue to favour the extremity to protect it from a second fracture.

Crutches

Crutches are prescribed for children for one of three reasons: to keep weight off one or both legs, to support weakened legs or to maintain balance. Usually, a physiotherapist measures crutch length and gives instruction in

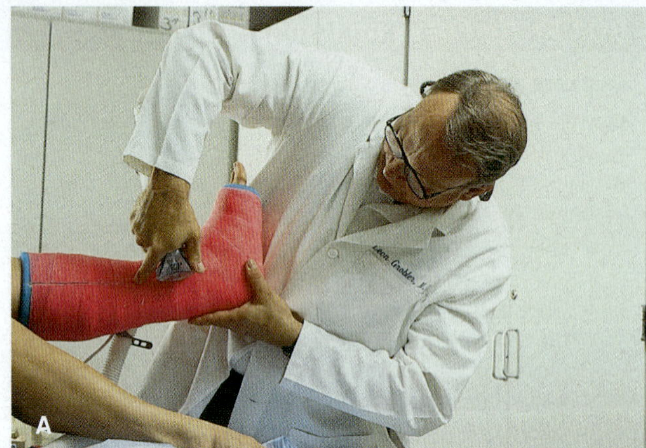

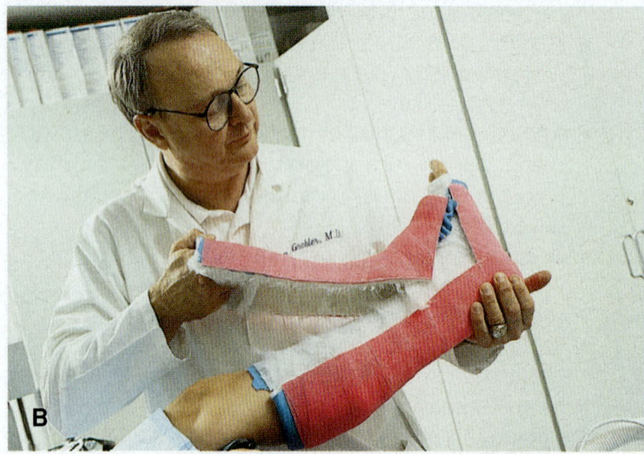

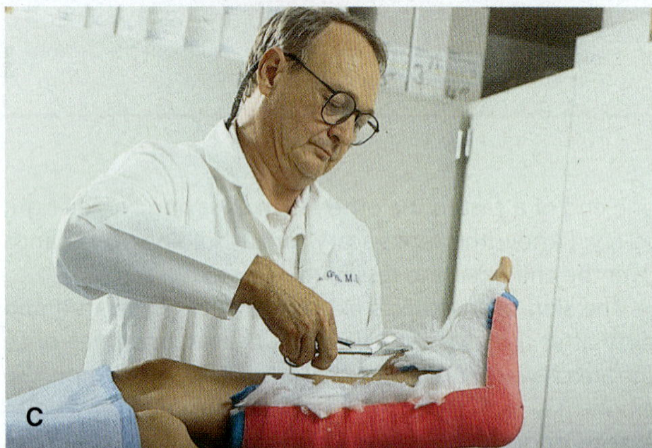

FIGURE 51.3 Cast removal. (**A**) A cast cutter is used to begin the removal of a fibreglass cast on an adolescent's leg. (**B**) The fibreglass cast is lifted off the leg. (**C**) Underlying stockinette and padding are removed. (© Will and Deni McIntyre/Science Source/Photo Researchers.)

crutch-walking. Be familiar with measuring and supervising crutch-walking, so that you can offer emotional support to children as they learn to use crutches and can assess progress at follow-up visits.

Fit and adjustment

If crutches are properly fitted, there should be a space of 2–3 cm between the axilla crutch pad and the child's axilla. When the child stands upright and places his hands on the hand rests of the crutches, the elbows should flex about 20°. This degree of flexion ensures that, when the child bears weight on the crutch, the body weight will be borne by the arm, not the axilla. Pressure of a crutch against the axilla could lead to compression and damage of the brachial nerve plexus crossing the axilla, resulting in permanent nerve palsy. Teach children not to rest with the crutch pad pressing on the axilla but always to support their weight at the hand grip.

Always assess the tips of crutches to see that the rubber tip is intact and not worn through as the tip prevents the crutch from slipping. Be certain that the child is walking with the crutches placed about 15 cm to the side of the foot. This distance furnishes a wide, balanced base for support.

Explore with children any problems crutches may cause with their daily activities. If they carry books to school, for example, they may prefer to wear a backpack until they are free of crutches so their hands are free for the hand rests. Caution parents to clear articles such as throw rugs and small footstools out of the way at home. If there are small children at home, parents will need to keep traffic areas free of toys to prevent an accident.

Crutch-walking

Two main crutch-walking patterns are used (see Fig. 51.4). A two-point gait is used when a child needs support for weakened muscles or balance but may bear weight on both lower extremities. The child places the right crutch and left foot forwards followed by the left crutch and right foot forwards, and so on. Using the crutch opposite a foot provides a wider base of support than using the crutch next to the foot. Caution children to take small steps until they feel confident.

A three-point swing-through gait is used when no weight-bearing is allowed on one foot. For this, the crutches are both brought forwards. The weight of the body is then shifted forwards as both legs are swung through the crutches. The child bears weight on the unaffected (good) leg and moves the crutches forwards again. It takes strong arm support to bear full weight on crutches this way. Be certain the child is bearing weight on the hands and not on the axillae when swinging through. Some children use a swing-through gait rather recklessly and need to be advised to slow their pace to a safer one.

To walk downstairs using a swing-through gait, children place their crutches on the lower step, then swing the unaffected (good) foot forwards and down to that step. To go upstairs, they place their unaffected (good) foot on the elevated step, then raise the crutches onto the step and lift themselves up. To help children remember this pattern, a saying—"angels" (the good foot) go up; "devils" (the bad foot with the crutches) go down—is traditionally used.

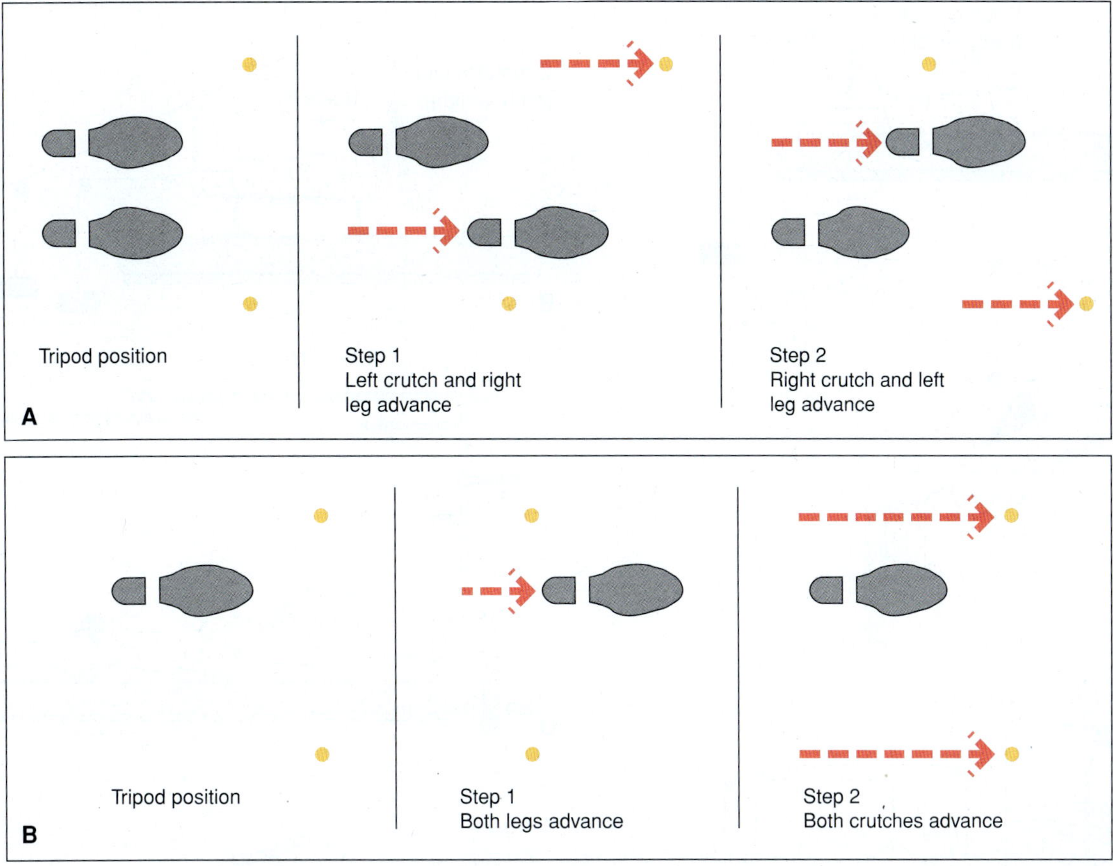

FIGURE 51.4 Crutch-walking patterns. (**A**) Two-point gait. (**B**) Swing-through gait.

✔ *Checkpoint question 51.1*

You are teaching a child to walk with crutches. Which is the best instruction?

a. He should bear weight on his armpits to keep stress off his arms
b. He should lean forwards at a 45° angle while walking
c. He should bear weight on his arms to avoid pressure on his axillae
d. It is unsafe to walk downstairs with crutches; upstairs is all right

Traction

Traction, which is used to reduce dislocations and immobilise fractures, involves pulling on a body part in one direction against a counterpull exerted in the opposite direction. Although still necessary for some conditions, the use of intermedullary rods replaces the need for this therapy for many conditions. In straight (running) traction, the child's body weight serves as the counterpull. In suspended or balanced traction, the body part is suspended by a sling and the counterpull and primary pull are accomplished by pulleys and weights. Either skin traction (in which skin provides the counterpull) or skeletal traction (in which bone provides the counterpull) may be used. Skin traction is used if only minimal traction is necessary; the child's skin must be in good condition for this procedure. Skeletal traction is used if a longer period of traction or a greater strength of traction pull is needed. Types of traction are illustrated in Figure 51.5. Use of traction in the home shortens hospital stays and enables a child to interact with family members, so it should be encouraged.

Skin traction

Skin traction involves a child's extremity being wrapped in a material such as a bandage and then suspended from a nearby pole or frame so the weight of the body part produces traction. Bryant's traction (or Gallow's traction), used for fractured femurs in children younger than 2 years of age, is an example of skin traction (see Fig. 51.6). It may also be used in preparation for surgical repair of congenital developmental disorders, such as developmental hip dysplasia (see Chapter 27). This type of traction is used less frequently now because the elevation of the extremities causes blood to pool at the hips. Another negative consequence of this therapy is the possible tourniquet effect of the traction strips, bandages and traction itself increase the risk for vasospasm and avascular hip necrosis.

Buck's extension is an example of skin traction used for immobilising lower-extremity fractures in older children.

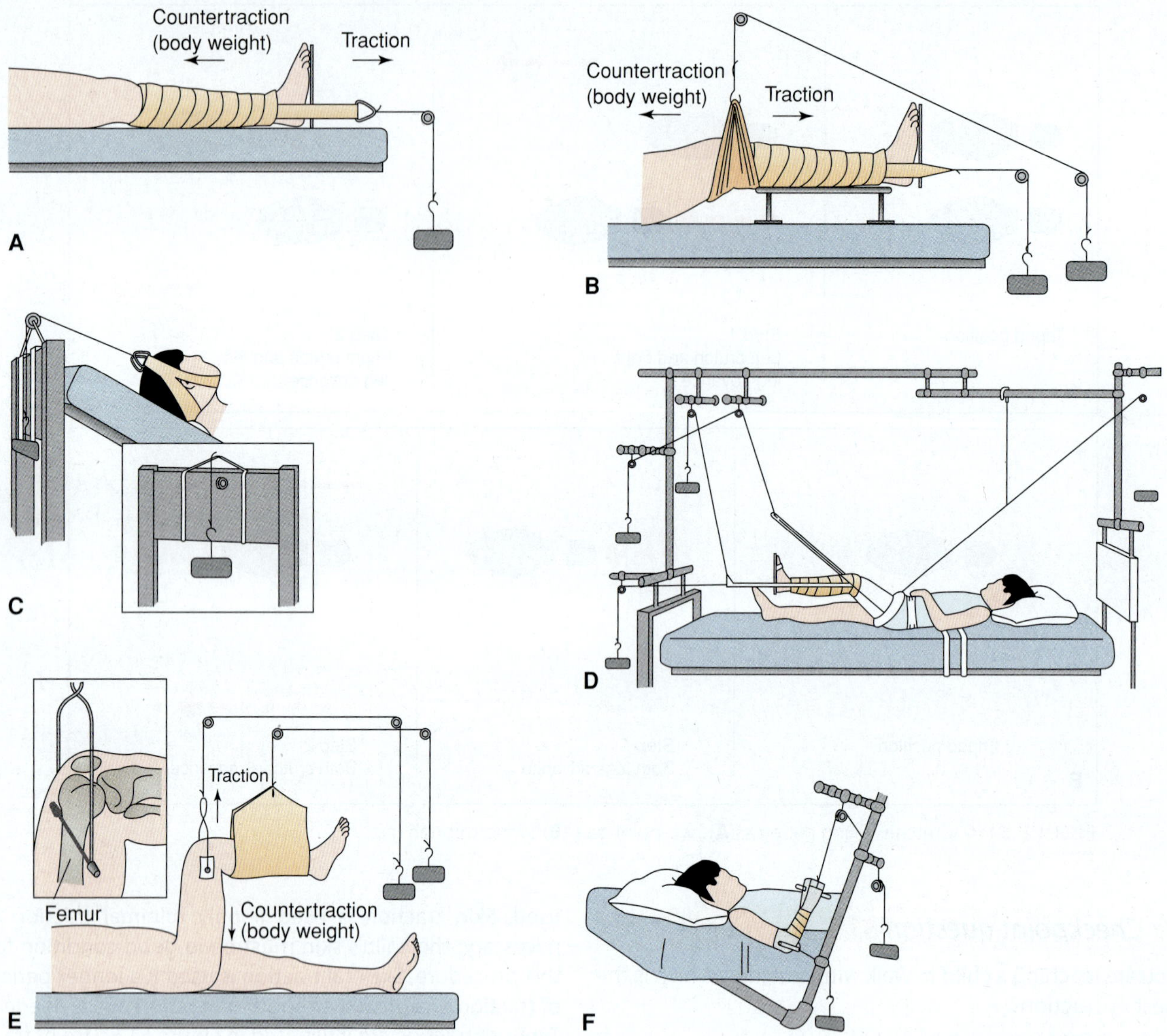

Countertraction (body weight) Traction

A

Countertraction (body weight) Traction

B

C

D

Traction

Femur

Countertraction (body weight)

E

F

FIGURE 51.5 Types of skin traction: (**A**) Buck's extension, (**B**) Russell, (**C**) Cervical skin traction. Types of skeletal traction: (**D**) Balanced suspension, (**E**) 90°, (**F**) Dunlop's traction with pin insertion.

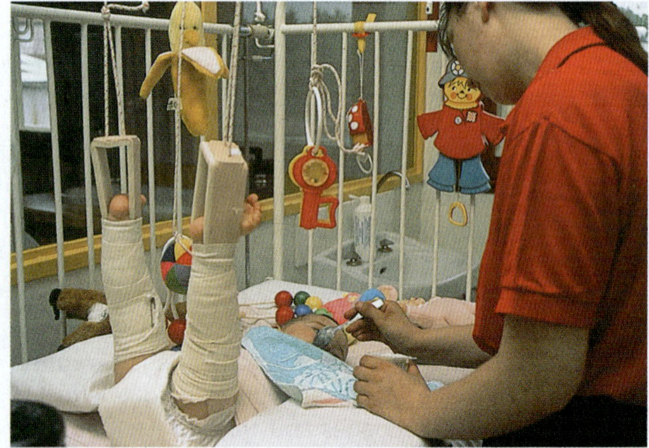

FIGURE 51.6 An infant in Bryant's traction. Here, the father feeds the infant while the infant is maintained in traction. (© BSIP/ Custom Medical Stock Photograph.)

Dunlop's traction is used to immobilise an upper extremity. Cervical skin traction may be used to decrease muscle spasms in the back. This type of traction uses a halter-type device attached to weights. With this type of traction, the head of the bed is elevated to provide some countertraction.

Skeletal traction

Skeletal traction involves the use of a pin, such as a Steinmann pin, or a wire, such as a Kirschner wire, that is passed through the skin into the end of a long bone. The pin or wire can be inserted in an emergency department under local anaesthesia if the child can hold absolutely still, but usually it is done under general anaesthesia in the operating room. With skeletal traction, ropes strung over pulleys and attached to weights exert a pull on the extremity at the pin site. The pins are to be observed for redness and any exudates. Pins are to be cleaned as per the hospital protocol. Be sure to observe the pin sites daily for drainage. Odorous or excessive drainage or erythema may be a sign of infection at the pin site.

Traction-related care

Children in traction need to be assessed carefully for neurovascular impairment. The extremity in traction should be checked every 15 minutes during the first hour, hourly for 24 hours, and every 4 hours thereafter. Signs of reduced neurovascular function include: pallor (or blueness), coolness, tingling, absent peripheral pulse, oedema or pain. Traction can lead to hypertension because the head typically is positioned lower than the lower extremities. Assess once a day for this possibility.

Be careful when changing a child's bed linen or carrying out nursing functions that you do not move the weights or interfere with the traction. Provide good skin care on the child's back, elbows and heels, which may become irritated due to prolonged periods of immobility. A trapeze bar suspended over the bed provides a great deal of mobility and assists children in using a bedpan and positioning themselves in bed.

Being in traction is not as dramatic for children as being placed in a cast. There is an unspoken feeling from other children that "if what you have is really serious, you'd have a cast". Explain to children why this type of treatment is best for them. Keep them informed of x-ray assessments (perhaps: "The fracture is being held in just the right position; the bone is beginning to re-form"). Although they cannot see progress, this information can help assure them that progress is occurring.

Children in traction usually are not "ill" children. They feel well except for the leg or arm being held in the correct position. Therefore, they have the energy and the need for stimulation of well children. Child life specialists or volunteers can be helpful to keep them occupied. Being certain that they are involved in activities (perhaps using a wireless computer or texting) is a major part of nursing care (see Fig. 51.7).

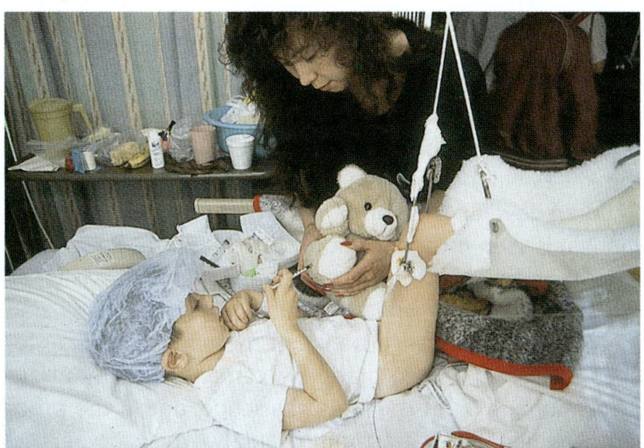

FIGURE 51.7 A child in skeletal traction engages in therapeutic play. (© Gary Wagner/Stock Boston.)

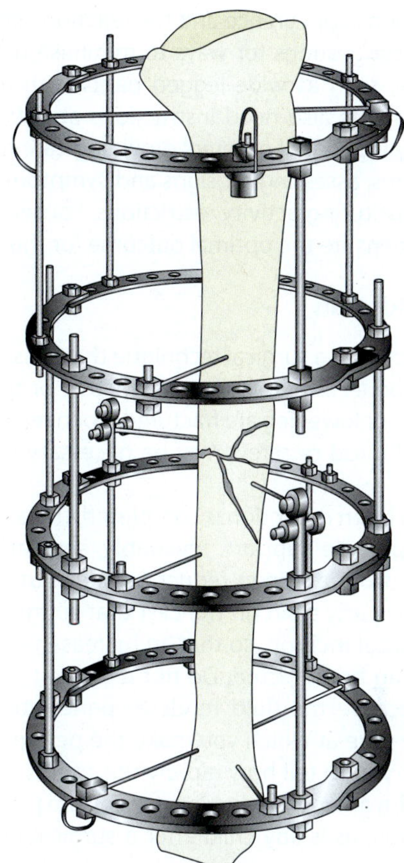

FIGURE 51.8 Ilizarov device in place to treat comminuted fracture.

Help children to maintain contact with their school friends through cards, letters or recorded messages. If hospitalised, their bed should be located so that they can see unit activities. Whether at home or in the hospital, encourage frequent visitors of their own age to help maintain peer relationships.

Distraction

Distraction involves the use of an external device to separate opposing bones, which encourages new bone growth. It can be used to lengthen a bone if one limb is shorter than the other. It can also be used to immobilise fractures or correct defects if the bone is rotated or angled.

A device such as the Ilizarov external fixator is used to achieve distraction (see Fig. 51.8). This device consists of wires that are inserted through the bone. The wires are attached to either full or half rings, which are secured to telescoping rods. For bone lengthening, the rods are adjusted approximately 1 mm each day to stimulate bone growth until the desired length is achieved. The device remains in place until consolidation is complete and there is no pain, limp or oedema. At this time, the bone is healed and can bear weight.

The child and parents need thorough preparation for the surgery and application of the device. Because the device is external, large and awkward, they need to be prepared for its appearance and the reactions of others to it. Provide suggestions for ways to minimise the device's appearance, such as wide-legged pants with adjustable closures. Parents also need instructions about: adjusting the telescoping rods, if ordered; providing care to the wire insertion sites; assessing for signs and symptoms of infection; and instituting activity restrictions. Follow-up care is essential to ensure the optimal outcome for the child.

Open reduction

Open reduction is a surgical technique that is used to align and repair bone. If there is a spinal fracture or both bones of a forearm or lower leg are fractured, open reduction and insertion of a rod or screw may be necessary to stabilise the bones.

Once an open reduction is completed, the area usually is cast to provide support. Invariably, serosanguineous fluid oozes from an open-reduction site. Outline with a ballpoint pen any stain on the cast that suggests oozing from a surgical incision, so that an increase in the size of the mark can be detected. Do not use a felt-tipped pen for this because the fluid tends to penetrate the cast. Noting the time at which you make the pen mark on the cast allows you to tell how rapidly the spot is increasing. Children with an open-reduction incision are prone to incision infection, as is any child after a surgical incision. Be aware of systemic symptoms (increased pulse, increased temperature, lethargy) and local signs (oedema, pain, tingling, blueness or coolness of the distal extremity) of infection.

DISORDERS OF BONE DEVELOPMENT

Many common musculoskeletal disorders in children are first noticed during routine physical assessments (see Box 51.2).

Flat feet (pes planus)

The term *"flat feet"* refers to relaxation of the longitudinal arch of the foot. Although it is rare, many parents worry that their children have this problem. Parents become concerned because a newborn's foot is normally flatter and proportionately wider than an adult's. A transverse arch is rarely visible and a longitudinal arch may not be present until the child has been walking for months. Parents notice that when their child leaves footprints in the sand or makes wet tracks on the bathroom floor, the track makes an impression of a "flat foot".

Evaluate children's feet by having them stand on tiptoe. In this position, a longitudinal arch should be visible. If they can stand on their heels with the soles of the feet off the ground, the feet are probably normal. Examine the ankle joint to be certain a full range of motion is present and to demonstrate that the Achilles tendon is not shortened. Tarsal and metatarsal joints should also show a full range of motion.

BOX 51.2 Assessment ✻ Assessing a child for possible signs and symptoms of a musculoskeletal disorder

Malaise, fever, irritability
Ptosis
Poor sucking
Muscle weakness
Spinal curvature
Pain (in hip joint)
Stiffness and swelling
Repeated fractures
External rotation
Knock-kneed or bowed legs
Waddling gait
Limp
Heel pain and tenderness
Flat feet
Pigeon toed

Some children experience foot pain at the end of the day. This likely occurs not from lack of a longitudinal arch, but from poor arch development. The arch can be strengthened and the pain usually can be eliminated if the child walks on tiptoe for 5 to 10 minutes daily or practices picking up marbles with the toes. For an older child, standing pigeon toed (toes pointed in) and throwing the weight forwards onto the lateral aspect of the feet tends to strengthen arches.

Teach parents that children do not need a high top or rigid shoe for foot development. If the child notices leg pain from poor arch support, a sneaker may correct the problem.

Bowlegs (genu varum)

Genu varum is lateral bowing of the tibia. If genu varum is present, the **malleoli** (rounded prominence on either side of the ankles) will be touching and the medial surfaces of the knees will be more than 5 cm apart (see Fig. 51.9A). Children develop this condition as part of normal development; it is seen most commonly in 2-year-olds. Record the extent of the bowing at health maintenance visits by approximating the medial malleoli of the ankles and measuring the distance between the patellas (knees) for changes. Genu varum gradually corrects itself by about 3 years of age or, at the latest, by school age. If the problem is unilateral, is becoming rapidly worse or persists beyond this time, the child requires referral to an orthopaedic specialist for further evaluation.

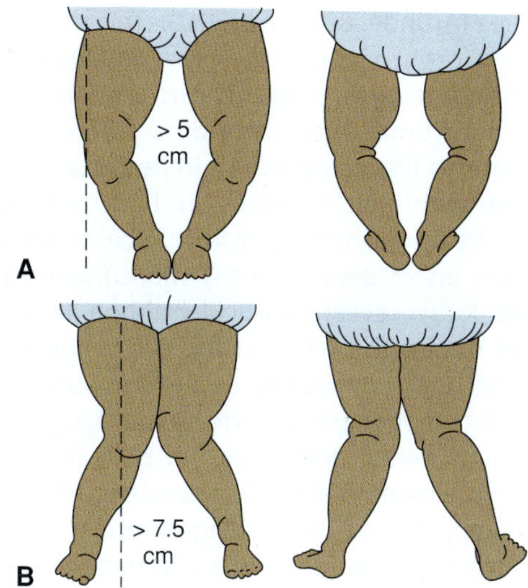

FIGURE 51.9 (**A**) Genu varum. (**B**) Genu valgum.

Knock knees (genu valgum)

Genu valgum, or "knock knee", appears as the opposite of genu varum. The medial surfaces of the knees touch and the medial surfaces of the ankle malleoli are separated by more than 7.5 cm (see Fig. 51.9B). This is seen most commonly in children 3 to 4 years old. No treatment is necessary for genu valgum. The problem tends to correct itself as the child grows. By school age, few children continue to have the problem. If the condition persists or the abnormality is unilateral or becoming more pronounced, the child should be referred to an orthopaedic specialist for further evaluation. The severity of the deformity can be measured at regular health maintenance visits by approximating the medial aspects of the knees and measuring the distance between the medial malleoli of the ankles.

Blount's disease (tibia vara)

Blount's disease is retardation of growth of the epiphyseal line on the medial side of the proximal tibia (inside of the knee) that results in bowed legs. Unlike the normal developmental aspect of genu varum, Blount's disease is a serious disturbance in bone growth that requires treatment (Birch, 2013). Because it is not possible to rule out Blount's disease by appearance alone, almost all children with bowed legs have an initial x-ray. In those with Blount's disease, the medial aspect of the proximal tibia will show a sharp, beak-like appearance on the x-ray. Bracing or osteotomy may be necessary to correct this deformity or prevent it from becoming more severe (Alsancak, Guner & Kinik, 2013). Explain to the parents why their child requires treatment or surgery when another child with a similar appearance (developmental genu varum) is expected to outgrow the problem.

Toeing-in

Toeing-in ("pigeon toe") in children may occur as a result of foot, tibial, femoral or hip displacement. Parents of children with these conditions often describe their child as "always falling over their feet" or "awkward". *Metatarsus adductus* is turning in of the forefoot. In this condition only the forefoot is turned in while the heel remains in good alignment. Metatarsus adductus may develop or become more pronounced in infants who sleep prone with the feet adducted and in older children who watch television by kneeling, resting on their feet and turning their feet in. If you stand the child on a copying machine and make a print, the turning in of the foot is well demonstrated.

Most instances of metatarsus adductus resolve without therapy. Those that persist beyond 1 year can be corrected by passive stretching exercises. A few infants with extremely rigid, incorrect foot posture may require casts or splints for correction. Early detection of these extreme instances is important as treatment for metatarsus adductus is most effective if it is commenced before an infant walks. With early treatment, the prognosis is excellent.

Inward tibial torsion also may be evidenced as toeing-in. This condition is diagnosed when a line drawn from the anterior superior iliac crest through the centre of the patella intersects the fourth or fifth toe (or a position even more lateral; see Fig. 51.10). Ordinarily, such a line should intersect the second toe. Tibial torsion usually improves as the tibia grows and requires no treatment. Parents need a good explanation of why no treatment is necessary. Reassure them at periodic health maintenance visits that patience and time will correct tibial torsion (Bazner-Chandler & Brady, 2013).

Inward femoral torsion can be detected if you ask a child to lie supine and attempt to rotate the leg internally and then externally at the hip. Normally, internal rotation is about 30° and outward rotation is about 90°. With inward femoral torsion, the internal rotation is closer to 90°. In some children, the femur rotates so far that the patellar bones face each other. As with tibial torsion, no

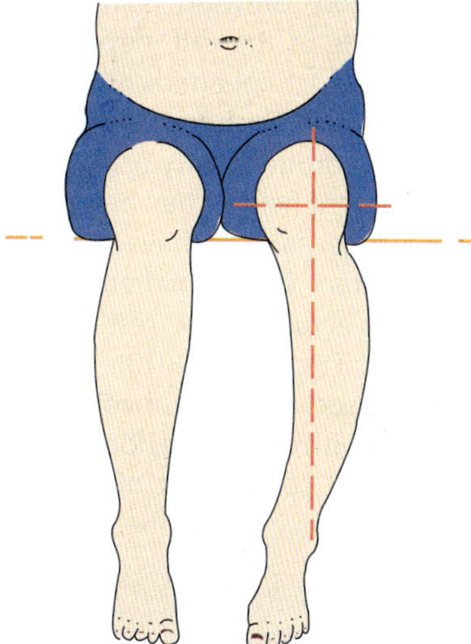

FIGURE 51.10 Toeing-in caused by inward tibial torsion. In good alignment, a line drawn from the anterosuperior iliac crest through the patella should intersect the second toe.

treatment is necessary. Inward femoral rotation will not correct itself, but a compensating tibial torsion will develop and make feet appear straight.

A fourth cause of toeing-in may be improper hip placement or developmental hip dysplasia, a problem that is very serious and needs early therapy for correction (see Chapter 27).

Limps

Observation of a child's gait should form part of every health assessment. Gait is a variable characteristic; however, limping is never normal. Although limping may reflect a simple problem such as a recently stubbed toe or a shin splint from excessive running, it may also reflect serious bone or muscle involvement, such as occurs with osteomyelitis or cerebral palsy.

History is important in determining the cause of a limp. When children have pain in a lower extremity, they protect the extremity by limping—stepping gingerly and quickly on the affected leg. Although children may seem to be favouring an ankle or a knee, ask them specifically what hurts. For example, a child may be experiencing hip pain and as a result they may be walking gingerly on the leg resulting in a presentation of knee pain (Jacob & Rammya, 2014).

The lower extremities need careful, thoughtful examination, including inspection, measurement of leg length, range of motion, palpation and a neurological examination. Radiography or a bone scan may be necessary to rule out a pathological process.

Growing pains

Listen to parents carefully when they state that their child has "growing pains". What they are reporting may be symptoms indicative of insidious conditions such as rheumatic fever or juvenile arthritis (JA) rather than a simple, transient phenomenon. Growing pains occur most frequently in the muscle of the calf, never in a joint. They occur in preschool and school-aged children, who wake at night because of the pain. Such cramping usually is associated with a day of vigorous activity or wearing new shoes with a heel of a different height than before. Children with genu varum (bowlegs) tend to have more of such pain than do other children. Some children reported to have growing pains may actually have restless leg syndrome (Walters, Gabelia & Frauscher, 2013). Restless leg syndrome (insomnia associated with involuntary leg movements) is associated with decreased dopamine production. As iron is an essential component of dopamine, a daily vitamin supplement with iron may help relieve the condition (Amos et al., 2014).

Osteogenesis imperfecta

Osteogenesis imperfecta is a connective tissue disorder in which fragile bone formation leads to increased susceptibility to fractures (Arundel & Bishop, 2010). This disease occurs in two main forms: a severe autosomal dominant form that is recognised at birth (osteogenesis imperfecta type 1) and an autosomal recessive form where symptoms develop later in life (osteogenesis imperfecta type 3).

Children with type 1 disease are born with countless fractures already present from the force of birth. These children go on to develop many more fractures during childhood. X-rays reveal a particular ribbon-like or mosaic pattern in bones. The sclera of the eye is unusually blue because of poor connective tissue formation. Children with type 3 osteogenesis imperfecta may have associated deafness and dental deformities. In both instances, the major clinical manifestation is a tendency for bones to fracture easily due to poor collagen formation. In some children, the bones are so fragile that fractures can result not only from trauma, such as a fall, but from daily activities as simple as walking. Because the child has such frequent injuries, parents may be accused of child abuse before the child's condition is diagnosed and documented.

As the child grows older, the multiple breaks tend to cause limb and spinal column deformities, interfering with alignment or growth. Children with this condition should be assessed to ensure they have sufficient dietary calcium and 25-hydroxy vitamin D intake. Several therapies, such as growth hormone to stimulate growth and bisphosphonates to increase bone mass, may be prescribed, although no therapy is curative (Harrington, Sochett & Howard, 2014). Non-surgical interventions include protecting children from trauma, effective fracture correction and undertaking activities (e.g. physiotherapy) to develop muscle strength, range of motion and generally improve functional ability. Lightweight leg braces or new intermedullary rod insertion techniques are available to strengthen bones (Monti et al., 2010).

Always be careful when caring for a child with this disorder not to cause any trauma to bones. Be sure to raise side rails on cots or beds. Keep floors dry and remove objects that could cause falls. Always lift children gently and avoid lifting them by a single arm or leg, to avoid placing strain on a single area.

Legg-Calvé-Perthes disease (coxa plana)

Legg-Calvé-Perthes disease (or Perthes' disease) is avascular necrosis of the proximal femoral epiphysis. While several strong associations have been identified relating to age, gender, ethnicity, sociocultural/environmental factors and some clinical conditions, the exact aetiology of the disease remains undetermined (Chaudhry, Phillips & Feldman, 2014). Legg-Calvé-Perthes disease occurs more often in boys than in girls and has a peak incidence between 4 and 8 years of age. It usually occurs unilaterally but may occur bilaterally. Only one hip is affected in over three-quarters of children.

The child notices pain in the hip joint accompanied by spasm and limited motion. X-ray studies are used to distinguish between Legg-Calvé-Perthes disease and simple synovitis (inflammation of the hip joint), which begins with the same symptoms. Radiographic changes may not be apparent when a child is first seen, but appear after about 3 weeks. For this reason, most children seen for synovitis of the hip joint are asked to return in 3 weeks for a repeat film.

Children with Legg-Calvé-Perthes disease pass through four stages. First is the synovitis stage, or period of painful inflammation. Next is a necrotic stage, during which bone in the femur head shrinks in size and shows increased density on radiography, lasts 6–12 months. The third stage is a fragmentation stage; resorption of dead bone occurs over a 1- to 2-year period. The fourth stage, a reconstruction stage, marks final healing, with deposition of new bone.

Treatment for Legg-Calvé-Perthes disease focuses on pain reduction with non-steroidal anti-inflammatory medications (NSAIDs) and on keeping the head of the femur within the acetabulum, which acts as a mould to preserve the shape of the femoral head and maintain range of motion.

Initially, rest is used to reduce inflammation and restore motion. To keep the head of the femur correctly positioned within the acetabulum, "containment" devices, such as abduction braces, casts or leather harness slings, or non-weight-bearing devices, such as abduction ambulation braces or casts (after bed rest and traction), may be used. Reconstructive surgery (an osteotomy to centre the femur head in the acetabulum followed by cast application) is most often used today. This technique returns the child to normal activity within 3 to 4 months in contrast to many months of restricted activity required by non-weight-bearing devices.

Parents and children need thorough education about treatment and care because most of it occurs on an ambulatory basis. It can be difficult for children to accept the extended treatment period involved with this disorder. Be certain that parents and children both understand the long-term consequences. Without treatment, the femur head tends to remould in a mushroom shape, making the hip unstable thereafter. Because this shape does not conform well to the acetabulum, degenerative changes may occur later in life, leading to chronic pain, reduced mobility of the hip joint and possibly permanent disability. Parents may need assistance with devising appropriate activities for the child during the time that activity is limited and weight-bearing is not allowed.

Osgood-Schlatter disease

Osgood-Schlatter disease is thickening and enlargement of the tibial tuberosity resulting from microtrauma. Children notice pain and swelling over the tibia tubercle that is aggravated by running and squatting. This disease is associated with growth spurts and is more common in boys than girls. (Weiler, Ingram & Wolman, 2011). Therapy depends on the extent of the bone changes. Administration of NSAIDs, ice and limiting strenuous physical exercise may be all that is necessary. Occasionally, immobilisation of the leg in a walking cast or immobiliser for around 6 weeks may be required.

Slipped upper femoral epiphysis (SUFE)

Slipped epiphysis (coxa vera) is, as the name implies, a slipping of the femur head in relation to the neck of the femur at the epiphyseal line. The proximal femoral head displaces posteriorly and inferiorly. An avascular necrosis similar to that observed in Legg-Calvé-Perthes disease may occur. The cartilage covering the femur head may be destroyed and permanent loss of motion of the femoral head may result (Loder & Dietz, 2012). Surgical reconstruction of the hip joint is necessary to correct the problem.

This disorder occurs most frequently in pre-adolescence. The exact cause of this condition is not known, but there may be a link between increased weight and puberty hormones. A SUFE is not usually associated with an injury. It occurs mostly in boys. It is most common in obese or rapidly growing children. This suggests that it occurs because of the influence of growth hormone and excessive weight-bearing in the pre-adolescent child.

The onset of symptoms is gradual. On inspection, children are often observed to be limping and holding their leg externally rotated to relieve stress and pain in the hip joint. They may report pain first in the knee because favouring the hip joint puts abnormal stress on the knee. On physical examination, internal rotation of the hip is difficult and painful. X-rays reveal the slipped epiphysis at the femoral head.

Early detection is important as correction is easiest in the earlier stages of the condition. Surgery with pinning or external fixation, such as with skeletal traction, is used to stabilise the femur head. After surgery, the child may have activity restrictions or be confined to bed. Because the disease is most common in pre-adolescence, these children need continued support. Although they may not like being restricted or confined in this way, supportive communication and education can help them accept this treatment as necessary to maintain good healing and function of the hip joint. Help them to understand the potential seriousness of the condition. Encourage frequent visits and telephone calls with friends to provide optimal growth and development.

Although this condition usually is unilateral, some affected children later develop the same condition in the opposite hip. All children with a slipped epiphysis, therefore, need follow-up care, with careful attention to the condition of the opposite hip.

What if...

Will's parents report that he has been waking up at night because of "growing pains"? Is there such a thing?

INFECTIOUS AND INFLAMMATORY DISORDERS OF THE BONES AND JOINTS

All bone infections are potentially dangerous because bones have rich blood supplies, so infection can easily spread and become septicaemia.

Osteomyelitis

Osteomyelitis is infection of the bone. It is most often caused by *Staphylococcus aureus* in older children and by *Streptococcus pyogenes* in younger children. Children with sickle cell anaemia have a special susceptibility to *Salmonella* invasion in long bones. Organisms are carried to the bone site by septicaemia (blood infection). It may occur after extensive impetigo, burns or something as simple as a furuncle (skin abscess). Osteomyelitis may also result directly by outside invasion from a penetrating injury or surgery (Aytaç et al., 2014).

Osteomyelitis begins typically as a metaphyseal infection because the blood supply is sluggish in that portion of the bone. An abscess forms and spreads along the shaft of the bone under the periosteum, possibly extending to and penetrating the bone marrow. Sinuses may form between the marrow and the periosteum, or between the infected bone and the skin above. If the epiphyseal plate is infected, altered bone growth may result.

Osteomyelitis usually begins with acute symptoms. Children show systemic malaise, fever and irritability. They may have sharp pain at the bone metaphysis. By the second day, the area of skin over the infected bone feels warm to the touch; oedema is present. Oedema reduces the blood supply to vast expanses of bone, causing death of bone tissue. This dead bone tissue, which appears dense on x-rays, is called **sequestrum**.

Blood studies reveal an increased white blood cell count, C-reactive protein level and sedimentation rate; blood culture results usually are positive. Computed tomography may demonstrate early-stage bone changes. Simple x-rays, however, may not reveal bone changes (formation of sequestrum) until 5–10 days after the beginning of the infection. Some children with osteomyelitis are not seen at healthcare facilities as soon as they should be because parents account for the pain as "growing pains". Children with systemic symptoms, such as fever, malaise and joint pain, must be evaluated carefully so that developing osteomyelitis, if present, can be detected early.

Medical therapy includes limitation of weight-bearing on the affected part, bed rest, immobilisation and administration of an IV antibiotic, as indicated by the blood culture. This therapy is usually initiated in the hospital and then continued at home for as long as 2 weeks; often an intermittent infusion device or peripherally inserted central catheter is used. After this, the child is prescribed an oral antibiotic for 3 to 4 more weeks. Additional therapy may include administration of bisphosphonates to help reduce bone loss (Simm, Allen & Zacharin, 2008).

If pus forms under the periosteum, it may be aspirated using a technique similar to bone marrow aspiration. After the procedure, a tube may be inserted into the area for instillation of an antibiotic solution. A drainage tube may be inserted and attached to suction to evacuate the subperiosteum area.

Parental health-seeking behaviours related to care of the child with osteomyelitis

When planning for care of a child with osteomyelitis, be certain that the long-term immobilisation necessary for care is considered. Parents may need to make major changes in their lifestyle if their child remains in hospital or if they need to give care at home for an extended period.

Parents have many questions when osteomyelitis is diagnosed, especially considering the defect does not show on x-rays initially. They may be startled to hear their doctor talking about the need for 6 weeks of antibiotic therapy. They may be suspicious, anxious and afraid that hospitalisation and administration of IV antibiotics are really unnecessary. Often, at the point at which x-rays reveal the process, they become more supportive and understanding of the care needed for their child.

Handle the extremity gently when giving care as the affected area is extremely sensitive. Provide instructions to the parents about good food sources of calcium and protein for bone healing. Keep in mind that young children are active, even if they are on bed rest. If a child had surgery and drainage tubes are in place, institute infection-control precautions because the drain evacuates infected material.

Most children with osteomyelitis (in developed countries) recover however time between hospital onset of symptoms and seeking medical attention can result in a slower recovery (Peltola & Pääkkönen, 2014). When the child is discharged from hospital, be sure to inform parents about the importance of follow-up antibiotic care at home, even though the child's symptoms may have completely disappeared. Review measures to care for a PICC line and techniques for antibiotic administration if required. Also review the signs and symptoms of re-infection, measures for wound care and infection control, and possible adverse effects of antibiotic treatment. A referral for home care follow-up is important to ensure continued support and education.

If osteomyelitis is not entirely eradicated with the initial treatment, it will return and result in a chronic infectious process with open, draining sinuses and bone deformity in years to come. Growth plates can be destroyed, leading to shortening of an extremity.

✔ Checkpoint question 51.2

When caring for Will, who has osteomyelitis, which of the following would be your most important intervention?

a. Maintain an intravenous antibiotic therapy infusion
b. Alert his parents that the infection was caused by food poisoning
c. Restrict fluid to encourage red blood cell production
d. Assist the child with moderate weight-bearing activities

Synovitis

Synovitis, an acute, non-purulent inflammation of the synovial membrane of a joint, occurs most commonly in the hip joint in children. While this condition can occur in toddlers and adolescents, most children presenting with this condition are between 3 and 8 years of age (Cook, 2014). Children notice pain in the groin, in the lower portion of the thigh or knee or in the buttocks. Pain is intense and is most noticeable in the morning, when children first wake. Children may wake from their sleep, crying from the pain of turning over. Pain again becomes worse later in the day, when the child becomes tired.

Aside from the localised pain, children feel well except that they usually hold the joint flexed in a position of comfort. On physical examination, range-of-motion exercises cause discomfort. An x-ray or MRI may reveal capsular swelling at the involved joint.

The treatment of synovitis is prescription of an NSAID such as ibuprofen (Nurofen) and limited activity until muscle spasm from pain has passed. In most children, 3 days of rest reduces the synovitis. However, some children may need 10 to 14 days and a short course of oral corticosteroids as well.

Synovitis must be differentiated from septic arthritis. With septic arthritis, a child tends to be systemically ill and blood studies reveal an increased white blood cell count. It is a serious orthopaedic condition that requires immediate medical attention (Cook, 2014).

It is important that children and parents understand that synovitis is a simple inflammation process that will heal without sequelae. The importance of rest for recovery must be emphasised.

Apophysitis

Adolescents who are growing rapidly and are physically active are prone to apophysitis or inflammation of the epiphysis of a heel bone (Tu & Bytomski, 2011). The heel feels tender and pain on walking may be acute.

Pain usually can be relieved by adding a lift to the heel of the adolescent's shoe, reducing the tension on the heel cord and bone. After the pain has subsided, the adolescent may need to practise exercises to stretch the heel cord. This can be accomplished by standing on a slanting board that elevates the foot and toes above the level of the heel for 20 minutes three times a day.

Apophysitis is an annoying condition, particularly for adolescents who enjoying participating in sports. They need assurance that, although this annoying pain may persist for weeks, it is not a serious disorder. It helps to put the slant board in front of the television or located where the child will be reminded of it daily. Many adolescents believe that they are too busy and do not have the time for such an exercise three times a day, unless they can combine it with another activity such as talking on the telephone or watching television.

DISORDERS OF SKELETAL STRUCTURE

Spinal disorders in children may include kyphosis (an outward curvature of the spine) or lordosis (an inward curving of the spine), but scoliosis (a sideways curve) is the most commonly seen disorder.

Functional (postural) scoliosis

Scoliosis is a lateral (sideways) curvature of the spine. It may involve all or only a portion of the spinal column. It may be functional (a curve caused by a secondary problem) or structural (a primary deformity).

Functional scoliosis occurs as a compensatory mechanism in children who have unequal leg lengths, in children with ocular refractive errors that cause them constantly to tilt their head sideways or children with accompanying neuromuscular disorders such as cerebral palsy. The pelvic tilt caused by unequal leg length or muscle strength results in a spinal deviation because this is necessary for the child to stand upright. The curve that occurs in functional scoliosis tends to be a C-shaped curve, whereas that in structural scoliosis tends to be S-shaped (composed of two separate curves). With functional curves, there is little change in the shape of the vertebrae on x-ray.

Children with non-correctable neuromuscular conditions may need spinal fusion but to rectify the simplest forms of functional scoliosis, the difficulty causing the spinal curvature can be corrected, eliminating the difficulty (D'Amico et al., 2012). Leg length is measured from the anterior iliac spine to the bottom of the medial malleolus; a lift inserted in one shoe corrects unequal leg length. Correction of ocular refractive errors improves problems caused by head tilt. In addition, children must be reminded to maintain good posture during everyday activities. Walking with a book on the head for 10 minutes, three times a day, or hanging by the hands from a door frame (chinning themselves) stretches the back and is often helpful. Sit-ups and push-ups are good exercises. Swimming is also good exercise because the reaching involved stretches the spine.

Parents and children need to be reassured that functional scoliosis is a disorder that can be corrected. Children need to be aware of this to prevent problems with self-esteem and body image. Caution parents about nagging children to do exercises or maintain good posture. Puberty is an age of rebellion and exertion of independence. Excessive reminders can lead to the child ignoring the parents' requests. Let children know that you understand that children of their age believe they do not have to do everything their parents want them to do. Help them to find alternative, more positive ways to exert their independence.

Structural scoliosis

Structural scoliosis is idiopathic, permanent curvature of the spine accompanied by damage to the vertebrae. The spine assumes a primary lateral curvature. To allow the child to hold the head level, a compensatory second curve develops, giving the spine an S-shaped appearance (see Fig. 51.11). The primary curve is often a right thoracic convexity. As the original curve becomes severe, rotation and angulation of vertebrae occur. The thoracic rib cage rotates to become very protuberant on the convex curve. Vertebral growth may halt because of extreme pressure changes.

A family history of curvature of the spine is found in up to 30% of children with scoliosis, although no specific inheritance pattern has been documented. It is five times more common in girls than in boys and has a peak incidence at 8 to 15 years of age. As long as the child is growing, the spinal curves will become more severe. This is why the symptoms become most marked at prepuberty, a time of rapid growth.

Children older than 10 years of age should be assessed for scoliosis at all health assessment visits. Often, the condition develops insidiously and is prominent before it is noticed because of the pre-adolescent's and adolescent's need for privacy and the lack of pain that accompanies the condition. A parent might notice when doing laundry that a daughter's bra straps are adjusted to unequal lengths. A girl may find it difficult to buy jeans that fit correctly because of uneven iliac crests, or she may notice that her skirts and dresses hang unevenly. If the child bends forwards, the curve becomes even more noticeable.

A scoliometer is a commercial device that can be used to document the extent of a spinal curve. With this device (a type of protractor), a reading greater than 7° equals a 20° scoliotic curve detected by x-ray. X-rays and photographs are helpful in estimating the extent of the deformity and provide a baseline description. If the child has a vertebral rotation causing rib imbalance, pulmonary function studies and a chest x-ray may be obtained to provide further baseline information. Children's bone age is established by radiography of the wrists or iliac bones. If bone growth is complete or almost complete, little more deformity will result, so no correction may be necessary. If the child has 1 to 2 years of bone growth remaining, some correction will most likely be undertaken.

Usually, if the spinal curve is less than 20°, no therapy is required except for close observation until the child reaches about 18 years of age. If the curve is greater than 20°, treatment may consist of a conservative, non-surgical approach using a body brace or traction, or it may include surgery or a combination of both surgical and non-surgical measures. Curves greater than 40° require surgery with spinal fusion. Regardless of the type of treatment chosen, a child must be prepared for long-term treatment. The

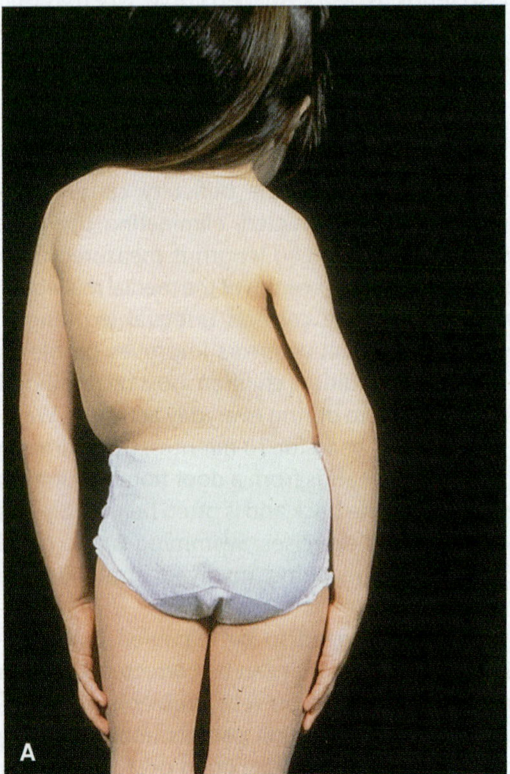

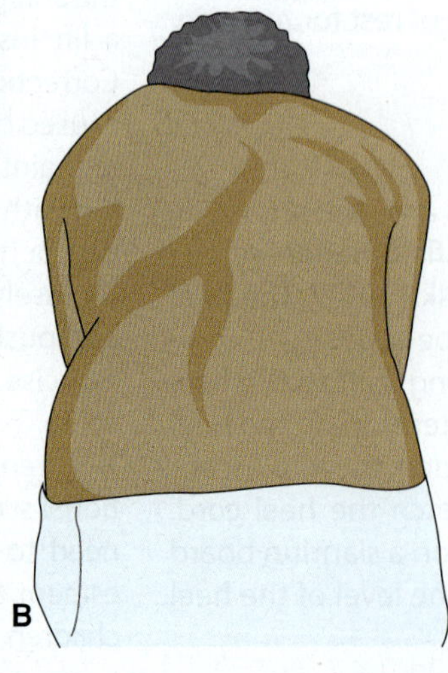

FIGURE 51.11 Assessing scoliosis. (**A**) Child with scoliosis (standing). (**B**) Child with scoliosis (bending over). (SIU Biomedical Communications/ Custom Medical Stock Photograph.)

goal of both surgery and mechanical bracing is to maintain spinal stability and prevent further progression of the deformity until bone growth is complete.

During prepuberty and adolescence, children are very concerned about body image and are very impatient with scoliosis correction, often wanting their problem to be corrected immediately. They need a great deal of support at healthcare visits to help them cope with the time needed for correction.

Bracing

If the spinal curve is greater than 20° but less than 40° and the child is still skeletally immature, bracing is still a prime intervention (Weiss & Werkmann, 2012). The Milwaukee brace was the first type used for this purpose so, although today's braces look much different, they may still be referred to by this name. Originally these braces extended to the neck and were almost impossible to conceal under clothing; today, they are underarm thoracolumbar supports that are worn under clothing (see Fig. 51.12). The brace is worn for 23 hours per day to be removed only for showering or participation in a structured athletic program. At night, the child may wear a Charleston Bending Brace that confines the spine to an overcorrected position.

Children and parents need thorough instruction on how to apply these braces. Frequent follow-up healthcare visits are necessary to check the fit of the device, making sure that it fits snugly without rubbing on bony prominences, such as the iliac crests. Caution children and parents to notify their healthcare providers if rubbing occurs. Also caution them not to loosen straps to decrease the discomfort. This makes the brace fit loosely and it will not exert adequate compression and traction.

During the first couple of weeks of wearing a brace, children may notice slight muscle aches resulting from the new alignment. If neck and pelvic traction were applied beforehand, this aching is minimised. A mild analgesic such as paracetamol (Panadol) will decrease the discomfort in most children. Rest also provides considerable relief. Caution children not to remove the brace during this time, because taking it off will compound the problem of discomfort by prolonging the period of adjustment. Braces should be worn over a t-shirt to prevent the plastic pads from touching skin surfaces and causing skin excoriation. Children should remove the brace to bathe or shower.

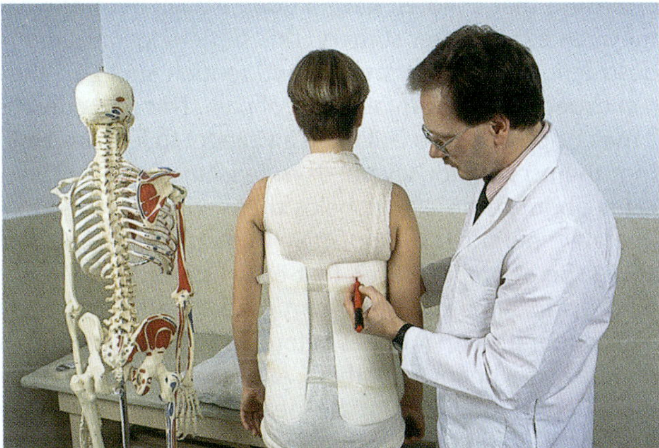

FIGURE 51.12 A teenage girl is fitted with a thoracic-lumbar-sacral orthotic device for treatment of scoliosis. (© Aaron Haupt/Science Source/Photo Researchers.)

Situational low self-esteem related to obviousness of the brace

It is easier for children to accept bracing today because the braces are more compact and teenage clothing now tends to be more casual and looser. Although choosing clothes is easier than it once was, it may still be a major problem for some children. They need time at healthcare visits to voice concerns about their appearance. Encourage children to explain what it feels like to have to constantly wear a brace of this size. Help them to concentrate on things they can do, such as having a friend over or going to the movies, rather than those things they cannot do because of the brace (play a contact sport).

Encourage children wearing scoliosis braces to remain as socially active as possible. They may comment at first that they feel awkward or "so much taller" that they are afraid they will fall. The only way to get comfortable with a brace is to walk and get used to the new sensation of actually being a little taller. Braces may be awkward at school if chairs are attached to desks. Advocate for the child with the school staff for seating arrangements that are comfortable.

Friends typically ask questions about what happened to the child. The sooner children expose themselves wearing a brace to friends and family, the sooner these questions will cease. A brace may need adjustment about every 3 months to accomplish more alignment, and frequent visits may be required so that children can express the problems they are having with social and school adjustment. However, do not underestimate an adolescent's ability to adjust to new situations. Children can see by looking in a mirror that their spine is curved and they want this corrected. They will endure necessary discomfort if they have hope that they will emerge at the end of the correction period without an obvious physical deformity.

In some instances, parents must be firm about insisting that the child wear the brace continuously. If bracing does not work, the child must have spinal alignment and fusion surgery. Be certain that children do not think spinal surgery is a simple, quick procedure, similar to an appendectomy, and therefore preferable to bracing. If they believe this, they may avoid wearing the brace, hoping that surgery will then be prescribed. However, be mindful of how surgery is depicted. In some children, the scoliosis continues to worsen despite good bracing, and surgery will still be necessary.

A scoliosis brace typically is worn until the child's spinal growth stops (at about 14½ years of age in girls, 16½ years in boys), as demonstrated by spinal radiographs. Bracing is not discontinued abruptly, however. The child is weaned from the brace gradually because some demineralisation of vertebrae may have occurred during the long period of bracing. Gradual resumption of activity allows remineralisation and continued spinal support. Adolescents may continue to wear the brace at night for an additional period (6 months).

Halo traction

Halo traction is the use of opposing forces to straighten and reduce spinal curves that are severe when first diagnosed (over 80°) or that progress despite bracing. Halo traction is achieved using a ring of metal (a halo) held in place with about four stainless steel pins inserted into the skull bones (Koller et al., 2012). Countertraction is applied by pins inserted into the distal femurs or iliac crests (see Fig. 51.13). A halo traction apparatus is bulky and looks frightening. Children may be afraid that, when the pins are inserted into their skull (under general anaesthesia), they will slip and penetrate their brain. They may worry that the apparatus will be so heavy that it will strain or break their neck.

Halo traction is typically used for children who have such severe scoliosis they experience respiratory involvement, cervical instability, a high thoracic deformity or decreased vital capacity from severe spinal curvature and rotation. Children need to see photographs of the apparatus or talk to other children who have the apparatus in place before having it applied. They need time to express their feelings about being placed in such a cumbersome device. Children may react to the apparatus physically, such as with nausea or diarrhoea, or emotionally, such as with chronic sadness, until they see that they can adjust to it. Orientation must be as thorough for the parents as it is for the child. Parents may show symptoms similar to those of the child for the first few days after the application of such traction. During the first week, they usually feel unsure about how to care for their child. Therefore, they need support to parent during this time.

Halo traction is prescribed for about 3 months. Careful explanations about the child's care before it is given helps to reduce anxiety. Stressing positive aspects, such as what the child can do, and explaining that the traction will help the spinal curvature, may encourage acceptance of such extreme traction.

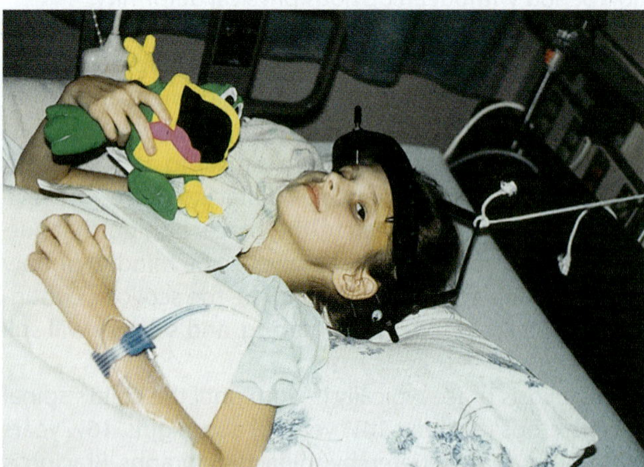

FIGURE 51.13 A 9-year-old girl in halo traction. (© Caroline Brown, RNC, MS, DEd.)

For the first 24 hours after the apparatus is applied, most children experience a nagging level of pain at the pin insertion sites. A generalised headache may occur, requiring analgesia. Accepting halo traction is difficult, even without this pain. Offer adequate analgesia for comfort.

Children in halo traction need frequent hair care to keep the pin sites clean. Crusting around the pin sites can be reduced by cleaning the pin insertion sites daily with half-strength hydrogen peroxide or another appropriate solution. Encourage children to be as self-sufficient as possible. Be certain that parents or children have a telephone number they can call for advice or if they have questions once they return home.

After optimal spinal correction has been achieved, halo traction equipment is easily removed. The pin sites in the skull heal within 1 week without obvious scarring.

Surgical intervention: Spinal instrumentation

Surgical correction usually is necessary if the spinal curvature is greater than 40°. Instruments, such as rods, screws and wires, are placed next to the spinal column to provide firm reduction of the curvature; the spine is then fused in the corrected position. A disadvantage of fusion is that it prevents further spinal growth, a concern that can be solved by the use of fusionless interventions such as intervertebral stapling or expandable rods (Laituri, Schwend & Holcomb, 2012).

Preoperative nursing care

Before spinal instrumentation, extensive x-rays are taken to plan the exact location of the rods or staples. Introduce children to the postoperative deep-breathing exercises and incentive spirometry they will need to perform. Deep-breathing exercises are particularly important for children whose scoliosis has caused chronically reduced lung capacity.

Ensure that children have a good explanation of what they can expect after surgery. This surgery involves bone destruction and major muscle and tendon shifts, so they can expect a significant amount of pain. This procedure is a major operation, so children can expect to feel tired and "not themselves" for several days. Teaching young adolescents about these events helps them adjust to the postoperative period. It is productive to treat adolescents like adults. Be aware, however, that early adolescents are not adults, and, although they seem eager to breathe deeply and cooperate with routines before surgery, these requests may be overwhelming for them. As a result postoperatively their behaviour may not be nearly as mature as they anticipate. Epidural anaesthesia offers a great deal of pain relief. Allowing children to use an IV or epidural patient-controlled analgesia system offers both pain relief and a feeling of control.

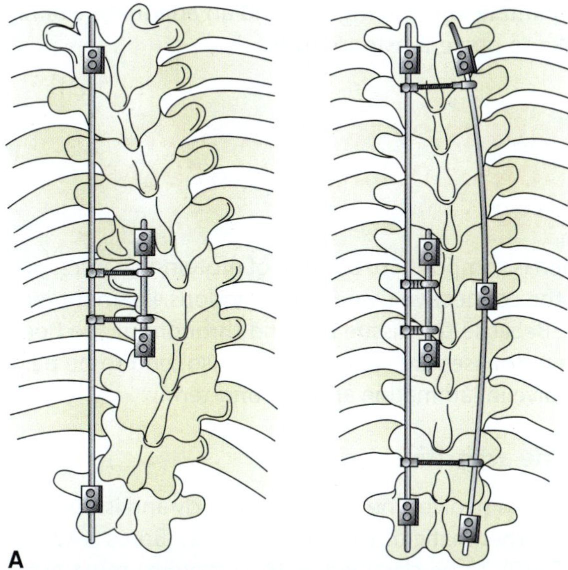

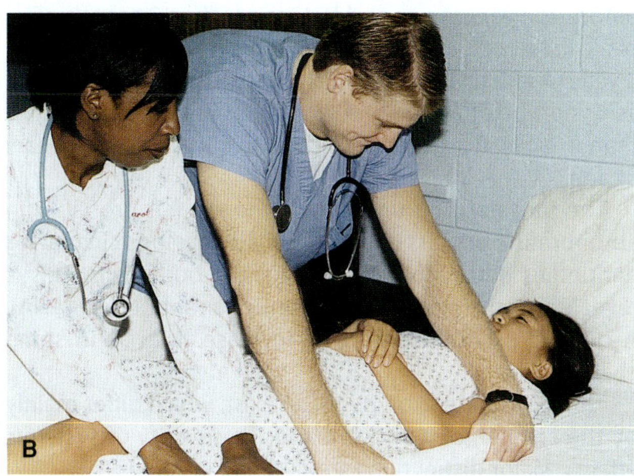

FIGURE 51.14 (**A**) Cotrel-Dubousset rods to correct scoliosis. A short distraction rod is linked to a longer one to correct the major curve. A convex rod is then applied. (**B**) Preparing to log roll. Two nurses use a drawsheet to roll the child in one coordinated movement to the side-lying position.

The type of rods used depends on the degree of spinal curvature and the age of the child. Harrington rods were the first such rods manufactured, so the surgery is frequently referred to as Harrington rod placement, although newer types of rods are now more commonly used. Luque rods and Wisconsin segmental spinal instrumentation use a segmental approach. Cotrel-Dubousset rods also are commonly used. These are attached to the vertebrae using hooks or screws (see Fig. 51.14A).

Postoperative care

After surgery, the head of the child's bed must not be raised because, once rods are in place and the spinal fusion has been done, the child's back must not be bent. Tape the latch of the bed in place or unplug electric controls so the head of the bed cannot be raised by accident by a parent or auxiliary personnel. A nasogastric tube usually is inserted before surgery to prevent abdominal distension as major surgery may cause temporary paralytic ileus and lack of bowel tone.

Depending on the type of rods inserted, when the child returns from surgery they may need to lie flat and be log-rolled (always by two people) to a side-lying position every 2 hours to enhance respiratory function (see Fig. 51.14B). Neurological dysfunction may result from bleeding or compression caused by a bone particle dislodged during the spinal fusion. Perform neurovascular assessment of lower-extremity function every hour for the first 24 hours. Assess lower extremities for warmth and sensation (whether the child can feel you touch a foot and wiggle the toes). Circulatory pressure changes resulting from realignment of the chest cage and reduced rotation of the spine may result in circulatory impairment so assess and record vital signs carefully. There is usually extensive blood loss during spinal fusion surgery. The procedure itself or the blood loss may cause shock and hypotension. A drainage system, such as a Hemovac, may be inserted next to the incision to evacuate any accumulating drainage.

The child will be prescribed nothing by mouth until bowel sounds return (usually 12–24 hours). An indwelling urinary catheter is usually left in place for 24 hours, because voiding may be difficult because of the horizontal position that must be maintained and the oedema at the lower spinal cord innervation points.

Although the child's parents have been prepared for the fact that spinal fusion is major surgery, they may be shocked by the child's appearance after surgery. This can cause them to be afraid to touch the child to provide comfort at a time when the child would probably enjoy being touched because of feeling so ill and frightened. Explaining that major surgery is frightening for everyone can help the parents feel more comfortable.

As soon as bowel sounds are present, a child can take fluids and then solids. Remaining flat can result in rapid release of calcium from bones. Calcium intake should, therefore, be moderate at first rather than extensive, to prevent renal calculi.

By 24–48 hours after surgery, children are allowed out of bed to sit up with a brace in place. They may feel dizzy at first and must get used to sitting by attempting it for short periods at a time. Then activity is increased to a normal level with few restrictions.

Because removing rods is as extensive a procedure as inserting them, instrumentation rods are left in place permanently unless they cause irritation later. The average child becomes unaware that the rods are in place. However, the child must always be conscious of good posture such as not slumping in chairs and stooping and not bending to pick up objects from the floor. Extremely active gymnastics, football or trampoline play is contraindicated. The rods do not interfere with other sports.

Children may be afraid to move freely after spinal fusion because, if they have had a brace applied beforehand, they have been in some type of restraining device for a long time. They may need to be reassured frequently that, with the spinal fusion, their problem finally is corrected. No further curvature can occur after this point, so it is safe for them to be without support.

Correction of scoliosis may have taken years. After surgery, children need an opportunity to talk at healthcare assessments about how they feel to be free of this problem. If the correction was not as complete as the child wished (children with severe scoliosis cannot expect 100% correction), they need time to talk about their disappointment and to adjust to their new appearance. They may believe their disorder has caused them to miss adolescence or "the best time of their lives". Emphasise positive experiences and point out positive attributes to help the adolescent gain self-esteem. Assure a child that with a straightened back, the best years are still to come.

What if...

Will, who has scoliosis, says to you, "Will I ever get better or will I be a cripple for the rest of my life?" How would you answer him?

Osteoporosis

Osteoporosis is loss of bone mass that leaves bones brittle and easily fractured. Stress on weakened spinal vertebrae can result in a severe kyphosis. Osteoporosis tends to occur most often in postmenopausal Caucasian women as their oestrogen levels decrease with ageing. Although osteoporosis is not a disease of adolescence, adolescents need education about it because adolescence is the time when most bone density is massed (Schoenfeld et al., 2010). Urge adolescent girls to begin a program of weight-bearing physical exercise, a dietary calcium intake of 1200 mg/day and an adequate vitamin D intake to prevent osteoporosis.

DISORDERS OF THE JOINTS AND TENDONS: COLLAGEN-VASCULAR DISEASE

Collagen is composed of bundles of protein-rich fibres and forms the connective tissue of the tendons, ligaments and bones. Because this tissue is found throughout the body, collagen diseases are systemic. They also tend to be painful, involve inflammation and are long-term.

Juvenile arthritis

JA primarily involves the joints of the body and is the most common rheumatic disease in childhood (Boros & Whitehead, 2010). To be classified as JA, symptoms must begin before 16 years of age and last longer than 3 months. The peak incidence occurs at two times in childhood: 1 to 3 years and 8 to 12 years. It can occur in children as young as 6 months of age and is slightly more common in girls than in boys. Acute changes rarely continue past 19 years of age.

The cause of JA is unknown, although it is probably an autoimmune process in which a child develops circulating antibodies (immunoglobulins) against body cells. This is revealed by the presence of antinuclear antibodies (ANA). A genetic predisposition may increase the risk in some children.

Three separate subtypes of JA exist, which differ mainly by the type of joint affected and the severity of systemic effects. Major distinctions are outlined in Table 51.1.

TABLE 51.1 Comparing different types of juvenile arthritis

Characteristic	Polyarticular	Pauciarticular	Systemic onset
Number of joints involved	Five or more	Four or less	Any number
Joints affected	Usually small joints of fingers and hands Also possibly weight-bearing joints Often same joint on both sides of body	Usually large joints, such as knees, ankle or elbow Usually particular joint on one side of body	Any joint
Gender affected	More girls than boys	More girls than boys (most common type)	Boys and girls equally
Body temperature	Low-grade fever	Low-grade fever	High spiking fever lasting for weeks or months
Other symptoms	Stiffness and minimal joint swelling, leading to limited motion Rheumatoid nodules or bumps on elbow or other body area receiving pressure from chairs, shoes or other object (+)Rheumatoid factor (in approximately 20% of children) (+)ANA titre (possible) Elevated white blood cell count, complement and sedimentation rate	Iridocyclitis (eye inflammation) Painless joint swelling with little redness (+)ANA titre (possible) (+)HLA antigen (possible in boys)	Macular rash on chest, thighs Inflammation of heart and lungs Anaemia Enlarged lymph nodes, liver and spleen Rarely + rheumatoid factor and ANA titre Elevated white blood cell count

Assessment

Children with systemic JA may be brought to a healthcare provider because of a persistent fever and rash, symptoms that are present even before joint involvement. When arthritis is diagnosed, parents may be surprised, believing that arthritis is a disease confined to older adults. Regardless of the type of JA, assess children for the effect their disease is having on self-care. Do they need help eating, dressing, ambulating or toileting? An activity such as sitting on the toilet may be uncomfortable if hip and knee joints are painful. An elevated toilet seat can be helpful because it reduces bending. Children may be unable to dress themselves independently because they cannot manage buttons or zippers with painful finger joints. Modifying these activities by using loops or Velcro strips not only helps children feel good about themselves but increases their overall level of activity.

Also assess the child's and parents' understanding of the illness and planned therapy, because children and parents typically bear the major responsibility for carrying out therapy at home and evaluating symptoms (see Fig. 51.15). Children with pauciarticular arthritis need screening with a slit-lamp examination every 6 months for uveitis (inflammation of the iris, ciliary body and choroid membrane of the eye). Severe uveitis can lead to blindness (Soep, 2012).

Because JA is a chronic illness, therapy includes a balanced program of exercise, rest and medication administration to relieve pain, restore function and maintain joint mobility.

Therapeutic management

Exercise

There is little documentation that exercise makes a long-term difference, but to preserve muscle and joint function, children are prescribed a set program of daily range-of-motion exercises to strengthen muscles and put joints through their full range of motion (Takken et al., 2008). It is best if these exercises can be incorporated into a dance routine or a game, such as "Simon Says". This not only makes exercises enjoyable, but it also can make the exercise a family participation time to be anticipated rather than a dull routine that must be followed. Swimming and tricycle or bicycle riding are excellent activities because they provide smooth joint action. Also encourage children to do as much self-care as they can because the natural motions of activities such as dressing and brushing teeth exercise joints. In contrast, to reduce joint destruction, activities that place excessive strain on joints, such as running, jumping, prolonged walking and kicking, should be avoided. School-aged children can cooperate to avoid these activities. Parents of preschool children need to create interesting alternative activities so that the child avoids such motions.

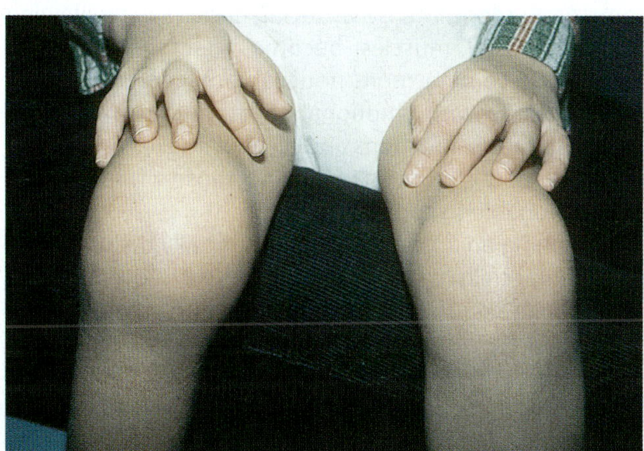

FIGURE 51.15 The knees of a child with juvenile arthritis. Note the degree of joint enlargement and swelling. (Photograph courtesy of A. I. duPont Institute, Children's Hospital, Wilmington, DE.)

Children should continue to attend school because active children tend to show fewer contractures and less decalcification of bones than do inactive children. Children with JA fatigue easily so they may need a shorter school day. If the school day is to be shortened, it is often better if the starting time is moved to mid-morning. This allows a child time for a warm bath in the morning before school, an activity that reduces the pain and increases movement of involved joints.

Heat application

Heat reduces pain and inflammation in joints and increases comfort and motion. Heat can be applied by the use of warm water soaks for 20 to 30 minutes. Paraffin soaks can be useful for wrist and finger inflammation.

Splinting

Splinting, once used extensively to immobilise inflamed joints in good body alignment, is rarely prescribed today because NSAIDs are effective and efficient in reducing joint inflammation.

Nutrition

Children with JA, like those with other chronic diseases, may eat poorly because of joint pain and fatigue. Some children experience mild gastric irritation from NSAID therapy. Help parents time mealtimes with "best times" of the day to overcome these problems.

Medication

NSAIDs such as ibuprofen (Nurofen) or naproxen (Naprosyn) are the medications of choice for children with JA. They are prescribed one to four times a day. They not only control pain and inflammation, thereby reducing joint swelling, joint discomfort and morning stiffness, but they may contribute to improvement in malaise and irritability. NSAIDs must be taken for at least 6 to 8 weeks to ensure effectiveness.

Because NSAIDs can cause gastrointestinal upset and bleeding, advise parents always to give the medication with food. Most parents think of NSAIDs as a medication to give children only when they have pain. Teach that they should continue to give the medication even if the child has no noticeable pain at the time of administration because the medication's anti-inflammatory action is just as important as preventing pain.

Slow-acting antirheumatic medication (SAARDs), also called disease-modifying antirheumatic medication (DMARDs), are used if NSAIDs are ineffective. In contrast to the immediate pain relief or anti-inflammatory effect of NSAIDs, these medications modify the natural progress of the disease over weeks to months (Beukelman et al., 2012).

Methotrexate, a cytotoxic drug, is the second drug usually prescribed. Steroids, such as prednisone, are only added to the medication therapy if the disease is extremely severe or is an incapacitating systemic disease that has not responded to other anti-inflammatory agents. Newer therapies include the administration of medications called tumour necrosis factor (TNF) inhibitors (Leblanc et al., 2012). These drugs reduce inflammation by blocking the action of TNFs, which cause inflammation.

Deficient knowledge related to care necessary to control disease symptoms

Help parents and children to understand the necessity for them to take an active role in therapy. Advise them to plan exercise and medication programs around school and other activities. Children with JA commonly experience irritability and fatigue, which may interfere with daily activities. Assist them with devising a schedule that allows for a balance of rest periods with exercise to maximise the possibility of success.

Children with JA need ongoing follow-up care to evaluate the disease and how they view themselves. Assist them with measures that allow them to view themselves as well again after such a long period of pain and illness. The few children who are left with joint contractures may require soft-tissue surgery, such as contracture release, tendon reconstruction and synovectomy, or orthopaedic surgery, such as equalisation of leg length and orthoplasty, at a later date. Surgery may be delayed until growth is complete so that further growth will not influence the outcome.

About half of children with JA recover without chronic joint involvement. The others continue to have the disease into adulthood. Until the disease does reach remission, children need a great deal of support to perform exercises and take daily medication as prescribed.

CASE STUDY QUESTION

3. Will's sister has juvenile arthritis. What is a common method used to reduce pain with this disorder?
   a. Apply ice to painful joints to reduce inflammation
   b. Have the joints scraped during an arthroscopy
   c. Apply hydrocortisone ointment to affected joints
   d. Take a non-steroidal anti-inflammatory medication daily

DISORDERS OF THE SKELETAL MUSCLES

Myasthenia gravis

For nerve conduction to cause muscles to contract effectively, a neurotransmitter, acetylcholine (ACh), must be released at synaptic junctions. ACh release is governed by the enzyme cholinesterase. With myasthenia gravis, there is interference in ACh processing, which leads to symptoms of progressive muscle weakness. The fault may be impaired synthesis or storage of ACh, insufficient ACh release, inadequate ACh receptors present at motor end plates, opposition of ACh by an ACh factor or excessive cholinesterase. In adults, the defect is probably most often a motor end plate insufficiency (decreased number of ACh receptors present). In children, the disorder most likely occurs from an autoimmune process (autoantibodies may block receptor sites for ACh). Myasthenia gravis occurs in three forms in childhood: neonatal transient myasthenia, congenital myasthenia and juvenile myasthenia.

With neonatal transient myasthenia, the mother has myasthenia gravis and the infant demonstrates transient disease symptoms at birth because of the transfer of antibodies from the mother. The newborn appears "floppy", sucks poorly and has weak respiratory effort. Ptosis (drooping eyelids) may be present. The symptoms disappear within 2 to 4 weeks, but if they are not recognised when present, they could prove fatal because of respiratory muscle dysfunction.

Congenital myasthenia is an inherited disorder that results in faulty ACh transmission or reception. Juvenile myasthenia gravis is an autoimmune process; it occurs most typically at 10–13 years of age and in girls more frequently than boys. Most children with this form have thymus hypertrophy; this sign helps document the autoimmune process (Bernard et al., 2012).

With all forms of this disease, children gradually begin to develop double vision (diplopia). Ptosis is present because of weakness of the extra ocular muscles. Symptoms grow more intense as facial, neck, jaw, swallowing and intercostal muscles become affected. Fatigue is extreme, becoming more noticeable by the day. Symptoms increase with emotional stress, fatigue, menstruation, respiratory infections and alcohol intake. In the most severe form, all muscles, including those of respiration, become unable to contract.

Obtaining an accurate history, especially documenting whether a child can perform repetitive movements, is important. Ask a child to look upwards and hold that position. Children with myasthenia gravis, unlike others, will gradually demonstrate ptosis. Other repetitive motions such as walking up stairs may also be tested although the time spent doing this should not be prolonged as it is tiring and does not reveal a significant amount of clinical information for the effort involved. Most children have myography performed to document their poor muscle function. Chest x-rays and computed tomography demonstrate the enlarged thymus gland. Administration of edrophonium (Tensilon), which prolongs the action of ACh and therefore increases muscle strength, renews exhausted muscles in a few minutes. If this occurs, the diagnosis is positive for myasthenia gravis (McKenna & Mirkov, 2014).

Myasthenia gravis is treated by the administration of neostigmine (Prostigmin) or pyridostigmine bromide (Mestinon), acetylcholinesterase inhibitors that prolong the action of ACh (see Box 51.3). The dosage of these agents must be individually determined. If toxicity occurs, symptoms similar to those of the original disease recur as excessive ACh leads to continued neurotransmitter stimulation and inability of muscles to repolarise for a new contraction. In some children, prednisone may be added to their medication regimen to decrease the amount of anticholinesterase medication required. In other children, plasmapheresis to remove immune complexes from the bloodstream or administration of intravenous immunoglobulin to provide immune suppression will reduce symptoms (Weeks, 2012).

Teach parents and children that symptoms become worse under stress, so parents need to prepare children well for new experiences such as menstruation, high school, a parental divorce or surgery in order to minimise stress. Help children plan their day to include rest periods, possibly advocating for a special school schedule if necessary. If chewing and swallowing are difficult, ensure a rest period before meals. Children may need to eat a soft diet and learn to eat slowly and cautiously to avoid choking and aspiration. Scheduling medication administration for about 1 hour before a mealtime is often helpful. If symptoms of muscle weakness suddenly become very severe, the child should be seen at a healthcare facility because loss of function of intercostal muscles may lead to respiratory arrest. Atropine, an anticholinergic agent and the antidote for an overdose of anticholinesterase medications, should be available to administer as necessary.

Dermatomyositis

Dermatomyositis occurs from degeneration of skeletal muscle fibres. The cause of the disorder is unknown, although an autoimmune basis is suspected. It is more common in girls and occurs between the ages of 5 and 14 years.

Symptoms usually begin insidiously, with muscle weakness that prevents children from performing tasks that they could manage previously, such as competing in gym classes, lifting objects or climbing onto a high stool. Muscle pain is infrequent. Skin symptoms such as swollen upper eyelids, a confluent rash on the cheeks that increases to become telangiectatic and scaling begin to develop. Subcutaneous calcifications may appear, making the skin feel unusually firm. Muscle breakdown leads to the appearance of creatinine in the urine. A muscle biopsy reveals lack of electrical activity in muscle fibres (Ruhlman, Otten & Colella, 2014).

BOX 51.3 * Focus on pharmacology

Neostigmine (Prostigmin)

Classification: Neostigmine is a cholinesterase inhibitor that acts as an antimyasthenic agent.

Action: Neostigmine increases the concentration of acetylcholine at nerve endings, prolonging and exaggerating its effects and facilitating neuromuscular transmission. (McKenna & Mirkov, 2014)

Pregnancy risk category: C

Dosage: Orally, 2 mg/kg daily in divided doses every 3 to 4 hours; or 0.01 to 0.04 mg/kg per dose intramuscularly, intravenously or subcutaneously every 2 to 3 hours, as needed

Neostigmine methylsulfate

Action: Cholinesterase inhibitor. Inhibits destruction of acetylcholine released from parasympathetic and somatic efferent nerves.

Pregnancy risk category: B2

Dosage: *Treatment of myasthenia gravis:* Children 0.01 to 0.04 mg/kg/dose IM or SC q 2 to 3 hrs, as needed.

Diagnosis of myasthenia gravis: Children 0.025 to 0.04 mg/g IM after 0.011 mg/kg atropine sulfate SC (McKenna & Mirkov, 2014).

Possible adverse effects: Salivation, dysphagia, nausea, vomiting, increased peristalsis, abdominal cramps, cardiac arrhythmias, increased respiratory secretions, urinary frequency, pupil constriction and diaphoresis.

Nursing implications

- If the drug is to be given intravenously, administer the dose slowly, directly into a vein or into the tubing's injection port of an intravenous infusion.
- Assess the child for increased muscle weakness, indicating possible cholinergic crisis. Keep atropine sulfate readily available as the antidote.
- If giving neostigmine orally, administer the drug with food or milk to minimise gastrointestinal upset. Instruct parents to administer the drug exactly as prescribed.
- Plan to administer larger portions of the divided doses approximately one half hour before anticipated times of greater fatigue.
- Review possible adverse effects with parents and child. Advise parents to watch for signs of excessive salivation, emesis or frequent urination and to notify the healthcare provider if any occur.
- Encourage parents to control the child's environmental temperature as much as possible, to prevent diaphoresis from too hot or too humid an environment.
- Inform parents that an increase in muscle weakness may be related to drug overdose or exacerbation of the disease. Urge them to report any signs of increased weakness to their healthcare provider.

High-dose corticosteroids or methotrexate are prescribed to improve muscle strength. Specific immunosuppressants may also be helpful (Zaba & Fiorentino, 2012). Children who survive beyond the first year after diagnosis have a good prognosis for prolonged remissions.

Muscular dystrophies

Muscular dystrophies are a group of inherited disorders that lead to progressive degeneration of skeletal muscles from lack of proteins necessary for muscle contraction (Mercuri & Muntoni, 2013).

Types

Muscular dystrophies seen in children are classified into three types: congenital myotonic dystrophy, facioscapulohumeral muscular dystrophy and pseudohypertrophic muscular dystrophy (Duchenne's disease).

Congenital myotonic dystrophy

Congenital myotonic dystrophy is inherited as an autosomal dominant trait. Because the disease process begins in utero, the infant may already have severe myotonia (muscle weakness) at birth. Muscle degeneration continues until adequate respiratory muscle movement becomes difficult. Diagnosis is by serum enzyme analysis and muscle biopsy. Most of these infants die before they are 1 year old because they cannot sustain respiratory function.

Facioscapulohumeral muscular dystrophy

Facioscapulohumeral muscular dystrophy is inherited as a dominant trait, carried on chromosome 4. Symptoms begin after the child is 10 years old. The predominant symptom is facial weakness. The child becomes unable to wrinkle the forehead and cannot whistle. Serum enzyme analysis and muscle biopsy are used in diagnosis. The symptoms usually progress so slowly that a normal life span is possible.

Pseudohypertrophic muscular dystrophy (Duchenne's disease)

Duchenne's disease, the most common form of muscular dystrophy, is inherited as a sex-linked recessive trait. Therefore, it occurs only in boys. Symptoms are usually apparent by 3 years of age.

Assessment

Children with Duchenne's muscular dystrophy usually have a history of meeting motor milestones, such as sitting, walking and standing, but they reach these milestones later than the average infant. By about 3 years of age, symptoms become acute and obvious as boys develop a waddling gait and have difficulty climbing stairs. They can rise from the floor only by rolling onto their stomachs and then pushing themselves to their knees. To stand, they press their hands against their ankles, knees and thighs (they "walk up their front"); this is Gower's sign. They may walk on their toes, which leads to the development of a short heel cord. Speech and swallowing become difficult. It can be hard to lift a young child with this condition by placing your hands under the axillae as the child seems to slip through your hands because of the lax shoulder muscles. In contrast, calf muscles are hypertrophied (measure larger than normal) because the muscles become so degenerated that they are replaced by fat and connective tissue.

As the disease progresses, muscle weakness becomes more pronounced. Scoliosis of the spine and fractures of long bones may occur from abnormal muscle tension and lack of muscle support. By early high school age, most boys become wheelchair dependent. Tachycardia occurs as the heart muscle weakens and enlarges. Pneumonia develops easily as the child's cough reflex becomes weak and ineffective. Death from pulmonary dysfunction tends to occur at about 20 years of age (Brown & Amato, 2012).

The diagnosis is based on the history and physical findings, a muscle biopsy showing fibrous degeneration and fatty deposits, electromyography showing a decrease in amplitude and duration of motor unit potentials and an increased concentration of serum creatine phosphokinase.

Therapeutic management

Encourage boys with muscular dystrophy to remain ambulatory for as long as possible. To do this, help the child and family plan a program of active and passive daily range-of-motion exercises. Splinting and bracing may be necessary to maintain lower-extremity stability and avoid contractures. If children become overweight, remaining ambulatory becomes more difficult for them. Therefore, encourage a low-kilojoule, high-protein diet to avoid excessive weight gain. In addition, to prevent constipation, encourage a high intake of fibre and fluids. Advocate for a stool softener if necessary. Drugs or enzymes to help activate dystrophin are being investigated (Abdel-Hamid & Clemens, 2012). In the interim corticosteroid therapy is helpful to increase function and strength at least on a short-term basis. In the future, stem cell therapy is a strong possibility (Tedesco & Cossu, 2012).

Because the disease is progressive, assist the child and family with achieving the optimal level of activity within the child's limitations. Provide support for parents, to assist them with coping because they can become depressed as disease symptoms progress.

Help children and parents locate a parent support group such as the Muscular Dystrophy Association <www.mda.org.au>.

✔ *Checkpoint question 51.3*

What is an important nursing intervention for children with muscular dystrophy?

a. Urge them to rest most of the day to avoid fatigue
b. Guide them to avoid weight gain so they can be mobile longer
c. Caution them not to eat meat and legumes in the same meal
d. Encourage a diet rich in calcium to prevent osteoporosis

INJURIES OF THE EXTREMITIES

Finger injuries

A common finger injury for a child to sustain is an injury from a slammed car door. This injury, which causes a crushing blow to the tip of the finger, is excruciatingly painful. The fingernail may be lacerated and detached. As blood accumulates under an attached fingernail, pain continues to increase. An incision under the distal end of the nail or a puncture through the attached nail helps to relieve pain. Fingernails often are lost after these injuries, but they grow back readily with little scarring. Reassure parents that, although the fingernail may be lost, the cosmetic effect will invariably not be a problem.

Parents may feel embarrassed and guilty when they bring a child to a healthcare facility for this type of injury. The accident usually occurred because they closed a door without looking for the child's finger. They appreciate how much this hurts and are angry with themselves for being so careless. Reassure parents that this is a common childhood injury.

An x-ray of the fingertip may be obtained to make certain that the tip of the distal phalanx is not broken. The rule, "If the child can bend it, it's not broken," does not apply to this injury because the fracture is distal to the last phalangeal joint. Any open wound must be cleaned well. If the distal phalanx is fractured, a splint is applied to the finger. A follow-up visit is necessary to ensure that healing has occurred.

Bicycle-spoke injuries

Children who ride in child bicycle seats or over the back wheel of a bicycle can catch a foot or ankle between the spoke and the frame of the bicycle, resulting in a crushing, lacerating injury that quickly becomes oedematous. Children can also injure their fingers in bicycle spokes. An x-ray is needed to rule out a fracture.

The wound, which usually is contaminated with spoke grease, needs cleaning with an antiseptic. It may be necessary to soak the area first with a solution of lignocaine, a local anaesthetic, because of the amount of pain that quickly occurs from oedema and ecchymosis. Sutures and a splint may be necessary. If it is a foot injury, the child may need to limit weight-bearing by using crutches.

Soft-tissue injuries continue to be painful. Elevating the body part on pillows helps to reduce both the pain and oedema. Such a major tissue injury may take up to 6 weeks to heal. Advise parents of this at the time of the injury. Otherwise, they may worry that the child's injury is not healing well. Because of the increase in the use of helmets, concussion or skull fracture from bicycle injuries are less commonly seen (Karkhaneh et al., 2013).

Fractures

A **fracture** is a break in the continuity or structure of bone. Because children experience falls during their growth years, fractures of long bones are common childhood injuries. Various types are described in Table 51.2. Fractures in children tend to be different from adults because:

- Bone in childhood is fairly porous allowing bones to bend rather than break
- The periosteum is thick so the bone may not break all the way through

TABLE 51.2 Common fractures in children

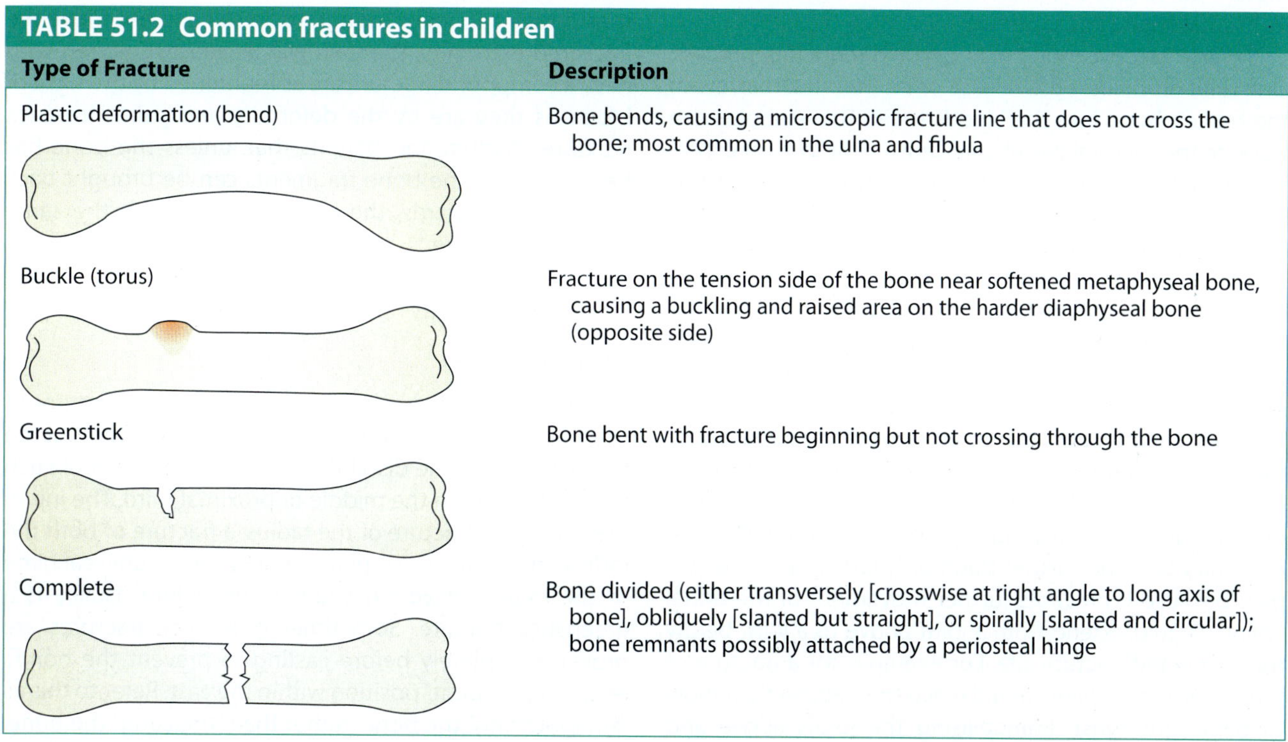

Type of Fracture	Description
Plastic deformation (bend)	Bone bends, causing a microscopic fracture line that does not cross the bone; most common in the ulna and fibula
Buckle (torus)	Fracture on the tension side of the bone near softened metaphyseal bone, causing a buckling and raised area on the harder diaphyseal bone (opposite side)
Greenstick	Bone bent with fracture beginning but not crossing through the bone
Complete	Bone divided (either transversely [crosswise at right angle to long axis of bone], obliquely [slanted but straight], or spirally [slanted and circular]); bone remnants possibly attached by a periosteal hinge

- Epiphyseal lines may cushion a blow so that the bone does not break
- Healing is rapid as a result of overall increased bone growth.

Because of the high resilience of immature bone, many fractures in early childhood are of the greenstick variety (one side of a bone is broken; the other is only bent). These fractures cause minimal pain, swelling or deformity, the usual hallmarks of fracture.

Many fractures in children, however, occur at the epiphyseal line. These are serious injuries because bone growth occurs at this point. Damage to the area can lead to undergrowth, overgrowth or uneven growth, resulting in angulation. If a fall occurred from a high distance or was caused by a violent force, such as a speeding motor vehicle, breaks may be complex, or the formation may be compounded (the bone pierces the skin) or comminuted (parts of the bone are fragmented). These injuries are always serious as well because the severed bone may lacerate nerves or blood vessels. The open wound may become infected and correction will most likely involve surgery with the risks of anaesthesia.

Fractures heal relatively slowly compared with other body injuries. Immediately after a fracture, a haematoma forms at the site of the break; over the next several days, granulation tissue is laid down. Over the next several weeks, osteoblasts invade this new tissue and calcium is deposited (termed *callus*) to form new bone. By the time callus formation is extensive (enough for movement at the fracture site to be impossible), clinical healing or clinical union has occurred. Complete healing does not occur until all the temporary callus formation has been replaced by mature bone cells and the bone has once more regained its normal shape and contour.

Several complications may occur during this process. One is fat embolus—the release of fat from the marrow of the broken bone into the bloodstream. This embolus can travel to the cerebral vessels and cause symptoms of confusion or hallucinations as the oxygen supply to brain cells is shut off. It also could become a pulmonary embolus, producing dyspnoea, tachycardia and cyanosis. A second problem is compartment syndrome, which was covered earlier in this chapter. A long-term complication of fracture may be interference with growth if the growth plate was involved. Some children need bone-lengthening or bone-shortening procedures later in life to correct this problem.

When children are seen in an emergency department for multiple trauma, the extremities should be observed closely for the hallmark signs of fracture (deformity, oedema and pain). If a fracture is suspected, splint the extremity to avoid further trauma. Splinting also reduces pain because it prevents further movement of the bone. Splints should extend from a joint above to a joint below the suspected fracture site. For example, for a fracture of the forearm, the splint should reach from above the elbow to below the wrist. Immobilising the joints above and below the injury in this way prevents movement and muscle tension with further dislocation of the fracture. If the extremity is so seriously deformed by the break that it will not conform to the contour of a splint, do not attempt to move it into a splint position. Immobilise the extremity by placing sandbags on the sides of the arm or leg and leave it in that position. Take a thorough history of the accident. Some fractures in childhood occur from child abuse. This must be ruled out with all accidents.

All children with a suspected fracture will need an x-ray to confirm the diagnosis and to determine the alignment and **apposition** (the amount of end-to-end contact of the bone fragments) of the fractured segments of bone. Apposition is not as important in children as it is in adults. Bayonet or side-to-side apposition may be established or left in children up to 10 to 12 years old because, as the child grows and remodelling occurs, the bone will develop with normal contour and length. Side-to-side apposition results in a rapid, strong union and actually is the preferred position for some fractures.

If skin has been broken, the child may need tetanus prophylaxis. A haematocrit determination to estimate blood loss and cross-matching for replacement therapy may be necessary. An IV line is usually established to provide a route for fluid or blood replacement or for administration of an IV antibiotic to reduce the possibility of infection through the open wound.

All children with fractures are in some pain. Usually, they are frightened not only from the pain, the appearance of the fracture and their inability to use the extremity, but also from the traumatic situation that led to the fracture such as a fall from a bunk bed or a motor vehicle accident. Spend time comforting and helping children to realise that they are now safe and will not be injured further. If they can relax enough to lie still and not move the fractured extremity, the pain will decrease. Children who have a compound fracture are as frightened by the sight of blood as they are by the deformity and pain. However, reassure children and parents that, unless the bone has been crushed, the bone fragments can be brought back into line. Afterwards, the bone will heal with the same strength as before.

Types of fractures

Forearm fractures

Children often fall on an outstretched arm, so fractures of the forearm are common. In children, most fractures of the forearm involve the distal third; a smaller number of such accidents occur in the middle or proximal third. The injury may involve a fracture of the radius, a fracture of both the radius and ulna, or a displacement of the epiphyseal plate of the radius. In young children, the injury usually is a greenstick fracture. Sometimes greenstick fractures are broken completely before casting to prevent the bone's resuming its "bent" position within the cast. Refer to this as "straightening" the bone, rather than "breaking" the bone.

If a greenstick fracture is slight so that the degree of angulation is not great, it may not be reduced or brought into a straight line; as callus is formed and the bone remodels itself, it will naturally straighten into good alignment.

If the fracture is complete and overriding is excessive, traction to the fingers may be used as a part of the cast. This "banjo" traction is cumbersome and limits the child's use of that hand. The hand is covered up to the first phalangeal knuckle to prevent the child from moving the hand excessively and damaging the edge of the cast, which would loosen it and pull the arm into poor alignment.

Elbow fractures

If a child falls and stops the fall with a hand, the elbow may hyperextend, transmitting the force of the blow to the distal humerus and causing a supracondylar fracture of the humerus. Fractures of the humerus are reduced and stabilised with an arm cast, a splint or traction, depending on the position of the fracture (Yaokreh et al., 2012). Elevating the cast on pillows or suspending the hand by a strip of gauze or traction apparatus reduces oedema. Although the fracture may be minor, the child needs to be assessed carefully for signs of blood vessel or nerve compression (Volkmann's contracture).

Volkmann's ischaemic contracture

When an arm is flexed and put into a cast, the radial artery and nerve may be compressed at the elbow, causing nerve injury or severe impairment of circulation. If the fracture is in the proximal third of the radius, parents need to assess for signs of circulatory or nerve impairment for 24 hours.

If symptoms of compression are present but not detected within 6 hours, Volkmann's contracture and possible permanent damage to the arm will result. The arm is left permanently flexed at the elbow. The wrist is hyperextended and the fingers assume a flexed, claw-like, useless position. If a child is going to be discharged after application of a cast, inform parents about the symptoms of compression so that its development can be detected. If a child is admitted to the hospital for 24 hours, the radial pulse (if palpable at the edge of the cast) should be taken hourly, along with checks for coldness, blanching and colour of the fingers, for the first 8 hours. In some instances, a cast is applied incompletely for 24 hours, the elbow portion being simply splinted and wrapped with elastic bandages. After 24 hours, when oedema has subsided and the chance of compression is less, the rest of the arm is casted.

Epiphyseal separations of the radius

If a child breaks a fall with an outstretched arm, a separation of the epiphysis of the distal radius may result. When this occurs, the wrist must be casted to restabilise the epiphysis. Although epiphyseal injuries are always serious, distal radial injury rarely causes serious sequelae in children. However, advise parents that it is important to keep appointments for follow-up visits, so that growth disturbances can be detected early and correction started. Stapling the epiphysis is an intervention that may be required to arrest abnormal growth if it occurs. Stimulation of the epiphyseal line may increase growth if growth restriction occurs.

Clavicle fractures

When young children fall and catch themselves with an outstretched arm, the force of the blow may be transmitted to the clavicle, causing fracture of the clavicle or dislocation at the sternal joint (Stewart & Van Klompenberg, 2008). Clavicles also may be fractured during birth or be a mark of child abuse.

Swelling is often present at the site of the break. In the newborn, a Moro reflex can only be demonstrated on the unaffected side. An older child refuses to use the arm, leaving it hanging at the side. Crepitus (crackling) can be felt over the clavicle. After x-ray diagnosis, the child is placed in a commercially manufactured or figure-of-eight splint of stockinette placed over the shoulders and under the axilla, keeping the arm adducted and flexed across the chest. This is left in place for about 3 weeks, during which time the wrap tends to look soiled. The child should keep the splint dry—no swimming or showering during this time. The parent often needs to tighten the splint every morning to keep it firmly in place. Parents are usually apologetic about the appearance of the stockinette when they return for a repeat x-ray after 3 weeks. They may be worried that the soiled appearance of the splint reflects the quality of their housekeeping or child care. Assure them that the soiled splint proves that they followed instructions well and left the splint in place for the required time.

Parents may need reassurance that this splint is adequate therapy. They may ask, "The bone is broken, after all—why is my child not being placed in a cast?" Acknowledge their concern by stating that most people think that when there is a broken bone, a cast is needed, however this injury is an exception. Doing so allows parents to voice their worries and receive necessary assurance.

Fracture of the femur

Children who are involved in motor vehicle accidents or who fall from considerable heights and land on their feet may suffer a fractured femur. Child abuse should be considered in an infant who sustains a fractured femur because there are few normal instances when a fracture of this magnitude occurs in an infant.

Even with closed femoral fractures, blood loss can be extensive because of the size of the bone broken. As the child lies on the examining table in the emergency department, the child tends to hold the leg externally rotated; the thigh may appear abnormally short or deformed. Often, the child is in a great deal of pain, possibly with signs of shock from pain and blood loss. Children are frightened as well by the force of the accident that caused such a severe injury.

In the past, fractured femurs were not casted immediately because strong tendon spasm causes poor alignment and overriding of the femur segments. Only after muscle spasm had been reduced enough by skeletal or Bryant's traction to allow close approximation of the bone edges (7 to 14 days) was the child removed from traction and placed in a hip spica cast. Today, a child may be taken to surgery immediately to have an intramedullary rod placed to align and stabilise the fracture. No cast may be required. Help the child and family identify ways for the child to continue contact with friends during any time of restricted activity.

Dislocation of the radial head

If a small child is lifted by one hand, as happens when a parent pulls on one arm to lift the child over a curb or up a step, the head of the radius may escape the ligament surrounding it and become dislocated ("nursemaid's elbow"; see Box 51.4). The child holds the arm flexed at the elbow with the forearm pronated. The child winces with pain when the radial head is palpated. A simple dislocation of the radial head can be reduced by a doctor, using gentle pressure on the radial head while the arm is flexed and supinated. Relief of pain is immediate and the child begins to use the arm again.

Parents feel guilty because they caused this dislocation. Reassure parents that this is a common injury in small children. They rarely need to be cautioned that lifting a child in this manner is not wise. Be aware, however, that a dislocation of the radial head can occur from extremely rough handling, as is seen in child abuse. Investigate the circumstances of the injury closely.

BOX 51.4 * Focus on evidence-based practice

Dislocation of the radial head

Young children frequently sustain dislocation of the radial head at the elbow when a parent or carer lifts them by an arm. To discover what are the most frequent activities that cause this, researchers studied the records of 2011 children seen at an urban tertiary care emergency department for this type of traction injury. The median age of children was 2.1 years; 59% of them were female. Activities that most frequently led to the traction and dislocation were lifting the child by the arms (28.3%), "wrestling" (12.3%), swinging the child by the arms (9.2%) and placing the child into and out of a seat (4.3%). Male carers were more likely to be involved when a child was swung by the arms, lifted or "wrestled" with. Injury tended to most often happen with female carers when the child pulled away, tripped or was in the process of getting dressed.

How could you use the results of the above study to improve how you educate new parents?

Source: Rudloe, T. F., Schutzman, S., Lee, L. K., et al. (2012). No longer a "nursemaid's" elbow: Mechanisms, caregivers, and prevention. *Pediatric Emergency Care, 28*(8), 771–774.

Athletic injuries

Although participating in athletics promotes growth and development, it can also lead to injury. Playing on backyard trampolines, in particular, is associated with a significant number of injuries in children (Klimek et al., 2013). Strategies to prevent sports injuries include: pre-participation health examinations, medical coverage at sporting events, proper coaching, adequate hydration, competent officiating, and proper equipment and field or surface playing conditions.

Knee injuries

Participation in sports such as football, skiing, soccer and athletics are frequent causes of knee injuries in children. These injuries usually involve the ligaments surrounding the knee—the medial, lateral, posterior or cruciate ligaments (figure-eight ligaments that stabilise the knee). After the injury, the child has severe pain in the knee with localised oedema. An x-ray or MRI will be taken to rule out fracture (Hoetzel et al., 2014).

If the injury is mild (only a few torn fibres), bed rest with ice applied to the knee is often the only therapy needed. Local infiltration of an anaesthetic may be necessary to minimise pain. After 24 hours, heat is applied to the knee to hasten healing. If the injury is more severe, the knee joint may fill with fluid. The child will need bed rest and ice applied to the joint. The abnormal synovial fluid will be aspirated and a compression dressing will be applied to discourage accumulation of further fluid. After 24 hours, heat treatments will be started to hasten healing. If the injury is severe, arthroscopy may be done to visualise and surgically repair the knee ligaments. Arthroscopic surgery makes repair of ligaments or cartilage a minor procedure and limits the necessity for immobilisation and a cast.

A severe twisting motion to the knee can cause a dislocation of the kneecap (it moves to the posterior surface of the knee). The knee appears deformed and the child is in acute pain. Immediate treatment for a dislocated kneecap is to slide it again to the front of the knee. After this realignment, the child usually has to use a leg immobiliser for 1 week. If the problem is chronic or occurs frequently, surgery to strengthen the ligaments may be necessary. Quadriceps exercises (straight-leg raising) are important to prevent the dislocation reoccurring.

Throwing injuries

Throwing places repeated stress on an upper extremity, particularly the elbow joint. The injury tends to occur during the forward motion of the arm or during the follow-through. After the injury, the child is unable to extend the elbow completely because of minute tears and fibrous contractures in the muscle. The child notices pain and tenderness and has loss of complete elbow extension for 24 to 48 hours after the injury. Resting the arm and applying icepacks for 15 to 20 minutes three times a day relieves the pain. An anti-inflammatory agent may be helpful. A limited number of cortisone injections into the elbow musculature may be helpful. Exercises to strengthen flexor muscles help to prevent this type of injury.

Children who participate in sports need time for proper warm-up.

Strains and sprains

A **strain** is a muscle-tendon injury. A **sprain** is a ligament injury. Strained or sprained ankles are common but difficult childhood injuries. The joint is painful and swollen. Such injuries typically occur from inline skating or snow- or skateboarding. When x-ray reveals no fracture, a child may feel as though someone has said that the injury is not serious but "just a sprain". This makes the extent of the swelling and pain baffling. Some children may be accused by parents of "putting on" pain because the injury is "only a sprain".

Help the child and parents to understand that strains and sprains are truly painful. Because a cast is not used and the ankle is not immobilised completely, strains and sprains can be more painful than fractures, which are casted.

If the injury is recent, an icepack should be applied for approximately 20 minutes at a time to reduce oedema at the site. An elastic bandage may be applied for firm support. The child may be given crutches to limit weight-bearing for the next 3 or 4 days. Make certain that the parents of the child understand how the elastic bandage is applied so that it can be rewrapped if it loosens and be sure that the child is using the crutches properly before being discharged from the emergency department.

✔ *Checkpoint question 51.4*

Why is casting an elbow a potentially dangerous type of cast application?

a. It prevents the ulna and radius from continuing to grow
b. Oedema at the elbow can cause permanent nerve damage
c. Holding the arm bent at the elbow causes low-grade pain
d. These casts get dirty and so lead to humeral osteomyelitis

Key points for review

- Bone and muscle disorders tend to be long-term conditions. Help children and their families to think about how the disorder will affect tasks of daily living to help a child better adjust to interventions such as a cast or brace. Assist children plan self-diversional activities as necessary, so they continue to grow developmentally while confined to a cast or traction.
- As a rule, children with a broken bone need additional calcium in their diet to aid bone healing. If they are on strict bed rest, however, this should only be a moderate addition to their diet, to prevent renal calculi from forming.
- Many children have casts applied to allow broken bones to heal. If broken bones are not easily aligned, children are placed in traction.
- Developmental disorders that occur in children include flat feet (pronation), genu varum (bowlegs) and genu valgum (knock knees). The majority of these disorders are corrected naturally by normal growth.
- Slipped epiphysis is slipping of the femur head in relation to the neck of the femur at the epiphyseal line. It occurs most frequently in obese or rapidly growing boys.
- Osteomyelitis is infection of the bone. It can result in extensive destruction of the bone. Antibiotic therapy is necessary to combat the infection.
- Scoliosis is a lateral curvature of the spine. It is treated by bracing or surgery.
- Juvenile arthritis occurs in several different forms: polyarticular, pauciarticular and systemic onset. Therapy includes exercise, heat application and administration of medications such as NSAIDs or methotrexate.
- Myasthenia gravis can occur in three types: neonatal transient myasthenia, congenital myasthenia and juvenile myasthenia. Anticholinesterase medications such as neostigmine, which prolong acetylcholine action, are used.
- Muscular dystrophies are a group of disorders that lead to progressive degeneration of skeletal muscles. Different types can occur, including congenital myotonic, facioscapulohumeral and pseudohypertrophic. Children and parents need support throughout this long-term illness.
- A fracture or bruise of soft tissue can result from any trauma, including child abuse. Be certain to secure a detailed history of an injury to be sure that the history is consistent with the degree of injury.
- Volkmann's ischaemic contracture is a complication that occurs when an arm is casted in a bent position and the radial artery and nerve are compressed at the elbow. Frequent assessments of finger colour and warmth are safeguards to detect if this is occurring.

CASE STUDY QUESTIONS

4. How would you explain to Will's mother what has happened to him?
5. Suppose Will, who has scoliosis, was prescribed a brace to wear 23 hours a day for treatment a month ago. During the last month, he dropped out of the school band and the one after-school club to which he belonged. He tells you he is dropping activities "to have more time to study". Would you be concerned about him? What areas would you need to assess and how would you intervene?
6. Will's sister has juvenile arthritis. You notice when she returns for a follow-up visit to the arthritis clinic that the inflammation in her joints is worse than at her last visit and she says she has more pain. Her mother tells

you she has been giving her acetaminophen instead of her prescribed NSAID because she read that NSAIDs cause stomach irritation and heart disease. Was she wise to substitute another medication this way? How would you suggest she proceed at this point?

Resources

For an extensive range of additional resources to enhance teaching and learning and to facilitate understanding of this chapter, please see the text's accompanying website located on thePoint at http://thepoint.lww.com.

References

Abdel-Hamid, H. & Clemens, P. R. (2012). Pharmacological therapies for muscular dystrophies. *Current Opinion in Neurology, 25*(5), 604–608.

Alsancak, S., Guner, S. & Kinik, H. (2013). Orthotic variations in the management of infantile tibia vara and the results of treatment. *Prosthetics and Orthotics International, 37*(5), 375–383.

Amos, L. B., Grekowicz, M. L., Kuhn, E. M., et al., (2014). Treatment of pediatric restless legs syndrome. *Clinical Pediatrics, 53*(4), 331–336.

Arundel, P. & Bishop, N. (2010). Diagnosing osteogenesis imperfecta. *Paediatrics and Child Health, 20*(5), 225–231.

Aytaç, S., Schnetzke, M., Swartman, B., et al. (2014). Posttraumatic and postoperative osteomyelitis: surgical revision strategy with persisting fistula. *Archives of Orthopaedic and Trauma Surgery, 134*(2), 159–165.

Bazner-Chandler, J. & Brady, M. A. (2013). Musculoskeletal disorders. In E. E. Burns, A. M. Dunn & M. A. Brady et al. (Eds.), *Pediatric Primary Care* (5th ed., pp. 928–960). Philadelphia: Elsevier/Saunders.

Bernard, T. J., Knupp, K., Yang, M. L., et al. (2012). Neurologic & muscular disorders. In W. W. Hay et al. (Eds). *Current Diagnosis & Treatment Pediatrics* (21st ed., pp. 740–829). New York: McGraw-Hill/Lange.

Beukelman, T., Ringold, S., Davis, T. E., et al. (2012). Disease-modifying antirheumatic drug use in the treatment of juvenile idiopathic arthritis: A cross-sectional analysis of the CARRA registry. *Journal of Rheumatology, 39*(9), 1867–1874.

Birch, J. (2013). Blount disease. *Journal of the American Academy of Orthopaedic Surgeons, 21*(7), 408–418.

Boros, C. & Whitehead, B. (2010). Juvenile idiopathic arthritis. *Australian Family Physician, 39*(9), 630–636.

Brenner, A., Koshy, J., Morey, J., et al. (2012). The bone scan. *Seminars in Nuclear Medicine, 42*(1), 11–26.

Brown, R. H. Amato, A. A. & Mendell, J. R. (2008). Muscular dystrophies and other muscle diseases. In A. S. Fauci et al. (Eds). *Harrison's Principles of Internal Medicine*. Columbus, OH: McGraw-Hill.

Chaudhry, S., Phillips, D. & Feldman, D. (2014). Legg-Calvé-Perthes disease: An overview with recent literature. *Bulletin of the Hospital for Joint Diseases, 72*(1), 18–27.

Cook, P. C. (2014). Transient synovitis, septic hip, and Legg-Calvé-Perthes disease: An approach to the correct diagnosis. *Pediatric Clinics of North America, 61*(6), 1109–1118.

D'Amico, M., Roncoletta, P., Di Felice, F., et al. (2012). Leg length discrepancy in scoliotic patients. *Studies in Health Technology and Informatics, 176*(1), 146–150.

Harrington, J., Sochett, E. & Howard, A. (2014). Update on the evaluation and treatment of osteogenesis imperfecta. *Pediatric Clinics of North America, 61*(6), 1243–1257.

Hellmann, D. B. & Imboden, J. B. (2009). Musculoskeletal & immunologic disorders. In S. J. McPhee & M. A. Papadakis (Eds). *Current Medical Diagnosis & Treatment*. Columbus, OH: McGraw-Hill.

Hoetzel, J., Preiss, A., Heitmann, M. A., et al. (2014). Knee injuries in children and adolescents. *European Journal of Trauma and Emergency Surgery, 40*(1), 23–36.

Jacob, N. C. & Rammya, M. (2014). The limping child. *InnovAiT, 7*(12), 744–749.

Karkhaneh, M., Rowe, B. H., Saunders, L. D., et al. (2013). Trends in head injuries associated with mandatory bicycle helmet legislation targeting children and adolescents. *Accident; Analysis and Prevention, 59*, 206–212.

Klimek, P. M., Juen, D., Stranzinger, E., et al. (2013). Trampoline related injuries in children: Risk factors and radiographic findings. *World Journal of Pediatrics, 9*(2), 169–174.

Koller, H., Zenner, J., Gajic, V., et al. (2012). The impact of halo-gravity traction on curve rigidity and pulmonary function in the treatment of severe and rigid scoliosis and kyphoscoliosis: A clinical study and narrative review of the literature. *European Spine Journal, 21*(3), 514–529.

Kontulainen, S. A., Kawalilak, C. E., Johnston, J. D., et al. (2013). Prevention of osteoporosis and bone fragility: A pediatric concern. *American Journal of Lifestyle Medicine, 7*(6), 405–417.

Laituri, C. A., Schwend, R. M. & Holcomb, G. W. (2012). Thoracoscopic vertebral body stapling for treatment of scoliosis in young children. *Journal of Laparoendoscopy & Advanced Surgical Techniques, 22*(8), 830–833.

Leblanc, C. M., Lang, B., Bencivenga, A., et al., (2012). Access to biologic therapies in Canada for children with juvenile idiopathic arthritis. *Journal of Rheumatology, 39*(9), 1875–1879.

Loder, R.T. & Dietz, F. R. (2012). What is the evidence for the treatment of slipped capital femoral epiphysis? *Journal of Pediatric Orthopedics, 32* (Suppl. 2), S158–S165.

Mercuri, E. & Muntoni, F. (2013). Muscular dystrophies. *The Lancet, 381*(9869), 845–860.

McKenna, L. & Mirkov, S. (2014). *McKenna's Drug Handbook for Nursing and Midwifery* (7th ed.). Lippincott Williams & Wilkins.

Monti, E., Mottes, M., Fraschini, P., et al., (2010). Current and emerging treatments for the management of osteogenesis imperfecta. *Therapeutics and Clinical Risk Management, 6*, 367–381.

Najarian, S. L. (2013) Compartment syndrome. In D. Cline & O. J. Ma (Eds.), *Tintinalli's Emergency Medicine* (pp. 615–616). New York: McGraw-Hill.

Peltola, H. & Pääkkönen, M. (2014). Acute osteomyelitis in children. *New England Journal of Medicine, 370*(4), 352–360.

Rudloe, T. F., Schutzman, S., Lee, L. K., et al. (2012). No longer a "nursemaid's" elbow: Mechanisms, caregivers, and prevention. *Pediatric Emergency Care, 28*(8), 771–774.

Ruhlman, D., Otten, C. & Colella, C. (2014). Dermatomyositis. *The Journal for Nurse Practitioners, 10*(9), 674–681.

Schoenfeld, R. et al., (2010). Using the internet to educate adolescents about osteoporosis: Application of a tailored web-education system, *Health Promotion Practice, 11*(1), 104–111.

Simm, P. J., Allen, R. C. & Zacharin, M. R. (2008). Bisphosphonate treatment in chronic recurrent multifocal osteomyelitis. *Journal of Pediatrics, 152*(4), 571–575.

Soep, J. B. (2012). Rheumatic diseases. In W. W. Hay et al. (Eds), *Current Diagnosis & Treatment Pediatrics* (21st ed., pp. 889–896). New York: McGraw-Hill Lange.

Stewart, D. P. & Van Klompenberg, L. H. (2008). Posterior dislocation of the clavicle at the sternoclavicular joint. *American Journal of Emergency Medicine, 26*(1), 108–111.

Takken, T., van Brussel, M., Engelbert, R. H., et al. (2008). Exercise therapy in juvenile idiopathic arthritis. *Cochrane Database of Systematic Reviews*, (4), (CD005954).

Tedesco, F. S. & Cossu, G. (2012). Stem cell therapies for muscular disorders. *Current Opinion in Neurology, 25*(5), 597–603.

Tu, P. & Bytomski, J. R. (2011). Diagnosis of heel pain. *American Family Physician, 84*(8), 909–916.

Walters, A. S., Gabelia, D. & Frauscher, B. (2013). Restless legs syndrome (Willis-Ekbom disease) and growing pains: Are they the same thing? A side-by-side comparison of the diagnostic criteria for both and recommendations for future research. *Sleep Medicine, 14*(12), 1247–1252.

Weeks, B. H. (2012) Myasthenia gravis: Helping patients have better outcomes. *The Nurse Practitioner, 37*(9), 30–36.

Weiler, R., Ingram, M. & Wolman, R. (2011). 10-Minute Consultation. Osgood-Schlatter disease. *British Medical Journal, 343*, d4534.

Weiss, H. & Werkmann, M. (2012). Soft braces in the treatment of Adolescent Idiopathic Scoliosis (AIS) - Review of the literature and description of a new approach, *Scoliosis*, *7*(1), 11–12.

Yaokreh, J. B., Gicquel, L., Schneider, L., et al. (2012). Compared outcomes after percutaneous pinning versus open reduction in paediatric supracondylar elbow fractures. *Orthopaedics & Traumatology: Surgery & Research*, *98*(6), 645–651.

Zaba, L. C. & Fiorentino, D. F. (2012). Skin disease in dermatomyositis. *Current opinion in rheumatology*, *24*(6), 597–601.

Suggested readings

Arthritis Australia. <www.arthritisaustralia.com.au>.

Griffin, S. (2013). Primary prevention of osteoporosis, *InnovAiT*, *6*(3), 148–154.

Hart, E. S. (2012). The power of remodeling bones in children. *Orthopaedic Nursing*, *31*(3), 187–189.

Heikkinen, K., Salanterä, S., Suomi, R., et al. (2011). Ambulatory orthopaedic surgery patient education and cost of care. *Orthopaedic Nursing*, *30*(1), 20–28.

Merenda, L., Costello, K., Santangelo, A. M., et al. (2011). Perceptions of self-image and physical appearance: Conversations with typically developing youth and youth with idiopathic scoliosis. *Orthopaedic Nursing*, *30*(6), 383–390.

Muscular Dystrophy Australia. <www.mda.org.au>.

Osteogenesis Imperfecta Society of Australia. <www.oiaustralia.org.au>.

Reed, C., Carroll, L., Baccari, S., et al. (2011). Spica cast care: A collaborative staff-led education initiative for improved patient care. *Orthopaedic Nursing*, *30*(6), 353–358.

Scoliosis Australia. <www.scoliosis-australia.org>.

Scoliosis Kids Australia. <www.scoliosiskidsaustralia.com.au/halo_traction.php>.

Secor-Turner, M., Scal, P., Garwick, A., et al. (2011). Living with juvenile arthritis: Adolescents' challenges and experiences. *Journal of Pediatric Health Care*, *25*(5), 302–307.

The Children's Hospital at Westmead. Bones and muscles fact sheets. <http://kidshealth.schn.health.nsw.gov.au/fact-sheets#Bones & Muscles>.

Vialle, R., Thévenin-Lemoine, C. & Mary, P. (2013). Neuromuscular scoliosis. *Orthopaedics & Traumatology: Surgery & Research*, *99*(1 Suppl), S124–S139.

Chapter 52

Nursing care of a family when a child has an unintentional injury

Previous chapters described the growth and development of well children and care of children with disorders of specific body systems. This chapter adds information about the characteristic changes, both physical and psychosocial, that occur when children experience an unintentional injury.

LEARNING OBJECTIVES

After mastering the contents of this chapter, you should be able to:

1. Describe the causes and consequences of common accidents and injuries in childhood and measures to prevent them.
2. Analyse ways that care of children with unintentional injuries can be more family-centred.
3. Identify key assessment needs of a child who is unintentionally injured from an accident.
4. Establish expected outcomes for an unintentionally injured child.
5. Plan nursing care related to an unintentionally injured child.
6. Implement nursing care for a child with an unintentional injury, such as providing pain relief.
7. Identify areas related to care of children with unintentional injuries that could benefit from additional nursing research or application of evidence-based practice.
8. Integrate knowledge of unintentional injuries in childhood with nursing process to achieve quality child and family healthcare.

KEY TERMS

- coma
- contrecoup injury
- debridement
- drowning
- grafting
- near drowning
- otorrhoea
- rhinorrhoea
- stupor

CASE STUDY

Jason, a 5-year-old boy, is seen in the emergency department after a car accident. He is crying and upset, although the only visible signs of trauma are a reddened and oedematous area on the middle of his forehead. Vital signs reveal: temperature, 37.5°C; respirations, 18 breaths per minute; pulse, 62 beats per minute; and blood pressure, 110/62 mmHg. His left pupil is more dilated than his right and it reacts sluggishly to light. His Glasgow Coma Scale (GCS) score is 10. His mother tells you, "I'm sure he's not injured badly. He was wearing his seatbelt."

CASE STUDY QUESTIONS

1. Consider how assessment and care would be prioritised if Jason and his family presented to a rural setting. You might like to consider the differences in areas, according to hospital location and resources.
2. Outline your initial assessment encompassing the primary and secondary surveys as a basic prioritisation format.

CARE OF A CHILD WITH AN UNINTENTIONAL INJURY

Assessment

Because the emergency department or clinic nurse is often the first person who sees a child after an injury, be ready to make a preliminary assessment of the extent of a child's injuries before a doctor arrives. Remember that children may be seriously hurt but not crying because they are in shock. They may be haemorrhaging, but, if they are bleeding internally, the blood may not be visibly evident. Accidents become fatal when lung, heart or brain function becomes inadequate. These three body systems, therefore, must be evaluated first (Airway, Breathing, Circulation and Disability, or an ABCD evaluation). Table 52.1 lists signs and symptoms to assess when determining the respiratory, cardiovascular and neurological status of an injured child.

While conducting a preliminary assessment of a child's major body systems, take a brief history of the accident. What happened? How long ago did it happen? Was the child using protective equipment such as a helmet or a secured seatbelt? What have the parents done? If the child fell, how far was the fall? On what body part did the child land? Ask the carer what they think are their child's major injuries. Evaluating children in an emergency department is difficult because they may be too young to communicate, unconscious, or they are so frightened that they cannot stop crying to report which body parts are painful or to indicate which parts should be assessed first. Spend a few minutes attempting to calm children and get them past this initial fright, unless symptoms of major body system disturbances require that you direct your immediate efforts elsewhere. Parents need frequent explanations of care given or planned, because as long as they are worried and tense, children cannot be calmed easily.

TABLE 52.1 Important assessments on initial examination of an injured child

Body system	Assessment
Respiratory system	Quality of respirations Rate of respirations Sound of obstruction (wheezing, stridor, retractions, coughing?) Colour (cyanotic?) Oxygen hunger (restlessness, inability to lie flat?)
Cardiovascular system	Colour (pallor from haemorrhage or cardiovascular collapse?) Gross bleeding Pulse rate (increases with haemorrhage) Blood pressure (decreases with haemorrhage) Feeling of apprehension from altered vascular pressure
Nervous system	Level of consciousness (child answers questions coherently, infant attunes to parent's voice?) Pupils (equal and reacting to light?) Bumps or bruises on head or spinal column Loss of motion or sensory function in a body part

A proportion of unintentional injuries in children result from child abuse. Conflicting histories or a parent and child recounting different stories is a hallmark of this. Always ask yourself if this could be a possibility and make a referral to appropriate services as determined by local health policy.

Nursing considerations

The nursing considerations most frequently identified with injured children are related to pain. Depending on the particular injury, several other nursing considerations are relevant, as are those that relate to the suffering that parents experience when their child is injured. Examples of possible nursing considerations are:

- Pain related to fractured tibia from sports injury
- Ineffective airway clearance related to burned oesophageal tissue
- Impaired physical mobility related to severe burn injury
- Disturbed body image related to change in physical appearance from thermal injury
- Parental fear related to outcome after head injury in child
- Interrupted family processes related to child's unintentional injury
- Anxiety related to apprehension and lack of knowledge regarding medical treatment of child.

A key component of nursing intervention in an emergency department is to help parents understand why an injury happened and plan ways to make their immediate or community environment safe for children. The extent of a child's injury depends on the injuring agent, the part of the body that was injured and often the immediate care, including both physical and psychological management that a child receives. The diameter of the airway in children is smaller than in adults, so an injury to this body area almost always results in a greater danger of airway closure. This could happen from the child inhaling a substance, such as water, that directly obstructs the airway or from inhaling toxic fumes that cause inflammation along the lining of the airway, resulting in obstruction. A blow to the neck can result in oedema of surrounding tissues, causing the airway to close.

Injuries may involve some blood loss. Fortunately, a child's circulatory system is capable of rapid compensation for blood loss by vasoconstriction. Because the total volume of blood in a child is reduced, however, blood loss in children is always potentially serious. Because of this, many hospitals have standing orders that allow emergency care nurses to begin intravenous normal saline boluses on children with obvious blood loss.

Often, in the emergency department, large portions of the child's body must be exposed to view so that care can be given easily. This means that rapid cooling can occur. Because of the large body surface area of children in relation to weight, always be conscious of body temperature and take active measures to decrease cooling by keeping a child covered as much as possible during examinations.

Standard infection precautions must be maintained in emergency situations, the same as at any other time. Parental consent must be obtained for treatment procedures even in an emergency, except for life-saving actions, such as cardiopulmonary resuscitation. In these instances, action can and should be taken to save a child's life with or without parental permission (it is assumed that parents would consent to life-saving procedures). Delaying emergency procedures until parents can be located may result in permanent disability or death.

After an injury, children need follow-up care to be certain that the immediate interventions were adequate and that healing is taking place. Home visits or outpatient appointments are also the time to determine whether the child's environment has been changed and is safer now than at the time of the accident (if applicable).

If an injury could not have been anticipated, parents appreciate hearing that such an accident could not have been avoided and that they are good parents. This helps them maintain adequate self-esteem to continue to function well as parents.

Examples of expected outcomes suggesting achievement of goals are:

- Child swallows fluids without distress after oesophageal burns
- Child states pain is at tolerable level within 30 minutes
- Child demonstrates full range of motion in hand after thermal injury

- Child states he understands that wearing a seatbelt is an important safety measure
- Child states she will wear helmet when riding bicycle in the future.

Reflect on your initial nursing assessment and care and now consider ongoing management.

HEAD TRAUMA

Children receive head injuries when they are involved in multiple-trauma accidents, such as motor vehicle accidents. Falls from swings, verandahs and bunk beds also cause many head injuries. Other children are injured by being struck on the head by an object, such as a ball, rock or hockey puck, or by falling from a bicycle especially if they're not wearing a protective helmet (Persaud et al., 2012).

Head injuries are always potentially serious not only because they can cause an immediate threat to the life of the child, but also because several complications may follow. With a depressed skull fracture, for example, recurrent seizures can occur. Many of these children show focal abnormalities on an electroencephalogram (EEG) because of scar tissue formation. Some children experience memory deficits or minor personality changes after head injury (Yeates et al., 2012). Symptoms such as headache, irritability and postural vertigo (sensation of feeling faint or the inability to maintain normal balance—also known as post-traumatic syndrome) also may occur. Behavioural manifestations may include aggressiveness or poor school performance. It is often difficult to determine whether these symptoms are organic or the result of being treated differently from usual by anxious parents.

Immediate assessment

All children with head trauma require immediate and ongoing neurological assessment to detect signs and symptoms of raised intracranial pressure (ICP). Increasing pressure puts stress on the respiratory, cardiac and temperature centres, causing dysfunction in these areas. With increased pressure, the pupils become slow or unable to react immediately. Level of consciousness and motor ability decrease; pulse and respiratory rates decrease; and temperature and pulse pressure increase.

Assess vital signs to detect these changes and observe children's pupils to be certain that they are equal and react to light. Assess children's level of consciousness and motor function. Instigate cervical precautions until cervical trauma has been ruled out.

Immediate management

After a head injury, brain oedema is likely because fluid rushes into the inflamed and bruised area. Both central venous and central arterial lines may be inserted. ICP monitoring may be initiated (see Chapter 49). A computed tomography (CT) scan or magnetic resonance imaging (MRI) will be ordered to determine areas of oedema or bleeding. An attempt may be made to decrease brain oedema by intravenous (IV) administration of a hypertonic solution, such as mannitol. This will increase intravascular pressure and shift the oedema fluid back into the blood vessels. Steroids such as dexamethasone may be added to decrease inflammation and oedema. Keeping the head elevated is also effective in reducing ICP, however ensure this is in line with cervical precautions.

Skull fracture

A skull fracture is a crack in the bone of the skull (Mandt & Grubenhoff, 2012). Recognising skull fractures in children is important because associated cerebral injury often occurs under the fracture. Many skull fractures are simple linear types, most often involving the parietal bones. In some children, the skull does not fracture, but the suture lines separate.

If the base of the skull is fractured, **rhinorrhoea** or **otorrhoea** (clear fluid draining from the nose or ear, respectively) may be present and reflects escaping cerebrospinal fluid (CSF). Test the fluid discharge with a glucose reagent strip if there is doubt about the source of the drainage. CSF will test positive for glucose, whereas the clear, watery drainage from an upper respiratory tract infection will not.

Take a careful history of the accident, so that the strength of the blow to the head can be judged. Shock with hypotension rarely occurs with an isolated head injury. If a child is in shock, investigate for bleeding points other than the head injury. Skull fractures are confirmed by skull x-ray.

If a skull fracture is linear with no underlying pathology, no treatment except observation and prescription of an analgesic is necessary. In about 3 weeks, a repeat x-ray will be needed to confirm that healing has taken place. Parents can be reassured that a second x-ray this soon is not harmful but necessary. If a fracture is depressed (a bone fragment is pressing inward) or compounded (bone is broken into pieces), surgery will be necessary to remove or repair broken fragments. If CSF is draining from the nose hospital admission for observation is needed. Ensure cervical precautions are followed and once clearance is given keep the child in a semi-Fowler's position so that fluid drains out, not inwards, to reduce the possibility of introducing infection. Make certain that children do not attempt to hold their nose or pack their nostrils with something to halt the drainage. Because coughing and sneezing may allow air to enter the meningeal space, coughing may be suppressed by medication. Children may be prescribed a prophylactic antibiotic to reduce the risk of meningitis. If the drainage does not stop within a few days, surgery will be necessary to repair the fracture and reduce the danger of meningitis. Air that enters intracranial spaces usually is absorbed rapidly. If x-rays at 72 hours still show air in the cerebral

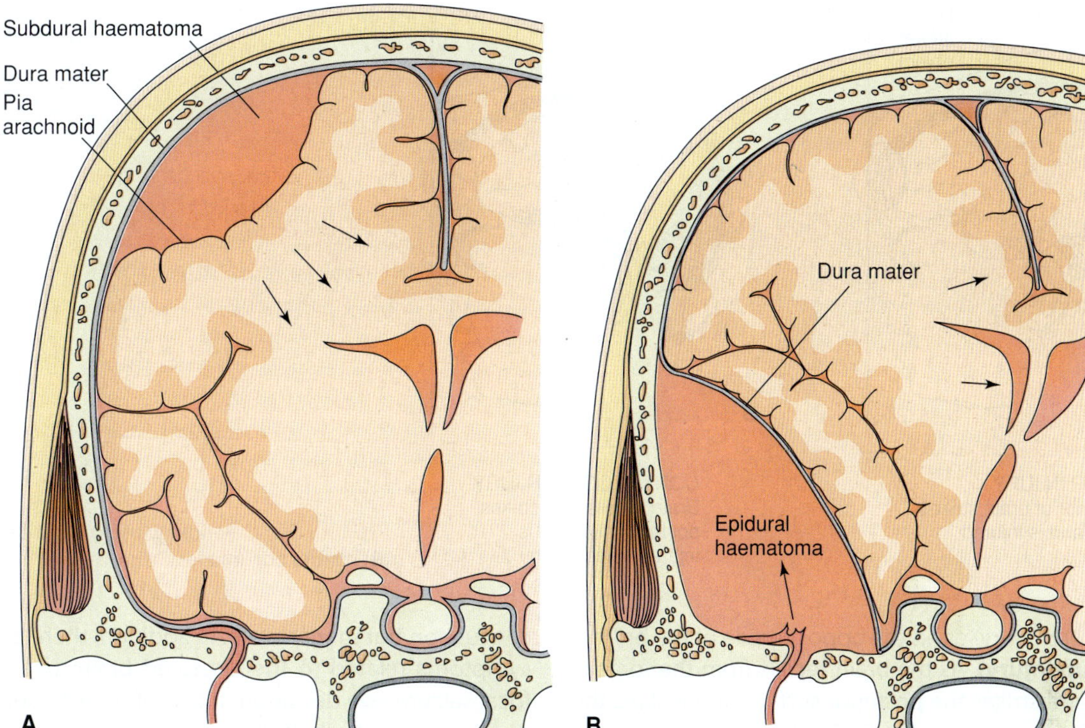

FIGURE 52.1 (**A**) Subdural haematoma. The red area in the upper left area of the drawing is the haematoma. Note the shift of structures. (**B**) Epidural haematoma. The red area in the lower left area of the drawing is the haematoma. Note the broken blood vessel and the shift of midline structures.

spaces, it implies that a skull defect remains and surgery may be indicated to close the defect.

Subdural haematoma

Subdural haematoma is venous bleeding into the space between the dura and the arachnoid membrane (see Fig. 52.1A). It occurs when head trauma lacerates minute veins in this area (Nickels et al., 2013). The collection of blood is usually bilateral. Subdural haematomas tend to occur in infants more often than in older children. Symptoms may occur within 3 days or as late as 20 days after trauma. Infants usually have symptoms of increased ICP. Seizures, vomiting, hyperirritability and enlargement of the head may occur. Anaemia caused by the substantial blood loss is a prominent sign. Angiography or ultrasound reveals the extent of the haematoma. In infants, accumulated subdural blood may be removed by a subdural puncture through the lateral aspect of a patent anterior fontanelle. Once the space is empty, expanding brain tissue will naturally occlude it. If the space has not been occluded after 2 weeks of daily punctures and active bleeding is still present, surgery usually is necessary to reduce the space and halt bleeding. In older children, surgery usually is necessary because the anterior fontanelle is closed and the space cannot be reached by puncture.

Epidural haematoma

Epidural haematoma is bleeding into the space between the dura and the skull (see Fig. 52.1B). This happens when head trauma is severe. Subdural haemorrhage is usually venous bleeding, but epidural haemorrhage is usually a result of rupture of the middle meningeal artery and is, therefore, arterial bleeding. It usually is intense and causes rapid brain compression. At the time of the injury, children become momentarily unconscious. They then regain consciousness and, to the untrained eye, appear to be well for minutes or hours. Then signs of cortical compression—vomiting, loss of consciousness, headache, seizures or hemiparesis (paralysis on one side)—are observed. On physical examination, unequal dilation or constriction of the pupils may be present. Decorticate posturing (see Chapter 49) may be seen, indicating extreme pressure on upper cortical centres. If the pressure is allowed to continue unchecked, cortical compression may be so great that brainstem, respiratory or cardiovascular function becomes impaired. As a rule, the closer to the time of the injury that symptoms of compression occur, the more extreme is the amount of blood loss. The treatment is surgical removal of the accumulated blood and cauterisation or ligation of the torn artery. The earlier the process is recognised and treated, the less the chance of residual damage from extreme pressure or anoxia to the involved portion of the brain.

Concussion

Concussion is the temporary and immediate impairment of neurological function caused by a hard, jarring shock (Purcell, 2012). It may occur on the side of the skull that was

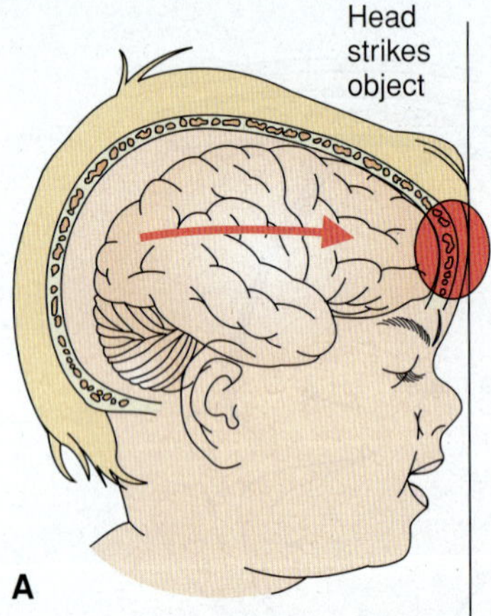

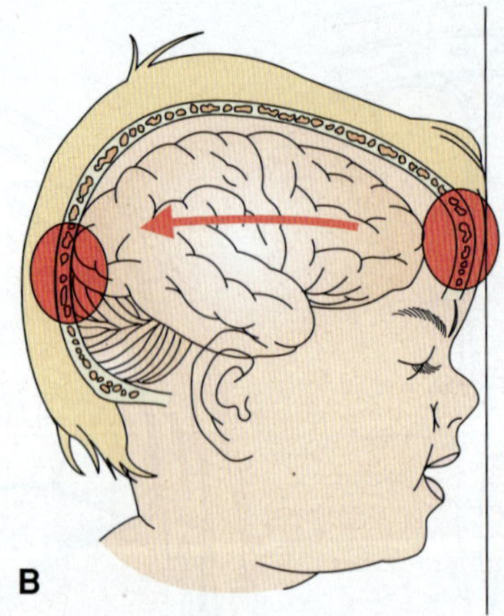

FIGURE 52.2 Aetiology of (**A**) coup and (**B**) contrecoup injuries.

struck (a *coup injury*) or on the opposite side of the brain (a **contrecoup injury**). As the brain recoils from the force of the blow and strikes the posterior surface of the skull, this second injury occurs (see Fig. 52.2). Children have at least a transient loss of consciousness at the time of the injury. They may vomit and may show irritability after regaining consciousness. They typically have no memory (amnesia) of the events leading up to the injury or of the injury itself. For some children, this makes being asked questions about the accident extremely upsetting because they do not remember anything that happened and feel a frightening loss of control. The child requires a skull x-ray to rule out skull fracture and observation for 24 hours to rule out severe brain trauma, oedema or laceration. A child usually can be observed at home by the parents, who are instructed to check the child's level of consciousness every 1–2 hours while the child is awake. Parents usually are instructed not to keep waking children during the night because this is disorienting and thus can be confused with unconsciousness. Parents should wake the child at least once during the night, however, and assess that the pulse rate is greater than 60 beats per minute.

To be certain that children are alert, parents can ask them to name a familiar object, such as a favourite toy, or to name the colour of an object shown to them. Telling parents their name or where they live is equally revealing. Give parents the telephone number to call if they have any questions about their child's care. Advise them to call if their child's behaviour changes in any way that seems worrisome. Many parents need to set an alarm clock to wake themselves during the night to assess their child's status. Be certain they understand that it is all right for children to sleep, but they must wake them at least once to assess their status.

Contusion

A brain contusion occurs when there is tearing or laceration of brain tissue. The symptoms are the same type as for concussion but more severe. In addition, there are specific symptoms related to the lacerated brain area such as a focal seizure, eye deviation or loss of speech. Surgery may be necessary to halt bleeding. The child's prognosis depends on the extent of the injury and effectiveness of therapy.

> ***What if...***
>
> In the emergency department, Jason's parents state that since his head injury he has been vomiting? Is it more likely that the vomiting is a result of the head injury, or that he has contracted a gastrointestinal infection?

Coma

Coma (unconsciousness from which a child cannot be roused) or **stupor** (grogginess from which a child can be roused) may be present in children after severe head trauma. Coma and stupor are both symptoms of underlying disorders; a history of the injury must be obtained so that treatment can be directed specifically towards the cause.

Obtain a history to determine the circumstances immediately before the time the child became comatose. Assess children in coma carefully and completely, so that the cause of the decreased consciousness can quickly be determined. Undress the child completely so that all body parts can be inspected, but maintain dignity and privacy. Establish baseline values; a child with increased ICP, for example, will show decreased pulse and respiratory rates and increased blood pressure.

If bulbar (brainstem) compression is present, a child cannot swallow effectively or safely. If this is suspected, turn the child on the side to prevent aspiration. Observe the eyes for signs of increased ICP. If both pupils are dilated, irreversible brainstem damage is suggested, although such a finding may also be present with poisoning from an atropine-like drug. Pinpoint pupils suggest barbiturate or opiate intoxication. One pupil dilated more than the other suggests third cranial nerve compression. An eye may be deviated downward and laterally as well. This situation requires immediate surgery to correct temporal compression.

The retina of the eye should be examined for papilloedema, which will be present if increased pressure is long-standing (more than 24 to 48 hours). Lack of a doll's eye reflex suggests that compression of the oculomotor nerves (third, fourth or sixth) or of the brainstem is involved. Observe for posturing, such as decerebrate posturing, which suggests cerebral compression and dysfunction.

Laboratory studies assessed include blood glucose, blood electrolytes, blood urea nitrogen (BUN), liver function tests, blood gas studies, lumbar puncture and toxicology tests may be ordered to rule out possible causes such as bacterial meningitis or haemorrhage. CT or MRI will be done if a head injury is the most likely cause (Isaacs, 2013).

Coma is usually graded according to a standard scale so that changes in the level of consciousness can be evaluated accurately. Ensure an age-appropriate GCS is used to undertake neurological assessment. An example is seen in Box 52.1. A score of 3 to 8 on the scale suggests severe trauma (a number less than 5 suggests a very severe prognosis); a score of 9 to 12, moderate trauma; and 13 to 15, slight trauma.

If children are unconscious for longer than a transient period, they usually are admitted to an observation unit for further assessment. Unless cervical precautions are in place, a child who is comatose is to be placed on their left side to reduce the risk of aspiration. Oral suctioning to remove mucus from the mouth and pharynx may be necessary, with extreme caution if potential skull or mandular fractures present. If a child has acute signs of respiratory compromise they may require upper airway protection and/or endotracheal intubation and ventilation.

An IV route is established so that, when specific measures such as blood replacement, electrolyte replacement or fluid replacement are needed, a route for immediate administration will be available. Blood will be drawn for a complete blood count, electrolyte determination, toxicology tests and cross-matching. If the cause of the coma is unknown, a lumbar puncture and EEG may be done. Skull x-ray, CT scan or MRI may be also performed.

Lumbar puncture has little value at first in predicting the severity of a head injury and is contraindicated if raised ICP is suspected. Obtain the child's vital signs and assess neurological status, such as state of consciousness and the ability of pupils to react to light, every 15 to 20 minutes or as ordered.

BOX 52.1 * Scoring for Glasgow Coma Scale

Eye opening

4. Child opens eyes spontaneously when you approach.
3. Child opens eyes in response to speech (spoken or shouted).
2. Child opens eyes only in response to painful stimuli, such as pressure on a nail bed.
1. Child does not open eyes in response to painful stimuli.

Motor response

6. Child can obey a simple command such as "hand me a toy" (infant smiles or attunes).
5. Child moves an extremity to locate a painful stimulus applied to the head or trunk and attempts to remove the source.
4. Child attempts to withdraw from the source of pain.
3. Child flexes arms at the elbows and wrists in response to painful stimuli to the nail beds (decorticate rigidity).
2. Child extends arms (straightens the elbows) in response to painful stimuli (cerebrate rigidity).
1. Child has no motor response to pain on any extremity.

Verbal response

5. Child is oriented to time, place and person (child >4 years old knows name, date and where he or she is; infant appears to recognise parent).
4. Child is able to converse, although not oriented to time, place or person (does not know who or where he or she is; infant says words but does not appear to differentiate parents from others).
3. Child speaks only in words or phrases that make little or no sense ("I want frazzle no"; infant's vocabulary is less than it is normally).
2. Child responds with incomprehensible sounds, such as groans.
1. Child does not respond verbally at all.

Modified from Teasdale, G. & Bennett, B. (1974). Assessment of coma and impaired consciousness: A practical scale. *Lancet, 2*(7872), 81–84.

Life-threatening and risk-taking behaviours or games

The incidences of high-risk and life-threatening adolescent activities are increasing and accentuated by social norms and social media networks. Peer pressure, including cyber bullying, is expanding the age ranges and incidences of extreme activities inflicted upon oneself or others. Examples of these activities include "choking games" which aim to elicit a euphoria by inducing a partial or complete loss of consciousness. This is done by intentionally depriving the brain of oxygen for a short period of time by strangulation or hanging or reducing the oxygen able to reach the nose by some technique such as pulling a plastic bag over the head. Extreme hyperventilation to induce hypocapnia is another technique. Unfortunately, the game can result in injury and death. The majority of deaths have occurred while the adolescent was alone; over 90% of the parents of the deceased children were unaware of the game (CDC, 2008a).

Other common life-threatening games and behaviours include "planking," which involves pivoting the body horizontally on a narrow vertical surface, as well as train jumping when a person intentionally jumps off moving trains.

ABDOMINAL TRAUMA

Assessment

Abdominal trauma results from an object striking the abdomen, such as a cricket bat, a seatbelt drawn tight in a motor vehicle accident or bicycle handlebar injuries. Child maltreatment is another cause (Klimek et al., 2013). Assess vital signs frequently until they are stable. Hypotension (less than 80 mmHg systolic pressure in an older child; less than 60 mmHg in an infant) usually suggests haemorrhage, which may be hidden abdominal bleeding. In addition, children may have increasing pallor and rapid respirations. If internal bleeding is present, blood pressure will show little improvement when IV fluid is administered.

If abdominal trauma is suspected, once cervical and skull fractures are excluded an NG tube is passed and stomach contents are aspirated to be checked visually for blood and to test for occult blood. Attach the tube to low intermittent suction if the presence of blood is established. An indwelling urinary (Foley) catheter is also inserted to evaluate urine for blood and urine output. Evidence of blood in the urine or decreased output may indicate accompanying kidney or bladder trauma. Be aware that having NG tubes or catheters passed is always frightening for a child. After an accident, when they are already frightened, they and their parents need a great deal of support to accept these procedures.

An abdominal x-ray or ultrasound may be ordered to rule out a fractured pelvis, a condition that could contribute to blood loss. Air under the diaphragm on the x-ray suggests gastric or intestinal rupture with escape of air from these organs into the peritoneal cavity. Free fluid in the abdomen, shown on the x-ray when the child is turned on the side, suggests leakage of bowel fluid or splenic rupture and pooling of blood. Parents often find it difficult to appreciate the seriousness of abdominal trauma because the signs are not as dramatic or obvious as those of fractured extremities or lacerations. Some parents may not bring their child to an emergency department immediately after abdominal trauma because they are unaware that serious injury can result to this part of the body. Without frightening them, explain that an injury need not be obvious at first glance to be serious and need care. They may ask why an x-ray is necessary. When their child is asked to turn on the x-ray table so that an abdominal fluid level can be revealed, they may perceive this as unnecessary manipulation of an injured child.

Splenic rupture

In children, the spleen is the most frequently injured organ in abdominal trauma because it is usually palpable under the lower left ribs (McCance & Huether, 2015). It is frequently injured by inappropriately applied seatbelts in motor vehicles and by handlebar injuries in bicycle accidents. Children with splenic injury have tenderness in the left upper quadrant, especially on deep inspiration, when the diaphragm moves down and touches the spleen. They may hold their left shoulder elevated, so that the diaphragm is raised on the left side, to keep this from happening. Occasionally, a child notices radiated left shoulder pain while lying in a supine position (Kehr's sign). An x-ray will show little about the spleen itself but may reveal a broken rib over the spleen, suggesting the extent of the trauma to that area.

An IV line is begun immediately for fluid replacement and an IV pyelogram or MRI will be done to rule out damage to the left kidney, which, because of its location just behind the spleen, may also have suffered trauma. A complete blood count is done to estimate the extent of the blood loss. Blood is typed and cross-matched, so that blood for replacement can be readied if necessary. The child will be admitted to an observation unit if the blood loss from the rupture appears to be mild. If bleeding is severe, immediate surgery, such as a partial or total splenectomy, may be necessary to halt bleeding and save the child's life. After a splenectomy, children are very susceptible to infection, particularly pneumococcal infections. Therefore, a large percentage of children are managed expectantly to see if the bleeding will halt without spleen removal (Lippert et al., 2013). Children who have their spleen removed are offered the pneumococcal vaccine to protect them from pneumococcal infections.

Liver rupture

Livers are also more prone to rupture in children than in adults because the liver, like the spleen, is not completely sheltered by the rib cage in children (Shao et al., 2013). Children with liver rupture or laceration usually have severe abdominal pain that is most marked on inspiration, when the diaphragm descends and touches the liver. They show symptoms of blood loss, including tachycardia, hypotension, anxiety and pallor. The haematocrit will be low or falling. Such children need to be prepared for immediate surgery because the liver is a highly vascular organ and blood loss from it is acute and possibly life-threatening.

Occasionally, a communication between an artery and the bile duct occurs at the time of trauma. In this situation, symptoms are not immediate, but gastrointestinal (GI) bleeding, such as haematemesis or melena, may occur in a few days. The child may have colicky upper abdominal pain that is relieved by emesis. Liver studies, such as a liver arteriogram, are necessary to reveal the extent of the problem.

After either liver or spleen surgery, children need careful observation for return of bowel function, assessment for the possibility that peritonitis may develop and careful reintroduction of oral nutrition. You may want to consider the complexity of the abdominal assessment in a young person in order to successfully undertake an accurate assessment, including such aspects as pain relief and diversional therapy.

DENTAL TRAUMA

Injuries to teeth occur most often from falls in which a child strikes the upper front incisors, or from blows to the face by objects such as tennis racquets or hockey sticks. Such accidents are always potentially serious because they can lead to aspiration of the injured teeth or misalignment of future teeth. Permanent teeth that have been knocked out recently can be washed with saline in the emergency department and replaced; there is a good chance that they will re-implant successfully. If a tooth is knocked out, parents should rinse the tooth in water, drop it in a salt solution or milk and bring it to the emergency department (Idzik & Krauss, 2013). Some dentists advocate immersing the tooth in an antiseptic and then in an antibiotic solution before replacing it. If a tooth is replaced, it usually is wired into place to hold it in good alignment. The child receives a course of oral antibiotics to prevent infection. Only soft food must be eaten until the tooth has firmly adhered (approximately 2 weeks) (Namdev et al., 2014).

If a blow to a child's teeth was extensive, an x-ray may be taken to rule out a mandibular or maxillary fracture. If a portion of a tooth cannot be located, the possibility of aspiration must be considered and confirmed or ruled out by a chest x-ray. In young children, often a tooth is not knocked out but is pushed back up into the gum. These teeth gradually regrow and, although they may darken in colour, they usually are healthy. If the affected tooth is a deciduous tooth, the permanent tooth is rarely injured even though it is already formed in the gum. At the appropriate time, the permanent tooth will erupt normally. Education to the child and parents is critical in dental discharge activities with correlated outcomes evident from good education (Namdev et al., 2014).

NEAR DROWNING

Drowning is death caused by suffocation from submersion in liquid. Inhaled water fills the lungs and therefore blocks the exchange of oxygen in the alveoli. The term **near drowning** is used to describe the child with a submersion injury who requires emergency treatment and who survives the first 24 hours after injury. Most infant drownings occur in bathtubs; 1- to 4-year-old children most frequently drown in artificial pools; older children most frequently drown in bodies of fresh water. The majority of drowning accidents that take place outside the home occur in the summer months, when more children are swimming and boating. Particularly at risk are male adolescents.

Emergency management

When a child is pulled from the water after near drowning, mouth-to-mouth or mouth to mask resuscitation should be started at once. If cardiac arrest has occurred from hypoxia, simultaneous measures to initiate cardiac action must be taken.

Assuming that cardiopulmonary resuscitation is effective, the child needs follow-up care at a healthcare facility because the child is certain to be acidotic from accumulated carbon dioxide and hypoxia (resulting from lack of oxygen because of the water in the alveoli) and is at risk of respiratory infection from contaminants in the water. Follow-up care aims to increase the child's oxygen and carbon dioxide exchange capacity, using the lung areas that are not filled with water. Typically, a child is intubated with a cuffed intratracheal tube; mechanical ventilation may be necessary to force air into the alveoli. Because water has been swallowed, vomiting usually occurs as the child is revived. The cuff of the intratracheal tube prevents vomitus from being aspirated. The child is given 100% oxygen so that as much space as possible in the available lung alveoli can be used. An NG tube is inserted to decompress the stomach. Usually, salbutamol is administered by aerosol to prevent bronchospasm and, again, to allow the child to make maximum use of the oxygen administered. If the child aspirated salt water, plasma may be administered to replace protein being lost into the lungs and prevent hypovolaemia. If the child's body temperature is very low, gradual warming (not using a warming blanket) is advised so that the metabolic requirement does not rise sharply before alveolar space is ready to accommodate this need. Extracorporeal membrane oxygenation may be used.

POISONING

Poisoning is a significant cause of serious injuries in children younger than 6 years of age; more than 1 million episodes occur internationally every year (Rumack & Dart, 2012). Common household agents are often the cause despite child-resistant packaging requirements. The home environment may still contain products that can be hazardous and poisonous to children if handled improperly. Plants, cosmetics and cleaning products can be dangerous to children if ingested or absorbed through the skin. Poisoning occurs most commonly in children between the ages of 2 and 3 years. Be aware that when poisoning occurs in an older child, it may not be poisoning but a suicide attempt. When strategically assessing possible poisoning incidents, you may want to consider in your approach issues that extend beyond the individual, i.e. other siblings or a family as a whole. Take the opportunity to involve allied health services such as social workers and counsellors. This encompasses a comprehensive multidisciplinary team assessment.

Emergency management of poisoning at home

If poisoning occurs, parents should telephone their local poison control centre to ask for advice. Information parents need to provide includes:

- Child's name, telephone number, address, weight, age and what the child swallowed
- How long ago the poisoning occurred

- The route of poisoning (oral, inhaled, ingested, sprayed on skin)
- How much of the poison the child took (the bottle should say how many pills or how much liquid it originally held)
- If the poison was in pill form, whether there are pills scattered under a chair or if they are all missing and presumed swallowed
- What was swallowed; if the name of a medicine is not known, what it was prescribed for and a description of it (colour, size, shape of pills)
- The child's present condition (sleepy? hyperactive? comatose? vomiting?).

If one child has swallowed a poison, parents should investigate whether other children have also poisoned themselves, because a preschooler often shares "lollies" with a younger sibling.

Emergency management of poisoning at the healthcare facility

In the emergency department, the best method to deactivate a swallowed poison is the administration of activated charcoal, either orally or by way of an NG tube. It is supplied as a fine black powder that is mixed with water for administration. A sweet syrup may be added to the mixture to make it more palatable. Caution parents that, as the charcoal is excreted through the bowel over the next 3 days, stools will appear black.

Always follow emergency measures to neutralise a poison with an education program for the family to prevent poisoning from happening again. For example, see the NSW Health emergency assessment and management guidelines for poisoning available at <www0.health.nsw.gov.au/policies/gl/2014/pdf/GL2014_007.pdf>. Specific measures for each age group are discussed in previous chapters, along with problems and concerns of that age group.

Caustic poisoning

Ingestion of a strong alkali, such as is often contained in toilet bowl cleaners or haircare products, may cause burns and tissue necrosis in the mouth, oesophagus and stomach. It is important that the parents do not try to make a child vomit after ingestion of these substances because they can cause additional burning as they are vomited (Australian and New Zealand Resuscitation Councils, 2011). After a caustic ingestion, the child has immediate pain in the mouth and throat and drools saliva. The mouth instantly turns white from the burn. Later, the mouth turns brown as oedema and ulceration occur. There may be such marked oedema of the lips and mouth that it is difficult to examine them. The child may immediately vomit blood, mucus and necrotic tissue. The loss of blood from the denuded, burned surface may lead to systemic signs of tachycardia, tachypnoea, pallor and hypotension.

A chest x-ray may be ordered to determine whether pulmonary involvement has occurred from any aspirated poison or whether an oesophageal perforation has allowed poison to seep into the mediastinum. An oesophagoscopy under conscious sedation may be done to assess the oesophagus, although this test may be omitted because of the possibility that an oesophagoscope might perforate the burned oesophagus. After 2 weeks, a barium swallow or oesophagoscopy may be performed to reveal the final extent of the oesophageal burns.

When parents call a poison information centre to ask for advice on how to proceed, they will be advised to immediately take the child to a healthcare facility for treatment. Be aware that pharyngeal oedema may obstruct the child's airway within 20 minutes (or sooner) after the burn. To detect respiratory interference, assess vital signs closely, especially the respiratory rate. In infants, increasing restlessness is an important accompanying sign of oxygen want. In the emergency department, intubation may be necessary to provide a patent airway. Assess the child also for the degree of pain involved. A strong analgesic, such as morphine, may need to be ordered and administered to achieve pain relief.

Pesticide poisoning

Pesticide poisoning can occur by accidental ingestion or through skin or respiratory tract contact when children play in an area that has recently been sprayed. Long-term exposure may result from exposure to a parent's clothing if the parent comes home covered with pesticide spray. Although pesticide poisoning was once thought to be only a rural problem, the increase in the use of lawn sprays by commercial lawn care companies now makes this a suburban problem as well.

Many pesticides have an organophosphate base that causes acetylcholine to accumulate at neuromuscular junctions; this accumulation leads to muscle paralysis. Within a few minutes to 2 hours after exposure, children develop nausea and vomiting, diarrhoea, excessive salivation, weakness of respiratory muscles, confusion, depressed reflexes and possibly seizures. In the emergency department, activated charcoal may be administered if the pesticide was swallowed. If clothing is contaminated, remove it and wash the child's skin and hair. To prevent coming in contact with the pesticide yourself, wear gloves while bathing the child.

Poisoning by drugs of abuse

Adolescents and even pre-adolescent children are brought to healthcare facilities by parents or friends because of a drug overdose or a "bad trip" caused by an unusual reaction or the effect of an unfortunate combination of drugs. Typical drugs involved include codeine and antidepressant drugs. Frequently, the drugs taken were prescription drugs removed from the family medicine cabinet (Viana et al., 2012).

Children are often extremely disoriented after this form of ingestion. They may be having hallucinations. Obtaining a history may be difficult because children may have no idea what they took except that it was a red or a yellow capsule. They may know but may be reluctant to name a drug if it was obtained illegally. Although a child may not appear to hear well or may not seem coherent, try to elicit a history.

Expect to obtain blood specimens for electrolyte levels and a toxicology screen. If the child is vomiting, save any vomitus for analysis. Try to determine whether the ingestion was an accident (perhaps the child was unaware that two drugs would react this way or took a wrong dose) or whether the child was actually attempting suicide. All poisonings or drug ingestions in children older than 7 years of age should be considered as potential suicides until established otherwise. If the ingestion was an accident, the child will need counselling to avoid drug use or about which drugs do not mix. If the incident was an attempted suicide, the child will need observation, possible mental health consultation and counselling about more effective coping mechanisms.

Children need supportive measures for their specific symptoms, including oxygen administration, electrolyte replacement (particularly if there is accompanying nausea and vomiting) and perhaps IV fluid administration in an attempt to dilute the drug. Children who have swallowed a drug of abuse need immediate treatment followed by investigation into the events leading to the poisoning. This potentially lethal ingestion may act as a turning point in the child's life, possibly alerting the child and family to a drug problem and the need for help. Factors such as reduction of fear and anxiety, increased coping mechanisms, knowledge of the effects of drug use and availability of referral sources for a drug problem are important areas to address.

FOREIGN BODY OBSTRUCTION

Foreign bodies can become lodged in children's oesophagus, ear canals or noses, causing stasis of secretions and infection. Direct obstruction or laceration of the mucous membrane may also result, leading to serious consequences. Whether a foreign substance is inhaled or embedded elsewhere, nursing interventions should focus first on comforting the child and aiding in removal of the substance, and then on teaching the child and parents ways to avoid such occurrences in the future.

Foreign bodies in the ear

Any child with a history of draining exudate from the ear canal needs an otoscopic examination to establish the reason for the drainage. In toddlers and preschoolers, the drainage often is the result of a foreign body in the ear canal. The object might be a small piece of a toy, a piece of paper, a small battery, or food, such as a peanut that was pushed into the ear canal (Sharpe, Rochette & Smith, 2012). Removal of a foreign body from the ear is difficult because children are afraid that the instrument used will hurt them, so they have difficulty lying still for the procedure. If there is reason to think that the tympanic membrane is intact, irrigating the object from the ear canal with a syringe and normal saline may be possible. This should not be done if the object is one that will swell when wet, such as a peanut. If it is possible that the tympanic membrane is ruptured, the ear canal must not be irrigated or fluid will be forced into the middle ear, possibly introducing infection (otitis media). Often, it is better to wait for an otolaryngologist to treat the child because trauma to the ear canal during an attempt to remove a foreign body will increase the oedema and make removal even more difficult.

Foreign bodies in the nose

Foreign objects stuffed into the nose eventually cause inflammation and purulent discharge from the nares. The odour from the impaction is often the first sign noticed by a parent. Objects may be removed with forceps and a local antibiotic might be necessary after removal if ulceration resulted from the local irritation.

Foreign bodies in the oesophagus or stomach

Children tend not to chew food well or to swallow portions that are too big to pass safely through the oesophagus. Lollies are common objects caught in the oesophagus in young children. Orthodontic appliances may become dislodged and swallowed. Intense pain at the site where the object is lodged will result. If it is an object that will dissolve, such as a lolly or a piece of digestible meat, offer the child fluid to drink to help flush the object into the stomach. Even after the object dissolves or passes into the stomach, the child will feel transient pain at the original site of the obstruction. Lithium button batteries, like those in watches, hearing aids and even children's toys, are also frequently swallowed by young children. These need to be removed by endoscopy as soon as possible as they can lead to bowel perforation or volvulus (Thabet et al., 2013). Objects, such as a part of a toy or a cooked chicken bone, that will not dissolve and should not be passed, are also removed by endoscopy.

BITES

Children receive bites from snakes, spiders, jellyfish and domestic animals such as dogs or even from other children. The source of a bite needs to be documented as human bites can also result from sexual abuse.

Mammalian bites

All bites can cause abrasions, puncture wounds, lacerations and crushing injuries related to the size of the animal and the location of the bite (Jacobs, Guglielmo & Chin-Hong, 2009). The biggest concerns associated with non-venomous animal bites are the possibility of long-term scarring and disfigurement as well as infection from the presence of microorganisms in the animal's mouth. Be mindful children are at greater risk of larger envenomation doses due to their smaller size.

Snake bite

Australia has an extensive array of venomous snakes, including but not limited to the tiger snake, brown snake, death adder and copper head. The only snake identified within New Zealand boundaries is the sea snake (see Sea snakes below). Envenomation by venomous snakes will result in varying degrees of localised and life-threatening systematic presentations. This may include paralysis and coagulopathy disorders which may become the most potentially life-threatening. In addition to primary or secondary renal damage, generalised symptoms include headache, vomiting, abdominal pain, collapse and convulsions. Localised irritation, swelling redness and bruising may be seen even if a non-definitive puncture mark is identifiable.

Emergency management at the scene

Basic first aid includes airway and breathing maintenance if indicated, as well as pressure immobilisation technique including splinting the affected limb. Do not wash or clean the wound. Keep the child still and transfer urgently for medical review (NSW Health, 2014).

Emergency management at the healthcare facility

Dependent on the child's presentation, the maintenance of airway, breathing and circulation will be a priority, as well as symptom management for paralysis and coagulopathy disorders. All possible snakebite victims should be monitored for at least 12 hours (see the NSW Health emergency clinical guidelines available at <www0.health.nsw.gov.au/policies/gl/2014/pdf/GL2014_007.pdf>; NSW Health, 2014).

Sea snakes

Australia has several known sea snakes and there are two species infrequently found off the north island of New Zealand. Sea snakes are highly venomous, although envenomation is rare. As with all snakebites, however, there is the potential for lethal envenomation and therefore first aid, including pressure immobilisation, is recommended as well as antivenom if indicated (NSW Health, 2014; Ministry of Health New Zealand, 2009).

Spider bite

Funnel-web spider

The funnel-web spider is found predominately on the east coast as well as in some other isolated pockets of Australia. It is classified as having the most rapid lethal envenomation progressions of all Australian spiders. The mouse spider has been classified with the same venom toxicity, however, limited bites have been reported (NSW Health, 2014).

On presentation there may be fang marks and localised pain at the site. While not all bites inflict venom, any suspected bite should be observed for a 6 hour period. Antivenom is available and implemented in conjunction with life-saving interventions as indicated. The only spider bite in Australia and New Zealand for which pressure bandaging is indicated is the funnel web spider. Nursing assessment includes observing for potential allergic reaction signs or symptoms as well as rapid systemic deterioration (NSW Health, 2014).

Redback spider

Redback spiders are prevalent across Australia and in small pockets of New Zealand. New Zealand also has a spider known as the Katipo which has similar presentation and management as for redback spider bites (Australian Resuscitation Council, 2011; Ministry of Health New Zealand, 2009). Redback spider bites inflict diffuse intense localised pain as well as generalised abdominal and neck or head pain. These may all be misinterpreted as other clinical presentations such as an acute abdomen. The onset of pain is usually within 15 minutes of the bite with diffuse symptoms seen within 1 to 24 hours. Treatment includes first aid and symptom relief such as analgesia and cool pack. Pressure bandaging is not indicated due to the localised nature of the affects and it has been found to increase localised pain (Australian Venom Research Unit, 2014). Antivenom is available and can be given in standard doses to paediatric clients (NSW Health, 2014).

Other animal bites and stings

Marine injuries

There is a wide variety of marine animals (particularly in the tropical areas of Australia) including blue-ringed octopus, cone snails, fish, jellyfish, sea snakes and sting rays that can cause significant injury, disability and even death. Pressure immobilisation technique is indicated for bites and stings from blue-ringed octopus, cone snails and sea snakes but is not indicated in jellyfish or fish stings (Australian Venom Research Unit, 2014; Australian Resuscitation Council, 2010 & 2011).

Stings cause immediate sharp pain and acute inflammatory skin reaction. In tropical regions these stings may be life-threatening and require immediate first aid and life-saving interventions. In non-tropical areas first aid is required, however, life-threatening injury generally only occurs following an allergic reaction.

The two most venomous jellyfish species in the world live in the tropical regions of Australia. There is no single nationwide first aid recommendation for marine envenomation by jellyfish because of the differences between jellyfish species around Australia. In most cases, first-aid providers are unlikely to be able to identify the jellyfish. In the tropics, because of the risk of a potentially lethal jellyfish sting, the priority is to preserve life. If the species cannot be clearly identified as harmless or as a bluebottle, it is safer to treat the victim with vinegar. However, vinegar is not recommended with jellyfish found outside the tropical regions of Australia as it has been found to increase toxin discharge. Outside the tropics and extending into New Zealand, where huge numbers of non-threatening stings occur, the primary objective is pain relief, with an initial application of sea water and removal of any remaining tentacles, then preferably the application of hot water (to 45°C only to avoid thermal injury), such as in a hot shower or bath (Australian Venom Research Unit, 2014; Australian Resuscitation Council, 2010).

Scorpions, centipedes and insects (including bee, wasp and ant stings)

There is a wide variety of scorpions, centipedes and insects in Australia that can inflict localised painful bites. The pain may vary from mild to severe, requiring analgesia and application of hot or cold packs. Pressure immobilisation technique is not indicated. Secondary infection may require antibiotic treatment. In hypersensitive individuals allergic reactions may occur and even progress to anaphylaxis. Analgesia or topical anaesthetic agents may be required in extreme cases (Australian Venom Research Unit, 2014).

When dealing with a bite, you must never disregard that the bite origin or bite wound may not be evident or obvious. Bee or wasp bites must be inspected to ensure the sting apparatus has been removed from the site. If not, gently scrape it to the side to remove it. Do not squeeze the skin or it will force more fluid into the site (Australian Venom Research Unit, 2014).

THERMAL INJURIES

Thermal injuries include those caused by either cold (frostbite) or by excessive heat (burns).

Frostbite

Frostbite is a tissue injury caused by freezing cold. Cold exposure leads to peripheral vasoconstriction, cutting off the oxygen supply to surrounding cells. In children, the body parts involved usually are the nose, fingers or toes. Cells at the site can be so injured that they die (see Table 52.2). The affected body part appears white or erythematous; oedema is present and it feels numb. Explore the cause of frostbite by careful history taking. It occurs most frequently in children who have been skiing, snowmobiling or snowboarding for long periods. If parents failed to provide adequate clothing because they underestimated the degree of cold outside, the possibility of neglect or child abuse must be ruled out as a cause.

Always warm frostbitten areas gradually. Sudden warming increases the metabolic rate of cells; without adequate blood flow to the area because of still-present vasoconstriction, additional damage can occur. Administration of a vasodilator and use of hyperbaric oxygen may help reduce the effect on body cells.

TABLE 52.2 Degrees of frostbite

Degree	Description
First	Mild freezing of epidermis; appears erythematous with oedema
Second	Partial- or full-thickness injury; appears erythematous with blisters and pain occurring after rewarming
Third	Full-thickness injury (epidermis, dermis, and subcutaneous tissue); appears white
Fourth	Complete necrosis with gangrene and possible ultimate loss of body part

Burns

Burns are injuries to body tissue caused by excessive heat (heat greater than 40°C). Such injuries commonly occur in children of all ages after infancy. Toddlers are often burned by pulling pans of scalding water off the stove and onto themselves or from bath water that is too hot (ACI Statewide Burn Injury Service, 2014). They can bite into electrical cords. Older children are more likely to suffer burns from open flames such as heaters or a fireplace, touching a hot iron, or playing with matches or lighted candles. Burn injuries tend to be more serious in children than in adults because the same size burn covers a larger surface of a child's body.

Assessment

When children are brought to a healthcare facility with a burn injury, the first questions must be, "Where is the burn and what is its extent and depth?" Burns are classified as severe, moderate or minor (see Table 52.3) (McCance & Huether, 2015). Refer to local policy guidelines including transfer criteria based on local agreements and requirements.

Along with the size and depth, be certain to assess and document the location of the burn. Face and throat burns

TABLE 52.3 Classification of burns

Classification	Description
Minor	First-degree burn or second- degree burn <10% of body surface or third-degree burn <2% of body surface; no area of the face, feet, hands or genitalia burned
Moderate	Second-degree burn between 10% to 20% or on the face, hands, feet or genitalia or third-degree burn <10% of body surface or if smoke inhalation has occurred
Severe	Second-degree burn >20% of body surface or third-degree burn >10% of body surface

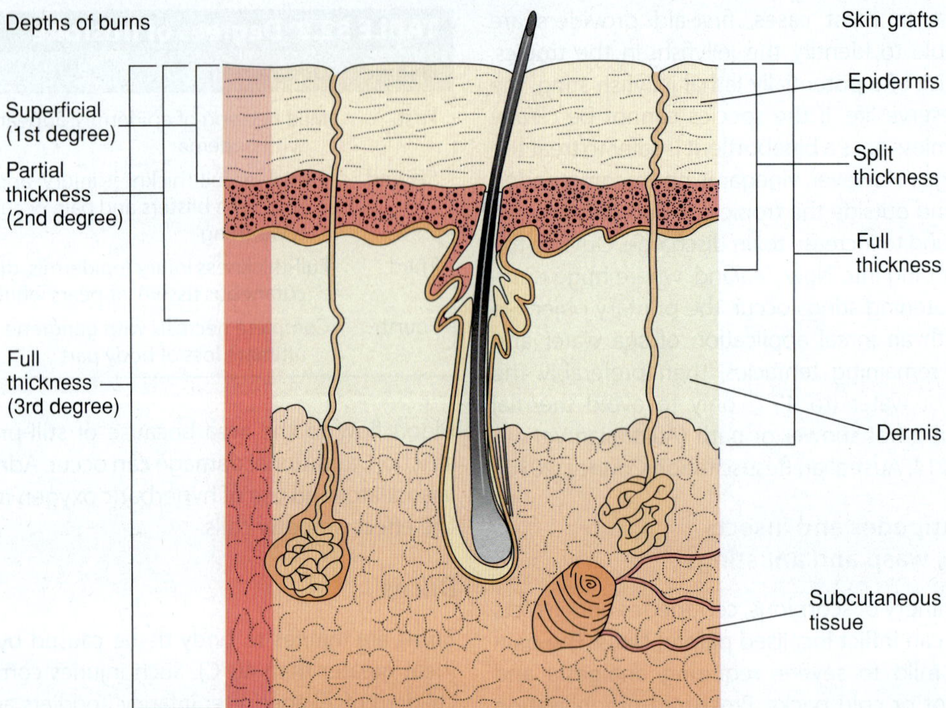

FIGURE 52.3 Depths of burns.

are particularly hazardous because there may be accompanying, but unseen, burns in the respiratory tract. Resulting oedema could lead to respiratory tract obstruction. Hand burns are also hazardous because, if the fingers and thumb are not positioned properly during healing, adhesions will inhibit a full range of motion in the future. Burns of the feet and genitalia carry a high risk of secondary infection. Genital burns are also hazardous because oedema of the urinary meatus may prevent a child from voiding.

With adults, the "rule of nines" is a quick method of estimating the extent of a burn. For example, each upper extremity represents 9% of the total body surface; each lower extremity represents two 9s, or 18%, and the head and neck represent 9%. Because the body proportions of children are different from those of adults, this rule does not always apply and is misleading in the very young child. For every year of life after 12 months take 1% from the head and add half a percent to each leg until the age of 10 years when adult proportions are used (ACI NSW Agency for Clinical Innovation, 2014).

Depth of burn

When estimating the depth of a burn, use the appearance of the burn and the sensitivity of the area to pain as criteria (see Fig. 52.3). *Partial-thickness* burns include first- and second-degree burns. A first-degree burn involves only the superficial epidermis (see Fig. 52.4A and Table 52.4). A second-degree burn involves the entire epidermis. Sweat

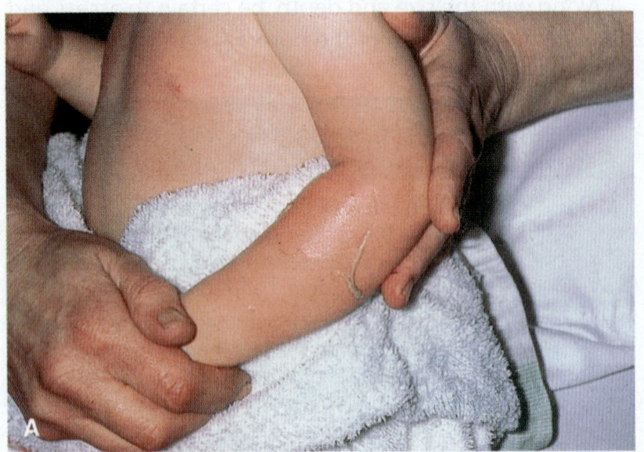

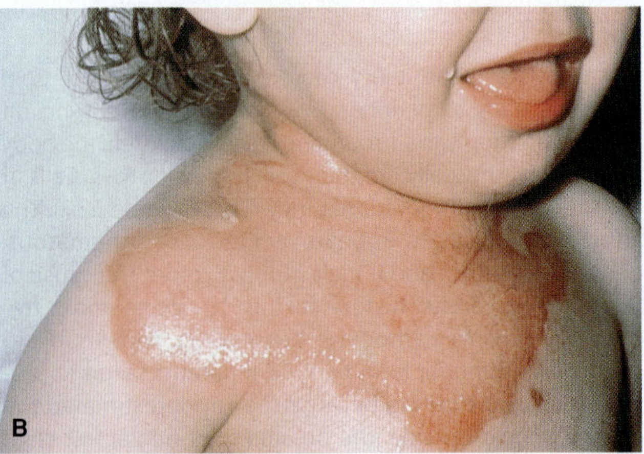

FIGURE 52.4 Partial-thickness burns. (**A**) An infant with a first-degree burn on the arm and chest caused by scalding with hot water. (**B**) A toddler with a second-degree burn caused by scalding. The area appears severely reddened and moist with some blistering. (**A**, © Dr. P. Marazzi/SPL/Science Source/Photo Researchers. **B**, © NMSB/Custom Medical Stock Photograph.)

TABLE 52.4 Characteristics of burns

Severity	Depth of tissue involved	Appearance	Example
First degree (partial thickness)	Epidermis	Erythematous, dry, painful	Sunburn
Second degree (partial thickness)	Epidermis Portion of dermis	Blistered, erythematous to white	Scalds
Third degree (full thickness)	Entire skin, including nerves and blood vessels in skin	Leathery; black or white; not sensitive to pain (nerve endings destroyed)	Flame

glands and hair follicles are left intact (see Fig. 52.4B and Table 52.4). A third-degree burn is a full-thickness burn, involving both skin layers, epidermis and dermis. It may also involve adipose tissue, fascia, muscle and bone (see Fig. 52.5 and Table 52.4).

Undress children with burns completely so the entire body can be inspected. A first-degree burn is painful, whereas a third-degree burn is not. Therefore, a child may be crying from a superficial burn that is obvious on the arm, although the condition needing the most immediate attention is a third-degree burn on the chest, which is covered by a jacket. Be certain to ask what caused the burn because different materials cause different degrees of burn. Hot water, for example, causes scalding, a generally lesser degree of burn than one caused by flaming clothing. Ask where the fire happened. Fires in closed spaces are apt to cause more respiratory involvement than fires in open areas. Ask whether the child has any secondary health problem. In their anxiety over the present burn, parents may forget to report important facts, such as the child has diabetes or is allergic to a common medication. After a fire, parents may pick up a burned child and bring the child to a healthcare facility, leaving other children unprotected at home. Ask about other children and where they are. Parents may have burned hands from putting out the fire on the child's clothes and need equal care, but in their anxiety about the child's condition, they do not mention this. Ask who put out the fire. Were any other family members or animals hurt? Does anyone else need care?

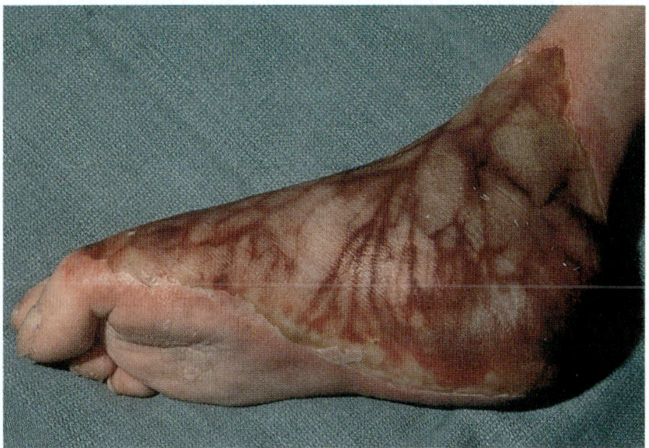

FIGURE 52.5 Full-thickness (third-degree) burn of the foot. Both layers of skin are involved with this type of burn. (© Dr Michael English/Custom Medical Stock Photograph.)

Emergency management of burns

All burns need immediate care because of the pain involved (Mandt & Grubenhoff, 2012).

Minor burns

Although minor burns (typically first-degree partial-thickness burns) are the simplest type of burn, they involve pain and death of skin cells, so they must be treated seriously. Immediately apply ice to cool the skin and prevent further burning. Application of an analgesic–antibiotic ointment and a gauze bandage to prevent infection is usually the only additional treatment required. The child should have a follow-up visit in 2 days to have the area inspected for a secondary infection and dressing changed. Caution parents to keep the dressing dry (no swimming or getting the area wet while bathing for 1 week). A first-degree burn heals in about that time.

Moderate burns

Moderate or second-degree burns may have blisters. Do not rupture them because doing so invites infection. The burn will be covered with a topical antibiotic such as silver sulfadiazine and a bulky dressing to prevent damage to the denuded skin. The child usually is asked to return in 24 hours to assess that pain control is adequate and there are no signs and symptoms of infection. Broken blisters may be debrided (cut away) to remove possible necrotic tissue as the burn heals.

Severe burns

The child with a severe burn is critically injured and needs swift, sure care, including fluid therapy, systemic antibiotic therapy, pain management and physiotherapy, to survive the injury without a disability caused by scarring, infection or contracture.

Electrical burns of the mouth

If a child puts the prongs of a plugged-in extension cord into the mouth or chews on an electrical cord, the mouth will be burned severely. Electrical current from the plug is conducted for a distance through the skin and underlying tissue, so a tissue area much larger than where the prongs or cord actually touched is involved, leaving a raw and inflamed ulcer (Yeroshalmi et al., 2011). If blood vessels were burned, active bleeding will be present.

The immediate treatment for electrical burns of the mouth is to unplug the electrical cord and control bleeding. Pressure applied to the site with gauze is usually effective. Most children are admitted to a hospital for at least 24 hours in an observation unit because oedema in the mouth can lead to airway obstruction. Supply adequate pain relief as long as necessary. Clean the wound about four times a day with an antiseptic solution, such as half-strength hydrogen peroxide, or as otherwise ordered to reduce the possibility of infection (a real danger in this area because bacteria are always present in the mouth). Eating will be a problem for the child because the mouth is so sore. However, the child may be able to drink fluids from a cup. Bland fluids, such as artificial fruit drinks or flat ginger ale, are best.

Electrical burns of the mouth turn black as local tissue necrosis begins. They heal with white, fibrous scar tissue, possibly causing a deformity of the lip and cheeks. This can be minimised by the use of a mouth appliance, which helps maintain lip contour. Some children have difficulty with speech sounds because of resulting lip scarring. They need follow-up care by a plastic surgeon to restore their lip contour. Obviously, you need to review with parents the importance of not leaving "live" electrical cords where young children can reach them.

Nursing considerations

Ineffective breathing patterns related to respiratory oedema

To help rule out smoke inhalation, obtain a history to assess whether the fire occurred in a closed space, such as a garage. Assess for burns of the face, neck or chest, which would indicate that the fire was near the nose and respiratory tract. Assess the quality of the child's voice (it will be hoarse if the throat is irritated from smoke). Carefully monitor the respiratory rate of all burned children because respiratory rate increases with respiratory obstruction. A child's respiratory rate should remain within 16 to 20 breaths per minute; lung auscultation should reveal no crackles and normal work of breathing evident.

A child also may become restless and thrash about because of lack of oxygen. Measurement of blood gases will demonstrate the degree of hypoxia present from carbon monoxide intoxication. Administration of 100% oxygen is the best immediate therapy for displacing carbon monoxide and providing adequate oxygenation to cells. The child may need emergency intubation to secure the airway as well as assisted ventilation to improve gaseous exchange.

Impaired urinary elimination

Blood volume must be maintained by IV fluid administration to establish good urinary output once more. Urine output should be 1 mL/kg of body weight per hour. The specific gravity of urine also should be monitored to determine whether the kidneys can concentrate urine to conserve body fluid. If free haemoglobin from destroyed red blood cells plugs kidney tubules (acute tubular necrosis), urine colour will be red to black because of the haemoglobin present.

An indwelling urinary catheter should be inserted in the emergency department and an immediate urine specimen should be obtained for analysis. A diuretic, such as mannitol, may be administered to flush haemoglobin from the kidneys. If this is effective, the urine returns to its usual straw colour. Throughout the child's hospital stay, observing urinary output is a major nursing responsibility.

Injury related to effects of burn, denuded skin surfaces and lowered resistance to infection

There appears to be some defect in the ability of neutrophils to phagocytise bacteria after burn injury. Nose, throat and wound cultures may be done immediately and then daily. Bacteria and fungi can penetrate the burn eschar readily, so this tissue offers little protection from infection. Fortunately, granulation tissue, which forms under the eschar 3–4 weeks after the burn, is resistant to microbial invasion.

Systemic antibiotics are not very effective in controlling burn-wound infection, probably because the burned and constricted capillaries around the burn site cannot carry the antibiotic to the area. For this reason, any equipment used with the child must be sterile to avoid introducing infection. Children are placed on a sterile sheet on the examining table. Personnel caring for the severely burned child should wear caps, masks, gowns and gloves, even for emergency care. Ensure the child's temperature remains in normal range and the skin surrounding the burned areas shows no signs of erythema or warmth.

Therapy for burns

Second- and third-degree burns may receive open treatment, leaving the burned area exposed to the air, or a closed treatment, in which the burned area is covered with an antibacterial cream and many layers of non-adherent dressing. A synthetic skin covering, artificial skin or amniotic membrane from placentas can be used to help decrease infection and protect granulation tissue. As a rule, burn dressings are applied loosely for the first 24 hours to prevent interference with circulation as oedema forms. Be certain not to allow two burned body surfaces, such as the sides of fingers or the back of the ears and the scalp, to touch because, as healing takes place, a webbing will form between these surfaces. Do not use adhesive tape to anchor dressings to the skin; it is painful to remove and can leave excoriated areas, which provide additional entry for infection. Netting is useful to hold dressings in place because it expands easily and needs no additional tape.

Topical therapy

Silver sulfadiazine is the topical drug of choice for burn therapy to limit infection at the burn site for children after burns specialist review. It is applied as a paste to the burn and the area is then covered with a non-adhesive dressing.

Silver sulfadiazine is an effective agent against both gram-negative and gram-positive organisms and even against secondary infectious agents, such as *Candida*. It is soothing when applied and tends to keep the burn eschar soft, making debridement easier. It does not penetrate the eschar well, which is its one drawback. If a burned area, such as the female genitalia, cannot be readily dressed, the area can be left exposed. The danger of this method is the potential invasion of pathogens.

Escharotomy

An eschar is the tough, leathery scab that forms over moderately or severely burned areas. Fluid accumulates rapidly under eschars, putting pressure on underlying blood vessels and nerves. If an extremity or the trunk has been burned so that both anterior and posterior surfaces have eschar formation, a tight band may form around the extremity or trunk, cutting off circulation to distal body portions. Distal parts feel cool to the touch and appear pale. The child notices tingling or numbness. Pulses are difficult to palpate and capillary refill is slow (longer than 5 seconds). To alleviate this problem, an *escharotomy* (cut into the eschar) is performed (Moelleken, 2009). Some bleeding will occur after escharotomy. Packing the wound and applying pressure usually relieves this.

Debridement

Debridement is the removal of necrotic tissue from a burned area. Debridement reduces the possibility of infection because it reduces the amount of dead tissue present on which microorganisms could thrive. Children usually have 20 minutes of hydrotherapy before debridement to soften and loosen the eschar, which then can be gently removed with forceps and scissors. Debridement is painful and some bleeding occurs. Medicate the child with a prescribed analgesic and help them use a distraction technique during the procedure to reduce the level of pain. Transcutaneous electrical nerve stimulation (TENS) therapy or patient-controlled analgesia may also be helpful. Praise any degree of cooperation. Plan an enjoyable activity afterward to aid in pain relief and also to help re-establish some sense of control over the situation.

Grafting

Grafting is the placement of skin (sterilised and frozen).

Nursing considerations

Deficient diversional activity related to restricted mobility after severe burn

Remember that, even if a child's chest, abdomen and hands are burned, they do not stop thinking so children who are burned need stimulation in their environment. A television is good for passing time but should not be the child's main communication with the outside world. Listening to favourite CDs, having stories read to them, talking about what is going on at home or what they normally do at school and doing schoolwork are also important. It is important to make toys and play materials available. Make certain to visit the child just to talk to him or come to play a game at times other than procedure or treatment sessions. The child may be hospitalised for a long time. He needs to view the nursing staff as friends and carers. Frequent visits convey that he is not alone and that others are aware of his important needs.

Disturbed body image related to changes in physical appearance

When children see others on the unit with burn scars, they begin to realise what healing will look like. Depending on the extent and the site of the burn, parents and children have varying degrees of difficulty accepting this reality. It can cause them to lose confidence in healthcare personnel.

Returning to school can be difficult for children who have been hospitalised or have been receiving home care for a long time. They look different if they have burn scars. The appearance of scar formation can be improved by the application of pressure dressings that the child wears 24 hours a day. If the child has facial burns, seeing friends with a compression bandage in place or returning for laser therapy to reduce burn scarring may be difficult. They need a great deal of support from healthcare personnel to be able to endure this. Sometimes children need referral for formal counselling. Parents may need formal counselling also, to help them accept their child's changed appearance.

✔ *Checkpoint question 52.1*

A 10-year-old girl has third-degree burns on her legs from lighting a fire to burn leaves. She will probably have a lengthy hospitalisation and may need skin grafts to improve healing. What precautions does this child need to prevent infection until healing is complete? What areas of care would you plan to address during the hospitalisation?

✔ *Checkpoint question 52.2*

If a 5-year-old spilled scalding hot water on his hand, which of the following would be the best emergency action?

a. Apply an ice compress to his hand
b. Pour vegetable oil over his hand
c. Cover his hand with a gauze dressing
d. Apply hand lotion to keep the area moist

Key points for review

- Children need total body assessment after an unintentional injury because they may be unable to describe other injuries besides the primary one they have suffered.
- Be aware that some trauma in children occurs as a result of child abuse. Screen for this through history-taking and physical examination.

- Use aseptic technique when caring for trauma victims, so that the child does not develop an additional unnecessary infection.
- Head injuries are always potentially serious in children. Skull fractures, subdural haematomas, epidural haematomas, concussions and contusions can occur. Coma may be present after severe head trauma.
- Abdominal trauma resulting in rupture of the spleen or liver may occur in connection with multiple trauma.
- Near drowning can occur in salt or fresh water. The physiological basis for complications after drowning differs depending on the type of water.
- Common substances children swallow that result in poisoning include paracetamol, caustic substances and hydrocarbons. Teach parents to keep the number of the local poison control centre next to their telephone and always to call first before administering an antidote for poisoning.
- Burns are classified as mild, moderate and severe and can be divided into three types—first, second and third degree—depending on the depth of the burn. Burns produce systemic body reactions and require long-term nursing care.

CASE STUDY QUESTIONS

3. Given Jason's vital signs and GCS score, as the triage nurse would you rate him as a child to be seen immediately, or could he be given second priority?
4. Jason's twin sister was seen in the emergency department for paracetamol poisoning last month. Her father tells you they normally lock all medicine away carefully. His wife left paracetamol on the counter because she had a bad headache. Would you want to discuss the necessity of poisoning prevention with these parents, or should they have learned from this experience that their actions were not safe?

Resources

For an extensive range of additional resources to enhance teaching and learning and to facilitate understanding of this chapter, please see the text's accompanying website located on thePoint at http://thepoint.lww.com.

References

ACI NSW Agency for Clinical Innovation. (2014). ACI Statewide burn injury service. Accessed 14 March 2015, <www.aci.health.nsw.gov.au/__data/assets/pdf_file/0016/250009/Clinical_Practice_Guidelines_Summary_of_Evidence_ACI_Statewide_Burn_Injury_Service.pdf>.

Australian Resuscitation Council. (2010). Guideline 9.4.5: Envenomation: Jellyfish Stings. Accessed 12 March 2015, <http://resus.org.au/?wpfb_dl=41>.

Australian Resuscitation Council. (2011). Guideline 9.4.8: Envenomation: Pressure Immobilisation Technique. Accessed 12 March 2015, <http://resus.org.au/?wpfb_dl=44>.

Australian Resuscitation Council & New Zealand Resuscitation Council. (2011). Guideline 9.5.1: Emergency management of a victim who has been poisoned. Accessed 12 March 2015, <http://resus.org.au/?wpfb_dl=82>.

Australian Venom Research Unit (AVRU) (2014). Accessed 14 March 2015, <www.avru.org/reference/reference_main.html>.

Centers for Disease Control and Prevention. (2008a). Unintentional strangulation deaths from the "choking game" among youths aged 6–19 years—United States, 1995–2007. *Morbidity and Mortality Weekly Report*, *57*(06), 141–144.

Idzik, S. & Krauss, E. (2013). Evaluating and managing dental complaints in primary and urgent care. *The Journal for Nurse Practitioners*, *9*(6), 329–338.

Isaacs, D. (2013). *Evidenced-based Neonatal Infections*, pp. 56–69, Wiley-Blackwell.

Jacobs, R. A., Guglielmo, B. J. & Chin-Hong, P. V. (2009). Infectious diseases: Common problems and antimicrobial therapy. In S. J. McPhee & M. A. Papadakis (Eds). *Current Medical Diagnosis and Treatment*. Columbus, OH: McGraw-Hill.

Klimek, P. M., Lutz, T., Stranzinger, E., et al. (2013). Handlebar injuries in children. *Pediatric Surgery International*, *29*(3), 269–273.

Lippert, S. J., Hartin, C. W., Jr., Ozgediz, D. E., et al. (2013). Splenic conservation: Variation between pediatric and adult trauma centers. *Journal of Surgical Research*, *182*(1), 17–20.

Mandt, M. J. & Grubenhoff, J. A. (2012). Emergencies & injuries. In W. W. Hay et al. (Eds), *Current Diagnosis & Treatment Pediatrics* (21st ed.). New York: McGraw-Hill/Lange.

McCance, K. L. & Huether, S. E. (2015). *Pathophysiology* (7th ed.). St Louis: Mosby.

Ministry of Health New Zealand. (2009). Spiders in New Zealand: What to look out for and keeping yourself safe. (HE1424). Accessed 13 March 2015, <www.cph.co.nz/files/SAF0055.pdf>.

Moelleken, R. R. (2009). Environmental disorders. In S. J. McPhee & M. A. Papadakis (Eds). *Current Medical Diagnosis and Treatment*. Columbus, OH: McGraw-Hill.

Namdev, R., Jindal, A., Bhargava, S., et al. (2014). Awareness of emergency management of dental trauma. *Contemporary Clinical Dentistry*, *5*(4), 507–513.

NSW Health, (2014). *NSW Rural Paediatrics Emergency Clinical Guidelines*. (2nd ed.). Accessed 13 March 2015, <www.health.nsw.gov.au/policies/gl/2014/pdf/GL2014_007.pdf>.

Nickels, D., Patel, T., Merhar, G., et al. (2013). Core curriculum illustration: Subdural hematoma. *Emergency Radiology*, *20*(1), 85–86.

Persaud, N., Coleman, E., Zwolakowski, D., et al. (2012). Nonuse of bicycle helmets and risk of fatal head injury: A proportional mortality, case-control study. *Canadian Medical Association Journal*, *184*(17), E921–E923.

Purcell, L. K. (2012). Evaluation and management of children and adolescents with sports-related concussion. *Paediatrics & Child Health*, *17*(1), 31–32.

Rumack, B. H. & Dart, R. C. (2012). Poisoning. In W. W. Hay et al. (Eds), *Current Diagnosis & Treatment Pediatrics* (21st ed.). New York: McGraw-Hill/Lange.

Shao, Y., Zou, D., Li, Z., et al. (2013). Blunt liver injury with intact ribs under impacts on the abdomen: A biomechanical investigation. *PLoS One*, *8*(1), e52366.

Sharpe, S. J., Rochette, L. M. & Smith, G. A. (2012). Pediatric battery related emergency department visits in the United States, 1990–2009. *Pediatrics*, *129*(6), 1111–1117.

Siskind, V. & Scott, D. (2013). Injuries leading to hospitalisation in the first year of life: Analysis by trimester of age using coded data and textual description. *Australian and New Zealand Journal of Public Health*, *37*, 168–172.

Thabet, M., Basha, M. & Askar, S. (2013). Button battery foreign bodies in children: Hazards, management, and recommendations. *BioMed Research International*, 2013, Article ID 846091.

Viana, A. G., Trent, L., Tull, M. T., et al. (2012). Non-medical use of prescription drugs among Mississippi youth: Constitutional, psychological, and family factors. *Addictive Behavior*, *37*(12), 1382–1388.

Yeates, O., Taylor, G., Rusin, J., Bangert, B., Dietrich, A., Nuss, K. & Wright, M. (2012). Premorbid child and family functioning as predictors of post-concussive symptoms in child with mild traumatic brain injuries. *International Journal of Developmental Neuroscience*, *30*(3), 231–237.

Yeroshalmi, F., Sidoti, E. J., Jr., Adamo, A. K., et al. (2011). Oral electrical burns in children—A model of multidisciplinary care. *Journal of Burn Care & Research*, *32*(2), e25–e30.

Suggested readings

ACI burns management guidelines: <www.aci.health.nsw.gov.au/__data/assets/pdf_file/0020/162344/HSS11-057_ACI-BurnsMoC_Web.pdf>.

Centers for Disease Control and Prevention. (2012). *Childhood lead poisoning data, statistics, and surveillance.* Atlanta, GA: Author.

Koestner, A. L. (2012). ThinkFirst for teens: Finding an injury-prevention approach for teenagers. *Journal of Trauma Nursing*, *19*(4), 227–231.

Lawton, L. (2012). Development of guidelines for nurse-led discharge of children presenting with toxic ingestion. *Emergency Nurse*, *20*(7), 27–29.

Mazotas, I. G., Hamilton, N. A., McCubbins, M. A., et al. (2012). The long-term outcome of retained foreign bodies in pediatric gunshot wounds. *Journal of Trauma Nursing*, *19*(4), 240–245.

Medlin, S. (2012). Nutrition for wound healing. *British Journal of Nursing*, *21*(12), S11–S15.

Riesch, S. K., Kedrowski, K., Brown, R. L., et al. (2013). Health-risk behaviors among a sample of US pre-adolescents: Types, frequency, and predictive factors. *International Journal of Nursing Studies*, *50*(8), 1067–1079.

White, R., Swales, B. & Butcher, M. (2012). Principles of infection management in community-based burns care. *Nursing Standard*, *27*(2), 64–68.

WA health information sheet on ingestion of lithium button batteries: <www.healthnetworks.health.wa.gov.au/docs/injury_button_battery.pdf>.

Chapter 53

Nursing care of a family when a child has cancer

Previous chapters described the growth and development of well children and disorders associated with specific body systems. This chapter adds information about the dramatic changes, both physical and psychosocial, that occur when children develop a malignancy, a phenomenon that can present in any body system. Such information forms a base for care and health teaching.

LEARNING OBJECTIVES

After mastering the contents of this chapter, you should be able to:

1. Describe normal cellular growth and theories that explain how cells alter to become cancerous in children.
2. Suggest ways that nursing care for a child with cancer can be more family-centred.
3. Explain why chemotherapy destroys cancer cells.
4. Identify components of an effective care plan for a child with cancer.

KEY TERMS

- biopsy
- chemotherapeutic agent
- chemotherapy
- Ewing's sarcoma
- histocompatible
- leukaemia
- lymphoma
- neoplasm
- nephroblastoma
- neuroblastoma
- oncogenic virus
- osteogenic sarcoma
- rhabdomyosarcoma
- sarcoma
- tumour staging

CASE STUDY

Tom is a 6-year-old boy you meet at a healthcare clinic. He is there for a routine check-up. His mother tells you that Tom wakes up every morning with a headache and then vomits. Immediately after that he is fine. The problem began just after he started a new school, so she is certain it is related to this. His teacher has suggested that Tom needs an eye examination because he cocks his head to see the whiteboard. You notice that he has lost weight. "What do I do for school phobia?" his mother asks you.

CASE STUDY QUESTIONS

1. Is Tom's mother describing school phobia?
2. What additional questions would you want to ask her to help discover whether this is something more serious?

The terms *malignant* and *cancerous* describe cells that are growing and proliferating in a disorderly, chaotic fashion. In adults, cancer usually occurs in the form of a solid tumour. In children, the most frequent type of cancer is that of immature white blood cell (WBC) overgrowth or **leukaemia** (Brown & Hunger, 2014).

Many parents assume that a diagnosis of cancer means that their child's life will be very limited. Because of the tremendous advances in cancer research and treatment over the past 20 years, however, the prognosis for children and the chances for a cure improve daily. For example, 95% of children with leukaemia can expect to be cured.

CARE OF A CHILD WITH CANCER

Assessment

The symptoms of malignancy in children are often insidious and difficult to define (see Box 53.1). Headaches or pain at a particular body site can often be the result of sports injuries or general fatigue. Weight loss, however, is a common symptom of cancer and is never normal in healthy children. Therefore, at every healthcare visit, record a child's height and weight. Be sure to refer children with swelling or pain of major joints to their general practitioner for further assessment so that bone tumours will not go undetected.

Nursing diagnoses

A nursing care plan addresses specific symptoms caused by a cancer and/or the side effects of treatment, it should also include the family/primary carer's response. Examples are:

- Pain
- Weight loss
- Risk of infection
- Disturbed body image
- Compromised family coping.

Nursing a child with cancer includes supporting the child and parents from the time of diagnosis through treatments such as surgery, radiation therapy and chemotherapy. This is a stressful and long-term process. Chemotherapy may be continued for 2 to 3 years after diagnosis. Increasingly, cancer treatment is offered on an ambulatory basis to keep hospitalisation to a minimum. Education of parents/carers and

BOX 53.1 ✻ Warning symptoms and signs of malignancy

General symptoms
- Unexplained weight loss
- Fever
- Fatigue
- Pain
- Skin changes (itching, darkening, reddening, hairiness)

General signs
- A change in bowel habits or bladder function
- Non-healing sores
- White patches inside the mouth or white spots on the tongue
- Unusual bleeding or discharge
- A thickening or lump in the breast or other body part
- Indigestion or difficulty swallowing
- An obvious change in a wart or mole
- A nagging cough or persistent hoarseness

the child about possible side effects of treatment and how to manage these at home is required.

Keep in mind that the stress of long-term treatment may put the child and family at risk of developmental or family coping problems. Nurses can be a positive force in encouraging healthy adaptation to the demands of the child's illness. Providing comfort and alleviating pain are primary concerns in oncology nursing. Measures for pain relief are discussed in Chapter 39.

Because cancer therapy includes long-term care, children need to be reviewed periodically by the treating team. Returning for treatment follow-up visits may cause anxiety for both the child and the parents/carers. Most children with cancer, even if no cure is possible, will be cared for at home rather than being hospitalised. Their parents/carers will need support from the treating team to feel confident in caring for a dying child (see Chapter 4). The treating team needs to maintain close contact with healthcare personnel to prevent feeling abandoned. If the child dies, the parents may feel a need to return to their primary carer for support. This provides an opportunity to evaluate their adjustment to the child's death and offer support if needed. For the child with a terminal diagnosis the decision as to where he or she dies (at home or in hospital) is a complex one and needs to be discussed thoroughly with the family and child well before the child enters the terminal phase of their illness (see Chapter 56).

HEALTH PROMOTION

Childhood cancers are not usually a direct result of environmental exposure as is the case with adult cancers. Therefore methods to reduce the risk are not as well defined. Reminding parents to reduce children's exposure to secondary cigarette smoke and urging adolescents not to begin smoking (including the use of flavoured tobacco products) can help reduce the incidence of lung cancer when they reach adulthood. Applying sunscreen and limiting the overall time of sun exposure for children can help reduce the development of skin cancer in later life. Children who receive chemotherapy or radiation for one cancer have a higher incidence of developing another cancer later in life. Therefore, reinforcing the need for children to continue health reviews so that any additional cancer development can be discovered is another important preventive measure. Reminding parents to obtain the vaccine against human papillomavirus (HPV), which leads to cervical cancer, is an important preventive measure for adolescent girls.

Parents of a child with cancer may seek medical advice or evaluation for their other children more often than other parents would. This is because they are worried that what seems just a minor symptom is actually a sign of cancer in that child also. They may need greater amounts of reassurance that their other children are well.

NEOPLASIA

Normally, the body is able to maintain the proliferation necessary to replace old cells that die plus producing new cells for physical growth needs. Cancer is a disease which disrupts the normal process of replacing worn out cells with new cells. Cancerous cells grow and proliferate in an abnormal way which can interfere with the normal functioning of the body.

People have many different beliefs around what cancer is and what it means to be diagnosed with a cancer. It is very important to talk to the parents and the child about what they understand is the cause of their cancer which can make explanations of therapy more meaningful to the parents and child.

The word **neoplasm** means "new growth"; it usually refers to a new *abnormal* growth that does not respond to normal growth-control mechanisms. Whether this process is one that produces a solid tumour or one that involves blood-forming elements, the process of abnormal cell growth begins insidiously. It may have been developing for some time before the parents or child realise that it is present. Even after they are aware that a change exists, some time may pass before they realise that it is serious enough to require medical attention, particularly if symptoms are not obvious.

Although cancer in children is rare, it is the leading cause of death from disease among children younger than 15 years of age. Australia has one of the highest incidences of childhood cancer in the world. Cancer is the leading cause of death by disease in Australian children, with 3 children dying from cancer every week (*Kids' Cancer in Australia Today*, The Kids Cancer Project, 2012). Leukaemia is the most common of all childhood cancers. Cancer is one of the Australian Government's nine National Health Priority Areas. For more information on cancer statistics, risk factors and publications, see <www.aihw.gov.au/cancer>. In New Zealand, approximately 150 children are diagnosed with cancer each year. Although childhood cancer is rare (1% of the total of newly diagnosed New Zealanders with cancer; <www.kidshealth.org.nz/childrens-cancer-services-new-zealand>), a recent Adolescents and Young Adults (AYA) Cancer Services review showed that there is a significant lag in five-year survival rates for AYA cancer patients in New Zealand, particularly in certain age ranges and ethnic groups, compared to countries such as Australia. Most significant is the survival rate for Māori and Pacifika, which is lower than for other ethnicities (<www.canteen.org.nz/about/news-and-media/youth-cancer-review-uncovers-troubling-statistics>).

Knowing the processes involved in the development of cancer and being able to explain it in a clear and concise manner is essential to help parents understand what is happening to their child and why specific treatment measures are necessary.

Cell growth

The normal cell cycle consists of two main divisions: an interphase (resting phase) and a mitosis (dividing phase). Body cells have the ability to recognise their own tissue type, possibly by recognising surface enzymes or glucose particles on cell membranes. Normally cells of like type do not migrate away from each other because they recognise and adhere to each other. In neoplastic cells, the ability to adhere can be defective in subsets of the tumour population (they are autonomous). This may be related to decreased calcium in the cell membrane or to an increased negative charge that repels other cells rather than bonding them together.

Normally, like cells are able to recognise when they are being crowded for the space they must occupy, and can signal with one another to halt growth. Neoplastic cells may not respond to this communication. By the time a tumour mass is detected, it is likely to be about 30 times the size of its original aberrant cell.

Neoplastic growth

Neoplasms can be either *benign* (is encapsulated and will not spread to other regions) or *malignant* (has the ability to metastasise i.e. spread to other parts of the body). Even when a tumour is benign, however, it may not be completely harmless. It can cause damage by pressing on adjacent tissue. For example, brain tumours in children are often benign but they can cause extensive respiratory depression from increased pressure on the respiratory centre.

Causes of neoplastic growth

The exact origin of many cancers is usually unknown and may potentially involve more than one cause. As more research is accomplished on the nature of genes, specific markers in tumours that fail to suppress or stimulate cancer-causing genes are being identified; almost all childhood cancers have such markers, a genetic trigger or predisposition to cancer (Graham et al., 2014; Virshup, 2012). In adults, tumours may grow because normal cell growth has been altered by environmental irritation, such as chronic exposure to chemical irritants or cigarette smoke. Cancers of the skin, bladder, lung and intestines involve organs exposed to such outside influences and irritation. In children, cancers most frequently occur in organs that are not directly exposed to the environment such as leukaemia (a cancer of white blood cells), nephroblastoma of the kidney, brain tumours or neuroblastoma in the abdomen. Because many tumours occur in children younger than 5 years of age, exposure to environmental carcinogens is limited, so environmental cause of tumours is probably not a major contributor to the development of the cancer although exposure to harmful substances in utero may be a cause (Sato et al., 2011). Two substances that lead to lung cancer and to which children may be exposed are secondary smoke and asbestos. Asbestos is a particular problem if a child's school or home is insulated with this material or a parent works in asbestos removal and brings home asbestos particles on their clothing.

A child who has survived one cancer is at a higher than normal risk of developing a second cancer, such as bone cancer. Radiation exposure used to treat the first malignancy may be responsible for this. In addition, there may be a predisposition to cancer in some families (Kurt et al., 2008).

One explanation of why cancers develop is the cell mutation theory. This model suggests that carcinogenic agents and hereditary susceptibility combine to alter the nature of cells, leading to abnormal growth. A first stage of initiation may mark the cells for abnormal growth. A second stage of promotion actually begins the abnormal growth. Carcinogenic agents can be living (viral), physical (radiation) or chemical. Radiation during intrauterine life is a documented cause of leukaemia. Radiation of the thyroid in infancy can cause thyroid cancer later in life. Use of androgenic steroids may lead to hepatocellular cancer.

This theory shows why the growth of neoplastic cells is irreversible (the cells cannot return to a normal state because they are intrinsically changed) and why neoplasms occur in some people but not in others (both an intrinsic and an extrinsic factor, or an inherited tendency and an environmental insult must be present). It is difficult to document this process because it stipulates that two separate steps are necessary for a cell to become cancerous. If there is a lengthy time span between these steps, the cause-and-effect relationship is difficult to trace (McCance & Huether, 2013).

Viruses play an important role in the development of some types of cancer. **Oncogenic viruses** have the ability to change the structure of cell DNA or RNA. C-type RNA viruses may be implicated in leukaemia. Epstein-Barr virus, a DNA virus, may be associated with Burkitt's lymphoma. This theory is supported by the fact that an immunodeficient state increases the risk of development of a cancer. When both viral surveillance and removal of abnormal cells are lost, virus invasion and abnormal cell growth is free to begin.

ASSESSING CHILDREN WITH CANCER

The incidence of various types of childhood cancers is shown in Figure 53.1. Because these cancers involve different body systems, signs and symptoms can vary greatly (see Box 53.2).

History

Cancer in children has usually been developing for some time before a child is brought for treatment because the symptoms (bruising, nosebleeds, headache, pain in a knee, constipation) are not perceived initially as significant by the parents/carers. Thorough assessment, including a history, can help reveal these symptoms so that a child can be further evaluated. As malignant cancers develop, they can cause systemic effects. Cachexia (loss of weight, anorexia) occurs if the tumour is growing so rapidly that it takes nutrients from normal cells. Excessive hormone production (overproduction of antidiuretic, thyroid or adrenocorticotropic hormone) may occur because of tumour growth in a specific body area that leads to systemic symptoms.

Physical and laboratory examination

To identify a cancer correctly requires a thorough physical examination. Assessing the height and weight of children is an important component. To confirm a diagnosis, several diagnostic procedures may be used, including x-ray, ultrasound, magnetic resonance imaging (MRI), blood analysis and biopsy.

Biopsy

A **biopsy** is the surgical removal of tissue cells for laboratory analysis. Most children with a possible diagnosis of cancer will have a biopsy performed to confirm their initial diagnosis (McLean & Wofford, 2015). Parents/carers and children need thorough preparation for the biopsy procedure and the care the child will need after the procedure. Anxious parents do not "hear" well and may need to have postoperative instructions repeated. Bone marrow aspiration is a frequent type of biopsy used with children. Although this can be done with only local anaesthesia, it is equally frightening (see Chapter 44).

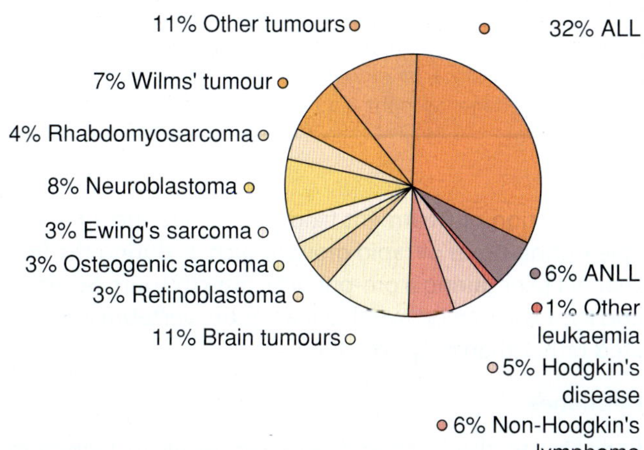

FIGURE 53.1 Approximate incidence of common childhood cancers. ALL, acute lymphocytic leukaemia; ANLL, acute non-lymphocytic leukaemia.

BOX 53.2 Assessment Assessing a child for signs of cancer

History

Chief concern: Weight loss, loss of appetite, easy bruising, swelling in a body part, headache, eye deviations.

Past medical history: Family member with a history of cancer.

Physical examination

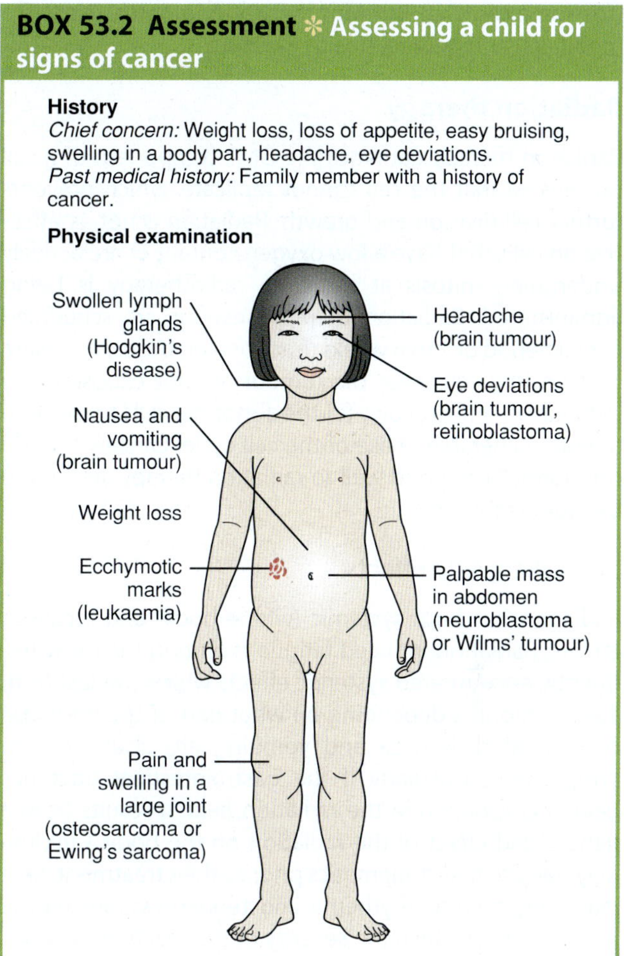

Tumour staging

Tumour staging is a process by which a cancer's spread and tissue type are identified. Knowing the stage of a tumour helps the treating team develop an effective treatment program, establish a prognosis and evaluate the progress or regression of the disease once treatment has commenced.

OVERVIEW OF CANCER TREATMENT MEASURES USED WITH CHILDREN

Therapy for a child with cancer focuses on killing the cancer cells while preserving as many healthy cells as possible. This is achieved using a combination of surgery, radiation therapy, chemotherapy, bone marrow transplantation (for some cancers), immunotherapy (biological response modifiers) and general health measures.

Radiation therapy

Radiation therapy damages the DNA component of a cell nucleus so that the cell cannot replicate, which prevents further cell division and growth. Radiation is not as effective on cells that have a low oxygen content or are actively undergoing mitosis at the time radiotherapy is being administered. Radiation therapy sessions are scheduled over a period of 1 to 6 weeks (fractionated doses) to ensure that healthy cells near the tumour are not exposed to a lethal dose. It also allows for the abnormal cells to move to a more vulnerable phase of the cell cycle. Cancers that do not normally respond well to radiation therapy are said to be radio-resistant.

Immediate side effects

Radiation has both systemic (whole body) and localised effects. Radiation-induced fatigue is among the most frequently encountered systemic effects which can last from days to months depending on what part of the body has been treated. Nausea and vomiting are also common symptoms, particularly if the gastrointestinal tract has been incorporated in the radiation field. It results from a generalised effect of the radiation on the body. Children may need to take antiemetics prior to their treatment. Skin reactions, such as erythema and tenderness, are typical local effects in which the severity of the reaction depends on the sensitivity of the skin area included in the field and the total amount of radiation the area receives.

Long-term side effects

The long-term side effects of radiation are becoming more apparent with the increased survival rate in children who have undergone intense radiation therapy. Long-term side effects once again depend on the total amount of radiation received and the target area and may include an increasing susceptibility to developing a secondary cancer. As therapies are becoming more targeted long-term side effects are becoming less common.

Possible short-term and long-term radiation side effects

It is important to remember that these side effects are only potential and as treatments become more targeted they are less likely to occur and clinicians have to be very careful how they describe treatment options because they can easily frighten parents and children who may feel that unproven treatments (that offer little hope of effectiveness) are the safer and therefore the wiser option (see Box 53.3).

Bone development

Asymmetrical growth of bones, easy fracturing, scoliosis, kyphosis or spinal shortening can occur without careful consideration of treatment fields. Bones are most vulnerable during times of rapid growth, such as during the first year of life or during a pre-pubertal growth spurt. Scoliosis and kyphosis can be avoided if an entire vertebra is irradiated rather than only one side.

Hormones

Radiation to the head and neck can result in long-term thyroid, hypothalamic and pituitary gland dysfunction. This may result in a growth hormone deficiency or hypothalamic-pituitary stimulation to the thyroid gland. Children's

BOX 53.3 ✻ Focus on communication

Tim Miller a 6-year-old boy, was diagnosed with a brain tumour 3 months ago. His mother brings him into the emergency room because of a severe nosebleed. While you are putting pressure on his nose, you notice that one eye seems to have poor alignment.

Less effective communication

Nurse: Is Tim still having chemotherapy, Mrs Miller?
Mrs Miller: No. He's in remission.
Nurse: Is he taking anything that would lower his platelet count or clotting factors?
Mrs Miller: All he takes is asparagus powder we get from Mexico.
Nurse: From Mexico?
Mrs Miller: It's a new treatment that's not legal here.
Nurse: Has he been back to clinic here for a checkup or follow-up?
Mrs Miller: No. Asparagus powder is a kind of chemotherapy.
Nurse: Well, let's focus right now on getting this bleeding stopped.

More effective communication

Nurse: Is Tim still having chemotherapy, Mrs Miller?
Mrs Miller: No. He's in remission.
Nurse: Is he taking anything that would lower his platelet count or clotting factors?
Mrs Miller: All he takes is asparagus powder we get from Mexico.
Nurse: From Mexico?
Mrs Miller: It's a new treatment that's not legal here.
Nurse: Are you worried that he still has so many new black and blue marks?
Mrs Miller: No, asparagus powder is a kind of chemotherapy.
Nurse: Well, let's get this nosebleed stopped. Then we can take a minute to talk about what chemotherapy means.

Of all known diseases, no other disease has as many false "cures" as cancer. When talking with parents, see if they are using any of these unproven methods. Some of them do no harm, so parents can continue to give them along with proven therapies. Others actually interfere with the action of a chemotherapy drug and are contraindicated. In the above scenario, the parent has chosen an unproven regimen. Ignoring the possibility that this choice may be an unhelpful one and denying a potential recurrence of cancer or other problem is not therapeutic and could be detrimental in the long term.

growth and thyroid function should be evaluated every 6 months for the next 3 years after therapy to detect these changes (if hormone-producing glands are included in the field). Both hypothyroidism and hypopituitary growth failure can be treated with hormone replacement in coming years.

Radiation to the ovaries or testes can result in infertility. In girls, normal oestrogen production may lag or fail, preventing the development of secondary sexual changes. In boys, testosterone production rarely fails. However, pre-treatment sperm banking may be advocated for a boy past puberty before he undergoes radiation to the testes.

Nervous system

Long-term effects of radiation to the brain can include demyelination and necrosis of the white matter. This can result in symptoms of lethargy, sleepiness and seizures. Effects on the grey matter can result in learning disabilities. There may be abnormal electroencephalograph tracings; a child may have low-intensity headaches, cataracts, salivary gland damage and a chronic change in or loss of taste. With careful planning these side effects can be significantly reduced.

Effects on the organs of the chest and abdomen

Because of the dangers of radiation damage the organs of the chest and abdomen are carefully shielded during radiation therapy.

- Radiation to the lungs may result in a chronic pneumonitis and/or pulmonary fibrosis
- Radiation to the heart may cause pericardial thickening and reduced heart expandability
- Radiation to the gastrointestinal system may result in chronic malabsorption from changes in the intestinal villi
- Radiation to the liver may cause hepatic fibrosis which may result in reduced liver function
- Radiation to the kidney and bladder may result in nephritis and chronic cystitis.

The possibility of these long-term effects of radiation should be explained to parents when radiation therapy is initially discussed, as a part of obtaining informed consent. At the early stage of diagnosis, however, parents rarely are concerned with these long-term effects. Their thoughts are understandably focused on short-term outcomes such as the achievement of a cure.

Chemotherapy

Chemotherapy is the common name used to describe a large variety of chemical agents used to treat cancer. Most chemotherapeutic regimens use several different types of medications which decreases the likelihood that the cancer can be resistant to all medications. Cells that are actively reproducing are more susceptible to chemotherapy. The various chemotherapies target specific aspects of the DNA or the components of the cell which enables cell division to take place.

Immunotherapy

Immunotherapy mobilises the body's immune system to target cancer cells. Interferon is an antiviral agent that prevents growth of viruses; stimulation of interferon or interferon therapy may be used to encourage the immune system to identify and halt malignant cell growth. Neuroblastoma is an example of a childhood cancer that appears to respond to antibody-based therapy (Parry & Engh, 2013).

Possible side effects of chemotherapy

All **chemotherapeutic agents** have side effects and toxic effects (see Box 53.4). Malnutrition, nausea and vomiting, hair loss, stomatitis, constipation, diarrhoea, cushingoid effects and susceptibility to infection are common side effects. It is not uncommon for a child receiving treatment for cancer to become malnourished. Nausea and vomiting resulting from chemotherapy can make it difficult to maintain an adequate kilojoule intake. If stomatitis occurs as a result of chemotherapy, eating becomes difficult because of mouth pain (see Box 53.5). Stomach and intestinal ulcers can interfere with absorption. Changes in fatty acid metabolism may alter the responsiveness of body cells to insulin metabolism. Unable to use glucose effectively, cells cannot function at an optimum level. This may account for the sense of fatigue that children with cancer frequently report.

BOX 53.4 ✻ Focus on evidence-based practice

Handling chemotherapy drugs at home

Following hospital discharge, parents assume the responsibility of administering chemotherapy at home. To see whether parents followed adequate protection for themselves while handling chemotherapy drugs, researchers asked 50 parents of children with acute lymphoblastic leukaemia to fill in a questionnaire asking about their experience with chemotherapy drugs. Seventy-two percent of parents reported receiving instruction on safe handling of oral chemotherapy. However, 90% reported they did not use protective gear such as gloves during preparation of oral chemotherapy. Although tablet crushers were designated for use with oral chemotherapy by 61% of parents, 22% used the same device to crush other non-chemotherapy medications. More than 50% of parents disposed of medication waste with regular garbage or poured the remainder down the sink.

How would the results of this study help in your education of parents whose children are to receive chemotherapy at home?

Source: Held, K., Ryan, R., Champion, J. M., et al. (2012). Caregiver survey results related to handling of oral chemotherapy for pediatric patients with acute lymphoblastic leukemia. *Journal of Pediatric Hematology & Oncology.* Advance online publication.

BOX 53.5 ✻ Focus on family teaching

Tips for relieving the discomfort of stomatitis

Q. Tim's father tells you, "Our son has developed ulcers in his mouth from the chemotherapy. What can we do to help him feel more comfortable?"

A. Continuing oral care despite discomfort is important to minimise the number of germs in the mouth and ideally prevent infection. Here are some tips for relieving the discomfort:

- Use a soft toothbrush.
- Make oral hygiene fun. Invent a game about mouth care that the whole family can play.
- Serve soft foods like mashed potatoes and pudding, rather than hard ones, such as toast crusts or crunchy cereal, to avoid further abrasions to tender gum lines.
- Encourage your child to rinse his mouth with lukewarm water three times a day (half-strength hydrogen peroxide may be prescribed), both for comfort and to encourage healing.
- Provide non-acidic foods, such as gelatine instead of orange juice, which can sting if sores are present.
- Encourage your child to drink as much fluid as possible because proper hydration helps to keep lips from cracking.
- Keep lips well lubricated with petroleum jelly or a commercial product. This care also prevents cracking.

Anorexia may occur from a hormone produced by the tumour that acts directly on the centre for hunger in the hypothalamus, reducing appetite and altering taste perception. Cyclophosphamide, a commonly used chemotherapeutic agent, is associated with taste alterations. Chemotherapy can also cause food to taste different. Many children report that foods taste bitter; they do not describe foods as sweet until they are very sweet. Because of these taste changes, foods the child used to enjoy are no longer enjoyable. Unwilling to try new foods, the child decreases oral intake (see Fig. 53.2).

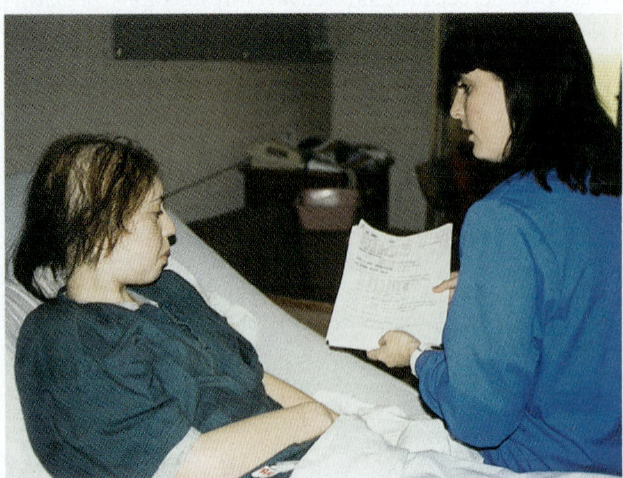

FIGURE 53.2 Children receiving radiation or chemotherapy often have reduced appetites. Here, a nurse discusses nutrition and food choices with a 15-year-old with leukaemia. (© Caroline Brown, RNC, MS, DEd.)

To counteract these taste changes, you may need to suggest different foods or methods of food preparation. Dieticians are usually part of the multidisciplinary team caring for patients and need to be contacted for advice.

Nausea and vomiting are common side effects of chemotherapy. Cells lining the stomach are fast-growing and therefore very susceptible to damage from chemotherapy. Nausea and vomiting can often be prevented by administering antiemetics before treatment is commenced.

Because chemotherapy causes changes in body appearance, both children and their parents can benefit from discussions of feelings about these changes. This can help to maintain self-esteem.

Alopecia, or hair loss, is a side effect that occurs with most chemotherapeutic medications; because hair cells are fast-growing they are very susceptible to the effects of chemotherapy. Even when forewarned that such a consequence is likely, most children and parents are surprised at the suddenness of the hair loss (a child can become totally bald in 2–3 days after some chemotherapy regimens). Hair loss can sometimes be a bigger problem for the parents than the child. Hats, caps, scarves or bandannas can be worn to protect the scalp and improve the appearance of a child who suffers from hair loss (see Fig. 53.3).

Children receiving long-term corticosteroid (prednisone) therapy develop a typical "moon face", red cheeks and a stocky build. Like the loss of body hair, a cushingoid appearance can be devastating to children. Ulceration of the gum line and mucous membranes of the mouth often occurs with administration of chemotherapy. The child may need a soft or light diet because chewing is painful. Brushing the teeth with a soft swab rather than a brush or just rinsing the mouth are options to reduce pain.

Some chemotherapeutic agents, particularly vincristine, can cause constipation. Anticipate the need for a stool softener, to prevent hard stools from exacerbating rectal ulcers. Diarrhoea may occur from the effects of chemotherapeutic agents on the absorptive surfaces of

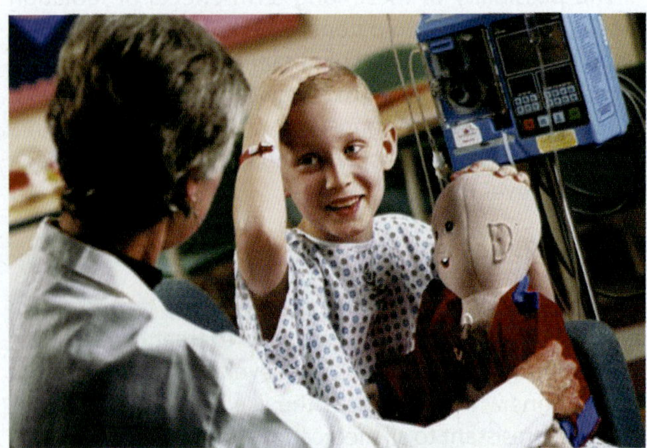

FIGURE 53.3 A nurse uses a doll to help prepare a child for the hair loss that accompanies chemotherapy.

the intestine. If diarrhoea is present, intravenous fluid will usually be prescribed to supplement fluid loss. Diarrhoea can be frightening for children because of the loss of control they experience.

Most children receiving chemotherapy experience fatigue and are unable to participate in their usual activities. Diversional therapists can be very helpful in suggesting ways for children to occupy themselves when their energy levels are low.

Vincristine, a chemotherapeutic agent that is often used for childhood leukaemia, results in specific neurological symptoms, such as weakness, tingling and numbing of the extremities and sometimes an inability to walk. Children may be unable to hold a pen or pencil or manoeuvre small parts of toys because their fingers are so affected. These symptoms subside after the medication is discontinued.

Children with cancer are very susceptible to infection, not only because their immune system is depressed by chemotherapy but also because they develop a degree of malnutrition that decreases the effectiveness of macrophage and phagocytosis functions, and possibly the production of interferon, which is important for destroying viral invaders. A malignant process in the body decreases the body's overall ability to recognise foreign invaders and respond with the usual efficient rejection process. Frequent insertion of intravenous devices, the development of dry and cracking mucous membranes, and ulcer formation throughout the gastrointestinal tract provide ready sites for the entrance of microorganisms (see Box 53.6).

When infection occurs, it may be difficult to recognise because common findings such as local erythema (redness), swelling, systemic fever and swollen lymph glands may not be present because of the immunosuppressive effects of treatment. Although not well studied in children, administration of colony-stimulating factors such as filgrastim (Neupogen) can help the body to quickly begin replacing damaged WBCs (McKenna & Mirkov, 2014). Even with the use of this agent, bacterial infections are common. Gram-negative bacteria such as *Escherichia coli, Pseudomonas aeruginosa* and *Klebsiella pneumoniae* and gram-positive bacteria such as *Staphylococcus aureus* and streptococci are common organisms responsible for causing infections. Viral infections such as varicella (chickenpox), varicella zoster (shingles), herpes simplex, viral hepatitis and cytomegalovirus are also common causes of infection.

When children are treated with immunosuppressive medications, protozoal infections, such as *Pneumocystis carinii* pneumonia (normally a very rare pneumonia), may occur. To compound the problem, treating bacterial infections with antibiotics can cause overgrowth of fungal infections such as candidiasis or aspergillosis. If infection is discovered in a child with cancer, the causative agent is identified by taking a culture. Specific antibiotics are then prescribed.

BOX 53.6 * Focus on family teaching

Preventing infection in the child with neutropenia

Q. Tim's mother asks you, "What special things should I do to help prevent my child from developing an infection until his WBC count returns to normal?"

A. Here are some suggestions to help prevent infections:

- Arrange for your child to sleep in a single bed and room, if possible, to avoid close contact with other family members who may be developing upper respiratory tract infections.
- Limit the child's exposure to large crowds, such as those at movie theatres.
- Screen and prohibit visitors who have signs of infection such as runny nose, oral herpes or rashes; who have been exposed to a communicable disease, such as chickenpox; or who have recently been vaccinated.
- Wash your hands frequently before child care and after handling potentially contaminated items such as tissues, nappies, or other containers of body secretions or fluids.
- Urge the child to wash hands well after using a bathroom and before eating.
- Keep child's immediate surroundings free of plants, flowers and goldfish, all of which could harbour mould spores.
- Be sure the child has a daily bath or shower. Clean mouth with soft toothbrush to reduce opportunity for bacteria, always present in the mouth, to invade.
- Inspect mouth daily for breaks in the tissue, bleeding or white patches that suggest oral thrush (*Monilia*) infection. Apply a moisturising and protective barrier, such as KY Jelly, to the lips to help prevent them from cracking.
- Take pulse and respiratory rate and temperature daily. Avoid taking rectal temperatures, to protect against injuring rectal tissue.
- Inspect all skin surfaces daily for scratches that could become entrances for infection. Include IV or IM injection sites, venous access device insertion sites and the nappy area.
- Administer stool softeners, if prescribed, to promote soft stools and bowel movements and avoid rectal tears.
- Provide high-kilojoule, high-protein foods and food supplements to help rebuild WBCs. Do not serve the child fresh fruits and vegetables because they have more potential to harbour infectious organisms than cooked foods.
- Assess for respiratory tract infection by listening for cough and throat clearing; inspect throat for redness and nasal passage for discharge. Keep child active and moving through playing a game, such as "Simon Says", that encourages deep breathing.
- Assess for possible genitourinary tract infections. Note the colour, clarity, frequency and concentration of urine. If necessary, obtain a urine specimen using a clean-catch method for testing. Promote increased fluid intake to keep urine flowing. Advise girls to wipe from front to back after voiding or defecating, to avoid bringing organisms forwards to the urethra. If a girl is menstruating, sanitary napkins do not have the potential to harbour as many germs as tampons do; urge her to change pads frequently (every 4 hrs).
- Question the administration of any vaccine made with a live virus until the child's WBC count returns to normal.

What if...

Tom's mother tells you that she does not want her child to have an antiemetic medication before chemotherapy because she sees the nausea and vomiting as proof that the chemotherapy is working? Would you give the medication?

Bone marrow transplantation

Transplantation of bone marrow that was previously harvested from a child with cancer or transplantation of marrow from a well person to a child with cancer has become a frequently used treatment for children. This can allow higher doses of chemotherapy and radiation to be used because, in the event of severe bone marrow depression, the child can have healthy marrow restored. Immune cells in the transplanted marrow may actually help to kill remaining cancer cells in the child's circulation.

If the child's own marrow is used, the procedure is called an *autologous* transfusion. Bone marrow may be donated by someone who is **histocompatible** (immune compatible) with the child; this is an *allogeneic* transplant. A *syngeneic* transplant is one between twins.

Before transplantation, the child receives a chemotherapy agent, such as cyclophosphamide, and total-body irradiation to kill as many marrow cells as possible, suppress the child's immune response to the transplanted tissue, and create space in the bone marrow to allow the newly-transplanted cells a place to grow.

Pain assessment

Because growing tumours displace cells, causing anoxia to those cells, pain is a common symptom experienced by children with cancer. Methods to assess pain and interventions to help children deal with pain are discussed in Chapter 39.

THE LEUKAEMIAS

Leukaemia is the distorted and uncontrolled proliferation of WBCs (leucocytes) and is the most frequently occurring type of cancer in children.

Acute lymphocytic (lymphoblastic) leukaemia

Acute lymphocytic leukaemia (ALL) accounts for 75% of leukaemia (Brown & Hunger, 2014) and involves lymphoblasts or immature lymphocytes. With the rapid proliferation of immature lymphocytes, the production of red blood cells and platelets falls, and invasion of body organs by the rapidly increasing WBC elements begins. Because the abnormally proliferating cells are so immature, they may be identifiable only at the immature "blast cell" or "stem cell" stage.

The highest incidence of ALL is in children between 2 and 6 years of age. The prognosis in children younger than 1 year or older than 10 years at the time of first occurrence is not as good as in those between 2 and 10 years of age. The incidence of ALL is slightly higher in boys than in girls, and the disease is seen more often in white children than in children of other races (McLean & Wofford, 2015).

Although it can be shown that leukaemia in mice and cats is of viral origin, the cause of leukaemia in children is unknown. Radiation, exposure to chemicals or genetic factors may have some influence on the occurrence. Children with Down syndrome or Fanconi syndrome are more likely to develop leukaemia than are other children. If a twin has leukaemia, the other twin (as opposed to a non-twin sibling) is more susceptible to the disease. Bone irradiation may be implicated, so children should be submitted to as few x-rays as possible, including while in utero. An association between magnetic fields or power lines and leukaemia is disputed because different studies show different results (Miller & Green, 2010).

Up to 95% of children will have a first remission. If a child experiences a relapse, the chances of long-term survival are reduced to approximately 70%. Although remission can be reinduced, the length of each subsequent remission tends to be shorter and less effective.

✔ *Checkpoint question 53.1*

Parents are often unaware that their child is developing leukaemia. What are the first signs commonly seen in a child with acute lymphocytic leukaemia (ALL)?

a. Nodules and pink rash
b. Headaches and sleepiness
c. Fatigue and bruising
d. Joint pain and coughing

Cure as goal

The goal of therapy for leukaemia is complete cure, based on the use of **chemotherapeutic agents** (see Table 53.1). A chemotherapy program is aimed at: first, achieving a complete remission or absence of leukaemia cells (induction phase); second, preventing leukaemia cells from invading or growing in the central nervous system (sanctuary or consolidation phase); third, administering delayed intensive therapy; and fourth, maintaining the original remission (maintenance phase).

Chemotherapy in children is often administered by means of a central venous catheter or port because administration of medications into a major vessel helps prevent irritation to the vessel walls. These access devices have the secondary advantage of being able to be clamped or "trapped" so that the child can be ambulatory between treatments.

Maintenance and monitoring

Maintenance chemotherapy aims to eliminate completely any remaining leukaemic cells, so that the child's immune system can complete the eradication. This is continued for 2–3 years.

TABLE 53.1 Commonly used chemotherapeutic agents

Drug	Classification	Side effects and toxic effects	Special considerations
Colasplase (Leunase)	Enzyme; deprives leukaemic cells of asparagine, leading to cell death	Anorexia, weight loss, nausea, vomiting, hepatotoxicity, central nervous system toxicity, anaphylactic reaction	Staying with child for first hour of infusion is important; take vital signs q15 min for first hour to detect anaphylactic reaction.
Carmustine (BCNU; BiCNU)	Nitrosourea compound; crosses blood–brain barrier	Nausea, vomiting, bone marrow depression (after 3–4 wk), hepatotoxicity	Child may notice burning sensation along vein during administration because of alcohol diluent.
Chlorambucil (Leukeran)	Nitrogen mustard derivative	Bone marrow depression	Monitoring of white blood cell count is necessary.
Cisplatin (Platinol)	Alkylating agent; reacts with and injures cell nucleus	Bone marrow depression, nephrotoxicity (renal dysfunction), nausea, vomiting, loss of taste, tinnitus, high-frequency hearing loss	Infusion bottle must be covered with aluminum foil to keep out light, or decomposition will result.
Cyclophosphamide (Cycloblastin)	Alkylating agent (nitrogen mustard derivative)	Bone marrow depression, anorexia, nausea, vomiting, stomatitis, alopecia, cystitis, (haemorrhagic) hepatotoxicity	Fluid intake is encouraged; maintain IV line to limit bladder irritation; test urine for blood and specific gravity.
Dacarbazine (DTIC)	Alkylating agent	Bone marrow depression	Extravasation causes severe tissue damage.
Dactinomycin (Cosmegan)	Antibiotic; inhibits DNA synthesis	Nausea, vomiting, bone marrow depression, stomatitis	Tissue inflammation occurs if it extravasates into tissue.
Daunorubicin	Antibiotic; vesicant	Alopecia, bone marrow depression	Extravasation causes severe tissue damage.
Etoposide	Mitotic inhibitor; inhibits DNA synthesis	Fatigue, alopecia, nausea and vomiting	Slow IV administration is necessary to avoid irritation.
Doxorubicin (Adriamycin)	Antibiotic; inhibits DNA synthesis; vesicant	Nausea, vomiting, bone marrow depression, alopecia, stomatitis, possible heart toxicity	Urine may turn red; take pulse for full minute to detect arrhythmia; tissue necrosis occurs if extravasated.
Ifosfamide (Holoxan)	Alkylating agent; interferes with DNA synthesis	Leucopenia, alopecia, haemorrhagic cystitis	Maintaining hydration is important to prevent cystitis.
Lomustine (CCNU; CeeNu)	Alkylating agent (nitrosourea compound)	Nausea, vomiting in 6 hr, bone marrow depression (after 3–4 wks)	Administration on an empty stomach enhances absorption.

(continued)

TABLE 53.1 Commonly used chemotherapeutic agents *(Continued)*

Drug	Classification	Side effects and toxic effects	Special considerations
Mercaptopurine (Purinethol)	Antimetabolite (purine analogue)	Bone marrow depression, nausea, vomiting, stomatitis, hepatotoxicity	Allopurinol delays the degradation of mercaptopurine and thus increases toxicity; question order if both are to be administered.
Methotrexate	Antimetabolite	Stomatitis, bone marrow depression, nausea, vomiting, alopecia, hepatotoxicity, nephrotoxicity at high dosage	Decreased effect occurs if administered with salicylates; often followed by leucovorin to decrease toxicity to normal cells.
Prednisone	Corticosteroid; suppresses lymphocyte production	Weight gain, cushingoid facies, depressed systemic response to infection	Child needs support to accept changed appearance.
Procarbazine (Natulan)	Antineoplastic; interferes with DNA and RNA synthesis	Nausea, vomiting, bone marrow depression	Drug may cause blurriness of vision; avoid foods with high tyramine content.
Thioguanine (Lanvis)	Antimetabolite	Bone marrow suppression	Monitoring of hepatic function tests is necessary.
Vincristine (Oncovin)	Plant alkaloid; vesicant	Constipation, alopecia, joint and muscle pain, muscle weakness	Paraesthesia of fingers and toes, foot drop may occur; may need stool softener; tissue necrosis occurs if infiltrated.
Additional agents			
Allopurinol (Zyloprim)	Antigout agent	Nausea, vomiting	Prevents uric acid formation from destroyed cells.
Bacillus Calmette-Guérin (BCG) vaccine*	Vaccine	Local inflammation	Stimulates immune system.
Leucovorin	Folic acid derivative		Neutralises the toxicity of methotrexate.
Interferon	Antiviral agent	Fever	Blocks virus replication.
Filgrastim (Neupogen)	Granulocyte colony-stimulating factor	Nausea, vomiting	Leucocyte count increases.
Epoetin alfa (Eprex)	Recombinant human erythropoietin	Hypertension; headache	Red blood cell count increases.

*Otherwise used to vaccinate against tuberculosis.

Complications

Throughout therapy, the treating team and family need to be alert for possible complications of therapy. Among these problems are central nervous system, renal and reproductive system disorders.

Central nervous system involvement

If central nervous system involvement occurs, it can become severe and intense. Blindness, hydrocephalus and recurrent seizures are possible.

Renal involvement

Kidney involvement, resulting from invasion of leukaemia cells, is another serious complication. The kidneys may enlarge and their function will be impaired.

Testicular invasion

In boys, leukaemic cells tend to invade the testes. Unless this problem is specifically addressed, these cells will not be destroyed by chemotherapy. As a result, once chemotherapy is halted, the leukaemic cells may grow and proliferate again. In most boys, therefore, the testes will be irradiated to destroy this sanctuary site for cells. This treatment leads to sterilisation. If a boy is past puberty and is forming sperm, sperm banking might be suggested before chemotherapy and radiation to preserve sperm for reproduction later in life.

Acute myeloid leukaemia

Acute myeloid leukaemia (AML) involves the over proliferation of granulocytes (neutrophils, basophils and eosinophils). It is most often seen in adults so accounts for only about 20% of all childhood leukaemia. The frequency of the disorder increases in late adolescence as children reach adulthood. With AML, granulocytes grow so rapidly that they are often forced out into the bloodstream while still in the blast stage. As with ALL, the over proliferation of granulocytes limits the production of red blood cells (RBCs) and platelets.

Assessment

Children with AML have the same symptoms as those with ALL. Because they do not have mature granulocytes, they are susceptible to infection and may have experienced many recent upper respiratory tract infections before the time of diagnosis. Diagnosis is established by bone marrow aspiration and biopsy. After diagnosis, chemotherapy to effect remission begins. Remission is more difficult to achieve in children with AML than in those with ALL, and if one is achieved, it may be brief. Bone marrow transplantation may be attempted after the initial remission to ensure new growth of normal granulocytes.

THE LYMPHOMAS

Lymphomas are malignancies of the lymph or reticuloendothelial system; they account for about 15% of all malignancies and are categorised as Hodgkin's or non-Hodgkin's lymphomas. Although Hodgkin's disease is better known, non-Hodgkin's lymphomas are more common worldwide in children (about 60% versus 40%). They both occur more frequently in males than in females (Copeland & Younes, 2012).

Hodgkin's disease

With Hodgkin's disease, lymphocytes proliferate in the lymph glands, and special *Reed-Sternberg cells* (large, multinucleated cells that are probably non-functioning monocyte-macrophage cells) are found. As with all neoplastic diseases, the aetiology of Hodgkin's disease is unknown, but both genetic and environmental factors probably play a part. It is rarely seen in children younger than 7 years of age. The incidence increases greatly during adolescence and young adulthood. Metastasis is through lymphatic channels.

Symptoms of Hodgkin's disease usually begin with only one painless, enlarged, rubbery-feeling lymph node, usually a cervical node. Other nodes then become involved, along with the liver, spleen, bone marrow, and eventually, the central nervous system. The child usually has accompanying symptoms of anorexia, malaise, night sweats and loss of weight. Fever may be present. It is confirmed by biopsy of the lymph nodes. Further studies are done to classify the clinical stage of the disorder (see Table 53.2).

Treatment depends on the clinical stage of the disease at the time of diagnosis. Although Hodgkin's disease was once treated mainly with radiation therapy, children today in all stages but stage 1, receive chemotherapy. Current therapy results in a 90% 5-year survival rate for children with stage I or stage II disease, and 60% to 90% for more advanced disease. If a relapse occurs, additional chemotherapy, radiation therapy or bone marrow transplantation will be scheduled. Children need conscientious follow-up for symptoms of Hodgkin's disease relapse during adult life. A relapse is often retreatable, using a chemotherapy course different from that used initially.

TABLE 53.2 Stages of Hodgkin's disease

Stage	Extent of disease
I	Disease affects single lymph node or single extra-lymphatic organ or site.
II	Disease affects two or more lymph node regions on the same side of the diaphragm, or there is localised involvement of an extralymphatic organ or site.
III	Disease affects lymph node regions on both sides of the diaphragm, or there is localised involvement of an extralymphatic organ or site.
IV	There is diffuse or disseminated involvement of extralymphatic organs with or without associated lymph node involvement.

Non-Hodgkin's lymphoma

Non-Hodgkin's lymphomas are malignant disorders of the lymphocytes. They involve stem cells and lymphocytes in varying degrees of differentiation. Unlike Hodgkin's disease, they are spread through the bloodstream rather than directly by lymph flow. The course of the disease is therefore unpredictable. Metastatic spread to the central nervous system tends to occur early in the disease. The most common age of occurrence is 5 to 15 years.

The cause of non-Hodgkin's lymphomas may be an oncogenic virus because they occur with increased frequency in children with agammaglobulinaemia or acquired immunodeficiency syndrome (AIDS) and in those who are receiving long-term immunosuppressive therapy, such as would be given after organ transplantation. Such immunosuppressed states may reduce the body's ability to recognise and destroy oncogenic viruses or malignant cells.

Non-Hodgkin's lymphomas of the lymphoblastic type most commonly involve the lymph glands of the neck and chest, although axillary, abdominal or inguinal nodes may be the first involved. To establish the diagnosis, biopsy of the affected lymph nodes and bone marrow is performed. Non-Hodgkin's lymphomas are treated with systemic chemotherapy, similar to that used for ALL. The initial phase of therapy is an induction phase (a time during which the child is put into remission, or no tumour can be detected by clinical means); this is followed by a maintenance phase, up to 2 years long.

Autologous bone marrow transfusion (using bone marrow removed at diagnosis, before the disease has spread to the marrow, and then replaced after blood components have been destroyed by chemotherapy) allows more aggressive chemotherapy to be used than formerly. Between 80% and 90% of children with non-Hodgkin's lymphoma with minimal symptoms achieve remission.

Burkitt's lymphoma

Burkitt's lymphoma (a non-Hodgkin's lymphoma) is a specifically named but rare form of cancer in Australia and New Zealand; it is much more commonly seen in Africa. When this lymphoma does occur, however, it tends to affect children. Children from 2 to 14 years of age have the highest incidence, with a peak at 7 years. An association between Burkitt's lymphoma and Epstein-Barr virus, which causes infectious mononucleosis, exists. It is also associated with HIV-positive individuals. The first indication of disease is an enlarged lymph node of the neck or abdomen. It is usually painless unless it blocks some body system.

A Burkitt's lymphoma is a rapidly growing tumour; the cell mass may double in size in 24 hours so early diagnosis and treatment is important. Surgery is used to remove the primary tumour and this is followed by chemotherapy. Because Burkitt's lymphomas are such rapidly growing tumours, they respond dramatically to chemotherapy (the cells are almost always in a susceptible state).

✔ *Checkpoint question 53.2*

An adolescent has been diagnosed as having Hodgkin's disease. How would you explain this disease to him? He is active in a school sports program and works part-time in a supermarket. How will you answer if he asks you whether he should stop these activities?

NEOPLASMS OF THE BRAIN

Brain tumours are the second most common form of cancer in children and the most common solid tumour form. Tumours tend to occur between 1 and 10 years of age, with 5 years being the peak age of incidence. In children, brain tumours tend to occur at the midline in the brainstem or cerebellum.

Types of brain tumours

Common sites for brain tumours in children are shown in Figure 53.4. The most common brain tumours are cerebellar astrocytomas, medulloblastomas and brainstem tumours.

- Astrocytomas are slow-growing, cystic tumours that arise from the glial or support tissue of neural cells. They account for about one-quarter of all brain tumours in children. The peak age of incidence is 5 to 8 years.
- Medulloblastomas are fast-growing tumours found most commonly in the cerebellum. The peak age of incidence is 5 to 10 years. Usually found at the midline, they cause fourth-ventricle compression and disturbances in the flow of cerebrospinal fluid.
- Brainstem tumours arise from the support tissue of the neural cells. They often cause paralysis of the fifth, sixth, seventh, ninth and tenth cranial nerves. They may

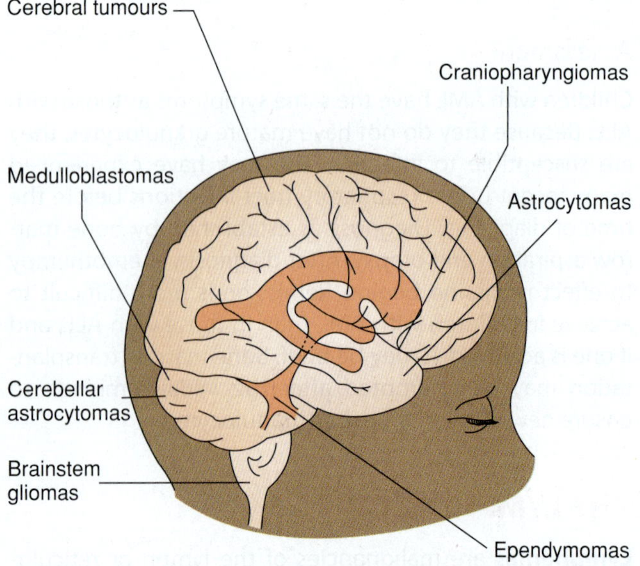

FIGURE 53.4 Common sites for brain tumours in children.

produce symptoms of ataxia, nystagmus and changes in respiratory and pulse findings because of pressure on these centres.

Children with a brain tumour develop symptoms of increased intracranial pressure: headache, vision changes, vomiting, an enlarging head circumference or papilloedema. Lethargy, projectile vomiting and coma are late signs. With some tumours the pain is occipital. This is an important finding, because this is an unusual location for a headache from any other cause.

Vomiting, like headache, most commonly occurs on arising. Unlike the child who vomits because of gastrointestinal distress, the child with a brain tumour is not usually nauseated and will eat immediately afterward. The vomiting pattern occurs morning after morning. It will eventually become projectile after a long time, but projectile vomiting is not an initial symptom.

Apart from these generalised symptoms of increased intracranial pressure, a growing tumour produces specific localised signs, such as nystagmus (constant horizontal movement of the eye), cranial nerve paralysis or visual field defects. Tumours of the cerebellum cause a definite head tilt because of vision suppression. As tumour growth continues, symptoms of ataxia, personality change (emotional lability, irritability), and seizures may occur.

Therapy for brain tumours includes a combination of surgery, radiation therapy and chemotherapy, depending on the location and extent of the tumour. Because they are located so deeply, most tumours cannot be completely removed in children; this makes radiation and chemotherapy increasingly important. Radiation therapy may be intense because if tumour tissue is not rapidly proliferating, cells are not easily destroyed. Chemotherapy is limited because many chemotherapeutic agents do not cross the blood–brain barrier. Administration of a medication directly into the ventricular system via a reservoir (Ommaya) may increase medication effectiveness (see Fig. 53.5). The diagnosis of a brain tumour at any age is always a serious one and causes significant stress for parents (Aminoff, 2009).

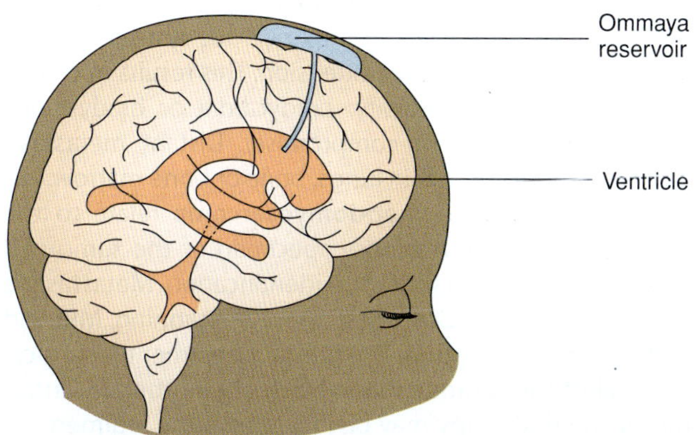

FIGURE 53.5 An Ommaya reservoir. Medication injected into the reservoir flows down to the ventricle and enters the cerebrospinal fluid.

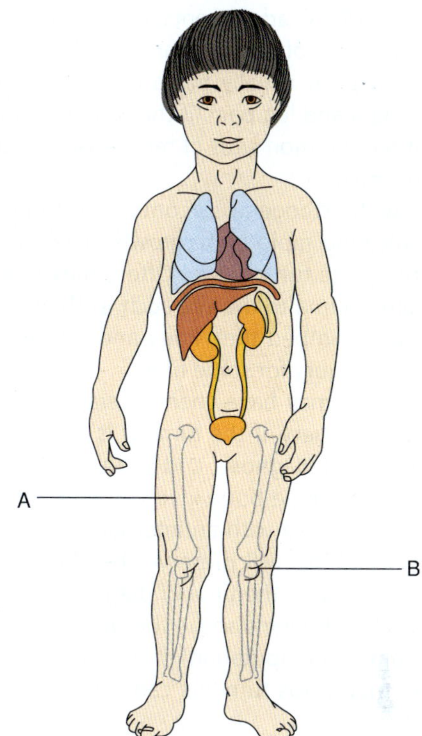

FIGURE 53.6 (A) The diaphysis (midshaft) is one of the most frequent sites of Ewing's sarcoma. (B) The epiphysis of a bone is a common site of osteogenic sarcoma.

BONE TUMOURS

Tumours derived from connective tissue, such as bone and cartilage, muscle, blood vessels or lymphoid tissue are called **sarcomas**. They are the second most frequently occurring neoplasms in adolescents (only lymphomas occur more frequently). Bone tumours may arise during adolescence because rapid bone growth is occurring at this time. Because girls have a puberty growth spurt earlier than boys, bone tumours tend to occur slightly earlier in girls than in boys (13 years for girls compared with 14 or 15 years for boys). The two most frequently occurring types are osteogenic sarcoma and **Ewing's sarcoma** (see Fig. 53.6).

Osteogenic sarcoma

An **osteogenic sarcoma** is a malignant tumour of long bone involving rapidly growing bone tissue (mesenchymal-matrix forming cells). It tends to occur more commonly in boys than in girls. The most common sites of occurrence are the distal femur (40–50%), the proximal tibia (20%), and the proximal humerus (10–15%) (Roth, Mirochna & Harsha, 2012). Osteogenic sarcoma can occur in children who have had radiation for other malignancies as a later life effect. Children with retinoblastoma have a higher incidence than normal of osteosarcoma, so a hereditary influence may be present.

Although bones do not have a lymphatic system, metastasis occurs early because of the extensive vascular system in bones. Metastasis to the lungs is the most common site;

as many as 25% of adolescents have lung metastasis already by the time of initial diagnosis. When this is present, the adolescent usually has a chronic cough, dyspnoea, chest pain and leg pain (if the tumour originates in the leg). Other common sites of metastasis are brain and other bone tissue.

Children with osteogenic sarcoma are often taller than average, indicating rapid bone growth. They notice pain and swelling at the tumour site. Often, they report a history of recent trauma to the site such as they fell playing basketball and bumped their knee and attribute pain in the knee to this injury for some time.

An adolescent may have chemotherapy to shrink the tumour before surgery. If the tumour is in the leg and is small at the time of diagnosis, and if the child has reached adult height, the single bone involved may be surgically removed and replaced with an internally placed bone or metal prosthesis. This will preserve the child's leg. If the tumour is extensive at the time of diagnosis, the leg may be amputated at the joint above the tumour (this usually involves a total hip amputation). If the cancer has spread to the lung, metastasis tumours can usually be removed by thoracotomy.

Only a few years ago, a diagnosis of osteogenic sarcoma was ominous; few children survived into adulthood. Today, 70% of adolescents in whom an early diagnosis is made and who are treated rigorously can be cured (Brown & Hunger, 2014).

What if...

A parent tells you his son developed an osteosarcoma from falling while playing basketball? Is that a possible cause of bone cancer?

OTHER CHILDHOOD NEOPLASMS

Neuroblastoma

Neuroblastomas are tumours that arise from the cells of the sympathetic nervous system; cells are highly undifferentiated and invasive, occurring most frequently in the abdomen near the adrenal gland or spinal ganglia. They are the most common abdominal tumour in childhood (Davenport, Blanco & Sandler, 2012). Neuroblastoma occurs primarily in infants and preschool children; it is slightly more common in boys than in girls. These tumours may occur so early in life that they are detected by fetal ultrasound or at birth. There may be an association between the development of neuroblastomas and fetal alcohol syndrome or cigarette or marijuana smoking by parents. Common sites of metastasis include the bone marrow, liver and subcutaneous tissue.

Tumours are classified as stage I to stage IV (see Table 53.3). If the tumour is localised (stage I), therapy will consist of surgical removal of the primary tumour. If the tumour is stage II to IV, surgery will be followed by chemotherapy. A subsequent surgical procedure may be scheduled within several months to determine the effectiveness of therapy and to attempt the possible removal of further tumour. If aggressive chemotherapy is not effective, bone marrow transplantation to restore functioning bone marrow may be scheduled.

TABLE 53.3 Staging neuroblastoma

Stage	Extent of disease
I	Tumour is well encapsulated and completely removed by surgery.
II	Tumour cannot be completely removed by surgery or disease extends to lymph nodes.
III	Tumour extends beyond the midline; regional lymph nodes may be involved bilaterally.
IV	Distant metastases; bone, eyes or liver involved.
IVs	Metastasis is present in child <1 year old.

Overall, children with neuroblastoma have a 5-year survival rate of 70% to 90%. Although most children have a positive initial response to therapy, recurrence is common within the first year. The prognosis is better in children diagnosed before 1 year of age.

✔ Checkpoint question 53.3

A 2-year-old child is going to be receiving chemotherapy after surgery for a neuroblastoma. How would you prepare the child for chemotherapy? What activities would you propose to keep the child occupied while an intravenous solution is infusing?

Rhabdomyosarcoma

A **rhabdomyosarcoma** is a tumour of striated muscle (Arndt et al., 2012). It arises from the embryonic mesenchyme tissue that forms muscle, connective and vascular tissue. The peak age of incidence of these tumours is 2 to 6 years, with a second peak occurring during puberty. Common sites of occurrence include the eye orbit, paranasal sinuses, uterus, prostate, bladder, retroperitoneum, arms and legs (see Table 53.4). Central nervous system invasion occurs from direct tumour extension. This results in cranial nerve palsy, nuchal rigidity, bradycardia or bradypnoea (because of brainstem compromise). Distant metastasis most commonly occurs in lungs, bone or bone marrow.

The symptoms of **rhabdomyosarcoma** relate to the site of the tumour. A biopsy specimen of the tumour is taken and examined for tissue identification. Metastasis is ruled out by bone scan, chest x-ray, CT scanning, MRI and bone marrow aspiration. The primary treatment is surgical removal of the tumour, followed by chemotherapy. Intrathecal chemotherapy may be included in the regimen.

A child's prognosis depends on the size of the tumour and whether metastasis was present at the time of initial diagnosis. If the entire tumour was removed and no lymph

TABLE 53.4 Common sites and associated symptoms of rhabdomyosarcoma

Site of tumour	Symptoms
Orbit	Proptosis (extruding eye); visible and palpable conjunctival or eyelid mass
Neck	Hoarseness, dysphagia; visible and palpable mass in neck
Nasopharynx	Airway obstruction, epistaxis, dysphagia, visible mass in nasal or nasopharyngeal passages
Paranasal sinuses	Swelling, pain, nasal discharge, epistaxis
Middle ear	Pain, chronic otitis media, hearing loss, facial nerve palsy, mass protruding into external ear canal
Bladder and prostate	Dysuria, urinary retention, haematuria, constipation, palpable lower abdominal mass
Vagina	Mass protruding from uterus or cervix into vagina, abnormal vaginal bleeding
Trunk, extremities	Visible and palpable soft-tissue mass
Testicles	Visible and palpable soft-tissue mass

node metastasis has occurred, the chances are as high as 80% that the tumour will not recur. If some of the tumour had to be left because of its size or location, the chance of recurrence rises to about 50%. If metastasis to the lungs or bone was present at the time of the initial diagnosis, the prognosis drops still further; about 20% of children in this situation have long-term survival. Among children who do survive, long-term complications such as cardiomyopathy and infertility may occur from the side effects of chemotherapy.

Nephroblastoma (Wilms' tumour)

Nephroblastoma (Wilms' tumour) is a malignant tumour that rises from the metanephric mesoderm cells of the upper pole of the kidney (Romão et al., 2012). It accounts for 20% of solid tumours in childhood; there is no increased incidence based on sex or race. It occurs in association with congenital anomalies.

A nephroblastoma is usually discovered early in life (6 months to 5 years; peak at 3 to 4 years), although it apparently arises from an embryonic structure present in the child before birth. Nephroblastomas distort the kidney anteriorly so that the tumour is felt as a firm, non-tender abdominal mass. A CT scan or ultrasound reveals the primary tumour and any points of metastasis. Kidney function studies, such as glomerular filtration rate or blood urea nitrogen, will be carried out to assess function of the kidneys before surgery. Little time, however, can be allotted for preoperative testing because these tumours metastasise rapidly as a result of the large blood supply to the kidneys and adrenal glands.

TABLE 53.5 Staging nephroblastoma (Wilms' tumour)

Stage	Description
I	Tumour confined to the kidney and completely removed surgically
II	Tumour extending beyond the kidney but completely removed surgically
III	Regional spread of disease beyond the kidney with residual abdominal disease postoperatively
IV	Metastases to lung, liver, bone, distant lymph nodes or other distant sites
V	Bilateral disease

Nephroblastomas are staged to predict therapy and prognosis (see Table 53.5). Therapy for nephroblastoma is so effective that about 90% of children who had no metastatic spread at diagnosis survive for at least 5 years.

Retinoblastoma

Retinoblastoma is a malignant tumour of the retina of the eye (Nagarkatti-Gude et al., 2012). A rare tumour, it accounts for only 1–3% of childhood malignancies. In about 10% of children, these tumours develop because of an inherited autosomal dominant pattern that causes an alteration of chromosome 13. Because of the dominant pattern of inheritance, a person who survives retinoblastoma has a 90% chance of having a child with a similar tumour. Parents who may be carriers, or a parent who has survived the disease, need genetic counselling so that they are aware of the risk to their children. The 5-year survival rate for children with retinoblastoma is at least 90%. Retinoblastoma occurs most often, however, as spontaneous development, not the inherited type. Children with the inherited type tend to develop bilateral disease; those with the spontaneous type may or may not have the tumour in both eyes.

Retinoblastoma occurs early in life, from about 6 weeks of age through the preschool period. It occurs equally in boys and girls, and there is no preference for either the right or the left eye. One tumour or many individual tumours may be present. Tumours are located on the retina or in the vitreous fluid or extend backwards into the choroid, the optic nerve and the subarachnoid space.

Retinoblastomas are serious tumours involving the retina of the eye; allowed to grow, they cause blindness. If the tumour is very small at the time of diagnosis, it may be treated with cryosurgery (freezing the tumour to destroy local cells). This will preserve partial vision in the eye. Photocoagulation using laser surgery to destroy the blood vessels supplying the tumour may be used. Localised radioactive applicators or plaques sutured to the sclera over the tumour may also be used. Such plaques remain in place for 4 to 7 days. The child may also receive radiation treatment and chemotherapy If the tumour is large when first discovered, removal of the eye (enucleation) may be necessary.

The long-term survival rate for children with retinoblastoma is as high as 90%. Evaluation of the child after retinoblastoma must include not only whether metastasis can be detected but whether the child is adjusting to the loss of sight in one or both eyes. If radiation was used for therapy, cataracts may develop several years later.

Skin cancer

Two in three Australians will be diagnosed with skin cancer by the time they are 70 years of age (Cancer Council Australia, 2015). The most common types involved are melanoma (the most dangerous form of skin cancer) and non-melanoma skin cancer (basal cell carcinoma and squamous cell carcinoma).

- A *malignant melanoma* is a tumour originating in melanocytes or nevi that appears as a mole changing in appearance.
- A *basal cell carcinoma* is a surface epithelial growth that appears as a small ulcer that does not heal.
- A *squamous cell carcinoma* is a tumour of the epidermis that appears as a white scaly lesion.

All three types of skin cancer are increasing in incidence and although the symptoms usually do not appear until late adolescence, the chief cause (excessive sun exposure) begins in childhood (Nicole & Huether, 2012).

Malignant melanoma

Malignant melanoma is usually evaluated according to the mnemonic ABCDE: A for asymmetrical; B for borders that are irregular (uneven or notched); C for colour variations; D for diametre exceeding 3 to 6 mm; and E for elevated, not flat (Lewis & Foley, 2014). Danger signs of malignant melanoma include any of these factors. However, smaller areas may indicate early stage melanomas. Other warning signs include itching, tenderness or pain, and a change in size or bleeding of a mole. New pigmentations are also warning signs (Cancer Council Australia, 2015).

Melanomas are treated with surgery, radiation and adjuvant interferon-α2b or ipilimumab (immunotherapy) to improve overall survival. Nurses can play a major role in helping to reduce the incidence of skin cancer by teaching parents, children and adolescents ways to identify these malignancies and better protect against excessive sun exposure using measures, such as:

- Apply a sunscreen or wear protective clothing if a child will be out in the sun for longer than 20 minutes
- Avoid indoor tanning beds or ultraviolet light—if used, maintain the same precautions as with sunlight
- Avoid sunburn because there is a direct association between two or more episodes of sunburn in adolescence and the development of malignant melanoma in young adulthood (ACS, 2012).

BOX 53.7 ✻ Focus on family teaching

Q. A mother asks you what she can do to help protect her baby from the harmful rays of the sun.

A. Here are some suggestions for minimising sun exposure in babies:

- Where possible, plan activities to avoid being outside in the middle of the day when UV levels are at their most intense.
- Cover as much of the baby's skin as possible with loose-fitting clothes or wraps made from closely woven fabrics.
- Choose a hat that protects the baby's face, neck and ears.
- Create shade for the baby's stroller and use a play area that has shade.
- Apply a broad-spectrum, water-resistant sunscreen to small areas of the baby's skin that cannot be protected by clothing, such as the face, ears, neck and hands and reapply every 2 hours.

Cancer Council Australia (2015) advises that there is no evidence to suggest that using sunscreen on babies is harmful. However, some babies may develop a minor skin irritation; if this occurs, try using a sunscreen for sensitive skin, which is less likely to irritate the skin.

Evidence suggests that childhood sun exposure contributes significantly to the lifetime risk of skin cancer. Cancer Council Australia (2015) recommends keeping babies out of the sun as much as possible for the first 12 months. Box 53.7 outlines other measures that parents and carers can take to minimise sun exposure in babies.

Nurses can give younger children the following physical reference when doing health promotion on safe sun exposure. Tell the child, "Play outside only when your shadow is taller than you are". The child's shadow will be "taller" before 10 a.m. and after 2 p.m. The nurse can demonstrate this concept by placing a ruler on end and shining a bright light over it. As the nurse moves the light, the child will see the ruler's shadow lengthen (Ricci and Kyle, 2012).

✔ Checkpoint question 53.4

What is an important intervention to take for a child with nephroblastoma (Wilms' tumour)?

a. Post a sign over the cot: "No abdominal palpation"
b. Alert the mother that her child will be infertile after surgery
c. Be certain the child eats no red vegetables before surgery
d. Record a head circumference in the nursing care plan

Key points for review

- After a diagnosis of malignancy, parents and children need help to change their perception of cancer as an always painful, fatal disease to viewing it as a condition for which there is therapy and hope.

- Because the therapy for cancer involves so many health-care visits and so much parental concern, the siblings of children with cancer may feel excluded from family activities. Remind parents to incorporate the entire family into activities whenever possible, to help them grow as a family during the course of therapy.
- Radiation is an important treatment modality in cancer therapy. Immediate side effects include anorexia, nausea, vomiting and hair loss if radiation is to the head. Long-term effects may include growth restriction or learning disabilities.
- A chemotherapeutic agent is capable of destroying malignant cells. Common side effects of chemotherapy are the same as those for radiation therapy. Help children to use time during chemotherapy treatments in constructive ways, such as playing a game, to keep them mentally stimulated yet quiet.
- Leukaemia is the distorted and uncontrolled proliferation of WBCs and is the most frequently occurring type of cancer in children. About 90–95% of children with an initially good prognosis now have long-term survival.
- Hodgkin's disease and non-Hodgkin's lymphomas are malignancies of the lymphatic system. Hodgkin's disease occurs most often in adolescents; the initial symptom is often one painless, enlarged lymph node. Therapy is radiation and chemotherapy.
- Brain tumours are the most common solid tumours occurring in childhood. Beginning symptoms are usually those of increased intracranial pressure. Therapy may include a combination of surgery followed by radiation and chemotherapy.
- Bone tumours occur in two main forms: osteogenic sarcoma and Ewing's sarcoma. These tumours tend to be fast growing because of the ready blood supply to bone. Therapy consists of surgery followed by radiation and chemotherapy.
- Neuroblastomas are tumours that arise from the cells of the sympathetic nervous system. They are the most common abdominal tumour in childhood. Therapy is surgery and chemotherapy.
- Rhabdomyosarcomas are tumours of striated muscle. The peak age of incidence is 2 to 6 years. Therapy is surgery and chemotherapy.
- Nephroblastoma (Wilms' tumour) is a malignancy that arises from the metanephric mesoderm cells of the kidney. It is usually discovered early in life. Therapy is surgery followed by radiation and chemotherapy.
- Retinoblastoma is a malignant tumour of the retina of the eye. It may be inherited as an autosomal dominant pattern. Therapy involves surgery, radiation, chemotherapy, and possibly, enucleation if the tumour is large.
- Skin cancer is a type of malignancy that can be prevented beginning in childhood. Cautioning children about sensible sun exposure can be an important health promotion role for nurses.

CASE STUDY QUESTION

3. Tom's mother told you that he wakes up every morning with a headache and then vomits. She says this pattern began just after school started, so she is certain it is related to school. His teacher has suggested that Tom have an eye examination. What are some additional questions you would want to ask to determine whether you should pursue this concern further?

Resources

For an extensive range of additional resources to enhance teaching and learning and to facilitate understanding of this chapter, please see the text's accompanying website located on thePoint at http://thepoint.lww.com.

References

Aminoff, M. J. (2009). Neurology. In S. J. McPhee & M. A. Papdakis (Eds). *Current Medical Diagnosis and Treatment*. Columbus, OH: McGraw-Hill.

Arndt, C. A., Rose, P. S., Folpe, A. L., et al. (2012). Common musculoskeletal tumors of childhood and adolescence. *Mayo Clinical Proceedings*, *87*(5), 475–487.

Brown, P. & Hunger, S. P. (2014). Acute leukemia in children. In E. T. Bope & R. D. Kellerman (Eds). *Conn's Current Therapy 2015*. Philadelphia: Elsevier/Saunders.

Cancer Council Australia. (2015). About skin cancer, accessed 17 June 2015, <www.cancer.org.au/cancersmartlifestyle/SunSmart/Aboutskincancer.htm>.

Copeland, A. & Younes, A. (2012). Current treatment strategies in Hodgkin lymphomas. *Current Opinion in Oncology*, *24*(5), 466–474.

Davenport, K. P., Blanco, F. C. & Sandler, A. D. (2012). Pediatric malignancies: Neuroblastoma, Wilms' tumor, hepatoblastoma, rhabdomyosarcoma, and sacroccygeal teratoma. *Surgery Clinics of North America*, *92*(3), 745–767.

De Bolle, M., et al. (2008). Self- and parental perspectives on quality of life in children with cancer. *Journal of Psychosocial Oncology*, *26*(2), 35–47.

Graham, D. K., Maloney, K., Quinones, R. R., et al. (2014). Neoplastic disease. In W. W. Hay et al. (Eds). *Current Diagnosis & Treatment Pediatrics* (22nd ed.), New York: McGraw-Hill/Lange.

Kurt, B. A., et al. (2008). Primary care management of the childhood cancer survivor. *Journal of Pediatrics*, *152*(4), 458–466.

Lewis, D. & Foley, P. (2014). *Health Assessment in Nursing* (2nd ed.). Sydney: Lippincott Williams & Wilkins.

McCance, K. L. & Huether, S. E. (2013). *Pathophysiology* (7th ed.). New York: Elsevier Publishing.

McKenna, L. & Mirkov, S. (Eds.). (2014). *McKenna's Drug Handbook for Nursing and Midwifery* (7th ed.). Sydney: Lippincott Williams & Wilkins.

McLean, T. W. & Wofford, M. M. (2015). Oncology. In K. J. Marcdante, R. M. Kliegman, et al. (Eds). *Nelson Essentials of Pediatrics* (7th ed.), Philadelphia: Saunders/Elsevier.

Miller, A. B. & Green, L. M. (2010). Electric and magnetic fields at power frequencies. *Chronic Diseases in Canada*, *29*(Suppl. 1), 69–83.

Nagarkatti-Gude, N., Wang, Y., Ali, M. J., et al. (2012). Genetics of primary intraocular tumors. *Ocular Immunology & Inflammation*, *20*(4), 244–254.

Nicole, N. H. & Huether, S. E. (2012). Structure, function and disorders of the integument. In S. E. Huether & K. L. McCance (Eds), *Understanding Pathophysiology* (5th ed., pp. 1038–1065). Philadelphia: Elsevier Mosby.

Parry, P. V. & Engh, J. A. (2013). Antibody-based therapeutic targeting of human neuroblastoma. *Neurosurgery*, *72*(2), N16–N17.

Ricci, S. S., Kyle, T. & Carman, S. (2012). *Maternity and Pediatric Nursing* (2nd ed.). Philadelphia: Lippincott Williams & Wilkins.

Romão, R. L., Pippi Salle, J. L., Shuman, C., et al. (2012). Nephron sparing surgery for unilateral Wilms tumor in children with predisposing syndromes: Single center experience over 10 years. *Journal of Urology, 188*(4, Suppl.), 1493–1498.

Roth, E., Mirochna, M. & Harsha, D. (2012). Adolescent with knee pain. *American Family Physician, 86*(6), 569–570.

Sato, Y., Izumi, Y., Minegishi, K., et al. (2011). Prenatal findings in congenital leukemia: A case report. *Fetal Diagnosis & Therapy, 29*(4), 325–330.

Virshup, D. M. (2012). Biology, clinical manifestations & treatment of cancer. In S. E. Huether & K. L. McCance (Eds). *Understanding Pathophysiology* (5th ed., pp. 222–248). Philadelphia: Elsevier Mosby.

Suggested readings

Cancer Council Australia. (2015). Cancer facts and figures, accessed 15 June 2015. <www.cancer.org.au/about-cancer/what-is-cancer/facts-and-figures.html>.

Cancer Society of New Zealand. (2015). Cancer information, accessed 15 June 2015. <www.cancernz.org.nz/information/>.

Gibbins, J., Steinhardt, K. & Beinart, H. (2012). A systematic review of qualitative studies exploring the experience of parents whose child is diagnosed and treated for cancer. *Journal of Pediatric Oncology Nursing, 29*(5), 253–271.

Jones, B. L. (2012). The challenge of quality care for family caregivers in pediatric cancer care. *Seminars in Oncology Nursing, 28*(4), 213–220.

Jones, S. (2012). Brain tumours and cancer: Insights as a parent and a nurse. *Nursing of Children & Young People, 24*(7), 14–17.

Rowland, E. & Metcalfe, A. (2013). Communicating inherited genetic risk between parent and child: A meta-thematic synthesis. *International Journal of Nursing Studies, 50*(6), 870–880.

Unit 8

The nursing role in restoring and maintaining the mental health of young people and families

Chapter 54

Nursing care of a family when a young person has an intellectual or a mental health disorder

Previous chapters described the growth and development of well children and the care of children with physiological disorders. This chapter adds information about the dramatic changes that occur when children demonstrate a cognitive or mental health disorder. Such information builds a base for care and health teaching.

LEARNING OBJECTIVES

After mastering the contents of this chapter, you should be able to:

1. Describe common intellectual and mental health disorders that occur in young people.
2. Assess and analyse ways that care of a young person with an intellectual or mental health disorder can be more family-centred.
3. Formulate nursing principles related to the intellectual or mental health disorders.
4. Establish expected outcomes and develop a care plan.
5. Implement and evaluate outcomes of nursing care for a young person with an intellectual or mental disorder.
6. Integrate knowledge of childhood intellectual and mental disorders to achieve quality family nursing care.

KEY TERMS

- binge eating
- complex vocal tics
- coprolalia
- dyslexia
- echolalia
- hyperactivity
- labile mood
- motor tics
- palilalia
- purging
- vocal tics

CASE STUDY

You are working as a school nurse and you meet Henry, in Year 2, who was diagnosed with attention-deficit/hyperactivity disorder (ADHD) 6 months ago. You observe Henry colouring, running to the door and opening and closing the door and then throwing pamphlets around. His mother tells you she is "at her wits' end" because Henry's attention span is short and his behaviour is disruptive. His father tells you he's proud that his son is "all boy".

CASE STUDY QUESTIONS

1. How can you help Henry's family?
2. What additional education do they need?

Children and young people who have good mental health successfully master the tasks of each developmental phase of childhood, they develop the ability to trust adults and grow up to possess a positive self-concept. Promoting healthy family functioning, providing guidance for parents about developmental milestones and needs, and listening carefully to both the young person and their parents are important in fostering the physical and mental health of young people.

Mental health implies that a child is able to use adaptive coping mechanisms appropriately to meet the normal stressors of life. This is one of the reasons why providing age-appropriate stimulation is an essential nursing responsibility. Some stressors in life, however, go beyond what is considered "the norm". Acute illness, hospitalisation and a natural disaster such as a flood are examples of increased stress. Chronic illness often provides greater emotional stress. Nurses must recognise the effects of illness and hospitalisation on a young person and their families and provide interventions to prevent maladaptive coping mechanisms (Eisendrath & Lichtmacher, 2009).

Children and young people can develop the same mental disorders that affect adults such as anxiety or depression. Several disorders such as Autistism Spectrum Disorder begin in childhood. Some problems, such as separation anxiety, may consist of behaviour that is considered normal at one stage of development (infancy) but pathological at another (adolescence). Current research attributes some of these disorders to genetic vulnerability, disruption in family life, trauma and attachment difficulties. Children and young people with mental illness must be assessed and treated by specialists in the mental health field as early as possible. The child health nurse is often the first to become aware of such problems and can be instrumental in helping the young person and their family understand and adjust to the disorder.

Mental health is one of the Australian Government's nine National Health Priority Areas. For more information on mental health statistics, associated indicators and risk factors across the Australian population, as well as relevant publications, see <www.aihw.gov.au/mental-health>.

CARE OF A YOUNG PERSON WITH AN INTELLECTUAL OR MENTAL DISORDER

Assessment

A child or young person's personality and intellectual development are influenced by several factors, including genetic makeup, cultural background, family environment and community resources. All of these need to be considered when assessing a young person's intellectual functioning and mental health. If a problem is suspected, obtain a detailed history of the presenting problem, the young person's school and social history, the developmental and family history, and the current family functioning.

Nursing considerations

Nursing considerations established for children and young people should address mental health and the response of the young person and their families to their condition and treatment. Examples of these considerations are:

- Anxiety/powerlessness related to a hospital experience
- Low self-esteem related to disfiguring scars after an accident
- Hopelessness related to prolonged caretaking responsibilities.

Additional nursing considerations are appropriate if an intellectual or mental health problem is present. For example:

- Risk of deliberate self-harm
- Impaired social interaction related to short attention span
- Interrupted family processes related to the inability of the young person to follow instructions
- Impaired communication skills.

Although the diagnosis of a mental disorder or referral to a child and youth mental health service does not carry the stigma it once did, many parents still believe a referral is a sign of inadequacy or failure as parents. Help parents to see that this type of referral is no different from one to a cardiologist or paediatrician. Remind parents that everyone recognises the pressures and stresses on young people today.

Parents find it reassuring that their contact with mental health services will be kept confidential.

Organisations that might be helpful for information include:

- Australian Advisory Board on Autism Spectrum Disorders <www.autismadvisoryboard.org.au>
- Australia and New Zealand Academy for Eating Disorders <www.anzaed.org.au>
- Autism New Zealand <www.autismnz.org.nz>
- Down Syndrome Association of Queensland <www.dsaq.org.au>
- Down Syndrome South Australia <www.downssa.asn.au/dsssa/index.php>
- Down Syndrome Victoria <www.downsyndromevictoria.org.au>
- Down Syndrome WA <http://dsawa.asn.au>
- Mental Health Australia <www.mhca.org.au>
- Mental Health Foundation of New Zealand <www.mentalhealth.org.nz/page/27-welcome>
- New Zealand Down Syndrome Association <www.nzdsa.org.nz/contacts.htm>
- Tourette Syndrome Association of Australia <www.tourette.org.au>.

What parents and young people require when an intellectual or mental disorder is identified is an empathetic person to listen to their story and provide support. The young person needs ongoing evaluation and assessment by healthcare professionals. It is important to determine whether any circumstances that might have led to a temporary problem have been corrected or superficially changed. If the circumstances remain the same, the child's problem may return or manifest later in another way.

Examples suggesting achievement of expected outcomes are:

- The young person's deliberate self-harm decreases in coming months
- Parents state they are better able to cope and manage their child's disruptive behaviour.

Health promotion

Nurses play a key role in assessing and promoting the mental and intellectual health of young people and their families. A working knowledge of growth and development

TABLE 54.1 Guidelines for the mental health interview of a child or young person

Observational data	Examples of possible findings
General appearance	Height, weight, grooming and hygiene, nutrition, physical health, distinguishing features (deformities, tics), maturity level
Motor behaviours	Fine and gross balance, bizarre motor activity
Speech and language	Receptive, expressive; content, tone and articulation
Affect	Range of emotion, predominant emotion (depressed, angry, anxious, happy, irritable, labile), emotional reactions to process and/or content of interview (appropriate, inappropriate)
Thought process	Estimated intellectual level via language and knowledge base (organisation and thought content), orientation (to person, place, time), perceptual distortions (hallucinations, illusions, tangentiality, obsessions, delusions), attention span, learning disabilities
Ability to relate to evaluator	Eye contact, attitude towards interviewer (negative, positive, shy, suspicious, withdrawn, friendly, self-centred)
Behaviours displayed during interview	Impulsivity, aggression, inhibition, distractibility, low frustration tolerance, ability to have fun, sense of humour, creativity
Interview data	
Interpersonal relationships	Attitudes towards and perceptions of family, siblings, peers, transitional objects (inanimate objects used to allay anxiety), pets; social skills with peers, best friend; relationships with family, siblings and peers; conflicts; behavioural problems; adjustment to changes in routine or new situations
Self-concept and image	Self-appraisal (does child like self?), comparison of self with others (siblings, peers), what does child like most about self? What would the child like to change about self? Sense of pride in accomplishments, sex role and gender identity
Conscience	Understands right and wrong, is able to express common judgements or values.

of a child provides the basis for assessment. Young people cope with stress differently. Acting as an educator, facilitator and advocate, nurses can assist children and families to identify their needs and implement measures to meet them. Various factors have been associated with an increased risk of mental disorders in young people:

- Trauma or neglect
- Attachment problems
- Experience of major losses
- Physical illnesses
- Exposure to high-risk activities, such as drug and alcohol abuse
- Poverty and homelessness
- Parental substance abuse
- Parental mental illness/disorder
- Isolation—rural and remote.

A thorough assessment of the young person and family can assist in identifying risk factors and strategies can be suggested to reduce their impact (see Table 54.1). If a young person develops an intellectual or mental disorder, nurses can act as advocates, obtaining referrals to support services and early intervention programs.

CLASSIFICATION OF MENTAL HEALTH DISORDERS

The *Diagnostic and Statistical Manual of Mental Disorders* (5th ed.), published by the American Psychiatric Association (APA), provides a standardised classification system that can be used by all members of the mental healthcare team (American Psychiatric Association, 2013).

NEURODEVELOPMENTAL DISORDERS

Neurodevelopmental disorders, although not related by aetiology, typically share a common feature in that there is a delay in one or more areas of development. These areas include attention, cognition, language, affect and social and moral behaviour. Because these behaviours are interrelated, a delay in one area may interfere with development in another. Developmental disorders include intellectual disability, autism spectrum disorder, attention deficit/hyperactivity disorder and specific developmental disorders such as learning, motor skills (developmental coordination) and language disorders.

Intellectual disability

Intellectual disability involves impairments of general intellectual abilities that impact adaptive functioning in three domains, or areas. These domains determine how well an individual copes with everyday tasks:

- The **conceptual** domain includes skills in language, reading, writing, maths, reasoning, knowledge and memory.
- The **social** domain refers to empathy, social judgement, interpersonal communication skills, the ability to make and retain friendships, and similar capacities.

BOX 54.1 * Common causes of intellectual disability

- Chromosomal abnormalities such as Down syndrome and fragile X syndrome
- Infection in utero, such as rubella or cytomegalic inclusion disease
- Anoxia at birth from such causes as umbilical cord compression
- Fetal alcohol syndrome
- Inherited metabolic disorders such as phenylketonuria
- Head trauma
- Lead poisoning
- Hypothyroidism
- Brain malformations such as anencephaly
- Very low birth weight
- Infections such as measles encephalitis.

- The **practical** domain centres on self-management in areas such as personal care, job responsibilities, money management, recreation, and organising school and work tasks.

While intellectual disability does not have a specific age requirement, an individual's symptoms must begin during the developmental period and are diagnosed based on the severity of deficits in adaptive functioning. The disorder is considered chronic and often co-occurs with other mental conditions such as depression, attention-deficit/hyperactivity disorder and autism spectrum disorder (American Psychiatric Association, 2013).

Approximately 2% of children have an intellectual disability. This is not the result of a single cause but of conditions such as genetic abnormalities, like fragile X syndrome, Down syndrome (trisomy 21) and metabolic disorders such as phenylketonuria (see Box 54.1).

Classification

Diagnosis is based on both clinical assessment and standardised testing of intelligence with the severity of impairment based on adaptive functioning rather than IQ test scores alone (American Psychiatric Association, 2013). Intellectual disability is considered to be approximately two standard deviations or more below the population, which equals an IQ score of about 70 or below (American Psychiatric Association, 2013).

Mild

About 85% of children who have an intellectual disability fall into this category. The child's IQ is between 50 and 70 (American Psychiatric Association, 2013). During early years, these children learn social and communication skills and are often not distinguishable from average children. They are able to learn academic skills up to about year six. As adults, they can usually achieve social and vocational skills adequate for minimum self-support. They may need guidance and assistance when faced with new situations or unusual stress.

Moderate

Children in this category have an IQ between 35 and 49. About 10% of children with an intellectual disability fall into this category (American Psychiatric Association, 2013). During preschool years, these children learn to talk and communicate, but have poor awareness of social conventions. They can learn some vocational skills during young adulthood and can learn to take care of themselves with moderate supervision. As adults, they may contribute to their own support by performing unskilled or semi-skilled work under close supervision.

Severe

Children in this group have an IQ between 20 and 34. About 4% of children with an intellectual disability fall into this category (American Psychiatric Association, 2013). During the preschool period, these children develop minimal speech. They usually have poor motor development. During school years, they may learn to talk and can be trained in basic hygiene and dressing skills. As adults, they need constant supervision for safety.

Profound

The IQ of children in this group is less than 20. Less than 1% of children with an intellectual disability fall into this group (American Psychiatric Association, 2013). During the preschool period these children show only minimal capacity for sensory motor functioning. They need a highly structured environment and a constant level of help and supervision. Some children respond to training in minimal self-care.

Assessment

Assessment of whether a child has an intellectual disability is carried out by history taking and IQ testing. Early assessment is vital. Assessment also allows parents to look at the things children can do, to maintain hope and optimism, so they can assist their child in achieving their highest level of functioning.

Intelligence is routinely measured with standardised tests. Adaptive behavioural functioning, which may vary in different environments, is judged according to several methods, including standardised instruments for assessing social maturity and adaptive skills. A picture of life functioning is drawn from these multiple sources.

Parents may react to the diagnosis of intellectual disability in the same way as parents who have been told that their child has a chronic or fatal illness—with a grief reaction. This may be manifested as disbelief, anger or sorrow. Work with the family to develop realistic plans. A child cannot achieve more than an individual disability will allow, but you can help parents better accept the child's limited capabilities.

Therapeutic management

To aid in planning, parents need a realistic prognosis for their child or young person. This is difficult to offer in early life, because infant intelligence tests are not accurate and more sophisticated tests are difficult to administer until the preschool years. Once parents have a realistic expectation based on the best judgement possible, they are ready, with guidance, to help their child achieve their full potential.

Parents have several important decisions to make concerning the care of their child.

Ongoing care

Institutional care is no longer an option in many countries, and parents are encouraged to provide and maintain a home and school environment that is as normal as possible. Parents carry a great responsibility to provide constant care, especially for a child with problems affecting their judgement. This responsibility increases as the child and parents grow older. The parents may spend so much time with the child that other children in the family feel left out or unloved. Services and online support are available to assist and support parents and siblings, such as the Women's and Children's Health Network: Child and Youth Health (<www.cyh.com>).

If parents are unable to care for a child at home, out of home care may be an option, although is generally only considered when unmanageable behaviours exist. There are organisations that offer respite care. As the child enters adulthood it may be possible for them to move to more independent living, depending on their level of functioning. Halfway houses or group homes can provide a home atmosphere and community experiences.

Before giving advice to any family about a child or young person, consider the individual circumstances of the family. Every family has its own coping mechanisms and individual parents may be at different stages of acceptance and coping, especially during the first year after the birth of a child with a disability.

Health maintenance needs

Children who have an intellectual disability need the same health maintenance supervision as other children. At healthcare visits, parents may need reinforcement and review of precautions against accidents. Remind them to treat children according to their intellectual age, not their chronological age.

Illness

It can be difficult to detect illness in children who have an intellectual disability because they are often unable to describe the problem. For example, children experiencing pain may respond to it by crying, as infants do. Parents must observe their child closely for symptoms such as tugging at an ear, refusing to swallow food or rapid breathing, because these symptoms will help localise the discomfort. Help parents become advocates for their child. They know their child better than anyone else.

When children and young people with an intellectual disability are seen in an emergency department or an outpatient clinic, they need simple explanations of what will happen. A child who has an intellectual disability may be unable to make an association between a thermometer and what you are going to do. Your explanation is the first introduction to the event. Ensure it is adequate. When children are admitted to hospital, nursing care must meet the needs of a child's intellectual age. The explanations and preparations for procedures must be geared to the child's intellectual age.

Education

Most children who have an intellectual disability do well in preschool programs, giving them a head start in learning to socialise with peers and develop motor coordination. The school chosen for the child will depend on the degree of intellectual impairment. Children should be included in mainstream classes as much as possible. These classes offer stimulation and help children reach their best potential. Children who have an intellectual disability need an individualised education plan (IEP) based on the child's individual learning style, current and projected capabilities.

Self-care activities

Children and young people who have an intellectual disability need to learn the maximum amount of self-care possible. Doing so provides a sense of control and accomplishment. Assess whether children need special aids to achieve such skills as brushing teeth, combing hair, taking a bath and eating. After children learn how to perform these skills, they may need continued reminders to carry them out because they are unaware of the reason for the skill.

Play

Children with an intellectual disability enjoy play like any other child. Guide parents to choose toys that are appropriate for their child's developmental, not chronological, age.

Social relationships

The ability to communicate may be delayed in children and young people who have an intellectual disability because the ability to develop language is often delayed. Speech therapy may be necessary to help articulate correct sounds.

Teaching early social behaviour, such as saying "thank you" and "excuse me", and taking turns, is important to help children relate to others. Providing good role models is effective in teaching social behaviour. Encourage parents to enrol children in preschool programs. For a school-aged child and young person, participating in organised groups such as Scouts, Girl Guides, dance and drama, is an important way to learn to interact with others and feel successful.

Preparation for adulthood

As children who have an intellectual disability reach adolescence, they benefit from orientation to sexual responsibility. Girls can understand a simple explanation of menstruation and necessary menstrual hygiene. Both boys and girls need explanations of how pregnancy occurs and the measures they need to take to prevent this. Help them understand socially acceptable sexual activities.

What if...

A 15-year-old girl who has a mild intellectual disability comes to your school office? During your conversation she asks you if she should have a baby. How would you respond?

✔ Checkpoint question 54.1

A 3-year-old child who is cognitively challenged is critically ill with pneumonia. The mother did not recognise how ill the child was and delayed bringing the child in for treatment. What reasons might explain a parent reacting in this way?

Autism spectrum disorder (ASD)

Autism spectrum disorder (ASD) occurs in 16–40 out of 10,000 children (Stafford, Talmi & Burstein, 2014). ASD is more common in boys than girls and may have a genetic cause (Volkmar, 2008). Up to 50% of children with the disorder may also have an intellectual disability. As many as 20% may have coexistent mental health diagnoses (Mouridsen et al., 2008).

Classification

A child or young person with ASD may present with one or more of the following, depending on the severity of the disorder:

A. Persistent deficits in social communication and social interaction across multiple contexts

1. Deficits in social-emotional reciprocity, ranging, for example, from abnormal social approach and failure of normal back-and-forth conversation, to reduced sharing of interests, emotions or affect, to failure to initiate or respond to social interactions.
2. Deficits in non-verbal communicative behaviours used for social interaction, ranging, for example, from poorly integrated verbal and non-verbal communication, to abnormalities in eye contact and body language or deficits in understanding and use of gestures, to a total lack of facial expressions and non-verbal communication.
3. Deficits in developing, maintaining and understanding relationships, ranging, for example, from difficulties adjusting behaviour to suit various social contexts, to difficulties in sharing imaginative play or in making friends, to absence of interest in peers.

B. Restricted, repetitive patterns of behaviour, interests or activities

1. Stereotyped or repetitive motor movements, use of objects or speech (e.g. simple motor stereotypes, lining up toys or flipping objects, echolalia, idiosyncratic phrases).
2. Insistence on sameness, inflexible adherence to routines or ritualised patterns of verbal/non-verbal behaviour (e.g. extreme distress at small changes, difficulties with transitions, rigid thinking patterns, greeting rituals, need to take same route or eat food every day).
3. Highly restricted, fixated interests that are abnormal in intensity or focus (e.g. strong attachment to or preoccupation with unusual objects, excessively circumscribed or perseverative interest).
4. Hyper- or hypo-reactivity to sensory input or unusual interests in sensory aspects of the environment (e.g. apparent indifference to pain/temperature, adverse response to specific sounds or textures, excessive smelling or touching of objects, visual fascination with lights or movement).

Intellectual disability and autism spectrum disorder frequently co-occur. Severity is based on social communication impairments and restricted, repetitive patterns of behaviour (American Psychiatric Association, 2013).

Assessment

A comprehensive biopsychosocial assessment is required and this should include patterns of attachment. Normal attachment behaviour tends not to develop due to impaired social skills (see Box 54.2). Although ASD is not diagnosed until the child is 2 to 3 years of age, parents report worries much earlier because their infant may fail to cuddle, make eye contact or exhibit facial responsiveness. Infants may not reach to be picked up and are unable to play cooperatively.

Impairment in communication is shown in verbal and non-verbal skills. Language may be totally absent. There is an inability to name objects (nominal aphasia) and an abnormal speech melody, such as question-like rises at the end of statements. Echolalia (repetition of words or phrases spoken by others) and concrete interpretation may also be present.

Bizarre responses to the environment may include intense reactions to minor changes (perhaps screaming if a toy box is moved across the room) and attachment to

BOX 54.2 ✻ Common symptoms in the child with autism spectrum disorder

- Failure to develop social relations
- Stereotyped behaviours such as hand gestures
- Extreme resistance to change in routine
- Abnormal responses to sensory stimuli
- Decreased sensitivity to pain
- Inappropriate or decreased emotional expressions
- Specific, limited intellectual problem solving abilities
- Stereotyped or repetitive use of language
- Impaired ability to initiate or sustain a conversation.

odd objects such as always carrying a string or a shoe. Repetitive hand movements, rocking and rhythmic body movements are often observed. Children are intensely preoccupied by objects that revolve, such as a fan or spinning top. Music often holds a special interest for them. Hitting, head banging and biting may also be present. Children with autism are said to have a **labile mood** (crying occurs suddenly and is followed by giggling or laughing). They may be over-responsive to sensory stimuli (e.g. light or sound), but then be unaware of major events (e.g. the sound of a fire alarm).

In contrast to these mannerisms, long-term memory and "savant" skills (exceptional skills such as virtuoso piano playing) may be excellent (Nicholas et al., 2008). Children with ASD can often recall dates and spoken words from conversations years earlier. Excellent memory previously led to the belief that most young people with ASD have normal intelligence. The level of intelligence varies across the population of those with ASD. Intelligence testing can be difficult because some young people with ASD do not respond well to test situations and they score poorly on the verbal parts of these tests. Tasks requiring manipulative or visual skills or immediate memory may be performed at above-normal levels.

Therapeutic management

ASD is a perplexing condition. Parents need education and support to understand their child's behaviour and foster acceptance. Behavioural interventions may be effective in controlling some of the bizarre mannerisms that accompany ASD. Various medications, such as SSRIs (selective serotonin reuptake inhibitors) have been tried, because of their potential to alleviate anxiety and reduce behavioural rigidity. However, no medications specific for ASD are, as yet, effective.

As children mature, they develop greater awareness of and attachment to parents and other familiar adults. Some children may be able to lead independent lives, although social ineptness and awkwardness may remain, especially if accompanied by cognitive challenges.

CASE STUDY QUESTION

3. Suppose Henry had symptoms of autism spectrum disorder. Which of these symptoms is common in autism?
   a. Lack of short-term memory
   b. Hallucinations (hearing voices)
   c. Constant whirling around in a circle
   d. Severe depression or feelings of sadness

Learning and communication disorders

Learning disorders occur in approximately 5% of children. Learning disorders may involve dyslexia (reading reversal), or problems with mathematics or writing. Children may develop low self-esteem and deficits in social skills (American Psychiatric Association, 2013). Children require individualised educational plans to help them reach their potential.

Communication disorders involve problems of speech (motor aspect) or language (formulation and comprehension of verbal communication). Examples include expressive disorders, phonological disorders and stuttering. These conditions can cause low self-esteem in a child if they do not have the support and encouragement of family, teachers and healthcare professionals. If a learning or communication disorder is suspected the child or young person requires a comprehensive speech and occupational therapy (OT) assessment and may require ongoing intervention.

The International Classification of Diseases (ICD 10) by the World Health Organization (WHO) describes learning disorders as Specific Developmental Disorders of Scholastic Skills. Children and young people who meet the criteria for specific developmental disorders of scholastic skills have specific and significant impairment in learning. There are four types: specific reading disorder, specific spelling disorder, specific disorder of arithmetical skills and mixed disorder of scholastic skills.

Specific reading disorder

The main feature of this disorder is the specific and significant impairment in the development of reading skills. Reading performance should be significantly below the level expected on the basis of age, general intelligence and school placement. There may also be deficits in reading comprehension. Reading disorder is almost always the result of deficits in processing sound units and sound symbol relationships. Children and young people with reading disorder have difficulty with phonological processing.

Specific spelling disorder

There is a specific and significant impairment in the development of spelling skills. Ability to spell orally and to write out words correctly are both affected. It may be associated with grammatical errors, punctuation errors, poor paragraph organisation and poor handwriting.

Specific disorder of arithmetical skills

The child or young person's mathematical performance should be significantly below what is expected on the basis of age, general intelligence and school placement. The mathematical difficulties may include: failure to understand the basic concepts of mathematical operations, lack of understanding of mathematical terms or signs, failure to recognise numerical symbols, poor spatial organisation of mathematical calculations, difficulty in properly aligning numbers and inability to learn mathematical tables satisfactorily.

Mixed disorder of scholastic skills

Reading, spelling and mathematical skills are significantly impaired in these children.

Attention-deficit/hyperactivity disorder

Attention-deficit and disruptive behaviour disorders may begin with behavioural problems that are no different from what most families experience. Parents may be unaware of the need for intervention initially and by the time they seek help, they may be extremely distressed about the seeming unmanageability of their child. These disorders need to be diagnosed early, before the child's behaviour leads to low self-esteem, compromised social skills and complications in family functioning.

ADHD is a persistent pattern of inattention and/or hyperactivity-impulsiveness revealed before the age of 12 years (American Psychiatric Association, 2013). It is estimated to occur in about 3–7% of school-aged children and a proportion of these will have the disorder through to adulthood. Males are affected more than females. The cause is unknown; however, it occurs more frequently in some families, indicating a possible genetic aetiological component. Both medication and behavioural intervention methods have been used with success.

The disorder is characterised by inattention, impulsiveness and hyperactivity (Sykora, 2008). Inattention makes children and young people unable to complete tasks effectively. They become distracted and do not seem to listen. Impulsiveness causes them to act before they think and have difficulty with tasks such as waiting their turn at games. With **hyperactivity**, children may shift excessively from one activity to another, exhibiting excessive muscular activity such as constant fidgeting and aimless running.

Classification

The nine inattentive symptoms are:

1. Fails to give close attention to details or makes careless mistakes in schoolwork, work or during other activities (e.g. overlooks or misses details, work is inaccurate)
2. Has difficulty sustaining attention in tasks or play activities (e.g. has difficulty remaining focused during lectures, conversations or lengthy reading)
3. Does not seem to listen when spoken to directly (e.g. mind seems elsewhere, even in the absence of any obvious distraction)
4. Does not follow through on instructions and fails to finish schoolwork, chores or duties in the workplace (e.g. starts tasks but quickly loses focus and is easily side-tracked)
5. Has difficulty organising tasks and activities (e.g. difficulty managing sequential tasks; difficulty keeping materials and belongings in order; messy, disorganised work; has poor time management; fails to meet deadlines)
6. Avoids or is reluctant to engage in tasks that require sustained mental effort (e.g. schoolwork or homework; for older adolescents and adults, preparing reports, completing forms, reviewing lengthy papers)
7. Loses things necessary for tasks or activities (e.g. school materials, pencils, books, tools, wallets, keys, paperwork, eyeglasses and mobile telephones)
8. Easily distracted by extraneous stimuli (e.g. for older adolescents and adults may include unrelated thoughts)
9. Forgetful in daily activities (e.g. doing chores, running errands) (American Psychiatric Association, 2013).

The nine hyperactive-impulsive symptoms are:

1. Fidgets with or taps hands or squirms in seat
2. Leaves seat in situations when remaining seated is expected (e.g. leaves his place in the classroom, in the office or workplace, or in other situations that require remaining in place)
3. Runs about or climbs in situations where it is inappropriate (In adolescents or adults, this may be limited to feeling restless)
4. Unable to play or engage in leisure activities quietly
5. "On the go" acting as if "driven by a motor" (e.g. is unable to be or uncomfortable being still for extended time, as in restaurants, meetings; may be experienced by others as being restless or difficult to keep up with)
6. Talks excessively
7. Blurts out answers before questions have been completed (e.g. completes people's sentences; cannot wait for turn in conversation)
8. Has difficulty waiting turn (e.g. while waiting in line)
9. Interrupts or intrudes on others (e.g. butts into conversations, games or activities; may start using other people's things without asking or receiving permission; for adolescents and adults, may intrude into or take over what others are doing) (American Psychiatric Association, 2013).

Assessment

ADHD may be diagnosed by 36 months of age, although parents may excuse the behaviours as "active" or "always on the go" until school-age, when it is apparent that the child cannot sit still or concentrate on problem solving for long periods. When the disorder is first suspected, a thorough initial history to reveal the extent of the problem needs to be obtained.

Review the developmental history and a typical day for the child. Hyperactivity is a term commonly carelessly used by parents to describe any active child. Have the parent give an exact description of what the child is unable to do, such as sitting still long enough to finish a full meal, to document that hyperactivity actually exists.

Assess for activity that is not only excessive but also disorganised. For example, in a school room, children with ADHD may run from the back of the room to the front of the room to the window. They perform repetitive activities such as pencil tapping and finger tapping. At home, they may leave a project they are working on or a television program they are watching intently and run to the window, unaware of why they are running. This is driven or compulsive behaviour. Variability is another important symptom. Everyone has days when they perform at their peak and days when their performance is less than optimal. Children with ADHD may have behaviour so variable that they have good and bad moments. This type of variability causes them to lose track of systems and methods, not just answers, so school performance may falter.

A high level of impulsiveness can cause children to make statements without thinking, to touch objects they have just been told not to touch, or to speak or act before they have time to think about what they want to say or do. Children with ADHD seem to have an "all-or-nothing" reaction to stimuli. They may block out all incoming stimuli so do not hear their parents or a teacher calling them. At other times, they may be unable to suppress any incoming stimuli. This may be reported by parents or teachers as an exceedingly short attention span.

Children with ADHD may also have difficulty with concepts such as right and left, before and after, in front of and behind, and yesterday and tomorrow, because these concepts call for sequencing, the process of relating things to one another in time or space. They can have difficulty with common tasks such as washing their hands because they never know which way to turn a tap.

Children with ADHD may have difficulty learning to read. To read words of more than one syllable, they must sound the first syllable, and then retain that sound in their mind while they sound the second syllable. If they have difficulty retaining the first syllable long enough to connect it with the second, they cannot construct the word. Similarly, they can have difficulty with mathematics and spelling.

Children with ADHD do not have a deficit in intelligence, although they may seem to because of their impulsive behaviour. On physical assessment, these children often show many "soft" neurological signs, such as an inability to use a pencil. A thorough neurological examination is often difficult because their attention span is so short. Testing children through the use of games may be necessary so that their attention is maintained long enough to complete the assessment. IQ testing is used to document intelligence. The Wechsler Intelligence Scale for Children (WISC) is often chosen, consisting of a verbal scale and a performance scale.

Children with ADHD are often referred to a health professional because they are not achieving at school. Parents may need time to accept that their child has a condition that interferes with learning.

Therapeutic management

A variety of treatment methods are used for children with ADHD.

Environment

A stable learning environment is crucial for children and young people with ADHD. This may include special instruction, free from the distractions of an entire class. Parents may need help seeing that their child's condition is interfering with intellectual functioning and that a special program must be constructed for their child to succeed.

At home, parents need to construct an environment that is as free from stimulating distractions as possible. Parents who are experiencing difficulty at home with discipline and management often appreciate support and advice. Encourage them to be fair but firm and to set consistent limits.

Young people who are easily distracted have difficulty completing chores such as picking up their toys. Teach parents to give instructions slowly and to make certain that they have their child's attention before beginning the instructions. Breaking down a chore into several steps may help.

Children and young people with ADHD often have difficulty telling a story or repeating a joke told to them. Suggest that parents help them by asking questions such as "Why?" " Where?" or "Who?" to reach the point of the story.

Medication

Several medications are helpful in reducing the excessive activity of children with ADHD and in lengthening their attention span or decreasing their distractibility so that they can function in normal classrooms. These medications have advantages and disadvantages.

Methylphenidate hydrochloride (Ritalin, Concerta [extended-release form]) is frequently prescribed for this disorder. Other medications that may be useful are atomoxetine, noradrenaline reuptake inhibitors and tricyclics antidepressants (Goldson & Reynolds, 2014).

Family support

A responsive, listening ear is crucial to the ability of parents to handle the challenge of raising a child with these symptoms. Any parents can grow short-tempered and irritable at times with a child who does not seem to hear them or follow what they say. Although hyperactivity fades, some children with ADHD continue to experience problems with impulsivity and inattention into adulthood.

TIC DISORDERS

Tic disorders are abnormalities of semi-involuntary movement that are thought to result from dysfunction in the basal ganglia. Tics are rapid, repetitive muscle movements, such as rapid eye blinking or facial twitching. They usually become more pronounced during periods of stress and diminish during sleep. **Motor tics** include eye blinking, neck jerking and facial grimacing. Simple **vocal tics** include coughing, throat clearing, snorting and barking. Complex motor tics include facial gestures, grooming behaviours, jumping, touching and smelling objects.

Children are most prone to these disorders between the ages of 9 and 13 years. They occur more frequently in boys, and more frequently in children who demonstrate obsessive-compulsive behaviour. Some instances tend to be familial, possibly because of dopamine receptor inhibition. Tic disorders are sub classified into Tourette's syndrome, chronic motor or vocal tic disorder and transient tic disorder. They occur so frequently that as many as 15% of children experience some form of transient tic disorder.

Because transient tics are associated with high stress, treatment usually focuses on reducing areas of stress.

Tourette's syndrome

Tourette's syndrome is an inherited syndrome of motor and phonic vocal tics (Xia & Rao, 2011). It occurs three times more frequently in boys than in girls and often there is some other form of tic in other family members. **Complex vocal tics** include the repeated use of words or phrases out of context—specifically, **coprolalia** (use of socially unacceptable words, usually obscenities), **palilalia** (repeating one's own words) and **echolalia** (repeating others' words). The age of onset is around 7 years, with motor tics usually occurring before vocal tics. Although most children can suppress their tics for short periods, the syndrome lasts a lifetime.

Tourette's syndrome responds to the administration of neuroleptic agents.

DISRUPTIVE, IMPULSE-CONTROL AND CONDUCT DISORDERS

Intermittent explosive disorder (IED)

Intermittent explosive disorder is a rapid onset of recurrent, impulsive, verbally or physically aggressive outbursts typically lasting less than 30 minutes, usually in response to minimal provocation by an intimate or associate, causing marked impairment in functioning or legal consequences. The prevalence of this disorder is approximately 3% of the population. It has an earlier onset and higher incidence in males.

Therapeutic management

Cognitive behaviour therapy (CBT), education for the young person and their family, and some medications, such as SSRIs, are used to treat the disorder.

Oppositional defiant disorder (ODD)

Oppositional defiant disorder (ODD) is a childhood behavioural problem characterised by constant disobedience and hostility. Around one in 10 children under the age of 12 years are thought to have ODD, with males outnumbering females by two to one. Early intervention and treatment are important, since children with untreated ODD may continue to be difficult and antisocial into their adult years. This can impact on their relationships, career prospects and quality of life. Some children with ODD will develop the more serious conduct disorder (CD), which is characterised by aggressive law-breaking and violent behaviours.

ODD behaviours usually surface when the child is at primary school, but the disorder can be found in children as young as three years of age. A child with ODD may:

- Become easily angered, annoyed or irritated
- Have frequent temper tantrums
- Argue frequently with adults, particularly the most familiar adults in their lives such as parents
- Refuse to obey rules
- Seem to deliberately try to annoy or aggravate others
- Have low self-esteem
- Have a low frustration threshold
- Seek to blame others for any accidents or bad behaviour.

The cause of disruptive behaviour disorders is unknown, but the quality of the child's family life seems to be an important factor in the development of ODD. Some studies have found that certain environmental factors in the family increase the risk of disruptive behaviour disorders. These include:

- Poor parenting skills (inadequate supervision, harsh or inconsistent discipline, rejection)
- Marital conflict
- Domestic violence
- Physical abuse
- Sexual abuse
- Neglect
- Poverty
- Substance misuse by parents or carers.

Therapeutic management

Treatment options for ODD may include the following:

- Parental training—to help the parents better manage and interact with their child, including behavioural techniques that reinforce good behaviour and discourage bad behaviour. Social support is increased if the parents are trained in groups with other parents who have children with ODD
- Functional family therapy—to teach all family members to communicate and problem-solve more effectively
- Consistency of care—all carers of the child (including parents, grandparents, teachers, childcare workers and so on) need to be consistent in the way they manage the child.

Conduct disorder (CD)

Conduct disorder (CD), is characterised by a repetitive and persistent pattern of behaviour, in which the basic rights of others or major age-appropriate societal norms or rules are violated (American Psychiatric Association, 2013). The disorder occurs in about 5% of children (Scott, 2007). It is seen more frequently in males than in females, however, the prevalence of conduct disorders in girls is increasing. Several factors have been described for this disorder including genetic predisposition, neurological deficit correlates, and sociological factors related to poverty and cultural disadvantage. The home environment is frequently characterised by rejection, frustration, and harsh and inconsistent discipline. Parents may have marital conflicts or substance abuse problems or children may have had a series of inconsistent carers (American Psychiatric Association, 2013).

Around one-third of children with CD also have attention deficit hyperactivity disorder (ADHD). One in five children with CD are depressed. CD is typically diagnosed when the child is between 10 and 16 years of age.

Assessment

Diagnosis is made if the disturbance in behaviour causes clinically significant impairment in social, academic or occupational functioning (American Psychiatric Association, 2013). The child or young person may display several of the following:

Aggression to people and animals

- Bullies, threatens or intimidates others
- Initiates physical fights
- Has used a weapon that can cause serious physical harm to others (e.g. a bat, brick, broken bottle, knife, gun)
- Has been physically cruel to people
- Has been physically cruel to animals
- Has stolen while confronting a victim (e.g. mugging, purse snatching, extortion, armed robbery)
- Has forced someone into sexual activity.

Destruction of property

- Has deliberately engaged in fire setting with the intention of causing serious damage
- Has deliberately destroyed others' property (other than by fire setting).

Deceitfulness or theft

- Has broken into someone else's house, building or car
- Often lies to obtain goods or favours or to avoid obligations (i.e. "cons" others)
- Has stolen items of non-trivial value without confronting a victim (e.g. shoplifting, but without breaking and entering; forgery).

Serious violations of rules

- Often stays out at night despite parental prohibitions, beginning before the age of 13
- Has run away from home overnight at least twice while living in the parental or parental surrogate home, or once without returning for a lengthy period
- Is often truant from school, beginning before the age of 13.

Therapeutic management

Treatment depends on the individual but may include:

- Behaviour therapy
- Cognitive behavioural therapy (CBT)
- Anger management
- Stress management
- Social skills training
- Special education program
- Parent management training
- Family therapy
- Multisystemic therapy
- Integrated approach by family, teachers and other carers
- Management of any co-existing problems
- Medication (in case of co-existing depression or ADHD).

Therapy for children with conduct disorders focuses on modifying the home environment and training the child in social and problem-solving skills. Social skills training teaches children to recognise how their behaviour affects others. Problem-solving skills training teaches children to generate alternative solutions to situations, sharpen their thinking about the consequences of choices and evaluate their responses. Parental education is also important. Medications such as carbamazepine (Tegretol), propranolol (Inderal) and lithium carbonate may reduce the aggressive behaviour. Long-term therapy, with an agent such as buspirone (BuSpar), may be effective in helping children control temper or explosive outbursts.

CASE STUDY QUESTION

4. Children like Henry, with ADHD, have difficulty with concepts such as before and after. This difficulty reflects which underlying problem?

   a. Not being able to sequence
   b. Not hearing equally in both ears
   c. Feeling chronically depressed
   d. Being too hyperactive to care

ANXIETY DISORDERS

Anxious feelings, worries or fears are common among children and young people. Many children experience a normal amount of apprehension in certain situations, whether it is about an upcoming test at school or a thunderstorm. Anxiety disorders are caused by a combination of life events, genetic and biochemical factors.

Some children, however, experience these types of situations with an overwhelming sense of fear and dread. No amount of reassurance seems to help. These children may tend to get "stuck" on their worried thoughts and have a hard time doing normal daily functions like going to school, playing, sleeping or trying new things. Getting "stuck", when it begins to interfere with daily functioning, is the key. This is what separates normal, fluctuating worries of childhood from an anxiety disorder that requires professional intervention.

All anxiety-related problems share four common features (American Psychiatric Association, 2013):

- The anxiety is often an inexplicable fear or preoccupation that interferes with the child's or adolescent's ability to enjoy life or to complete daily routines or to do the things they are expected to do
- The anxiety is often as puzzling to the child as it is to their parents

- The anxiety does not respond to, or diminish, after logical explanations
- The anxiety problem can be helped.

Types of anxiety disorder

There are several different types of anxiety disorder, including generalised anxiety, social anxiety, separation anxiety, obsessive-compulsive symptoms, phobias and panic. All of these disorders cause significant distress and a reduced level of functioning and competency for children and young people (American Psychiatric Association, 2013). Common symptoms of anxiety include:

- Feeling nervous or "on edge"
- Unfounded or unrealistic fears
- Trouble separating from parents
- Sleep disturbance
- Obsessive thoughts and/or compulsive behaviours
- Trembling, sweating, shortness of breath, stomach-aches, headaches and/or muscle tension or other physical symptoms.

Generalised anxiety disorder

Generalised anxiety disorder is an excessive worry and/or apprehension about a number of events or activities. These feelings occur almost all the time and are not triggered by any one specific issue. Rather, the worry seems to float in a more generalised way, from one topic to the next. Some examples include: fear of failure or poor performance, worries about the child's and/or family's safety, worries about thunderstorms or wars, worries about what others will think of them and apprehension about new situations.

Phobias

Phobias are highly specific and exclusive fears. The child or young person functions normally until confronted by the dreaded object, event or situation. Some examples include fears of bugs, heights or flying in an aeroplane.

Separation anxiety disorder

Separation anxiety disorder is the child or young person's excessive worry and apprehension about being away from their parents. Children with separation anxiety disorder often fear that their parents will be harmed in some way or will not return to them as promised. Separation anxiety disorder is often seen in preschoolers, but it is also seen in older children and adolescents in response to stressful life events.

Obsessive-compulsive disorder

Obsessive-compulsive disorder is a condition involving obsessions and compulsions. Obsessions are recurrent thoughts, impulses, or images that are difficult to control and cause significant distress. Compulsions are behaviours that the child engages in (such as hand washing, checking, redoing, etc.) to make the distress feel better. Some examples of obsessive-compulsive disorder may include excessive concerns about germs or lucky/unlucky numbers.

Panic disorder

Panic disorder is characterised by discrete and intense periods of anxiety that occur unexpectedly, without warning, and are not always linked to a specific place or situation. With panic disorder, there is often no warning, and therefore it is harder to predict when it may occur. Children and young people with panic symptoms may experience high anxiety, have difficulty breathing, feel as if everything around them is closing in and may experience feelings of impending doom.

Post-traumatic stress disorder

Post-traumatic stress disorder is an intense re-experiencing of a traumatic event by distressing recollections, dreams, and/or associations (such as things or situations that remind the child or adolescent of the traumatic event). Some examples include witnessing or experiencing a natural disaster, being in a serious car accident or witnessing a crime.

Assessment

The first step to successful treatment begins with a comprehensive evaluation of your child. This evaluation would include:

- A review of current symptoms and concerns, their duration and level of intensity
- A thorough review of the child or young person's developmental history
- Past medical and psychiatric history
- Important family background as well as family psychiatric history
- A mental status examination.

Parents and guardians are included in the evaluation process to obtain background information and history as well as to participate in treatment planning.

Therapeutic management

The treatment plan for an anxiety disorder may include a combination of the following:

- Cognitive behavioural therapy
- Medication
- Family therapy
- Parent education and support.

Group programs for parents and children (e.g. Cool Kids program <www.centreforemotionalhealth.com.au/pages/cool-kids-program.aspx>) and online interventions for teens (e.g. Chilled Plus Online Program <www.centreforemotionalhealth.com.au/pages/chilledplus.aspx>) have proven efficacy in the treatment of anxiety.

FEEDING AND EATING DISORDERS

Feeding and eating disorders include the following diagnoses: pica, rumination disorder, avoidant/restrictive food intake disorder (ARFID), anorexia nervosa, bulimia nervosa and binge eating disorder (BED) (American Psychiatric Association, 2013).

Pica

Children who persistently eat non-food substances such as dirt, clay, paint chips, crayons, wool or paper are said to have pica (Starn & Udall, 2008). The primary danger lies in the possibility of accidental poisoning. Other complications include constipation, gastrointestinal malabsorption, faecal impaction and intestinal obstruction. The disorder is seen predominantly between the ages of 2 and 6 years, although it may be present into adolescence. The incidence of pica increases in children who are intellectually impaired. An individualised treatment plan needs to be devised to meet the child's needs until the phenomenon fades. Keeping the child safe from ingesting inedible substances is a major responsibility until then.

Rumination disorder of infancy

Rumination disorder is the act of regurgitating and then re-swallowing previously ingested food. It is a rare disorder affecting infants between 3 and 12 months. It is seen most often in children who are intellectually impaired (Lyons et al., 2007). Both organic and environmental theories have been explored to explain the disorder. Attachment between the child and the parents may be at risk because of the anxiety the parents experience from their infant's constant regurgitation of food and lack of growth. Parents may need support, reassurance and education to help them maintain or re-establish this bond.

Avoidant/restrictive food intake disorder

Avoidant/restrictive food intake disorder (ARFID) is an eating or feeding disturbance (e.g. apparent lack of interest in eating or food; avoidance based on the sensory characteristics of food; concern about aversive consequences of eating) as manifested by persistent failure to meet appropriate nutritional and/or energy needs associated with one (or more) of the following:

- Significant weight loss (or failure to achieve expected weight gain or faltering growth in children)
- Significant nutritional deficiency
- Dependence on enteral feeding or oral nutritional supplements
- Marked interference with psychosocial functioning.

Individuals who meet the criteria for ARFID have developed some type of problem with eating (or for very young children, a problem with feeding). As a result of the eating problem, the person isn't able to take in adequate calories or nutrition through their diet. There are many types of eating problems that might warrant an ARFID diagnosis—difficulty digesting certain foods, avoiding certain colours or textures of food, eating only very small portions, having no appetite, or being afraid to eat after a frightening episode of choking or vomiting.

Anorexia nervosa

Anorexia nervosa is characterised by a refusal to maintain normal body weight because of a disturbance in perception of the size or appearance of the body (Zandian et al., 2007). It includes self-induced starvation; a relentless drive for thinness, a fear of fatness, or both; and medical signs and symptoms resulting from starvation.

Classification

To be diagnosed as having anorexia nervosa a young person must display:

- Persistent restriction of energy intake leading to significantly low body weight (in context of what is minimally expected for age, sex, developmental trajectory and physical health)
- Either an intense fear of gaining weight or of becoming fat, or persistent behaviour that interferes with weight gain (even though significantly low weight)
- Disturbance in the way one's body weight or shape is experienced, undue influence of body shape and weight on self-evaluation, or persistent lack of recognition of the seriousness of the current low body weight.

Specific characteristics of a child or young person with anorexia nervosa include:

- Body mass index (BMI) less than 17.5 or less than 85% of expected weight
- Fear of gaining weight or becoming fat even though underweight
- Severely distorted body image
- Refusal to acknowledge seriousness of weight loss
- Amenorrhoea (in girls).

Anorexia nervosa occurs most often in girls during adolescence between 13 and 20 years of age. The disorder may be manifested as severe weight restriction controlled by limiting food intake, by excessive exercise, or by binge eating or purging—episodes of uncontrollable intake of large amounts of food over a specified period of time **(binge eating)** followed by self-induced vomiting or the use of laxatives, enemas or diuretics **(purging)** (Latner & Clyne, 2008).

Children who develop eating disorders have a genetic susceptibility. Stressors in the environment such as parental divorce, social pressure to lose weight and personal psychological trauma can set into motion a chain reaction that leads to the development of eating disorders. Children may have a poor self-image and excessive dieting gives them a sense of control over their own body.

Lack of nutrition becomes so extreme that it causes delayed psychosexual development. With a lean, almost starved appearance, girls do not appear as sexually developed or as old as their chronological age. They may have significant symptoms of dehydration and acidosis because of starvation. They may develop severe osteoporosis from loss of calcium (Jayasinghe, Grover & Zacharin, 2008).

Assessment

By the time most young people are seen at healthcare facilities, they are already extremely underweight, pale and lethargic. Amenorrhea is commonly present. Often the parents have tried various methods of getting the child to eat and, as a result, parent–child relationships may be strained.

Therapeutic management

Planning and outcome identification for a child or young person with anorexia nervosa need to be realistic. Although the condition began as a psychosocial problem, by the time a child is seen for care, physical starvation and its effects may have become evident. Therapeutic interventions include:

- Medications such as antidepressants
- Review by a paediatrician
- Family therapy (Maudsley Model–utilised extensively in Australia and New Zealand, see <www.thenewmaudsleyapproach.co.uk>
- Review by a dietician.

Gradual weight gain is recommended, with weight being measured weekly by a dietician. Children who have had anorexia nervosa usually require long-term therapy (see Fig. 54.1).

Bulimia nervosa

To be diagnosed as having bulimia nervosa a young person must display recurrent episodes of binge eating. An episode of binge eating is characterised by both of the following:

- Eating, in a discrete period of time (e.g. within any 2-hour period) an amount of food that is definitely larger than most people would eat during a similar period of time and under similar circumstances.
- A sense of lack of control over eating during the episode (e.g. a feeling that one cannot stop eating or control what or how much one is eating).

Recurrent inappropriate compensatory behaviour in order to prevent weight gain, such as self-induced vomiting; misuse of laxatives, diuretics or other medications; fasting; or excessive exercise must also be present. For a diagnosis of bulimia nervosa the binge eating and inappropriate compensatory behaviours must both occur, on average, at least once a week for three months with the young person's self-evaluation being unduly influenced by body shape and weight (American Psychiatric Association, 2013).

A period of depression or guilt usually follows the period of bingeing. Bulimia is typically seen in adolescent girls. The disorder may last for months or years. Periods of normal eating may be interspersed with bingeing. Food consumed during a binge often has high kilojoule content. It may be eaten secretly, such as late at night or in the privacy of a bedroom. After ingestion of this food, abdominal pain develops and the teenager will vomit to decrease the physical pain of abdominal distension and to improve self-image.

Young people with bulimia may abuse purgatives, laxatives and diuretics to aid in weight control (Sigel, 2014). The combination of frequent vomiting and the use of these medications can result in serious physical complications, notably electrolyte abnormalities, which can lead to cardiac arrest. Adolescents with bulimia may develop severe erosion of their teeth because of the constant exposure to acidic gastrointestinal juices from vomiting. Oesophageal tears may also result (Baron, 2009).

The sufferers exhibit great concern about their weight and overall body image. Most of those with bulimia are only slightly underweight or are of average weight and therefore may be discounted as merely slim unless a thorough history is obtained.

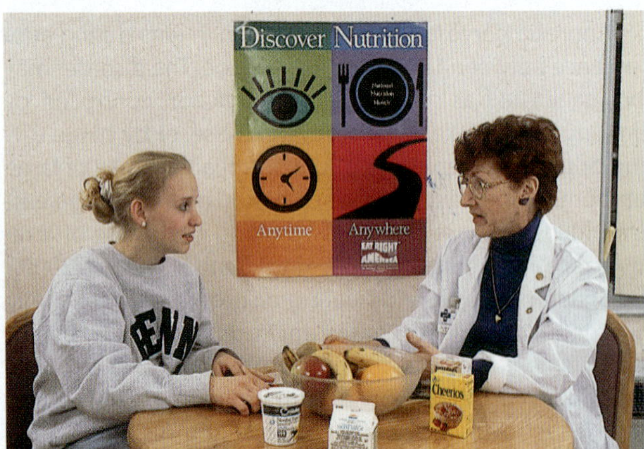

FIGURE 54.1 A young person recovering from anorexia, who is in the later stages of treatment, continues to meet with a counsellor to discuss her food choices, exercise program and overall well-being. (© Barbara Proud.)

Binge eating disorder

To be diagnosed as having binge eating disorder a young person must display recurrent episodes of binge eating. An episode of binge eating is characterised by eating, in a discrete period of time (e.g. within any 2-hour period), an amount of food that is definitely larger than most people would eat during a similar period of time and under similar circumstances. There must also be a sense of lack of control over eating during the episode (e.g. a feeling that one cannot stop eating or control what or how much one is eating). The binge eating episodes must be associated with three or more of the following:

- eating much more rapidly than normal
- eating until feeling uncomfortably full
- eating large amounts of food when not feeling physically hungry
- eating alone because of feeling embarrassed by how much one is eating
- feeling disgusted with oneself, depressed or very guilty afterwards.

The person must show marked distress regarding the binge eating and the binge eating should occur, on average, at least once a week for three months.

Binge eating disorder is less common but much more severe than overeating. Binge eating disorder is associated with more subjective distress regarding the eating behaviour and commonly other co-occurring psychological problems (American Psychiatric Association, 2013).

✔ Checkpoint question 54.2

Which child is most likely to have anorexia nervosa?

a. Nathan, a 7-year-old boy whose parents are divorced
b. Susie, a 15-year-old girl who has poor self-image
c. Josh, a 14-year-old boy who plays various sports
d. Georgia, a 13-year-old girl who is overweight

ELIMINATION DISORDERS

Elimination disorders include functional enuresis (involuntary loss of urine) and encopresis (involuntary loss of faeces).

Encopresis

Loss of faeces is *encopresis* if there is repeated passage of faeces, at least once a month, in places where it is not culturally appropriate. It is considered primary, if the child was never fully toilet-trained and secondary, if the problem began after effective toilet training (Culbert & Banez, 2007). Encopresis is considered to exist only after medical causes have been ruled out. It is more common in boys.

Isolated occurrences of encopresis may happen when a sibling is born or when a child is visiting a strange house or new school. Encopresis is a distressing condition for children. In a few instances, encopresis occurs because of extreme constipation. Because it hurts to move the bowels, children avoid bowel movements, leading to chronically distended rectums. They are then no longer able to sense when they need to defecate, so involuntary or overflow defecation occurs (Philichi, 2008).

Assessment

To document encopresis, take a thorough history, including usual bowel evacuation habits, the number of bowel accidents and the times at which they occur. Investigate any recent changes or stress factors in the child's environment.

Therapeutic management

Therapy is based on the cause. If children evacuate their bowels before they leave for school in the morning, they are less likely to experience encopresis and embarrassment at school. Arranging to have children attempt to evacuate their bowels about two times daily may create "habit" periods for them. Allowing children adequate time to sit on the toilet or encouraging them to take the time to defecate may be helpful.

Emphasise to parents that children should not be punished. Encourage them to pay as little attention as possible to bowel accidents and to give praise for days when encopresis does not occur.

Enuresis

Enuresis is defined as repeated involuntary or intentional urination during the day or at night after an age at which a child should have attained control over bladder function, when there is no organic cause (American Psychiatric Association, 2013). Most children outgrow the problem by adolescence. As with encopresis, the most serious result of enuresis is related to the child's feelings of failure with each occurrence and associated rejection by peers, parents or other carers. All this contributes to a lowered sense of self-esteem.

PSYCHIATRIC DISORDERS AFFECTING CHILDREN AND YOUNG PEOPLE

Depression

Young people can have depressive episodes similar to those experienced by adults (Kaplan & Love-Osborne, 2014). Depression is becoming an increasing concern in our society due to the escalating suicide rate among young people (see Fig. 54.2). A young person is considered to be depressed when symptoms such as significant weight loss or decrease in appetite (more than 5 percent of body weight in a month), insomnia or hypersomnia, psychomotor agitation or retardation, fatigue or lack of energy, feelings of worthlessness or guilt, decreased concentration or indecisiveness, or recurrent thoughts of death or suicide exist for 2 weeks or longer (American Psychiatric Association, 2013). A history should be taken from the young person as well as from their parents. Symptoms cause significant distress or impairment in functioning. Depression Scales such as the Beck Depression Inventory, Children's Depression Inventory or the Reynolds Adolescent Depression Inventory can be used to establish severity, baseline functioning and to monitor the progress of treatment.

Young people who are depressed need to be referred to an appropriate health professional for assessment and cognitive behaviour therapy (CBT). Many require antidepressant therapy, such as a selective serotonin reuptake inhibitor, to relieve the symptoms. Family or individual

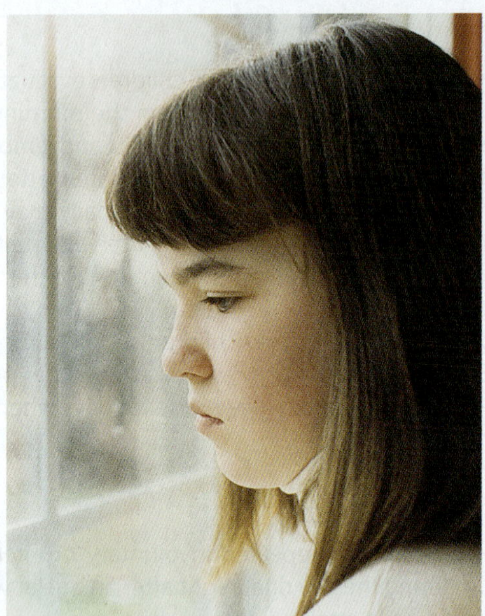

FIGURE 54.2 Symptoms of depression are easily missed in school-aged children unless history taking is thorough. (© Caroline Brown, RNC, MS, DEd.)

counselling may be necessary to help the young person regain self-esteem and the family to understand the level of depression. Few antidepressants are approved for children, and when a young person is prescribed these drugs, attempts at suicide have been noticed to rise dramatically—possibly because at the point at which the child feels less depressed, increased ability to act makes a suicide attempt possible (Simon, 2008).

Schizophrenia spectrum and other psychotic disorders

Psychosis is the term used to describe a state of mind in which the individual experiences a distortion or loss of contact with reality, without clouding of consciousness. This mental state is characterised by the presence of delusions, hallucinations and/or thought disorder. As well as these symptoms, referred to as positive symptoms, negative symptoms such as affective blunting and loss of motivation can also occur (American Psychiatric Association, 2013). In addition, there are a number of other secondary features that can present during a psychotic episode such as depression, anxiety, sleep disturbance, social withdrawal and impaired role functioning (see Box 54.3).

Psychosis can be caused by a complex interaction of biological, psychological, social and environmental factors. Organic factors such as drug intoxication, metabolic conditions and infection can play a significant role. Sole precipitants are less likely for functional disorders such as brief reactive psychosis, schizophrenia, bipolar disorder, schizophreniform, delusional disorder and schizoaffective disorder (Early Psychosis Prevention and Intervention Centre).

Psychotic disorders are of major social and public health importance. These conditions affect around 2% of the population. The incidence of psychosis in children under 12 is estimated to be around 1 in every 10,000. A number of theories have been suggested as to what causes psychosis. There is some indication that psychosis is caused by a poorly understood combination of biological factors that create a vulnerability to experiencing psychotic symptoms during adolescence or early adult life. These symptoms often emerge in response to stress, drug abuse or social changes (Early Psychosis Prevention and Intervention Centre).

The causes of first-episode psychosis can be particularly unclear. It is therefore necessary for the young person to have a thorough examination to rule out potential medical causes and to help make the diagnosis as clear as possible. This usually involves medical tests, as well as a detailed interview with a mental health specialist. The course and outcome vary from person to person. Recovery is likely, with most people experiencing a cessation of positive symptoms within 12 weeks from the acute onset,

BOX 54.3 ✻ Common symptoms of a young person with a psychotic disorder

Confused thinking	Everyday thoughts become confused or don't join up properly. Sentences are unclear or don't make sense. A person may have difficulty concentrating, following a conversation or remembering things. Thoughts seem to speed up or slow down.
False beliefs	It is common for a person experiencing a psychotic episode to hold false beliefs, known as *delusions*. They may be so convinced of their delusion that the most logical argument cannot make them change their mind. Common delusions may include: paranoia, where the young person may believe that they are being watched or followed, or others want to harm them; grandiosity, where a person believes they have special abilities or powers. *Hallucinations*-In a state of psychosis, the person sees, hears, feels, smells or tastes experiences that are not actually occurring, but the sensation that these experiences are real can be quite overwhelming.
Changed feelings	How someone feels may change for no apparent reason. They may feel strange and cut off from the world with everything moving in slow motion. Mood swings are common and they may feel unusually excited or depressed. People's emotions seem dampened, they feel less than they used to, or show less emotion to those around them.
Changed behaviour	People experiencing psychosis behave differently from the way they usually do. They may be extremely active or lethargic. They may laugh inappropriately or become angry or upset without apparent cause. Often changes in behaviour are associated with the symptoms already described above.

if adequately treated (Early Psychosis Prevention and Intervention Centre).

Early intervention is aimed at shortening the course and decreasing the severity of the initial psychotic episode, thereby minimising the many complications that can arise from untreated psychosis. Early intervention is providing information, assessment and treatment at the earliest possible stage of someone experiencing psychotic symptoms. This can happen at the "at-risk" stage, as well as once a psychotic episode has developed (Early Psychosis Prevention and Intervention Centre).

Young people most at risk of developing a psychosis may include those with a family history of psychosis, particularly in first degree relatives, and those with schizotypal, schizoid and paranoid personality disorders. The onset and course of psychosis is determined by an underlying vulnerability to psychosis coupled with the impact of environmental stressors which may then trigger active psychotic symptoms. An estimated 80% of people affected by psychosis experience their first episode between the ages of 15–30 years. Psychosis does not discriminate; it affects people of all nationalities, all social standings and all intelligence levels, as well as both young males and females (Early Psychosis Prevention and Intervention Centre).

Assessment

Everyone's experience of psychosis is different and attaching a specific name or label to the psychotic illness is not always useful for a young person in the early stages. However, when a young person is experiencing an episode of psychosis, a diagnosis of a particular type of psychotic illness is usually given. A diagnosis should not, however, be "set in stone". Treating clinicians should always be open to reviewing, and if necessary, changing the diagnosis as the episode of illness progresses (Early Psychosis Prevention and Intervention Centre).

The particular type of illness is identified by the symptoms experienced. Formulating a diagnosis will also depend on what brought on the illness and how long the symptoms last. Diagnoses include:

- Schizophrenia
- Schizophrenaform disorder
- Schizoaffective disorder
- Drug intoxication
- Delusional disorder
- Bipolar disorder
- Major depression with psychotic features
- Brief reactive psychosis
- Medical illnesses that resemble a psychiatric disorder.

Therapeutic management

Effective treatments are readily available for psychotic illnesses. The earlier treatment is started, the quicker and better the recovery. With appropriate treatment the majority of young people who experience a psychotic illness will recover. However, for some young people, psychosis can become an episodic problem through their lives.

Treatment for psychosis involves the use of antipsychotic medication, individual counselling, family support and counselling, practical support, and involvement in a recovery program which focuses on helping a young person attain social recovery in particular. The focus of treatment is to control and minimise symptoms, to assist the young person to make sense of and overcome any associated trauma, and to prevent relapse through decreasing risk factors such as stress, substance abuse, family conflict and stigma. Treatment also focuses on recovery by identifying the young person's protective factors such as secure accommodation and income; engagement in work or study; developing coping strategies to deal with stress; strong social networks and family supports; and adherence to medication (Early Psychosis Prevention and Intervention Centre).

Nursing considerations

Young people experiencing a psychotic disorder are not always willing to explain or able to understand what is happening to them. Most fear they will be labelled as "mad" and may not seek help on their own. Professionals working with young people may be in a position to identify a young person experiencing a psychotic disorder and assist the young person to get the help they need (Early Psychosis Prevention and Intervention Centre).

✔ *Checkpoint question 54.3*

The parents of an adolescent tell you that he seems increasingly depressed, so much so that he sleeps almost all day on weekends. Does this adolescent need a referral or is he simply demonstrating usual adolescent behaviour? What questions would you want to ask to be able to tell?

Key points for review

- Both cognitive and mental health disorders pose care concerns for young people and their families.
- For children who are intellectually impaired, a stigma may still be present in many communities. Parents may have a more difficult time accepting this diagnosis than they would a physical illness. Mental health disorders often begin subtly in children and are often first manifested as behavioural problems in school. Assess thoroughly any child who is referred for disruptive behaviour.
- Autistic disorder is a pervasive developmental disorder that has a syndrome of behaviours, including fascination with movement, impairment of communication skills and insensitivity to pain.
- Attention-deficit and disruptive behaviour disorders, such as oppositional defiant and conduct disorders, may occur in childhood. Children with ADHD may be treated with medication to reduce the hyperactivity and allow them to achieve better outcomes and interact successfully.

- Eating disorders seen in childhood include pica, rumination, anorexia nervosa and bulimia. All of these disorders can lead to loss of weight and electrolyte imbalances if left unrecognised and untreated.
- Tic disorders such as Tourette's syndrome are abnormalities of semi-involuntary movement that are thought to result from dysfunction of the basal ganglia or distorted dopamine reception.
- Encopresis is the repeated passage of faeces in places not appropriate for that purpose. Therapy is both physiological and psychological.
- Children who are depressed are at high risk of committing suicide. They need thorough assessment and close observation.
- Schizophrenia spectrum and other psychotic disorders may occur in childhood. This usually presents as disorganised behaviour. Long-term therapy is necessary.

CASE STUDY QUESTION

5. Henry's mother feels "at her wits' end" because his attention span is so short and his behaviour so disruptive. His father is proud of his behaviour. What suggestions could you make to his parents to help them to adjust better to his behaviour?

Resources

For an extensive range of additional resources to enhance teaching and learning and to facilitate understanding of this chapter, please see the text's accompanying website located on thePoint at http://thepoint.lww.com.

References

American Psychiatric Association (2013). *Diagnostic and Statistical Manual of Mental Disorders (5th ed.).* Washington, DC: American Psychiatric Association.

Baron, R. B. (2009). Nutritional requirements and disorders. In S. J. McPhee & M. A. Papdakis (Eds). *Current Medical Diagnosis and Treatment.* Columbus, OH: McGraw-Hill.

Culbert, T. P. & Banez, G. A. (2007). Integrative approaches to childhood constipation and encopresis. *Paediatric Clinics of North America, 54*(6), 927–947.

Early Psychosis Prevention and Intervention Centre (EPPIC). Psychosis. Accessed 17 March 2015, <http://eppic.org.au/psychosis>.

Eisendrath, S. J. & Lichtmacher, J. E. (2009). Psychiatry. In S. J. McPhee & M. A. Papdakis (Eds). *Current Medical Diagnosis and Treatment.* Columbus, OH: McGraw-Hill.

Goldson, E. & Reynolds, A. (2014). Child development and behaviour. In W. W. Hay et al. (Eds). *Current Paediatric Diagnosis and Treatment* (22nd ed.). Columbus, OH: McGraw-Hill.

Jayasinghe, Y., Grover, S. R. & Zacharin, M. (2008). Current concepts in bone and reproductive health in adolescents with anorexia nervosa. *BJOG: An International Journal of Obstetrics & Gynaecology, 115*(3), 304–315.

Kaplan, D. W. & Love-Osborne, K. (2014). Adolescence. In W. W. Hay et al. (Eds). *Current Paediatric Diagnosis and Treatment* (22nd ed.). Columbus, OH: McGraw-Hill.

Latner, J. D. & Clyne, C. (2008). The diagnostic validity of the criteria for binge eating disorder. *International Journal of Eating Disorders, 41*(1), 1–14.

Lyons, E. A., et al. (2007). Brief functional analysis and supplemental feeding for post meal rumination in children with developmental disabilities. *Journal of Applied Behavior Analysis, 40*(4), 743–747.

Mouridsen, S. E., et al. (2008). Psychiatric disorders in individuals diagnosed with infantile autism as children: A case control study. *Journal of Psychiatric Practice, 14*(1), 5–12.

Nicholas, J. S., et al. (2008). Prevalence and characteristics of children with autism-spectrum disorders. *Annals of Epidemiology, 18*(2), 130–136.

Philichi, L. (2008). When the going gets tough: Pediatric constipation and encopresis. *Gastroenterology Nursing, 31*(2), 121–130.

Scott, S. (2007). Conduct disorders in children. *British Medical Journal, 334*(7595), 646.

Sigel, E. J. (2014). Eating disorders. In W. W. Hay et al. (Eds). *Current Pediatric Diagnosis and Treatment* (22nd ed.). Columbus, OH: McGraw-Hill.

Simon, G. (2008). Antidepressants and suicide. *British Medical Journal, 336*(7643), 515–516.

Stafford, B., Talmi, A. & Burstein, A. (2014). Child and adolescent psychiatric disorders and psychosocial aspects of paediatrics. In W. W. Hay et al. (Eds). *Current Paediatric Diagnosis and Treatment* (22nd ed.). Columbus, OH: McGraw-Hill.

Starn, A. L. & Udall, J. N. (2008). Iron deficiency anemia, pica, and restless legs syndrome in a teenage girl. *Clinical Pediatrics, 47*(1), 83–85.

Sykora, W. S. (2008). Disruptive behavioral disorders in children. In J. E. South-Paul, S. C. Matheny & E. L. Lewis (Eds). *Current Diagnosis and Treatment in Family Medicine* (2nd ed.). Columbus, OH: McGraw-Hill.

Volkmar, F. R. (2008). Autism and the pervasive developmental disorders. In M. H. Ebert et al. (Eds). *Current Diagnosis and Treatment: Psychiatry* (2nd ed.). Columbus, OH: McGraw-Hill.

World Health Organization (WHO). (2011). International statistical classification of diseases and related health problems (10th revision). Accessed 17 March 2015, <www.who.int/classifications/icd/ICD10Volume2_en_2010.pdf?ua=1>.

Xia, Y. & Rao, G. (2011). Movement disorders. In J. E. South-Paul, S. C. Matheny & E. L. Lewis (Eds). *Current Diagnosis and Treatment in Family Medicine* (3rd ed.). Columbus, OH: McGraw-Hill.

Zandian, M., et al. (2007). Cause and treatment of anorexia nervosa. *Physiology and Behavior, 92*(1–2), 283–290.

Suggested readings

Australia and New Zealand Academy for Eating Disorders <www.anzaed.org.au>.

Australian Advisory Board on Autism Spectrum Disorders <www.autismadvisoryboard.org.au>.

Chilled Plus Online Program <www.centreforemotionalhealth.com.au/pages/chilledplus.aspx>.

Cool Kids Program <www.centreforemotionalhealth.com.au/pages/cool-kids-program.aspx>.

Dossetor, D. (2013). Intellectual disability and autism spectrum disorder: Psychiatric comorbidities in adolescence. In M. Kang, S. R. Skinner, L. A. Sanci & S. M. Sawyer (Eds), *Youth health and adolescent medicine*, pp. 104–128. Melbourne: IP Communications.

Dossetor, D., White, D. & Whatson, L. (Eds). (2011). *Mental Health of Children and adolescents with Intellectual and Developmental Disabilities: A Framework for Professional Practice.* Melbourne: IP Communications.

Early Psychosis Prevention and Intervention Centre (EPPIC) <www.eppic.org.au>.

Headspace National Youth Mental Health Foundation <www.headspace.org.au>.

Mental Health Australia <www.mhca.org.au>.

Mental Health Foundation of New Zealand <www.mentalhealth.org.nz>.

Norgate, K. (2012). EMDR for post-traumatic stress and other psychological trauma. *Nursing Times, 108*(44), 24–26.

Sadock, B. J. & Sadock, V. A. (2014). *Kaplan and Sadock's Synopsis of Psychiatry: Behavorial Sciences/Clinical Psychiatry* (11th ed.). Philadelphia: Lippincott Williams & Wilkins.

Chapter 55

Nursing care of a family in crisis: Abuse and violence in the family

This chapter includes information about the effect on children when abuse occurs in a family.

LEARNING OBJECTIVES

After studying the contents of this chapter, you should be able to:

1. Discuss and define the types of abuse seen in Australian and New Zealand families.
2. Analyse ways that nurses can help make care more family-centred and so ideally help to prevent family abuse.
3. Assess a child who is physically or emotionally abused.
4. Develop an understanding of nursing responsibilities related to a child who has experienced abuse.
5. Discuss positive outcomes for a child who has experienced abuse.
6. Identify nursing care for a family in which abuse has occurred.
7. Identify health promotion and preventive measures nurses can implement for a child who has experienced abuse.
8. Identify areas related to care of a child who has experienced abuse that could benefit from additional nursing research or application of evidence-based practice.

KEY TERMS

- abuse
- domestic violence
- mandatory reporting
- neglect
- physical abuse
- psychological harm
- sexual abuse

CASE STUDY

Lily is a 3-year-old you see in an emergency department. Her mother tells you Lily fell off a swing in the back yard. Lily has a broken forearm, a broken rib and multiple bruises on her chest and back. You notice in her chart that Lily was seen in the same emergency department a month ago for a burn on the palm of her hand. When you mention to her mother that Lily's injuries seem extreme for a simple fall, her mother says, "Lily is very clumsy and always injuring herself".

CASE STUDY QUESTION

1. You suspect that Lily is a victim of child abuse. What additional questions would you want to ask her mother to help determine whether this is so?

Child abuse is estimated to affect between 5% and 10% of Australian and New Zealand children (Australian Institute of Family Studies, 2013). During 2012–2013, 184,216 Australian children were suspected of being harmed or at risk of harm from abuse and/or neglect, resulting in 272,980 notifications being issued by state and territory authorities. The number of notifications has increased by more than 35,000 over the last 3 years (AIHW, 2014). In New Zealand on average one child is killed every 5 weeks as a result of child abuse. Most of these children are under 5 years of age and in 90% of cases the perpetrator is someone the child knew. Child abuse is estimated to cost New Zealand about $2 billion each year <www.childmatters.org.nz/55/learn-about-child-abuse/facts>.

Abuse is associated with stress and has been linked to an inability of a family to handle external and internal stressors. Accordingly, abuse in a family is rarely an isolated event but rather an indication of how much the family needs care overall.

Abuse takes several forms: child abuse, which can be physical or emotional and includes neglect and sexual abuse; and domestic violence (otherwise known as family violence). The World Health Organization (2015) provides current thinking in their definition of child abuse. "Child maltreatment, sometimes referred to as child abuse and neglect, includes all forms of physical and emotional ill-treatment, sexual abuse, neglect and exploitation that results in actual or potential harm to the child's health, development or dignity. Within this broad definition, five subtypes can be distinguished—physical abuse; sexual abuse; neglect and negligent treatment; emotional abuse; and exploitation."

Maternity, child health and family care nurses need to be especially observant for signs of possible abuse in a family and prepared to handle this highly emotional and complex problem objectively. The victim's safety is paramount, but ensuring this safety must be done with sensitivity to the importance of maintaining and improving overall family functioning. Abuse has long-term consequences, because as many as 30% of children from abusive families become abusive parents themselves (Lang et al., 2010; Valentino et al., 2012). It also may lead to a post-traumatic stress disorder with long-term effects (Ullman, 2007).

CARE OF A FAMILY THAT EXPERIENCES ABUSE

Assessment

Commonly, nurses are the first individuals to identify symptoms of possible abuse in a family, because they are often the first to see a child undressed at a healthcare visit and recognise significant bruising, and they are often the person in whom a pregnant woman or child confides about the problem (see Box 55.1). Nurses are often the first to notice inconsistencies in a child's story. This will then be compared with the history of injury reported by the parent. If there are differences in the parent's and child's explanation of an injury or you are concerned or suspect abuse it is important that you refer to current health facility work place policy. The Australian Nursing and Midwifery Federation (2013) states in its policy on child abuse and neglect that "nurses and midwives working with children, young people and families should have the necessary skill to assess, identify, report and implement early intervention strategies in the management of any case of suspected child abuse and/or neglect. It's important then that nurses are familiar with their role to ensure that the evidence is substantiated with objective data." The Australian Nursing and Midwifery Federation is clear in reassuring nurses that all healthcare organisations are responsible for ongoing education and awareness raising regarding the impact of abuse and neglect on the child and the need for correct criminal history checks on all those working with children. This combination of responsibilities then ensures that the child and family experiencing abuse are then provided the care required based on the most recent evidence-based practice professional standards.

BOX 55.1 Assessment ✻ Assessing a child for signs and abuse

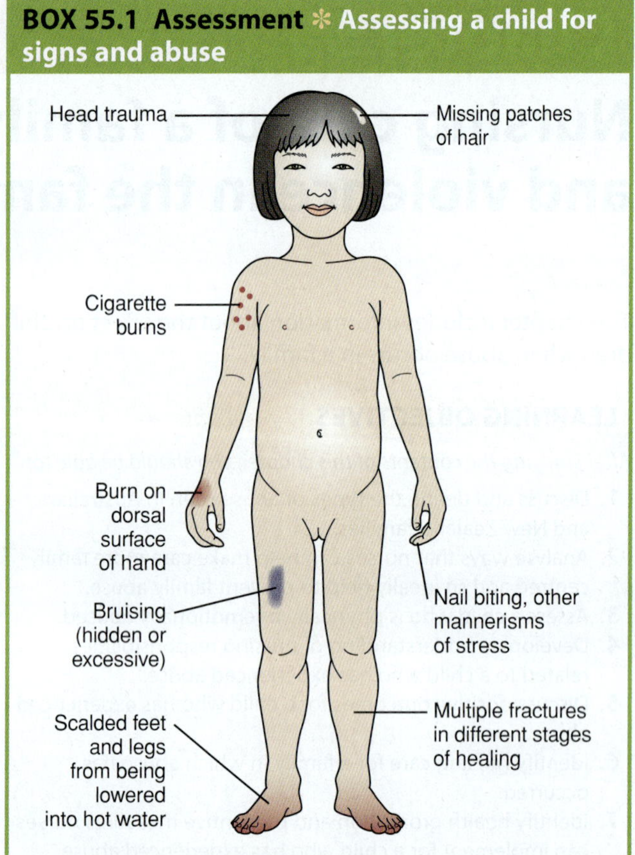

Nursing considerations

Nursing care associated with abuse should take into consideration a holistic approach to addressing the needs of families suffering abuse. Some examples of these needs are:

- Pain, injury and disability
- Psychological injury related to previous abuse
- Learned abusive behaviour
- Impaired parenting related to high level of stress
- Compromised family coping abilities
- Low self-esteem
- Risk of sexual abuse.

Planning nursing care must centre first on ensuring the safety of the abused family member and minimising the effects of trauma. Second, it is concerned with reporting the discovery to authorities. *Nurses are mandated by law to report child abuse*; identifying and reporting this problem are important nursing actions. Long-term planning includes identifying services and organisations that can help an abused family member find safe refuge and re-establishing self-esteem through a self-help or advocacy program. Teaching empowerment, or the ability to take charge of one's life, is particularly important for members of abusive families. In addition, the abuser needs a program of therapy to help prevent future abuse.

The following organisations are helpful for referral or further information on abuse and violence in families:

- Australian Childhood Foundation <www.childhood.org.au/home>
- Australian Women Against Violence Alliance <www.awava.org.au>
- The Campaign for Action on Family Violence <www.areyouok.org.nz>
- Child Abuse Prevention Service <www.childabuseprevention.com.au>
- Education Centre Against Violence <www.ecav.health.nsw.gov.au>
- Families Commission (Kōmihana a Whānau) <www.justice.govt.nz/publications/global-publications/d/directory-of-official-information-2013/alphabetical-list-of-entries/f/families-commission>
- Family Relationships Online <www.familyrelationships.gov.au/Pages/default.aspx>
- Jigsaw <www.jigsaw.org.nz>
- Kids Helpline <www.kidshelp.com.au>
- Mensline Australia <www.mensline.org.au>
- Shine <www.2shine.org.nz>.

HEALTH PROMOTION AND PREVENTION

Prevention must be the most important goal of healthcare providers to reduce the incidence of child abuse (see Box 55.2). Because many child abusers were abused themselves, stopping child abuse in any one generation helps prevent it in the next and promotes family health.

Nurses can do much in all settings through serving as a role model or providing education to promote healthy patterns of childrearing and optimal ways of handling family stress. They can be particularly observant for families who seem to be at risk of abusive behaviour, but also be alert to possible abuse in families that are not showing obvious signs. Further education is an intervention that can help parents who may not recognise their children's needs or normal child behaviour. Lecturing is not a useful intervention, but supportive education can be extremely valuable.

Abuse and pregnancy

Identifying parents who are potential abusers is a necessary step in prevention. Some parents can be identified as potential abusers during pregnancy. Listen carefully to the way pregnant women or their partners talk about the child they are expecting. Prenatal concerns of abuse that may occur in the postnatal period include: failure to attend clinic visits; history of domestic violence; homelessness; developmental disability or mental health issues in the parents; maternal depression; hazardous drug and alcohol issues during pregnancy; and previous reports of child abuse or neglect.

BOX 55.2 * Measures to prevent child abuse

1. Advocate for high school courses on parenting and growth and development of children.
2. Help children learn problem-solving techniques so they are not overwhelmed by mounting problems as adults.
3. Foster high self-esteem in children so they are not dependent on others but are assertive (they will not become passive observers of abuse).
4. Help parents with responsible reproductive planning, so children are desired.
5. Help parents locate support people in their community, such as support groups or church or social contacts.
6. Teach children to verbalise their problems and to seek help for problems so problems do not mount to overwhelming proportions.
7. Role model caring behaviours with children for parents.
8. Identify children who may be viewed as special in some way by parents such as those who were separated from the family at birth, were premature or are physically challenged.
9. Identify parents who were abused as children and offer specific help to them to break the cycle of child abuse.
10. Suggest that potential abusers join Parents Anonymous, an effective support group.

BOX 55.3 * Characteristics of parents at high risk of causing child abuse or neglect

1. Frequent changes of address in the year before child's birth
2. Past or present treatment for mental illness
3. Emotional problems
4. Lack of intellectual ability
5. Unrealistic expectations of the new baby
6. Changed decision about adoption
7. Abuse or neglect of a previous child
8. History of parental violence or neglect in childhood
9. Low self-esteem
10. Unable to earn independent income
11. Parent has a new co-partner

Abuse and the postnatal period

Identifying a potential child at risk in the early postnatal period is difficult. However, risk factors are similar to those identified in the prenatal period, in addition to failure to engage with the baby and leaving the baby alone for long periods. Remember, though, that not all parents immediately bond or react warmly to their newborns. They may only tentatively touch or pick up their infant. Risk factors during pregnancy and the early postpartum period are summarised in Box 55.3.

Parents may also be identified as potential abusers during child and family health nurse visits for an infant. By the time a baby has an early childhood healthcare visit (usually within 3 days of discharge from the maternity unit), a good parent–child interaction should have begun. A thorough assessment of early family development is important in identifying indicators of possible abusive situations and to ensure strategies can be implemented to prevent physical and **psychological harm** to individual family members.

Helping parents to seek assistance from support people is another necessary step in prevention of abuse. Interventions to reduce family abuse include home visits, family counselling and therapy. Nurses can be proactive in implementing health promotion programs to improve family health, such as parenting classes, educating on child growth and development, and building self-esteem classes.

CHILD ABUSE

Parenting is not an easy task and effective parenting is not an automatic or truly instinctive ability, thus children in every community are injured because of abuse. Abuse may be physical (the child is beaten or burned) or it may be **neglect** (the child is not fed, clothed, supervised properly or offered medical care or educational opportunities). Abuse may also be psychological or emotional (a child is made to feel unintelligent or inadequate). In some instances, women who threatened the health of their fetus by drug abuse during pregnancy have been viewed by the courts as child abusers (Goodwin, 2011).

Abuse not only places a child at immediate risk of harm but can also lead to long-term effects. For example, children who have been physically abused are found to be more angry, non-compliant and hyperactive than others; they may demonstrate poor self-control and low self-esteem. Children whose parents do not interact with them (emotional abuse) are apt to be more withdrawn and to have a flatter affect than others. Because the abusive family is a disrupted one, children often have undiagnosed medical problems, such as anaemia, otitis media, lead poisoning or sexually transmitted infections. Children who suffer sexual abuse can have long-term effects of depression, guilt and difficulty enjoying sexual relations (Hornor, 2010).

It must be remembered that most toddlers have some ecchymotic spots on their legs from bumping into tables or chairs during normal toddler walking. Some childhood diseases, such as leukaemia or purpura, begin with easy bruising. Children with osteogenesis imperfecta have frequent broken bones as a natural consequence of their disease. Because of inadequate fact-finding in these instances, false reports do occur. This can lead to severe stress in a family that has been falsely accused and can interfere with the relationship between the parents of an ill child and the nurse.

In addition, when children reach adulthood and begin parenting, they tend to rear their children in basically the same way as they were reared. Parents who themselves received little love or were abused as children may never form a basic sense of trust, and this may cause them to have parenting difficulties themselves.

Providing consistent care and support for the child who has experienced abuse

A major nursing role is supplying a consistent, caring adult presence for a child who has experienced abuse or furnishing a relationship that the child has never enjoyed. Use a primary or case management type of nursing care assignment with children who have experienced abuse, to offer them consistency and the security of a one-to-one relationship. Many children who have experienced abuse are not used to playing for their own enjoyment but only to the point at which a parent wants to play a game; this means that they may watch you carefully for signs that you approve of their behaviour. They may not be used to activities such as rocking or talking. Be careful when asking questions not to imply that any one answer is the correct one or they will supply what they think you want to hear rather than the truth. (A question such as, "That feels better, doesn't it?" may be followed by an instant "yes" even though the child feels no improvement in symptoms.)

It is important to care for the child *and* family in a non-judgemental way. It is not up to the team caring for the child to pass judgement; rather our role is to support the child and family until child protection services investigate or take action.

Mandatory reporting

In Australia, legislation for reporting is different in each state and territory, however, there is now a national framework that guides the protection of children (Mitchell & Ellis, 2011). Nurses are included in the **mandatory reporting** category in most states; this means they must report suspected child abuse when they identify it. It is important that nurses working with children and young people understand the concept of abuse, recognise the signs of abuse and neglect and potential for abuse, and are able to respond appropriately to children who are at risk of being abused (Mitchell & Ellis, 2011). The fact that the information was given in a confidential interview does not free a nurse from this responsibility (Mathews & Kenny, 2008). The NSW Government website Keep Them Safe, A Shared Approach to Child Wellbeing <www.keepthemsafe.nsw.gov.au> provides answers to the many questions posed by nurses in regard to professional responsibilities and displays strategies that can be implemented to safeguard children who are at risk.

In New Zealand, if nurses and other carers are concerned about a child, they are advised not to worry about categorising the particular type of abuse but instead to concentrate on noticing a pattern forming or multiple signs that are of concern, as these factors could be indications that something is wrong. The cluster of signs includes physical signs, behavioural concerns, developmental delays, the child talking about things that may indicate abuse, and the family environment (Child Youth & Family NZ, 2011).

Documenting suspected cases of child abuse

Child abuse is a crime. Objective data assessment and reporting is an essential nursing care skill. Nursing documentation can be subpoenaed and displayed in court. Be certain when charting information related to child abuse that you make specific and factual notes (observations, not interpretations), such as "Parent spoke loudly and slurred his words" rather than "Parent was intoxicated" or "Mother stated, 'This child is nothing but trouble'", not "I think this mother dislikes this child". Record conversations with parents using exact quotations, if possible. Photographs of physical abuse enhance the strength of the evidence of abuse, so these are usually taken.

Physical abuse

Physical abuse is the action of a carer that causes injury to a child. It is commonly revealed by burns or by injuries to the head or hands. Always ask parents to account for any injury to a child's body. Remember, however, that most childhood injuries are the result of unintentional injuries caused by the child's inability to distinguish safe situations from dangerous ones or by parents overestimating their child's abilities.

If a child has been physically abused, the injury is usually out of proportion to the history of the injury given by the parent. The parent may report, for example, that the child was playing underneath the coffee table when he reared up quickly and hit his head, sustaining a large haematoma and temporary loss of consciousness or that an infant "rolled off the couch" and now has two broken arms. In other instances, the parents may give conflicting stories (the mother says that the child fell, but the father says that the child broke his arm throwing a ball) or they may give no reason for the injury ("He woke up from his nap and couldn't move his arm; I don't know what could have happened").

When questioned about the injury, children who have experienced abuse often repeat the parent's story; this loyalty to parents seems misplaced, but they may fear further beatings or simply believe that living with such parents is better than not having anyone. It is essential that the nurse asks about behavioural problems at school, because the constant stress under which these children live frequently results in disruptive school behaviour.

Physical examination

When children are examined, be certain to remove all bandages and Band-Aids so that the entire body can be observed. Delays in growth may suggest neglect so assessment of height and weight on a standard growth chart is important to display this.

Several injuries in children clearly signal child abuse. Most parents protect their children's hands carefully; children who are abused have a higher incidence of hand injury than others. Children who are beaten with electrical cords, belts or clotheslines have peculiar circular and linear lesions (see Fig. 55.1D). Children who are beaten with a belt buckle have additional curved lacerations from the imprint of the buckle; few other weapons produce such contusions. Abrasions or ecchymotic areas on the wrists or ankles may be present if the child was tied to a bed or against a wall (see Fig. 55.1C).

Burns or scalds are frequent injuries in children who have experienced abuse. The peak age at which children accidentally burn themselves is 2 years; that of burns related to abuse is closer to 3 years. When children burn their hand by accident, they usually burn the palm; burns from abuse are often on the dorsal surface. Scalding with hot water can occur from a child pulling a hot drink off a

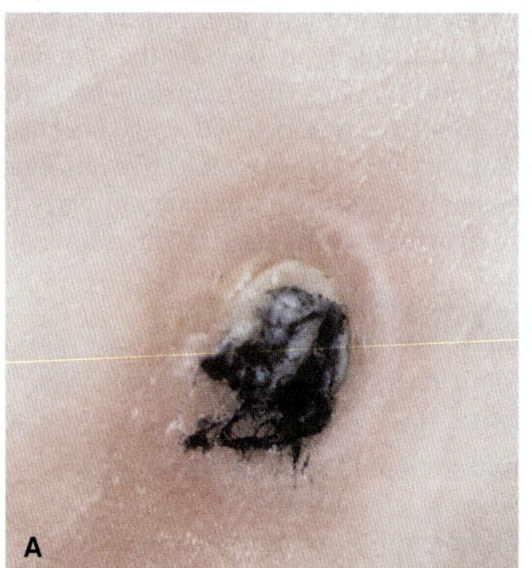

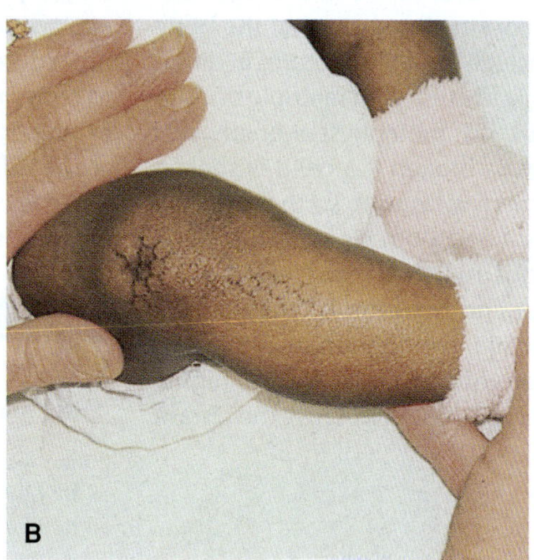

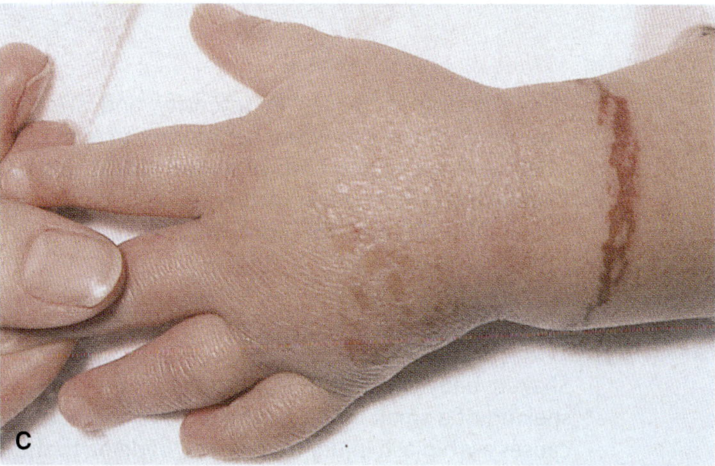

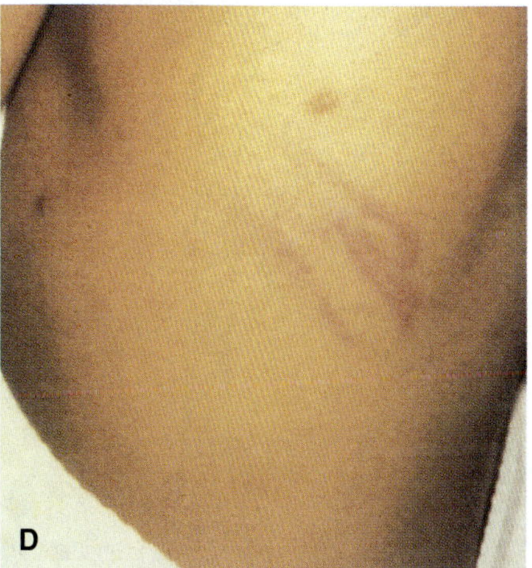

FIGURE 55.1 (**A**) Cigarette burn on child's foot. (**B**) Branding injury showing imprint of radiator cover. (**C**) Rope burn with oedema and skin breakdown from being tied to cot rails. (**D**) Imprint marks from beating with a looped electrical cord. (From Zitelli, B. J. & Davis, H. W. (1997). *Atlas of pediatric physical diagnosis* (3rd ed.). St. Louis: Mosby–Year Book, Inc.)

table. It is often, though, a signal of child abuse (an adult deliberately scalded the child). A child who is placed in a bath of hot water buttocks first may have no burn in the centre of the buttocks because they touched the bath; the result is a ring of burns causing a "doughnut-hole" effect. Young children do accidentally step into baths containing water that is hot enough to burn. When this happens, however, the child usually falls forwards and so also has burns on the hands and splash marks on the chest or face. If a child is lowered into scalding water as punishment, only the feet and the skin up to the knees are scalded.

Cigarette burns are another common finding on the bodies of children who have experienced physical abuse. A fresh cigarette burn causes a blister that resembles the scab of impetigo (see Fig. 55.1A); differentiation at this stage is often difficult. Impetigo lesions, however, heal without scarring. Cigarette burns heal with a definite circular scar.

Human bites or chunks of hair pulled off the scalp may be present. Head injury is common. Broken bones are another frequent finding. Children who are of preschool age and younger usually do not fall far enough in normal accidents to break bones; a broken bone at this age suggests the child was thrown or struck so hard that the bone broke. Common findings include multiple fractures in different stages of healing, a single fracture with multiple bruises, rib or occipital fractures and metaphyseal-epiphyseal injuries. Bones are not always broken if a child is shaken roughly, but the periosteum may be torn, so that an x-ray reveals a strange haziness along both sides of the bone shaft. Tibial torsion (twisting) is also often seen (see Fig. 55.2). Deliberate poisoning is yet another form of child abuse; this usually occurs in a child younger than 2½ years. Bruises on a child who is too young to walk are also highly suspicious (Chiesa & Sirotnak, 2014; see Fig. 55.3): the phrase "Doesn't cruise, can't bruise" can be helpful to remember here.

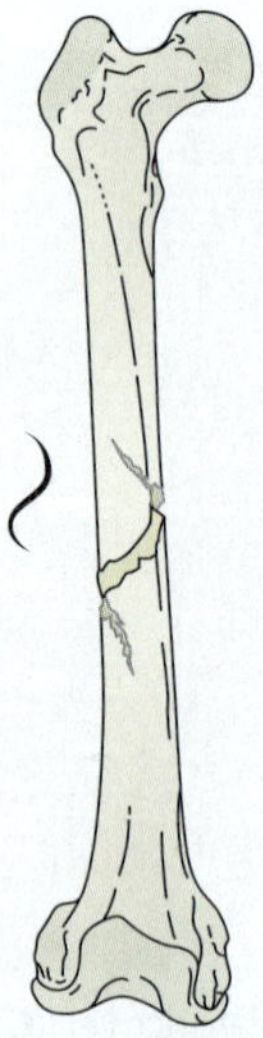

FIGURE 55.2 A spiral fracture around the bone is caused by a wrenching force and is frequently associated with child abuse.

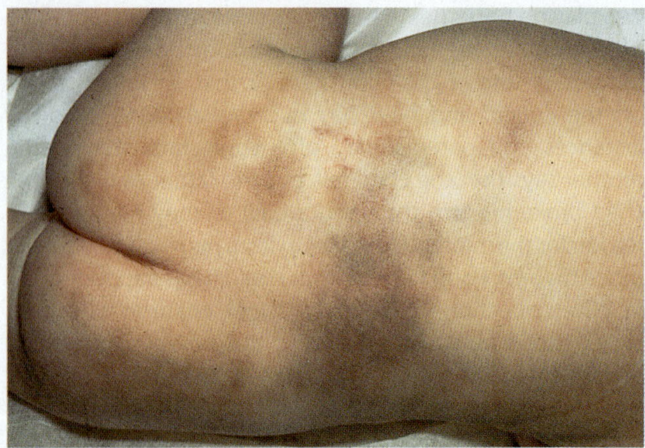

FIGURE 55.3 Large bruises on a child's body. With this type of injury, carefully assessing the history of the traumatic event would be essential. (© Biophoto Associates/Photograph Researchers.)

Listen to children while they are being examined. If they did not hear the parent's explanation of the accident, they may say something that is inconsistent with the parent's explanation. They may cry little in response to a painful procedure, such as an injection, because they are not used to receiving comfort for pain. They may draw back from an examiner more than the average child would because they are afraid of adults. These are very subjective observations, however, because children react in different ways to the fear produced by a recent injury or a health examination.

CASE STUDY QUESTION

2. Which finding in Lily's background is a typical finding of child abuse?
   a. Lily's mother describes her as "not pretty".
   b. Lily's birthday is in autumn.
   c. Lily's mother works part-time for low pay.
   d. Lily's father smokes a pack of cigarettes a day.

What if...

Lily's crying increases in intensity and she clearly becomes distressed when her mother tries to comfort her? Is this a typical sign of abuse? Could this be too subjective? Reflect on strategies you could use to assess this situation for more objective data.

Shaken baby syndrome

Shaken baby syndrome is caused by repetitive, violent shaking of a small infant by the arms or shoulders, which causes a whiplash injury to the neck, oedema to the brainstem and distinct retinal haemorrhages (Hitchcock, 2012). This is a particularly insidious form of child abuse, because the damage inflicted on the infant is not readily apparent.

Increased use of computed tomography (CT) scans and magnetic resonance imaging (MRI) is helping to detect children with these internal symptoms. Parents have sometimes used covert recordings to reveal that a carer or an adult not related to the child but living in the house shook a baby in this way.

Physical neglect

Physical neglect is a more subtle form of abuse than physical abuse, but it can be just as damaging to a child's welfare. A neglected child may appear unwashed, thin and malnourished or be dressed inappropriately, such as without a coat or shoes in cold weather. In some families, no one has a warm coat to wear or receives enough food because there is no money for these things; that is different from the family in which parents do have these things, but the children or a particular child does not. This type of abuse may be overlooked because, if you never see the other members of the family, it is easy to believe that all are dressed poorly.

Failing to bring a child for immunisations and failing to seek early medical care for an infection are other signs of neglect. Not requiring a child to attend school, deliberately keeping a child out of school without setting up a home school program or allowing a child to go unsupervised after school may also be interpreted as neglect.

Neglect may be wilful or it may occur if parents simply do not realise the normal needs of a child. Such parents need guidance from healthcare personnel to understand their child's needs.

Psychological abuse

Psychological abuse includes constant belittling or threatening, rejecting, isolating or exploiting a child. Psychological neglect is the absence of positive parenting. Children who are psychologically abused are likely to have difficulty becoming emotionally confident adults. This type of abuse is the most difficult form of abuse to detect because it may occur only in the home, and its effects, although severe, may be subtle. However, it can be just as damaging to the child's ability to achieve as physical abuse.

The parent who uses only negative terms to describe a child may be psychologically abusing the child. Be sure to include enough growth and development questions during a health assessment to reveal this, and observe the parent–child interaction to determine whether it is positive and healthy or negative and potentially unhealthy.

Ritual abuse

Ritual abuse is cult-based or religiously, spiritually or satanically motivated. It can involve physical, sexual or psychological abuse with bizarre or ceremonial activities. With this type of abuse, multiple perpetrators may abuse multiple victims over an extended period (Schwecke, 2011).

CASE STUDY QUESTION

3. If Lily had been abused as an infant, she might have experienced "shaken baby" syndrome. Which of the following is a usual finding with this syndrome?

a. A baby is fearful of strangers
b. Retinal haemorrhages develop
c. A baby develops Crohn's disease
d. A major bone, such as a femur, is broken

SEXUAL ABUSE

Sexual abuse occurs when a person uses power or authority over a child to involve the child in sexual activity and the child's parent or carer has not protected the child. Physical force is sometimes involved. Child sexual abuse involves a wide range of sexual activity, including: fondling of the child's genitals; masturbation; oral sex; vaginal or anal penetration by a penis, finger or other object; or exposure of the child to pornography (Department of Human Services Victoria, 2013).

Adolescents and older children may also be perpetrators. Sexual abuse involves the coercion of children who are dependent, developmentally immature or adolescents in sexual activities that they do not fully comprehend, to which they are unable to give informed consent or that violate the social taboos of family roles. Adolescents have a higher rate of rape or sexual abuse than any other age group (8% to 10%) (Howard et al., 2007). Remember that boys, as well as girls, can be sexually abused (Holmes, 2008). Abusers may contact children online through chat rooms making the monitoring of websites an important preventive measure for parents (Wolak et al., 2008).

Child sexual abuse is the least reported of any form of child abuse in Australia; however, population studies indicate that the incidence is much higher than that reported (ECAV, 2010).

Sexual abuse is physically and emotionally destructive; it leaves children unable to trust others, and may result in a sense of ambivalence towards intimacy and an overall sense of worthlessness. Children should be taught at an early age that their bodies are their own and to report anyone who tries to touch them in a way they do not like. Children who have been sexually abused may have a sexual vocabulary beyond that expected in a child of their age.

Types of sexual abuse

Sexual abuse involves both non-contact forms of harm as well as contact behaviours. Non-contact sexual abuse includes flashing, posing a child in a sexual manner, exposure to pornography and communication of graphic sexual material (including via SMS or email). Contact sexual abuse includes kissing, touching or fondling the child in a sexual manner, penetration of anus or vagina or coercing the child to perform any such act on themselves or others.

Children may be sexually abused by family members, by acquaintances or by strangers. It occurs in all types of families, regardless of culture, economic status or education level. Children of all ages may be sexually abused and it may occur once or many times over months or even years. Perpetrators are usually male (>90%) and the victims are three times more likely to be female. Generally, girls are more likely to be abused by a family member whereas boys are usually abused by either a family friend or acquaintance, or another adult in a position of trust. Grooming behaviours, such as special treats or attention and keeping secrets from parents, as well as creating a sense of trust or reliance in parents are insidious ways to isolate the child from assistance (ECAV, 2010).

Nursing considerations

Signs of sexual abuse are listed in Box 55.4. Symptoms of sexual abuse may be revealed by a health history such as a young girl worrying that she is pregnant; it may also be revealed by a child's abnormal anxiety about a parent returning home from a hospital stay or anxiety about being left with a particular individual in the family (see Box 55.5). Young children who are the victims of this type of abuse often have been threatened or bribed to keep the secret; they have extremely low self-esteem and may think that they are so bad that they deserve to be treated this way. Allowing young children to play with anatomically correct dolls is a common way of determining whether sexual abuse is occurring. For example, the average reaction of a preschooler or young school-age child who has not been abused is to undress the dolls, giggle for a moment or two about how they look, and then redress or put them aside. The child who is involved in an incestuous relationship is more apt to make the dolls perform a sexual act, such as placing the male doll's penis into the female doll's mouth. The use of such dolls is controversial because there is a concern that without a common protocol for their use, the child's actions could be over-interpreted. Asking the child to draw a picture of what happened may also be an effective way of revealing abuse.

Parents may need as much counselling as the child, so that they can help the child work through feelings about this situation. In many instances, the offender is a family member, such as an uncle, stepfather or older brother. Often the behaviour has been occurring for some time before it is reported. The parents may feel guilty that they allowed the family member to have access to the child or did not listen to a child's protestations that being alone with this family member was uncomfortable for them. If incest involves a parent, it may be extremely difficult for the parents to continue to relate to each other effectively

BOX 55.4 ✻ Focus on family teaching

Identifying signs of sexual abuse

Q. A grandmother asks you, "What signs should I look for if I suspect my granddaughter is being sexually abused?"

A. Here are some general indications that a child is being sexually abused:

- Verbal reports of sexual activity with an adult
- An awareness of sex and sexual vocabulary beyond age expectations
- Participation in sexual expression with dolls
- Pregnancy in a girl younger than 15 years
- Perineal, vaginal or anal inflammation
- Vaginal tears or anal fissures
- Pain on going to the toilet
- Presence of a sexually transmitted infection or urinary tract infection
- Symptoms of increased anxiety, such as sleep disturbance, development of tics, nail biting or stuttering
- Change in school performance, school phobia or truancy
- Fear of being left alone with a certain adult
- Vague abdominal pain or acting-out behaviour

BOX 55.5 ✻ Focus on communication

You notice during history taking that a 4-year-old girl uses several four-letter words to describe where she hurts.

Less effective communication

Nurse: Mrs Holly, your daughter seems to know some words that are unusual for a 4-year-old.
Mrs Holly: She gets that from watching cartoons on TV.
Nurse: Cartoon characters don't usually use the words she uses.
Mrs Holly: We're proud she's advanced for her age.
Nurse: Okay. I just want you to know I think her vocabulary is advanced. Here is the medicine to apply to her bottom.

More effective communication

Nurse: Mrs Holly, your daughter seems to know some words that are unusual for a 4-year-old.
Mrs Holly: She gets that from watching cartoons on TV.
Nurse: Cartoon characters don't usually use the words she uses.
Mrs Holly: We're proud she's advanced for her age.
Nurse: Using words with sexual connotations doesn't necessarily mean her vocabulary is advanced. It means she most likely keeps company with an adult who talks to her that way.
Mrs Holly: That's probably her uncle. He babysits for us once a week.
Nurse: Does she mind staying with him?
Mrs Holly: A free babysitter doesn't happen every day.
Nurse: Let's talk some more about her vocabulary, especially in the light of her infection.

It is often very difficult for families to face the fact that a family member could be guilty of child sexual abuse. In these instances, it is necessary to pursue the subject, rather than let yourself be distracted, to help a parent examine what could be happening.

enough to help the child. Encourage parents to teach children simple rules to help them avoid sexual abuse (see Chapter 32).

✔ Checkpoint question 55.1

Physical examination determines that a 4-year-old girl has a purulent vulvovaginitis. A culture reveals this infection is gonorrhoea. What questions would you want to ask her to determine how she contracted this infection? Suppose her parents are influential people in your community. Would this fact influence what questions you ask?

DOMESTIC VIOLENCE

Domestic violence is abuse by a family member against another adult living in the household, such as a spouse or significant other. That spouse abuse and child abuse may both exist in a family strengthens the importance of providing family-centred nursing care so that both these situations can be identified and halted. Approximately 23–34% of women experience violence from an intimate partner at some time during the relationship (Drabsch, 2007). Screening for domestic violence is important when parents bring children for healthcare visits.

Domestic violence occurs at a higher rate during pregnancy than other times (Shoffner, 2008). Homicide from partner abuse is the number-one cause of death in pregnant women. Abused women may have an unintended and unwanted pregnancy because they were unable to resist sexual advances from their abusive partner. Another woman may desire the pregnancy very much even with such a poor beginning because she believes having a child will change the partner and make him a better person. Women can also be grateful for the pregnancy, thinking that by having an infant she will have someone to love her.

Although it is impossible to predict how any individual woman will respond, pregnant abused women may demonstrate behaviours that reveal abuse. A woman may come for care late in pregnancy or not at all, for example, because her partner controls her transportation or money; she may fear that a healthcare provider will identify and report the abuse.

When undressed for a physical examination, there may be bruises or lacerations on her breasts, abdomen or back she cannot explain. Her neck may reveal linear bruises from strangulation. It is important to develop good communication skills with any woman with bruises to account for them. Determine whether the explanation correlates with the extent and placement of a bruise or laceration (see Box 55.6).

A woman who has experienced abuse may be anxious to listen to the baby's heartbeat at prenatal visits because her partner recently punched or kicked her in the abdomen and she is worried the fetus has been hurt. If abdominal trauma is suspected, an ultrasound may be done

BOX 55.6 Assessment ✻ Assessing the pregnant woman for intimate partner abuse

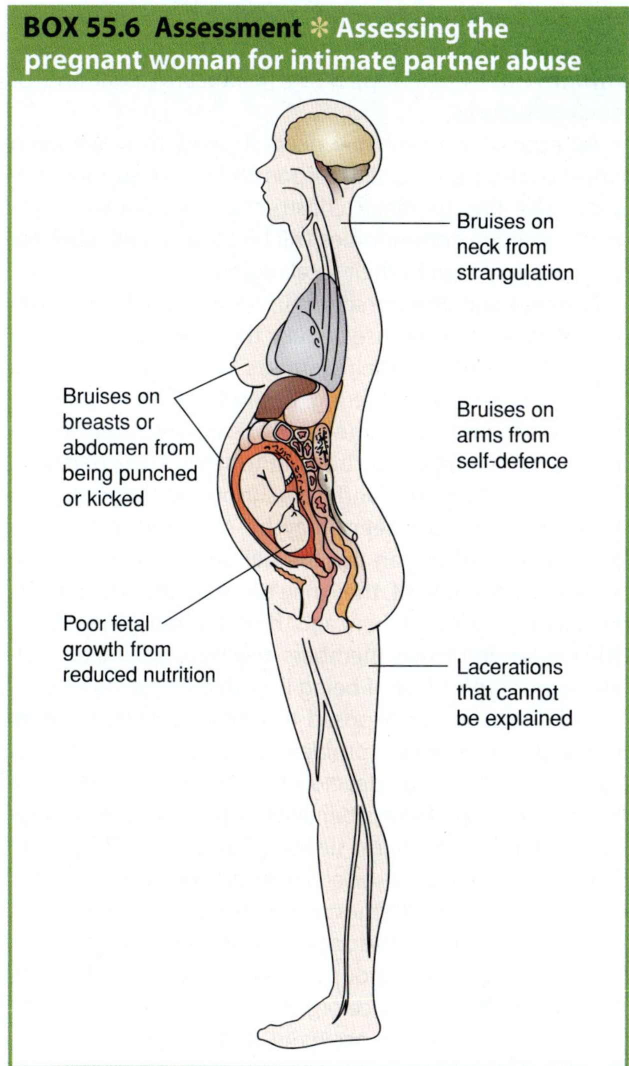

because this is the most accurate method of assessing fetal health after trauma.

Nursing considerations for an abused woman should take a holistic approach and address the physical injuries sustained, the emotional manifestations of abuse and environmental circumstances. Some examples include:

- Powerlessness within the relationship
- Fear related to constant threat of violence
- Social isolation related to client's need to hide evidence of her abuse
- Denial related to inability to face the fact partner is abusive
- Compromised family coping mechanisms.

It may be difficult to work with an abused woman who will not leave an abusive relationship because it is so hard to understand why she stays in the situation. A common finding is that a woman cannot leave because of fear of the abusive person (he has threatened that if she leaves, he will find her and kill her) and the guilt and low self-esteem she feels (he has told her so many times this is her fault and she deserves to be treated in this way that she believes it). To free herself from this emotional paralysis, a women will need supportive healthcare, legal and/or family structures.

An abused woman may need support to make even simple decisions. A nursing responsibility is to support any ability she has to make constructive decisions. Nurses working within communities will be familiar with shelters for abused women in their local region.

Battered and emotionally abused individuals are often so immobilised by a sense of guilt: they believe that if they were better people, their partners would not resort to beatings or verbal badgering. Because victims may have no access to money and no skills to earn any, they need a great deal of support to be able to leave their partners. Even if they have a skill and have supported themselves in the past, their self-esteem may be so low that they no longer believe they can put the skill to use. As the abuse becomes more violent, they may be afraid that their abusers will follow and kill them and their children if they leave. Other extended family members may be unwilling to shelter the victims for fear of being included in the violence.

Children who are exposed to domestic violence may demonstrate conduct problems, non-compliance and aggression. They may develop low levels of empathy or they may display distress behaviours such as clinging, crying, abdominal pain or sleeping disorders. They may regress in language or social developmental milestones.

Like child abuse, domestic violence affects all cultural and social groups. If it appears to be more prevalent in lower socioeconomic groups, it is because these families are more visible to service organisations and law enforcement officials. When it occurs in middle-class or upper-class families, the tendency is to keep the violence hidden.

Key points for review

- Child abuse can exist in many forms. It may be physical, emotional or sexual and may encompass neglect.
- A high suspicion of child abuse should be present if burns, head injury or rib fractures are present or if the history of the accident seems out of proportion to the injury.
- Shaken baby syndrome involves repetitive, violent shaking of a small infant by the arms or shoulders, causing a whiplash injury to the neck, oedema to the brainstem and distinct retinal haemorrhages.
- Children who comfort parents in emergency settings may just be sensitive children or they may be demonstrating role reversal, a behaviour characteristic of children who have experienced abuse.
- In families in which a child is abused, a parent may also be a victim of abuse. Screening for domestic violence is indicated.
- Child abuse is reportable by law. Nurses in Australia are identified as mandatory reporters and must be familiar with the reporting processes.
- Methods to prevent abuse in which nurses can actively participate include teaching about the expected growth and development of children, educating parents for parenting roles, and teaching empowerment or a sense that children and adults have control of their own lives.
- Sexual abuse of children can be prevented by teaching children to recognise abnormal advances and to know it is right to speak out about wrongs against them.
- Abuse is a family problem, not an individual problem. Therapy must include all family members to be effective.
- Pregnant women with traumatic injuries need to be carefully assessed to determine if domestic violence was the cause of the trauma.

CASE STUDY QUESTIONS

4. Although Lily's mother told you that Lily fell from a swing, Lily has a broken forearm, a broken rib and multiple bruises on her chest and back. Her mother tells you, "I guess she's also clumsy". What additional questions would you want to ask to determine whether Lily has been abused?
5. What would be a possible research topic to explore that would be applicable to Lily's family and also advance evidence-based practice?

Resources

For an extensive range of additional resources to enhance teaching and learning and to facilitate understanding of this chapter, please see the text's accompanying website located on thePoint at http://thepoint.lww.com.

References

Australian Institute of Family Studies. (2013). The prevalence of child abuse and neglect. CFCA Resource Sheet, accessed 6 March 2015, <www3.aifs.gov.au/cfca/publications/prevalence-child-abuse-and-neglect>.

Australian Institute of Health and Welfare (AIHW). (2014). *Child Protection Australia 2012–2013*, accessed 6 March 2015 <www.aihw.gov.au/publication-detail/?id=60129547965>.

Australian Nursing and Midwifery Federation. (2013). ANMF position statement on child abuse and neglect, accessed 6 March 2015 <http://anmf.org.au/documents/policies/PS_Child_abuse_and_neglect.pdf>.

Chiesa, A. & Sirotnak, A. P. (2014). Child abuse and neglect. In W.W. Hay, et al. (Eds). *Current Paediatric Diagnosis and Treatment* (22nd ed.). Columbus, OH: McGraw-Hill.

Child Youth & Family NZ. (2011). Working together to keep children and young people safe (Me mutu tā tātou tūkino tamariki), Ministry of Social Development, accessed 9 March 2015 <www.cyf.govt.nz/documents/about-us/publications/27713-working-together-3-0-45ppi.pdf>.

Department of Human Services Victoria. (2013). What is child abuse?, accessed 9 March 2015, <www.dhs.vic.gov.au/for-individuals/children,-families-and-young-people/child-protection/about-child-abuse/what-is-child-abuse>.

Drabsch, T. (2007). Domestic Violence in NSW. Briefing Paper 7/07. NSW Parliamentary Library Research Service, accessed 9 March 2015, <www.parliament.nsw.gov.au/prod/parlment/publications.nsf/0/c943ee514205619bca2572f4000c56fc/$FILE/DomesticViolence Final&index.pdf>.

ECAV Education Centre Against Violence. (2010). NSW Health child protection and child wellbeing training: Identifying and responding to children and young people at risk of harm. DVD, accessed 18 March 2015, <www.ecav.health.nsw.gov.au/online-shop/dvds-cd-roms-videos/identifying-and-responding-to-children-and-young-people-at-risk-of-harm>.

Goodwin, M. B. (2011). Precarious moorings: Tying fetal drug law policy to social profiling. *Rutgers Law Journal*, *42*(3), 659–694.

Hitchcock, J. (2012). The debate over shaken baby syndrome. *Journal of Neonatal Nursing*, *18*(1), 20–21.

Holmes, W. C. (2008). Men's self-definitions of abusive childhood sexual experiences, and potentially related risky behavioral and psychiatric outcomes. *Child Abuse and Neglect, 32*(1), 83–97.

Hornor, G. (2010). Child sexual abuse: Consequences and implications. *Journal of Pediatric Health Care*, *24*(6), 358–364.

Howard, D. E., Wang, M. Q. & Yan, F. (2007). Prevalence and psychosocial correlates of forced sexual intercourse among U.S. high school adolescents. *Adolescence, 42*(168), 629–643.

Kralik, D. & van Loon, A. (2011) *Community Nursing in Australia* (2nd ed.). Sydney: John Wiley & Sons.

Lang, A. J., Garstein, M. A., Rodgers, C. S., et al. (2010). The impact of maternal childhood abuse on parenting and infant temperament. *Journal of Child and Adolescent Psychiatric Nursing*, *23*(2), 100–110.

Mathews, B. & Kenny, M. C. (2008). Mandatory reporting legislation in the United States, Canada and Australia: a cross-jurisdictional review of key features, differences and issues. *Child Maltreatment, 13*(1), 50–63.

Mitchell, C. & Ellis, I. (2011). Promoting family and child health. In D. Kralik & A. van Loon. (2011) *Community Nursing in Australia* (2nd ed.). Sydney: John Wiley & Sons.

Nusbaum, M. R. H. & Katsufrakis, P. J. (2008). Adolescent sexuality. In J. E. South-Paul, S. C. Matheny & E. L. Lewis (Ed). *Current Diagnosis and Treatment in Family Medicine* (2nd ed.). Columbus, OH: McGraw-Hill.

Schwecke, L. H. (2011). Beyond childhood sexual abuse: Ritual abuse—Torture and human trafficking. *Journal of Psychosocial Nursing and Mental Health Services*, *49*(1), 8–10.

Shoffner, D. H. (2008). We don't like to think about it: Intimate partner violence during pregnancy and postpartum. *Journal of Perinatal and Neonatal Nursing, 22*(1), 39–48.

Ullman, S. E. (2007). Relationship to perpetrator, disclosure, social reactions, and PTSD symptoms in child sexual abuse survivors. *Journal of Child Sexual Abuse, 16*(1), 19–36.

Valentino, K., Nuttall, A. K., Comas, M., et al. (2012). Intergenerational continuity of child abuse among adolescent mothers: Authoritarian parenting, community violence, and race. *Child Maltreatment*, *17*(2), 172–181.

Wolak, J., et al. (2008). Online "predators" and their victims: Myths, realities, and implications for prevention and treatment. *American Psychologist, 63*(2), 111–128.

World Health Organization. (2015). Child maltreatment, accessed 5 March 2015, <www.who.int/topics/child_abuse/en/>.

Zitelli, B. J. & Davis, H. W. (1997). *Atlas of Pediatric Physical Diagnosis* (3rd ed.). St Louis: Mosby.

Suggested readings

Australian Childhood Foundation <www.childhood.org.au/home>.

Australian Women Against Violence Alliance <www.awava. org.au>.

Child Abuse Prevention Service <www.childabuseprevention.com.au>.

Child matters: Educating to prevent child abuse: <www.childmatters.org.nz>.

Child, Youth and Family NZ <www.cyf.govt.nz>.

Keep Them Safe <www.keepthemsafe.nsw.gov.au>.

Kids Helpline <www.kidshelp.com.au>.

Mensline Australia <www.mensline.org.au>.

Shine <www.2shine.org.nz>.

The Campaign for Action on Family Violence <www.areyouok.org.nz>.

Underwood, L. (2010). Recession shakes the nation but not our babies. *Journal of Obstetric, Gynecologic & Neonatal Nursing*, *39*(Suppl. 1), S47.

Widom, C. S., Czaja, S., Wilson, H. W., et al. (2013). Do the long-term consequences of neglect differ for children of different races and ethnic backgrounds? *Child Maltreatment*, *18*(1), 42–55.

Chapter 56

Nursing care of a family when a child has a long-term or terminal illness

Previous chapters described the growth and development of well children and the care of children with specific disorders. This chapter adds information about the care of chronically and terminally ill children.

LEARNING OBJECTIVES

After mastering the contents of this chapter, you should be able to:

1. Describe common concerns of parents of children with a long-term or terminal illness.
2. Describe ways that nursing care of a child with a long-term or terminal illness can be more family-centred.
3. Have an understanding of the coping mechanisms that a child or family with a long-term or terminal illness may use.
4. Identify expected outcomes for effectiveness of care.
5. Integrate knowledge of long-term and terminal illness in children to achieve quality child and family health nursing care.

KEY TERMS

- anticipatory grief
- complicated grief
- death
- grief process
- grief response
- vulnerable children

CASE STUDY

Charlie is a 3-year-old who has had a relapse after 18 months of chemotherapy for leukaemia. You meet him in the emergency department because he has developed a severe cough and high fever. He is diagnosed as having pneumonia. "He's been sick for so long", his mother tells you. "We're all so tired and he's been through so much. How could he develop something else?"

CASE STUDY QUESTIONS

1. How could you best help Charlie's parents?
2. What would be important topics to talk to them about?

When children have acute illnesses, both they and their parents become frightened by the sudden onset and severity of symptoms. Because human beings have a great capacity for coping with stress, however, as long as they are given adequate support, they can usually adjust to the strain of disrupted daily routines, hospital visits and home care. When a child's illness becomes long-term or is one that is projected to have a terminal outcome, a family's capacity to cope can become stretched beyond its limits. Coordinated multi-disciplinary support is essential for such a family if it is to survive under this level of pressure and stress (Epelman, 2012; Nikkola et al., 2013).

People cope with situations depending on their perception of the event, the type and kind of support they receive from people around them, and the ways that they have found to be successful in coping with stressful situations in the past. When working with parents of a child with a long-term or terminal illness, discovering how the parents perceive the problem, what resources they have available and how they plan to use these resources are crucial in planning effective nursing care.

Whether the medical diagnosis involves a permanent impairment or impending death, parents' first response may be grief. The parents have either lost the "perfect" child imagined during pregnancy or the well child they had up to the time of diagnosis. Depending on their age and maturity, children may also experience a **grief response**.

THE CHILD WITH A LONG-TERM ILLNESS

Because families have different resources and everyone reacts to situations differently, each child with a long-term illness and the family need to be assessed for their potential to cope with the illness and provide necessary care. Through such assessment, appropriate interventions to help the family adapt can be started early in the course of the illness (Longden, 2011).

The parents' adjustment

Children have difficulty adjusting to stressful events without good role modelling from their parents. Therefore, an assessment begins with an examination of how well the parents are responding to the diagnosis of a long-term illness.

The grief response

Parents can be expected to experience a **grief process**, or the regulated steps in grieving, when they are told their child will be physically or cognitively challenged or is terminally ill. The most commonly accepted steps or stages of grief are those outlined by Kübler-Ross (1969). Table 56.1 summarises these stages. Many parents with a child who is

TABLE 56.1 The stages of grief

Stage	Parents' reaction	Description
1	Denial	Parents have difficulty realising what has occurred. They ask, "How could this have happened?"
2	Anger	Parents react to the injustice of being singled out this way. They say, "It isn't fair this is happening."
3	Bargaining	Parents attempt to work out a "deal" to buy their way out of the situation. They say, "If my child gets well, I'll devote the rest of my life to doing good."
4	Depression	Parents begin to face what is happening. They feel sad and unprotected.
5	Acceptance	Acceptance is being able to say, "Yes, this is happening, and it is all right it is happening." With a child who has a long-term illness, parents may never reach this stage but will always remain in the chronic sorrow of the depression stage.

Based on Kübler-Ross, E. (1969). *On Death and Dying*. New York: Macmillan.

physically or cognitively challenged never arrive at the final stage of acceptance or they spend years with chronic sorrow (also called **complicated grief**) (Whittingham et al., 2013). For parents with a terminally ill child, acceptance may come only with the child's death. Reaching a final stage may be particularly difficult when parents grieve in different ways or at different paces (Wender, 2012).

Factors influencing parental adjustment

Certain circumstances appear to increase parents' difficulty in adjusting to a disabling or long-term illness in their child. These include the degree and timing of the illness, the experience of the parents, the availability of support people and the ability to make long-term plans.

Degree of illness

The seriousness of an illness obviously affects the ability of parents to adjust (Eddy & Engel, 2008). A child who needs total care, for example, requires a much more radical readjustment of the parents' lives than a child who only needs additional speech therapy for an hour a day. In most instances, the parents' perception of the child's illness is as important as the child's condition itself (see Fig. 56.1).

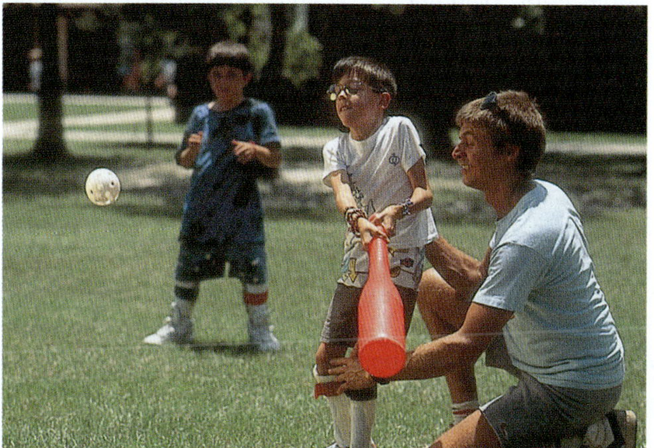

FIGURE 56.1 A parent's perception of a child's disability is important to how well the family adjusts. Often it is easier to accept an impairment that allows for greater functioning in everyday activities. (© Bachman/Science Source/Photo Researchers.)

Whether an illness is noticeable (spastic cerebral palsy) or not noticeable (controlled seizures) can also make a difference to how parents adjust. A mother who takes her child with cerebral palsy shopping (a child who walks unsteadily and knocks over a display) may hear other shoppers say, "Wouldn't you think a mother would watch her child more carefully?" On days that her child uses a wheelchair, however, shoppers' comments are more apt to be, "Poor little thing. Isn't it wonderful that his mother brings him shopping with her?" She is happy to have a signal (the wheelchair) that announces that her child is different and cannot be held to the same standards as other children. Other parents might be more grateful that a child's illness is not a visible one: it makes the illness seem lesser in extent and therefore easier for them to accept.

Onset of the illness

Whether a condition is apparent at birth (such as a myelomeningocele) or occurs at a later time (following an accident) may make a difference in the parents' ability to adjust. For some parents, never having had a well child can make the child's illness easier to accept. In any event, the need for long-term care of a child can totally change the parents' lifestyle.

Availability of support people

A family that has few close friends and lives some distance from relatives is apt to have more difficulty adjusting to illness in a child than a family which has close support people. People who have secondary support systems in the community, such as an organisation for parents of children who are physically or cognitively challenged or a local church or synagogue, usually do better than parents who are without these resources. People who are able to use healthcare resources effectively adjust more easily than those who cannot do so. The ability to use healthcare resources depends on several factors, including:

1. Transportation
2. Language barriers
3. Past experience with healthcare providers.

TABLE 56.2 Factors that ease parental adjustment to a child's long-term illness

Factor	Rationale
Support people are available.	Caring for a child is a series of crises during which support people become very important.
A strong marital bond exists between the parents.	A marriage partner can serve as the strongest support person.
A good relationship exists between the child's parents and their parents.	The parents (because they had good care) have a firm sense of trust and the ability to give care to another.
The child is other than the first-born.	The parents have had practice parenting.
The family lives close to shopping, schools and transportation.	The family is not isolated.
The family has a strong religious faith.	Secondary support systems are important in times of stress.
The parents are told of the child's disability as soon as possible.	A disability is easier to accept if the parents never thought of the child as totally well.

Life events

A child's illness usually appears to be more acute at times when the child would normally reach developmental milestones than at other times: at 12 months, for example, when the baby should be taking a first step; 5 years, when the child should begin school; time for learning to drive; or voting age. When the child does not reach these milestones, parents are reminded of the illness in a particularly painful way.

Factors that indicate that a family will probably be able to adjust to caring for a child with a long-term illness are summarised in Table 56.2.

✔ Checkpoint question 56.1

What factor is most apt to help parents accept long-term illness in their child?

a. The parents believe in alternative therapies and consequently have many options.
b. Both parents have a good relationship with their own parents.
c. The parents are wealthy, so are not distressed by the cost of the child's care.
d. The family is private, so they cannot compare their child's condition to other ill children.

The child's adjustment

A child's reaction to being physically or cognitively challenged or having a long-term illness is strongly influenced by the family's reaction to the illness. Family reactions may range from over-protectiveness to rejection. The child's adjustment may also be influenced by peers and other support people, such as school personnel or healthcare providers. Social exclusion, discrimination and physical barriers at school make it difficult for a child to adjust to a physical challenge or long-term illness. On the other hand, inclusion in school and social activities, acceptance by peers and support people and the ability to function as normally as possible help the child adjust.

A child's ability to cope is further influenced by personal attitude and temperament, self-concept, age and development, understanding of the condition and degree of the disorder. As the child grows and life situations change, the ability to cope may improve or worsen. For example, an adolescent who is physically challenged may become more optimistic about her condition because she is successfully working at her first job; another adolescent may become angered by his deteriorating condition because he is suddenly confined to a wheelchair. The degree of fatigue that a child experiences is also instrumental to how well a child adjusts to a chronic illness as chronic fatigue can play a large role, making even simple tasks seem monumental (Eddy & Cruz, 2007).

Siblings' adjustment

Siblings' reactions to a child with a long-term or life-limiting illness are influenced by individual circumstances; however, their chief reaction is most profoundly affected by the reactions and perceptions of the parents. Without counselling, siblings may react with jealousy, anger, hostility, resentment, competition, guilt or withdrawal. They may feel that they take second place to the child who needs more care. These reactions are common when parents focus most of their attention on the ill child, allow the health problem and its treatment to disrupt family life significantly, or grant the ill child special privileges and minimal discipline.

With counselling and appropriate support, however, siblings can develop acceptance, care, concern and cooperation (Vermaes et al., 2012). Such reactions are common when parents make it a point to set aside time each day for special activities with the well siblings such as playing a board game, walking in the park, teaching a child to swim, carefully explaining the condition and the necessity for special care, including siblings in the care of the ill child, providing siblings with respite from care if needed and establishing realistic rules for all family members.

At any one time, the siblings may experience a mixture of feelings. For example, if a boy's parents must take his sister for chemotherapy during his swimming carnival, the boy may feel both resentment that his parents missed the carnival and sadness that his sister could not also compete.

The nurse and the ill child

Caring for children with long-term illnesses can be a stressful role for nurses (Pontin & Lewis, 2008). To help the parents and child with a long-term illness, learn specific aspects of the child's condition and the possible complications that could occur. Over a period of years, parents become experts on the care of a child with a particular condition. This can make them grow frustrated with healthcare providers who appear to be unaware of things that they know well.

Developmental tasks

Children with long-term illnesses often do not meet developmental milestones on schedule; achieving developmental tasks can be difficult. The unique concerns of children who are physically or cognitively challenged and ways to help them achieve developmental tasks are discussed in Chapters 29 to 33. For healthcare providers, exposing them to usual events during a hospital stay or an ambulatory healthcare visit can help expand their world (see Fig. 56.2).

Education

Children with a long-term illness often need special education programs or at least separate hours of individualised instruction to achieve at school. Most children benefit from preschool programs; these programs offer them a head start on school adjustment and learning. Children with a long-term illness tend to miss school more often than do their healthier classmates because of healthcare visits and exacerbations of the illness. This can cause them to fall behind at school unless individualised plans to keep them with their school group are made.

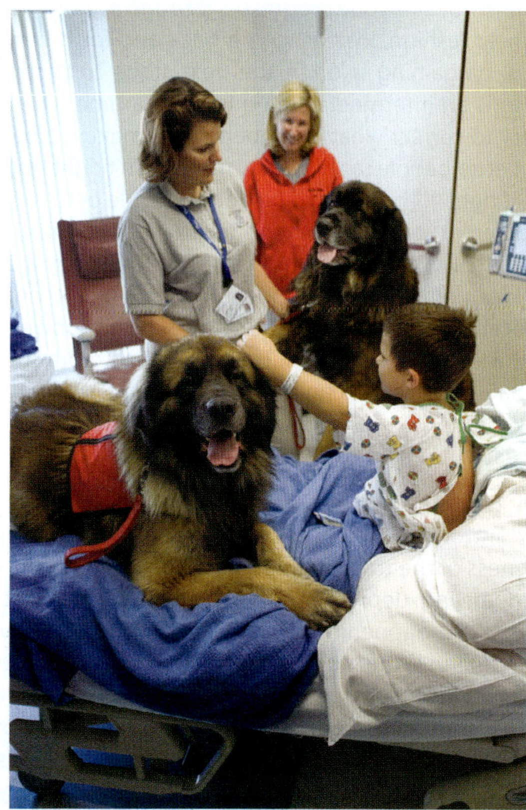

FIGURE 56.2 Therapy dogs can be helpful to keep children with long-term illnesses active and in touch with usual events. (© Marmaduke St John/Alamy.)

Home care

Most children with a long-term illness receive care at home today (Remke & Chrastek, 2007). Planning for home care is discussed in Chapter 4. Important aspects to consider include: the best school setting (home or away?); ways to involve the family in community activities; ways to include the child in a play group if possible (children as young as preschool age may not choose an ill child as a playmate unless urged to do so); how much self-care the child can achieve; and future plans, such as preparing a child for puberty or enrolling in university. Home care or community health nurses can be instrumental in planning this type of care (Peacock & Stanik-Hutt, 2013).

Many parents today seek complementary or alternative therapies for children with long-term illnesses.

> ***What if...***
>
> You arrange for Charlie's mother to spend an afternoon shopping so she can have some respite time away from her ill child, but she spends the time cleaning her kitchen cupboards instead? Would you consider this a good use of respite time?

THE CHILD WHO IS TERMINALLY ILL

Death comes suddenly to some families, such as when an adolescent commits suicide or is killed in a car accident, providing no time for parents to prepare for the death (Carr et al., 2012). Most people are brought up to accept the fact that elderly people die, but such people have also lived a long life. Most people can accept the death of middle-aged people with the same philosophy—they experienced at least a portion of their life. It is often more difficult to accept the death of children because they have had so little opportunity to live. This can make it difficult to work though feelings about a child's death (see Box 56.1).

Parental grief responses

The way that death is viewed and the manner in which people express grief differ greatly across cultures. Some people are very expressive with grief; some are very restrained. The way a child's body is handled after death also differs. Some religions, for example, forbid organ donations or transplants. Autopsies are not approved of because it is important that children be buried quickly after death. Cremation is not permitted. Being aware that

BOX 56.1 ✻ Focus on evidence-based practice

The death of a child

Helping parents survive the death of a child can be a challenging experience in nursing. To investigate what role parents wanted to most play in the care of their terminally ill children, researchers interviewed the parents of 18 children who had recently died in a paediatric intensive care unit. Results of the interviews revealed that parents most wanted to be able to continue to be "good parents" through such means as providing love, comfort and care; creating security and privacy for the family; and exercising responsibility for procedures or therapy that their child was receiving.

How might you use the results of this study to help parents whose child was nearing the end of life?

Source: McGraw, S. A., Truog, R. D., Solomon, M. Z. et al., (2012). "I was able to still be her Mom". Parenting at end of life in the PICU. *Pediatric Critical Care Medicine, 13*(6), e350–e356.

people have different expectations for final care and that grief is expressed differently by different cultures enables better understanding of parents' concerns and reactions during a child's terminal illness and when death occurs. Although reactions to learning that a child has a terminal illness are strongly culturally influenced, each family reacts in a unique way.

Denial

A parent's usual response to the diagnosis of a terminal illness in a child is denial. Although people are aware that children die, most proceed through life thinking, "It won't happen to my child". When they learn it may, they often respond with disbelief or denial.

How the parents handle this initial disbelief has a great deal to do with their relationship with healthcare personnel. If they have trusted healthcare personnel up to this point, they may be able to accept the diagnosis. Only after people can grasp that the illness is definitely present can they begin to accept that the disease will ultimately prove fatal.

During this stage of denial, parents' actions may be inappropriate to the child's condition. They may talk of an "upset stomach from the flu" when the child is vomiting blood or "his cold" when the child has cystic fibrosis. Denial can be seen as a temporary coping mechanism that is a necessary step on the way to acceptance.

Anger

Parents can be expected to become angry—a change from "Surely not me" to "It's not right that this is happening to me". When parents are angry about a diagnosis, they may be unable to direct their anger appropriately. They may find themselves angry with the child (scolding the child for crying during a painful procedure). One parent may be angry with the other parent (criticising the other for reckless driving or for eating a fattening food for lunch). They may direct their anger towards: doctors; nurses; x-ray, laboratory and dietary staff; or the entire healthcare system.

Parents' reaction will depend to a great extent on their experience with death in the past and the meaning this child has to them. Because grandparents live longer today, for some parents fatal illness in a child is their first contact with death. Another influential factor is that different children mean different things to parents. A child born to them at a happy time can represent all that is good and happy in their life, so loss of that child could also mean loss of all the joy the child represents.

When you ask grieving parents to talk, therefore, they may talk not about the child, but about how they felt when a parent died, how hard their job is for them or how they feel that their marriage is failing. This is part of grief: gathering resources, reworking stress from the past and arming themselves to face stress in the near future. Parents often receive support from other parents whose children are also terminally ill. They are helped by seeing parents of other children adjusting to approaching death—or, if not adjusting, at least functioning in what passes for a normal manner.

Bargaining

Although not everyone progresses through a grief response in a linear fashion, instead going back and forth between phases, bargaining is often the next stage to occur. Bargaining is an intermediate step in grief, a time when parents try to correct what is happening by making a bargain to be better people (a change from "This isn't right" to "I can make it right"). They vow to be better people or to function in a different way in exchange for their child's life. When parents realise that bargaining is ineffective, they are at a very low point: they have been let down not only by healthcare providers but also by the superior power with whom they tried to bargain. They may need more support after bargaining fails than at any other point.

Depression

When parents have passed through phases of denial, anger and bargaining, a further step occurs: developing awareness of the true meaning of what is happening, with accompanying depression. This is a change from "I can keep it from happening" to "It is happening". Behaviour such as crying is the most common sign that this stage has been reached. Parents may ask more questions about care, procedures or medications than before. Parents, for example, may ask why a child must have continuous dialysis not to criticise care, but because this is the first time they are fully aware of its serious implications.

Parents may work through the expected loss of a child by talking about their plans for the child or how the child was doing in school. They may suddenly shower the child with expensive gifts or trips. On the surface, this reaction appears to be a step backwards (they were accepting the diagnosis so well; now they seem demanding and overwhelmed by it). Actually, this is the first time they have actually begun to appreciate the diagnosis and what it means.

At about this time, parents need to think about preparing other children in the family for the death of the ill child. If the ill child is hospitalised and siblings have not been allowed to visit, they may feel excluded at not having been given a chance to be with their brother or sister.

Some siblings feel responsible for the death of the ill child. They may have wished the child dead, for example, so that they could have a room to themselves or so they could have the child's bicycle. They were told not to wrestle with the ill sibling and they did anyway. These children need reassurance that wishing for something does not make it come true and that the sibling's death is uncontrollable: it will happen no matter what they or their parents did or will do.

Acceptance

The acceptance stage of the grief process is resolution that the child will die (a change from "This is happening" to "It's all right that this is happening"). Few parents reach this point by the time of the child's death.

CASE STUDY QUESTION

3. Charlie's parents are starting to grieve because they fear he will not survive this recurrence of his illness. During which stage of grief do parents usually feel saddest?
   a. The first stage, because everything is such a shock
   b. The last stage, because they fully accept the death
   c. The fourth stage, as they realise death is happening
   d. The stage at which the child talks about death

Parental coping responses

Throughout the phases of the child's illness, parents are developing important coping mechanisms to see them through this crisis. They may have already learned to cope positively with their child's illness and treatment measures, but the determination that the illness is terminal requires yet another step. Promoting the development of positive coping strategies while being sensitive to the unique needs of each family member is an important aspect of care. It may be difficult to determine when a coping strategy is truly helpful and when it has become maladaptive. For instance, seeking information, such as surfing the Internet and asking to have medical library access, is generally a very useful strategy for parents with ill children: knowing what to expect reduces anxiety. Some parents, however, continue these seeking procedures past the point at which the information is helpful to them. They may believe that if they look hard enough, they'll discover a way to cure their child or they may "over-intellectualise" their child's illness and impending death to block feelings of sadness.

Problem-solving is always an effective coping strategy as long as the parents are realistic about which problems they can solve. Seeking the support of others, including healthcare providers and families with similar needs, is another positive strategy to encourage; providing the names of support groups or individual families (with their permission) who have gone through similar experiences can also be helpful. Nurses may also need to help parents who are not comfortable accepting the help of others to learn how to do so or simply learn how to feel comfortable expressing their feelings to others.

Assuring parents that their child will be kept comfortable and will not die in pain can be extremely comforting. Parents may also be able to cope by searching for the meaning of their child's impending death in philosophical, spiritual or religious terms. For these parents, body organ donation may be a meaningful way to give themselves some solace that their child will in some way continue to live and contribute to others.

Anticipatory grief

Parents who have some warning that death is expected may begin a preparatory or **anticipatory grief** phase in which they gradually incorporate the reality of their child's fate into their thoughts. Anticipatory mourning prepares parents for their child's death and spares them the abrupt, devastating, intolerable grief reaction that comes to parents whose child dies suddenly from trauma, such as a car accident or sudden infant death syndrome.

Although anticipatory grief does not shield parents from experiencing grief once their child has died, it can be a useful process for them. A danger of anticipatory grief is that a parent may reach the acceptance stage of the grief process too far in advance of the child's death. If this happens, parents may accept the child's death so thoroughly that they begin to treat the child as if the child has already died. They stop visiting, or when they do visit, spend most of their time visiting other children or talking to other parents. Whereas they once spent time comforting their child, now they may fail to rock or touch the child as much. They may clean out the child's room and throw out or give away toys. Gradually they are drawing back from emotional attachment, to shield themselves from the abrupt, stabbing pain that death will bring. Children need a great deal of support if this happens. For some parents, when the child actually dies, the event seems anticlimactic. They have anticipated death for so long that, when it does occur, they cannot believe that it has actually happened.

The vulnerable or fragile child syndrome

When anticipatory grief proceeds so effectively that parents begin to think of a child as already dead but then the child does not die, parents may find that their grief reaction was so complete that they are unable to reverse it; they cannot view the child as they did before. They begin to treat the child in a cold and unfeeling way, as if the child were not really there but actually did die. Such children are termed **vulnerable children** or fragile children (Green & Solnit, 1964). These children may develop behaviour problems as they grow older (acting-out behaviour such as temper tantrums, stealing at school, shoplifting as adolescents) as if to say, "Notice me! I'm not dead".

Children's reactions to impending death

Children's reactions to death are strongly influenced by their previous experiences and the family's attitudes towards death. If children have had little or no exposure to death, it can be a strange and frightening phenomenon. This often happens when children are reared without pets or older relatives, forbidden to visit a dying relative, excluded from the rites of death or discouraged from discussing the death of a loved one. To help ease the fear of death, encourage parents to maintain an open attitude, even if it is painful or uncomfortable. Children's reactions to death are also influenced by their stage of development and cognitive ability.

Infants and toddlers

Infants and toddlers are certainly too young to appreciate that their death is about to occur. If the person who cared for them dies, they experience deep loss and a void in their life. If such a loss interferes with the development of a sense of trust, its implications for the child's ability to achieve warm, close relationships could last a lifetime.

Preschoolers

Preschoolers usually learn about the concept of death when a pet dies or they discover a dead bird or mouse. They envision death as temporary, however, and appear to have little of adults' fear of it. This casualness towards death is sometimes interpreted as callousness. For example, the first response of a child who is told that his brother has just been killed in a car accident might be to ask if he can have his brother's toys. This happens because he thinks of his brother as being gone for only a short time, making this a chance to take advantage of his property. This concept is strengthened by children's cartoons, in which characters are frequently killed and then immediately revive and go on with the story.

Because preschoolers fear separation greatly, they are stunned by the death of a parent. If children grasp the concept that they are dying, their major worry might be that they will be alone and separated. These children may need someone to stay with them constantly to reassure them that they are not alone.

School-aged children

School-aged children begin to have additional experience with death, so their knowledge of it as a final measure increases. They may think of it, however, as something that happens only to adults. Some children's books deal only shallowly with the subject, although many books that deal specifically with death are available for children (see Box 56.2). As children near 8 or 9 years of age, they begin to appreciate that death is permanent. It is the same lonely feeling they experienced when their parents left them at camp or went away for a weekend, but this time the separation will be permanent.

Most children of school age are aware of what is happening to them when their disorder has a fatal prognosis. They may learn from other children receiving treatment ("Are you the kid who's dying?"), from their parents' strange responses to questions, or from overhearing snatches of conversation about reports or physical findings. Children, however, are accustomed to meeting new situations—starting school, visiting a museum for the first time, boarding an aeroplane for the first time—and they cope with these experiences very well, as long as they know that someone they care about will be there to support them. Dying can be viewed in this same light, as another new experience for them.

Many children associate death with sleep (perhaps that was the explanation they were given for a grandparent's death), so they may be afraid to fall asleep without someone near them. They may need the light left on to fall asleep because death is associated with darkness. They may need to have you sit with them while they fall asleep.

BOX 56.2 ✻ Books about death for children

Bradbury, M. T. (2004). *My Friend Christopher is Dead*. Frederick, MD: Publish America Incorporated.

Farrant, N. (2013). *After Iris*. New York: Dial Press.

Isherwood, S. & Isherwood, K. (2000). *Remembering Granddad*. London: Oxford Press.

Koppens, J. & van Lindenhuizen, E. (2013). *Goodbye, Fish*. New York: Clavis Publishing.

Millis, J. C. (2003). *Gentle Willow: A Story for Children about Dying*. Warminster, PA: Marco Publishers.

Spergel, H. & Stylou, G. (2013). *Cloud City: A Child's Journey through Bereavement*. Upper Montclair, NJ: Turn the Page Publishing.

Varley, S. (2013). *Badger's Parting Gifts*. Atlanta, GA: Andersen.

Adolescents

Although adolescents have an adult concept of death, they also may feel immune to death. Risky activities such as driving at high speeds reflect this judgement. They may deny symptoms for longer than usual because they believe it is impossible that anything serious could be happening to them. They appreciate time provided for discussion about how they view death and the ways they have contributed to their family even though they are dying young. Continuing to participate in typical activities helps them maintain a sense of control.

Environment for death

The environment in which children die can influence their acceptance and their family's acceptance of death.

The hospital

A few children who have a terminal illness need such a great deal of physical or specialised care (have a new tracheotomy, need lung ventilation) that they may remain in a hospital for care rather than at home.

The home

Today, most children with terminal illnesses are not kept in the hospital past the time when it is determined that therapy is no longer effective. Many families prefer that a child die at home, surrounded by family and familiar possessions, rather than in a hospital. Time spent talking about arrangements—such as who the parents should contact if the child suddenly becomes more ill than usual, how they will manage periodic check-ups or how they will purchase medicine or supplies—are important preparations for home care. Assess how the family will schedule time to have some leisure periods free so they can balance the care of the ill child in their lives.

Home care can be an extremely satisfying experience, both for a child who is dying and for the family, as long as safeguards exist for protecting the carers' health and for providing good care for the child. This is discussed further in Chapter 4.

The hospice

In 1967, St Christopher's Hospice in London opened as a facility for people who wanted to die in a homelike setting while still receiving skilled professional healthcare.

In a hospice, friends, family, and even younger children and pets are allowed unlimited visiting time. Children are invited to bring possessions with them that are important to them. The philosophy of hospice care is that death is an extension or part of life, not a separate entity; therefore, it can be accepted not with separate or awkward rituals, but with the same warm concern as other situations in everyday life. For many children, hospice care is furnished as part of home care, so that they are not separated from their families (Robert et al., 2012).

Preparation for a nursing role with dying children and their families

Caring for dying children can be an emotionally draining experience for healthcare providers as well as family members (Hogan, 2007).

Self-awareness

Before you can offer support to children in any circumstance, it helps to be aware of your own reactions and feelings.

Fear

Fear is a natural response to death because the phenomenon is new and strange. People who have never seen someone die are often afraid that the moment of death will be terrifying to watch. Death usually occurs gently, however, with body functioning gradually lessening until it stops in a pain-free, quiet manner. People who have been declared dead and were then resuscitated by heroic measures report that death was not frightening but involved a feeling of exceptional calm and comfort (Belanti et al., 2008).

Failure

Some healthcare professionals find themselves drawing back from caring for dying children because death symbolises failure to them. This can make children feel as if they have failed—they have not been able to keep their body from dying despite everyone's best efforts.

Grief

Nursing care is so intense that the relationship formed may be closer than you realise until a child is diagnosed as having a terminal illness or dies; only then do you experience the depth of the relationship. Because nurses develop such close bonds with terminally ill children, they may experience profound grief when a child dies or no longer requires their care.

Acceptance

The average person can reach a stage of acceptance in grief because people are subjected to few true losses in a lifetime. As a nurse on a unit where many terminally ill children come for care, you may find yourself facing loss or death repeatedly. Therefore, a stage of acceptance may never be reached. A carer who cannot reach a stage of acceptance is left in a stage of depression and has extreme difficulty functioning.

To achieve acceptance, you may need to modify what it is you are trying to accept. You cannot accept the unfairness of death in children, but you can accept your ability to offer care that gives death dignity and compassion.

> ***What if...***
>
> While caring for Charlie for an extended period, you notice yourself making poor judgements in your personal life such as not following through on projects or spontaneous buying? Could this be an expression of grief?

Caring for the dying child

A child may live for days, weeks or even months in a "dying phase". Attentive physical and emotional care is essential to a child maintaining a sense of security and positive self-esteem during this time. It is also essential to the grieving

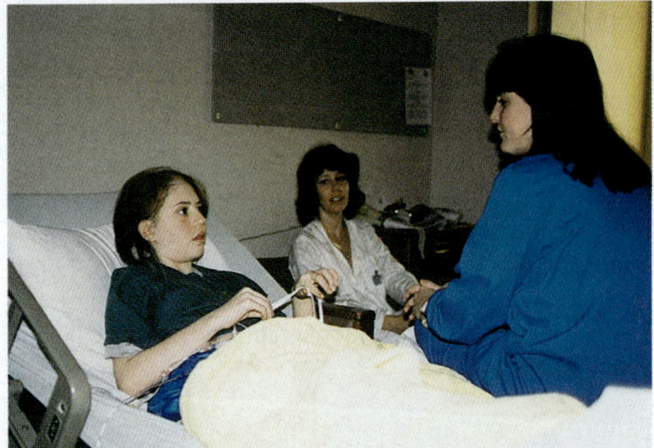

FIGURE 56.3 Good communication skills help build a trusting relationship, allowing a child to share feelings about being terminally ill. (© Caroline Brown, RNC, MS, DEd.)

process for both the child and the child's family. Frequent and substantive communication is a major part of providing this care. Children, like their parents, need the opportunity to talk about their fears and feelings about death. Practising good communication skills when providing any care, such as when administering pain relief, starting intravenous lines or providing basic comfort measures such as a bath, help to establish a trusting relationship with the child, making the child feel more comfortable about sharing feelings with you (see Fig. 56.3). Box 56.3 provides some specific guidelines about communicating with a child who is dying.

The child's family

For many children, terminal illness involves a series of hospital admissions interspersed with ambulatory care or home visits. Parents need time during these visits to talk about the problems they are having, not only with physical care (Should the child attend regular school? Could the child come on holidays? How many times a day are they supposed to give the child the immunosuppressant?) but also about how it feels to live with a child who is dying (How should they answer the child's or siblings' questions about dying?). Although many parents are reluctant to tell a child that they are dying, this is probably the soundest course once the child can see that their condition is deteriorating. There is often less anxiety in knowing what is happening than in hearing people whispering or spelling out words around you.

The onset of death

As death nears in children, physiological changes, such as slowed metabolism, decreased cell oxygenation and cell dysfunction, begin to occur, changing their appearance. Stroke volume of the heart decreases, so the power to circulate blood is reduced. The child's skin feels cool and may appear mottled or cyanotic because blood can no longer be pushed to distal sites. Just before death, blood begins to pool in dependent body parts, making them appear purple. Medications usually taken orally may need to be administered subcutaneously or intravenously to have an effect.

As peripheral circulation fails, less heat is lost from the body and the internal temperature rises. The child's body compensates for this by increased perspiration to increase heat loss through evaporation. This makes the child's skin feel cool and damp.

Slowed respirations lead to increased secretions in the lungs and the onset of rales, the sound of air being pulled through fluid in the alveoli. To compensate for a few minutes of very slow respirations, a child may take several quick or extremely deep inhalations periodically. Be certain the child's chest is not compressed so that the child has optimal lung expansion to do this.

A decrease in muscular function leads to severe weakness and fatigue. More and more, children maintain the exact position into which they are placed. As the throat muscles become lax, the possibility of aspiration increases.

As children grow closer and closer to death, they begin to demonstrate a lessened level of consciousness, although

BOX 56.3 * Approaches to communicating with dying children

1. *Continue active conversation.* Children who are dying need to receive stimulation in as near normal a way as possible.
2. *Use moments of silence therapeutically.* Such moments occur normally just as speech occurs normally. Do not feel you have to chatter to fill quiet intervals.
3. *Use the words death and dying as appropriate in conversation.* Trying to avoid a word makes interchanges awkward. Statements such as, "These flowers are dying", "That's a dead-end job" or "I'm dying to try that" may make it acceptable for the child you are caring for to voice for the first time what is happening—"I'm dying, too; let me tell you about dead-ending".
4. *Preserve dying children's defences.* If they are using denial or bargaining, do not try to push them to the next step of grieving by confrontation. Children will move on to the next step when they are psychologically ready.
5. *Remember that many children assume that they will die at night.* Therefore, night is "owned" by the dying. A child may talk more freely at night about fears or an unfulfilled life ambition than during the day. Children may also be more frightened at night and enjoy having someone sit beside them until they fall asleep.
6. *Be supportive, not trite.* A statement such as "All of us are dying" is true but not helpful. A supportive statement such as, "This must be hard for you" is better.
7. *Be aware that not all people's beliefs are the same as yours.* A statement such as, "God works in mysterious ways" may explain death for you but can be of little comfort to a family who does not envision that as true. A statement such as, "I believe God made some children die early to teach us to appreciate life" may evoke an angry response such as, "Who could believe in a God like that?" rather than be comforting.

they may remain perfectly alert until seconds before death. Vision apparently blurs, because children tend to turn their head towards a light. Touch seems to remain intact, because they often quiet to a gentle stroking of the arm or shoulder; they grasp your hand meaningfully, as if touch is appreciated and felt. Hearing remains intact; continue to explain procedures to unconscious children as if they were conscious, because they undoubtedly do hear you. Never make any comment in their presence that you would not make if they were alert. Continue to use the same gentle touch and non-verbal communication motions, such as holding a hand or brushing hair from the forehead, as if children were fully conscious. They may be fully aware of your actions even though they can give no indication of it.

Digestion slows as total body metabolism slows. Constipation because of poor bowel tone and decreased peristaltic action will occur. The abdomen may become distended from intestinal flatus. Mouth dryness will lead to cracking and secondary infection and pain; prevent this by frequent cleaning of the mucus membrane with clear water and applications of a lubricant to the lips.

Documentation of death

Defining when death occurs is controversial and involves both legal and ethical issues. Signs of death in a child not receiving ventilatory or mechanical assistance are the same as in adults:

- Absence of respirations
- No audible heart sounds by stethoscope
- No pulse by palpation
- No apparent blood pressure
- Absence of body movement or reflexes
- Dilated, fixed pupils.

Death is officially determined by unreceptivity and unresponsivity; no spontaneous muscular movement or breath; no reflex responses.

Organ donation

Parents may be asked by their doctor or by a specifically designated transplantation team before a child's death to grant permission for body organs to be transplanted into other children after death occurs (Brierley & Hasan, 2012). This is particularly important for liver and kidney transplants, because it is difficult to transplant adult-size organs into children. The donation of body organs may help parents accept their child's death more easily, because they can feel their child has helped another person live. However, donating their child's organs is not a practice for everyone (Siebelink et al., 2012).

Aftercare

Before beginning any aftercare for a child who has died in a healthcare facility or at home, check with family members to see if they want to spend a few minutes with the child or if there are any religious rites they want to complete before the body is transported to the morgue. Some parents need this time to comprehend that death has really occurred. Some people have special prayers they want to say; others want to say a final, private goodbye.

Remain in the room with the family in case they need your support, but be unobtrusive. Some parents fear touching a child's body after death, but touch is a strong and intimate communication technique that a family member may appreciate being shown how to use.

As a rule, crying is helpful for parents. You may need to tell them that it is all right to cry. On the other hand, do not interpret a lack of tears as a lack of feeling, because crying is not everyone's response to death. It is not unprofessional for nurses to cry when a child dies. A parent's warmest memory of a hospital experience may be that a nurse cried as she said goodbye to their child—the implication being that the child made an important impact on people other than family.

Autopsy permission

If a child's death is a result of homicide, suicide, death within 24 hours of a hospital admission, suspected harmful death, or death in an institution or home where the child was not under a doctor's care, an autopsy is required by law.

✓ Checkpoint question 56.2

Suppose parents are told their child will die, but then the child does not die. What is an unexpected consequence of anticipatory grieving?

a. It has no effect, because the child does not die.
b. It can disrupt the parent–child relationship.
c. It teaches the child that parents can be wrong.
d. It breaks parents' confidence in their religion.

Key points for review

- Factors that make it easier for parents to accept a long-term illness in a child include having support people present and being told about the child's condition as early as possible.
- Long-term illness in a child is often most difficult for parents to accept at times when the child would have been achieving specific milestones of development. Extra support for both the parents and the child may be necessary at these times.
- Help children to do as much care for themselves as possible within the limits of their illnesses. Self-care empowers them to be as independent as possible.
- Children are about 9 years old before they are able to understand the meaning of death and that it is permanent. A child and parents can be expected to move through the stages of grief (denial, anger, bargaining, depression and acceptance) on learning about a potentially fatal diagnosis.

- Children and parents are apt to need help to face a terminal diagnosis in a child. Urge the parents and the child to ask for help to see them through this very difficult time in their lives.

CASE STUDY QUESTIONS

4. Charlie's parents tell you that Charlie's disease has put them through a great deal of strain. What would be important topics to discuss with these parents?
5. Charlie's parents are both 50 years old and live on a farm; finances are tight and they have no health insurance. Two grown children have expressed resentment at their parents for spending so much time and money trying to find a cure for Charlie. What risk factors do this family have that might make adjusting to a child with a long-term illness more difficult than usual?
6. You notice Charlie's parents in the waiting room of the hospital comforting parents whose child was just hit by a car and killed instantly; you hear them say that losing a child suddenly is better than what they are experiencing. Why do you think these parents feel this way? What stage of grief could they be experiencing? How could you help them with their feelings?

Resources

For an extensive range of additional resources to enhance teaching and learning and to facilitate understanding of this chapter, please see the text's accompanying website located on thePoint at http://thepoint.lww.com.

References

Belanti, J., Perera, M. & Jagadheesan, K. (2008). Phenomenology of near-death experiences: A cross-cultural perspective. *Transcultural Psychiatry, 45*(1), 121–133.

Brierley, J. & Hasan, A. (2012). Aspects of deceased organ donation in paediatrics. *British Journal of Anaesthesia, 108* (Suppl. 1), i92–i95.

Carr, B. G., Nance, M. L., Branas, C. C., et al. (2012). Unintentional firearm death across the urban-rural landscape in the United States. *Journal of Trauma & Acute Care Surgery, 73*(4), 1006–1010.

Eddy, L. & Cruz, M. (2007).The relationship between fatigue and quality of life in children with chronic health problems: A systematic review. *JSPN: Journal for Specialists in Pediatric Nursing, 12*(2), 105–114.

Eddy, L. L. & Engel, J. M. (2008). The impact of child disability type on the family. *Rehabilitation Nursing, 33*(3), 98–103.

Epelman, C. L. (2012). End-of-life management in pediatric cancer. *Current Oncology Reports, 14*(2), 191–196.

Green, M. & Solnit, A. (1964). Reactions to the threatened loss of a child: A vulnerable child syndrome. *Pediatrics, 34*(6), 58.

Hogan, M. (2007). Children with severe chronic conditions increasingly dying at home instead of in the hospital. *Oncology Times, 29*(14), 47–48.

Kübler-Ross, E. (1969). *On Death and Dying.* New York: Macmillan.

Longden, J. V. (2011). Parental perceptions of end-of-life care on paediatric intensive care units: a literature review. *Nursing Critical Care, 16*(3), 131–139.

McGraw, S. A., Truog, R. D., Solomon, M. Z. et al., (2012). "I was able to still be her Mom" Parenting at end of life in the PICU. *Pediatric Critical Care Medicine, 13*(6), e350–e356.

Nikkola, I., Kaunonen, M. & Aho, A. L. (2013). Mother's experience of the support from a bereavement follow-up intervention after the death of a child. *Journal of Clinical Nursing, 22*(7–8), 1151–1162.

Peacock, J. & Stanik-Hutt, J. (2013). Translating best care practices to improve nursing documentation regarding pediatric patients dependent on home mechanical ventilation and tracheostomy tube support: a quality improvement initiative. *Home Healthcare Nurse, 31*(1), 10–17.

Pontin, D. & Lewis, M. (2008). Managing the caseload: A qualitative action research study exploring how community children's nurses deliver services to children living with life-limiting, life-threatening, and chronic conditions. *Journal for Specialists in Pediatric Nursing, 13*(1), 26–35.

Remke, S. S. & Chrastek, J. R. (2007). Hospice and palliative care. Improving care in the home for children with palliative care needs. *Home Healthcare Nurse, 25*(1), 45–53.

Robert, R., Zhukovsky, D. S., Mauricio, R., et al. (2012). Bereaved parents' perspectives on pediatric palliative care. *Journal of Social Work in End of Life & Palliative Care, 8*(4), 316–338.

Siebelink, M. J., Albers, M. J., Roodbol, P. F., et al. (2012). Children as donors: A national study to assess procurement of organs and tissues in pediatric intensive care units. *Transplant International, 25*(12), 1268–1274.

Vermaes, I. P., van Susante, A. M. & van Bakel, H. J. (2012). Psychological functioning of siblings in families of children with chronic health conditions: A meta-analysis. *Journal of Pediatric Psychology, 37*(2), 166–184.

Wender, E. (2012). Supporting the family after the death of a child. *Pediatrics, 130*(6), 1164–1169.

Whittingham, K., Wee, D., Sanders, M. R., et al. (2013). Predictors of psychological adjustment, experienced parenting burden and chronic sorrow symptoms in parents of children with cerebral palsy. *Child: Care, Health & Development, 39*(2), 366–373.

Suggested readings

Cant, R., Cooper, S., Chung, C., et al. (2012). The divided self: Near death experiences of resuscitated patients—A review of literature. *International Emergency Nursing, 20*(2), 88–93.

Cook, K. A., Mott, S., Lawrence, P., et al. (2012). Coping while caring for the dying child: Nurses' experiences in an acute care setting. *Journal of Pediatric Nursing, 27*(4), e11–e21.

Goldman, A. (Ed.) (2012). *Oxford Textbook of Palliative Care for Children.* Oxford: Oxford University Press.

Kars, M. C., Grypdonck, M. H., & van Delden, J. J. (2011). Being a parent of a child with cancer throughout the end-of-life course. *Oncology Nursing Forum, 38*(4), E260–E271.

Kirk, S., Beatty, S., Callery, P., et al. (2012). Perceptions of effective self-care support for children and young people with long-term conditions. *Journal of Clinical Nursing, 21*(13–14), 1974–1987.

Lago, P. M., Nilson, C., Pedro Piva, J., et al. (2012). Nurses' participation in the end-of-life process in two paediatric intensive care units in Brazil. *International Journal of Palliative Nursing, 17*(6), 264–270.

Macconnell, G., Aston, M., Randel, P., et al. (2013). Nurses' experiences providing bereavement follow-up: An exploratory study using feminist poststructuralism. *Journal of Clinical Nursing, 22*(7–8), 1094–1102.

Palliative Care Australia. (2010). *Journeys: Palliative Care for Children and Teenagers* (2nd ed.), accessed 5 March 2015 <www.palliativecare.org.au/Portals/46/JOURNEYS/Journeys%202010%20full%20document.pdf>.

Price, J., Dornan, J. & Quail, L. (2012). Seeing is believing—Reducing misconceptions about children's hospice care through effective teaching with undergraduate nursing students. *Nurse Education in Practice.* Advance online publication.

Warnock, C., Siddall, J., Freeman, J., et al. (2013). Emerging nursing roles for late effects care for children and young adults with cancer. *European Journal of Oncology Nursing, 17*(2), 242–249.

Appendix A
Drug effects in pregnancy and breastfeeding

In Australia, drugs are classified according to poisons schedules which differ depending on the geographical area. Scheduling of drugs is regulated by jurisdictions; thus, each state or territory has a set of poisons schedules from 1 to 8 or 9.

Schedule 1 is intentionally left blank. Subsequent schedules consist of drugs or poisons of increasing potency, with a corresponding tightening of regulations governing their sale and use:

- Schedules 2 and 3 include therapeutic substances available without a prescription
- Schedule 4 consists of restricted substances, such as prescription drugs whose use must follow certain regulatory requirements
- Schedules 5 and 6 include domestic, industrial, agricultural and veterinary products
- Schedule 7 covers dangerous poisons whose sales are restricted because of their potency
- Schedule 8 consists of narcotic substances governed by many regulations because of their potential for addiction, dependence or both
- Schedule 9, used in certain states, covers prohibited poisons and drugs of abuse.

For further information on drug schedules, please see the website of the Australian Therapeutic Goods Administration (TGA) at <www.tga.gov.au/industry/scheduling.htm>. The TGA site includes information on the Australian categorisation system for prescribing medicines in pregnancy. For further information on this, please see the TGA site at <www.tga.gov.au/hp/medicines-pregnancy.htm>.

In New Zealand, the *Medicines Act* defines three classification categories: Prescription Medicine, Restricted Medicine and Pharmacy-only Medicine. For further information on medications in New Zealand, please see the website of the New Zealand Medicines and Medical Devices Safety Authority, Medsafe, at <www.medsafe.govt.nz/>. The site also features links to a wide range of information on medications in pregnancy, which may be found at <www.medsafe.govt.nz/search/query.asp>.

Drug effects in breastfeeding	
Women who are breastfeeding should ask their healthcare providers about the safety of any medicine or alternative therapy during breastfeeding.	
Adrenergics	Parenteral adrenalin is excreted in breast milk; the status of other adrenergic bronchodilators is not known. Albuterol (Proventil, Ventolin) has tumorigenic effects in animals; if considered necessary, breastfeeding should be discontinued. Oral drugs used as nasal decongestants (e.g. pseudoephedrine [Sudafed], others) are contraindicated in nursing mothers because of higher than usual risks to infants from sympathomimetic drugs.
Analgesics	Most non-steroidal anti-inflammatory drugs, such as ibuprofen (Motrin, Advil), are excreted in breast milk, and nursing is not recommended. However, occasional use of therapeutic doses is probably acceptable. Acetaminophen (Tylenol) is excreted in breast milk in low concentrations. No adverse effects have been reported, and it is probably the analgesic-antipyretic drug of choice for nursing mothers. Salicylates (e.g. aspirin) are excreted in breast milk in small amounts. Adverse effects on nursing infants have not been reported but are a potential risk. Narcotic analgesics such as meperidine (Demerol) are excreted in breast milk, but amounts may not be enough to cause adverse effects in the nursing infant. Some authorities recommend waiting 4 to 6 hours after a dose before nursing. Alfentanil (Alfenta) should probably not be given. Significant amounts have been found in breast milk 4 hours after a dose.
Angiotensin-converting enzyme (ACE) inhibitors	Captopril (Capoten) is excreted in breast milk, but effects on the infant are unknown. It is not known whether enalapril (Vasotec) or lisinopril (Prinivil, Zestril) is excreted in breast milk. In general, nursing is not recommended while taking these drugs. Anti-anginal agents (nitrates) safety for use in the nursing mother has not been established.
Anti-anxiety and sedative-hypnotic agents (benzodiazepines)	Diazepam (Valium) and other benzodiazepines should generally be avoided. They are excreted in breast milk and may cause lethargy and weight loss in the infant. The drugs and their metabolites may accumulate to toxic levels in neonates because of slow drug metabolism.

(*continued*)

Drug effects in breastfeeding *(Continued)*

Anti-arrhythmics	When these agents are required for a nursing mother, breastfeeding should generally be discontinued. Quinidine (Quinaglute), disopyramide (Norpace), and mexiletine (Mexitil) are excreted in breast milk; it is unknown whether procainamide (Pronestyl, Procan), lignocaine (Xylocaine), and flecainide (Tambocor) are excreted. Potential exists for serious adverse effects in infants.
Antibiotics	Read the labelling on all antibiotics, antifungals and antivirals to be certain they are safe for lactating women and infants. Examples of those commonly prescribed for women are: *Penicillins* which are excreted in breast milk in low concentrations and may cause diarrhoea, candidiasis or allergic responses in nursing infants. *Cephalosporins* are excreted in small amounts and may alter bowel flora, cause pharmacological effects and interfere with interpretation of culture reports with fever or infection. *Aztreonam* (Azactam) is excreted in small amounts; discontinuing breastfeeding temporarily is probably indicated. It is unknown whether imipenem/cilastatin (Primaxin) is excreted. The aminoglycosides netilmicin (Netromycin) and streptomycinare are excreted in small amounts. Because these drugs are nephrotoxic and ototoxic, the immature kidney function of neonates and infants should be considered. Tetracyclines are excreted in breast milk and should be avoided. Sulfonamides are excreted and generally contraindicated. They may cause kernicterus in the neonate and diarrhoea and skin rash in the nursing infant. Erythromycinis is excreted and may become concentrated in breast milk. No adverse effects on nursing infants have been reported. However, the potential exists for alteration in bowel flora, pharmacological effects and interference with fever workup. Nitrofurantoin (Macrodantin) is excreted in very small amounts. However, safety for use in nursing mothers has not been established and infants with glucose-6-phosphate dehydrogenase (G-6-PD) deficiency may be adversely affected. Clindamycin (Cleocin) is excreted. Breastfeeding is probably best discontinued if the drug is necessary, to avoid potential problems in the infant. Cinoxacin (Cinobac) and norfloxacin (Noroxin) are probably excreted, and there is a potential for severe adverse effects in nursing infants. Depending on the mother's need for the drug, either the drug or breastfeeding should be discontinued. Isoniazid (INH) and rifampin (Rifadin) are excreted in breast milk, and nursing infants should be observed for adverse drug effects. Trimethoprim (Proloprim, Bactrim) is excreted and may interfere with folic acid metabolism in the infant.
Anticholinergics	Atropine and others are excreted and may cause infant toxicity or decreased breast milk production. Safety for use is not established.
Anticoagulants	Heparin is not excreted in breast milk; warfarin (Coumadin) is excreted, but some evidence suggests no harm to the nursing infant. More data is needed, and heparin is preferred if anticoagulant therapy is required.
Anticonvulsants	Phenytoin (Dilantin) and other hydantoins are excreted and may cause serious adverse effects in nursing infants. The drug or breastfeeding should be discontinued. Phenobarbitone is excreted in small amounts and may cause drowsiness in the infant.
Antidepressants	Tricyclic antidepressants such as amitriptyline (Elavil) and others are excreted in small amounts; effects on nursing infants are not known. Other antidepressants have not been established as safe for use.
Antidiabetic drugs	Insulin does not enter breast milk and is not known to affect the nursing infant. However, insulin requirements of the mother may be decreased while breastfeeding. Oral agents chlorpropamide (Diabinese) and tolbutamide (Orinase) are excreted in breast milk; the status of other sulfonylureas is unknown. There is a potential for hypoglycaemia in nursing infants.
Antidiarrhoeals	Diphenoxylate (Lomotil) and loperamide (Imodium) should be used cautiously during lactation; effects on the nursing infant are unknown.
Antiemetics	Although information is limited, most of the drugs (e.g. phenothiazines such as promethazine [Phenergan] and antihistamines such as dimenhydrinate [Dramamine]) are apparently excreted in breast milk and may cause drowsiness and possibly other effects in nursing infants. Antihistamines used for antiemetic effects also may inhibit lactation. Metoclopramide (Reglan) is excreted and concentrated in breast milk; it should be used cautiously, if at all.
Antihistamines	Histamine 1 receptor antagonists such as diphenhydramine (Benadryl) may inhibit lactation by their drying effects and may cause drowsiness in nursing infants. For most of the commonly used drugs, including over-the-counter allergy and cold remedies, little information is available about excretion in breast milk or effects on nursing infants. Histamine 2 receptor antagonists such as cimetidine (Tagamet) and ranitidine (Zantac) are excreted in breast milk. Famotidine (Pepcid) is excreted in animals, but it is not known whether it is excreted in human breast milk. It is generally recommended that either the drug or nursing be discontinued.

Drug effects in breastfeeding *(Continued)*	
Antihypertensives	Beta-adrenergic blocking agents should generally be avoided by nursing mothers. Propranolol (Inderal) and metoprolol (Lopressor) are excreted in low concentrations; acebutolol (Sectral) and its major metabolite are excreted; it is unknown whether nadolol (Corgard) and timolol (Blocadren) are excreted. Methyldopa (Aldomet) is excreted; effects on nursing infants are unknown. It is unknown whether hydralazine (Apresoline) is excreted; safety for use is not established. Captopril (Capoten), clonidine (Catapres), guanabenz (Wytensin), and guanfacine (Tenex) are not generally recommended, because information about effects on nursing infants is limited. Calcium channel blocking drugs should not be given to nursing mothers. Verapamil (Calan) and diltiazem (Cardizem) are excreted in breast milk.
Antimanic agent	Lithium is excreted in breast milk and reaches about 40% of the mother's serum level. Infant serum and milk levels are about equal. If the drug is required, nursing should be discontinued.
Antipsychotic drugs	Little information is available considering the extensive use of these drugs. Chlorpromazine (Thorazine) and haloperidol (Haldol) have been detected in breast milk in small amounts. Safety has not been established.
Antithyroid drugs	Nursing is contraindicated for clients on the antithyroid drugs propylthiouracil and methimazole (Tapazole).
Beta-adrenergic blocking agents	See Antihypertensives.
Bronchodilators (Xanthine)	Theophylline (Theo-Dur) enters breast milk readily; use with caution.
Calcium channel blocking agents	See Antihypertensives.
Corticosteroids	Prednisone (Deltasone), dexamethasone (Decadron) and others appear in breast milk and could suppress growth, interfere with endogenous corticosteroid production or cause other adverse effects in nursing infants. Advise mothers taking pharmacological doses not to breastfeed.
Digitalis	Digoxin (Lanoxin) is excreted. However, infants receive very small amounts, and no adverse effects have been reported.
Diuretics	If diuretic drug therapy is required, nursing mothers should discontinue breastfeeding. Thiazide diuretics such as hydrochlorothiazide (HydroDIURIL) and the loop diuretic furosemide (Lasix) are excreted in breast milk. It is unknown whether bumetanide (Bumex) and ethacrynic acid (Edecrin) are excreted. Little information is available about potassium-sparing diuretics, such as amiloride (Midamor), triamterene (Dyrenium, Dyazide, Maxide) and spironolactone (Aldactone). They are not recommended for use.
Laxatives	Cascara sagradais is excreted in breast milk and may cause diarrhoea in the nursing infant. It is not known whether docusate (Colace) is excreted.
Non-steroidal anti-inflammatory drugs	See Analgesics.
Thyroid hormones	Small amounts are excreted in breast milk. The drugs are not associated with adverse effects on nursing infants but should be used with caution in nursing mothers.

References:

McKenna, L. & Lim, A. (2014). *Pharmacology for Nursing & Midwifery* (2nd ed.). Sydney: Lippincott Williams & Wilkins.

McKenna, L. & Mirkov, S. (Eds). (2014). *Australia New Zealand Nursing & Midwifery Drug Handbook* (7th ed.). Sydney: Lippincott Williams & Wilkins.

MIMS Australia, accessed on 12 June 2012, <www.mims.com.au>.

The Royal Women's Hospital. Breastfeeding: Best practice guidelines. (2004). Accessed 12 June 2012, <http://www.thewomens.org.au/uploads/downloads/HealthProfessionals/CPGs/BreastFeeding/Breastfeeding_Best_Practice_Guidelines_2004.pdf>.

Appendix B

Growth charts

Birth to 36 months: Boys
Length-for-age and Weight-for-age percentiles

NAME ____________________

RECORD # ____________

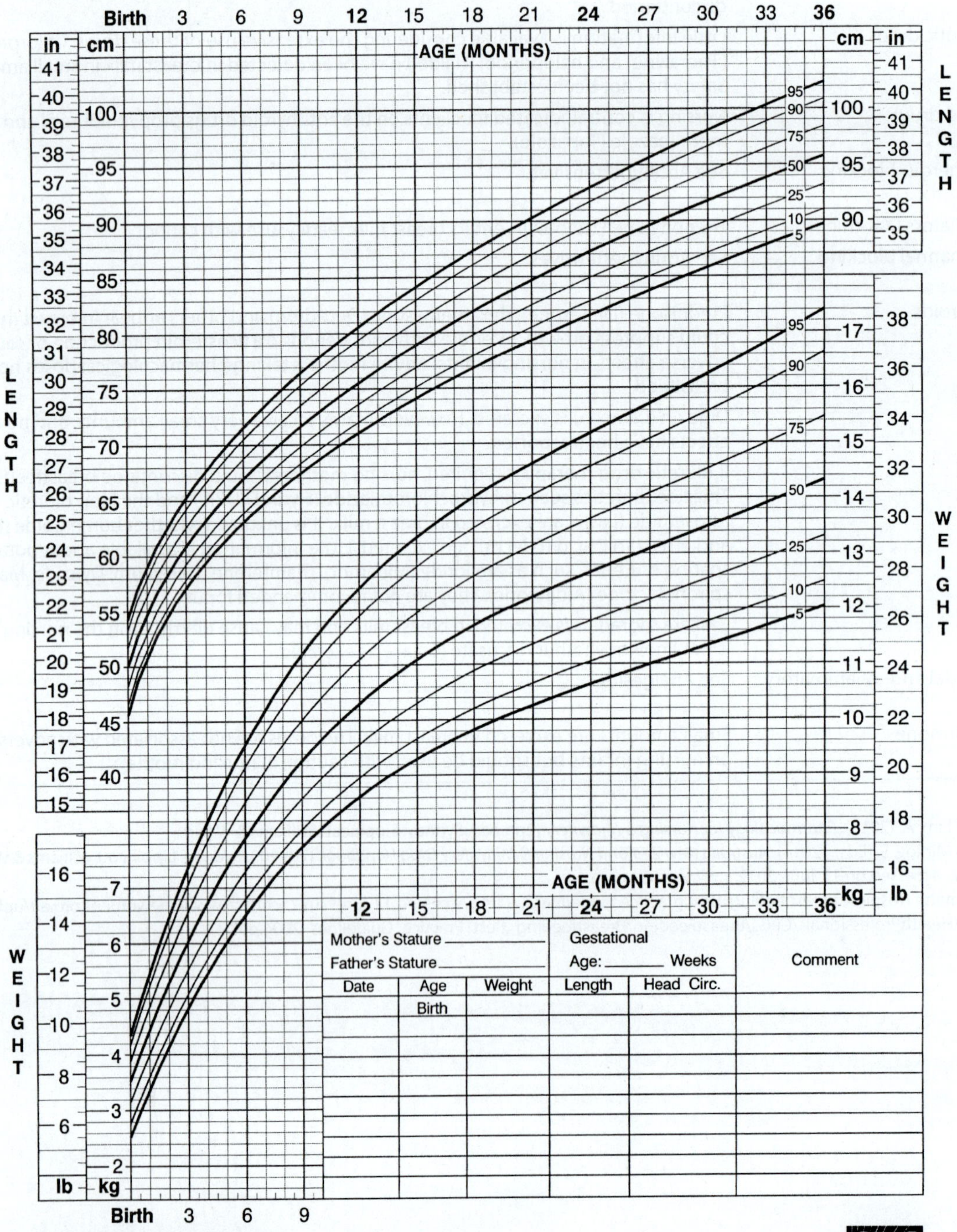

AGE (MONTHS)

Birth 3 6 9 12 15 18 21 24 27 30 33 36

LENGTH

WEIGHT

Mother's Stature ____________

Father's Stature ____________

Gestational Age: ______ Weeks

Comment

Date	Age	Weight	Length	Head Circ.
	Birth			

Published May 30, 2000 (modified 4/20/01).
SOURCE: Developed by the National Center for Health Statistics in collaboration with the National Center for Chronic Disease Prevention and Health Promotion (2000).
http://www.cdc.gov/growthcharts

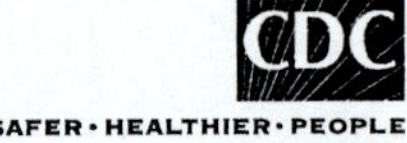

Birth to 36 months: Boys
Head circumference-for-age and Weight-for-length percentiles

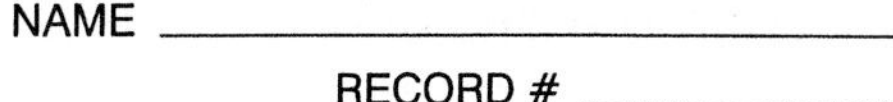

Birth 3 6 9 **12** 15 18 21 **24** 27 30 33 **36**

AGE (MONTHS)

HEAD CIRCUMFERENCE

in: 12 13 14 15 16 17 18 19 20

cm: 30 32 34 36 38 40 42 44 46 48 50 52

Percentiles: 95 90 75 50 25 10 5

WEIGHT

lb: 2 4 6 8 10 12 14 16 18 20 22 24 26 28 30 32 34 36 38 40 42 44 46 48 50

kg: 1 2 3 4 5 6 7 8 9 10 11 12 13 14 15 16 17 18 19 20 21 22

LENGTH

cm: 46 48 50 52 54 56 58 60 62 64 66 68 70 72 74 76 78 80 82 84 86 88 90 92 94 96 98 100

in: 18 19 20 21 22 23 24 26 27 28 29 30 31 32 33 34 35 36 37 38 39 40 41

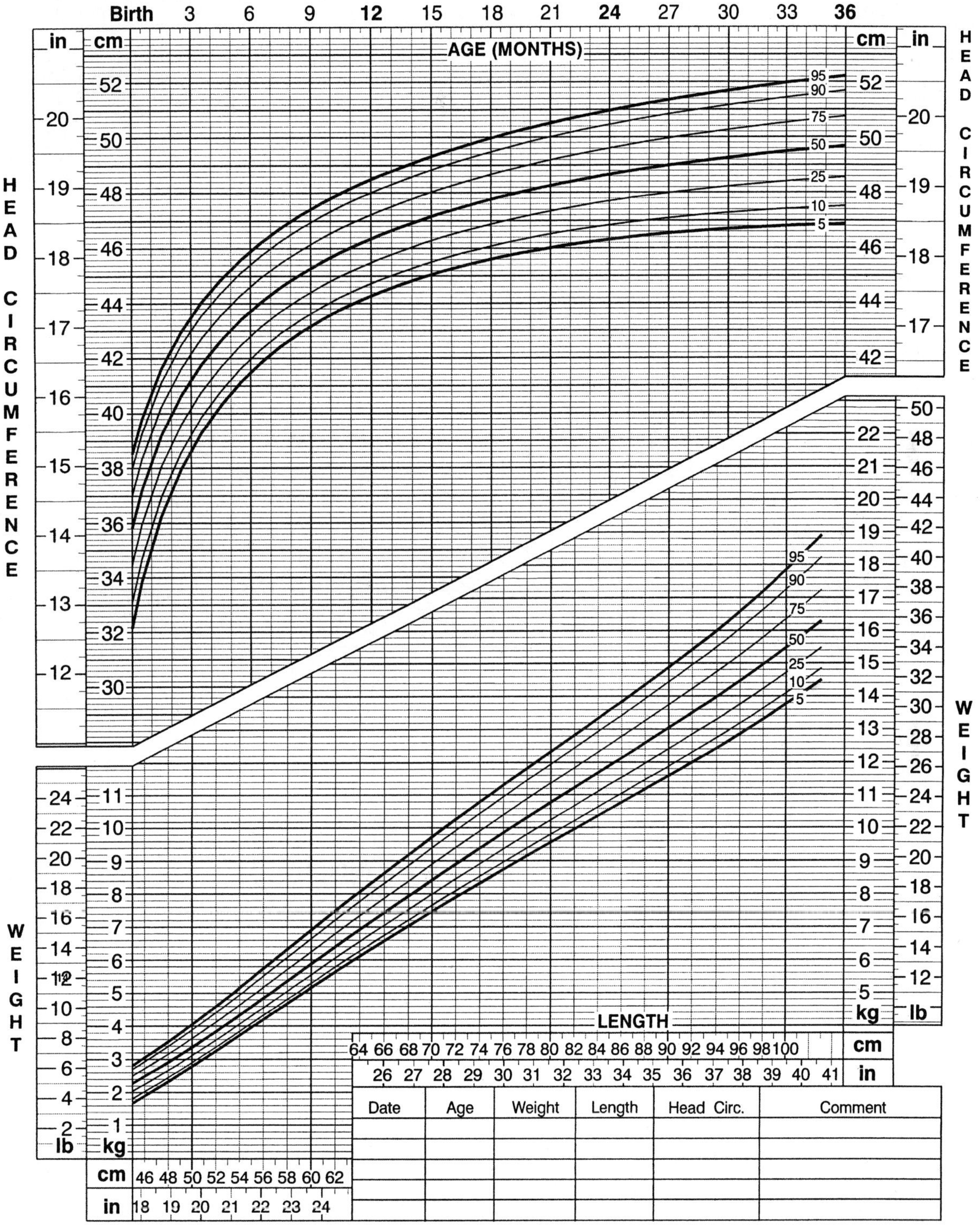

Date	Age	Weight	Length	Head Circ.	Comment

Published May 30, 2000 (modified 10/16/00).
SOURCE: Developed by the National Center for Health Statistics in collaboration with the National Center for Chronic Disease Prevention and Health Promotion (2000).
http://www.cdc.gov/growthcharts

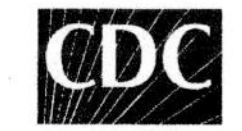

SAFER • HEALTHIER • PEOPLE™

Birth to 36 months: Girls
Length-for-age and Weight-for-age percentiles

NAME ______________________

RECORD # ______________

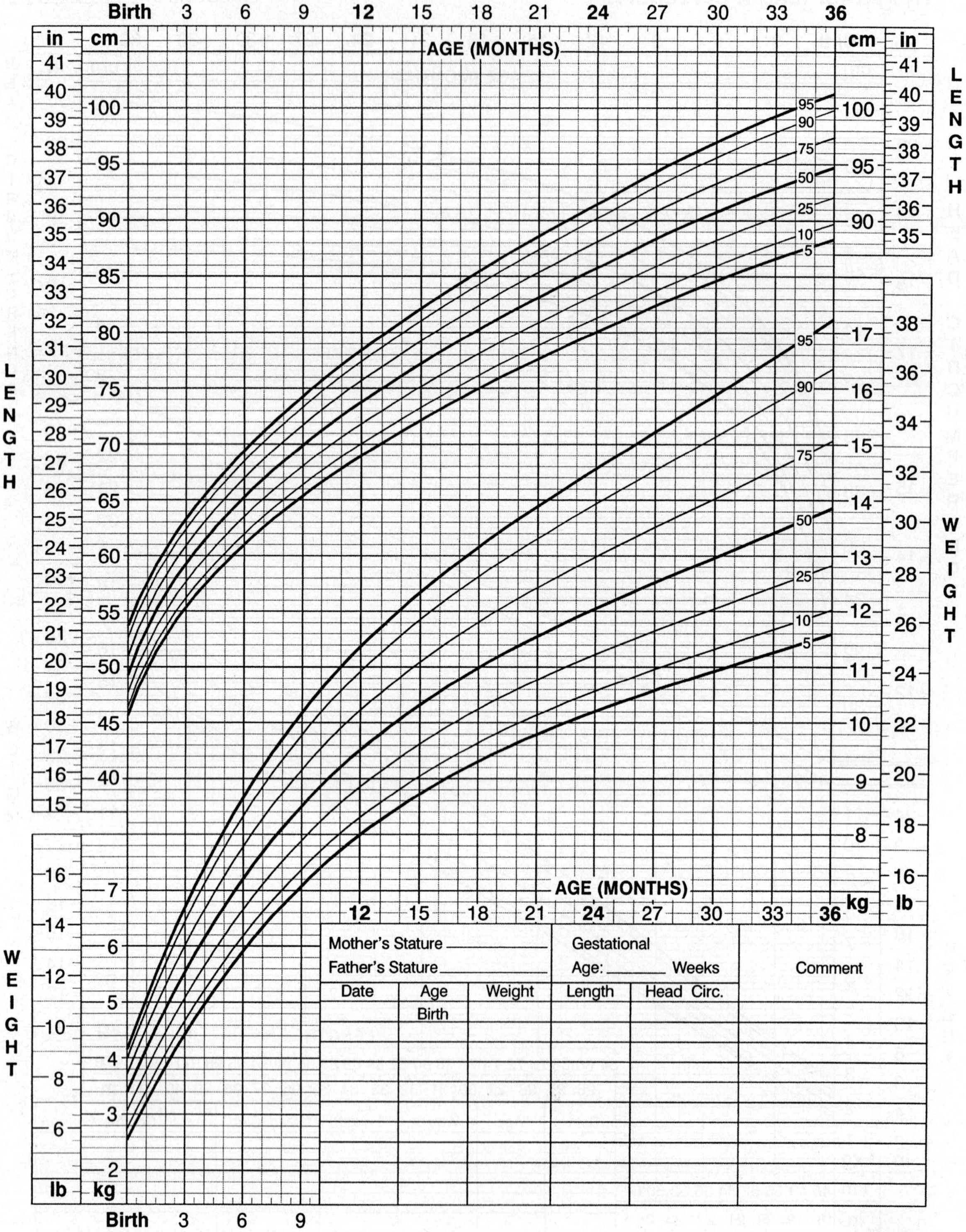

AGE (MONTHS)

Birth 3 6 9 12 15 18 21 24 27 30 33 36

LENGTH (in / cm)

WEIGHT (lb / kg)

Mother's Stature ________			Gestational		Comment
Father's Stature ________			Age: ______ Weeks		
Date	Age	Weight	Length	Head Circ.	
	Birth				

Published May 30, 2000 (modified 4/20/01).
SOURCE: Developed by the National Center for Health Statistics in collaboration with the National Center for Chronic Disease Prevention and Health Promotion (2000).
http://www.cdc.gov/growthcharts

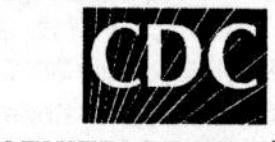

SAFER • HEALTHIER • PEOPLE™

Birth to 36 months: Girls
Head circumference-for-age and Weight-for-length percentiles

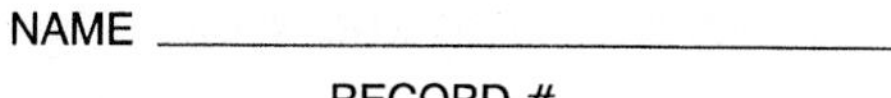

Birth 3 6 9 12 15 18 21 24 27 30 33 36

AGE (MONTHS)

HEAD CIRCUMFERENCE

in: 12 13 14 15 16 17 18 19 20

cm: 30 32 34 36 38 40 42 44 46 48 50 52

Percentiles: 95 90 75 50 25 10 5

WEIGHT

lb: 2 4 6 8 10 12 14 16 18 20 22 24 26 28 30 32 34 36 38 40 42 44 46 48 50

kg: 1 2 3 4 5 6 7 8 9 10 11 12 13 14 15 16 17 18 19 20 21 22

LENGTH

cm: 46 48 50 52 54 56 58 60 62 64 66 68 70 72 74 76 78 80 82 84 86 88 90 92 94 96 98 100

in: 18 19 20 21 22 23 24 26 27 28 29 30 31 32 33 34 35 36 37 38 39 40 41

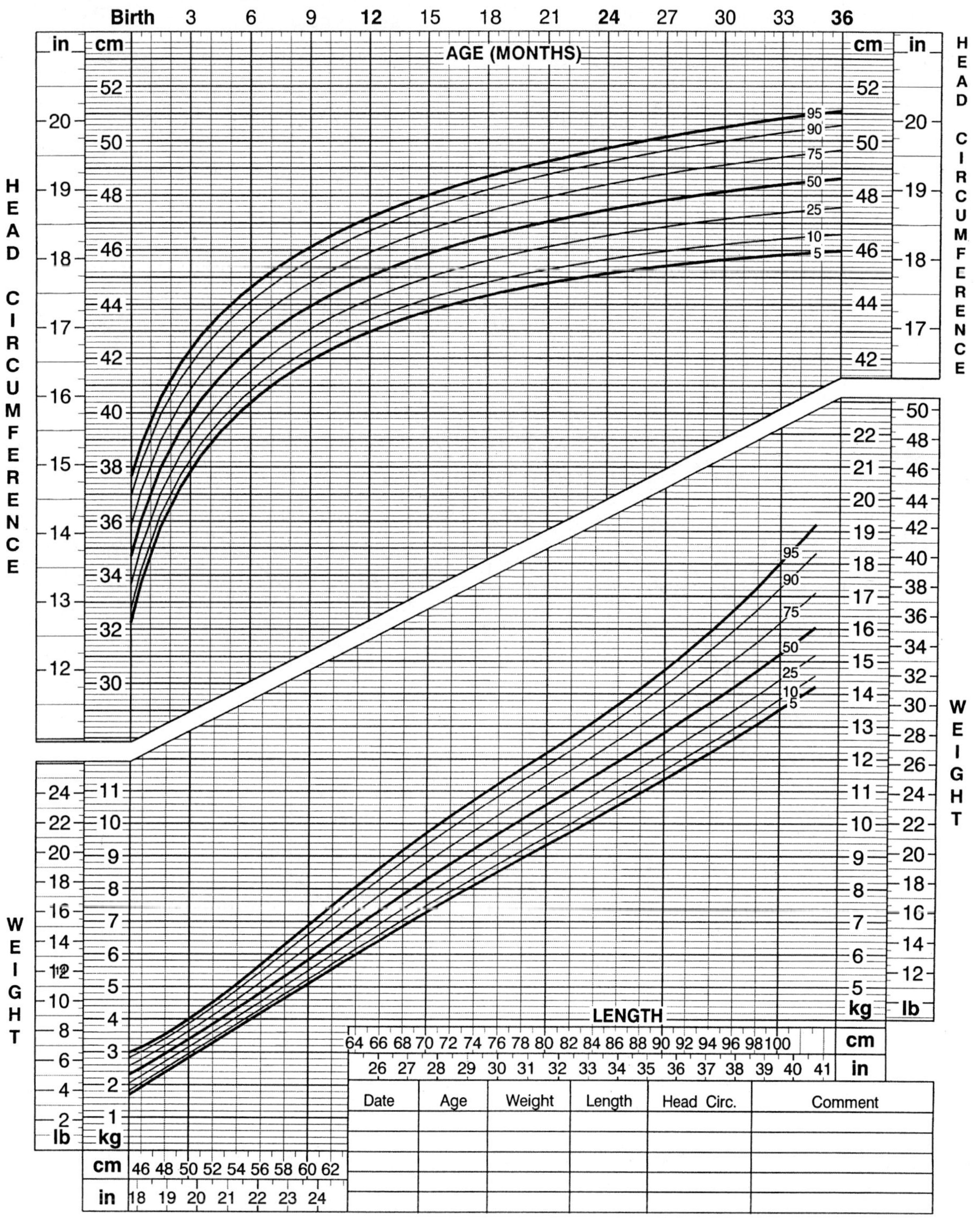

Date	Age	Weight	Length	Head Circ.	Comment

Published May 30, 2000 (modified 10/16/00).
SOURCE: Developed by the National Center for Health Statistics in collaboration with the National Center for Chronic Disease Prevention and Health Promotion (2000).
http://www.cdc.gov/growthcharts

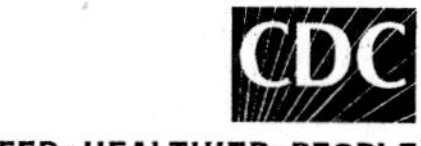

2 to 20 years: Boys
Stature-for-age and Weight-for-age percentiles

NAME ____________________

RECORD # ____________

Mother's Stature __________ Father's Stature __________

Date	Age	Weight	Stature	BMI*

***To Calculate BMI**: Weight (kg) ÷ Stature (cm) ÷ Stature (cm) x 10,000
or Weight (lb) ÷ Stature (in) ÷ Stature (in) x 703

AGE (YEARS)

STATURE

WEIGHT

Published May 30, 2000 (modified 11/21/00).
SOURCE: Developed by the National Center for Health Statistics in collaboration with the National Center for Chronic Disease Prevention and Health Promotion (2000).
http://www.cdc.gov/growthcharts

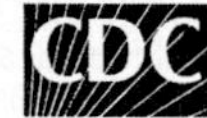

SAFER • HEALTHIER • PEOPLE

2 to 20 years: Boys
Body mass index-for-age percentiles

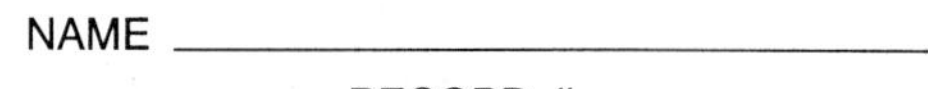
NAME ______________________

RECORD # ____________

Date	Age	Weight	Stature	BMI*	Comments

***To Calculate BMI**: Weight (kg) ÷ Stature (cm) ÷ Stature (cm) x 10,000
or Weight (lb) ÷ Stature (in) ÷ Stature (in) x 703

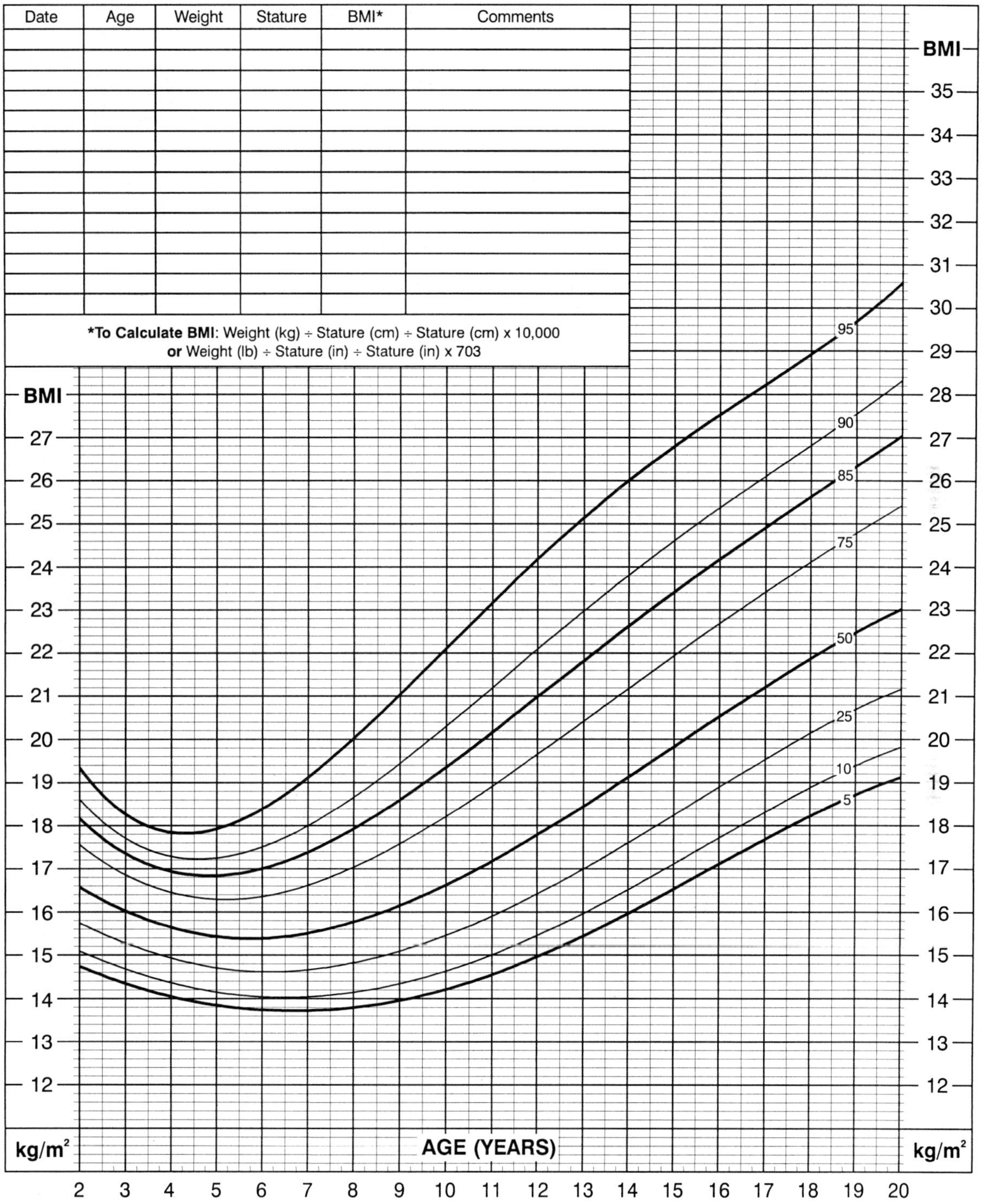

BMI

35 34 33 32 31 30 29 28 27 26 25 24 23 22 21 20 19 18 17 16 15 14 13 12

95 90 85 75 50 25 10 5

kg/m² AGE (YEARS) kg/m²

2 3 4 5 6 7 8 9 10 11 12 13 14 15 16 17 18 19 20

SOURCE: Developed by the National Center for Health Statistics in collaboration with
the National Center for Chronic Disease Prevention and Health Promotion (2000).
http://www.cdc.gov/growthcharts

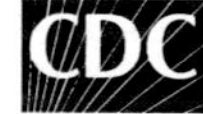

2 to 20 years: Girls
Stature-for-age and Weight-for-age percentiles

NAME ____________

RECORD # ____________

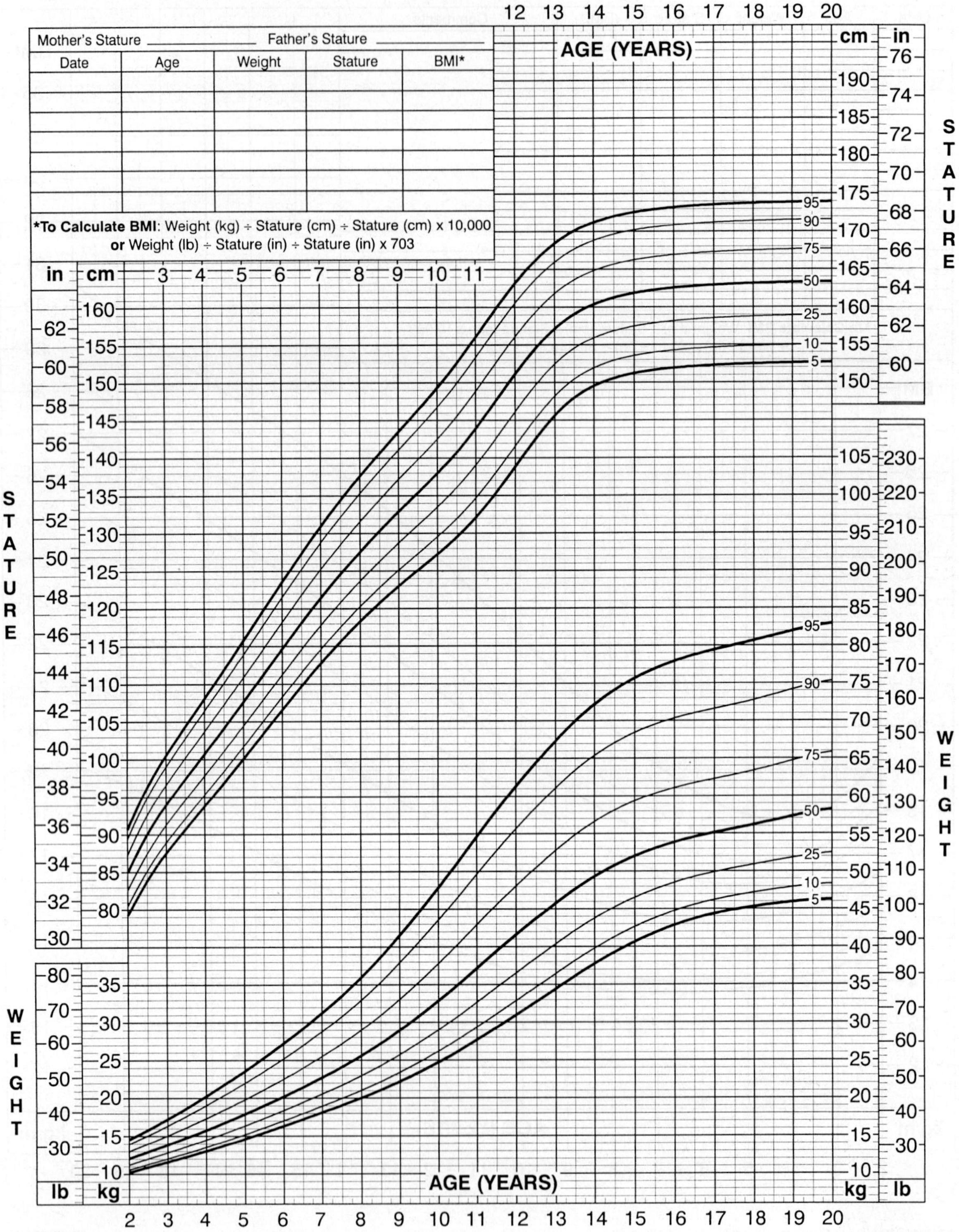

Mother's Stature ____________ Father's Stature ____________

Date	Age	Weight	Stature	BMI*

***To Calculate BMI**: Weight (kg) ÷ Stature (cm) ÷ Stature (cm) x 10,000
or Weight (lb) ÷ Stature (in) ÷ Stature (in) x 703

Revised and corrected November 21, 2000.
SOURCE: Developed by the National Center for Health Statistics in collaboration with the National Center for Chronic Disease Prevention and Health Promotion (2000).
http://www.cdc.gov/growthcharts

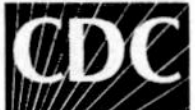

2 to 20 years: Girls
Body mass index-for-age percentiles

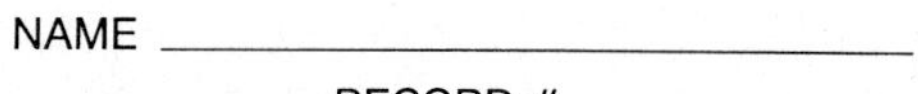

RECORD #

Date	Age	Weight	Stature	BMI*	Comments

***To Calculate BMI**: Weight (kg) ÷ Stature (cm) ÷ Stature (cm) x 10,000
or Weight (lb) ÷ Stature (in) ÷ Stature (in) x 703

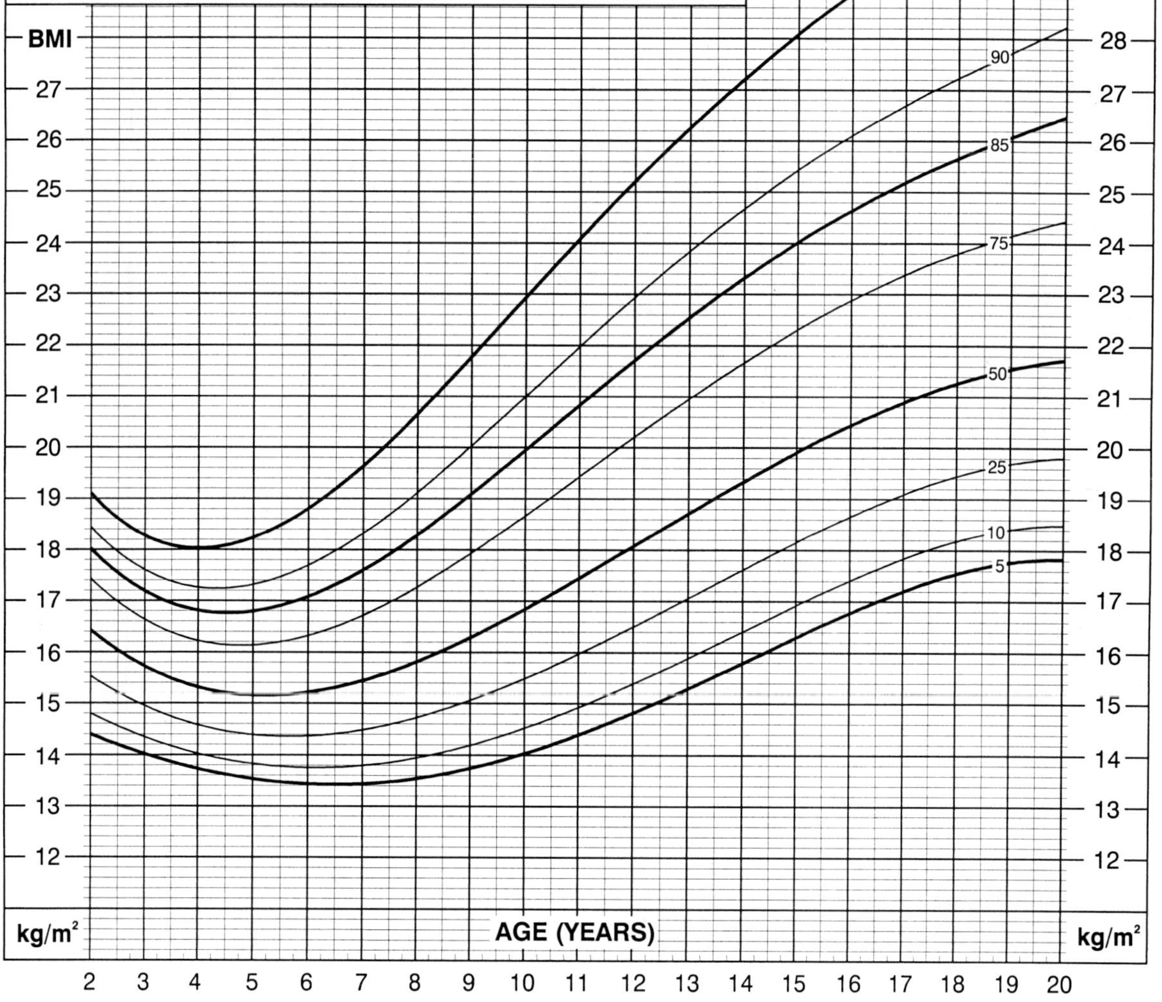

BMI
35
34
33
32
31
30
29
28
27
26
25
24
23
22
21
20
19
18
17
16
15
14
13
12
kg/m²

95
90
85
75
50
25
10
5

AGE (YEARS)
2 3 4 5 6 7 8 9 10 11 12 13 14 15 16 17 18 19 20

SOURCE: Developed by the National Center for Health Statistics in collaboration with the National Center for Chronic Disease Prevention and Health Promotion (2000).
http://www.cdc.gov/growthcharts

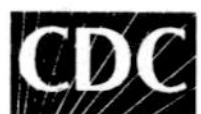

Appendix C

Denver II

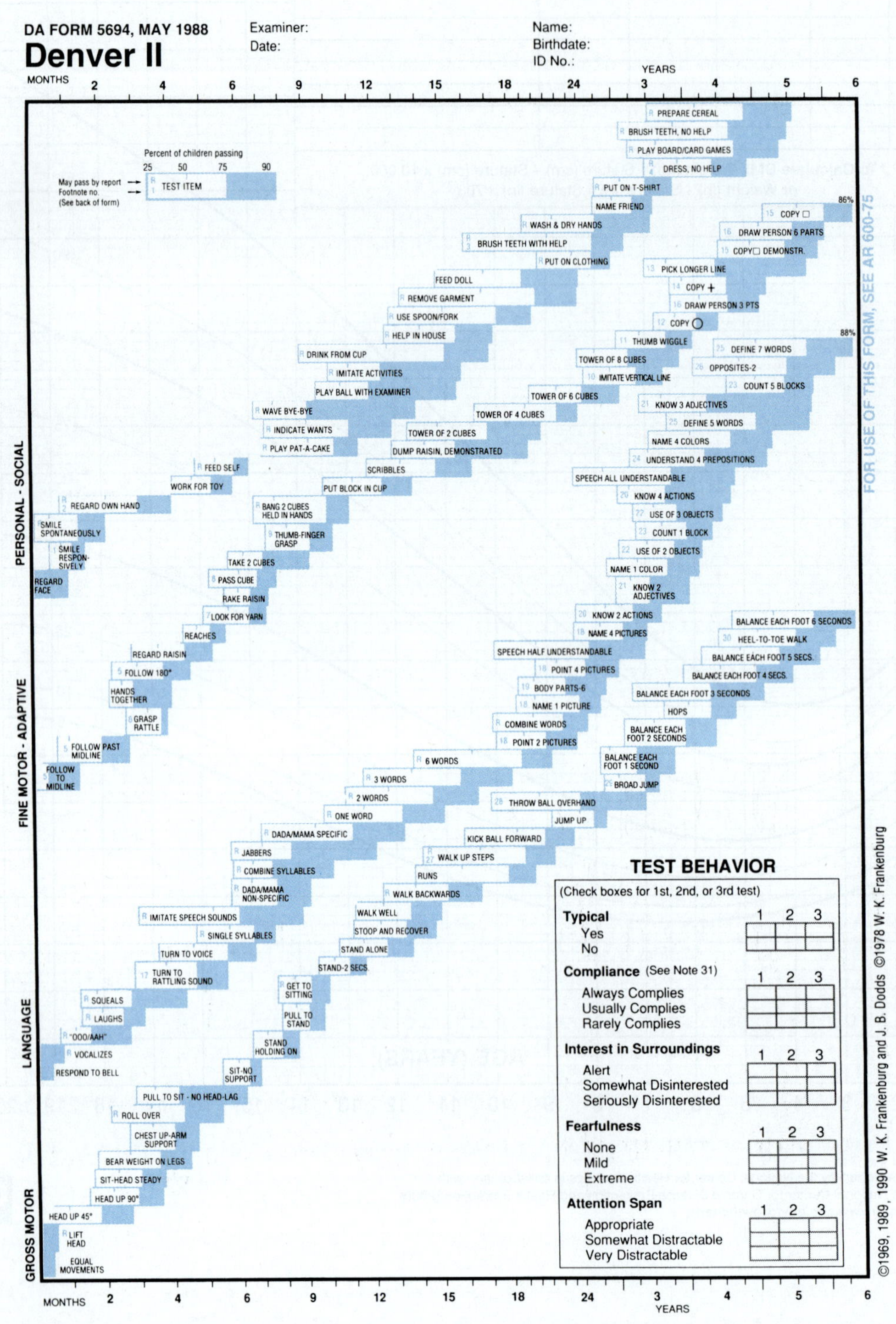

DIRECTIONS FOR ADMINISTRATION

1. Try to get child to smile by smiling, talking, or waving. Do not touch him/her.
2. Child must stare at hand several seconds.
3. Parent may help guide toothbrush and put toothpaste on brush.
4. Child does not have to be able to tie shoes or button/zip in the back.
5. Move yarn slowly in an arc from one side to the other, about 8" above child's face.
6. Pass if child grasps rattle when it is touched to the backs or tips of fingers.
7. Pass if child tries to see where yarn went. Yarn should be dropped quickly from sight from tester's hand without arm movement.
8. Child must transfer cube from hand to hand without help of body, mouth, or table.
9. Pass if child picks up raisin with any part of thumb and finger.
10. Line can vary only 30 degrees or less from tester's line.
11. Make a fist with thumb pointing upward and wiggle only the thumb. Pass if child imitates and does not move any fingers other than the thumb.

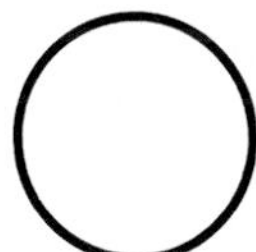

12. Pass any enclosed form. Fail continuous round motions.

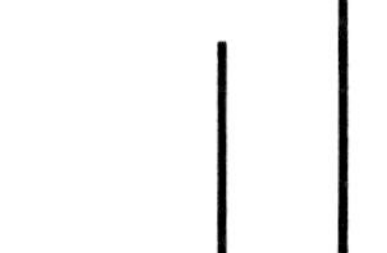

13. Which line is longer? (Not bigger.) Turn paper upside down and repeat. (pass 3 of 3 or 5 of 6)

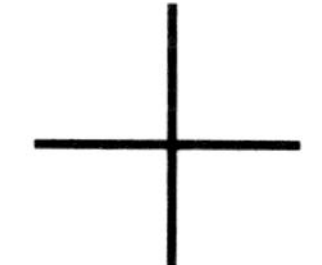

14. Pass any lines crossing near midpoint.

15. Have child copy first. If failed, demonstrate.

When giving items 12, 14, and 15, do not name the forms. Do not demonstrate 12 and 14.

16. When scoring, each pair (2 arms, 2 legs, etc.) counts as one part.
17. Place one cube in cup and shake gently near child's ear, but out of sight. Repeat for other ear.
18. Point to picture and have child name it. (No credit is given for sounds only.)
    If less than 4 pictures are named correctly, have child point to picture as each is named by tester.

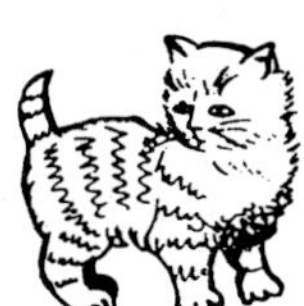

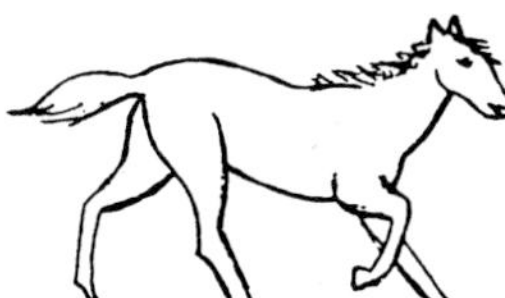

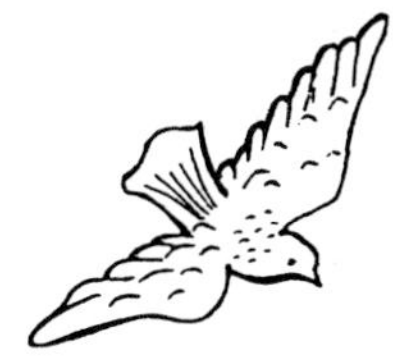

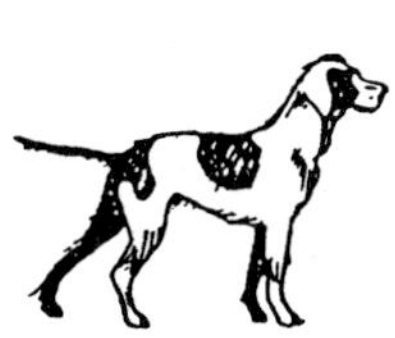

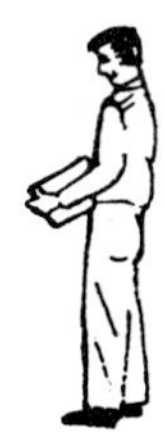

19. Using doll, tell child: Show me the nose, eyes, ears, mouth, hands, feet, tummy, hair. Pass 6 of 8.
20. Using pictures, ask child: Which one flies?... says meow?... talks?... barks?... gallops? Pass 2 of 5, 4 of 5.
21. Ask child: What do you do when you are cold?... tired?... hungry? Pass 2 of 3, 3 of 3.
22. Ask child: What do you do with a cup? What is a chair used for? What is a pencil used for?
    Action words must be included in answers.
23. Pass if child correctly places and says how many blocks are on paper. (1, 5).
24. Tell child: Put block **on** table; **under** table; **in front of** me, **behind** me. Pass 4 of 4.
    (Do not help child by pointing, moving head or eyes.)
25. Ask child: What is a ball?... lake?... desk?... house?... banana?... curtain?... fence?... ceiling? Pass if defined in terms of use, shape, what it is made of, or general category (such as banana is fruit, not just yellow). Pass 5 of 8, 7 of 8.
26. Ask child: If a horse is big, a mouse is __? If fire is hot, ice is __? If the sun shines during the day, the moon shines during the __? Pass 2 of 3.
27. Child may use wall or rail only, not person. May not crawl.
28. Child must throw ball overhand 3 feet to within arm's reach of tester.
29. Child must perform standing broad jump over width of test sheet (8 1/2 inches).
30. Tell child to walk forward, → heel within 1 inch of toe. Tester may demonstrate.
    Child must walk 4 consecutive steps.
31. In the second year, half of normal children are non-compliant.

OBSERVATIONS:

Appendix D

PEDS

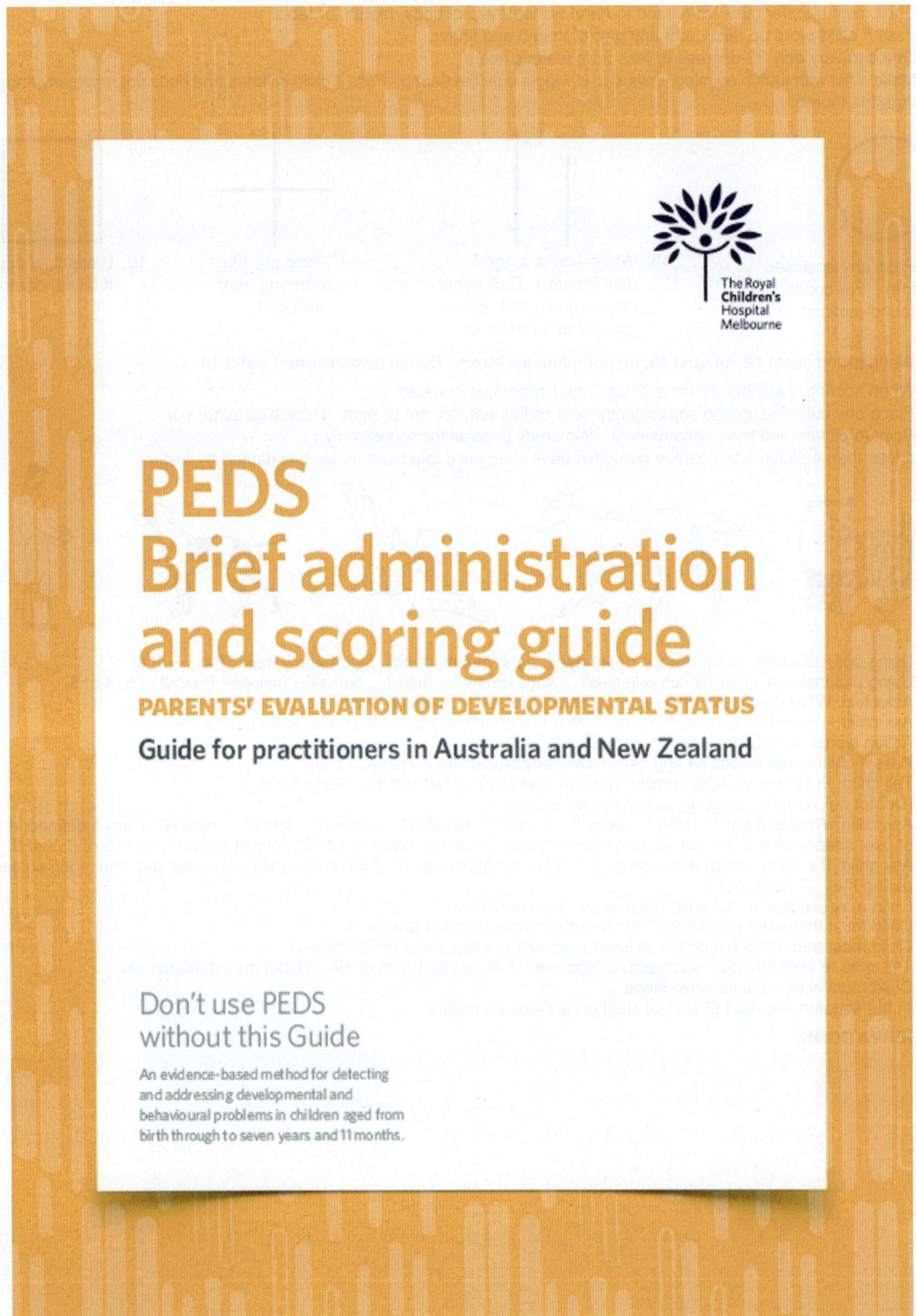

Parents' Evaluation of Developmental Status (PEDS)

Response form

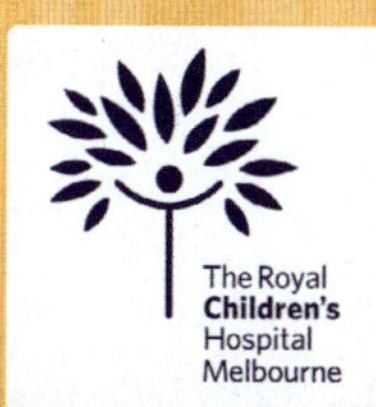

Child's name *Mohammed* Parent's name *Azhaar*

Child's date of birth *26 / 5 / 2013* Child's age Today's date *28 / 11 / 2014*

Please list any concerns about your child's learning, development and behaviour.

Do you have any concerns about how your child talks and makes speech sounds?

Select one: ☑ No ○ Yes ○ A little Comments:

Do you have any concerns about how your child understands what you say?

Select one: ○ No ○ Yes ☑ A little Comments:

Mohammed doesn't listen

Do you have any concerns about how your child uses his or her hands and fingers to do things?

Select one: ☑ No ○ Yes ○ A little Comments:

Do you have any concerns about how your child uses his or her arms and legs?

Select one: ☑ No ○ Yes ○ A little Comments:

Mohammed likes to run and climb

Do you have any concerns about how your child behaves?

Select one: ○ No ○ Yes ☑ A little Comments:

Mohammed can be naughty, runs away when I call him

Do you have any concerns about how your child gets along with others?

Select one: ☑ No ○ Yes ○ A little Comments:

Do you have any concerns about how your child is learning to do things for himself/herself?

Select one: ○ No ○ Yes ☑ A little Comments:

Mohammed took ages to walk

Do you have any concerns about how your child is learning preschool or school skills?

Select one: ☑ No ○ Yes ○ A little Comments:

Please list any other concerns.

Mohammed has had lots of ear infections

To re-order visit **www.peds.org.au** For PEDS training visit **www.learninghub.org.au**

ERC 150212 March 2015

Parents' Evaluation of Developmental Status (PEDS)

Score form

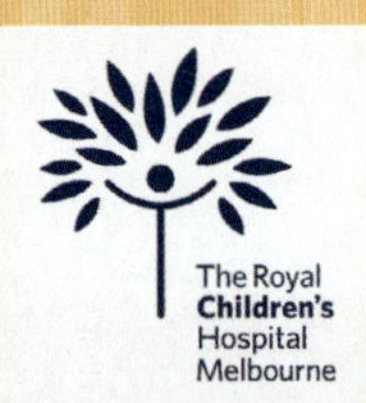

Child's name Mohammed

Child's date of birth 26/ 5 / 2013 **Today's date** 28 / 11 / 2014

You must refer to the PEDS Brief Administration and Scoring Guide in order to correctly administer, score and interpret PEDS.

Child's age in months	0-3	4-5	6-11	12-14	15-17	18-23	24-35	36-47	48-53	54-71	72-83	84-96
Global/cognitive	○	○	○	○	○	○	○	○	○	○	○	○
Expressive language and articulation	○	○	○	○	○	○	○	○	○	○	○	○
Receptive language	□	□	□	□	□	✔	○	Mohammed doesn't listen				○
Fine motor	□	□	□	□	□	□	□	□	□	○	○	○
Gross motor	□	□	□	□	□	✔	□	Took ages to walk				○
Behavior	□	□	□	□	□	✔	□	Can be naughty. Runs away when I call him.				□
Social-emotional	○	○	○	○	○	□	□	□	□	□	□	□
Self-help	□	□	□	□	□	□	□	□	□	□	□	□
School	□	□	□	□	□	□	□	□	□	○	○	○
Other	○	○	○	○	○	✔	○	Lots of ear infections				○

Count the number of small circles with checkmarks and place the total in the large circle below.

Child's age in months	0-3	4-5	6-11	12-14	15-17	18-23	24-35	36-47	48-53	54-71	72-83	84-96
	○	○	○	○	○	2	○	○	○	○	○	○

If the number shown in the large circle is 2 or more, follow **Path A** on the PEDS Interpretation Form. If the number shown is exactly 1, follow **Path B**. Then count the number of small boxes and place the total in the large box below.

Child's age in months	0-3	4-5	6-11	12-14	15-17	18-23	24-35	36-47	48-53	54-71	72-83	84-96
	□	□	□	□	□	2	□	□	□	□	□	□

If the number shown in the large box is 1 or more, also follow **Path C**. If the number 0 is shown, consider **Path D** if relevant. Otherwise, follow **Path E**.

To re-order visit **www.peds.org.au** For PEDS training visit **www.learninghub.org.au**

ERC 150212 March 2015

Parents' Evaluation of Developmental Status (PEDS)
Interpretation form

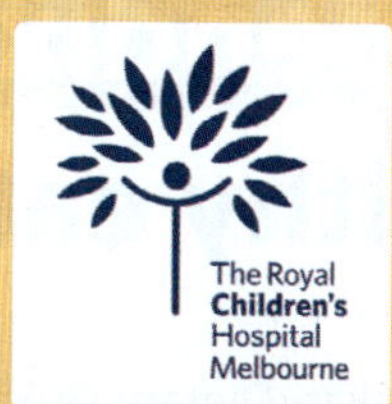

Child's name *Mohammed* Child's date of birth *26 / 5 / 2013*

Path A
Two or more predictive concerns? → Yes → Two or more concerns about self-help, social, school or receptive language skills?
- Yes → Refer for audiological and speech-language testing. Use professional judgement to decide if referrals are also needed for social work, occupational/physiotherapy, mental health services etc.
- No → Refer for intellectual and educational assessments. Use professional judgement to decide if speech-language, audiological, or other evaluations are also needed.

Path B
One predictive concern? → Yes → Health concerns only?
- Yes → Screen for health/sensory problems, consider second-stage developmental screen.
- No → Administer second-stage developmental screen.
  - If screen is passed, counsel in areas of concern and watch vigilantly.
  - If screen is failed, refer for testing in areas of difficulty.

Path C
Non-predictive concerns? → Yes → Counsel in areas of difficulty and follow up in several weeks. → If unsuccessful, screen for emotional/behavioral problems and refer as indicated. Otherwise refer for parent training, behavioral intervention etc.
If concerns still exist at age 4 ½ and older, refer for mental health services.

Path D
Parental difficulties communicating? → Yes → Foreign language a barrier?
- Yes → Use foreign language versions; send PEDS home in preparation for a second visit; seek an interpreter; or refer for screening elsewhere.
- No → Use a second screen that directly elicits children's skills or refer for screening elsewhere.

Path E
No concerns? → Yes → Elicit concerns at next checkpoint. → No → Use PEDS between checkpoints (eg sick or return visit).

Specific decisions

0-3 months	24-35 months
4-5 months	36-47 months
6-11 months	48-53 months
12-14 months	54-71 months
15-17 months	72-83 months
18-23 months *Pathways A and C. See notes re advice and referral option.*	84-96 months

Appendix E

Healthy eating for children

The Australian Dietary Guidelines provide advice on the amount and types of foods we need to eat to stay healthy. The guidelines of most relevance to children are:

- Guideline 1: Children and adolescents should eat sufficient nutritious foods to grow and develop normally. They should be physically active every day and their growth should be checked regularly.
- Guideline 2: Children should enjoy a wide variety of foods from these five food groups every day: vegetables and legumes/beans; fruit; grains; lean meats and poultry, fish, eggs, tofu, nuts and seeds; milk, yoghurt, cheese and their alternatives. Sample serving sizes are given in the table below.
- Guideline 3: Limit intake of foods containing saturated fats, added salt, added sugars and alcohol.
- Guideline 4: Encourage, support and promote breastfeeding.
- Guideline 5: Care for your food; prepare and store it safely.

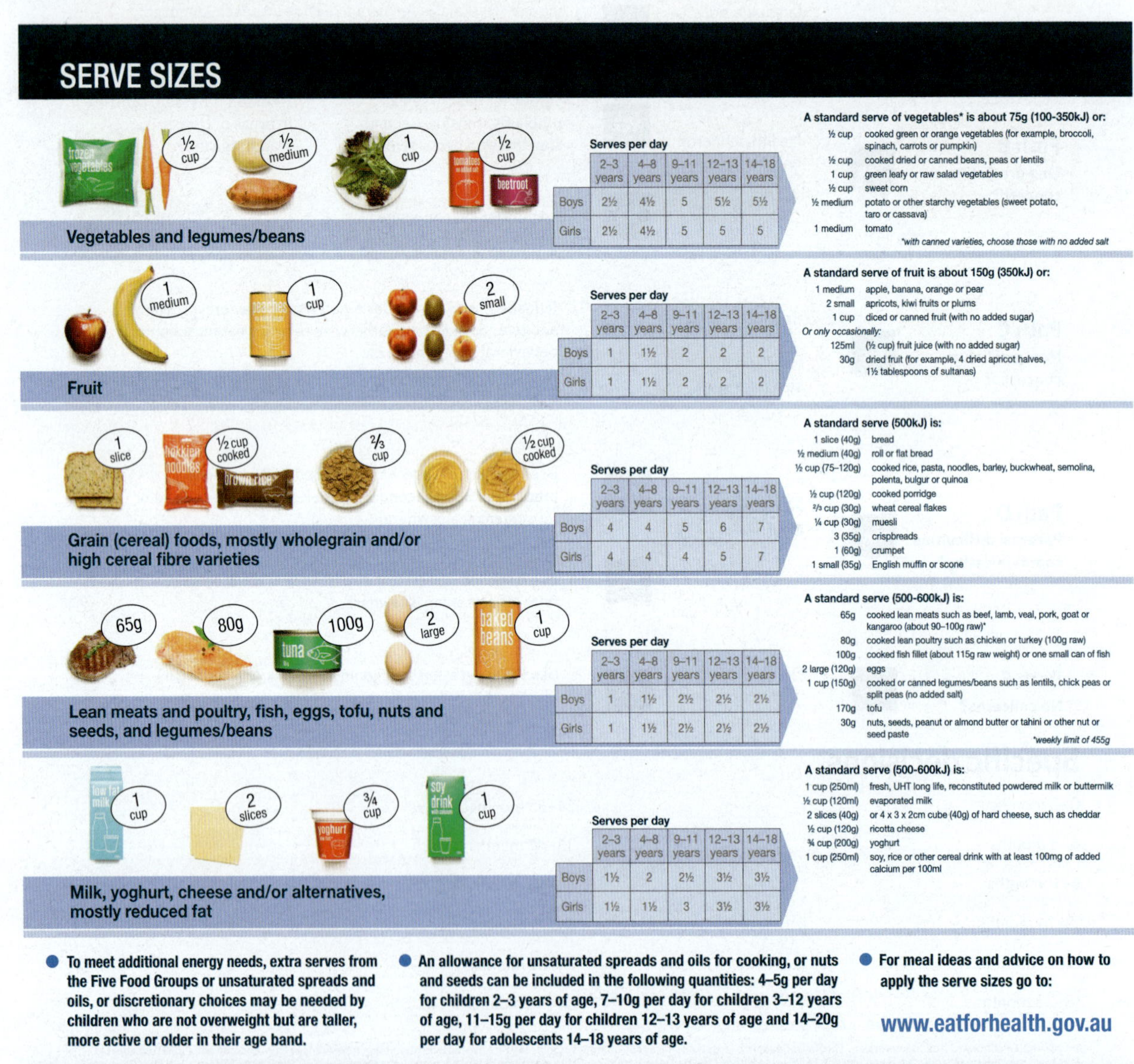

SERVE SIZES

Vegetables and legumes/beans

Serves per day

	2–3 years	4–8 years	9–11 years	12–13 years	14–18 years
Boys	2½	4½	5	5½	5½
Girls	2½	4½	5	5	5

A standard serve of vegetables* is about 75g (100-350kJ) or:

½ cup	cooked green or orange vegetables (for example, broccoli, spinach, carrots or pumpkin)
½ cup	cooked dried or canned beans, peas or lentils
1 cup	green leafy or raw salad vegetables
½ cup	sweet corn
½ medium	potato or other starchy vegetables (sweet potato, taro or cassava)
1 medium	tomato

**with canned varieties, choose those with no added salt*

Fruit

Serves per day

	2–3 years	4–8 years	9–11 years	12–13 years	14–18 years
Boys	1	1½	2	2	2
Girls	1	1½	2	2	2

A standard serve of fruit is about 150g (350kJ) or:

1 medium	apple, banana, orange or pear
2 small	apricots, kiwi fruits or plums
1 cup	diced or canned fruit (with no added sugar)
Or only occasionally:	
125ml	(½ cup) fruit juice (with no added sugar)
30g	dried fruit (for example, 4 dried apricot halves, 1½ tablespoons of sultanas)

Grain (cereal) foods, mostly wholegrain and/or high cereal fibre varieties

Serves per day

	2–3 years	4–8 years	9–11 years	12–13 years	14–18 years
Boys	4	4	5	6	7
Girls	4	4	4	5	7

A standard serve (500kJ) is:

1 slice (40g)	bread
½ medium (40g)	roll or flat bread
½ cup (75–120g)	cooked rice, pasta, noodles, barley, buckwheat, semolina, polenta, bulgur or quinoa
½ cup (120g)	cooked porridge
⅔ cup (30g)	wheat cereal flakes
¼ cup (30g)	muesli
3 (35g)	crispbreads
1 (60g)	crumpet
1 small (35g)	English muffin or scone

Lean meats and poultry, fish, eggs, tofu, nuts and seeds, and legumes/beans

Serves per day

	2–3 years	4–8 years	9–11 years	12–13 years	14–18 years
Boys	1	1½	2½	2½	2½
Girls	1	1½	2½	2½	2½

A standard serve (500-600kJ) is:

65g	cooked lean meats such as beef, lamb, veal, pork, goat or kangaroo (about 90–100g raw)*
80g	cooked lean poultry such as chicken or turkey (100g raw)
100g	cooked fish fillet (about 115g raw weight) or one small can of fish
2 large (120g)	eggs
1 cup (150g)	cooked or canned legumes/beans such as lentils, chick peas or split peas (no added salt)
170g	tofu
30g	nuts, seeds, peanut or almond butter or tahini or other nut or seed paste

**weekly limit of 455g*

Milk, yoghurt, cheese and/or alternatives, mostly reduced fat

Serves per day

	2–3 years	4–8 years	9–11 years	12–13 years	14–18 years
Boys	1½	2	2½	3½	3½
Girls	1½	1½	3	3½	3½

A standard serve (500-600kJ) is:

1 cup (250ml)	fresh, UHT long life, reconstituted powdered milk or buttermilk
½ cup (120ml)	evaporated milk
2 slices (40g)	or 4 x 3 x 2cm cube (40g) of hard cheese, such as cheddar
½ cup (120g)	ricotta cheese
¾ cup (200g)	yoghurt
1 cup (250ml)	soy, rice or other cereal drink with at least 100mg of added calcium per 100ml

- **To meet additional energy needs, extra serves from the Five Food Groups or unsaturated spreads and oils, or discretionary choices may be needed by children who are not overweight but are taller, more active or older in their age band.**
- **An allowance for unsaturated spreads and oils for cooking, or nuts and seeds can be included in the following quantities: 4–5g per day for children 2–3 years of age, 7–10g per day for children 3–12 years of age, 11–15g per day for children 12–13 years of age and 14–20g per day for adolescents 14–18 years of age.**
- **For meal ideas and advice on how to apply the serve sizes go to:**

www.eatforhealth.gov.au

Source: National Health and Medical Research Council. (Available from <www.nhmrc.gov.au/_files_nhmrc/publications/attachments/n55a_australian_dietary_guidelines_summary_131014.pdf>.)

Appendix F

Australian Guide to Healthy Eating

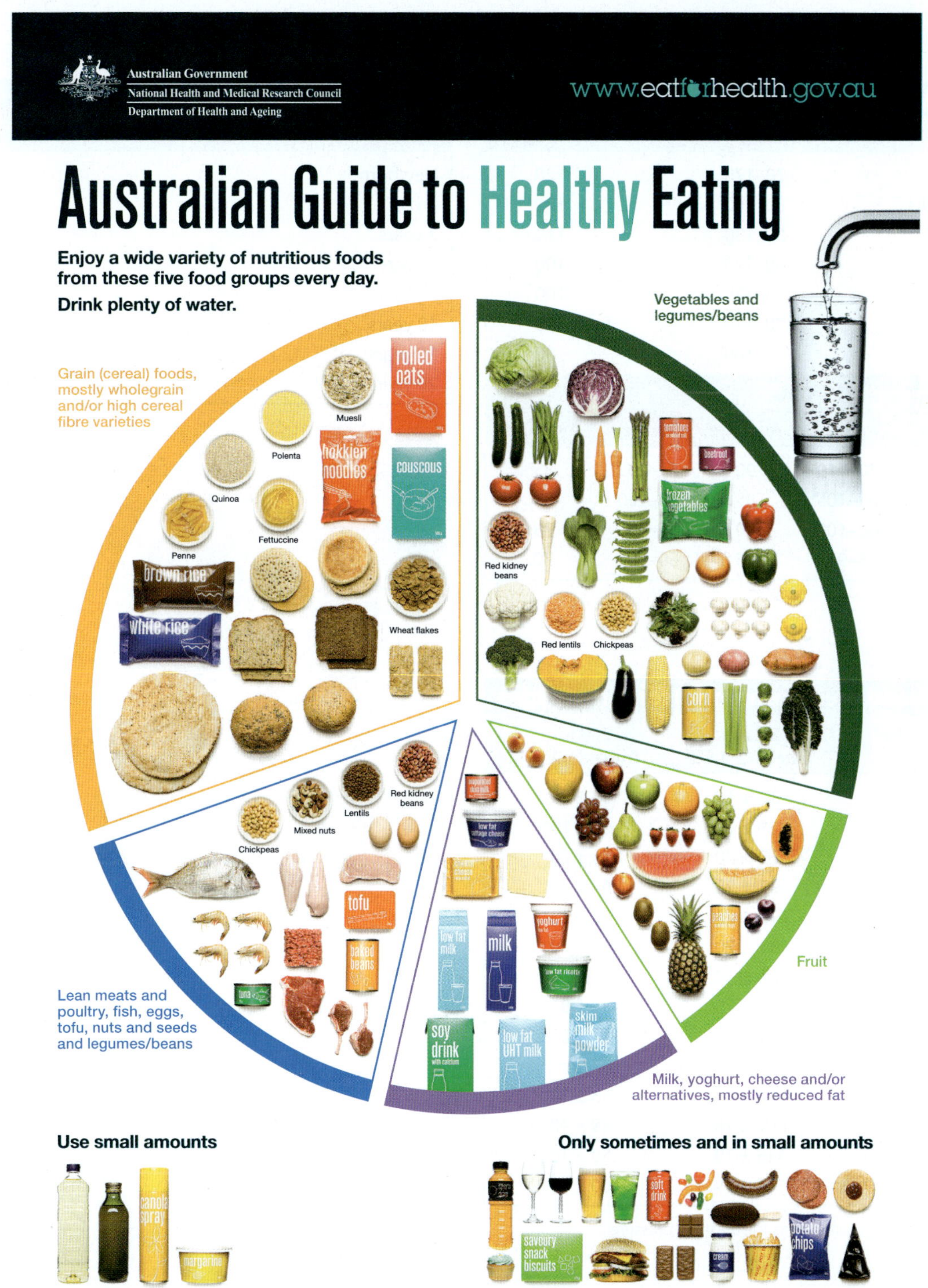

Source: National Health and Medical Research Council.

Appendix G

Pulse, respiration and blood pressure values

Pulse rate (bpm) at various ages

Age	Range	Average
Newborn	70–170	120
1–11 months	80–160	120
2 years	80–130	110
4 years	80–120	100
6 years	75–115	100
8 years	70–110	90
10 years	70–100	90

	Girls		Boys	
	Range	Average	Range	Average
12 years	70–110	90	65–105	85
14 years	65–105	85	60–100	80
16 years	60–100	80	55–95	75
18 years	55–95	75	50–90	70

Variations in respirations with age

Age	Rate per minute
Newborn	40–90
1 year	20–40
2 years	20–30
3 years	20–30
5 years	20–25
10 years	17–22
15 years	15–20
20 years	15–20

Normal blood pressure (mmHg) for various ages

Age	Systolic (mean ± 2 SD)	Diastolic (mean ± 2 SD)
Newborn	80 ± 16	46 ± 16
6 months–1 year	89 ± 29	60 ± 10*
1 year	96 ± 30	66 ± 25*
2 years	99 ± 25	64 ± 25*
3 years	100 ± 25	67 ± 23*
4 years	99 ± 20	65 ± 20*
5–6 years	94 ± 14	55 ± 9
6–7 years	100 ± 15	56 ± 8
8–9 years	105 ± 16	57 ± 9
9–10 years	107 ± 16	57 ± 9
10–11 years	111 ± 17	58 ± 10
11–12 years	113 ± 18	59 ± 10
12–13 years	115 ± 19	59 ± 10
13–14 years	118 ± 19	60 ± 10

*The point of muffling is shown as the diastolic pressure.

Appendix H

Standard infection guidelines

ADHA* and NZMOH† infection control guidelines

Standard precautions

Assume that every person is potentially infected or colonised with an organism that could be transmitted in the healthcare setting, and apply the following infection control practices during the delivery of healthcare.

Hand hygiene

- During the delivery of healthcare, avoid unnecessary touching of surfaces in close proximity to the patient to prevent both contamination of clean hands from environmental surfaces and transmission of pathogens from contaminated hands to surfaces.
- When hands are visibly dirty, contaminated with proteinaceous material, or visibly soiled with blood or body fluids, wash hands with either a non-antimicrobial soap and water or an antimicrobial soap and water.
- If hands are not visibly soiled, or after removing visible material with non-antimicrobial soap and water, decontaminate hands in the clinical situations described later. The preferred method of hand decontamination is with an alcohol-based hand rub. Alternatively, hands may be washed with an antimicrobial soap and water. Frequent use of alcohol-based hand rub immediately following hand washing with non-antimicrobial soap may increase the frequency of dermatitis. Perform hand hygiene
  - Before having direct contact with patients
  - After contact with blood, body fluids or excretions, mucous membranes, non-intact skin or wound dressings
  - After contact with a patient's intact skin (e.g. when taking a pulse or blood pressure or lifting a patient)
  - If hands will be moving from a contaminated body site to a clean body site during patient care
  - After contact with inanimate objects (including medical equipment) in the immediate vicinity of the patient
  - After removing gloves
- Wash hands with non-antimicrobial soap and water or with antimicrobial soap and water if contact with spores (e.g. *Clostridium difficile* or *Bacillus anthracis*) is likely to have occurred. The physical action of washing and rinsing hands under such circumstances is recommended because alcohols, chlorhexidine, iodophors and other antiseptic agents have poor activity against spores.
- Do not wear artificial fingernails or extenders if duties include direct contact with patients at high risk for infection and associated adverse outcomes (e.g. those in ICUs or operating rooms).
  - Develop an organisational policy on the wearing of non-natural nails by healthcare personnel who have direct contact with patients outside of the groups specified in the preceding text.

Personal protective equipment (PPE)

- Observe the following principles of use:
  - Wear PPE (gloves, gown, plastic aprons eye and/or facial protection) when the nature of the anticipated patient interaction indicates that contact with blood or body fluids may occur.
  - Prevent contamination of clothing and skin during the process of removing PPE.
  - Before leaving the patient's room or cubicle, remove and discard PPE.

Gloves

- Wear gloves when it can be reasonably anticipated that contact with blood or other potentially infectious materials, mucous membranes, non-intact skin or potentially contaminated intact skin (e.g. of a patient incontinent of stool or urine) could occur.
- Wear gloves with fit and durability appropriate to the task.
  - Wear disposable examination gloves for providing direct patient care.
  - Wear disposable examination gloves or reusable utility gloves for cleaning the environment or medical equipment.
- Remove gloves after contact with a patient and/or the surrounding environment (including medical equipment) using proper technique to prevent hand contamination. Do not wear the same pair of gloves for the care of more than one patient. Do not wash gloves for the purpose of reuse since this practice has been associated with transmission of pathogens.
- Discard single-use gloves as soon as they are damaged.
- Change gloves during patient care if the hands will move from a contaminated body site (e.g. perineal area) to a clean body site (e.g. face).

Gowns/plastic apron

- Wear a gown/plastic apron that is appropriate to the task, to protect skin and prevent soiling or contamination of clothing during procedures and patient care activities when contact with blood, body fluids, secretions, or excretions is anticipated.
  - Wear a gown/plastic apron for direct patient contact if the patient has uncontained secretions or excretions.
  - Remove gown/plastic apron and perform hand hygiene before leaving the patient's environment.
- Do not reuse gowns/plastic aprons, even for repeated contacts with the same patient.
- Routine donning of gowns/plastic apron upon entrance into a high-risk unit (e.g. ICU, NICU, or HSCT$^{\Delta}$ unit) is not indicated.

*ADHA: Australian Department of Health and Ageing; †NZMOH: New Zealand Ministry of Health.

(continued)

ADHA* and NZMOH† infection control guidelines *(Continued)*

Mouth, nose, eye protection

- Use PPE to protect the mucous membranes of the eyes, nose and mouth during procedures and patient care activities that are likely to generate splashes or sprays of blood, body fluids, secretions and excretions. Select masks, surgical face masks, respirators, goggles, face shields and combinations of each according to the need anticipated by the task performed.
- During aerosol-generating procedures (e.g. bronchoscopy, suctioning of the respiratory tract [if not using in-line suction catheters], endotracheal intubation) in patients who are not suspected of being infected with an agent for which respiratory protection is otherwise recommended (e.g. *Mycobacterium tuberculosis*, SARS‡, or haemorrhagic fever viruses), wear one of the following: a face shield that fully covers the front and sides of the face, a mask with attached shield, or a mask and goggles (in addition to gloves and gown).

Respiratory hygiene/cough etiquette

- Educate healthcare personnel on the importance of source control measures to contain respiratory secretions to prevent droplet and fomite transmission of respiratory pathogens, especially during seasonal outbreaks of viral respiratory tract infections (e.g. influenza, RSV§, adenovirus, parainfluenza virus) in communities.
- Implement the following measures to contain respiratory secretions in patients and accompanying individuals who have signs and symptoms of a respiratory infection, beginning at the point of initial encounter in a healthcare setting (e.g. triage, reception and waiting areas in emergency departments, outpatient clinics, and doctors' offices).
  - Post signs at entrances and in strategic places (e.g. lifts, cafeterias) within ambulatory and inpatient settings with instructions to patients and other persons with symptoms of a respiratory infection to cover their mouths/noses when coughing or sneezing, to use and dispose of tissues, and to perform hand hygiene after hands have been in contact with respiratory secretions.
  - Provide tissues and no-touch receptacles (e.g. pedal-operated lid or open, plastic-lined waste basket) for disposal of tissues.
  - Provide resources and instructions for performing hand hygiene in or near waiting areas in ambulatory and inpatient settings; provide conveniently located dispensers of alcohol-based hand rubs and, where sinks are available, supplies for hand washing.
  - During periods of increased prevalence of respiratory infections in the community (e.g. as indicated by increased school absenteeism or increased number of patients seeking care for a respiratory infection), offer masks to coughing patients and other symptomatic persons (e.g. persons who accompany ill patients) upon entry into the facility or medical office and encourage them to maintain special separation, ideally a distance of at least 1 metre, from others in common waiting areas. Some facilities may find it logistically easier to institute this recommendation year-round as a standard of practice.

Patient placement

- Include the potential for transmission of infectious agents in patient placement decisions. Place patients who pose a risk for transmission to others (e.g. uncontained secretions, excretions or wound drainage; infants with suspected viral respiratory or gastrointestinal infections) in a single-patient room when available.
- Determine patient placement based on the following principles:
  - Route(s) of transmission of the known or suspected infectious agent
  - Risk factors for transmission in the infected patient
  - Risk factors for adverse outcomes resulting from an HAI§§ in other patients in the area or room being considered for patient placement
  - Availability of single-patient rooms
  - Patient options for room sharing (e.g. cohorting patients with the same infection)

Patient care equipment and instruments/devices

- Establish policies and procedures for containing, transporting and handling patient care equipment and instruments/devices that may be contaminated with blood or body fluids.
- Remove organic material from critical and semicritical instrument/devices using recommended cleaning agents before high-level disinfection and sterilisation to enable effective disinfection and sterilisation processes.
- Wear PPE (e.g. gloves, gown), according to the level of anticipated contamination, when handling patient care equipment and instruments/devices that are visibly soiled or may have been in contact with blood or body fluids.

Care of the environment

- Establish policies and procedures for routine and targeted cleaning of environmental surfaces as indicated by the level of patient contact and degree of soiling.
- Clean and disinfect surfaces that are likely to be contaminated with pathogens, including those that are in close proximity to the patient (e.g. bed rails, overbed tables) and frequently touched surfaces in the patient care environment (e.g. door knobs, surfaces in and surrounding toilets in patients' rooms), on a more frequent schedule compared to that for other surfaces (e.g. horizontal surfaces in waiting rooms).
- Use hospital-grade disinfectants that have microbiocidal (i.e., killing) activity against the pathogens most likely to contaminate the patient care environment, in accordance with the manufacturer's instructions.
  - Review the efficacy of in-use disinfectants when evidence of continuing transmission of an infectious agent (e.g. rotavirus, *C. difficile*, norovirus) may indicate resistance to the in-use product and change to a more effective disinfectant as indicated.

‡SARS: Severe Acute Respiratory Syndrome; HSCT: Haematopoietic Stem Cell Transplant
§RSV: Respiratory Syncytial Virus
§§HAI: Healthcare Associated Infections

ADHA* and NZMOH[†] infection control guidelines *(Continued)*

- In facilities that provide healthcare to paediatric patients or have waiting areas with child's play toys (e.g. obstetric/gynaecology rooms and clinics), establish policies and procedures for cleaning and disinfecting toys at regular intervals. Use the following principles in developing this policy and procedures:
  - Select toys that can be easily cleaned and disinfected
  - Do not permit use of stuffed furry toys if they will be shared
  - Clean and disinfect large stationary toys (e.g. climbing equipment) at least weekly and whenever visibly soiled
  - If toys are likely to be mouthed, rinse with water after disinfection; alternatively, wash in a dishwasher
  - When a toy requires cleaning and disinfection, do so immediately or store in a designated labelled container separate from toys that are clean and ready for use
- Include multiuse electronic equipment in policies and procedures for preventing contamination and for cleaning and disinfecting, especially those items that are used by patients, those used during delivery of patient care, and mobile devices that are moved in and out of patient rooms frequently (e.g. daily).
  - No recommendation for use of removable protective covers or washable keyboards. *Unresolved issue.*

Textiles and laundry

- Handle used textiles and fabrics with minimum agitation to avoid contamination of air, surfaces and persons.
- If laundry chutes are used, ensure that they are properly designed, maintained and used in a manner to minimise dispersion of aerosols from contaminated laundry.

Safe injection practices

The following recommendations apply to the use of needles, cannulas that replace needles and, where applicable, intravenous delivery systems.

- Use aseptic technique to avoid contamination of sterile injection equipment.
- Do not administer medications from a syringe to multiple patients, even if the needle or cannula on the syringe is changed. Needles, cannulas and syringes are sterile, single-use items; they should not be reused for another patient or used to access a medication or solution that might be intended for a subsequent patient.
- Use fluid infusion and administration sets (i.e. intravenous bags, tubing and connectors) for one patient only, and dispose of appropriately after use. Consider a syringe or needle/cannula contaminated once it has been used to enter or connect to a patient's intravenous infusion bag or administration set.
- Use single-dose vials for parenteral medications whenever possible.
- Do not administer medications from single-dose vials or ampules to multiple patients or combine leftover contents for later use.
- If multidose vials must be used, both the needle or cannula and syringe used to access the multidose vial must be sterile.
- Do not keep multidose vials in the immediate patient treatment area and store in accordance with the manufacturer's recommendations; discard if sterility is compromised or questionable.
- Do not use bags or bottles of intravenous solution as a common source of supply for multiple patients.

Infection control practices for special lumbar puncture procedures

- Wear a surgical mask when placing a catheter or injecting material into the spinal canal or subdural space (i.e. during myelograms, lumbar puncture and spinal or epidural anaesthesia).

Worker safety

- Adhere to federal and state requirements for protection of healthcare personnel from exposure to bloodborne pathogens.

Australian Commission on Safety and Quality in Healthcare. (2010). *Australian Guidelines for the Prevention and Control of Infection in Healthcare.* Commonwealth of Australia. New Zealand Ministry of Health (NZMOH). (2007). *Guidelines for the control of multidrug-resistant organisms in New Zealand.* Wellington: Ministry of Health.

Appendix I

Primary and secondary skin lesions

PRIMARY SKIN LESIONS

Primary skin lesions are original lesions arising from previously normal skin.

Description	Examples	Illustration	Photograph
Macule, patch • Flat, non-palpable skin colour change (skin colour may be brown, white, tan, purple, red) • Macule: <1 cm, circumscribed border • Patch: >1 cm, may have irregular border	• Freckles • Flat moles • Petechiae • Rubella • Vitiligo • Port-wine stains • Ecchymosis	Macule	Rubella. (*Source:* Goodheart, H. G. [2009]. *Goodheart's Photoguide to Common Skin Disorders: Diagnosis and Management* [3rd ed.]. Philadelphia: Lippincott Williams & Wilkins.)
		Patch	Port-wine stain. (*Source:* Weber, J. & Kelley, J. [2003]. *Health Assessment in Nursing* [2nd ed.]. Philadelphia: Lippincott Williams & Wilkins.)
Papule, plaque • Elevated, palpable, solid mass; circumscribed border • Papule: <0.5 cm • Plaque: >0.5 cm (may be coalesced papules with flat top)	Papules: • Elevated naevi • Warts • Lichen planus	Papule	Warts, circumscribed elevations caused by a virus. (Courtesy of Reed and Carnick Pharmaceuticals.)

Description	Examples	Illustration	Photograph
	Plaques: • Psoriasis • Actinic keratosis	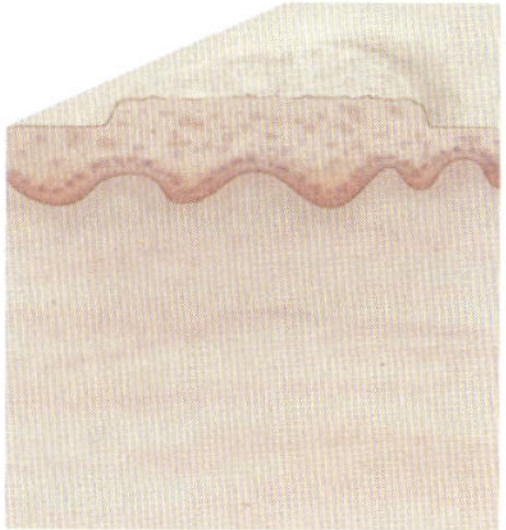 Plaque	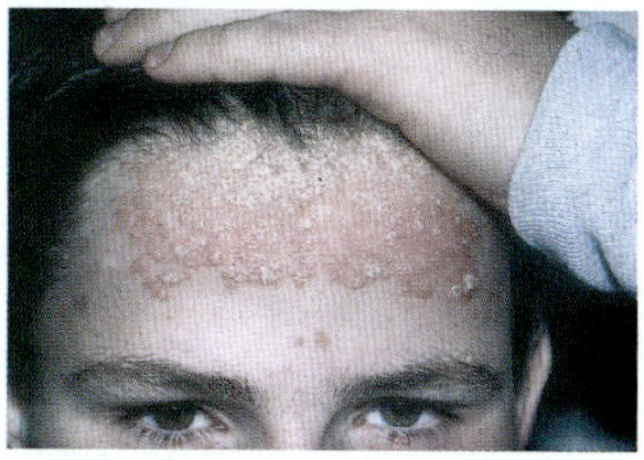 Psoriasis vulgaris. (*Source:* Goodheart, H. G. [2009]. *Goodheart's Photoguide to Common Skin Disorders: Diagnosis and Management* [3rd ed.]. Philadelphia: Lippincott Williams & Wilkins.)
Nodule, tumour • Elevated, solid, palpable mass • Extends deeper into dermis than a papule • Nodule: 0.5–2 cm; circumscribed • Tumour: >1–2 cm; does not always have sharp borders	Nodules: • Lipoma • Squamous cell carcinoma • Poorly absorbed injection • Dermatofibroma	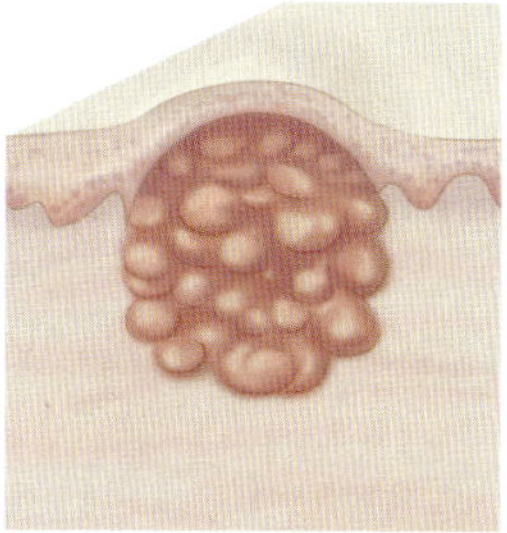 Nodule	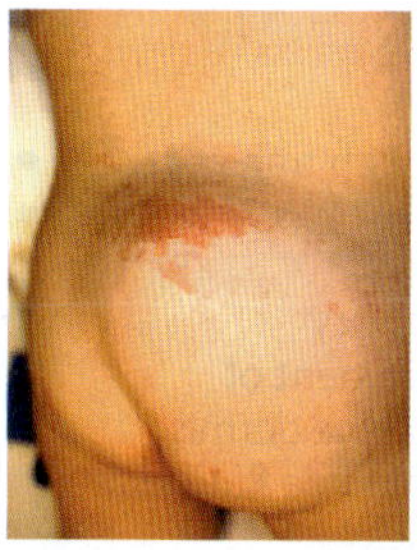 Subcutaneous lipoma. (*Source:* Cover Mechanicals.)
	Tumours: • Larger lipoma • Carcinoma	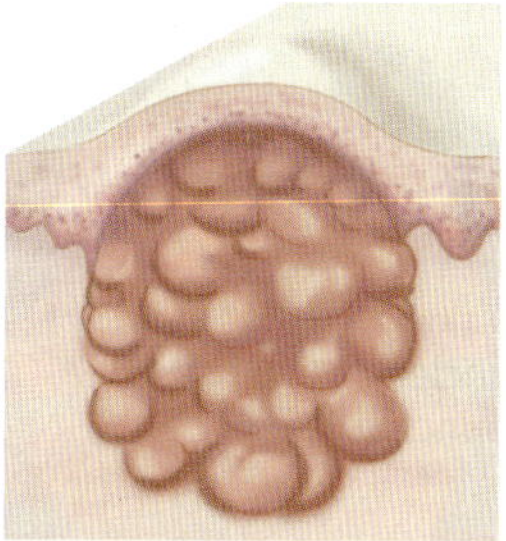 Tumour	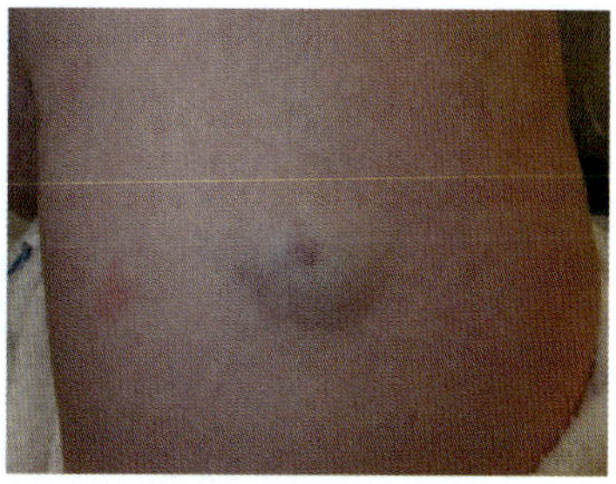 Haemangioma of infancy: back. (*Source:* Stedman's.)
Vesicle, bulla • Circumscribed elevated, palpable mass containing serous fluid • Vesicle: <0.5 cm • Bulla: >0.5 cm	Vesicles: • Herpes simplex/ zoster • Varicella (chickenpox) • Poison ivy • Second-degree burn	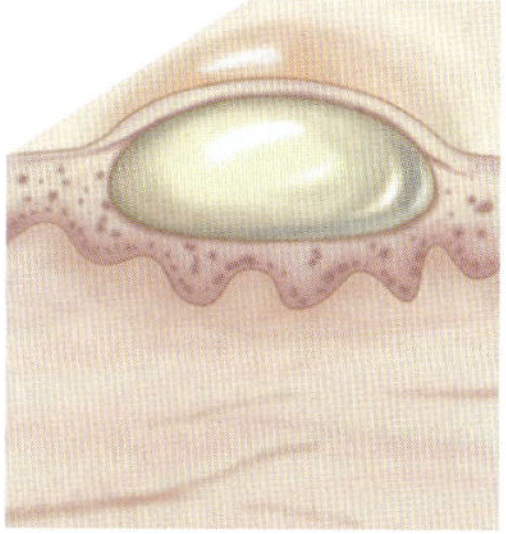 Vesicle	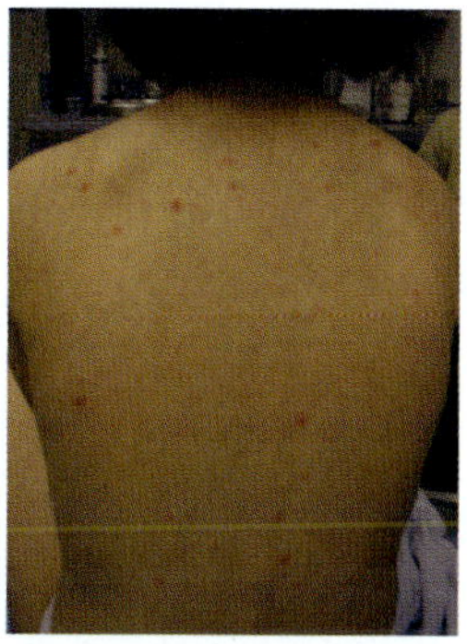 Varicella. Vesicles and crusts. (*Source:* Stedman's.)

(*continued*)

Description	Examples	Illustration	Photograph
	Bulla: • Pemphigus, contact dermatitis, large burn blisters, poison ivy, bullous impetigo	Bulla	Bullous impetigo. Lesions appear crusted, scabbed, bullous or covered with calamine lotion. (*Source:* Fleisher, G.R., Ludwig, W. & Baskin, M.N. [2004]. *Atlas of Pediatric Emergency Medicine*. Philadelphia: Lippincott Williams & Wilkins.)
Wheal • Elevated mass with transient borders • Often irregular • Size and colour vary • Caused by movement of serous fluid into the dermis • Does not contain free fluid in a cavity (e.g. vesicle)	• Urticaria (hives) • Insect bites	Wheal	Urticaria. (*Source:* Hall, B. J., & Hall, J. C. [2010]. *Sauer's Manual of Skin Diseases* [10th ed.]. Philadelphia: Lippincott Williams & Wilkins.)
Pustule • Pus-filled vesicle or bulla	• Acne • Impetigo • Furuncles • Carbuncles	Pustule	Inflammatory acne lesions. Papules, pustules and closed comedones are all present on this patient. (*Source:* Goodheart, H.G. [2009]. *Goodheart's Photo Guide of Common Skin Disorders*. Philadelphia: Lippincott Williams & Wilkins.)

Description	Examples	Illustration	Photograph
Cyst • Encapsulated fluid-filled or semisolid mass • Located in the subcutaneous tissue or dermis	• Sebaceous cyst • Epidermoid cyst	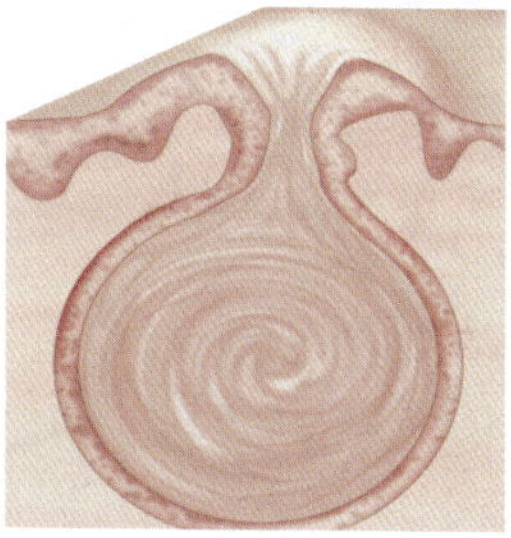 Cyst	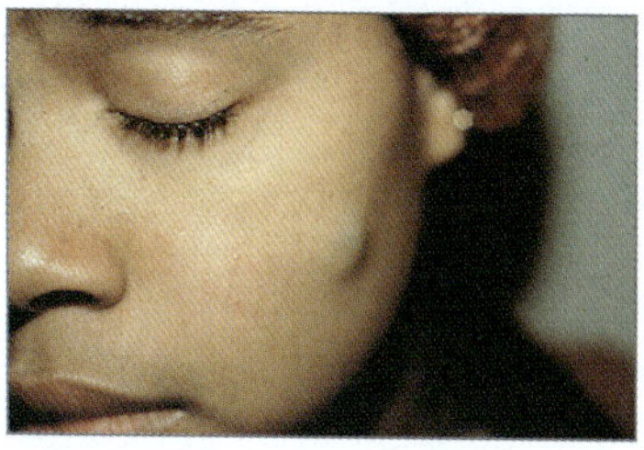 Epidermoid cysts are nodular.

SECONDARY SKIN LESIONS

Secondary skin lesions result from changes in primary lesions.

Description	Examples	Illustration	Photograph
Erosion • Loss of superficial epidermis • Does not extend to the dermis • Depressed, moist area	• Rupture vesicles • Scratch marks • Aphthous ulcer	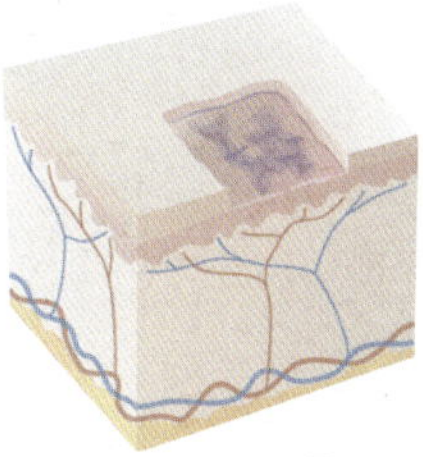 Erosion	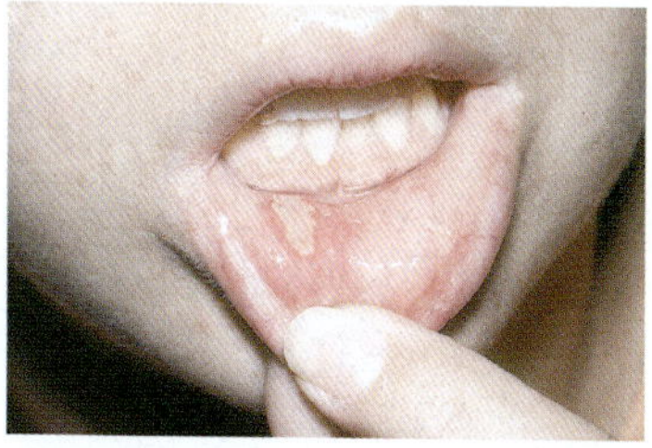 Aphthous ulcer. (*Source:* Goodheart, H. G. [2009]. *Goodheart's Photoguide to Common Skin Disorders: Diagnosis and Management* [3rd ed.]. Philadelphia: Lippincott Williams & Wilkins.)
Scar (cicatrix) • Skin mark left after healing of wound or lesion • Represents replacement by connective tissue of the injured tissue • Young scars: red or purple • Mature scars: white or glistening	• Healed wound • Healed surgical incision	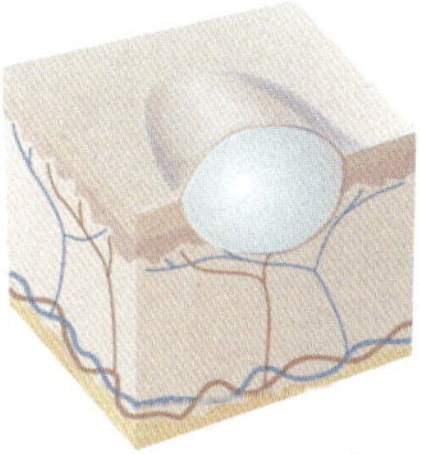 Scar	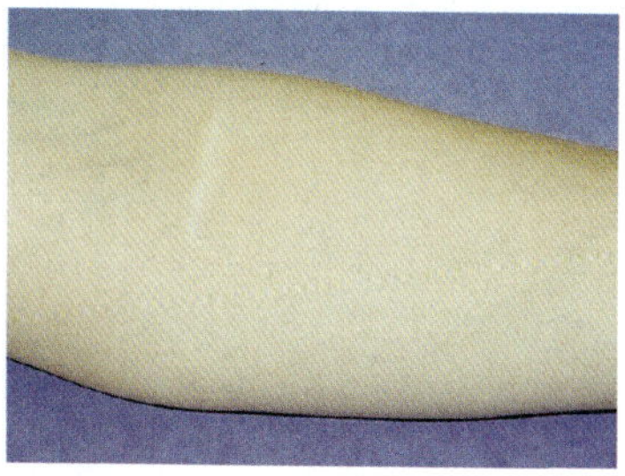 Mature healed wound.
Fissure • Linear crack in the skin • May extend to the dermis	• Chapped lips or hands • Athlete's foot	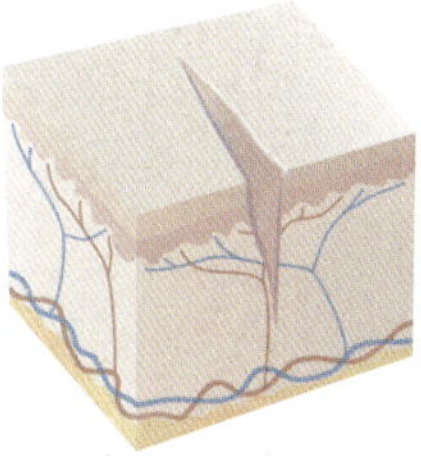 Fissure	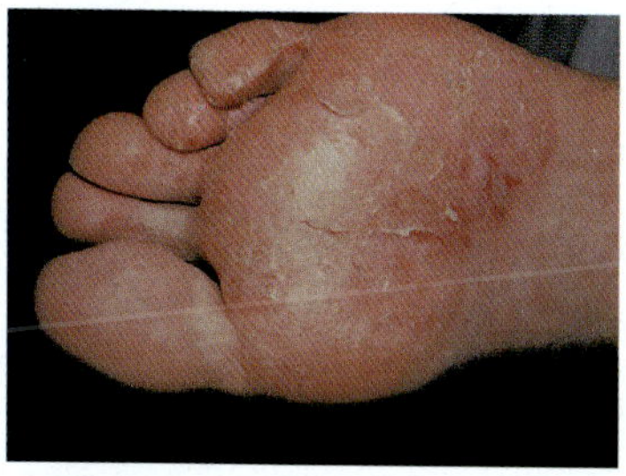 Athlete's foot

Source: Lewis, P. & Foley, D. (2014). *Health Assessment in Nursing* (2nd ed.). Sydney: Lippincott Williams & Wilkins.

Glossary

abdominal palpation: pressing a hand against the abdominal wall in order to determine areas of tenderness

Aboriginal: Indigenous Australian

abortion: any interruption of a pregnancy before the fetus is viable (a stage of development that will enable the fetus to survive outside the uterus if born at that time)

absorption: transfer of a medication from its point of entry in the body into the bloodstream

abstinence: refraining from sexual intercourse

abstract thought: final stage in cognitive thought processes; allows problem solving and creating hypotheses

abuse: wilful injury by one person of another

accommodation: adjustment of the eye to focus on a close image (ophthalmology); the ability to adapt thought processes to fit what is perceived (Piaget)

acrocyanosis: cyanosis (blue colour) in the feet and hands

adolescence: the time period between the age of 13 years and 18–20 years

adventitious sounds: extra or abnormal breathing sounds

advocacy: a political process by an individual or a large group which aims to influence public policy and resource allocation

affective learning: learning that involves a change in attitude

allergen: antigen that causes the release of mediating substances causing tissue injury and allergic symptoms

allogeneic transplantation: transfer of body tissues from an immune-compatible (histocompatible) donor

Alport's syndrome: a progressive chronic glomerulonephritis inherited as an autosomal dominant disorder

amblyopia: reduced vision in one eye; "lazy eye"

amenorrhoea: absence of a menstrual flow

amniocentesis: the withdrawal of amniotic fluid from the uterus by means of introduction of a needle through the abdominal and uterine wall

amniotic fluid embolism: condition in which amniotic fluid is forced into maternal circulation and travels to the lungs as small emboli

amniotic membrane: the innermost layer of the placenta

anaemia: a decrease in haemoglobin in the blood to levels below the normal range

anaesthesia: the absence of all sensation, especially sensitivity to pain, as induced by an anaesthetic substance

analgesia: a medication that reduces or decreases awareness of pain

anaphylactic shock: a severe and sometimes fatal systemic reaction to a substance such as a drug, vaccine, food, serum, allergen extract, insect venom or chemical

ankle clonus: continued motion of the foot

ankyloglossia: a condition where the bottom of the tongue is attached to the floor of the mouth; sometimes known as tongue tie

anovulation: faulty or inadequate release of ova

anoxia: an abnormal condition characterised by a local or systemic lack of oxygen in body tissues

antigen: any foreign substance (molecule) capable of stimulating an immune response

apnoea: pause in respiration longer than 20 seconds with accompanying bradycardia

apposition: the amount of end-to-end contact of bone fragments

areola: the pigmented circle surrounding the nipple

arthroscopy: direct visualisation of a joint with a fibreoptic instrument

artificial insemination: the introduction of semen into the vagina or uterus by mechanical or instrumental means

aspiration: inhalation of a foreign object into the airway

assimilation: changing a situation or one's perception of it to fit one's thoughts

aspiration studies: studies involving the removal of body fluids by such techniques as lumbar puncture or bone marrow aspiration

astereognosis: difficulty identifying objects placed in the hand when the eyes are closed

astigmatism: congenital or acquired unevenness of the curvature of the cornea

atelectasis: collapse of alveoli

atresia: complete closure of a body opening

attitude: the degree of head flexion a fetus assumes during labour, or the relation of the fetal parts to each other

augmentation of labour: assisting labour that has started spontaneously to be more effective

auscultation: listening with the aid of a stethoscope

autologous transplantation: transplantation using the person's own previously removed tissue

automatisms: complex purposeless movements, such as lip smacking or fumbling hand movements

autonomic dysreflexia: a powerful sympathetic reflex reaction that causes signs of hypertension, tachycardia, flushed face and severe occipital headache

autonomy: independence

azotaemia: accumulation of nitrogen waste in the bloodstream

baby-bottle syndrome: decay of all the upper teeth and the lower posterior teeth, usually due to repeatedly putting an infant to bed with a bottle

balloon angioplasty: procedure usually by way of cardiac catheterisation in which a catheter with an uninflated balloon at its tip is inserted and passed through the heart into a stenosed valve. As the balloon is inflated, it breaks valve adhesions and may relieve the stenosis

ballottement: a technique of palpating an organ or floating structure by bouncing it gently and feeling it rebound

barium contrast studies: x-ray involving the use of barium, a radiopaque substance to outline the gastrointestinal tract

barrier methods: a method of reproductive life planning in which sperm are prevented from entering the cervix

battledore placenta: a placenta with the cord inserted marginally rather than centrally

behaviour therapy: type of psychotherapy that attempts to modify maladjusted patterns of behaviour by substituting a new set of responses to a particular stimulus

bifidus factor: specific growth-promoting factor for the bacteria *Lactobacillus bifidus* whose presence in breast milk interferes with colonisation of pathogenic bacteria in the gastrointestinal tract

binge eating: episodes of uncontrollable intake of large amounts of food over a specified period of time

binocular vision: ability to fuse two images into one

biological gender: a person's chromosomal sexual designation of being male (XY) or female (XX)

biopsy: surgical removal of tissue cells for laboratory analysis

birth centre: a health facility where antenatal, intrapartum and postnatal care is provided predominantly by midwives in consultation with other health professionals

birthing bed: a bed specifically prepared for birth

birthing chair: a chair used in labour and birth

birthing room: a specifically prepared room for aiding comfort, safety and conduct of birth

blood dyscrasias: haematological disorders

blood transfusion: administration of whole blood or a component such as packed red cells, to replace blood lost through trauma, surgery or disease

body mass index: determination of body weight by comparing height to weight (weight divided by height squared)

bone marrow: specialised tissue filling the spaces in cancellous bone of the epiphyses

Braxton Hicks contractions: painless, erratic uterine contractions that occur towards the end of pregnancy. They ready the cervix for labour, but cervical dilation does not occur with them.

breech presentation: fetal presentation in which either the buttocks or feet are the first body parts to contact the cervix

broken fluency: repetition and prolongation of sounds, syllables and words

bronchoscopy: a procedure in which a bronchoscope, a specially designed tube, is passed through the nose or mouth to observe the larynx, trachea, bronchi and alveoli

brown fat: the special tissue present in newborns to maintain body temperature

bruxism: grinding the teeth during sleep

caesarean birth: birth accomplished through an abdominal incision into the uterus

caput succedaneum: oedema of the scalp at the presenting part of the head

cardiac catheterisation: a procedure in which a small radiopaque catheter is passed through a major vein in the arm, leg or neck into the heart to secure blood samples or inject dye, to evaluate cardiac function

cardiopulmonary arrest: a sudden cessation of cardiac output and effective circulation

cartilage: connective tissue

catarrhal stage: inflammation of the nose and throat during infectious diseases

catatonia: immobility

cavities: progressive, destructive lesions or decalcification of the tooth enamel and dentin

central cyanosis: cyanosis of the trunk

centring: the action or process of placing something in the middle of something else

cephalhaematoma: a collection of blood under the periosteum of the skull bone

cephalic presentation: fetal presentation in which the head is the body part that first contacts the cervix

cervical cerclage: suturing of the cervix to maintain a pregnancy to prevent premature cervical dilatation

Chadwick's sign: discolourisation of vaginal walls from pink to violet

chemotherapeutic agent: one that is capable of destroying malignant cells

chief concern: the reason the parents or individual has come to the healthcare agency

child and family health nursing: a form of nursing that focuses on promoting health and well-being as well as the prevention and management of disease with children and families

chloasma: extra pigment on the face

choreoathetosis: rapid, purposeless movements

choreoid: irregular and jerking movements

chorioamnionitis: infection of the fetal membranes and amniotic fluid

chorionic membrane: the outer fetal membrane

chorionic villi: projections of the trophoblast that produce human chorionic gonadotropin and begin osmosis of nutrients to the embryo

chromosomes: the structure that weaves genes into strands in the nucleus of all body cells

clarifying: repeating statements others have made so that you and they can be certain that you understood

class inclusion: the ability to understand that objects can belong to more than one classification

classic caesarean incision: an incision that is made vertically through both the abdominal skin and the uterus
cleft lip: failure of the maxillary and median nasal processes to fuse normally
cleft palate: an opening of the palate
client advocacy: a term frequently used to describe the nurse–client relationship
coeliac disease: a condition characterised by the inability to hydrolyse peptides contained in gluten
cognitive development: the acquisition of the ability to think and reason
cognitive learning: learning that involves a change in the individual's level of understanding or knowledge
coitus interruptus: a method of contraception in which the penis is withdrawn from the vagina before ejaculation
colonoscopy: a procedure in which a colonoscope, a specially designed tube, is passed through the anus to examine the rectum or colon
colostrum: a thin, watery, yellow fluid composed of protein, sugar, fat, water, minerals, vitamins and maternal antibodies that precedes breast milk
communication: the exchange of ideas between two or more persons
community: a limited geographical area in which the residents relate to and interact among themselves
community assessment: gathering information on the current strengths, concerns and conditions of children, families and the community
compartment syndrome: pathological condition caused by arterial compression and subsequent reduction of blood supply to a limb
complex vocal tics: repeated use of words or phrases out of context
complicated grief: chronic and long-lasting sorrow
computed tomography (CT): x-ray procedure in which many views of an organ or a body part are made to represent what the organ would look like if it were cut into thin slices
conduction: transfer of body heat to a cooler solid object in contact with the body
congestive heart failure (CHF): a condition in which the myocardium of the heart cannot pump and circulate enough blood to supply oxygen and nutrients to body cells
conjunctivitis: commonly called "pink eye" by parents; an infection of the conjunctiva that covers the eye
conservation: property of an object when a change in form does not equate to a change in size or amount
contraceptive planning: the process of considering the different options that are available to prevent pregnancy
contrecoup injury: an injury resulting from a blow to one side of the skull that causes the brain to rebound and then injure the opposite side
convalescent period: interval between when infectious symptoms begin to fade and the child returns to full wellness
convection: flow of heat from the body surface to cooler surrounding air
coprolalia: use of socially unacceptable words, usually obscenities
cottonwool children: a term used to describe children in contemporary society who are restricted from engaging in outdoor play
couvade syndrome: somatic symptoms experienced by the father during pregnancy simulating those of the pregnant mother
Couvelaire uterus: uteroplacental apoplexy due to blood entering the uterine musculature
crackles: the sound of rales
crowning: the appearance of the fetal head at the perineum just before birth
cryptorchidism: failure of one or both testes to descend from the abdominal cavity to the scrotum
cultural safety: the provision of effective healthcare to a person of a dissimilar culture that ensures that the care provided is not diminishing, demeaning or disempowering
culture: the learned way of life of a community or society
cyanosis: a blue tinge to the skin indicating hypoxia
cytogenetics: branch of genetics that studies the cellular constituents concerned with heredity
cytomegalovirus: a member of the herpes virus family; teratogen that can cause extensive damage to a fetus yet causes few symptoms in the woman
death: end of life; officially determined by unreceptivity and unresponsivity, no spontaneous muscular movement or breath, no reflex response and a flat electroencephalogram
débridement: the removal of foreign material from a burn or wound
decentring: to project the self into other people's situations and see the world from their viewpoint
decerebrate posturing: typical posture occurring when the midbrain is not functional; characterised by rigid extension and adduction of arms and pronation of the wrists with the fingers flexed, legs extended and the feet plantar-flexed
deciduas: the epithelial tissue of the endometrium lining the uterus
deciduous teeth: temporary teeth that are replaced by permanent teeth at around the age of 6 to 7 years
decorticate posturing: a child's arms adducted and flexed on the chest with wrists flexed, hands fisted; lower extremities extended and internally rotated; feet plantar-flexed; denotes brainstem involvement
deep vein thrombosis (DVT): formation of thrombus (blood clot) in the deep veins secondary to stasis, vessel damage and hypercoagulation
dehydration: an excessive loss of body water
demonstration: the showing of a procedure to stimulate learning
dermatoglyphics: the study of surface markings of the skin
development: an increase in ability (a qualitative change)

developmental milestones: major markers of normal development
developmental task: a skill or a growth responsibility arising at a particular time, the successful achievement of which will provide a foundation for the accomplishment of future tasks
dialysis: separation and removal of solutes from body fluid by diffusion through a semipermeable membrane
diaphragm: a mechanical barrier contraceptive device fitted over the cervix
diaphysis: central shaft of a long bone
diastasis: the forcible separation of two parts that are normally joined, such as parts of a bone at an epiphysis
dilatation: widening of the opening of the cervix in labour
diplegia: (paraplegia); paralysis of the lower extremities
diplopia: double vision
discipline: setting rules so people know what is expected
discrimination: the act of distinguishing or differentiating
distraction: a technique that allows the cells of the brainstem that register an impulse as pain to be preoccupied with other stimuli so the pain impulse cannot register; use of an external device to separate opposing bones, thus encouraging new bone growth
distribution: movement of a drug through the bloodstream to the specific site of action
diversity: being composed of different elements
domestic violence: physical and or emotional abuse of one spouse or partner by another
domiciliary midwives: midwives who are employed to provide a range of midwifery services to mothers and infants upon their discharge from hospital
doula: a person without professional experience who guides and assists a woman in labour
drowning: asphyxiation because of submersion in a liquid
dysfunctional labour: a labour that is abnormal in that it does not meet the milestones that define a normal labour; for example, lack of progressive cervical dilatation or lack of descent of the fetus
dyskinetic: disordered muscle tone
dyslexia: reading impairment disorder in which letters or words are reversed
dysmenorrhoea: painful menstruation
dyspareunia: pain on sexual intercourse
dystocia: difficult labour
early pregnancy failure: also known as blighted ovum or anembryonic gestation; a common cause of miscarriage that happens when a fertilised egg implants in the uterus but the resulting embryo either stops developing or does not form at all
echolalia: repetitive words or phrases spoken by others
eclampsia: development of a seizure from hypertension in pregnancy
ecomap: a diagram of the family's interactions within the community
ectomorphic: having a slim body build
ectopic pregnancy: one in which implantation occurs outside the uterine cavity
effacement: thinning of the cervix in labour
egocentrism: perceiving that one's thoughts and needs are better or more important than those of others
eighth-month anxiety: fear of strangers that peaks during a baby's eighth month
elective termination of pregnancy: termination of a pregnancy by medical intervention
electrical impulse studies: those that include electrical conduction
emancipated minor: a person before the age of majority who is free from the custody, care, and control of their parents and is capable of healthcare decisions; a pregnant adolescent
embryo: the intrauterine growth period from the time following implantation until organogenesis is complete (tenth day to 5 to 8 weeks)
empathy: the ability to put yourself in another's place and experience a feeling as that person does
empowerment: refers to increasing the spiritual, political, social, educational and economic strength of individuals and communities
enanthem: rash on the mucus membrane
endocervix: the inner surface of the cervix
endometriosis: abnormal growth of extrauterine endometrial cells, often in the cul-de-sac of the peritoneal cavity, the uterine ligaments and the ovaries
endometritis: an infection of the endometrium, the lining of the uterus
endomorphic: having a large body build
endorphins: naturally occurring opiate-like substances in the body
endoscopy: a procedure in which an endoscope, a specially-designed tube, is passed through the mouth to examine the gastrointestinal tract
engagement: settling of the fetal head into the pelvis during labour
engorgement: breast distension with swelling caused by vascular and lymphatic congestion arising from an increase in the blood and lymph supply to the breasts
enucleation: eye removal
enuresis: involuntary passage of urine past the age when a child should be expected to have attained bladder control
environmental control: as many common allergens as possible are removed from the environment
epidural anaesthesia: a type of anaesthesia block in which a local anaesthetic is injected into the epidural space
epidural analgesia: injection of an analgesic agent into the epidural space just outside the spinal canal, to provide analgesia to the lower body for 12 to 24 hours
epiphyseal plate: area where the increase in the length of long bones occurs
epiphysis: rounded end portion of a long bone

episiotomy: surgical incision of the perineum to prevent tearing and to release pressure on the fetal head with birth

epispadias: opening of the urinary meatus on the dorsal or superior surface of the penis

equity: fairness

erectile dysfunction: impotence; the inability to achieve erection in order to complete a sex act

erosion: inflammation of the epithelium of the cervical canal spreading onto the area surrounding the os, giving the cervix a reddened appearance

erythema toxicum: newborn rash that usually appears in the 1st to 4th day of life; sometimes called a flea-bite rash

esotropia: condition in which the eye is always turning in

estimated date of birth: the predicted date on which a baby will be born

ethnicity: the cultural group into which a person is born

ethnocentrism: the belief that one's own values or beliefs are superior to others

evaporation: loss of heat through conversion of a liquid to a vapour

evidence-based practice: the use of research or controlled investigation of a problem using a scientific method in conjunction with clinical expertise as acquired through experience and practice as a foundation for action

Ewing's sarcoma: malignant tumour occurring most often in the bone marrow of the diaphyseal area (midshaft) of long bones

exanthem: a skin rash

excretion: elimination of raw drug or drug metabolites, a process that largely prevents properly-administered medications from becoming toxic

exophthalmos: protrusion of the eyeballs

exotropia: condition in which the eye is always turning outwards

exstrophy of the bladder: midline closure defect occurring during the embryonic period of gestation (first 8 weeks) and resulting in the bladder lying open and exposed on the abdomen

external cephalic version: turning of a fetus from a breech to a cephalic position before birth

extrusion reflex: a tongue reflex in infants that expels solid objects from the mouth; fades at 4 months of age

family: two or more people who live in the same household (usually), share a common emotional bond and perform certain interrelated social tasks

family nursing: the concept that clients do not exist outside a family; the family rather than an individual is considered the client

family of orientation: one's birth family: oneself, mother, father and siblings

family of procreation: one's marriage family: oneself, spouse and children

family theory: a way of analysing problems or concerns from a family's point of view

feedback: a reply to communication indicating that the message has been received and interpreted

female condom: a thin polyurethane device designed to act as a well-lubricated secondary vagina

fertile days: the days during the menstrual cycle when a woman is most likely to fall pregnant

fertilisation: the union of male and female gametes to form a zygote from which an embryo develops

fertility rate: the proportion of women who could have babies who are having them

fetal alcohol syndrome: condition associated with an infant born to a woman who uses alcohol during pregnancy; infant typically is small for gestational age, cognitively challenged and has a characteristic craniofacial deformity including short palpebral fissures, thin upper lip and upturned nose

fetal descent: sinking of the fetus in the birth canal just prior to birth (one of six cardinal movements of labour)

fetus: the developing structure from the eighth week postfertilisation until birth

fever: an elevation of temperature above the normal circadian range as a result of a rise in the body's core temperature

fistula: abnormal opening

flat affect: not revealing feelings

focusing: helping a person to centre on a subject

food standards: government requirements under which foods must be processed and sold

foramen ovale: an opening between the atria of the heart during intrauterine life

forceps birth: birth using forceps (steel double-bladed instruments used to prevent pressure on the fetal head); forceps outlet procedure is when the forceps are applied after the fetal head reaches the perineum

formal operational thought: final stage of cognitive development, involving the ability to think in abstract terms and use the scientific method to arrive at conclusions

fovea centralis: (the centre of the macula); an area of closely-packed cones on the retinas where colour is best perceived

fracture: break in the continuity or structure of bone

frenulum: the membrane attached to the lower anterior tip of the tongue

gastro-oesophageal reflux: (commonly called achalasia in infants) a neuromuscular disturbance in which the gastro-oesophageal (cardiac) sphincter and the lower portion of the oesophagus are lax, allowing easy regurgitation of gastric contents into the oesophagus

gastrostomy tube feeding: the introduction of a nutrient solution through a tube that has been surgically inserted into the stomach

gender identity: the inner sense of being male or female, which may be the same as or different from biological gender

gender role: the behaviour a person conveys about being male or female

genes: basic units of heredity that determine both the physical and mental characteristics of people

genetic counselling: providing information regarding the occurrence or risk of occurrence of a genetic disorder in a family

genetics: study of how and why chromosomal disorders occur; the science of heredity

genogram: a diagram of family structure depicting essential family relationships; the interactive roles that exist in a family

genome: complete set of genes present

genotype: actual gene composition

gestational age: number of weeks fetus remained in utero

gestational trophoblastic disease: proliferation and degeneration of the trophoblastic villi

glomerular filtration rate: rate at which substances are filtered from the blood to the urine

glomerulonephritis: inflammation of the glomeruli of the kidney

glycosuria: excess glucose in the urine

glycosylated haemoglobin: measure of the amount of glucose attached to haemoglobin

goniotomy: surgical procedure used to treat congenital glaucoma

Goodell's sign: softening of the cervix; a probable sign of pregnancy

grafting: surgical transplantation of living tissue

graphaesthesia: ability to recognise a shape that has been traced on the skin

gravida: number of times a woman has been pregnant, including the present pregnancy; a pregnant woman

grief: pattern of physical and emotional responses to bereavement, separation or loss

grief process: the regulated steps in grieving

grief responses: symptoms associated with extreme sorrow or loss, specifically the death of a loved one

growth: an increase in size; a quantitative change

guided imagery: therapeutic technique for relieving pain or anxiety and for promoting relaxation where the person is encouraged to concentrate on an image

gynaecomastia: enlargement of the breasts; excess development of male breast tissue; a transient occurrence in normal adolescence

haematological: relating to the scientific study of blood and blood-forming tissues in health and disease

haemophilia: bleeding disorder characterised by a deficiency of one of the factors necessary for the coagulation of blood

haemorrhage: a loss of a large amount of blood in a short period either externally or internally

haemosiderosis: deposition of iron in body tissues

hand regard: infants holding their hands in front of their face and studying their fingers for long periods of time

health assessment: an evaluation of the health status of an individual by performing a physical examination after obtaining a health history

health education: an educational program directed at the general public that attempts to improve, maintain and safeguard the health of the community

health literacy: an individual's ability to read, understand and use health information in order to make decisions and follow advice

health promotion: the promotion of good health and prevention of disease

heartburn (pyrosis): a painful burning sensation in the oesophagus just below the sternum

Hegar's sign: softening of the lower uterine segment; a probable sign of pregnancy

HELLP syndrome: a variation of hypertension of pregnancy named for the common symptoms that occur: haemolysis, elevated liver enzymes and low platelets

hermaphrodite: having both ovaries and testes

hiatal hernia: intermittent protrusion of the stomach up through the oesophageal opening in the diaphragm

high-risk pregnancy: one in which a concurrent disorder, pregnancy-related complication or external factor jeopardises the health of the mother and/or fetus

Homans' sign: pain in the calf on dorsiflexion of the foot

hormones: chemicals produced by ductless glands of the endocrine system

hydramnios: an excessive amount of amniotic fluid (generally over 2000 millilitres)

hydrocele: collection of fluid in the scrotal sac

hydrocephalus: an excess of cerebrospinal fluid (CSF) in the ventricles and subarachnoid spaces of the brain

hydronephrosis: enlargement of the pelvis of the kidney with urine as a result of back-pressure in the ureter

hyperactivity: excess movement

hyperbilirubinaemia: increased serum bilirubin

hyperemesis gravidarum: an abnormal condition of pregnancy characterised by protracted vomiting

hyperglycaemia: increased blood glucose level

hyperopia: farsightedness

hypersensitivity: excessive antigen-antibody response when the invading organism is an allergen rather than a simple immunogen

hypodermoclysis: subcutaneous infusion

hypoglycaemia: decreased blood glucose level

hyposensitisation: immunotherapy; a process to diminish an allergic response

hypospadias: urethral defect in which the urethral opening is not at the end of the penis but on the ventral (lower) aspect of the penis

hypotonic uterine contractions: the number of contractions are low, infrequent (not increasing beyond two or three in a 10-minute period) or ineffective

hypoxia: inadequate oxygenation of body tissue

identity: developmental task of adolescence; determining who one is

imitation: copying or trying to be the same as

immunisation: a process by which resistance to an infectious disease is induced or augmented

immunity: the ability to destroy invading antigens

implantation: nidation; the attachment of the zygote to the uterine endometrium

incubation period: time between the invasion of an organism and the onset of symptoms of infection

Indigenous: native to or occurring naturally in a specified area or environment

induction of labour: labour that is artificially started

infant mortality rate: percent of infants who die during the first year of life per 1000 births

infantile spasms: a form of generalised seizures—"salaam" and "jackknife"—or infantile myoclonic seizures, characterised by very rapid movements

infertility: the inability to produce children

initiative: readiness to take the first step

innocent heart murmur: heart murmur of no significance; also called insignificant or functional heart murmur

inspection: visual observation to determine health

intercostal spaces: spaces between the ribs

intermittent infusion: an infusion that occurs at intervals

intrauterine device (IUD): a contraceptive device inserted into the uterine cavity

intrauterine growth restriction or retardation (IUGR): failure to grow at the expected rate in utero

intuitive thought: a stage of preschool thinking in which children can only see one characteristic of an object (centring)

intussusception: invagination of one portion of the intestine into another

in-vitro fertilisation (IVF): a method of fertilising human ova outside the body

involution: the process whereby the reproductive organs return to their non-pregnant state

irritable bowel syndrome: presence of either intermittent episodes of loose and normal stools or recurrent abdominal pain

isoimmunisation: production of antibodies against Rh positive blood in a fetus by a woman's immunologic system

jaundice: yellowing of the skin

karyotype: a visual presentation of chromosomes

kernicterus: permanent brain cell damage secondary to elevated bilirubin levels

ketoacidosis: a lowered serum pH resulting from accumulation of ketones

kilojoule counting: counting the number of kilojoules that a person ingests in 1 day

kinaesthesia: ability to distinguish movement

Koplik's spots: small, irregular, bright red spots with a blue-white centre point, appearing on the buccal membrane with measles

kwashiorkor: disease caused by protein deficiency

labile mood: sudden mood changes (e.g. crying occurs, followed immediately by giggling or laughing)

lactoferrin: iron-binding protein in breast milk that interferes with growth of pathogenic bacteria

lanugo: fine, downy hair that covers a newborn's shoulders, back and upper arms

laparoscopy: examination of the abdominal cavity and organs by insertion of a surgical instrument through the anterior abdominal wall

large for gestational age (LGA): an infant who falls above the 90th percentile in weight

latchkey children: children who are without adult supervision for a part of each day

latent tetany: neuromuscular irritability associated with hypocalcaemia

left-to-right shunts: heart or circulatory anomalies that involve blood movement from the arterial to the venous system (oxygenated to unoxygenated blood)

let-down reflex: collecting sinuses of the mammary glands contract, forcing milk forward through the nipples, thus making it available for the baby

letting-go phase: the third phase of the postpartum period in which the woman redefines her new role

leucopoenia: a decrease in the number of white blood cells

leucorrhoea: a whitish, viscous vaginal discharge or an increase in the amount of normal vaginal secretions

leukaemia: distorted and uncontrolled proliferation of white blood cells (leukocytes)

lie: the relationship between the long axis of the fetus and the long axis of the mother

light refraction: manner that light is bent as it passes through the lens of the eye

lightening: descent of the fetus into the pelvis at about 2 weeks prior to birth; also called engagement

linea nigra: a dark line appearing longitudinally on the abdomen of a pregnant woman during the last 24 weeks of pregnancy

liver transplantation: surgical replacement of a malfunctioning liver by a donor liver

lochia: the discharge that flows from the vagina after childbirth

lordosis: forward curve of the spine

low segment incision: an incision made horizontally across the abdomen just over the symphysis pubis and also horizontally across the uterus just over the cervix

low-birth-weight infant: infant weighing under 2500 g

lymphoma: malignancy of the lymph or reticuloendothelial system

lysozyme: enzyme found in breast milk that apparently actively destroys bacteria by lysing (dissolving) their cell membranes, possibly increasing the effectiveness of antibodies

magnetic resonance imaging (MRI): combination of a magnetic field, radio frequency and computer technology to produce diagnostic images

male condom: a thin sheath that covers the penis during intercourse; it protects against pregnancy and sexually-transmitted infection (STI)

malleoli: a rounded bony process such as the protuberance on each side of the ankle

mandatory reporters: persons who are required to report suspected child abuse when they identify it

manifest tetany: muscular twitching and carpopedal spasms from hypocalcaemia

mastitis: infection of the breast

maternal mortality rate: the number of maternal deaths per 100,000 live births

McDonald's rule: the fundus-to-symphysis distance in centimetres is equal to the week of gestation between the 20th to 31st week of pregnancy

mechanism of labour: the typical sequence of positions assumed by the fetus as it descends through the pelvis during labour and birth

Meckel's diverticulum: a congenital condition where an anomalous sac protrudes from the wall of the ileum

meconium: a sticky, tarlike, blackish-green, odourless material formed from mucus, vernix, lanugo, hormones and carbohydrates that accumulates during intrauterine life in the intestine

meconium plug: extremely hard portion of meconium that completely obstructs the intestinal lumen, causing bowel obstruction

megakaryocytes: immature thrombocytes

megaloblastic anaemia: enlarged red blood cells

melasma: excessive body pigment on the face that occurs during pregnancy

menarche: the first menstrual period

menopause: the cessation of ovarian function

menorrhagia: an abnormally heavy menstrual flow

metabolism: conversion of a medication into an active form (biotransformation) or an inactive form (inactivation)

metaphysis: a region of a growing long bone in which diaphysis and epiphysis converge

metrorrhagia: bleeding between menstrual periods

mid-stream urine specimen: a urine specimen collected during the middle of a flow of urine

minority: the smaller number or part

miscarriage: term used in preference to abortion in a clinical situation

mittelschmerz: abdominal pain during ovulation from the release of accompanying prostaglandins

Montgomery's tubercles: sebaceous glands of the areola of the breast

motor tics: eye blinking, neck jerking and facial grimacing

moulding: change in shape of the fetal skull due to uterine contractions pressing the vertex against the not-yet-dilated cervix

multiculturalism: the acknowledgement and promotion of cultural diversity

multipara: a woman who has given birth to more than one child past the age of viability

myopathy: disease of the muscular system

myopia: nearsightedness

nasogastric tube feedings: a method of feeding liquid diet through a tube inserted through the nostrils to the stomach

natal teeth: teeth present at birth

natural family planning: contraception involving no medical devices or chemicals

neck-righting reflex: turning of shoulders, trunk and pelvis in the same direction when the infant turns their head to the side

neglect: a condition that occurs when a parent or guardian fails to provide minimal physical and emotional care for a child or other dependent person

neonatal teeth: teeth erupting in the first 4 weeks of life

neoplasm: new growth, usually referring to new abnormal growth that does not respond to normal growth-control mechanisms

nephroblastoma: a malignant neoplasm of the kidney occurring in young children

nephrosis: altered glomeruli permeability due to fusion of the glomeruli membrane surfaces causing abnormal loss of protein in urine

neuroblastoma: tumour that arises from the cells of the sympathetic nervous system

newborn: recently born

non-therapeutic communication: communication that lacks deliberate purpose (e.g. socialising)

nursing research: controlled investigation of problems that have implications for nursing practice

nystagmus: rapid, irregular eye movement

obese: a body mass index over 30.0 or, in a child, a weight over the 90th percentile on a weight chart

object permanence: awareness that an object exists even when it is out of sight

oligohydramnios: a decreased amount of amniotic fluid

omphalocele: protrusion of abdominal contents through the abdominal wall at the point of the junction of the umbilical cord and abdomen

oncogenic virus: virus associated with causing cancer due to their ability to change the structure of DNA or RNA

operculum: the mucus plug formed in the cervix

orchiectomy: removal of the testis

organic heart murmur: murmur occurring as the result of heart disease or a congenital defect

orthopnoea: position with the head and chest elevated to ease breathing

orthoptics: eye exercises

osteogenic sarcoma: malignant tumour of long bone involving rapidly growing bone tissue (mesenchymal-matrix forming cells)

ostomy care: the management of a person with a surgical opening created in the bladder, ileum or colon for the temporary or permanent passage of urine or faeces

otorrhoea: discharge from the external ear

oxytocin: a pituitary hormone that initiates or sustains uterine contractions

pain: an unpleasant sensation caused by pressure, injury or tissue anoxia; whatever the person experiencing it says it is and existing whenever he or she says it does

palilalia: repeating one's own words

palpation: an assessment technique that yields information on warmth and oedema through touching

pancytopenia: reduction of all blood cell components

para: number of children above the age of viability a woman has previously given birth to

paracervical block: a form of regional anaesthetic in which a local anaesthetic is injected into each side of the uterine cervix to block nerves innervating the uterine cervix

parallel play: playing alongside, not with, other children; characteristic of toddlers

paraphrasing: restating what a person has said not only to assure the person that you have heard correctly (as in clarifying), but to help explain what the person was trying to say

paraplegia (diplegia): paralysis of the lower extremities

paroxysmal coughing: series of expiratory coughs after a deep inspiration

paroxysmal nocturnal dyspnoea: suddenly waking at night short of breath

patent urachus: failure of the urachus (narrow tube that joins the bladder to the umbilicus in utero) to close properly during embryologic development, leading to the development of a fistula between the bladder and umbilicus

pathological retraction ring: a type of contraction ring that occurs at the juncture of the upper and lower uterine segments; a warning sign that severe dysfunctional labour is occurring

patient-controlled analgesia (PCA): form of administration that allows self-administration of IV boluses of medication, usually opioids, with a medication pump

pelvic inflammatory disease (PID): infection of the pelvic organs: the uterus, fallopian tubes, ovaries and their supporting structures

perception checking: documenting a feeling or emotion

percussion: a chest physiotherapy technique that uses a cupped or curved palm against the chest; an assessment technique that helps determine the consistency of tissue beneath the surface area

periosteum: outside sensitive layer covering of central shafts of long bones

peripartum cardiomyopathy: myocardial failure apparently due to the effect of the pregnancy on the circulatory system

peritonitis: infection of the peritoneal cavity

permanence: the awareness that objects exist when out of sight

petechiae: pinpoint, macular, purplish-red spots caused by intradermal or submucus haemorrhage

pharmacokinetics: the way a medication is absorbed, distributed throughout the body, metabolised, inactivated and excreted

photophobia: sensitivity to light

physical abuse: one or more episodes of aggressive behaviour usually resulting in physical injury

pica: indiscriminate eating of non-food substances

pincer grasp: ability to bring the thumb and first finger together to pick up small objects

placenta accreta: an unusually deep attachment of the placenta to the uterine myometrium

placenta circumvallata: the fetal side of the placenta is covered with chorion membrane

placenta marginata: the fold of chorion reaches just to the edge of the placenta

placenta praevia: low implantation of the placenta

placenta succenturiata: one or more accessory lobes connected to the main placenta by blood vessels

play therapy: a psychoanalytic technique used by psychiatrists to help children better understand their feelings, thoughts and motivations

pneumothorax: the presence of atmospheric air in the pleural space

point of maximum impulse (PMI): the point on the chest where the apical heartbeat can be heard best

polycystic kidney: large, fluid-filled cysts forming in place of normal kidney tissue

polydactyly: presence of one or more additional fingers

polydipsia: excessive thirst

polyuria: excessive urination

position: the relationship of a specific fetal part to the maternal pelvis

positive reinforcement: rewarding someone for demonstrating desired behaviour

positron emission tomography (PET): a medical imaging procedure that can provide information about how an organ or body system is working

postpartum depression: overall feeling of sadness in a woman accompanied by extreme fatigue, an inability to stop crying, increased anxiety about her own or her infant's health, insecurity (unwilling to be left alone or unable to make decisions), psychosomatic symptoms, and either depressive or manic mood fluctuations during the first year following birth

postpartum psychosis: psychiatric illness occurring during the postpartum period

postterm pregnancy: a pregnancy that lasts more than 42 weeks

postural proteinuria: also called postural albuminuria; condition in which albumin spills into the urine when children stand upright for an extended period and decreases when resting in the supine position

precipitate labour: uterine contractions so strong that the woman gives birth with only a few rapidly occurring contractions

preeclampsia: in pregnancy-induced hypertension, the phase before the pregnant woman experiences a seizure

prejudice: an unreasonable opinion formed for or against anything

premature cervical dilatation: previously termed an incompetent cervix; refers to a cervix that dilates prematurely and therefore cannot hold a fetus until term

premature ejaculation: deposition of sperm before vaginal penetration or the full enjoyment of the sexual partner

premature separation of the placenta: also called abruptio placentae; separation of the placenta before birth of the fetus

premenstrual dysphoric disorder (PDD): condition occurring in the luteal phase of the menstrual cycle and relieved by the onset of menses that has both behavioural and physiologic symptoms
preterm infant: infant born before term (less than the full 37th week of pregnancy)
preterm labour: labour that occurs before the end of week 37 of gestation
preterm rupture of membranes: rupture of fetal membranes with loss of amniotic fluid during pregnancy
primary healthcare (PHC): essential healthcare that is accessible, affordable, acceptable and available
primary nursing: a nursing pattern in which one nurse assumes complete responsibility for the care of a client
primigravida: a woman during her first pregnancy
primipara: a woman who experiences pregnancy for the first time
prodromal period: a time between the beginning of nonspecific symptoms and specific infectious symptoms
proteinuria: protein in the urine
prune belly syndrome: severe urinary tract dilation that develops as early as intrauterine life from an unknown cause
pseudohermaphrodite: a child with some external features of both sexes, although only either ovaries or testes (or neither) are present
psychological harm: any detrimental effect of a significant nature on a person's emotional psychological health
psychomotor learning: the acquisition of ability to perform motor skills
ptosis: drooping of the eyelid
puberty: the stage at which a person first becomes capable of sexual reproduction
pudendal nerve block: the injection of a local anaesthetic near the right and left pudendal nerves at the level of the ischial spine
puerperium period: the time after childbirth, lasting approximately 6 weeks during which the anatomical and physiological changes brought about by pregnancy resolve
pulse pressure: the gap between systolic and diastolic blood pressure
punishment: a consequence that results from a breakdown in discipline (disregarding the rules)
purging: self-induced vomiting or the use of laxatives, enemas or diuretics
purpura: haemorrhagic rash or small haemorrhages occurring in the superficial layer of skin
quadriplegia: paralysis of all four extremities
quickening: the first movement of the fetus perceived by the mother
racism: discriminatory behaviour motivated by racial stereotypes
radiation: transfer of body heat to a cooler solid object not in contact with the baby
radiopharmaceuticals: radioactive-combined substances that, when given orally or by injection, flow to designated body organs
recurrent pregnancy loss: having three spontaneous miscarriages that occurred at the same gestation age in three pregnancies
reflecting: technique for therapeutic communication that involves restating the last word or phrase a person has said
registered midwife: a person registered to practice in the nursing and midwifery profession
remodelling: new bone tissue replacing old bone tissue
resorption: the breakdown of bone cells
resources: materials or assets that are transformed to produce benefit
respect: imparting a positive feeling of esteem or deference to a person or entity
retractions: indentation of intercostal spaces reflecting difficulty breathing
reversibility: the ability to retrace steps
Rh incompatibility: an Rh-negative mother (one negative for a D antigen or one with a dd genotype) is carrying a fetus with an Rh-positive blood type (DD or Dd genotype)
rhabdomyosarcoma: tumour of striated muscle
rhinorrhoea: discharge from the nose
right-to-left shunt: cardiac anomaly when blood is shunted from the venous to the arterial system as a result of abnormal communication between the two (deoxygenated blood to oxygenated blood)
ripening of the cervix: softening of the cervix with the approach of labour
role confusion: characteristic of people who do not develop a sense of identity; uncertainty about what kind of person one is
role fantasy: a method of thinking that changes perceptions to how the child would like things to turn out (magical thinking)
rooming-in: a hospital pattern in which an infant stays in the room with the mother
sadomasochism: a personality disorder characterised by traits of sadism and masochism
sarcoma: tumour derived from connective tissue, such as bone and cartilage, muscle, blood vessels or lymphoid tissue
schemas: the means by which thoughts are organised (Piaget)
scope of practice: range of activity
seborrhoea: a scaly scalp condition, often called cradle cap
secondary stuttering: stuttering that develops after a child learns to speak without stuttering
sensorimotor stage: the period from birth to 2 years of age (Piaget)
sensory deprivation: loss of environmental stimuli
sensory overload: receiving more stimulation than can be tolerated or processed
separation anxiety: fear and apprehension caused by separation from familiar surroundings and significant people

sequestrum: dead bone tissue detached from adjoining healthy bone

sexual abuse: the sexual mistreatment of another person by fondling, rape or forced participation in unnatural sex acts or other perverted behaviour

sexually-transmitted infections (STIs): those spread through sexual contact with an infected partner

shoulder presentation: the part of the fetus that occupies the centre of the birth canal

Sims' position: turned to the left side with the weight of the uterus resting on the bed

single-photon emission computerised tomography (SPECT): CT scan involving the use of an injectable iodine-based contrast medium

sinus arrhythmia: a marked heart rate increase occurring as the child inspires and a marked decrease in heart rate as the child expires

sleep deprivation: lack of adequate amount of sleep leading to difficulty in concentrating and episodes of disorientation and misperception

small for gestational age (SGA): an infant who falls below the 10th percentile of weight for age

social determinants of health: social factors that bring about a change in health: these factors can be socioeconomic, biological or related to the physical environment

social-ecological approach: a framework that recognises the interwoven relationship that exists between the individual and their environment

social justice: a term based on the concept of human rights and equality

social smile: a definite response (smiling) to an interaction occurring at about 6 weeks of age

sperm motility: whether sperm are seen to be active

spermatogenesis: production of sperm cells

spina bifida: Latin for "divided spine"; most often used as a collective term for all spinal cord disorders

sprain: a traumatic injury to the tendons, muscles or ligaments surrounding a joint

standard of care: written statement describing the rules, actions or conditions that direct client care

station: the relationship of the presenting part of the fetus to the level of the ischial spines

status epilepticus: a seizure that lasts continuously for more than 30 minutes or a series of seizures from which the child does not return to their previous level of consciousness

steatorrhoea: large, bulky, greasy stools

stem cells: cells whose daughter cells may give rise to other cell types

stenosis: narrowing

stereognosis: the ability to recognise an object by touch

stereopsis: depth perception; the ability to locate an object in space relative to another object

stereotyping: applying a fixed conception

strabismus: crossed eye

strain: to exert physical force in a manner that may result in injury, usually muscular

striae gravidarum: reddish steaks appearing on the abdominal wall during pregnancy

stridor: a harsh, strident breath sound on inspiration

stupor: lethargy and unresponsiveness

substance abuse: the use of chemicals to improve a mental state or induce euphoria

substance dependent: when a person has withdrawal symptoms following discontinuation of the substance, and such activities as abandonment of important activities, spending increased time in activities related to substance use, using substances for a longer time than planned and continued use despite the existence of worsening problems due to substance use

sudden infant death syndrome (SIDS): the unexpected and sudden death of an infant that occurs during sleep

surfactant: a lipoprotein secreted by the alveoli cells to reduce surface tension in alveoli

syndactyly: fusing of the fingers

synergeneic transplant: transplant between a donor and recipient who are genetically identical (i.e. identical twins)

tachypnoea: an increased respiratory rate

taking-hold phase: the second phase of the postpartum period where the woman begins to initiate action

taking-in phase: the first phase of the postpartum period experienced when the woman is reflective and plays a largely passive role

teaching plan: a design of content to be taught and the teaching–learning techniques to be used

temperament: a child's innate behavioural characteristics such as activity level, rhythmicity, tendency to approach or withdraw and adaptability to situations

teratogen: substance that causes fetal harm

therapeutic communication: an interaction between two people that is planned, has structure, and is helpful and constructive

therapeutic play: play technique that can be used by nurses to better understand children's feelings and thoughts and relieve their anxiety

thrombocytopenia: decreased platelet count

thrombophlebitis: inflammation of the lining of a blood vessel with the formation of blood clots

thumb opposition: ability to bring the thumb and fingers together

tocolytic agent: a drug to halt labour

tolerance: a state of not responding to an allergen

total parenteral nutrition (TPN): concentrated hypertonic solutions of intravenous fluid containing glucose, vitamins, electrolytes, trace minerals, fats and proteins to meet all of the child's nutritional needs

toxic shock syndrome (TSS): an infection usually caused by toxin-producing strains of Staphylococcus aureus organisms

toxoplasmosis: a protozoan infection spread most commonly through contact with uncooked meat; also contracted through handling cat stool in soil or cat litter

tracheostomy: an opening into the trachea to create an artificial airway

tracheotomy: procedure to create an airway

traction: pulling on a body part in one direction against a counterpull exerted in the opposite direction to reduce dislocations and immobilise fractures

transcutaneous electrical nerve stimulation (TENS): a method of pain control involving the application of electrical impulses to the nerve endings

transition: the end of the first stage of labour, just before the woman experiences pushing sensations

transsexual: a person of one sex whose perceived identity is of the opposite sex

transvestite: a person who engages in the practice of dressing in the clothes of the opposite sex for sexual gratification

trophoblast: the outer layer of the blastocyst

tubal ligation: a method of contraception in which the fallopian tubes are cauterised, tied or clamped to prevent sperm from reaching the discharged oocyte

tumour staging: procedure by which a malignant tumour's extent and progress are determined

turgor: skin characteristic reflecting the amount of fluid in body tissue

tympanocentesis: withdrawal of fluid from the middle ear through the tympanic membrane

ultrasound: painless diagnostic procedure in which pictures of internal tissue and organs are produced by high-frequency sound waves

umbilical cord: the structure composed of one vein and two arteries that connects the placenta to the fetus

umbilical cord prolapse: a loop of the umbilical cord slipping down in front of the presenting fetal part

uterine atony: relaxation of the uterus in the postpartum period

uterine inversion: a rare phenomenon in which the uterus turns inside out

vacuum extraction: birth of a fetus by means of vacuum pressure

vaginal birth after caesarean birth (VBAC): a vaginal birth in a woman who previously had a child by caesarean

vaginal ring: a device designed to provide controlled release of drugs for intravaginal administration over extended periods of time

vaginismus: painful, involuntary spasms of the vagina

varicocele: abnormal dilation of the veins of the spermatic cord

vascular access port (VAP): small device (infusion port) implanted under the skin, usually on the anterior chest just under the clavicle to allow for circulatory access

vasculitis: inflammation of blood vessels

vasectomy: a surgical ligation of the vas deferens that results in male sterility

vesicoureteral reflux: retrograde flow of urine from the bladder into the ureters

vital signs: the measurements of pulse rate, blood pressure, respiration rate and body temperature

vitamin K deficiency bleeding (VKDB): formerly known as haemorrhagic disease of the newborn results from a deficiency of vitamin K dependent clotting factors in the newborn

vocal tics: coughing, throat clearing, snorting, and barking

volvulus: a twisting of the bowel causing obstruction

voyeurism: the practice of obtaining sexual pleasure by looking at the nude body of another person

vulnerable children: children whose parents were told they would die, but who lived and are treated in a cold and unfeeling way—as if they actually did die

vulvovaginitis: inflammation of the vulva or vagina

wheezing: whistling expiratory sound

xenophobia: an anxiety disorder characterised by fear or uneasiness in the presence of strangers

zygote: a fertilised ovum

Index

Page numbers followed by b indicate box; those followed by f indicate figure; those followed by t indicate table.

D

E

F

G

H

I

R